July 1999

Volume 212 • Number 1

RADLAX 212 (1) 1–296

Radiology

Editorial	1
Special Report	4
State of the Art	5
Genitourinary Imaging	19
Nuclear Medicine	35
Obstetric Imaging	43
Thoracic Imaging	49
Signs in Imaging	67
Cardiac Imaging	69
Ultrasonography	75
Experimental Studies	79
Musculoskeletal Imaging	103
Emergency Radiology	117
Diagnosis Please: Case 16	126
Case 12 Answer	129
Neuroradiology	133
Radiation Oncology	155
Vascular and Interventional Radiology	159
Health Policy and Practice	181
Breast Imaging	189
Computer Applications	195
Gastrointestinal Imaging	213
Pediatric Imaging	249
Technical Developments	265
Letters to the Editor	291

RSNA® **85th Scientific Assembly and Annual Meeting**
Chicago, November 28–December 3, 1999

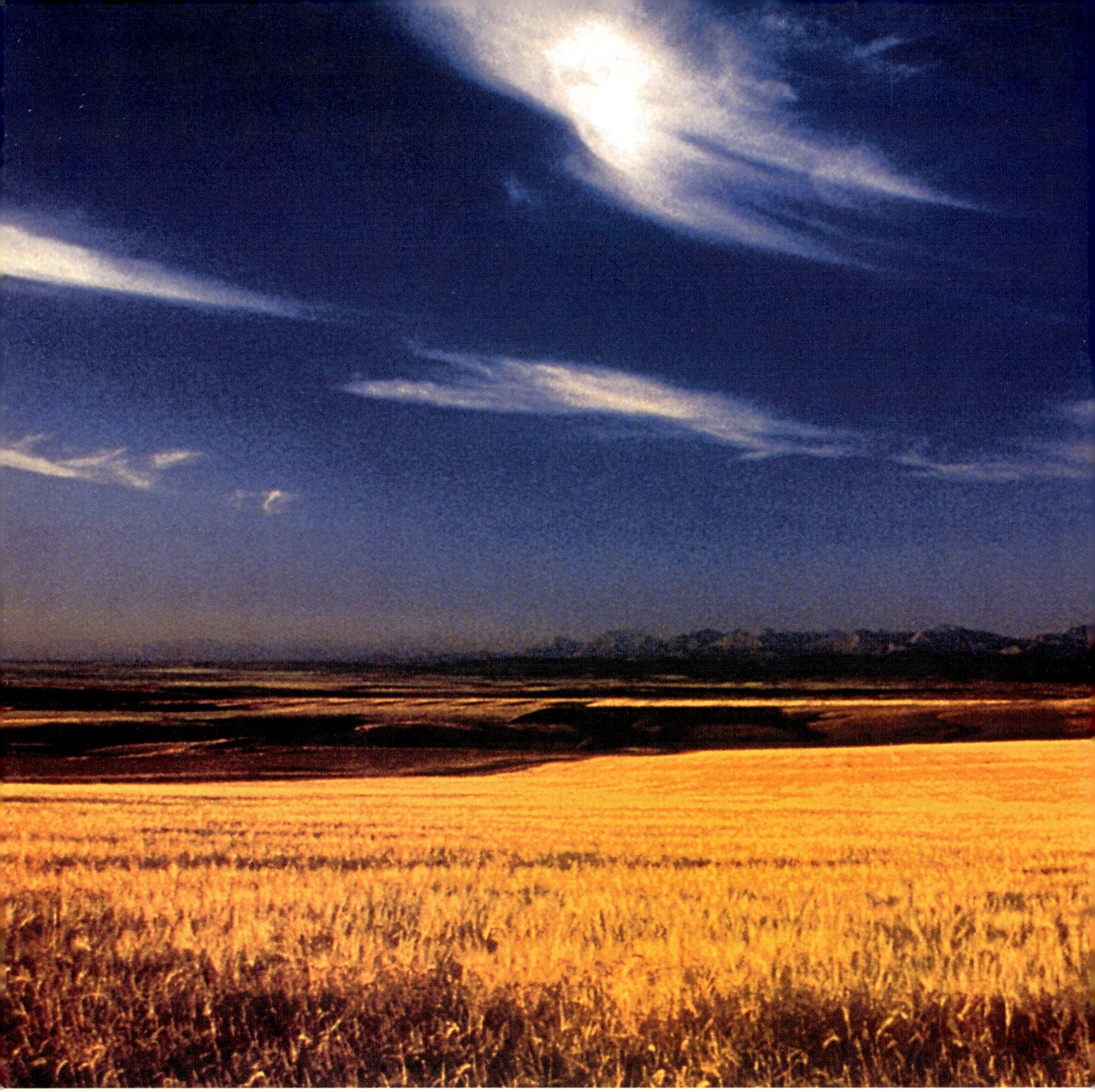

Introducing the FCR 5000 Series from Fuji.

A CENTURY OF RESEARCH & EDUCATION
RSNA 1999

Radiological Society of North America
85th Scientific Assembly and Annual Meeting
November 28–December 3, 1999
McCormick Place, Chicago

New Realities in Radiology: Multidisciplinary Strategies for Compliance

Associated Sciences Program at RSNA 1999

Workshop: Saturday, Nov. 27, 1999 10:15 am - 4:00 pm, McCormick Place South

Refresher Courses: Sunday, Nov. 28, through Friday, Dec 3, 1999

Credits: 5 hours

Welcome and Introduction
10:15 am
Samuel L. Hissong, MD, Chair, Associated Sciences Consortium and Committee
JoAnn Belanger, RN, CRN, Coordinator, Associated Sciences Consortium

Keynote Presentation
10:30 am - 11:50 am
Compliance, Audits and Radiology: The Art of Survival (AHRA)
Karol Handrahan RT(R)

Break
11:50 am - 12:10 pm

Special Luncheon Program
12:10 - 1:20 pm
Uncle Sam Strikes Back: Medicine in the Enforcement Age (RBMA)
Tom Hoffman

Break
1:20 - 1:30 pm

Panel Presentation
1:30 - 4:00 pm
(Break 2:45 pm - 3:00 pm)
Practicum (SROA)
Andrew Woods, Esq.
Gadi Weinreich, Esq.
Bruce Freid, Esq.

AAPM/RSNA Basic Physics Lecture for the Radiologic Technologists: Digital Imaging: What You Need to Know Now and What You Need to Know Next
Organized by
Gerald A. White, Jr., MS
3:00 - 4:30 pm
1½ hours credit

Refresher Courses

(Each Refresher Course is approved for 1½ hours credit)

Sunday RC 124
Organizational Culture and Health System Change
Sponsored by the Associated Sciences Consortium
Paula Maramonte, MEd, RT(R) (AERS) Coordinator
Cornelius J. Rater, MD (AERS)
Harry J. Granito, MS (RBMA)
Susan K. Snyder, BS, EdD (ASRT)

Monday RC 224
Asset Management for High-Technology Systems
Sponsored by the Associated Sciences Consortium
Chester T. Szerlag, MBA (SROA) Coordinator
Tim Guertin (SROA)
Sheila M. Sferrella (AHRA)
Dennis A. Bair, RT(R)(CV) (AVIR)

Monday RC 324
Economic Implications of Regulatory Change
Sponsored by the Associated Sciences Consortium
DuVonne Campbell (ASRT) Coordinator
Cherrill Farnsworth (AHRA)
Sherry Makely, PhD (ASRT, SNM)
Donna L. Wright, EdD, RT(R) (AERS)

Tuesday RC 424
Managing a Multisite Radiology Network
Sponsored by the Associated Sciences Consortium
Kathryn J. Canny, (RBMA) Coordinator
Larry A. Ranahan, MBA (RBMA) Moderator
Charles Deschamps RT(R)(MR) (SMRT)
Scott Seberg, MS (RBMA)
Chester T. Szerlag, MBA (RBMA)

Wednesday RC 524
Current Challenges in Radiology and Planning and Design
Sponsored by the Associated Sciences Consortium
Morris A. Stein (AIA-AAH) Coordinator
Bill Rostenberg (AIA-AAH)
Jerry W. Froelich, MD (AIA-AAH)
Eliot L. Siegel, MD (AIA-AAH)

Thursday RC 624
Specialized Accreditations: A Cost of Doing Business
Sponsored by the Associated Sciences Consortium
Luann J. Culbreth, MEd, RT(R) (SMRT) Moderator
John Kovelski, RT(R) (SMRT)
Karol Handrahan, RT(R) (SMRT)
Sandra Katanick, RN, RVT (SDMS)
Ronald F. Bernardi, BA, RT(R) (AHRA)

Thursday RC 724
Multidisciplinary Standards for the New Millennium
Sponsored by the Associated Sciences Consortium
Susan S. Weiss, CNMT (SNM-TS) Moderator
William R. Poller, MD (SNM-TS)
Michael R. Bloyd, RT(R), BSN (ASRT)
Sue M. Smith, RT(R)(CV)(M), FAVIR (AVIR)

Friday RC 824
Marketing Radiology: Getting the Message Out
Sponsored by the Associated Sciences Consortium
Ronald F. Bernardi, BA, RT(R) (AHRA) Moderator
Cherrill Farnsworth (AHRA)
Michael R. Favreau (AHRA)

Registration Information

Advance registration for the RSNA Scientific Assembly ends October 29. Onsite registration begins at 12:00 noon on Saturday, November 27, at McCormick Place. RSNA shuttle bus service to McCormick Place will be available beginning at 10:00 am on Saturday. Advance registration is not required for the Saturday workshop; however, to receive continuing education credit, you must register.

Advance registration information appears in the July issue of *Radiology*. Brochures are also available from your association or from the RSNA, 820 Jorie Boulevard, Oak Brook, IL 60523-1860. Phone: 630/571-7852.

Registration for the RSNA Scientific Assembly includes registration for the Associated Sciences Workshop. A box lunch will be available for purchase to facilitate your attendance at the workshop. These lunches must be purchased with your advance registration for the RSNA Meeting. **If you wish to purchase a box lunch, please check the appropriate box on the RSNA Advance Registration form and enclose your $11.50 payment.**

If you would like a copy of the published Associated Sciences Proceedings, please call 630/571-7874

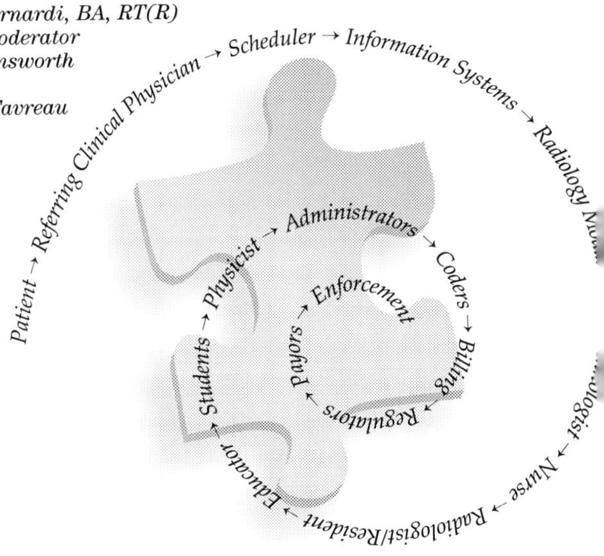

Sponsoring Organizations

- American Healthcare Radiology Administrators (AHRA)
- American Institute of Architects — Academy on Architecture for Health (AIA-AAH)
- American Radiological Nurses Association (ARNA)
- American Society of Radiologic Technologists (ASRT)
- Association of Educators in Radiological Sciences, Inc. (AERS)
- Association of Vascular and Interventional Radiographers (AVIR)
- Radiology Business Management Association (RBMA)
- Society for Radiation Oncology Administrators (SROA)
- Society of Diagnostic Medical Sonographers (SDMS)
- Section for Magnetic Resonance Technologists (SMRT-ISMRM)
- Society of Nuclear Medicine — Technologists Section (SNM-TS)

RSNA® Radiological Society of North America Founded in 1915
820 Jorie Boulevard
Oak Brook, Illinois 60523-1860
630/571-2670 FAX: 630/571-7837
www.rsna.org

Radiology

July 1999
Volume 212
Number 1

RSNA®
A monthly journal devoted to clinical radiology and allied sciences, owned and published by THE RADIOLOGICAL SOCIETY OF NORTH AMERICA, INC.
http://www.rsna.org

July 1999
Volume 212 • Number 1

Radiology

A monthly journal devoted to clinical radiology and allied sciences, owned and published by the Radiological Society of North America, Inc.

RSNA

Editorial

1 Pulmonary Emphysema: Imaging Assessment of Lung Volume Reduction Surgery
John H. M. Austin

Special Report

4 Paula J. Woodward, MD
Armed Forces Institute of Pathology 1999–2000 Distinguished Scientist
Melissa L. Rosado-de-Christenson

State of the Art

5 Tissue Characterization in the Female Pelvis by Means of MR Imaging
Evan S. Siegelman and Eric K. Outwater

The purpose of this article is to review the ability of MR imaging to help characterize tissue in the female pelvis.

Genitourinary Imaging

19 Diagnosis and Staging of Ovarian Cancer: Comparative Values of Doppler and Conventional US, CT, and MR Imaging Correlated with Surgery and Histopathologic Analysis—Report of the Radiology Diagnostic Oncology Group
Alfred B. Kurtz, John V. Tsimikas, Clare M. C. Tempany, Ulrike M. Hamper, Peter H. Arger, Robert L. Bree, Richard J. Wechsler, Isaac R. Francis, Janet E. Kuhlman, Evan S. Siegelman, Donald G. Mitchell, Stuart G. Silverman, Douglas L. Brown, Sheila Sheth, Beverly G. Coleman, James H. Ellis, Robert J. Kurman, Daryl J. Caudry, and Barbara J. McNeil

Because of the importance of not understaging abdominal malignancy as disease limited to the pelvis, if stage III cancer is not detected at initial abdominal US, CT or MR imaging should be performed because of their higher sensitivities in staging.

28 Renal Neoplasms Amenable to Partial Nephrectomy: MR Imaging
E. Scott Pretorius, Evan S. Siegelman, Parvati Ramchandani, Thomas Cangiano, and Marc P. Banner

Contrast-enhanced, surface-coil MR imaging is well suited for evaluating renal lesions in which partial nephrectomy is being considered.

Nuclear Medicine

35 Pheochromocytomas: Imaging with 2-[Fluorine-18]fluoro-2-deoxy-D-glucose PET
Barry L. Shulkin, Norman W. Thompson, Brahm Shapiro, Isaac R. Francis, and James C. Sisson

FDG PET helps localize the majority of pheochromocytomas.

Obstetric Imaging

43 **Congenital Chest Lesions: Diagnosis and Characterization with Prenatal MR Imaging**
Anne M. Hubbard, N. Scott Adzick, Timothy M. Crombleholme, Beverly G. Coleman, Lori J. Howell, John C. Haselgrove, and Saroosh Mahboubi
In this series, MR imaging helped further characterize the fetal chest lesions and confirm or change the prenatal diagnosis.

Thoracic Imaging

49 **Advanced Emphysema: Preoperative Chest Radiographic Findings as Predictors of Outcome Following Lung Volume Reduction Surgery**
Daniel D. Maki, Wallace T. Miller, Jr, Judith M. Aronchick, Warren B. Gefter, Wallace T. Miller, Sr, Robert M. Kotloff, and Gregory Tino
High disease heterogeneity on standard chest radiographs is strongly predictive of a favorable outcome following lung volume reduction surgery.

56 **Lung Cancer Staging and Management: Comparison of Contrast-enhanced and Nonenhanced Helical CT of the Thorax**
Edward F. Patz, Jr, Jeremy J. Erasmus, H. Page McAdams, John E. Connolly, Edith M. Marom, Philip C. Goodman, Richard A. Leder, Mary T. Keogan, and James E. Herndon
Nonenhanced thoracic CT through the adrenal glands is sufficient for successful radiologic staging in patients with newly diagnosed lung cancer.

61 **Detection Failures in Spiral CT Screening for Lung Cancer: Analysis of CT Findings**
Ryutaro Kakinuma, Hironobu Ohmatsu, Masahiro Kaneko, Kenji Eguchi, Tsuguo Naruke, Kanji Nagai, Yutaka Nishiwaki, Akira Suzuki, and Noriyuki Moriyama
Minute nodules of lung cancer that are near the threshold of detectability may be overlooked at spiral CT screening.

Signs in Imaging

67 **The Signet Ring Sign**
Hugue Ouellette
The signet ring sign is a CT finding in patients with bronchiectasis.

Cardiac Imaging

69 **Pericardial Sinuses and Recesses: Findings at Electrocardiographically triggered Electron-Beam CT**
Reinhard Groell, Gottfried J. Schaffler, and Rainer Rienmueller
Knowledge of the location of these structures [pericardial sinuses and recesses] helps the radiologist avoid a misdiagnosis of lymphadenopathy or other mediastinal disease processes.

Ultrasonography

75 **Clinically Suspected Pulmonary Embolism: Use of Bilateral Lower Extremity US as the Initial Examination—A Prospective Study**
Robert G. Sheiman and Colin R. McArdle
If lower extremity US is contemplated as the initial examination in patients suspected of having pulmonary embolism, it should be applied only in those patients who also have deep venous thrombosis symptoms or risk factors.

Experimental Studies

79 **Stenosis of the Main Artery Supplying an Organ: Effect of End-Organ Vascular Resistance on the Poststenotic Peak Systolic Velocity in an in Vitro Hydraulic Model at Doppler US**
Ronald O. Bude, Ronald G. Larson, Wilmer W. Nichols, and Jonathan M. Rubin
Poststenotic peak systolic velocity decreases only mildly with increasing vascular resistance distal to the stenosis for stenoses at both ends of the hemodynamic spectrum (low- and high-grade stenoses).

Continued—

Radiology is published monthly by the Radiological Society of North America, Inc, 820 Jorie Boulevard, Oak Brook, IL 60523-2251 (ISSN 0033-8419). Printed in USA. Periodical class postage paid at Oak Brook, Ill, and additional mailing offices. The nonmember subscription rate for the USA is $215.00 per year; for all other countries, $260.00 (includes postage). Information about subscription rates for residents is available on request. (Air freight is available; rates are furnished on request.) Single copies are $25.00 ($36.00 to a non-U.S. address). Notice of missing issues or change of address (include old mailing label and new address) should be sent to RSNA Subscriptions Department, 820 Jorie Boulevard, Oak Brook, IL 60523-2251. Inquiries via e-mail should be directed to *subscrib@rsna.org*. POSTMASTER: Send address correction "changes" to: *Radiology*, RSNA, 820 Jorie Boulevard, Oak Brook, IL 60523-2251.

Claims for copies lost in the mail are allowed within 90 days of the date of issue. Claims are not allowed for issues lost as a result of insufficient notice of change of address.

Membership in the Radiological Society of North America is by formal application. Membership information should be secured from the Executive Director, the Radiological Society of North America, Inc, 820 Jorie Boulevard, Oak Brook, IL 60523-2251. Dues are payable annually in January. In accordance with U.S. postal regulations, $107.50 of active membership dues is allocated to a subscription to *Radiology*.

88 **Shark Liver Oil–induced Lipoid Pneumonia in Pigs: Correlation of Thin-Section CT and Histopathologic Findings**
Joon Beom Seo, Jung-Gi Im, Woo Sun Kim, Chang Kyu Seong, Jae Woo Song, and Jin Haeng Chung
The serial thin-section CT findings of exogenous lipoid pneumonia after a single endobronchial administration of oil in pigs were ground-glass opacity and airspace consolidation, followed by complete or incomplete resolution with lobular volume loss and septal thickening.

97 **Contrast Medium–induced Pulmonary Edema Is Aggravated by Silicone Contamination in Rats**
Toshiaki Sendo, Masaaki Hirakawa, Kaori Fujie, Yasufumi Kataoka, and Ryozo Oishi
Although in this experiment it was not possible to match conditions, such as the dose and rate of injection of contrast medium, the results raise the possibility that the incidence of pulmonary edema could be increased in patients who are examined by using contrast medium contaminated with silicone.

Musculoskeletal Imaging

103 **Iliotibial Band Friction Syndrome: MR Imaging Findings in 16 Patients and MR Arthrographic Study of Six Cadaveric Knees**
Claus Muhle, Joong Mo Ahn, LeeRen Yeh, Gabrielle A. Bergman, Robert D. Boutin, Mark Schweitzer, Jon A. Jacobson, Parviz Haghighi, Debra J. Trudell, and Donald Resnick
With MR imaging, poorly defined signal intensity abnormalities or a circumscribed fluid collection located in a compartmentlike space medial to the iliotibial tract with obliteration of the fatty layer distal to the vastus lateralis muscle may allow the diagnosis of iliotibial band friction syndrome in patients with corresponding clinical symptoms.

111 **Bicipitoradial Bursitis: MR Imaging Findings in Eight Patients and Anatomic Data from Contrast Material Opacification of Bursae Followed by Routine Radiography and MR Imaging in Cadavers**
Abdalla Y. Skaf, Robert D. Boutin, Robert Weiber M. Dantas, Andrew W. Hooper, Claus Muhle, David S. Chou, Nittaya Lektrakul, Debra J. Trudell, Parviz Haghighi, and Donald L. Resnick
MR imaging is a useful diagnostic method for evaluating bicipitoradial bursitis and its effect on adjacent structures.

Emergency Radiology

117 **Cervical Spine Screening with CT in Trauma Patients: A Cost-effectiveness Analysis**
C. Craig Blackmore, Scott D. Ramsey, Frederick A. Mann, and Richard A. Deyo
On the basis of our cost-effectiveness analysis, CT should be considered as the primary cervical spine screening modality in selected victims of major trauma who are examined in high-volume urban emergency departments and trauma centers.

Diagnosis Please

126 **Case 16**
Lawrence E. Ginsberg and Franco DeMonte

129 **Case 12: Mazabraud Syndrome**
Mark J. Kransdorf and Mark D. Murphey
The identification of a well-defined soft-tissue mass with a fluidlike signal intensity and multiple bone lesions compatible with fibrous dysplasia established the diagnosis of Mazabraud syndrome.

Neuroradiology

133 **Central Nervous Pathway for Acupuncture Stimulation: Localization of Processing with Functional MR Imaging of the Brain—Preliminary Experience**
Ming-Ting Wu, Jen-Chuen Hsieh, Jing Xiong, Chien-Fang Yang, Huay-Ban Pan, Yin-Ching Iris Chen, Guochuan Tsai, Bruce R. Rosen, and Kenneth K. Kwong
Given that the hypothalamus and limbic system provide multidimensional integration of neuroendocrinal and autonomic homeostasis, our finding that acupuncture activates the hypothalamus and limbic system also may provide a basis for the versatility of acupuncture for use in conditions other than pain disorders, such as management of nausea and vomiting, asthma, and substance addiction.

143 **Stereotactic Radiosurgical Pallidotomy and Thalamotomy with the Gamma Knife: MR Imaging Findings with Clinical Correlation—Preliminary Experience**
David P. Friedman, H. Warren Goldman, Adam E. Flanders, Stephen M. Gollomp, and Walter J. Curran, Jr
Findings in our pilot study show that radiosurgical thalamotomy with the gamma knife is a promising treatment for patients with medically refractory tremor.

Continued—

151 MR Imaging of Intraventricular Silicone: Case Report
Robert L. Williams, Randall L. Beatty, Emanuel Kanal, and Jane L. Weissman
MR imaging demonstrated, in a patient who was treated for retinal detachment with intravitreous silicone, intraocular and intraventricular silicone oil, as confirmed by identical signal intensity characteristics and chemical shifts in the two locations.

Radiation Oncology

155 Localization of the Apex of the Vagina: Implications for Radiation Therapy Planning
Choong R. Kim, Beverly A. Eaton, and Kenneth R. Stevens, Jr
The vaginal rod causes displacement of the vaginal apex during the simulation performed to establish the locations of small boost irradiation fields.

Vascular and Interventional Radiology

159 Transrectal versus Transvaginal Abscess Drainage: Survey of Patient Tolerance and Effect on Activities of Daily Living
David M. Hovsepian, Joseph R. Steele, Celette Sugg Skinner, and Eric S. Malden
Prior to pelvic abscess drainage, especially by means of the transvaginal route, patients and referring physicians should be made well aware of the potential for discomfort and severe limitations on activities of daily living.

165 Transthoracic Needle Aspiration Biopsy: Variables That Affect Risk of Pneumothorax
Joseph E. Cox, Caroline Chiles, Christopher M. McManus, Suzanne L. Aquino, and Robert H. Choplin
The only factors that independently altered the risk of pneumothorax were size of the lesion and presence of emphysema.

169 Descending Thoracic Aortic Aneurysm: Thoracic CT Findings after Endovascular Stent-Graft Placement
Toyohiko Sakai, Michael D. Dake, Charles P. Semba, Tetsuhisa Yamada, Akihiko Arakawa, Stephen T. Kee, Nobushige Hayashi, Mahmood K. Razavi, and Daniel Y. Sze
Thoracic CT is useful in the treatment of patients after stent-graft insertion for management of descending thoracic aortic aneurysm.

175 Treatment of Hemodialysis-related Central Venous Stenosis or Occlusion: Results of Primary Wallstent Placement and Follow-up in 50 Patients
Patrick Haage, Dierk Vorwerk, Werner Piroth, Karl Schuermann, and Rolf W. Guenther
Initial Wallstent deployment is effective in the treatment of central venous stenosis or occlusion and shows improved long-term patency rates as compared with those of other therapeutic modalities (eg, percutaneous balloon angioplasty alone).

Health Policy and Practice

181 Core-Needle and Surgical Breast Biopsy: Comparison of Three Methods of Assessing Cost
Jeffrey H. Burkhardt and Jonathan H. Sunshine
We calculated costs in three different ways—in terms of input resource costs, actual payments, and billed charges–and found remarkable consistency in relative costs among the measures, with surgical biopsy, including needle localization, uniformly costing two and a half to three times as much as core-needle biopsy.

Breast Imaging

189 Follow-up of Breast Lesions Diagnosed as Benign with Stereotactic Core-Needle Biopsy: Frequency of Mammographic Change and False-Negative Rate
Carol H. Lee, Liane E. Philpotts, Laura J. Horvath, and Irena Tocino
We believe that 6-month follow-up mammography for cases with nonspecific benign diagnoses and routine yearly screening mammography for cases with specific benign histologic results is a reasonable management strategy.

Computer Applications

195 Display Modes for CT Colonography Part I. Synthesis and Insertion of Polyps into Patient CT Data
Chandu Karadi, Christopher F. Beaulieu, R. Brooke Jeffrey, Jr, David S. Paik, and Sandy Napel
Our polyp synthesis and insertion method allows the generation of a variety of realistic colonic polyps that could not be distinguished from real lesions by experienced observers and, therefore, can facilitate the comparison of display techniques.

Continued—

TO SEE IS TO BELIEVE.

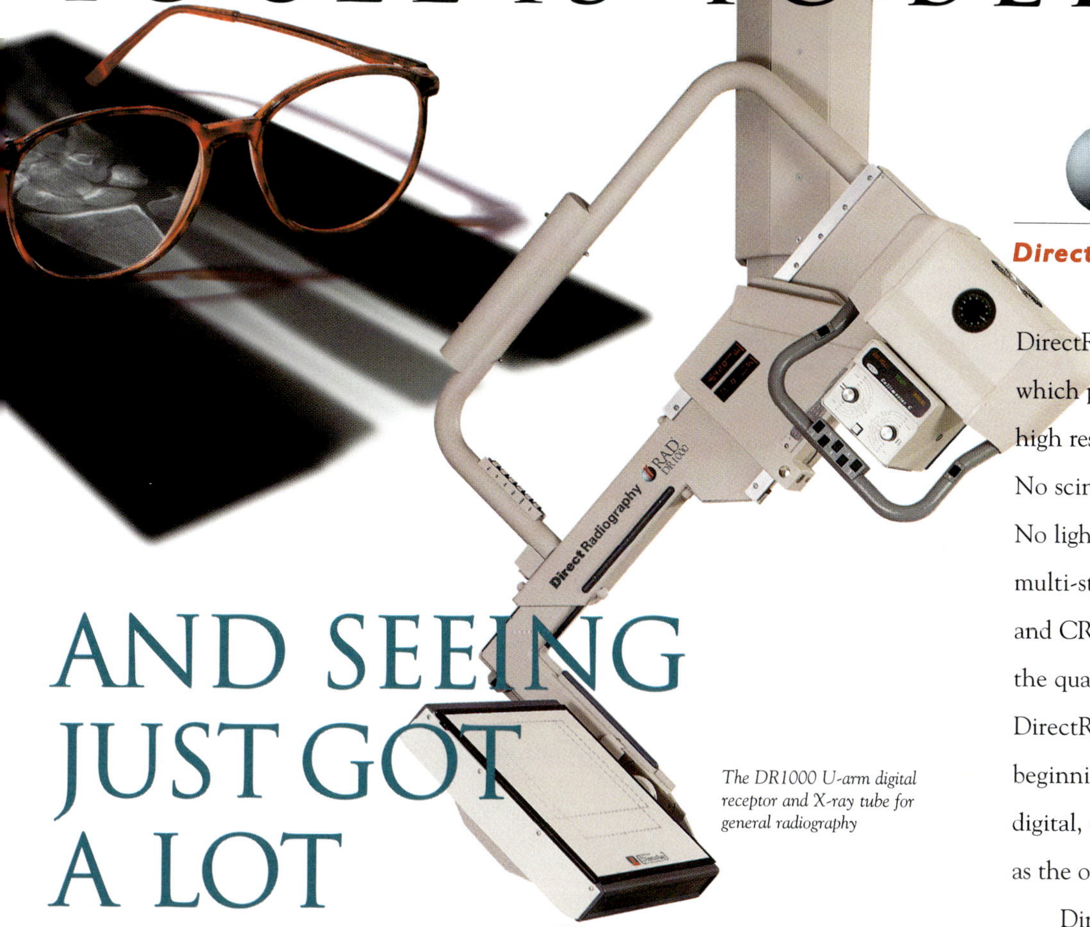

iiRAD™

Direct-to-digital X-ray systems with DirectRay®

DirectRay is a direct capture process which produces sharp, high-quality, high resolution images. No phosphors. No scintillators. No intermediate steps. No light to diffuse or scatter. Unlike multi-step processes such as screen-film and CR, there is nothing to degrade the quality of the digital signal. DirectRay is sharp and clear from the beginning, and because the original is digital, every copy has the same quality as the original.

DirectRay technology is available in the DR1000, a general radiography X-ray system, and the DR1000C, a dedicated chest system.

Ask your Sterling representative for an *ii*RAD data sheet and a side-by-side comparison of DirectRay versus CR or screen-film images. See for yourself how easy it is to improve your vision digitally with DirectRay. Or visit our Web site at http://www.DirectRadiography.com.

The DR1000 U-arm digital receptor and X-ray tube for general radiography

AND SEEING JUST GOT A LOT EASIER.

Quality diagnosis comes from seeing all of the right information. The more information you see in an image, the more confidence you have in your diagnosis. DirectRay, patented and clinically proven, produces digital X-ray images that are better than or equal to the best screen-film systems. And, as DirectRay images are captured digitally, these originals can be sent through your network for soft or hard copy review. *ii*RAD™ X-ray systems with DirectRay are a necessary step in the transition process to the all-digital department. Combine *ii*RAD with the Sterling *ii*SYS™ PACS and *ii*LINX™ printer systems for a completely integrated digital image and information system.

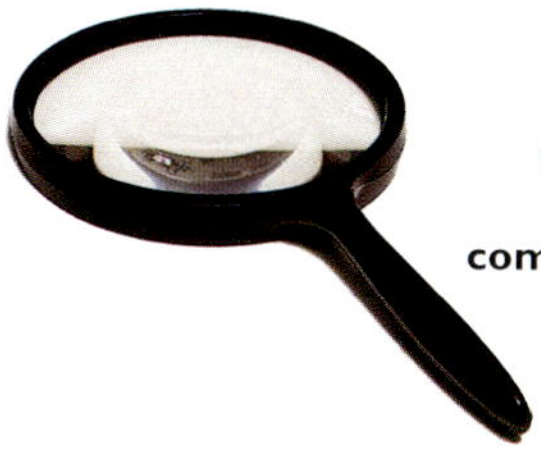

[DirectRay]®

Direct Radiography Corp.

Direct Radiography Corp. • Glasgow Business Community, Route 896 • P.O. Box 6020 • Newark, Delaware 19714-6020 USA
(800) 252 9099, then 7 • http://www.DirectRadiography.com • *DirectRay@DirectRadiography.com*

203 Display Modes for CT Colonography Part II. Blinded Comparison of Axial CT and Virtual Endoscopic and Panoramic Endoscopic Volume-rendered Studies
Christopher F. Beaulieu, R. Brooke Jeffrey, Jr, Chandu Karadi, David S. Paik, and Sandy Napel
Our panoramic rendering technique significantly increased the sensitivity for polyp detection above that of a display mode in which a conventional virtual camera is used, by increasing the percentage of displayed surface area.

Gastrointestinal Imaging

213 Pancreatic Carcinoma versus Chronic Pancreatitis: Dynamic MR Imaging
Pamela T. Johnson and Eric K. Outwater
The similar gradual pattern of enhancement and overlap in peak enhancement preclude distinction of the two entities on the basis of gadolinium-enhanced MR findings.

219 Pancreatic CT Imaging: Effects of Different Injection Rates and Doses of Contrast Material
Tonsok Kim, Takamichi Murakami, Satoru Takahashi, Atsuya Okada, Masatoshi Hori, Yoshifumi Narumi, and Hironobu Nakamura
Both a higher dose and a faster rate for the injection of contrast material thus appear to increase the maximum pancreatic enhancement.

227 Hepatic Iron Concentration: Noninvasive Estimation by Means of MR Imaging Techniques
Herbert L. Bonkovsky, Richard B. Rubin, Edward E. Cable, Ashley Davidoff, Tammo H. Pels Rijcken, and David D. Stark
Rapid gradient-recalled-echo MR imaging at high magnetic field strength is a sensitive, accurate, and noninvasive modality for the estimation of hepatic iron concentration and for ruling out clinically important hepatic iron overload (ie, greater than three times the upper limit of normal).

235 Hepatocellular Carcinoma: Association with Increased Iron Deposition in the Cirrhotic Liver at MR Imaging
Katsuyoshi Ito, Donald G. Mitchell, Toshifumi Gabata, Hie-Won L. Hann, Pyo N. Kim, Takeshi Fujita, Hitomi Awaya, Kazumitsu Honjo, and Naofumi Matsunaga
The occurrence of hepatocellular carcinoma (HCC) may be associated causally with iron deposition in large regenerative nodules in patients with cirrhosis, and MR imaging is a useful modality for assessing iron deposition in these regenerative nodules as a possible risk factor for the development of HCC.

241 Low-Grade Gastric Mucosa-associated Lymphoid Tissue Lymphoma: Correlation of Radiographic and Pathologic Findings
Young H. Kim, Hyo K. Lim, Joon K. Han, Byung I. Choi, Yong I. Kim, Won J. Lee, and Seung H. Kim
Low-grade gastric mucosa-associated lymphoid tissue lymphomas manifested as mucosal nodularity, either shallow or deep ulcers, and rugal thickening at upper gastrointestinal examination and showed similar findings to those of gastric carcinoma and *Helicobacter pylori* gastritis.

Pediatric Imaging

249 MR Cholangiography in the Evaluation of Neonatal Cholestasis
Twei-Shiun Jaw, Yu-Ting Kuo, Gin-Chung Liu, Shaou-Hsium Chen, and Chien-Kuo Wang
MR cholangiography can be used to depict the major biliary structures of neonates and small infants, and it can be used to accurately exclude biliary atresia as the cause of neonatal cholestasis by allowing visualization of the biliary tract.

257 Autoimmune Lymphoproliferative Syndrome: A Syndrome Associated with Inherited Genetic Defects That Impair Lymphocytic Apoptosis—CT and US Features
Nilo A. Avila, Andrew J. Dwyer, Janet K. Dale, Uri A. Lopatin, Michael C. Sneller, Elaine S. Jaffe, Jennifer M. Puck, and Stephen E. Straus
Patients with autoimmune lymphoproliferative syndrome demonstrate nonspecific imaging findings of lymphoproliferative disorders (adenopathy, splenomegaly, thymic enlargement, and hepatomegaly); the stability of the clinical findings over months to years and the pattern of lymph node echogenicity may suggest the diagnosis.

Technical Developments

265 MR Colonography: Optimized Enema Composition
Wolfgang Luboldt, Johannes M. Frohlich, Nicole Schneider, Dominik Weishaupt, Franziska Landolt, and Jorg F. Debatin
Iron glycerophosphate seems to be a feasible alternative to gadopentetate dimeglumine as a contrast enema in MR colonography.

270 Volumetric Imaging with Ultrasonic Spiral CT
Haim Azhari and Didi Sazbon
Findings in this study demonstrate that spiral ultrasonic CT is feasible.

Continued—

276 **Virtual CT Intravascular Endoscopy of the Aorta: Pierced Surface and Floating Shape Thresholding Artifacts**
Emanuele Neri, Davide Caramella, Fabio Falaschi, Paola Sbragia, Claudio Vignali, Edoardo Laiolo, Adriano Viviani, and Carlo Bartolozzi
Knowledge about segmentation pitfalls can help avoid the appearance of artifacts on virtual CT intravascular endoscopic images, thus preventing wrong interpretations of endoluminal findings.

280 **Gadolinium-based Contrast Agents as an Alternative at Vena Cavography in Patients with Renal Insufficiency: Early Experience**
John A. Kaufman, Stuart C. Geller, Hasan Bazari, and Arthur C. Waltman
Findings in this small series suggest that gadolinium-based contrast agents are suitable as an alternative at digital subtraction vena cavography in patients with renal insufficiency, particularly when a limited volume of contrast agent is needed.

285 **Head and Neck Cancer: Detection of Recurrence with Three-dimensional Principal Components Analysis at Dynamic FDG PET**
Yoshimi Anzai, Satoshi Minoshima, Gregory T. Wolf, and Richard L. Wahl
Findings in this study demonstrate improved distinction of tumors in the head and neck regions with principal components analysis images as compared to that with conventional standardized uptake value images.

Letters to the Editor

291 **Can Inversion-Recovery Gradient- and Spin-Echo T2-weighted MR Imaging Be an Alternative to Fast Spin-Echo Imaging with Fat Suppression?**
Masayuki Kanematsu and Hiroaki Hoshi

291 **Reply**
Martin N. J. M. Wasser, Milan E. J. Pijl, Els L. van Persijn van Meerten, Jan-Willem C. Gratama, and Johan L. Bloem

292 **Audience Preference for Scientific Presentation Method**
Edward I. Bluth and Kent Nash

Book Reviews

42 Imaging in Oncology. 2 Vols.
74 Guidelines and Gamuts in Musculoskeletal Ultrasound
164 Vascular Brachytherapy. 2nd ed.
202 PACS: Basic Principles and Applications

Interludes

142 Left Ventricular Mouse
226 Before Biopsy: A Worried Hepatocellular Carcinoma
264 An Egg-ceptional Dissection of the Ascending Aorta

Departments

293 Abstracts of Current Literature
16A Advertisers' Index
19A Announcements and Books, Audiovisual Materials, and Software Received
2A Associated Sciences Workshop 1999
43A Classified Services
24A Continuing Medical Education
36A Copyright and Certifications Agreement
37A Publication Information for Authors
63A *Radiology* Business Information
41A *Radiology* Manuscript Categorization Terms
65A RSNA Bulletin Board
15A RSNA Quick Reference

RSNA® Radiological Society of North America Founded in 1915

820 Jorie Boulevard
Oak Brook, Illinois 60523-2251
630/571-2670
FAX: 630/571-7837

Quick Reference

RSNA PURPOSE

The purpose of the Radiological Society of North America is to promote and develop the highest standards of radiology and related sciences through education and research. The Society seeks to provide radiologists and allied health scientists with educational programs and materials of the highest quality, and to constantly improve the content and value of these educational activities. The Society seeks to foster closer fellowship among all radiologists and greater cooperation among radiologists and members of other branches of medicine and allied health care professionals.

RSNA OFFICERS FOR 1999

President, **Seymour H. Levitt, MD**, Minneapolis, MN

President-Elect, **C. Douglas Maynard, MD**, Winston-Salem, NC

First Vice-President, **William M. Thompson, MD**, Minneapolis, MN

Second Vice-President, **J. Frank Wilson, MD**, Milwaukee, WI

Third Vice-President, **Stephen Balter, PhD**, New York, NY

Secretary-Treasurer, **David H. Hussey, MD**, Iowa City, IA

Historian, **William R. Eyler, MD**, Beverly Hills, MI

RSNA BOARD OF DIRECTORS FOR 1999

Jerry P. Petasnick, MD, Chairman of the Board, Chicago, IL

David H. Hussey, MD, Secretary-Treasurer, Iowa City, IA

Brian C. Lentle, MD, Liaison for Education, Vancouver, BC

R. Nick Bryan, MD, PhD, Liaison for Publications and Educational Materials, Bethesda, MD

Peggy J. Fritzsche, MD, Liaison for Communications and Corporate Relations, Riverside, CA

Robert R. Hattery, MD, Liaison Designate for Publications and Educational Materials, Rochester, MN

Seymour H. Levitt, MD, President, Minneapolis, MN

C. Douglas Maynard, MD, President-Elect, Winston-Salem, NC

Delmar J. Stauffer, Executive Director

RSNA IMPORTANT TELEPHONE NUMBERS

MAIN TELEPHONE	(630) 571-2670	MEMBERSHIP	(630) 571-7873 e-mail: membersh@rsna.org
FAX	(630) 571-7837	RESEARCH DEVELOPMENT	(630) 368-3756
ACCOUNTING	(630) 571-7812	PROGRAM SERVICES	(630) 571-7874
EXECUTIVE	(630) 571-7866	RESEARCH & EDUCATION FOUNDATION	(630) 571-7816
LEARNING CENTER	(630) 368-3753	ADVERTISING	(630) 571-7817
MARKETING COMMUNICATIONS	(630) 571-7830	CLASSIFIED ADVERTISING	(630) 571-7817
MEETINGS	(630) 571-7850	RSNA LINK	http://www.rsna.org
PERMISSIONS	(630) 571-7829	SUBSCRIPTIONS	(630) 571-7873 e-mail: subscrib@rsna.org

RSNA MEETING DATES AND LOCATIONS

1999 November 28 to December 3
McCormick Place, Chicago

2000 November 26 to December 1
McCormick Place, Chicago

2001 November 25 to November 30
McCormick Place, Chicago

RSNA YEAR-AT-A-GLANCE

July 1, 1999
Deadline for Receipt of Derek Harwood-Nash Fellowship Application

September 15, 1999
Third Seed Grant Deadline

September 17–19, 1999
RSNA Board of Directors Meeting

October 1, 1999
Deadline for Non–North American Advance Registration for RSNA Scientific Assembly

October 29, 1999
Deadline for North American Advance Registration for RSNA Scientific Assembly

November 28 to December 3, 1999
RSNA 85th Scientific Assembly and Annual Meeting

January 1, 2000
Call for Scientific Papers, Scientific Exhibits, and *info*RAD Exhibits

January 8, 2000
Deadline for Receipt of all RSNA R&E Foundation Grant Materials

January 15, 2000
First Seed Grant Deadline

February 18–20, 2000
RSNA Board of Directors Meeting

March 1, 2000
Roentgen Centennial Fellow "Preliminary Letter of Interest" Deadline

April 12–13, 2000
R&E Foundation Trustee Meeting

April 15, 2000
Deadline for Submission of Scientific Paper, Scientific Exhibit, and *info*RAD Applications

May 1, 2000
Deadline for Receipt of Editorial Fellowship Applications

May 15, 2000
Second Seed Grant Deadline

June 8–10, 2000
RSNA Board of Directors Meeting

Advertisers' Index

RSNA Advertising Policy

According to the advertising policy of the Radiological Society of North America, the information describing radiological equipment, products, and services offered by vendors in their advertisements should be ethical, educational, professional, of value in furthering the radiologic evaluation and treatment of patients and furthering the education of the radiologists and allied scientists. The guidelines below should be followed for advertising in RSNA journals.

- All advertising must be directed to radiologic diagnosis, therapy, research, communication and/or to the professional and managerial roles of radiologists and allied scientists. Advertising material should be consistent with the highest standards of professionalism.
- RSNA reserves the right to reject copy which, in its opinion, is not in good taste, is unprofessional, or is inappropriate for a radiology publication, or offers products or services not in the best interest of the patient or the Society. Advertisements that are constructed to resemble the journal's editorial pages will not be accepted in that form.
- Acceptance of advertising does not mean endorsement by RSNA of the products or services advertised, the advertisers, or the claims made.

For media kits and questions about advertising ONLY, contact:

Jim Drew, *Director of Advertising*
RSNA Publications
820 Jorie Boulevard
Oak Brook, IL 60523-2251
(630) 571-2670
FAX (630) 571-7837

For all other RSNA department telephone numbers, see "RSNA Quick Reference"; consult "Departments" in the Table of Contents for page.

Aloka 27A
American College of Radiology 28A
Bioscan 20A
C.B. Fleet 25A
Cejka & Company 58A
CompHealth 47A
Daniel & Yeager 45A
Diversified Diagnostic Products, Inc 21A, 32A
East Texas Medical Center 47A
Eastern Regional Health Board 56A
Franciscan Skemp Healthcare 51A
Fuji Medical Systems IFC–1A
GE Medical Systems OBC
Hitachi Medical Systems America 22A–23A
The Hospital for Sick Children 59A
Interim Physicians 49A
J & C Nationwide 56A
Karmanos Cancer Institute 55A
Lahey Clinic 57A
Mount Sinai School of Mediciene 55A, 61A
New York Medical College 53A
Penn State Geisinger Health System 53A
Philips Medical Systems 29A
RadioGraphics 34A
RSNA Associated Sciences 2A
RSNA International Programs 31A
RSNA Learning Center 67A–70A
RSNA Resident Membership 17A–18A
RSNA Scientific Assembly and Annual Meeting IBC
S&S X-Ray Products Inc 33A
W.B. Saunders Company 35A
Siemens Medical Systems, Inc 9A
Staff Relief, Inc 58A
Staten Island University Hospital 28A
Sterling Diagnostic Imaging 11A
Synarc 13A
Temple University School of Medicne 52A
Toshiba 4A
Trex Medical Corporation 7A
University of Pittsburgh Medical Center 51A
Vista Staffing Solutions 49A

Announcements and Books, Audiovisual Materials, and Software Received

Announcements

Associated Sciences to Present Program at RSNA '99

The RSNA Associated Sciences Consortium is sponsoring a workshop on Saturday, November 27, 1999, from 10:15 AM to 4:00 PM during the RSNA Scientific Assembly in Chicago. The theme for the workshop is "New Realities in Radiology: Multidisciplinary Strategies for Compliance." Five speakers will discuss a variety of issues currently affecting radiology departments. The keynote presentation, "Compliance, Audits, and Radiology: The Art of Survival," will be given by Karol Handrahan, RT(R).

Tom Hoffman, senior attorney for the American College of Radiology, will present a luncheon program entitled "Uncle Sam Strikes Back: Medicine in the Enforcement Age."

The afternoon practicum will include three associates from the law firm of Shaw and Pittman, Washington, DC. They are Mr Andrew Woods, who will speak on the topic of legislative policy; Mr Gadi Weinreich, an expert on Medicare fraud, abuse, and compliance plan development; and Mr Bruce Freid, formerly of the Health Care Financing Administration, who will discuss outpatient hospital reimbursement changes affecting radiology and radiation oncology. A question and answer session will occur after the presentation.

The Associated Sciences program also includes a series of eight refresher courses of interest to managers and supervisors of radiology departments and radiologists. Three new courses will be introduced this year: "Economic Implications of Regulatory Change," "Asset Management," and "New Challenges in Radiology Planning and Design."

The consortium is composed of the American Healthcare Radiology Administrators, American Institute of Architects—Academy of Architecture for Health, American Radiological Nurses Association, American Society of Radiologic Technologists, Association of Educators in Radiological Sciences, Radiology Business Management Association, Society of Diagnostic Medical Sonographers, Society of Nuclear Medicine—Technologists Section, Society for Radiation Oncology Administrators, Association of Vascular and Interventional Radiographers, and Section for Magnetic Resonance Technologists of the International Society for Magnetic Resonance in Medicine.

Members of the participating organizations, physicians, physicists, and exhibitors are encouraged to attend the Associated Sciences Program. Registration for the RSNA Scientific Assembly and Annual Meeting (November 27 to December 3) is required for admission. Registration may be made in advance by mail before October 24 or at the assembly. Advance registration brochures will be available through the office of each association beginning the 1st week in July. Free bus transportation is provided by the RSNA from all hotels to McCormick Place beginning Saturday morning.

Detailed information about the Associated Sciences Program will appear in this issue of *Radiology* and in the RSNA Scientific Program, a supplement to the November issue of *Radiology*.

Free Radiology Review Course for Residents

The Department of Radiology of New Jersey Medical School/UMDNJ (University of Medicine and Dentistry of New Jersey) will hold its 2nd annual radiology review course for residents on July 31 to August 1, 1999, on its campus in Newark, NJ. The conference is ideal for residents who are preparing for their board examinations. Course chairman: Wolansky. Faculty: Baker, Berdon, Kalisher, Lang, Sider, Wojtowycz, Wolansky. Tuition is free, but places are limited and preregistration is essential. For further information, contact Leo J. Wolansky, MD, Department of Radiology, UH C-320, New Jersey Medical School/UMDNJ, 150 Bergen St, Newark, NJ 07103; telephone (973) 972-5149; fax (973) 972-7429; *e-mail LWolansky@aol.com.*

CAS '99

The Institute of Medical Physics of the University of Erlangen is sponsoring the 5th International Workshop on Computer Assisted Surgery and Rapid Prototyping in Medicine (CAS '99) on October 14–16, 1999, at the Congress Center, Erlangen, Germany. This workshop is designed to provide a forum for and by experts in the fields of medicine, clinical research, and basic sciences, as well as physicians, engineers, computer scientists, and physicists, to exchange their views and experiences. Topics include technical and clinical aspects of medical imaging, simulation and planning, image processing and virtual endoscopy, surgical navigation systems and neurosurgery, robotics, orthopedic surgery, and rapid prototyping in medicine. Fee: DM 250 until July 31, DM 300 thereafter (DM 125 [DM 150] for students). For further information, contact Willi A. Kalender, PhD, Institute of Medical Physics, University of Erlangen, Krankenhausstrasse 12, 91054 Erlangen, Germany; telephone 49 9131 85 223 10; fax 49 9131 85 228 24; e-mail *cas99@imp.uni-erlangen.de; http://www.imp.uni-erlangen.de/cas99/.*

First International Radiologic Pathology Course

The First International Radiologic Pathology Course will be held on October 18–21, 1999, at the Riyadh Armed Forces Hospital, Riyadh, Saudi Arabia. For further information, contact the Department of Postgraduate and Academic Affairs, Riyadh Armed Forces Hospital, PO Box 7897, Riyadh 11159, Saudi Arabia; telephone 966 1 477 7714, ext 4933 or 4937; fax 966 1 476 0853 or 966 1 478 4057.

9th International Symposium of Nephrology at Montecatini

The 9th International Symposium of Nephrology at Montecatini will take place on October 25–27, 1999, at the Terme Tamerici, Montecatini Terme, Italy. The theme of this year's symposium is "Kidney, Proteins and Growth Factors." It is devoted to the discussion of advances in hormonal and nonhormonal protein research, proteinuria (pathophysiology and management), mechanisms of progression of chronic renal disease, growth factors in the progression and therapy of kidney disease, tubular hypermetabolism, and new methods for analysis of proteins. Advances in the assessment of kidney function will also be addressed. The official language of the symposium is English. Chairmen: Bianchi, Drüeke, Kanwar, Locatelli, Rabkin. Fee: $210. For further information, contact Professor Claudio Bianchi, University of Pisa, U.O. Nefrologia Universitaria, Ospedale S. Chiara, 56100 Pisa, Italy; telephone 39 050 992573; fax 39 050 553414 or 39 050 993110.

Books, Audiovisual Materials, and Software Received

Radiology carries a complete listing of all books, CD-ROMs, and other material received by the Radiological Society of North America. If the material is later reviewed, the reviews of books will be printed in *Radiology* and the reviews of CD-ROMs and electronic material will appear in *RadioGraphics*.

Send publications for review to Richard A. Szucs, MD, Book Review Editor, *Radiology* Editorial Office, 1001 E Broad St, Suite 310, Richmond, VA 23219.

Arteriovenous Malformations in Functional Areas of the Brain. Edited by Shokei Yamada, MD, PhD. Hardcover, $145.00; 276 pp, 114 illustrations. ISBN: 0-87993-424-7. Armonk, NY: Futura, 1999.

Classic Radiologic Signs: An Atlas and History. Michael E. Mulligan. Hardcover, $49.95; 208 pp, 222 illustrations. ISBN: 1-85070-664-6. Pearl River, NY: Parthenon, 1997.

Announcements and Books, Audiovisual Materials, and Software Received

Diagnostic Ultrasound. Essentials of Medical Imaging series. Stewart C. Bushong, ScD. Softcover, $19.95; 160 pp, illustrations. ISBN: 0-07-012017-X. Blacklick, Ohio: McGraw-Hill, 1999.

Disorders of the Pancreas: Current Issues in Diagnosis and Management. Edited by Gerard P. Burns, MCh, FRCS, Simmy Bank, MD, FRCP. Hardcover, $82.00; 524 pp, 98 illustrations. ISBN: 0-07-105402-2. Blacklick, Ohio: McGraw-Hill, 1999.

Early Breast Cancer from Screening to Multidisciplinary Management. Edited by M. W. E. Morgan, FRCS, R. Warren, FRCP, FRCR, G. Querci della Rovere, MD, FRCS. Hardcover, $95.00; 288 pp, 366 illustrations. ISBN: 90-5702-469-1. Amsterdam, the Netherlands: Harwood Academic Publishers, 1998.

Felson's Principles of Chest Roentgenology: A Programmed Text. 2nd ed. Lawrence R. Goodman, MD. Softcover, $35.00; 261 pp, 193 illustrations. ISBN: 0-7216-7685-5. Philadelphia, Pa: Saunders, 1999.

Patient Care. Essentials of Medical Imaging series. Erica Koch Williams, MEd, RT(R)(M), Stewart C. Bushong, ScD. Softcover, $19.95; 159 pp, illustrations. ISBN: 0-07-070632-8. Blacklick, Ohio: McGraw-Hill, 1999.

Patient Positioning. Essentials of Medical Imaging series. Mark J. Schubert, RT(R), Stewart C. Bushong, ScD. Softcover, $19.95; 108 pp, illustrations. ISBN: 0-07-058067-7. Blacklick, Ohio: McGraw-Hill, 1999.

Pocket Guide to Body CT Differential Diagnosis. Richard M. Slone, MD, Andrew J. Fisher, MD. Softcover, $35.00; 380 pp. ISBN: 0-07-134435-7. Blacklick, Ohio: McGraw-Hill, 1999.

Radiation Protection. Essentials of Medical Imaging series. Stewart C. Bushong, ScD. Softcover, $19.95; 155 pp, illustrations. ISBN: 0-07-012013-7. Blacklick, Ohio: McGraw-Hill, 1999.

Radiology and Imaging for Medical Students. 7th ed. David Sutton, MD, FRCP, FRCR. Softcover, $36.00; 279 pp, 246 illustrations. ISBN: 0-443-05917-9. Philadelphia, Pa: Churchill Livingstone, 1998.

Thoracic Imaging: A Practical Approach. Richard M. Slone, MD, Fernando R. Gutierrez, MD, Andrew J. Fisher, MD. Hardcover, $89.00; 383 pp, 376 illustrations. ISBN: 0-07-058223-8. Blacklick, Ohio: McGraw-Hill, 1999.

Ultrasound Atlas of Vascular Diseases. Carol A. Krebs, RT, RDMS, RVT, Vishan L. Giyanani, MD, Ronald L. Eisenbery, MD. Hardcover, $175.00; 448 pp, 724 illustrations. ISBN: 0-8385-9244-9. Stamford, Conn: Appleton & Lange, 1998.

Vascular and Interventional Radiology. Karim Valji, MD. Hardcover, $140.00; 509 pp, 578 illustrations. ISBN: 0-7216-7003-2. Philadelphia, Pa: Saunders, 1999.

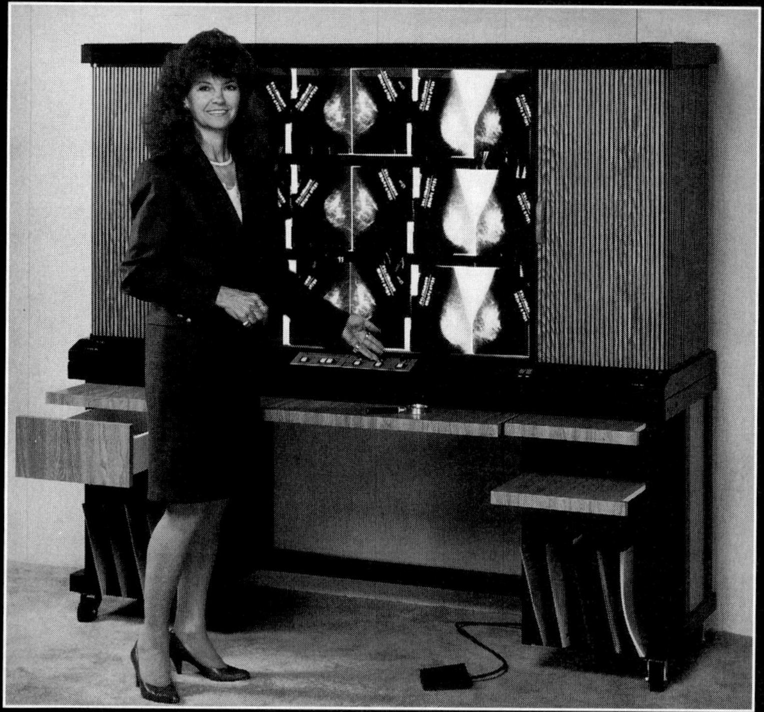

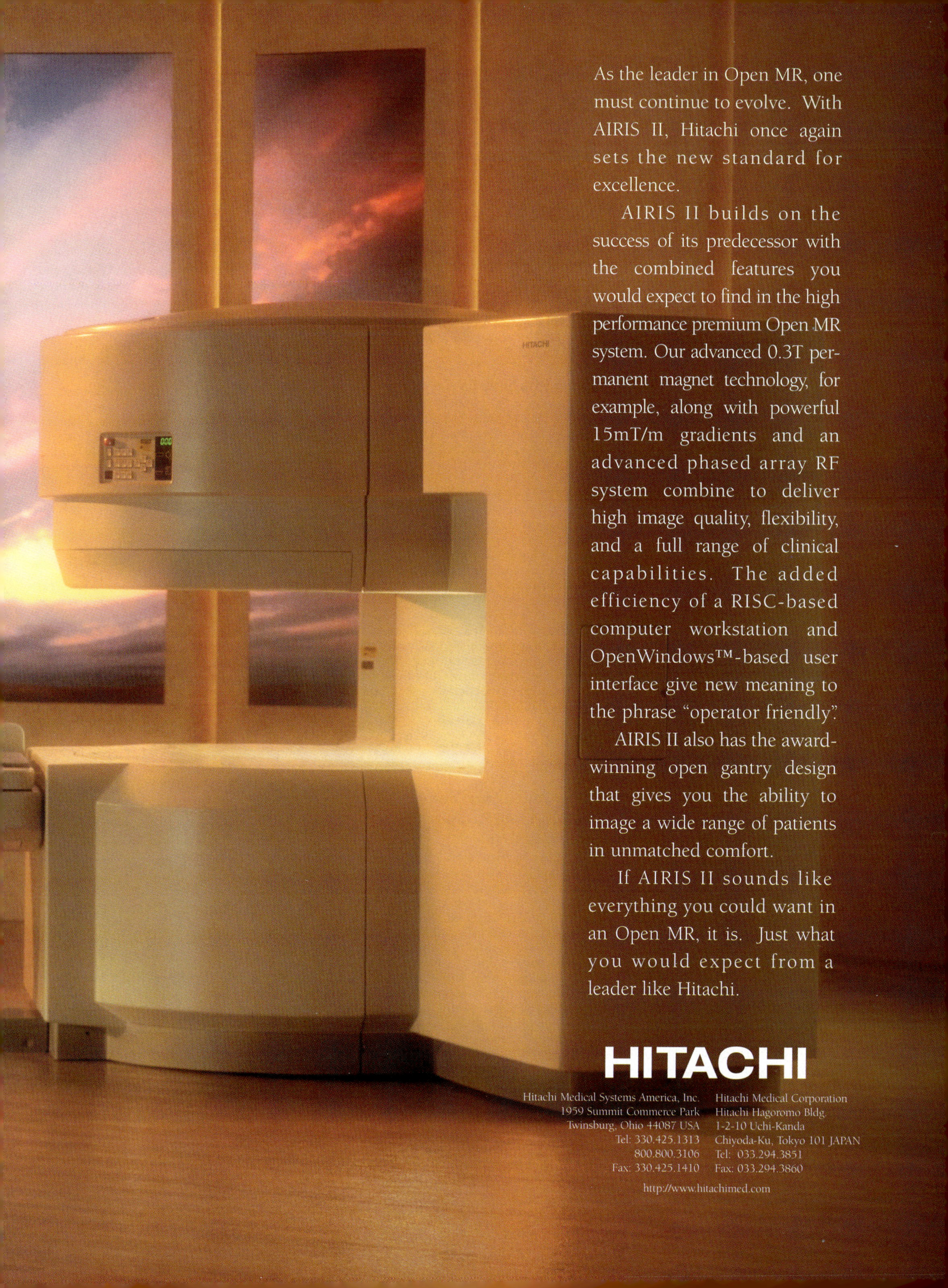
HITACHI
As the leader in Open MR, one must continue to evolve. With AIRIS II, Hitachi once again sets the new standard for excellence.
AIRIS II builds on the success of its predecessor with the combined features you would expect to find in the high performance premium Open MR system. Our advanced 0.3T permanent magnet technology, for example, along with powerful 15mT/m gradients and an advanced phased array RF system combine to deliver high image quality, flexibility, and a full range of clinical capabilities. The added efficiency of a RISC-based computer workstation and OpenWindows™-based user interface give new meaning to the phrase "operator friendly".
AIRIS II also has the award-winning open gantry design that gives you the ability to image a wide range of patients in unmatched comfort.
If AIRIS II sounds like everything you could want in an Open MR, it is. Just what you would expect from a leader like Hitachi.
HITACHI
Hitachi Medical Systems America, Inc.
1959 Summit Commerce Park
Twinsburg, Ohio 44087 USA
Tel: 330.425.1313
800.800.3106
Fax: 330.425.1410
Hitachi Medical Corporation
Hitachi Hagoromo Bldg.
1-2-10 Uchi-Kanda
Chiyoda-Ku, Tokyo 101 JAPAN
Tel: 033.294.3851
Fax: 033.294.3860
http://www.hitachimed.com

Continuing Medical Education

NOTE: Notices of continuing medical education programs will be considered for publication in *Radiology* if the program is directly relevant to medical imaging and if the following information is included: (*a*) dates and location, (*b*) a brief description of the course, (*c*) a listing of local and visiting faculty, (*d*) fees, and (*e*) number of category 1 credits that are available. Such notices should be submitted *at least* 5 months before the meeting date. Announcements of CME programs we consider not pertinent will not be published. We assume no responsibility for the content of CME programs appearing here. **Address announcements to** Julie Pietryla, RSNA Publications, 820 Jorie Blvd, Oak Brook, IL 60523.

Continuing medical education programs are listed according to diagnostic discipline; interdisciplinary programs are grouped under the predominant or first-listed specialty.

Diagnostic Imaging

Radiology Refresher Course

A "Radiology Refresher Course," sponsored by the Department of Radiology, University of Minnesota, will take place on August 22–25, 1999, at the Silverado Country Club and Resort, Napa Valley, Calif. This course is designed to provide an overview of philosophy and up-to-date techniques used in everyday clinical practice. After attending the course, participants will be able to identify current applications of ultrasonography, computed tomography, and magnetic resonance imaging in radiology and demonstrate effective imaging approaches to common clinical situations. Course directors: Engeler, Everson, Thompson, Trenkner, Truwit. Fee: $695; 18 hours of category 1 credit will be available. For further information, contact the Office of Continuing Medical Education, University of Minnesota, 615 Washington Ave SE, Suite 107, Minneapolis, MN 55414; telephone (800) 776-8636 or (612) 626-7600; fax (612) 626-7766; *http://www.med.umn.edu/cme/*.

8th Annual Pulmonary and Mediastinal Radiology Course

The "8th Annual Pulmonary and Mediastinal Radiology Course," sponsored by the Armed Forces Institute of Pathology/American Registry of Pathology, will be held on September 18–19, 1999, at the Washington Marriott Hotel, Washington, DC. This course is designed to provide radiologists, thoracic surgeons, and pulmonary medicine physicians a review of current thoracic imaging. The morphologic, physiologic, and pathologic basis of disease will be emphasized and correlated with abnormal radiologic findings in chest radiography, computed tomography, and magnetic resonance imaging. Faculty: Abbott, Galvin, Gefter, McAdams, Rosado de Christenson, Strollo, Templeton. Fee: $300 until September 7, $330 thereafter ($180 [$210] for residents; $125 for military personnel); 13.25 hours of category 1 credit will be available. For further information, contact Earlene Turner, Department of Radiologic Pathology, Armed Forces Institute of Pathology/American Registry of Pathology, 14th and Alaska Ave NW, Washington, DC 20306-6000; telephone (202) 782-2438; fax (202) 782-8124; e-mail *turnere@afip.osd.mil; http://www .afip.org*.

Organ Imaging Review

The Department of Medical Imaging, Faculty of Medicine, of the University of Toronto is sponsoring an "Organ Imaging Review" on October 3–7, 1999, at the Toronto Marriott Eaton Centre Hotel, Toronto, Ontario, Canada. This review will focus on subjects of interest to both general radiologists and radiologists in training. Participants will be able to enhance their knowledge of thoracic, abdominal, neuroradiologic, musculoskeletal, biliary, and luminal gastrointestinal imaging, as well as imaging of infertility and stroke. Newer modalities and state-of-the-art imaging will be emphasized. Course director: Rappaport. Fee: Can $800 (U.S. $550) until September 17, Can $850 (U.S. $590) thereafter; 27.5 hours of category 1 credit will be available. For further information, contact the Office of Continuing Education, Faculty of Medicine, University of Toronto, FitzGerald Bldg, Rm 121, 150 College St, Toronto, Ontario, Canada M5S 3E2; telephone (416) 978-2719; fax (416) 971-2200; e-mail *a.lind@utoronto.ca; http://www.cme .utoronto.ca*.

24th Annual San Diego Postgraduate Radiology Review Course

The 24th Annual San Diego Postgraduate Radiology Review Course, sponsored by the University of California–San Diego School of Medicine, will be held on October 4–8, 1999, at the Hotel del Coronado, San Diego, Calif. This course, intended for practicing radiologists, will be a comprehensive review of the recent advances and most difficult subject material within each subspecialty. Emphasis is placed on practical and useful clinical information and understanding clinical problems. Fee: $995 ($700 for residents, fellows, and technologists); 39 hours of category 1 credit will be available. For further information, contact Ryals & Associates, Inc, PO Box 1925, Roswell, GA 30077-1925; telephone (770) 641-9773; fax (770) 552-9859; e-mail *webmaster@ryalsmeet.com; http://www.ryalsmeet.com*.

Mt Sinai 1999 Body Imaging Update

The "Mt Sinai 1999 Body Imaging Update," sponsored by the International Institute for Continuing Medical Education, will be held on October 9–12, 1999, at the Plaza Hotel, New York, NY. This is a comprehensive course that covers current imaging concepts of the most important subspecialty areas in the field of body imaging. Basic anatomy and recent advances in the various subspecialty areas will be reviewed. Emphasis will be placed on the practical relationship between imaging and the clinical problems presented by patients. Program directors: Drayer, Som. Fee: $775 ($550 for residents, fellows, and technologists); 22.5 hours of category 1 credit will be available. For further information, contact Ryals & Associates, Inc, PO Box 1925, Roswell, GA 30077-1925; telephone (770) 641-9773; fax (770) 552-9859; e-mail *webmaster@ryalsmeet .com; http://www.ryalsmeet.com*.

Breast Imaging

Breast Imaging and Interventions Update

The University of California–San Diego is sponsoring a "Breast Imaging and Interventions Update" course on October 1–3, 1999, at the Hotel del Coronado, San Diego, Calif. This course will provide a practical overview of breast imaging and interventions by leaders in the field. Topics include evaluation of the male breast, fine- and core-needle biopsy, and diagnosis of breast disease with mammography, ultrasonography, and magnetic resonance imaging. Fee: $475 ($350 for residents, fellows, and technologists); 15 hours of category 1 credit will be available. For further information, contact Ryals & Associates, Inc, PO Box 1925, Roswell, GA 30077-1925; telephone (770) 641-9773; fax (770) 552-9859; e-mail *webmaster@ryalsmeet.com; http://www .ryalsmeet.com*.

Computed Tomography

Clinical Essentials of CT and MRI

"Clinical Essentials of CT and MRI," a course sponsored by the Institute for Advanced Medical Education, will take place on October 27–31, 1999, at the Renaissance Hotel, Chicago, Ill. This is a weekend course designed for practicing radiologists and technologists who want to gain practical knowledge of computed tomography and magnetic resonance imaging. Fee: $745; 18 hours of category 1 credit will be available. For further information, contact Cheryl Ann

Continued

DeLena, Institute for Advanced Medical Education, 14 Elm Pl, Rye, NY 10580; telephone (914) 921-5700; fax (914) 921-6048; e-mail *info@iame.com; http://www.iame.com.*

Interventional Radiology

Practical Training in Interventional Radiology

A course entitled "Practical Training in Interventional Radiology," sponsored by the University of Texas–M. D. Anderson Cancer Center, will take place on October 4–8, 1999, at the University of Texas–M. D. Anderson Cancer Center, Houston, Tex, and on October 11–15, 1999, at University Hospital Sart Tilman, Liège, Belgium. This course is designed to teach technical skills to physicians who perform minimally invasive vascular and nonvascular procedures and to acquaint them with products currently available for the performance of these procedures. The course will incorporate 5 days of hands-on training using the pig as a model. Fee: $2,500 (includes all course materials and lunch); 40 hours of category 1 credit will be available. For further information, contact Ken Wright, PhD, or Sidney Wallace, MD, M. D. Anderson Cancer Center, 1515 Holcombe Blvd, Houston, TX 77030; telephone (713) 792-2733; fax (713) 745-3034; e-mail *kwright@di.mdacc.tmc.edu*; or Robert Dondelinger, MD, or Laurent Dorthu, MD, Department of Medical Imaging, University Hospital Sart Tilman, Domaine Univ du Sart Tilman B35, 4000 Liège, Belgium; telephone 32 4 366 7259; fax 32 4 366 7224; e-mail *rdondelinger@chu.ulg.ac.be; http://rpiwww.mdacc.tmc.edu/di/ditraining.html.*

19th Annual Comprehensive Review of Vascular and Interventional Radiology

The 19th Annual Comprehensive Review of Vascular and Interventional Radiology, sponsored by the University of California–San Diego, will take place on October 8–10, 1999, at the Hotel del Coronado, San Diego, Calif. This course is designed to provide a comprehensive review of vascular and interventional radiology. It is intended for interventionists and interventional fellows, general radiologists who perform invasive procedures, and radiology residents. Program directors: D'Agostino, Oglevie. Fee: $550 ($375 for residents, fellows, and technologists); 18.75 hours of category 1 credit will be available. For further information, contact Ryals & Associates, Inc, PO Box 1925, Roswell, GA 30077-1925; telephone (770) 641-9773; fax (770) 552-9859; e-mail *webmaster@ryalsmeet.com; http://www.ryalsmeet.com.*

Interventional Radiology and Vascular Imaging 1999

The Department of Radiology, University of Pennsylvania, is sponsoring the "Interventional Radiology and Vascular Imaging 1999" course, which will be held on October 17–20, 1999, at the University of Pennsylvania Medical Center, Philadelphia, Pa. This course will provide a thorough and intensive review of magnetic resonance angiography and interventional radiology throughout the body. Fundamentals of well-established procedures and the latest developments in new techniques will be reviewed by a faculty of nationally known experts. Course directors: Haskal, Soulen. Fee: $750 ($495 for residents and fellows); 24 hours of category 1 credit will be available. For further information, contact Janice Ford Benner, Department of Radiology, University of Pennsylvania Medical Center, 3400 Spruce St, 1 Founders Bldg, Philadelphia, PA 19104; telephone (215) 662-7825; fax (215) 349-5925.

Neuroradiology

AFIP Neuroradiology Weekend

The Armed Forces Institute of Pathology/American Registry of Pathology is sponsoring the "AFIP Neuroradiology Weekend," to take place on August 28–29, 1999, at the Wyndham Emerald Plaza Hotel, San Diego, Calif. This weekend course is designed to provide radiologists, neurologists, neurosurgeons, and pathologists a basic review and update of neuroradiology. The essential morphologic and physiologic principles that create the diagnostic image will be emphasized. Important radiologic-pathologic concepts will be illustrated through the use of magnetic resonance imaging, computed tomography and conventional modalities. A series of unknown cases will be discussed at the end of each session. Faculty: Barakos, Berger, Koeller, Osborn, Ross, Smirniotopoulos, Smoker. Fee: $300 until August 18, $330 thereafter ($180 [$210] for residents; $125 for military personnel); 15.5 hours of category 1 credit will be available. For further information, contact Earlene Turner, Department of Radiologic Pathology, Armed Forces Institute of Pathology/American Registry of Pathology, 14th and Alaska Ave NW, Washington, DC 20306-6000; telephone (202) 782-2438; fax (202) 782-8124; e-mail *turnere@afip.osd.mil; http://www.afip.org.*

Mt Sinai 1999 Brain, Spine, Neurovascular and ENT Imaging Update

The International Institute for Continuing Medical Education is sponsoring the "Mt Sinai 1999 Brain, Spine, Neurovascular and ENT Imaging Update" on October 13–17, 1999, at the Plaza Hotel, New York, NY. This course is designed for neuroradiologists, general radiologists, and clinicians who are interested in imaging of the brain, spine, heart, and neck. Case material will include examples of common and uncommon diseases that affect these areas. Program directors: Drayer, Som. Fee: $795 ($550 for residents, fellows, and technologists); 25.5 hours of category 1 credit will be available. For further information, contact Ryals & Associates, Inc, PO Box 1925, Roswell, GA 30077-1925; telephone (770) 641-9773; fax (770) 552-9859; e-mail *webmaster@ryalsmeet.com; http://www.ryalsmeet.com.*

Nuclear Medicine

Nuclear Cardiology Symposium and Workshop

A "Nuclear Cardiology Symposium and Workshop," co-sponsored by the Department of Continuing Medical Education of the University of Wisconsin Medical School and Heart Care Associates, will take place on October 22–23, 1999, at the Sheraton Milwaukee Airport Hotel, Milwaukee, Wis. This course will provide an update and review of many topics related to nuclear cardiology. Fee: $495 ($295 for technologists); 14 hours of category 1 credit will be available. For further information, contact Sarah Aslakson, Department of Continuing Medical Education, University of Wisconsin Medical School, 2715 Marshall Ct, Madison, WI 53705; telephone (608) 263-2856; fax (608) 262-8421; e-mail *aslakson@facstaff.wisc.edu; http://www.medsch.wisc.edu/cme/cme.html.*

Southeastern Chapter, Society of Nuclear Medicine

The Southeastern Chapter of the Society of Nuclear Medicine is holding its 40th Annual Meeting on October 29–31, 1999, at the Wynfrey Hotel, Birmingham, Ala. This year's course is entitled "Imaging and Therapeutic Advances in Nuclear Medicine." Topics include oncology, cardiology, ventilation perfusion versus computed tomography for detection of pulmonary embolus, and carotid balloon occlusion testing in neurovascular disease. Gastrointestinal infection in children, deep venous thrombosis imaging, and dealing with imaging artifacts will also be discussed. Approximately 35 companies will exhibit their nuclear medicine–related instrumentation, radiopharmaceuticals, and supplies. Program committee: Halliburton, Martin. Fee: $150 for physician nonmembers, $100 for physician members ($85 for residents and technologist nonmembers; $60 for

technologist members); category 1 accreditation pending. For further information, contact Vincent J. Sodd, PhD, executive director, Southeastern Chapter, SNM, Inc, 5987 Turpin Hills Dr, Cincinnati, OH 45244-3946; telephone (513) 231-6955.

Ultrasonography

Principles and Instruments

"Principles and Instruments," a course sponsored by and being held at the Center for Medical Ultrasound, Wake Forest University School of Medicine, will take place on September 8–10, 1999. This introductory course, intended for beginning physicians and allied health students, will provide participants with an understanding of the physical principles and instruments of ultrasonography and how these principles apply to clinical practice. Topics include transducers, spectral and color-flow Doppler instruments, artifacts, performance, and safety. Fee: $495; 16 hours of category 1 credit will be available. For further information, contact the Center for Medical Ultrasound, Wake Forest University School of Medicine, Medical Center Blvd, Winston-Salem, NC 27157-1039; telephone (800) 277-7654 or (336) 716-4505; fax (336) 716-4204; e-mail *cmu@wfubmc.edu; http://www.wfubmc.edu/bgsm/ultrasound.*

Obstetrical Ultrasound

"Obstetrical Ultrasound," a course sponsored by and being held at the Center for Medical Ultrasound, Wake Forest University School of Medicine, will take place on September 13–17, 1999. About 15 hours are dedicated to lectures by experienced sonologists, with the remaining time spent in scanning laboratories with obstetric and gynecologic patients. Fee: $945; 30 hours of category 1 credit will be available. For further information, contact the Center for Medical Ultrasound, Wake Forest University School of Medicine, Medical Center Blvd, Winston-Salem, NC 27157-1039; telephone (800) 277-7654 or (336) 716-4505; fax (336) 716-4204; e-mail *cmu@wfubmc .edu; http://www.wfubmc. edu/bgsm/ultrasound.*

Adult Echocardiography

"Adult Echocardiography," a course sponsored by and being held at the Center for Medical Ultrasound, Wake Forest University School of Medicine, will take place on September 20–24, 1999. This course will provide an introduction to basic cardiac ultrasonography techniques, including two-dimensional and m-mode echocardiography and spectral and color Doppler flow imaging. While brief overviews of advanced techniques such as transesophageal and stress echocardiography are provided, emphasis will be placed on fundamental and practical aspects of adult echocardiography. Several small scanning laboratory sessions will be conducted, featuring up-to-date equipment from many major manufacturers, to provide practical hands-on experience. Fee: $895; 32 hours of category 1 credit will be available. For further information, contact the Center for Medical Ultrasound, Wake Forest University School of Medicine, Medical Center Blvd, Winston-Salem, NC 27157-1039; telephone (800) 277-7654 or (336) 716-4505; fax (336) 716-4204; e-mail *cmu@wfubmc.edu; http://www.wfubmc .edu/bgsm/ultrasound.*

Neurovascular Ultrasound

"Neurovascular Ultrasound (Carotid and TCD)," a course sponsored by and being held at the Center for Medical Ultrasound, Wake Forest University School of Medicine, will take place on September 27 to October 1 and December 13–17, 1999. This course will

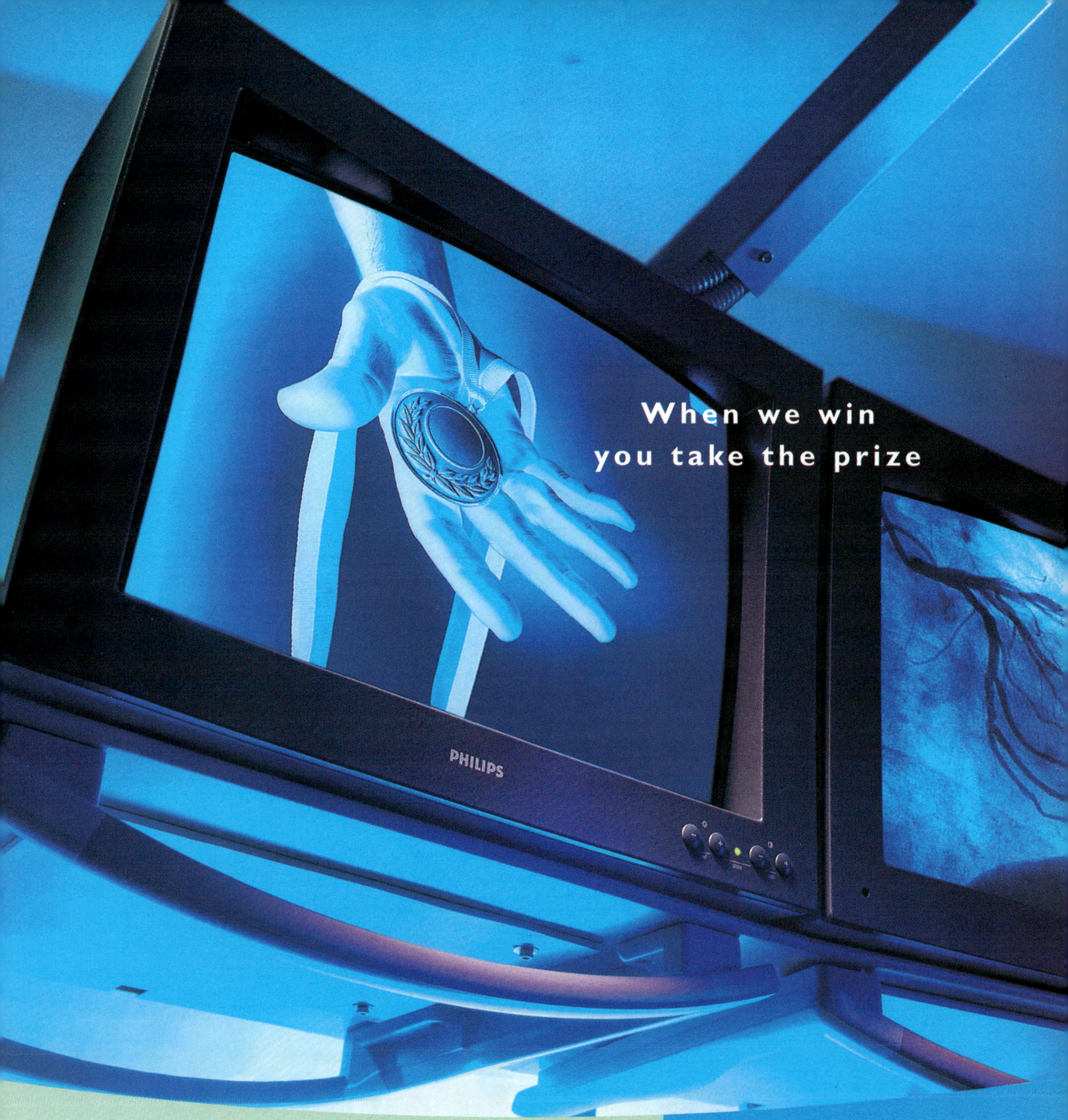
When we win
you take the prize
PHILIPS

present the basic principles of ultrasonographic (US) physics and technology, as well as anatomy, pathophysiology, and hemodynamics with regard to extra- and intracranial cerebral circulation. Duplex US, color-flow imaging, transcranial Doppler imaging, and new developments will be discussed during lectures and hands-on scanning laboratory sessions. Fee: $895; 32 hours of category 1 credit will be available. For further information, contact the Center for Medical Ultrasound, Wake Forest University School of Medicine, Medical Center Blvd, Winston-Salem, NC 27157-1039; telephone (800) 277-7654 or (336) 716-4505; fax (336) 716-4204; e-mail *cmu@wfubmc .edu; http://www.wfubmc .edu/bgsm/ultrasound.*

Fetal and Maternal Ultrasound 1999

"Fetal and Maternal Ultrasound 1999," a course sponsored by the Institute for Advanced Medical Education, will take place on October 1–3, 1999, at the Loews L'Enfant Plaza Hotel, Washington, DC. This program will review state-of-the-art fetal evaluation of the pregnant and nonpregnant patient with the use of real-time and Doppler ultrasonography. Participants will have the opportunity for discussion with the faculty during panel discussions, case review sessions, and live demonstrations. Fee: $445; 16 hours of category 1 credit will be available. For further information, contact Cheryl Ann DeLena, Institute for Advanced Medical Education, 14 Elm Pl, Rye, NY 10580; telephone (914) 921-5700; fax (914) 921-6048; e-mail *info@iame.com.*

Peripheral Vascular Ultrasound

"Peripheral Vascular Ultrasound," a course sponsored by and being held at the Center for Medical Ultrasound, Wake Forest University School of Medicine, will take place on October 4–7, 1999. Participants will learn how ultrasonography is used to detect and evaluate disorders of the blood vessels of the extremities and abdomen. Topics include interpretation of test results, clinical manifestations of peripheral arterial and venous diseases, and vascular anatomy and physiology. Fee: $795; 27 hours of category 1 credit will be available. For further information, contact the Center for Medical Ultrasound, Wake Forest University School of Medicine, Medical Center Blvd, Winston-Salem, NC 27157-1039; telephone (800) 277-7654 or (336) 716-4505; fax (336) 716-4204; e-mail *cmu@wfubmc .edu; http://www.wfubmc.edu/bgsm/ultrasound.*

Course and Symposium on Infant Hip Dysplasia

The Page and William Black Post-Graduate School of the Mount Sinai School of Medicine is sponsoring a didactic and practical course entitled "Ultrasonographic Diagnosis of Infant Hip Dysplasia," to be held on October 13–15, 1999, and a symposium entitled "Current Concepts of Ultrasonographic Screening of Infant Hip Dysplasia," to be held on October 16, 1999. They will take place at the Mount Sinai School of Medicine, New York, NY. The 3-day course will focus on the theory and practice of neonatal hip ultrasonography (US) and its use as a tool for the diagnosis and management of developmental dysplasia of the hip. The symposium will discuss the efficacy, practicality, implications, and cost-effectiveness of US screening for infant hip dysplasia. Course director: Graf. Fee: not available; 27.5 hours of category 1 credit will be available. For further information, contact the Page and William Black Post-Graduate School for Continuing Medical Education, Mount Sinai School of Medicine, 1 Gustave L. Levy Pl, Box 1193, New York, NY 10029; telephone (212) 241-6737.

Current Practice of Vascular Ultrasound

The Institute for Advanced Medical Education is sponsoring a course entitled "Current Practice of Vascular Ultrasound: Carotid and Transcranial Doppler," which will take place on October 15–17, 1999, at the Renaissance Hotel, Washington, DC. This program will emphasize carotid, peripheral, and abdominal applications, and it will include individual hands-on instruction and live demonstrations using the latest in ultrasonographic equipment. Physician interpretation sessions include panel discussions and practice cases, and live scanning of patients with known disease is featured. Fee: $525; 21 hours of category 1 credit will be available. For further information, contact Cheryl Ann DeLena, Institute for Advanced Medical Education, 14 Elm Pl, Rye, NY 10580; telephone (914) 921-5700; fax (914) 921-6048; e-mail *info@iame .com; http://www.iame.com.*

Advanced Applied Ultrasound in Obstetrics

"Advanced Applied Ultrasound in Obstetrics," a course sponsored by and being held at the Center for Medical Ultrasound, Wake Forest University School of Medicine, will take place on October 28–30, 1999. This course, designed, for experienced sonographers and sonologists, will provide an update on the use of ultrasonography (US) in the evaluation of fetal anomalies. Emphasis will be placed on assessing fetal well-being and reviewing current issues with regard to the use of US during pregnancy. Fee: $595 ($495 for residents and sonographers); 13 hours of category 1 credit will be available. For further information, contact the Center for Medical Ultrasound, Wake Forest University School of Medicine, Medical Center Blvd, Winston-Salem, NC 27157-1039; telephone (800) 277-7654 or (336) 716-4505; fax (336) 716-4204; e-mail *cmu@wfubmc.edu; http://www .wfubmc.edu/bgsm/ultrasound.*

Transfer of Copyright and Certifications Agreement

Manuscript No. (for Editorial Office use only)________________________

Complete copyright to the article entitled:

____

____

is hereby transferred to the Radiological Society of North America (for **U.S. government employees:** to the extent transferable), effective if and when the article is accepted for publication in ***Radiology***, printed or electronic format. In the case of authors who are officers or employees of the U.S. government, the Radiological Society of North America recognizes that works prepared by them as part of their official government duties are in the public domain.

Authors reserve the following rights:

A. Other than copyright, all proprietary rights including patent rights relating to the subject matter of the article.
B. The license for personal use in lectures, lecture notes, and exhibits.

Please return this form as soon as possible. The signed statement **must** be received by the Editor **before** the manuscript can be processed for publication.

A. All authors certify that this material or similar material has not been and will not be submitted by them or by colleagues in their institution to any other publication prior to its appearance in ***Radiology.***

B. All authors certify that they have read the Publication Information for Authors found in the most recently published issue of ***Radiology*** at the time the manuscript is submitted. They further certify their compliance with the various requirements found therein.

C. All authors certify that they have submitted all required permissions and that all required statements have been inserted in the text where appropriate.

D. All authors certify that all individuals who have participated sufficiently in the conception and design of this work, in the analysis of the data, and in the writing of the manuscript have been listed as authors. All authors further certify that they have read the final version of the manuscript and approve it for submission for publication.

E. All authors certify that the Editor may correspond with the designated *corresponding author* regarding acceptance, rejection, revision of the manuscript and that the corresponding author is responsible for informing all other authors of the same.

F. All authors certify that responses, revisions received by the Editor from the designated *corresponding author* will be treated as if from all authors and that the corresponding author is responsible for informing all other authors of the same.

G. All authors certify that: **(must check one)**

- ❒ they have no direct or indirect financial interest in the products under investigation or subject matter discussed in this manuscript, or
- ❒ one or more (please name) authors do have a direct or indirect financial interest in the products under investigation or subject matter discussed in this manuscript. A separate statement is attached that details this proprietary interest, and the authors hereby grant permission to publish this information or an appropriate summary thereof with the manuscript if the manuscript is published.

TO BE SIGNED BY ALL AUTHORS:

Name (print) (First) ______________________ Signature ______________________

Name (print) ______________________ Signature ______________________

Name (print) ______________________ Signature ______________________

Name (print) ______________________ Signature ______________________

Name (print) ______________________ Signature ______________________

Name (print) ______________________ Signature ______________________

Use additional page if necessary.

This signed form (a photocopy is acceptable) must be submitted with all proffered works.

Radiology Publication Information for Authors

Radiology is published under the supervision of the Board of Directors of the Radiological Society of North America, Inc, which appoints the Editor who selects all material submitted for publication, including advertisements. No responsibility is accepted by the Board of Directors or the appointed Editor for the opinions expressed by the contributors. Please note that the instructions below are in accord with the *Uniform Requirements for Manuscripts Submitted to Biomedical Journals* (*Annals of Internal Medicine* 1997; 126:36-47). Although *Radiology* will receive material prepared and submitted according to these instructions, the right is reserved to introduce any changes necessary to make the contributions conform to the individual editorial standards of this Journal.

Full manuscripts should be addressed to:
Anthony V. Proto, MD—Editor, *Radiology*
Radiology Manuscripts • RSNA Publications
820 Jorie Boulevard • Oak Brook, IL 60523-2251 USA
FAX (630) 571-7837

All other submissions and correspondence concerning accepted or published material should be addressed to:
Anthony V. Proto, MD—Editor, *Radiology*
Radiology Editorial Office • 1001 East Broad Street
Suite 310 • Richmond, VA 23219
(804) 644-5667 FAX (804) 644-5672
e-mail: *proto@rsna.org*

Assistant to the Editor: Deborah L. Hogan
Office Coordinators: Tonya R. Emerson, Donna L. Schulze

Inquiries about manuscript status and preparation, as well as letters to the editor, can be directed to *radiolog@ rsna.org*

The page containing advertising information (Advertisers' Index) may be located by consulting the Departments section in the Table of Contents.

■ TRANSFER OF COPYRIGHT AND CERTIFICATIONS AGREEMENT

Please send the copyright and certifications agreement with the initial submission of all proffered works. This may be accomplished by using a copy of the form that appears in this issue. **All** authors of any single composition must sign this agreement. In the case of officers or employees of the U.S. government, the Society recognizes that works prepared as part of their official government duties are in the public domain, but they must still sign the copyright and certifications agreement.

■ FINANCIAL INTEREST

Authors must describe any direct or indirect financial interest they may have in the subject matter of a submitted manuscript, and they must authorize the Society to publish this financial disclosure with the article if deemed appropriate. The Society's Financial Disclosure policy is as follows:

"Each author shall describe (*a*) any direct financial interest that author has in the subject matter discussed in the submitted manuscript, and (*b*) any affiliation or financial involvement that author has with or in any organization having a direct financial interest in the subject matter discussed in the submitted manuscript. Such information will be held in the confidence of the journal Editor during the review process. If necessary, in the Editor's view, this information may be shared with reviewers after discussion between the Editor and author. The submission of a manuscript to *Radiology* grants permission for RSNA to publish the financial information described above, or an appropriate summary thereof, with the manuscript if the manuscript is accepted for publication."

■ MANUSCRIPT PREPARATION

Original writings will be accepted only with the understanding that they are contributed solely to *Radiology*. Manuscripts should be typewritten and **double-spaced (all pages)** on only one side of the paper with at least 3-cm margins. Each manuscript component should begin on a **new page** in this order: title pages, abstract, text, acknowledgments, references, tables (each on a separate page), and captions for illustrations. The title pages and abstract page should not be numbered. Sequential numbering should begin with the text. To ensure anonymity in the review process, authors' names should appear on only the full title page; names of authors or the institution should **not** be given in the text or on the illustrations. **Three copies** of the manuscript and three complete sets of mounted illustrations should be submitted. The author should retain a complete copy of the manuscript, since accepted manuscripts will not be returned and only the illustrations of rejected manuscripts will be returned. All manuscripts are acknowledged; please allow 2-3 weeks from the time you mailed the manuscript for receipt of an acknowledgment.

■ TITLE PAGES, AUTHOR CONTRIBUTIONS

***Full Title Page*:** This page should include the title of the manuscript, the first and last names, middle initials, and degrees of all authors, the name and street address (not a postal box) of the institution from which the work originated, the telephone number, the FAX or Telex number, and the e-mail address (if available) of the **corresponding author**, and information concerning grants. The address for reprint requests should include

(continued)

the **complete** name, street address (not a postal box), and zip code. It is important to indicate on this title page whether your paper has been presented at an RSNA meeting (please give year) or has been accepted for presentation at a future meeting.

Abbreviated Title Page: This page should include only the title of the manuscript so as to allow for anonymity during the review process.

Author Contributions: Authors are required to identify their manuscript contributions, for which they are responsible. The author(s) responsible for the integrity of the entire study should also be identified. Please list the following phrases on a separate page, to follow the *"Abbreviated Title Page,"* and beside each indicate the name(s) of the author(s) to whom these phrases apply:

- guarantor of integrity of entire study
- study concepts
- study design
- definition of intellectual content
- literature research
- clinical studies
- experimental studies
- data acquisition
- data analysis
- statistical analysis
- manuscript preparation
- manuscript editing
- manuscript review

For those phrases that do not apply, please list them and so indicate.

■ ABSTRACT, KEY WORDS, CATEGORIZATION TERMS, AND SUMMARY STATEMENT

An abstract of 200 words or less must be submitted with each manuscript of a major paper. The abstract must be divided into four paragraphs with the following headings.

PURPOSE: State the hypothesis being tested or the procedure being evaluated.

MATERIALS AND METHODS: Briefly state what was done and what materials were used, including number of subjects. Also include the methods used to assess the data and to control bias.

RESULTS: Provide the findings of the study, including indicators of statistical significance. Include actual numbers, as well as percentages.

CONCLUSION: Summarize in one or two sentences the conclusion made on the basis of the findings.

Below the abstract, please list three to six key words as derived from the terms used in the most recent 3-year *RSNA Index to Imaging Literature*. Also, on the Manuscript Categorization Terms form provided at the end of these instructions, please select as many terms as are appropriate for your manuscript. It is important that you comply with this request, since the terms you select are utilized to match your manuscript with the appropriate reviewers.

On the reverse side of the Manuscript Categorization Terms form, the *author should reproduce from the text the one statement that best conveys or summarizes the message of the study*.

An abstract of 60 words or less must be submitted for each case report or Technical Developments paper. The abstract must state (*a*) what was done, (*b*) what was found, and (*c*) what was concluded.

■ TEXT

The text of observational and experimental studies is arranged in sections with the headings Introduction, Materials and Methods, Results, and Discussion. Lengthy papers may need subheadings within some sections to clarify their content, especially within the Results and Discussion sections.

Introduction: Clearly state the hypothesis or purpose of the study. Give only strictly pertinent references, and do not review the literature extensively.

Materials and Methods: Describe clearly the number and selection of the subjects studied (patients or experimental animals, including controls). Identify the methods, instrumentation (manufacturer's name and address in parentheses), and procedures in sufficient detail to allow other workers to reproduce the results. To ensure anonymity in the review process, do **not** include the name of the institution where the work was performed, either within the text or at the top of each manuscript page. Give references to established methods, including statistical methods that have been published but are not well known; describe new or substantially modified methods and give reasons for using these techniques. Include numbers of observations and the statistical significance of the findings when appropriate. Detailed statistical analyses, mathematical derivations, and the like should be presented in one or more appendixes.

Results: Present the results in logical sequence in the text, along with tables, and illustrations. Do not repeat in the text all the data in the tables and/or illustrations; summarize only important observations.

Discussion: Emphasize the new and important aspects of the study and conclusions that follow from them. Do not repeat in detail the data given in the Results section. Include in the Discussion the implications of the findings and their limitations, in particular with reference to the use of modified methods, statistical or otherwise. Relate the observations to other relevant studies. Link the conclusions with the goals of the study, but avoid unqualified statements and conclusions not supported completely by the data. Avoid claiming priority and alluding to work that has not been completed. State new hypotheses when warranted, but clearly label them as such. Recommendations, when appropriate, may be included.

For experimental studies, please describe the potential importance of your conclusions as they relate to future practical applications. Please identify this paragraph with the title "Practical Application(s)."

■ ACKNOWLEDGMENTS

List here those who have contributed substantially to the work reported in the manuscript, such as editorial and writing assistance, but who are not authors of the study. Authors are expected to obtain written permission of those acknowledged, and to submit the same, as readers might interpret that those acknowledged agree with the data and conclusions of the study.

■ REFERENCES

Number references consecutively in the order in which they are first mentioned. The abbreviations used for periodicals cited in the references should follow the style of *Index Medicus*. For journal articles, list surnames and initials of all authors when six or less, such as:

1. Stuart MJ, Elrad H, Graeber JE, Hakanson DO, Sunderji SG, Barvinchak MK. Increased synthesis of prostaglandin endoperoxides and platelet hyperfunction in infants of mothers with diabetes mellitus. J Lab Clin Med 1979; 94:12–26.

When seven or more authors are listed, only the first three names need to be identified, followed by "et al," such as:

1. Hibbard CT, Campbell S, Sabbagha RE, et al. Demonstration of tissue interfaces within the body by ultrasonic echo sounding. Br J Radiol 1961; 34:539–549.

Abstracts, editorials, and letters to the Editor should be noted as such. In the case of books, the authors of a chapter, title of the chapter, editor(s), title of the book, edition, city, publisher, year, and specific pages must be provided.

1. Brown M, Gray L. Indications for hematology. In: Wintrobe MM, ed. Clinical hematology. 3rd ed. Philadelphia, Pa: Lea & Febiger, 1975; 1146–1167.

It is the responsibility of the author(s) to ensure that all references are listed accurately.

■ TABLES

Tables should be numbered in Arabic numerals and should have a title. All abbreviations used in the table should be explained in a footnote.

Tables should be presented in the style used in recent issues of the Journal. No vertical lines or shading should be included. Avoid excessive use of horizontal lines within the table.

■ CAPTIONS FOR ILLUSTRATIONS

A caption must be supplied for each illustration, including drawings and graphs. It should not duplicate text material and should follow the style used in recent issues of the Journal. All captions should appear collectively on one or more pages separate from the text, and each caption should also appear below the corresponding illustration. It is essential that the caption describes all labels placed on the print of an illustration.

■ ILLUSTRATIONS

Illustrations should be limited to those required to show the essential features described in the manuscript. Space constraints prevent us from publishing redundant or excessive illustrations. Unretouched glossy prints no larger than 12.7 × 17.8 cm (5 × 7 inches) are desirable. Prints to be combined into one array, such as posteroanterior and lateral views, should be the same height or the same width to facilitate reproduction. They should correspond in appearance to the tonal relations of the original radiograph (ie, showing the bones white on a dark background, with the patient's right to the observer's left; computed tomograms and MR images should employ the "view from below"). If an image has been enhanced electronically, explain the alterations that have been made and send an original image along with the enhanced one. Drawings and charts should be rendered professionally in India ink on white paper. In computer-generated artwork, shading should be done in continuous tones (ie, solid black, solid gray, solid white): **Do not use dotted shadings.**

Since the size of the illustration printed in the Journal is typically smaller than that submitted by the author(s), it is essential that each submitted illustration show only the area(s) of interest with enough surrounding area for orientation puposes (e.g., to illustrate a cavity at the right lung apex, show only that area with enough surrounding area for orientation, rather than the entire chest).

All illustrations must be numbered and the top indicated on the back. For protection against loss or damage, each illustration should then be neatly attached to paper (one illustration per page), and the number and top should be reindicated on this page. For attachment, **avoid using glue, staples, or corner mounts.** Because it holds the illustration securely to the page without damage, we recommend Scotch Removable Magic Tape (3M, St Paul, Minn). **Please** do not add letters or numbers to the **face** of the illustration to identify the figure (such as 1A or 1B).

Arrows and other labels should be placed only on the final print, should be of professional quality, and should be **removable.** Professional artist service for such items is available to authors without charge. The desired additions may simply be indicated on tissue or a transparent overlay attached securely to the print.

Illustrations of accepted manuscripts become the property of the RSNA and will be stored for 2 years after publication. Illustrations will be returned only upon receipt of a written request from the corresponding author. We suggest that authors make and keep a set of illustrations in addition to the three sets submitted to the Journal.

■ UNITS AND ABBREVIATIONS

Radiation measurements and laboratory values should be given in the *International System of Units (SI)* (resources: SI Units in Radiation Protection and Measurements, NCRP Report no. 82 [August 1985]; "Now Read This: The SI Units Are Here," *JAMA* 1986; 255:2329–2339). Abbreviations should be spelled out when first used in the text, such as "cerebrospinal fluid (CSF)." Laboratory slang, clinical jargon, and uncommon abbreviations should be avoided.

■ INFORMED CONSENT

Manuscripts reporting the results of experimental studies on human subjects must include a statement in Materials and Methods to the effect that informed consent was obtained after the nature of the procedure(s) had been fully explained. In addition, a statement affirming approval of the appropriate institutional review board is required. If a review board does not exist, then the Declaration of Helsinki principles should be followed and a statement affirming the same should be made (41st World Medical Assembly. Declaration of Helsinki: recommendations guiding physicians in biomedical research involving human subjects. Bull Pan Am Health Organ 1990; 24: 606-609).

The maintenance and care of experimental animals to provide humane treatment and to ensure reliable results are described in the National Institutes of Health guidelines for use of laboratory animals. Authors must affirm compliance with these guidelines or approval of the appropriate institutional review board in the Materials and Methods section.

■ RIGHTS AND PERMISSIONS

Written permission (we require a copy) must be granted by the publisher and author to reproduce any previously published figures, including permission to reproduce in both print and electronic formats; any such material must be clearly noted and its source given in the manuscript. A signed letter of permission must be included with your manuscript for any individual who might be identified due to written descriptions, photographs (masking the eyes in photographs is not sufficient protection of anonymity), or otherwise. Informed consent, which requires that the individual be shown the manuscript, should be affirmed in the Materials and Methods section.

If reference is made in the text to personal communication (oral or written) as a source of information, a signed statement of permission is required from each such source.

■ AUTHOR RESPONSIBILITY

Authors must be certain that no manuscript on the same or similar material has been or will be submitted to another journal by themselves or others at their institution before their work appears in *Radiology*. The submission by authors of similar material to advertising media must be indicated at the time *Radiology* receives the manuscript.

■ ELECTRONIC SUBMISSION OF ACCEPTED MANUSCRIPTS

Text File: Manuscripts that have been accepted for publication must be submitted on computer disk (required for text, desirable for illustrations). Submit text on a 3½-inch diskette prepared in WordPerfect or Microsoft Word format for Windows or Macintosh. A hard copy should accompany the diskette and should match the diskette file exactly. The diskette should be labeled with its assigned manuscript number, the first author's last name, the word processing program used, and the file name.

The entire article should be submitted as a single text file, with the elements in the standard order: title pages, abstract, text, acknowledgments, references, tables, captions. *Do not embed illustrations.* Only the final version of the article should be on the submitted disk. Keep the text file as free from formatting codes as possible: Do not use boldface, italic, underlining, strange fonts, codes for centering, unnecessary line spacing, etc. Use the default settings of the word-processing program; especially do not use right-justified margins. Use tabs to indent at the beginnings of paragraphs, and insert only one space after end punctuation marks. Use hard returns only at the ends of paragraphs or between sections of the manuscript; do not insert them mid-paragraph. Do not insert tabs in references; use only one hard return at the end of each reference.

Illustrations File: Although not required, submission of illustrations on 3½-inch disk, ZIP disk, or CD is acceptable. All image files should be in PC tif or eps format. Do not sumbit images in bitmap, jpeg, or gif format. *Do not embed images in the text file.*

For black and white images, we require that they be submitted in PC tif or PC eps format with a dot range of 5% Highlight to 95% Shadow and resolution of 500 dpi. Four-color images should also be PC tif or PC eps format with a maximum of 280% total tonal density and resolution of 300 dpi. Note that when your RGB files are converted to CYMK, there will be less color due to conversion. Images should be supplied as close as possible to print size: 2¼ inches wide for one column, 3¼ inches wide for 1½ columns, 4⅝ inches wide for two columns.

Each image file should be named, and with the diskette or cartridge the following should be provided: a hard-copy inventory with specific information on the image, two sets of proofs obtained at 800–1,800 dpi, and one set of proofs obtained with a laser printer to be used as a reference set.

■ BOOK REVIEWERS

Any person who would like to help in reviewing books for *Radiology* should contact

Richard A. Szucs, MD, Book Review Editor
Radiology Editorial Office
1001 E Broad St
Suite 310
Richmond, VA 23219

■ BOOKS FOR REVIEW

Publishers wishing to have books reviewed should send them to the address above.

✔ **Checklist of Requirements:**

- ❐ 1. Send 3 copies of manuscript and 3 copies of illustrations.
- ❐ 2. Mount each illustration on a separate page, 8½ × 11 inches. Indicate figure number and top.
- ❐ 3. Double space all parts of manuscript.
- ❐ 4. Send copyright and certifications agreement with signatures of all authors.
- ❐ 5. Send institutional affiliation for each author and corresponding author's name, address, phone number, FAX or Telex number, and e-mail address.
- ❐ 6. Send a **brief** abstract: 200 words or less for regular articles, 60 words or less for case reports and Technical Developments papers.
- ❐ 7. Give SI units for radiation measurements and laboratory values.
- ❐ 8. Send copy of letter of permission to reprint any figure that was published previously or for any other reasons as noted in the instructions found above.
- ❐ 9. Send a completed copy of the Manuscript Categorization Terms form. Please remember to reproduce from the text the one statement that best conveys or summarizes the message of your study.

Radiology Manuscript Categorization Terms

Please PRINT your name: ____________________

Please print the title of your manuscript ____________________

____

For each section, please categorize your manuscript by checking off **as many terms as are appropriate.**

Modalities/Techniques

___ Absorptiometry/ Bone Densitometry
___ Angiography
___ Arthrography
___ Conventional Radiography
___ CT
___ CT-Angiography
___ CT-Electron Beam
___ CT-High Resolution
___ CT-Spiral
___ Dacryocystography
___ Defecography
___ Digital Radiography
___ Echocardiography
___ Fluoroscopy
___ Hysterosalpingography
___ Image Manipulation/ Reconstruction
___ Lymphography
___ MR-Angiography
___ MR-Diffusion/Perfusion
___ MR-Functional Imaging
___ MR-Imaging
___ MR-Spectroscopy
___ Neural Networks
___ PACS
___ PET
___ Radionuclide Studies
___ Sialography
___ SPECT
___ Ultrasound
___ Ultrasound-Color Doppler
___ Ultrasound-Doppler
___ Ultrasound-Power Doppler
___ Ultrasound-Spectral Doppler

Procedures

___ Angioplasty
___ Angioscopy
___ Balloon Insertions
___ Biopsy/Drainage
___ Dilation
___ Embolization
___ Endoscopy
___ Filter Insertions
___ Interventional Other ____________
___ Intraoperative
___ Laser
___ Lithotripsy
___ Localization
___ Myelography
___ Percutaneous
___ Radiation Therapy/Oncology
___ Radionuclide Therapy
___ Shunts
___ Stents
___ Thrombolysis

Areas/Systems

___ Abdomen
___ Biliary
___ Breast
___ Cardiac
___ CNS
___ Ear/Nose/Throat
___ Genital/Reproductive
___ GI
___ Head/Neck
___ Hematologic
___ Lymphatic
___ Muscular
___ Nervous-Peripheral
___ Skeletal-Appendicular
___ Skeletal-Axial
___ Soft Tissues/Skin
___ Thorax
___ Urinary
___ Vascular

Structures

___ Adrenal
___ Ankle
___ Anus
___ Aorta
___ Appendix
___ Arteries
___ Bile Ducts
___ Bladder
___ Brain/Brain Stem
___ Breast
___ Cervix
___ Diaphragm
___ Duodenum
___ Ear
___ Elbow
___ Esophagus
___ Extremities
___ Eye
___ Face
___ Fallopian Tubes
___ Foot
___ Gallbladder
___ Hand
___ Heart
___ Hip
___ Jaw
___ Joints
___ Kidney
___ Knee
___ Lacrimal Glands
___ Large Bowel
___ Larynx
___ Ligaments
___ Liver
___ Long Bones
___ Lung
___ Marrow
___ Mediastinum
___ Meninges
___ Mesentery
___ Omentum
___ Orbit
___ Ovaries
___ Pancreas
___ Paranasal Sinuses
___ Parathyroid
___ Pelvis
___ Pelvocalyceal
___ Penis
___ Pericardium
___ Peritoneum
___ Pharynx
___ Pineal
___ Pituitary
___ Pleura
___ Prostate
___ Pylorus
___ Rectum
___ Retina
___ Retroperitoneum
___ Ribs
___ Salivary Glands
___ Scrotum
___ Shoulder
___ Skull
___ Small Bowel
___ Spinal Cord
___ Spine-Cervical
___ Spine-Lumbar

Continued

Structures, continued

___ Spine-Sacrum/Coccyx
___ Spine-Thoracic
___ Spleen
___ Stomach
___ Tendons
___ Testes
___ Thymus
___ Thyroid
___ Tongue
___ Tracheobronchial Tree
___ Ureters
___ Urethra
___ Uterus
___ Vagina
___ Valves
___ Veins
___ Vena Cava
___ Wrist

Topics

___ Abscess
___ Acceptance Testing
___ Acute
___ Adults
___ AIDS
___ Anatomy
___ Aneurysms
___ Animal Investigations
___ Arteriosclerosis
___ Arthritides
___ Artifacts
___ Atelectasis
___ Athletic Injuries
___ AVM
___ Axilla
___ Biological Effects
___ Biostatistics
___ Blood
___ Calcifications/Calculi
___ Cardiac Assist Devices
___ Catheters
___ Cavitation
___ Cerebral Palsy
___ Chemistry
___ Chronic Obstructive Airways Disease
___ Cirrhosis
___ Comparative Studies
___ Complications
___ Computer Applications-3D
___ Computer Applications-Teleradiology
___ Computer Applications-Virtual Imaging
___ Computer Applications-Other______________
___ Congenital
___ Connective Tissue Disorders
___ Contrast Agents-Intravenous
___ Contrast Agents-Oral
___ Cost-effectiveness
___ CSF
___ Cysts
___ Dementia
___ Demineralization-Bone
___ Dilatation
___ Dissection
___ Diverticula
___ Dosimetry
___ Drugs/Reactions
___ Dysplasias
___ Eating Disorders
___ ECMO
___ Edema
___ Education
___ Efficacy Studies
___ Embolism
___ Endocrine Disorders
___ Equipment
___ Ethics
___ Experimental Investigations
___ Fetus
___ Fistula
___ Foreign Bodies
___ Forensics
___ Genetic Defects
___ Grafts
___ Health Policy and Practice
___ Hemangioma
___ Hematologic Diseases
___ Hemodynamics/Flow Dynamics
___ Hemorrhage
___ Hernia
___ History
___ Hyperplasia/Hypertrophy
___ Hypertension
___ Imaging Sequences
___ Infection
___ Inflammation
___ Instrumentation
___ Ischemia/Infarction
___ Laboratory Tests
___ Leukemia
___ Lymphoma
___ Medicolegal Issues
___ Metabolic Disorders
___ Metastases
___ Monoclonal Antibodies
___ Motility
___ Neoplasms-Primary
___ Normal Variants
___ Observer Performance
___ Obstetrics
___ Obstruction/Occlusion
___ Occupational/Environmental Hazards
___ Outcomes Analysis
___ Parasites
___ Pathology
___ Pediatric Population-Adolescents
___ Pediatric Population-Children
___ Pediatric Population-Infants
___ Pediatric Population-Neonates
___ Physics
___ Physiological Studies
___ Pregnancy
___ Prostheses
___ QA/QC
___ Radiation Effects
___ Radiation Safety
___ Radiobiology
___ Safety
___ Screening
___ Sedation
___ Seizure Disorders
___ Socioeconomic Issues
___ Speech Disorders
___ Staging
___ Statistics
___ Surgery
___ Technical Aspects
___ Technology Assessments
___ Tissue Characterization
___ Transplantation
___ Trauma
___ Treatment Effects
___ Tropical Diseases
___ Varices
___ Volvulus

Please reproduce here the **one sentence** from the text that best conveys or summarizes the message of your study.

____

____

Please provide author initials by appropriate author contribution category.

________ Guarantor of integrity of entire study
________ Study concepts
________ Study design
________ Definition of intellectual content
________ Literature research
________ Clinical studies
________ Experimental studies
________ Data acquisition
________ Data analysis
________ Statistical analysis
________ Manuscript preparation
________ Manuscript editing
________ Manuscript review

This form *must be* included with your manuscript submission.

John H. M. Austin, MD

Pulmonary Emphysema: Imaging Assessment of Lung Volume Reduction Surgery[1]

Now in its 7th year, modern lung volume reduction surgery for treatment of severe pulmonary emphysema has achieved results that appear to be impressive: The results of many studies (1–13) have shown symptomatic and functional improvement after this procedure. However, on review of Medicare data, the U.S. Health Care Financing Administration (HCFA) found that 215 (30%) of 722 patients who underwent lung volume reduction surgery in 1995–1996 died within 18 months of the procedure (14). The disparity between the HCFA data and that in the peer-reviewed literature led to the current National Emphysema Treatment Trial (NETT).

When lung volume reduction surgery does work, what does it do? Downsizing the thorax to a normal or nearly normal configuration probably reduces dyspnea by unloading thoracic stretch receptors and allowing respiratory muscles to again contract at optimal points along their length-tension curves (2,6,15). Removing nonfunctional and minimally functional lung tissue improves many aspects of lung function. Results include decreased air trapping, increased elastic recoil, and increased maximum expiratory airflow (1–13).

What is the role of imaging in lung volume reduction surgery? The answer is simple: Imaging is central. Clearly, the assessment of severe pulmonary emphysema in vivo depends on modern imaging, but the roles of chest radiography, computed tomography (CT), and other imaging modalities in confirming the diagnosis, finding target sites for resection, and excluding coexistent morbidity are timely issues that need careful investigation in patients who are candidates for lung volume reduction surgery.

Is the distribution of emphysema a predictor of success after lung volume reduction surgery? Virtually every day, radiologists see chest radiographs that show opacification of upper lung zone vessels, which is the most common chest radiographic sign of the characteristic upper zone distribution of centrilobular pulmonary emphysema in tobacco abusers. The path-setting work of Cooper et al (1) suggested that this population, whose lower lung regions are mostly intact, would be the obvious group to benefit from lung volume reduction surgery. Support for this concept came in 1997 from three separate series, in which CT and radiographic data showed the best outcomes after lung volume reduction surgery in patients with predominantly heterogeneously distributed emphysema, which was predominantly in the upper lung zones and associated with both compressed lung and sizable zones of normal or mildly emphysematous lung tissue (7–9). Although the more heterogeneous the distribution of emphysema, the better the results of lung volume reduction surgery, some patients with homogeneous disease do show some decreased dyspnea and some improvement in pulmonary function after lung volume reduction surgery (9,13).

Are chest radiographic findings alone a satisfactory predictor of outcome after lung volume reduction surgery? The data of Slone et al (8) in 1997 suggested this possibility, which is now supported by the results of an outcome study by Maki et al (16), from the Hospital of the University of Pennsylvania, Philadelphia, which is published in this issue of *Radiology*. The results of Maki et al appear to be compelling: High levels of heterogeneity of emphysema and unequivocal compression of lung parenchyma at inspiratory chest radiography both were 100% predictive of a 30% or greater forced expiratory volume in 1 second (FEV_1). Their definition of heterogeneity is the difference between the maximal upper lung zone score and minimal lower lung zone score—a measure of predominant upper zone disease. On the other hand, they found that low heterogeneity and a lack of lung compression strongly (94% and 92%, respectively) indicated that the postoperative FEV_1 would not increase by at least 30%.

What is "heterogeneous" distribution of pulmonary emphysema? Investigators have been struggling with its definition. While Maki et al (16) compared scores in one zone with those in another, others have compared differences within zones—for example, severely destroyed "target areas" in regions of mild emphysema (8,17) have been described—or they have compared differences in the extent of emphysema among adjacent segments (9,13). To compound matters, investigators' subjective rating systems vary, using three- to 10-point scales (8,9,13,16,17). Investigative radiologists are still groping

Index terms:
Editorials
Emphysema, pulmonary, 60.751
Lung, radiography, 60.11
Lung, surgery
Lung, ventilation, 60.1295

Radiology 1999; 212:1–3

[1] From the Department of Radiology, Columbia-Presbyterian Medical Center, 622 W 168th St, New York, NY 10032-3270. Received February 4, 1999; accepted February 5. **Address reprint requests to** the author. (e-mail: *jha3@columbia.edu*).

See also the article by Maki et al (pp 49–55) in this issue.

for a workable measure to assess nonhomogeneous disease. Will quantitative CT assessment be needed (10,18)? The work of Slone et al (8) and now that of Maki et al (16) suggest that fairly simple chest radiographic assessments may suffice.

A methodologic analogy to the pneumoconioses may be useful to consider. The analytic scales that Maki et al used were short: a two-point scale (all or nothing) for compression and a four-point scale for heterogeneity. However, only after the scale for chest radiographic evaluation of pneumoconiosis was expanded from four points (absent, mild, moderate, severe) to 10 points (absent, possibly mild, probably mild, mild, possibly moderate, etc) did the radiologic data correlate positively with nonradiologic variables (19). It might be advisable to consider a comparable analysis of the conventional radiographic findings of compression and heterogeneity in candidates for lung volume reduction surgery.

What about hyperinflation? The study results of Slone et al (8) and Maki et al (16) failed to show hyperinflation as a predictor of outcome after lung volume reduction surgery. However, nearly all patients with severe pulmonary emphysema have hyperinflated lungs. As both groups of authors appropriately suggest, demonstration of hyperinflation with imaging appears to be too nonspecific to be helpful. Rather, the aspect of hyperinflation that appears to be most important is the functional aspect: The higher the ratio of residual volume to total lung capacity, the better the functional results after lung volume reduction surgery, as measured by using vital capacity and the residual volume–to–total lung capacity ratio (13).

What about exercise capability? The two major clinical tests of breathlessness are the 6-minute walk test and dyspnea index (20). Unfortunately, Maki et al (16) found weak correlations between 6-minute walk test results and both compression and heterogeneity; they did not analyze the dyspnea index. The FEV_1, as Maki et al (16) appropriately state, is an exceedingly well established test for patients with pulmonary emphysema. However, as they also indicate, other tests, such as the dyspnea index, ultimately may become accepted as the most valuable tests in assessing the outcome of lung volume reduction surgery (21).

What about chest radiographs obtained in inspiration and expiration? Expiratory chest radiographs to assess the variables of respiratory motion before and after lung volume reduction surgery were not included in the study of Maki et al. The inspiratory chest radiographs obtained by Takasugi et al (11) before and after bilateral lung volume reduction surgery showed decreased heights of each lung postoperatively. However, a diaphragmatic excursion of less than 3 cm before lung volume reduction surgery, which is a finding that one might expect to be a predictor of favorable outcome, was not reported as a predictor in a major series in which upper lobe heterogeneous distribution was a favorable predictor (7).

What about CT? Certainly, chest CT is an appropriate preoperative test in this population. The diagnosis of emphysema needs to be confirmed, bronchiectasis and other airway diseases need to be excluded (22), and in 2%–5% of patients, CT may help to detect incidental stage I peripheral "early" lung cancer, which is appropriate for excision during lung volume reduction surgery (23,24). CT also has investigative uses. By using inspiration and expiration CT, Becker et al (10) assessed each lung separately in patients who had undergone unilateral and bilateral lung volume reduction surgery and found that the magnitude of the response to lung volume reduction surgery was comparable in all operated lungs—that is, "a lung's response to LVRS [lung volume reduction surgery] was independent from that of the contralateral lung."

The results of quantitative CT analysis have shown that lung volume reduction surgery is associated with increases in airflow, improved 6-minute walk test results, and decreases in lung volumes and imaging indexes of emphysema (10,25,26). Another use of CT findings as predictors may be to combine them with the results of tests of airway obstruction. For example, in a small series, Hunsaker et al (26) described a combination of CT assessment of emphysema and measurements of inspiratory resistance; the high-resistance cohort fared poorly after lung volume reduction surgery.

What about magnetic resonance (MR) imaging? MR imaging is an excellent tool for comparing thoracic dimensions in inspiration and expiration; however, its uses in lung volume reduction surgery patients are likely to be only investigational. Gierada et al (27) reported that MR images showed decreases in pulmonary dimensions in all three planes after lung volume reduction surgery, especially in expiration.

What about lung scanning? Perfusion scintigraphy "may help to identify target areas for resection" (13), but in that same series, assessment of heterogeneity with CT was found to be superior to that with scintigraphy in helping to predict the outcome after lung volume reduction surgery. Wang et al (17) found that preoperative perfusion scintigraphy "can provide modest prognostic information" and noted, as a scintigraphic antecedent for the study of Maki et al (16), that upper lobe predominance of emphysema and heterogeneous distribution of emphysema were major predictors of postoperative increases in FEV_1, albeit with a fairly wide scatter in their data. As for ventilation-perfusion scanning, which would seem like an excellent tool to help identify abnormal regions of the lung for resection in a disease of abnormal ventilatory function, to my knowledge, no series has yet been published.

What will happen with the NETT? Currently under way in 17 centers in the United States, the NETT was designed as a prospective randomized trial to compare lung volume reduction surgery and contemporary nonsurgical management of pulmonary emphysema (14,28). Lung volume reduction surgery does have major implications as a source of health care expenditures (29). Its role in nonheterogeneous emphysema is especially uncertain (3,13). Cooper and Lefrak (5) have questioned the ethical appropriateness of a trial that assigns half of the subjects to a nonsurgical arm. Yang (28) has called the ethical issue of randomization "unsettling." Other investigators (14,30), however, believe that a randomized trial is the best way to clarify the issues. The NETT is designed to continue for a number of years. How the NETT data will place in the debate between the peer-reviewed literature data and HCFA data will be important for patients and health care providers.

What is the take-home message? Long-term data are not yet in, but lung volume reduction surgery has certainly improved the lives of many patients. Although we are clearly still on a learning curve in predicting the outcome after lung volume reduction surgery, because of the relative simplicity of the old-fashioned chest radiograph, it may yet turn out to be as important a tool as the CT scan.

References

1. Cooper JD, Trulock EP, Triantafillou AN, et al. Bilateral pneumectomy (volume reduction) for chronic obstructive pulmonary disease. J Thorac Cardiovasc Surg 1995; 109:106–119.
2. Sciurba FC, Rogers RM, Keenan RJ, et al. Improvement in pulmonary function and elastic recoil after lung-reduction surgery for diffuse emphysema. N Engl J Med 1996; 334:1095–1099.
3. Cooper JD, Patterson GA, Sundaresan RS, et al. Results of 150 consecutive bilateral

lung volume reduction procedures in patients with severe emphysema. J Thorac Cardiovasc Surg 1996; 112:1319–1330.
4. Gelb AF, Brenner M, McKenna RJ Jr, Zamel N, Fischel R, Epstein JD. Lung function 12 months following emphysema resection. Chest 1996; 110:1407–1415.
5. Cooper JD, Lefrak SS. Is volume reduction surgery appropriate in the treatment of emphysema? Yes. Am J Respir Crit Care Med 1996; 153:1201–1204.
6. Martinez FJ, Montos de Oca M, Whyte RI, Stetz J, Gay SE, Celli BR. Lung-volume reduction improves dyspnea, dynamic hyperinflation, and respiratory muscle function. Am J Respir Crit Care Med 1997; 155:1984–1990.
7. McKenna RJ Jr, Brenner M, Fischel RJ, et al. Patient selection criteria for lung volume reduction surgery. J Thorac Cardiovasc Surg 1997; 114:957–967.
8. Slone RM, Pilgram TK, Gierada DS, et al. Lung volume reduction surgery: comparison of preoperative radiologic features and clinical outcome. Radiology 1997; 204:685–693.
9. Weber WR, Thurnheer R, Stammberger U, Burge M, Russi EW, Bloch KE. Radiologic emphysema morphology is associated with outcome after surgical lung volume resection. Ann Thorac Surg 1997; 64:313–320.
10. Becker MD, Berkmen YM, Austin JHM, et al. Lung volumes before and after lung volume reduction surgery: quantitative CT analysis. Am J Respir Crit Care Med 1998; 157:1593–1599.
11. Takasugi JE, Wood DE, Godwin JD, Richardson ML, Benditt JO, Albert RK. Lung-volume reduction surgery for diffuse emphysema: radiologic assessment of changes in thoracic dimensions. J Thorac Imaging 1998; 13:36–41.
12. O'Brien GM, Furukawa S, Kuzma AM, Cordova F, Criner GJ. Improvements in lung function, exercise, and quality of life in hypercapnic COPD patients after lung volume reduction surgery. Chest 1999; 115:75–84.
13. Thurnheer R, Engel H, Weder W, et al. Role of lung perfusion scintigraphy in relation to chest computed tomography and pulmonary function in the evaluation of candidates for lung volume reduction surgery. Am J Respir Crit Care Med 1999; 159:301–310.
14. Shelala DE. Health Care Financing Administration, Department of Health and Human Services report to Congress, 1998: lung volume reduction surgery and Medicare coverage policy—implications of recently published evidence. Washington, DC: Department of Health and Human Services, 1998; 1–66.
15. Benditt JO, Wood DE, McCool FD, Lewis S, Albert RK. Changes in breathing and ventilatory muscle recruitment patterns induced by lung volume reduction surgery. Am J Respir Crit Care Med 1997; 155:279–284.
16. Maki DD, Miller WT Jr, Aronchick JM, et al. Advanced emphysema: preoperative chest radiographic findings as predictors of outcome following lung volume reduction surgery. Radiology 1999; 212: 49–55.
17. Wang SC, Fischer KC, Slone RM, et al. Perfusion scintigraphy in the evaluation of lung volume reduction surgery: correlation with clinical outcome. Radiology 1997; 205:243–248.
18. Bae KT, Slone RM, Gierada DS, Yusen RD, Cooper JD. Patients with emphysema: quantitative CT analysis before and after lung volume reduction surgery—work in progress. Radiology 1997; 203: 705–714.
19. Liddell FDK, Lindars DC. An elaboration of the I.L.O. classification of simple pneumoconiosis. Br J Ind Med 1969; 26:89–100.
20. Sweer L, Zwilich CW. Dyspnea in the patient with obstructive pulmonary disease. Clin Chest Med 1990; 11:417–445.
21. Teramoto S, Matsuse T, Ouchi Y. Is the symptomatic improvement after lung volume reduction surgery correlated with FEV1 in patients with diffuse emphysema? Chest 1997; 111:1144–1145.
22. Gückel C, Hansell DM. Imaging the "dirty lung": has high-resolution computed tomography cleared the smoke? Clin Radiol 1998; 53:717–722.
23. Pigula FA, Keenan RJ, Ferson PF, Landreneau RJ. Unsuspected lung cancer found in work-up for lung reduction operation. Ann Thorac Surg 1996; 61:174–176.
24. Rozenshtein A, White CS, Austin JHM, Romney BM, Protopapas Z, Krasna MJ. Incidental lung carcinoma detected at CT in patients selected for lung volume reduction surgery to treat severe pulmonary emphysema. Radiology 1998; 207:487–490.
25. Holbert JM, Brown ML, Sciurba FC, Keenan RJ, Landreneau RJ, Holzer AD. Changes in lung volume and volume of emphysema after unilateral lung reduction surgery: analysis with CT lung densitometry. Radiology 1996; 201:793–797.
26. Hunsaker A, Ingenito E, Topal U, Pugatch R, Reilly J. Preoperative screening for lung volume reduction surgery: usefulness of combining thin-section CT with physiologic assessment. AJR 1998; 170:309–314.
27. Gierada DS, Hakimian S, Slone RM, Yusen RD. MR analysis of lung volume and thoracic dimensions in patients with emphysema before and after lung volume reduction surgery. AJR 1998; 170:707–714
28. Yang SC. Lung volume reduction surgery: let the trials begin. Radiology 1997; 204: 613–615.
29. Huizenga HF, Ramsey SD, Albert RK. Estimated growth of lung volume reduction surgery among Medicare enrollees: 1994 to 1996. Chest 1998; 114:1583–1587.
30. Weinmann GG, Hyatt R. Evaluation and research in lung volume reduction surgery. Am J Respir Crit Care Med 1996; 154:1913–1918.

Melissa L. Rosado-de-Christenson, Col, USAF, MC

Paula J. Woodward, MD Armed Forces Institute of Pathology 1999–2000 Distinguished Scientist[1]

Paula J. Woodward, MD, will serve as Distinguished Scientist in the Department of Radiologic Pathology at the Armed Forces Institute of Pathology (AFIP) from July 1, 1999, to June 30, 2000. Dr Woodward is an associate professor of radiology and the director of the radiology residency program at the University of Utah School of Medicine, Salt Lake City. Her area of expertise is abdominal imaging, with special interest in genitourinary radiology. She obtained her medical degree from the University of Colorado, Denver, in 1984, and completed a diagnostic radiology residency at the Wilford Hall United States Air Force (USAF) Medical Center, Lackland Air Force Base, Tex, in 1990. After her training, she served as staff radiologist in the abdominal imaging section of the same institution from 1990 to 1992. Her military career also included a tour of duty as a flight surgeon at the Dover USAF Hospital, Del, and military deployment in support of Operation Desert Storm.

Index terms:
Armed Forces Institute of Pathology
Radiology and radiologists
Special reports

Radiology 1999; 212:4

[1] From the Department of Radiologic Pathology, Armed Forces Institute of Pathology, Bldg 54, Rm M-121, 14th St and Alaska Ave, Washington, DC 20306-6000. Received March 18, 1999; accepted April 23. **Address reprint requests to** the author (e-mail: *rosado@afip.osd.mil*).

The opinions and assertions contained herein are the private views of the author and are not to be construed as official or as reflecting the views of the Department of the Air Force or the Department of Defense.

Dr Woodward is active in numerous national and international radiologic societies, including the Radiological Society of North America, the American College of Radiology, the American Roentgen Ray Society, the American Institute for Ultrasound in Medicine, the Society of Radiologists in Ultrasound, the American Association for Women Radiologists, and the Association of Program Directors in Radiology. She is a reviewer for the *Journal of Magnetic Resonance, Cancer*, and the *International Journal of Radiation Oncology, Biology, Physics* and has served as guest editor for *Seminars in Ultrasound, CT and MRI*.

She has authored or co-authored 20 original publications and book chapters. She is well known for her outstanding teaching abilities and has a reputation as an enthusiastic and gifted lecturer. In fact, she was selected "Teacher of the Year" for her department on three separate occasions. Her expertise in abdominal imaging and genitourinary radiology will greatly enhance the fulfillment of the mission of the AFIP. As Distinguished Scientist, Dr Woodward will participate in all educational and research activities of the Department of Radiologic Pathology at the AFIP, thus making a major contribution to the education of radiology residents and practicing radiologists in the United States and throughout the world.

The Distinguished Scientist program was first established in 1983 and is now an integral part of the Department of Radiologic Pathology. The position receives federal funding through the American Registry of Pathology. Funding is also provided by several other organizations: the American College of Radiology, the American Roentgen Ray Society, the Radiological Society of North America, the Association of University Radiologists, and the American Osteopathic College of

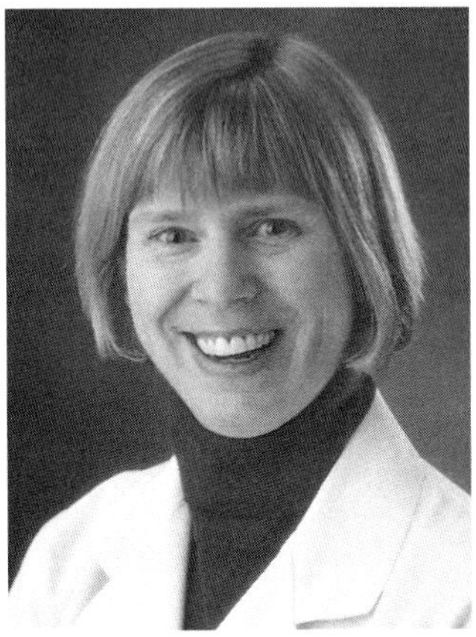

Paula J. Woodward, MD

Radiology. Representatives from each of these organizations, together with a representative from the Association of Program Directors in Radiology, form the Conjoint Committee for Radiologic Pathology at the AFIP and are responsible for selecting the Distinguished Scientist each year. The committee strongly considers the projected needs of the Department of Radiologic Pathology and the AFIP when selecting the Distinguished Scientist.

Any established academic radiologist interested in spending a year studying the correlation between abnormal radiologic images and their underlying pathologic processes is welcome to apply. Those wishing to apply should submit a letter of interest outlining the projects they would pursue during their time at the AFIP and an updated copy of their curriculum vitae to Melissa L. Rosado-de-Christenson at the address listed herein. Applications for the AFIP Distinguished Scientist position for the 2001–2002 academic year must be received by January 15, 2000.

Evan S. Siegelman, MD
Eric K. Outwater, MD

Index terms:
Magnetic resonance (MR), tissue characterization, 85.121412, 85.121413, 85.121414
Pelvic organs, MR, 85.121412, 85.121413, 85.121414
State-of-art reviews

Radiology 1999; 212:5–18

Abbreviations:
GRE = gradient-recalled echo
RARE = rapid acquisition with relaxation enhancement
SE = spin echo
STIR = short inversion time inversion recovery

[1] From the Department of Radiology, University of Pennsylvania Medical Center, 1st Floor Silverstein, 3400 Spruce St, Philadelphia, PA 19104-4283 (E.S.S.), and the Department of Radiology, Thomas Jefferson University Hospital, Philadelphia, Pa (E.K.O.). Received July 16, 1998; revision requested August 28; revision received October 13; accepted February 10, 1999. **Address reprint requests to** E.S.S. (e-mail: *siegelm@oasis.rad.upenn.edu*).

Tissue Characterization in the Female Pelvis by Means of MR Imaging[1]

Pelvic imaging techniques such as computed tomography and ultrasonography provide a limited capability for tissue characterization. Fat, fluid, and calcification, for example, can be identified on the basis of parameters such as x-ray attenuation, echogenicity, and sound attenuation. Because of the many tissue parameters, such as T1, T2, magnetic susceptibility, and chemical shift, that contribute to signal intensity, magnetic resonance (MR) imaging may afford an ability to identify a wider array of specific tissues. The purpose of this article is to review the ability of MR imaging to help identify various types of soft tissue and to provide an approach to interpretation of MR images of the female pelvis through tissue characterization. Lipid, fluid, hemorrhage, smooth muscle, fibrosis, solid malignant tissue, and hydrated soft tissue (including edema, mucin, and myxomatous tissue) have typical MR imaging properties, and their presence in a mass can often be established on MR images. Consideration of the tissue composition of various pathologic processes in the pelvis can result in more systematic approaches to image interpretation and thus narrow the differential diagnosis.

Magnetic resonance (MR) imaging is emerging as a cost-effective technique for the evaluation of a variety of disorders of the female pelvis (1), including endometriosis (2) and cervical cancer (3). MR imaging of the pelvis in some clinical situations can obviate surgery or change a planned surgical procedure, alter medical treatment, and decrease health care costs (4), particularly after an inconclusive (5) sonogram of the adnexa has been obtained (4–6). Reviews of MR imaging of the female pelvis have detailed routine MR techniques and time-efficient protocols that use fast spin-echo (SE) sequences obtained in multiple planes and T1-weighted imaging with contrast material enhancement in selected cases (7–9).

The purpose of this article is to review the ability of MR imaging to help characterize tissue in the female pelvis. Our goal is to present a systematic approach to image interpretation through tissue characterization and not to describe an encyclopedic list of pelvic masses as seen on MR images. When interpreting an MR study of a female pelvis, one should often be able to determine what tissues are likely to compose a pathologic process. Tissue characterization is an important function of diagnostic radiologists ("the issue is tissue"); it is this aspect of image interpretation that often affects patient care. Computer-assisted MR tissue segmentation techniques have been developed that can anatomically locate and characterize specific soft-tissue types from a set of MR images (10–12). Similar analyses can often be done by radiologists when evaluating MR studies. The soft tissues that can often be characterized in the female pelvis include fluid, hemorrhage, lipid, smooth muscle, fibrosis, solid malignant tissue, and hydrated soft tissue (including mucin, myxoid tissue, and edematous tissue) (Table).

TISSUE CHARACTERIZATION IN THE FEMALE PELVIS

MR imaging findings other than size, location, and cystic solid composition are important in lesion characterization. What are the relative T1 and T2 signal intensities? What is the morphology of the mass? Is there loss of signal on fat-suppressed or chemical shift images? Is there signal loss from magnetic susceptibility effects on T2*-weighted images? Is enhancement present, and if so, what portions of the lesion enhance? Is there ascites and peritoneal enhancement? Assimilating the answers to the above questions can often determine what tissue(s) composes a detected abnormality.

Summary of MR Characteristics of Pelvic Soft Tissues

Tissue	T1 Signal Intensity*	T2 Signal Intensity*	Enhancement	Examples Where Tissue May Be Present
Fat	High†	Intermediate‡	None	Mature teratoma, lipoma, normal pelvic fat
Noncomplicated fluid	Low	High§	None	Urine, spinal fluid, serous ascites, ovarian follicles
Blood				
Methemoglobin	Very high	Very low or high‖	None	Subacute hematomas, ectopic pregnancy, endometriomas, ovarian torsion
Ferritin or hemosiderin	Low	Very low	None	In the rim of maturing hematomas and endometriomas
Fibrous tissue or smooth muscle	Isointense	Low	Variable	Leiomyomas, adenomyosis, scar, solid endometriosis, ovarian fibroma, and Brenner tumor
Mucin	Low to high#	High	Peripheral with or without lacelike	Mucinous cystic ovarian neoplasms, pseudomyxoma peritonei, other mucinous adenocarcinomas
Myxomatous tissue	Low to isointense	High	Present but variable	Aggressive angiomyxoma, myxoid degeneration of a leiomyoma
Solid malignant tissue	Isointense	Isointense	Present	Endometrial, cervical, and ovarian carcinoma

* Signal intensity relative to that of the outer myometrium.
† Lower signal intensity on fat-suppressed T1-weighted images and/or opposed-phase T1-weighted GRE images (see text for details).
‡ Higher on fast SE images than on conventional T2-weighted images.
§ Persistently high signal intensity on heavily T2-weighted images (MR hydrography).
‖ Very low = intracellular methemoglobin; high = extracellular methemoglobin.
\# There is variable T1 shortening, which depends on the amount of hydration of the mucinous tissue.

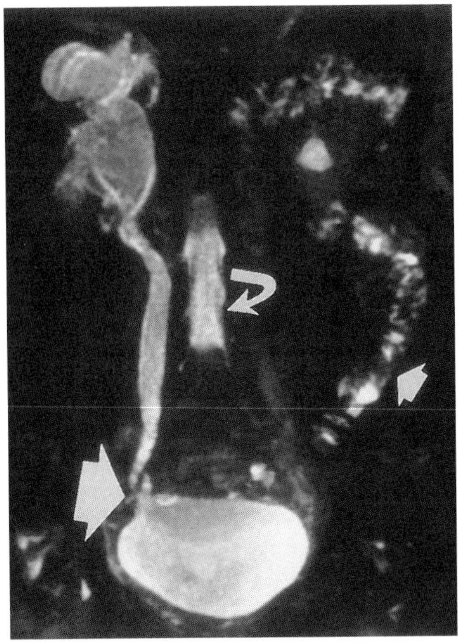

Figure 1. MR urography demonstrates obstruction of the distal ureter in a 49-year-old woman with surgically proved cervical carcinoma with parametrial invasion. Coronal maximum intensity projection MR urogram (∞/100) shows a dilated right collecting system and ureter to the level of the right ureterovesical junction (large straight arrow). Other fluid-containing structures include spinal fluid (curved arrow) and bowel (small straight arrow).

Fluid

Fluid has characteristic imaging findings independent of its location in the body. Simple fluid has the longest T1 and longest T2 of any other tissue. Thus, static fluid has very low signal intensity on T1-weighted images and very high signal intensity on T2- and heavily T2-weighted images. By using a very long effective echo time with a T2-weighted sequence, fluid-containing structures in the pelvis remain hyperintense, while all other soft tissues show very low relative signal intensity. Such MR hydrograms (13), which can be obtained by using T2-weighted half-Fourier rapid acquisition with relaxation enhancement (RARE) imaging, are useful in the rapid evaluation of postoperative fluid collections and in the detection of an obstructed ureter (Fig 1) (14).

Blood

The MR imaging findings of hemorrhage and hematomas have been described for the central nervous system (15), chest (16–18), and pelvis (19,20). Blood shortens the T1 and T2 of water. High signal intensity on T1-weighted images in regions of hemorrhage primarily results from the paramagnetic effects of methemoglobin. The T2-weighted signal intensity of methemoglobin depends on whether it is in an intracellular or extracellular location; the former results in low signal intensity (profound T2 shortening), while the latter results in high signal intensity (less T2 shortening). Iron in intracellular ferritin or hemosiderin in the walls of mature hematomas results in marked signal loss on T2- and T2*-

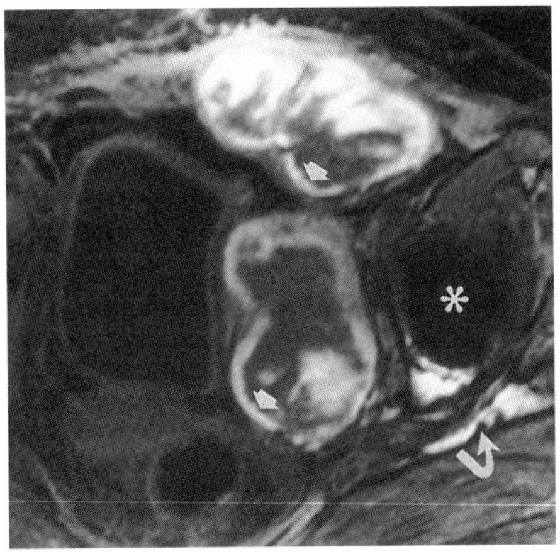

Figure 2. Blood within a subacute hematoma of rectus sheath and pelvis in a 76-year-old woman with atrial fibrillation who was being treated with oral anticoagulants. Axial fat-suppressed T1-weighted GRE image (300/1.7, 90° flip angle) shows typical left-sided rectus sheath and pelvic sidewall hematomas with a very high-signal-intensity outer rim (straight arrows) characteristic of methemoglobin. Magnetic susceptibility artifact (*) is present in the left femoral head from prior joint replacement. The unsuppressed fat (curved arrow) in the posterior acetabulum and deep gluteal soft tissues should not be interpreted as an additional site of hemorrhage.

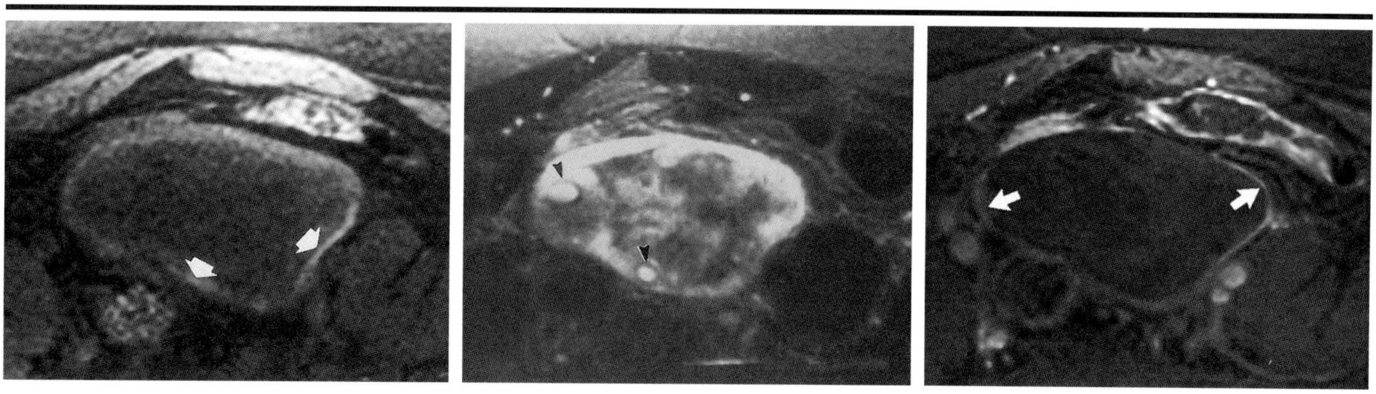

a. b. c.

Figure 3. Blood present within an adnexal mass in a 17-year-old girl with ovarian torsion. Hemorrhagic infarction of the left ovary was confirmed at surgery. **(a)** Axial T1-weighted, fat-suppressed, spoiled GRE image (280/1.7, 90° flip angle) shows a 10-cm left adnexal mass that has a high-signal-intensity rim (arrows), suspicious for subacute hemorrhage. **(b)** Axial fat-suppressed T2-weighted fast SE image (4,600/98) obtained slightly higher throughout the mass shows scattered subcentimeter cysts (arrowheads) representing ovarian follicles. The remainder of the ovary is composed of low- to intermediate-signal-intensity material, likely representing deoxyhemoglobin. **(c)** Axial gadopentetate dimeglumine–enhanced, T1-weighted, fat-saturated GRE image obtained with identical imaging parameters as in **a** shows only faint rim enhancement (arrows) of the ovary. The remainder of the ovary shows no perfusion.

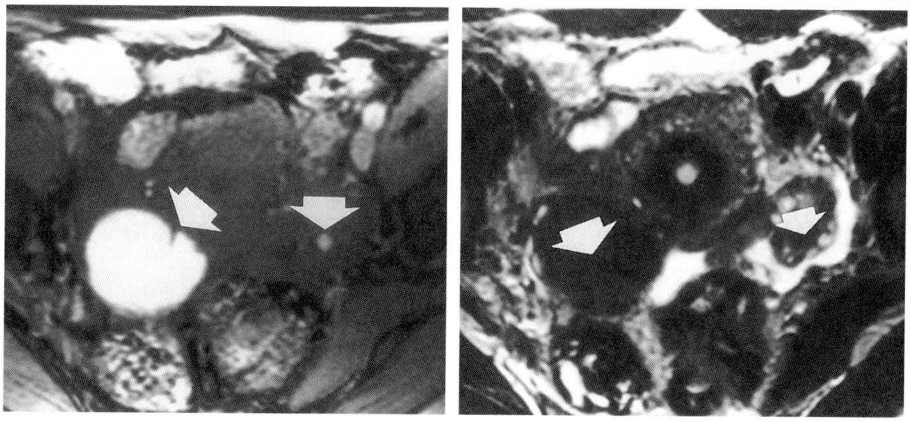

a. b.

Figure 4. Adnexal endometrial cysts in a 37-year-old woman with surgically confirmed endometriosis. **(a)** Axial fat-suppressed T1-weighted GRE image (120/2.6, 60° flip angle) shows bilateral high-signal-intensity adnexal lesions (arrows). **(b)** Axial T2-weighted fast SE image (5,000/108) shows that the lesions are of low-signal-intensity "shading" (arrows). Bilateral adnexal lesions with high signal intensity on T1-weighted images and low signal intensity on T2-weighted images have high specificity for endometriosis.

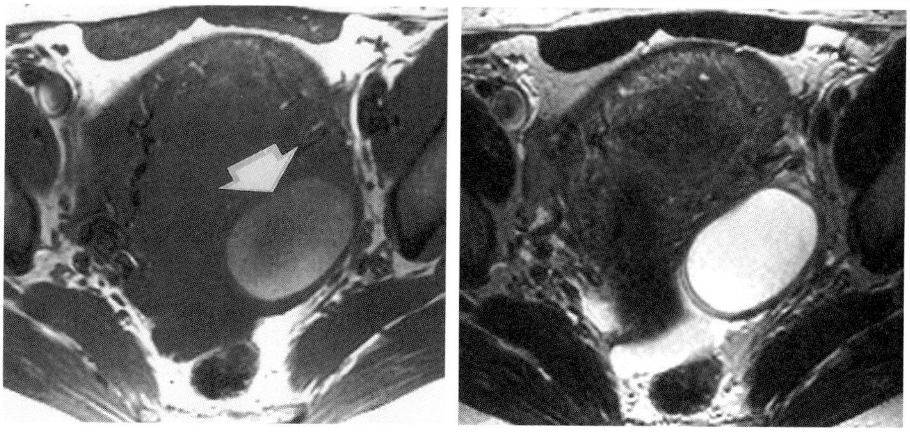

a. b.

Figure 5. Hemorrhagic corpus luteum cyst in a 41-year-old woman. **(a)** Axial T1-weighted SE image (500/16) shows a cyst with high signal intensity (arrow) in the left ovary. **(b)** Axial T2-weighted fast SE image (3,600/119) shows high signal intensity of the cyst. This combination of short T1 and long T2 is suggestive, but not diagnostic, of hemorrhagic functional cysts since some endometriomas can have a similar appearance (33). In our experience, the degree of T1 shortening is greater for endometriomas (Fig 4a) than for hemorrhagic functional cysts.

weighted images from magnetic susceptibility effects.

Fat-saturated T1-weighted images are recommended for the detection and characterization of hemorrhagic foci for several reasons. First, fat suppression decreases potential motion artifact from subcutaneous and intraabdominal fat. Second, a fat-saturated image distinguishes between fatty and hemorrhagic masses. Third, fat suppression improves the dynamic range of the image, with superior ability to distinguish small differences in signal intensity.

Characteristic MR imaging findings of a subacute hematoma has been termed the "concentric ring sign" (21–23). Often best delineated on fat-suppressed T1-weighted images, the concentric ring consists of an inner band of high signal intensity from methemoglobin and an outer low-signal-intensity rim from ferritin within macrophages. The outer low-signal-intensity ring is absent in early hematomas and in intraperitoneal hematomas (Figs 2, 3) (24,25). The ring sign is also absent in other hemorrhagic masses such as endometriomas and hemorrhagic functional cysts.

Pelvic hematomas.—Pelvic hematomas tend to have loculations with different rates of clot maturation that result in a heterogeneous appearance on MR images (25). The concentric ring sign, when present, has high specificity for a subacute to chronic hematoma (21). Foci of very high signal intensity on T1-weighted images representing methemoglobin may be present within the hematoma, although in various amounts and distribution. Even with such signal heterogeneity, the MR imaging diagnosis is often straightforward. Computed tomography is less sensitive and specific in the diagnosis of hematomas (26,27).

Subacute hematomas are commonly detected in the female pelvis in women after surgery (ie, cesarean delivery or oophorectomy) (28) and in women receiving anticoagulation therapy who present with pelvic pain and/or a palpable mass (Fig 2). In some postoperative patients, it can be difficult, if not impossible, to determine whether a hematoma is infected; aspiration and/or culture may be necessary in some patients. Subacute hematomas have also been described in women with ectopic pregnancy (29,30).

It has been suggested that in the setting of a pelvic hematoma, a hemorrhagic neoplasm should be excluded (30). However, hemorrhagic pelvic malignancies also contain solid, vascularized tissue and are distinguishable from masslike foci of bland hemorrhage (31).

Endometriosis.—Hemorrhagic foci within the ovary and pelvis are most commonly encountered in endometriosis. MR imaging can depict the presence of blood products within endometrial cysts (32) and usually distinguishes them from other hemorrhagic adnexal masses (33,34). The most common and specific appearance of endometrioma is a relatively homogeneous, high-signal-intensity cyst on T1-weighted images with low signal intensity on T2-weighted images (termed "shading") (Fig 4). Endometrial cysts are very hyperintense on T1-weighted images, similar to fat. The reasons for the characteristic low signal intensity of endometriomas on T2-weighted images may be related to their high iron content, which is 10–20 times the concentration of whole blood (35). Sugimura et al (35) found that 15 endometriomas had an iron concentration between 320 and 5,720 µg/dL (57 and 1,024 µmol/L), while the iron content of whole blood varied between 40 and 175 µg/dL (7 and 31 µmol/L). Increasing iron content of endometriomas corresponds with higher signal intensity on T1-weighted images (35) and lower signal intensity on T2-weighted images relative to the signal intensity of muscle (36).

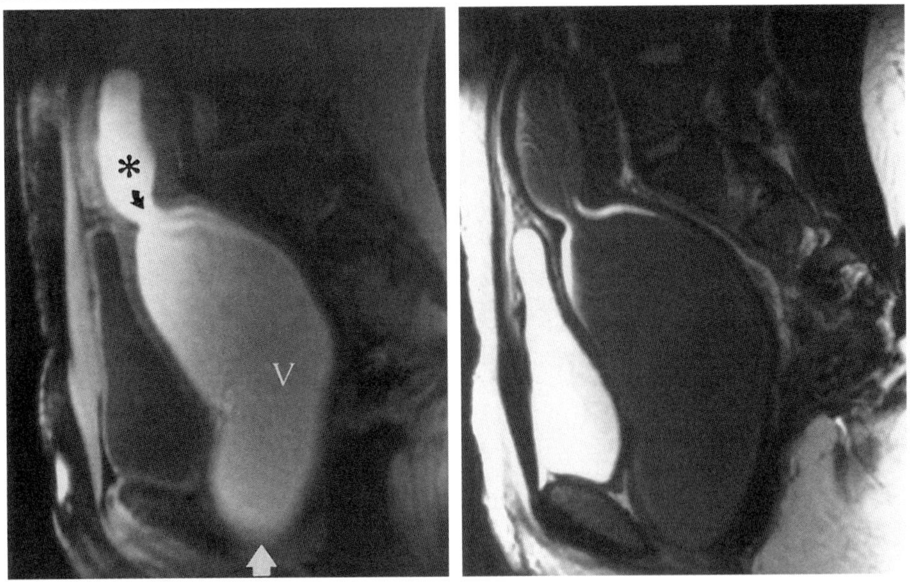

a. b.

Figure 6. MR imaging demonstration of blood within a distended vagina and endocervical and endometrial canal in a 12-year-old girl with primary amenorrhea, pelvic pain, and a palpable pelvic mass. An obstructing low transverse vaginal septum was confirmed surgically. **(a)** Sagittal T1-weighted, fat-suppressed, GRE image (250/7, 90° flip angle) shows distention of the endometrial (*), endocervical (black arrow), and vaginal (*V*) canals by very high-signal-intensity material representing subacute blood. The level of the obstruction lies below the symphysis pubis, near the introitus (white arrow). **(b)** Sagittal T2-weighted fast SE image (4,000/105) shows low-signal-intensity "shading" of the hematometrocolpos. It can be difficult to differentiate an imperforate hymen from a low transverse septum at MR imaging.

A single ovarian lesion with high signal intensity on T1-weighted images and high signal intensity on T2-weighted images could either represent an endometrioma, hemorrhagic cyst, or ovarian neoplasm (33,37–39). Multiple or bilateral adnexal lesions, cul-de-sac lesions, or a dilated fallopian tube with high signal intensity on T1-weighted images favor the diagnosis of endometriosis (34,40). Fat-saturated T1-weighted techniques improve the sensitivity for detecting small foci of endometriosis and help differentiate endometrial cysts from fat-containing dermoids (41,42).

Whereas pelvic hematomas have a variable appearance on both T1- and T2-weighted images as described above, hematomas will not mimic a typical endometrioma with diffusely high signal intensity on T1-weighted images and low signal intensity on T2-weighted images at any stage in development (25).

Hemorrhagic functional cysts and corpus luteum cysts.—High signal intensity on T1-weighted images in an ovarian cyst is not diagnostic of an endometrioma and is commonly seen in functional cysts. Hemorrhagic corpus luteum cysts are not uncommon in premenopausal women. MR imaging findings suggestive of a corpus luteum cyst include a unilateral, uni-

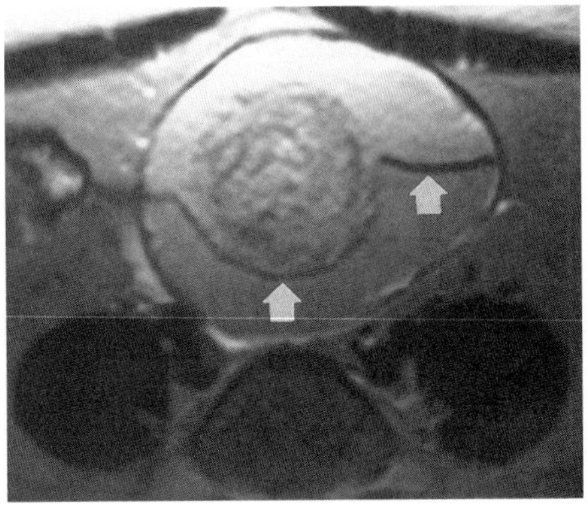

Figure 7. Fat within a left adnexal mass in a 37-year-old woman with a surgically confirmed mature teratoma. Axial T2-weighted fast SE image (5,000/102) shows a complex mass with a meniscoid tissue–fluid level that is separated by a low-signal-intensity boundary (arrows). The latter likely represents a chemical shift in the frequency-encoding direction (anterior-to-posterior) at a fat-water interface. A spherical central portion of the mass is present. This sequence alone, while sufficient to establish a diagnosis of a teratoma, should be confirmed with either a fat saturation, water saturation, or chemical shift technique.

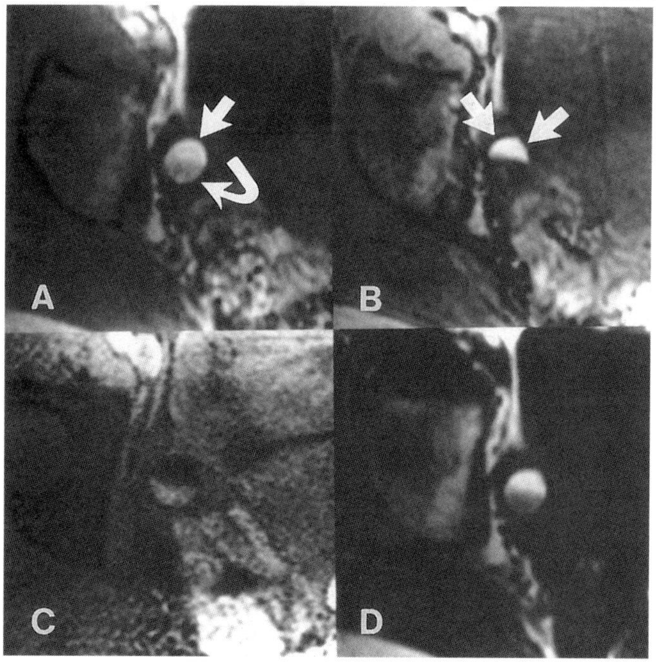

Figure 8. Varying amounts of fat within a right-sided mature teratoma in a 41-year-old woman. *A,* Axial T1-weighted, in-phase, spoiled GRE image (120/4.2, 90° flip angle) shows a right adnexal mass with a very high-signal-intensity anterior component (straight arrow) and an intermediate- to high-signal-intensity posterior component (curved arrow). *B,* Axial T1-weighted, opposed-phase, spoiled GRE image (120/2.1, 90° flip angle) shows marked signal loss in the posterior portion of the mass, establishing the presence of microscopic lipid. While there is no signal loss of the anterior component of the mass, there is a subtle etching artifact at the border between the anterior aspect of the mass and the surrounding ovarian and paraovarian tissue (arrows). *C,* Axial T1-weighted, fat-saturated, opposed-phase, spoiled GRE image (120./2.1, 90° flip angle) shows marked loss of signal in the anterior portion of the mass, establishing the presence of macroscopic fat. Compared to the in-phase image in *A,* it is difficult to appreciate any change in signal intensity in the posterior portion of the mass. *D,* Axial T1-weighted, water-saturated spoiled GRE image (120/4.2, 90° flip angle) shows the macroscopic fat anteriorly and microscopic lipid posteriorly. This mature teratoma in a 41-year-old woman illustrates the complementary use of fat saturation and in-phase–opposed-phase chemical shift techniques in the characterization of lipid-containing masses.

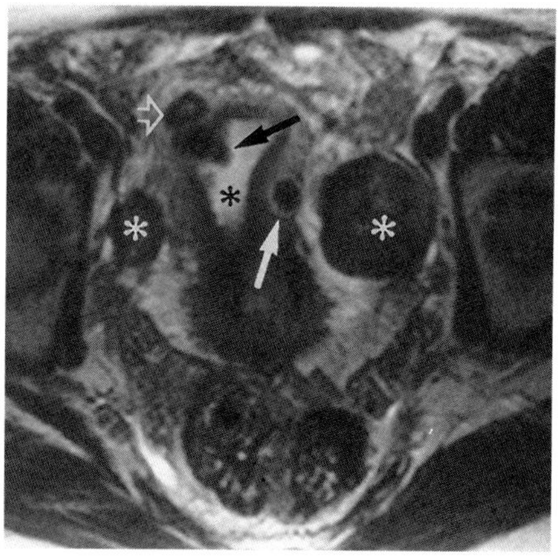

Figure 9. MR imaging demonstration of fibrotic bilateral adnexal masses and smooth-muscle myometrial masses in a 73-year-old woman with bilateral fibrothecomas, endometrial hyperplasia, and uterine leiomyomas. Axial T2-weighted fast SE image (5,000/136) shows bilateral adnexal masses (white *) whose signal intensity is lower than that of the outer myometrium and isointense to minimally hyperintense compared with the normal junctional zone and pelvic musculature. There is a widened endometrial complex (black *) and clear definition of the inner and outer myometrium, both of which are suggestive of hormonal production by the tumors in this postmenopausal woman. Three well-circumscribed, low-signal-intensity myometrial masses are present. One has a submucosal component (black arrow), another has a high-signal-intensity rim (solid white arrow), and the third has high signal intensity internally (open white arrow).

focal ovarian lesion and the presence of high signal intensity on T2-weighted images (Fig 5). The reason for the relative high signal intensity on T2-weighted images within hemorrhagic functional and corpus luteum cysts (as opposed to the lower signal intensity on T2-weighted images within endometriomas) presumably relates to the lower protein and iron content of the former, which results in minimal T2 shortening. Unlike endometrial cysts, corpus luteum cysts contain a layer of luteinized cells that line the cyst wall and that can appear thickened on MR imaging studies (7).

Ovarian torsion.—The MR imaging appearance of ovarian torsion depends on the severity and chronicity of vascular compromise. If a twisted ovary remains untreated, it can progress to hemorrhagic infarction. One MR imaging appearance of an ovary with hemorrhagic infarction is that of an enlarged ovary with displaced follicles and low signal intensity on T2-weighted images due to interstitial hemorrhage. A thin rim of high signal intensity on T1-weighted images that demonstrates no enhancement after administration of contrast material may also be seen (43) (Fig 3). Typical endometriomas and corpus luteum cysts do not have methemoglobin isolated to the rim and do not usually involve the entire ovary. In adults, the majority of ovaries that twist are not normal; the most common associated instigating masses are benign cysts or neoplasms, particularly, cystic teratoma. Malignant lesions account for less than 10% of twisted tumors and are usually present in older women (44,45).

Adenomyosis.—Adenomyosis represents the presence of ectopic endometrial glands and stroma in the uterine myometrium (see "Smooth Muscle"). While less frequent than the ectopic endometrial glands of endometriosis, adenomyotic glands can bleed and result in high signal intensity on T1-weighted images (46,47).

Hematometrocolpos.—MR imaging is useful in the evaluation of primary amenorrhea and developmental uterine anomalies (48–50). Hematometrocolpos is the result of an imperforate hymen, transverse vaginal septum, or other obstruction to menstrual blood flow. MR imaging can noninvasively delineate the location and amount of retained blood (49,50) (Fig 6) and identify endometrial implants in the peritoneal cavity from retrograde menstruation. Blood in the dilated vagina or uterus with or without associated endometriosis (from retrograde menstruation) shows typical shading due to its chronic accumulation (Fig 6b).

Lipid

Efficient T1 relaxation occurs when a proton interacts with a magnetic field that is fluctuating near the Larmor frequency (51). Water protons tumble rapidly and are inefficient at T1 relaxation, accounting for the very low signal intensity of fluid on T1-weighted images. Protons within macroscopic fat rotate near the Larmor frequency and therefore are very efficient at T1 relaxation, which results in high signal intensity on T1-weighted images. The signal of fat on T2-weighted images is of intermediate intensity relative to muscle on conventional T2-weighted images and is of high signal intensity relative to muscle on fast SE images. Fast SE sequences minimize the signal loss in fat from dephasing effects of J-coupling, and relative signal loss from magnetization transfer effects is minimal (52–54).

Almost all lipid-containing masses within the adnexa are teratomas. Approximately 99% of teratomas are mature cystic teratomas (dermoid cysts) (55). The lipid content of dermoid cysts is largely sebaceous liquid material and less commonly adipose tissue. Immature teratomas are large cystic and solid tumors of children and young women and may also show small foci of fat.

Several techniques are available to characterize fat-containing structures in the pelvis. One method for establishing that tissue is composed of fat is through recognition of chemical shift misregistration in the frequency-encoding direction on

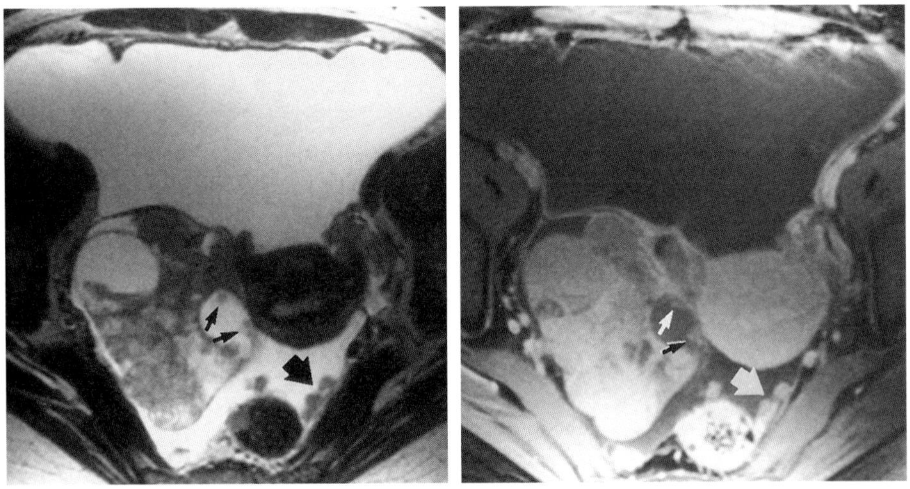

a. b.

Figure 10. MR imaging demonstration of enhancing solid cancer with spread to the peritoneum in a 41-year-old woman with a surgically confirmed malignant epithelial ovarian neoplasm with peritoneal spread of disease. **(a)** Axial T2-weighted fast SE image (5,800/126) shows a large complex right adnexal mass with both cystic and solid components. The solid components are of higher signal intensity than that of the uterine myometrium. Solid projections of tissue (small arrows) within one of the intratumoral cysts and nodules of soft-tissue signal intensity (large arrow) are present in the cul-de-sac. **(b)** Axial gadopentetate dimeglumine–enhanced fat-saturated GRE image (400/2.9, 90° flip angle) shows enhancing intracystic solid tissue (small arrows) and peritoneal implants (large arrow).

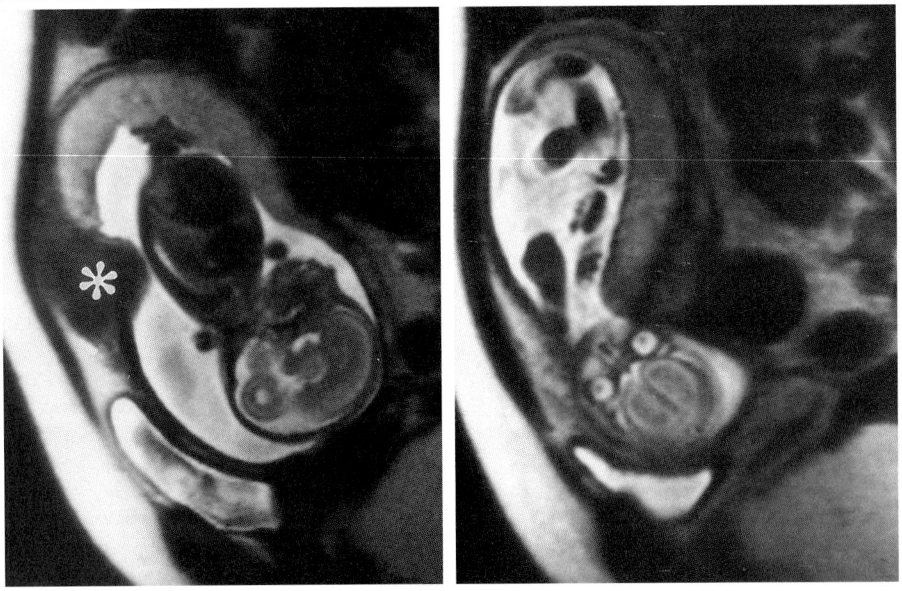

a. b.

Figure 11. MR imaging demonstration of a focal myometrial contraction. **(a, b)** Sagittal T2-weighted half-Fourier RARE images (∞/96) obtained 25 minutes apart in a 32-year-old woman shows fetal head, chest, and abdominal contents to good advantage. A transient low-signal-intensity mass of the anterior uterine wall (*) represents a focal myometrial contraction. Half-Fourier RARE techniques have allowed one to obtain fetal MR images that are relatively free of motion artifacts (79,80).

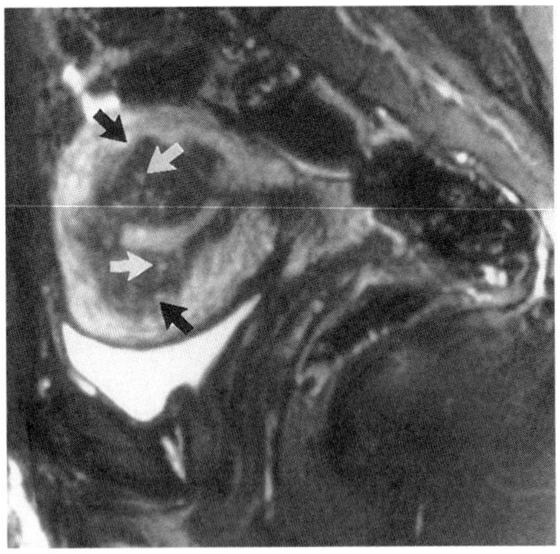

Figure 12. MR imaging demonstration of diffuse smooth-muscle proliferation within the inner myometrium in a 36-year-old woman with adenomyosis. Sagittal T2-weighted fast SE image (4,200/108) shows diffuse asymmetric thickening of the inner myometrium by a relatively low-signal-intensity process (black arrows) compared to the outer myometrium. Punctate foci of high signal intensity (white arrows) are present. The diffuse area of low signal intensity within the myometrium represents reactive smooth-muscle proliferation. The ectopic intramyometrial endometrial glands have high signal intensity on this T2-weighted image.

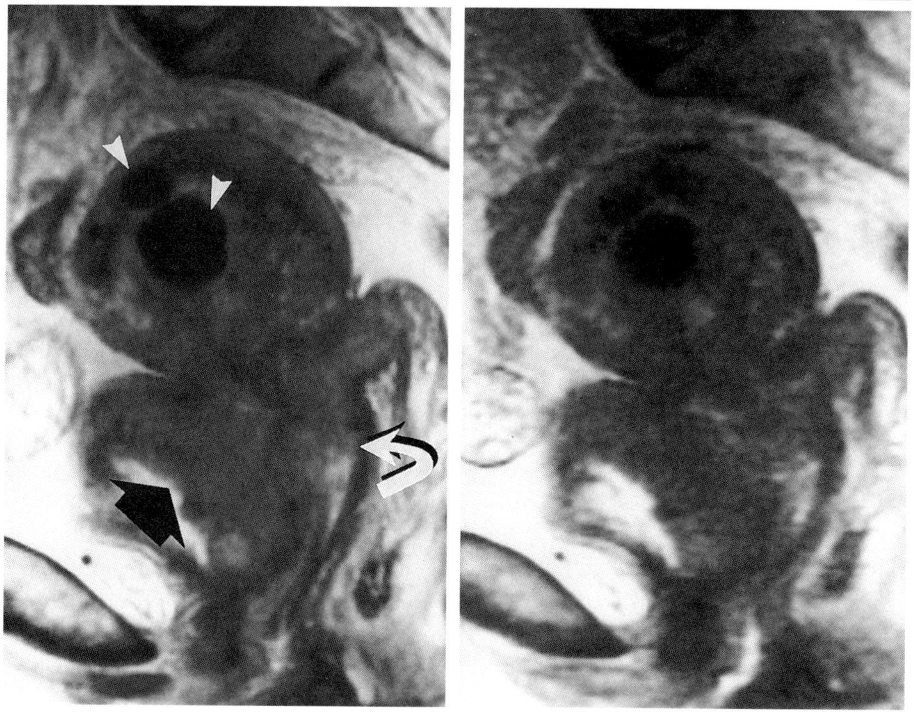

a. b.

Figure 13. Invasive squamous cell carcinoma of the cervix in a 64-year-old woman with vaginal bleeding . (a) Sagittal T2-weighted fast SE image (3,500/90) shows an infiltrative intermediate-signal-intensity cervical mass that invades the vagina (white arrow), posterior bladder wall (black arrow), and uterine body. Two low-signal-intensity leiomyomas (arrowheads) are clearly delineated. (b) Sagittal T2-weighted half-Fourier RARE image (∞/98) shows blurring of the margins of the cancer and the leiomyomas, secondary to T2 decay during the long echo train (83,84). An optimized fast SE sequence is preferred to a corresponding half-Fourier RARE sequence in the evaluation of normal uteri, because of the latter sequence's limitations on contrast and signal-to-noise ratio (85). However, a diagnosis of bladder invasion can still be established in this instance.

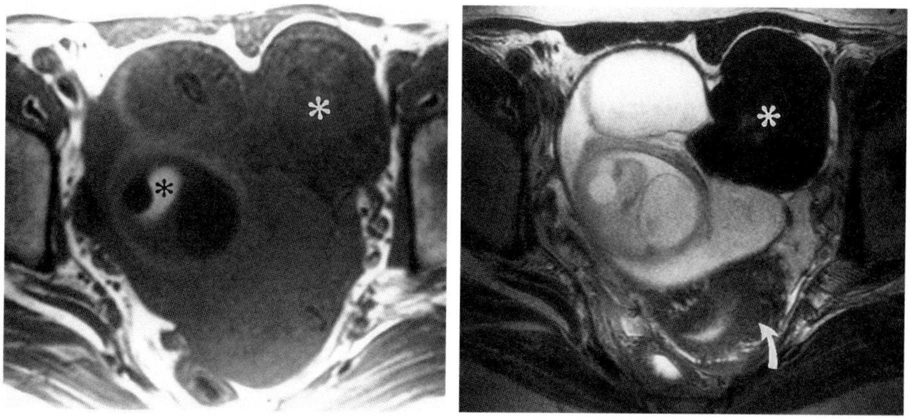

a. b.

Figure 14. MR imaging demonstration of fibrous tissue and mucin within a complex left adnexal mass in a 51-year-old woman. At surgery, the fibrous mass was a Brenner tumor and the mucin-containing mass was a borderline mucinous tumor. (a) Axial T1-weighted SE (400/10) and (b) T2-weighted fast SE (4,700/85) images show a large pelvic mass that displaces the uterus (curved arrow in b) posteriorly. The mass has two components. Anteriorly and laterally, there is a well-circumscribed, 6.5-cm mass (white ∗) that has low signal intensity on both the T1- and T2-weighted images. The remainder of the mass has low-, intermediate-, and high- (black ∗ in a) signal-intensity components relative to muscle on the T1-weighted image and intermediate- to high-signal-intensity components on the T2-weighted image. (MR images courtesy of Bohyun Kim, MD, Samsung Medical Center, Seoul, Korea.)

SE images (56). Such a chemical shift effect with an SE sequence establishes that the boundary phenomenon is occurring at a fat-water interface (Fig 7). A second method for establishing the lipid content of a pelvic mass is to compare T1-weighted images obtained before and after a proton-selective fat saturation or water saturation pulse. If a mass loses signal after fat saturation or has persistent signal after water saturation, then the mass contains fat. Both fat (Fig 8c) and water saturation techniques (Fig 8d) (57) enable detection and characterization of dermoid cysts and distinguish them from other processes that have high signal intensity on T1-weighted images (38,58–61).

Short inversion time inversion-recovery (STIR) techniques have been used as a method to suppress fat. By selecting an appropriate inversion time (ie, 150 msec at 1.5 T) before the application of the repetition time pulse, the signal from fat will be nulled. However, any other tissue with a similar short T1 value will also be suppressed with the STIR technique; thus, it is not specific in the characterization of fatty tissue (62). Hemorrhagic masses could have components with similar T1 values as fat and therefore also "suppress" on STIR images.

Some cystic teratomas do not have abundant lipid but instead contain smaller amounts of adipocytes or tissue with intracellular lipid (63). Chemical shift imaging using GRE techniques is a more sensitive method for detecting the presence of small amounts of lipid within such masses (64) (Fig 8a, 8b). By demonstrating loss of signal on an opposed-phase image compared to an in-phase image, chemical shift MR imaging techniques can depict the lipid content of teratomas (7) and perform as well as standard fat-saturation techniques (65). The latter methods result in greater signal loss in masses composed almost entirely of fat, while the former methods are more sensitive for suppressing microscopic lipid.

Macromolecules

To understand the relative signal intensity of tissues composed of macromolecules, a brief review of the biologic states of water is necessary (66–69). Water can exist in either a free or bound state. Free water has unrestricted motion, whereas bound water (for example water molecules that are associated with intracellular proteins) has restricted motion. The hydrogen protons of bound water tumble with a frequency closer to the Larmor frequency and are more efficient at T1 relaxation and T2 decay. This results in shortening of both the T1 and T2 relaxation times of the water. While this mechanism of T1 and T2 shortening occurs to some extent in all tissues, there are several subtypes of soft tissue, such as muscle and fibrous tissue, that are composed of a large proportion of macromolecules. Their relative signal intensities may provide insight into their tissue components.

Magnetization transfer effects are a second phenomenon that results in lower signal intensity of macromolecular-rich soft tissues on T2-weighted images, especially when using fast SE techniques that employ multiple refocusing pulses. The latter pulses result in increased off-resonance radiofrequency energy, which saturates protons bound to macromolecules (43,62).

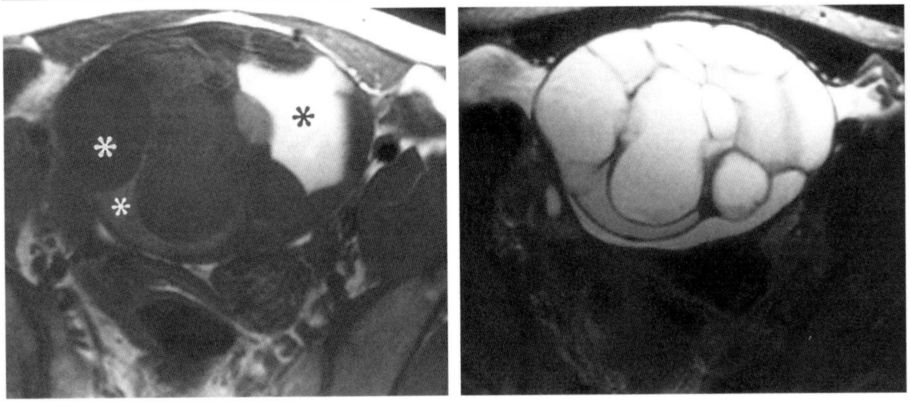

a. b.

Figure 15. MR imaging demonstration of various concentrations of mucin within a mucinous neoplasm of low malignant potential of the right ovary in a 37-year-old woman. **(a)** Axial T1-weighted SE image (600/12) demonstrates a large multilocular cystic mass with varying signal intensities that are hypointense (large white *), minimally hyperintense (small white *), and markedly hyperintense (black *) relative to muscle. **(b)** Axial T2-weighted fast SE image (6,000/126) shows that the majority of the locules are moderately hyperintense to muscle. The lack of solid components, ascites, or peritoneal implants suggests a benign diagnosis.

Smooth Muscle

Compared to other soft tissues in the body, both smooth muscle and skeletal muscle have low signal intensity on T2-weighted images, which results from the T2 shortening effects of intramuscular actin, myosin, and collagen and decreased extracellular fluid compared with surrounding tissues (70–72). Normal structures in the pelvis that have very low signal intensity on T2-weighted images include the junctional zone of the uterus; the vaginal, urethral, and rectal muscularis; and the bladder detrusor muscle.

The smooth-muscle composition of the uterine myometrium has been studied with MR imaging. The junctional zone (inner myometrium) of the uterus is both functionally and structurally different from the outer myometrium (73). The normal junctional zone has lower signal intensity on T2-weighted images than that of the adjacent outer myometrium (Figs 4, 9, 10). The outer myometrium has higher signal intensity because of less compact smooth muscle, greater extracellular matrix, increased water content, and more numerous venous structures (74,75). Focal myometrial contractions cause more compact smooth muscle with compressed venous structures and thus can mimic either leiomyoma or focal adenomyosis on MR imaging studies (76). Situations in which contractions are seen are during pregnancy (77) and less typically during any phase of the menstrual cycle (78). Documenting the transient nature of the pseudomass will establish the diagnosis (Fig 11).

Adenomyosis.—The ectopic endometrial glands and stroma of adenomyosis are surrounded by dense proliferation of smooth-muscle cells (47). This reactive proliferation results in apparent thickening of the junctional zone and is a sensitive MR imaging finding of adenomyosis. More specific findings include a junctional zone of at least 12 mm (76,81), focal thickening of the junctional zone, ill-defined spiculated low-signal-intensity masses, and sub-

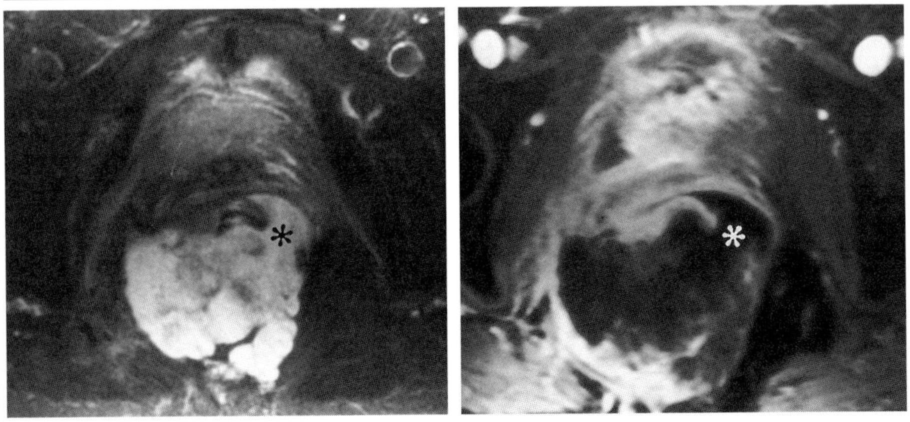

a. b.

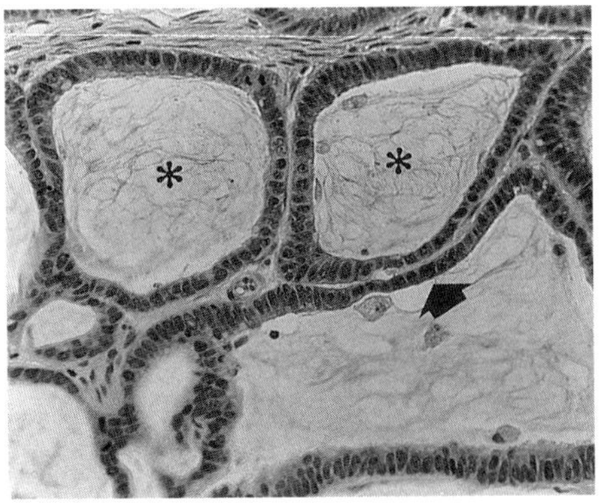

c.

Figure 16. MR imaging demonstration of mucin within recurrent mucinous adenocarcinoma of the rectum in a 65-year-old woman. **(a)** Axial fat-suppressed T2-weighted fast SE (3,000/99) and **(b)** gadopentetate dimeglumine–enhanced fat-saturated GRE (200/2.9, 90° flip angle) images show an infiltrative heterogeneous mass that has high signal intensity on the T2-weighted image; the center of the mass is in the rectal bed. There is a fistula to the left vaginal fornix (*). There is heterogeneous peripheral enhancement and patchy internal enhancement that distinguishes this process from a postprocedural fluid collection. Both the high signal intensity of the rectal tumor on the T2-weighted image and the irregular rim enhancement are very suggestive of a mucinous subtype of rectal carcinoma (110). **(c)** Histologic section of the mass shows glandular epithelium (arrow) with abundant extracellular mucin (*). (Hematoxylin-eosin stain; original magnification, ×20.)

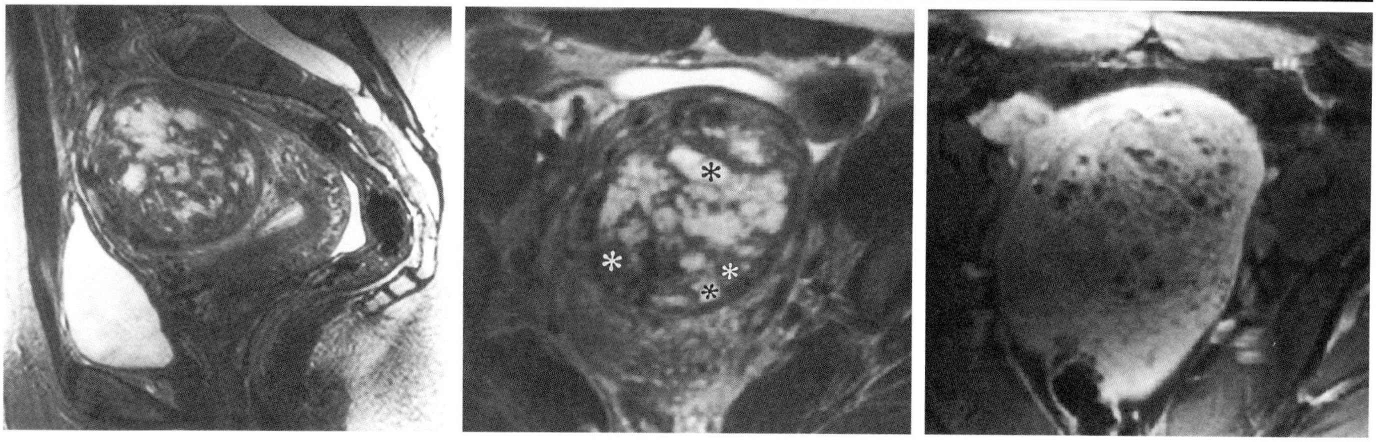

a. b. c.

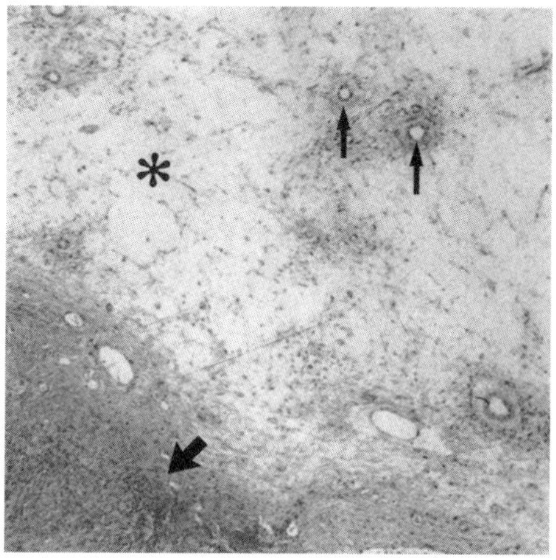

d.

Figure 17. Myxoid tissue in a degenerated leiomyoma in a 49-year-old woman. **(a)** Sagittal and **(b)** axial T2-weighted fast SE images (5,300/126) show a well-circumscribed mass of the anterior uterus that has both low- (white * in **b**) and high- (black * in **b**) signal-intensity components compared to the outer myometrium. **(c)** Gadopentetate dimeglumine–enhanced fat-saturated GRE image (500/3.3, 90° flip angle) obtained at the same level as **b** shows that some of the intratumoral tissue with high signal intensity on the T2-weighted image enhances, indicating that it does not represent intratumoral cysts or necrosis. **(d)** Histologic section of a different myxoid leiomyoma shows the loose, water-laden myxoid tissue (*) contrasted with the denser smooth-muscle bundles of the leiomyomas (thick arrow). Myxoid degeneration is not necrosis; several vessels (thin arrows) still course through the myxoid tissue. (Hematoxylin-eosin stain; original magnification, ×40.)

centimeter foci of high signal intensity representing imbedded endometrial glands on T2-weighted images (46,47) (Fig 12).

Leiomyomas.—The vast majority of leiomyomas appear as well-circumscribed, homogeneous low-signal-intensity masses on T2-weighted images (Figs 9, 13) (82–85). This appearance results from densely arranged myoma cells with intervening collagen (86,87). Commonly, hyaline degeneration and/or calcification also contributes to the low signal intensity of myomas (82,88). Degenerated leiomyomas may also show foci of high signal intensity that correspond to a combination of edematous swelling of myoma cells from ischemia (87), cystic change, and/or myxoid degeneration (see "Myxoid Tissue").

Fibrosis

Relatively acellular regions of fibrous tissue (with a large proportion of collagen and few cells and vessels) will, like compact smooth muscle, have intermediate signal intensity on T1-weighted images and low signal intensity on T2-weighted images. The cervix, like the uterine corpus, has a zonal anatomy that is well depicted on T2-weighted images. The cervical fibromuscular stroma is one component of the cervix that is composed mostly of fibrous connective tissue (89–91). Similar to the uterine myometrium, the cervical fibromuscular stroma has two discernible layers on T2-weighted images—an inner low-signal-intensity layer and an outer low- to intermediate-signal-intensity layer. MR imaging–histologic correlation suggests that the inner layer has an increased number of fibroblasts and muscle cells that likely explains the differences in T2 signal intensity (90). Various amounts of fibrous tissue are commonly present in tumors (eg, metastases, stromal tumors), but the following are masses in which fibrosis can be a dominant component.

Solid masses of endometriosis.—Solid fibrotic masses or nodules of endometriosis are composed of reactive fibrosis surrounding glands of endometriosis. They appear as spiculated masses that have low signal intensity on T2-weighted images sometimes with punctate high signal intensity on T1-weighted images (92). Fibrotic masses of endometriosis affect the cul-de-sac, bladder, and rectum and are also encountered in the anterior abdominal wall in women after a cesarean delivery (93).

Fibromas and fibrothecomas.—Fibromas are composed of spindle cells that produce a variable amount of collagen and are not hormonally active. Fibrothecomas contain both fibrous tissue and theca cells and are often hormonally active. The fibrous tissue that composes the majority of most of these tumors is responsible for the low signal intensity delineated on both T1- and T2-weighted images (Fig 9). Intratumoral edema is also common in larger fibromas, which explains why many fibromas are not uniformly hypointense on T2-weighted images (94). A widened endometrial stripe in association with an ovarian mass with low signal intensity on T2-weighted images can suggest a diagnosis of functioning fibrothecoma with endometrial hyperplasia (95) (Fig 9).

Cystadenofibroma.—Cystadenofibromas are a subset of epithelial ovarian neoplasms that are usually benign. The presence of rims, plaques, or nodules that have low signal intensity on T2-weighted images and that range in size between 2 mm and 4 cm within a multiloculated cystic ovarian mass can suggest the diagnosis (95). As is the case for fibromas, the low-signal-intensity foci correspond to intratumoral regions of dense fibrous tissue.

Brenner tumor.—Benign transitional cell (Brenner) tumors of the ovary compose approximately 2% of epithelial ovarian neoplasms. Brenner tumors are often discovered incidentally at surgery or pathologic examination because they are small and asymptomatic (96). In 30% of cases, Brenner tumors are associated with an epithelial ovarian neoplasm of either the ipsilateral or contralateral ovary (Fig 14). Brenner tumors contain abundant fibrous stroma (96), which accounts for the low signal intensity on T2-weighted images in those masses visible on MR images (Fig 14) (97). Brenner tumors also contain small epithelial nests that are too small to visualize as high-signal-intensity foci on T2-weighted images.

Fibrotic masses after radiation therapy or surgery.—Patients with pelvic cancer who have been treated with surgery and/or radiation therapy may have scarring that is masslike, mimicking recurrent tumor. Initial reports suggested that if the mass had low signal intensity on T2-weighted images, then tumor recurrence could be excluded with relative high specificity (98,99), especially in patients who have been evaluated after 12 months (100). Unfortunately, subsequent studies have documented that recurrent malignancies with a desmoplastic reaction can have relatively low signal intensity on T2-weighted images (101). Thus, both treatment-related scarring and tumors have low signal intensity that is related to the amount of fibrosis present. Analysis of lesion morphology can help distinguish the two; posttreatment fibrosis or scar often has angular margins, whereas recurrent malignancy is usually round (102). Tissue sampling may be necessary in some instances (103).

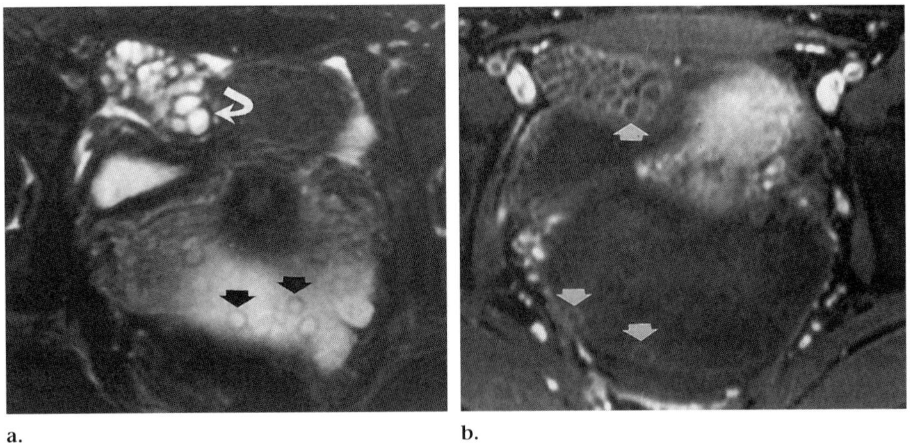

a. b.

Figure 18. MR imaging appearance of ovarian edema without hemorrhage in a 16-year-old girl with pelvic pain. At subsequent surgery, a partially twisted, viable left ovary (massive ovarian edema) was present. **(a)** Fat-suppressed, T2-weighted fast SE image (4,600/133) shows a large left adnexal mass that contains multiple follicles (black arrows), identifying it as the left ovary. A prominent right ovary (white arrow) is also present. **(b)** Gadopentetate dimeglumine–enhanced axial fat-suppressed T1-weighted spoiled GRE image (150/2.9, 90° flip angle) shows enhancing follicles within both ovaries (arrows). No high signal intensity was present on the T1-weighted images before administration of contrast material (not shown) to suggest hemorrhagic infarction (see Fig 3).

HYDRATED TISSUE

Mucin

Mucin is a secretion that contains carbohydrate-rich glycoproteins. Hydrated mucinous tissue is of low viscosity and in general has low signal intensity on T1-weighted images and high signal intensity on T2-weighted images. In desiccated mucinous secretions, the decrease in free water can result in marked T2 shortening (68), which can be so pronounced that it also results in very low signal intensity on T1-weighted images (104). This latter phenomenon has not been encountered in the pelvis but has been documented in the paranasal sinuses (105).

Mucinous ovarian neoplasms.—Mucinous neoplasms of the ovary compose approximately one-third of epithelial ovarian tumors, and approximately 80% are benign (89). Benign tumors are commonly large, so size does not strongly correlate with the probability of malignancy in this type of tumor. At gross examination, mucinous neoplasms are multilocular and the cyst contents vary from a low-viscosity waterlike consistency to a thick viscous material from concentrated mucin. The latter cyst contents can result in variable T1 shortening within some locules. T2 shortening is usually slight (Figs 14, 15). Unilocular mucinous neoplasms may be indistinguishable from other adnexal cysts.

Pseudomyxoma peritonei.—Pseudomyxoma peritonei is a subtype of mucinous neoplasm that has typical imaging features, including appendiceal and ovarian masses with associated mucinous ascites and peritoneal implants. The appendix is the primary neoplasm in the majority of patients with ovarian metastases (106,107). Imaging the primary tumor of the appendix has not been emphasized in the imaging literature (108). The gelatinous mucin present in both the primary tumor and in the complex ascites results in intermediate to high signal intensity on T2-weighted images (109). Pseudomyxoma shows mass effect and a fine network of strands and septations that enhance with contrast material, features not usually seen in nonmucinous ascites.

Other mucin-producing adenocarcinomas.—Mucin-producing adenocarcinomas show high signal intensity on T2-weighted images from the extracellular mucin of the primary lesion (Fig 16). Nonmucinous adenocarcinomas have substantially lower signal intensity than that of mucinous tumors on T2-weighted images, although they still are of higher signal intensity than that of skeletal muscle (110). After administration of contrast material, mucinous malignancies show lacelike internal enhancement, which distinguishes them from cysts or abscesses. This is most conspicuous with fat-suppressed T1-weighted techniques.

Myxoid Tissue

Myxomatous tissue is composed of stellate cells in a background of abundant hyaluronic acid–rich mucopolysaccharides, resembles primitive mesenchymal tissue (111), and has a gelatinous texture at gross examination (112). Myxomatous tissue has a very high water content. Intramuscular myxomas and other neoplasms that have a large proportion of myxoid elements can mimic complex cysts on MR images because of the low signal intensity on T1-weighted images and high signal intensity on T2-weighted images of the myxomatous tissue (113–115). Myxomas show enhancement after administration of contrast material, which distinguishes them from cysts. Pure intramuscular myxomas are rare neoplasms that most often involve the extremities (116).

Angiomyxoma.—Angiomyxoma is an unusual neoplasm that characteristically arises within the mesenchymal tissues of the pelvis and perineum of young women. The tumor is benign but often recurs locally.

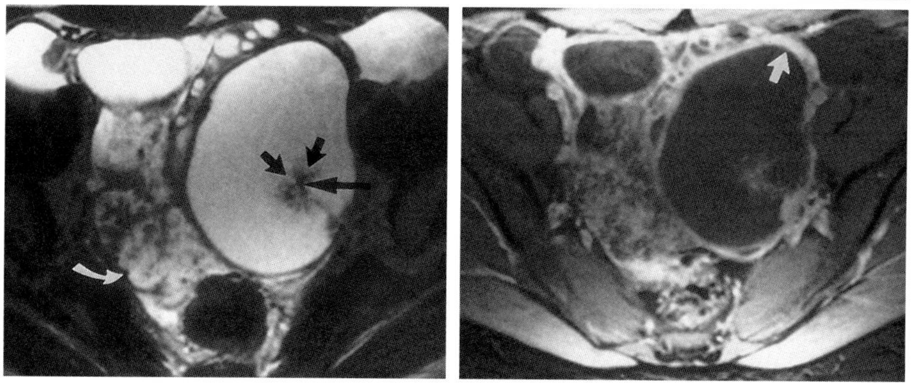

a. b.

Figure 19. MR imaging demonstration of papillary projections in a papillary serous borderline tumor in a 19-year-old woman. **(a)** Axial T2-weighted fast SE image (4,000/126) shows a complex multiloculated pelvic mass that contains multiple papillary projections. The projections in the left cyst are composed of a central fibrous core (long black arrow) surrounded by edematous stroma (short black arrows). The right-sided mass (curved white arrow) is a cyst filled entirely with papillary projections. **(b)** Corresponding axial gadopentetate dimeglumine–enhanced fat-saturated GRE image (250/2.9, 90° flip angle) shows enhancement of the cyst wall (arrow) and papillary projections. The fluid that makes up the remainder of the tumor does not enhance.

A suggestive MR imaging finding is that of an infiltrative soft-tissue mass of the female pelvis and/or perineum of very high signal intensity on T2-weighted images that tends to displace, but not invade, adjacent soft-tissue structures (49,117,118).

Myxoid degeneration of uterine leiomyomas.—Myxomatous change is one subtype of degeneration that occurs in uterine leiomyomas, especially in larger masses (112,119) (Fig 17). Myxoid change appears as a geographic patchwork of very high signal intensity within a leiomyoma. Characterization of the subtypes of degeneration within uterine leiomyomas is often not necessary for lesion characterization. However, knowledge of the degree and subtype of degeneration may influence the decision to treat a symptomatic women with medical therapy. Degenerated tumors do not respond to medical therapy, whereas nondegenerated leiomyomas shrink in size (86).

Edematous Tissue

Edema is an accumulation of an excessive amount of water in cells or tissues. Thus, edema within pelvic soft tissues results in lower signal intensity on T1-weighted images and higher signal intensity on T2-weighted images. Within the normal female pelvis, tissue with increased water content is present within the uterine endometrium and within ovarian medulla. Uterine endometrium in premenopausal woman both increases in thickness and increases in signal intensity on T2-weighted images from the early proliferative phase to the midsecretory stage of menstruation (120–122). The increase in signal intensity corresponds to the endometrial stromal edema that is derived from plasma transudate and glandular secretions (123). This cyclic effect on the endometrium is absent or blunted in postmenopausal women and in woman taking oral contraceptives.

The normal ovary has a zonal anatomy consisting of an outer ovarian cortex and central ovarian medulla that along with the follicles compose the internal contents of the ovary. In premenopausal patients, ovarian zonal anatomy is distinguishable on T2-weighted images (39,124). At histologic examination, ovarian stroma in the cortex is more cellular (125), while medullary stroma is composed of looser, vascularized connective tissue with a higher free water content, thus explaining the difference in contrast on T2-weighted images (39).

Massive edema of the ovary.—In a subset of intermittently or partially twisted, viable ovaries, a characteristic appearance of enlargement from ovarian edema without hemorrhage is termed "massive ovarian edema" (126–129). Similar to adnexal torsion, follicles are displaced peripherally, but unlike torsion, the ovarian stroma is edematous and of high signal intensity on T2-weighted images (Fig 18). In these women, laparoscopic oophoropexy can be performed instead of an oophorectomy, thus preserving fertility (130).

Papillary projections of ovarian neoplasms.—Papillary projections are specific features of epithelial ovarian neoplasms (Fig 19). Large papillary projections show two distinct tissue types at T2-weighted MR imaging–pathologic correlation. Edematous papillae have an area of high signal intensity that surrounds a low-signal-intensity fibrous stalk (37). Distinct low- and high-signal-intensity components are not discernible within smaller papillary projections. Papillary projections enhance after contrast material administration, thus facilitating differentiation from intracystic clot or debris.

SOLID MALIGNANT TISSUE

Malignant tissue has increased amounts of both intracellular and extracellular water, which results in increased T1 and T2 relaxation times of malignant tissue (66,131) (Figs 10, 13, 19). However, whether this results in a relatively higher signal intensity on T2-weighted images compared to the signal intensity of background tissue depends on the comparison tissue. For example, endometrial cancer usually has lower signal intensity compared with that of normal endometrium. On fast SE images, fat signal intensity is typically equal to or higher than the signal intensity of malignant tissue. The relative T2 signal intensity of soft tissue is also dependent on the degree of T2 weighting. For example, when performing heavily T2-weighted sequences (MR hydrography [13]), most soft tissues are of very low signal intensity with minimal or no difference in tissue contrast (Fig 1). Therefore, one cannot always rely on the relative T2 signal intensity of a mass to suggest malignancy. However, many organs in the female pelvis contain a layer with low signal intensity on T2-weighted images—for example, uterine junctional zone, cervical stroma (132), urethral muscularis (133), and bladder wall (Fig 13) (134,135)—so that malignancies show higher signal intensity than these structures. Masses that extend through these low-signal-intensity mural layers are suggestive of invasive disease.

In addition to evidence of invasion, the presence of serosal implants suggests a diagnosis of malignancy and excludes benign disease. Gadolinium-enhanced, breath-hold, fat-saturated T1-weighted gradient-echo imaging performed after the ingestion of a dilute barium suspension has been shown to accurately detect serosal disease from pelvic malignancies (double contrast MR imaging) (136,137). It is still unclear whether intraluminal barium improves sensitivity since similar detection rates of serosal disease have also been demonstrated with an identical sequence without an orally administered contrast material (138) (Fig 10). Peritoneal disease with a pelvic mass does not necessarily indicate spread of pelvic malignancy, however, and can be seen in endometriosis and borderline tumors.

When evaluating adnexal masses specifically, the presence of papillary projections adds high specificity for an epithelial ovarian neoplasm (Fig 19) (7,37). The presence and quantity of papillary projections can suggest the degree of tumor invasiveness. Papillary projections are usually absent in benign epithelial neoplasms and abundant within borderline tumors. Solid tumor is usually present in greater proportion than papillary projections within ovarian malignancies (139,140).

CONCLUSION

This article provides an approach to interpretation of MR images of the female pelvis through tissue characterization. Fluid, blood, lipid, smooth muscle, fibrous tissue, mucin, myxomatous tissue, and solid neoplastic tissue have typical signal intensity and enhancement patterns that can be recognized. Identification of these tissue types in a mass can narrow the differential diagnosis. It is our hope that the MR imaging information of tissue composition of various pathologic processes in the pelvis can result in more systematic approaches to diagnosis.

References

1. Yu KK, Hricak H. Can MRI of the pelvis be cost effective? Abdom Imaging 1997; 22:597–601.
2. Sugimura K, Imaoka I, Okizuka H. Pelvic endometriosis: impact of magnetic resonance imaging on treatment decisions and costs. Acad Radiol 1996; 3(suppl 1): S66–S68.
3. Hricak H, Powell CB, Yu KK, et al. Invasive cervical carcinoma: role of MR imaging in pretreatment work-up—cost minimization and diagnostic efficacy analysis. Radiology 1996; 198:403–409.
4. Schwartz LB, Panageas E, Lange R, Rizzo J, Comite F, McCarthy S. Female pelvis: impact of MR imaging on treatment decisions and net cost analysis. Radiology 1994; 192:55–60.
5. Yamashita Y, Hatanaka Y, Torashima M, Takahashi M, Miyazaki K, Okamura H. Characterization of sonographically indeterminate ovarian tumors with MR imaging: a logistic regression analysis. Acta Radiol 1997; 38:572–577.
6. Medl M, Kulenkampff KJ, Stiskal M, Peters-Engl C, Leodolter S, Czembirek H. Magnetic resonance imaging in the preoperative evaluation of suspected ovarian masses. Anticancer Res 1995; 15: 1123–1125.
7. Outwater EK, Dunton CJ. Imaging of the ovary and adnexa: clinical issues and applications of MR imaging. Radiology 1995; 194:1–18.
8. Outwater EK, Mitchell DG. Magnetic resonance imaging techniques in the pelvis. Magn Reson Imaging Clin N Am 1994; 2:481–488.
9. Lipson SA, Hricak H. MR imaging of the female pelvis. Radiol Clin North Am 1996; 34:1157–1182.
10. Brown HK, Hazelton TR, Fiorica JV, Parsons AK, Clarke LP, Silbiger ML. Composite and classified color display in MR imaging of the female pelvis. Magn Reson Imaging 1992; 10:143–154.
11. Brown HK, Hazelton TR, Parsons AK, Fiorica JV, Berman CG, Silbiger ML. PC-based multiparameter full-color display for tissue segmentation in MRI of adnexal masses. J Comput Assist Tomogr 1993; 17:993–1005.
12. Vinitski S, Gonzalez C, Mohamed F, et al. Improved intracranial lesion characterization by tissue segmentation based on a 3D feature map. Magn Reson Med 1997; 37:457–469.
13. Jara H, Barish MA, Yucel EK, Melhem ER, Hussain S, Ferrucci JT. MR hydrography: theory and practice of static fluid imaging. AJR 1998; 170:873–882.
14. Roy C, Saussine C, Guth S, et al. MR urography in the evaluation of urinary tract obstruction. Abdom Imaging 1998; 23:27–34.
15. Bradley WG Jr. MR appearance of hemorrhage in the brain. Radiology 1993; 189: 15–26.
16. Seelos KC, Funari M, Chang JM, Higgins CB. Magnetic resonance imaging in acute and subacute mediastinal bleeding. Am Heart J 1992; 123:1269–1272.
17. Bluemke DA. Definitive diagnosis of intramural hematoma of the thoracic aorta with MR imaging (editorial). Radiology 1997; 204:319–321.
18. Takahashi N, Murakami J, Murayama S, Sakai S, Masuda K, Ishida T. MR evaluation of intrapulmonary hematoma. J Comput Assist Tomogr 1995; 19:125–127.
19. Di Cesare E, Di Renzi P, Pavone P, et al. Evaluation of hematoma by MRI in follow-up of aorto-femoral bypass. Magn Reson Imaging 1991; 9:247–253.
20. Yamashita Y, Torashima M, Harada M, Yamamoto H, Takahashi M. Postpartum extraperitoneal pelvic hematoma: imaging findings. AJR 1993; 161:805–808.
21. Hahn PF, Saini S, Stark DD, Papanicolaou N, Ferrucci JT Jr. Intraabdominal hematoma: the concentric-ring sign in MR imaging. AJR 1987; 148:115–119.
22. Hahn PF, Stark DD, Vici LG, Ferrucci JT Jr. Duodenal hematoma: the ring sign in MR imaging. Radiology 1986; 159:379–382.
23. Siegelman ES, Outwater EK. The concentric-ring sign revisited (letter). AJR 1996; 166:1493.
24. Cirillo RL, Bennett WF, Vitellas KM, Poulos AG, Bova JG. Pathology of the adrenal gland: imaging features. AJR 1998; 170:429–435.
25. Yamashita Y, Hatanaka Y, Torashima M, Takahashi M. Magnetic resonance characteristics of intrapelvic haematomas. Br J Radiol 1995; 68:979–985.
26. Swensen SJ, McLeod RA, Stephens DH. CT of extracranial hemorrhage and hematomas. AJR 1984; 143:907–912.
27. Lenchik L, Dovgan DJ, Kier R. CT of the iliopsoas compartment: value in differentiating tumor, abscess, and hematoma. AJR 1994; 162:83–86.
28. Mitchell DG, Outwater EK. Benign gynecologic disease: applications of magnetic resonance imaging. Top Magn Reson Imaging 1995; 7:26–43.
29. Kobayashi K, Matsuo M, Matsuki M, Kuroida Y. The role of MR imaging in diagnostic aids for ectopic pregnancy (abstr). Radiology 1997; 205(P):378.
30. Kuhl CK, Heuck A, Kreft BP, Luckhaus S, Reiser M, Schild HH. Combined intrauterine and ovarian pregnancy mimicking ovarian malignant tumor: imaging findings. AJR 1995; 165:369–370.
31. Panicek DM, Casper ES, Brennan MF, Hajdu SI, Heelan RT. Hemorrhage simulating tumor growth in malignant fibrous histiocytoma at MR imaging. Radiology 1991; 181:398–400.
32. Bis KG, Vrachliotis TG, Agrawal R, Shetty AN, Maximovich A, Hricak H. Pelvic endometriosis: MR imaging spectrum with laparoscopic correlation and diagnostic pitfalls. RadioGraphics 1997; 17: 639–655.
33. Outwater E, Schiebler ML, Owen RS, Schnall MD. Characterization of hemorrhagic adnexal lesions with MR imaging: blinded reader study. Radiology 1993; 186:489–494.
34. Togashi K, Nishimura K, Kimura I, et al. Endometrial cysts: diagnosis with MR imaging. Radiology 1991; 180:73–78.
35. Sugimura K, Takemori M, Sugiura M, Okizuka H, Kono M, Ishida T. The value of magnetic resonance relaxation time in staging ovarian endometrial cysts. Br J Radiol 1992; 65:502–506.
36. Takahashi K, Okada S, Okada M, Kitao M, Kaji Y, Sugimura K. Magnetic resonance relaxation time in evaluating the cyst fluid characteristics of endometrioma. Hum Reprod 1996; 11:857–860.
37. Outwater EK, Huang AB, Dunton CJ, Talerman A, Capuzzi DM. Papillary projections in ovarian neoplasms: appearance on MRI. JMRI 1997; 7:689–695.
38. Occhipinti KA, Frankel SD, Hricak H. The ovary: computed tomography and magnetic resonance imaging. Radiol Clin North Am 1993; 31:1115–1132.
39. Outwater EK, Mitchell DG. Normal ovaries and functional cysts: MR appearance. Radiology 1996; 198:397–402.
40. Outwater EK, Siegelman ES, Chiowanick P, Dunton CJ, Talerman A. Dilated fallopian tubes: MR imaging characteristics. Radiology 1998; 208:463–469.
41. Ascher SM, Agrawal R, Bis KG, et al. Endometriosis: appearance and detection with conventional and contrast-enhanced fat-suppressed spin-echo techniques. JMRI 1995; 5:251–257.
42. Ha HK, Lim YT, Kim HS, Suh TS, Song HH, Kim SJ. Diagnosis of pelvic endometriosis: fat-suppressed T1-weighted vs conventional MR images. AJR 1994; 163: 127–131.
43. Kawakami K, Murata K, Kawaguchi N, et al. Hemorrhagic infarction of the diseased ovary: a common MR finding in two cases. Magn Reson Imaging 1993; 11:595–597.
44. Lee CH, Raman S, Sivanesaratnam V.

Torsion of ovarian tumors: a clinicopathological study. Int J Gynaecol Obstet 1989; 28:21–25.
45. Sommerville M, Grimes DA, Koonings PP, Campbell K. Ovarian neoplasms and the risk of adnexal torsion. Am J Obstet Gynecol 1991; 164:577–578.
46. Togashi K, Ozasa H, Konishi I, et al. Enlarged uterus: differentiation between adenomyosis and leiomyoma with MR imaging. Radiology 1989; 171:531–534.
47. Outwater EK, Siegelman ES, Van Deerlin V. Adenomyosis: current concepts and imaging considerations. AJR 1998; 170: 437–441.
48. Reinhold C, Hricak H, Forstner R, et al. Primary amenorrhea: evaluation with MR imaging. Radiology 1997; 203:383–390.
49. Siegelman ES, Outwater EK, Banner MP, Ramchandani P, Anderson TL, Schnall MD. High-resolution MR imaging of the vagina. RadioGraphics 1997; 17:1183–1203.
50. Pellerito JS, McCarthy SM, Doyle MB, Glickman MG, DeCherney AH. Diagnosis of uterine anomalies: relative accuracy of MR imaging, endovaginal sonography, and hysterosalpingography. Radiology 1992; 183:795–800.
51. Elster AD. Questions and answers in magnetic resonance imaging. Philadelphia, Pa: Mosby, 1994.
52. Constable RT, Anderson AW, Zhong J, Gore JC. Factors influencing contrast in fast spin-echo MR imaging. Magn Reson Imaging 1992; 10:497–511.
53. Listerud J, Einstein S, Outwater E, Kressel HY. First principles of fast spin echo. Magn Reson Q 1992; 8:199–244.
54. Henkelman RM, Hardy PA, Bishop JE, Poon CS, Plewes DB. Why fat is bright in RARE and fast spin-echo imaging. JMRI 1992; 2:533–540.
55. Talerman A. Germ cell tumors of the ovary. In: Kurman RJ, ed. Pathology of the female genital tract. New York, NY: Springer-Verlag, 1994; 849–914.
56. Yamashita Y, Torashima M, Hatanaka Y, et al. Value of phase-shift gradient-echo MR imaging in the differentiation of pelvic lesions with high signal intensity at T1-weighted imaging. Radiology 1994; 191:759–764.
57. Kier R, Mason BJ. Water-suppressed MR imaging of focal fatty infiltration of the liver. Radiology 1997; 203:575–576.
58. Imaoka I, Sugimura K, Okizuka H, Iwanari O, Kitao M, Ishida T. Ovarian cystic teratomas: value of chemical fat saturation magnetic resonance imaging. Br J Radiol 1993; 66:994–997.
59. Mitchell DG. Chemical shift magnetic resonance imaging: applications in the abdomen and pelvis. Top Magn Reson Imaging 1992; 4:46–63.
60. Kier R, Smith RC, McCarthy SM. Value of lipid- and water-suppression MR images in distinguishing between blood and lipid within ovarian masses. AJR 1992; 158:321–325.
61. Stevens SK, Hricak H, Campos Z. Teratomas versus cystic hemorrhagic adnexal lesions: differentiation with proton-selective fat-saturation MR imaging. Radiology 1993; 186:481–488.
62. Krinsky G, Rofsky NM, Weinreb JC. Nonspecificity of short inversion time inversion recovery (STIR) as a technique of fat suppression: pitfalls in image interpretation. AJR 1996; 166:523–526.
63. Yamashita Y, Hatanaka Y, Torashima M, Takahashi M, Miyazaki K, Okamura H. Mature cystic teratomas of the ovary without fat in the cystic cavity: MR features in 12 cases. AJR 1994; 163:613–616.
64. Earls JP, Krinsky GA. Abdominal and pelvic applications of opposed-phase MR imaging. AJR 1997; 169:1071–1077.
65. Belley G, Reinhold C, Gallix BP, Wang L, Atri M, Bret PM. Comparison of in- and opposed-phase gradient-echo seqeunces versus T1-weighted spin echo seqeunce without and with fat saturation in diagnosing ovarian dermoids (abstr). Radiology 1997; 205(P):378.
66. Mitchell DG, Burk DL Jr, Vinitski S, Rifkin MD. The biophysical basis of tissue contrast in extracranial MR imaging. AJR 1987; 149:831–837.
67. Cameron IL, Ord VA, Fullerton GD. Characterization of proton NMR relaxation times in normal and pathological tissues by correlation with other tissue parameters. Magn Reson Imaging 1984; 2:97–106.
68. Fullerton GD, Potter JL, Dornbluth NC. NMR relaxation of protons in tissues and other macromolecular water solutions. Magn Reson Imaging 1982; 1:209–226.
69. Wehrli FW, MacFall JR, Shutts D, Breger R, Herfkens RJ. Mechanisms of contrast in NMR imaging. J Comput Assist Tomogr 1984; 8:369–380.
70. Misra LK, Kim EE, Hazlewood CF, Todd LE, Elizondo-Riojas G. Characterization of skeletal muscles by MR imaging and relaxation times. Physiol Chem Phys Med NMR 1990; 22:219–228.
71. Scholz TD, Fleagle SR, Burns TL, Skorton DJ. Tissue determinants of nuclear magnetic resonance relaxation times: effect of water and collagen content in muscle and tendon. Invest Radiol 1989; 24:893–898.
72. Polak JF, Jolesz FA, Adams DF. NMR of skeletal muscle. Differences in relaxation parameters related to extracellular/intracellular fluid spaces. Invest Radiol 1988; 23:107–112.
73. Brosens JJ, de Souza NM, Barker FG. Uterine junctional zone: function and disease. Lancet 1995; 346:558–560.
74. Brown HK, Stoll BS, Nicosia SV, et al. Uterine junctional zone: correlation between histologic findings and MR imaging. Radiology 1991; 179:409–413.
75. McCarthy S, Scott G, Majumdar S, et al. Uterine junctional zone: MR study of water content and relaxation properties. Radiology 1989; 171:241–243.
76. Kang S, Turner DA, Foster GS, Rapoport MI, Spencer SA, Wang JZ. Adenomyosis: specificity of 5 mm as the maximum normal uterine junctional zone thickness in MR images. AJR 1996; 166:1145–1150.
77. Togashi K, Kawakami S, Kimura I, et al. Sustained uterine contractions: a cause of hypointense myometrial bulging. Radiology 1993; 187:707–710.
78. Lyons EA, Taylor PJ, Zheng XH, Ballard G, Levi CS, Kredentser JV. Characterization of subendometrial myometrial contractions throughout the menstrual cycle in normal fertile women. Fertil Steril 1991; 55:771–774.
79. Levine D, Barnes PD, Sher S, et al. Fetal fast MR imaging: reproducibility, technical quality and conspicuity of anatomy. Radiology 1998; 206:549–554.
80. Yamashita Y, Namimoto T, Abe Y, et al. MR imaging of the fetus by a HASTE sequence. AJR 1997; 168:513–519.
81. Reinhold C, McCarthy S, Bret PM, et al. Diffuse adenomyosis: comparison of endovaginal US and MR imaging with histopathologic correlation. Radiology 1996; 1996:151–158.
82. Hricak H, Tscholakoff D, Heinrichs L, et al. Uterine leiomyomas: correlation of MR, histopathologic findings, and symptoms. Radiology 1986; 158:385–391.
83. Mulkern RV, Wong ST, Winalski C, Jolesz FA. Contrast manipulation and artifact assessment of 2D and 3D RARE sequences. Magn Reson Imaging 1990; 8:557–566.
84. Constable RT, Gore JC. The loss of small objects in variable TE imaging: implications for FSE, RARE, and EPI. Magn Reson Med 1992; 28:9–24.
85. Gryspeerdt S, Van Hoe L, Bosmans H, Baert AL, Vergote I, Marchal G. T2-weighted MR imaging of the uterus: comparison of optimized fast spin-echo and HASTE sequences with conventional fast spin-echo sequences. AJR 1998; 171:211–215.
86. Yamashita Y, Torashima M, Takahashi M, et al. Hyperintense uterine leiomyoma at T2-weighted MR imaging: differentiation with dynamic enhanced MR imaging and clinical implications. Radiology 1993; 189:721–725.
87. Okizuka H, Sugimura K, Takemori M, Obayashi C, Kitao M, Ishida T. MR detection of degenerating uterine leiomyomas. J Comput Assist Tomogr 1993; 17: 760–766.
88. Zaloudek C, Norris HJ. Mesenchymal tumors of the uterus. In: Kurman RJ, ed. Blaustein's pathology of the female genital tract. 4th ed. New York, NY: Springer-Verlag, 1994; 487–528.
89. Ferenczy A, Wright TC. Anatomy and histology of the cervix. In: Kurman RJ, ed. Blausteins's pathology of the female genital tract. 4th ed. New York, NY: Springer-Verlag, 1994; 185–201.
90. Scoutt LM, McCauley TR, Flynn SD, Luthringer DJ, McCarthy SM. Zonal anatomy of the cervix: correlation of MR imaging and histologic examination of hysterectomy specimens. Radiology 1993; 186:159–162.
91. Danforth DN. The distribution and functional activity of the cervical musculature. Am J Obstet Gynecol 1954; 68: 1261–1271.
92. Siegelman ES, Outwater E, Wang T, Mitchell DG. Solid pelvic masses caused by endometriosis: MR imaging features. AJR 1994; 163:357–361.
93. Yu CY, Perez-Reyes M, Brown JJ, Borrello JA. MR appearance of umbilical endometriosis. J Comput Assist Tomogr 1994; 18:269–271.
94. Troiano RN, Lazzarini KM, Scoutt LM, Lange RC, Flynn SD, McCarthy S. Fibroma and fibrothecoma of the ovary: MR imaging findings. Radiology 1997; 204:795–798.
95. Outwater EK, Siegelman ES, Talerman A, Dunton C. Ovarian fibromas and cystadenofibromas: MRI features of the fibrous component. JMRI 1997; 7:465–471.
96. Russel P. Surface epithelial-stromal tu-

mors of the ovary. In: Kurman RJ, ed. Blaustein's pathology of the female genital tract. 4th ed. New York, NY: Springer-Verlag, 1994; 705–782.
97. Outwater EK, Siegelman ES, Kim B, Chiowanick P, Kilger A, Dunton CJ. Ovarian Brenner tumors: MR imaging characteristics. Magn Reson Imaging 1999; 16:1147–1153.
98. Ito K, Kato T, Tadokoro M, et al. Recurrent rectal cancer and scar: differentiation with PET and MR imaging. Radiology 1992; 182:549–552.
99. Krestin GP, Steinbrich W, Friedmann G. Recurrent rectal cancer: diagnosis with MR imaging versus CT. Radiology 1988; 168:307–311.
100. Ebner F, Kressel HY, Mintz MC, et al. Tumor recurrence versus fibrosis in the female pelvis: differentiation with MR imaging at 1.5 T. Radiology 1988; 166: 333–340.
101. DeLange EE, Fechner RE, Wanebo HJ. Suspected recurrent rectosigmoid carcinoma after abdominoperineal resection: MR imaging and histopathologic findings. Radiology 1989; 170:323–328.
102. Markus J, Morrissey B, deGara C, Tarulli G. MRI of recurrent rectosigmoid carcinoma. Abdom Imaging 1997; 22:338–342.
103. Blomqvist L, Frannson P, Hindmars T. The pelvis after surgery and radio-chemotherapy for rectal cancer studied with Gd-DTPA-enhanced fast dynamic MR imaging. Eur Radiol 1998; 8:781–787.
104. Som PM, Dillon WP, Fullerton GD, Zimmerman RA, Rajagopalan B, Marom Z. Chronically obstructed sinonasal secretions: observations on T1 and T2 shortening. Radiology 1989; 172:515–520.
105. Dillon WP, Som PM, Fullerton GD. Hypointense MR signal in chronically inspissated sinonasal secretions. Radiology 1990; 174:73–78.
106. Ronnett BM, Kurman RJ, Zahn CM, et al. Pseudomyxoma peritonei in women: a clinicopathologic analysis of 30 cases with emphasis on site of origin, prognosis, and relationship to ovarian mucinous tumors of low malignant potential. Hum Pathol 1995; 26:509–524.
107. Ronnett BM, Shmookler BM, Diener-West M, Sugarbaker PH, Kurman RJ. Immunohistochemical evidence supporting the appendiceal origin of pseudomyxoma peritonei in women. Int J Gynecol Pathol 1997; 16:1–9.
108. Walensky RP, Venbrux AC, Prescott CA, Osterman FA Jr. Pseudomyxoma peritonei. AJR 1996; 167:471–474.
109. Buy JN, Malbec L, Ghossain MA, Guinet C, Ecoiffier J. Magnetic resonance imaging of pseudomyxoma peritonei. Eur J Radiol 1989; 9:115–118.
110. Hussain SM, Outwater EK, Siegelman ES. Mucinous versus nonmucinous rectal carcinomas: differentiation with MR imaging. 1999; Radiology (in press).
111. Stout AP. Myxoma: the tumor of primitive mesenchyma. Ann Surg 1948; 127: 706–719.
112. Prayson RA, Hart WR. Pathologic considerations of uterine smooth muscle tumors. Obstet Gynecol Clin North Am 1995; 22:637–657.
113. Ma LD, McCarthy EF, Bluemke DA, Frassica FJ. Differentiation of benign from malignant musculoskeletal lesions using MR imaging: pitfalls in MR evaluation of lesions with a cystic appearance. AJR 1998; 170:1251–1258.
114. Abdelwahab AF, Kenan S, Hermann G, Lewis MM, Klein MJ. Intramuscular myxoma: magnetic resonance features. Br J Radiol 1992; 65:485–490.
115. Peterson KK, Renfrew DL, Feddersen RM, Buckwalter JA, el-Khoury GY. Magnetic resonance imaging of myxoid containing tumors. Skeletal Radiol 1991; 20:245–250.
116. Benign soft tissue tumors of uncertain type. In: Enzinger RM, Weiss SW, eds. Soft tissue tumors. 3rd ed. Philadelphia, Pa: Mosby, 1995; 1039–1066.
117. Davani M, Chablani VN, Saba PR. Aggressive angiomyxoma of pelvic soft tissues: MR imaging appearance. AJR 1998; 170: 1113–1114.
118. Outwater EK, Marchetto BE, Wagner BJ, Siegelman ES. Aggressive angiomyxoma: findings on CT and MRI. AJR 1999; 172:435–438.
119. Clement PB, Young RH, Scully RE. Diffuse, perinodular, and other patterns of hydropic degeneration within and adjacent to uterine leiomyomas: problems in differential diagnosis. Am J Surg Pathol 1992; 16:26–32.
120. Haynor DR, Mack LA, Soules MR, Shuman WP, Montana MA, Moss AA. Changing appearance of the normal uterus during the menstrual cycle: MR studies. Radiology 1986; 161:459–462.
121. McCarthy S, Tauber C, Gore J. Female pelvic anatomy: MR assessment of variations during the menstrual cycle and with use of oral contraceptives. Radiology 1986; 160:119–123.
122. Lee JK, Gersell DJ, Balfe DM, Worthington JL, Picus D, Gapp G. The uterus: in vitro MR-anatomic correlation of normal and abnormal specimens. Radiology 1985; 157:175–179.
123. Ferenczy A. Anatomy and histology of the uterine corpus. In: Kurman RJ, ed. Blausteins's pathology of the female geneital tract. 4th ed. New York, NY: Springer-Verlag, 1994; 327–366.
124. Outwater EK, Schiebler ML. Magnetic resonance imaging of the ovary. Magn Reson Imaging Clin N Am 1994; 2:245–274.
125. Clement PB. Anatomy and histology of the ovary. In: Kurman RJ, ed. Blausteins's pathology of the female genital tract. 4th ed. New York, NY: Springer-Verlag, 1994; 563–595.
126. Nogales FF, Martin-Sances L, Mendoza-Garcia E, Salamanca A, Gonzalez-Nunez MA, Pardo Mindan FJ. Massive ovarian oedema. Histopathology 1996; 28:229–234.
127. Lee AR, Kim KH, Lee BH, Chin SY. Massive edema of the ovary: imaging findings. AJR 1993; 161:343–344.
128. Hall BP, Printz DA, Roth J. Massive ovarian edema: ultrasound and MR characteristics. J Comput Assist Tomogr 1993; 17:477–479.
129. Kramer LA, Lalani T, Kawashima A. Massive edema of the ovary: high resolution MR findings using a phased-array pelvic coil. JMRI 1997; 7:758–760.
130. Nagel TC, Sebastian J, Malo JW. Oophoropexy to prevent sequential or recurrent torsion. J Am Assoc Gynecol Laparosc 1997; 4:495–498.
131. Martin AJ, Poon CS, Thomas GM, Kapusta LR, Shaw PA, Henkelman RM. MR evaluation of cervical cancer in hysterectomy specimens: correlation of quantitative T2 measurement and histology. JMRI 1994; 4:779–786.
132. Hricak H, Lacey CG, Sandles LG, Chang YC, Winkler ML, Stern JL. Invasive cervical carcinoma: comparison of MR imaging and surgical findings. Radiology 1988; 166:623–631.
133. Siegelman ES, Banner MP, Ramchandani P, Schnall MD. Multicoil MR imaging of symptomatic female urethral and periurethral disease. RadioGraphics 1997; 17:349–365.
134. Siegelman ES, Schnall MD. Contrast-enhanced MR imaging of the bladder and prostate. Magn Reson Imaging Clin N Am 1996; 4:153–169.
135. Barentsz JO, Ruijs SH, Strijk SP. The role of MR imaging in carcinoma of the urinary bladder. AJR 1993; 160:937–947.
136. Low RN, Barone RM, Lacey C, Sigeti JS, Alzate GD, Sebrechts CP. Peritoneal tumor: MR imaging with dilute oral barium and intravenous gadolinium-containing contrast agents compared with unenhanced MR imaging and CT. Radiology 1997; 204:513–520.
137. Low RN, Francis IR. MR imaging of the gastrointestinal tract with i.v., gadolinium and diluted barium oral contrast media compared with unenhanced MR imaging and CT. AJR 1997; 169:1051–1059.
138. Low RN, Sigeti JS. MR imaging of peritoneal disease: comparison of contrast-enhanced fast multiplanar spoiled gradient-recalled and spin-echo imaging. AJR 1994; 163:1131–1140.
139. Krigman H, Bentley R, Robboy SJ. Pathology of epithelial ovarian tumors. Clin Obstet Gynecol 1994; 37:475–491.
140. Wagner BJ, Buck JL, Seidman JD, McCabe KM. Ovarian epithelial neoplasms: radiologic-pathologic correlation. RadioGraphics 1994; 14:1351–1374; quiz 1375–1356.

Diagnosis and Staging of Ovarian Cancer: Comparative Values of Doppler and Conventional US, CT, and MR Imaging Correlated with Surgery and Histopathologic Analysis—Report of the Radiology Diagnostic Oncology Group[1]

Alfred B. Kurtz, MD
John V. Tsimikas, PhD[2]
Clare M. C. Tempany, MD
Ulrike M. Hamper, MD
Peter H. Arger, MD
Robert L. Bree, MD
Richard J. Wechsler, MD
Isaac R. Francis, MD
Janet E. Kuhlman, MD[3]
Evan S. Siegelman, MD
Donald G. Mitchell, MD
Stuart G. Silverman, MD
Douglas L. Brown, MD
Sheila Sheth, MD
Beverly G. Coleman, MD
James H. Ellis, MD
Robert J. Kurman, MD
Daryl J. Caudry, MS[2]
Barbara J. McNeil, MD, PhD[2]

Index terms:
Computed tomography (CT), comparative studies, 852.1211, 852.12112, 852.12115
Magnetic resonance (MR), comparative studies, 852.1214, 852.121415, 852.12143
Ovary, neoplasms, 852.32
Receiver operating characteristic curve (ROC)
Ultrasound (US), comparative studies, 852.1298
Ultrasound (US), Doppler studies, 852.12984

Radiology 1999; 212:19–27

[1] From the Dept of Radiology, Jefferson Medical College and Thomas Jefferson University Hospital, Gibbon Bldg 3350AB, 111 S 11th St, Philadelphia, PA 19107 (A.B.K., R.J.W., D.G.M.); the Dept of Health Care Policy, Harvard Medical School, Boston, Mass (J.V.T., D.J.C., B.J.M.); the Dept of Radiology, Brigham and Women's Hospital and Harvard Medical School, Boston (C.M.C.T., S.G.S., D.L.B.); the Depts of Radiology (U.M.H., S.S., J.E.K.) and Pathology (R.J.K.), Johns Hopkins Hospital, Baltimore, Md; the Dept of Radiology, Hospital of the University of Pennsylvania, Philadelphia (P.H.A., E.S.S., B.G.C.); and the Dept of Radiology, University of Michigan Medical Center, Ann Arbor (R.L.B., I.R.F., J.H.E.). Received Jun 26, 1998; revision requested Aug 6; revision received Oct 15; accepted Dec 16. Supported in part by Public Health Service grant U01 CA59401 from the National Cancer Institute. **Address reprint requests to** A.B.K. (e-mail: *alfred.b.kurtz@mail.tju.edu*).

[2] Current address: Dept of Mathematics and Statistics, University of Massachusetts at Amherst.

[3] Current address: Dept of Radiology, University of Wisconsin Medical School, Madison.

Author contributions:
Guarantor of integrity of entire study, A.B.K.; study concepts, A.B.K.; study design, A.B.K., J.V.T., B.J.M., C.M.C.T., U.M.H., R.L.B., P.H.A., D.J.C.; definition of intellectual content, A.B.K., C.M.C.T.; literature research, J.V.T., R.J.W., A.B.K., C.M.C.T., I.R.F.; clinical studies, A.B.K., C.M.C.T., U.M.H., P.H.A., R.L.B., R.J.W., I.R.F., J.E.K., E.S.S., D.G.M., S.G.S., D.L.B., S.S., B.G.C., J.H.E., R.J.K.; data acquisition and analysis, J.V.T., B.J.M., D.J.C.; statistical analysis, J.V.T., B.J.M., D.J.C.; manuscript preparation, all authors; manuscript editing, A.B.K., B.J.M., J.V.T., C.M.C.T.; manuscript review, A.B.K., C.M.C.T.

PURPOSE: To determine the optimal imaging modality for diagnosis and staging of ovarian cancer.

MATERIALS AND METHODS: Two hundred eighty women suspected to have ovarian cancer were enrolled in a prospective study before surgery. Doppler ultrasonography (US), computed tomography (CT), and magnetic resonance (MR) imaging were used to evaluate the mass; conventional US, CT, and MR imaging were used to stage spread.

RESULTS: All three modalities had high accuracy (0.91) for the overall diagnosis of malignancy. In the ovaries, the accuracy of MR imaging (0.91) was higher than that of CT and significantly higher than that of Doppler US (0.78). In the extraovarian pelvis and in the abdomen, conventional US, CT, and MR imaging had similar accuracies (0.87–0.95). In differentiation of disease confined to the pelvis from abdominal spread, the specificity of conventional US (96%) was higher than that of CT and significantly higher than that of MR imaging (88%), whereas the sensitivities of MR imaging (98%) and CT (92%) were significantly higher than that of conventional US (75%).

CONCLUSION: MR imaging is superior to Doppler US and CT in diagnosis of malignant ovarian masses. There is little variation among conventional US, CT, and MR imaging as regards staging.

Ovarian cancer is the second most common gynecologic malignancy in the United States with 25,400 new cases detected yearly (1,2), 70% in advanced stages. The prognosis is considerably changed by the extent of spread: The 5-year survival rate is 85% if the cancer is confined to the ovaries (stage I), 55% if the cancer has spread into the pelvis (stage II), 14% for stage III abdominal spread, and 4% for stage IV more distant spread. There are two major diagnostic challenges when an ovarian mass is detected: the determination of malignancy and the evaluation of tumor extent (staging). Diagnostic studies that allow accurate confirmation of benignity might reduce unnecessary surgery. Diagnostic studies that allow accurate cancer staging should help determine surgical and chemotherapeutic planning.

Bimanual pelvic examination and serum CA-125 levels have failed to allow consistent detection of ovarian malignancy. Because the sensitivities of these techniques are often below 50% (2–4), imaging modalities, particularly ultrasonography (US), computed tomography (CT), and magnetic resonance (MR) imaging, have become indispensable. US performed with transabdominal and endovaginal techniques has demonstrated accuracies of up to 80% in evaluation of ovarian masses; US is better in detection of masses than in diagnosis of malignancy (5–9). Abdominal spread has not been evaluated with US, to our knowledge. Spectral analysis of Doppler waveforms (Doppler US), which is often directed by color Doppler US, allows detection of tumor flow. Doppler US has not demonstrated consistency in diagnosis of malignancy (10–15). Studies of contrast material–enhanced CT and MR imaging have shown accuracies of almost 80% in diagnosis of cancer and 80%–90% in detection of abdominal spread (16–22).

In general, comparison studies of US and MR imaging have shown MR imaging to be better in differentiation of benign from malignant masses on the basis of accurate identification of fat and hemorrhage in benign tumors (23–27). In one study, US and CT performed equally well in detection of masses; CT was superior in diagnosis of malignancy (28).

To our knowledge, only one study has compared all three of these modalities in diagnosis of ovarian cancer and its spread (29). This study evaluated conventional US, nonenhanced CT, and low-field-strength MR imaging. In 75 patients with 29 cancers, these modalities demonstrated accuracies of only 60% or lower. Because of advances in technology, a larger study that evaluated state-of-the-art techniques was thought to be needed.

The Radiology Diagnostic Oncology Group performed a 3-year, five-institution, prospective study of nearly 300 patients with ovarian masses. We evaluated the results of Doppler and conventional US, CT, and MR imaging and compared their performances in diagnosis of a malignant ovarian mass and staging of its spread.

MATERIALS AND METHODS

Patient Population

From May 1, 1993, to April 30, 1996, all eligible patients were referred by participating gynecologic oncologists. The participating institutions were Brigham and Women's Hospital, University of Michigan Hospitals, Hospital of the University of Pennsylvania, Johns Hopkins Hospital, and Thomas Jefferson University Hospital.

Women over 18 years of age were admitted to the study if they were suspected to have ovarian cancer on the basis of abnormal results of a pelvic physical examination and/or a preliminary pelvic US study. Abnormal results of a physical examination were defined as detection of an enlarged ovary or an adnexal mass, sometimes with satellite pelvic nodularity. Abnormal US results were defined as detection of a complex (noncystic) and/or solid ovarian or adnexal mass, which was 5 cm or larger along its longest axis in a premenopausal woman and of any size in a postmenopausal woman. Complex and solid characteristics included heterogeneous and/or hyperechoic internal echoes, a wall thickness of 3 mm or greater, wall nodularity, solid components, and internal septa at least 2 mm thick.

When the results of physical examination and pelvic US were equivocal or negative, an additional inclusion criterion could be detection of complex ascites (internal echoes, septa) at US. The serum CA-125 level was not an inclusion criterion but was recorded when available.

Each patient had to be enrolled in at least two and ideally all three of the imaging modalities within 4 weeks before pelvic-abdominal surgery. The protocol and consent forms were approved by the institutional review board at each hospital. For evaluation of the ovarian or adnexal abnormality, the performances of Doppler US, CT, and MR imaging in diagnosis of malignancy were compared. Conventional US could not be included in this analysis because abnormal results at conventional US were an admission criterion. For evaluation of spread into the extraovarian pelvis and the abdomen, the performances of conventional US, CT, and MR imaging were compared.

Women were excluded from the study if they could not provide informed medical consent or if they were not a candidate for or did not need complete pelvic-abdominal surgical exploration. Other exclusion criteria were pregnancy and prior pelvic-abdominal laparoscopy or surgery within 6 months of entry into the study.

Of the 310 patients considered for the study, 30 were excluded because they had medical contraindications (n = 19), did not need extensive surgery (n = 6), refused surgery (n = 4), or had no disease (n = 1). The remaining 280 patients made up the study group. They ranged in age from 19 to 82 years with a mean age of 52.0 years and a median age of 51.5 years.

Conventional and Doppler US Protocol

State-of-the-art commercially available US equipment was used. The systems used were the UltraMark 9 HDI and HDI 3000 platforms (Advanced Technology Laboratories, Bothell, Wash) and the model 128XP and 128 XP/10 platforms (Acuson, Mountain View, Calif). All machines had transabdominal and endovaginal probes with maximal frequencies of 2–5 MHz and 5–7 MHz, respectively. All machines had both color and pulsed Doppler capability. Whenever possible, Doppler US of the ovarian or adnexal abnormality was performed endovaginally; transabdominal Doppler US of the abnormality was reserved for studies with nondiagnostic results. Premenopausal women were scheduled for US within 8 days of the start of their menstrual cycles (30). The extraovarian pelvis was evaluated with combined endovaginal and transabdominal US, whereas the abdomen was analyzed transabdominally.

CT Protocol

The CT scanners used were the Somatom Plus and Plus-S units (Siemens Medical Systems, Iselin, NJ) and the 9800 Advantage and Hi Speed Advantage units (GE Medical Systems, Milwaukee, Wis). The scanners were used in a dynamic or spiral mode with 2-second scanning times and suspended respiration. After opacification of the gastrointestinal tract, the pelvis was examined during peak arterial enhancement after the start of an injection of 150 mL of 60% contrast material (ionic or nonionic). The pelvis was scanned with 5-mm collimation; spiral CT was performed with a 5 mm/sec table speed and 5-mm reconstruction thickness, and incremental CT was performed with contiguous scans obtained at 10 scans per minute. In the abdomen, spiral CT and incremental CT were performed with 5-mm collimation at 8–10-mm intervals.

MR Imaging Protocol

All sites used 1.5-T units (Signa; GE Medical Systems). MR imaging was performed with a multicoil array or a built-in body coil. Whenever possible, the multicoil array was used for pelvic imaging with the body coil reserved for abdominal imaging. However, the body coil alone was used for imaging the pelvis and abdomen in the following situations: a mass larger than 15 cm in diameter or a patient with severe obesity or ascites. All patients were requested to fast for at least 3 hours before MR imaging and received 1 mg of intramuscularly administered glucagon (unless contraindicated) before MR imaging.

The pelvis was imaged with an axial fast spin-echo T2-weighted sequence (5,000–6,000/102–126 [repetition time msec/echo time msec]) with an echo train length of 16, a 5–10-mm section thickness, and a 0–2.5-mm intersection gap. The matrix size was 256 × 256 with two signals acquired. This sequence was repeated in the coronal and sagittal planes as indicated. An axial T1-weighted spin-echo sequence (600–800/11–20) with spatial resolution similar to that of the T2-weighted sequence was then performed. The T1-weighted sequence was repeated with fat suppression after intravenous injection of 10–20 mL of gadolinium chelate.

The remainder of the abdomen and pelvis was imaged with an axial T2-weighted fast spin-echo sequence and an axial fat-suppressed T1-weighted spin-echo sequence. The T2-weighted sequence (4,000/102–126) had an echo train length of 16, an 8–10-mm section thickness, and a 1.0–2.5-mm gap. The matrix was 256 × 192 or 256 with two to four signals acquired. This sequence was repeated in the coronal and sagittal planes as indicated. The T1-weighted sequence (400–600/11–20) had an 8–10-mm section thickness with a 2-mm gap. The matrix was 256 × 128–192 with two signals acquired.

Quality Control

Uniform standards were provided for all institutions and all imagers at the onset of the study and at routine intervals throughout the study. These standards covered hard-copy and recorded assessment; test objects, distance, resolution, and penetration for US; test patterns and low-contrast detection for CT; and phantoms and surface coil assessment for MR imaging.

Interpretation of Studies

Three radiologists (one for each modality) from each institution read the protocol imaging studies. They read studies only from their own institution. The readers had access to all clinical information, available laboratory test results, and admitting imaging studies; they had no knowledge of the results of the other protocol imaging studies or of surgery and histopathologic analysis.

In the analysis of the ovary and adnexa, Doppler US was used to evaluate the arterial flow of the detected complex and solid components of one or two masses. Up to three spectral arterial waveform samples were taken from thick walls, thick septa, and solid components (when present). If possible, three waveform samples were also obtained from both ovaries (normal or abnormal). For each waveform, a pulsatility index and resistive index were calculated; thresholds for malignancy were a pulsatility index of less than 1.0 and a resistive index of less than 0.4 (10,11). To increase the likelihood of diagnosing malignancy, only the lowest values of these indexes were used. Each waveform was also analyzed for the presence of a diastolic notch, a finding thought by some to be diagnostic of benign lesions. Analysis of the ovaries and adnexa with CT and MR imaging involved measurement and characterization of one or two complex and/or solid masses for all components ranging from cystic to solid, including identification of necrosis and fat. Both ovaries (normal or abnormal) were also analyzed.

Malignant spread into the remainder of the pelvis and into the abdomen was defined as complex and/or solid masses and/or complex fluid on US, CT, and MR images. In the pelvis, all organs and regions were evaluated including the fallopian tubes, uterus, parametrium, cul-de-sac, pelvic side walls, vagina, and lymph nodes. In the abdomen, all organs; the bowel; the mesenteric, omental, and peritoneal regions; and the lymph nodes were evaluated. Complex ascites in both the pelvis and abdomen and pleural effusions were noted. A total of 59 sites were evaluated including five peritoneal, three mesenteric, nine intestinal, and eight nodal regions.

The presence or absence of every finding was evaluated with the following five-point scale: 0 = normal, 1 = probably normal, 2 = indeterminate, 3 = probably abnormal, and 4 = abnormal. Each radiologist then determined a final stage based on the modified International Federation of Gynecology and Obstetrics staging classification (31) (Table 1).

Surgical and Histopathologic Correlation

Findings from protocol imaging studies were used to plan each patient's surgical procedure. Patients underwent complete resection of the primary tumor and a debulking or staging procedure when indicated. Adequate exploration of all structures was attempted with resection of the known gross tumor and associated lymph nodes, when possible by means of en bloc excision. If tissues could not be resected, multiple biopsies were performed. Ascites was submitted for cytologic examination.

Pathologists from each institution performed the interpretation in a routine manner using the revised World Health Organization histologic classification for ovarian neoplasms (32,33). For the primary ovarian tumor, a minimum of one block per centimeter of the greatest tissue diameter was examined along with additional specimens if the tumor extended to the surface. If there was ambiguity about the histologic type, another pathologist made the final decision.

The standard of reference was a combination of surgical and histopathologic results, which were classified according to the modified International Federation of Gynecology and Obstetrics staging classification (Table 1). Although there are different types of ovarian malignancies, all are similarly staged. Patients who had nonovarian cancer with spread to the ovaries were evaluated as if they had primary ovarian cancer. For example, a primary malignancy of the appendix with spread to the ovaries was classified as stage III disease because ovarian cancer with appendiceal spread would have been classified as stage III ovarian cancer.

Quality Review Committee

The quality review committee consisted of four radiologists (A.B.K., P.H.A., D.G.M., E.S.S.) from two institutions; two of the radiologists had expertise in US and CT, and two had expertise in MR imaging. They assessed the studies for quality and adherence to study protocols (without reinterpreting the studies) in their areas of expertise no later than 3 months after the start of patient accrual and at regular intervals thereafter.

Statistical Methods

The abilities of the three modalities to allow discrimination between benign cases and those with cancer in any anatomic region of the pelvis and abdomen were assessed. As previously stated, Doppler US, CT, and MR imaging were used to evaluate the ovaries and adnexa for malignancy; conventional US, CT, and MR imaging were used to evaluate the extraovarian pelvis and abdomen for spread.

For each institution, the accuracies of the modalities were measured by estimating the area under the receiver operating characteristic (ROC) curve, and homogeneity among the five institution-specific areas under the ROC curve was tested with the χ^2 method. Modality-specific areas under the ROC curve were estimated by pooling the institution-specific area estimates by means of weighted averages. Pairwise comparisons between modalities were performed for each institution by testing the difference between areas under the ROC curve obtained for each modality pair. Thus, whereas overall estimated areas were determined for each modality across institutions, comparisons between modalities were made by comparing results in the subset of patients who underwent both modalities. Modality-specific differences were addressed by pooling these differences across institutions. Estimation and comparison of the areas under the ROC curve were based on the nonparametric approach of DeLong et al (34).

The accuracy of each modality in detection of malignancy was estimated separately for the three anatomic regions (ovaries and adnexa, extraovarian pelvis, abdomen and beyond) by computing the relevant areas under the ROC curve. For detection of malignancy in the ovaries and adnexa, the accuracies of Doppler US, CT, and MR imaging were compared. For detection of spread into the extraovarian pelvis and abdomen and beyond, the accuracies of conventional US, CT, and MR imaging were compared. For the ovaries and adnexa, the accuracy of detection was based on the presence or absence of malignancy in the ovaries and adnexa. For the extraovarian pelvis, the accuracy of detection was based on the presence or absence of extraovarian pelvic disease without consideration of the presence or absence of disease in the ovaries and adnexa or in the abdomen. For the abdomen and beyond, the accuracy of detection was based on the presence or absence of disease in this area without consideration of the presence or absence of disease in the pelvis. Analysis of each specific pelvic and abdominal site, however, was beyond the scope of the study.

For all ROC curve analyses, modality-specific parametric ROC curves were obtained by fitting an ordinal regression model, accounting for institution-specific cutoff points on the latent variable scale (35). Both empiric institution-specific ROC curves and smooth parametric curves were generated.

Agreement between the results of imaging and the standard of reference (surgical and histopathologic analysis) was based on the reader's final assessment and was measured with κ statistics. The stages of disease were grouped as follows in a 3 × 3 table: benign lesions and stage I cancer, stage II cancer, and stage III or IV cancer. Benign lesions and stage I cancer were grouped to assess the abilities of the imaging modalities to allow distinction between disease confined to the ovaries and spread of cancer (stage II to IV). Cases of nonadvanced disease (benign lesions, stage I and II cancer) were grouped to assess the abilities of the imag-

TABLE 1
Modified International Federation of Gynecology and Obstetrics Staging Classification for Ovarian Cancer (1986)

Stage	Criteria
I	Growth limited to the ovaries
IA	Growth limited to one ovary; no ascites; no tumor on the external surfaces, capsule intact
IB	Growth limited to both ovaries; no ascites; no tumor on the external surfaces, capsule intact
ICa	Tumor stage IA or IB but with tumor on the surface of one or both ovaries, with capsule ruptured, with ascites containing malignant cells, or with positive peritoneal washings
II	Growth involving one or both ovaries with pelvic extension
IIA	Extension or metastases to the uterus or tubes
IIB	Extension to other pelvic tissues
IICa	Tumor stage IIA or IIB with tumor on the surface of one or both ovaries, with capsule ruptured, with ascites containing malignant cells, or with positive peritoneal washings
III	Tumor involving one or both ovaries with peritoneal implants outside the pelvis or positive retroperitoneal or inguinal nodes; superficial hepatic metastases equal stage III; tumor is limited to the true pelvis but with histologically verified malignant extension to the small bowel or omentum
IIIA	Tumor grossly limited to the true pelvis with negative nodes but with histologically confirmed microscopic seeding of abdominal peritoneal surfaces
IIIB	Tumor of one or both ovaries; histologically confirmed implants of abdominal peritoneal surfaces, none exceeding 2 cm in diameter; nodes negative
IIIC	Abdominal implants greater than 2 cm in diameter or positive retroperitoneal or inguinal nodes
IV	Growth involving one or both ovaries with distant metastases; if pleural effusion is present, there must be positive cytologic test results to allot a case to stage IV; parenchymal hepatic metastases equal stage IV

Source.—Reference 31.

TABLE 2
Surgically and Histopathologically Confirmed Diagnoses by Institution

Institution	Benign Lesion	Ovarian Cancer by Stage			Total
		I	II	III or IV	
A	28	5	1	9	43
B	41	6	3	12	62
C	42	11	2	23	78
D	23	8	2	16	49
E	28	5	5	10	48
Total	162	35	13	70	280

TABLE 3
Estimated Areas under the ROC Curve for the Overall Detection of Ovarian Cancer

Institution	Doppler or Conventional US	CT	MR Imaging
A	0.95	0.74	0.95
B	0.89	0.86	0.96
C	0.89	0.94	0.96
D	0.92	0.89	0.90
E	0.96	0.97	0.77
Pooled	0.91*	0.91†	0.91*

Note.—The pooled area estimates are weighted averages of the institution-specific area estimates.
* The 95% CI was 0.87, 0.95.
† The 95% CI was 0.86, 0.95.

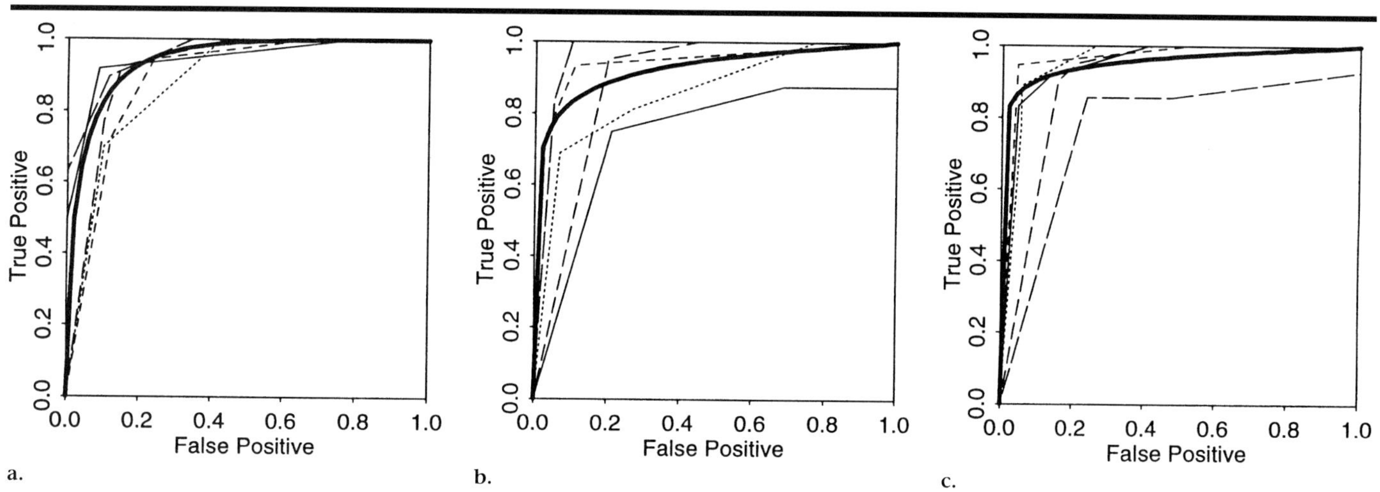

Figure 1. ROC curves for the overall detection of ovarian cancer by imaging modality: (a) Doppler US, (b) CT, and (c) MR imaging. For each modality, the five institution-specific ROC curves are shown as interrupted or thin lines; the bold, smooth curves are the modality-specific ROC curves obtained by means of an ordinal regression fit to the data from all five institutions.

ing modalities to demonstrate abdominal spread (stage III and IV) because the surgical approach is different. This issue was addressed by using the radiologist's final assessment of disease stage to estimate and compare modality-specific sensitivities and specificities by means of the McNemar test for correlated proportions.

RESULTS

Ovarian masses were surgically removed in all 280 patients; the masses were solitary in 189 patients and bilateral in 91. The masses ranged in diameter from 1.3 to 30.0 cm with a mean diameter of 9.9 cm ± 5.4 (SD); there was no statistically significant difference in diameter between benign and malignant lesions. All masses were correctly identified with all three modalities.

Of the 280 patients, 118 (42.1%) had malignancies (Table 2): 87 primary ovarian, 27 metastatic (nonovarian) with spread to the ovaries, and four metastatic but with concomitant benign ovarian disease. The cancers were staged as follows: 35 confined to the ovaries (stage I), 13 involving the ovaries and adjacent pelvic structures (stage II), and 70 with abdominal spread (stage III or IV).

The other 162 patients (57.9%) had benign neoplasms (n = 104) or nonneoplasms, mostly endometriomas (n = 58) (Table 2). There was no statistically significant difference between institutions as regards the actual histopathologically determined disease stage (P = .48 [χ^2 test]).

According to the inclusion criteria, all patients had to be enrolled in at least two modalities. However, not all patients completed their studies due to noncompliance or physical disability, which was often caused by advanced disease. The results of all completed studies were included in the evaluation. All three modalities were performed in 103 patients (36.8%). Only two modalities were performed in 170 patients (60.7%): Doppler and conventional US and CT in 97, Doppler and conventional US and MR imaging in 60, and CT and MR imaging in 13. Only one modality was performed in seven patients (2.5%): Doppler and conventional US in four and MR imaging in three. In summary, the modality accuracy estimates and the statistical analyses were based on the results of 264 Doppler and conventional US examinations, 213 CT examinations, and 179 MR imaging examinations.

In discrimination between cases of benign and cases of malignant disease in any region of the pelvis and abdomen, all three modalities had approximately equal overall pooled areas under the ROC curve of 0.91 (95% CI = 0.87, 0.95) (Table 3, Fig 1). There was a statistically significant difference between institutions only for MR imaging, with the institution-specific areas ranging from 0.77 to 0.96 (P = .045) because of a considerably smaller area for institution E. Although the range for CT was larger, from 0.74 to 0.97, no statistically significant difference between institutions was detected.

For diagnosis of disease in the three anatomic regions (ovaries and adnexa, extraovarian pelvis, abdomen and beyond) separately, the results varied by institution and by modality (Table 4, Fig 2). For diagnosis of malignancy in the ovaries and adnexa, MR imaging yielded a higher pooled area under the ROC curve than did the other two modalities. The difference in accuracy between MR imaging (0.91) and Doppler US (0.78) was statistically significant (P < .01) (Tables 4, 5). Among the pairwise comparisons between institutions for this anatomic area, only institution B showed a statistically significant intermodality difference, which was between Doppler US (0.63) and MR imaging (0.96) (P = .014). Use of information about the presence of a diastolic notch did not improve diagnostic accuracy, although the presence of such a notch slightly favored the diagnosis of benign disease.

For diagnosis of malignancy in the extraovarian pelvis and in the abdomen and beyond, MR imaging yielded higher pooled areas under the ROC curve than did US and CT. However, these differences were not statistically significant in either the extraovarian pelvis (range, 0.87–0.91) or the abdomen and beyond (range, 0.90–0.95) (Table 4). Statistically significant differences (P < .01) in areas under the ROC curve between institutions were detected only for the following modality–anatomic area combinations: (*a*) US in detection of malignancy in the abdomen and beyond (range, 0.82–0.97); (*b*) MR imaging in detection of malignancy in the extraovarian pelvis (range, 0.81–0.98); and (*c*) MR imaging in detection of malignancy in the abdomen and beyond (range, 0.93–0.99).

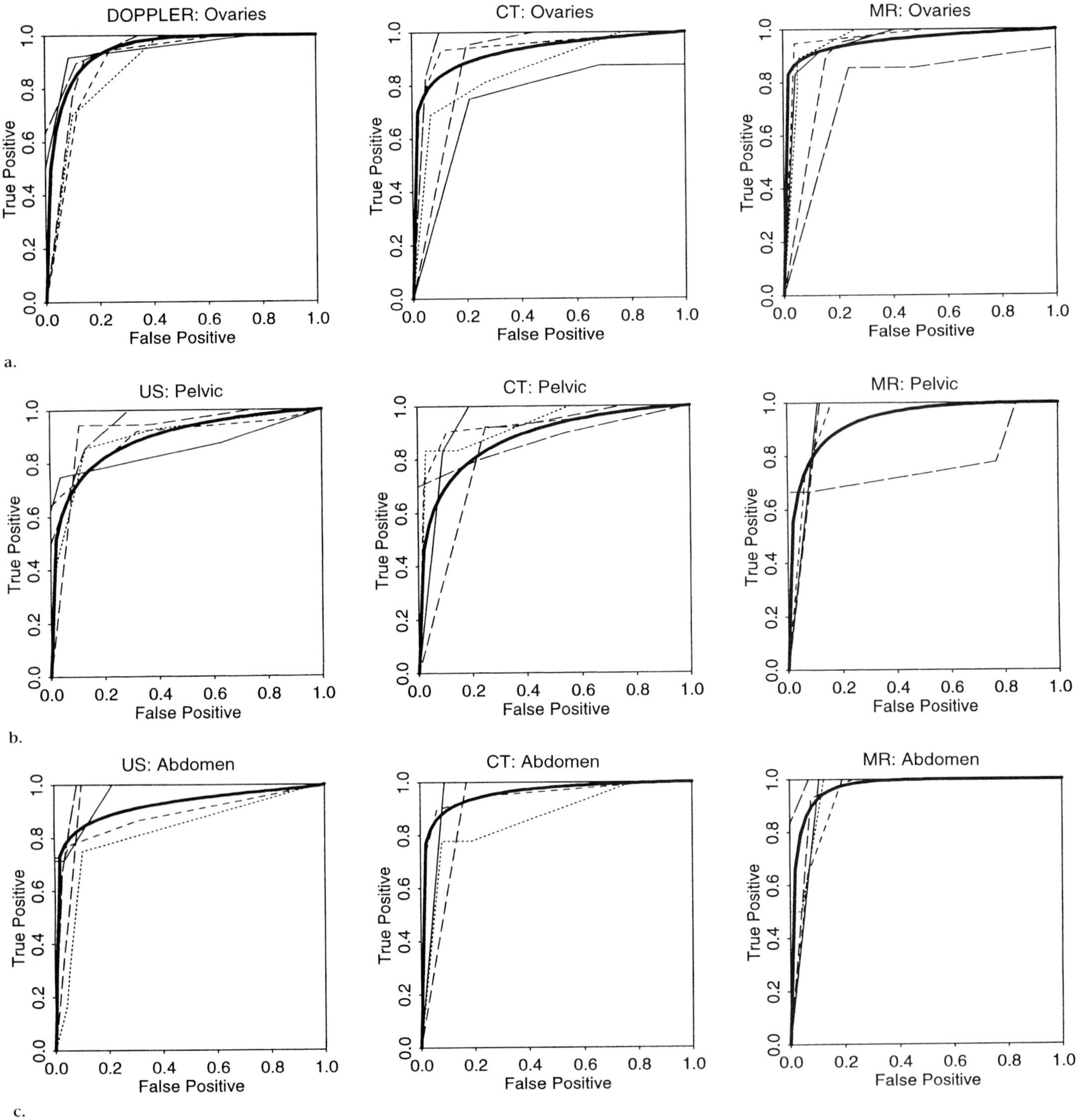

Figure 2. ROC curves for the detection of malignancy by anatomic region and modality: In **a–c**, results of analysis of the **(a)** ovaries, **(b)** other pelvic sites, and **(c)** abdomen and beyond with US (left graph), CT (middle graph), and MR imaging (right graph) are shown. For each anatomic region and modality combination, the five institution-specific ROC curves are shown as interrupted or thin lines; the bold, smooth curves are the modality-specific ROC curves obtained by means of an ordinal regression fit to the data from all five institutions.

The κ statistics for agreement between the results of a modality (based on the readers' final evaluation) and the standard of reference were similar for staging with US, CT, and MR imaging: 0.66 for US (95% CI = 0.56, 0.74); 0.65 for CT (95% CI = 0.55, 0.75); and 0.70 for MR imaging (95% CI = 0.60, 0.81).

In the differentiation of nonadvanced disease (benign lesions, stage I and II cancers) from advanced malignancy (stage III and IV cancers) with US, eight of 197 cases of nonadvanced disease were overstaged as advanced malignancy (false-positive rate = 0.041) and 17 of 67 cases of advanced malignancy were understaged as stage I or II (false-negative rate = 0.254) (Table 6). With CT, 17 of 161 cases

TABLE 4
Estimated Areas Under the ROC Curve within Anatomic Regions

Institution	Doppler or Conventional US*			CT			MR Imaging		
	Ovaries and Adnexa	Extra-ovarian Pelvis	Abdomen and Beyond	Ovaries and Adnexa	Extra-ovarian Pelvis	Abdomen and Beyond	Ovaries and Adnexa	Extra-ovarian Pelvis	Abdomen and Beyond
A	0.75	0.88	0.96	0.74	0.92	0.95	0.94	0.93	0.95
B	0.63	0.92	0.82	0.83	0.91	0.86	0.96	0.98	0.96
C	0.82	0.89	0.89	0.88	0.88	0.95	0.95	0.95	0.93
D	0.82	0.83	0.95	0.88	0.83	0.91	0.89	0.90	0.95
E	0.88	0.88	0.97	0.82	0.75	1.00	0.80	0.81	0.99
Pooled†	0.78	0.88	0.90	0.85	0.87	0.93	0.91	0.91	0.95

Note.—The pooled area estimates are weighted averages of the institution-specific area estimates.
* Doppler US was used to evaluate the ovaries and adnexa; conventional US was used to evaluate the extraovarian pelvis and the abdomen and beyond.
† The 95% CIs were 0.72, 0.84 for 0.78; 0.84, 0.93 for 0.88; 0.85, 0.95 for 0.90; 0.80, 0.91 for 0.85; 0.81, 0.92 for 0.87; 0.89, 0.98 for 0.93; 0.87, 0.96 for 0.91 (ovaries and adnexa); 0.86, 0.96 for 0.91 (extraovarian pelvis); and 0.92, 0.98 for 0.95.

TABLE 5
***P* Values for Pairwise Comparisons of Modalities**

Modality Pair	Ovaries and Adnexa	Extraovarian Pelvis	Abdomen and Beyond
Doppler US vs CT	.17	. . .	. . .
Doppler US vs MR imaging	.01*	. . .	. . .
CT vs MR imaging	.16	.10	.83
Conventional US vs CT	. . .	.55	.91
Conventional US vs MR imaging	. . .	.36	.11

* Statistically significant difference.

of nonadvanced disease were overstaged as advanced malignancy (false-positive rate = 0.106) and four of 50 cases of advanced malignancy were understaged as stage I or II (false-negative rate = 0.080). With MR imaging, 17 of 139 cases of nonadvanced disease were overstaged as advanced malignancy (false-positive rate = 0.122) and one of 41 cases of advanced malignancy was understaged as stage I or II (false-negative rate = 0.024). Five cases were overstaged with both CT and MR imaging. In summary, the specificity was 96% for US, 89% for CT, and 88% for MR imaging and the sensitivity was 75% for US, 92% for CT, and 98% for MR imaging. On the basis of the common cases for each modality pair, the following differences were statistically significant: (*a*) the difference in specificity between US and MR imaging (P = .018), with US more specific; (*b*) the difference in sensitivity between US and CT (P = .014), with CT more sensitive; and (*c*) the difference in sensitivity between US and MR imaging (P = .003), with MR imaging more sensitive.

The number of misinterpreted studies was relatively small. Nevertheless, review of these studies suggested that cancer spread was understaged with US primarily because of the inability to consistently identify abnormality in the omentum, pelvic side walls, colon, paracolic gutters, and iliac and paraaortic lymph nodes. There were no predominant sites of overstaging with US. Conversely, overstaging with CT and MR imaging appeared to occur because subtle areas and benign variants were misinterpreted as malignant, particularly in the paracolic gutters, subdiaphragmatic areas, colon, iliac and paraaortic lymph nodes, and hepatic surface. A statistical analysis for each individual organ was not feasible due to the limited number of cases of disease. Further studies of individual peritoneal sites, lymph nodes, and organ involvement are under way.

DISCUSSION

This prospective study addressed the issues of differentiating benign from malignant ovarian masses and evaluating cancer spread. We enrolled patients from five institutions, evaluated all three imaging modalities currently used for staging, used state-of-the-art equipment in all centers, and correlated the imaging results with the results of surgery and histopathologic analysis performed in a close temporal relationship (<1 month apart).

The percentage of stage III and IV cancers was high, almost 60% (70 of 118 cases). However, the malignancy rate of 42.1% was more than double those in previous studies (36,37). This result was likely due to the referral source, which was specialists in gynecologic oncology.

There was remarkably little variability among participating institutions and modalities. Recruitment patterns were similar with no statistically significant differences in the percentages of ovarian cancers and their stages (Table 2). This fact suggests that the results are reproducible and can likely be generalized to other centers.

The three imaging modalities yielded similar estimated areas under the ROC curve for discrimination between benign disease and cancer in all regions, with a mean area of 0.91 for all three modalities (Table 3). Although differentiation of benign from malignant disease is obviously clinically important and these detection rates are higher than those previously reported, they are likely still not high enough for surgery to be avoided in most cases.

For the ovaries and adnexa, the intent of this study was not to evaluate the efficacy of screening or mass detection. Rather, because all of the patients had a mass detected at US, the intent was to evaluate the abilities of Doppler US, CT, and MR imaging to allow diagnosis of malignancy in the mass. For this application, the estimated areas under the ROC curve for each modality revealed that MR imaging and CT were superior to Doppler US (Table 4). It is unfortunate (but un-

TABLE 6
Results of Staging Ovarian Cancer with Imaging versus Surgery and Histopathologic Analysis

Surgery and Histopathologic Analysis	Doppler or Conventional US*: Benign Lesion or Stage I	Doppler or Conventional US*: Stage II	Doppler or Conventional US*: Stage III or IV	CT: Benign Lesion or Stage I	CT: Stage II	CT: Stage III or IV	MR Imaging: Benign Lesion or Stage I	MR Imaging: Stage II	MR Imaging: Stage III or IV
Benign lesion or stage I	167	12	6	128	8	14	114	3	15
Stage II	5	5	2	7	1	3	3	2	2
Stage III or IV	8	9	50	3	1	46	0	1	40

Note.—Values are numbers of cases. These results are based on the radiologists' final assessment of stage for each case; conversely, the ROC curve results in Tables 3 and 4 were based on the rating scales.

* Doppler US was used to evaluate the ovaries and adnexa for malignancy; conventional US was used to evaluate the extraovarian pelvis, abdomen, and beyond for spread.

avoidable) that our study design did not allow statistical evaluation of the performances of CT and MR imaging versus that of combined Doppler and conventional US (38).

The relatively poor performance of Doppler US has been discussed without identification of a unifying cause (13–15,39). The neovascular response of ovarian cancer may be incomplete or nonspecific; thus, when intratumoral arterial flow is detected with Doppler US, differentiation of benign from malignant processes is often not possible. It has been suggested that central flow, increased impedance, elevated peak systolic velocity, loss of the diastolic notch, and low Doppler US indexes favor malignancy. None of these have shown a high enough diagnostic accuracy. Therefore, whatever the reason, the present lack of specificity makes Doppler US a poor diagnostic tool. It is possible that different numeric cutoff values for the Doppler indexes (40–42) may provide more encouraging results, although the considerable overlap of the indexes in benign and malignant tumors makes this possibility unlikely. Perhaps use of intravenous contrast agents to enhance the tumor and its vascularity may improve diagnostic accuracy (43,44).

Areas under the ROC curve reflect the tendencies of readers to overstage and understage disease. However, these areas do not reveal differences in overstaging and understaging at the routine interpretative cutoffs used by most readers. Thus, we also analyzed the data according to the way they are actually received and used by the referring clinicians (Table 6). Although trends were difficult to discern because the "off-diagonal" numbers were small (Table 6), the data suggest the following: (*a*) For pelvic spread (stage II cancers), there was considerable understaging (false-negative cases) and overstaging (false-positive cases) with all three modalities. (*b*) For differentiation of pelvic malignancy (stage I or II) from abdominal spread (stage III or IV), abdominal spread was more likely to be understaged with US and pelvic malignancy was more likely to be overstaged with CT and MR imaging.

There are problems with both overstaging and understaging. Overstaging leads to a wider surgical approach but makes it more likely that malignancy will not be overlooked; understaging causes extension of the originally planned pelvic surgery with the potential for tumor to be overlooked. The extent of surgical expertise devoted to the case may also be affected. In most centers, the greater the suspicion of abdominal spread, the more likely it is that a specialist in gynecologic oncology will perform the exploration. This point is important because surgery by specialists leads to better staging and maximal debulking (cytoreduction) and to longer survival (45–48). Although one could argue that it is always better to overstage so that malignancy is not overlooked, it is more important to accurately distinguish malignancy that has spread into the abdomen (stage III or IV) from malignancy confined to the pelvis (stage I or II).

Our results show remarkable accuracy in demonstrating the extent of malignant spread for all three imaging modalities. Although US, CT, and MR imaging may have demonstrated disease in different sites (eg, the mesentery rather than paracolic gutters), all three modalities had high staging accuracies at ROC curve analysis of 0.91. It is therefore difficult to suggest a simple algorithm for evaluation of women with ovarian masses. However, US is often the initial imaging study in evaluation of a suspected ovarian abnormality. If a complex or solid ovarian mass and abdominal spread are detected with US, our data support the accuracy of a diagnosis of stage III disease. Similarly, CT and MR imaging allow accurate diagnosis of a complex or solid ovarian mass with stage III spread. Because of the importance of not understaging abdominal malignancy as disease limited to the pelvis, if stage III cancer is not detected at initial abdominal US, CT or MR imaging should be performed because of their higher sensitivities in staging. Whatever the modality used, it is hoped that correct staging of advanced disease will lead to appropriate referral to a specialist in gynecologic oncology.

Acknowledgments: The Radiology Diagnostic Oncology Group includes the following: Eric Outwater, MD, John A. Carlson, Jr, MD, Charles J. Dutton, MD, Alexander Talerman, MD, PhD, Neil B. Rosenshein, MD, Edward L. Trimble, MD, Michael B. Dillon, MD, Cynthia I. Caskey, MD, James A. Roberts, MD, Thomas S. Frank, MD, Gregory T. Sica, MD, Steven E. Seltzer, MD, Douglass F. Adams, MD, Ramin Khorasani, MD, Christopher P. Crum, MD, Ross S. Berkowitz, MD, Ellen E. Sheets, MD, Michael G. Muto, MD, Sara Feldman, MD, Stephen C. Rubin, MD, Mark Morgan, MD, A. Virginia LiVolsi, MD, Constantine Gatsonis, PhD, Christina Fu, PhD, Jane Z. Dumsha, Mary C. Pyles, Victoria Trapanotto, MS, BS, RDMS, Manette London, CCRC, Bronwyn Head, Susan Calder, Lisa Herman, and Alexandra Kilger.

References

1. Cancer facts and figures 1998. Atlanta, Ga: American Cancer Society, 1998.
2. Taylor K, Schwartz P. Screening for ovarian cancer. Radiology 1994; 192:1–10.
3. Creasman W, DiSaia P. Screening in ovarian cancer. Am J Obstet Gynecol 1991; 165:7–10.
4. Droegumueller W. Screening for ovarian carcinoma: hopeful and wishful thinking. Am J Obstet Gynecol 1994; 170:1095–1098.
5. Mendelson EB, Bohm-Velez M, Joseph N, Neiman HL. Gynecologic imaging: comparison of transabdominal and transvaginal sonography. Radiology 1988; 166:321–325.
6. Leibman A, Kruse B, McSweeney MB. Transvaginal sonography: comparison with transabdominal sonography in the

diagnosis of pelvic masses. AJR 1988; 151: 89–92.
7. Rulin M, Preston A. Adnexal masses in postmenopausal women. Obstet Gynecol 1987; 70:578–581.
8. Sassone AM, Timor-Tritsch IE, Artner A, Westhoff C, Warren W. Transvaginal sonographic characterization of ovarian disease: evaluation of a new scoring system to predict ovarian malignancy. Obstet Gynecol 1991; 78:70–76.
9. Benacerraf BB, Finkler NJ, Wojciechowski RN, Knapp RC. Diagnosis of ovarian masses. J Reprod Med 1990; 35:491–495.
10. Bourne T, Campbell S, Steer C, Whitehead M, Collins W. Transvaginal colour flow imaging: a possible new screening technique for ovarian cancer. Br Med J 1989; 299:1367–1370.
11. Kurjak A, Zalud I, Alfirevic Z. Evaluation of adnexal masses with transvaginal color ultrasound. J Ultrasound Med 1991; 10: 295–297.
12. Jain K. Prospective evaluation of adnexal masses with endovaginal gray-scale and duplex and color Doppler US: correlation with pathologic findings. Radiology 1994; 191:63–67.
13. Brown D, Frates M, Laing F, et al. Ovarian masses: can benign and malignant lesions be differentiated with color and pulsed Doppler US? Radiology 1994; 190:333–336.
14. Stein SM, Laifer-Narin S, Johnson MB, et al. Differentiation of benign and malignant adnexal masses: relative value of gray-scale, color Doppler, and spectral Doppler sonography. AJR 1995; 164:381–386.
15. Fleischer A, Rodgers WH, Kepple DM, Williams L, Jones HW. Color Doppler sonography of ovarian masses: a multiparameter analysis. J Ultrasound Med 1993; 12:41–48.
16. Forstner R, Hricak H, Occhipinti KA, Powell CB, Frankel SD, Stern JL. Ovarian cancer: staging with CT and MR imaging. Radiology 1995; 197:619–626.
17. Ghossain MA, Buy NJ, Ligneres C, et al. Epithelial tumors of the ovary: comparison of MR and CT findings. Radiology 1991; 181:863–870.
18. Meyer J, Kennedy AW, Friedman R, Ayoub A, Zepp RC. Ovarian carcinoma: value of CT in predicting success of debulking surgery. AJR 1995; 165:875–878.
19. Buist MR, Golding RP, Buger CW, et al. Comparative evaluation of diagnostic methods in ovarian carcinoma with emphasis on CT and MRI. Gynecol Oncol 1994; 52:191–198.
20. Steven S, Hricak H, Stern J. Ovarian lesions: detection and characterization with gadolinium-enhanced MR imaging at 1.5 T. Radiology 1991; 181:481–488.
21. Semelka RC, Lawrence PH, Shoenut JP, Heywood M, Kroeker MA, Lotocki R. Primary ovarian cancer: prospective comparison of contrast-enhanced CT and pre- and postcontrast, fat-suppressed MR imaging, with histologic correlation. JMRI 1993; 3:99–106.
22. Outwater EK, Siegelman ES, Wilson KM, Mitchell DG. Benign and malignant gynecologic disease: clinical importance of fluid and peritoneal enhancement in the pelvis at MR imaging. Radiology 1996; 200:483–488.
23. Yamashita Y, Torashima M, Hatanaka Y, et al. Adnexal masses: accuracy of characterization with transvaginal US and precontrast and postcontrast MR imaging. Radiology 1995; 194:557–565.
24. Komatsu T, Konishi I, Mandai M, et al. Adnexal masses: transvaginal US and gadolinium-enhanced MR imaging assessment of intratumoral structure. Radiology 1996; 198:109–115.
25. Hata K, Hata T, Manabe A, Sugimura K, Kitao M. A critical evaluation of transvaginal Doppler studies, transvaginal sonography, magnetic resonance imaging, and CA 125 in detecting ovarian cancer. Obstet Gynecol 1992; 80:922–926.
26. Jain K, Friedman DL, Pettinger TW, Alagappan R, Jeffrey RB Jr, Sommer FG. Adnexal masses: comparison of specificity of endovaginal US and pelvic MR imaging. Radiology 1993; 186:697–704.
27. Jain K, Jeffrey RB Jr. Evaluation of pelvic masses with magnetic resonance imaging and ultrasonography. J Ultrasound Med 1994; 13:845–853.
28. Buy JN, Ghossain MA, Sciot C, et al. Epithelial tumors of the ovary: CT findings and correlation with US. Radiology 1991; 178:811–818.
29. Smith FW, Cherryman GR, Bayliss AP, et al. A comparative study of the accuracy of ultrasound imaging, x-ray computerized tomography, and low field MRI diagnosis of ovarian malignancy. Magn Reson Imaging 1988; 6:225–227.
30. Steer CV, Campbell S, Pampiglione JS, Kingsland CR, Mason BA, Collins WP. Transvaginal colour flow imaging of the uterine arteries during the ovarian and menstrual cycles. Hum Reprod 1990; 5:391–395.
31. Forstner R, Chen M, Hricak H. Imaging of ovarian cancer. JMRI 1995; 5:606–613.
32. Robboy SJ, Kraus FT, Kurman RJ. Gross description, processing, and reporting of gynecologic and obstetric specimens. In: Kurman RJ, ed. Blaustein's pathology of the female genital tract. 3rd ed. New York, NY: Springer-Verlag, 1987; 925–940.
33. Talerman A. Ovarian pathology. Curr Opin Obstet Gynecol 1992; 4:608–615.
34. DeLong ER, DeLong DM, Clarke-Pearson DL. Comparing the areas under two or more correlated ROC curves: a nonparametric approach. Biometrics 1988; 44:837–845.
35. Gatsonis C. Random-effects models for diagnostic accuracy data. Acad Radiol 1995; 2(suppl 1):S14–S21.
36. Valentin L. Gray scale sonography, subjective evaluation of the color Doppler image, and measurement of blood flow velocity for distinguishing benign and malignant tumors of suspected adnexal origin. Eur J Obstet Gynecol Reprod Biol 1997; 72:63–72.
37. Rehn M, Lohmann K, Rempen A. Transvaginal ultrasonography of pelvic masses: evaluation of B-mode technique and Doppler ultrasonography. Am J Obstet Gynecol 1996; 175:97–104.
38. Buy JN, Ghossain MA, Hugol D, et al. Characterization of adnexal masses: combination of color Doppler and conventional sonography compared with spectral Doppler analysis alone and conventional sonography alone. AJR 1996; 166:385–393.
39. Hamper UM, Sheth S, Abbas FM, Rosenshein NB, Aronson D, Kurman RJ. Transvaginal color Doppler sonography of adnexal masses: differences in blood flow impedance in benign and malignant lesions. AJR 1993; 160:1225–1228.
40. Bromley B, Goodman H, Benacerraf B. Comparison between sonographic morphology and Doppler waveform for the diagnosis of ovarian malignancy. Obstet Gynecol 1994; 83:434–437.
41. Wu CC, Lee CN, Chen TM, Lai JI, Hsieh CY, Hsieh FJ. Factors contributing to the accuracy in diagnosing ovarian malignancy by color Doppler ultrasound. Obstet Gynecol 1994; 84:605–608.
42. Tepper R, Lerner-Geva L, Altaras M, et al. Transvaginal color flow imaging in the diagnosis of ovarian tumors. J Ultrasound Med 1995; 14:731–734.
43. Kedar RP, Cosgrove D, McCready VR, Bamber JC, Carter ER. Microbubble contrast agent for color Doppler US: effect on breast masses. Radiology 1996; 198:679–686.
44. Goldberg BB, Liu JB, Forsberg F. Ultrasound contrast agents: a review. Ultrasound Med Biol 1994; 20:319–333.
45. Nguyen HN, Averette HE, Hoskins W, Penalver M, Sevin BU, Steren A. National survey of ovarian carcinoma. V. The impact of physician's specialty on patients' survival. Cancer 1993; 72:3663–3670.
46. Puls LE, Carrasco R, Morrow MS, Blackhurst D. Stage I ovarian carcinoma: specialty-related differences in survival and management. South Med J 1997; 90:1097–1100.
47. Mayer AR, Chambers SK, Graves E, et al. Ovarian cancer staging: does it require a gynecologic oncologist? Gynecol Oncol 1992; 47:223–227.
48. Chen SS, Bochner R. Assessment of morbidity and mortality in primary cytoreductive surgery for advanced ovarian carcinoma. Gynecol Oncol 1985; 20:190–195.

E. Scott Pretorius, MD
Evan S. Siegelman, MD
Parvati Ramchandani, MD
Thomas Cangiano, MD
Marc P. Banner, MD

Index terms:
Angiomyolipoma, 81.3141
Kidney, cysts, 81.311
Kidney neoplasms, 81.321, 81.324
Kidney neoplasms, MR, 81.121412, 81.121415, 81.12142
Oncocytoma, 81.3239
von Hippel-Lindau disease

Radiology 1999; 212:28–34

Abbreviation:
GRE = gradient-recalled echo

[1] From the Departments of Radiology (E.S.P., E.S.S., P.R., M.P.B.) and Surgery, Division of Urology (T.C., M.P.B.), University of Pennsylvania Medical Center, 3400 Spruce St, Philadelphia, PA 19104. From the 1997 RSNA scientific assembly. Received March 25, 1998; revision requested June 19; revision received September 8; accepted December 9. **Address reprint requests to** E.S.S.

Author contributions:
Guarantors of integrity of entire study, E.S.P., E.S.S., P.R., M.P.B.; study concepts and design, E.S.P., E.S.S., P.R., T.C., M.P.B.; definition of intellectual content, E.S.P., E.S.S., P.R., T.C., M.P.B.; literature research, E.S.P., E.S.S., P.R., M.P.B.; clinical studies, E.S.P., E.S.S., P.R., M.P.B.; data acquisition and analysis, E.S.P., E.S.S., P.R., M.P.B.; manuscript preparation, editing, and review, E.S.P., E.S.S., P.R., M.P.B.

Renal Neoplasms Amenable to Partial Nephrectomy: MR Imaging[1]

PURPOSE: To determine the magnetic resonance (MR) imaging characteristics of renal lesions in patients who undergo technically successful partial nephrectomy.

MATERIALS AND METHODS: Between February 1991 and September 1997, 38 patients (41 lesions) who underwent partial nephrectomy at a single institution were preoperatively evaluated with contrast material–enhanced, multiplanar, surface-coil MR imaging. Imaging findings that could affect the decision to perform partial nephrectomy were retrospectively evaluated: tumor size; tumor location; presence of pseudocapsule; suspected tumor invasion of renal sinus fat, renal collecting system, renal vein, or perinephric fat; and morphologic and physiologic status of the contralateral kidney. Correlation was made with surgical and pathologic findings.

RESULTS: Thirty-three of 41 lesions (80%) were renal cell carcinomas, five were oncocytic neoplasms (12%), two were hemorrhagic cysts (5%), and one was an angiomyolipoma (2%). Twenty-four of 41 (59%) lesions had pseudocapsules. In most cases, the perinephric fat (n = 38 [93%]), the renal sinus fat (n = 31 [76%]), and the renal collecting system (n = 39 [95%]) were correctly interpreted as being uninvolved by tumor.

CONCLUSION: Renal neoplasms amenable to partial nephrectomy can be identified and characterized with contrast-enhanced, multiplanar, surface-coil MR imaging.

Partial nephrectomy is advocated for the management of select renal neoplasms, particularly in patients with diminished renal function, a solitary kidney, or bilateral renal malignancy (1,2). Increasing utilization of and technical improvements in cross-sectional imaging have led to the detection of many renal neoplasms of small size and early stage. Although controversy remains regarding the use of partial nephrectomy for localized, incidentally discovered small renal neoplasms in patients with a normal contralateral kidney (3), physicians at many centers, including our own, sometimes perform elective partial nephrectomy in this clinical situation.

Imaging findings that suggest that a renal lesion can be successfully and completely removed at partial nephrectomy include tumor smaller than 3 cm; peripheral location of the tumor; lack of invasion of the renal sinus fat, perinephric fat, or renal collecting system; presence of a pseudocapsule; lack of renal venous involvement; and absence of lymphadenopathy or distant metastases. Larger tumors and lesions that are locally invasive of the renal sinus fat, renal collecting system, or perinephric fat may be removed at partial nephrectomy if there are compelling reasons (ie, limited renal function, bilateral renal malignancies, or tumor in a solitary kidney).

The intrinsic soft-tissue contrast and direct multiplanar imaging capabilities of magnetic resonance (MR) imaging make it well suited for detecting and characterizing small renal lesions, as well as for determining the extent of local tumor invasion. To determine the MR imaging characteristics of lesions in patients who subsequently underwent technically successful partial nephrectomy, we retrospectively reviewed the MR images from 38 patients (41 lesions).

MATERIALS AND METHODS

Sixty-three patients underwent partial nephrectomy at our institution between February 1991 and September 1996. Of these, 38 patients (41 renal lesions) were preoperatively

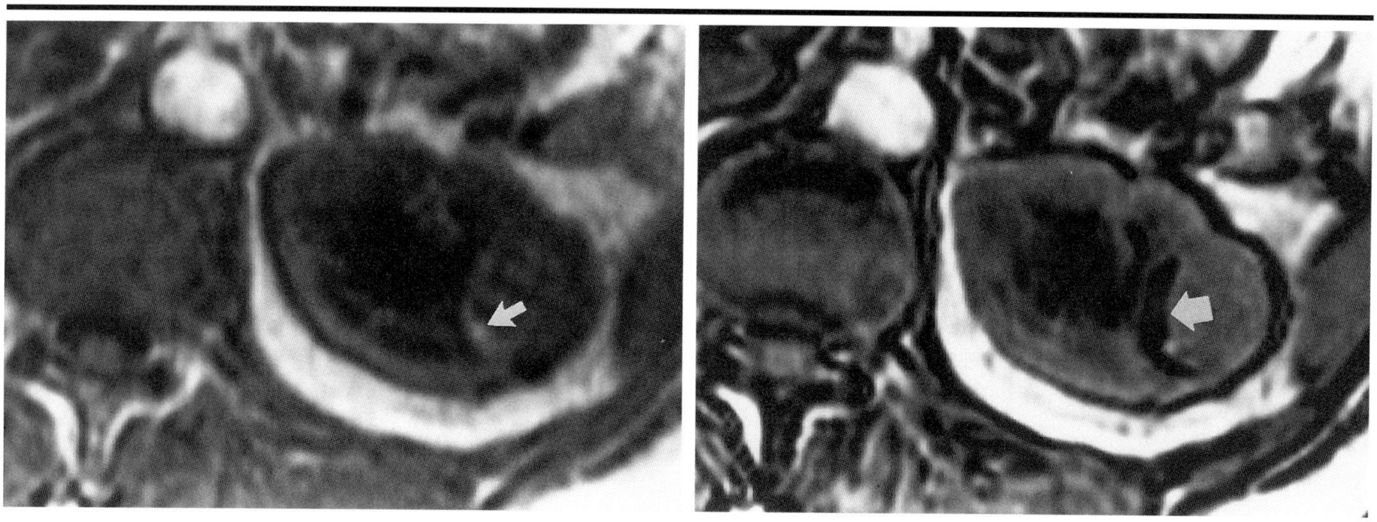

a. b.

Figure 1. Angiomyolipoma misinterpreted as a renal cell carcinoma in a 67-year-old woman. (a) Axial in-phase spoiled GRE image (220/4.2; flip angle, 90°). The area of high signal intensity (arrow) was prospectively thought to represent renal sinus fat invasion by a probable renal cell carcinoma. (b) Axial out-of-phase spoiled GRE image (220/2.1; flip angle, 90°). In fact, this area (arrow), which loses signal intensity on this opposed-phase image, was fat within an angiomyolipoma.

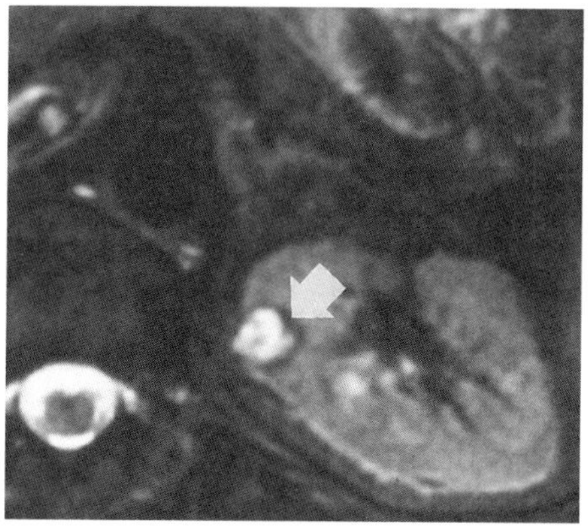

Figure 2. Pseudocapsule in peripheral renal cell carcinoma in a 38-year-old man. Axial fast spin-echo T2-weighted fat-suppressed image (4,000/102 [effective]) demonstrates a hypointense rim (arrow) around this small renal cell carcinoma.

evaluated with contrast material–enhanced, surface-coil MR imaging performed by using a 1.5-T Signa MR imager (GE Medical Systems, Milwaukee, Wis).

The mean patient age at the time of surgery was 60 years (age range, 28–82 years). Two patients had von Hippel-Lindau syndrome. Nine additional patients had previously undergone nephrectomy: seven for renal cell carcinoma and two for transitional cell carcinoma. The mean preoperative serum creatinine level was 1.2 mg/dL (106 µmol/L; range, 0.6–4.3 mg/dL [53–380 µmol/L]). Five patients had a serum creatinine level of 1.5 mg/dL (133 µmol/L) or greater.

Our standard protocol for evaluating a renal lesion evolved over the time encompassed by this study. We obtained a series of coronal localizer images, followed by nonenhanced T1-weighted breath-hold spoiled gradient-recalled-echo (GRE) images (100–240/2.1 and 4.2 [repetition time msec/echo time msec]; 90° flip angle; 256 × 128–192 matrix; one signal acquired; field of view, three-fourths in the phase-encoding direction and sized to the patient; 6-mm section thickness; and 1-mm section interval, with a bandwidth of ±16 or ±32 kHz). For patients unable to undergo breath-hold imaging, we employed the following T1-weighted sequence: 300–600/9–14 (effective), two signals acquired. T2-weighted images were obtained with an axial fat-suppressed, respiratory-triggered fast spin-echo sequence (3,000–9,000/102–155 [effective] [the repetition time was dependent on the respiratory rate]; 256 × 192–256 matrix; two signals acquired; other parameters similar to those for the T1-weighted GRE sequence). Breath-hold coronal, T1-weighted, fat-suppressed, spoiled GRE imaging was performed before, immediately after, and then 45 seconds after the intravenous administration of 0.1 mmol of gadopentetate dimeglumine (Magnevist, Berlex Laboratories, Wayne, NJ; or Omniscan, Nycomed, Princeton, NJ) per kilogram of body weight. Imaging parameters included 68–130/1.6–2.9; 60°–90° flip angle; 256 × 128 matrix; two signals acquired (no phase wrap); 20–26-cm field of view; 4–6-mm section thickness; and a 1-mm section interval, with a bandwidth of ±32 kHz. Finally, we obtained delayed axial fat-suppressed spoiled GRE images by using parameters similar to those used to obtain the precontrast images.

All images were retrospectively reviewed by two or more conferring staff radiologists (E.S.S., P.R., M.P.B.) with an interest in urologic imaging who were unaware of the surgical and pathologic outcomes. Retrospective MR interpretation was by consensus.

Image reviewers noted the location of the lesion, the imaging plane in which the lesion was best delineated, whether the lesion was of primarily homogeneous or heterogeneous signal intensity, and whether the lesion appeared cystic or solid. Reviewers also compared the signal intensity of the lesion with that of the normal renal cortex on T1-weighted, T2-weighted, dynamic, and delayed postgadolinium images.

Imaging findings that could affect the decision to perform partial nephrectomy were evaluated. These included tumor size in three planes; tumor location within the kidney; presence of a pseudocapsule (a thin band of fibrous tissue and compressed renal parenchyma surrounding the lesion); tumor invasion of the renal sinus fat, collecting system, renal vein, or perinephric fat; presence of lymphadenopathy; and morphologic and physiologic status of the contralateral kidney. Partial nephrectomy was accomplished by means of either wedge resection, guillotine excision (removal of a renal pole), or tumor enucleation. Imaging findings were correlated with surgical and pathologic data.

RESULTS

On MR images, the 41 renal lesions were 0.9–5.8 cm, with a mean size of 2.5 × 2.6 × 2.5 cm. Fifteen lesions (37%) were in the upper pole, 13 (32%) in the interpolar region, and 13 (32%) in the lower pole. Two lesions (5%) were primarily exophytic, six (15%) were primarily intrarenal, and 33 (80%) had both exophytic and intrarenal components.

Twenty of 38 (53%) patients had an absolute indication for partial nephrectomy: bilateral neoplasms (*n* = 11 [27%]) or tumor in a solitary kidney (*n* = 9 [22%]). Bilateral synchronous renal neoplasms were accurately diagnosed in 11 of the 11 patients (100%), including both patients with von Hippel-Lindau syndrome. All 11 of these patients underwent radical nephrectomy and contralateral partial nephrectomy. Of these 11 patients, 10 (91%) had renal cell carcinomas, while one (9%) had a renal cell carcinoma and a contralateral transitional cell carcinoma. The nine additional patients (22%) for whom partial nephrectomy was absolutely indicated had previously undergone nephrectomy and subsequently developed lesions in the remaining solitary kidney.

Of the remaining 18 (44%) patients in our study, two (5%) had renal insufficiency (serum creatinine level >1.5 mg/dL [>133 µmol/L]), a relative indication for partial nephrectomy. Partial nephrectomy in the remaining 16 (39%) patients was performed on an elective basis.

Prior to MR imaging, 25 of 38 patients (66%) had undergone computed tomography (CT). Most of these examinations were performed at other institutions, and many were not performed with a dedicated renal protocol: thin-section (5-mm-section) renal imaging before and after the power-injected, bolus administration of iodinated contrast material. CT images from 16 (64%) of the 25 patients were prospectively interpreted as being diagnostic of renal cell carcinoma, and MR imaging was performed to resolve issues of staging. In the nine (36%) remaining patients, MR imaging was performed to characterize lesions detected at earlier cross-sectional imaging.

Thirteen of our 38 patients (34%) had not previously undergone CT. These were largely patients who had had prior renal cell carcinomas who were unable or unwilling to receive iodinated contrast material.

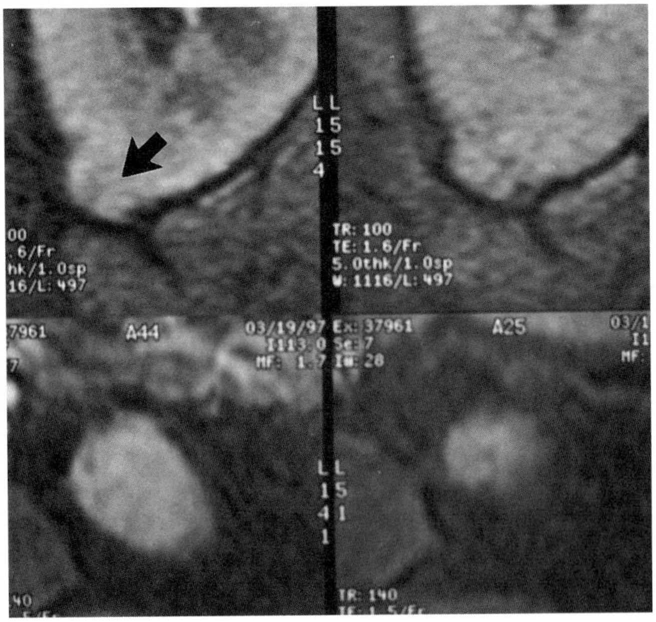

Figure 3. Exophytic lower-pole renal cell carcinoma in a 62-year-old man. Top: Coronal breath-hold T1-weighted fat-suppressed spoiled GRE images (100/1.6). Bottom: Axial fat-suppressed delayed spoiled GRE images (140/1.5). The coronal images reveal a small, slightly exophytic renal cell carcinoma (arrow). The polar lesion is difficult, if not impossible, to appreciate on the corresponding axial images.

Thirty-three of the lesions (80%) were renal cell carcinomas, five (12%) were oncocytic neoplasms, two (5%) were hemorrhagic cysts, and one (2%) was an angiomyolipoma (Fig 1).

Thirty-six of the 41 lesions (88%) were of heterogeneous signal intensity with at least one pulse sequence, while five (12%) were homogeneous with all pulse sequences. Three lesions (7%) were considered primarily cystic, and each of these proved to be cystic renal cell carcinoma.

On T1-weighted images, 21 of the 41 lesions (51%) were primarily hypointense to the normal renal cortex, 15 (37%) lesions were isointense, and five (12%) were hyperintense.

On T2-weighted images, 20 of the 41 lesions (49%) were hyperintense to the normal cortex, 15 lesions (37%) were hypointense, and six (15%) were isointense.

T1-weighted fat-suppressed spoiled GRE images obtained during dynamic gadopentetate dimeglumine injection showed that 30 of 40 lesions (75%) enhanced to a lesser degree than the normal renal parenchyma. Ten of the 40 lesions (25%) were isointense to the normal cortex on these images, and no lesions were hyperintense. Dynamic imaging of one lesion was not performed.

On delayed postgadolinium images, 33 of the 41 lesions (80%) continued to enhance less than normal renal parenchyma. Six lesions (15%) remained isointense, and two lesions (5%) became hyperintense.

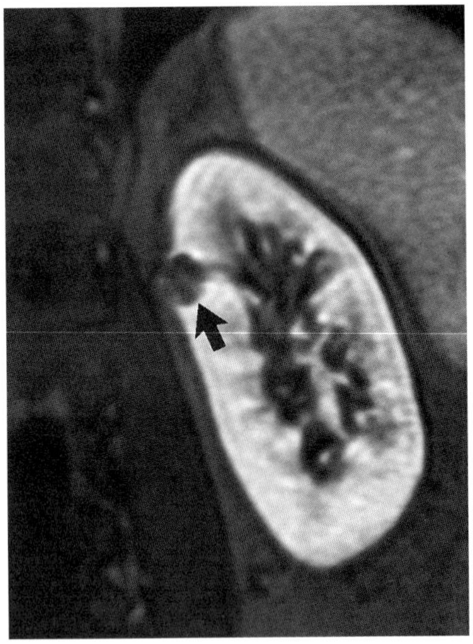

Figure 4. Peripheral renal cell carcinoma in a 38-year-old man. Coronal spoiled GRE image (125/2.9; flip angle, 90°) obtained following the dynamic administration of gadopentetate dimeglumine. The 1-cm peripheral, medial renal cell carcinoma (arrow) did not invade the perinephric fat, the renal sinus fat, or the renal collecting system.

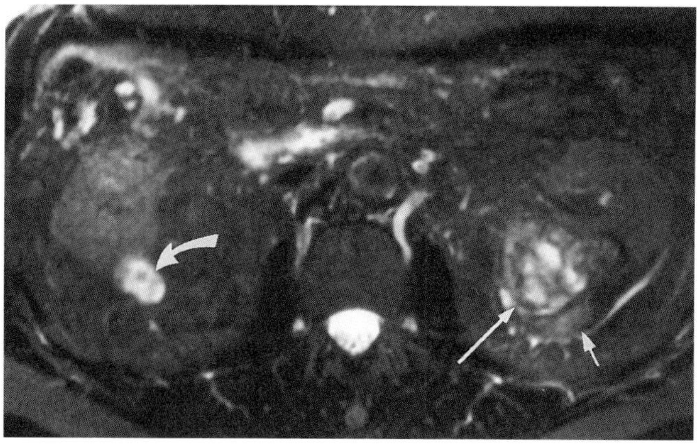

Figure 5. Bilateral renal cell carcinoma in a 71-year-old man. Axial fast spin-echo T2-weighted fat-suppressed image (7,058/120 [effective]). The large left renal cell carcinoma (long straight arrow) was excised at radical nephrectomy. Pathologic sectioning revealed the suspected left perinephric fat invasion (short straight arrow). The smaller, right-sided renal cell carcinoma (curved arrow) was also excised at partial nephrectomy.

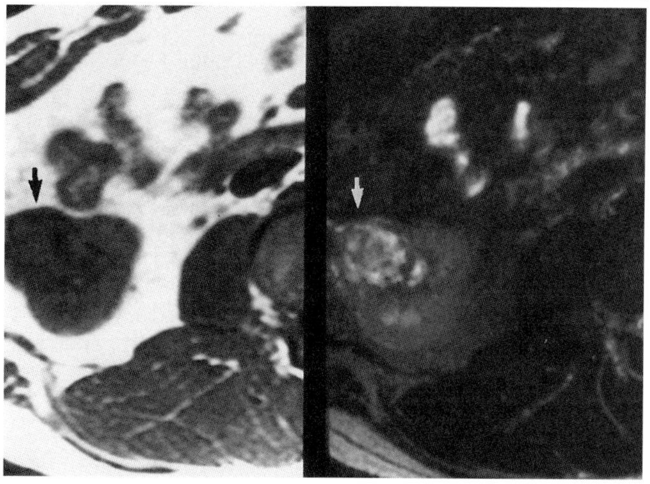

Figure 6. Suspected renal collecting system invasion by renal cell carcinoma in a 44-year-old man. Left: Axial T1-weighted image (450/10). Right: Axial fast spin-echo fat-suppressed T2-weighted image (4,500/153 [effective]). This renal cell carcinoma (arrow) was thought to invade the renal collecting system. At pathologic sectioning, the tumor was immediately adjacent to the renal collecting system, without invasion.

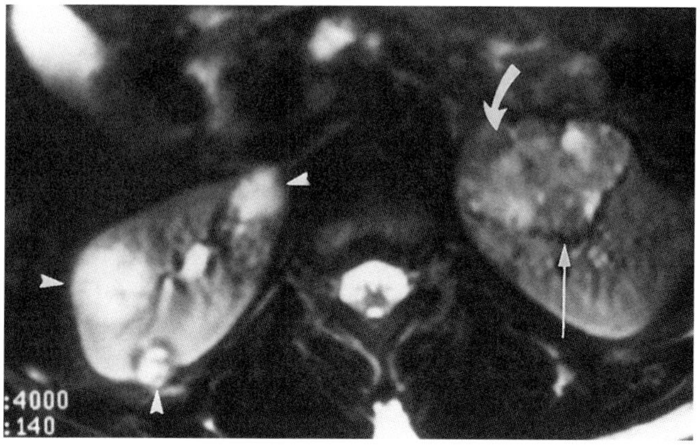

Figure 7. Bilateral renal cell carcinomas in a 28-year-old man with von Hippel-Lindau syndrome. Axial fast spin-echo T2-weighted fat-suppressed image (4,000/140). This patient had three renal cell carcinomas in the right kidney (arrowheads), which necessitated radical nephrectomy. The large left renal cell carcinoma (curved arrow), which displays a partial pseudocapsule (straight arrow), was excised at partial nephrectomy. Suspected invasion of the renal collecting system and renal sinus fat was pathologically confirmed.

On both T1- and T2-weighted images, both of the hemorrhagic cysts were hyperintense and enhanced less than the surrounding renal parenchyma.

The appearance of the oncocytomas was variable. Two of the five (40%) were primarily homogeneous in signal intensity, while three of the five (60%) were heterogeneous. On T1-weighted images, three oncocytomas (60%) were hypointense, and two (40%) were isointense; on T2-weighted images, three (60%) were hyperintense, and two (40%) were hypointense. In the dynamic postgadolinium phase, three (60%) were isointense, and two (40%) were hypointense. In the delayed phase, one lesion (20%) remained isointense, while four (80%) were hypointense.

The angiomyolipoma was heterogeneous in appearance and was isointense on T1-weighted images but hypointense on T2-weighted and on postgadolinium images (Fig 1).

Twenty-four of 41 lesions (59%) exhibited a pseudocapsule (Fig 2). Pseudocapsules were identified in 20 of 33 renal cell carcinomas (61%), two of five oncocytic neoplasms (40%), one of two hemorrhagic cysts (50%), and one of one angiomyolipoma (100%). Pseudocapsules were best seen on T2-weighted images (13 of 24 [54%]) and on postgadolinium spoiled GRE images (10 of 24 [42%]). One pseudocapsule (4%) was best seen on nonenhanced T1-weighted images.

Dynamic and delayed postcontrast images were most helpful in lesion identification and characterization. Approximately half of the lesions were best seen in the axial plane (19 of 41 lesions [46%]), and half were best seen in the coronal plane (22 of 41 lesions [54%]), although most lesions were conspicuous in all imaging planes. Sagittal imaging was performed in two patients with polar masses. In these cases, sagittal and coronal images were judged to be more useful than axial images (Fig 3).

Lesion extent also was best defined on gadolinium-enhanced axial and coronal images. The perinephric fat was correctly demonstrated to be uninvolved by tumor in 38 cases (true-negative findings, 93%) (Fig 4). One case of suspected perinephric fat invasion was not confirmed with pathologic evaluation (false-positive finding, 2%). Two cases (true-positive finding, 5%) of suspected perinephric fat invasion were confirmed at pathologic review (Fig 5).

The renal collecting system was accurately shown to be uninvolved by parenchymal tumor in 39 cases (true-negative

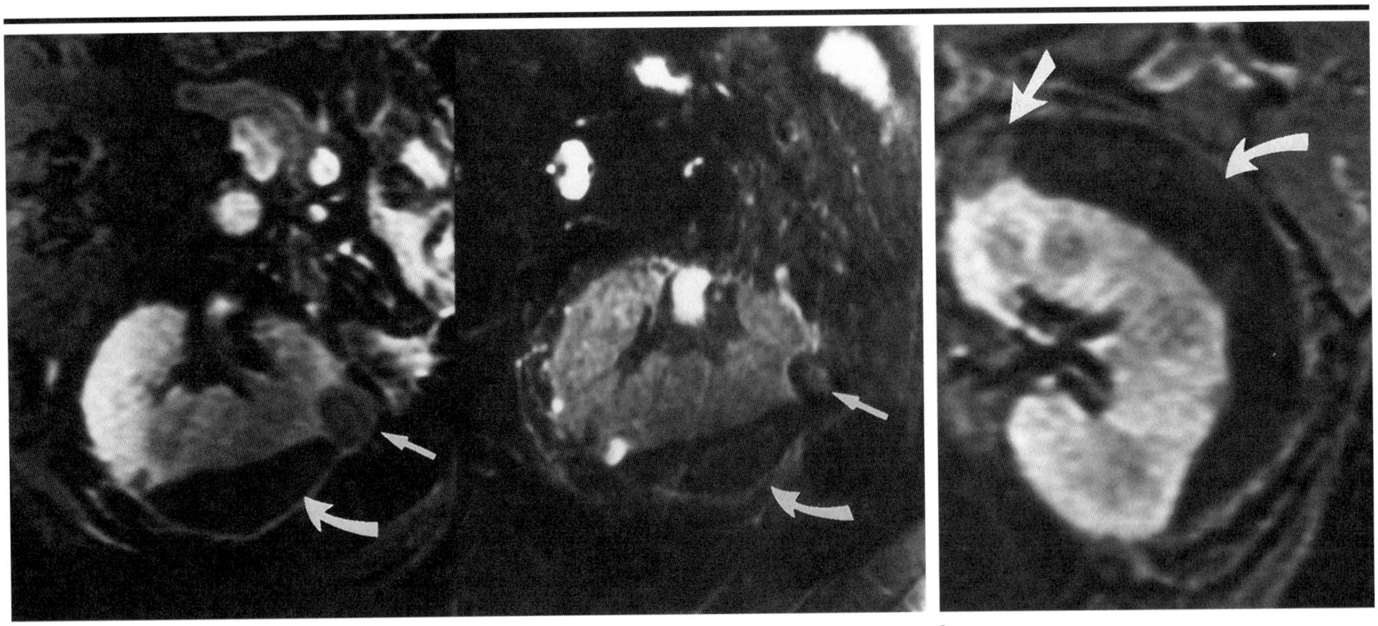

a. b.

Figure 8. Multifocal renal cell carcinoma complicated by subcapsular hemorrhage in a 59-year-old man. **(a)** Left: Axial postgadolinium fat-suppressed spoiled GRE image (100/1.6). Right: Axial fast spin-echo fat-suppressed T2-weighted image (6,666/140 [effective]). The exophytic renal cell carcinoma in the left interpolar region (straight arrow), complicated by subcapsular hemorrhage (curved arrow), was identified at MR imaging. At the time of partial nephrectomy, however, only an upper pole lesion was identified at intraoperative ultrasonography, and only this lesion was excised at partial nephrectomy. This interpolar lesion was seen again at follow-up imaging, which necessitated radical nephrectomy. Although tumor multifocality was not appreciated at the time of prospective reading, in retrospect, multifocality was depicted on the initial study. **(b)** Coronal postgadolinium spoiled GRE T1-weighted image (80/1.6; flip angle, 80°) demonstrates the upper pole lesion (straight arrow) not identified at the initial interpretation. Subcapsular hemorrhage (curved arrow) complicated lesion detection.

findings, 95%). One case of collecting system invasion was correctly identified (true-positive finding, 2%), but a second case of suspected invasion was not confirmed pathologically (false-positive finding, 2%) (Fig 6).

The renal sinus fat adjacent to the lesion was correctly shown to be uninvolved by tumor in 31 cases (true-negative findings, 76%). Three cases of renal sinus fat invasion were correctly identified (true-positive findings, 7%). Two of these patients had von Hippel-Lindau syndrome, and one had limited renal function; so, partial nephrectomy was performed despite suspected renal sinus fat invasion (Fig 7). In six additional cases, suspected renal sinus fat invasion was not confirmed (false-positive findings, 15%). One case of renal sinus fat invasion was not identified at MR imaging (false-negative finding, 2%).

The renal veins were correctly shown to be free of tumor involvement in all cases. Retroperitoneal lymph nodes larger than 1.0 cm in short-axis diameter were seen in one case involving the inferior aortocaval and the ipsilateral common iliac chains. These nodes were unchanged in size at a 1-year follow-up examination and are presumed to be reactive.

Surgery was technically successful in all cases; tumor removal was performed by means of wedge resection in 25 of 41 cases (61%), guillotine excision in 14 cases (34%), and enucleation in two cases (5%). Surgical resection margins were clear in all cases.

Follow-up imaging was available in 34 of 35 patients (97%) who had renal cell carcinomas or oncocytic neoplasms: by means of MR imaging in 31 and by means of CT in three (mean follow-up, 19.7 months; range, 1–71 months). Thirty-one of these 34 patients (91%) had no evidence of residual tumor or tumor recurrence. One patient with von Hippel-Lindau syndrome developed an ipsilateral renal cell carcinoma 31 months after partial nephrectomy, which necessitated subsequent radical nephrectomy. Another patient developed a metachronous renal cell carcinoma in the contralateral kidney that was identified 21 months following partial nephrectomy. On the third patient's initial MR image, the renal neoplasm was complicated by extensive subcapsular hemorrhage. A baseline MR imaging examination following partial nephrectomy demonstrated multifocal renal cell carcinoma, which necessitated subsequent radical nephrectomy. In retrospect, the multifocality of this patient's disease was identifiable on the initial MR image (Fig 8).

DISCUSSION

As radiation therapy and chemotherapy are of limited therapeutic utility for renal cell carcinoma (4,5), surgery has long been the mainstay of treatment for patients with localized disease. For many years, radical nephrectomy has been the accepted urologic standard of care.

Recently, investigators in several studies have examined the efficacy of partial nephrectomy for select renal neoplasms, namely, those which occur in solitary kidneys, synchronously in both kidneys, or in those patients with poor renal function. Rates of local tumor recurrence following partial nephrectomy range from 4% to 10% (6), but overall patient survival has not substantially differed from that of patients with similar-stage disease who have undergone radical nephrectomy (7–12).

These findings have stimulated interest in performing elective partial nephrectomy in patients with small renal neoplasms and normal contralateral kidneys.

Arguments against this therapeutic philosophy are based on the known 7%–11% incidence of tumor multifocality and the potential of incomplete resection of the malignancy (13,14). However, the rate of local tumor recurrence following partial nephrectomy has been shown to be approximately 2% at 3–6 years and is similar to the rate of metachronous renal cell carcinoma in the contralateral kidney following radical nephrectomy (15,16). Furthermore, the rate of multicentricity for tumors 3 cm or smaller has been shown to be less than 3% (14), which makes partial nephrectomy a reasonable treatment for patients with small renal neoplasms.

CT and MR imaging are both effective modalities for staging renal cell carcinoma. MR imaging has been shown to be slightly more accurate in staging than CT, especially for the evaluation of tumor involvement of the perinephric fat, the renal vein, and the adjacent organs (17,18). US, although useful in screening for the presence of renal tumors, is limited in the staging of renal cell carcinoma because of the difficulty in assessing retroperitoneal lymphadenopathy (19).

Thin-section, helical CT can be used to accurately stage renal cell carcinoma. Although CT cannot be used to reliably differentiate stage I disease (tumor confined by the renal capsule) from stage II disease (tumor spread to the perinephric fat), this distinction has not historically been critical, as the perinephric fat is routinely excised as part of a radical nephrectomy (19). If, however, partial nephrectomy is contemplated, it is desirable to know preoperatively if the perinephric fat is invaded by cancer, as this may affect the surgical approach. Findings of one study (20) have shown MR imaging to be slightly superior to CT in making this determination.

The detection of tumor thrombus involving the renal vein and inferior vena cava excludes the possibility of a curative partial nephrectomy. In one study, CT was 78% accurate for the detection of tumor in the renal vein and 96% accurate for the detection of involvement of the inferior vena cava (21). MR imaging is generally considered to be superior to CT in the evaluation of these venous structures (17,19,22), although achieved results are highly dependent on equipment and technique. Although tumor thrombus may be suspected on conventional T1- and T2-weighted images, nonenhanced or contrast-enhanced MR angiographic sequences can be used to confirm the presence of renal venous or inferior vena caval thrombus.

Identification of small synchronous renal cell carcinomas has proved difficult. Intraoperative US is no more sensitive than preoperative CT scanning for detection of small lesions (23). Tumors smaller than 1 cm have not been reliably detected and characterized with either CT or MR imaging (24), although there were limitations in several studies with high failure rates for the radiologic detection of synchronous renal cell carcinoma. Investigators in one such study found that neither MR nor CT could reliably depict multifocality if lesions were smaller than 2 cm, although dynamic postgadolinium images were not obtained (24). In another study, radiologically undetected multifocal disease was reported in half of all nephrectomized kidneys in patients who would have been candidates for partial nephrectomy; however, the authors (25) fail to mention which radiologic studies were obtained and how they were performed.

Contrast-enhanced, surface-coil MR imaging is well suited for evaluating renal lesions in which partial nephrectomy is being considered. The direct multiplanar imaging capabilities of MR imaging make tumor size easily measurable in three planes. In particular, the relationship of polar lesions to the normal adjacent renal parenchyma can be difficult to define on axial images, whether they be CT or MR images (Fig 3). Sagittal and coronal images considerably assist in defining the relationship of polar masses to the adjacent normal renal parenchyma.

Lesion conspicuity on dynamic and delayed postgadolinium images is generally very high, owing to both the differential enhancement of tumor and normal renal parenchyma and to the inherently high soft-tissue MR imaging contrast. Tumor heterogeneity, thought to represent hemorrhage or necrosis (26), also adds to lesion conspicuity.

In our study, MR imaging had reasonable accuracy for evaluating possible involvement of perinephric fat, renal sinus fat, and the renal collecting system. MR imaging was particularly accurate in identifying the true-negative findings in the group, correctly depicting the perinephric fat (38 of 38 cases [100%]), the renal sinus fat (31 of 34 cases [91%]), and the renal collecting system (39 of 39 cases [100%]) to be uninvolved by parenchymal tumor. Among our patients, microscopic infiltration of the renal sinus fat by renal cell carcinoma was not appreciated in one patient, who thus had a false-negative diagnosis. This patient nevertheless underwent a technically successful partial nephrectomy with clear tumor margins and underwent an unremarkable follow-up MR imaging examination at 6 months.

Only one false-negative finding was generated, and that was of microscopic renal sinus fat invasion not detected on MR images. Therefore, in our patient population, the negative predictive value of MR imaging was 100% for invasion of the perinephric fat (38 of 38 cases) and for the collecting system (39 of 39 cases) and 97% (31 of 32 cases) for involvement of the renal sinus fat.

Several false-positive diagnoses were made (perinephric fat, one of 41 cases [2%]; renal sinus fat, six of 41 cases [15%]; collecting system, one of 41 cases [2%]). As with all imaging modalities, it is extremely difficult with MR imaging to determine whether malignant tissue and normal tissue are merely adjacent to one another or local invasion has occurred.

No attempt was made to define the sensitivity and specificity of MR imaging for the determination of invasion of the perinephric fat, the renal sinus fat, and the collecting system. The population chosen for this study is not appropriate for such evaluation, as patients with clear invasion of these tissues on preoperative imaging studies would generally not have been considered for partial nephrectomy unless other circumstances forced consideration of partial nephrectomy. Also, at our institution, renal lesions preoperatively evaluated with MR imaging tend to be "problem" lesions, those in which diagnosis or staging is uncertain at contrast-enhanced CT.

Twenty-four of 41 lesions (59%) studied demonstrated a pseudocapsule, or a thin, hypointense rim surrounding the lesion (Fig 2). Pseudocapsules consist of fibrous tissue and compressed renal parenchyma and have been associated with lower tumor grades. Findings of several studies have demonstrated that pseudocapsules are most often seen on T2-weighted images (27,28). Our study findings confirm this. When a pseudocapsule was present, it was best seen on T2-weighted images (13 of 24 lesions [54%]). A minority of pseudocapsules were best seen on postgadolinium spoiled GRE images (10 of 24 lesions [42%]). One pseudocapsule (one of 24 lesions [4%]) was best delineated on nonenhanced T1-weighted images.

Although most of the lesions in our series were renal cell carcinomas (33 of 41 lesions [80%]), several other lesions were also excised. Five were oncocytic neoplasms, which are considered radiologically indistinguishable from renal cell carcinomas (3,29). The oncocytomas we studied displayed no MR imaging characteristics that would have allowed them to have been reliably distinguished from renal cell carcinomas. However, all of the oncocytic neoplasms in our study displayed cellular atypia, and partial nephrectomy has been advocated as the treatment of choice (22).

Two hemorrhagic cysts were removed by means of partial nephrectomy in our study. Both of these lesions were prospectively and retrospectively suspected to be hemorrhagic cysts at MR imaging, although a small focus of renal cell carcinoma could not be radiologically excluded. In the patients with these lesions, the contribution of MR imaging to patient treatment was the confirmation that these lesions could be excised by using partial nephrectomy.

Stage III or IV renal cell carcinoma is also well depicted on MR images (22). In particular, MR imaging has advantages over CT in evaluating the renal vein and inferior vena cava for tumor thrombus (17,30). In all of our cases, the renal vein was well seen and was correctly shown to be free of thrombus.

Lymph nodes larger than 1 cm were present in one case. Because these were inferior to the renal hilum and in the ipsilateral common iliac chain, they were thought to be in a distribution atypical for metastatic renal cell carcinoma. The patient's renal cell carcinoma was successfully extirpated at partial nephrectomy, and these nodes have been stable for the ensuing 4 years.

The contrast-enhanced, surface-coil MR imaging characteristics of lesions amenable to partial nephrectomy have been described. Although our evaluation is retrospective, in many cases the patients in this study underwent partial nephrectomy because preoperative MR images suggested that the renal lesions could be safely extirpated in this fashion. Heightened interest in the urologic community in partial nephrectomy will make it increasingly important for radiologists to determine preoperatively if a lesion can be successfully removed by means of partial nephrectomy. Contrast-enhanced MR imaging seems well suited for making that determination with a reasonable degree of accuracy.

References

1. Block NL, Ciancio G. Conservative surgical treatment of renal cell carcinoma: the University of Miami experience. J Fla Med Assoc 1995; 82:607–611.
2. Polascik TJ, Pound C, Meng MV, Partin AW, Marshall FF. Partial nephrectomy: technique, complications and pathological findings. J Urol 1995; 154:1312–1318.
3. Ornstein DK, Arcangeli CG, Andriole GL. Renal masses: urologic management. Magn Reson Imaging Clin N Am 1997; 5:1–12.
4. Yagoda A, Abi-Rached B, Petrylak D. Chemotherapy for advanced renal cell carcinoma: 1983–1993. Semin Oncol 1995; 22:42–60.
5. DeKernion JB, Mukamel E. Selection of initial therapy for renal cell carcinoma. Cancer 1987; 60:539–546.
6. Motzer RJ, Bander NH, Nanus DM. Renal cell carcinoma. N Engl J Med 1996: 335: 865–875.
7. D'Armiento M, Damiano R, Feleppa B, Perdona S, Oriani G, De Sio M. Elective conservative surgery for renal carcinoma versus radical nephrectomy: a prospective study. Br J Urol 1997; 79:15–19.
8. Morgan WR, Zincke H. Progression and survival after renal-conserving surgery for renal cell carcinoma: experience in 104 patients and extended follow-up. J Urol 1990; 144:852–857.
9. Steinbach F, Stöckle M, Hohenfellner R. Current controversies in nephron sparing surgery for renal cell carcinoma. World J Urol 1995; 13:163–165.
10. Provet J, Tessler A, Brown J, Golimbu M, Bosniak M, Morales P. Partial nephrectomy for renal cell carcinoma: indications, results, and implications. J Urol 1991; 145:472–476.
11. Licht MR, Novick AC, Goormastic M. Nephron-sparing surgery in incidental versus suspected renal cell carcinoma. J Urol 1994; 152:39–42.
12. Steinbach F, Stöckle M, Müller SC, et al. Conservative surgery of renal cell tumors in 140 patients: 21 years of experience. J Urol 1992; 148:24–29.
13. Saiki S, Kinouchi T, Meguro N, et al. Multicentricity and concomitant tumors in renal cell carcinoma: analysis by serial section of resected kidneys. Hinyokika Kiyo 1995; 41:725–729. [Japanese]
14. Nissenkorn I, Bernheim J. Multicentricity in renal cell carcinoma. J Urol 1995; 153: 620–622.
15. Motzer RJ, Bander NH, Nanus DM. Renal cell carcinoma. N Engl J Med 1996; 335: 865–875.
16. Herr HW. Partial nephrectomy for renal cell carcinoma with a normal opposite kidney. Cancer 1994; 73:160–162.
17. Semelka RC, Shoenut JP, Magro CM, Kroeker MA, MacMahon R, Greenberg HM. Renal cancer staging: comparison of contrast-enhanced CT and gadolinium-enhanced fat-suppressed spin-echo and gradient-echo MR imaging. JMRI 1993; 3:597–602.
18. Patel SK, Stack CM, Turner DA. Magnetic resonance imaging in staging of renal cell carcinoma. RadioGraphics 1987; 7:703–728.
19. Bechtold RE, Zagoria RJ. Imaging approach to staging of renal cell carcinoma. Urol Clin North Am 1997; 24:507–522.
20. Fein AB, Lee JDT, Balfe DM, et al. Diagnosis and staging of renal cell carcinoma: a comparison of MR imaging and CT. AJR 1987; 148:749–753.
21. Johnson CD, Dunnick NR, Cohan RH, et al. Renal adenocarcinoma: CT staging of 100 tumors. AJR 1987; 148:59–63.
22. Choyke PL. Detection and staging of renal cancer. Magn Reson Imaging Clin North Am 1997; 5:29–47.
23. Campbell SC, Fichtner J, Novick AC, et al. Intraoperative evaluation of renal cell carcinoma: a prospective study of the role of ultrasonography and histopathological frozen sections. J Urol 1996; 155:1191–1195.
24. Gschwend JE, Vogel U, Bader C, Mattfeldt T, Hautmann RE. Predictive value of magnetic resonance imaging and computerized tomography for conservative renal surgery in an ex vivo tumor enucleation study followed by step-sectioning. J Urol 1996; 155:451–454.
25. Lerner SE, Tsai H, Flanigan RC, Trump DL, Fleischmann J. Renal cell carcinoma: considerations for nephron-sparing surgery. Urology 1991; 45:574–577.
26. Wagner BJ. The kidney: radiologic-pathologic correlation. Magn Reson Imaging Clin North Am 1997; 5:13–28.
27. Takahashi S, Ueda J, Furukawa T, et al. Renal cell carcinoma: preoperative assessment for enucleative surgery with angiography, CT, and MRI. J Comput Assist Tomogr 1996; 20:863–870.
28. Yamashita Y, Honda S, Nishiharu T, Urata J, Takahashi M. Detection of pseudocapsule of renal cell carcinoma with MR imaging and CT. AJR 1996; 166:1151–1155.
29. Licht MR. Renal adenoma and oncocytoma. Semin Urol Oncol 1995; 13:262–266.
30. Narumi Y, Hricak H, Presti JC Jr, et al. MR imaging evaluation of renal cell carcinoma. Abdom Imaging 1997; 2:216–225.

Pheochromocytomas: Imaging with 2-[Fluorine-18]fluoro-2-deoxy-D-glucose PET[1]

Barry L. Shulkin, MD
Norman W. Thompson, MD
Brahm Shapiro, MD
Isaac R. Francis, MD
James C. Sisson, MD

Index terms:
Adrenal gland, emission CT (ECT), 86.12161, 86.12162, 86.12163
Fluorine, radioactive metaiodobenzylguanidine (MIBG)
Pheochromocytoma, 67.3163, 86.328

Radiology 1999; 212:35–41

Abbreviations:
FDG = 2-[fluorine-18]fluoro-2-deoxy-D-glucose
MIBG = metaiodobenzylguanidine
SUV = standardized uptake value

[1] From the Departments of Internal Medicine, Division of Nuclear Medicine (B.L.S., B.S., J.C.S.), Surgery (N.W.T.), and Radiology (I.R.F.), University of Michigan Medical Center, 1500 E Medical Center Dr, Ann Arbor, MI 48109. Received July 9, 1998; revision requested August 18; revision received September 16; accepted December 16. Supported in part by grant CA54216 from the National Cancer Institute and grant MO1 RR 00042 from the University of Michigan Clinical Research Center. **Address reprint requests to** B.L.S. (e-mail: *bshulkin@umich.edu*).

Author contributions:
Guarantor of integrity of entire study, B.L.S.; study concepts, B.L.S., J.C.S.; study design, B.L.S.; definition of intellectual content, B.L.S., J.C.S.; literature research, B.L.S., I.R.F.; clinical studies, B.L.S., J.C.S., B.S., N.W.T.; data acquisition, B.L.S., J.C.S., N.W.T.; data analysis, B.L.S., J.C.S., B.S.; statistical analysis, B.L.S.; manuscript preparation, editing, and review, all authors.

PURPOSE: To assess the sensitivity of positron emission tomography (PET) with 2-[fluorine-18]fluoro-2-deoxy-D-glucose (FDG) in pheochromocytomas and, secondarily, to compare images obtained with FDG PET to those obtained with metaiodobenzylguanidine (MIBG) scintigraphy.

MATERIALS AND METHODS: Twenty-nine patients with one or more known or subsequently proved pheochromocytomas underwent FDG PET (35 scans) and MIBG scintigraphy (35 scans). Tumor uptake of FDG was quantified on positive PET scans.

RESULTS: Tumor uptake of FDG was detected in 22 of 29 patients. Most benign (seven of 12 patients) and most malignant (15 of 17 patients) pheochromocytomas and their metastases avidly concentrated FDG. In four patients whose pheochromocytomas failed to accumulate MIBG, uptake of FDG in the tumors was intense. For the majority of the 16 patients whose tumors concentrated both agents, however, ratings for MIBG images compared to FDG PET images for delineation of the tumor in comparison to background and normal organ accumulation were superior for nine patients (56%) and as good or better for 14 (88%).

CONCLUSION: Most pheochromocytomas accumulate FDG. Uptake is found in a greater percentage of malignant than benign pheochromocytomas. FDG PET is especially useful in defining the distribution of those pheochromocytomas that fail to concentrate MIBG.

Pheochromocytomas are tumors derived from the sympathetic nervous system and related structures (1–4). Pheochromocytomas cause hypertension, along with a variety of signs and symptoms of catecholamine excess, and subsequent morbidity from the direct effects of the tumor secretory products dopamine, norepinephrine, and epinephrine. If the pheochromocytomas are identified, the attendant disorders are usually curable by means of surgical resection of the tumor. If undiagnosed or improperly treated, pheochromocytoma can be fatal. Thus, its detection is critical to patient treatment. The presence of pheochromocytoma is established biochemically by measuring plasma and urine catecholamines and their metabolites (1–4).

A variety of imaging techniques have been used to locate pheochromocytoma, each of which exhibits important drawbacks. Since approximately 90% of pheochromocytomas occur within the adrenal glands, computed tomography (CT) of the adrenal glands has been found efficacious (5,6). However, CT depicts only anatomic abnormalities. Occasional false-positive studies can lead to unnecessary surgery (7). Although CT in the past has been less accurate than other approaches for the detection of extraadrenal lesions, to our knowledge, there are no recent studies comparing the accuracy of CT with that of other imaging techniques. Magnetic resonance (MR) imaging, like CT, provides excellent anatomic detail and has the advantages of lack of ionizing radiation, the potential for better tissue characterization, and the capacity for imaging in multiple planes without the need for intravenous iodinated contrast material (8,9). The effect of new, shorter imaging sequences has yet to be determined.

The procedure of choice for the localization of pheochromocytoma is currently scintigraphy with metaiodobenzylguanidine (MIBG) (9–13). Not all pheochromocytomas concentrate MIBG, however, and MIBG uptake can be adversely affected by a variety of medications. Thus, there is a need for another procedure that has either a higher sensitivity or will at least supplement currently available techniques (14). Our preliminary experience

TABLE 1
Benign Pheochromocytomas

Patient No./ Age (y)	Comparison	Findings	SUV	Tumor-to–Reference-Organ Ratio		Better Images	Diameter (cm) of Principal Tumor
				FDG	MIBG		
1/21	^{131}I MIBG planar	False-negative MIBG scan; uptake of FDG into right adrenal pheochromocytoma; reference organ, liver	8.1	3.1	NA	FDG	4.0
2/70	^{123}I MIBG SPECT	False-negative FDG scan; uptake of MIBG into right adrenal pheochromocytoma; reference organ, liver	NA	NA	1.0	MIBG	5.0
3/78	^{123}I MIBG SPECT	Uptake of both FDG and MIBG into into left adrenal pheochromocytoma; reference organ, liver	5.8	1.3	2.1	MIBG	4.0
4/75	^{123}I MIBG SPECT	Uptake of both FDG and MIBG into left adrenal pheochromocytoma; reference organ, liver	3.7	1.2	2.9	MIBG	5.0
5/48	^{123}I MIBG SPECT	False-negative FDG scan; slight uptake of MIBG into right adrenal pheochromocytoma; reference organ, liver	NA	NA	0.9	MIBG	2.0
6/81	^{123}I MIBG SPECT	False-negative FDG scan; uptake of MIBG into right adrenal pheochromocytoma; reference organ, liver	NA	NA	1.8	MIBG	3.0
7/26	^{123}I MIBG SPECT	Uptake of both FDG and MIBG into cardiac pheochromocytoma; reference organ, lung	11.8	8.8	2.6	MIBG	4.0
8/25	^{131}I MIBG planar	False-negative FDG scan; uptake of MIBG into left adrenal pheochromocytoma; reference organ, liver	NA	NA	0.9	MIBG	5.0
9/46	^{123}I MIBG SPECT	False-negative MIBG scan; uptake of FDG into periaortic pheochromocytoma adjacent to left kidney; reference organ, liver	13.4	5.5	NA	FDG	2.5
10/32	^{123}I MIBG SPECT	Uptake of both FDG and MIBG into pheochromocytoma at aortic bifurcation; reference organ, abdominal soft tissue	2.6	2.4	2.1	FDG	3.0
11/51	^{123}I MIBG SPECT	False-negative FDG scan; uptake of MIBG into right adrenal pheochromocytoma; reference organ, liver	NA	NA	1.1	MIBG	1.5
12/76	^{123}I MIBG SPECT	Uptake of both FDG and MIBG into right adrenal pheochromocytoma; reference organ, liver	4.6	2.6	1.9	MIBG	3.0

Note.—NA = not applicable.

suggests that positron emission tomography (PET) with 2-[fluorine-18]fluoro-2-deoxy-D-glucose (FDG) has promise, and we previously reported the depiction with FDG PET of two pheochromocytomas that did not accumulate MIBG (15). The purpose of this study was to estimate the sensitivity of FDG PET for pheochromocytomas and to compare findings with MIBG scintigraphy to demonstrate the complementary role of FDG PET.

MATERIALS AND METHODS

Patients

This study was approved by our institutional review board. Twenty-nine patients with one or more known or subsequently proved pheochromocytomas (35 FDG PET scans) were the subjects of this study. Patients and their studies are described in Tables 1–4. Twelve patients had benign pheochromocytoma (patients 1–12 [four men, eight women; age range, 21–81 years; mean age, 52.4 years]). Seventeen patients had malignant pheochromocytoma (patients 13–29 [14 male and three female patients; age range, 16–72 years; mean age, 40.4 years]). Patients 13, 15, 18, 20, 21, and 26 were examined twice. None of the patients were receiving medications known to interfere with the uptake of MIBG (14).

PET Examinations

The procedure was explained, and written informed consent was obtained from the adult patients or from a parent of the pediatric patient 15. After an overnight or 4-hour fast, patients were placed within the PET scanner (models CTI 931-08/12 or Exact; Siemens Medical Systems, Hoffman Estates, Ill) with the principal tumor centered in the field of view. Positioning was accomplished on the basis of physical findings and in conjunction with findings at CT, MR imaging, and MIBG scintigraphy. After acquisition of a 10–20-minute transmission scan for attenuation correction, with use of retractable germanium 68 sources, 370 MBq (10 mCi) FDG was administered intravenously (16). Patient 15 received 305 MBq (8 mCi) FDG.

Images of the tumor were acquired dynamically for 50–60 minutes (patients 1–7, 13, 15, 18, and 29). Data obtained with the dynamic sequence were reconstructed into transverse cross-sectional images by means of filtered back projection and a

TABLE 2
Findings at FDG PET and MIBG Scintigraphy in Benign Pheochromocytomas

FDG	MIBG Positive	MIBG Negative
Positive	5	2
Negative	5	0

Note.—Data are the number of patients.

TABLE 3
Malignant Pheochromocytomas

Patient No./ Age (y)	Comparison	Findings	SUV	Tumor-to-Reference-Organ Ratio		Better Images	Diameter (cm) of Principal Tumor
				FDG	MIBG		
13/41	^{131}I MIBG planar, ^{123}I MIBG SPECT	False-negative MIBG scans; FDG PET depicted pheochromocytoma arising from heart (reference 15); reference organ, lung	NAC	NAC	NA	FDG	8
13/45	^{111}In octreoscan SPECT	Tumor recurrence; moderate uptake on octreoscan and intense uptake of FDG; reference organ, lung	7.0	17.0	2.6*	FDG	4
14/43	^{123}I MIBG SPECT	False-negative FDG scan; MIBG uptake in middle of abdomen; reference, organ lung	NA	NA	3.1	MIBG	6
15/16	^{131}I MIBG planar	Uptake of FDG and MIBG in metastases in tibia; reference organ, muscle	4.0	3.6	2.4	MIBG	Bone†
15/16	^{131}I MIBG planar	Uptake of FDG and MIBG in metastases in tibia after ^{131}I MIBG therapy, reference organ, muscle	3.9	2.9	3.2	MIBG	Bone†
16/52	^{123}I MIBG planar	False-negative MIBG scan; FDG uptake in metastases to spine; reference organ, liver	3.8	4.5	NA	FDG	Bone†
17/72	^{131}I MIBG planar	Uptake of both MIBG and FDG into large right adrenal pheochromocytoma; reference, organ liver	4.6	4.3	2.5	Equal	10
18/37	^{123}I MIBG SPECT	Lung and liver metastases after adrenalectomy; faint FDG uptake; reference organ, lung	1.6	5.0	2.3	MIBG	2
18/39	^{131}I MIBG planar	Hepatic and mediastinal metastases 1.5 y after surgery; false-negative FDG scan; reference organ, lung	NA	NA	2.4	MIBG	2
19/48	^{131}I MIBG planar	Cervical, mediastinal, and retroperitoneal metastases; reference organ, neck muscles	7.9	5.1	1.4	FDG	4
20/32	^{131}I MIBG planar	Lower thoracic and middle abdominal lesions; before ^{131}I MIBG therapy; reference organ, liver	13.3	6.1	1.4	Equal	10
20/32	^{131}L MIBG planar	Lower thoracic and middle abdominal masses; 4 months after ^{131}I MIBG therapy; reference organ, liver	6.3	3.6	1.1	Equal	9
21/52	^{123}I MIBG SPECT	Extensive mediastinal and abdominal metastases; before ^{131}I MIBG therapy; reference organ, liver	NA	NA	1.4	MIBG	8
21/52	^{131}I MIBG	No uptake of FDG despite tumor growth; reference organ, liver	NA	NA	1.0	MIBG	8
22/38	^{123}I MIBG SPECT	Widespread skeletal metastases not visualized with FDG PET; reference organ, lung	NA	NA	1.8	MIBG	Lung, 2.5 Skull, 5
23/34	^{123}I MIBG SPECT	Abdominal metastases; reference organ, liver	10.7	4.9	1.2	MIBG	
24/42	^{131}I MIBG planar	Thoracic and abdominal metastases; reference organ, contralateral abdomen	8.0	11.7	1.6	FDG	7
25/51	^{123}I MIBG SPECT	Liver and lung metastases; reference organ, liver	4.6	2.0	2.1	MIBG	8
26/25	^{123}I MIBG SPECT	Large liver metastasis prior to surgical reduction; reference organ, liver	11.4	4.9	3.6	Equal	9
26/25	^{131}I MIBG planar	Large liver metastasis was surgically debulked 8 months earlier; reference organ, liver	8.3	3.0	2.1	Equal	5
27/36	^{131}I MIBG planar	Multiple skeletal metastases; reference organ, lung	2.8	4.7	3.2	MIBG	Bone†
28/66	^{131}I MIBG planar	Vertebral and pelvic metastases; reference organ, pelvic soft tissue	5.8	5.1	3.3	Equal	Bone†
29/66	^{131}I MIBG planar	Mediastinal and pelvic metastases; reference organ, lung	6.5	5.0	NA	MIBG	2.5

Note.—NA = not applicable, NAC = not attenuation corrected.
* Value for radiolabeled octreotide scan. MIBG scintigraphy not performed.
† Size of tumors in bone could not be reliably determined.

Hann filter with a cutoff frequency of 0.35 cycles per projection ray. From the transverse images, attenuation-corrected images were constructed in the coronal and sagittal planes. In addition, in most studies, limited "whole-body" views of the chest and abdomen were obtained to screen for metastatic disease. These views consisted of sequential acquisitions covering 40–60 cm in the z axis. The data from the whole-body acquisition were stacked in a three-dimensional volume and forward projected into images every 10° to allow viewing as a rotating cine display of 32 images.

In patients 9–13 and 15–28, images were acquired on an Exact PET scanner beginning 45 minutes after FDG injection. This device contains three rotating ^{68}Ge rods, which allow performance of emission scanning followed by transmission scanning for attenuation correction. This method does not eliminate contamination for the emission events but does reduce its effect, and the resultant scan values do not differ by more than 5% from those corrected on the basis of standard preinjection transmission scans (17).

MIBG Scintigraphy

Iodine 131 MIBG.—In 14 patients (patients 1, 8, 13, 15, 17–21, 24, 26–29), planar scintigraphy with ^{131}I MIBG was performed as previously described (18). In brief, overlapping anterior and poste-

TABLE 4
Findings at FDG PET and MIBG Scintigraphy in Malignant Pheochromocytomas

	MIBG	
FDG	Positive	Negative
Positive	15 (12)	2 (2)
Negative	5 (4)	0 (0)

Note.—Data are the number of scans. Data in parentheses are the number of patients.

rior images from the top of the head to the knees were acquired for 100,000 counts or 20 minutes, whichever came first, at 24, 48, and 72 hours after administration of 19 MBq (0.5 mCi) or 38 MBq (1 mCi) ^{131}I MIBG (the higher dose was administered to patients with malignant pheochromocytoma who were undergoing evaluation for possible ^{131}I MIBG therapy). Data were acquired with a gamma camera with a large field of view and a high-energy collimator interfaced with a computer.

Iodine 123 MIBG.—In 19 patients (patients 2–7, 9–14, 16, 18, 21–23, 25, 26), ^{123}I MIBG was used and was preferred whenever possible. After the intravenous administration of 370 MBq (10 mCi) ^{123}I MIBG, both planar and tomographic images were obtained (19).

Planar images.—Anterior views from the head to the knees and posterior views of the chest and abdomen were obtained at 18–24 and 48 hours. Each image was acquired for 10 minutes with use of a gamma camera with a large field of view and a low-energy collimator interfaced to a computer.

Tomographic images.—Single photon emission CT (SPECT) was performed at 24 hours with use of a single or multihead rotating gamma camera with one or more low-energy collimators. The camera was rotated through 360° with 64 stops of 20 seconds each. Data were reconstructed by means of filtered back projection and a Butterworth filter with a cutoff frequency of 0.2–0.5 Nyquist.

In most patients, findings at CT (models CT/T 8800 or 9800; GE Medical Systems, Milwaukee, Wis) of the principal tumor were available for confirmation. An intravenous bolus of approximately 150 mL of ionic (Conray 60; Mallinckrodt Medical, St Louis, Mo) or nonionic (Omnipaque 300; Nycomed-Amersham, Princeton, NJ) contrast material was administered at a rate of 2 mL/sec followed by acquisition of 10-mm-thick contiguous axial sections through the thorax, abdomen, or pelvis depending on the site of the principal tumor. Both α- and β-adrenergic blockades were used when necessary to prevent contrast media–induced hypertensive crises.

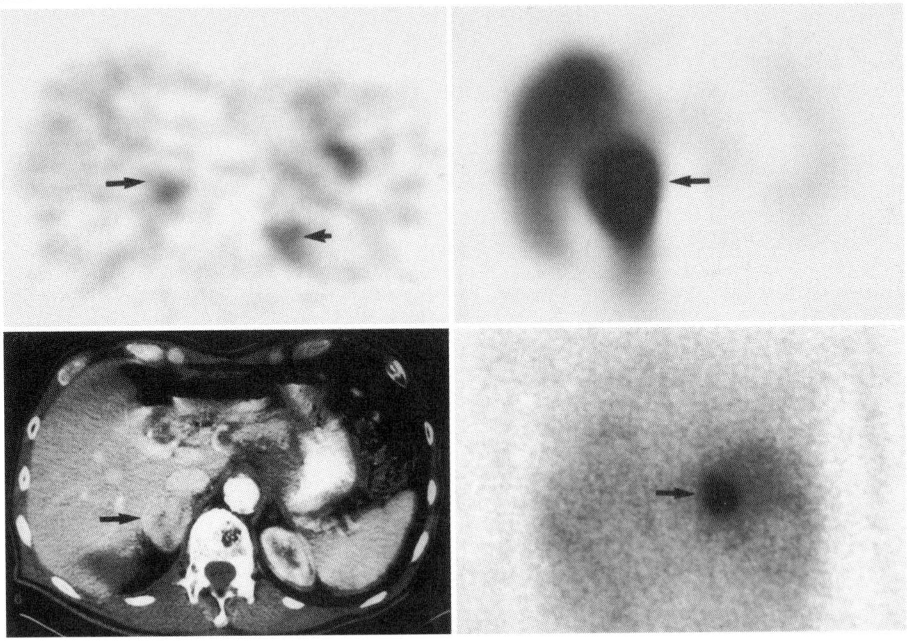

Figure 1. Patient 12. Benign pheochromocytoma (FDG positive, MIBG positive) in a 76-year-old man with recent history of prostate cancer. Abdominal CT depicted a right adrenal mass. Urinary catecholamine metabolites were elevated. Top left: PET scan (transverse plane) shows mildly increased accumulation of FDG in the region of the right adrenal gland (long arrow). A small amount of tracer is present in the left kidney (short arrow). Top right: SPECT scan (transverse plane) shows increased uptake (arrow) of ^{123}I MIBG in the same location as in the PET scan. Bottom left: CT scan shows enlargement of the right adrenal gland (arrow). Bottom right: Posterior planar view of ^{123}I MIBG scan at 24 hours shows markedly increased uptake in the right adrenal mass (arrow). The adrenal gland was removed and pheochromocytoma confirmed pathologically.

Image Analysis

Images were reviewed by three nuclear imaging physicians (B.L.S., B.S., J.C.S.) by consensus. The images for each patient were presented in random order, with the FDG PET images of a patient analyzed immediately before the MIBG images of the same patient. Any identifying information on each image was masked. Results of other studies (eg, bone scanning, MR imaging, biochemistry) were not revealed prior to analysis of the FDG PET and MIBG images. Tumor uptake of FDG and MIBG was assessed both qualitatively and semiquantitatively.

Qualitative analysis.—Organs that normally accumulate the tracers were identified by means of visual inspection. Sites of accumulation that did not conform to the usual anatomic configurations of normal sites of radiotracer accumulation were considered abnormal. A scale was used to visually assess tumor uptake with reference to the surrounding background: 0, no uptake; 1, faint uptake less than that of the surrounding background; 2, uptake equal to that of the background; and 3, uptake greater than that of the background. FDG and MIBG images were then compared for overall quality and clarity of tumor definition, and the set of images was selected that was considered to better depict the tumors.

Semiquantitative analysis.—On images obtained 50–60 minutes after injection of FDG, regions of interest were placed over the tumor and identifiable noninvolved organs to serve as reference organs. For chest lesions, the reference organ was the lung; for abdominal lesions, the liver; and for extremity lesions, the surrounding muscle. Irregular regions of interest were constructed around the entire tumor, and a region of interest of approximately the same size was placed over the reference organs. Tumor-to–reference-organ ratios of radioactivity were calculated for those sets of images on which both the tumor and reference organ were within the attenuation-corrected field of view. Regions of interest of similar size and shape were

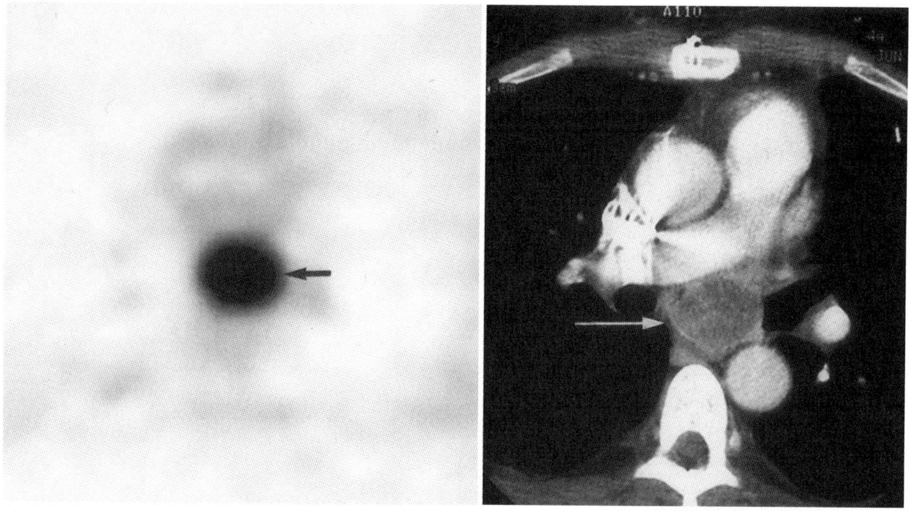

Figure 2. Patient 13. Malignant pheochromocytoma (FDG positive, MIBG positive) in a 45-year-old woman with a history of cardiac pheochromocytoma removed 4 years previously (described in reference 15) and seen now with recurrence. Multiple prior MIBG scans (not shown) were negative, and MIBG scintigraphy was not repeated for this recurrence. Left: FDG PET scan (transverse plane) shows increased uptake (arrow) in the middle of the chest. Right: CT scan shows a heterogeneous 3 × 4-cm subcarinal mass (arrow). Scintigraphy with ^{111}In pentetreotide (not shown) demonstrated moderate uptake in the mass. The lesion was subsequently removed and recurrence of pheochromocytoma confirmed.

drawn on SPECT images, and tumor-to–reference-organ ratios were calculated. Standardized uptake values (SUVs) were derived from 3 × 3-pixel regions of interest centered over areas of greatest FDG accumulation within the tumor at 50–60 minutes. Tumor-to–reference-organ ratios for planar MIBG studies were derived from the geometric mean of the tumor activity divided by the geometric mean of the reference organ uptake and for SPECT studies from regions of interest of the same size and shape as those on the PET studies.

Biochemical Characterization

At the time of FDG PET, approximately 10 mL of blood was withdrawn via an indwelling intravenous catheter after the patient lay recumbent for 20 minutes. Plasma was separated and analyzed for catecholamines by means of high-performance liquid chromatography.

The 12- or 24-hour urine was collected for analysis of catecholamines—norepinephrine and epinephrine—and catecholamine metabolites—normetanephrine and metanephrine—by means of high-performance liquid chromatography and vanillylmandelic acid by means of column extraction.

RESULTS

Findings in patients 1 and 13 have been reported previously (15). FDG PET and MIBG findings in patients with benign pheochromocytomas (patients 1–12) are given in Tables 1 and 2 and in patients with malignant pheochromocytomas (patients 13–29) are given in Tables 3 and 4.

Benign Pheochromocytomas

Qualitative analysis.—For the 12 benign tumors (Fig 1), uptake of FDG was seen in seven (58%) and of MIBG in 10 (83%). The pheochromocytomas in five of these patients accumulated both FDG and MIBG (Table 2), whereas those in the remaining seven patients accumulated either one or the other tracer but not both. The tumors that failed to accumulate MIBG avidly concentrated FDG (15). Each of the tumors that did not accumulate FDG was visualized with MIBG scintigraphy. For four of the five patients whose tumors accumulated both agents, MIBG images were ranked superior to FDG images.

Semiquantitative analysis.—In the tumors that accumulated FDG (n = 7), SUVs ranged from 2.6 to 13.4 (mean, 7.1 ± 4.1 [SD]). The corresponding tumor-to–reference-organ ratios for FDG ranged from 1.2 to 8.8 (mean, 3.5 ± 2.7). The tumor-to–reference-organ ratios for the tumors that accumulated MIBG (n = 10) ranged from 0.9 to 2.9 (mean, 1.7 ± 0.7).

Malignant Pheochromocytomas

Findings in malignant pheochromocytomas are presented in Figures 2–4.

Qualitative analysis.—Among the 17 patients with malignant pheochromocytomas, tumors in 14 (82%) concentrated FDG and in 15 (88%) concentrated MIBG (Table 3). Two patients had tumors that did not accumulate MIBG, and four had tumors that did not accumulate FDG. This included tumors in two patients that increased in diameter while being studied. The tumors in patient 21 did not concentrate sufficient FDG for visualization either before or after therapy with ^{131}I MIBG, despite evidence of tumor progression. The tumor in patient 18, however, showed weak uptake of FDG prior to therapy with ^{131}I MIBG but no uptake of FDG following therapy with ^{131}I MIBG. Among the 12 patients whose tumors concentrated both FDG and MIBG, MIBG images were ranked as better than FDG images in six, MIBG and FDG images were equal in five, and FDG images were better than MIBG images in one. FDG and MIBG uptake in metastatic disease was similar to that in the principal tumor.

Semiquantitative analysis.—SUVs for positive FDG PET scans (n = 14 [only the initial study was used in patients examined more than once]) ranged from 1.6 to 13.3 (mean, 6.6 ± 3.4). Tumor-to–reference-organ ratios for FDG ranged from 2.0 to 17.0 (mean, 6.0 ± 3.8) and for MIBG (n = 16 [only the initial study was used in patients examined more than once]) ranged from 1.0 to 3.6 (mean, 2.2 ± 0.8).

In both benign and malignant pheochromocytomas, FDG uptake was unrelated to tumoral catecholamine production.

DISCUSSION

FDG PET has been found to localize many different types of tumors, including those of the central nervous system, breast, lung, and colon. We previously reported successful localization of pheochromocytomas in two patients whose tumors failed to concentrate MIBG (15). In this study, we found that FDG PET localized the majority of pheochromocytomas, both benign or malignant and intraadrenal or extraadrenal. Overall sensitivity for tumor detection on a patient-by-patient basis was 72% (21 of 29 patients). The sensitivity in other series might be less because our patient population contained a large number of patients with malignant pheochromocytomas, which may accumulate FDG more frequently than do benign pheochromocytomas. In most positive cases, uptake was intense and impressive.

Semiquantitative analysis on the basis of SUVs and tumor-to–reference-organ ratios did not distinguish benign from malignant pheochromocytomas. The tumor-to–reference-organ index was calculated for FDG to allow comparison with that of MIBG, since the usually accepted quantification of FDG, the SUV, is based on very small regions of interest and may not reflect global tumor FDG uptake. Tumor-to–reference-organ SUVs for benign and malignant pheochromocytomas that accumulated FDG were in the range described for common malignant neoplasms. However, pheochromocytomas in eight (28%) of the 29 patients in this series did not show FDG uptake. SUV determinations are dependent on multiple factors, including time after injection, plasma glucose levels, recovery coefficients, and partial volume effects (20). Thus, different values might be found in different laboratories depending on the protocol and equipment used.

It is unclear why some pheochromocytomas, which appear clinically and histologically indistinct from tumors that concentrate FDG, do not concentrate the tracer. It is believed that increased glucose use by tumor cells may be due to a combination of factors—overexpression of glucose transporter proteins, elevated concentrations of hexokinase, and decreased rates of glucose-6-phosphate dephosphorylation (21–23). However, some pheochromocytomas that accumulate MIBG poorly were well visualized with FDG and all that fail to concentrate FDG were well visualized with MIBG in this study. We have yet to encounter a pheochromocytoma that cannot be localized with one tracer or the other. FDG uptake appears unrelated to the secretory status of the tumor.

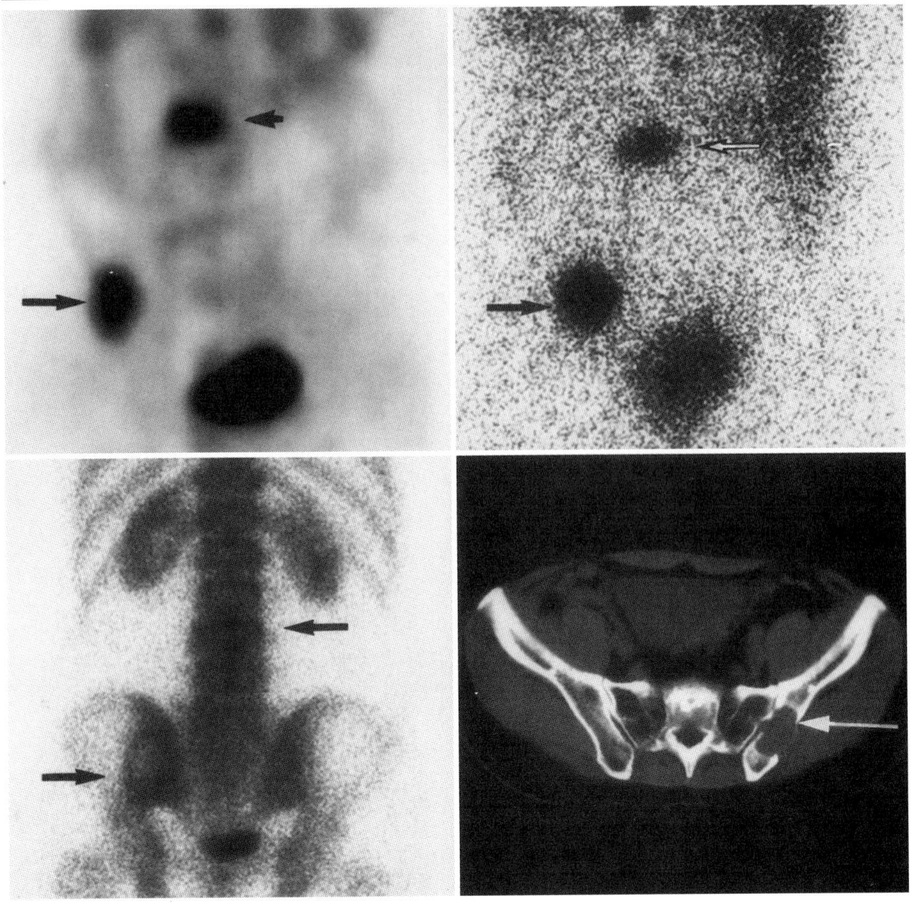

Figure 3. Patient 28. Malignant pheochromocytoma (FDG positive, MIBG positive) in a 66-year-old man with pheochromocytoma metastatic to bone. Top left: Posterior projection image from PET scan of the lower abdomen and pelvis demonstrates increased accumulation of FDG in the middle of the lumbar spine (short arrow) and left ilium (long arrow). Bladder activity is seen inferiorly in the midline. Top right: Posterior image from ^{131}I MIBG scan of the lower abdomen and pelvis at 48 hours also shows uptake in the middle of the lumbar spine (white arrow) and left ilium (black arrow) corresponding to the foci identified on the PET scan. Bladder activity from MIBG excreted into the urinary tract is also noted. Bottom left: Posterior image of the lower thorax, abdomen, and pelvis from bone scan (made by means of computer-assisted stacking of posterior abdominal and pelvic images) 3 hours after intravenous administration of 25 mCi technetium-99m methylene diphosphonate demonstrates that the lesions depicted on the FDG PET and ^{131}I MIBG scans are metastases (arrows) within bone. Bottom right: CT scan shows destruction of the left ilium (arrow) and L3 (not shown).

There are multiple single photon and positron emitting tracers available for detecting pheochromocytoma. After the first reports of ^{131}I MIBG scintigraphy to detect pheochromocytoma, this agent has been used widely and found effective for the localization of benign pheochromocytomas and for the localization and monitoring of malignant pheochromocytomas. This technique uses a guanethidine analogue, MIBG, and the specific catecholamine uptake transport system of tissues of the sympathetic nervous system to concentrate the radiopharmaceutical within the tumor. Whole-body screening allows the detection of both intraadrenal and extraadrenal pheochromocytomas. Although ^{123}I MIBG is not widely available in the United States, it is commercially available in Europe and is synthesized for local use at several large academic facilities in the United States.

The principal advantage to use of ^{123}I MIBG is in image quality (ie, images have much higher counts) and the ability to perform high-quality SPECT. Radiation dosimetry for ^{123}I MIBG (10 mCi) is favorable, and this allows approximately 20-fold greater activity to be administered for radiation exposure similar to that with ^{131}I MIBG (0.5 mCi) (24). In patients with disseminated neuroblastoma, more lesions may be identified with ^{123}I MIBG than with ^{131}I MIBG, but this does not affect staging (25). To our knowledge, comparison data are not available in patients with pheochromocytoma, but our experience suggests that only very rarely can a pheochromocytoma be visualized with ^{123}I MIBG and not with ^{131}I MIBG (26). Thus, we pooled the ^{131}I MIBG and ^{123}I MIBG data for analysis.

We previously observed approximately 12% false-negative studies with MIBG scintigraphy and reported successful localization at FDG PET of two pheochromocytomas that did not concentrate MIBG (15). These observations provided the foundation for this more extensive investigation of the uptake of FDG by pheochromocytomas regardless of their MIBG avidity. Indium 111 pentetreotide depicts most pheochromocytomas, although results with this agent are inferior to those with MIBG for localizing pheochromocytomas (27). Other positron emitting tracers of the sympathetic nervous system

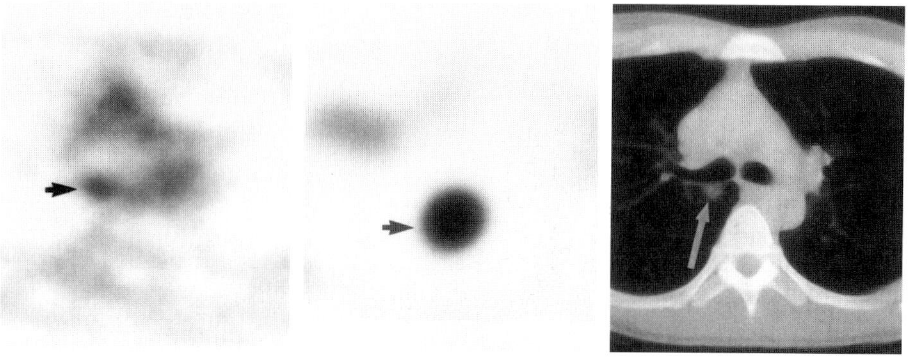

a. b. c.

Figure 4. Patient 18. Malignant pheochromocytoma (MIBG positive, FDG positive) in a 37-year-old man with pheochromocytoma metastatic to the lungs. **(a)** FDG PET scan (transverse plane) shows minimally increased uptake (arrow). **(b)** SPECT ^{123}I MIBG scan at 24 hours (transverse plane) shows abnormal uptake (arrow) in the right middle lung field. **(c)** For comparison, the CT scan shows a 1-cm-diameter right-side peribronchial mass (arrow).

have been evaluated and found to be concentrated within pheochromocytomas. These are carbon 11 metahydroxyephedrine, which is a norepinephrine analogue that shows excellent and rapid localization of pheochromocytoma, and ^{11}C epinephrine (28,29). Like MIBG, these tracers use the catecholamine uptake pathway and catecholamine storage mechanisms characteristic of neuroendocrine tumors, especially pheochromocytomas and neuroblastomas. These agents may also be subject to interference from agents that inhibit uptake of MIBG. A similar number of false-negative studies might be expected with use of these positron emitting tracers of the sympathetic nervous system, although direct comparison studies would be required for certainty.

Though most histologically benign tumors can be distinguished from malignant neoplasms at FDG PET, we found that most pheochromocytomas, whether benign or malignant, are metabolically active and thus concentrate FDG (30,31). On the other hand, a minority of either benign or malignant pheochromocytomas did not accumulate FDG, even when clinical evidence suggested growth and uptake of FDG was expected. Thus, caution is warranted against concluding that absence of uptake of FDG excludes pheochromocytoma.

FDG PET helps localize the majority of pheochromocytomas. Because its sensitivity is slightly less than that of MIBG and its specificity is considerably lower due to uptake of FDG by a variety of other neoplastic and nonneoplastic processes, FDG PET is not recommended as a first line method to localize pheochromocytomas. However, the technique is a useful adjunct to MIBG scintigraphy and is of most value in the localization of pheochromocytomas when other methods have failed.

Acknowledgments: The authors thank Laurie Enz for typing the manuscript for this article; Shirley Zempel, RNC, and Sharon Stetz, RNC, for assistance in patient care; Christine Allman, CNMT, Todd Hauser, CNMT, Paul Kison, CNMT, Edward McKenna, CNMT, Jill Rothley, CNMT, and Andrew Weeden, CNMT, for technologic expertise and support; Robert Koeppe, PhD, David E. Kuhl, MD, and Donald M. Wieland, PhD, for stimulating discussions; the cyclotron chemistry staff for the production of FDG; and William H. Beierwaltes, MD, without whose longstanding interest in the imaging of pheochromocytoma this work would not have been possible.

References

1. Bravo EL. Evolving concepts in the pathophysiology, diagnosis, and treatment of pheochromocytoma. Endocr Rev 1994; 15:356–368.
2. Gifford RW Jr, Manger WM, Bravo EL. Pheochromocytoma. Endocrinol Metab Clin North Am 1994; 23:387–404.
3. Werbel SS, Ober KP. Pheochromocytoma: update on diagnosis, localization, and management. Med Clin North Am 1995; 79:131–153.
4. Ram CV, Fierro-Carrion GA. Pheochromocytoma. Semin Nephrol 1995; 15:126–137.
5. Stewart BH, Bravo EL, Haaga J, Meaney TF, Tarazi R. Localization of pheochromocytoma by computed tomography. N Engl J Med 1978; 299:460–461.
6. Francis IR, Glazer GM, Shapiro B, Sisson JC, Gross BH. Complementary roles of CT and ^{131}I-MIBG scintigraphy in diagnosing pheochromocytoma. AJR 1983; 141:719–725.
7. Connor CS, Hermreck AS, Thomas JH. Pitfalls in the diagnosis of pheochromocytoma. Am Surg 1988; 54:634–636.
8. Quint LE, Glazer GM, Francis IR, Shapiro B, Chenevert TL. Pheochromocytoma and paraganglioma: comparison of MR imaging with CT and I-131 scintigraphy. Radiology 1987; 165:89–93.
9. Velchik MG, Alavi A, Kressel HY, Engelman K. Localization of pheochromocytoma: MIBG, CT, and MRI correlation. J Nucl Med 1989; 30:328–336.
10. Chatal JF, Charbonnel B. Comparison of iodobenzylguanidine imaging with computed tomography in locating pheochromocytoma. J Clin Endocrinol Metab 1985; 61:769–772.
11. Bomanji J, Conry BG, Britton KE, Reznek RH. Imaging neural crest tumours with ^{123}I-metaiodobenzylguanidine and x-ray computed tomography: a comparative study. Clin Radiol 1988; 39:502–506.
12. Samaan NA, Hickey RC. Pheochromocytoma. Semin Oncol 1987; 14:297–305.
13. Shapiro B, Copp JE, Sisson JC, Eyre PL, Wallis J, Beierwaltes WH. Iodine-131 meta-iodobenzylguanidine for the locating of suspected pheochromocytoma: experience in 400 cases. J Nucl Med 1985; 26:576–585.
14. Solanki KK, Bomanji J, Moyes J, et al. A pharmacological guide to medicines which interfere with biodistribution of radiolabelled metaiodobenzylguanidine (MIBG). Nucl Med Comm 1992; 13:513–521.
15. Shulkin BL, Koeppe RA, Francis IR, Deeb GM, Lloyd RV, Thompson NW. PET FDG localization of pheochromocytomas which fail to accumulate MIBG. Radiology 1993; 186:711–715.
16. Hamacher K, Coenen HH, Stocklin G. Efficient stereospecific synthesis of no-carrier-added 2-[18F]-fluro-2-D-deoxyglucose using aminopolyether supported nucleophilic substitution. J Nucl Med 1986; 27:235–238.
17. Shulkin BL, Hutchinson RJ, Castle VP, Yanik GA, Shapiro B, Sisson JC. Neuroblastoma: positron emission tomography with 2-[fluorine-18]fluoro-2-deoxy-D-glucose compared with metaiodobenzylguanidine scintigraphy. Radiology 1996; 199:743–750.
18. Shapiro B, Copp JE, Sisson JC, Eyre PL, Wallis J, Beierwaltes WH. Iodine-131 meta-iodobenzylguanidine for the locating of suspected pheochromocytoma: experience in 400 cases. J Nucl Med 1985; 26:576–585.
19. Lynn MD, Shapiro B, Sisson JC, et al. Pheochromocytomas and the normal adrenal medulla: improved visualization with I-123-MIBG scintigraphy. Radiology 1985; 156:789–792.
20. Keyes JW Jr. SUV: standard uptake or silly useless value (editorial). J Nucl Med 1995; 36:1836–1839.
21. Brown RS, Wahl RL. Overexpression of glut-1 glucose transporter in human breast cancer. Cancer 1993; 72:2979–2785.
22. Paul R, Johansson R, Kellokumpu-Lehtinen PL, Soderstrom KO, Kangas L. Tumor localization with 18F-2-fluoro-2-deoxy-D-glucose: comparative autoradiography, glucose 6-phosphatase histochemistry, and histology of renally implanted sarcoma of the rat. Res Exp Med (Berl) 1985; 185:87–95.
23. Graham MM, Spence AM, Muzi M, Abbott GL. Deoxyglucose kinetics in rat brain tumor. J Cereb Blood Flow Metab 1989; 9:315–322.
24. Shulkin BL, Shapiro B. Current concepts on the diagnostic use of MIBG in children. J Nucl Med 1998; 39:679–688.
25. Gelfand MJ. I-123-MIBG and I-131-MIBG imaging in children with neuroblastoma (abstr). J Nucl Med 1996; 37 (suppl):35P.
26. Shulkin BL, Shapiro B, Francis I, Dorr R, Sisson JC. Primary extraadrenal pheochromocytoma: a case of positive ^{123}I-MIBG scintigraphy with negative ^{131}I-MIBG scintigraphy. Clin Nucl Med 1986; 11:851–854.
27. Tenenbaum R, Lumbroso J, Schlumberger M, et al. Comparison of radiolabeled octreotide and meta-iodobenzylguanidine (MIBG) scintigraphy in malignant pheochromocytoma. J Nucl Med 1995; 36:1–6.
28. Shulkin BL, Wieland DM, Schwaiger M, et al. PET scanning with hydroxyephedrine: an approach to the localization of pheochromocytoma. J Nucl Med 1992; 33:1125–1131.
29. Shulkin BL, Wieland DM, Shapiro B, Sisson JC. PET epinephrine studies of pheochromocytoma (abstr). J Nucl Med 1995; 36(suppl): 22P–23P.
30. Lowe VJ, Hoffman JM, DeLong DM, Patz EF, Coleman RE. Semiquantitative and visual analysis of FDG-PET images in pulmonary abnormalities. J Nucl Med 1994; 35:1771–1776.
31. Gupta NC, Frank AR, Dewan NA, et al. Solitary pulmonary nodules: detection of malignancy with PET with 2-[F-18]-fluoro-2-deoxy-D-glucose. Radiology 1992; 184:441–444.

Book Review

Imaging in Oncology. 2 Vols.

Edited by Janet E. S. Husband and Rodney H. Reznek
Oxford, England: Isis Medical Media, 1998. ISBN 1-899066-48-9.
Hardcover, £180.00 ($295.00); pp 1,057; 863 figures; tables.

This two-volume set comes from England with contributions from the United States, France, and Greece. The first volume covers general principles of oncology and the primary evaluation and staging of tumors. The second volume covers hematologic malignancies, pediatric neoplasms, metastases, tumors related to acquired immunodeficiency syndrome, and the assessment of treatment and complications. Individual chapters discuss tumors of specific anatomic areas such as the lung, stomach, kidney, prostate, breast, and thyroid.

Key points and topic summaries are highlighted on almost every page with the use of colored boxes (eg, "Drug-Related Pulmonary Toxicity," p 934; "Contrast Medium Enhancement of Metastases [Liver]," p 790; and "Key Points: Renal Cell Carcinoma," p 207). Not only is this method attractive, but it makes these points easier to remember and find again when one returns to a particular chapter.

The real beauty of *Imaging in Oncology* is the simplicity with which this complex topic is presented. The editors have produced a reference not just for oncologists but also for general and subspecialty radiologists who see patients with neoplasms. Each chapter discusses the epidemiology, clinical presentation, staging, and treatment of a specific cancer. The roles of the various imaging modalities are also presented, which may be of particular interest to residents and nonradiologists. All the major tumor groups are included. There are even short sections on trophoblastic disease and adamantinoma. The chapter on second malignancies discusses the most commonly linked malignancies and possible etiologies. Bibliographies at the end of each chapter cite references from the last 10 years.

The rich, concise text is complemented by good-quality images drawn by Dee McLean. Several examples of the same neoplasm are demonstrated with different modalities. Abundant radiographs as well as ultrasonographic, computed tomographic, and magnetic resonance images illustrate the concepts of tumor staging, treatment, and complications. Many helpful and pleasing diagrams depict normal anatomy and tumor staging.

This two-volume set has all the characteristics of a best seller. If you work in a clinic or hospital with cancer patients, get these books!

Reviewed by Bernice Capusten, MD

Anne M. Hubbard, MD
N. Scott Adzick, MD
Timothy M. Crombleholme, MD
Beverly G. Coleman, MD
Lori J. Howell, RN, MS
John C. Haselgrove, PhD
Saroosh Mahboubi, MD

Index terms:
Fetus, MR, 856.121411, 856.121416
Fetus, neoplasms, 856.872, 856.875
Fetus, respiratory system, 856.8754, 875.8755, 875.8756, 875.8759
Fetus, US, 856.12981
Magnetic resonance (MR), comparative studies

Radiology 1999; 212:43–48

Abbreviations:
BPS = bronchopulmonary sequestration
CCAM = congenital cystic adenomatoid malformation
RARE = rapid acquisition with relaxation enhancement

[1] From the Departments of Radiology (A.M.H., J.C.H., S.M.) and Surgery (N.S.A., T.M.C., L.J.H.), Children's Hospital of Philadelphia, 34th and Civic Center Blvd, Philadelphia, PA 19104, and the Department of Radiology, University of Pennsylvania Medical Center, Philadelphia (B.G.C.). Received March 25, 1998; revision requested June 18; revision received September 8; accepted December 21. **Address reprint requests to** A.M.H. (e-mail: *Hubbard@email.chop.edu*).

Author contributions:
Guarantor of integrity of entire study, A.M.H.; study concepts and design, A.M.H.; definition of intellectual content, A.M.H.; literature research, all authors; clinical studies, A.M.H., S.M.; data acquisition, A.M.H., L.J.H.; data analysis, A.M.H., S.M.; manuscript preparation and editing, A.M.H.; manuscript review, all authors.

Congenital Chest Lesions: Diagnosis and Characterization with Prenatal MR Imaging[1]

PURPOSE: To evaluate prenatal magnetic resonance (MR) imaging for diagnosis of fetal chest masses and to determine if MR imaging provides information in addition to that of ultrasonography (US).

MATERIALS AND METHODS: Eighteen pregnant women were referred for MR imaging of possible fetal chest tumors seen at US (16 congenital cystic adenomatoid malformation [CCAM], two bronchopulmonary sequestration [BPS]). The presence, position, size, and characteristics of masses were determined and correlated with postnatal results.

RESULTS: The MR imaging diagnoses were three cases of congenital diaphragmatic hernia, nine of CCAM, two of BPS, and one each of foregut cyst, lung atresia, tracheal atresia, and bronchial stenosis. MR imaging results were in agreement with US results in nine fetuses and in disagreement in nine. MR imaging diagnoses were confirmed at surgery or autopsy in 17 fetuses. MR imaging results led to an error in diagnosis in one fetus with BPS.

CONCLUSION: Fetal chest masses had characteristic MR imaging appearances. MR imaging was accurate for distinguishing congenital diaphragmatic hernia from CCAM and was useful for less common diagnoses and determination of the origin of very large chest tumors. Prenatal diagnosis was changed in some patients owing to MR results and affected treatment and counseling of parents. MR imaging is a valuable adjunct to US for prenatal diagnosis of fetal chest masses.

Marked improvements in the resolution of ultrasonography (US) in the past 10 years have increased our ability to diagnose fetal anomalies in utero. US also has allowed the variable prenatal natural history of many lesions to be characterized. Congenital lung tumors may enlarge rapidly in utero, grow commensurately with the fetus, or involute. The most common masses seen in the chest are congenital diaphragmatic hernia, congenital cystic adenomatoid malformation (CCAM), and bronchopulmonary sequestration (BPS) (1). All represent a risk of fetal death or life-threatening respiratory compromise after birth. Recent development of in utero treatment for chest masses has made the prenatal assessment of the fetus and the need for accurate prenatal diagnosis even more important (2,3).

Magnetic resonance (MR) imaging has been used to evaluate uterine and fetal anatomy. Until the advent of fast MR imaging, however, the images were severely degraded owing to fetal motion. Maternal sedation or in utero paralysis of the fetus by means of intramuscular injection of pancuronium into the fetus was frequently needed (4). With the advent of fast MR imaging, prenatal imaging has entered a new age. Prenatal MR imaging has been successfully performed by using echo-planar imaging, as well as rapid acquisition with relaxation enhancement (RARE) imaging (5–8).

The purpose of this study was to compare the diagnostic utility of prenatal MR imaging and US for evaluation of chest tumors and to determine if MR imaging could provide additional valuable information.

MATERIALS AND METHODS

Eighteen pregnant women were referred for prenatal MR imaging because of an abnormal pregnancy in which a primary fetal chest tumor (16 CCAM tumors, including eight on the left, six on the right, and two bilateral; two BPS tumors) was diagnosed at US. US had been performed at multiple institutions, mainly by obstetricians trained in maternal and fetal medicine. MR imaging was performed as part of the clinical evaluation of an abnormal fetus and was not part of a research protocol. Thus, institutional review board approval was not required. However, informed consent was obtained from all mothers prior to the examination. The mean gestational age of the fetuses was 26 weeks (gestational age range, 21–32 weeks).

MR imaging was performed with a 1.5-T magnet (Vision; Siemens Medical Systems, Iselin, NJ) equipped with a phased-array body coil. The nonsedated mother was positioned either supine or in a partial left lateral decubitus position. The following imaging sequences were performed: RARE (HASTE; Siemens Medical Systems) imaging (4.4/64 [repetition time msec/effective echo time msec]; flip angle, 120°; section thickness, 6 mm) in the sagittal, coronal, and axial planes relative to the fetal chest; two-dimensional fast low-angle shot imaging (174/4.1 [repetition time msec/echo time msec]; flip angle, 80°; section thickness, 6 mm) in the sagittal and coronal planes relative to the fetus; turbo fast low-angle shot imaging (11/5.3 [effective]; flip angle, 20°; section thickness, 5 mm) in the axial plane relative to the fetus; and echo-planar free induction decay imaging (0.8/56; flip angle, 90°; section thickness, 5 mm) in the axial plane. For each sequence, 4–20 seconds were needed to acquire 20 anatomic images.

All MR studies were interpreted by one radiologist (A.M.H.), who also knew the results of US. MR imaging results were compared with the US report; US images were not available for review. The presence, position, size, and signal intensity characteristics of the masses were determined and correlated with findings from postnatal studies, including postmortem, surgical, or pathologic results.

RESULTS

Eighteen fetuses were imaged. Congenital diaphragmatic hernia was diagnosed on the basis of MR imaging findings in three fetuses, (two right-sided lesions, one left-sided lesion); CCAM, in nine fetuses; BPS, in two fetuses; and foregut cyst, bronchial stenosis, lung atresia, and tracheal atresia, in one fetus each. MR imaging diagnoses were in agreement with prenatal US diagnoses in nine fetuses and in disagreement in nine fetuses.

At follow-up, the MR imaging diagnoses were confirmed with either surgical or histopathologic results in 17 fetuses. In one case, a large CCAM lesion was predicted on the basis of both US and MR imaging results, but at pathologic examination the lesion was diagnosed as BPS. One lesion had been diagnosed as BPS at MR imaging and as mixed BPS and CCAM at pathologic examination. MR imaging substantially augmented US in terms of localization of masses relative to the lobar anatomy of the lung and other chest structures, particularly in very large lesions. With MR imaging, we were able to assess the volume of normal ipsilateral and contralateral lung.

The imaging characteristics of the chest lesions were variable. Normal lung tissue was homogeneous and of moderately high signal intensity, with markedly higher signal intensity than that of chest wall muscle (Fig 1). The signal intensity of compressed but otherwise normal lung was intermediate and lower than that of noncompressed normal lung (Fig 2).

The appearance of pathologically proved CCAM lesions varied, depending on whether the lesion was macrocystic or microcystic. CCAM lesions had markedly higher signal intensity than did the remaining normal lung and manifested either as multiple large cysts with discrete walls that could be identified or as more solid-appearing lesions with a few small cysts scattered throughout (Figs 2, 3). The signal intensity was higher in lesions with more macrocysts.

Both BPS lesions were left lower lobe masses with high signal intensity. The mass was homogeneous and had a well-defined margin (Fig 4). No anomalous vessels could be identified on MR images.

The bronchial stenosis involved the right middle lobe and had signal intensity higher than that of surrounding normal lung, although not as high as that of the CCAM lesions, especially in CCAM lesions as large as this mass (Fig 5). The lesion also had homogeneous signal intensity.

Tracheal atresia manifested as uniform very high signal intensity throughout both lungs, with fluid in the dilated trachea and eversion of the diaphragm. In the fetus with lung atresia, uniform moderate signal intensity was seen in the remaining lung, with a shift of the mediastinal structure toward the atretic side.

The foregut cyst manifested as a single large homogeneous cyst of high signal

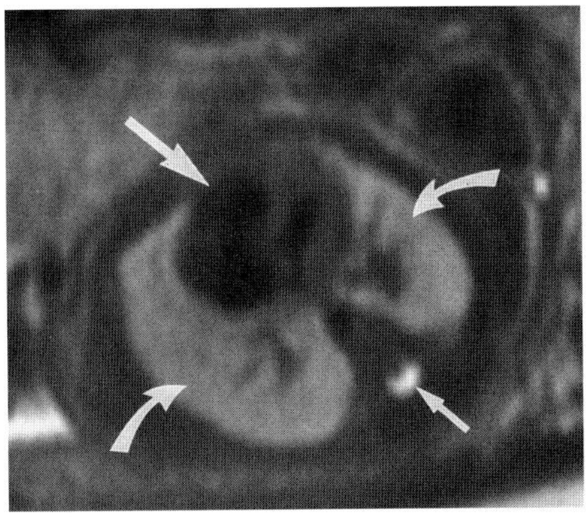

Figure 1. Axial RARE MR image (4.4/64 [effective], 120° flip angle, 6-mm section thickness) through the level of the heart (large straight arrow) shows a normal chest in a fetus at 30 weeks gestational age. The spinal canal (small straight arrow) is shown posteriorly. The lungs (curved arrows) are homogeneous and high in signal intensity.

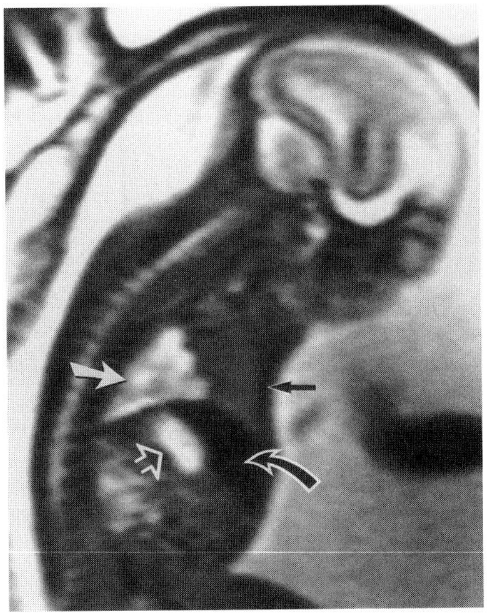

Figure 2. CCAM in a fetus of 23 weeks gestational age. Sagittal RARE MR image (4.4/64 [effective], 120° flip angle, 6-mm section thickness) through the left side of the chest. A well-defined, slightly heterogeneous high-signal-intensity mass (solid white arrow) is shown originating from the left lower lobe. The normal lung (straight black arrow) is visible in the anterior portion of the chest and is notably lower in signal intensity than the CCAM. The left lobe of the liver (curved arrow) has very low signal intensity, and the fluid-filled stomach (open arrow) has high signal intensity.

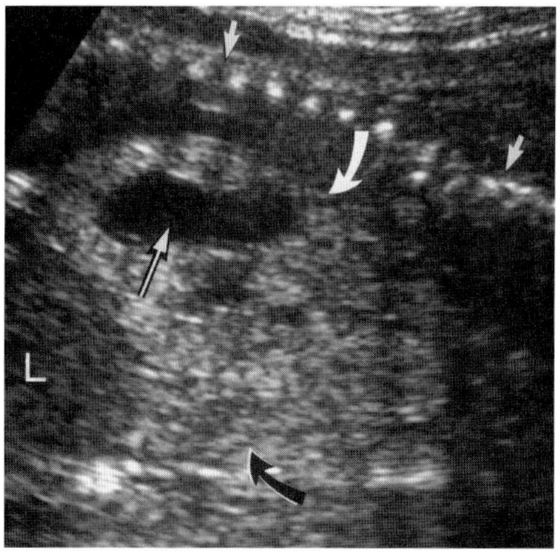

a.

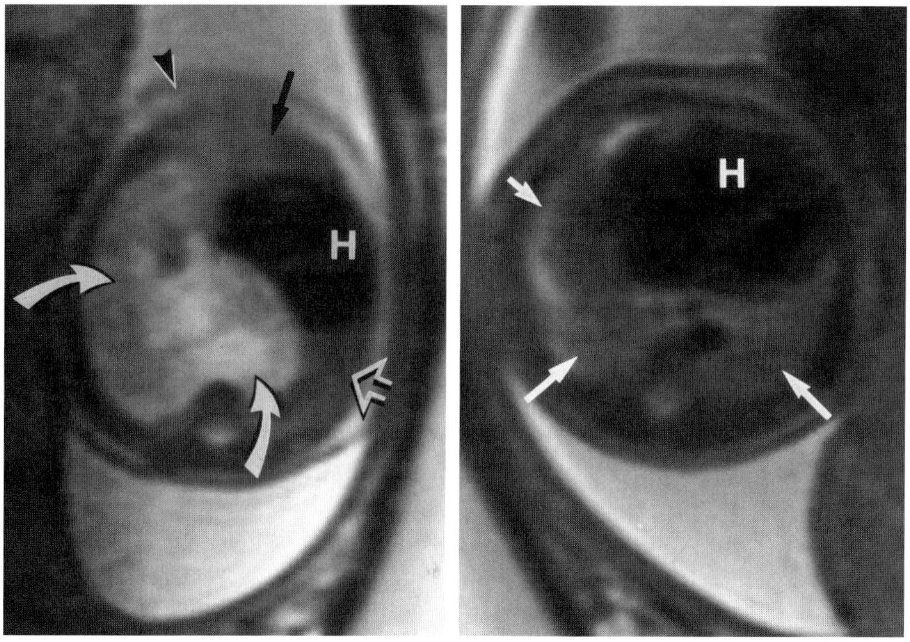

b. c.

Figure 3. CCAM in a fetus of 29 weeks gestational age. **(a)** Sagittal US image through the fetus with the spine (small straight arrows) directed toward the transducer. There is a large hyperechoic mass (curved arrows) in the right side of the chest. A large, dominant cyst (long straight arrow) is present within the hyperechoic lesion. The lung lesion is substantially more echogenic than the liver (*L*). **(b)** Axial RARE MR image (4.4/64 [effective], 120° flip angle, 6-mm section thickness) through the chest at the level of the heart (*H*) shows a large high-signal-intensity heterogeneous mass (curved arrows) arising from the right lung and crossing the midline. A small amount of normal right lung (black arrow) can be seen anterior to the heart, which is shifted to the left. The left lung (open arrow) can be seen posterior to the heart. There also is marked subcutaneous edema (arrowhead), consistent with hydrops. **(c)** Axial RARE MR image (4.4/64 [effective], 120° flip angle, 6-mm section thickness) obtained through the chest at the level of the heart (*H*) at gestational age of 32 weeks, 3 weeks after in utero removal of the CCAM lesion, shows marked growth of both lungs (long arrows). A small amount of right-sided pleural fluid (short arrow) is present.

intensity, with a small tail of cystic tissue that extended into the mediastinum, posterior to the carina and anterior to the spine (Fig 6). Vertebral body anomalies were not demonstrated, but severe kyphosis of the upper thorax was present. One fetus was imaged twice at 3-week intervals after in utero removal of a CCAM lesion. MR imaging demonstrated lung growth and allowed differentiation of effusion and hemorrhage from normal lung tissue (Fig 3c).

Images from all MR sequences were evaluated at the same time. The RARE sequence provided the best overall image quality and produced the least amount of artifact due either to motion or susceptibility effects. Image quality was usually very good with the RARE sequence. The image quality was decreased when the mother was obese, because the size of the maternal abdomen limits the field of view that can be used. The quality also was decreased in cases of polyhydramnios, which allows increased fetal motion.

The prenatal US studies had been performed at several institutions. This made comparison of the US and MR images somewhat difficult. The quality of the US images generally was good. Most incorrect diagnoses were due to a misinterpretation of the US findings. The lesions that were misdiagnosed on the basis of US results were three congenital diaphragmatic hernias (two on the right side, one on the left side), which were diagnosed as CCAM; one tracheal atresia, diagnosed as bilateral CCAM; one pulmonary agenesis, diagnosed as CCAM; one neurenteric cyst, diagnosed as CCAM; one bronchial stenosis, diagnosed as CCAM; one very large CCAM, diagnosed as bilateral CCAM; and one BPS, diagnosed as CCAM.

DISCUSSION

To our knowledge, this is the first report of the use of fast MR imaging for prenatal evaluation of fetuses with a chest tumor. Fetal survival after birth is greatly dependent on adequate in utero development of the lungs. Factors that influence normal fetal lung growth include adequate size and shape of the fetal thorax, fetal breathing movements, and adequate volume of amniotic fluid. Pulmonary hypoplasia can occur when any of these factors are abnormal but is most commonly seen when the lesion occupies intrathoracic space. The most common space-occupying lesions are congenital diaphragmatic hernia, CCAM, BPS, and fetal hydrothorax. The degree of hypoplasia is dependent on the gestational age at which the mass develops and the size of the mass.

At US, the normal fetal lung has a homogeneous and moderately hyperechoic appearance (1). The degree of echogenicity relative to that of the liver increases throughout gestation. The normal fetal lung on T2-weighted MR images has moderately high signal intensity (9) (Fig 1), with higher signal intensity than chest wall muscle but lower signal intensity than amniotic fluid. The compressed normal lung was not as high in signal intensity as was the normal noncompressed lung. This finding is probably secondary to decreased production of alveolar fluid in the compressed lung.

To date, to our knowledge US has not been useful for accurate predictions about fetal lung maturity (1). Preliminary MR imaging studies have been performed to evaluate changes in T1 and T2 signal intensity with increasing gestational age, but this approach has not yet proved to be a reliable method for assessment of fetal lung maturity (9). MR imaging can be used for accurate measurement of lung volumes and may prove to be helpful for prediction of whether sufficient lung tissue is present to sustain life after birth (10). The conspicuity of the signal intensity in fetal lung is high enough that, even in very large chest masses, small amounts of compressed normal lung can be visualized.

Accurate prenatal diagnosis of chest masses is important because the natural history of these lesions and their treatment vary substantially (11–13). We have previously shown (7) that MR imaging results can be used to easily diagnose congenital diaphragmatic hernia and differentiate it from primary chest tumors.

Because MR imaging relies on differences in tissue characteristics, a combination of fast imaging sequences with T1 and T2 weighting can be used to easily differentiate bowel and liver from lung. On two-dimensional fast low-angle shot MR images, which are T1-weighted images, the liver has very high signal intensity, and its position above or below the diaphragm can easily be determined (Fig 7). The MR signal intensity characteristics of the liver are very different from those of the lung. The US differentiation of liver from lung can be difficult. Meconium-filled distal bowel also has very high signal intensity on T1-weighted images. This may be helpful because, on US images, bowel loops that do not exhibit peristalsis may appear the same as a hyperechoic lung tumor.

CCAM of the lung is a rare lesion; it is characterized by a multicystic mass of pulmonary tissue with an abnormal proliferation of bronchial structures. A CCAM lesion communicates with the normal tracheal-bronchial tree and usually receives its blood supply from the pulmonary vessels. Stocker et al (14) categorized this lesion into three histologic types. Type 1 CCAM consists of large cysts, type 2 is composed of numerous cysts with a diameter of less than 1 cm, and type 3 CCAM is microcystic and generally appears as a solid mass at US. The appearance of type 1 and type 2 CCAM lesions on RARE MR images was of a mass with very high signal intensity, almost equal to that of the amniotic fluid and markedly higher than that of surrounding normal lung. Discrete cysts larger than 3 mm in diameter were easily seen (Fig 2). Type 3 CCAM lesions appeared on RARE MR images as moderately high-signal-intensity lesions, with signal intensity that was higher than that of normal lung but not as high as that of amniotic fluid. Type 3 lesions were relatively homogeneous.

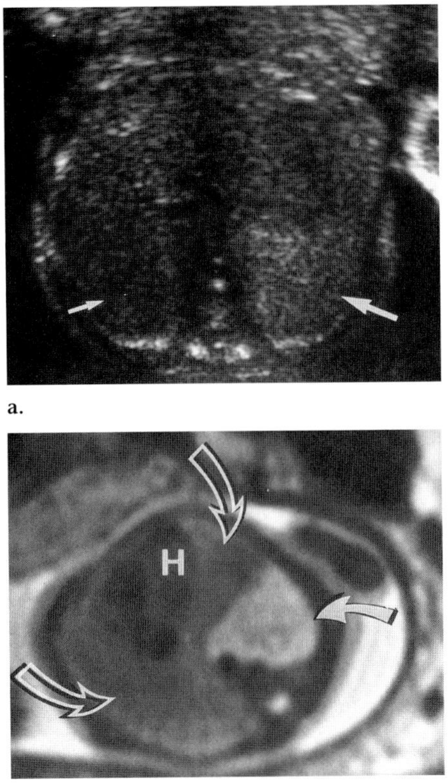

a.

b.

Figure 4. BPS in a fetus of 23 weeks gestational age. **(a)** Transverse US image through the lower portion of the chest demonstrates a hyperechoic lesion (large arrow) in the region of the left lower lobe. This lesion is more hyperechoic than the normal right lower lobe (small arrow). **(b)** Axial RARE MR image (4.4/64 [effective], 120° flip angle, 6-mm section thickness) through the chest at the level of the heart (*H*) demonstrates a well-defined lesion (solid arrow) with homogeneously high signal intensity involving the left lower lobe. The normal right and left lungs (open arrows) are shown.

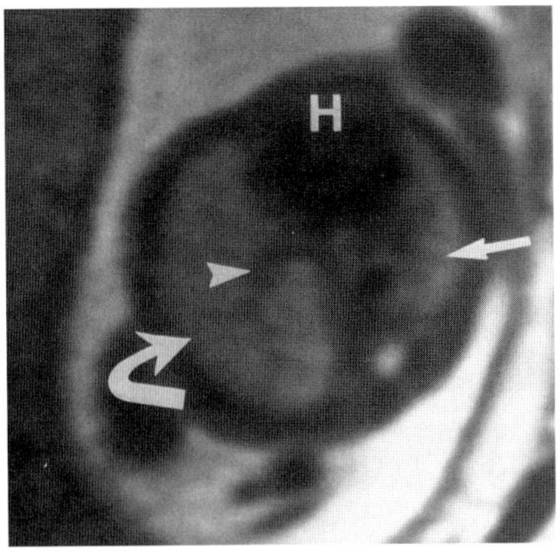

Figure 5. Bronchial stenosis of the right middle lobe in a fetus of 23 weeks gestational age. Axial RARE MR image (4.4/64 [effective], 120° flip angle, 6-mm section thickness) through the chest at the level of the heart (*H*) shows shift of the heart to the left side of the chest. The right middle lobe (curved arrow) is enlarged. A normal vessel can be seen coursing through the right lung (arrowhead). The markedly enlarged right middle lobe has homogeneous signal intensity that is only minimally higher than that of the left lung (straight arrow).

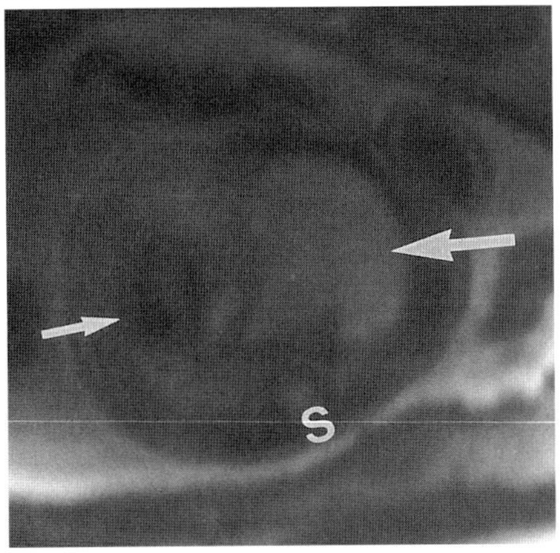

Figure 6. Foregut cyst in a fetus of 23 weeks gestational age. Axial RARE MR image (4.4/64 [effective], 120° flip angle, 6-mm section thickness) through the chest at the level of the heart (small arrow) shows marked shift of the heart to the right side of the chest. There is a large, homogeneous unilocular cyst (large arrow) occupying the left side of the chest and extending anterior to the spine (*S*) and posterior to the heart.

The natural history and prognosis of CCAM are variable (15). The prognosis associated with this lesion is dependent on the size, rather than the histologic type, of the lesion. Larger lesions are associated with a higher frequency of mediastinal shift, pulmonary hypoplasia, vascular compromise, and hydrops. Large lesions may also manifest with polyhydramnios, due probably to compression of the fetal esophagus by the mass and consequent interference with fetal swallowing of amniotic fluid. However, some CCAM lesions have been shown to involute in utero (15,16).

Hydrops is a harbinger of impending fetal death. Two of the fetuses with CCAM had hydrops at the time of imaging (Fig 3). One fetus had a large CCAM lesion associated with hydrops, abdominal ascites, and polyhydramnios. The ascites and hydrops resolved without intervention; however, the fetus died at birth because

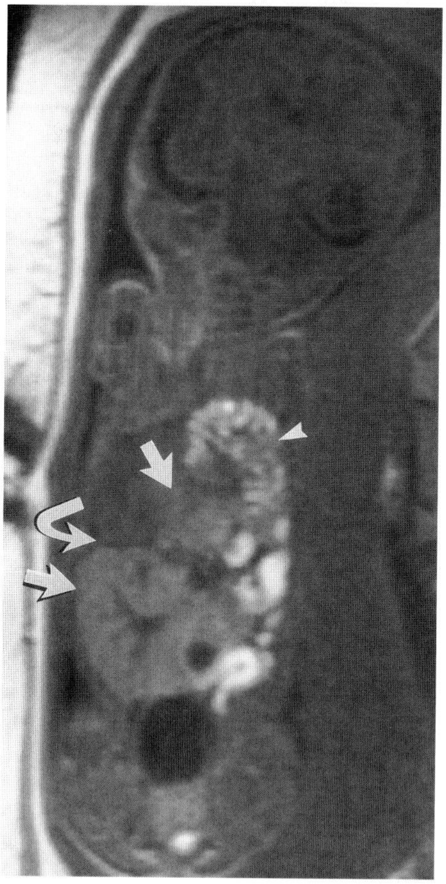

Figure 7. Left-sided congenital diaphragmatic hernia in a fetus of 22 weeks gestational age. Coronal T1-weighted fast low-angle shot MR image (174/4.1, 80° flip angle, 6-mm section thickness) shows the high-signal-intensity liver (straight arrows) extending into the chest above the diaphragmatic ridge (curved arrow). The meconium-filled bowel (arrowhead) has high signal intensity and extends to the apex of the chest.

of severe pulmonary hypoplasia. The second fetus had hydrops and a large CCAM lesion at the time of the mother's presentation; in utero removal of the CCAM was performed at 29 weeks gestation. The hydrops resolved in utero, and MR imaging demonstrated growth of both lungs. The fetus was born with mild respiratory distress syndrome.

It has been shown (2) that prenatal resection of a CCAM lesion may result in the survival of 60% of fetuses who develop hydrops. MR imaging findings were important for the planning of in utero removal of the tumor. MR imaging provided a large field of view and the ability to depict all of the fetal chest anatomy, including the size of the tumor, the remaining normal lung tissue, and the relationship to other chest structures, in a way that the pediatric surgeon could easily visualize.

BPS is a mass of nonfunctional lung tissue that does not communicate with the normal bronchial tree and receives its vascular supply from systemic arteries (1,17). BPS lesions may be extralobar or intralobar. The extralobar form is most commonly diagnosed in the prenatal and neonatal periods, whereas the intralobar form is more usually diagnosed in childhood. These lesions may involute in utero.

The prenatal US appearance of BPS is of a homogeneously hyperechoic mass in the lower lobe of a lung. MR imaging in the one fetus with BPS in our series demonstrated the lesion to be well defined with straight margins and very high signal intensity (Fig 4). In the one fetus with mixed BPS and CCAM, the lesion could no longer be demonstrated at US and was believed to have involuted. However, a mass of moderate size and very high signal intensity could still be demonstrated at MR imaging. US had the advantage of being able to demonstrate anomalous vessels in one of these cases and helped confirm the prenatal diagnosis of BPS. Although there are MR sequences capable of demonstrating blood flow, we could not demonstrate the anomalous vessels in two fetuses.

Although tracheal atresia is rare, this diagnosis should be considered when bilateral hyperechoic lung lesions are encountered at prenatal US. Although bilateral CCAM has been described (17), it is extremely uncommon, and it is more likely that uniformly echogenic lungs represent some form of occlusion of the trachea or larynx. When the trachea becomes obstructed, fetal lung fluid created by the alveoli becomes trapped, which causes hyperplasia of lung tissue and tracheal dilatation. Prenatal MR imaging demonstrated the lungs to have homogeneous high signal intensity, with obvious dilatation of the fluid-filled tracheobronchial tree. Such fetuses are at serious risk for development of hydrops due to cardiac compression and obstructed venous return. It is hoped that, in the future, the level of airway occlusion may be accurately identified at both US and MR imaging, so that in utero treatment or preparation for delivery with placental support (the ex utero intrapartum treatment, or EXIT, procedure) can be performed (18). The fetus in our series who had tracheal atresia was delivered with placental support and underwent tracheostomy in the delivery room.

Prenatal MR imaging was helpful for definition of the anatomy of very large chest masses and lesions that had an atypical US appearance. MR imaging clearly demonstrated a large foregut cyst and allowed differentiation of the cyst from a CCAM lesion. In another fetus, what appeared at US to be bilateral masses was seen at MR imaging to be a solitary CCAM that crossed the midline anterior to the heart (Fig 6).

Even at institutions where fetal surgery is not performed, MR imaging may be helpful for further definition of a chest mass and confirmation of the prenatal diagnosis. The accuracy of the prenatal diagnosis and the knowledge of the prenatal natural history of different chest masses can affect parental counseling. In many of the patients in our series, the wrong diagnosis had been established on the basis of the US findings, which would affect the counseling that a parent would receive. Several parents referred to our institution had been counseled that their fetus had a lethal chest lesion, even though the lesion was not causing substantial mass effect. These parents continued their pregnancies and delivered babies who required surgery, from which the babies quickly recovered.

Although a poor outcome for most fetal chest masses was predicted in the past, the results in more recent reports (11,15) have shown that most such lesions are not lethal. Counseling must include not only the diagnosis, natural history, and possible prenatal interventions, such as cyst aspiration or fetal surgery, but also planned delivery at an institution that is prepared to resuscitate and immediately perform surgery in a neonate who may be in severe respiratory distress. The surgeons at our institution found that MR images helped them mentally visualize a large fetal mass prior to delivery. MR imaging provides an image of the fetus that is easier to understand than the US image for physicians and patients not familiar with the performance and interpretation of the results of US.

In this study, we characterized the MR imaging appearance of common and uncommon congenital masses. With the use of US, more fetal chest lesions are being recognized, but they are not always accurately diagnosed. In this series, MR imaging helped further characterize the fetal chest lesions and confirm or change the prenatal diagnosis. MR imaging allowed clear differentiation of congenital diaphragmatic hernia from primary chest tumors. MR imaging was useful for defining tissue and anatomic effects of large and atypical chest masses. This information had an important effect on prenatal counseling and therapeutic planning.

References

1. Goldstein R. Ultrasound of the fetal thorax. In: Callen PW, ed. Ultrasonography in obstetrics and gynecology. 3rd ed. Philadelphia, Pa: Saunders, 1994; 333–346.
2. Adzick N, Harrison M, Flake A, Howell L, Golbus M, Filly R. Fetal surgery for congenital cystic adenomatoid malformation of the lung. J Pediatr Surg 1993; 28:806–812.
3. Harrison M, Adzick N, Flake A, et al. Correction of congenital diaphragmatic hernia in utero. IV. Hard-earned lessons. J Pediatr Surg 1993; 28:1411–1418.
4. Weinreb J, Lowe T, Cohen J, Kutler M. Human fetal anatomy: MR imaging. Radiology 1985; 157:715–720.
5. Mansfield P, Stehling M, Ordidge R, et al. Echo planar imaging of the human fetus in utero at 0.5T. Br J Radiol 1990; 63:833–841.
6. Levine D, Hatabu H, Gaa J, Atkinson MW, Edelman RR. Fetal anatomy revealed with fast MR sequences. AJR 1996; 167:905–908.
7. Hubbard AM, Adzick NS, Crombleholme TM, Haselgrove JC. Left-sided congenital diaphragmatic hernia: value of prenatal MR imaging in preparation for fetal surgery. Radiology 1997; 203:636–640.
8. Levine D, Barnes PD, Sher S, et al. Fetal fast MR imaging: reproducibility, technical quality, and conspicuity of anatomy. Radiology 1998; 206:549–554.
9. Gowland P, Moore R, Freeman A, et al. Monitoring fetal lung maturation using echo-planar magnetic resonance imaging (abstr). In: Proceedings of the Fourth Meeting of the International Society for Magnetic Resonance in Medicine. Berkeley, Calif: International Society for Magnetic Resonance in Medicine, 1996; 157.
10. Baker P, Johnson I, Gowland P, et al. Estimation of fetal lung volume using echo-planar magnetic resonance imaging. Obstet Gynecol 1994; 83:951–954.
11. Barret J, Chitayat D, Sermer M, et al. The prognostic factors in the prenatal diagnosis of the echogenic fetal lung. Prenat Diagn 1995; 15:849–853.
12. Achiron R, Strauss S, Seidman D, et al. Fetal lung hyperechogenicity: prenatal ultrasonographic diagnosis, natural history and neonatal outcome. Ultrasound Obstet Gynecol 1995; 6:40–42.
13. King S, Pilling D, Walkinshaw S. Fetal echogenic lung lesions: prenatal ultrasound diagnosis and outcome. Pediatr Radiol 1995; 25:208–210.
14. Stocker J, Madewell J, Drake R. Congenital cystic adenomatoid malformation of the lung: classification and morphologic spectrum. Hum Pathol 1977; 8:155–171.
15. MacGillivray P, Harrison M, Goldstein R, Adzick N. Disappearing fetal lung lesions. J Pediatr Surg 1993; 28:1321–1325.
16. Mashiach R, Hod M, Friedman S, Schoenfeld A, Ovadia J, Merlob P. Antenatal ultrasound diagnosis of congenital cystic adenomatoid malformation of the lung: spontaneous resolution in utero. J Clin Ultrasound 1993; 21:453–457.
17. Dolkart L, Reimers F, Wertheimer I, et al. Prenatal diagnosis of laryngeal atresia. J Ultrasound Med 1992; 11:496–498.
18. Mychaliska G, Bealer J, Graf J, Adzick N, Harrison M. Operating on placental support: the ex utero intrapartum treatment (EXIT) procedure. J Pediatr Surg 1997; 32:227–230.

Advanced Emphysema: Preoperative Chest Radiographic Findings as Predictors of Outcome Following Lung Volume Reduction Surgery[1]

Daniel D. Maki, MD
Wallace T. Miller, Jr, MD
Judith M. Aronchick, MD
Warren B. Gefter, MD
Wallace T. Miller, Sr, MD
Robert M. Kotloff, MD
Gregory Tino, MD

Index terms:
Emphysema, pulmonary, 60.751
Lung, diseases, 60.751
Lung, surgery
Lung, ventilation, 60.1295

Radiology 1999; 212:49–55

Abbreviation:
FEV_1 = forced expiratory volume in 1 second

[1] From the Departments of Radiology (D.D.M., W.T.M.Jr., J.M.A., W.B.G., W.T.M.Sr.) and Medicine, Pulmonary and Critical Care Division (R.M.K., G.T.), Hospital of the University of Pennsylvania, 1st Floor Silverstein, 3400 Spruce St, Philadelphia, PA 19104. From the 1997 RSNA scientific assembly. Received February 3, 1998; revision requested April 9; final revision received October 12; accepted December 16. **Address reprint requests to** W.T.M.Jr. (e-mail: *miller2@rad.upenn.edu*).

See also the editorial by Austin (pp 1–3) in this issue.

Author contributions:
Guarantor of integrity of entire study, D.D.M.; study concepts and design, D.D.M., W.T.M.Jr.; definition of intellectual content, D.D.M., W.T.M.Jr.; literature research, D.D.M., W.T.M.Jr.; clinical studies, all authors; data acquisition, D.D.M.; data and statistical analyses, D.D.M., W.T.M.Jr.; manuscript preparation, D.D.M., W.T.M.Jr.; manuscript editing and review, all authors.

PURPOSE: To determine whether preoperative chest radiographic findings alone can reliably predict which patients will achieve the best functional outcome of lung volume reduction surgery.

MATERIALS AND METHODS: The preoperative chest radiographs obtained in 57 patients who had undergone lung volume reduction surgery were retrospectively scored by five blinded readers for severity and distribution of emphysema, evidence of lung compression, disease heterogeneity, and other features. Comparisons were made with the 3–6-month postoperative functional outcome for each patient.

RESULTS: High disease heterogeneity (score >2) and unequivocal lung compression (score 1) both were 100% predictive of a favorable outcome (FEV_1 increase, ≥30%). Low heterogeneity (score <1) was 94% predictive of an unfavorable outcome (FEV_1 increase <30%), as was a lack of lung compression, which was 92% predictive of an unfavorable outcome. These two features also correlated with an improved 6-minute walk test result, although this correlation was weaker.

CONCLUSION: Chest radiography alone may be sufficient for initial screening. High disease heterogeneity and lung compression on chest radiographs are highly predictive of a favorable functional outcome.

Emphysema in its advanced form is a devastating pulmonary disease characterized by the loss of elastic recoil throughout the lungs, which manifests as hyperinflation and hindrance of expiratory airflow (1). Medical therapy that consists primarily of inhaled bronchodilators, corticosteroids, and supplemental oxygen provides limited symptomatic relief, particularly in patients with advanced disease (2). As a result, there has been renewed interest in surgical options for treatment of advanced emphysema. Although lung transplantation may ultimately provide the best long-term result in many patients, the supply of available organs is limited, and many patients are not candidates for transplantation because of coexistent disease or advanced age. Lung volume reduction surgery has thus attracted much attention in recent years. There is little disagreement that resection of large localized pulmonary bullae associated with compression and atelectasis is efficacious. However, the partial resection of nonbullous areas of the lung in patients with generalized emphysema has been much more controversial until recently (2).

In lung volume reduction surgery, which was described by Brantigan et al (3) in 1959, the overall lung volume is reduced by means of multiple nonsegmental wedge resections aimed at the most diseased areas of the lung when possible, with the purpose of decreasing the total lung volume by approximately 20%–30%. The theoretic basis of the procedure is that returning the lung to a more physiologic total volume may promote elastic recoil and enhance diaphragmatic function (4).

Lung volume reduction surgery has been shown to improve pulmonary function test results, exercise tolerance, and quality of life in many patients (5). However, the functional outcomes in most centers have varied, and it has been suggested that the outcome differences may be predicted preoperatively by using a variety of clinical, laboratory, and radiographic parameters (5–8). We set out to determine whether the functional outcome of patients who underwent lung volume reduction surgery at our institution could have been reliably predicted by using various objective findings on these patients' preoperative chest radiographs alone.

MATERIALS AND METHODS

Patient Population

Between September 1993 and January 1996, 120 patients (59 men, 61 women; mean age [± SD], 61.4 years ± 7.7) with severe emphysema underwent bilateral lung volume reduction surgery at our institution. The majority of these patients had smoking-related centrilobular emphysema, although several had a pattern that resembled panlobular emphysema. All of these patients had severe airflow obstruction, with a mean (± SD) forced expiratory volume in 1 second (FEV_1) of 0.73 L ± 0.25, which was 20%–30% of that predicted for their ages. After passing the initial screening, all patients underwent mandatory outpatient pulmonary rehabilitation for 6 weeks prior to surgery. Standard surgical methods and screening parameters, which have been previously described by Kotloff et al (9), were used. Six patients died within 30 days following surgery, and another six died prior to being discharged from the inpatient facility. The surviving patients underwent follow-up pulmonary function tests 3–6 months postoperatively. The in-house preoperative chest radiographs obtained in 57 patients were available for this retrospective review. The remaining patients were referred by outside physicians, so their preoperative radiographs were obtained at outside institutions and thus unavailable for this retrospective analysis.

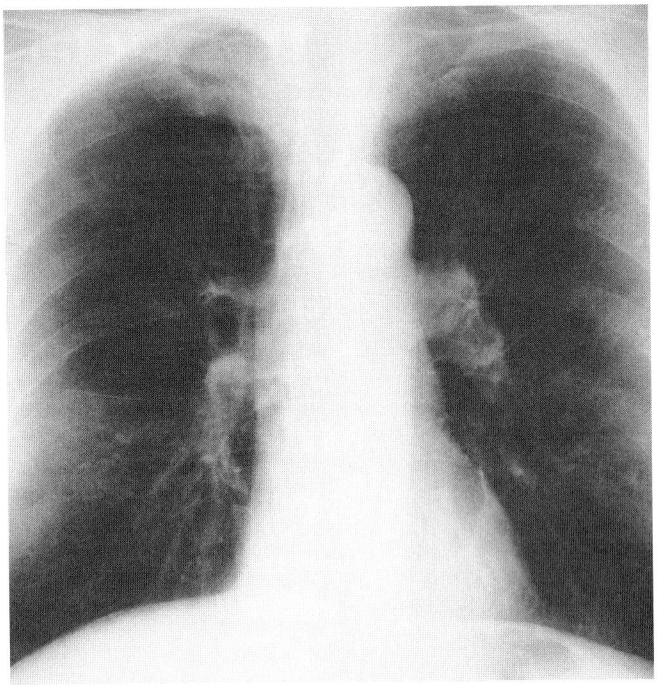

a.

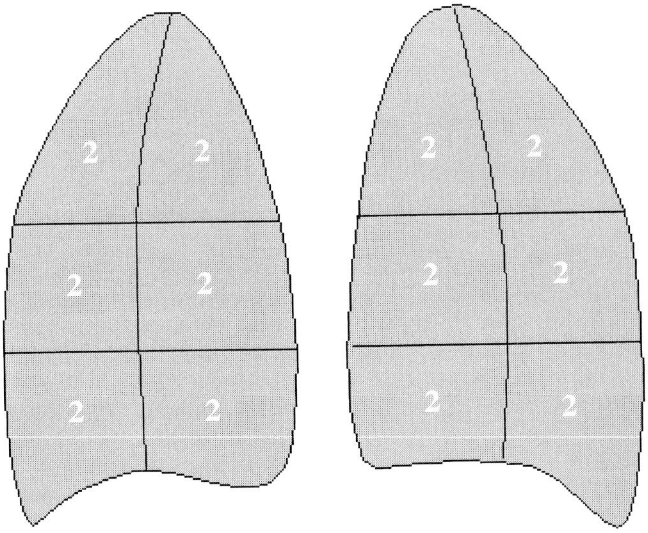

b.

Figure 1. **(a)** Posteroanterior radiograph obtained in a 79-year-old man with homogeneous emphysema demonstrates very little variability in disease from one area of the lung to the next. **(b)** One reader's scoring of the radiograph in **a**, which resulted in a heterogeneity score of 0. This patient's radiograph was given a negative score for lung compression.

Clinical Evaluation of Outcome

Pulmonary function testing, including spirometry and lung volume measurement, was performed preoperatively and 3–6 months postoperatively by using standard techniques (9). Body plethysmography was used to measure lung volumes because it is regarded by many to be the most accurate method. Exercise tolerance was assessed with the standardized 6-minute walk test, in a flat hallway without coaching, by using titrated supplemental oxygen to maintain the oxyhemoglobin saturation level at 90% or higher.

For outcome analysis, the percentage changes in FEV_1 and 6-minute walk test results were used, as opposed to the absolute values, to better standardize the relative magnitude of improvement or deterioration between patients with different baseline values.

Radiographic Evaluation and Scoring

Standard inspiratory posteroanterior and lateral chest radiographs were phototimed at 120 kVp, with use of a fixed grid

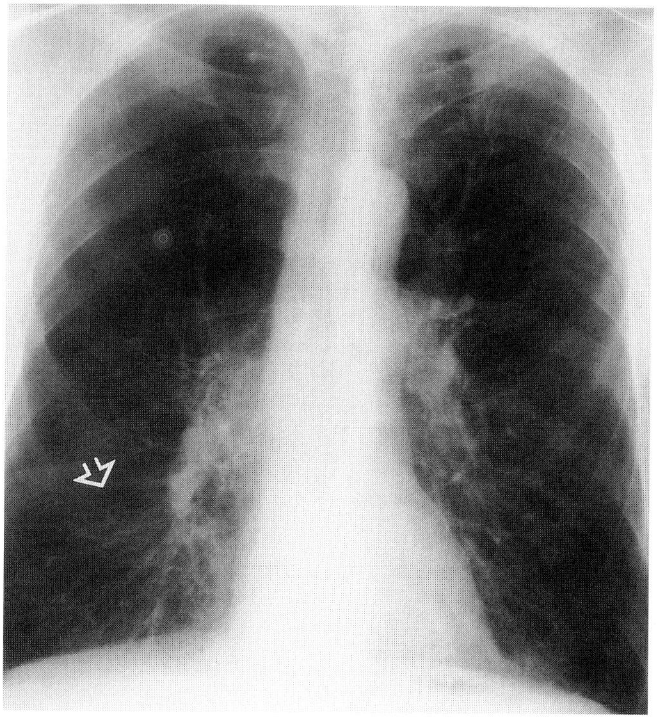

a.

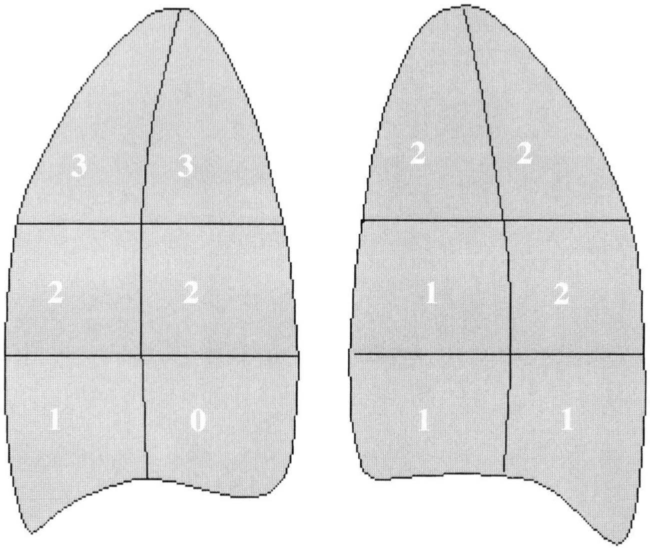

b.

Figure 2. **(a)** Posteroanterior radiograph obtained in a 66-year-old man with heterogeneous emphysema demonstrates severe disease in the right upper lobe, with relatively normal lung tissue in the right base. Vascular crowding (arrow) also is evident in the lower right lung medially compared with the upper zone vasculature. (The circle is a snap on the patient's clothing.) **(b)** One reader's scoring of the radiograph in **a**, which resulted in a heterogeneity score of 3. This patient's radiograph was given a positive score for lung compression.

and a wide-latitude screen-film system (Eastman-Kodak, Rochester, NY).

Radiographs were read and scored by five readers independently on different dates. Four of the readers (W.T.M.Jr., W.T.M.Sr., J.M.A., W.B.G.) were subspecialized thoracic radiologists, with levels of experience ranging from 7 to 40 years. The fifth reader (D.D.M.) was a diagnostic radiology resident. It was felt that these differing experience levels might provide insight into the variability and reproducibility of scoring. All of the radiologists were blinded to each patient's ultimate functional outcome. No time constraint for reading and scoring the images was provided. Individual cases and scoring were not discussed between radiologists.

No standard scores were provided, but the radiologists were asked to score the images as follows: A lung compression score of 1 (positive) was given if there were any signs of vascular crowding or atelectasis; otherwise a score of 0 (negative) was given. The severity of emphysema in various zones of each lung was scored on a scale of 0–3 as follows: 0, normal lung; 1, mild disease (<25% airspace replacement); 2, moderate disease (25%–75% airspace replacement); and 3, severe disease (>75% airspace replacement). Each lung was divided into six upper-, middle-, and lower-third zones and into medial versus lateral (central vs peripheral) divisions (Figs 1, 2). An overall severity score was calculated by adding the scores in the 12 individual zones.

Heterogeneity was assessed by constructing mathematical models that explored the differences and ratios between the most diseased and least diseased lung zones—for example, differences in disease severity between upper and lower zones and between peripheral and central zones. What will subsequently be referred to as the heterogeneity score is simply the difference between the maximum upper zone score and the minimum lower zone score, which yielded scores that ranged from 0 to 3. A peripheral versus central zone score, which represented the difference between the total peripheral zone scores and the total central zone scores, also was calculated.

Two examples of scoring are shown in Figures 1 and 2. Figure 1 shows very homogeneous emphysema; two radiologists gave all zones a score of 2, and three radiologists gave all zones a score of 3. This resulted in a heterogeneity score of 0 by all radiologists. No vascular crowding or atelectasis was present, so lung compression was scored as 0 (negative) by all five radiologists. Figure 2 demonstrates the lungs of a patient with heterogeneous disease. All five readers gave the right upper zones a score of 3 and the right base of the lung a score of either 0 or 1. This resulted in high heterogeneity scores of 3 from four readers and 2 from one reader. This patient's radiograph was given a lung compression score of 1 (positive) by all five radiologists, because there was vascular crowding just inferior to the severely diseased right upper lobe.

Several other parameters were scored

by two of the radiologists (W.T.M.Jr., D.D.M.). Hyperinflation was initially assessed by using two quantitative measurements. First, the angles of the anterior and posterior costophrenic sulci were measured in degrees and averaged to obtain the diaphragm angle score. Second, the anteroposterior/longitudinal chest wall diameter was calculated by dividing the maximal anteroposterior diameter, from pleural surface to pleural surface, by the maximal longitudinal dimension, from the apex to the dome of the higher hemidiaphragm on the lateral image. Finally, a subjective hyperinflation score of 0 (normal), 1 (mild), 2 (moderate), 3 (severe), or 4 (inversion of diaphragms) was assigned. The percentage of normal or minimally diseased lung also was estimated in each patient by these two radiologists. The other three readers were not asked to score these additional features, because the first two readers found them to be overly cumbersome and time-consuming to score.

Statistical Analyses

The Student *t* test, with a heteroscedastic one-tailed distribution, was used to compare scores between groups of patients, specifically those patients with a favorable outcome versus those who did poorly. A favorable outcome was defined as an increase of 30% or greater in postoperative FEV_1 over the preoperative baseline value, and a poor outcome was defined as a less than 30% increase in FEV_1. The 30% cutoff was chosen because it was thought to be a change that was not only reproducible and beyond the range of measurement error but also likely to represent a clinically important improvement. The nonsurvivors were excluded from analysis. A *P* value of less than .05 was considered to be statistically significant.

The predictive values, sensitivity, and specificity of the various predictive features studied were determined. In addition, Pearson correlation coefficients were used to test the correlation between various scored features and functional outcome. Tests for statistical significance and correlation coefficients were performed for each radiologist individually. In addition, statistical analyses were performed to determine the composite (mean) scores of all five radiologists. Interobserver variability was assessed by using receiver operating characteristic analysis and comparing the individual radiologists' scores and *P* values.

TABLE 1
Scored Radiographic Features versus Functional Outcomes Following Lung Volume Reduction Surgery

	Mean Scores (± SD)*		
Scored Radiographic Feature	Poor Outcome Group	Favorable Outcome Group	*P* Value
Heterogeneity			
Upper vs lower	0.64 ± 0.83	1.96 ± 0.32	<.001
Peripheral vs central	0.58 ± 0.59	1.34 ± 0.62	<.01
Compression	0.12 ± 0.23	0.67 ± 0.34	<.001
Estimated percentage of normal lung	15.2 ± 19.5	20.4 ± 18.9	.16
Overall severity of emphysema	24.8 ± 5.8	23.4 ± 4.4	.17
Hyperinflation			
Diaphragm angles	84.9 ± 9.7	84.3 ± 7.5	.25
Qualitative score	2.8 ± 0.9	2.6 ± 0.3	.25
Anteroposterior/longitudinal chest wall diameter	0.81 ± 0.11	0.79 ± 0.08	.22

* The poor outcome group consisted of 32 patients with increases in FEV_1 of less than 30%. The favorable outcome group consisted of 25 patients with increases in FEV_1 of 30% or greater.

TABLE 2
Discriminating Scores of Heterogeneity and Lung Compression for Prediction of Outcome Following Lung Volume Reduction Surgery

Scored Feature	No. of Patients	No. of Patients Who Did Poorly*	No. of Patients Who Did Favorably†
Heterogeneity‡			
Low	17	16 (94)	1 (6)
Moderate	25	16 (64)	9 (36)
High	15	0 (0)	15 (100)
Compression			
0 (unanimously negative)	25	23 (92)	2 (8)
Less than 0.5 but greater than 0	13	6 (46)	7 (54)
Less than 1 but greater than 0.5	9	3 (33)	6 (67)
1 (unanimously positive)	10	0 (0)	10 (100)

Note.—Numbers in parentheses are percentages.
* Patients with increases in FEV_1 of less than 30%.
† Patients with increases in FEV_1 of 30% or greater.
‡ Heterogeneity score is defined as the maximum upper zone score minus the minimum lower zone score. Low = mean heterogeneity score less than 1 but greater than or equal to 0. Moderate = score less than 2 but greater than or equal to 1. High = score greater than or equal to 2.

RESULTS

Complete preoperative data and 3–6-month postoperative follow-up data, including FEV_1 measurements, were available in all 57 patients. In addition, the 6-minute walk test results for 51 of the 57 patients were available. The poor outcome group (<30% FEV_1 increase) consisted of 32 patients, who had a mean (± SD) increase in FEV_1 of 9.2% ± 16.3 over the baseline; seven of these 32 patients experienced a postoperative decrease in FEV_1. In contrast, the favorable outcome group (≥30% FEV_1 increase) consisted of 25 patients with a mean increase in FEV_1 of 73.3% ± 26.8. The mean 6-minute walk test measurements for the two groups were 29.2% ± 43.5 and 30.3% ± 19.6, respectively, which were not significantly different.

As seen in Table 1, there was a highly significant difference in the mean heterogeneity score between the two outcome groups. Those with a poor outcome generally demonstrated a low heterogeneity score, in contrast to those with a favorable outcome, who consistently demonstrated high heterogeneity. Similarly, those patients who did favorably tended to have higher heterogeneity as measured by the peripheral zone versus central zone disease severity scores; these differences also were statistically significant. Table 2 shows the outcomes of patients with specific radiographic heterogeneity scores. Note that of those patients (n = 17) with very low heterogeneity (mean score <1),

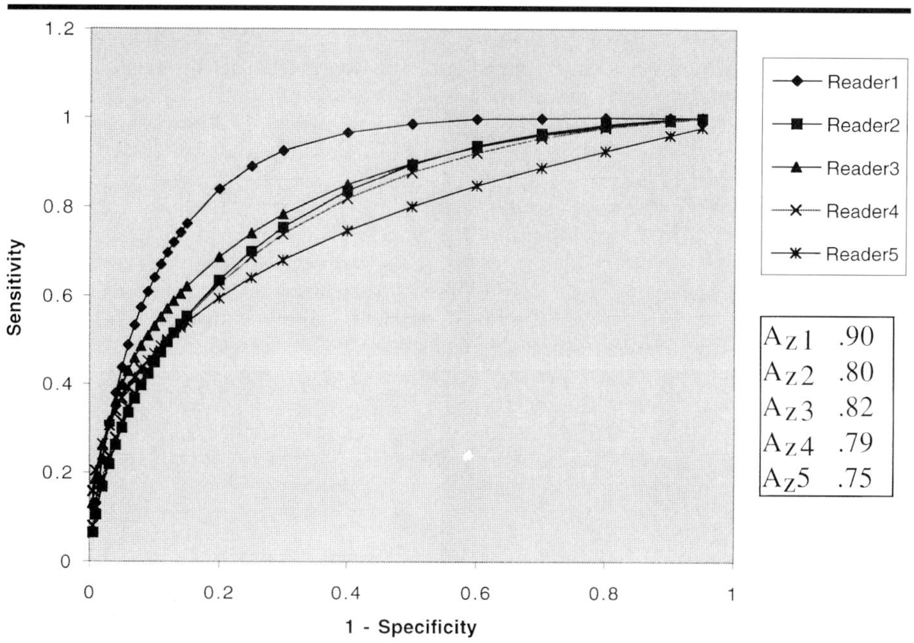

Figure 3. Receiver operating characteristic analysis of disease heterogeneity scores among five independent readers. Analysis results are plotted as the heterogeneity score versus the outcome, as measured by using the FEV_1. The A_z values (areas under the receiver operating characteristic curves) obtained by each reader are shown on the right. The similar high A_z values and highly concordant receiver operating characteristic curves indicate high performance and low inter-reader variability among the five readers despite their varying levels of experience.

TABLE 3
Correlation between Scored Features and Two Different Outcome Measures

Scored Radiographic Feature	FEV_1	6-Minute Walk Test
Heterogeneity		
Upper vs lower disease*	0.680	0.191
Peripheral vs central disease	0.469	0.016
Lung compression	0.718	0.195
Overall severity of emphysema	−0.029	0.189

Note.—Data are Pearson correlation coefficients.

* Maximum disease score in upper lung zone minus minimum disease score in lower lung zone.

16 (94%) did unfavorably, with a <30% increase in FEV_1. Similarly, by using the 6-minute walk test result as a measure of outcome, 15 (88%) of the 17 patients with a heterogeneity score of less than 1 were unable to increase their 6-minute walk test measurement to 30% or more over the baseline. On the contrary, all 15 (100%) of the patients with very high heterogeneity (mean score ≥2) did favorably, demonstrating a 30% or greater increase in FEV_1. By using the 6-minute walk test result as a measure of outcome, seven (47%) of the 15 patients whose radiographs were given a heterogeneity score of 2 or higher experienced an increase in the 6-minute walk test measurement of 30% or more over the baseline.

The majority of patients who did poorly had no evidence of lung compression, whereas the majority of those who did well had clear evidence of compression, as shown in Table 1. These differences were highly statistically significant. Table 2 shows the outcomes of patients with specific scores of lung compression. It is particularly noteworthy that of the 25 patients whose radiographs were unanimously given a negative score (ie, 0) for compression, 23 (92%) did poorly (increase of <30% over baseline FEV_1), whereas all 10 (100%) of the patients whose radiographs were unanimously given a positive score (ie, 1) for compression did well, with an increase of 30% or more over the baseline FEV_1. For those patients with available 6-minute walk test data, a similar, albeit weaker, correlation between the 6-minute walk test result and lung compression was found. Of the 25 patients whose radiographs were given a negative (ie, 0) lung compression score, 19 (77%) experienced an increase of less than 30% over the baseline 6-minute walk test measurement, whereas seven (71%) of the 10 patients whose radiographs were given a positive (ie, 1) score experienced an increase of 30% or more over the baseline 6-minute walk test measurement.

As shown in Table 1, the estimated percentage of normal lung, overall score of emphysema severity, and the various measures of hyperinflation were not significantly different between the two outcome groups.

Table 3 shows the Pearson correlation coefficients for each of the measured features in relation to FEV_1 and 6-minute walk test. Again, both heterogeneity and lung compression correlated strongly with increased FEV_1. Interestingly, these two features had a weaker correlation with the 6-minute walk test; however, as the data above demonstrate, a definite correlation between 6-minute walk test and these two features was present. The calculated overall disease severity showed no significant correlation with outcome.

Interradiologist variability of individual lung zone severity scores was high. The scores for individual lung zones commonly varied by one to two grades among the five readers, although the readers' scores never varied by greater than two grades. The resultant overall severity scores, or estimates of pulmonary reserve, were therefore also highly variable between different radiologists.

In contrast, interreader variability of heterogeneity and lung compression was minimal. Figure 3 illustrates the results of receiver operating characteristic analysis of the five independent radiologists' scores for heterogeneity, including the A_z value—that is, area under the receiver operating characteristic curve—for each radiologist. Receiver operating characteristic analysis could not be performed for lung compression, because this variable was discrete (ie, noncontinuous). However, there was unanimous agreement on compression in 35 of 57 cases and agreement among four of the five radiologists on another 10 of 57 cases. Put more simply, there was agreement on lung compression among at least four of the five readers in 79% of the cases.

DISCUSSION

Given the large number of patients with emphysema in the United States, the high cost of lung volume reduction surgery (10), and the variable outcomes of patients who undergo this procedure (9,11), there is a great deal of interest in identifying reliable clinical and radiologic predictors of outcome that could be used to aid patient selection. It is for this reason that a multicenter national trial was initiated by the National Institutes of Health and Health Care Financing Administration in 1998 to evaluate more than 4,800 patients in 17 selected medical centers. The results of this trial are not expected in the short-term, however, because the study has a 3–5-year follow-up after patient entry.

The work of Slone and colleagues (5,8) has provided an important foundation for the use of imaging techniques to help predict the outcome from lung volume reduction surgery. The results of their studies, which involved the use of inspiration and expiration chest radiography, chest computed tomography (CT), and nuclear medicine ventilation-perfusion scanning, suggest that high disease heterogeneity, evidence of lung compression, and higher residual normal lung are predictive of a favorable outcome. Our data confirm many of their conclusions; however, the results of our study suggest that conventional chest radiography alone is highly predictive, without the need for additional expensive or invasive imaging modalities.

The results of this study show that high disease heterogeneity on standard chest radiographs is strongly predictive of a favorable outcome following lung volume reduction surgery. Specifically, we found that a very high heterogeneity score (≥ 2) virtually guaranteed a favorable result (positive predictive value of 100%) in our patient population. In contrast, an extremely low heterogeneity score (<1) strongly correlated with a poor outcome and thus should be helpful in patient selection. In our study population, this criterion alone would have excluded 17 (30%) patients from eligibility for the procedure; only one could have done well (positive predictive value of 94%), as indicated by an increase in FEV_1 of 30% or more over the baseline.

We did not provide disease severity score standards for our radiologists, and thus the disease severity scores of individual lung zones varied among the different radiologists. However, the relative differences in disease severity between lung zones, which is what determined the heterogeneity, was very consistent between readers, as demonstrated by the highly concordant receiver operating characteristic curves. Thus, absolute standards may not be necessary for determining heterogeneity, because an internal standard of sorts exists within each case. However, standards may be of value for achieving better consistency in scoring overall disease severity (vs residual normal lung). This feature, often referred to as normal pulmonary reserve, is thought by some investigators (5) to be predictive of surgical mortality. If it were important to get a more consistent overall severity from reader to reader, a scoring strategy in which individual lung zones are scored as 0 for normal or near normal lung and as 1 for advanced disease could be devised. With such a strategy, one could expect much less interreader variability among individual and overall severity scores, but this might be at the expense of a loss in the predictive value of the heterogeneity score.

Lung compression should also be helpful in patient selection for lung volume reduction surgery. In our population, if those patients who indisputably had no lung compression (n = 25) had been denied lung volume reduction surgery, we would have prevented 44% of the candidates from undergoing this expensive operation and excluded only two who would have done well (positive predictive value of 92%). In contrast, the finding of indisputable lung compression provided a virtual guarantee of a favorable outcome (positive predictive value of 100%) in our population.

Our decision to use a 30% increase in FEV_1 as the cutoff for favorable versus unfavorable outcome may be subject to criticism. We believe, however, that this cutoff represents a magnitude of improvement that is well beyond the error of measurement of the test and, hence, statistically meaningful and reproducible. We also believe that this magnitude of change represents a clinically relevant improvement. Ultimately, it is necessary for individual surgeons and pulmonologists to decide which threshold represents a functional improvement that is substantial enough to warrant surgery at their particular center.

Although in our study the radiographic features of heterogeneity and lung compression were highly predictive of a postoperative increase in FEV_1, their correlation with the 6-minute walk time was somewhat weaker. Some have argued that the 6-minute walk time is a better functional evaluation than is FEV_1, which is more of a physiologic measure (5). In our population, the two measures did not correlate strongly. There is no clear explanation for this poor correlation, but it has been reported by other investigators (9,11,12). It may be because lung volume reduction surgery probably influences physiologic parameters that are not reflected in pulmonary function tests, such as gas exchange, cardiac function, and perceived dyspnea (2,9). There is probably no single test that best evaluates the overall outcome following lung volume reduction surgery. Inasmuch as we relied on FEV_1 as our primary measure of outcome, this may be considered a limitation of the study. However, the FEV_1 measurement is reproducible, standardized, and, in our opinion, not as prone to be influenced by motivation and psychologic factors. In addition, FEV_1 is one of the few objective measures that has been shown to correlate with mortality caused by emphysema (13).

Some may consider it a mistake to have included a resident as one of the five readers. However, we believed it was necessary to include one reader who was not subspecialized and, in fact, was considerably less experienced to see how a less specialized and less experienced reader would perform in the model. The resident's scores were not significantly different from those of the other four radiologists (Fig 3), which suggests that readings by general radiologists or experienced clinician readers may be as consistent and predictive of outcome in our model as those by subspecialized thoracic radiologists.

Twelve (10%) of the 120 patients in our initial population died within 90 days after the procedure. These patients were not included in the analysis. All 12 of the patients who died succumbed to infection or sepsis, which are complications that are not predictable by using preoperative radiography. The high mortality in this series may reflect the steep learning curve of performing lung volume reduction surgery; these were the first 120 patients to undergo this procedure at our institution. However, this was not a major limitation of our study, because mortality was not examined as an end point.

Roughly one-half of the patients who underwent lung volume reduction surgery at our institution during the study period had preoperative radiographs that were available for our analysis. Although this is a limitation of our study, it should be noted that the functional outcomes in our study group of 57 patients were virtually identical to those in the series studied by Kotloff et al (9). Specifically, one-third of our study patients demonstrated an increase of less than 20% over the baseline FEV_1, one-third demonstrated a 20%–60% increase in FEV_1, and one-third demonstrated a greater than 60% increase in FEV_1.

It seems counterintuitive that hyperinflation was not predictive, particularly given that the basis of the lung volume reduction procedure is a reduction in hyperinflation in the chest. This may derive from the fact that most patients who are chosen for lung volume reduction surgery already have substantial hyperinflation, and this may be why the variance in hyperinflation scores was small. However, an equally plausible explanation is that the findings of disease heterogeneity and lung compression are much more powerful predictors of outcome than is hyperinflation, and hyperinflation would have shown a predictive value with greater statistical power in a study with more patients.

Other investigators (14–16) have recently evaluated the role of other imaging modalities such as CT and ventilation-perfusion scanning in the preoperative examination of patients who are being considered for lung volume reduction surgery. The results of our study have shown that the findings on chest radiographs alone may be highly predictive of outcome in this population. Although further studies on the radiographic evaluation for lung volume reduction surgery are needed, the preliminary data on the radiographic prediction of outcome are compelling. Clearly, radiography will have an important role in patient selection for this promising but costly approach to the management of advanced emphysema in the years to come.

References

1. Snider GL, Kleinerman J, Thurlbeck WM, et al. The definition of emphysema: report of a National Heart, Lung, and Blood Institute Division of Lung Disease workshop. Am Rev Respir Dis 1985; 132:182–185.
2. Cooper JD, Trulock EP, Triantafillou AN, et al. Bilateral pneumectomy (volume reduction) for chronic obstructive lung disease. J Thorac Cardiovasc Surg 1995; 109:106–119.
3. Brantigan OC, Mueller E, Kress MB. A surgical approach to pulmonary emphysema. Am Rev Respir Dis 1959; 8:194–206.
4. Sciurba F, Rogers R, Keenan RJ, et al. Improvement in pulmonary function and elastic recoil after lung-reduction surgery for diffuse advanced emphysema. N Engl J Med 1996; 334:1095–1099.
5. Slone RM, Pilgram TK, Gierada DS, et al. Lung volume reduction surgery: comparison of preoperative radiologic features and clinical outcome. Radiology 1997; 204:685–693.
6. Szekely LA, Oelberg DA, Wright C, et al. Preoperative predictors of operative morbidity and mortality in COPD patients undergoing bilateral lung volume reduction surgery. Chest 1997; 111:550–558.
7. Yusen RD, Lefrak SS, Washington University Emphysema Study Group. Evaluation of patients with emphysema for lung volume reduction surgery. Semin Thorac Cardiovasc Surg 1996; 8:83–93.
8. Slone RM, Gierada DS. Radiology of pulmonary emphysema and lung volume reduction surgery. Semin Thorac Cardiovasc Surg 1996; 8:61–82.
9. Kotloff RM, Tino G, Bavaria JE, et al. Bilateral lung volume reduction surgery for advanced emphysema: a comparison of median sternotomy and thoracoscopic approaches. Chest 1996; 110:1399–1406.
10. Albert RK, Lewis S, Wood D, et al. Economic aspects of lung volume reduction surgery. Chest 1996; 110:1068–1071.
11. Yusen RD, Trulock EP, Pohl MS, Biggar DG, Washington University Emphysema Study Group. Results of lung volume reduction surgery in patients with emphysema. Semin Thorac Cardiovasc Surg 1996; 8:99–109.
12. Teramoto S, Matsuse T, Ouchi Y. Is the symptomatic improvement after lung volume reduction surgery correlated with FEV_1 in patients with diffuse emphysema? Chest 1996: 110:28–34.
13. Nocturnal Oxygen Therapy Trial Group. Continuous or nocturnal oxygen therapy in hypoxemic chronic obstructive lung disease: a clinical trial. Ann Intern Med 1980; 93:391–398.
14. Wang SC, Fischer KC, Slone RM, et al. Perfusion scintigraphy in the evaluation for lung volume reduction surgery: correlation with clinical outcome. Radiology 1997; 205:243–248.
15. Gierada DS, Hakimian S. Slone RM, Yusen RD. MR analysis of lung volume and thoracic dimensions in patients with emphysema before and after lung volume reduction surgery. AJR 1998; 170:707–714.
16. Bae KT, Slone RM, Gierada DS, Yusen RD, Cooper JD. Patients with emphysema: quantitative CT analysis before and after lung volume reduction surgery. Radiology 1997; 203:705–714.

Lung Cancer Staging and Management: Comparison of Contrast-enhanced and Nonenhanced Helical CT of the Thorax[1]

Edward F. Patz, Jr, MD
Jeremy J. Erasmus, MD
H. Page McAdams, MD
John E. Connolly, MD
Edith M. Marom, MD
Philip C. Goodman, MD
Richard A. Leder, MD
Mary T. Keogan, MD
James E. Herndon, PhD

Index terms:
Computed tomography (CT), comparative studies, 60.12111, 60.12112, 60.12115, 76.12111, 76.12112, 76.12115, 86.12111, 86.12112, 86.12115
Computed tomography (CT), helical, 60.12115, 76.12115, 86.12115
Lung, CT, 60.12111, 60.12112, 60.12115
Lung neoplasms, 60.321, 60.334, 60.3313, 60.3376, 60.3386
Lung neoplasms, staging, 60.33

Radiology 1999; 212:56–60

[1] From the Department of Radiology (E.F.P., J.J.E., H.P.M., J.E.C., E.M.M., P.C.G., R.A.L., M.T.K.) and Biometry Division, Community and Family Medicine (J.E.H.), Duke University Medical Center, Box 3808, Erwin Rd, Durham, NC 27710. Received May 20, 1998; revision requested June 18; final revision received September 2; accepted December 15. **Address reprint requests to** E.F.P. (e-mail: *patz0002@mc.duke.edu*).

Author contributions:
Guarantor of integrity of entire study, E.F.P.; study concepts, E.F.P., P.C.G.; study design, E.F.P., H.P.M., P.C.G.; definition of intellectual content, all authors; literature research, E.F.P., J.J.E., H.P.M.; clinical studies, all authors; data acquisition, E.F.P., J.J.E., H.P.M.; data analysis, all authors; statistical analysis, J.E.H.; manuscript preparation, editing, and review, all authors.

PURPOSE: To determine whether contrast material–enhanced helical computed tomography (CT) of the thorax and upper abdomen changes the tumor stage and management compared with nonenhanced helical CT in patients with newly diagnosed lung cancer.

MATERIALS AND METHODS: During 15 months, any patient in whom lung cancer was strongly suspected or newly diagnosed and who was scheduled for thoracic CT was considered eligible for the study. All patients underwent nonenhanced thoracic helical CT from the lung apices through the adrenal glands and then contrast-enhanced thoracic helical CT from the lung apices through the entire liver. Each study was read independently, and the thoracic radiologic stage was determined. Tissue sampling was performed and the final pathologic stage assigned.

RESULTS: Ninety-six patients had a final pathologic diagnosis of lung cancer. There was agreement in stage between the nonenhanced and contrast-enhanced examinations in 92 of the 96 patients. In three patients, the tumor stage at nonenhanced CT increased at contrast-enhanced CT, from IA to IIA ($n = 1$), IIB to IV ($n = 1$), and IIIB to IV ($n = 1$). In one patient, the tumor stage decreased from IIIB to IIB. There was no substantial change in management of any patient.

CONCLUSION: The results suggest that contrast-enhanced thoracic CT through the liver for staging lung cancer rarely changes the tumor stage determined with nonenhanced CT through the adrenal glands and does not substantially influence management decisions.

Computed tomography (CT) is the standard imaging modality used to radiologically stage lung cancer (1–7). CT protocols vary between institutions because the optimal and most cost-effective imaging parameters have not been rigorously established (8). Some radiologists prefer contrast material–enhanced studies through the chest and liver, whereas others prefer nonenhanced CT from the apices of the lungs through the adrenal glands. The former protocol covers a larger anatomic region and may demonstrate abnormalities that might not be seen with nonenhanced CT. This protocol, however, is subject to extra time, expense, and potential complications of intravenous contrast material administration. Furthermore, it is not clear whether the additional information results in more accurate radiologic staging or changes the management of patients with newly diagnosed lung cancer. We performed this study to compare the radiologic stage determined with nonenhanced helical CT with that determined by using contrast-enhanced helical CT of the thorax and upper part of the abdomen to determine whether the latter protocol would result in alterations in clinical management.

MATERIALS AND METHODS

During a 15-month period, all patients who presented to the radiology department for CT evaluation of newly diagnosed lung cancer or with chest radiographic findings strongly

Agreement between Pathologic Stage and Radiologic Stage before and after Contrast Material Administration

Stage at Contrast-enhanced CT	Stage at Nonenhanced CT*				
	I	II	IIIA	IIIB	IV
I	I (19) II (1) IIIB (1)				
II	IIIA (1)	II (2) IIIA (1) IV (1)		IIIA (1)	
IIIA			IIIA (15) IV (1)		
IIIB				IIIB (18)	
IV		IV (1)		IV (1)	IV (21)

* Stages given are the pathologic stage. Numbers in parentheses are the number of patients.

suggestive of lung cancer were considered eligible. Ultimately, only those patients with a pathologically proved diagnosis of lung cancer were included in the final analysis.

CT was performed with a CT HiSpeed Advantage scanner (GE Medical Systems, Milwaukee, Wis). The standard procedure at our institution was to perform nonenhanced helical CT from the lung apices through the adrenal glands by using the following imaging parameters: section collimation, 10 mm; pitch, 1; and reconstruction interval, 10 mm. Subsequently, each patient underwent contrast-enhanced helical CT with intravenous administration of 150 mL of iopamidol (Isovue 300; Bracco Diagnostics, Princeton, NJ) at a rate of 3 mL/sec from the lung apices through the lung bases beginning 25 seconds after the start of contrast enhancement; the imaging parameters were identical to those used for nonenhanced CT. Imaging of the liver began 70 seconds after intravenous administration of contrast material with a section collimation of 7 mm, a pitch of 1, and a reconstruction interval of 7 mm (8). Helical CT scans through the thorax were obtained in one breath hold, and a second set of images was obtained through the liver (also in one breath hold).

The scans were obtained by using a standard soft-tissue algorithm (window width, 350 HU; level, 40 HU) and a retrospective lung algorithm (window width, 1,500 HU; level, −600 HU). In addition, liver windows (nonenhanced CT: width, 160 HU; level, 40–60 HU; contrast-enhanced CT: width, 160 HU; level, 90–100 HU) were used to evaluate the abdominal images.

The nonenhanced CT scans of the chest were interpreted independently by at least two experienced thoracic radiologists (E.F.P., J.J.E., H.P.M., J.E.C., E.M.M., P.C.G.), and the abdominal images were interpreted independently by at least two experienced thoracic and/or abdominal radiologists (E.F.P., J.J.E., J.E.C., E.M.M., P.C.G., R.A.L., M.T.K.). Then, a radiologic stage was assigned by each reviewer. The contrast-enhanced scans were similarly interpreted independently and also assigned a radiologic stage by each reviewer. In patients with non–small cell lung cancer, disease was staged according to the newly revised International Staging System (9), and the local size and extension, regional lymph nodes, and distant sites of metastases were evaluated. For this study, lymph nodes larger than 1 cm in the short axis were considered positive. In patients with small cell lung cancer, disease was staged according to the guidelines of the Veterans Administration Lung Cancer Study Group (10). This classification system separates patients into two groups: those who have limited disease (tumor confined within a single radiation therapy port) and those who have extensive disease with distant metastases or noncontiguous metastases to the contralateral lung. Discrepancies in stage between reviewers were resolved by consensus.

Patient management was suggested independently for each nonenhanced and contrast-enhanced examination. If there was agreement in the radiologic stage determined with the nonenhanced and enhanced CT study, then management was, by definition, identical. If there was disagreement in the radiologic stage between the nonenhanced and enhanced CT study, then management decisions were typically as follows: Patients with stage I–IIIB disease underwent bronchoscopy or mediastinoscopy for airway evaluation and lymph node sampling, whereas patients with findings suggestive of metastatic disease underwent sampling of distant sites.

Pathologic sampling by means of transthoracic needle aspiration, bronchoscopy, mediastinoscopy, thoracotomy, or a combination of these procedures was used to determine the pathologic stage. Exact binomial CIs were computed for measures of agreement.

RESULTS

One hundred twenty-two patients were eligible for the study. Fourteen patients had diagnoses other than lung cancer, including aspergillosis (n = 1); lymphoma (n = 1); hamartoma (n = 2); fibrosis (n = 1); nonspecific inflammatory process, granuloma, or both (n = 5); actinomycosis (n = 1); tuberculosis (n = 1); pulmonary infarct (n = 1); and sarcoidosis (n = 1). A tissue diagnosis was not obtained in 12 patients. The remaining 96 patients had lung cancer, and they composed the study group.

Non–Small Cell Lung Cancer

Eighty-four patients (60 men, 24 women; mean age, 64 years; age range, 30–85 years) had non–small cell lung cancer. Twenty-four (29%) patients had squamous cell carcinoma, 21 (25%) had adenocarcinoma, three (4%) had large cell carcinoma, and 36 (43%) had unspecified non–small cell lung cancer.

There was complete agreement in the thoracic radiologic stage determined with nonenhanced and contrast-enhanced CT in 80 (95%) of the 84 patients (95% CI: 0.88, 0.99). Twenty-one patients had stage I disease, four had stage II disease, 16 had stage IIIA disease, 18 had stage IIIB disease, and 21 had stage IV disease. In the patients with stage IV disease, the sites of metastases included the liver (n = 8), lungs (n = 6), bone (n = 4), and adrenal glands (n = 5). There was agreement between the radiologic and pathologic stage in 75 (94%) of these 80 patients and disagreement in five (6%) (Table). Patients with radiologic stage I–IIIA disease underwent biopsy of the primary lesion, bronchoscopy, or mediastinoscopy, and patients with stage IIIB–IV disease underwent mediastinoscopy, bronchoscopy, or biopsy of distant sites so a final pathologic stage could be determined. Because there was agreement in radiologic stage between the nonenhanced and contrast-enhanced CT study, by definition there was no change in management.

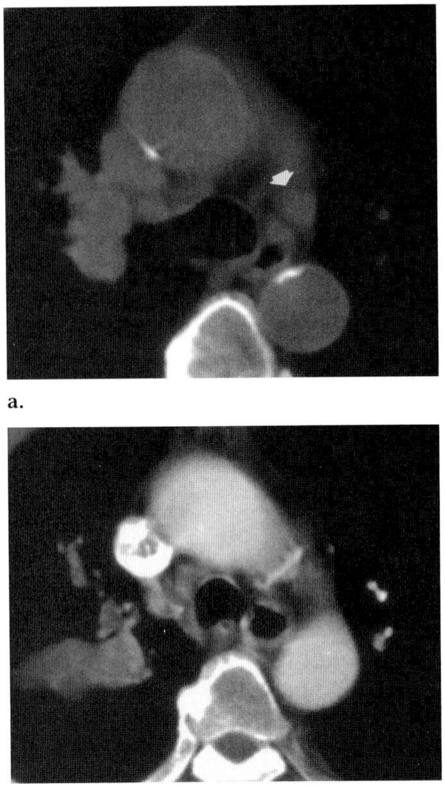

Figure 1. CT scans obtained in a 76-year-old man with a 4-cm mass in the right upper lobe of the lung. **(a)** Nonenhanced axial CT scan demonstrates a 1.5-cm, aortopulmonary window (level 5) lymph node (arrow). **(b)** Contrast-enhanced axial CT scan obtained at approximately the same level as **a** demonstrates no substantial aortopulmonary window adenopathy. No abnormalities were seen on any of the adjacent images. This patient underwent mediastinoscopy and had a right paratracheal (level 4R) lymph node positive for metastatic disease; stage IIIA non–small cell lung cancer was diagnosed.

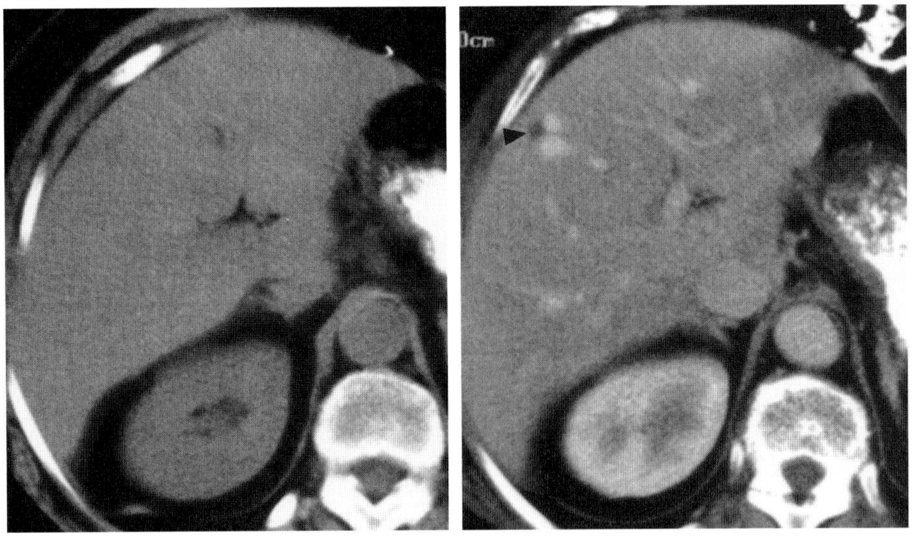

Figure 2. CT scans in a 71-year-old woman with a lobular right hilar mass. **(a)** Nonenhanced axial CT scan through the liver was interpreted as normal. **(b)** Contrast-enhanced axial CT scan through the liver obtained at approximately the same level as **a** demonstrates a 4-mm-diameter, low-attenuating lesion (arrowhead) that was too small to characterize any further. No abnormalities were seen on any of the adjacent scans. This patient underwent mediastinoscopy; N2 positive nodes and thus stage IIIA non–small cell lung cancer was diagnosed. The low-attenuating lesion in the liver was believed to be benign, and there were no changes in patient management.

There was disagreement in thoracic radiologic stage between nonenhanced and contrast-enhanced CT in four (5%) of the 84 patients. In three patients, the radiologic stage based on findings at contrast-enhanced CT was higher than that determined with nonenhanced CT. In one patient, the disease stage increased from IA (N0) to IIA (N1, hilar nodes); at mediastinoscopy, this patient had N2 disease (and, thus, stage IIIA disease) and was treated with chemotherapy and radiation therapy. In one patient, the disease stage increased from IIB to IV (possible small liver metastases); brain metastases were seen at head CT, which enabled us to confirm stage IV disease. In one patient, the disease stage increased from IIIB to IV (possible small liver metastases); bone metastases were seen on a bone scan, and stage IV disease was diagnosed at pathologic examination. In one patient, the radiologic stage decreased from IIIB (N3, aortopulmonary window nodes) to IIB (N1, hilar nodes) (Fig 1). At mediastinoscopy, this patient had N2 disease (and, thus, stage IIIA disease at pathologic examination) and was not considered a candidate for resection. In none of the patients was treatment changed because of the additional information noted at contrast-enhanced CT. Agreement between the thoracic radiologic stage and pathologic stage in all 84 patients is shown in the Table.

Eleven (13%) of the 84 patients with non–small cell lung cancer had at least one small (<5-mm) low-attenuating lesion in the liver that was considered unlikely to represent metastasis and therefore clinically unimportant (11). Four patients had liver lesions detected on both studies, and seven patients had lesions detected only on the contrast-enhanced studies (Fig 2). In no cases did the use of contrast material enable a more accurate characterization of liver lesions.

In six (six patients with bone metastases, two of which with both brain and bone metastases) of the 84 patients, extrathoracic metastases were demonstrated with additional radiologic studies performed preoperatively because of advanced disease or clinical symptoms. The thoracic radiologic stage in these patients before the discovery of metastatic disease was as follows: stage II (n = 1), stage IIIB (n = 1), and stage IV (n = 4).

Small Cell Lung Cancer

Twelve patients (seven men, five women; mean age, 64 years; age range, 47–80 years) had small cell lung cancer. There was complete agreement in the thoracic CT radiologic stage between the nonenhanced and contrast-enhanced studies in all cases. Seven patients had limited disease, and five had extensive disease.

In the patients with extensive disease, metastases were in the liver (n = 5) and bone (n = 2). One patient had additional liver lesions detected at contrast-enhanced CT, but this did not change the stage established at the nonenhanced examination. There was no change in pathologic stage or management decisions between the nonenhanced and enhanced studies in any case.

DISCUSSION

Lung cancer continues to be a major health problem. It is the most common malignancy in the United States and accounts for the greatest number of cancer-related deaths in both men and women (12). Unfortunately, because most patients have advanced disease at presentation, treatment options are limited to chemotherapy, radiation therapy, or both. Despite advances in these therapeutic regimens, the effect on the 5-year survival and disease-free interval has been minimal (12).

Many patients undergo extensive radiologic evaluation and laboratory studies to accurately define the clinical-radiologic stage before a final pathologic stage is determined with tissue sampling (1–7). Given the known patterns of metastases, imaging studies typically include thoracic CT through the adrenal glands and liver, radionuclide bone scanning, and head CT or magnetic resonance imaging. There is some doubt as to the usefulness of all of these studies, but various institutions use them routinely despite their high cost and questionable clinical benefit (5,6,13–16).

Thoracic CT is almost uniformly performed to stage lung cancer because it provides information about the primary lesion, thoracic lymph nodes, pleura, chest wall, and upper abdomen. What is uncertain is whether the routine use of intravenous contrast material or imaging of the entire contrast-enhanced liver is warranted. To our knowledge, there are no studies showing that additional information regarding the primary lesion, intrathoracic lymph nodes, or extrathoracic sites obtained with enhanced images has an effect on patient management.

In a number of studies, the use of contrast-enhanced CT for delineating and defining the primary lung mass in relationship to surrounding structures has been evaluated, but the additional information obtained with the routine use of contrast material does not appear to substantially change clinical treatment of the patient (1,4,5,17). Contrast-enhanced CT might permit identification of additional hilar or mediastinal lymph nodes, particularly for clinicians who do not routinely interpret these studies, but its findings do not necessarily reflect the true pathologic stage (7,18–20). In fact, some patients with small, normal-sized nodes at CT will have microscopic disease and, thus, disease will be understaged radiologically (20). Other patients will have enlarged reactive nodes and, thus, disease will be overstaged (1,6,18,19,21). In most series, CT is only 60% sensitive and specific for lymph node metastases (1,3,4). In one study, 37% of lymph nodes larger than 2 cm in diameter in patients with lung cancer were reactive and not neoplastic (22). Thus, tissue sampling should be performed in all surgical candidates to determine the pathologic stage. In the current study, enlarged abnormal lymph nodes were adequately seen with both CT examinations. Only two patients had a change in the nodal status (N0 to N1 and N3 to N1). This, however, did not alter patient treatment because, at our institution, patients who are candidates for resection undergo mediastinoscopy for pathologic staging.

Intraabdominal sites of lung metastases frequently include the adrenal glands and liver (23–25). The adrenal glands are equally well visualized on nonenhanced and contrast-enhanced images, although the results of many current studies suggest that characterization of adrenal abnormalities is, in fact, better with nonenhanced imaging (26–30). It is not clear at this time whether contrast-enhanced studies, even those performed with delayed imaging, will improve the characterization of adrenal abnormalities (31–34).

Although dedicated abdominal contrast-enhanced helical CT studies have yielded an increased rate of hepatic lesion detection (11,35–37), our literature search yielded no studies that addressed the clinical importance of lesions seen only at contrast-enhanced CT in patients with lung cancer. In our study, the metastatic status of patients did not change with contrast enhancement. When small (<5-mm) low-attenuating lesions in the liver that were too small to further characterize were demonstrated, they were considered to be benign, as suggested by results of prior investigations (11). All of the patients with small, low-attenuating lesions who underwent curative surgery were followed-up clinically or with CT (up to 5 months), and at the time this article was written, no case of hepatic metastasis had been detected. Furthermore, no patient with otherwise resectable disease has had pathologically proved isolated hepatic metastases that were seen only on contrast-enhanced images. All of the patients in our series who had hepatic metastases also had other pathologically documented disease in mediastinal lymph nodes, distant sites (including the brain, bone, or adrenal gland), or both. Thus, the frequency of true isolated hepatic metastases in patients who are candidates for surgery is probably rare. The detection of additional hepatic lesions in patients with liver metastases is of no clinical consequence because none of these patients would undergo resection.

There are several limitations to this study: There was minimal follow-up to ensure accurate staging in some patients, definitive tissue samples were not taken of all suspicious lesions, and there was the inherent selection bias of a tertiary care institution. In this study, however, we addressed a very specific question: Do stage and management change with use of contrast material? We believe the limitations of the study did not have a substantial effect on the outcome. We had to keep the study simple so that any institution can easily duplicate our results.

The results of our study suggest that nonenhanced thoracic CT through the adrenal glands is sufficient for successful radiologic staging in patients with newly diagnosed lung cancer. This has now become a standard procedure at our institution. Contrast-enhanced CT of the thorax did not substantially alter patient treatment, and routine contrast-enhanced CT through the liver is not required.

References

1. Webb WR, Gatsonis C, Zerhouni EA, et al. CT and MR imaging in staging non–small cell bronchogenic carcinoma: report of the Radiologic Diagnostic Oncology Group. Radiology 1991; 178:705–713.
2. Musset D, Grenier P, Carette MF, et al. Primary lung cancer staging: prospective comparative study of MR imaging with CT. Radiology 1986; 160:607–611.
3. Bragg DG. The diagnosis and staging of primary lung cancer. Radiol Clin North Am 1994; 32:1–14.
4. Klein JS, Webb WR. The radiologic staging of lung cancer. J Thorac Imaging 1991; 7:29–47.
5. Quint LE, Francis IR, Wahl RL, Gross BH, Glazer GM. Preoperative staging of non-small-cell carcinoma of the lung: imaging methods. AJR 1995; 164:1349–1359.
6. Dales RE, Stark RM, Raman S. Computed tomography to stage lung cancer. Am Rev Respir Dis 1990; 141:1096–1101.
7. Epstein DM, Stephenson LW, Gefter WB, van der Vorde F, Aronchik JM, Miller WT. Value of CT in the preoperative assessment of lung cancer: a survey of thoracic surgeons. Radiology 1986; 161:423–427.
8. Chen MY, Chiles C, Choplin RH, Aquino SL. Bronchogenic carcinoma: a survey of CT protocols for staging disease. Acad Radiol 1997; 4:687–692.
9. Mountain CF. Revisions in the international system for staging lung cancer. Chest 1997; 111:1710–1717.
10. Abrams J, Doyle LA, Aisner J. Staging, prognostic factors, and special considerations in small cell lung cancer. Semin Oncol 1988; 15:261–277.
11. Jones EC, Chezmar JL, Nelson RC, Bernardino ME. The frequency and significance of small (≤15 mm) hepatic lesions detected by CT. AJR 1992; 158:535–539.
12. Landis SH, Murray T, Bolden S, Wingo PA. Cancer statistics, 1998. CA Cancer J Clin 1998; 48:6–29.
13. Silvestri GA, Littenberg B, Colice GL. The clinical evaluation for detecting metastatic lung cancer. Am J Respir Crit Care Med 1995; 152:225–230.
14. Colice GL, Birkmeyer JD, Black WC, Littenberg B, Silvestri G. Cost-effectiveness

of head CT in patients with lung cancer without clinical evidence of metastases. Chest 1995; 108:1264–1271.
15. Silvestri GA, Lenz JF, Harper SN, Morse RA, Colice GL. The relationship of clinical findings to CT scan evidence of adrenal gland metastases in the staging of bronchogenic carcinoma. Chest 1992; 102: 1748–1751.
16. Primack SL, Lee KS, Logan PM, Miller RR, Müller NL. Bronchogenic carcinoma: utility of CT in the evaluation of patients with suspected lesions. Radiology 1994; 193:795–800.
17. McLoud TC. CT of bronchogenic carcinoma: indeterminate mediastinal invasion. Radiology 1989; 173:15–16.
18. Cascade PN, Gross BH, Kazerooni EA, et al. Variability in the detection of enlarged mediastinal lymph nodes in staging lung cancer: a comparison of contrast-enhanced and unenhanced CT. AJR 1998; 170:927–931.
19. Laissy J, Gay-Depassier P, Soyer P, et al. Enlarged mediastinal lymph nodes in bronchogenic carcinoma: assessment with dynamic contrast-enhanced MR imaging. Radiology 1994; 191:263–267.
20. Arita T, Kuramitsu T, Kawamura M, et al. Bronchogenic carcinoma: incidence of metastases to normal sized lymph nodes. Thorax 1995; 50:1267–1269.
21. Passlick B, Izbicki JR, Kubuschok B, Thetter O, Pantel K. Detection of disseminated lung cancer cells in lymph nodes: impact on staging and prognosis. Ann Thorac Surg 1996; 61:177–183.
22. McLoud TC, Bourgouin PM, Greenberg RW, et al. Bronchogenic carcinoma: analysis of staging in the mediastinum with CT by correlative lymph node mapping and sampling. Radiology 1992; 182:319–323.
23. Feld R, Rubinstein LV, Weisenberger TH, Lung Cancer Study Group. Sites of recurrence in resected stage I non-small-cell lung cancer: a guide for future studies. J Clin Oncol 1984; 2:1352–1358.
24. Winton TL. Staging for M disease. World J Surg 1993; 17:690–693.
25. Stenbygaard LE, Sørensen JB, Olsen JE. Metastatic pattern in adenocarcinoma of the lung. J Thorac Cardiovasc Surg 1995; 110:1130–1135.
26. Dunnick NR, Korobkin M, Francis I. Adrenal radiology: distinguishing benign from malignant adrenal masses. AJR 1996; 167: 861–867.
27. McNicholas MM, Lee MJ, Mayo-Smith WW, et al. An imaging algorithm for the differential diagnosis of adrenal adenomas and metastases. AJR 1995; 165:1453–1459.
28. Lee MJ, Hahn PF, Papanicolaou N, et al. Benign and malignant adrenal masses: CT distinction with attenuation coefficients, size, and observer analysis. Radiology 1991; 179:415–418.
29. Korobkin M, Brodeur FJ, Yutzy GG, et al. Differentiation of adrenal adenomas from nonadenomas using CT attenuation values. AJR 1996; 166:531–536.
30. Szolar DH, Kammerhuber F. Quantitative CT evaluation of adrenal gland masses: a step forward in the differentiation between adenomas and nonadenomas? Radiology 1997; 202:517–521.
31. Boland GW, Hahn PF, Peña C, Mueller PR. Adrenal masses: characterization with delayed contrast-enhanced CT. Radiology 1997; 202:693–696.
32. Korobkin M, Brodeur FJ, Francis IR, Quint LE, Dunnick NR. Delayed enhanced CT for differentiation of benign from malignant adrenal masses. Radiology 1996; 200: 737–742.
33. Korobkin M, Brodeur FJ, Francis IR, Quint LE, Dunnick NR, Londy F. CT time-attenuation washout curves of adrenal adenomas and nonadenomas. AJR 1998; 170:747–752.
34. Szolar DH, Kammerhuber FH. Adrenal adenomas and nonadenomas: assessment of washout at delayed contrast-enhanced CT. Radiology 1998; 207:369–375.
35. Oliver JH III, Baron RL, Federle MP, Jones BC, Sheng R. Hypervascular liver metastases: do unenhanced and hepatic arterial phase CT images affect tumor detection? Radiology 1997; 205:709–715.
36. Platt JF, Francis IR, Ellis JH, Reige KA. Liver metastases: early detection based on abnormal contrast material enhancement at dual-phase helical CT. Radiology 1997; 205:49–53.
37. Baker ME, Pelley R. Hepatic metastases: basic principles and implications for radiologists. Radiology 1995; 197:329–337.

Detection Failures in Spiral CT Screening for Lung Cancer: Analysis of CT Findings[1]

Ryutaro Kakinuma, MD
Hironobu Ohmatsu, MD
Masahiro Kaneko, MD
Kenji Eguchi, MD
Tsuguo Naruke, MD
Kanji Nagai, MD
Yutaka Nishiwaki, MD
Akira Suzuki, MD
Noriyuki Moriyama, MD

Index terms:
Cancer screening, 60.321
Diagnostic radiology, observer performance, 60.321
Lung neoplasms, CT, 60.12115, 60.12118
Lung neoplasms, diagnosis, 60.3211, 60.3212

Radiology 1999; 212:61–66

Abbreviation:
ALCA = Anti–Lung Cancer Association

[1] From the Department of Thoracic Oncology, National Cancer Center Hospital East, 6-5-1 Kashiwa-no-ha, Kashiwa 277-8577, Japan (R.K., H.O., K.N., Y.N.); the Departments of Endoscopy (M.K.), Surgery (T.N.), and Radiology (N.M.), National Cancer Center Hospital, Tokyo, Japan; the National Shikoku Cancer Center Hospital, Matsuyama, Japan (K.E.); and the Japan Anti-Tuberculosis Association, Shizuoka Branch, Japan (A.S.). Received April 3, 1998; revision requested June 5; revision received September 16; accepted December 9. Supported in part by a grant-in-aid for cancer research from the Ministry of Health and Welfare, by a grant for scientific research expenses for health and welfare programs from the Foundation for the Promotion of Cancer Research, and by the New 10-year Strategy for Cancer Control (researching new technology for diagnostic purposes). **Address reprint requests to** R.K. (e-mail: *rkaki@east.ncc.go.jp*).

Author contributions:
Guarantors of integrity of entire study, R.K., H.O., M.K., K.E., T.N., A.S., N.M.; study concepts and design, R.K., H.O., M.K., K.E.; literature research, R.K.; clinical studies, R.K., H.O., M.K., K.E.; data acquisition and analysis, R.K., H.O., M.K., K.E.; manuscript preparation, R.K., H.O., M.K., K.E.; manuscript editing, H.O., M.K., K.E.; manuscript review, K.N., Y.N.

PURPOSE: To clarify the computed tomographic (CT) findings and the progression of minute lung cancers that were missed at initial spiral CT screening but were later detected.

MATERIALS AND METHODS: The findings from seven patients with lung cancer that was missed at the initial spiral CT screening were reviewed. Retrospective CT findings, time to detection, cell type, and pathologic stage were evaluated.

RESULTS: Minute lung cancers missed at early spiral CT included a nodule among the shadows of old tuberculosis (n = 2), a faint nodule with high attenuation in the center of the nodule (n = 1), an increase in attenuation just adjacent to an axial peripheral pulmonary vessel (n = 1) and adjacent to a craniocaudal peripheral pulmonary vessel (n = 1), and a minute faint nodule (n = 2). The time to detection ranged from 6 to 18 months. At pathologic examination, six cancers were stage I, and one was stage II.

CONCLUSION: Minute nodules of lung cancer that are near the threshold of detectability may be missed at spiral CT screening. It is important to examine noncalcified nodules with thin-section CT even when lesions from prior disease, such as those from old tuberculosis, exist and to evaluate the shadows of pulmonary vessels carefully. A follow-up examination is highly recommended.

The findings from several recent studies of spiral computed tomographic (CT) screening for lung cancer have been published in Japan (1–5). Although chest CT is more sensitive for the detection of nodules of lung cancer than chest radiography is (1–3), the potential for missing minute cancerous lesions is a major shortcoming of chest CT (6,7). In September 1993, the Anti–Lung Cancer Association (ALCA), an organization in Japan, introduced low-dose spiral CT screening to detect lung cancer in its early stages (1). Between September 1993 and April 1996, lung cancer was detected by the ALCA in 22 patients out of a population of 1,443 persons who underwent screening. Of the 22 lung cancers, seven had been missed at early spiral CT screening.

The purpose of this study was to clarify the CT findings and the progression of minute lung cancers that were missed at early spiral CT screening, thereby improving the diagnostic criteria for detecting lung cancer.

MATERIALS AND METHODS

A total of 1,443 members of the ALCA underwent semiannual screening (1,273 men and 170 women). Nearly all members were heavy smokers and elderly. The mean age of the subjects was 60.7 years (age range, 40–85 years). Each screening consisted of a low-dose spiral CT examination, chest radiography, and cytologic studies of sputum. Between September 1993 and April 1996, a total of 5,418 CT examinations were performed on the 1,443 members.

The CT screening system used was a TCT-900S Superhelix (Toshiba Medical, Tokyo, Japan). The scanning parameters were 120 kVp, 50 mA, 10-mm collimation, one rotation of the x-ray tube per second, and a table speed of 20 mm/sec (pitch, 2:1). A thoracic area spanning 30 cm was scanned from a level 2 cm superior to the apex to the level of the diaphragm with a 15-second

Clinical and Imaging Characteristics of the Seven Patients

Patient No./ Age (y)/Sex	Diagnosis at Initial CT	CT Findings in Retrospect	Location*	Diameter (mm)	Interval to Detection (mo)	Diameter at Detection (mm)	Histologic Findings	Stage
1/85/M	Old tuberculoma	Noncalcified nodule	RUL	13	12	15	Adenocarcinoma	IA
2/63/M	Old tuberculoma	Noncalcified nodule	RLL	11	12	15	Adenocarcinoma	IA
3/69/M	Granuloma	Nodule with faint increase in attenuation	LLL	9	18	12	Adenocarcinoma	IA
4/65/M	Normal	Increase in attenuation adjacent to vessel	RLL	7	6	9	Squamous cell carcinoma	IA
5/77/M	Normal	Increase in attenuation adjacent to vessel	LUL	7	12	18	Squamous cell carcinoma	IIA
6/49/M	Normal	Minute and faint nodule	LUL	6	6	8	Adenocarcinoma	IA
7/63/M	Normal	Minute and faint nodule	RUL	4	18	5	Adenocarcinoma	IA

* LLL = left lower lobe, LUL = left upper lobe, RLL = right lower lobe, RUL = right upper lobe.

breath hold. Image reconstruction was performed with 180° linear interpolation at intervals of 1 cm.

All CT images were reviewed independently by four diagnostic experts (M.K., K.E., H.O., R.K.) who used both the cathode-ray–tube monitor and the hard-copy display. Display conditions were a window width of 2,000 HU and a window level of −700 HU. As part of the screening protocol, the diagnostic experts classified the images into four categories: (*a*) suspected lung cancer, (*b*) a benign tumor or an active inflammatory disease, (*c*) a scar lesion caused by a previous inflammatory episode, and (*d*) normal.

Thin-section CT was performed with the same CT scanner whenever lesions seen on CT scans, radiographs, or both were suggestive of lung cancer, or whenever the lesion seen was a solitary nodule without calcification, a nodule larger than 4.9 mm in diameter, or an area of localized opacification increasing in size with sequential comparison. The scanning parameters for thin-section CT were 120 kVp, 250 mA, 2-mm collimation, one rotation of the x-ray tube per second, a table speed of 2 mm/sec (pitch, 1:1), and a thin-section algorithm. Areas of opacification with calcification, multiple lesions confined to the same segment, linear shadows of focal collapsed lung, and shadows without any progressive change were considered benign (1).

Four authors (R.K., H.O., M.K., K.E.) together reviewed the CT images of the 22 patients with lung cancer to determine retrospectively when the cancers were first visible. Consensus opinion was used. Retrospective CT findings, the time to detection, and the pathologic stage of the lung cancer at detection were evaluated. The diameters of the nodules at the initial screening and at detection were assessed from the standpoint of conspicuity.

We classified nodules into two categories: conspicuous and inconspicuous. Conspicuous nodules were easily seen because they were well defined and had high attenuation. Inconspicuous nodules were not only smaller but also less well defined and had low attenuation. The diameters of the nodules were measured with a built-in program in the CT console by using digital data from the screening CT image stored on optical disks.

RESULTS

Of the 1,443 subjects screened between September 1993 and April 1996, lung cancer was detected in 22 patients. Among the 22 patients, 12 had lung cancer detected only with spiral CT. Among these 12 patients, six patients had cancers that were visible retrospectively on the images from an earlier spiral CT examination. Five of these six patients had adenocarcinoma, and one had squamous cell carcinoma. In another patient, squamous cell carcinoma, which was detected with frontal chest radiography and spiral CT, was visible retrospectively on the images from an earlier spiral CT examination. All seven patients with lung cancer visible retrospectively on earlier CT images were men. They ranged in age from 49 to 85 years (mean, 67 years).

The clinical and imaging characteristics of the seven patients are listed in the Table. In reviewing the original diagnoses from initial CT images, the nodule in patient 1 (Fig 1) was misdiagnosed as a lesion of old pulmonary tuberculosis because of an area of opacification that resembled calcification and pleural thickening. In patient 2, the nodule was also diagnosed as old pulmonary tuberculosis because of the coexistence of multiple lesions confined to the same segment and areas of opacification with calcification. In patient 3, the nodule was diagnosed as a granuloma (Fig 2) because of its high attenuation and relatively smooth edge.

In patients 4 and 5 (Fig 3), although increases in attenuation just adjacent to an axial peripheral pulmonary vessel (patient 4) and to a craniocaudal peripheral pulmonary vessel (patient 5) that were caused by lung cancer were detected retrospectively, the patients were classified as normal at the time of initial spiral CT screening. In patients 6 and 7, although minute and faint nodules of lung cancer were detected retrospectively, these patients also were classified as normal at the time of initial spiral CT screening.

We classified the seven patients into two groups on the basis of nodule conspicuity. In the first group (patients 1–3), the nodules were easily detected but were difficult to diagnose as lung cancer. In the second group (patients 4–7), the nodules were difficult to detect. The conspicuous nodules were at least 9 mm in diameter, while the inconspicuous nodules were at most 7 mm in diameter. The mean diameters of conspicuous nodules at initial CT screening and at detection were 11 and 14 mm, respectively. The mean diameters of inconspicuous nodules at initial CT screening and at detection were 6 and 10 mm, respectively. The time between initial CT screening and detection ranged from 6 to 18 months.

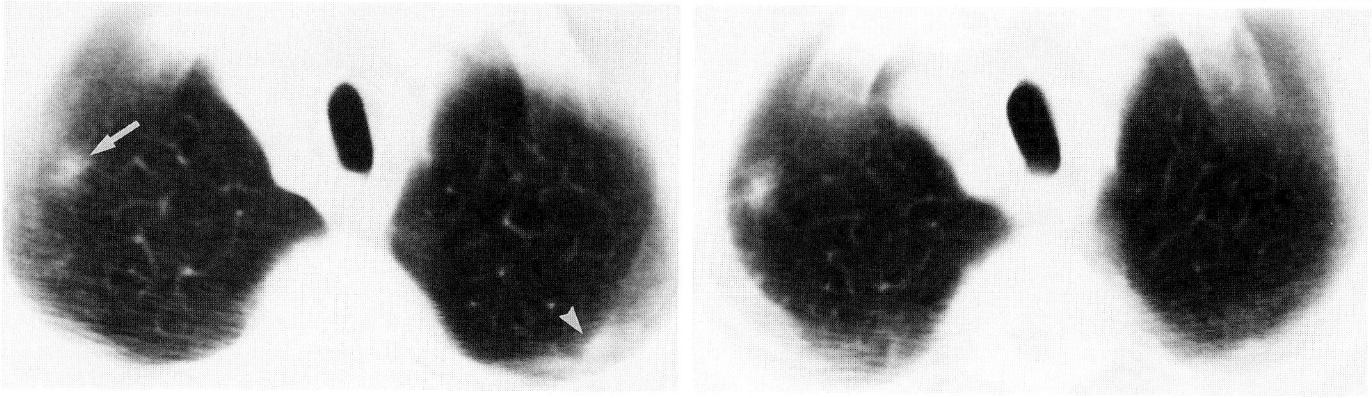

a. b.

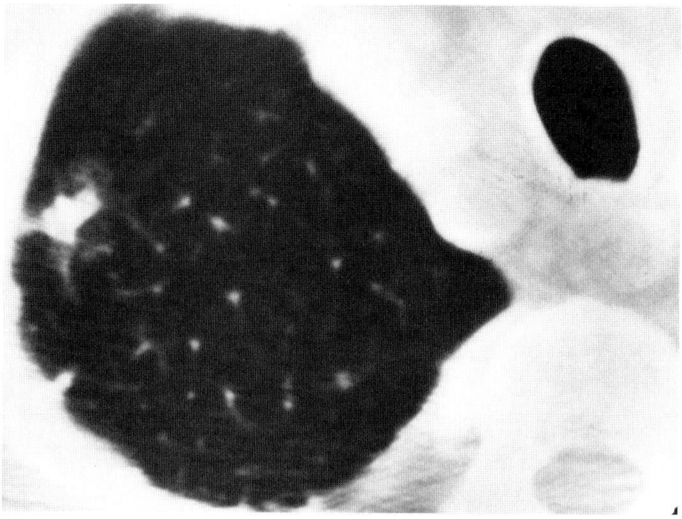

c.

Figure 1. Patient 1. Adenocarcinoma in an 85-year-old man. **(a)** CT image obtained in January 1994 shows high attenuation in the nodule (arrow), which was thought to represent calcification; the nodule was diagnosed as an old tuberculoma. Pleural thickening (arrowhead) was seen at the posterior wall of the left hemithorax. **(b)** CT image obtained in February 1995 shows nodule that was diagnosed as highly suggestive of lung cancer. **(c)** Thin-section CT image shows mixed areas of ground-glass opacity and consolidation.

The diagnoses at detection of lung cancer were classified into two groups. In the first group (patients 1 and 4–6), two diagnostic experts agreed that a nodule was highly suggestive of lung cancer. In the second group (patients 2, 3, and 7), one diagnostic expert diagnosed each nodule as highly suggestive of lung cancer, but the other diagnostic expert diagnosed the findings in patients 2 and 3 as scar lesions caused by previous inflammatory episodes and failed to detect the lesion in patient 7. In the second group, two lesions (in patients 2 and 7) were diagnosed on the cathode-ray–tube monitor as highly suggestive of lung cancer, and one lesion (in patient 3) was so diagnosed on the hard-copy display.

At the time of detection, the pathologic stages of the missed lung cancers were as follows: the six cancers detected only with spiral CT (ie, five adenocarcinomas [patients 1–3, 6, and 7] [Figs 1, 2] and one squamous cell carcinoma [patient 4]) were stage I, and the second squamous cell carcinoma (patient 5) (Fig 3), which was detected with frontal chest radiography and spiral CT, was stage II.

DISCUSSION

Lung cancers may be overlooked not only on chest radiographs (8–11) but also on CT images (6,7). White et al (6) reported that an endobronchial location and lower lobe predominance were the most common characteristics of overlooked lung cancer at CT. In our patients with squamous cell carcinoma (patients 4 and 5), a finding of increased attenuation just adjacent to axial (patient 4) and craniocaudal (patient 5) peripheral pulmonary vessels was detected retrospectively.

Saida et al (12) reported that more than half of the early squamous cell carcinoma lesions that showed polypoid growth or that reached the cartilaginous layer of the bronchial wall could be seen at CT with 5.0-mm, 3.0-mm, or 1.5-mm sections. However, in our study of spiral CT screening, we were not able to acquire images of peripheral bronchi in detail because the pitch was 2:1 and because image reconstruction was performed at intervals of 1 cm. We thought that in its early stages, the spread of squamous cell carcinoma to the outside of the bronchial wall looked like a slight increase in attenuation just adjacent to the peripheral pulmonary vessel, which led to the missed diagnosis of early squamous cell carcinoma. In patients 1 and 2, the reason why adenocarcinoma was missed was probably the presence of shadows of old pulmonary tuberculosis.

White et al (6) also reported that the presence of unrelated major abnormalities on CT images may contribute to diagnostic failure. In patient 3, the reason why the malignant nodule was missed was its close resemblance to a minute granuloma. However, the follow-up CT examinations revealed an increase in attenuation around the granuloma. The area of increased attenuation appeared as an area of ground-glass opacity at thin-section CT.

Pathologic examination of the specimen from patient 3 revealed that the granuloma-like appearance was caused by a fibrotic focus. In patient 3, this minute lung cancer already had fibrosis in the nodule. Jang et al (13) reported that focal areas of ground-glass opacity on thin-section CT images could be an early sign of localized bronchioloalveolar carcinoma. Yamada et al (14) reported that conventional and thin-section CT revealed "air-density lesions" in each of five resected minute lung cancers that measured less than 6 mm in diameter. Air

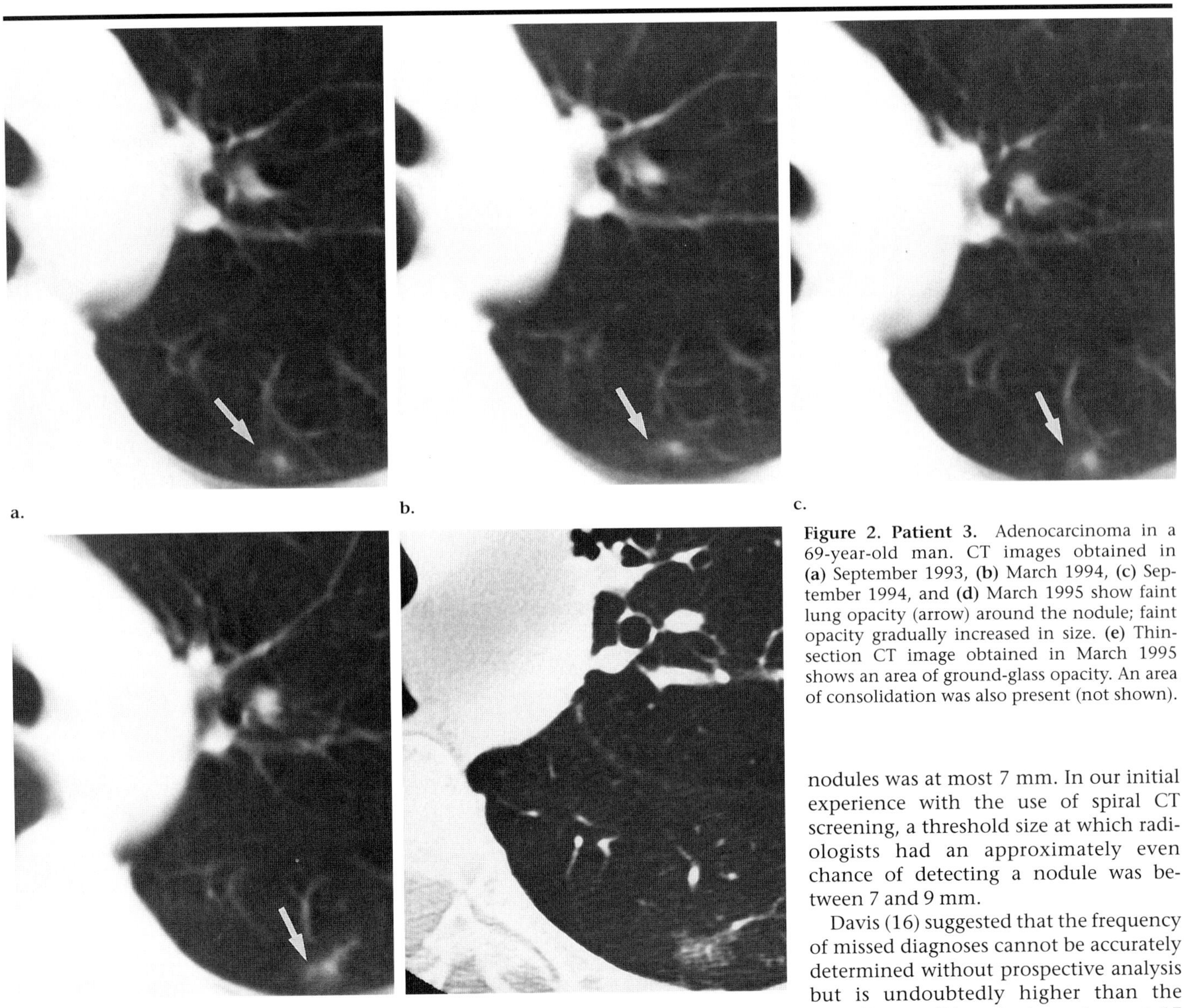

a. b. c. d. e.

Figure 2. Patient 3. Adenocarcinoma in a 69-year-old man. CT images obtained in **(a)** September 1993, **(b)** March 1994, **(c)** September 1994, and **(d)** March 1995 show faint lung opacity (arrow) around the nodule; faint opacity gradually increased in size. **(e)** Thin-section CT image obtained in March 1995 shows an area of ground-glass opacity. An area of consolidation was also present (not shown).

density is a synonym for ground-glass opacity.

In our patients with inconspicuous adenocarcinoma (patients 6 and 7), differences between localized faint increased attenuation and the attenuation of the surrounding lung were not clear enough to permit detection of these lesions with any degree of certainty. Furthermore, if these lesions were detected, it would be difficult to differentiate these lesions from other causes of a localized faint increase in attenuation, such as localized fibrosis, localized emphysema, or artifacts of spiral CT. Artifacts on spiral CT images are faint trapezoid-like increases in attenuation just inside the ribs and faint round or oval increases in attenuation between pulmonary vessels that run parallel.

Gurney (7) reported that all peripheral tumors that were missed were smaller than 3 mm in diameter and that such failure of detection was attributable primarily to the poor conspicuity of lesions. Naidich et al (15) reported that observers identified 1%, 48%, 82%, and 91% of the nodules that were less than 1.5 mm, 3.0 mm, 4.5 mm, and 7.0 mm in diameter, respectively, on 1.5-mm sections in a three-dimensional computer simulation. From these results, Gurney (7) proposed that 3 mm might be a threshold size at which an observer had an approximately even chance of detecting a nodule.

However, of the lung cancers that were missed in our study, the diameter of conspicuous nodules was at least 9 mm, whereas the diameter of inconspicuous nodules was at most 7 mm. In our initial experience with the use of spiral CT screening, a threshold size at which radiologists had an approximately even chance of detecting a nodule was between 7 and 9 mm.

Davis (16) suggested that the frequency of missed diagnoses cannot be accurately determined without prospective analysis but is undoubtedly higher than the 0.045% rate (14 patients underwent 17 examinations out of a total of 37,500 CT examinations) that can be estimated from the results of the study by White et al (6). In retrospect, as of April 1996, our results showed that the frequency of missed cancers during spiral CT screening was 0.26% (seven patients with missed lung cancer underwent a total of 14 CT examinations out of 5,418 CT examinations).

Despite the fact that lung cancer was missed in seven patients by using spiral CT screening, six of these cancers were pathologic stage I at detection, and one was pathologic stage II. Therefore, these cancers had the potential for cure.

At spiral CT, the pitch used was 2:1 (ie, 10-mm collimation and a table speed of 20 mm/sec), and the image reconstruction was performed at intervals of 1 cm. We previously evaluated the feasibility of using a 2.5:1 pitch on solitary and meta-

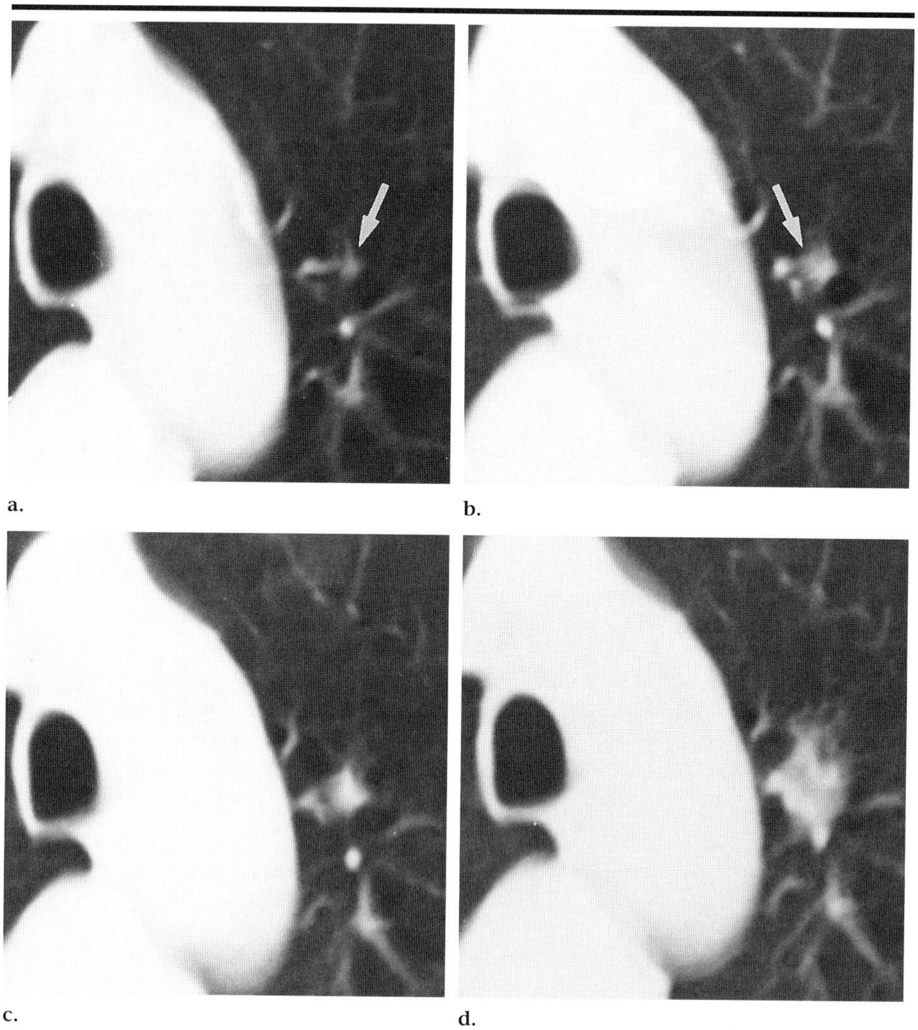

Figure 3. Patient 5. Squamous cell carcinoma in a 77-year-old man. **(a)** CT image obtained in September 1994 shows that one branch of the pulmonary vessel (arrow) appears to be normal. **(b)** CT image obtained in March 1995 shows an increase in opacity (arrow) just adjacent to the pulmonary vessel. **(c)** CT image obtained in September 1995 shows that the same area appears to be slightly larger. **(d)** CT image obtained in March 1996 shows that the nodule clearly increased in size.

static pulmonary nodules (17). Mori et al (18) reported that the optimal table speed and reconstruction image interval for helical CT that are needed to keep the detection sensitivity comparable with that of conventional CT are 20 mm/sec and 10-mm images. However, Wright et al (19) reported that the risk of understaging disease in patients with solitary nodules is greater with increasing pitch, and pitch should therefore be limited to no greater than 1.5 for initial staging of pulmonary metastatic disease.

Buckley et al (20) compared spiral CT with interscan spacing of 4 to 5 mm versus spacing of 8 to 10 mm with regard to the detection rate and the level of confidence in the diagnosis of pulmonary nodules. These investigators (20) concluded that increased reconstruction frequency of spiral CT volume data sets improves the detection of pulmonary nodules and enhances confidence in the diagnosis.

With regard to reading methods, we read static images on the cathode-ray–tube monitor and film display. Seltzer et al (21) compared cine viewing with film-based viewing at spiral CT of the chest and concluded that cine viewing of spiral CT images of the chest improves the ability of the radiologist to detect nodules.

Given these preliminary results, further research is needed to determine the most appropriate conditions for spiral CT screening, including pitch, viewing method, and reconstruction interval. We are now developing a computer-aided lung cancer diagnosis system that is based on spiral CT images (22,23) as a counterpart to the double-reading technique now used in our spiral CT screening program.

In conclusion, minute nodules of lung cancer that are near the threshold of detectability may be overlooked at spiral CT screening. It is important to examine noncalcified nodules with thin-section CT even when prior lesions, such as those of old tuberculosis, exist. It is also important to evaluate the shadows of pulmonary vessels carefully. To establish appropriate diagnostic criteria for minute lung cancer, we need to analyze the progression of many such minute lung cancers. Therefore, follow-up CT examination is highly recommended.

Acknowledgments: We thank the physicians and technical staff of the ALCA and also the excellent administrative work of Jun Misawa, head of the ALCA administration office in Tokyo.

References

1. Kaneko M, Eguchi K, Ohmatsu H, et al. Peripheral lung cancer: screening and detection with low-dose spiral CT versus radiography. Radiology 1996; 201:798–802.
2. Yasuda S, Shohtsu A, Ohkubo K, et al. Lung cancer screening with spiral CT. Jpn J Lung Cancer 1997; 37:433–439. [Japanese]
3. Mori K, Kishiro I, Yokoyama K, Onishi T, Tominaga K. Helical CT for secondary screening of lung cancer. Nippon Kyobu Shikkan Gakkai Zasshi 1995; 33:1475–1482. [Japanese]
4. Matusmoto M, Horikoshi H, Moteki T, et al. A pilot study with lung-cancer screening CT (LSCT) at the secondary screening for lung cancer detection. Nippon Acta Radiol 1995; 55:172–179. [Japanese]
5. Motoyama A, Kono M, Adachi S, et al. Secondary screening for lung cancer by helical CT. Jpn J Lung Cancer 1995; 35: 883–890. [Japanese]
6. White CS, Romney BM, Mason AC, Austin JHM, Miller BH, Protopapas Z. Primary carcinoma of the lung overlooked at CT: analysis of findings in 14 patients. Radiology 1996; 199:109–115.
7. Gurney JW. Missed lung cancer at CT: imaging findings in nine patients. Radiology 1996; 199:117–122.
8. Muhm JR, Miller WE, Fontana RS, Sanderson DR, Uhlenhopp MA. Lung cancer detected during a screening program using four-month chest radiographs. Radiology 1983; 148:609–615.
9. Heelan RT, Flehinger BJ, Melamed MR, et al. Non-small-cell lung cancer: results of the New York screening program. Radiology 1984; 151:289–293.
10. Woodring JH. Pitfalls in the radiologic diagnosis of lung cancer. AJR 1990; 154: 1165–1175.
11. Austin JHM, Romney BM, Goldsmith LS. Missed bronchogenic carcinoma: radiographic findings in 27 patients with a potentially resectable lesion evident in retrospect. Radiology 1992; 182:115–122.
12. Saida Y, Kujiraoka Y, Akaogi E, Ogata T, Kurosaki Y, Itai Y. Early squamous cell

carcinoma of the lung: CT and pathologic correlation. Radiology 1996; 201:61–65.
13. Jang HJ, Lee KS, Kwon OJ, Rhee CH, Shim YM, Han J. Bronchioloalveolar carcinoma: focal area of ground-glass attenuation at thin-section CT as an early sign. Radiology 1996; 199:485–488.
14. Yamada K, Kondou M, Katou Y, et al. Thin-section computed tomography analysis of resected small lung cancers measuring less than 6 mm in diameter. Jpn J Lung Cancer 1996; 36:375–384. [Japanese]
15. Naidich DP, Rusinek H, McGuinness G, Leitman B, McCauley DI, Henschke CI. Variables affecting pulmonary nodule detection with computed tomography: evaluation with three-dimensional computer simulation. J Thorac Imaging 1993; 8:291–299.
16. Davis SD. Through the "retrospectoscope": a glimpse of missed lung cancer at CT. Radiology 1996; 199:23–24.
17. Ohmatsu H, Eguchi K, Mori K, Kaneko M, Hirano H, Moriyama N. Feasibility study of helical-volume CT for the detection of peripheral lung nodules (abstr). Radiology 1992; 185(P):353.
18. Mori K, Sasagawa M, Moriyama N. Detection of nodular lesions in the lung using helical computed tomography: comparison of fast couch speed technique with conventional computed tomography. Jpn J Clin Oncol 1994; 24:252–257.
19. Wright AR, Collie DA, Williams JR, Hashemi-Malayeri B, Stevenson AJM, Turnbull CM. Pulmonary nodules: effect on detection of spiral CT pitch. Radiology 1996; 199:837–841.
20. Buckley JA, Scott WW, Siegelman SS, et al. Pulmonary nodules: effect of increased data sampling on detection with spiral CT and confidence in diagnosis. Radiology 1995; 196:395–400.
21. Seltzer SE, Judy PF, Adams DF, et al. Spiral CT of the chest: comparison of cine and film-based viewing. Radiology 1995; 197: 73–78.
22. Kakinuma R, Ohmatsu H, Kaneko M, Eguchi K, Niki N, Moriyama N. Computer-aided diagnosis system for lung cancer based on helical CT images (abstr). Radiology 1996; 202(P):563.
23. Kanazawa K, Kawata Y, Niki N, et al. Computer-aided diagnosis for pulmonary nodules based on helical CT images. Comput Med Imaging Graph 1998; 22:157–167.

Hugue Ouellette, MD

The Signet Ring Sign[1]

APPEARANCE

The signet ring sign is a finding seen on computed tomographic (CT) scans of the thorax. It consists of a small circle of soft-tissue attenuation that abuts a ring of soft-tissue attenuation surrounding a larger low-attenuating circle of air (Fig 1).

EXPLANATION

The ring of soft-tissue attenuation represents the wall of the dilated bronchus seen on a cross-sectional CT scan, whereas the low-attenuating circle of air represents air within the dilated bronchus. The circle of soft-tissue attenuation abutting the ring represents a cross-sectional image of the pulmonary artery that lies adjacent to the dilated bronchus.

DISCUSSION

The signet ring sign is a CT finding seen in patients with bronchiectasis (1–3). Bronchiectasis is defined as irreversible abnormal bronchial dilatation (Fig 2) (1). Dilatation of the bronchi usually is most extensive in medium-sized bronchi. In addition, bronchial muscle atrophy, bronchial wall destruction, peribronchial inflammation, and fibrosis may occur. Excess mucus accumulates in these dilated bronchi owing to impaired ciliary action and abnormal bronchial dynamics (4).

Bronchiectasis is most often due to bronchial wall damage after necrotizing viral or bacterial bronchitis, which usually occurs in early childhood (4). Bronchial dilatation also occurs distal to the bronchial obstruction when secretions accumulate in the bronchi distal to the obstruction and cause them to dilate. Traction on the bronchi in advanced pulmonary fibrosis or in radiation-induced lung injury also causes bronchiectasis. Cystic fibrosis; increased inflationary pressures, as seen in positive pressure ventilation; ciliary dysfunction, as in Kartagener syndrome; and various immunodeficiencies are similarly associated with dilated bronchi (4).

Bronchiectasis is commonly classified into three morphologic categories. Cylindrical bronchiectasis, the mildest form, is characterized by mildly and uniformly dilated bronchi. Varicose bronchiectasis is the term used to describe moderately dilated and irregularly beaded bronchi. Cystic bronchiectasis is the most severe: Marked cystlike dilatations of the bronchi are found, and these dilatations contain variable amounts of pooled secretions (3).

The clinical findings of bronchiectasis are often nonspecific. Chronic cough, excess sputum production, recurrent lung infections, and hemoptysis all may occur (4). Although chest radiography can demonstrate dilated bronchi, CT has improved our ability to detect them. In fact, CT has replaced bronchography as the diagnostic study of choice for evaluation of possible bronchiectasis (1). Thin-section CT has a sensitivity of 87%–97% and specificity of 93%–100% for the detection of bronchiectasis (1,5,6).

Chest radiographic findings of bronchiectasis include dilated air-filled bronchi, bronchial wall thickening, parenchymal volume loss, and bronchial crowding. Abnormal lung opacities, such as those due to pneumonia and fibrosis, also may be seen (4). At thin-section CT, bronchial dilatation, lack of bronchial tapering, bronchi that are visible within 1 cm of the pleura, bronchial wall thickening, and the signet ring sign all may be visualized (1). The bronchoarterial ratio varies with different parameters, such as the altitude at which CT is performed (7); therefore, depiction of only a bronchus larger in diameter than the adjacent artery is not sufficient for the diagnosis of bronchiectasis (8).

Several pitfalls in the CT-based diagnosis of bronchiectasis have been described, including artifact caused by respiratory motion or cardiac pulsations and technical factors related to collimation and windowing. Therefore, it is often necessary to perform thin-section CT to make the diagnosis of bronchiectasis.

Of interest is the term "signet ring sign" that is applied to the cross-sectional image of both the dilated bronchus and the adjacent pulmonary artery. The *New Lexicon Webster's Dictio-*

Index terms:
Bronchi, diseases, 60.26, 60.742
Bronchiectasis, 60.26, 60.742
Lung, CT, 68.12111, 68.12118

Radiology 1999; 212:67–68

[1] From the Faculty of Radiology, Ottawa Hospital, Civic Campus, 1053 Carling Ave, Ottawa, Ontario K1Y 4E9, Canada. Received December 1, 1997; revision requested January 15, 1998; final revision received July 28; accepted November 19. **Address reprint requests to** the author.

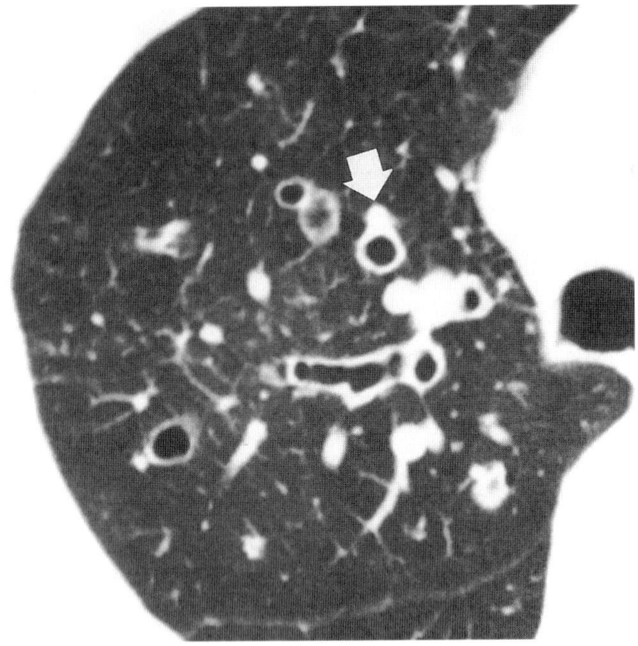

Figure 1. Cross-sectional CT scan of the right lung in a patient with bronchiectasis. The signet ring sign (arrow) consists of a small circle of soft-tissue attenuation that abuts a ring of soft-tissue attenuation surrounding a larger low-attenuating circle of air.

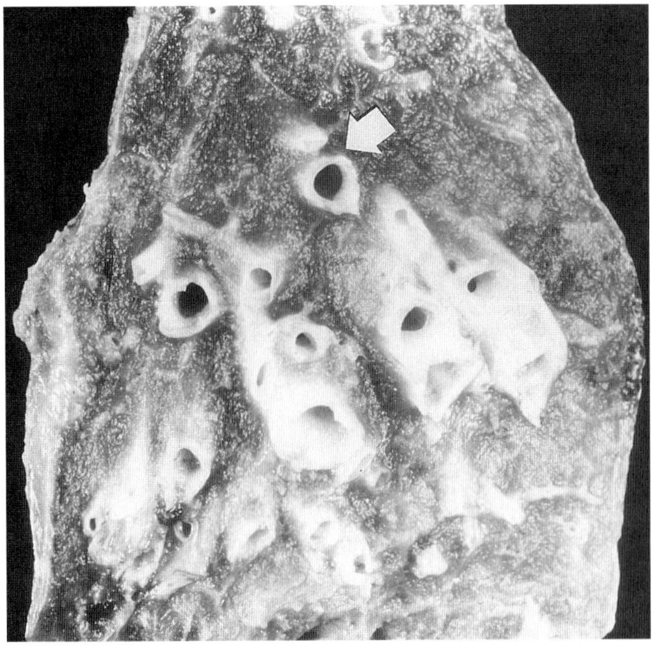

Figure 2. Gross pathologic lung specimen from a patient with bronchiectasis. Notice the small pulmonary artery abutting the much larger dilated bronchus (arrow), both of which are seen on a cross-sectional view.

nary of the English Language defines a signet ring as a "finger ring set or engraved with the monogram, sign or initials of the owner" (9). It further defines a signet as "a personal seal used to show authenticity of documents, often in addition to the signature" (9). The signet or seal appears to be a structure that is flat rather than elevated or somewhat rounded like the characteristic appearance of the pulmonary artery adjacent to the dilated bronchus. Is the term "signet ring sign" therefore a misnomer? Should the sign be termed instead the "*pearl* ring sign" to reflect the fact that the pulmonary artery in a living patient more closely resembles a pearl that may be variable in size (Fig 3)?

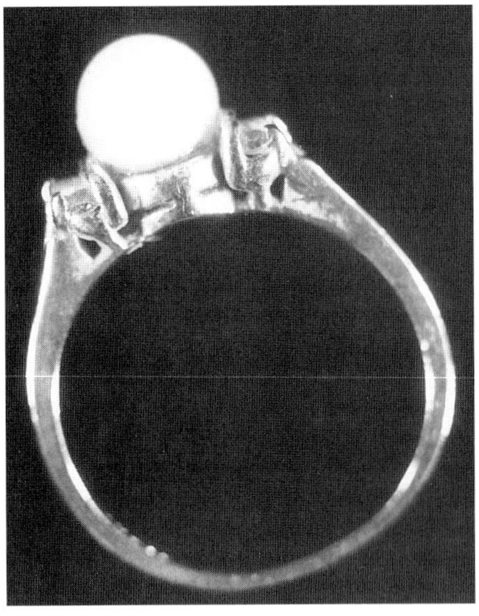

Figure 3. Photograph of a pearl ring. Does the pearl more closely simulate the pulmonary artery seen in Figure 1 than does the signet?

References

1. Kang EY, Miller RR, Muller NL. Bronchiectasis: comparison of preoperative thin-section CT and pathologic findings in resected specimens. Radiology 1994; 195:649–654.
2. Webb WR. High-resolution computed tomography of obstructive lung disease. Radiol Clin North Am 1994; 32:745–757.
3. McGuinnes G, Naidich DT, Leitman BS, McCauley DI. Bronchiectasis: CT evaluation. AJR 1993; 160:254–259.
4. Westcott JL. Bronchiectasis. Radiol Clin North Am 1991; 29:1031–1042.
5. Grenier P, Maurice F, Musset D, Menu Y, Nahum H. Bronchiectasis: assessment by thin-section CT. Radiology 1986; 161:95–99.
6. Young K. High-resolution CT and bronchography in the assessment of bronchiectasis. Acta Radiol 1991; 32:439–441.
7. Kim JS. Bronchoarterial ratio on thin-section CT: comparison between high altitude and sea level. J Comput Assist Tomogr 1997; 21:306–311.
8. Lynch DA, Newell JD, Tschomper BA, Cink TM, Newman LS, Bethel R. Uncomplicated asthma in adults: comparison of CT appearance of the lungs in asthmatic and healthy subjects. Radiology 1993; 188:829–833.
9. Lechner DE, ed. The new lexicon Webster's dictionary of the English language, encyclopedic edition. New York, NY: Lexicon Publications, 1987.

Reinhard Groell, MD
Gottfried J. Schaffler, MD
Rainer Rienmueller, MD

Index terms:
Computed tomography (CT), electron beam, 51.12112, 51.12114, 51.12118, 55.12112, 55.12114, 55.12118
Heart, anatomy, 51.92
Heart, CT, 51.12112, 51.12114, 55.12112, 55.12114
Pericardium
Pericardium, CT, 55.12112, 55.12114, 55.12118, 55.92

Radiology 1999; 212:69–73

[1] From the Department of Radiology, University Hospital Graz, Auenbruggerplatz 9, A-8036 Graz, Austria. Received April 14, 1998; revision requested May 29; final revision received October 30; accepted February 12, 1999. **Address reprint requests to** R.G.

Author contributions:
Guarantor of integrity of entire study, R.G.; study concepts, R.G., R.R.; study design, R.G., R.R.; definition of intellectual content, R.G., R.R.; literature research, R.G.; data acquisition and analysis, R.G., G.J.S.; manuscript preparation, editing, and review, R.G., R.R.

Pericardial Sinuses and Recesses: Findings at Electrocardiographically Triggered Electron-Beam CT[1]

PURPOSE: To evaluate the appearance of the pericardial sinuses and recesses at electrocardiographically triggered electron-beam computed tomography (CT).

MATERIALS AND METHODS: Findings in 100 patients without known pericardial disease were reviewed. The patients underwent electron-beam CT of the heart because of suspected coronary arterial disease. Incremental electrocardiographically triggered images were obtained with a 100-msec exposure time and 1.5-mm section thickness after intravenous administration of contrast material. The appearance of the pericardial sinuses and recesses was determined.

RESULTS: In each patient, at least one of the sinuses was visible at CT. The transverse and oblique sinuses (or one of their recesses) were depicted in 95 and 89 patients, respectively. The left pulmonic recess was depicted in 81 patients; inferior aortic recess, 80 patients; posterior pericardial recess, 67 patients; left pulmonic vein recess, 60 patients; right pulmonic recess, 51 patients; superior aortic recess, 47 patients; right pulmonic vein recess, 29 patients; and postcaval recess, 23 patients.

CONCLUSION: Pericardial sinuses and recesses are frequently depicted on electrocardiographically triggered electron-beam CT images. Knowledge of their locations is helpful in the differentiation of normal pericardium from pericardial effusions and mediastinal processes such as lymph nodes.

In their cross-sectional anatomic study, Vesely and Cahill (1) systematically described and named the pericardial recesses. In former computed tomographic (CT) studies (2–7), some of these recesses were identified with different frequencies as areas of water attenuation around the great mediastinal vessels. The knowledge of their location and appearance was considered to be helpful to the radiologist in avoiding the misdiagnosis of lymphadenopathy and other mediastinal disease processes. With the advent of fast imaging modalities that provide high temporal and spatial resolution, more and more recesses have been observed on imaging studies of the mediastinum. Although in most of the reports, the appearance of the cranial (superior aortic and left pulmonic) recesses was described, less is known about the caudal (inferior aortic, postcaval, and pulmonary vein) recesses. In our experience, some of these recesses, particularly the less well-known ones, have caused diagnostic problems in the evaluation of cardiac and pericardiac structures. This led us to review 100 consecutive thin-section, electrocardiographically triggered electron-beam CT images obtained in patients who had no known pericardial disease to evaluate the appearance of the pericardial sinuses and recesses.

MATERIALS AND METHODS

We reviewed 100 consecutive electron-beam CT images obtained in patients (56 men, 44 women; mean age ± SD, 52 years ± 11; age range, 27–88 years) who did not have clinical evidence of pericardial effusion, pericarditis, or mediastinal lymphadenopathy. The patients had been examined between November 1996 and December 1997 because they were clinically suspected of having coronary arterial disease. CT was performed with an

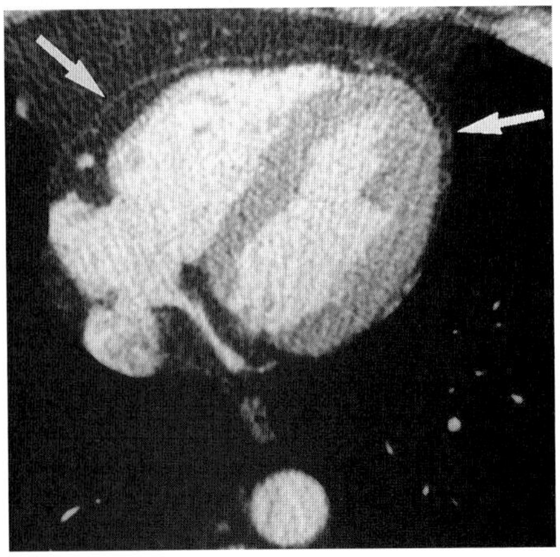

Figure 1. Electron-beam CT image of the mediastinum. The pericardium appears as a thin band (arrows) in the anterior mediastinum.

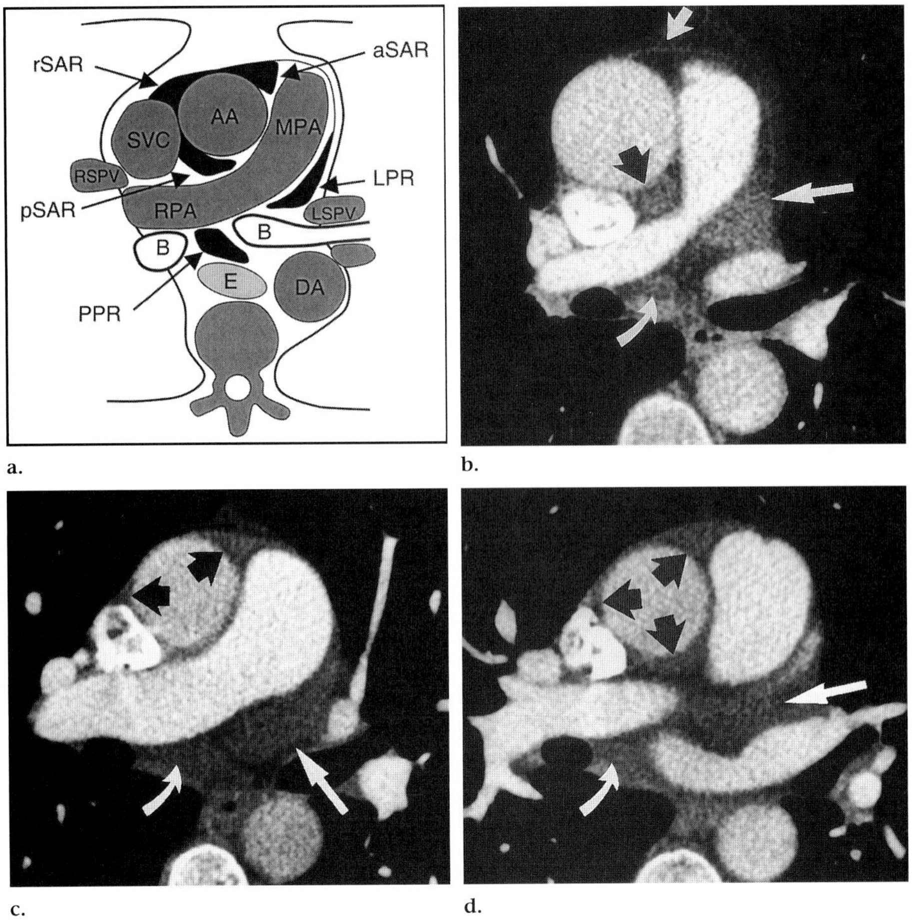

Figure 2. **(a)** Cross-sectional drawing of the pericardial sinuses and recesses and **(b–d)** corresponding electron-beam CT images (obtained in different patients) at the level of the right pulmonary artery (*RPA*). In **a**, *AA* = ascending aorta, *B* = bronchus intermedius, *DA* = descending aorta, *E* = esophagus, *LSPV* = left superior pulmonary vein, *MPA* = main pulmonary artery, *RSPV* = right superior pulmonary vein, *SVC* = superior vena cava. (See Key Box for abbreviation expansions not given here.) **(b)** The pericardium (short white arrow) is seen in the anterior mediastinum. **(b–d)** The left pulmonic recess (straight white arrow) lies lateral to the main pulmonary artery. The posterior pericardial recess (curved arrow) of the oblique sinus is posterior to the right pulmonary artery and medial to the bronchus. The anterior portion of the superior aortic recess, right lateral portion of the superior aortic recess, and posterior portion of the superior aortic recess (black arrows) also are seen.

Key Box for Abbreviations in Figures 2–4

Nomenclature of the Pericardial Cavity	Abbreviation
Pericardial cavity proper	. . .
Postcaval recess	PCR
Right pulmonic vein recess	RPVR
Left pulmonic vein recess	LPVR
Transverse sinus	TS
Superior aortic recess	SAR
Anterior portion	aSAR
Posterior portion	pSAR
Right lateral portion	rSAR
Inferior aortic recess	IAR
Right pulmonic recess	RPR
Left pulmonic recess	LPR
Oblique sinus	OS
Posterior pericardial recess	PPR

Sources.—Nomina Anatomica and reference 1.

electron-beam CT scanner (Evolution; Siemens, Erlangen, Germany). All patients were lying in the supine position, and the images were obtained in the middle of inspiration; in our experience, this enables patients to maintain a maximal breath hold. Forty to 60 contiguous, axial sections were obtained by using a collimation of 1.5 mm and exposure time of 100 msec. The images were cardiac gated at the end of diastole (at 80% of the RR interval) to minimize cardiac motion artifacts. Nonionic contrast material (120 mL of iopromide [Ultravist 300; Schering, Berlin, Germany]) was injected into an antecubital vein at a rate of 3 mL/sec. The scanning delay in each patient was individually determined after the administration of a test bolus of 10 mL of contrast material. Typically, the scanning delay range was 20–25 seconds. Because the examinations were performed to image the proximal 4–5 cm of the coronary arteries, the imaging extended from the top of the right pulmonary artery to the bottom of the left atrium (6–9 cm in the craniocaudal direction, depending on the heart size).

The nomenclature of the pericardial cavity, based on the Nomina Anatomica and work of Vesely and Cahill (1), is described in the Key Box. Three recesses of the pericardial cavity proper were named as follows: postcaval recess, left pulmonic vein recess, and right pulmonic vein recess. The transverse sinus was divided into the following four recesses: the superior aortic recess, inferior aortic recess, left pulmonic recess, and right pulmonic recess. In addition, we added the following subdivisions to the descriptions of the sinuses and recesses that had been suggested previously by Kubota et al (2): The superior aortic recess was divided into the anterior, posterior, and right lateral portions. The posterior pericardial recess was described as part of the oblique sinus.

To distinguish pericardial sinuses and recesses from lymphatic tissue or soft tissue, we, like others before us, used the criterion of sharply outlined structures with uniform water-equivalent attenuation without walls or rims in the expected anatomic locations to define sinuses and recesses (3). To evaluate the frequency of the depiction of the sinuses and recesses, all images were reviewed by two radiologists (R.G., G.J.S.) in a consensus reading.

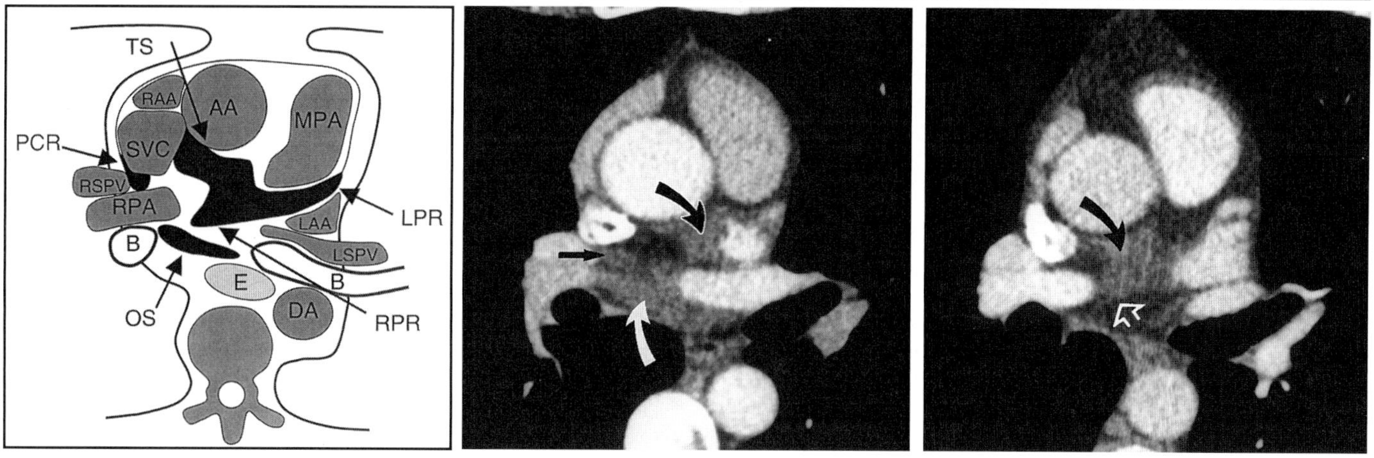

a. b. c.

Figure 3. **(a)** Cross-sectional drawing of the pericardial sinuses and recesses and **(b, c)** corresponding electron-beam CT images (obtained in different patients) below the level of the right pulmonary artery (*RPA*). In **a**, *AA* = ascending aorta, *B* = bronchus intermedius, *DA* = descending aorta, *E* = esophagus, *LAA* = left atrial appendage, *LSPV* = left superior pulmonary vein, *MPA* = main pulmonary artery, *RAA* = right atrial appendage, *RSPV* = right superior pulmonary vein, *SVC* = superior vena cava. (See Key Box for abbreviation expansions not given here.) **(b)** The oblique sinus (curved white arrow) is posterior to the right pulmonary artery and left atrium. The postcaval recess (straight black arrow) may be seen at the same level lateral and posterior to the superior vena cava. **(b, c)** The transverse sinus (curved black arrow) lies posterior to the ascending aorta. **(c)** The right pulmonic recess (open arrow) extends posteriorly below the right pulmonary artery.

RESULTS

All 100 electron-beam CT images were included in the evaluation, because there were no limiting factors that might reduce image quality such as beam-hardening or motion artifacts. The pericardium had the appearance of a thin band in the anterior mediastinum (Fig 1).

In each patient, at least one of the sinuses or recesses could be identified. Figures 2–4 are drawings of the sinuses and recesses and the corresponding CT images. Note that all of the CT images were obtained in different patients. The transverse sinus or one of its recesses was depicted in 95 patients, and the oblique sinus, including the posterior pericardial recess, was depicted in 89 patients. The pericardial recesses were depicted as follows: the left pulmonic recess was demonstrated in 81 patients; inferior aortic recess, in 80 patients; posterior pericardial recess, in 67 patients; left pulmonic vein recess, in 60 patients; right pulmonic recess, in 51 patients; superior aortic recess, in 47 patients; right pulmonic vein recess, in 29 patients; and postcaval recess, in 23 patients.

DISCUSSION

The pericardium consists of an outer fibrous layer (the fibrous pericardium) and an inner serous sac (the serous pericardium) (8). The serous pericardium consists of an inner visceral layer (the epicardium), which is intimately connected to the heart and the epicardial fat, and an outer parietal layer, which lines the fibrous pericardium. The visceral layer is reflected from the heart and the root of the great vessels onto the inner surface of the fibrous pericardium to become continuous with the parietal layer. The pericardial cavity lies between these two layers of the serous pericardium. Under physiologic conditions, it contains 20-25 mL of serous fluid; however, the amount of fluid may vary considerably among individuals, particularly in children and infants (9). These differences may explain, at least in part, why in some patients, sinuses or recesses may or may not be seen. Moreover, clinically asymptomatic patients can have large pericardial fluid collections, especially when it accumulates over long periods, and it may be found incidentally.

At the reflections of the serous pericardium between the great vessels at the base of the heart, the pericardial cavity forms the pericardial sinuses, which are not separate compartments, but rather they represent extensions of the pericardial cavity. The Nomina Anatomica labels them the transverse sinus and oblique sinus. As the pericardium extends onto the roots of the great vessels, the pericardial cavity proper and the sinuses form recesses, as described by Vesely and Cahill (1). Because there is no histologic difference between the layers of the sinuses and those of the recesses, their differentiation is based on topographic landmarks (1).

Recesses of the Pericardial Cavity Proper

The postcaval recess (Fig 3) is an extension of the pericardial cavity proper that lies behind and on the right lateral aspect of the superior vena cava. The right and left pulmonic vein recesses (Fig 4) are between the superior and inferior pulmonic veins on both sides. In our series, these three recesses of the pericardial cavity proper were usually small, with diameters of up to approximately 1 cm. The left pulmonic vein recess was depicted at CT more often (in 60 [60%] of 100 patients) than was the right pulmonic vein recess and postcaval recess, which were depicted in 29% and 23% of patients, respectively. These recesses are located in the venous reflection zone of the pericardium where the pericardium is attached to the adventitia of the superior vena cava and the pulmonary veins, with no fat tissue between these structures. Vesely and Cahill (1) demonstrated the close relationship between the bronchopulmonary lymph nodes and these recesses.

Transverse Sinus

The transverse sinus (Fig 3) is posterior to the ascending aorta and pulmonary

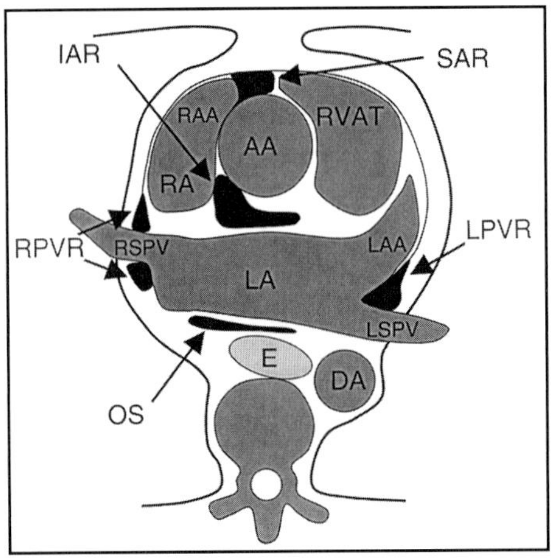

a.

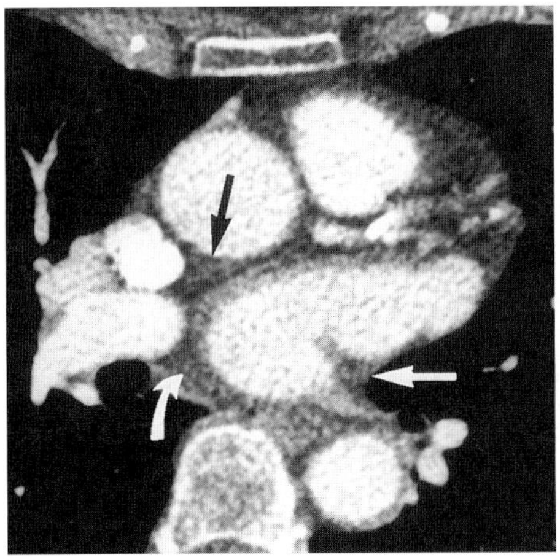
b.

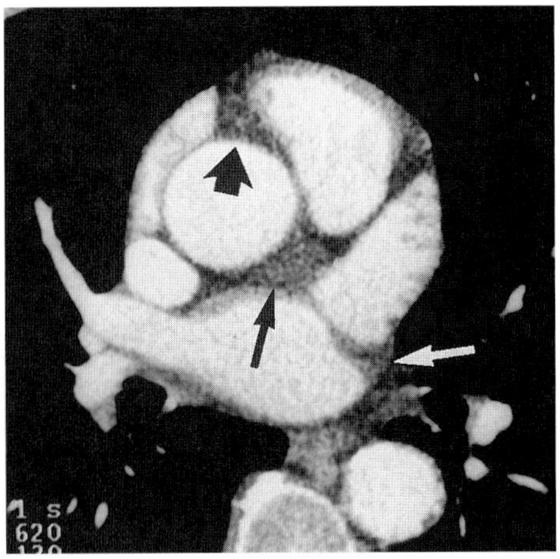
c.

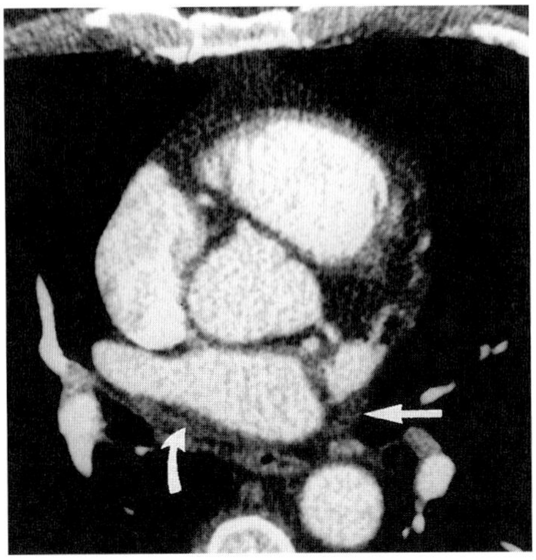
d.

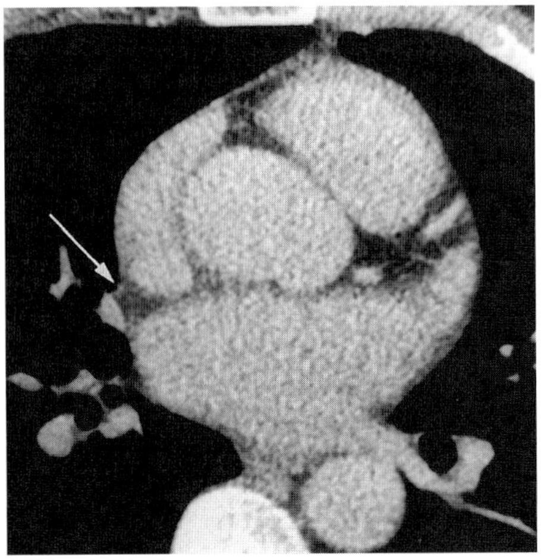
e.

Figure 4. (a) Cross-sectional drawing of the pericardial sinuses and recesses and **(b–e)** corresponding electron-beam CT images (obtained in different patients) at the level of the left atrium (*LA*). In **a**, *AA* = ascending aorta, *DA* = descending aorta, *E* = esophagus, *LAA* = left atrial appendage, *LSPV* = left superior pulmonary vein, *RA* = right atrium, *RAA* = right atrial appendage, *RSPV* = right superior pulmonary vein, *RVAT* = right ventricular outflow tract. (See Key Box for abbreviation expansions not given here.) **(b–d)** The inferior aortic recess (straight black arrow in **b** and **c**) extends downward behind the ascending aorta. The superior aortic recess (short arrow in **c**) also is seen. The left pulmonic vein recess (straight white arrow) is between the left pulmonic veins. The oblique sinus (curved arrow in **b** and **d**) lies posterior to the left atrium. **(e)** The right pulmonic vein recess (arrow) is adjacent to the right pulmonic veins.

trunk and above the left atrium. Between the ascending aorta and superior vena cava, it is connected with the pericardial cavity proper. However, this connection was not depicted on the electron-beam CT images in this study. The transverse sinus was identified in 95 (95%) patients. It extends upward along the ascending aorta, where it forms the superior aortic recess (Figs 2, 4). The superior aortic recess is frequently depicted on CT images and was one of the first recesses described in CT studies of the mediastinum (4–6). Other authors (2) previously divided the superior aortic recess into anterior, posterior, and right lateral portions. Although the communication between the anterior portion and right lateral portion was sometimes visible in our study, we could never clearly identify the connection between the right lateral portion and posterior portion that runs between the ascending aorta and superior vena cava. Occasionally, the anterior portion extended downward to the level of the right atrium (Fig 4). The anterior and right lateral portions are directly related to the thymus, and the posterior portion is related to the tracheobronchial lymph nodes.

On nonenhanced CT images and magnetic resonance images, the superior aortic recess may also simulate aortic dissection or thrombus (3,6). The left pulmonic recess (Figs 2, 3) is situated below the left pulmonary artery and posterolateral to the proximal portion of the right pulmonary artery. Protopapas and Westcott (3) demonstrated the different appearances of this recess and discussed the diagnostic problems that may lead to a misdiagnosis of lymphadenopathy. The right pulmonic recess (Fig 3) lies below the right pulmonary artery and above the left atrium. Its posterior circumference is directly related to the inferior tracheobronchial lymph nodes. The inferior aortic recess (Fig 4) lies between the ascending aorta and either the inferior portion of the vena cava superior or the right atrium. Vesely and Cahill (1) demonstrated that the inferior aortic recess extends down to the level of the aortic valve. However, in our series, we could not identify this recess to that extent.

At the arterial reflections of the pericardium, the superior aortic recess is directly attached to the aortic wall. Posterior to the ascending aorta and main pulmonary artery, there may be a variable amount of epicardial fat. At CT, this was frequently seen as a fat space between these vessels on the one hand, and the transverse sinus, inferior aortic recess, and left pulmonic recess on the other. Only the right-sided entrance of the transverse sinus always directly attached to the posterior aspect of the ascending aorta. Often, there was a clear separation by fat between the left pulmonic recess and either the main pulmonary artery or the left atrial appendage.

Oblique Sinus

The oblique sinus (Figs 3, 4) is located behind the left atrium. In its cranial portion, it is separated from the transverse sinus by a double reflection of the pericardium between the right and left superior pulmonic veins. At CT, the transverse sinus, including the right and left pulmonic recesses, was always clearly separated from the oblique sinus, including the posterior pericardial recess, by a fat plane (Figs 2, 3). The upper right lateral extension of the oblique sinus is the posterior pericardial recess (Fig 2), which lies behind the distal right pulmonary artery and medial to the bronchus intermedius. In a former radiology report (2), the oblique sinus and posterior pericardial recess were seen at CT in less than 10% of patients. We observed them in 89 (89%) and 67 (67%) of 100 patients, respectively. The esophagus runs posterior to the oblique sinus, and the inferior tracheobronchial lymph nodes are in close proximity to these structures. The upper circumference of the oblique sinus and posterior pericardial recess is frequently surrounded by fatty tissue. In the present study, at CT, this often delineated these structures from the right pulmonary artery and right bronchus intermedius, and from the upper portion of the left atrium. More caudally, the oblique sinus is attached to the adventitia of the left atrium. Because the pericardium is separated from the esophagus by loose connective tissue, the esophagus was frequently separated from the oblique sinus by a fat space on the CT images in this study.

Summary

With the advent of fast imaging methods that provide high temporal and spatial resolution, the pericardial sinuses and recesses have been more frequently identified on imaging studies of the mediastinum. In general, pericardial sinuses and recesses may be difficult to differentiate from lymph nodes, esophageal or thymic processes, or vascular abnormalities. Rarely, pericardial cysts or tumors, which can mimic cardiac tumors, may develop in these sinuses and recesses (9).

In former studies (3,4,6), the more cranial recesses such as the superior aortic and left pulmonic recesses mainly were described. Less attention was paid to the caudal aspects of the sinuses—that is, the right pulmonic recess, inferior aortic recess, oblique sinus, and pulmonary vein recesses. This may be because the caudal recesses are more affected by heart motion than are the superior recesses—that is, the superior aortic recess and left pulmonic recess. In addition, the superior recesses are largely surrounded by fatty tissue, which makes them more delineated. The inferior recesses are often close to the esophagus or surrounded mainly by cardiac chambers, which makes the exact delineation of these structures more difficult. In general, the more mediastinal fat present, the better one can see the sinuses and recesses at CT.

In the present study, separations by fat planes were frequently observed between the sinuses or recesses and the intrapericardial structures (eg, between the transverse sinus and main pulmonary artery or between the left pulmonic recess and main pulmonary artery) and between the sinuses or recesses and the extrapericardial structures (eg, between the right pulmonic recess and right pulmonary artery or between the oblique sinus and esophagus). However, there were certain locations where the sinuses and recesses always directly abutted the adjacent intrapericardial structures—for example, between the superior aortic recess and ascending aorta, between the pulmonary vein recesses and proximal pulmonary veins, between the postcaval recess and superior vena cava, and between the right-sided entrance of the transverse sinus and the posterior aspect of the ascending aorta. In this context, it should be stated that the transition from water to fat was not always clearly identifiable, but rather it was occasionally blurred by image noise, especially in patients with a large volume of adipose tissue.

Soulen et al (10) described changes in pericardial fluid distribution due to heart motion and respiratory maneuvers in dogs with pericardial effusion. Because the pericardial sinuses and recesses are extensions of the pericardial cavity proper, it is very likely that pericardial fluid might move from one area to another during the cardiac cycle or during respiration (3). However, this was not investigated in our study, because we used constant conditions, with the CT images obtained at the end of diastole and in the middle of inspiration.

In conclusion, when electrocardiographically triggered electron-beam CT is performed, the pericardial sinuses and recesses are frequently observed on images of the heart. Knowledge of the location of these structures helps the radiologist avoid a misdiagnosis of lymphadenopathy or other mediastinal disease processes.

References

1. Vesely TM, Cahill DR. Cross-sectional anatomy of the pericardial sinuses, recesses and adjacent structures. Surg Radiol Anat 1986; 8:221–227.
2. Kubota H, Sato C, Ohgushi M, Haku T, Sasaki K, Yamaguchi K. Fluid collection in the pericardial sinuses and recesses: thin-section helical computed tomography observations and hypothesis. Invest Radiol 1996; 31:603–610.
3. Protopapas Z, Westcott JL. Left pulmonic recess of the pericardium: findings at CT and MR imaging. Radiology 1995; 196: 85–88.
4. Aronberg DJ, Peterson RR, Glazer HS, Sagel SS. The superior sinus of the pericardium: CT appearance. Radiology 1984; 153:489–492.
5. Levy-Ravetch M, Auh YH, Rubenstein WA, Whalen JP, Kazam E. CT of the pericardial recesses. AJR 1985; 144:707–714.
6. Chiles C, Baker ME, Silverman PM. Superior pericardial recess simulating aortic dissection on computed tomography. J Comput Assist Tomogr 1986; 10:421–423.
7. Choe YH, Im JG, Park JH, Han MC, Kim CW. The anatomy of the pericardial space: a study in cadavers and patients. AJR 1987; 149:693–697.
8. Shabetai R. Anatomy. In: The pericardium. New York, NY: Grune & Stratton, 1981; 1–32.
9. Moncada R, Baker M, Salinas M, et al. Diagnostic role of computed tomography in pericardial heart disease: congenital defects, thickening, neoplasms, and effusions. Am Heart J 1982; 103:263–282.
10. Soulen RL, Lapayowker MS, Cortes FM. Distribution of pericardial fluid: dynamic and static influences. AJR 1968; 103:583–588.

Book Review

Guidelines and Gamuts in Musculoskeletal Ultrasound

Edited by Rethy K. Chhem, MD, PhD, and Etienne Cardinal, MD
New York, NY: Wiley, 1998. ISBN 0-471-19755-6.
Hardcover, $100.00; pp 408, 251 figures; tables.

Few subjects in musculoskeletal imaging cause as much anxiety for radiologists as the topic of musculoskeletal ultrasonography (US). Few of us, even those who have been trained recently, receive any instruction in musculoskeletal US during our residencies or fellowships, a fact pointed out by Dr Donald Resnick in his forward to this volume. The current situation is not unlike the one that accompanied the advent of musculoskeletal magnetic resonance imaging in the 1980s. The era of musculoskeletal US is only just arriving, and it is driven partially by technologic advances in instrumentation and partially by a growing body of published literature on musculoskeletal US applications. Most of the major contributions to the development of the field have come from outside of the United States, where these applications are more widely practiced. This book aims to remedy the deficiencies that most of us have in our training in musculoskeletal US and provide a "hands-on" manual for the radiologist.

The intended audience is radiologists and other physicians who are involved in imaging of the musculoskeletal system. The book will be especially appreciated by anyone who has a need to master the techniques of musculoskeletal US quickly. The editors have done an outstanding job of synthesizing the vital information needed to rapidly develop proficiency in applying these new techniques. They provide a concise, clear, lavishly illustrated, step-by-step instruction manual complete with checklists to verify that each key structure has been identified and evaluated, that each clinical issue is taken in turn, and that nothing is overlooked. Common pathologic conditions are well illustrated, and lists of differential diagnostic possibilities (ie, "gamuts") with concise discussions of each of these possibilities are provided. The superb anatomic line drawings that accompany the US images assist in orienting the reader to the appearance of musculoskeletal anatomy.

The editors are Canadian radiologists who are skilled in the depiction of musculoskeletal disease with the use of multiple modalities, and both are internationally known experts in musculoskeletal US imaging. The 19 contributors from the United States and abroad include many leaders in the field. Although it is concise, the book represents an authoritative review and thus can serve as both an excellent introductory textbook and an exceptional long-term reference resource.

The book is well written, well indexed, and succinct. It is organized into 11 major chapters that include the evaluation of bone and joints, muscles and fascia, ligaments and tendons, and soft-tissue masses. The 11th chapter is dedicated to soft-tissue imaging in pediatrics. A possible omission, which may have been deliberate, is a chapter on the use of Doppler US, which would have required color illustrations. Although Doppler US applications are discussed in several chapters, the book provides no color plates.

The US images are gray scale and include black-and-white photographs and line drawings of the anatomy, all of very good quality. An excellent appendix of US-oriented anatomy contains line drawings and is organized primarily as a guide to evaluation. All figures and illustrations are printed on good-quality, low-gloss paper and serve to greatly enhance and amplify the content of the text.

In conclusion, this outstanding textbook will be useful to anyone who wishes to perform clinical musculoskeletal US and interpret findings, regardless of the reader's level of experience. It will be of particular value to radiologists who are beginners in the application of this modality. It compares very favorably in price and quality with a similar, earlier textbook by a leading sonologist in the United States. *Guidelines and Gamuts in Musculoskeletal Ultrasound* is probably the better value in that it offers a broader scope and more immediate utility than previous textbooks at a similar price. At $100, the price is very reasonable for a textbook of this scope and quality.

Reviewed by Michael A. Bruno, MD

Robert G. Sheiman, MD
Colin R. McArdle, MD

Index terms:
Embolism, pulmonary, 60.72
Extremities, thrombosis, 93.751
Thrombosis, US, 93.1298, 93.12983, 93.751
Ultrasound (US), Doppler studies, 93.12983
Veins, thrombosis, 93.751

Radiology 1999; 212:75–78

Abbreviations:
DVT = deep venous thrombosis
PE = pulmonary embolism

[1] From the Department of Radiology, Beth Israel Deaconess Medical Center and Harvard Medical School, 330 Brookline Ave, Boston, MA 02215. Received October 2, 1998; revision requested November 19; revision received December 17; accepted January 27, 1999. **Address reprint requests to** R.G.S. (e-mail: *rsheiman@caregroup.harvard.edu*).

Author contributions:
Guarantor of integrity of entire study, R.G.S.; study concepts and design, R.G.S.; definition of intellectual content, R.G.S., C.R.M.; literature research, R.G.S.; clinical studies, R.G.S., C.R.M.; data acquisition, R.G.S.; data analysis, R.G.S., C.R.M.; manuscript preparation, R.G.S.; manuscript editing and review, R.G.S., C.R.M.

Clinically Suspected Pulmonary Embolism: Use of Bilateral Lower Extremity US as the Initial Examination—A Prospective Study[1]

PURPOSE: To determine the prevalence of deep venous thrombosis (DVT) and evaluate the use of symptoms and risk factors as selection criteria in the patient population undergoing lower extremity ultrasonography (US) as an initial examination for suspected pulmonary embolism (PE).

MATERIALS AND METHODS: One hundred eighty-two consecutive patients referred for bilateral lower extremity US as the first examination for suspected PE were evaluated prospectively for predisposing factors and symptoms of DVT. Patients were placed into four groups: group 1, no symptoms or risk factors; group 2, both symptoms and risk factors; group 3, only risk factors; group 4, only symptoms. The prevalence of DVT detected at lower extremity US in each group was determined.

RESULTS: There were 89 patients in group 1, 12 in group 2, 43 in group 3, and 38 in group 4, with a DVT prevalence of 0%, 25%, 14%, and 24%, respectively. There was no significant difference in DVT prevalence between groups with symptoms or risk factors but a significant difference between these groups and the group lacking both symptoms and risk factors.

CONCLUSION: Lower extremity US as the initial examination in patients suspected of having PE should be used only in those patients who have symptoms or risk factors for DVT. This would substantially decrease the number of examinations performed without a decline in DVT detection.

Performing lower extremity ultrasonography (US) for assessment for deep venous thrombosis (DVT) has become an important step in the current noninvasive work-up for pulmonary embolism (PE). Although there has been agreement as to its value, its location in the algorithm for PE assessment is variable. Many authors (1–3) have reserved this examination for the selected patient population with an initial ventilation-perfusion scan deemed to have indeterminate results. Performance of lower extremity US in this scenario also has been shown to be cost-effective, as positive study results eliminate the need for pulmonary angiography (2,4). To improve pretest probability in the setting of a nonconclusive ventilation-perfusion scan, Rosen et al (5) advocated its application in only those patients who have risk factors for or symptoms of DVT.

At our institution (Beth Israel Deaconess Medical Center) and others (6,7), US assessment for lower extremity DVT is becoming the initial study requested for clinically suspected PE. This is likely owing to the well-documented association of lower extremity DVT and PE, the high sensitivity and specificity of US for DVT, and the availability and noninvasive nature of this test. However, when used as a screening study for all patients suspected of having a PE, lower extremity US no longer is being applied in the preselected population with an indeterminate ventilation-perfusion scan. Initial assessment for lower extremity DVT in all patients suspected of having PE, therefore, includes patients who otherwise would not have undergone DVT examination because of a ventilation-perfusion scan with normal or high-probability results.

Spiral computed tomographic (CT) angiography of the pulmonary arteries has become another noninvasive tool for PE assessment and demonstrates sensitivities above 90% and a specificity of 78% or greater for PE up to the segmental level (8,9). In a recent theoretic evaluation of multiple algorithms for the work-up for PE (10), which included pulmonary CT angiography and a D-dimer test, lower extremity US, followed by pulmonary CT angiography, was identified as the most cost-effective initial approach for the evaluation for PE. Other investigators (11) have advocated lower extremity US as the initial screening examination for PE when concomitant lower extremity symptoms of DVT exist. On the basis of these recent publications and our experience, it is expected that the use of US for DVT detection as the first-line examination for PE will increase.

To our knowledge, the application of lower extremity US for DVT in patients who are suspected of having PE and who have not undergone any preselection has not been evaluated prospectively. Therefore, we sought to determine the prevalence of DVT in this patient population and whether DVT symptoms or risk factors may be applied as selection criteria to improve the pretest probability of lower extremity US when used as the initial examination for PE assessment.

MATERIALS AND METHODS

Between December 1997 and August 1998, a prospective evaluation was performed in all patients referred for lower extremity US as the initial examination for clinically suspected PE. All examinations were bilateral according to our protocol for PE work-up. Patients either were referred from our emergency department or were inpatients at our institution. Clinical suspicion was based on the acute onset of shortness of breath, an abnormal arterial-alveolar gradient, chest pain, new onset of atrial fibrillation, or any combination of these. All patients for whom assessment for DVT was the major indication for study performance were excluded. A total of 182 patients were identified and formed our study cohort (78 men, 104 women; age range, 18–90 years; mean age, 61 years).

At the time US was performed, each patient was examined by a resident or staff physician for symptoms of acute DVT, which included lower extremity pain, swelling, erythema, or any combination of these, and each patient's clinical history was reviewed for risk factors for DVT. Leg swelling was determined subjectively and on the basis of direct comparison of both legs when swelling was unilateral or was considered bilateral if thought to be present by the patient or the referring physician. Risk factors were elicited directly from the patient and from chart review and included underlying malignancy, hypercoagulable state, prior DVT, pregnancy, prolonged travel or immobility, and recent surgery. When present, symptoms were documented as unilateral, including which extremity, or bilateral. For each patient, data were recorded on a work sheet completed before leaving the US suite and were verified later at the time of chart review.

All examinations were performed on a model 128XP/10 (Acuson Computed Sonography, Mountain View, Calif) or Ultramark 9 or HDI 3000 (Advanced Technology Laboratories, Bothell, Wash), all with color Doppler and duplex capabilities and with the appropriate 5-, 7-, or 10-MHz linear array transducer. Examinations included gray-scale, color Doppler, and spectral evaluation of the common femoral, saphenous, superficial femoral, popliteal, and proximal calf veins in the longitudinal and transverse planes. Vessels were assessed for compressibility and intraluminal filling defects on gray-scale scans, presence or absence of flow voids on color Doppler scans, and spectral evaluation of blood flow characteristics, which included augmentation with calf compression. Patients were examined by staff sonographers and then reexamined by a staff radiologist to confirm all findings before patient discharge from the vascular laboratory.

Positive diagnosis of thrombus was based on lack of complete lumen obliteration with compression, flow void on color Doppler scans, and lack of flow detection at spectral analysis. The last two criteria alone were applied to the adductor canal because assessment for compressibility cannot be performed in this area. Intraluminal filling defects on gray-scale scans and luminal expansion, if present, helped to confirm the finding of thrombus. Chronic thrombus, as defined by vessel noncompressibility, wall thickening, and luminal contraction with or without flow at spectral analysis and color Doppler, was not considered a positive study result for the sake of statistical analysis.

Patients were placed into one of four groups according to the presence or absence of DVT symptoms and risk factors as follows: group 1, no symptoms or risk factors; group 2, both symptoms and risk factors; group 3, only DVT risk factors; group 4, only symptoms. Groups were then compared for the prevalence of DVT by using the Fleiss method of multiple pairwise comparison of proportions. A P value less than .05 was considered to indicate a statistically significant difference. This allowed us to determine the potential utility of using DVT symptoms and risk factors as selection criteria for using lower extremity US for screening in patients suspected of having a PE. In addition, the prevalence of US-detectable DVT in the entire patient population in our study was calculated. Finally, we noted if patients underwent any additional evaluation for PE; however, we made no attempt to determine the final disposition or prevalence of PE in the population of patients in our study, as this was not the focus of our study.

RESULTS

One hundred eighty-two bilateral lower extremity examinations were performed as the initial study for clinically suspected PE in 182 patients. DVT was identified in 18 patients for a prevalence of 10%. Eighty-nine patients presented with neither risk factors nor symptoms of DVT (group 1), 12 patients had both symptoms and risk factors (group 2), 43 patients had only risk factors (group 3), and 38 patients had only DVT symptoms (group 4). No patients in group 1 had DVT, while the diagnosis of DVT was made in three patients (25%) in group 2, six (14%) in group 3, and nine (24%) in group 4 (Table). Overall, there was no significant difference in the prevalence of DVT between the groups of patients with symptoms or risk factors for DVT. However, a significant difference in DVT prevalence was found between each of these patient groups when compared with group 1, the set of patients lacking both symptoms and risk factors for DVT.

Fifty-four patients (30%) had additional work-up for PE after their lower extremity US, while in the remaining 128 patients (70%) no additional testing was performed. Of the 18 patients with documented DVT, only five had their evaluation for PE terminated after initial DVT identification. Therefore, of the 128 patients in whom the PE work-up ended after lower extremity US, 123 had no evidence of DVT.

Of the nine patients with DVT who presented with only symptoms, all presented with unilateral symptoms and had DVT only in the symptomatic leg. No

Prevalence of DVT by Group

Group	No. of Patients	Symptoms	DVT Risk Factors	DVT*	*P* Value†
1	89	No	No	0 (0)	. . .
2	12	Yes	Yes	3 (25)	<.001
3	43	No	Yes	6 (14)	<.01
4	38	Yes	No	9 (24)	<.001

* Data are the number of patients. Data in parentheses are percentages.

† The *P* value represents the difference in DVT prevalence between group 1 compared with groups 2, 3, or 4. No difference in DVT prevalence between groups 2, 3, and 4 was identified.

patient with bilateral symptoms was found to have DVT.

DISCUSSION

Our goal was to prospectively determine the prevalence of US-detectable DVT in patients suspected of having PE and also to identify whether DVT symptoms, risk factors, or both can be applied as selection criteria when lower extremity US is used as the initial study in this scenario. We believe that we have demonstrated that in patients without symptoms or risk factors for DVT, the use of US as the initial examination to evaluate for PE is of little utility. These studies almost invariably have normal results and do not offer any additional useful information. Our data also indicate that application of symptoms or risk factors as selection criteria could have almost doubled the prevalence of DVT in the patient population in our study from 10% (18 of 182) to 19% (18 of 93) without missing a single DVT. More important, use of these criteria could have decreased the number of US examinations by 49% (89 of 182).

Multiple retrospective studies support our results, although none focused formally on the use of both DVT symptoms and risk factors as selection criteria for the application of lower extremity US to screen for PE. Eze et al (6) found lower extremity DVT in only 10% (31 of 306) of patients referred for US for the work-up for PE, and this declined to 7% (22 of 306) when patients with isolated calf clot were excluded. However, when patients were stratified according to the presence or absence of unilateral symptoms of DVT, the prevalence of DVT was 40% (10 of 25) and 5% (15 of 281), respectively. Unlike in our study, these investigators did not define DVT symptoms or discuss how they assessed for DVT symptoms. This study also differs from ours in that no attempt was made to assess for risk factors for DVT, which may explain why DVT was found in the 5% of patients without lower extremity symptoms. Of interest was the lack of further evaluation for PE in 66% of their patients, similar to our findings (70%).

Bendick et al (12) retrospectively evaluated 507 patients who underwent lower extremity US for DVT assessment who were referred for suspected PE. Seventy-six percent (384) of these patients had no symptoms or risk factors for DVT, and clot above the knee was identified in only one patient (0.3% prevalence). Conversely, 44 (36%) of 123 patients with symptoms or risk factors were found to have DVT. This study, however, included all patients who underwent lower extremity US as part of their work-up for PE and did not focus solely on patients in whom lower extremity US was the initial examination for suspected PE.

Finally, Lipski et al (13) reviewed the records of 450 patients suspected of having PE who were referred for lower extremity testing for DVT. No stratification concerning lower extremity symptoms or risk factors for DVT was performed because these investigators were concerned with the effect of lower extremity US on the management of suspected PE rather than the development of selection criteria for the use of lower extremity US in this clinical scenario. In 171 of the patients in their study, US was the first-line examination, and DVT was identified in only 13 for a prevalence of 8%.

Although we know of no other study that prospectively evaluated the frequency of DVT in patients clinically suspected of having a PE, a theoretic calculation of this can be estimated. In their study modeling the cost-effectiveness of spiral CT angiography for suspected PE, van Erkel et al (10) combined data from multiple published reports to derive a pretest probability of 24% for PE in patients clinically suspected of having PE and a probability of 65% for detectable DVT in patients with documented PE. On the basis of these values, theoretically only 15.6% of all patients suspected of having PE should have demonstrable DVT. This is slightly higher than our findings and is likely owing to their use of the upper limit quoted in the literature for the probability of DVT when PE is documented. Still, this implies, as is exemplified by our data, that the majority of examinations for DVT performed for suspected PE are negative. We believe that the number of studies with normal results can be substantially reduced by using DVT symptoms and risk factors as selection criteria.

As mentioned, 70% of the patients in our study had no additional work-up for PE, and within this subgroup 96% had normal examination results. This would indicate that the suspicion for PE in the patient population in our study was low. It is likely that the combination of low clinical suspicion for PE and normal bilateral US results allayed the fears of PE. However, this type of logic, which was put forth in a recent publication (14), seems neither safe nor cost-effective. We and others (11,13,15) point out the shortcoming of terminating the pursuit of PE after normal lower extremity US results owing to the frequent absence of DVT in cases of documented PE. As stated by Cronan (16), ". . .the absence of a positive US study should not be used to exclude the diagnosis of PE."

Also, we point out that quantifying the clinical suspicion for PE, once the question of PE has been raised, is difficult. This is exemplified by the Prospective Investigation of Pulmonary Embolism Diagnosis, or PIOPED, study (17) in which clinical suspicion for PE was graded as noncommittal in the majority (64% [569 of 887]) of cases. This is why we made no attempt to formally quantify the level of clinical suspicion for PE in this study and do not believe that the lack of doing so led to any selection bias. We believe, however, that on the basis of our findings, if such an approach is to persist, the selection criteria put forth here for the use of lower extremity US should be applied.

Within the group of patients with only lower extremity symptoms, all cases of DVT were unilateral, with thrombus identified only in the symptomatic extremity. No DVT was found in any asymptomatic extremity or in any patient with bilateral symptoms. This is in accord with our previous findings (18,19). These data support performance of a larger prospective study focused on the utility of performing a bilateral examination in the patient who has unilateral DVT symptoms and who is undergoing lower extremity US for suspected PE.

In conclusion, if lower extremity US is contemplated as the initial examination in patients suspected of having PE, it should be applied only in those patients who also have DVT symptoms or risk factors. In this way, DVT detection can be optimized and the maximum number of patients eliminated from further work-up for PE. In patients who are suspected of having PE and who have no symptoms or risk factors, our data indicate that screening US is of no clinical utility, and an alternative noninvasive examination such as pulmonary CT arteriography should be contemplated. In addition, our results indicate that the diagnosis of PE is often not pursued once an initial lower extremity US examination shows normal results. Because DVT is frequently absent with documented PE, lower extremity US should not be ordered as a first-line study for PE if a normal result will terminate additional work-up.

Acknowledgment: We thank Bernard Ransil, MD, for statistical evaluation of our data.

References

1. Smith LL, Iber C, Sirr S. Pulmonary embolism: confirmation with venous duplex US as adjunct to lung scanning. Radiology 1994; 91:143–147.
2. Beecham RP, Dorfman GS, Cronan JJ, Spearman MP, Murphy TP, Scola FH. Is bilateral lower extremity compression sonography useful and cost-effective in the evaluation of suspected pulmonary embolism? AJR 1993; 161:1289–1292.
3. Hull RD, Raskob GE, Ginsberg JS, et al. A noninvasive strategy for the treatment of patients with suspected pulmonary embolism. Arch Intern Med 1994; 154:289–297.
4. Oudkerk M, vanBeek EJ, vanPutten WL, Buller HR. Cost-effectiveness analysis of various strategies in the diagnostic management of pulmonary embolism. Arch Intern Med 1993; 153:947–954.
5. Rosen MP, Sheiman RG, Weintraub J, McArdle C. Compression sonography in patients with indeterminate or low-probability lung scans: lack of usefulness in the absence of both symptoms of deep-vein thrombosis and thromboembolic risk factors. AJR 1996; 166:285–289.
6. Eze AR, Comerota AJ, Kerr RP, Harada RN, Domeracki F. Is venous duplex imaging an appropriate initial screening test for patients with suspected pulmonary embolism? Ann Vasc Surg 1996; 10:220–223.
7. Matteson B, Langsfeld M, Schermer C, Johnson W, Weinstein E. Role of venous duplex scanning in patients with suspected pulmonary embolism. J Vasc Surg 1996; 24:768–773.
8. van Rossum AB, Pattynama PMT, Ton ERTA, et al. Pulmonary embolism: validation of spiral CT angiography in 149 patients. Radiology 1996; 201:467–470.
9. Remy-Jardin M, Remy J, Deschildre F, et al. Diagnosis of pulmonary embolism with spiral CT: comparison with pulmonary angiography and scintigraphy. Radiology 1996; 200:699–706.
10. van Erkel AR, van Rossum AB, Bloem JL, Kievit J, Pattynama PMT. Spiral CT angiography for suspected pulmonary embolism: a cost-effectiveness analysis. Radiology 1996; 201:29–36.
11. Goodman LR, Lipchik RJ. Diagnosis of acute pulmonary embolism: time for a new approach. Radiology 1996; 199: 25–27.
12. Bendick PJ, Catto S, Cornelius P, Burr MO, Ryan R, Glover JL. Outcome of duplex ultrasound testing for DVT relative to referral source. J Vasc Tech 1994; 18:5–8.
13. Lipski DA, Shepard AD, McCarthy BD, Ernst CB. Noninvasive venous testing in the diagnosis of pulmonary embolism: the impact on decision making. J Vasc Surg 1997; 26:757–763.
14. Goldhaber SZ. Pulmonary embolism. N Engl J Med 1998; 339:93–104.
15. Killewich LA, Nunnelee JD, Auer AI. Value of lower extremity venous duplex examination in the diagnosis of pulmonary embolism. J Vasc Surg 1993; 17:934–938.
16. Cronan JJ. Venous thromboembolic disease: the role of US. Radiology 1993; 186:619–630.
17. The PIOPED Investigators. Value of the ventilation/perfusion scan in acute pulmonary embolism: results of the prospective investigation of pulmonary embolism diagnosis (PIOPED). JAMA 1990; 263: 2753–2759.
18. Sheiman RG, McArdle CR. Bilateral lower extremity US in the patient with unilateral symptoms of deep venous thrombosis: assessment of need. Radiology 1995; 194:171–173.
19. Sheiman RG, Weintraub JL, McArdle CR. Bilateral lower extremity US in the patient with bilateral symptoms of deep venous thrombosis: assessment of need. Radiology 1995; 196:379–381.

Stenosis of the Main Artery Supplying an Organ: Effect of End-Organ Vascular Resistance on the Poststenotic Peak Systolic Velocity in an in Vitro Hydraulic Model at Doppler US[1]

Ronald O. Bude, MD
Ronald G. Larson, PhD
Wilmer W. Nichols, PhD
Jonathan M. Rubin, MD, PhD

Index terms:
Blood, flow dynamics, 961.72
Renal arteries, flow dynamics, 961.72
Renal arteries, stenosis or obstruction, 961.72
Renal arteries, US, 961.12983, 961.12984
Test objects, 961.12983, 961.12984, 961.72

Radiology 1999; 212:79–87

Abbreviations:
PSV = peak systolic velocity
RI = resistive index

[1] From the Department of Radiology, TC 2910K, University of Michigan Medical Center, 1500 E Medical Center Dr, Ann Arbor, MI 48109-0326 (R.O.B., J.M.R.); the Department of Chemical Engineering, University of Michigan, Ann Arbor (R.G.L.); and the Division of Cardiology, Department of Medicine, University of Florida, College of Medicine, Gainesville (W.W.N.).
Received June 3, 1998; revision requested July 15; revision received August 25; accepted November 25.
Address reprint requests to R.O.B. (e-mail: *ronbude@umich.edu*).

Author contributions:
Guarantor of integrity of entire study, R.O.B.; study concepts, R.O.B., R.G.L., W.W.N.; study design, R.O.B.; definition of intellectual content, R.O.B., J.M.R.; literature research, R.O.B.; experimental studies, R.O.B.; data acquisition, R.O.B.; data analysis, R.O.B., J.M.R.; manuscript preparation, R.O.B.; manuscript editing, R.O.B., J.M.R., W.W.N.; manuscript review, all authors.

PURPOSE: To test the hypothesis that increased end-organ vascular resistance reduces blood flow to the kidney, thus reducing the mean velocity in the renal artery and secondarily lowering the peak systolic velocity (PSV).

MATERIALS AND METHODS: An in vitro hydraulic model with a pulsatile pump, blood-mimicking fluid, interchangeable stenoses, and variable compliance and resistance was used to investigate the relationship between end-organ vascular resistance and poststenotic PSV.

RESULTS: Poststenotic PSV was mildly dependent on end-organ vascular resistance and decreased with increasing resistance.

CONCLUSION: The results help explain some of the reported variability from using poststenotic PSV to detect hemodynamically significant renal arterial stenoses, but the effect is not great enough to completely explain the variability. Other factors not investigated in this study must be at work as well.

Variable results have been reported for the detection of hemodynamically significant renal arterial stenosis through evaluation of the poststenotic peak systolic velocity (PSV) (1–19), with sensitivities ranging from 0% (2) to 98% (11). We postulated that renal end-organ vascular resistance might be responsible for some of this variability by causing the poststenotic PSV to decrease as increasing end-organ resistance reduces the blood flow to the kidney, thus reducing the mean velocity in the renal artery.

If this postulate is true, since renal vascular resistance varies from individual to individual (especially in those with renal disease), depending on the end-organ resistances, stenoses of the same geometric severity might produce different PSVs in different individuals. An in vitro hydraulic model was developed, and experiments were performed to evaluate the effect of end-organ vascular resistance on the poststenotic PSV.

MATERIALS AND METHODS

Hydraulic Model

The model (Fig 1) was constructed to study the effect of end-organ vascular resistance on the poststenotic PSV of a stenotic artery that supplies an organ, such as the kidney. A pulsatile pump supplied flow through a single tube that branched, which represented the descending aorta; one branch simulated blood flow to the kidney, and the other branch simulated blood flow to the rest of the body. (These components are referred to as "aorta," "renal" or "kidney," and "body" for clarity and brevity, although we acknowledge this is an in vitro and not an in vivo study.)

This setup allowed the flow to be diverted from the kidney to the rest of the body as end-organ vascular resistance increased, as this happens in vivo. Four experimental trials were performed; two were performed with a low-grade stenosis, and two were performed with a high-grade stenosis (discussed later) that was inserted into the renal branch.

For each stenosis, PSVs were obtained immediately downstream of the stenosis with end-organ resistances that ranged from "normal" to infinite (complete occlusion of the distal artery) and with two degrees of distal vascular compliance (vascular compliance downstream of the stenosis; described later): compliance that simulated normal in vivo compliance and compliance lower than the compliance that is possible in vivo (referred to as very low compliance).

Pump and pump output tubing.—A constant-volume pump (model 1421; Harvard Apparatus, Holliston, Mass) supplied pulsatile flow through a single $\frac{3}{8}$-inch (9.53-mm)–inside diameter, $\frac{9}{16}$-inch (1.43-cm)–outside diameter vinyl tube at fixed settings throughout the experiment: 60 strokes per minute; 10 mL per stroke; with a duty cycle, or systolic fraction of the cardiac cycle, of 0.3.

Because the pump output was very pulsatile without diastolic flow, the fluid-flow analogue of a resistive-capacitive circuit (20) was installed immediately downstream of the pump to modify the pump output waveform. By moving the clamps up or down the tubing to adjust the position and by tightening or loosening the clamp to adjust the degree of the stenoses on the two parallel lengths of gum rubber tubing ($\frac{5}{16}$-inch [7.94-mm] inner diameter, $\frac{7}{16}$-inch [1.11-cm] outer diameter; 24 and 45 cm long) (Fig 1) that composed this network, it was possible to produce diastolic flow in the renal arterial waveform, so each experimental trial started with as nearly the same prestenotic renal arterial resistive index (RI) as possible (actual RIs measured 0.52 or 0.53).

Aorta, renal branch, and body branch.—After the resistive-capacitive network, the descending aorta was simulated with $\frac{1}{4}$-inch (6.35-mm)–inner diameter, $\frac{3}{8}$-inch (9.53-mm)–outer diameter vinyl tubing that bifurcated into the body branch (and that was entirely composed of the same tubing that formed the aorta) and the renal branch (discussed later).

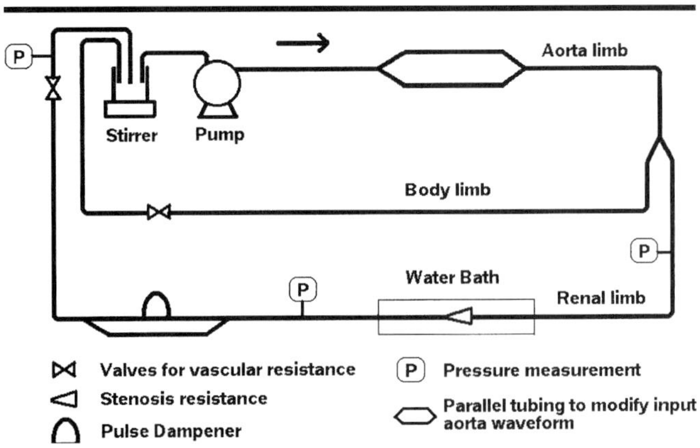

Figure 1. Schematic diagram of the experimental design.

Needle valves (catalog no. 6393-60; Cole-Parmer Instrument, Vernon Hills, Ill) near the ends of these branches simulated the total vascular resistances of the body and kidney. Initially, these valves were set so the mean pressure was as close to physiologic pressure as the model allowed (pressure ranged from 58 to 90 mm Hg for all experimental trials and increased with increasing renal end-organ resistance), and so approximately 10% of pump output flowed through the renal branch, since the normal kidney receives approximately 10% of the cardiac output (21). Renal volume flows for the four trials were as follows: for high-grade stenosis with normal compliance, 9.68% (0.70 mL/sec flow to the kidney ÷ [0.70 mL/sec flow to the kidney + 6.53 mL/sec flow to the body]); for low-grade stenosis with very low compliance, 9.92% (0.72 mL/sec ÷ [0.72 mL/sec + 6.54 mL/sec]); for low-grade stenosis with normal compliance, 9.94% (0.77 mL/sec ÷ [0.77 mL/sec + 6.98 mL/sec]); and for high-grade stenosis with very low compliance, 10.1% (0.68 mL/sec ÷ [0.68 mL/sec + 6.08 mL/sec]) (Table).

Once set at the beginning of the first trial, the valve on the body side was not readjusted throughout the remainder of the experiment. When stenoses were interchanged for a new experimental trial, the renal resistance valve was readjusted until renal flow was approximately 10% of pump output at the beginning of that trial.

The proximal renal branch, which extended from the aorta through the stenotic region, was composed of the same vinyl tubing that formed the aorta and was the branch through which Doppler ultrasonography (US) was successfully performed. The remainder of the renal branch was composed of stiff polypropylene tubing to simulate as closely as possible zero compliance in this portion; the tubing was so stiff that intraluminal signals could not be obtained because the ultrasound beam could not sufficiently penetrate the tubing. The polypropylene tubing had a $\frac{1}{4}$-inch (6.35-mm) inner diameter and a $\frac{3}{8}$-inch (9.53-mm) outer diameter, except in the following regions (discussed later): the stenoses; the compliance region (Fig 1); a 27-cm segment of vinyl tubing immediately proximal to the distal resistance valve that provided an insonation port, when necessary; and the short lengths of vinyl tubing that allowed leak-free placement of pressure monitor needles (silicone caulk prevented leakage from the vinyl tubing, but no method could be found to prevent leakage with the polypropylene tubing) and that allowed the clamps to occlude flow, when flow was diverted from the compliance region, because the polypropylene tubing was too stiff to clamp effectively (the polypropylene tubing was so stiff that it could not be perceptibly compressed by hand). The tubing was bent to fit the model by softening it in nearly boiling water and by allowing it to cool and to set in place.

Flow through the body and renal branches returned to a common reservoir that was placed on a magnetic stirrer (Magnestir; A.S. Aloe, St Louis, Mo). Renal arterial pressures upstream of the stenosis, downstream of the stenosis but upstream of the renal vascular resistance valve, and downstream of the renal vascular resistance valve were measured with pressure transducers (Transpac IV; Abbott Laboratories, Hospital Products, North Chicago, Ill) (Fig 1) that were connected to a monitor (model 78354A; Hewlett-Packard, Bad Homburg, Germany).

Experimental Data

Stenosis	Poststenotic PSV (cm/sec)	Aortic PSV (cm/sec)	Poststenotic PSV Normalized to Aortic PSV	Renal Volume Flow (%)
High-grade				
Very low compliance	633 ± 21	70.0 ± 0.8	9.04	10.1
	609 ± 11	70.1 ± 0.8	8.69	8.22
	546 ± 23	69.4 ± 1.0	7.87	6.54
	528 ± 20	69.2 ± 0.8	7.63	3.74
	473 ± 37	68.0 ± 1.4	6.96	1.59
	421 ± 24	67.6 ± 1.5	6.23	0.00
Normal compliance	599 ± 5	62.1 ± 1.0	9.65	9.68
	580 ± 11	63.0 ± 0.6	9.21	7.65
	*	62.3 ± 1.1	†	6.54
	619 ± 23	61.2 ± 1.1	10.1	3.66
	559 ± 11	63.3 ± 1.0	8.83	2.09
	552 ± 9	63.4 ± 1.1	8.71	0.00
Low-grade				
Very low compliance	62.6 ± 1.0	63.7 ± 0.9	0.98	9.92
	60.5 ± 2.3	67.4 ± 0.7	0.90	7.56
	53.4 ± 1.7	65.6 ± 0.3	0.81	5.78
	48.6 ± 1.3	59.2 ± 0.6	0.82	3.38
	35.0 ± 2.4	63.6 ± 0.7	0.55	1.97
	35.6 ± 3.2	63.0 ± 1.3	0.57	0.00
Normal compliance	93.0 ± 2.4	56.8 ± 0.5	1.64	9.94
	77.0 ± 1.9	54.7 ± 0.4	1.41	7.40
	72.2 ± 1.2	53.4 ± 1.3	1.35	6.30
	60.0 ± 1.6	53.9 ± 0.6	1.11	3.78
	55.1 ± 2.1	53.1‡	1.04	1.80
	51.8 ± 1.3	52.3 ± 0.8	0.99	0.00

Note.—Decreasing renal volume flow percentages indicate increasing vascular resistances. Data are the mean ± SD.

* This value was inadvertently not obtained.

† Could not be calculated because poststenotic PSV was not obtained.

‡ This value also was inadvertently not obtained. Since the aortic PSV did not vary much in this run, the value listed is an interpolation between adjacent aortic PSV values.

Interchangeable renal arterial stenoses.—Two renal arterial stenoses were made with 23-mm-long segments of copper tubing with 0.7- and 2.5-mm inner diameters, which produced 61% diameter ([6.35 mm − 2.5 mm]/6.35 mm) and 89% diameter ([6.35 mm − 0.7 mm]/6.35 mm) stenoses in the ¼-inch (6.35-mm)–inner diameter vinyl tubing. These stenoses were glued into centrally drilled holes in 2-cm lengths of 5⁄16-inch (7.94-mm)-diameter wooden dowel, which was carefully painted to preclude water absorption or exudation, so that the tubing edges extended from the cut surfaces of the dowel plugs approximately 1.5 mm on each side.

Spectral Doppler US was performed immediately distal to the copper-tubing edges, which could be clearly seen at US. Color or power Doppler US of the poststenotic jet was performed to correctly determine the insonation angle. The 5⁄16-inch (7.94-mm)–outer diameter wooden dowel segments slid into the ¼-inch (6.35-mm)–inner diameter vinyl tubing, which facilitated stenosis interchanges, to produce a watertight fit.

At the beginning of the experiment, pressure gradients across the stenoses and across the renal resistance valve were measured to determine the relative hemodynamic significance of the stenoses. The pressure gradients across the 61% diameter stenosis and across the renal resistance valve were 6 and 53 mm Hg, respectively, which gave a ratio of the stenotic pressure gradient to the total renal arterial pressure gradient of 10% (6 mm Hg/[6 mm Hg + 53 mm Hg]). The pressure gradients across the 89% diameter stenosis and across the renal resistance were 39 and 30 mm Hg, respectively, which gave a ratio of the stenotic pressure gradient to the total renal arterial pressure gradient of 57% (39 mm Hg/[39 mm Hg + 30 mm Hg]).

In the typical human, the mean arterial pressure is approximately 100 mm Hg (22). Therefore, a pressure gradient of 10% in the human renal artery would give a 10 mm Hg pressure gradient for our 61% diameter stenosis (10% × 100 mm Hg = 10 mm Hg), and a pressure gradient of 57% in the human renal artery would give a 57 mm Hg pressure gradient for our 89% diameter stenosis (57% × 100 mm Hg = 57 mm Hg).

In our institution, University of Michigan, Ann Arbor, a 10 mm Hg transstenotic renal arterial pressure gradient is the threshold level for angioplasty or the placement of stents, whereas a 57 mm Hg transstenotic pressure gradient is so high that it is not often encountered. On the basis of these results, we refer to these stenoses as low- and high-grade stenoses throughout this article.

Renal arterial compliance.—A pulse dampener (catalog no. 07596-20; Cole-Parmer Instrument), which is a hollow plastic container roughly the shape of a half sphere that rests on its flat surface (Fig 1), was used to provide finite compliance downstream of the stenosis, which simulated the normal compliance of the renal vasculature. Air that is introduced through a valve that is inserted into the top of this device collects at the top, while liquid flows, unmixed with air, through the base. The entrapped air compresses during systole and expands during the lower pressure of diastole, thus absorbing some of the flow pulsatility. If the quantity of air is large enough, highly pulsatile flow can be completely converted to steady, nonpulsatile flow. This device is a windkessel, which is well known in the physiology literature and which was first described by Hales near the turn of the 18th century (23).

Trial-and-error adjustment of the amount of air in the pulse dampener revealed that 1.3 mL of air for the low-grade stenosis and 3.0 cm^3 of air for the high-grade stenosis were sufficient to damp the input renal arterial RI from the initial value of 0.52 or 0.53 to 0.20, or near nonpulsatility (Fig 2). An RI of 0.20 was chosen rather than an RI of 0 because at very low RIs it is extremely difficult to measure the RI accurately and because an RI of 0.20 was so nearly nonpulsatile that it was considered adequate to simulate the degree of pulsatility damping that happens when flow progresses from the pulsatile renal arteries to the essentially nonpulsatile capillaries. Yet, the flow was still pulsatile enough to be measured and reproduced accurately.

These amounts of air were used in the pulse dampener for the normal compliance trials, since they produce approximately the same amount of pulsatility damping that occurs in vivo. For the very low compliance trials, clamps diverted flow away from the pulse dampener through polypropylene tubing (Fig 1).

Inlet lengths of tubing.—A flow perturbation (eg, bifurcation, stenosis, tight turn) transiently alters the flow profile for a variable distance, up to a maximal length known as the inlet length (24). Since the nonpulsatile laminar–flow inlet length is longer than the inlet lengths for other types of flow, it was used to ensure that the Doppler measurements were obtained in areas of stable flow. All US and pressure measurements were obtained at least one inlet length from any flow perturbation, except for the poststenotic PSV, which was obtained in the poststenotic jet at the distal orifice of the stenosis. The nonpulsatile laminar–flow inlet length is defined as follows: $L = 2kvr^2/\upsilon$, where L is the inlet length in centimeters, k is an experimentally derived constant with a value of 0.08, v is the mean velocity in centimeters per second, r is the tube radius in centimeters, and υ is the kinematic viscosity in stokes (centimeters squared per second) (24).

Blood-mimicking liquid.—The model was filled with 1,500 mL of a solution with the mean viscosity of blood (2.5 centipoise [25]) that was composed of 35 mL of glycerol and 0.67 g of microparticles (Sephadex G-50; Sigma Chemical, St Louis, Mo) as ultrasound scatterers for every 100 mL of water (26). Green food coloring tinted the fluid, so air bubbles could be seen and eliminated from the nearly opaque white tubing, since bubbles cyclically changed in volume with the cardiac cycle and caused undesirable and unmeasurable compliance.

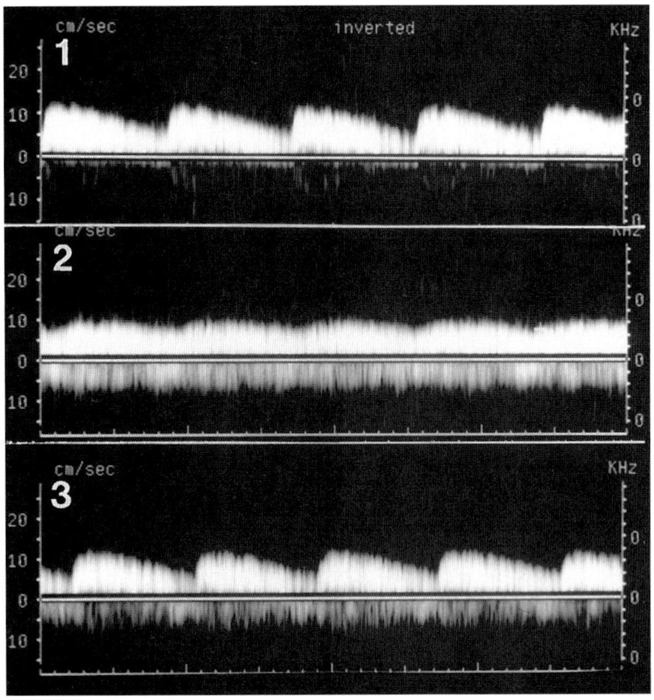

Figure 2. Waveforms used to validate normal and very low compliances used with low-grade stenosis. *1,* Input waveforms in the renal artery upstream of the stenosis, without compliance. Mean RI is 0.53 ± 0.02. *2,* Nearly nonpulsatile waveforms downstream of the stenosis, with compliance. Mean RI was 0.20, which indicates a large portion of the pulsatility was damped by the compliance. *3,* Waveforms downstream of the stenosis, with flow diverted past the compliance through a diverting tube (Fig 1). Mean RI is 0.48 ± 0.03. Very slight change in RIs between the waveforms in *1* and *3* suggests our model had very little compliance in the very low compliance mode.

Measuring Renal Vascular Resistance

The fluid-flow analogue of the Ohm law ($P = QR$, where P is the transstenotic pressure gradient, Q is the volume flow rate, and R is the resistance) was not used to calculate vascular resistance. This is because the Ohm law applies to steady flow, but it might not apply to pulsatile flow (27,28). Since the only variable altered, once the compliance and stenosis were selected during each experimental trial, was the degree of stenosis of the renal resistance valve (described in a subsequent section), renal resistance was assumed to be related to the ratio of the flow rate at increased resistance to the baseline flow rate, with this ratio decreasing with increasing renal resistance because the flow to the kidney decreased with increasing renal resistance. This is the same method used by Norris and Barnes (29) in an in vivo dog study in which they investigated the relationship between RI and vascular resistance.

Doppler US

A freestanding aluminum frame supported the US transducers (Spectra; Diasonics Vingmed Ultrasound, Santa Clara, Calif). Doppler waveforms were obtained with 5.0-MHz curvilinear transducers (Doppler frequency, 4.0 MHz) at gains at which noise first became apparent and at pulse repetition frequencies that were sufficient to prevent aliasing. Waveforms were obtained at the aorta (48° insonation angle, 2.9–4.0-kHz pulse repetition frequency, 75–105-Hz wall filter), in the renal artery proximal to the stenosis (48°–53° insonation angle, 1.4-kHz pulse repetition frequency, 35-Hz wall filter), at the distal orifice of the low-grade stenosis (43°–51° insonation angle, 2.9–6.0-kHz pulse repetition frequency, 75–160-Hz wall filter), and at the distal orifice of the high-grade stenosis (59°–70° insonation angle, 14.2–22.2-kHz pulse repetition frequency, 375–590-Hz wall filter).

Color and power Doppler US ensured accurate angle correction for spectral Doppler US in the poststenotic jet. The large insonation angles for the high-grade stenosis were needed to prevent aliasing in the very high velocity jet. Renal arterial US was performed in a water bath (wallpaper soaking tray); water-filled plastic bags (acting as interfaces between the transducer and tubing) and US gel were used for US elsewhere. A sound-absorbent material (70-durometer Sorbothane; Sorbothane, Kent, Ohio) was interposed between the tubing and its resting surfaces to reduce ultrasound reverberations.

PSVs and RIs were measured by hand using calipers, with RIs calculated according to the following formula: $RI = (S - D)/S$, where S is the height of the systolic peak and D is the height of the end-diastolic trough. All reported PSVs and RIs were means and were obtained by averaging the values for four to five consecutive waveforms (RIs) or five consecutive waveforms (PSVs). The Doppler scale that produced the largest possible waveform without aliasing was used to decrease measurement error.

Validation That the Model, Downstream of the Stenosis and without the Windkessel, Had Very Little Compliance

Vascular compliance is defined as dV/dP, where V is the volume and P is the pressure. It is a dynamic phenomenon that could not be measured in our model. Therefore, an indirect method was used to determine if our model had appreciable compliance in the very low compliance mode. Vascular compliance, in conjunction with vascular resistance, causes the progressive dampening of pulsatility that occurs as flow progresses from the highly pulsatile central arteries to the essentially nonpulsatile capillaries (30–33).

Therefore, our model, in the very low compliance mode (in the absence of the pulse dampener) can be assumed to have very low compliance, which is lower than that which can occur in vivo if the RI in the distal renal artery just proximal to the resistance valve (which, in terms of the distal RI, corresponds to the small arteriolar or capillary region) is nearly the same as the RI in the proximal renal artery during maximal flow.

Waveforms at the input and output portions of the renal segment of our model, with the low-grade stenosis in the very low compliance mode at a 10% renal volume flow, had RIs of 0.53 ± 0.02 (SD) and 0.48 ± 0.03, respectively (Fig 2), which indicated the compliance in this mode was very low, much lower than that which occurs in vivo.

Experimental Trials

Four experimental trials were performed; two trials each were performed with 61% and 89% diameter stenoses. For each stenosis, trials were performed with normal and very low compliances by varying the flow into the renal branch from a baseline of approximately 10% of pump output to complete occlusion of flow in five increments, for a total of six measurements per trial (Table). This was done by progressively tightening the distal renal resistance valve, which produced increasing renal end-organ resistances. Since the purpose of the experiment was to show the relationship of PSV to end-organ resistance, initial input flows were adjusted to be very nearly the same; they ranged from 9.68% to 10.1% (Table), but they were not adjusted until they were all exactly 10.0%.

The upstream compliance assembly was adjusted so that each trial commenced with a renal arterial RI, as measured on the monitor of the US unit, of 0.53 (which measured 0.53 for three of the trials and 0.52 for the trial with high-grade stenosis and normal compliance at subsequent measurement with hand calipers on the hard-copy images at the time of data analysis). This RI value was chosen because it is within the in vivo range and because it was the maximal value the model could achieve. PSVs immediately distal to the stenoses and in the aorta were obtained at each flow increment (Table).

Data Analysis

Since the aortic PSV varied slightly during the experiment (Table), and since this in turn affected the poststenotic PSV, all poststenotic PSVs were normalized to the aortic PSV by dividing the poststenotic PSV by the aortic PSV to alleviate this effect. Normalized poststenotic PSVs were plotted against the renal flow percentage for each trial (Fig 3).

RESULTS

The data for the four experimental trials are presented in the Table and in Figures 3–5. Note that the poststenotic PSV decreased with increasing end-organ vascular resistance for both stenoses, with both normal and very low vascular compliances. Poststenotic waveforms for the high-grade stenosis are shown in Figures 4 and 5.

From the linear regressions, we determined that the calculated poststenotic PSVs decreased from normal renal end-organ resistance (10% volume flow through the kidney) to infinite resistance (complete occlusion of distal renal vasculature) as follows: 42% decrease ([{1.60 calculated normalized PSV − 0.93 calculated normalized PSV at infinite resistance} ÷ 1.60 calculated normalized PSV] × 100) for the low-grade stenosis and normal compliance, 44% decrease ([{1.00 − 0.56} ÷ 1.00] × 100) for the low-grade stenosis and very low compliance, 8% decrease ([{9.69 − 8.96} ÷ 9.69] × 100) for the high-grade stenosis and normal compliance, and 29% decrease ([{9.04 − 6.41} ÷ 9.04] × 100) for the high-grade stenosis and very low compliance.

For the high-grade stenosis with normal compliance, the very slight PSV decrease with increasing end-organ resistance is better depicted on the graph (Fig 3a) than in the waveform illustrations (Fig 4). The major visual alterations of the waveforms are a decrease in the width of the systolic pulse with increasing end-organ vascular resistance and a progressive loss of antegrade diastolic flow, which culminated in reversed diastolic flow at high (infinite) end-organ vascular resistance (Fig 4). A similar pattern (not illustrated) was seen with the low-grade stenosis.

For the high-grade stenosis with very low compliance, the poststenotic PSV progressively decreased with increasing end-organ vascular resistance. The progressive narrowing of the systolic pulse and the loss of antegrade diastolic flow that were noted at normal compliance were again present, but they were more pronounced (Fig 5). At infinite end-organ vascular resistance (complete occlusion of flow through the renal artery) (Fig 5, part *6*), the width of the systolic pulse was extremely narrow. Even at infinite resistance, however, with a system as noncompliant as possible (the model at very low compliance had a compliance that is much lower than that which occurs in vivo), the poststenotic PSV was still relatively preserved when compared with the marked overall change in waveform morphology that occurred. Similar results were again seen with the low-grade stenosis.

DISCUSSION

Hemodynamically significant renal arterial stenoses can be detected by measuring the jet of increased velocity that the stenosis causes. Many investigators (1–14) have evaluated the PSV of the stenotic jet for this purpose. Unfortunately, widely disparate results have been reported in the detection of hemodynamically significant stenoses; results range from 0% sensitivity and 37% specificity (2) to 98% sensitivity and 98% specificity (11).

Technical factors, such as obesity and bowel gas, preclude visualization of the renal artery. Also, accessory arteries, which may be stenotic, occur in up to approximately 20% of kidneys and are often not appreciated during US (2,3,34). These factors limit the usefulness of this technique, but they do not completely explain the discrepant results. Furthermore, a large range of PSV thresholds has been suggested for stenosis detection, with values ranging from 100 to 350 cm/sec advocated (1–14).

As renal end-organ vascular resistance increases, flow is shunted from the kidney to the aorta, thus reducing the volume of flow passing through the stenosis.

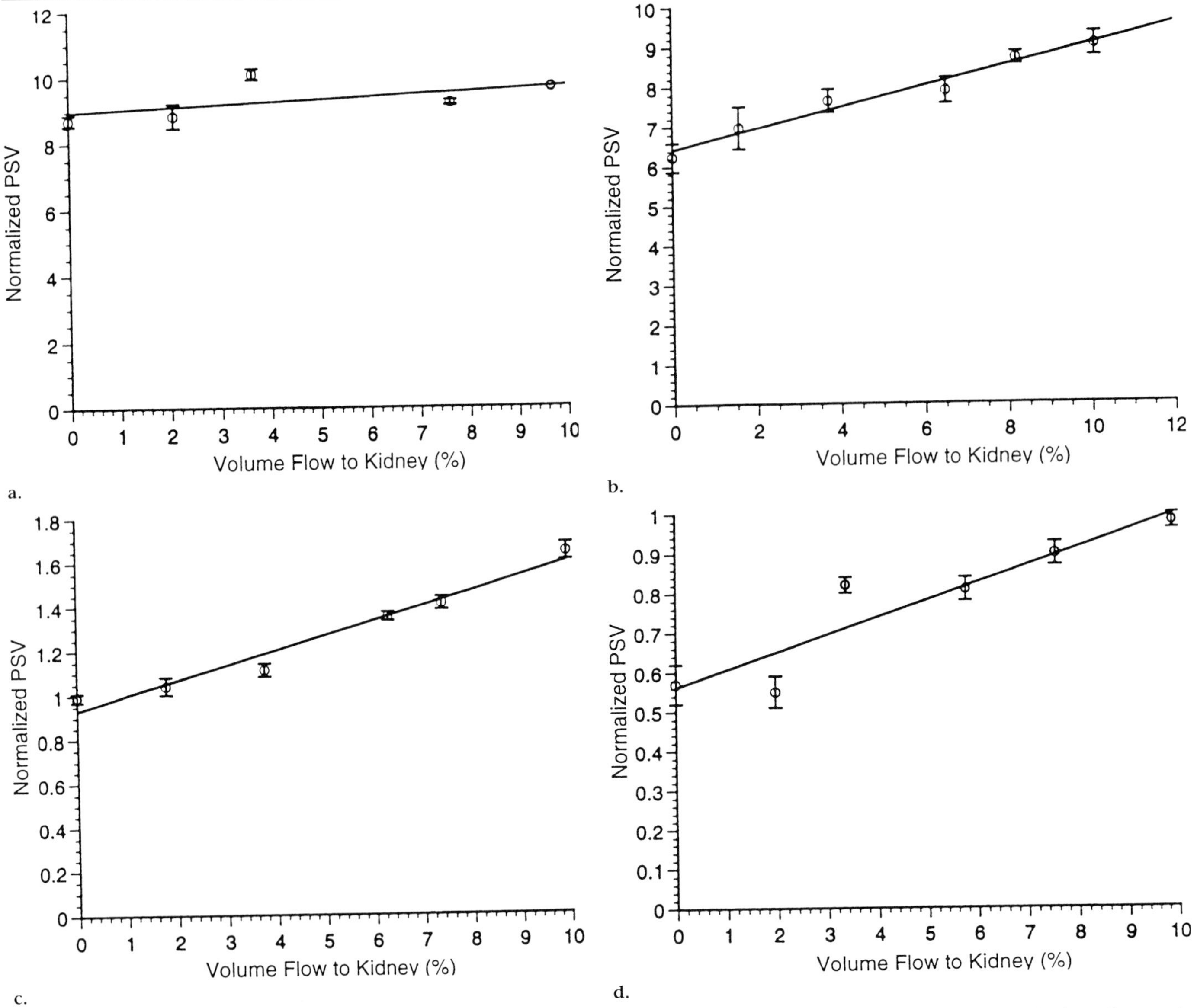

Figure 3. Normalized PSV versus volume flow percentage to the kidney for **(a)** high-grade stenosis and normal compliance, **(b)** high-grade stenosis and very low compliance, **(c)** low-grade stenosis and normal compliance, and **(d)** low-grade stenosis and very low compliance. Error bars (± 1 SD) are not visible at the highest volume flow percentage in **a** because the SD is very small (0.08). Linear regression lines have been plotted. PSV decreases mildly with increasing vascular resistance for all four modes of the experiment.

We believed this reduced flow might decrease the stenotic PSV and might help explain the variable thresholds that have been reported. Since end-organ renal vascular resistance varies from individual to individual due to physiologic variation and renal disease, stenoses of the same degree of hemodynamic severity might, therefore, produce different PSVs in different individuals, if our hypothesis is correct.

To test this hypothesis in vitro, we studied the effect of varying the renal resistance from normal to infinite. We did this using two values of vascular compliance, normal and very low, which span a range of compliances that are greater than that possible in vivo. We did this not to completely study the effect of compliance, but to determine if compliance substantially modifies the effect of end-organ vascular resistance. (To study completely the effect of compliance alone, an experiment in which end-organ vascular resistance is held constant while the compliance is varied through a large range is required.)

Our results show poststenotic PSV decreases only mildly with increasing vascular resistance distal to the stenosis for stenoses at both ends of the hemodynamic spectrum (low- and high-grade stenoses). This is true for both normal and very low vascular compliance. We found it surprising that the decrease in PSV for both stenotic grades was not much more substantial, especially at infinite end-organ vascular resistance (absence of net flow through the kidney), not only with normal compliance, but especially with very low compliance.

It is likely this occurs because the compliance (the normal ability of the artery to respond to the pressure gradient between systole and diastole by expanding

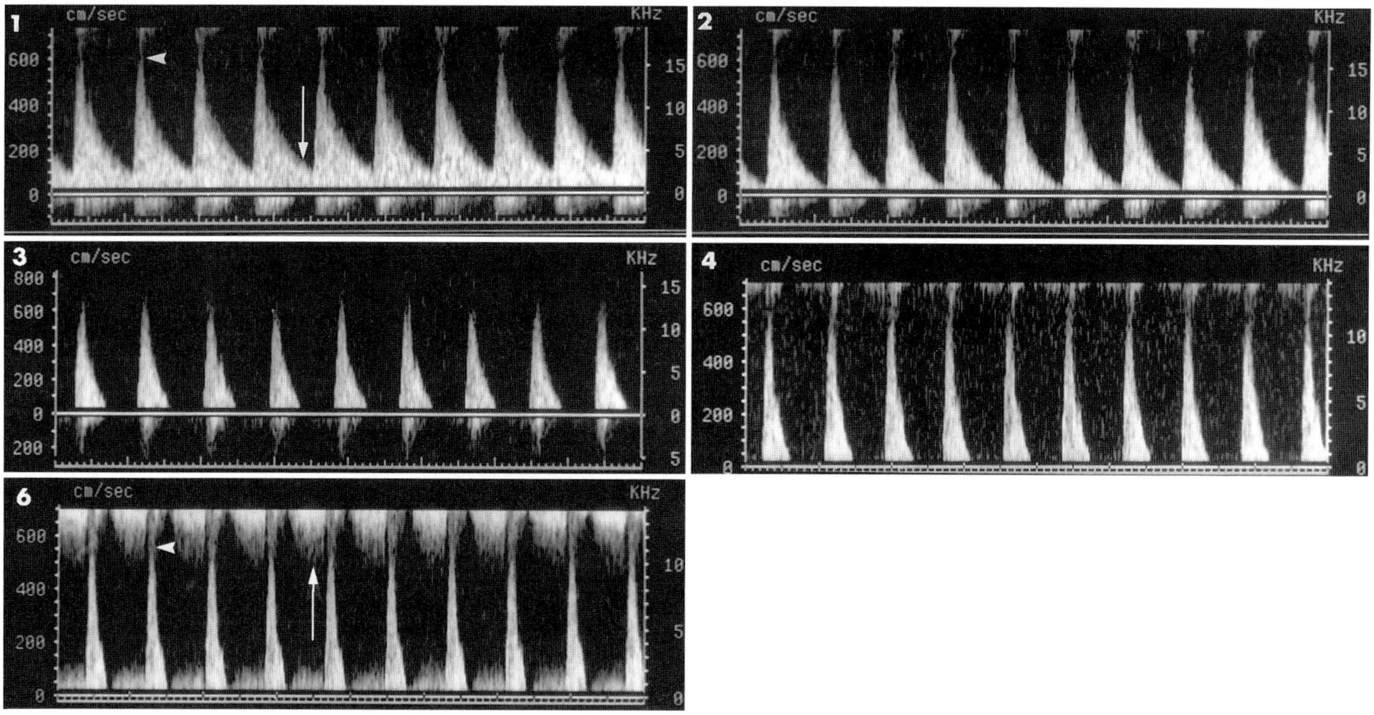

Figure 4. Sequence of poststenotic Doppler waveforms, with the high-grade stenosis and normal vascular compliance, from lowest (part *1*) to highest (part *6*) vascular resistance. The fifth set of waveforms was inadvertently not obtained due to experimental error. Note the progressive narrowing of the systolic peak (arrowhead in *1* and *6*) and the progressive loss of antegrade diastolic flow (arrow in *1* and *6*) as vascular resistance increases, with relative preservation of the PSV and with reversed diastolic flow (aliased) at complete distal vascular occlusion (part *6*). (Reversed diastolic flow is analogous to the reversed flow that occurs in vivo in renal vein thrombosis.) The amplitudes of the waveforms in *3* appear artifactually lower than those of the other waveforms owing to a larger velocity scale. In *6*, diastolic aliasing could not be eliminated, because displaying the baseline higher than the bottom of the image would result in aliasing of the systolic peak and also because the waveform scale could not be made any larger due to the insonation angle required by the stenotic jet.

in systole and by relaxing in diastole) allows the artery to accommodate enough of the systolic jet so PSV is only mildly affected, even when the compliance is much smaller than that which occurs in vivo. Rather than substantially reducing the PSV, the main effect of increasing end-organ resistance is both progressively reducing diastolic flow and progressively narrowing the width of the systolic pulse (Fig 4). Halpern et al (35) have shown similar results regarding the PSV in vessels without proximal stenosis.

Our results also likely apply to another parameter that is used to detect hemodynamically significant stenoses and that incorporates the poststenotic PSV: the ratio of the renal arterial PSV to the aortic PSV (RAR, or its closely related variant in renal transplants, the ratio of the renal arterial PSV to the iliac arterial PSV), where RAR is stenotic PSV/aortic PSV (15–19).

Variable results have been reported for the detection of hemodynamically significant renal arterial stenoses with this parameter, as well; results range from 71% sensitivity and 91% specificity (19) to 91% sensitivity and 95% specificity (18). Our results help explain some of this variability because variations in end-organ resistance change the poststenotic PSV, but it is known experimentally that the aortic PSV is essentially independent of increases in peripheral vascular resistance in vivo (36). Thus, the ratio of the renal arterial PSV to the aortic PSV should change with changes in end-organ vascular resistance, as the PSV does.

Even though PSV is only mildly dependent on end-organ vascular resistance, the dependence is still important. Consider a stenosis at the threshold of hemodynamic significance (10 mm Hg pressure gradient in vivo), as modeled by our low-grade stenosis. At normal compliance in our model, a vascular resistance high enough to decrease the volume of blood flowing to the kidney by 50% (reduction from 10% to 5% volume flow) decreases the normalized PSV from 1.60 to 1.27 (Fig 3c), a decrease of 21%.

If a velocity threshold of 100 cm/sec is used for stenosis detection at normal compliance, any stenosis that produces a PSV of up to 127 cm/sec at normal end-organ resistance produces a PSV of less than 100 cm/sec at the higher resistance (127 cm/sec × [100% − 21%] = 100 cm/sec). Therefore, in our model, any stenosis at normal renal resistance that gives a PSV in the 100–127 cm/sec range will give a spuriously normal PSV at the higher resistance.

These results may, therefore, help to explain some of the false-negative results that occur from using PSV to detect hemodynamically significant stenoses. They do not, however, provide a complete explanation, since the reported PSV thresholds for detecting hemodynamically significant stenoses vary substantially more than this (eg, 100–350 cm/sec). Other factors not investigated in our study must be at work, as well.

Although end-organ vascular resistance exerts much the same effect on high-grade and low-grade stenoses, the effect on a high-grade stenosis is inconsequential. This is because in vivo, a high-grade stenosis often has a very high PSV that far exceeds the threshold for stenosis detection. Even if this PSV is lowered by the maximal amount demonstrated in our

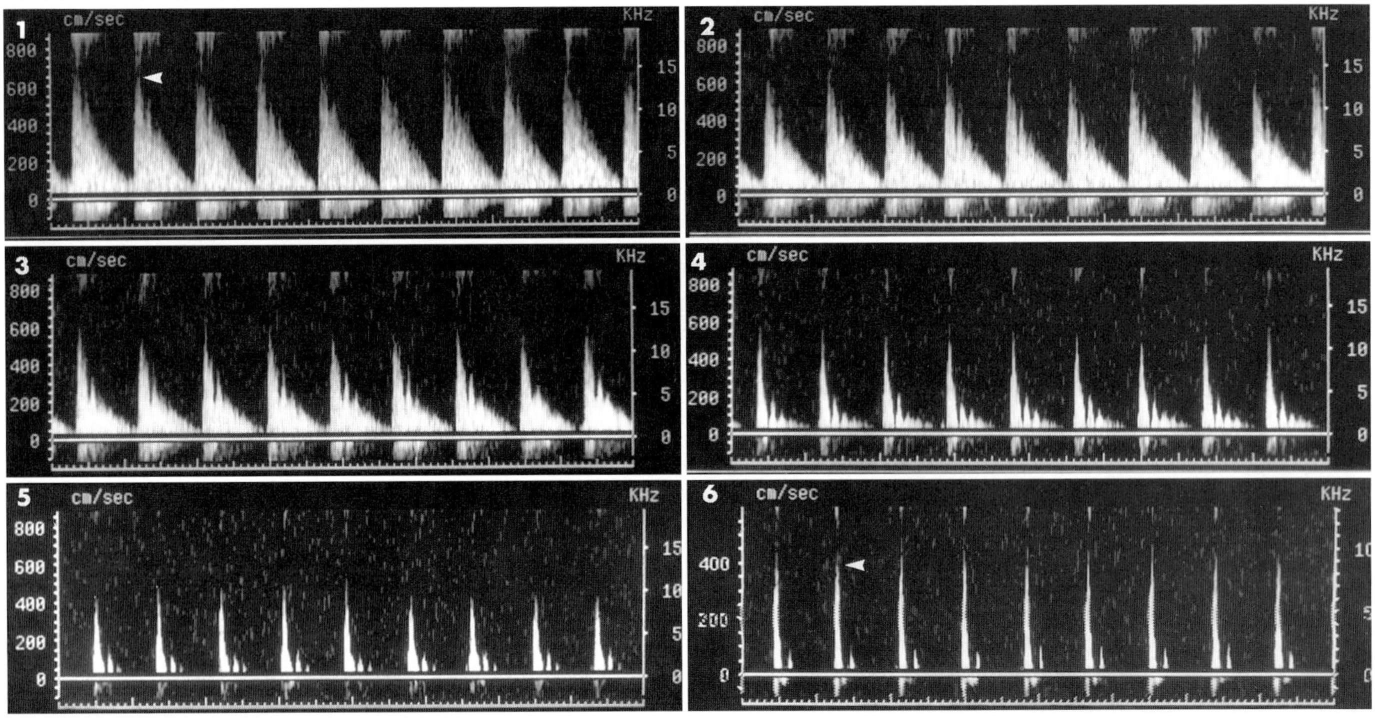

Figure 5. Sequence of poststenotic Doppler waveforms, with the high-grade stenosis and very low vascular compliance, from lowest (part *1*) to highest (part *6*) vascular resistance. Note the waveforms in *6* have a smaller velocity scale than that of the other waveforms. PSV (arrowhead in *1* and *6*) of the waveforms in *6* was the lowest of the series. (Retrograde diastolic flow is not depicted at infinite resistance probably because the flow entering the nearly noncompliant vessel during systole is so small that retrograde diastolic flow is lost in the wall filter.)

experiment (a resistance increase from normal to infinite), it is reduced by only 8% at normal compliance and by 29% at very low compliance (see Results) and should still exceed the PSV threshold and not escape detection on that basis alone.

Another feature of the waveforms in our experiment needs to be addressed: the small component of reversed flow during systole in many of the waveforms (Figs 4, 5). The cause is uncertain, but it may be related to the following. The Doppler sample gate included the entire width of the systolic jet, as determined with color Doppler US. Since blooming causes overestimation of vessel size at color Doppler US, the sample volume probably included areas of fluid adjacent to but not actually in the jet. Since eddy currents occur at substantial flow boundaries, it is possible that the eddy currents adjacent to the jet were included in the Doppler sample volume and caused the low-amplitude reversed systolic flow.

A limitation of our model is it only mimics in vivo conditions. It does not simulate the autoregulatory ability of the kidney. However, autoregulation changes renal vascular resistance, and even if a kidney autoregulates, the relationship we have shown between PSV and end-organ resistance still applies.

Practical application: A greater understanding of the effect of end-organ resistance on the stenotic PSV may enable future studies in which end-organ resistance is taken into account to better use the PSV to detect hemodynamically significant stenoses. The effect of end-organ resistance also helps explain the morphology of the stenotic jet Doppler waveform.

Acknowledgments: The authors acknowledge the help of the two research assistants in this project, Lois Otte Bude, BS, and Doris Otte Tomlin, BS. Without their assistance, this project could not have been completed.

References

1. Avasthi PS, Voyles WF, Greene ER. Noninvasive diagnosis of renal artery stenosis by echo-Doppler velocimetry. Kidney Int 1984; 25:824–829.
2. Berland LL, Koslin DB, Routh WD, Keller FS. Renal artery stenosis: prospective evaluation of diagnosis with color duplex US compared with angiography—work in progress. Radiology 1990; 174:421–423.
3. Desberg AL, Paushter DM, Lammert GK, et al. Renal artery stenosis: evaluation with color Doppler flow imaging. Radiology 1990; 177:749–753.
4. Duda SH, Erley CM, Wakat JP, et al. Posttransplant renal artery stenosis: outpatient intraarterial DSA versus color aided duplex Doppler sonography. Eur J Radiol 1993; 16:95–101.
5. Kliewer MA, Tupler RH, Carroll BA, et al. Renal artery stenosis: analysis of Doppler waveform parameters and tardus-parvus pattern. Radiology 1993; 189:779–787.
6. Saarinen O, Salmela K, Edgren J. Doppler ultrasound in the diagnosis of renal transplant artery stenosis: value of resistive index. Acta Radiol 1994; 35:586–589.
7. Baxter GM, Ireland H, Moss JG, et al. Colour Doppler ultrasound in renal transplant artery stenosis: which Doppler index? Clin Radiol 1995; 50:618–622.
8. Gottlieb RH, Lieberman JL, Pabico RC, Waldman DL. Diagnosis of renal artery stenosis in transplanted kidneys: value of Doppler waveform analysis of the intrarenal arteries. AJR 1995; 165:1441–1446.
9. Hélénon O, El Rody F, Correas JM, et al. Color Doppler US of renovascular disease in native kidneys. RadioGraphics 1995; 15:833–854.
10. Hoffmann U, Edwards JM, Carter S, et al. Role of duplex scanning for the detection of atherosclerotic renal artery disease. Kidney Int 1991; 39:1232–1239.
11. Olin JW, Piedmonte MR, Young JR, DeAnna S, Grubb M, Childs MB. The utility of duplex ultrasound scanning of the renal arteries for diagnosing significant renal artery stenosis. Ann Intern Med 1995; 122:833–838
12. Strotzer M, Fellner CM, Geissler A, et al. Noninvasive assessment of renal artery stenosis: a comparison of MR angiography, color Doppler sonography, and intraarterial angiography. Acta Radiol 1995; 36:243–247.
13. Miralles M, Cairols C, Cotillas J, Gimenez A, Santiso A. Value of Doppler parameters in the diagnosis of renal artery stenosis. J Vasc Surg 1996; 23:428–435.

14. van der Hulst VPM, van Baalen J, Kool LS, et al. Renal artery stenosis: endovascular flow wire study for validation of Doppler US. Radiology 1996; 200:165–168.
15. Merkus JW, Hoitsma AJ, van Asten WN, et al. Echo-Doppler diagnosis of renal allograft artery stenosis. Clin Transplant 1995; 9:383–389.
16. Taylor DC, Kettler MD, Moneta GL, et al. Duplex ultrasound scanning in the diagnosis of renal artery stenosis: a prospective evaluation. J Vasc Surg 1988; 7:363–369.
17. Hansen KJ, Tribble RW, Reavis SW, et al. Renal duplex sonography: evaluation of clinical utility. J Vasc Surg 1990; 12:227–236.
18. Kohler TR, Zierler RE, Martin RL, et al. Noninvasive diagnosis of renal artery stenosis by ultrasonic duplex scanning. J Vasc Surg 1986; 4:450–456.
19. Halpern EJ, Needleman L, Nack TL, East SA. Renal artery stenosis: should we study the main renal artery or segmental vessels? Radiology 1995; 195:799–804.
20. Bude RO, Rubin JM, Platt JF, Fechner KP, Adler RS. Pulsus tardus: its cause and potential limitations in detection of arterial stenosis. Radiology 1994; 190:779–784.
21. Folkow B, Neil E. General principles. In: Circulation. New York, NY: Oxford University Press, 1971; 10.
22. Nichols WW, O'Rourke MF. The nature of flow of a fluid. In: Nichols WW, O'Rourke MF, eds. McDonald's blood flow in arteries: theoretical, experimental and clinical principles. 4th ed. New York, NY: Oxford University Press, 1998; 11.
23. Nichols WW, O'Rourke MF. Introduction. In: Nichols WW, O'Rourke MF, eds. McDonald's blood flow in arteries: theoretical, experimental and clinical principles. 4th ed. New York, NY: Oxford University Press, 1998; 1.
24. Nichols WW, O'Rourke MF. The nature of flow of a fluid. In: Nichols WW, O'Rourke MF, eds. McDonald's blood flow in arteries: theoretical, experimental and clinical principles. 4th ed. New York, NY: Oxford University Press, 1998; 40–47.
25. Duck FA. Mechanical properties of tissue. In: Physical properties of tissue. San Diego, Calif: Academic Press, 1990; 161.
26. Weast RC. Handbook of chemistry and physics: a ready-reference book of chemical and physical data. 48th ed. Cleveland, Ohio: Chemical Rubber, 1967; D191–D192.
27. Gould KL. Dynamic coronary stenosis. Am J Cardiol 1980; 45:286–292.
28. Nichols WW, O'Rourke MF. The nature of flow of a fluid. In: Nichols WW, O'Rourke MF, eds. McDonald's blood flow in arteries: theoretical, experimental and clinical principles. 3rd ed. Philadelphia, Pa: Lea & Febiger, 1990; 26.
29. Norris CS, Barnes RW. Renal artery flow velocity analysis: a sensitive measure of experimental and clinical renovascular resistance. J Surg Res 1984; 36:230–236.
30. Nichols WW, O'Rourke MF. Introduction. In: Nichols WW, O'Rourke MF, eds. McDonald's blood flow in arteries: theoretical, experimental and clinical principles. 4th ed. New York, NY: Oxford University Press, 1998; 3.
31. Nichols WW, O'Rourke MF. Coupling of the left ventricle with the systemic circulation: implications to cardiac failure. In: Nichols WW, O'Rourke MF, eds. McDonald's blood flow in arteries: theoretical, experimental and clinical principles. 4th ed. New York, NY: Oxford University Press, 1998; 295–296.
32. McDonald DA, Taylor MG. The hydrodynamics of the arterial circulation. Prog Biophys Chem 1959; 9:107–173.
33. Halpern EJ, Deane CR, Needleman L, Merton DA, East SA. Normal renal artery spectral Doppler waveform: a closer look. Radiology 1995; 196:667–673.
34. Merklin RJ, Michels NA. The variant renal and suprarenal blood supply with data on the inferior phrenic, ureteral, and gonadal arteries. J Int Coll Surg 1958; 29: 41–76.
35. Halpern EJ, Merton DA, Forsberg F. Effect of distal resistance on Doppler US flow patterns. Radiology 1998; 206:761–766.
36. Westerhof N, Sipkema P, Bos GC, van den Elzinga Z. Forward and backward waves in the arterial system. Cardiovasc Res 1972; 6:648–656.

Joon Beom Seo, MD[2]
Jung-Gi Im, MD
Woo Sun Kim, MD
Chang Kyu Seong, MD
Jae Woo Song, MD
Jin Haeng Chung, MD[3]

Shark Liver Oil–induced Lipoid Pneumonia in Pigs: Correlation of Thin-Section CT and Histopathologic Findings[1]

Index terms:
Computed tomography (CT), experimental, 60.12111, 60.12118
Computed tomography (CT), thin-section, 60.12118
Lung, CT, 60.12111, 60.12118
Lung, diseases, 60.214, 60.253
Pneumonitis, aspiration, 60.214

Radiology 1999; 212:88–96

[1] From the Department of Radiology and Institute of Radiation Medicine (J.B.S., J.G.I., W.S.K., C.K.S.), and Department of Pathology (J.H.C.), Seoul National University College of Medicine, 28 Yongon-dong, Chongno-gu, Seoul 110-744, South Korea; and Department of Radiology, Seoul City Boramae Hospital, Seoul (J.W.S.). Received May 27, 1998; revision requested July 16; final revision received November 2; accepted February 12, 1999. **Address reprint requests to** J.G.I. (e-mail: *imjg@radcom.snu.ac.kr*).

[2] Current address: Department of Radiology, Gachon Medical College, Gil Medical Center, Inchon, Korea.

[3] Current address: Department of Pathology, Korea Cancer Center Hospital, Seoul.

PURPOSE: To evaluate sequential changes in thin-section computed tomographic (CT) findings after inducement of lipoid pneumonia and provide the histopathologic bases of these findings.

MATERIALS AND METHODS: Shark liver oil was administered to 12 sites in seven pigs. Thin-section CT scans were obtained within 1 hour and at 1 week, 2 weeks, 4 weeks, 8 weeks, 12 weeks, and 16 weeks after oil administration. Scans were assessed for opacity, distribution, location at the lobular level, extent, and volume of the lesions. The CT number in consolidation areas also was measured. Findings at CT were correlated with those in the histopathologic specimens.

RESULTS: Diffuse ground-glass opacity was noted on all immediately obtained scans. The opacity of the lesions was highest at 1 week; then it decreased gradually to an area of ground-glass opacity. The extent and volume of the lesions decreased at follow-up CT. Histopathologically, the lesions showed a lobular distribution sharply demarcated from the normal lungs. The lobules of decreased volume showed residual thickening of the alveolar walls with bronchiolectasis and mild collagen deposition of the interlobular septa. Pathologic examination of the low-attenuating consolidation area at CT revealed evidence of partial aeration.

CONCLUSION: Thin-section CT findings of lipoid pneumonia include ground-glass opacity and airspace consolidation, followed by complete or incomplete resolution with volume loss and septal thickening. Low-attenuating consolidation at CT does not always indicate the presence of fat.

Exogenous lipoid pneumonia is an uncommon condition that results from aspiration or inhalation of fatlike material. After Laughlen (1) in 1925 described exogenous lipoid pneumonia when he reported discovering oil droplets in the lungs during the autopsies of three children and one adult who had received mineral oil nose drops or oral laxatives, many clinical and experimental studies were conducted until the 1950s (2–9). Lipoid pneumonia has been encountered in patients who used mineral oils such as liquid paraffin, which is used in laxatives and nose drops (6,9–11); animal oils such as cod liver oil, which is commonly given to children (2,5); and vegetable oils such as sesame oil, which is used in medical suspensions (12,13). Several cases of lipoid pneumonia have originated from the use of traditional folk remedies (14–19). Currently, several cases of lipoid pneumonia caused by various materials are reported in the literature annually. Squalene is a lipid derived from shark liver oil. In some Asian countries, squalene is taken as a traditional folk remedy. Similar to the symptoms in most cases of oil aspiration, symptoms of shark liver oil–induced lipoid pneumonia are either absent or nonspecific, and the radiologic findings can simulate those of other diseases (16,19).

Lipoid pneumonia is difficult to diagnose because it mimics various diseases. In chest radiographic studies (8,14,20–25), various findings, from diffuse bilateral infiltration to solitary lung nodules that mimic neoplasm, have been described. Efforts were made to classify these radiographic findings and understand those that manifest as sequential

Author contributions:
Guarantors of integrity of entire study, J.G.I., J.B.S.; study concepts, J.G.I., J.B.S., W.S.K.; study design, J.G.I., J.B.S.; definition of intellectual content, J.G.I., J.B.S., W.S.K.; literature research, J.B.S.; experimental studies, J.B.S., C.K.S.; data acquisition, J.B.S., C.K.S.; data analysis, J.G.I., J.B.S., J.W.S., J.H.C.; manuscript preparation and editing, J.B.S., J.G.I.; manuscript review, J.B.S., J.G.I., W.S.K., J.H.C.

changes after aspiration (20,21,23,24), but these efforts were limited owing to the lack of pathologic correlation. Depiction of low-attenuating consolidation at CT has been suggested as a diagnostic clue in lipoid pneumonia (10,15,16,26,27).

Although lipoid pneumonia is a well-recognized entity, our literature search disclosed that reports on the radiologic-pathologic correlation of this disease are limited (20,22,28). The purpose of this study was to evaluate the sequential changes in thin-section CT findings after inducement of lipoid pneumonia with shark liver oil and provide the histopathologic bases of these findings by correlating them with histopathologic findings.

MATERIALS AND METHODS

Selection of Animals and Lipid Material

This study was approved by the animal research committee at our institution. Pigs were chosen for this study because their secondary lobules are well developed, similar to those in humans, and the size of their lungs is suitable for both handling and imaging (29). Seven 10–12-week-old Yorkshire pigs (15–20 kg) were used. Shark liver oil (Shark King Capsule; Banner Pharmacaps, Elizabeth, NJ) was selected as the lipid material because of our knowledge of its components, its convenience of preparation, and the recent increase in the number of clinical cases associated with use of this material in Korea. The capsule consists of 99.26% squalene and 0.74% vitamin E. The oil material in the capsule was aspirated with needle puncture, and 10 mL of the substance was prepared for each site.

Animal Preparation

The pigs were not allowed to eat for 6 hours before anesthesia was induced, and they were injected intramuscularly with 0.5 mg of atropine (Daehan Atropine; Daehan Pharmaceutical, Seoul, Korea) just before anesthesia. Anesthesia was induced with an intramuscular injection of 10 mg/kg ketamine hydrochloride (Ketara; Yuhan Yanhang, Seoul, Korea) and 4 mg/kg xylazine hydrochloride (Rompun; Bayer Korea, Seoul, Korea), and it was maintained with an intravenous injection of 5–10 mg/kg thiopental sodium (Pentothal; Choong Wae Pharmacy, Seoul, Korea). The animals were intubated with a 6.5-mm inside-diameter endotracheal tube after being paralyzed with an intravenous injection of 1 mg/kg succinylcholine chloride (Quelin; Abbott Laboratories, Chicago, Ill).

Administration of Shark Liver Oil

With fluoroscopic guidance, we introduced a 5.5-F balloon catheter (Selection Multi-Catheter; Clinical Supply, Hashimagun, Japan) at the level of the lower lobar bronchus by using a guide wire with the pig in a semierect prone position. The balloon was inflated to prevent spillover of oil into the trachea or contralateral lung. Five milliliters of the prepared oil was injected slowly by hand. The animals were hyperventilated with a ventilator bag (Ambu bag; Ambu, Linthicum, Md) after the balloon was deflated to promote migration of the oil into the distal airspace. After keeping the animals in a semierect prone position for 15–20 minutes, we repeated the above procedure. Thus, a total dose of 10 mL was injected per site. In the first two pigs, oil was administered to the unilateral lung to compare it with the contralateral lung. The oil was administered bilaterally in the remaining five pigs.

CT Scanning

Contiguous thick-section (ie, 5-mm collimation, 5-mm intervals, standard algorithm, through the thorax) and thin-section CT scans were obtained immediately (ie, within 1 hour) and at 1 week after the administration of oil in 12 sites in seven pigs, at 2 weeks in 10 sites in six pigs, at 4 weeks in eight sites in five pigs, at 8 weeks in six sites in four pigs, at 12 weeks in four sites in three pigs, and at 16 weeks in two sites in two pigs. The CT scans were obtained with a CT HiSpeed Advantage scanning system (GE Medical Systems, Milwaukee, Wis). Initially, thick-section CT scans were obtained for overall assessment of the lung lesions and selection of the appropriate level for thin-section CT. Thin-section CT scans were obtained at contiguous 30-mm lengths in a spiral mode with 1-mm collimation and 1-mm table speed and reconstructed at 1-mm intervals by using a high-spatial-frequency algorithm. The scanning parameters were 120 kVp, 230 mA, a 1-second rotation time, a 15–17-cm field of view, and a 512 × 512 matrix. At follow-up CT, the level of the thin-section CT scan was adjusted to that in the initial study.

All pigs were examined in the prone position. Both mediastinal window (width, 400 HU; level, 10 HU) and lung window (width, 1,500 HU; level, −700 HU) scans were obtained. All scans were obtained during suspended respiration at resting end expiration (functional residual capacity), which was induced by muscular paralysis with an intravenous injection of 1 mg/kg succinylcholine chloride, after hyperventilation with a ventilator bag, because suspended respiration at functional residual capacity was easy to maintain in animals with muscular paralysis. The animals were bred during follow-up periods. No complications such as infection or aspiration occurred. None of the pigs involved in this study died unexpectedly.

Lung Fixation, Radiography of Specimens, and Histologic Section Preparation

After all scheduled follow-up CT scans were obtained, the pigs were sacrificed by intravenously administering an excessive dose of thiopenthal sodium. The lungs were removed from the thorax, with care taken not to tear the visceral pleura. This procedure was performed within 2 hours after the final CT scans were obtained. Lung fixation and inflation was performed by using the method of Markarian and Dailey (30). A total of 12 sites of lipoid pneumonia were prepared: 1 week after oil administration, two sites from one pig were prepared; at 2 weeks, two sites from one pig; at 4 weeks, two sites from one pig; at 8 weeks, two sites from one pig; at 12 weeks, two sites from one pig; and at 16 weeks, two sites from two pigs.

Following fixation, the specimens were cut into 10-mm slices that corresponded to the section at in vivo thin-section CT, and radiographs of each specimen slice were obtained. A soft x-ray radiographic unit (Faxitron 43805N; Hewlett-Packard, Sunnyvale, Calif) and X-Omat V film (Kodak, Rochester, NY) were used to perform radiography of the specimens. Subsequently, thin 2–3-mm sections were obtained from the thick 10-mm slices, and radiographs of the specimens were obtained with technical parameters of 25 kVp, 3 mA, and 3–4-minute exposure. Six-micron-thick, 12 × 8-cm giant microscopic section slides from the selected 2–3-mm-thick sections were prepared with hematoxylin-eosin stain. Additional giant section slides from 12-week follow-up specimens were prepared with Masson trichrome stain to evaluate the deposition of collagen fibers.

Analyses of Thin-Section CT Scans

The CT scans were reviewed by three radiologists (J.G.I., J.W.S., J.B.S.). The lung window and mediastinal window images were analyzed together. Conclusions were made in consensus. The CT scans were assessed specifically for the intensity, distribution, and extent of opacification. The opacification was classified as ground-glass opacity or airspace consolidation. The distribution of the opacification was classified as either dependent or nondependent. Because the CT scans were obtained with the patient in the prone position, the anterior portion of the lung corresponded to the dependent area, and the posterior portion, to the nondependent area. The location of the lesion at the lobular level also was assessed. The opacity, extent of opacification, and volume of the affected area on follow-up CT scans were evaluated and compared with the findings in the same region on initial CT scans.

To measure the CT number in the consolidated lung, the data were transferred to an Advantage Windows workstation (GE Medical Systems, Milwaukee, Wis). The scans were magnified four times. Measurements of the consolidation area were obtained on mediastinal window images. Care was taken to avoid the air-attenuation area within the region-of-interest circles. We could measure the attenuation on all CT scans obtained 1–8 weeks after oil administration and that in five sites on the scans obtained immediately after administration, where the consolidation areas were detected. We regarded −10 HU as the threshold value of low-attenuating consolidation that was sufficient for the detection of fat on CT scans. The attenuation values of subcutaneous fat, lobar arteries, and oil in the squalene capsule also were measured for comparison.

The findings on thin-section CT scans were correlated with those on radiographs of the specimens and on giant microscopic slide specimens by two radiologists (J.G.I., J.B.S.) and one pathologist (J.H.C.) in consensus.

RESULTS

Thin-Section CT Findings

Areas of diffuse centrilobular or panlobular ground-glass opacity were seen on the CT scans obtained immediately after the administration of oil (Fig 1b). An area of low-attenuating consolidation in the dependent (anterior) portion was noted in five of 12 sites. One week after oil administration, consolidation in the dependent area was seen in all sites (Fig 1c). The degree of opacity decreased on CT scans at 2–4 weeks after the oil administration (Fig 1d). The opacity changed mostly to ground-glass opacity at 12–16 weeks after the oil administration (Table 1), with panlobular distribution in the dependent area and centrilobular distribution in the nondependent area (Fig 1). The extent of the lesions decreased with time, especially in the nondependent area. Thickening of the interlobular septa in the areas of intermediate and ground-glass opacity was observed at the 2-, 4-, and 8-week follow-up CT examinations (Table 1; Figs 1d, 2a). Smooth thickening of the interlobular septa was observed in the cleared lung on CT scans obtained 4–16 weeks after oil administration (Figs 1d, 1e, 3a). The affected lung decreased in volume gradually, with pleural retraction and crowding of the bronchovascular bundle and bronchiolectasis (Fig 1d–f).

The measured CT attenuation value of the oil in the capsule ranged from −210 to −200 HU, whereas that of the subcutaneous fat and lobar arteries ranged from −120 to −40 HU and from 0 to 40 HU, respectively. The measured CT attenuation value of the consolidated lung ranged from −150 to 50 HU (Fig 4a). In all sites, within the airspace consolidation areas, an area of low attenuation below −10 HU was identified. The attenuation value of the low-attenuating portion of the consolidated lung measured immediately after oil administration was markedly low, with a range of −150 to −120 HU. The attenuation of the consolidation was highest on the CT scans obtained 1 week after oil administration and reflective of the extensive inflammatory process involving the alveolar spaces and alveolar wall.

Correlation of Thin-Section CT with Radiography of Pathologic Specimens and Histopathology

The histopathologic findings of airspace consolidation that were visible at 1- and 2-week follow-up CT were exudate of lipid droplets, lipid-laden macrophages, and polymorphonuclear leukocytes in the alveolar space, along with thickening of the alveolar walls with cellular infiltrates (Table 2, Fig 4c). Areas of ground-glass opacity on CT scans were seen as areas of fine reticular opacity on radiographs of the specimens, which corresponded to the "washout" of alveolar space with a variable degree of residual intraalveolar exudate and the thickened alveolar wall with residual cellular infiltrates and activation of pneumonocytes (Fig 2b). Thickening of the alveolar wall decreased in severity over time (Fig 3b), which explains the gradual decrease in the intensity of the opacification on sequential CT scans.

The well-demarcated lobular opacity at CT corresponded to a lobular distribution of cellular infiltrates, whereas the centrilobular opacity in the nondependent area at CT and radiography of the specimens corresponded to peribronchiolar infiltration by inflammatory cells (Fig 5).

Thickened interlobular septa in the area of opacification corresponded to collagen fiber deposition with infiltration by lymphocytes, young fibroblasts, and histiocytes, with telangiectatic change in the capillaries of the septa (Fig 2b). The smooth thickening of the septa surrounding the normal lung during the late phase (4–16 weeks after oil administration) corresponded to dilated lymphatics and capillaries and residual cellular infiltrates (Table 2, Fig 3b). Histologic examination of specimens prepared with Masson trichrome stain revealed deposition of collagen fibers in the septa.

The decreased volume of the involved lung at CT corresponded to lobular volume loss with retraction of the overlying pleura and thickening of the interlobular septa at radiography of the specimens (Fig 6a). Histologic examination with Masson trichrome stain revealed evidence of fibrosis in the interlobular septa and pleura. There was no area of collagen fiber deposition in the alveolar wall. Areas of lobular collapse were seen on 8- and 12-week follow-up histologic specimens (Fig 6b).

The area of low attenuation on CT scans contained both fat and partly aerated alveoli at pathologic examination. However, the aeration was not seen at CT, even after magnification and modification of the window settings on the workstation.

DISCUSSION

In our study, the earliest CT finding of lipoid pneumonia was diffuse ground-glass opacity, which was prominent in the dependent area and had a centrilobular or panlobular distribution (Fig 1b). The centrilobular opacities were due to peribronchiolar airspace consolidation, which may correspond to the "acinar pattern" on radiographs previously described by Weill et al (22), who produced

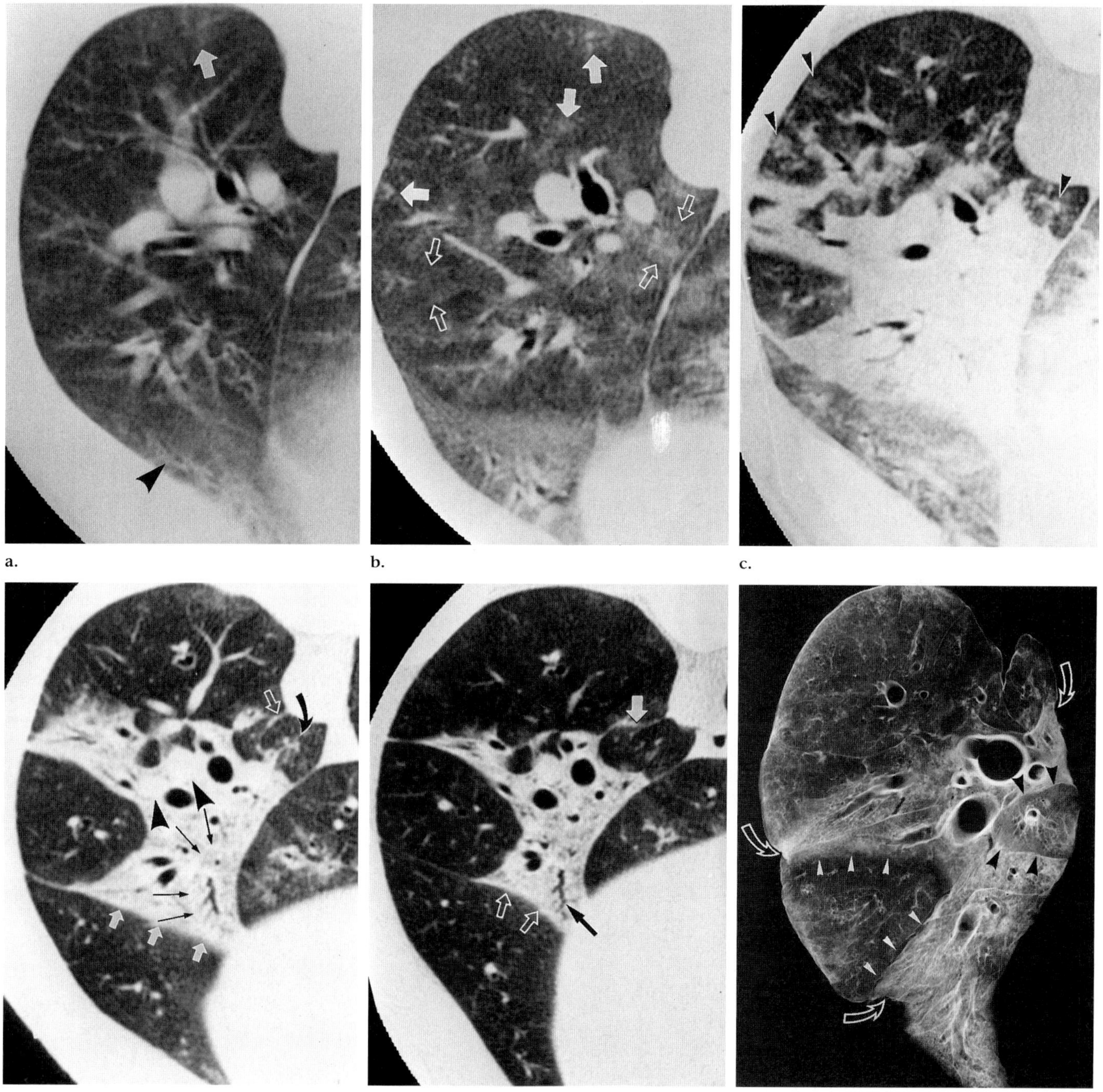

a. b. c. d. e. f.

Figure 1. Serial axial CT scans at the level of the lower lobe of the left lung in a pig in the prone position obtained **(a)** before and **(b–e)** after endobronchial administration of shark liver oil, and **(f)** radiograph of a sliced specimen obtained at the same level. **(a)** CT scan obtained with 5-mm collimation before the oil injection shows the lung is clear except for a nonspecific ill-defined opacity (arrow) in the nondependent area and a peribronchial infiltration (arrowhead) in the dependent area, into which oil was not injected. **(b)** CT scan obtained immediately after oil administration shows diffuse ground-glass opacity in the lung. The areas of opacification are distributed mainly in the dependent (anterior) portion. Note the segmental or lobular distribution of the lesions (open arrows). Areas of ill-defined centrilobular ground-glass opacity (solid arrows) are noted in the nondependent area. **(c)** CT scan obtained 1 week after oil administration shows airspace consolidation in the dependent area. Note also the areas of centrilobular lesions (arrowheads) in the nondependent area. **(d)** CT scan obtained 4 weeks after oil administration shows a decreased degree of opacity. The opacity obscures the small lobular vessels but not the larger pulmonary vessels (arrowheads). The fine linear structures in the area of opacification represent thickening of interlobular septa (thin black arrows). Note the decreased extent of centrilobular opacity with areas of residual peribronchiolar opacification (curved arrow). Smooth thickening of the interlobular septum (open arrow) between the normal lobules also is noted. Note the straightening of the interlobar fissure (solid white arrows) compared with the bulging appearance of the corresponding interlobar fissure in **b** and **c**; the change in the fissure from bulging to straight suggests volume loss in the affected lung. **(e)** CT scan obtained 12 weeks after oil administration shows further volume decrease in the affected lung. Note the crowding of bronchovascular bundles within the lesion and the retraction of the interlobar fissure (open arrows). The attenuation of the lesion has decreased. The bronchiole (black arrow) in the area of opacification is irregular and slightly dilated. Smooth thickening of an interlobular septum (white arrow) is still seen. **(f)** Contact radiograph of the resected and sliced lung at a level similar to that in **e** shows retraction of the lung surface (curved arrows), which represents a volume decrease caused by lipoid pneumonia. Compared with the size of the adjacent normal lobule (white arrowheads), that of the affected lobule (black arrowheads) is markedly smaller.

the "rosette and stippled" patterns of lipoid pneumonia by using intrabronchial instillation of mineral oil in anesthetized dogs and in clinical cases.

The airspace consolidation on CT scans at 1 week was due to the filling of the alveolar space with exudate and inflammatory cells, which is associated with thickening of the alveolar wall (Fig 4c). The degree of opacification decreased on 2- and 4-week follow-up studies and changed to ground-glass opacity. Histologically, a marked decrease in the extent of intraalveolar lipid droplets, lipid-laden macrophages, and inflammatory cells was noted. These changes were considered to be due to expectoration of lipid droplets and inflammatory cells and drainage through the lymphatic vessels.

The thickening of interlobular septa in the opacified area of the lungs in our study was mainly due to cellular infiltrates (Fig 2b). The smooth septal thickening surrounding the resolved lung on 4-week or later follow-up CT scans (Fig 3a) was due to ectatic changes in the lymphatics and capillaries, with residual cellular infiltrates and fibrosis (Fig 3b). We suggest that this finding may reflect lymphostasis induced by increased absorption of lipid droplets or lipid-laden macrophages, because the lymphatic channels are believed to be the route of clearance of exudates accumulated in the alveolar and interstitial spaces (2,3,6,7,31). Another possible theory is the proximal obstruction of lymphatics by large lipid droplets. Brody and Levin (28) reported interlobular septal thickening that manifested as Kerley B lines on the chest radiographs obtained in four patients with pathologically confirmed lipoid pneumonia.

The combination of ground-glass opacity and thickened interlobular septa can mimic alveolar proteinosis, which is a form of endogenous lipoid pneumonia (Fig 2a) (32). Recently, Lee et al (33) and Franquet et al (34) reported the crazy-paving pattern at CT in patients with exogenous lipoid pneumonia. In our experimental study, the partial filling of alveolar space with intraalveolar exudate, thickening of the alveolar wall with cellular infiltrates, and activation of pneumonocytes, combined with the thickening of interlobular septa with dilatation of the lymphatics, cellular infiltrates, and a varied degree of fibrosis were the histopathologic bases of the crazy-paving pattern at CT (Fig 2b).

The decreased volume of the affected lung on CT scans during the later stage (ie, 14–16 weeks after oil administration)

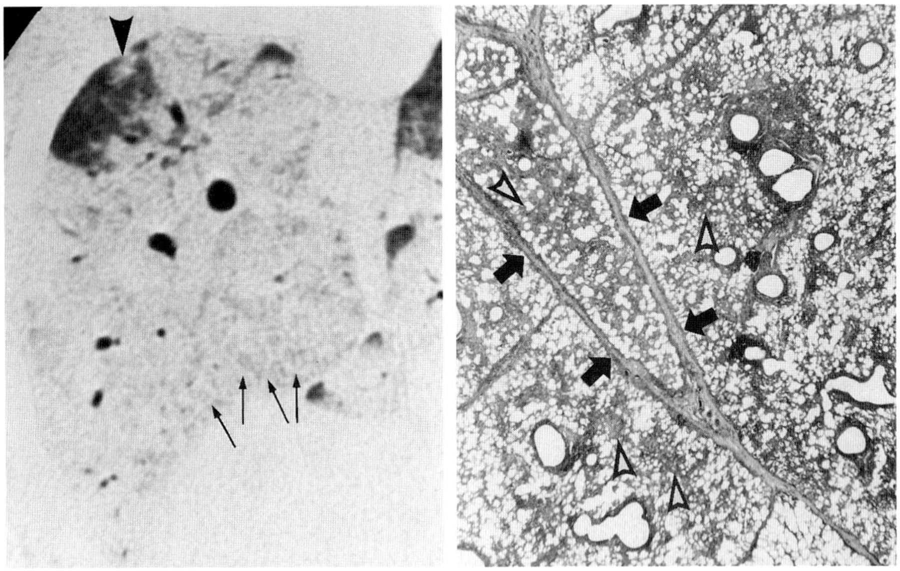

a. b.

Figure 2. Histopathologic bases of thickening of interlobular septa at CT in the early phase (2–8 weeks after oil administration) of lipoid pneumonia in a pig. **(a)** Axial CT scan at the level of the lower lobe of the left lung obtained 2 weeks after oil administration shows airspace consolidation. Note the areas of faint linear opacification (arrows) in the consolidated lung. Ill-defined centrilobular opacity (arrowhead) is seen in the nondependent area. **(b)** Corresponding photomicrograph demonstrates thickened interlobular septa (arrows) with cellular infiltrates of lymphocytes, histiocytes, and young fibroblasts, and telangiectatic change in the capillaries. Note the alveolar wall thickening and the inflammatory exudate filling the alveolar spaces (arrowheads). (Hematoxylin-eosin stain; original magnification, ×10.)

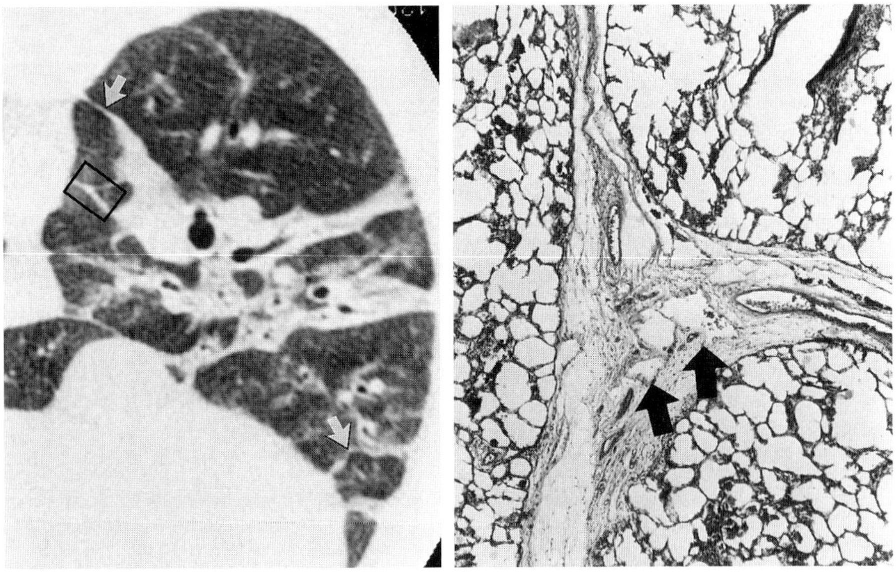

a. b.

Figure 3. Histopathologic bases of interlobular septa seen on CT scans in the later phase (4–16 weeks) of lipoid pneumonia in a pig. **(a)** Axial CT scan at the level of the lower lobe of the right lung obtained 8 weeks after endobronchial administration of shark liver oil shows smooth thickening of the interlobular septa (boxed area and arrows) in the aerated portion of the lung. Also note the lobular airspace consolidation with volume loss. **(b)** Photomicrograph of a resected specimen from the boxed area in **a** demonstrates widening of the interlobular septum with ectatic lymphatic channels and capillaries (arrows); there are residual cellular infiltrates in the septum. (Hematoxylin-eosin stain; original magnification, ×40.) The residual thickening of the alveolar walls explains the ground-glass opacity seen at CT (boxed area in **a**). Photomicrograph of the specimen prepared with Masson stain (not shown) showed wavy, green-stained linear structures in the septa, which confirmed collagen fibers.

TABLE 1
Changes in Thin-Section CT Findings after Endobronchial Administration of Shark Liver Oil

CT Finding	Time of Examination after Oil Administration (wk)*						
	Immediately	1	2	4	8	12	16
Opacification pattern†							
Ground-glass opacity	++++	+	+	++	++	++++	++++
Airspace consolidation	+	+++	+++	+++	+++	–	–
Distribution in lobular unit†							
Panlobular	++	+++	+++	++++	++++	++++	++++
Centrilobular	+++	++	++	+	+	–	–
Random	–	+	+	–	–	–	–
Changes over time‡							
Opacity	NA	↑↑	↓↓	↓	→, ↓	↓	↓
Extent	NA	↓, ↓↓	↓	↓	→, ↓	→, ↓	↓
Volume	NA	→	→, ↓	↓	→, ↓	→, ↓	→, ↓
Septal thickening							
In area of opacification	NA	–	○	○	○	–	–
In cleared lung	NA	–	–	○	○	○	○

Note.—NA = not applicable, – = not seen, ○ = seen.

* CT scans were obtained immediately and 1 week after the administration of shark liver oil in 12 sites in seven pigs, 2 weeks after oil administration in 10 sites in six pigs, 4 weeks after oil administration in eight sites in five pigs, 8 weeks after oil administration in six sites in four pigs, 12 weeks after oil administration in four sites in three pigs, and 16 weeks after oil administration in two sites in two pigs.

† Extent of lesion. + = small lesion occupying less than 10% of area of opacification, ++ = lesion occupying more than 10% but less than 50% of area of opacification, +++ = lesion occupying more than 50% but less than 90% of area of opacification, ++++ = large lesion occupying more than 90% of area of opacification.

†† Sequential changes in lesion opacity, extent, and volume compared with these lesion characteristics on previously obtained CT scans. ↓ = mild decrease (≤25%) in lesion opacity, extent, or volume; ↓↓ = marked decrease (>25%) in lesion opacity, extent, or volume; ↑↑ = marked increase (>25%) in lesion opacity, extent, or volume; → = no change.

TABLE 2
Radiologic-Histopathologic Correlation of Shark Liver Oil–induced Lipoid Pneumonia

CT Finding	Histopathologic Finding
Consolidation	Exudate of lipid droplets, lipid-laden macrophages, and polymorphonuclear leukocytes in alveolar space along with widening of alveolar wall with cellular infiltrate
Intermediate and ground-glass opacity	Alveolar wall thickening and variable degree of residual intraalveolar exudate
Lobular opacity	Cellular infiltration that occupies entire lobule and is sharply demarcated from normal lung by interlobular septa
Centrilobular opacity	Cellular infiltration next to the bronchiole in central area of lobule
Volume decrease	Decreased size of affected lobule with residual alveolar wall thickening and mild fibrosis of septum; collapse of lobular unit with cellular infiltrate
Septal thickening in area of opacification	Thickening of interlobular septum caused by telangiectatic change in capillaries and infiltrates of histiocytes, lymphocytes, and young fibroblasts
Septal thickening in cleared lung	Widening of interlobular septa with ectatic lymphatic channels and capillaries and deposition of collagen fibers

was due to fibrosis of the interlobular septa and pleura, with residual thickening of the alveolar wall without fibrosis (Fig 3b). Another explanation for the volume decrease was lobular collapse, which was detected in 8- and 12-week follow-up specimens (Fig 6b).

In 1932, Pierson (20) performed a systematic evaluation of radiographic findings by correlating them with clinical data and performing a gross inspection of autopsy specimens. He reported that pathologic changes register on radiographs and that radiologic findings vary according to the different phases of the disease. In 1937, Ikeda (6) introduced an adult form of lipoid pneumonia that resembles chronic granulomatous pneumonitis or tumor, which is different from the acute bronchopneumonic form that occurs in children. He suggested that although the same material is aspirated, the difference in the amount of oil, the manner and duration of its administration, and the character of the local inflammatory reaction cause the discrepancy. Hampton et al (21) and Kennedy et al (24) used this concept in assessing radiologic findings.

Recently, Lee et al (33) analyzed thin-section CT findings of pathologically or clinically confirmed shark liver oil–induced lipoid pneumonia in 25 patients. Six of ten patients with a diffuse ground-glass opacity pattern at CT had a recent history of taking a large amount of squalene through the nose, whereas seven patients who had a consolidation pattern had a history of taking squalene for several months. All of the five patients who had an interstitial thickening pattern had a history of taking squalene for more than 1 year.

There are several reports on the usefulness of CT in diagnosing lipoid pneumonia by detecting areas of low attenuation that range from 140 HU to −17 HU in the consolidation or mass (10,15,16,26,27). There was wide variation in the CT numbers of the consolidated lungs in our study. The CT numbers ranged from −150 HU to 50 HU, which is a higher range of attenuation than that in the oil in the capsule (−210 to −200 HU). As Joshi and Cholankeril (27) stated earlier, and as we confirmed with histologic studies, the inflammation surrounding the oil material in the lung can account for a higher CT attenuation value. In our study, the attenuation of the consolidation was highest on CT scans obtained 1 week after oil administration, which reflected the extensive inflammatory process involving the alveolar spaces and alveolar wall. However, even on 1-week follow-up CT scans, an area of low attenuation below −10 HU was identified in the airspace consolidation in all sites.

Another point to keep in mind when regarding the low-attenuating consolidation as a sign of lipoid pneumonia is that partial volume averaging of the partly aerated alveoli can also appear as low-attenuating consolidation. To avoid this artifact, we magnified the images on the monitor four times and reviewed both the mediastinal window and lung window images when localizing the region-of-interest circles. However, pathologic review of the area of consolidation at CT

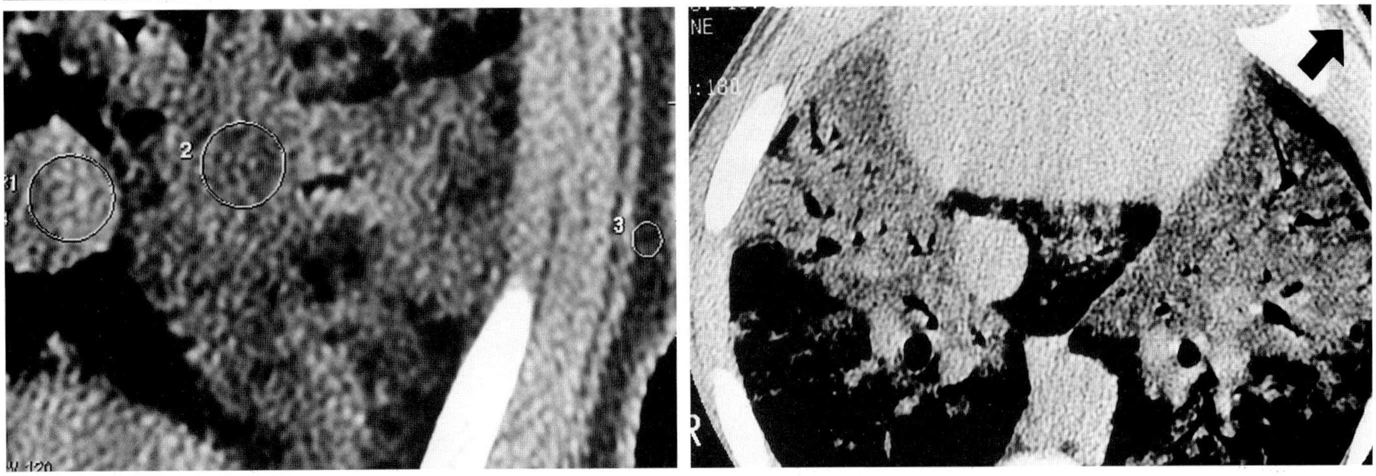

a. b.

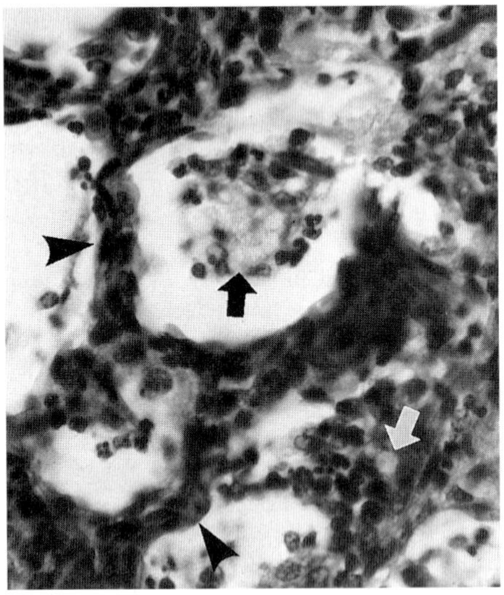

c.

Figure 4. **(a, b)** Axial CT scans and **(c)** photomicrograph of shark liver oil–induced lipoid pneumonia in the earlier phase obtained in a pig 1 week after oil administration. **(a)** The measured CT numbers of the inferior vena cava (circle 1), consolidated lung (circle 2), and subcutaneous fat (circle 3) are 26 HU, −17 HU, and −65 HU, respectively. **(b)** The attenuation of the consolidated lung in the dependent area is low (arrow), similar to that of the subcutaneous fat. The measured CT number is −85 HU. **(c)** Photomicrograph of the area in **b** shows intraalveolar lipid droplets (arrows) surrounded by numerous macrophages and polymorphonuclear lymphocytes filling most of the alveolar spaces. In this case, one can regard the low attenuation of the consolidation in **b** as fat without a CT number measurement. Note the widening of the alveolar walls (arrowheads), with infiltration by inflammatory cells. This finding explains the nature of the consolidation in **a** and **b**. (Hematoxylin-eosin stain; original magnification, ×400.)

where we measured the CT numbers showed evidence of partial aeration. We think that the measurement of attenuation for the diagnosis of lipoid pneumonia should be limited to the area of a masslike lesion in the chronic stage and to areas of compact consolidation in the earlier stage—that is, from immediately to about 1 week after aspiration of lipid materials, when most of the alveolar spaces are filled with lipid material and inflammatory exudate (Fig 4).

There have been several case reports of magnetic resonance (MR) imaging findings of lipoid pneumonia (10,35–37). In three reports (10,35,36) in which MR imaging findings of spin-echo sequences were described, both T1- and T2-weighted images displayed a high signal intensity that was equal to or slightly less than that of the subcutaneous fat. However, these signal intensity changes cannot always represent a fat component, because animal fat is more likely to produce necrotizing hemorrhagic pneumonia owing to its higher content of free fatty acid (3,5,7), and the signal intensity of blood can be high on both T1- and T2-weighted images. Recently, Cox et al (37) reported on the usefulness of chemical shift imaging in the diagnosis of lipoid pneumonia.

The degree and quality of tissue reaction to aspirated oil are quite variable and depend on the quality and frequency of aspiration, the chemical characters of the oil itself, and the effects of other substances that may be aspirated at the same time (3,5,7). In our study, the reaction of parenchyma after injection of shark liver oil was similar to those previously reported, but it was milder than the reaction after instillation of other animal fats. There was no area of alveolar hemorrhage or necrosis on histologic studies in the earlier stage, and mild septal fibrosis without distortion of the alveolar structures was noted in the later stage. Although squalene is extracted from shark liver oil, it is an intermediate form of biosynthetic cholesterol and different from common animal fat, which can be hydrolyzed into fatty acid by using lipase (38). A small amount of administered oil may be another explanation for the absence of a severe inflammatory reaction.

The method of lipid administration in our study was different from that in clinical settings; we made a single intrabronchial injection rather than repeated aspirations of small amounts. However, because the basic pathologic changes in the lung after oil administration in humans seem similar to those seen in our study, we think that the serial thin-section CT findings that correlated with the histopathologic findings in our study could be referred to when treating patients with squalene-induced pneumonia. Another shortcoming of our study is that the follow-up after administration of oil did not exceed 16 weeks. Thus, we can provide data on only the acute and subacute stages of lipoid pneumonia. Finally, all of the CT scans were obtained at functional residual capacity rather than at full inspiration. However, when the CT scans were compared with the corresponding contact radiographs of inflated and sliced specimens, there was no abnormal opacification that was thought to be due to the difference in the degree of inflation. We obtained CT scans before the oil injection in all of the pigs at functional residual capacity and could not find an area of substantially abnormal opacity that affected the CT findings of lipoid pneumonia (Fig 1a).

At first, we injected the oil endobronchially with the pig in a supine position by using a catheter without a balloon.

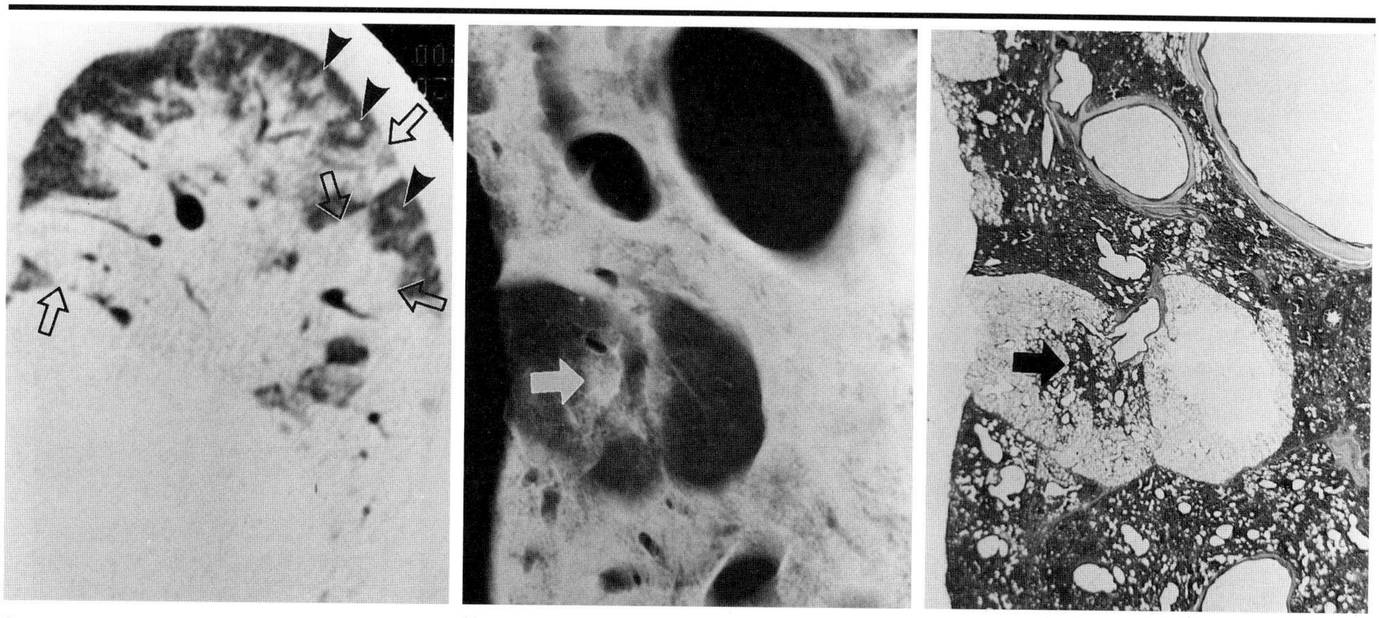

a. b. c.

Figure 5. Lobular distribution of shark liver oil–induced lipoid pneumonia in a pig. **(a)** Axial CT scan of the right lung obtained 1 week after administration of shark liver oil demonstrates airspace consolidation (arrows) with lobular or segmental distribution in the dependent area and areas of centrilobular opacity (arrowheads) in the nondependent area. **(b)** Close-up view of the corresponding area on the contact radiograph of a specimen from the lung shows a lobule (arrow) with centrilobular peribronchiolar airspace consolidation. Also note the consolidation of the surrounding lung. **(c)** Photomicrograph of the area in **b** shows centrilobular airspace consolidation (arrow) with cellular infiltrates adjacent to the bronchiole. The adjacent cellular infiltrates occupying whole lobules correspond to the lobular or segmental consolidation in **a** and **b**. (Hematoxylin-eosin stain; original magnification, ×4.)

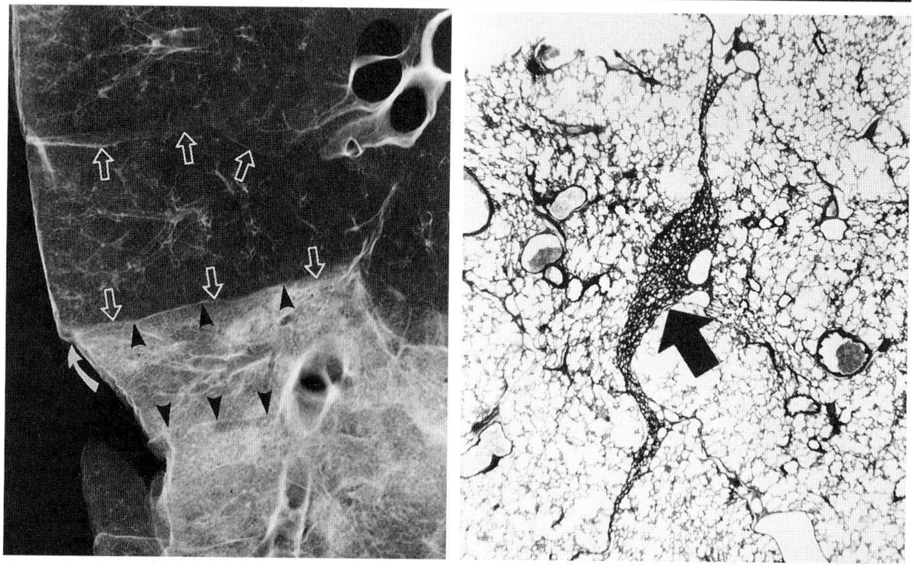

a. b.

Figure 6. **(a)** Contact radiograph (axial plane) and **(b)** photomicrograph of a porcine lung specimen show the bases of volume decreases in shark liver oil–induced pneumonia at CT. **(a)** Close-up view on the contact radiograph of the specimen obtained 4 weeks after endobronchial administration of oil shows the decreased size of the pulmonary lobule (arrowheads) in the affected lung compared with the size of that in the adjacent normal lung (open arrows). Also note the retraction of the surface (curved arrow) of the affected lobule. The increased opacity was due to residual wall thickening of the alveoli at histologic examination (see Fig 3b). **(b)** Photomicrograph of a specimen from the pig, which was sacrificed 8 weeks after oil administration, shows a diamond-shaped area (arrow) demarcated sharply by interlobular septa. This area represents total collapse of a secondary pulmonary lobule. (Hematoxylin-eosin stain; original magnification, ×10.)

The CT scans obtained immediately after the administration of oil showed dissemination of the oil into the upper and contralateral areas of the lung. We then placed the animal in a semierect prone position and used a balloon catheter to prevent regurgitation of the oil. We added a hyperventilation procedure with a ventilator bag just after the administration of oil to promote migration of the oil into the distal airspace. This modification allowed us to localize the pneumonic process to the unilateral lower lobe. We think localization of pneumonia is important for comparing the affected and normal lungs in the same animal and for decreasing the rate of mortality and morbidity. By using this model, it is feasible to produce pneumonia induced by various agents such as gastric juice in the pig; this may be useful for studying the pathophysiologic and radiologic changes of aspiration pneumonia.

In conclusion, the serial thin-section CT findings of exogenous lipoid pneumonia after a single endobronchial administration of oil in pigs were ground-glass opacity and airspace consolidation, followed by complete or incomplete resolution with lobular volume loss and septal thickening.

Practical application: These results provide basic knowledge of serial changes in

CT findings in cases of exogenous lipoid pneumonia and provide the histopathologic background of the CT findings. The results of our study also show that low-attenuating consolidation as a sign of lipoid pneumonia should be considered carefully, because partial volume averaging of partly aerated lung can cause a false-positive interpretation.

Acknowledgments: We express our gratitude to Sung Hwan Hong, MD, Sun Won Park, MD, and Hyuk Jae Choi for their technical assistance with the animal experiments and management and to Eun Hoi Goo for his help in CT scanning. We also thank Jeong Wook Seo, MD, for advice in histopathologic interpretations.

References

1. Laughlen GF. Studies on pneumonia following nasopharyngeal injections of oil. Am J Pathol 1925; 1:407–415.
2. Pinkerton H. Oils and fats: their entrance into and fate in the lungs of infants and children—a clinical and pathologic report. Am J Dis Child 1927; 33:259–285.
3. Pinkerton H. The reaction to oils and fats in the lung. Arch Pathol 1928; 5:380–401.
4. Graef I. Pulmonary changes due to the aspiration of lipids and mineral oil. Am J Pathol 1935; 11:862–868.
5. Ikeda K. Oil aspiration pneumonia (lipoid pneumonia): clinical, pathologic and experimental considerations. Am J Dis Child 1935; 49:985–1006.
6. Ikeda K. Lipoid pneumonia of the adult type (paraffinoma of the lung): report of five cases. Arch Pathol 1937; 23:470–492.
7. Paterson JLH. An experimental study of pneumonia following the aspiration of oily substances: lipoid cell pneumonia. J Pathol Bacteriol 1938; 46:151–164.
8. Volk BW, Nathanson L, Losner S, Slade WR, Jacobi M. Incidence of lipoid pneumonia in a survey of 389 chronically ill patients. Am J Med 1951; 10:316–324.
9. Jampolis RW, McDonald JR, Clagett OT. Mineral oil granuloma of the lung: an evaluation of methods for identification of mineral oil in tissue. Int Abs Surg 1953; 97:105–119.
10. Bréchot JM, Buy JN, Laaban JP, Rochemaure J. Computed tomography and magnetic resonance findings in lipoid pneumonia. Thorax 1991; 46:738–739.
11. Brown AC, Slocum PC, Puthoff SL, Wallace WE, Foresman BH. Exogenous lipoid pneumonia due to nasal application of petroleum jelly. Chest 1994; 105:968–969.
12. Brody H. Focal lipid granulomatosis of the lung following instillation of ionized poppyseed oil. Arch Pathol 1943; 35:744–749.
13. Storrs RP, McDonald JR, Good CA. Lipoid granuloma of the lung following bronchography with iodized oil. J Thorac Surg 1949; 18:561–568.
14. Annobil SH, Ogunbiyi AO, Benjamin B. Chest radiographic findings in childhood lipoid pneumonia following aspiration of animal fat. Eur J Radiol 1993; 16:217–220.
15. de Oliveira GA, Del Caro SR, Bender Lamago CM, Mercon de Vargas PR, Vervloet VEC. Radiographic plain film and CT findings in lipoid pneumonia in infants following aspiration of mineral oil used in the treatment of partial small bowel obstruction by *Ascaris lumbricoides*. Pediatr Radiol 1985; 15:157–160.
16. Lee KS, Müller NL, Hale V, Newell Jr JD, Lynch KA, Im JG. Lipoid pneumonia: CT findings. J Comput Assist Tomogr 1995; 19:48–51.
17. Hugosson CO, Riff EJ, Moore CCM, Akhtar M, Tufenkeji HT. Lipoid pneumonia in infants: a radiographical-pathological study. Pediatr Radiol 1991; 21:193–197.
18. Balakrishman S. Lipoid pneumonia in infants and children in South India. Br Med J 1973; 4:329–331.
19. Asnis DS, Saltzman HP, Melchert A. Shark oil pneumonia: an overlooked entity. Chest 1993; 103:976–977.
20. Pierson JW. Some unusual pneumonias associated with the aspiration of fats and oils in the lungs. AJR 1932; 27:572–579.
21. Hampton SO, Bickham CE, Winship T. Lipoid pneumonia. AJR 1955; 73:938–949.
22. Weill H, Ferrans VJ, Gay RM, Ziskind MM. Early lipoid pneumonia: roentgenologic, anatomic, and physiologic characteristics. Am J Med 1964; 36:370–376.
23. Genereux GP. Lipids in the lungs: radiologic-pathologic correlation. J Can Assoc Radiol 1970; 21:2–15.
24. Kennedy JD, Costello P, Balikian JP, Herman PG. Exogeneous lipoid pneumonia. AJR 1981; 136:1145–1149.
25. Wright BA, Jeffrey PH. Lipoid pneumonia. Semin Respir Infect 1990; 5:314–321.
26. Wheeler PS, Stitik FP, Hutchins GM, Klinefelter HF, Siegelman SS. Diagnosis of lipoid pneumonia by computed tomography. JAMA 1981; 245:65–66.
27. Joshi RR, Cholankeril JV. Computed tomography in lipoid pneumonia. J Comput Assist Tomogr 1985; 6:211–213.
28. Brody JS, Levin B. Interlobular septa thickening in lipid pneumonia. AJR 1962; 88: 1061–1069.
29. Todo G, Herman PG. High-resolution computed tomography of the pig lung. Invest Radiol 1986; 21:689–696.
30. Markarian B, Dailey ET. Preparation of inflated lung specimens. In: Heitzman ER, ed. The lung: radiologic-pathologic correlations. 2nd ed. St Louis, Mo: Mosby–Year Book, 1984; 4–12.
31. French JE, Morris B. The uptake and storage of lipid particles in lymph-gland in the rat. J Pathol Bacteriol 1960; 79:11–19.
32. Godwin JD, Müller NL, Takasugi JE. Pulmonary alveolar proteinosis: CT findings. Radiology 1988; 169:609–613.
33. Lee JS, Im JG, Song KS, Seo JB, Lim TH. Exogenous lipoid pneumonia: high-resolution CT findings. Eur Radiol 1999; 9:287–291.
34. Franquet T, Giménez A, Bordes R, Rodríguez-Arias JM, Castella J. The crazy-paving pattern in exogenous lipoid pneumonia: CT-pathologic correlation. AJR 1998; 170:315–317.
35. Carrillon Y, Tixier E, Revel D, Cordier JF. MR diagnosis of lipoid pneumonia. J Comput Assist Tomogr 1988; 12:876–877.
36. Carette MF, Grivaux M, Monad B, Capeau F, Lebreton C, Bigot JM. MR findings in lipoid pneumonia. AJR 1989; 153:1097–1098.
37. Cox JE, Choplin RH, Chiles C. Chemical-shift MRI of exogeneous lipoid pneumonia. J Comput Assist Tomogr 1996; 20: 465–467.
38. Budavari S, ed. The Merck index. 11th ed. Rahway, NJ: Merck, 1989; 1383.

Toshiaki Sendo, PhD
Masaaki Hirakawa, BS
Kaori Fujie, MS
Yasufumi Kataoka, PhD
Ryozo Oishi, PhD

Index terms:
Animals
Contrast media, complications, 60.46, 60.711
Contrast media, experimental studies, 60.46, 60.711
Lungs, fluid, 60.46, 60.711
Silicone, 60.46

Radiology 1999; 212:97–102

Abbreviation:
USP = U.S. Pharmacopeia

[1] From the Department of Hospital Pharmacy, Faculty of Medicine, Kyushu University, 3-1-1 Maidashi, Higashi-ku, Fukuoka 812-8582, Japan. Received May 15, 1998; revision requested July 14; revision received October 26; accepted February 12, 1999. **Address reprint requests to** R.O.

Author contributions:
Guarantor of integrity of entire study, R.O.; study concepts, T.S., Y.K., RO.; study design, T.S., R.O.; definition of intellectual content, T.S., Y.K., R.O.; literature research, K.F., M.H.; experimental studies, T.S., K.F., M.H.; data acquisition, T.S., K.F., M.H.; data analysis, T.S., K.F.; statistical analysis, K.F., M.H.; manuscript preparation, T.S., K.F.; manuscript editing, T.S., Y.K., R.O.; manuscript review, Y.K., R.O.

Contrast Medium–induced Pulmonary Edema Is Aggravated by Silicone Contamination in Rats[1]

PURPOSE: To examine the effect of silicone contamination, which occurs in clinical settings during vial preparation with disposable syringes, on contrast medium–induced pulmonary edema in rats.

MATERIALS AND METHODS: Ioxaglate, ioversol, and iohexol, silicone-containing physiologic saline solutions, and three silicone-containing contrast media were separately, intravenously injected at 1.5 mL/min in rats. Pulmonary edema was evaluated as changes in the relative lung weight and in the water, sodium, and potassium contents of the lung.

RESULTS: Intravenous injection of ioxaglate induced marked pulmonary edema, even with a dose of only 4 g of iodine per kilogram of body weight. In contrast, ioversol and iohexol induced significant pulmonary edema only after the injection of large doses (6 g of iodine per kilogram; $P < .05$). The injection of 4 μL/mL silicone-containing physiologic saline at a dose of 18.75 mL/kg also produced marked pulmonary edema, whereas doses of 6.25 and 12.5 mL/kg showed no significant influence. The addition of an ineffective dose (12.5 mL of physiologic saline per kilogram of body weight) of silicone in contrast medium substantially aggravated the pulmonary edema induced by the contrast medium alone; this phenomenon was also confirmed with morphologic observation.

CONCLUSION: Ionic contrast media are more toxic to the endothelial cells than are nonionic contrast media. Silicone contamination might be one of the causes of pulmonary edema after intravenous injection. However, caution must be exercised in extrapolating these results to humans.

Parenteral solutions for intravenous injection are often contaminated with extrinsic foreign particles (1). Findings of animal studies have demonstrated that particles in parenteral solutions produce undesirable effects, such as particle-induced coronary vasoconstriction (2), embolization of arterioles in the kidney (3), and granulomas (4). Findings of some investigations (3,5,6) have also revealed the involvement of glass particles from the opening of the package and cotton fibers and other particles from the ambient air that enter the contrast medium.

In the case of vial preparations, contrast medium is transferred into disposable plastic syringes for injection. We (7) recently found a marked increase in the particle contamination of contrast media during the loading of disposable syringes due to silicone released from the inner surface and the rubber plunger. However, little is known about the harmful effects of the injection of contrast medium contaminated with silicone.

Pulmonary edema is a severe adverse reaction that sometimes occurs after the intravascular injection of a contrast medium and, although this is rare, might be the main cause of death related to contrast media (8). In the present study, therefore, we investigated the influence of silicone contamination in pulmonary edema induced by contrast media in rats.

MATERIALS AND METHODS

Animals

Specific pathogen–free male Sprague-Dawley rats weighing 200–250 g were obtained from the Laboratory of Animal Experiments, Faculty of Medicine, Kyushu University, Fukuoka, Japan. Animals were given free access to food and water before the experiments.

This study was reviewed by the ethics committee regarding animal experiments at the Faculty of Medicine, Kyushu University, and was performed according to the Guidelines for Animal Experiments in the Faculty of Medicine, Kyushu University, and the law (no. 105) and guidelines for notification (no. 6) from the Japanese government.

Administration of Contrast Media in Study Rats or Physiologic Saline in Control Rats

Each nonanesthetized rat was placed in a plastic restrainer (model KN-328; Natsume, Tokyo, Japan); ioxaglate (Hexabrix 320, lot no. 3100, ionic dimer containing 320 mg of iodine per milliliter; Mallinckrodt Medical, St Louis, Mo), ioversol (Optiray 320, lot no. 305465J, nonionic monomer containing 320 mg of iodine per milliliter; Mallinckrodt Medical), or iohexol (Omnipaque 300, lot no. FQ41, nonionic monomer containing 300 mg of iodine per milliliter; Daiichi Pharmaceutical, Tokyo, Japan) was injected into the tail vein with a 25-gauge butterfly needle connected to an injection pump (Terumo, Tokyo, Japan) at a rate of 1.5 mL/min. Silicone-free plastic syringes (20-mL capacity; Top, Tokyo, Japan) were used for injection.

Control animals received injections of physiologic saline. In the study animals, the dose of the contrast medium was adjusted with the injection volume. Contrast medium at a dose of 2, 4, or 6 g of iodine per kilogram of body weight or a volume of physiologic saline equal to the volume of a dose of contrast medium at 6 g of iodine per kilogram was injected. Volume-related effects between the control group and the contrast media groups can therefore be excluded.

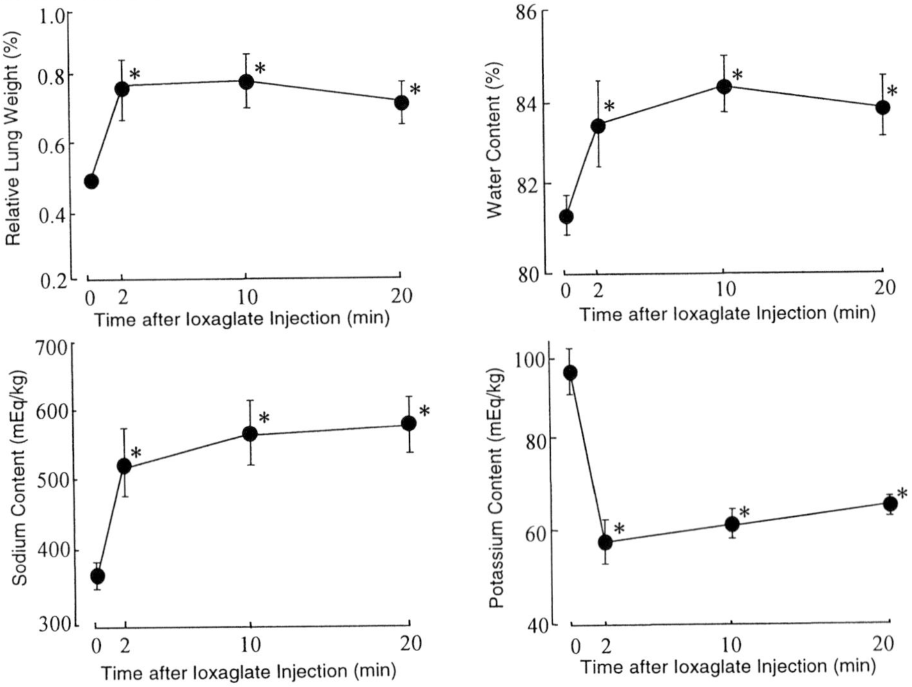

Figure 1. Graphs show the course of pulmonary edema development in rats after intravenous injection of ioxaglate. The maximum changes in the lung weight and potassium content were observed at 2 minutes after the injection, the maximum change in the water content was observed at 10 minutes, and the maximum change in the sodium content was observed at 20 minutes. Ioxaglate was intravenously injected at a dose of 6 g of iodine per kilogram and a rate of 1.5 mL/min. Each point with a vertical bar indicates the mean ± SEM for three to eight animals. Error bars are not shown when they are smaller than the symbols. * = $P < .05$ in a comparison with the value at 0 minute.

Preparation of Silicone-containing Contrast Media

Silicone-containing contrast media were prepared from commercially available contrast media by adding medical-grade silicone (silicone oil SH-200; Nacalai Tesque, Tokyo, Japan). Each silicone-containing solution was made on the basis of the number of contaminated particles in a previous report (7). Also, silicone (4 µL/mL) was added to the contrast media and physiologic saline. The solutions were filtered through a 5-µm membrane filter (Millex-SV; Millipore, Tokyo, Japan).

The degree of silicone contamination was evaluated by counting the particles derived from the interaction of the contrast media with silicone. Particle counting was performed with an automated light extinction method by using an automatic parenteral sampling system (Particle Measuring Systems, Boulder, Colo), as in a previous study (7). The prepared silicone-containing solutions of ioxaglate or ioversol were at 164% or 112%, respectively, of the U.S. Pharmacopeia (USP) acceptable limit of 6,000 pieces of 10 µm or larger per container; the solution of iohexol was at 76% of the USP limit. These differences among the three contrast media were based on the partition coefficient of their physicochemical properties (7).

To summarize, in the first experiment, we injected pure physiologic saline and pure contrast medium (ioxaglate, ioversol, or iohexol). In the second experiment, we injected pure physiologic saline and silicone-containing physiologic saline. In the third experiment, we injected pure contrast medium (4 g of iodine per kilogram) and silicone-containing contrast medium (4 g of iodine per kilogram).

Water Content of Lung

The rats were lightly anesthetized with ether and killed by means of cervical vertebra dislocation at an appropriate time after injection. The chest was opened, and the lungs were removed rapidly. The lungs were then placed on absorbent paper, and nonpulmonary tissue was carefully trimmed off. The lobes of each lung were separated, and all extralobar vessels were removed. Compression was avoided to prevent passive bleeding and fluid discharge from the lung. The wet weight was recorded after any visible blood stains were removed. The lobes were then placed in a drying oven at 100°C for 24 hours to measure the dry weight. The percentage

TABLE 1
Effect of Contrast Medium Dose on Development of Pulmonary Edema

Contrast Medium	Relative Lung Weight (%)	Water Content (%)	Sodium Content (mEq/kg Tissue)	Potassium Content (mEq/kg Tissue)
Ioxaglate				
Saline solution*	0.45 ± 0.02	81.6 ± 0.7	429.0 ± 3.3	85.7 ± 9.0
2 g I/kg	0.48 ± 0.02	81.8 ± 0.5	408.7 ± 19.5	74.4 ± 2.0
4 g I/kg	0.63 ± 0.09	84.0 ± 1.0†	642.1 ± 85.0†	66.0 ± 8.5†
6 g I/kg	0.81 ± 0.08†	85.0 ± 0.7†	597.3 ± 48.5†	62.2 ± 3.5†
Ioversol				
Saline solution‡	0.50 ± 0.02	82.0 ± 0.3	442.1 ± 14.9	76.6 ± 4.5
2 g I/kg	0.44 ± 0.01	81.1 ± 0.1	389.0 ± 12.0	68.9 ± 5.9
4 g I/kg	0.55 ± 0.05	81.6 ± 0.7	448.0 ± 62.3	63.1 ± 8.3†
6 g I/kg	0.60 ± 0.01†	83.3 ± 0.4†	488.7 ± 7.4	62.3 ± 4.1†
Iohexol				
Saline solution§	0.47 ± 0.02	80.8 ± 0.8	422.2 ± 43.7	73.5 ± 5.2
2 g I/kg	0.46 ± 0.01	81.2 ± 0.4	388.0 ± 12.4	76.5 ± 5.7
4 g I/kg	0.53 ± 0.04	82.3 ± 0.7	441.8 ± 31.9	63.0 ± 2.9
6 g I/kg	0.83 ± 0.07†	85.2 ± 0.7†	604.4 ± 34.9†	57.0 ± 5.2†

Note.—Each measurement was obtained at 10 minutes after injection. Each value represents the mean ± SEM for six animals.
* Volume of saline solution equal to the volume of ioxaglate at a dose of 6 g of iodine per kilogram of body weight.
† $P < .05$ in a comparison with respective saline solution–injected groups.
‡ Volume of saline solution equal to the volume of ioversol at a dose of 6 g of iodine per kilogram of body weight.
§ Volume of saline solution equal to the volume of iohexol at a dose of 6 g of iodine per kilogram of body weight.

of water content was calculated as [(wet weight − dry weight)100]/(wet weight).

Measurement of Sodium and Potassium Contents

The dry lung lobes were subjected to wet ashing with a mixture of nitric acid and perchloric acid (2:1, vol/vol). After centrifugation at 1,000 *g* for 10 minutes, the supernatant was diluted with distilled and deionized water. After this dilution, the sodium and potassium contents were measured by means of atomic absorption spectrophotometry (model AA-6400F; Shimadzu, Kyoto, Japan) by using diluted standard solutions (sodium standard solution, 997 mg of sodium per liter, and potassium standard solution, 1,000 mg of potassium per liter; Wako Pure Chemical Industries, Osaka, Japan). Results were obtained from triplicate assays and are expressed in milliequivalents per kilogram of dried lung.

Statistical Analysis

At least six rats were studied in each experimental group. All data are expressed as the mean ± SEM. Analysis of variance and then the Fisher protected least significant difference test were performed. Significance was indicated with a *P* value of less than .05.

RESULTS

Time Course of Pulmonary Edema Formation

At 0 minute after ioxaglate injection, the mean relative lung weights and water, sodium, and potassium contents in untreated rats were 0.50% ± 0.01, 81.7% ± 0.5, 381.8 mEq ± 8.1, and 97.1 mEq ± 5.2 per kilogram of tissue, respectively (Fig 1). The relative lung weights and water and sodium contents increased significantly, and the potassium content decreased significantly at 2, 10, and 20 minutes after the injection of ioxaglate (6 grams of iodine per kilogram). Although no significant differences in these parameters were noted among these three time points, the maximum changes in the lung weights and potassium contents were observed at 2 minutes after the injection, the maximum changes in the water content were observed at 10 minutes, and the maximum changes in the sodium content were observed at 20 minutes. No significant effects on these parameters were observed at 2, 10, or 20 minutes following the injection of a volume of physiologic saline equal to the volume of a dose of contrast material at 6 g of iodine per kilogram. In the subsequent experiments, therefore, the evaluation at the 10-minute observation point was assumed to be representative of the degree of pulmonary edema.

Contrast Medium-induced Pulmonary Edema

Table 1 summarizes the dose-dependent effects of the three contrast media on the relative lung weights and on the water, sodium, and potassium contents. The data obtained at 10 minutes after injection were chosen as a reference. The relative lung weights and water contents increased with increases in the doses of the three contrast media. The dose-dependent elevation in the relative lung weights became significant at the dose of 6 g of iodine per kilogram for all three contrast media.

In parallel with these changes, the water, sodium, and potassium contents also showed significant changes at the dose of 6 g of iodine per kilogram for iohexol. For ioxaglate, however, these parameters showed significant changes even at a dose of 4 g of iodine per kilogram. For ioversol, the potassium contents showed significant decreases at doses of 4 and 6 g of iodine per kilogram, but the sodium contents showed no significant changes.

Silicone-induced Pulmonary Edema

Table 2 summarizes the effects of the intravenous injection of silicone (4 µL/mL) in physiologic saline on the relative lung weights and on the water, sodium, and potassium contents in rats. Those values did not change significantly after the injection of 6.25 or 12.5 mL of silicone-containing solution (4 µL/mL) per kilogram. However, injection of 18.75 mL of solution per kilogram significantly increased the relative lung weights and water and sodium contents.

Pulmonary Edema Induced by Silicone-containing Contrast Media

Table 3 shows the effect of silicone on the pulmonary edema induced with contrast medium (4 g of iodine per kilogram). The dose of the silicone-containing contrast medium (silicone concentration, 4 µL/mL) was 12.5 mL/kg; at this dose, silicone showed little influence on the parameters of pulmonary edema (Table 2). In this experiment (Table 3), each contrast medium also showed pulmonary edema to an extent similar to that observed in the earlier experiments (Table 1). Silicone-containing contrast medium significantly increased the lung weights.

Silicone-containing iohexol induced maximum edema and also caused significant changes in all other indexes.

The aggravation of contrast medium–induced pulmonary edema by silicone was also clearly observed morphologically (Fig 2). A left lung 10 minutes after the injection of silicone at a dose of 12.5 mL/kg (Fig 2c) was morphologically similar to that in the control rat (Fig 2a). A lung was slightly but apparently enlarged with the injection of iohexol at a dose of 4 g of iodine per kilogram (Fig 2b). This phenomenon became more marked after the injection of silicone-containing iohexol (Fig 2d).

TABLE 2
Silicone-induced Pulmonary Edema

Injection Volume (mL/kg)	No. of Rats	Relative Lung Weight (%)	Water Content (%)	Sodium Content (mEq/kg Tissue)	Potassium Content (mEq/kg Tissue)
Saline solution: 18.75	16	0.49 ± 0.02	81.8 ± 0.4	414.5 ± 15.8	80.7 ± 3.0
Silicone-containing saline solution					
6.25	6	0.46 ± 0.02	81.1 ± 0.6	391.2 ± 12.0	78.6 ± 1.2
12.5	6	0.48 ± 0.02	80.9 ± 0.2	381.3 ± 3.8	79.2 ± 3.2
18.75	6	0.59 ± 0.02*	83.3 ± 0.4*	510.8 ± 27.0*	71.0 ± 3.0

Note.—Each measurement was obtained at 10 minutes after injection. Each value represents the mean ± SEM.
* $P < .05$ in a comparison with the group with pure saline solution injected.

TABLE 3
Effect of Silicone Contamination on the Pulmonary Edema Induced with Contrast Media

Substance Injected	Relative Lung Weight (%)	Water Content (%)	Sodium Content (mEq/kg Tissue)	Potassium Content (mEq/kg Tissue)
Ioxaglate	0.64 ± 0.07	84.4 ± 0.8	661.9 ± 63.3	64.3 ± 6.2
Silicone-containing ioxaglate	0.82 ± 0.06*	85.1 ± 0.6	693.1 ± 47.0	63.2 ± 2.8
Ioversol	0.55 ± 0.04	81.8 ± 0.6	447.6 ± 48.3	60.1 ± 7.1
Silicone-containing ioversol	0.70 ± 0.06*	84.5 ± 0.8*	532.1 ± 56.9	60.1 ± 3.9
Iohexol	0.54 ± 0.03	81.9 ± 0.9	434.9 ± 33.9	63.4 ± 2.4
Silicone-containing iohexol	0.90 ± 0.05*	85.9 ± 0.3*	667.4 ± 39.2*	54.8 ± 1.9*

Note.—The dose of all contrast media was 4 g of iodine per kilogram of body weight. The silicone concentration was 4 µL/mL. The dose of all silicone-containing contrast media was 12.5 mL/kg. Each measurement was obtained at 10 minutes after injection. Each value represents the mean ± SEM for six animals.
* $P < .05$ in a comparison with the respective pure contrast medium–injected groups.

DISCUSSION

These results clearly demonstrate that the intravenous injection of currently used contrast media produces pulmonary edema in rats and that the edema is markedly aggravated by the contamination of contrast medium with silicone. An increase in lung weight is caused mainly by the increase in extravascular lung water (9,10). Hayashi et al (11) presented histologic evidence, together with the evaluation of lung weights, that the increase in the relative lung weights closely correlates with perivascular edema. However, a change in the lung weight following an injection of contrast medium may not be distinguishable from the vascular engorgement or presence of contrast medium in the lung. Thus, we also determined the water, sodium, and potassium contents in the lung as better indications of pulmonary edema (12).

Time- and dose-dependency studies of pulmonary edema induced by contrast medium were also performed to decide the optimal time and dose for the evaluation of the effect of silicone contamination. The time course of the increase in the lung weight observed in the present study is in agreement with that reported by Mare and Violante (9). In addition, findings of the present investigation confirm that the substantial increases in lung weight are due to extravascular (interstitial or alveolar) fluid accumulation accompanied by disturbances of the ionic equilibrium, that is, sodium and water influx and potassium efflux. The water, sodium, and potassium contents are more sensitive than the lung weight in the detection of pulmonary edema induced by the ionic contrast medium ioxaglate.

Differences in the chemotoxicity and osmotoxicity of contrast media are considered to be responsible for the degree of pulmonary edema (13,14). In a Japanese prospective study of adverse reactions to intravenous contrast media (15), the incidences of severe reactions to ionic and nonionic contrast media were 0.22% and 0.04%, respectively, and the incidence of fatal reactions to ionic contrast media was 0.04%, while the incidence of fatal reactions to nonionic contrast media was 0%.

Beynon et al (16) reported that ioxaglate caused marked endothelial damage as an indication of chemotoxicity, while iohexol did not elicit substantial endothelial damage. In the present study, however, the large dose of iohexol of 6 g of iodine per kilogram produced the same degree of pulmonary edema as did ioxaglate. Therefore, it is suggested that large doses of the nonionic contrast media iohexol and ioversol can induce chemotoxic reactions. The very large doses of contrast media in the present study are well above clinically relevant doses, and results of this study are not immediately applicable to clinical conditions. However, since the larger doses of contrast media are clinically recommended for computed tomography and digital angiography (17), close attention should be paid to the risk of serious or fatal adverse reactions, including pulmonary edema.

Silicone, because of its inert biologic property (18), is supplied for manufacturing a variety of medical devices, such as intravenous tubing; pacemaker leads; joint prostheses; lens replacements; and mandibular, breast, and nasal implants. It has been reported that silicone elicits foreign body reactions such as granulomatous inflammation, fibrosis (19), and embolism (20–22).

We showed in this study that large amounts of silicone (18.75 mL/kg) produce pulmonary edema. Silicone alone, at the doses of 6.25–12.5 mL/kg set according to the injection volume, did not produce pulmonary edema. It is interesting that the addition of an ineffective dose (12.5 mL/kg) of silicone to all of the contrast media significantly aggravated the pulmonary edema induced by the contrast media alone. Significant changes in all indexes after the injection of silicone-containing iohexol were observed, even though the particle amounts were below the acceptable limit. These changes were also strongly supported by the morphologic findings of the swollen lungs.

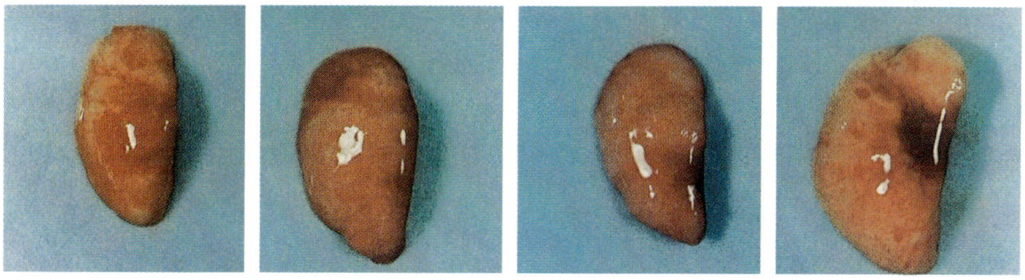

a. b. c. d.

Figure 2. Photographs of left lungs demonstrate morphology at 10 minutes after the injection of **(a)** physiologic saline at 18.75 mL/kg, **(b)** iohexol at 4 g of iodine per kilogram, **(c)** silicone at 12.5 mL/kg, and **(d)** iohexol at 4 g of iodine per kilogram with silicone-containing solution at 12.5 mL/kg. The preparation of silicone-containing solutions is described in the text. The lung in **a** was morphologically similar to a nontreated lung. The lungs in **b** and **c** were slightly enlarged after the injection of **(b)** iohexol and **(c)** silicone. The aggravation of iohexol-induced pulmonary edema by silicone was clearly shown by the morphologic finding of a swollen lung in **d**.

Ioxaglate did not show a notable effect of silicone contamination in a comparison with the nonionic contrast media. This might be because the inherent chemotoxicity of ionic contrast media is enough to induce the pulmonary changes (23).

The observed aggravation of pulmonary edema following the injection of silicone-containing contrast medium may be due to several mechanisms. In general, the foreign particles in the parenteral solution cause the vascular endothelial injury (24) and lodge in the vessels and disturb the pulmonary circulation, which leads to elevated pulmonary venous pressure (20–22,25). However, silicone has no effect on the capillary filtration coefficient, which is used as an index of alterations in microvascular permeability in the lungs (26).

Immiscible particles are derived from the interaction of the contrast medium with silicone. These particles may produce pulmonary edema due to vascular endothelial injury and/or disturbance of pulmonary circulation. Consequently, the aggravating effect of silicone on the pulmonary edema induced with contrast medium may result from the synergistic effect of the contrast medium and silicone. For further exploration of the actual mechanism of the pulmonary edema formation, histologic examinations are necessary.

Findings of our previous study (27) showed that an electronic counting method based on light extinction could be used to determine the number of silicone droplets present as particles in a contrast medium. The USP acceptable limit is based on counts of particles with a diameter of 10 µm or larger and of 25 µm or larger. Since pulmonary capillaries vary between 8 and 12 µm, any particles larger than 12 µm are likely to be trapped and retained in the pulmonary vascular bed (28). Findings of an animal experiment (29) in which microspheres have been intravenously injected indicate that small particles enter the system circulation and end up in organs. However, the clinical importance of silicone droplets that are too small to be retained in the lungs is uncertain. Abnormal liver function in some patients undergoing hemodialysis was speculated to be a result of silicone particles in the liver derived from siliconized peristaltic blood pumps (30). However, the count of particles in the circulating solution was not determined in that study.

Practical application: Silicone contamination aggravated pulmonary edema that occurred after the intravenous injection of contrast medium in rats. Although in this experiment it was not possible to match conditions such as the dose and rate of injection of contrast medium, the results obtained raise the possibility that the incidence of pulmonary edema could be increased in patients who are examined by using contrast medium contaminated with silicone.

References

1. Borchert SJ, Abe A, Aldrich DS, et al. Particulate matter in parenteral products: a review. J Parenter Sci Technol 1986; 40:212–224.
2. David JH, Cetin E, Lary AR, et al. Particle-induced coronary vasoconstriction during cardioplegic infusion. J Thorac Cardiovasc Surg 1985; 89:428–438.
3. Brekkan A, Lexow PE, Woxholt G. Glass fragments and other particles contaminating contrast media. Acta Radiol Diagn 1975; 16:600–608.
4. Garvan JM, Gunner BW. Particulate contamination of intravenous fluid. Br J Clin Pract 1971; 25:119–121.
5. Winding O. Foreign bodies in contrast media for angiography. Am J Hosp Pharm 1977; 34:705–708.
6. Markus K, Loh A, Israel D. Microscopic air embolism during cerebral angiography and strategies for its avoidance. Lancet 1993; 341:784–787.
7. Sendo T, Otsubo K, Hisazumi A, et al. Particle contamination in contrast media induced by disposable syringes. J Pharm Sci 1995; 84:1490–1491.
8. Lalli AF. Contrast media reactions: data analysis and hypothesis. Radiology 1980; 134:1–12.
9. Mare K, Violante M. Pulmonary edema induced by high intravenous doses of diatrizoate in the rat. Acta Radiol Diagn 1983; 24:419–424.
10. Mare K, Violante M, Fischer HW. Pulmonary edema following high intravenous doses of ionic contrast media: effect of the anion composition and concentration. Invest Radiol 1984; 19:188–191.
11. Hayashi H, Kumazaki T, Asano G. Pulmonary edema induced by intravenous administration of contrast media: experimental study in rats. Radiat Med 1994; 12:47–52.
12. Pearce M, Yamashita J, Beazell B. Measurement of pulmonary edema. Circ Res 1965; 16:482–485.
13. Wood BP, Smith WL. Pulmonary edema in infants following injection of contrast media for urography. Radiology 1981; 130: 377–379.
14. Borish L, Martloff SM, Findlay SR. Radiographic contrast media-induced noncardiogenic pulmonary edema: case report and review of the literature. J Allergy Clin Immunol 1984; 74:104–107.
15. Yamaguchi K, Katayama H, Takashima T, et al. Prediction of severe adverse reactions to ionic and nonionic contrast media in Japan: evaluation of pretesting—a report from the Japanese Committee on the Safety of Contrast Media. Radiology 1991; 178:363–367.
16. Beynon HLC, Walport MJ, Dawson P. Vascular endothelial injury by intravascular contrast agents. Invest Radiol 1994; 29(suppl):195–197.
17. Shehadi W, Toniolo G. Adverse reactions to contrast media. Radiology 1980; 137: 299–302.
18. Branley S. Chemistry and properties of medical grade silicones. J Macromol Sci Chem A 1970; 4:529–544.
19. Busch H. Silicone toxicology. Arthritis Rheum 1994; 24:11–17.
20. Williams MA, Stephens JF, Brunckhorst LF. Identification of silicone in retinal vessels by electron probe x-ray microanalysis. J Histochem Cytochem 1975; 24:149–151.
21. Orenstein JM, Aaron B, Buchholz B, et al. Microemboli observed in deaths following cardiopulmonary bypass surgery. Hum Pathol 1982; 13:1082–1090.
22. Rodriguez MA, Martinez MC, Lopez-Artiguez M, et al. Lung embolism with liquid silicone. J Forensic Sci 1989; 34:504–510.
23. Dawson P. Chemotoxicity of contrast media and clinical adverse effects: a review. Invest Radiol 1985; 20:52–59.
24. Dorris GG, Bivins BA, Rapp RP, et al. Inflammatory potential of foreign particu-

lates in parenteral drugs. Anesth Analg 1977; 56:422–428.
25. Morisette M, Gagnon R, Lamoureux J, et al. Effect of angiographic contrast media on colloid oncotic pressure. Am Heart J 1980; 100:319–324.
26. Townsley MI, Taylor GE, Korthuis RJ, et al. Promethazine or DPPD pretreatment attenuates oleic acid-induced injury in isolated canine lungs. J Appl Physiol 1985; 59:39–46.
27. Sendo T, Hirakawa M, Yaginuma M, et al. Quality evaluation of radiographic contrast media in large volume prefilled syringes and vials. Acad Radiol 1998; 5:444–447.
28. Kanke M, Simmons GH, Weiss DL, et al. Clearance of ^{141}Ce-labeled microspheres from blood and distribution in specific organs following intravenous and intraarterial administration in beagle dogs. J Pharm Sci 1980; 69:755–762.
29. Lyon TC, Beasley JD, Cutright DE. Particle contamination of dextran for intravenous use: an in vitro and in vivo study. Military Med 1974; 141:466–469.
30. Hunt J, Farthing MJG, Baker LRI. Silicone in the liver: possible late effects. Gut 1989; 30:239–242.

Iliotibial Band Friction Syndrome: MR Imaging Findings in 16 Patients and MR Arthrographic Study of Six Cadaveric Knees[1]

Claus Muhle, MD
Joong Mo Ahn, MD, PhD
LeeRen Yeh, MD
Gabrielle A. Bergman, MD
Robert D. Boutin, MD
Mark Schweitzer, MD
Jon A. Jacobson, MD
Parviz Haghighi, MD
Debra J. Trudell, RA
Donald Resnick, MD

Index terms:
Athletic injuries, 452.485
Iliotibial tract, 452.92
Joints, MR, 452.121411, 452.121412, 452.121415
Knee, injuries, 452.485
Knee, ligaments, menisci, and cartilage, 452.485, 452.92
Knee, MR, 452.121411, 452.121412, 452.121415
Magnetic resonance (MR), arthrography, 452.122

Radiology 1999; 212:103–110

Abbreviations:
ITBFS = iliotibial band friction syndrome
ITT = iliotibial tract

[1]From the Depts of Radiology (C.M., J.M.A., L.R.Y., D.J.T., D.R.) and Pathology (P.H.), Veterans Affairs Medical Center, 3350 La Jolla Village Dr, San Diego, CA 92161; Dept of Diagnostic Radiology, University of Kiel, Germany (C.M.); Dept of Radiology, Stanford University, Calif (G.A.B.); Dept of Radiology, Beth Israel Deaconess Medical Center, Boston, Mass (R.D.B.); Dept of Radiology, Thomas Jefferson Hospital, Philadelphia, Pa (M.S.); and Dept of Diagnostic Radiology, Henry Ford Hospital, Detroit, Mich (J.A.J.). Received May 1, 1998; revision requested Jul 6; final revision received Jan 22, 1999; accepted Jan 27. Supported in part by the Deutsche Forschungsgemeinschaft and Veterans Administration grant SA360. **Address reprint requests to** D.R.

Author contributions:
Guarantors of integrity of entire study, C.M., D.R.; study concepts, C.M., D.R.; study design, J.M.A., L.R.Y.; definition of intellectual content, C.M., J.M.A., D.R.; literature research, L.R.Y., C.M.; clinical studies, G.A.B., R.D.B.; experimental studies, C.M.; data acquisition, J.A.J., G.A.B., R.D.B., M.S.; data analysis, C.M., P.H., D.J.T.; statistical analysis, C.M.; manuscript preparation, D.J.T., C.M.; manuscript editing, C.M., D.R.; manuscript review, D.R.

PURPOSE: To define magnetic resonance (MR) imaging findings in patients with the iliotibial band friction syndrome (ITBFS) and to correlate these findings with anatomic features defined at magnetic resonance (MR) arthrography in cadavers.

MATERIALS AND METHODS: The anatomic relationship of the iliotibial tract (ITT) to the lateral recesses of the knee joint and the lateral femoral epicondyle was investigated with MR arthrography at full extension and at 30° and 60° of knee flexion in six cadaveric knees. Seventeen MR imaging studies in 16 patients with ITBFS were evaluated.

RESULTS: In the cadaveric study, no interference of the lateral synovial recess with the lateral femoral epicondyle at full extension and at 30° and 60° of knee flexion was observed. In all specimens, correlation of MR images with macroscopic and microscopic sections revealed no primary bursa between the lateral femoral epicondyle and the ITT. In clinical studies, MR imaging findings of poorly defined signal intensity abnormalities or circumscribed fluid collections were located in a compartmentlike space confined laterally by the ITT and medially by the meniscocapsular junction, the lateral collateral ligament, and the lateral femoral epicondyle.

CONCLUSION: MR imaging accurately depicts the compartmentlike distribution of signal intensity abnormalities in patients with ITBFS.

Iliotibial band friction syndrome (ITBFS) is a common cause of lateral knee pain that is often related to intense physical activity, as occurs in long-distance runners, cyclists, and American football players (1–6). The diagnosis of ITBFS is based on clinical examination, with tenderness over the lateral femoral epicondyle and reproducible pain during flexion and extension of the knee while the examiner exerts pressure over the lateral femoral epicondyle (7). In some patients, however, ITBFS can be misdiagnosed as some other derangement of the knee, such as a lateral meniscal tear, lateral collateral ligament sprain, popliteal tendon strain, or lateral hamstring strain (3). Although repetitive friction of the iliotibial tract (ITT) over the lateral femoral epicondyle at 30° of knee flexion is described as the main cause of ITBFS, no study, to our knowledge, has yet evaluated the relation of the ITT and the lateral femoral epicondyle during the critical range of knee motion between full extension and 60° of flexion.

The ITT is formed proximally at the level of the greater trochanter by the coalescence of the fascial investments of the tensor fasciae latae, the gluteus maximus muscle, and the gluteus medius muscle (Fig 1). Proximal to the knee joint, the ITT is attached to the supracondylar tubercle of the femoral condyle and the intermuscular septum, and it continues distally to attach to the Gerdy tubercle at the anterolateral aspect of the tibia (8,9). Proximal to the lateral femoral epicondyle, the ITT is separated from the femur by a wide layer of fatty tissue that extends to the vastus lateralis muscle.

At the level of the lateral femoral condyle, the ITT contacts the lateral femoral epicondyle and the inserting fibers of the lateral collateral ligament (Fig 2). With its tense fibers, the ITT moves forward in extension and backward in flexion. In flexion, the ITT, the popliteal tendon, and the lateral collateral ligament cross each other, which enhances their function as lateral stabilizers of the knee (10).

Ultrasonography (US) can be used for detection of soft-tissue abnormalities in patients with the ITBFS (2). The findings, however, are not specific. Bone scintigraphy may show abnormal radionuclide uptake about the lateral femoral condyle or near the lateral tibial tubercle in patients with this syndrome (11). Magnetic resonance (MR) imaging is superior to US and bone scintigraphy in the detection of ITBFS, but, to our knowledge, its role has been described only in a small number of patients (7,12,13). MR imaging findings include either ill-defined signal intensity alterations or a localized fluid collection deep to the ITT (7,12,13).

The purpose of our study was to describe the characteristic MR imaging findings in patients with ITBFS and to investigate the anatomic relationship of the ITT and the lateral femoral epicondyle during knee flexion by using MR arthrography in cadavers.

MATERIALS AND METHODS

Six human legs with preserved hemipelves were obtained from nonembalmed fresh cadavers (four men, two women; age range, 72–86 years at the time of death; mean age, 75 years) and were immediately deep-frozen at −40°C (Forma Bio-Freezer; Forma Scientific, Marietta, Ohio). The specimens were allowed to thaw for 24 hours at room temperature prior to imaging. All specimens were examined with routine radiography to exclude those with previous injuries.

MR images were obtained with a 1.5-T superconducting MR imager (Signa; GE Medical Systems, Milwaukee, Wis). The specimens were positioned supine inside a receive-only knee coil at full extension and at 30° and 60° of knee flexion by using precisely angled wooden bars. These angle positions were chosen because prior clinical studies (9,10) described the occurrence of ITBFS in knee positions that ranged from full extension to 60° of flexion. To determine the relation of the lateral synovial recess to the lateral femoral epicondyle during knee flexion, 60 mL of a 2 mmol/L gadopentetate dimeglumine solution (Magnevist [1 mL in 250 mL saline solution]; Schering, Berlin, Germany) was injected intraarticularly to simulate a joint effusion, following the protocol described by Engel (14). Gadolinium-enhanced MR arthrography was performed with T1-weighted spin-echo imaging in the axial and coronal planes. Images were acquired in both planes because of prior documentation that both are useful in the assessment of the ITT (6,7). The imaging parameters are listed in Table 1.

After MR imaging, the specimens were frozen at −60°C for more than 72 hours. Of the six cadaveric legs, two each were positioned at full extension (0°), 30° of flexion, and 60° of flexion and sectioned with a band saw parallel to the axial MR imaging plane into 4-mm thick slices. The anatomic sections were cleaned with running water for macroscopic inspection. Microscopic examination of the ITT at the level of the epicondyle was performed in four randomly selected specimens for correlation with the gross pathologic findings. All histologic slides were evaluated by an experienced pathologist (P.H.) blinded to the MR imaging findings and results of inspection of the anatomic sections.

In addition, MR imaging studies of 16 patients (six male patients, 10 female patients; age range, 17–54 years; mean age, 35 years) with ITBFS were obtained from five institutions and were analyzed. In each patient, available history and results of physical examination performed by one or more orthopedic surgeons provided evidence consistent with ITBFS. All patients were treated conservatively without surgical intervention.

All MR images were obtained with the knee placed supine and in extension inside a receive-only knee coil. The MR examinations were performed by using 1.0- or 1.5-T magnets (Signa, GE Medical Systems; Magnetom Expert, Siemens Medical Systems, Iselin, NJ) with the following sequences: fat-saturated T2-weighted fast spin-echo sequence, T1-weighted spin-echo sequence, T2*-weighted two-dimensional multiplanar gradient-recalled-echo sequence, and three-dimensional double-echo steady state sequence. The MR imaging protocol is summarized in Table 1.

The MR images were evaluated by consensus by two radiologists (C.M., J.M.A.) experienced in musculoskeletal imaging who used the following criteria (7,12,13): (*a*) poorly defined signal intensity abnormalities lateral, distal, or proximal to the lateral epicondyle; (*b*) signal intensity abnormalities superficial or deep to the ITT; (*c*) localized fluid collection lateral, distal, or proximal to the lateral epicondyle; (*d*) width of the ITT at the level of the lateral epicondyle; (*e*) joint effusion; and (*f*) additional findings (eg, meniscal tears).

To compare the width of the ITT in patients with that in a control group, 20 healthy subjects (10 male subjects, 10 female subjects; age range, 15–63 years; mean age, 37 years) were examined with the knee placed supine and in extension inside a receive-only knee coil by using a coronal T1-weighted spin-echo sequence (550/18 [repetition time msec/echo time msec]) with a 4-mm section thickness. The Student t test was used to evaluate statistically significant differences with regard to the width of the ITT between patients and healthy subjects. Significant results were assumed on the 5% level ($P < .05$).

RESULTS

Cadaveric Study

The ITT, the lateral collateral ligament, the popliteus tendon, and the insertion of the tendon of the biceps femoris muscle demonstrated complex anatomic interrelationships. The relationships among the ITT, the lateral synovial recess, and the lateral femoral epicondyle were visualized best on axial MR images. At extension, in this imaging plane, contact of the posterior fibers of the ITT with the lateral femoral epicondyle and the inserting fibers of the lateral collateral ligament was observed in four (66%) of six specimens. In two (33%) of six specimens, however, the ITT was located anterior to the femoral insertions of the popliteus tendon and the lateral collateral ligament. With further flexion, in all specimens the ITT moved posteriorly and came in contact with the lateral femoral epicondyle and the inserting fibers of the lateral collateral ligament below this epicondyle (Fig 3).

In contrast, in all specimens (100%) and knee positions the lateral recess of the knee joint extended anterior to the lateral epicondyle, with no contact with the lateral femoral epicondyle. In addition, at all three positions, a thin layer of high signal intensity, which correlated with yellow tissue at macroscopic examination, was found between the ITT and the lateral femoral epicondyle at MR imaging in five (83%) of six specimens.

At microscopic inspection, the layer of high signal intensity between the ITT and lateral femoral epicondyle represented fatty and vascular tissue with no evidence of a bursa (Fig 3e). The synovial lining of the lateral recess was found in all specimens to extend anterior and proximal to the lateral femoral epicondyle, without

TABLE 1
MR Imaging Sequences

Method	Sequence*	Imaging Plane	Section Thickness (mm)	Intersection Gap (mm)	Repetition Time (msec)	Echo Time (msec)	Flip Angle (degrees)	Number of Signals Acquired	Matrix Size (pixel)	Field of View (cm)
Cadaveric Studies										
MR Arthrography	T1-SE	Coronal, transaxial	3.0	1	600	20	90	2	256 × 192	16
Clinical Studies										
MR Imaging	T1-SE	Coronal	4.0	1	550	18	90	1	256 × 192	16
	FSE-T2 fat saturated	Coronal, transaxial	4.0	1	4,400	108	90	2	256 × 192	14
	MPGR	Coronal	4.0	1	600	15	30	2	256 × 192	14
	3D DESS	Transaxial	1.6	0	27	9	45	1	256 × 192	16

* FSE-T2 fat saturated = fast spin-echo T2-weighted fat-saturated, MPGR = multiplanar gradient-recalled echo, T1-SE = T1-weighted spin-echo, 3D DESS = three-dimensional double-echo steady state.

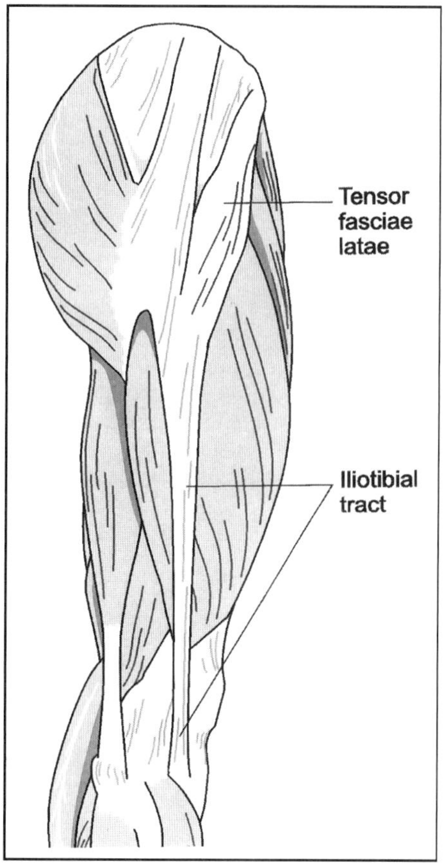

Figure 1. Drawing of the normal anatomy of the ITT as seen from the lateral aspect of the thigh.

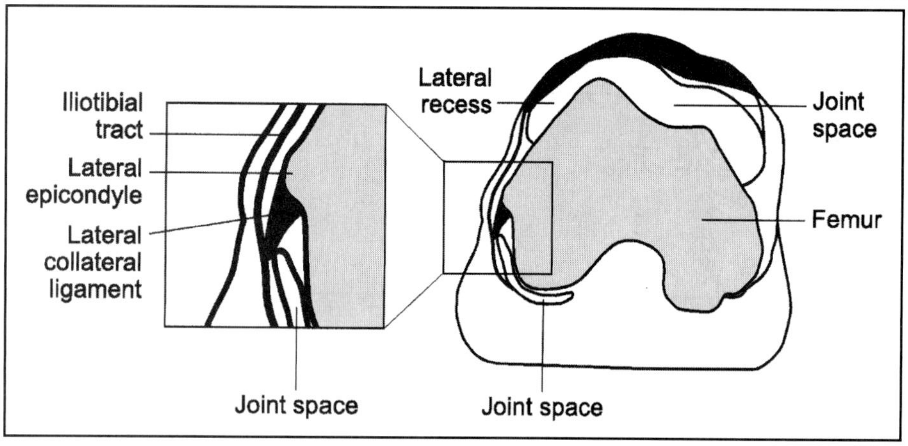

Figure 2. Drawing of the relationship of the ITT to the lateral epicondyle, the lateral collateral ligament, and the lateral recess of the knee joint in the axial plane.

any contact with the lateral femoral epicondyle.

Clinical Study

The clinical findings in 16 patients with ITBFS are summarized in Table 2. Poorly defined MR signal intensity abnormalities lateral, proximal, or distal to the lateral femoral epicondyle were found in 12 (75%) of 16 patients (Table 3). On coronal images, signal intensity changes were observed deep to the ITT proximal to the lateral femoral epicondyle in the fatty layer extending distal to the vastus lateralis muscle (Figs 4–6). On axial images, in four (23%) of 17 knees signal intensity abnormalities were located in the posterolateral aspect of the knee joint, in an area confined by the biceps femoris muscle and the femoral shaft. In six (35%) of 17 knees, signal intensity alterations were found distal to the lateral femoral epicondyle, bounded medially by the lateral collateral ligament and the meniscocapsular junction and laterally by the ITT. The ITT demonstrated normal signal intensity on all MR images. Signal intensity abnormalities were accompanied by a joint effusion in five (29%) of 17 knees and by meniscal tears in three (18%) of 17 knees. In the patient group, the mean width of the ITT at the level of the lateral femoral epicondyle was 2.3 mm ± 0.54 (1 SD). In comparison, the width of the ITT in healthy subjects was 2.0 mm ± 0.46 (1 SD). The difference in measurements between the two groups was not significant ($P = .8$).

A circumscribed fluid collection medial to the ITT was observed in five (31%) of 16 patients (Figs 7, 8). The size of this fluid collection varied from 1.0 × 0.5 × 0.5 cm to 5.0 × 1.5 × 5.0 cm. In two knees, the fluid collections extended distal to the lateral femoral epicondyle into the fatty layer located distal to the vastus lateralis muscle. In addition, in four knees the cystic lesions were located either lateral or proximal to the lateral femoral epicondyle of the femur.

DISCUSSION

Findings of previous studies (5,7,15) show that ITBFS is related to an inflamed bursa beneath the ITT caused by friction created when the ITT passes from anterior to posterior over the lateral femoral epicondyle during the early stages of knee flexion. Our results were derived from close

TABLE 2
Summary of Clinical Findings in Patients with ITBFS

Patient No./ Age (y)/Sex	Knee	Activity	Clinical History	Therapy*
1/28/M	Left	Long-distance running	Lateral knee pain with swelling and tenderness	Rest, NSAID, physical therapy
2/22/M	Left	Jogging	Anterolateral knee pain	Rest, ice, NSAID
3/34/F	Left	Marathon running	Lateral and anterior knee pain especially after long-distance running	Rest, NSAID, physical therapy
4/52/M	Left	Nonathlete	Lateral knee pain with tenderness over the lateral femoral epicondyle	Rest
5/37/F	Right	Walking	Lateral knee pain after walking	Rest, ice
6/32/M	Left	Roller blading	Anterolateral knee pain	Rest, NSAID, physical therapy
7/45/F	Right	Jogging	Lateral knee pain	Rest, physical therapy
8/34/M	Left	Nonathlete	Swelling with lateral knee pain after sports activity	Rest, ice, NSAID, physical therapy
9/20/M	Left	Hiking, rock climbing	Tenderness and pain over the lateral femoral epicondyle	Rest, ice, NSAID
10/17/F	Left	Soccer playing	Lateral knee pain, swelling, and tenderness of the lateral femoral epicondyle	Rest, ice, physical therapy
11/54/F	Left	Nonathlete	Anterolateral knee pain	Rest, ice
12/45/F	Left	Aerobics and walking	Lateral thigh and knee pain	Rest, NSAID, physical therapy
13/40/F	Left	Jogging	Anterolateral knee pain with tenderness and swelling	Rest, ice, NSAID, physical therapy
14/38/F	Left	Long-distance running	Lateral knee pain with tenderness above the lateral femoral epicondyle	Rest, NSAID, physical therapy
15/40/F	Left Right	Marathon running	Lateral knee pain on both sides	Rest, ice, NSAID, physical therapy
16/33/F	Right	Nonathlete	Anterolateral knee pain	Rest, physical therapy

* NSAID = nonsteroidal antiinflammatory drugs.

TABLE 3
Summary of MR Imaging Findings in Patients with ITBFS

Patient No./ Age (y)/Sex	Knee	Poorly Defined Signal Intensity Abnormalities in Relation to LFE*	Localized Fluid Collection		Signal Intensity Alterations in Relation to ITT	Width of the Iliotibial Band (mm)	Additional Findings
			Size (cm)	In Relation to LFE*			
1/28/M	Left	Lateral, proximal, distal	ND	. . .	Medial	2	Joint effusion
2/22/M	Left	Lateral, proximal, distal	ND	. . .	Medial	2	Medial meniscal tear
3/34/F	Left	Lateral, proximal	ND	. . .	Medial	3	Joint effusion
4/52/M	Left	Lateral, proximal, distal	ND	. . .	Medial, lateral	2.5	Joint effusion
5/37/F	Right	Lateral, proximal	ND	. . .	Medial	2	Joint effusion
6/32/M	Left	Lateral, proximal	ND	. . .	Medial	3	None
7/45/F	Right	Lateral, proximal, distal	ND	. . .	Medial	2.5	None
8/34/M	Left	Lateral, proximal	ND	. . .	Medial	2	None
9/20/M	Left	Lateral, proximal	ND	. . .	Medial	2	Joint effusion
10/17/F	Left	Lateral, proximal, distal	ND	. . .	Medial	2	Medial meniscal tear
11/54/F	Left	Lateral, proximal, distal	ND	. . .	Medial	3	None
12/45/F	Left	ND	$4.0 \times 1.5 \times 1.0$	Proximal	Medial	1.5	None
13/40/F	Left	Proximal	$5.0 \times 1.5 \times 5.0$	Lateral, proximal, distal	Medial	3.5	Lateral meniscal tear
14/38/F	Left	ND	$2.0 \times 1.0 \times 1.0$	Lateral, proximal, distal	Medial	1.5	None
15/40/F	Left	ND	$1.0 \times 0.5 \times 0.5$	Lateral	Medial	2.5	None
	Right	ND	$1.0 \times 1.5 \times 0.5$	Lateral	Medial	2	None
16/33/F	Right	ND	$1.0 \times 0.5 \times 0.5$	Proximal	Medial	2.5	None

Note.—ND = not detected.
* LFE = lateral femoral epicondyle.

correlation of the results of MR imaging and microscopic examination in cadavers and showed no bursa beneath the ITT (9,16). At microscopic inspection, in all specimens, a thin layer of fatty tissue was found between the ITT and the lateral femoral epicondyle. In addition, as demonstrated in our studies accomplished at full extension of the knee and at 30° and 60° of knee flexion and by corresponding microscopic examination, the lateral synovial recess was found in all specimens to be located anterior and proximal to the lateral femoral epicondyle.

These observations are in contrast to the findings of Nemeth and Sanders (15), who suggested that synovial tissue from the lateral recess insinuates itself under the ITT to become an interface between the ITT and the lateral femoral epicondyle and acts like a bursa and allows the ITT to move over the lateral femoral epicondyle with minimal shearing forces. This latter study (15), however, was performed only at full extension of the knee. Therefore, the relationships of the lateral recess to the lateral femoral epicondyle at different degrees of knee flexion were not evaluated.

While the ITBFS was previously thought to be related to either an invagination of the lateral recess of the knee joint under the ITT or inflammation of a primary bursa, the results of our cadaveric studies demonstrated additional information concerning the dynamic changes in the

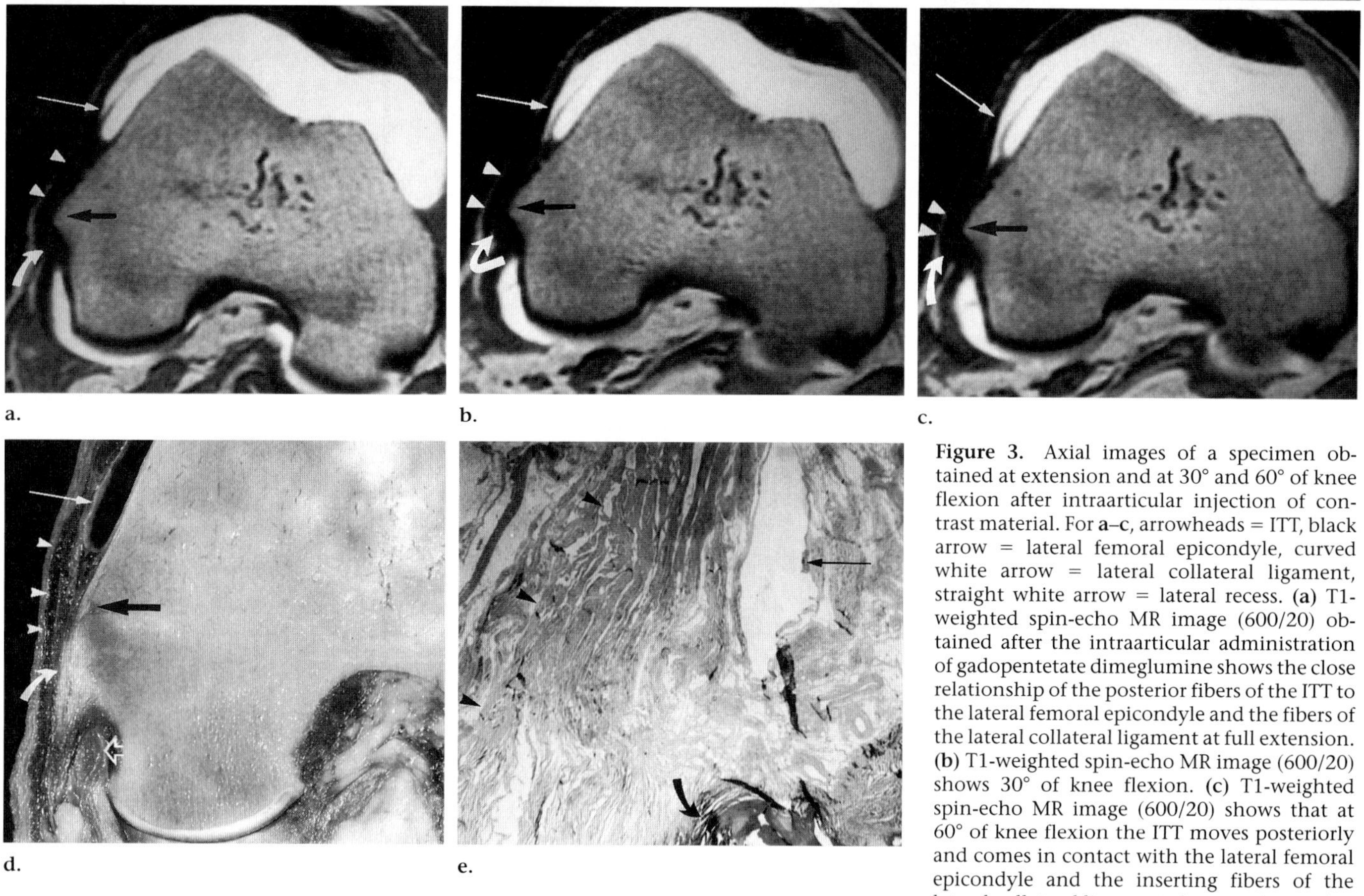

Figure 3. Axial images of a specimen obtained at extension and at 30° and 60° of knee flexion after intraarticular injection of contrast material. For **a–c**, arrowheads = ITT, black arrow = lateral femoral epicondyle, curved white arrow = lateral collateral ligament, straight white arrow = lateral recess. **(a)** T1-weighted spin-echo MR image (600/20) obtained after the intraarticular administration of gadopentetate dimeglumine shows the close relationship of the posterior fibers of the ITT to the lateral femoral epicondyle and the fibers of the lateral collateral ligament at full extension. **(b)** T1-weighted spin-echo MR image (600/20) shows 30° of knee flexion. **(c)** T1-weighted spin-echo MR image (600/20) shows that at 60° of knee flexion the ITT moves posteriorly and comes in contact with the lateral femoral epicondyle and the inserting fibers of the lateral collateral ligament. At extension and at 30° and 60° of knee flexion, the lateral recess extends anterior to the lateral femoral epicondyle. **(d)** Photograph of the corresponding macroscopic section reveals prominent inserting fibers of the lateral collateral ligament (curved white arrow) distal to the lateral femoral epicondyle (black arrow) in close proximity to the ITT (arrowheads). Straight white arrow = lateral recess, open arrow = popliteus tendon. **(e)** Photomicrograph shows layers of fatty tissue and vessels between the lateral femoral epicondyle (curved arrow) and the ITT (arrowheads). No bursa is identified. The lateral recess (straight arrow) extends anterior to the lateral femoral epicondyle (curved arrow). (Hematoxylin-eosin stain; original magnification, ×4.)

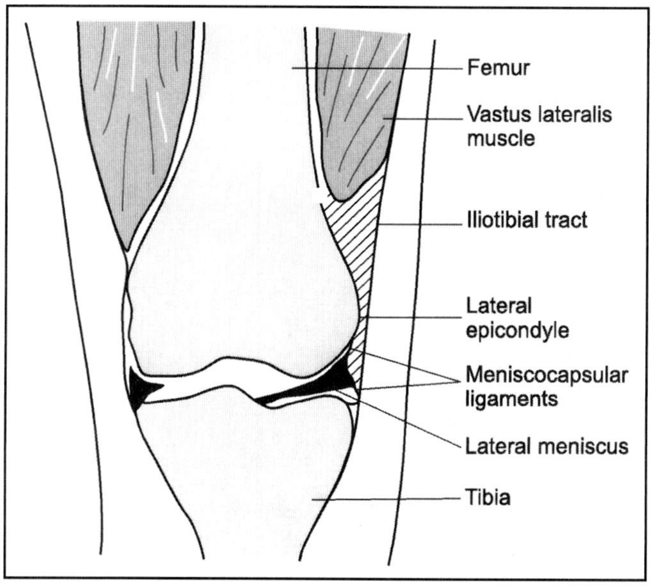

Figure 4. Drawing of the compartmentlike space in which signal intensity changes can be observed on coronal MR images in patients with ITBFS. The signal intensity abnormalities are located in the confines of a space demarcated laterally by the ITT and distally and medially by the meniscocapsular ligaments, the lateral meniscus, and the lateral femoral epicondyle. Proximal to the lateral femoral epicondyle, the signal intensity alterations extend into the fatty tissue distal to the vastus lateralis muscle.

lateral aspect of the knee during knee flexion. The ITT, the lateral collateral ligament, the popliteus tendon, and the insertion of the tendon of the biceps femoris muscle form a complex of tissues. In extension, the ITT is normally located anterior to the femoral insertion of the popliteus tendon and the lateral collateral ligament.

In some patients, however, posterior fibers of the ITT may remain in contact with the lateral femoral epicondyle in extension. When the knee flexes, the ITT

Figure 5. Patient 10. Images obtained in a 17-year-old soccer player with lateral knee pain for 6 weeks. (a) Coronal T2-weighted fat-saturated fast spin-echo MR image (4,400/108, 4-mm section thickness) reveals poorly defined high-signal-intensity alterations (straight arrows) medial to the ITT (arrowheads) that extend into the fatty layer distal to the vastus lateralis muscle (curved arrow). (b) Corresponding axial T2-weighted fat-saturated fast spin-echo MR image (4,400/108, 4-mm section thickness) demonstrates soft-tissue edema (arrows) between the ITT (arrowheads) and the femur.

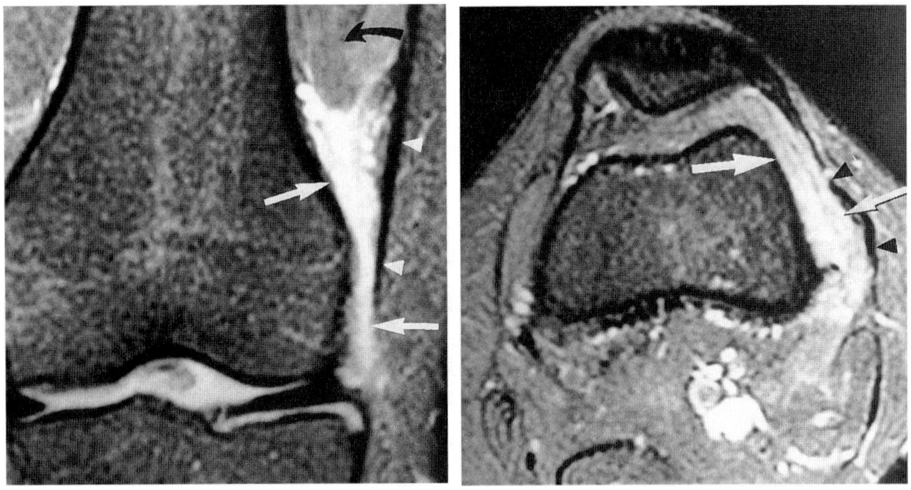

a. b.

Figure 6. Patient 9. Images obtained in a 20-year-old freehand rock climber with tenderness and pain over the lateral femoral epicondyle. (a) Coronal T1-weighted spin-echo MR image (550/18, 4-mm section thickness) shows poorly defined low-signal-intensity changes (straight arrows) medial to the ITT (arrowheads) and distal to the vastus lateralis muscle (curved arrow). (b) Corresponding coronal two-dimensional multiplanar gradient-recalled-echo image (600/15, 4-mm section thickness, 30° flip angle) shows high-signal-intensity alterations (arrows) that correspond to the low-signal-intensity changes in a. Arrowheads = ITT. (c) Axial T2-weighted fat-saturated fast spin-echo MR image (4,400/108, 4-mm section thickness) shows abnormal signal intensity alterations (white arrow) lateral to the lateral femoral epicondyle (black arrow). Arrowhead = ITT. (d) Axial T2-weighted fat-saturated fast spin-echo MR image (4,400/108, 4-mm section thickness) shows abnormal signal intensity alterations (solid arrows) medial to the ITT (arrowhead), adjacent to the biceps femoris muscle (open arrow) and femur.

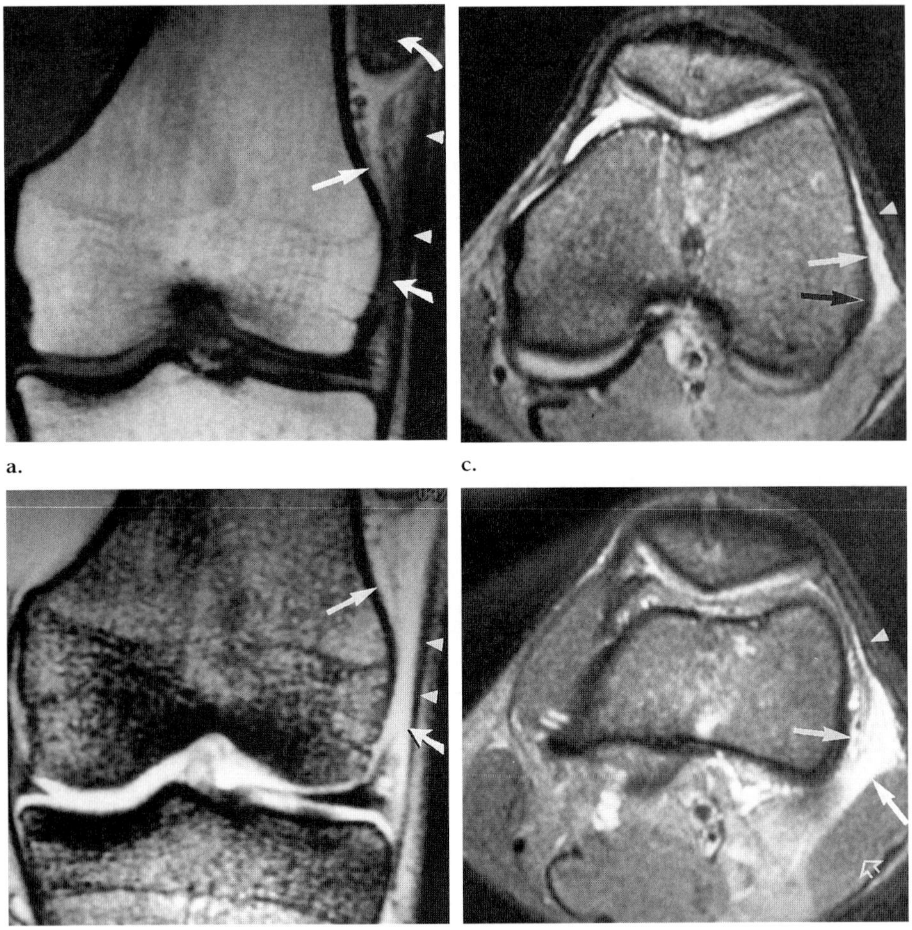

a. c. b. d.

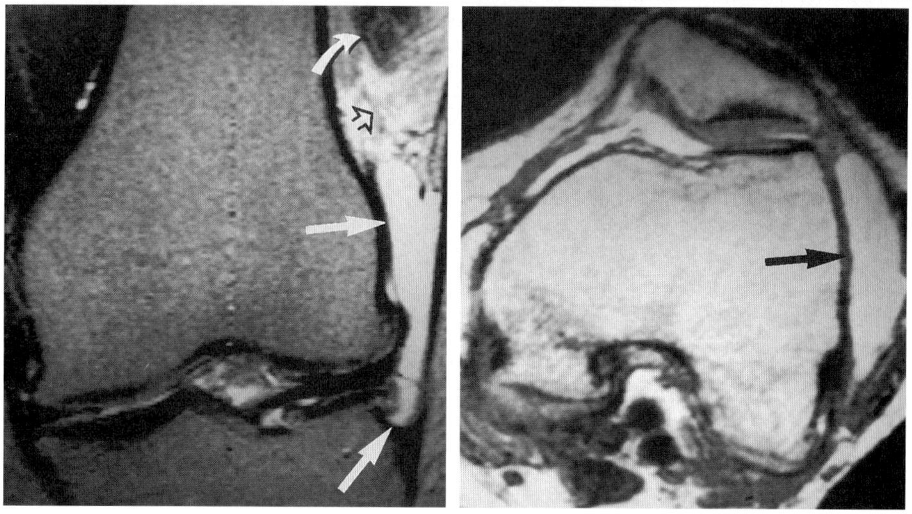

a. b.

Figure 7. Patient 13. Images obtained in a 40-year-old jogger with anterolateral knee pain, swelling, and tenderness. **(a)** Coronal T2-weighted fat-saturated fast spin-echo MR image (4,400/108, 4-mm section thickness) demonstrates a high-signal-intensity large cystic fluid collection (straight arrows) medial to the ITT and extending to the tibial plateau. The lesion extends proximal to the lateral femoral epicondyle with soft-tissue edema (open arrow) adjacent to the vastus lateralis muscle (curved arrow). **(b)** Axial three-dimensional double-echo steady state MR image (27/9, 1.6-mm section thickness, 40° flip angle) shows a well-circumscribed fluid collection (arrow) medial to the ITT.

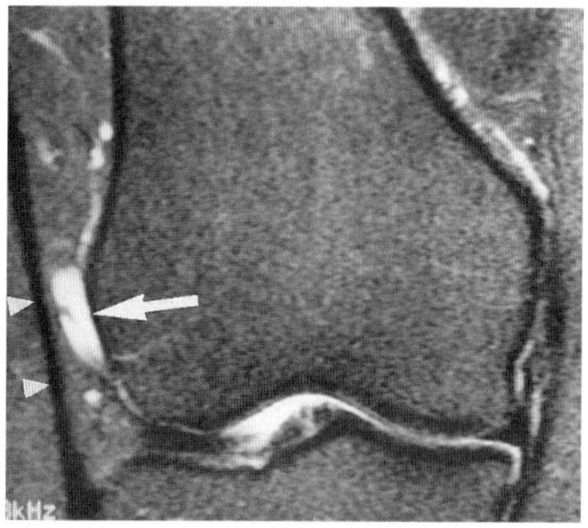

a.

Figure 8. Patient 15. Images obtained in a 40-year-old marathon runner with persistent bilateral knee pain and tenderness. **(a)** Coronal T2-weighted fat-saturated fast spin-echo MR image (4,400/108, 4-mm section thickness) demonstrates small cystic fluid collections (arrow), which are 1.5 × 1.0 cm, on the right side medial to the ITT (arrowheads) adjacent to the lateral femoral epicondyle. **(b)** Coronal T2-weighted fat-saturated fast spin-echo MR image (4,400/108, 4-mm section thickness) shows a similar cystic lesion (arrow), which is 1.0 × 0.5 cm, on the left side. The ITT (arrowheads) shows no signal intensity alterations or thickening.

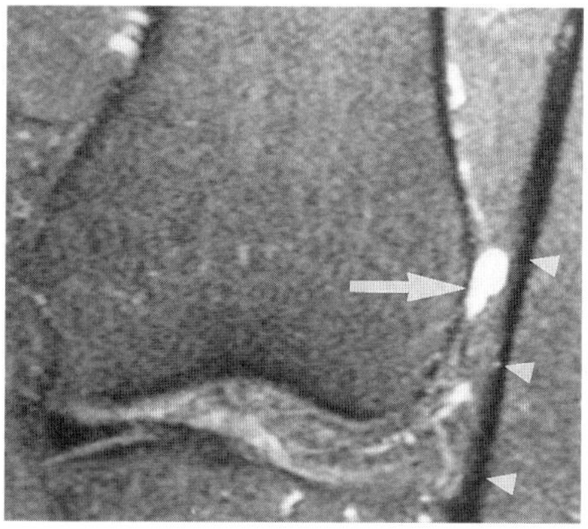

b.

begins to move posteriorly and comes in contact with the lateral femoral epicondyle and the inserting fibers of the lateral collateral ligament below this epicondyle (Fig 3). With further flexion, however, the ITT, the lateral collateral ligament, and the popliteus tendon cross each other at one point and result in further friction of the ITT during joint motion (10).

The MR imaging characteristics in the patients with ITBFS in our study were consistent with those found by Murphy et al (12) and Nishimura et al (13). Poorly defined signal intensity alterations were observed in the fatty tissue deep to the ITT in the majority of patients, except in one patient with additional signal intensity changes superficial to the ITT. In addition, in our study the signal intensity abnormalities (high signal intensity on T2-weighted and gradient-echo sequences and low signal intensity on T1-weighted sequences) were located within a compartmentlike space demarcated laterally by the ITT and distally and medially by the meniscocapsular junction of the lateral meniscus, the lateral collateral ligament, and the lateral femoral epicondyle. Proximal to this epicondyle, the signal intensity alterations extended into the fatty tissue distal to the vastus lateralis muscle. Posterolateral signal intensity alterations were seen in an area bounded by the ITT and the biceps femoris muscle.

In common with the findings of previous studies (7,12,13), circumscribed fluid collections at MR imaging were found in a minority of patients with ITBFS in our study. In addition, these well-defined fluid collections had the same compartmentlike distribution as the poorly defined soft-tissue edema described previously. The signal intensity characteristics were similar to those observed in patients with bursitis of the pes anserinus or the tibial collateral ligament (17–19). Our results support the findings of other anatomic investigations (5,8,16–22) that suggest the well-defined fluid collections are more likely to arise from chronic inflammation beneath the ITT with formation of a secondary, or adventitious, bursa, rather than from inflammation of a primary bursa. However, further studies are necessary to verify this hypothesis.

Our observations seem to be similar to findings in patients with amputations below the knee, in whom adventitious bursae develop over the head of the fibula and the tibial tubercle because of chronic friction and pressure caused by an unsatisfactory fit or malalignment or suspension of the prosthesis (20–22). However, solely on the basis of microscopic examination as performed in patients with ITBFS treated surgically, differentiation between a true bursa and bursalike reactive tissue is sometimes difficult (2,13,15).

In addition, our results indicate a normal width of the ITT in patients with early stages of ITBFS when compared with that in a healthy control group. Our findings are in contrast to those of Ekman and co-workers (7), who noted a thickened ITT in patients with ITBFS. However, thickening of the ITT may represent a chronic stage of ITBFS rather than an acute or subacute stage of this syndrome as seen in recreational athletes or even nonathletic persons with sudden onset of clinical symptoms.

Our study has several limitations. First, due to the inability to compare MR findings with clinical data such as the duration and the severity of symptoms, no predisposing factors for the development of an adventitious bursa could be established. Second, the relationships of the ITT to the lateral femoral epicondyle at full extension and at 30° and 60° of flexion were determined in cadavers rather than in living subjects, a situation that is not entirely analogous to the examination of patients. Third, artifacts produced by anatomic sectioning or freezing may have influenced the observations, although this appeared to be a minor problem. Fourth, as only a small number of specimens derived from elderly cadavers were included in this study, it is difficult to determine the relationship of the lateral recess to the lateral femoral epicondyle during knee motion and the prevalence of a primary bursa beneath the ITT in the general population.

In summary, with MR imaging, poorly defined signal intensity abnormalities or a circumscribed fluid collection located in a compartmentlike space medial to the ITT with obliteration of the fatty layer distal to the vastus lateralis muscle may allow the diagnosis of ITBFS in patients with corresponding clinical symptoms. Our results derived from cadaveric studies demonstrate a close relationship of the ITT to the lateral femoral condyle during knee flexion. Our results also suggest that localized fluid collections in patients with the ITBFS are more likely due to inflammation of a secondary, or adventitious, bursa rather than to inflammation of synovial tissue arising from the lateral recess of the knee joint or from a primary bursa.

Acknowledgment: The authors specially thank Gerd Baumer for the preparation of the positioning devices.

References

1. Orava S. Iliotibial tract friction syndrome in athletes: an uncommon exertion syndrome on the lateral side of the knee. Br J Sports Med 1978; 12:69–73.
2. Martens M, Libbrecht P, Burssens A. Surgical treatment of the iliotibial band friction syndrome. Am J Sports Med 1989; 17:651–654.
3. Noble CA. Iliotibial band friction syndrome in runners. Am J Sports Med 1980; 8:232–234.
4. McNicol K, Taunton JE, Clement DB. Iliotibial tract friction syndrome in athletes. Can J Appl Sport Sci 1981; 6:76–80.
5. Orchard JW, Fricker PA, Abud AT, Mason BR. Biomechanics of iliotibial band friction syndrome in runners. Am J Sports Med 1996; 24:375–379.
6. Pavlov H. Physical injury: sports related abnormalities. In: Resnick D, ed. Diagnosis of bone and joint disorders. 3rd ed. Philadelphia, Pa: Saunders, 1995; 3256–3257.
7. Ekman EF, Pope T, Martin DF, Curl WW. Magnetic resonance imaging of iliotibial band syndrome. Am J Sports Med 1994; 22:851–854.
8. Terry GC, Hughston JC, Norwood LA. The anatomy of the iliopatellar band and iliotibial tract. Am J Sports Med 1986; 14: 39–45.
9. Grana WA, Larson RL. Functional and surgical anatomy. In: Larson RL, Grana WA, eds. The knee: form, function, pathology, and treatment. Philadelphia, Pa: Saunders, 1993; 11–50.
10. Kaplan EB. Some aspects of functional anatomy of the human knee joint. In: DePalmer AF, ed. Clinical orthopaedics. Philadelphia, Pa: Lippincott, 1962; 18–29.
11. DeGreter F, De Neve J, VanSteelandt H. Bone scan in iliotibial band syndrome. Clin Nucl Med 1995; 20:550–551.
12. Murphy BJ, Hechtman KS, Uribe JW, Selesnick H, Smith RL, Zlatkin MB. Iliotibial band friction syndrome: MR imaging findings. Radiology 1992; 185:569–571.
13. Nishimura G, Yamato M, Tamai K, Takahashi J, Uetani M. MR findings in iliotibial band syndrome. Skeletal Radiol 1997; 26: 533–537.
14. Engel A. Magnetic resonance knee arthrography: enhanced contrast by gadolinium complex in the rabbit and in humans. Acta Orthop Scand 1990; 240(suppl): 1–57.
15. Nemeth WC, Sanders BL. The lateral synovial recess of the knee: anatomy and role in chronic iliotibial band friction syndrome. Arthroscopy 1996; 12:574–580.
16. Williams PL, Warwick R. Arthrology. In: Williams PL, Warwick R, eds. Gray's anatomy. 36th ed. Philadelphia, Pa: Saunders, 1980; 487.
17. Lee JK, Yao L. Tibial collateral ligament bursa: MR imaging. Radiology 1991; 178: 855–857.
18. LaPrade RF, Hamilton CD. The fibular collateral ligament-biceps femoris bursa: an anatomic study. Am J Sports Med 1997; 25:439–443.
19. Forbes JR, Helms CA, Janzen DL. Acute pes anserine bursitis: MR imaging. Radiology 1995; 194:525–527.
20. Ahmed A, Bayol MG, Ha DB. Adventitious bursae in below knee amputees: case report and a review of the literature. Am J Phys Med Rehabil 1994; 73:124–129.
21. Rubin G, Dixon M, Fischer E. Lower extremity amputation problems: etiology, manifestations, and prevention. Orthot Prosthet 1985; 39:47–61.
22. Kuhns JG. Adventitious bursas. Arch Surg 1943; 47:687–696.

Bicipitoradial Bursitis: MR Imaging Findings in Eight Patients and Anatomic Data from Contrast Material Opacification of Bursae Followed by Routine Radiography and MR Imaging in Cadavers[1]

Abdalla Y. Skaf, MD
Robert D. Boutin, MD
Robert Weiber M. Dantas, MD
Andrew W. Hooper, MD
Claus Muhle, MD
David S. Chou, MD
Nittaya Lektrakul, MD
Debra J. Trudell, RA
Parviz Haghighi, MD
Donald L. Resnick, MD

Index terms:
Bursa, 422.251
Bursitis, 422.251
Elbow, anatomy, 422.11, 422.121411, 422.121415, 422.12143, 422.251, 422.92
Elbow, MR, 422.121411, 422.121415, 422.12143

Radiology 1999; 212:111–116

[1] From the Departments of Radiology (A.Y.S., R.D.B., R.W.M.D., A.W.H., C.M., D.S.C., N.L., D.J.T., D.L.R.) and Pathology (P.H.), Veterans Affairs Medical Center and University of California San Diego, 3350 La Jolla Village Dr, San Diego, CA 92161. Received April 23, 1998; revision requested June 24; final revision received December 15; accepted January 15, 1999. Supported in part by Veterans Administration grant no. SA-360. **Address reprint requests to** D.L.R. (e-mail: *dresnick@ucsd.edu*).

PURPOSE: To use radiography and magnetic resonance (MR) imaging after contrast material opacification of the bursae in cadaveric specimens to demonstrate the anatomy of the bicipitoradial bursa and to report MR imaging findings in patients with bicipitoradial bursitis.

MATERIALS AND METHODS: Bicipitoradial bursa in eight cadaveric elbows were injected with a solution containing gadodiamide, iodinated contrast agent, and gelatin. Radiographs and MR images were obtained in each specimen, with both supination and pronation of the forearm. The morphology and relationships of the bursa were studied. Anatomic sections subsequently were obtained. MR imaging studies in eight patients with bicipitoradial bursitis were also evaluated.

RESULTS: The bicipitoradial bursa revealed a smooth outline and a wide base along the superficial aspect of the radius. The mean volume of contrast material that could be injected before extravasation was 4 mL. The mean size of the bursa was 1.8 × 2.5 cm. The bicipitoradial bursa enveloped the biceps tendon, with internal septation seen in two cases. Displacement of the superficial branch of the radial nerve by the bursa was found in two specimens. Communication between the bicipitoradial bursa and elbow joint was not observed. In patients, MR imaging demonstrated fluid collections in the bicipitoradial bursa in all cases, with compression of branches of the radial nerve in two cases.

CONCLUSION: The anatomy of the bicipitoradial bursa is demonstrated with radiography and MR imaging of bursae. MR imaging allows accurate diagnosis of bicipitoradial bursitis and its effects on adjacent structures.

Author contributions:
Guarantors of integrity of entire study, A.Y.S., D.L.R.; study concepts, D.L.R.; study design, A.Y.S., D.L.R.; definition of intellectual content, R.D.B., D.L.R.; literature research, A.Y.S., A.W.H.; clinical studies, R.D.B., C.M., R.W.M.D.; experimental studies, R.D.B., A.Y.S., R.W.M.D., D.J.T.; data acquisition, R.D.B., D.J.T.; data analysis, R.D.B., A.W.H., C.M., P.H., N.L.; manuscript preparation, N.L., A.Y.S., R.D.B.; manuscript editing, D.S.C., N.L., D.L.R., R.D.B.; manuscript review, N.L., D.L.R., R.D.B.

Bursal cavities are interposed between surfaces that move on each other and produce a friction force, such as sites where a tendon glides over a projecting bone surface (1). The bursae found in the cubital fossa (cubital bursae) consist of the bicipitoradial bursa and interosseous bursa (Fig 1), which occasionally communicate. When inflamed, the bursae may enlarge and produce symptoms. Patients with cubital bursitis present clinically with a mass in the cubital fossa, sensory and motor symptoms and signs resulting from nerve compression, or both. To our knowledge, few reports describing the anatomy (2–5) and magnetic resonance (MR) imaging (4–7) of the bicipitoradial bursa have been published.

The purpose of our study was twofold. First, our objective was to describe the normal imaging anatomy of the bicipitoradial bursa, including its relationship with the radial

Figure 1. **(a)** Diagram demonstrates the normal anatomy of the antecubital fossa in the coronal plane. The relationships between the bicipitoradial bursa, biceps tendon, and neural structures are shown. *Flex* = flexor. **(b)** Diagram shows that the bicipitoradial bursa (*BRB*) surrounds the biceps tendon (*BT*) in supination. In pronation, the radial tuberosity (*rt*) rotates posteriorly, which compresses the bicipitoradial bursa between the biceps tendon and the radial cortex; this consequently increases the pressure within the bursa. *R* = radius, *U* = ulna. **(c)** Photograph of a transaxial cadaveric section shows the exact location of the bicipitoradial bursa (long black arrow) between the biceps tendon (arrowheads) and the cortex of the radius (*R*) and its relationship with the adjacent neural structures. Also demonstrated are the median nerve (long white arrow), the superficial branch of the radial nerve (short black arrow), and the deep branch of the radial nerve (short white arrow).

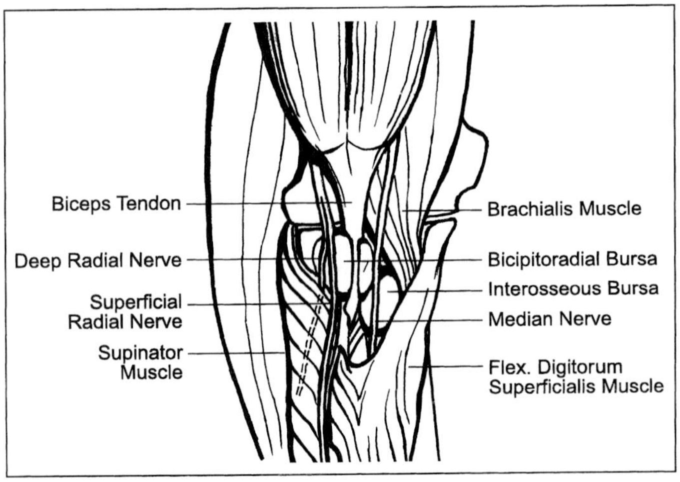

a.

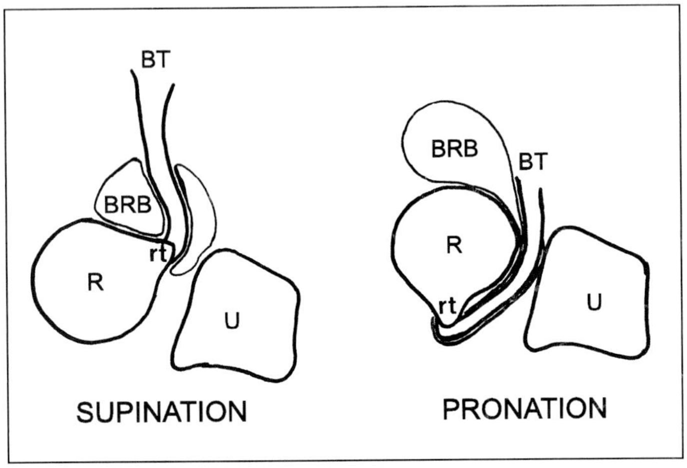

b.

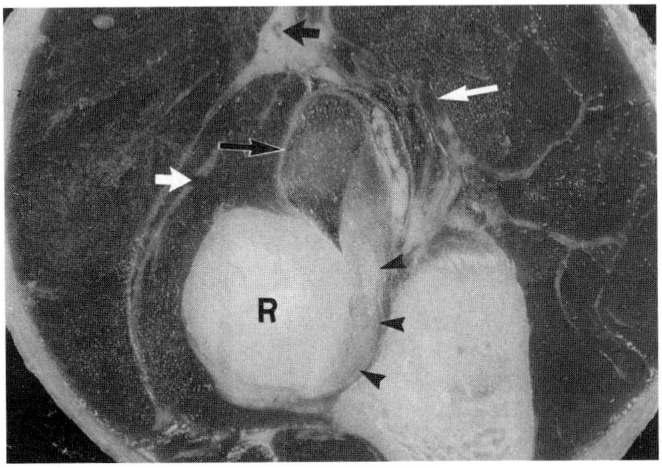

c.

insertion of the biceps tendon and the adjacent branches of the radial nerve, by using radiography and MR imaging after contrast material opacification of the bursa. Our second aim was to report the MR findings in eight patients with bicipitoradial bursitis.

MATERIALS AND METHODS

Cadaveric Study

Eight upper extremities (transected at the midhumeral level) containing the wrist and hand were obtained from fresh nonembalmed cadavers (four women, four men; age range at death, 75–88 years; mean age at death, 80 years) and were immediately deep-frozen at −40°C (Bio-Freezer; Forma Scientific, Marietta, Ohio). The specimens were allowed to thaw for 24 hours at room temperature prior to imaging. All specimens were examined with anteroposterior and lateral radiography to confirm the absence of arthritis or previous osseous injuries affecting the elbow.

Imaging of bursae.—A single-contrast technique was used for both radiography and MR imaging of bursae. The contrast material that was injected was a 3–6-mL mixture of iohexol (Omnipaque; Nycomed Amersham, Princeton, NJ), gadodiamide (Omniscan; Nycomed Amersham), and a 15% concentrated solution of gelatin. Gadodiamide was injected in a concentration of 2 mmol/L. To obtain this concentration, 2 mL of gadodiamide was added to 250 mL of a normal saline solution (7), and 5 mL of the resultant solution was mixed with 5 mL of iohexol and 5 mL of the gelatin solution. With fluoroscopic guidance, a 22-gauge (0.7 × 40.0-mm) needle was inserted obliquely through the skin from an anterior approach and advanced until the proximal portion of the radial tuberosity was contacted (Fig 2). The intrabursal position of the tip of the needle was verified with a test injection of a small amount of iohexol. The bursa was slowly and progressively distended until resistance to further injection was met. When the needle was withdrawn, pressure was maintained at the point of entry to prevent leakage of contrast material.

Elbow radiographs (radiographic unit manufactured by Siemens, Erlangen, Germany) obtained after the injection procedure included anteroposterior and lateral projections with supination and pronation of the forearm. The upper arm was fixed to a frame by Velcro straps to guide these movements.

The interval between radiography and MR imaging of bursae varied from 30 to 80 minutes. With the arm placed in extension, MR images were obtained by using two receive-only 3-inch extremity surface coils and a 1.5-T magnet (Signa; GE Medical Systems, Milwaukee, Wis). Imaging was performed in transaxial, coronal ob-

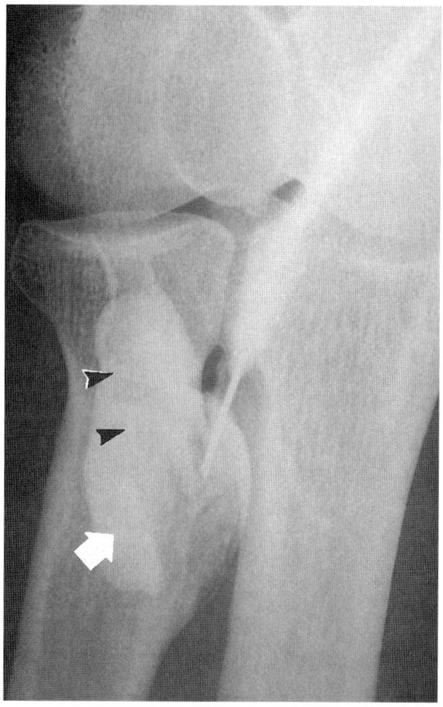

Figure 2. Anteroposterior radiograph of the bicipitoradial bursa in a cadaver. The needle is placed immediately superficial to the radial tuberosity. Contrast material outlines the bicipitoradial bursa (arrow) that surrounds the biceps tendon (arrowheads).

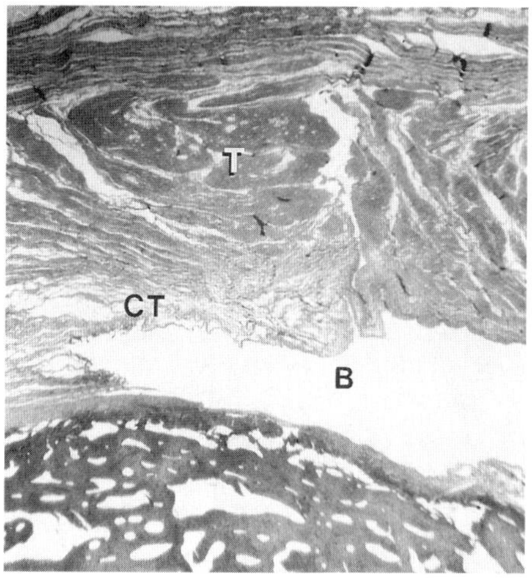

Figure 3. Photomicrograph. Bicipitoradial bursa (*B*) separates the biceps tendon (*T*) from the bone. There is a thin layer of irregular collagenous connective tissue (*CT*) between the tendon and the bursa. (Hematoxylin-eosin stain; original magnification, ×4.)

lique, and sagittal oblique planes. Transaxial and sagittal oblique images were obtained with supination and pronation of the forearm. The coronal oblique images were obtained only with supination of the forearm. T1-weighted spin-echo and fat-suppressed T1-weighted spin-echo sequences were obtained with these parameters: 500/15 msec (repetition time msec/echo time msec), two signals acquired, 12-cm field of view, 256 × 256 imaging matrix, and 3-mm section thickness, without an intersection gap.

Histology and radiography.—After MR imaging, the specimens were refrozen at −40°C and subsequently sectioned with a band saw into 3-mm sections that corresponded to the thickness of the images. The plane of anatomic section in each specimen corresponded to one of the imaging planes according to lines drawn on the specimen at the time of imaging. The sections were obtained in the transaxial plane in six specimens (three in pronation and three in supination) and in the sagittal and coronal oblique planes in one specimen each. Microscopic examination was performed by an experienced pathologist (P.H.) in four specimens to allow correlation with the macroscopic findings.

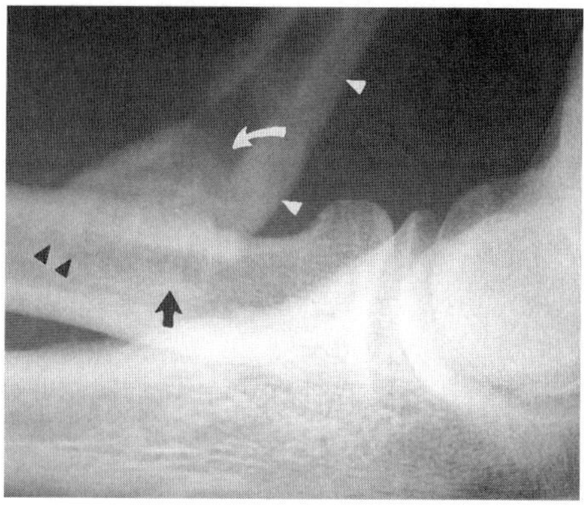

a.

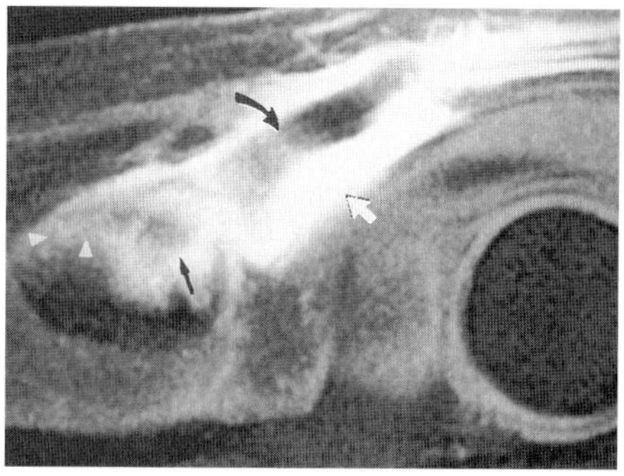

b.

Figure 4. (a) Radiograph of bursa in a cadaver shows the normal configuration of the bicipitoradial bursa (white arrowheads) in the lateral projection, with the arm supine. The tubular filling defect is the biceps tendon (curved arrow). Note the insertion of the biceps tendon (black arrowheads and straight arrow) into the radial tuberosity. (b) Sagittal T1-weighted fat-suppressed MR image (500/15) of the corresponding elbow. Note the bicipitoradial bursa (white straight arrow), biceps tendon (curved arrow), short head of the biceps tendon (arrowheads), and long head of the biceps tendon (black straight arrow).

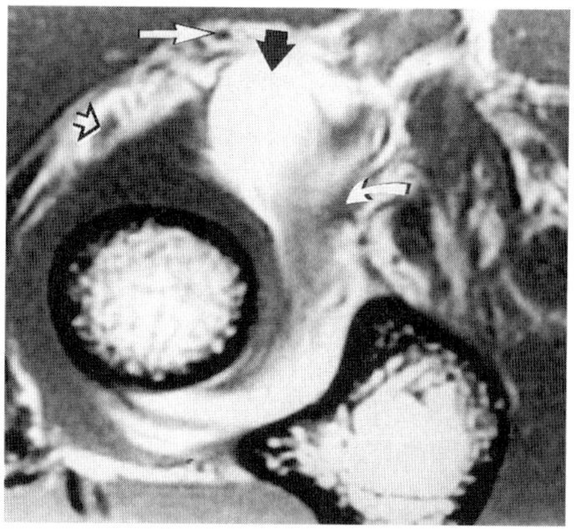

Figure 5. Transaxial T1-weighted spin-echo MR image (500/15) of the bursa in a cadaver. The distended bursa (black straight arrow) is in proximity with the superficial branch of the radial nerve (long white straight arrow) and may cause compression of the nerve. The short white straight arrow indicates the deep branch of the radial nerve, and the curved arrow indicates the biceps tendon.

Transaxial sections at the level of the radial insertion of the biceps tendon were imaged. A special radiographic unit (X-ray System 43805 N; Faxitron X-ray, division of Hewlett-Packard, Palo Alto, Calif) designed to examine sections of cadaveric specimens was then used after the injection of contrast material. Two musculoskeletal radiologists (A.Y.S., R.D.B.) evaluated these radiographs by consensus to determine the location and extent of the injected contrast material relative to the adjacent biceps tendon and radial tuberosity.

Clinical Study

We retrospectively reviewed MR images of the elbow obtained in eight patients (five men, three women; age range, 40–78 years; mean age, 52 years) with bicipitoradial bursitis for evaluation of their clinical manifestations. Two musculoskeletal radiologists (A.Y.S., R.D.B.) reviewed these images by consensus for the presence, extent, and appearance of any fluid collection in the expected position of the bicipitoradial bursa.

All MR images were obtained with the elbow in extension and the forearm in supination by using a pair of receive-only

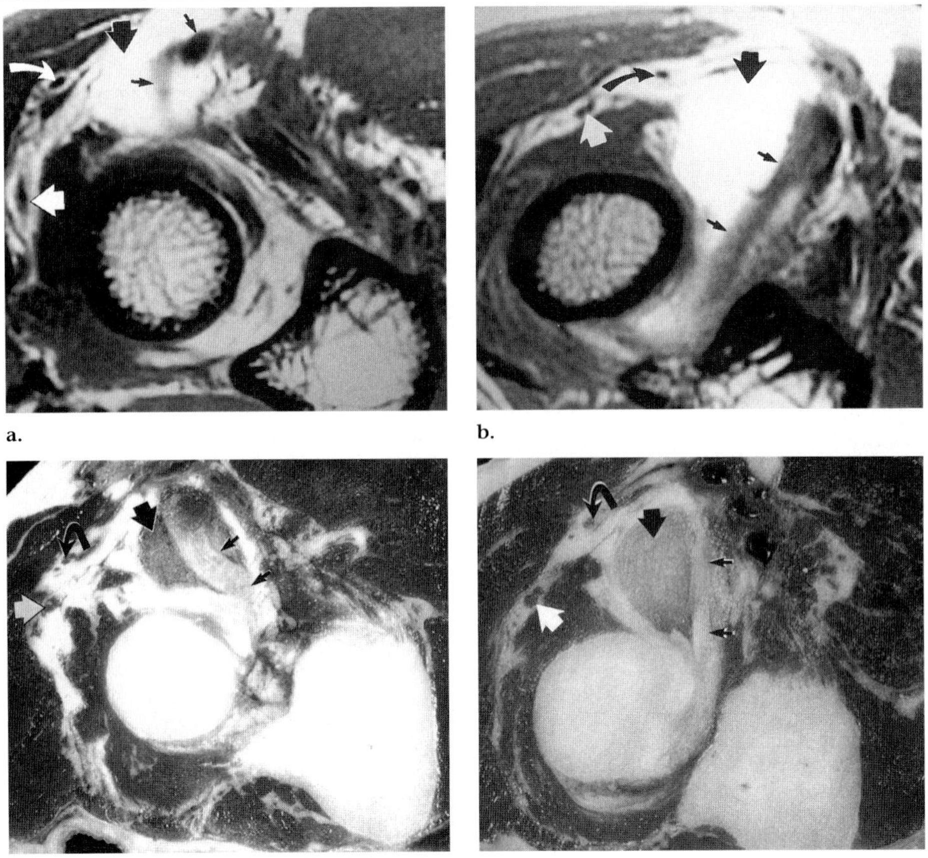

a. b. c. d.

Figure 6. In **a–d**, the large black straight arrow indicates the bicipitoradial bursa, the small black straight arrows indicate the biceps tendon, the curved arrow indicates the superficial branch of the radial nerve, and the white straight arrow indicates the deep branch of the radial nerve. **(a, b)** Transaxial T1-weighted MR images (500/15) with the forearm in **(a)** supination and **(b)** pronation. The bicipitoradial bursa changes shape with supination and pronation of the forearm. **(c, d)** Photographs of corresponding anatomic sections with the forearm in **(c)** supination and **(d)** pronation demonstrate similar findings, with the plane of section in the anatomic sample varying only slightly from that during MR imaging.

extremity surface coils placed dorsally and ventrally and a 1.5-T magnet (Signa, GE Medical Systems; Magnetom Vision, Siemens Medical Systems, Iselin, NJ). The sequences varied and consisted of T1-weighted spin-echo (300–500/15–20), T2-weighted fast spin-echo with or without fat suppression (2,500–4,800/40–112), and double-echo (intermediate-weighted and T2-weighted spin-echo; 3,000–4,600/17–20 and 90–110) imaging. The field of view was 12–15 cm, the section thickness was 2–4 mm, and the intersection gap was 1.0–2.5 mm, with two to four signals acquired.

RESULTS

Cadaveric Study

Imaging of bursae.—The bicipitoradial bursa was easily outlined by percutaneously injecting contrast material under fluoroscopic guidance between the biceps tendon anteriorly and the radial tuberosity posteriorly (Fig 3). In the transaxial plane, the bicipitoradial bursa had a wide base along the superficial aspect of the radius, with a mean dimension of 2.8 cm (range, 2.4–3.9 cm). In the sagittal oblique plane, the biceps tendon was partially enveloped by the bicipitoradial bursa for a mean length of 4.1 cm (range, 3.8–4.9 cm) proximal to the radial tubercle (Fig 4). The mean amount of contrast material that could be injected into the bursa without resistance was 4.1 mL (range, 3.6–5.3 mL). Extravasation occurred in one case after injection of 6.0 mL, with contrast material appearing adjacent to the paratenon of the biceps tendon.

With MR imaging of bursae, the bicipitoradial bursa was noted to have a smooth outline in six specimens. Septa were seen in only two cases with MR imaging of bursae. In all eight cases, no communication between the bicipitoradial bursa and the interosseous bursa or the elbow joint was observed. The biceps tendon was

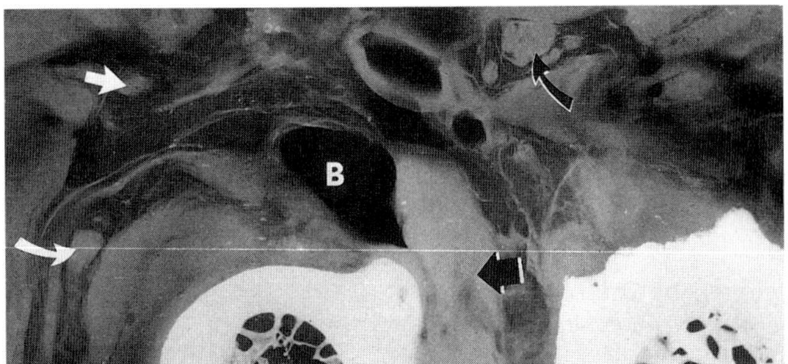

Figure 7. Faxitron radiograph in cadaver. Enthesopathic lesion (small black straight arrow) and cortical irregularity (arrowheads) of the radial tuberosity at the insertion site of the biceps tendon (large black straight arrow) may cause degenerative changes or biceps tendon bursitis. *B* indicates the bicipitoradial bursa, the straight white arrow indicates the superficial branch of the radial nerve, the curved white arrow indicates the deep branch of the radial nerve, and the curved black arrow indicates the median nerve.

Findings in Patients with Bicipitoradial Bursitis

Patient Age (y)/Sex	Elbow	Cause	Pain	Impairment of Movement	Palpable Mass in Cubital Fossa	Nerve Compression on MR Images	Extensor Muscle Weakness
49/F	Left	Rheumatoid arthritis	Yes	Yes	Yes	Superficial and deep branches of the radial nerve	Yes
78/M	Right	Partial tear of the biceps tendon	Yes	Yes	Yes	No	No
53/M	Right	Repetitive trauma	No	No	Yes	No	No
51/F	Right	Repetitive trauma	No	No	Yes	No	No
40/M	Right	Partial tear of the biceps tendon	Yes	No	Yes	No	No
48/M	Left	Partial tear of the biceps tendon	Yes	No	Yes	No	No
41/F	Left	Repetitive trauma	Yes	Yes	Yes	Superficial and deep branches of the radial nerve	Yes
56/M	Right	Partial tear of the biceps tendon	Yes	No	Yes	No	No

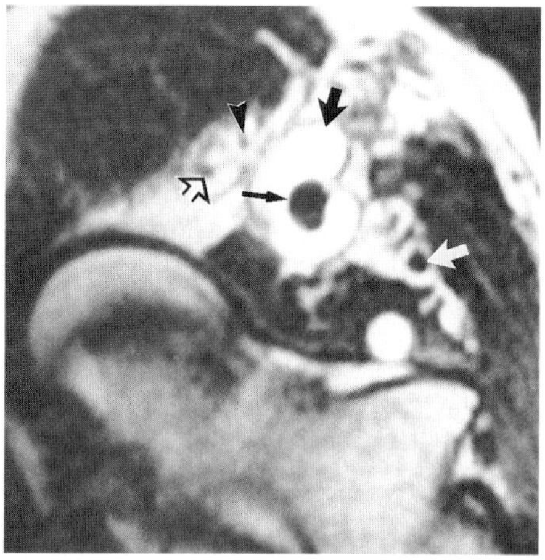

Figure 8. Transaxial fast T2-weighted MR image (4,800/112) obtained in a 53-year-old man with a palpable mass in the antecubital fossa shows the biceps tendon (small black solid arrow) completely enveloped by the bicipitoradial bursa (large black solid arrow). There is no direct contact of the bicipitoradial bursa with the median nerve (white solid arrow) or with the superficial (arrowhead) or deep (open arrow) branch of the radial nerve.

partially enveloped by the bicipitoradial bursa in six cases and was ensheathed completely by the bicipitoradial bursa in two cases.

After injection of 4.8 and 5.3 mL of solution, the superficial branch of the radial nerve was displaced volarly by the distended bicipitoradial bursa in the prone position (Fig 5), with the forearm in supination; no evidence of mass effect on the adjacent superficial branch of the radial nerve was observed. The deep branch of the radial nerve was not affected by the enlarged bursa in either pronation or supination (Fig 6).

Histology and Faxitron radiography.—The identification of anatomic structures with MR imaging was accurate, as confirmed with histologic examination. The distal tendon of the biceps brachii had no identifiable tendon sheath.

Faxitron radiographs demonstrated bone proliferation arising from the radial tuberosity at the biceps tendon insertion site in one specimen (Fig 7).

Clinical Study

Six of eight patients presented with pain in the cubital fossa. All patients had a palpable mass in this region at physical examination (Table). Two of these patients had additional weakness of the extensor muscles of the forearm, which correlated with nerve compression revealed at MR imaging.

MR imaging in all patients demonstrated distention of the bursa by fluid with hypointensity on T1-weighted images and hyperintensity on T2-weighted images. In three patients, the bicipitoradial bursa was noted to have a smooth outline; in the other three patients, the bicipitoradial bursa had an irregular outline. Septa within the bursa were seen in one patient; no communication between the bicipitoradial bursa and the interosseous bursa or the elbow joint was observed in any patient. The biceps tendon was partially enveloped by the bicipitoradial bursa in five patients; in the sixth patient, it was ensheathed completely by the bicipitoradial bursa (Fig 8). Direct contact of the superficial and deep branches of the radial nerve by the bicipitoradial bursa was found in two patients (Fig 9).

DISCUSSION

Bursae are located where structures that move relative to each other are in apposition, such as where tendons are deflected around bone or under retinacula in the vicinity of joints. At such sites, the bursa is composed of a simple flattened sac lined by a synovial membrane and supported by dense irregular connective tissue. The majority of bursae occur between a tendon and bone (eg, bicipitoradial bursa) and are termed "subtendinous bursae." Some bursae communicate with nearby joints such that the synovial membrane is continuous between the bursa and the articulation. Such communicating bursae may develop separately from the joint and only subsequently become connected with the articular cavity.

The role of the bicipitoradial bursa is to reduce friction between the biceps tendon and the tuberosity of the radius. In this fashion, the bicipitoradial bursa may allow free movement of the biceps tendon over a limited range of pronation and supination of the forearm (1). Sometimes the bicipitoradial bursa ensheaths the distal insertion of the biceps tendon for a short distance (1–3). Histologically, the bicipitoradial bursa contains a synovial lining, and its apposed walls are separated by a thin film of fluid. At histologic examination, the posterior wall of the bicipitoradial bursa is easily visualized close to the cortex of the radius, but the anterior wall is hard to distinguish from the paratenon of the biceps tendon.

The distal portion of the biceps tendon is formed by the union of two muscle bellies, the long and short heads of the biceps brachii; individual components of the biceps brachii can be readily separated until a level approximately 7 cm above the elbow joint, where they join and terminate in a flattened tendon that is attached to the rough posterior portion of the radial tuberosity (Fig 4). The distal tendon of the biceps brachii has no tendon sheath.

Bursitis leading to enlargement of the bicipitoradial bursa can result from a number of causes, but most frequently it results from repetitive mechanical trauma (8); other causes include infection, inflammatory arthropathy, chemical synovitis, bone proliferation, and synovial chondromatosis (3,4,8–10).

When the bicipitoradial bursa is enlarged, it often is palpable and can impair normal flexion and extension of the elbow. With pronation, the tuberosity of the radius rotates posteriorly, causing compression of the bursa between the biceps tendon and the radial tuberosity, consequently increasing the tension within the bursa (Figs 1, 6). With the accumulation of fluid in the bicipitoradial bursa, a mass effect in the cubital fossa may lead to compression of the adjacent nerves (4,8). Resultant symptoms depend on which nerve is compressed. When the superficial branch of the radial nerve is affected, the symptoms are sensory related; when the deep branch of the radial nerve (posterior interosseous nerve) is affected, the symptoms are motor related (weakness of the extensor muscles).

In all cadaveric and clinical cases, the median nerve was not compressed by the distended bursa and was medial to the bicipitoradial bursa. In our opinion, the median nerve is unlikely to be compressed unless there is substantial distention of the bicipitoradial bursa, an anatomic variation of the nerve, or intercommunication between the bicipitoradial bursa and interosseous bursa (4–6, 8–12).

MR imaging allows assessment of the relationship between the bicipitoradial bursa and the adjacent structures and, owing to the signal intensity characteristics of the bursal fluid, is helpful in defining cystic masses in this area, such as ganglion cysts (6). However, with MR imaging, it may be difficult to distinguish bicipitoradial bursitis from interosseous bursitis, especially in patients with a very enlarged bicipitoradial bursa.

Conservative treatment of bicipitoradial bursitis consists of aspiration of the bursa and injection of corticosteroid medications. Surgical resection may be required if failure of conservative treatment occurs, with recurrence of pain after aspiration, neurologic impairment, or mechanical limitation to flexion and extension of the elbow (4).

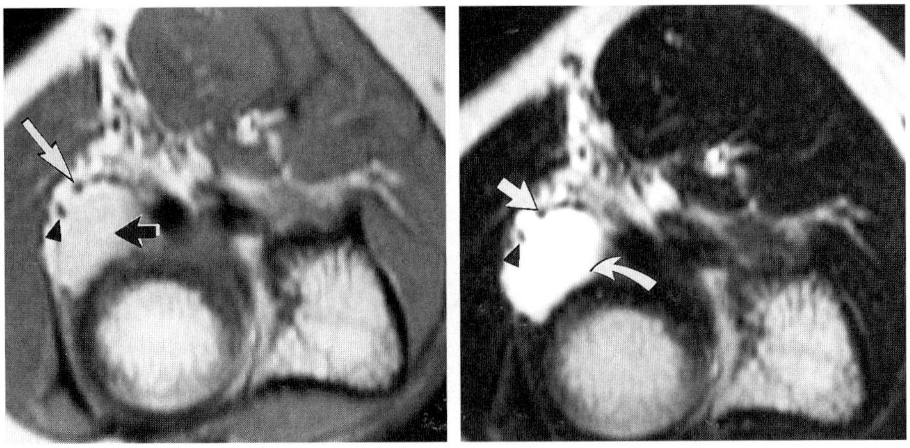

a. b.

Figure 9. Transaxial MR images obtained in a 41-year-old woman who presented with a palpable mass in antecubital fossa, pain, and weakness of the extensor muscles. **(a)** Intermediate-weighted MR image (4,600/17) shows enlargement of the bicipitoradial bursa (black arrow) directly contacting the superficial (white arrow) and deep (arrowhead) branches of the radial nerve. **(b)** T2-weighted fast spin-echo non–fat-suppressed MR image (4,600/102) shows enlargement of the bicipitoradial bursa (curved arrow) directly contacting the superficial (straight arrow) and deep (arrowhead) branches of the radial nerve. (Image courtesy of Mini Pathria, MD, San Diego, Calif).

In summary, the bicipitoradial bursa is a thin and delicate structure lined by a synovial membrane and is located between the radial insertion of the biceps tendon and the cortex of the radial tuberosity. Enlargement of the bicipitoradial bursa should be recognized as distinct from tenosynovitis or a ganglion cyst. MR imaging is a useful diagnostic method for evaluating bicipitoradial bursitis and its effect on adjacent structures.

References

1. Williams P, Warwick R, eds. Gray's anatomy. 36th ed. Philadelphia, Pa: Saunders, 1980; 522, 571–572, 1101–1102.
2. Toldt C. An atlas of human anatomy for students and physicians. 2nd ed. New York, NY: Macmillian, 1928; 321.
3. Treves F. Surgical applied anatomy. 12th ed. London, England: Cassell, 1952; 252.
4. Liessi G, Cesari S, Spaliviero B, Dell'Antonio C, Avventi P. The US, CT and MR findings of cubital bursitis: a report of five cases. Skeletal Radiol 1996; 25:471–475.
5. Cooney WP. Bursitis and tendinitis in the hand, wrist and elbow: an approach to treatment. Minn Med 1983; 66:491–494.
6. Kasarek FJ, Durham NC, Hoffman CJ, Martinez S. Distal bicipital bursitis: MR imaging characteristics (abstr). Radiology 1997; 205(P):398.
7. Kopka L, Funke M, Fisher V, Keating D, Detesmann J, Grabbe E. MR arthrography of the shoulder with gadopentetate dimeglumine: influence of concentration, iodinated contrast material, and time on signal intensity. AJR 1994; 163:621–623.
8. Karanja ND, Stiles PJ. Cubital bursitis. J Bone Joint Surg [Br] 1988; 70:832–833.
9. McCollam SM, Corley FG, Green DP. Posterior interosseous nerve palsy caused by ganglion of the proximal radioulnar joint. J Hand Surg [Am] 1988; 13:725–728.
10. El Hadidi S, Burke FD. Posterior interosseous nerve syndrome caused by a bursa in the vicinity of the elbow. J Hand Surg [Br] 1987; 12:23–24.
11. Spinner RJ, Lins RE, Collins AJ, Spinner M. Posterior interosseous nerve compression due to an enlarged bicipital bursa confirmed by MRI. J Hand Surg [Br] 1993; 18:753–756.
12. Matsumoto K, Hukuda S, Fujita M, Karimoto A, Tachibana S, Shiga O. Cubital bursitis caused by localized synovial chondromatosis of the elbow: a case report. J Bone Joint Surg [Am] 1996; 78:275–277.

Cervical Spine Screening with CT in Trauma Patients: A Cost-effectiveness Analysis[1]

C. Craig Blackmore, MD, MPH
Scott D. Ramsey, MD, PhD
Frederick A. Mann, MD
Richard A. Deyo, MD, MPH

Index terms:
Cost-effectiveness
CT, helical, 31.12115
Spine, CT, 31.12115
Spine, fractures, 31.41
Trauma

Radiology 1999; 212:117–125

Abbreviations:
ASIA = American Spinal Injury Association
QALY = quality-adjusted life year
RVU = relative value unit

[1] From the Department of Radiology, University of North Carolina–Chapel Hill School of Medicine, CB #7510, 508 Old Infirmary Bldg, Chapel Hill, NC 27599-7510 (C.C.B.), and the Robert Wood Johnson Clinical Scholars Program (C.C.B., R.A.D.), Department of Radiology, Harborview Medical Center (C.C.B., F.A.M.), and Department of Medicine (S.D.R., R.A.D.), University of Washington School of Medicine, Seattle. Received December 23, 1997; revision requested March 23, 1998; final revision received November 23; accepted January 8, 1999. C.C.B. supported by the Seattle Veterans Affairs Medical Center-Robert Wood Johnson Clinical Scholars Program. **Address reprint requests to** C.C.B., Department of Radiology, Harborview Medical Center, Box 359728, 325 Ninth Ave, Seattle, WA 98104-2499.

The opinions expressed are those of the authors and not necessarily those of the Robert Wood Johnson Foundation or the United States Veterans Administration.

Author contributions:
Guarantors of integrity of entire study, all authors; study concepts and design, all authors; definition of intellectual content, all authors; literature research, C.C.B., F.A.M.; clinical studies, C.C.B.; data acquisition, C.C.B.; data and statistical analyses, C.C.B., S.D.R.; manuscript preparation, C.C.B., F.A.M.; manuscript editing and review, all authors.

PURPOSE: To investigate the cost-effectiveness of computed tomography (CT) relative to radiography for cervical spine screening in trauma patients.

MATERIALS AND METHODS: A decision analysis model was constructed to compare the incremental cost-effectiveness of radiography and CT as primary cervical spine screening modalities in trauma patients. Analyses were performed from a societal perspective, and probability and cost estimates from the literature and institutional experience were used. In separate cost-effectiveness analyses, hypothetical cohorts of trauma patients from three defined clinical scenarios were considered: high, moderate, and low risk for cervical spine fracture. Outcome measures included cases of paralysis prevented, total cost of screening strategies, and incremental cost-effectiveness ratios.

RESULTS: In high-risk patients, screening with CT is a dominant strategy that prevents cases of paralysis and saves money for society. In moderate-risk patients, screening with CT is cost-effective with reference-case assumptions and within the range of most sensitivity analyses. In the low-risk group, CT screening helps prevent cases of paralysis, but the incremental cost-effectiveness ratio is high (>$80,000 per quality-adjusted life year).

CONCLUSION: CT is the preferred cervical spine screening modality in trauma patients at high and moderate risk for cervical spine fracture.

An estimated 10,000 persons sustain spinal cord injuries in the United States each year; this represents an incidence of approximately 40 injuries per million persons per year (1–3) at an estimated annual cost to society of $3.4 billion (4). The majority of these injuries are related to cervical spine fracture from motor vehicle accidents or falls (5,6). However, cervical spine fractures may not be clinically apparent, and progressive neurologic compromise, including paralysis and death, may develop if diagnosis of fracture is delayed (7–9). Accordingly, major trauma patients are considered to have unstable cervical spine injuries until proved otherwise (10). Patients in whom cervical spine fracture cannot be definitively excluded on the basis of clinical evaluation undergo a screening radiographic examination of the cervical spine, which is one of the most commonly ordered imaging procedures in the emergency department or trauma center. At our single urban trauma center, more than 3,000 patients undergo screening radiography of the cervical spine each year.

The standard method of screening the cervical spine is a conventional radiographic series, which typically consists of lateral, anteroposterior, and odontoid views. Nonetheless, 5%–8% of patients with fracture may have normal radiographs (11–16). In addition, particular difficulty in positioning multiple-trauma patients may lead to a large number of inadequate radiographic examinations (17).

Computed tomography (CT) has been proposed as a method of screening trauma patients to exclude cervical spine fracture (12,18). The sensitivity of screening cervical spine CT is higher than that of radiography (12,19,20). Furthermore, in some trauma centers, performing screening CT of the cervical spine at the time of head CT may allow a more rapid radiologic exclusion of cervical spine fracture than performing conventional radiography (12). Higher direct medical costs and variable availability are the primary disadvantages of screening the cervical spine with CT. However, associating screening cervical spine CT with the head CT commonly performed in trauma patients may mitigate these factors.

Current standards of care dictate that all patients at risk for cervical spine fracture undergo radiologic screening. However, it is possible to define groups of patients in whom there is a higher probability of injury. We previously reported on a clinical prediction rule that can be used to stratify patients into various groups according to their level of probability for injury (21,22). The prediction rule was based on a case-control study involving 168 patients with cervical spine fracture and 304 control patients. By using the relatively simple clinical factors of mechanism of injury, age, presence of severe head injury, and presence of focal neurologic deficit, patients can be separated into groups that have a broad range of probabilities of cervical spine fracture. The use of a clinical prediction rule enables the tailoring of cervical spine screening imaging in patients with different levels of injury probability rather than the use of the same strategy for all patients.

In this study, we used cost-effectiveness analyses to compare the use of screening CT with the use of the standard radiographic screening protocol in evaluating blunt trauma victims with possible cervical spine fracture. The target population was patients who are screened for possible cervical spine fracture in trauma centers or emergency departments and who are already scheduled to undergo CT scanning of the head. We performed separate analyses for patients with different levels of probability of injury. Our purpose was to compare the cost-effectiveness of CT with that of radiography in screening for possible cervical spine fracture in trauma patients.

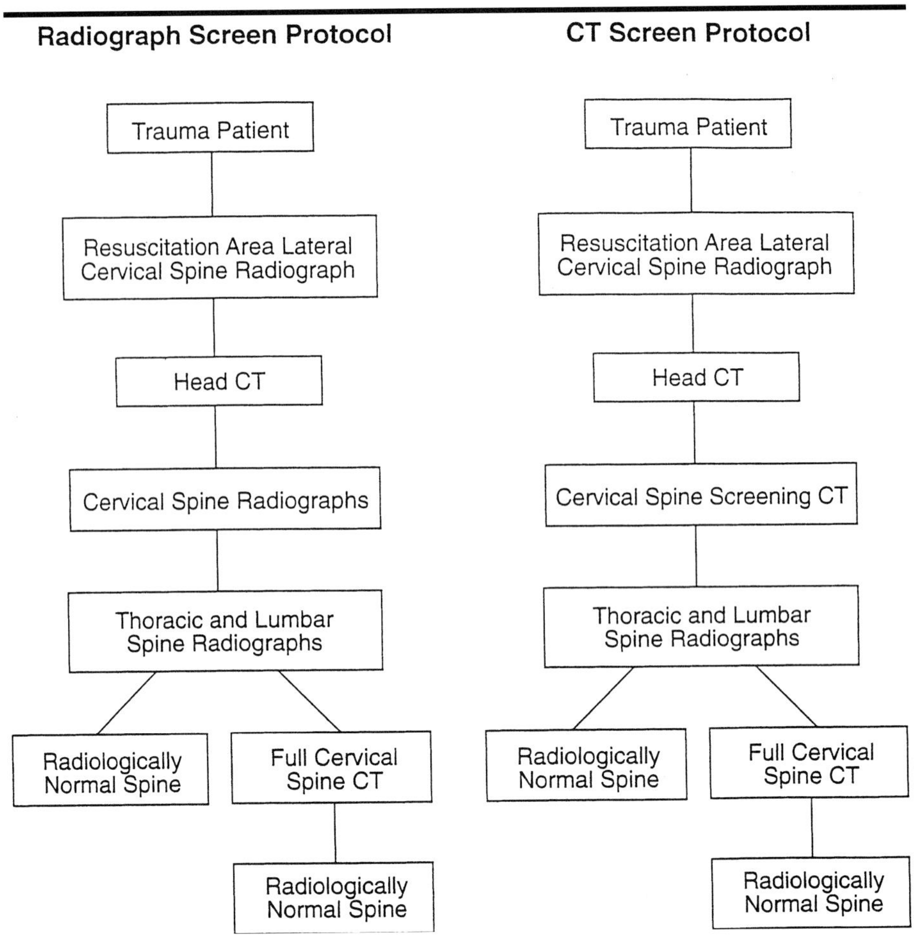

Figure 1. Flow sheet of radiographic and CT screening protocols. All patients are assumed to undergo lateral cervical spine radiography and head CT in the resuscitation area. Cervical spine screening with either radiography or CT follows head CT. If the radiograph or CT scan is inadequate or abnormal, then the patient will undergo a full CT examination after radiographic evaluation of the remainder of the spine.

MATERIALS AND METHODS

The institutional human subjects review committee at our institution approved the experimental procedures in this study. Because the study involved only retrospective chart review and analysis, with the patients' confidentiality preserved, the committee did not require patients to give informed consent.

For patients clinically deemed to require imaging of the cervical spine, we developed an imaging algorithm in which screening cervical spine CT would be substituted for conventional radiography (Fig 1). As described below (in the Probability Estimates section), three sample populations with different risks of cervical spine fracture were defined on the basis of the mechanism of injury and clinical factors that would be available to the emergency department or trauma center physician at the time of the imaging decision (Table 1). These clinical scenarios were determined by means of development and bootstrap validation of a clinical prediction rule from a previously reported retrospective case-control study (21) conducted at our institution. The scenarios selected represented a range of pretest probabilities for injury and thus were representative of the range of patients in whom CT screening might be considered. For each of these clinical scenarios, the cost-effectiveness of CT versus that of radiography for cervical spine screening in trauma patients was determined.

For each clinical scenario, the CT screening protocol was based on the assumptions that CT scanning is immediately available and the trauma patient will undergo CT of the head as part of the emergency evaluation. Screening CT of the cervical spine is then performed as a continuation of head CT; this protocol eliminates the need for additional patient transport and transfer and decreases the time required to position the patient and prepare the CT scanner. These time efficiencies distinguished screening CT from the full (ie, standard) CT examination that is performed as a separate study to evaluate a specific area of possible abnormality. Because the cost of screening CT in patients who are already scheduled to undergo head CT is different from that in those who are not, this analysis was restricted to the head CT group only. The screening CT technique in this study involved helical acquisitions at a 1:1 pitch and 5-mm axial section interval (12).

TABLE 1
Clinical Scenarios and Probabilities of Cervical Spine Fracture

Clinical Scenario Group*	Fracture Probability (%)	95% CI†
High-risk		
Focal neurologic deficit	31.1	19.8, 76.0
Severe head injury‡	11.2	9.4, 15.3
High-energy mechanism and age older than 50 years	14.8	6.2, 100
Moderate-risk		
High-energy mechanism and age 50 years or younger‡	4.2	2.7, 6.9
Moderate-energy mechanism and age older than 50 years	5.5	3.6, 10.1
Low-risk		
Moderate-energy mechanism and age 50 years or younger‡	2.1	1.6, 3.2
Low-energy mechanism	0.6	0.4, 0.9

* Severe head injury = skull fracture, intracranial hemorrhage, or injury causing unconscious state during emergency department evaluation. High-energy mechanism = high-speed motor vehicle accident (>30 mph) or pedestrian struck by car. Moderate-energy mechanism = motor vehicle accident of low or unknown speed, motorcycle accident of unknown speed, fall, or bicycle accident. Low-energy mechanism = blunt object trauma, other, or unknown mechanism.
† CI = confidence interval.
‡ Scenario used for reference case in cost-effectiveness analysis.

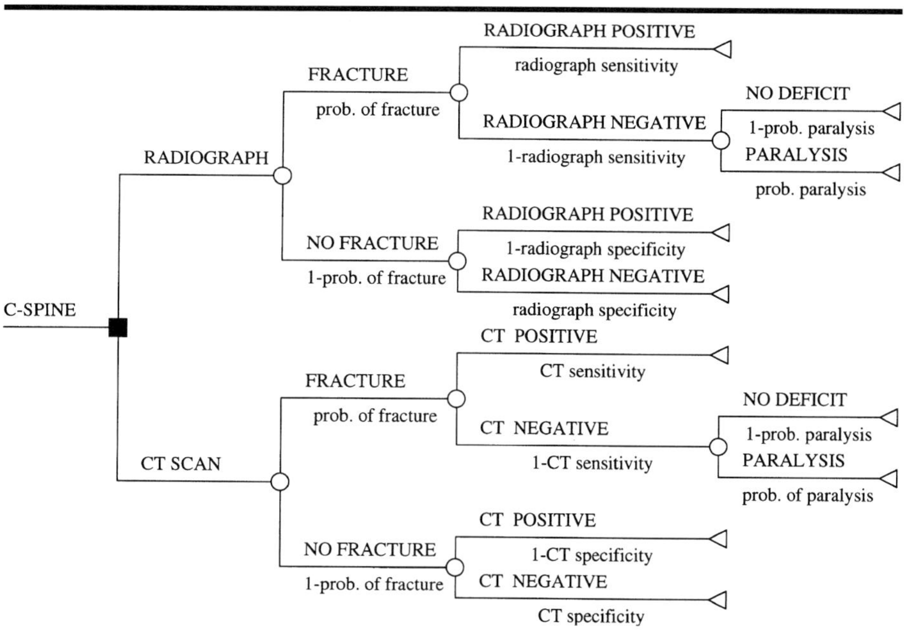

Figure 2. Decision analysis model demonstrates the options and outcomes of radiographic and CT screening strategies. A patient at risk of cervical spine injury may undergo either conventional radiographic screening or CT screening. After that decision is made, there are several possible outcomes. The patient may have a fracture that is either detected or missed at screening, as defined by the sensitivity of the test. Alternatively, the patient may not have a fracture, and the test results may be truly negative or falsely positive, as defined by the specificity of the test. Finally, if a fracture is missed, there is some probability that the patient will develop paralysis. The probability and costs of each of these outcomes determine the cost-effectiveness. Outcomes are noted in uppercase letters above the lines, and probabilities are in lowercase letters below the lines. This model is simplified: Outcomes not influencing the cost-effectiveness are excluded.

Decision Analysis Model

A computer-based decision analysis model (TreeAge Software, Williamstown, Mass) was constructed to compare the CT screening algorithm with the conventional radiographic screening protocol (Fig 2). By using probability and cost estimates for each possible outcome, incremental cost-effectiveness ratios were calculated for the use of screening CT compared with the use of radiography. The results were expressed as dollars per quality-adjusted life year (QALY), which represents the additional benefit in terms of longevity and quality of life per additional dollar spent on cervical spine screening when the CT scanning strategy is used.

In the decision analysis model (Fig 2), a patient in either protocol has a defined pretest probability of fracture, which represents the prevalence of fracture for that clinical scenario. The rates of true-positive and false-negative studies and of true-negative and false-positive studies are defined as the sensitivity and specificity, respectively, of the imaging study. In this model, we made the assumption that all cases of unstable cervical spine fracture eventually become evident and are treated identically in both protocols. The only additional cost associated with a false-negative screening study and the resultant delay in diagnosis is that which arises from any severe secondary neurologic deficits, which are defined as American Spinal Injury Association (ASIA) grade C or worse; in these abnormalities, most motor muscles below the level of the neurologic lesion are unable to oppose gravity. The probability of developing such a deficit was represented by the natural history of an undetected fracture. Minor secondary deficits were ignored. We also assumed that a false-positive screening study with either radiography or CT prompts additional diagnostic evaluation with full CT scanning.

Probability Estimates

The cost-effectiveness model was dependent on six probability estimates: probability of fracture, sensitivity of radiography, specificity of radiography, sensitivity of CT, specificity of CT, and probability of paralysis from undetected fracture. Sensitivity was defined as the ability of the screening examination to enable the identification of patients with fractures, or the number of true-positive results divided by the number of patients with fracture. Specificity, on the other hand, was defined as the ability of the screening test to enable correct classification of patients without fracture as individuals with normal spines, or the number of true-negative results divided by the total number of patients without disease (23). Probability estimates were derived from the medical literature and from the collection of original data, as described below. Because the cervical spine radiographic protocol is the current standard of care and the CT screening protocol is less well accepted, we intentionally chose values that are more favorable to radiography when uncertainty existed.

To determine the risk of cervical spine fracture, we adapted a clinical prediction rule that we had developed previously (21,22). The original clinical prediction rule was derived to estimate the risk of fracture in all trauma patients. However, for consideration of CT cervical spine screening in the present study, the relevant population consisted of only those patients scheduled to undergo head CT. To estimate the risk of fracture in the head CT population, we performed a case-control study with 224 patients (161 men and 63 women aged 18–88 years [mean age, 42.8 years]) with cervical spine fracture and 379 control patients (275 men and 104 women aged 18–94 years [mean age, 35.7 years]). The control patients were randomly selected from trauma patients who underwent head CT as part of their emergency department evaluation. Both groups were selected from victims of nonpenetrating trauma who were (*a*) examined at our institution between 1992 and 1995, (*b*) aged 18 years or older, and (*c*) not transferred from another institution. The purpose of this clinical prediction rule was to influence cervical spine imaging decision making at the initial patient presentation in the emergency department or trauma center. Therefore, the information used for the clinical prediction rule was only that which would be available at the initial evaluation.

Because patients who were transferred from another institution might have undergone a previous examination or intervention, there would be potential for selection bias if they were included. Accordingly, we included only those patients who had undergone the initial examination at our center and excluded all those who were transferred from another facility. One hundred twenty-three (55%) of the 224 patients and 76 (20%) of the 379 control subjects in this analysis also were included in the previous study from which the original clinical prediction rule was derived. For each case and control subject, information regarding the presence or absence of clinical predictors of cervical spine fracture was noted by one of two trained chart abstractors, who were one of the authors (C.C.B.) and a research assistant. To avoid ascertainment bias, we selected clinical predictors from information that is determined before the diagnosis of cervical spine fracture is made. These predictors included age, mechanism of injury, obvious head or facial injury, and loss of consciousness. Head injury was determined both clinically and with the findings of head CT, which would, by design, precede the screening cervical spine CT. To determine agreement, both reviewers assessed 29 (5%) of the 603 charts. Data from the chart review forms were then entered into a database by using double-key entry with verification.

The clinical prediction rule previously derived for all trauma patients was then applied to the trauma and head CT data set, and the odds ratio for cervical spine fracture was determined for several clinical scenarios. To calculate the absolute risk of fracture for each of the clinical scenarios, we used likelihood ratios adapted from the clinical prediction rule and the baseline probability of fracture in trauma patients who undergo head CT, which was directly measured at our institution. Confidence intervals (CIs) were calculated by using bootstrap modeling of the baseline risk of fracture and the likelihood ratios for each of the clinical scenarios. Bootstrap modeling is a method of randomly resampling from a given experimental sample to simulate the drawing of multiple samples from the underlying population. It is used to ensure that a clinical prediction rule is not overfit to the data from which it was derived but rather generalizable to other similar samples (24). On the basis of the clinical prediction rule results, we selected three clinical scenarios to represent conditions with high, moderate, and low risk for cervical spine fracture.

The sensitivity of cervical spine radiography was estimated on the basis of values from literature reports (11,14–16, 20,25). First, we used the χ^2 test to exclude heterogeneity ($P = .24$); then we pooled the reported sensitivities (26,27). A computerized search of the English-language literature was conducted. References of the located articles were then searched for additional relevant sources. For inclusion, the number of true-positive and false-negative images had to be reported in the study, and the eventual clinical presentation with fracture had to be used as the reference standard. Studies in which CT scanning was used as the reference standard were excluded, because, to our knowledge, there is no information on the natural history of such injuries. We do not know on the basis of the existing literature whether such injuries will become clinically relevant. Accordingly, fractures discovered at CT with no associated clinical findings were excluded from estimates of the sensitivity of radiography. By excluding these CT-based studies, the derived sensitivity of radiography was higher, and the bias was more conservative in favor of the radiographic protocol.

The specificity of cervical spine radiography was measured directly from the medical records of randomly selected trauma patients who were examined at our institution, fit into the described clinical scenarios, and had undergone cervical spine radiography. For each patient, we determined whether cervical spine CT had been performed and whether a cervical spine fracture had been identified at this examination. The group of patients who had undergone cervical spine CT but did not have fractures constituted the false-positive cases for specificity determination. This "false-positive" group was heterogeneous and included patients with equivocal or inadequate radiographs and patients in whom the radiographs were thought to be abnormal. However, because the radiographs obtained in all of these patients led to CT scanning, they were considered to be false-positive for decision-making purposes. This study has been reported in greater detail previously (17).

The sensitivity of CT was determined by reviewing the literature, with simple pooling of the available data. Research articles in which there was a defined cohort of patients who underwent screening CT were included in the analysis (12,18). In addition, because of the low number of published studies, we included unpublished data representing the continuation of the largest published series in which CT and radiography are directly compared (Nunez D.B., personal communication, May 1997). For determination of the sensitivity of CT, the eventual clinical presentation or identification of fracture by using any other imaging modality was considered the reference standard. To our knowledge, no estimates of the specificity of CT are available in the literature. An estimate of specificity was determined from the authors' experience and from consultations with physicians at other trauma centers. This estimate was tested over a broad range in the sensitivity analysis to allow for the added uncertainty of this method of estimation.

The probability of severe secondary deficit (ASIA grade C or worse) was obtained from the medical literature. Three studies (7,9,28,29) have been published encompassing 137 cervical spine fractures of which there was a delay in diagnosis. In these studies, a range in probability of severe neurologic sequelae of 0% to 18% is reported. Heterogeneity in the methodology of these studies limits the ability to combine the data. Accordingly, a conservative estimate between the measured probabilities (5%) was chosen as the reference value of probability, and a broad range was considered in the sensitivity analysis (1%–15%).

Cost Estimates

Cost estimates for radiologic procedures were derived from the 1995 Medicare relative value unit (RVU) reimbursement schedules (30). The reference-case estimate for the cost of cervical spine radiography was the global reimbursement for a four-view cervical spine study (1.38 RVUs); the reimbursement for two- and six-view studies were included in the sensitivity analysis. The cost of full cervical spine CT scanning, which was not performed in conjunction with head CT, also was determined from the RVU schedule (7.74 RVUs).

The Medicare RVU schedule does not have a code for screening cervical spine CT at the time of head CT. However, the assumption that the incremental cost of cervical spine CT at the time of head CT is less than that of the independently performed, full-cost cervical spine CT examination is a key component in the argument for cervical spine screening with CT. This economic advantage of performing more than one examination in a scanning session is recognized by the RVU schedule in other cases. For example, the RVU cost of one cervical spine examination, performed with and without contrast material, is considerably less than the sum of the costs of the individual studies performed independently. We estimated the incremental RVU technical cost of obtaining a CT scan of the cervical spine in a patient who is already positioned in the scanner for head CT to be 1.78 RVUs, which is equivalent to the incremental technical component of the RVU cost of obtaining a CT scan of the cervical spine without contrast material in a patient already positioned for CT of the cervical spine with contrast material. The professional component of the RVU cost of cervical spine CT is not affected by the method of acquiring the scan and therefore remains 1.75 RVUs. The total cost of screening cervical spine CT at the time of head CT is therefore the sum of the professional and technical components, or 3.53 RVUs. For sensitivity analysis, we tested the effect of a 50% over- or underestimation of the cost.

Estimates of the lifetime costs of spinal cord injury were derived from the literature (4,6,31–34). Direct medical costs in the 1st year and in all subsequent years, as well as rehabilitation and home care costs, were included. Indirect costs such as lost wages were excluded. All costs reported in the literature were adjusted to 1995 dollars by using the medical care consumer price index (U.S. Bureau of Labor Statistics) and a standard Medicare reimbursement rate of $34 per RVU. Costs occurring beyond the base year of the analysis were discounted by using a 3% discount rate (35,36).

Survival Analysis

The mean age of the patients with cervical spine fracture at our institution who were eligible for this study was 43 years. The life expectancy of a 43-year-old person in the United States who sustains a spinal cord injury is 14 years (37,38), which was used as the time horizon to estimate lifetime medical costs. The life expectancy of patients without spinal cord injury (39 years) was derived from life tables and used to estimate the number of years of life lost by sustaining a spinal cord injury.

Quality of Life Determination

The Health Utilities Index Mark 2 (39) was used to estimate the utility adjustment for life with a severe neurologic deficit. Six scenarios that typify the injury level and severity in patients with cervical spine fracture were devised. Three physiatrists with expertise in the care of patients with spinal cord injury were then asked to select the specific level of health status defined by the Health Utilities Index for each of seven attributes that is most representative of a typical patient's health status in a given scenario. The resultant levels of health status were converted into utility scores (39), which were then combined by using the relative population frequency of each of the scenarios for weighting. The average and range of the three physiatrists' scores were used as the utility adjustment reference standard and sensitivity analysis range, respectively.

QALYs were calculated from the measurements of life expectancy and utility adjustment for life with cervical spinal cord injury. To account for the time value of benefits and comply with the recent recommendations of the U.S. Public Health Service for the standardization of cost-effectiveness analysis methodology, QALYs, like costs, were discounted, with 3% as the reference-standard discount rate (35). The baseline utility in the absence of spinal cord injury was assumed to be 1.0. Because all patients may not be in perfect health, an estimated baseline utility of 0.9 was explored in the sensitivity analysis.

Sensitivity Analyses

Univariate sensitivity analyses were performed over the range of plausible estimates for all variables, including the discount rate. Table 2 lists the range of values included in the sensitivity analysis for each probability and cost estimate. In addition, we studied the effects of a systematic overestimation of the sensitivity and specificity of radiography and CT and of a systematic underestimation of the sensitivity and specificity of radiography and CT by using multivariate sensitivity analyses. Finally, to further test the stability of the results, we performed Monte Carlo simulations of 1,000 iterations by using triangular distributions for the major variables. This is a method of repeatedly testing the outcome of the simulation model by using random selection of a value for each of the variables from within their probable ranges (40).

RESULTS

The results of analyses performed by using the prediction rule to determine the probability of fracture are shown in Table 1. Agreement between the chart abstractors, as measured by using the κ statistic, was excellent (κ = 0.80) (41). Patients who sustained severe head injury were selected as the reference group at high risk for cervical spine fracture (fracture risk = 11.2%; 95% CI = 9.4%, 15.3%). Patients with focal neurologic deficit and those older than 50 years with a high-energy mechanism of injury were included in the high-risk group in the sensitivity analysis. Patients aged 50 years or younger with a high-energy mechanism were selected as the reference group at moderate risk for cervical spine fracture (fracture risk = 4.2%, 95% CI = 2.7%, 6.9%). Patients older than 50 years with a moderate-energy mechanism were included in the moderate-risk group in the sensitivity analysis. Finally, patients aged 50 years or younger with a moderate-energy mechanism were selected as the reference group at low risk for cervical spine fracture (fracture risk = 2.1%; 95% CI = 1.6%, 3.2%). Patients with a low-energy mechanism were included in the low-risk group in the sensitivity analysis. The results of the cost-effectiveness analysis of each reference-case clinical scenario are shown in Table 3; the incremental summary analysis, in Table 4; and the univariate sensitivity analysis, in Table 5.

High-Risk Patients

In the high-risk clinical scenario (severe head injury), use of screening cervical spine CT was a dominant strategy; it not only prevented cases of paralysis, but it also saved society money. In a hypothetical cohort of 100,000 high-risk patients, the screening CT protocol prevented 23 additional cases of paralysis and saved society $3.4 million. The dominance of this strategy held throughout the range of sensitivity analysis variables, except at the lowest probability of paralysis from a missed fracture, at the highest estimate of radiography sensitivity, and at the highest cost of screening CT. At the lowest probability of paralysis, the use of screening CT had an incremental cost-effectiveness ratio of $55,000 per QALY. Use of CT screening in high-risk patients also was dominant in the best- and worst-case multivariate analyses. In the Monte Carlo simulations, the CT strategy was dominant 84% of the time, and the incremental cost-effectiveness ratio for CT screening was less than $20,000 per QALY in 98% of the iterations.

TABLE 2
Reference Case and Sensitivity Analysis Estimates

Variable	Scenario Group*	Reference Case	Range	Reference
Radiography sensitivity (%)	All	94	92–96	11, 14–16, 20, 22
Radiography specificity (%)	High-risk	89	85–94	17, Institutional data
	Moderate-risk	89	80–98	17, Institutional data
	Low-risk	96	94–97	17, Institutional data
CT sensitivity (%)	All	98	96–100	12, 18
CT specificity (%)	All	95	90–100	Authors' experience
Probability of fracture (%)	High-risk	11	9–13	21, Institutional data
	Moderate-risk	4	3–7	21, Institutional data
	Low-risk	2	2–3	21, Institutional data
Probability of paralysis (%)	All	5	1–15	7, 9, 23, 24
Radiography cost				
In RVUs	All	1.38	0.94–1.70	25
In dollars	All	47	32–58	25
Screening CT cost				
In RVUs	All	3.53	2.43–5.33	25
In dollars	All	120	80–180	25
Full CT scanning cost				
In RVUs	All	7.74	6.19–9.29	25
In dollars	All	263	210–310	25
Paralysis cost ($)	All	405,000	350,000–500,000	4, 6, 26–29
Life expectancy (y)†	All	14	9.0–22.1	32, 33
Utility adjustment (QALY)†	All	0.516	.465–.611	34
Baseline utility (QALY)‡	All	1.0	0.9–1.0	NA
Discount rate (%)	All	3.0	0.0–5.0	30

* All indicates that data apply to all three scenario groups.
† With paralysis.
‡ Baseline utility in the absence of spinal cord injury was assumed to be 1.0.

Moderate-Risk Patients

In the moderate-risk group (high-energy mechanism and age 50 years or younger), the use of screening CT was more expensive than was the use of radiography at reference-case estimates. However, the CT screening strategy did prevent an additional 8.5 cases of paralysis at an incremental cost-effectiveness ratio of $16,500 per QALY. Throughout the range of the sensitivity analysis, the incremental cost-effectiveness ratio for screening CT in the moderate-risk group was less than $50,000 per QALY, except at the lowest estimate of paralysis risk and highest cost estimate for screening CT. At a probability of paralysis from missed fracture of 1%, the incremental cost-effectiveness ratio for screening CT scan was $180,000 per QALY. The incremental cost-effectiveness ratio for CT crossed the $50,000 per QALY mark at a probability of paralysis of approximately 2.8%.

At multivariate sensitivity analysis based on the highest estimates of sensitivity and specificity, screening CT in the moderate-risk group had an incremental cost-effectiveness ratio of $26,000 per QALY. At the lowest estimates of sensitivity and specificity, the cost-effectiveness ratio was $7,600 per QALY. The relatively low cost-effectiveness ratio in this worst-case scenario was primarily due to the lower sensitivity of radiography. Although this worst-case scenario also included low estimates for radiography specificity and for CT sensitivity and specificity, the most important factor was the lower radiography sensitivity, which caused the cost-effectiveness ratio to decrease. In the Monte Carlo simulations, the CT strategy was dominant in 380 (38%) of the 1,000 iterations, and the incremental cost-effectiveness ratio for screening with CT was less than $50,000 per QALY in 940 (94%) of the iterations.

Low-Risk Patients

On the basis of the data from this study, in the low-risk group—that is, those patients younger than 50 years with a moderate-energy mechanism—the use of CT screening is more expensive and prevents fewer additional cases of paralysis. In our hypothetical cohort of 100,000 low-risk patients, 4.2 additional cases of paralysis were prevented. The incremental cost-effectiveness ratio of such a strategy was $84,000 per QALY. Incremental cost-effectiveness ratios at extreme ranges of the sensitivity analysis varied from $12,000 to $526,000 per QALY. Finally, multivariate sensitivity analyses based on the highest and lowest sensitivity and specificity demonstrated cost-effectiveness ratios of $72,000 per QALY and $90,000 per QALY, respectively.

DISCUSSION

During the past 2 decades, CT has become an invaluable tool in the initial evaluation of trauma patients. CT is the standard of care for the evaluation of the head in trauma patients, and in many trauma centers, it is used as the primary modality to evaluate the chest, abdomen, and pelvis. The work of Nunez et al (12) demonstrates the technical and diagnostic efficacy of screening the cervical spine with CT. In this article, we explored the societal efficacy and demonstrated that screening with CT in high-risk groups can prevent cases of paralysis and save money for society. The cost savings is due to the lower sensitivity of radiography, which leads to the high cost of secondary development of paralysis, and to the low specificity of cervical spine radiography, which necessitates further imaging. The results of our analysis indicated that screening CT of the cervical spine is cost-effective and should be adopted for the initial evaluation of high-risk patients.

In the moderate-risk group, including younger patients with a high-energy

TABLE 3
Reference Case Results

Variable	High-Risk Group		Moderate-Risk Group		Low-Risk Group	
	CT	Radiography	CT	Radiography	CT	Radiography
Total cost ($)*	20,600,000	24,000,000	16,000,000	13,700,000	14,700,000	8,800,000
Total no. of cases of paralysis	11.2	34.1	4.2	12.7	2.1	6.3
Total disutility (QALY)	182	556	69	207	34.2	103

* Estimates are based on a hypothetical cohort of 100,000 patients.

TABLE 4
Incremental Summary Results

	High-Risk Group	Moderate-Risk Group	Low-Risk Group
Incremental cost of CT ($)*	−3,400,000	2,300,000	5,800,000
Incremental cases of paralysis†	−22.9	−8.5	−4.2
Incremental disutility (QALY)†	−373	−139	−69.0
Incremental cost-effectiveness ($/QALY)‡	Dominant§	16,500	84,000

Note.—Estimates are based on a hypothetical cohort of 100,000 patients.
* Negative number indicates cost savings with CT.
† Negative number indicates paralysis (disutility) prevented with CT.
‡ Incremental cost-effectiveness = (cost of CT − cost of radiography)/(effectiveness of CT − effectiveness of radiography).
§ Dominant indicates that strategy saves money and prevents paralysis (disutility).

mechanism of injury and older patients with a moderate-energy mechanism, screening CT was more expensive than radiography, with a cost-effectiveness ratio of $16,500 per QALY at the reference-case assumptions. The absolute threshold for what constitutes a cost-effective intervention remains controversial. However, society has expressed a willingness to fund interventions that cost less than $20,000 per QALY (42,43), and many authors would consider $50,000 per QALY a reasonable threshold (44,45). Because the cost per QALY in the moderate-risk group was less than $20,000 with the reference-case assumptions and less than $50,000 per QALY in most of the sensitivity analyses and Monte Carlo simulations, the bulk of the evidence supports CT screening in this group. However, in this group in particular, because the determination of the most cost-effective screening study is less well defined, the individual experience at each institution also is important for selection of the optimal imaging strategy.

Finally, although screening with CT continues to prevent cases of paralysis in the low-risk group, the cost to society is high. In the low-risk reference group and in most of the ranges explored in the sensitivity analysis in this study, the cost of screening with CT was in excess of that which society is likely to be willing to pay. Therefore, CT is not cost-effective for screening low-risk patients.

Because cost-effectiveness is dependent on risk of fracture, use of screening CT should be limited to patients at moderate or high risk of fracture. In this study, we examined only three scenarios in detail; however, the results may be extended to other clinical scenarios with known fracture risk. For example, in the moderate-risk group, we considered patients aged 50 years or younger with a high-energy mechanism; however, the results were also relevant to those patients older than 50 years with a moderate-risk mechanism, in whom the risk of fracture was 5.5% (Table 1). Although assigning an absolute value to a QALY is controversial, a cutoff of $20,000 per QALY as cost-effective yields a fracture risk threshold of approximately 4%, above which CT is the cost-effective imaging choice. In this study, we defined several scenarios that fit this criterion; therefore, these results may serve as a foundation for evidence-based guidelines for cost-effective imaging.

We note the limitations of this study. The complexities of each clinical scenario were necessarily simplified to allow analysis. For example, minor neurologic abnormalities such as mild motor or sensory deficits were ignored. We also ignored the effects of treatment of incidental or clinically unimportant findings in either screening protocol. In addition, we assumed that screening cervical spine CT at the time of head CT has less direct medical cost than does a separate cervical spine CT examination and that all patients would undergo head CT. Although all patients in the high-risk group do undergo head CT for evaluation of their head injuries, this assumption may not hold in the low-risk group. To be complete, we included low-risk patients in the decision analysis model. However, the results indicated that screening cervical spine CT is not cost-effective in this group, even when head CT is performed.

In addition, we considered only patients who are victims of blunt trauma, because the treatment of patients with penetrating neck trauma may be quite different. Investigation of the use of CT in victims of penetrating trauma was beyond the scope of this analysis. Finally, there are assumptions intrinsic to this analysis that must be acknowledged. For example, we assumed that all unstable cervical spine fractures eventually become evident and are treated. In addition, we assumed that the treatment of cervical spine fracture will not be related to the initial imaging study.

This study, like all decision analysis models, is dependent on estimates and assumptions derived from various sources. To maximize the accuracy of such estimates, we attempted to locate and include all relevant estimates from the medical literature and performed primary data collection where necessary. Furthermore, sensitivity analyses were broad where the uncertainty was the greatest—for example, for the probability of paralysis. Our estimates of sensitivity might be high, given that the published literature comes from academic institutions that specialize in trauma care; thus, they may not represent the values obtained in common practice. However, any overestimation of the sensitivity would be expected to oc-

TABLE 5
Results of Univariate Sensitivity Analyses

	High-Risk Group		Moderate-Risk Group		Low-Risk Group	
Variable	Estimate	Incremental Cost-effectiveness Ratio ($/QALY)*	Estimate	Incremental Cost-effectiveness Ratio ($/QALY)*	Estimate	Incremental Cost-effectiveness Ratio ($/QALY)*
Reference case	NA	Dominant	NA	16,400	NA	84,000
Sensitivity analysis						
Radiography sensitivity	92, 96	Dominant, 1,800	92, 96	5,200, 46,000	92, 96	76,000, 94,000
Radiography specificity	78, 89	Dominant, Dominant	80, 98	Dominant, 33,000	94, 97	76,000, 89,000
CT sensitivity	96, 100	Dominant, Dominant	96, 100	39,000, 5,200	96, 100	93,000, 76,000
CT specificity	90, 100	Dominant, Dominant	90, 100	25,000, 7,200	90, 100	103,000, 65,000
Probability of fracture	10, 16	Dominant, Dominant	3, 7	39,000, 400	2, 3	138,000, 46,000
Probability of paralysis	1, 15	55,000, Dominant	1, 15	180,000, Dominant	1, 15	526,000, 12,000
Radiography cost ($)	32, 58	Dominant, Dominant	32, 58	27,000, 8,600	32, 58	106,000, 68,000
Screen CT scan cost ($)	83, 181	Dominant, 7,200	83, 181	Dominant, 60,000	83, 181	30,000, 173,000
Paralysis cost (at 3% discount rate [$])	350,000, 500,000	Dominant, Dominant	350,000, 500,000	19,000, 11,000	350,000, 500,000	89,000, 78,000
Discount rate (%)	0, 7	Dominant, Dominant	0, 7	7,600, 32,000	0, 7	46,000, 151,000
Utility of paralysis (QALY)	0.47, 0.61	Dominant, Dominant	0.47, 0.61	15,000, 19,000	0.47, 0.61	77,000, 100,000
Baseline utility (QALY)	0.90	Dominant	0.90	19,000	0.90	96,000
Life expectancy (y)	9.0, 22.1	Dominant, Dominant	9.0, 22.1	15,000, 18,400	9.0, 22.1	79,000, 95,000

Note.—The lowest and highest value for each variable is given. Dominant indicates that the strategy saves money and increases QALYs. NA = not applicable.
* Added cost per unit of additional benefit.

cur for both radiography and CT, and we expected the relationship between them to be similar. We included multivariate sensitivity analyses to explore this possibility and demonstrated no major change from the reference-case analysis findings. The multiple sensitivity analyses and Monte Carlo simulations used in this analysis are a way of determining how robust the results are, and they have a role that parallels that of statistical hypothesis testing in more traditional research designs.

Additional technology assessment is needed to confirm the superior sensitivity of CT over that of radiography and determine the optimal technique for CT screening. Furthermore, validation of the injury risk prediction rule in different settings would be useful to ensure that the fracture probabilities reported in this study are generalizable beyond the major urban trauma center setting from which they were derived. However, one barrier to the broader use of CT has been the higher cost. The results of this analysis demonstrated that, on the basis of current knowledge, CT is cost-effective in high- and moderate-risk patients when all costs are considered. We believe that CT should be the initial screening modality of choice in selected patients at major trauma centers in the United States.

The greatest uncertainty in our decision analysis model was with regard to the probability of developing a severe neurologic deficit from an undiagnosed cervical spine fracture. We believe the estimates of Davis et al (9) and of Gerrelts et al (28) are most relevant because they were derived from trauma centers, where screening CT might be implemented. The pooled risk of paralysis from undetected fracture in these two studies was 15%. In both studies, roughly half of the injuries with diagnostic delay were missed on the initial radiographs, and in half, the delay was secondary to inadequate imaging. The rate of paralysis in both groups was similar. Davis et al (9) also reported that 71% of the missed injuries were unstable.

An Alberta, Canada study (29) involved patients who were transferred to a spine injury referral center. In that study, although 16 (14.2%) of 113 patients with a diagnostic delay developed secondary neurologic deficits, there were no severe deficits reported. However, those patients who were not transferred to the spinal injury center, including those who died as a result of the secondary deficit, those who sought care outside of the province, and those who could not be transferred because of other injuries, could have been missed. Although we believe that the Davis and Gerrelts study populations are more relevant to our analyses, to be conservative, we used a reference-case estimate of 5%, which is between that used in the Alberta study and that used in the Davis and Gerrelts studies (9,28,29). We used a wide range of estimates in the sensitivity analysis to accommodate the uncertainty in estimating this risk.

The estimate of the probability of developing a severe neurologic deficit was a key determinant of CT cost-effectiveness. However, in the high-risk group, the incremental cost-effectiveness of CT was still relatively low ($55,000 per QALY), even at the extreme of the sensitivity analysis range. In the moderate-risk group, the incremental cost-effectiveness ratio crossed out of the range that society would be willing to pay as the probability of paralysis decreased (<3%), which indicates that some uncertainty persists as to which strategy is favored in this group. Nonetheless, the best estimate of cost-effectiveness was that in the baseline case, which indicated that CT is the preferred strategy.

The standard of care has been radiography of the cervical spine; screening CT has been considered to be experimental. Therefore, in situations of substantial uncertainty, we selected estimates with a bias in favor of radiography. Furthermore, we ignored other possible advantages of CT scanning, including the decreased time required to "clear" the cervical spine of any fracture (12) and the possibility of clearing the spine in patients who are too unstable for prolonged examination in the radiography suite. Finally, we excluded lost wages from the cost analysis of spinal cord injury. In the high- and moderate-risk scenarios, CT was cost-effective, or dominant, despite this intentional bias.

In conclusion, the use of cervical spine

CT to screen high- and moderate-risk patients prevents cases of paralysis and may save money for society. On the basis of our cost-effectiveness analysis, CT should be considered as the primary cervical spine screening modality in selected victims of major trauma who are examined in high-volume urban emergency departments and trauma centers.

Acknowledgment: We are grateful to Diego B. Nunez, MD, University of Miami School of Medicine, Fla, for providing data critical to this analysis.

References

1. Bracken MB, Freeman DH, Hellenbrand K. Incidence of acute traumatic hospitalized spinal cord injury in the United States, 1970-1977. Am J Epidemiol 1981; 113: 615–622.
2. Fine PR, Kuhlemeier KV, DeVivo MJ, Stover SL. Spinal cord injury: an epidemiologic perspective. Paraplegia 1979; 17:237–250.
3. Shingu H, Ohama M, Ikata T, Katoh S, Akatsu T. A nationwide epidemiological survey of spinal cord injuries in Japan from January 1990 to December 1992. Paraplegia 1995; 33:183–188.
4. Berkowitz M. Assessing the socioeconomic impact of improved treatment of head and spinal cord injuries. J Emerg Med 1993; 1:63–67.
5. DeVivo MJ, Rutt RD, Black KJ, Go BK, Stover SL. Trends in spinal cord injury demographics and treatment outcomes between 1973 and 1986. Arch Phys Med Rehabil 1992; 73:424–430.
6. Kalsbeek WD, McLaurin RL, Harris BSd, Miller JD. The National head and spinal cord injury survey: major findings. J Neurosurg 1980; 31(suppl):19–31.
7. Reid DC, Henderson R, Saboe L, Miller JD. Etiology and clinical course of missed spine fractures. J Trauma 1987; 27:980–986.
8. Rogers WA. Fractures and dislocations of the cervical spine: an end-result study. J Bone Joint Surg [Am] 1957; 39:341–376.
9. Davis JW, Phreaner DL, Hoyt DB, Mackersie RC. The etiology of missed cervical spine injuries. J Trauma 1993; 34:342–346.
10. American College of Surgeons. Advanced Trauma Life Support. Chicago, Ill: American College of Surgeons, 1993.
11. Acheson MB, Livingston RR, Richardson ML, Stimac GK. High-resolution CT scanning in the evaluation of cervical spine fractures: comparison with plain film examinations. AJR 1987; 148:1179–1185.
12. Nunez DB, Ahmad AA, Coin CG, et al. Clearing the cervical spine in multiple trauma victims: a time-effective protocol using helical computed tomography. Emerg Radiol 1994; 1:273–278.
13. Woodring JH, Lee C. Limitations of cervical radiography in the evaluation of acute cervical trauma. J Trauma 1993; 34:32–39.
14. Streitwieser DR, Knopp R, Wales LR, Williams JL, Tonnemacher K. Accuracy of standard radiographic views in detecting cervical spine fractures. Ann Emerg Med 1983; 12:538–542.
15. Ringenberg BJ, Fisher AK, Urdaneta LF, Midthun MA. Rational ordering of cervical spine radiographs following trauma. Ann Emerg Med 1988; 17:792–796.
16. Borock EC, Gabram SG, Jacobs LM, Murphy MA. A prospective analysis of a two-year experience using computed tomography as an adjunct for cervical spine clearance. J Trauma 1991; 31:1001–1005.
17. Blackmore CC, Deyo RA. Specificity of cervical spine radiography: importance of clinical scenario. Emerg Radiol 1997; 4:283–286.
18. Link TM, Schuierer G, Hufendiek A, Horch C, Peters PE. Substantial head trauma: value of routine CT examination of the cervicocranium. Radiology 1995; 196:741–745.
19. Bachulis BL, Long WB, Hynes GD, Johnson MC. Clinical indications for cervical spine radiographs in the traumatized patient. Am J Surg 1987; 153:473–478.
20. Woodring JH, Lee C. The role and limitations of computed tomographic scanning in the evaluation of cervical trauma. J Trauma 1992; 33:698–708.
21. Blackmore CC, Emerson SS, Mann FA, Koepsell TD. Determination of fracture risk to improve cost-effective cervical spine imaging: a clinical prediction rule (abstr). Radiology 1997; 205(P):225.
22. Blackmore CC, Emerson SS, Mann FA, Koepsell TD. Cervical spine imaging in patients with trauma: determination of fracture risk to optimize use. Radiology 1999; 211:759–765.
23. Sox HC, Blatt MA, Higgins MC, Marton KI. Medical decision making. Boston, Mass: Butterworth, 1988.
24. Efron B, Tibshirani RJ. An introduction to the bootstrap. New York, NY: Chapman & Hall, 1993.
25. Clark CR, Igram CM, el Khoury GY, Ehara S. Radiographic evaluation of cervical spine injuries. Spine 1988; 13:742–747.
26. Light RJ, Pillemer DB. Reviewing research: the science of summing up. Cambridge, Mass: Harvard University Press, 1984.
27. Rockette HE, Gur D, Campbell WL, Thaete FL. Use of meta-analysis in the evaluation of imaging systems. Acad Radiol 1994; 1:63–69.
28. Gerrelts BD, Petersen EU, Mabry J, Petersen SR. Delayed diagnosis of cervical spine injuries. J Trauma 1991; 31:1622–1626.
29. University of Alberta Spine Trauma Study Group. Factors and outcomes of traumatic spine injuries treated at UAH 1983–1991: a prospectively gathered longitudinal database. Edmonton, Alberta, Canada: University of Alberta Spine Trauma Study Group, 1991.
30. Rules and regulations (part 414). Federal Register December 8, 1994; 59(235): 63463–63623.
31. Harvey C, Wilson SE, Greene CG, Berkowitz M, Stripling TE. New estimates of the direct costs of traumatic spinal cord injuries: results of a nationwide survey. Paraplegia 1992; 30:834–850.
32. Waters RL, Sie IH, Adkins RH. Rehabilitation of the patient with a spinal cord injury. Orthop Clin North Am 1995; 26: 117–122.
33. Webb SB Jr, Berzins E, Wingardner TS, Lorenzi ME. Spinal cord injury: epidemiologic implications, costs and patterns of care in 85 patients. Arch Phys Med Rehabil 1979; 60:335–340.
34. Cotler HB, Cotler JM, Alden ME, Sparks G, Biggs CA. The medical and economic impact of closed cervical spine dislocations. Spine 1990; 15:448–452.
35. Weinstein MC, Siegel JE, Gold MR, Kamlet MS, Russell LB. Recommendations of the panel on cost-effectiveness in health and medicine. JAMA 1996; 276:1253–1258.
36. Siegel JE, Weinstein MC, Russell LB, Gold MR. Recommendations for reporting cost-effectiveness analyses: panel on cost-effectiveness in health and medicine. JAMA 1996; 276:1339–1341.
37. Delisa JA, Gans BM. Rehabilitation medicine. 2nd ed. Philadelphia, Pa: Lippincott, 1993.
38. Smart CN, Sanders CR. The costs of motor vehicle related spinal cord injuries. Washington, DC: Insurance Institute for Highway Safety, 1976.
39. Torrance GW, Feeny DH, Furlong WJ, Barr RD, Zhang Y, Wang Q. Multiattribute utility function for a comprehensive health status classification system: health utilities index mark 2. Med Care 1996; 34:702–722.
40. Gold MR, Siegel JE, Russell LB, Weinstein MC. Cost-effectiveness in health and medicine. New York, NY: Oxford University Press, 1996.
41. Landis JR, Koch GG. The measurement of observer agreement for categorical data. Biometrics 1977; 33:159–174.
42. Laupacis A, Feeny D, Detsky AS, Tugwell PX. Tentative guidelines for using clinical and economic evaluations revisited. Can Med Assoc J 1993; 148:927–929.
43. Torrance GW. Measurement of health state utilities for economic appraisal. J Health Econ 1986; 5:1–30.
44. Hunink MG, Wong JB, Donaldson MC, Meyerovitz MF, de Vries J, Harrington DP. Revascularization for femoropopliteal disease: a decision and cost-effectiveness analysis. JAMA 1995; 274:165–171.
45. Goldman L, Gordon DJ, Rifkind BM, et al. Cost and health implications of cholesterol lowering. Circulation 1992; 85:1960–1968.

Lawrence E. Ginsberg, MD ■ Franco DeMonte, MD, FRCSC

Case 16[1]

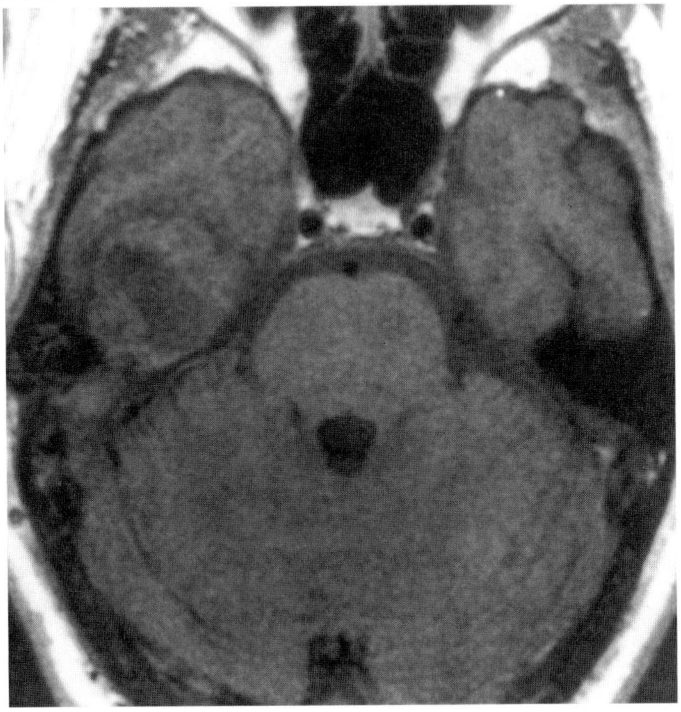

a.

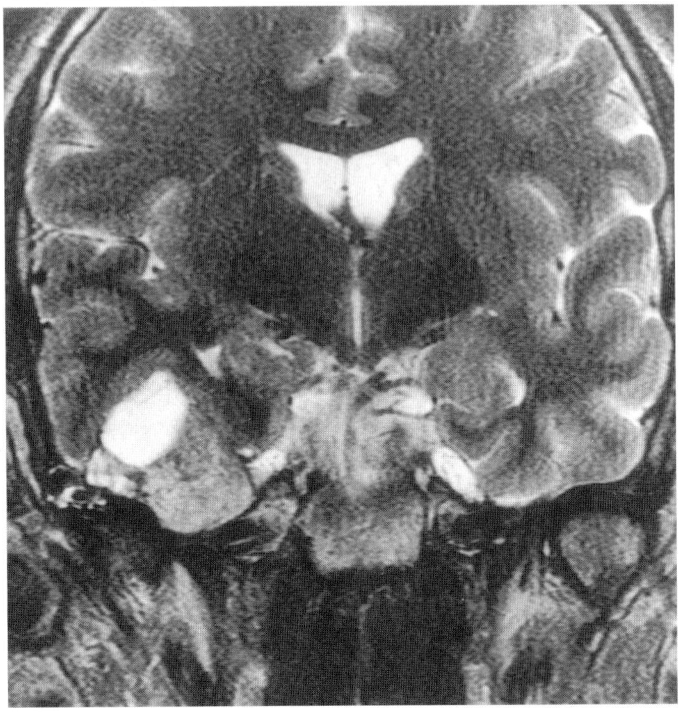

b.

Figure 1. **(a)** Axial T1-weighted 616/12 (repetition time msec/echo time msec) MR image. **(b)** Coronal fast spin-echo, T2-weighted (5,433/108) MR image (*Fig 1 continues*).

HISTORY

A 26-year-old man presented with a 6–8-month history of progressive right-sided facial weakness. This was preceded by dryness of the right eye. The patient also reported a sensation of fullness or fluid within his right ear, and he subsequently experienced decreased hearing in that ear.

Index term:
Diagnosis please

Radiology 1999; 212:126–128

[1] From the Departments of Diagnostic Radiology (L.E.G.) and Neurosurgery (F.D.), University of Texas M.D. Anderson Cancer Center, 1515 Holcombe Blvd, Houston, TX 77030. Received August 28, 1998; revision requested September 23; revision received October 8; accepted December 22. **Address reprint requests to** L.E.G. (e-mail: *lginsberg@di.mdacc.tmc.edu*).

E-mail the most likely diagnosis to *dxplease@rsna.org* (use ***only*** for submission of diagnosis). Include case number, your name (as you would want it to appear in the journal), address, phone and fax numbers. Only one case, one name, and one diagnosis per e-mail submission. Multiple diagnoses, multiple submissions, submissions without a case number will not be considered. ***Deadline:*** September 15, 1999. Answer will appear in the November issue. Authors wishing to submit cases for Diagnosis Please should first write to the Editor to obtain approval for the case and further information.

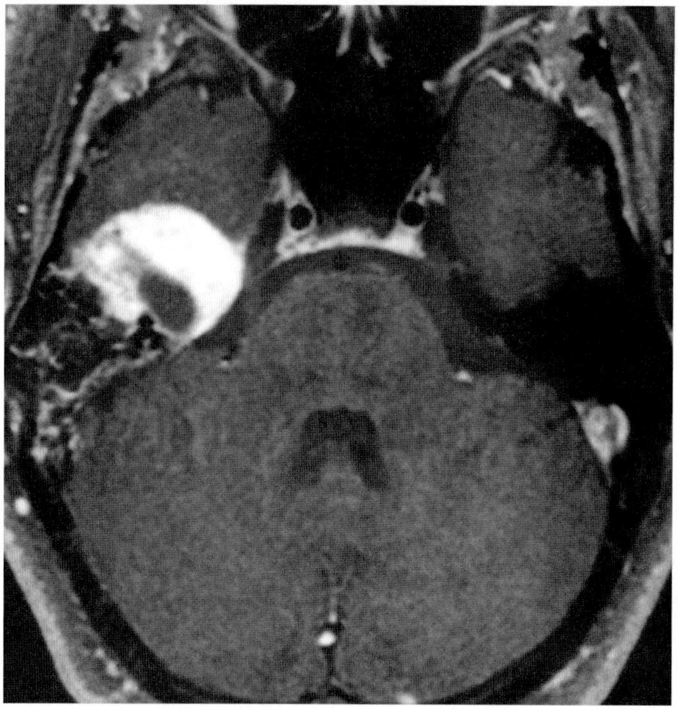

c.

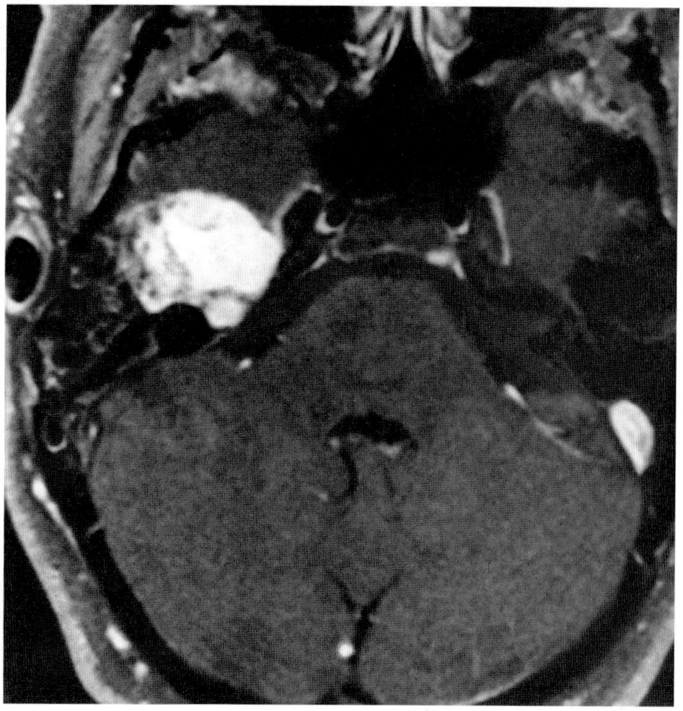

d.

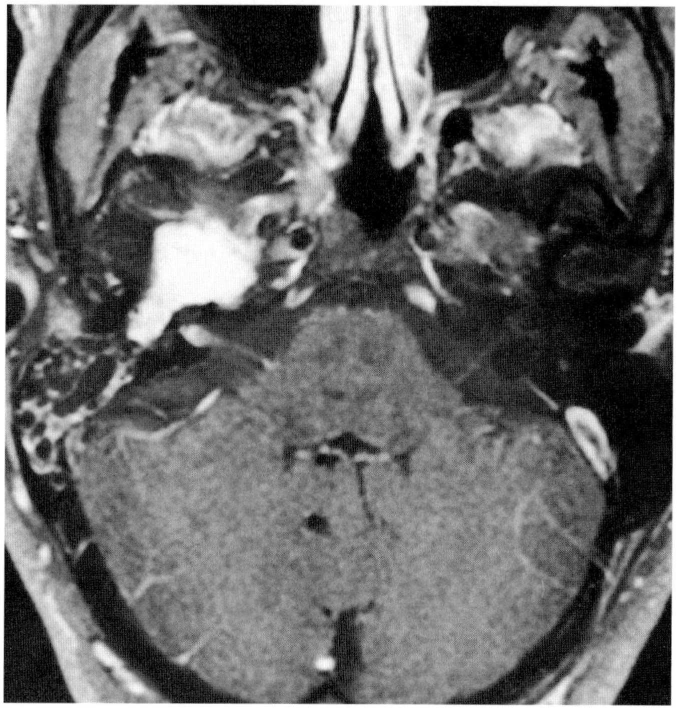

e.

Figure 1. (*continued*). **(c)** Axial T1-weighted (616/12), contrast material–enhanced, fat-suppressed MR image obtained at approximately the same level as **a**. **(d)** Axial T1-weighted (616/12), contrast-enhanced, fat-suppressed MR image obtained caudal to **c**. **(e)** Axial T1-weighted (616/12), contrast-enhanced, fat-suppressed MR image obtained caudal to **d**.

At physical examination, facial sensation and visual acuity were normal. There was a House grade III right-sided facial paresis. Audiometry revealed right-sided conductive hearing loss. The lower cranial nerves were intact, and other neurologic test results were unremarkable.

Magnetic resonance (MR) imaging (Fig 1) and computed tomography (CT) (Fig 2) were performed.

(*continued*)

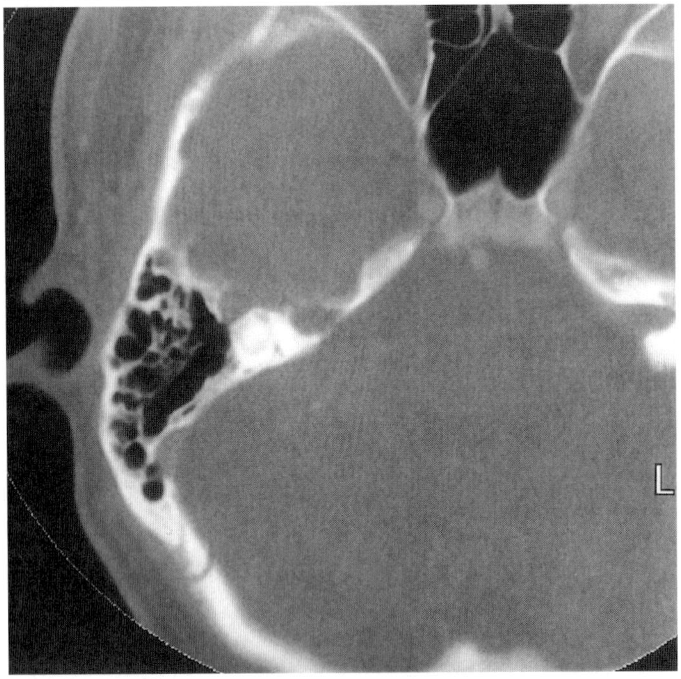

a.

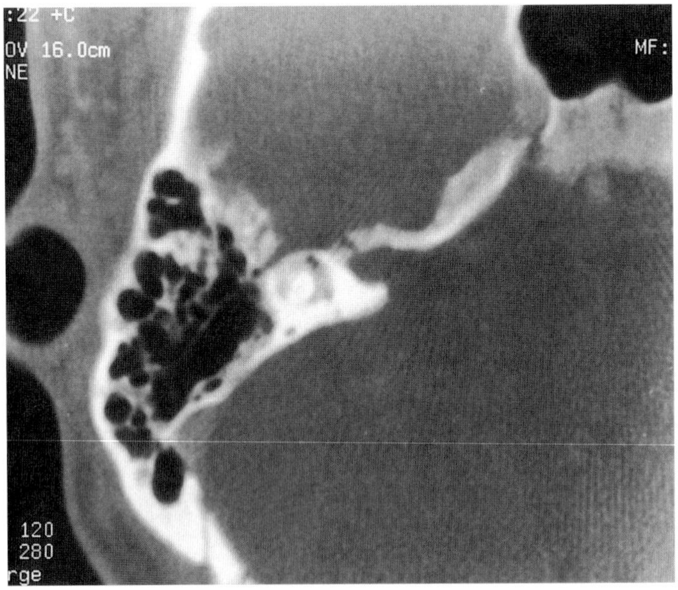

b.

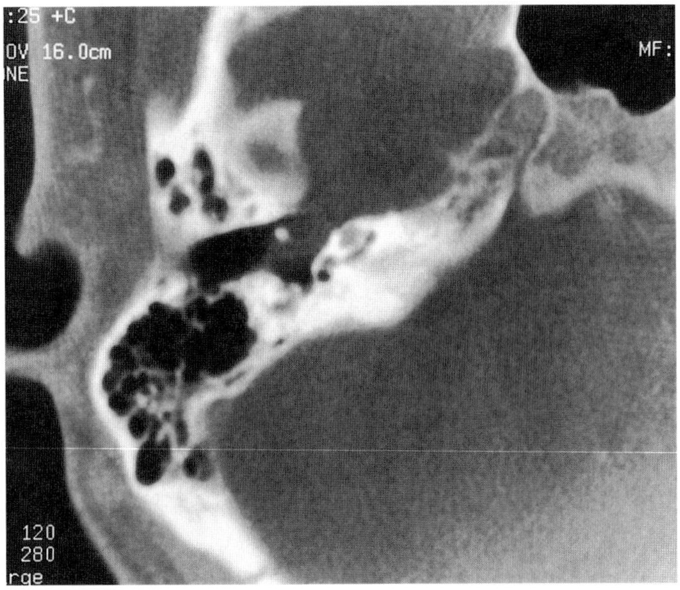

c.

Figure 2. (**a**) Axial CT image, bone technique. (**b**) Axial CT image, bone technique, obtained caudal to **a**. (**c**) Axial CT image, bone technique, obtained caudal to **b**.

Mark J. Kransdorf, MD
Mark D. Murphey, MD

Case 12: Mazabraud Syndrome[1]

HISTORY

A 34-year-old woman presented for evaluation of a soft-tissue mass in the lateral aspect of the right lower leg.

IMAGING FINDINGS

Magnetic resonance (MR) imaging of the right lower extremity showed a well-defined soft-tissue mass with a fluidlike signal intensity in the peroneus longus muscle (Fig 1). There was an expansile remodeled contour to the fibula, with diffuse replacement of the normal fatty marrow and tissue, which demonstrates a relatively homogeneous intermediate signal intensity on T1-weighted images and heterogeneous intermediate signal intensity on T2-weighted images. Imaging performed after the intravenous administration of contrast material showed moderate heterogeneous enhancement. Similar changes were seen in the tibia.

A radiograph of the right lower leg (Fig 2) showed areas of mild expansile remodeling of both the tibia and fibula, with endosteal scalloping and cortical thinning. There are regions of increased opacity to the bone that showed a ground-glass character. The identification of a well-defined soft-tissue mass with a fluidlike signal intensity and multiple bone lesions compatible with fibrous dysplasia established the diagnosis of Mazabraud syndrome.

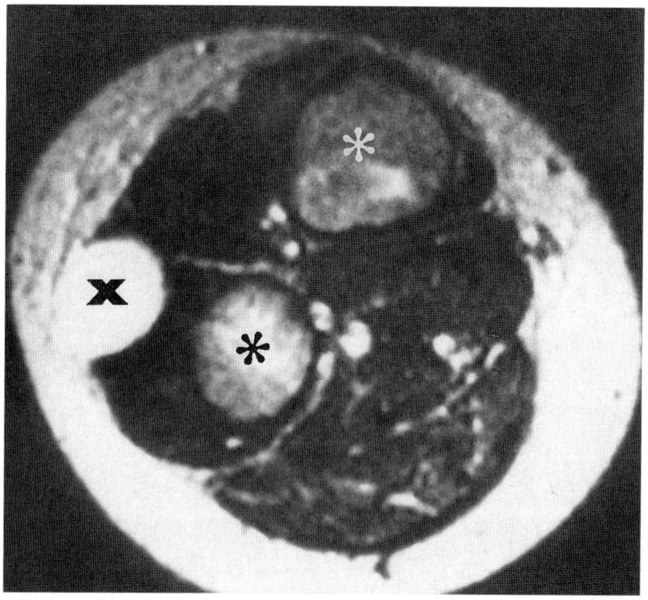

Figure 1. **(a)** Axial T2-weighted (1,800/80 [repetition time msec/echo time msec]) spin-echo MR image of the right lower leg at the level of the midcalf shows a well-defined soft-tissue mass (X) in the peroneus longus muscle with a signal intensity much greater than that of fat. Note the expansile remodeled contour to the fibula (black *) with a signal intensity slightly greater than that of skeletal muscle. There are similar but milder changes in the tibia (white *) (*Fig 1 continues*).

Index terms:
Bones, fibrous dysplasia, 45.355
Diagnosis please
Mazabraud syndrome, 45.31, 45.355
Myxoma, 45.31
Soft tissues, MR, 45.121411, 45.12143
Soft tissues, neoplasms, 45.355

Radiology 1999; 212:129–132

[1] From the Department of Radiology, Saint Mary's Hospital, 5801 Bremo Rd, Richmond, VA 23226 (M.J.K.); the Department of Radiologic Pathology, Armed Forces Institute of Pathology, Washington, DC (M.J.K., M.D.M.); the Department of Radiology and Nuclear Medicine, Uniformed Services University of the Health Sciences, Bethesda, Md (M.D.M.); and the Department of Radiology, University of Maryland School of Medicine, Baltimore, Md (M.D.M.). Received June 9, 1998; revision requested June 30; revision received July 22; accepted October 19. **Address reprint requests to** M.J.K.

The opinions or assertions contained herein are the private views of the authors and are not to be construed as official or as reflecting the views of the Department of the Army or the Department of Defense.

DISCUSSION

The key to the correct diagnosis is the identification of abnormalities in both the soft-tissue and osseous structures. Evaluation of the fibula (Fig 1b, 1c) shows moderate to marked expansile remodeling with extensive replacement of the normal marrow. There is no evidence of soft-tissue extension, and the area of marrow replacement enhances extensively after the administration of contrast material. The tibia shows similar marrow abnormalities. Although one is ill-advised to interpret musculoskeletal MR images without radiographs, the identification of multiple extensive diaphyseal lesions with expansile remodeling in long bones strongly suggests polyostotic fibrous dysplasia.

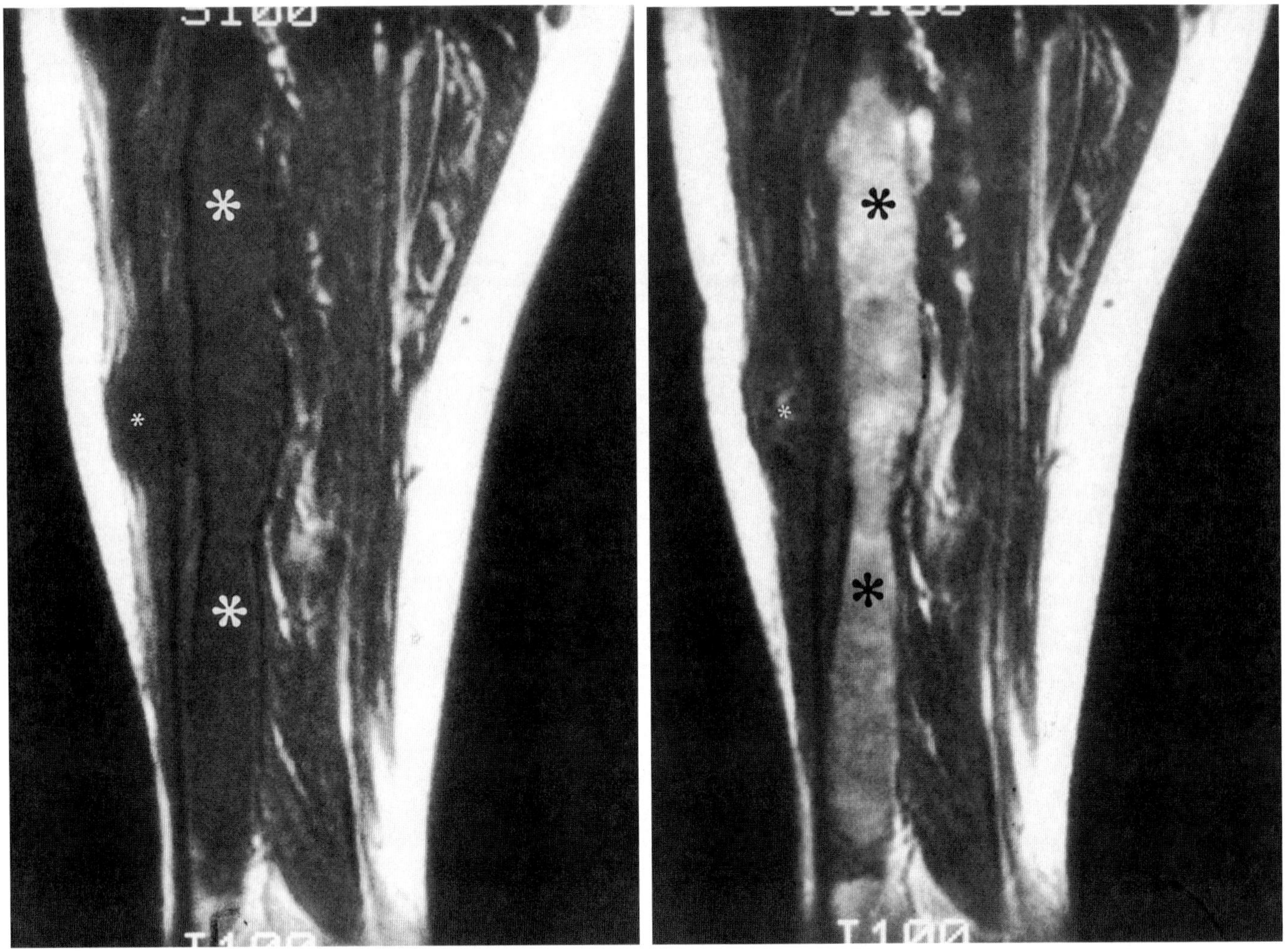

b. c.

Figure 1 (*continued*). **(b)** Coronal precontrast T1-weighted (700/20) spin-echo MR image of the right lower leg through the level of the fibula (large *) shows the soft-tissue mass (small *) to have a signal intensity less than that of skeletal muscle. There is replacement of the normal fatty marrow in the fibula with tissue with a signal intensity less than that of skeletal muscle. **(c)** Coronal postcontrast T1-weighted (700/20) spin-echo MR image of the right lower leg at the same position as in **b**. There is moderate heterogeneous enhancement of the fibula (large *), with less enhancement in the soft-tissue mass (small *).

The MR signal intensity of lesions in fibrous dysplasia is quite variable. On T2-weighted images, lesions are homogeneous to mildly heterogeneous, with about 60% of cases showing a signal intensity greater than that of fat. The remaining lesions will show either an intermediate or low signal intensity on T2-weighted images. All lesions demonstrate decreased signal intensity on T1-weighted images (1,2). The diagnosis of fibrous dysplasia is readily confirmed on the corresponding radiograph (Fig 2). The adjacent soft-tissue mass is located within the substance of the peroneus longus muscle. It shows a well-defined margin with a homogeneous signal intensity similar to that of fluid, with mild heterogeneous septumlike enhancement. These imaging characteristics strongly suggest a myxomatous mass.

The association of fibrous dysplasia with soft-tissue myxoma has been well established. This association was described by Henschen in 1926 (3), and it was emphasized by Mazabraud et al in 1967 (4) and is often referred to as "Mazabraud syndrome." Sundaram et al (5) reviewed the literature through 1987 and found a total of 17 reported cases. Soft-tissue myxoma is much more common with the polyostotic form of fibrous dysplasia but has been reported with monostotic involvement as well (5). The myxomas occur in the vicinity of the most severely affected bones and may be multiple (5,6). The association between these entities may be the result of a common origin for both fibrous dysplasia and myxoma (4), as well as a metabolic anomaly in the initial growth of both bone and soft tissue (7).

Malignant transformation in fibrous dysplasia is relatively uncommon, with a reported prevalence of approximately 0.5%, although two cases of malignant transformation have been reported in patients with Mazabraud syndrome (8). This suggests that patients with fibrous dysplasia and myxomas may be at greater risk for malignant transformation than are patients with fibrous dysplasia alone (8). Other diagnostic considerations for this case are quite limited. There are very few diseases in which there are multiple bone lesions with an associated soft-tissue tumor. Patients with neurofibromatosis

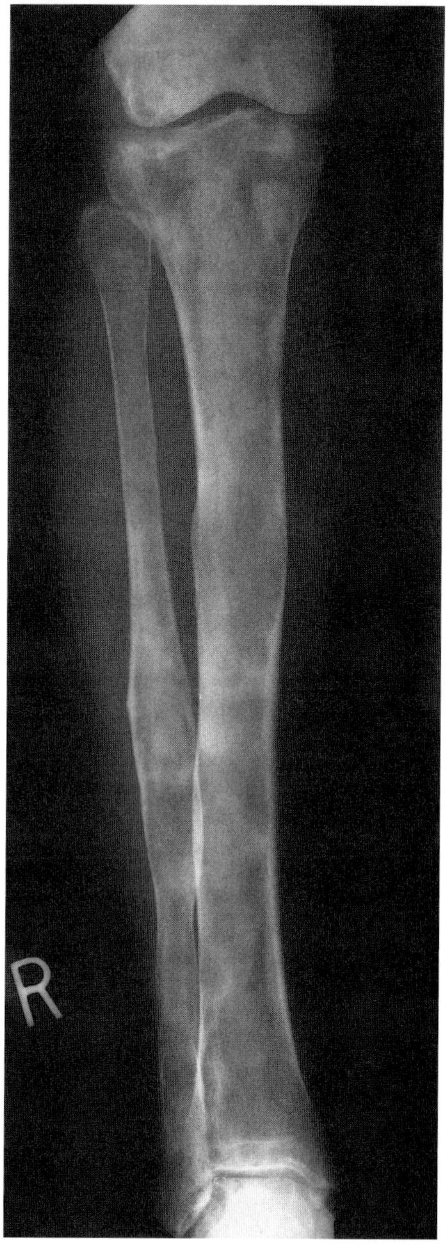

Figure 2. Anteroposterior radiograph of the right lower leg shows areas of mild expansile remodeling with endosteal scalloping and cortical thinning in both the tibia and fibula. There are regions of increased opacity to the bone that show a ground-glass character.

may show abnormalities of both bone and soft tissue. Osseous changes in neurofibromatosis reflect the underlying mesodermal dysplasia; show bowing, pathologic fracture, and pseudarthrosis; and are usually readily separable from those of fibrous dysplasia. Biopsy is not usually performed on intramedullary lesions in neurofibromatosis; however, limited histologic study has shown these typically to be fibroxanthomas (nonossifying fibromas).

Abnormalities of the bone and soft tissue should also suggest the possibility of metastases. The MR appearance of metastatic carcinoma typically is associated with peritumoral high signal intensity on T2-weighted images, in contradistinction to the well-defined margin seen in the current case. Extraosseous involvement in patients with multiple myeloma is also quite common and occurs in about half the patients (9). The skin is a frequent site of involvement and typically manifests subcutaneous nodules (10). Subcutaneous metastases are also commonly seen in patients with malignant melanoma (11). Focal intramuscular soft-tissue involvement is rare in these conditions.

Maffucci syndrome, consisting of enchondromatosis with associated soft-tissue hemangiomas, should also be considered in any patient with osseous and soft-tissue lesions; however, this diagnosis can be excluded on the basis of lesion morphology and signal intensities. Lymphoma could also be a consideration, but skeletal muscle involvement in this entity is quite rare and usually reflects diffuse involvement of multiple muscle groups (12,13). Focal muscle involvement has been reported, but is exceedingly rare, and the morphology of the bone and soft-tissue findings also exclude this diagnosis.

References

1. Utz JA, Kransdorf MJ, Jelinek JS, Moser RP, Berrey BH. MR appearance of fibrous dysplasia. J Comput Assist Tomogr 1989; 13:845–851.
2. Jee WH, Choi KH, Choe BY, Park JM, Shinn KS. Fibrous dysplasia: MR imaging characteristics with radiopathologic correlation. AJR 1996; 167:1523–1527.
3. Henschen F. Fall von ostitis fibrosa mit multiplen tumoren in der umgebenden muskulatur. Verh Dtsch Ges Pathol 1926; 21:93–97.
4. Mazabraud A, Semat P, Roze R. A propos de l'association de fibromyxomes des tissus mous a la dysplasie fibreuse des os. Presse Med 1967; 75:2223–2228.
5. Sundaram M, McDonald DJ, Merenda G. Intramuscular myxoma: a rare but important association with fibrous dysplasia of bone. AJR 1989; 153:107–108.
6. Abdelwahab IF, Kenan S, Hermann G, Lewis MM, Klein MJ. Intramuscular myxoma: magnetic resonance features. Br J Radiol 1992; 65:485–490.
7. Wirth WA, Leavitt D, Enzinger FM. Multiple intramuscular myxomas: another extraskeletal manifestation of fibrous dysplasia. Cancer 1971; 27:1167–1173.
8. Witkin GB, Guilford WB, Siegal GP. Osteogenic sarcoma and soft tissue myxoma in a patient with fibrous dysplasia and hemoglobins $J_{Baltimore}$ and S. Clin Orthop 1986; 204:245–252.
9. Kapadia SB. Multiple myeloma: a clinicopathological study of 62 consecutively autopsied cases. Medicine 1980; 59:380–392.
10. Moulopoulos LA, Granfield CAJ, Dimopoulos MA, Kim EE, Alexanian R, Libshitz HI. Extraosseous multiple myeloma: imaging features. AJR 1993; 161:1083–1087.
11. Patten RM, Shuman WP, Teefey S. Subcutaneous metastases from malignant melanoma: prevalence and findings on CT. AJR 1989; 152:1009–1012.
12. Lee VS, Martinez S, Coleman ER. Primary muscle lymphoma: clinical and imaging findings. Radiology 1997; 203:237–244.
13. Travis WD, Banks PM, Reiman HM. Primary extranodal soft tissue lymphoma of the extremities. Am J Surg Pathol 1987; 11:359–366.

Our congratulations to the 46 individuals who submitted the most likely diagnosis (Mazabraud syndrome) for Diagnosis Please, Case 12. Credit was given only if the syndrome was named or if both of its components (fibrous dysplasia and myxoma) were provided. The names and locations of the individuals, as submitted, are as follows:

Paul Aitchison, MD, *Charlottesville, Va*
William W. Atherton, DC, *Chesterfield, Mo*
Edward L. Baker, MD, *San Francisco, Calif*
Kenneth Baliga, MD, *Rockford, Ill*
Charles H. Bush, MD, *Gainesville, Fla*
Dr. V. N. Cassar-Pullicino, *Shropshire, United Kingdom*

Pierre Chevalier, *Belgium*
Marc G. de Baets, MD, *Lugano, Switzerland*
Felipe Esteban Alonso, *Madrid, Spain*
Russell C. Fritz, MD, *Mill Valley, Calif*
Akira Fujikawa, *Tokyo, Japan*
Mabel Gil Garcia, *Lerida, Spain*
Terrence M. Gross, MD, *Orlando, Fla*
Carlos Holguera Blazquez, MD, *Madrid, Spain*
Timothy D. Kadlecek, DO, *Granger, Ind*
Osamu Karakida, MD, *Matsumoto, Japan*
Alan Laorr, *Eden Prairie, Minn*
John Lin, MD, *Ann Arbor, Mich*
Jaume Llauger, *Barcelona, Spain*
Peter Miltner, MD, *Heidelberg, Germany*
Manabu Minami, MD, *Tokyo, Japan*
Hidetoshi Miyake, MD, *Oita, Japan*
Sergio J. Moguillansky, MD, *Rio Negro, Argentina*
Dr. Eduardo Mondello, *Buenos Aires, Argentina*
Philip J. Munschauer, DO, *Cincinnati, Ohio*
Dana Murakami, *Las Vegas, Nev*
Art Newberg, MD, *Boston, Mass*
Vung D. Nguyen, MD, *San Antonio, Tex*
Marcello H. Nogueira Barbosa, MD, *Ribeirão Preto, Brazil*
Narendrakumar Patel, MD, *Newburgh, NY*
Shawn P. Quillin, MD, *Charlotte, NC*
Matt Rheinboldt, MD, *Lafayette, La*
Derek J. Roebuck, FRACR, *Hong Kong, China*
David A. Rubin, MD, *St Louis, Mo*
Steven M. Schultz, MD, *Fort Worth, Tex*
Matt Shapiro, MD, *Boxborough, Mass*
Margaret A. Stull, MD, *Riverwoods, Ill*
Brian Sullivan, MD, *Wauwatosa, Wis*
Douglas L. Teich, MD, *Hermosa Beach, Calif*
John To, MD, *Iron Mountain, Mich*
Filip Vanhoenacker, *Duffel, Belgium*
Marnix van Holsbeeck, MD, *Detroit, Mich*
Joan C. Vilanova, MD, *Girona, Spain*
Craig W. Walker, MD, *Omaha, Neb*
Cecilia S. F. Wang, *Taiwan, ROC*
Michael G. Wysoki, MD, *Philadelphia, Pa*

There was one individual who submitted the highest number of most likely diagnoses. The name of this person will be announced in an upcoming issue of the journal.

Ming-Ting Wu, MD
Jen-Chuen Hsieh, MD, PhD
Jing Xiong, MD
Chien-Fang Yang, MD
Huay-Ban Pan, MD
Yin-Ching Iris Chen, PhD
Guochuan Tsai, MD, PhD
Bruce R. Rosen, MD, PhD
Kenneth K. Kwong, PhD

Index terms:
Acupuncture, 40.1299
Anesthesia, 10.459
Brain, function, 10.99
Brain, MR, 10.121412, 10.121413, 10.121419
Magnetic resonance (MR), functional imaging, 10.121419

Radiology 1999; 212:133–141

Abbreviation:
CNS = central nervous system

[1] From the Department of Radiology, Kaohsiung Veterans General Hospital, 386 Ta-chung 1st Rd, Kaohsiung 813, Taiwan (M.T.W., C.F.Y., H.B.P.); the NMR Center, Massachusetts General Hospital, Charlestown (M.T.W., J.X., Y.C.I.C., B.R.R., K.K.K.); the School of Medicine (M.T.W., J.C.H., C.F.Y., H.B.P., Y.C.I.C., G.T.) and Institute of Neuroscience, School of Life Science (J.C.H.), National Yang-Ming University, Taipei, Taiwan; the Laboratory of Functional Brain Imaging, Taipei Veterans General Hospital, Taiwan (M.T.W., J.C.H.); the Department of Radiology, National Defense Medical College, Taipei, Taiwan (C.F.Y.); and the Laboratory of Molecular and Developmental Neuroscience, Massachusetts General Hospital, Boston, (G.T.).
From the 1996 RSNA scientific assembly. Received July 20, 1998; revision requested August 26; revision received October 5; accepted January 20, 1999. M.T.W. supported in part by National Science Council (Taiwan) grant NSC 87-2314-B-075B-002 and National Health Research Institute (Department of Health, Taiwan) grant NHRI DOH88-HR-824.
Address reprint requests to M.T.W. (e-mail: *mtwu@isca.vghks.gov.tw*).

Author contributions:
Guarantor of integrity of entire study, M.T.W.; study concepts, M.T.W., C.F.Y., B.R.R.; study design, M.T.W., K.K.K., G.T.; definition of intellectual content, M.T.W., J.C.H., H.B.P.; clinical studies, M.T.W., J.X., K.K.K., Y.C.I.C.; data acquisition, M.T.W., J.X.; data analysis, M.T.W., Y.C.I.C.; statistical analysis, M.T.W.; manuscript preparation, M.T.W., J.X.; manuscript editing, M.T.W., J.C.H., G.T.; manuscript review, B.R.R., K.K.K., C.F.Y.

Central Nervous Pathway for Acupuncture Stimulation: Localization of Processing with Functional MR Imaging of the Brain—Preliminary Experience[1]

PURPOSE: To characterize the central nervous system (CNS) pathway for acupuncture stimulation in the human brain by using functional magnetic resonance (MR) imaging.

MATERIALS AND METHODS: Functional MR imaging of the whole brain was performed in two groups of nine healthy subjects during four stimulation paradigms: real acupuncture at acupoints ST.36 (on the leg) and LI.4 (on the hand) and control stimulations (minimal acupuncture and superficial pricking on the leg). Stimulations were performed in semirandomized, balanced order nested within two experiments. Psychophysical responses (pain, *De-Qi* effect [characteristic acupuncture effect of needle-manipulation sensation], anxiety, and unpleasantness) and autonomic responses were assessed. Talairach coordinates–transformed imaging data were averaged for a group analysis.

RESULTS: Acupuncture at LI.4 and ST.36 resulted in significantly higher scores for *De-Qi* and in substantial bradycardia. Acupuncture at both acupoints resulted in activation of the hypothalamus and nucleus accumbens and deactivation of the rostral part of the anterior cingulate cortex, amygdala formation, and hippocampal complex; control stimulations did not result in such activations and deactivations.

CONCLUSION: Functional MR imaging can demonstrate the CNS pathway for acupuncture stimulation. Acupuncture at ST.36 and LI.4 activates structures of descending antinociceptive pathway and deactivates multiple limbic areas subserving pain association. These findings may shed light on the CNS mechanism of acupuncture analgesia and form a basis for future investigations of endogenous pain modulation circuits in the human brain.

Acupuncture originated in ancient China and has been used to manage various clinical disorders. Acupuncture techniques are based on the theory of meridians and energy flow, which evolved after painstaking observation against a background of Chinese philosophy. However, acupuncture was not widely introduced as an alternative medicine in the West until the scientific basis of acupuncture analgesia began to be explored in the middle of the 1970s (1–5). In recent years, acupuncture has gained increasing popularity in modern health care and increasing support among scientific investigators (6–8).

Of the versatile clinical uses of acupuncture, acupuncture analgesia was one of the earliest, and so far most advanced, aspects to be explained on the basis of physiology and anatomy (1,9). Results from human and animal studies (2,9–13) suggest that acupuncture acts as a neuromodulating input into the central nervous system (CNS) that can activate multiple analgesia systems and stimulate pain modulation systems to release neurotransmitters such as endogenous opioids.

The exact CNS pathway mediating acupuncture analgesia has been explored in animal studies (2,4,9,14–17) with lesion creation or microinjection of naloxone hydrochloride (a narcotic antagonist) in a variety of hypothesized areas. Up to now, the most important and repeatedly demonstrated pathway has been the descending antinociceptive system, including the hypothalamus (the arcuate nucleus), the nucleus accumbens, and the mesencephalon (the periaqueductal gray matter and raphe nuclei) to the dorsal horn of the spinal cord (2,4,9,14–17). In addition, several areas of the limbic system have been found to participate in the nervous system circuit for acupuncture analgesia (17,18). Because it has long been hypothesized that limbic areas encode the affective-cognitive aspects of pain (19–23), the limbic system may be as important as the descending antinociceptive pathway for the CNS mechanism of acupuncture analgesia.

Although the underlying neurophysiologic mechanism remains unclear, it is generally accepted (2,4,5,24,25) that *De-Qi* (the acupuncture effect of characteristic needle-manipulation sensation, which manifests as numbness, heaviness, distention, and soreness, with spreading sensation) is the sine qua non of acupuncture for the achievement of a clinical therapeutic effect. Although the correlation between the stimulation of certain acupoints and human cortical activation has recently been explored (26), the CNS pathways that mediate *De-Qi* have not been characterized in the human brain.

Knowledge of how acupuncture stimulation proceeds centrally during the state of *De-Qi* may shed light on the CNS mechanism of acupuncture analgesia, as well as provide a common explanation for nonanalgesic effects of acupuncture. Because functional magnetic resonance (MR) imaging, a technique that is sensitive to changes in regional blood oxygenation as an index of neuronal activity (27), has been used with wide success in the mapping of human brain functions (28), we hypothesized that functional MR imaging may be useful for characterization of the CNS pathway for acupuncture stimulation. On the basis of results from the aforementioned animal studies of acupuncture analgesia, we hypothesized that acupuncture stimulation may activate the hypothalamus and limbic system to mediate the acupuncture effect (29).

In the present study, we performed functional MR imaging in healthy subjects to map the CNS pathway for real acupuncture at two acupoints, ST.36 and LI.4 (30), which are the two most widely used acupoints in experimental studies of acupuncture analgesia (2,14-18). In addition, two control stimulations were performed to test our hypothesis.

MATERIALS AND METHODS

Study Design

General protocol.—We used four stimulation paradigms nested within two experiments. In experiment 1, nine right-handed, healthy subjects (six men, three women; age range, 20–35 years) underwent two stimulation paradigms in a balanced, semirandomized order. Four subjects first underwent a real acupuncture paradigm at acupoint ST.36 (traditionally known as the *Zusanli* acupoint) (30) on the left leg; 20 minutes later, a control stimulation paradigm was performed, which consisted of superficial pricking of the skin at ST.36. The other five subjects underwent the same series of stimulations in reverse order. Experiment 2 was conducted in similar fashion: Another nine right-handed, healthy subjects (five men, four women; age range, 22–38 years) underwent a real acupuncture paradigm at acupoint LI.4 (traditionally, the *Hegu* acupoint) (30) on the left hand; 20 minutes later, a control stimulation paradigm, which consisted of minimal acupuncture (31,32) at a nonacupoint area near ST.36 on the left leg, was performed.

Acupoints ST.36 and LI.4 were chosen because they are the two most frequently used acupoints in experimental studies of acupuncture analgesia (2,14–18). Minimal acupuncture and superficial pricking were used as the control stimulations for the ST.36 stimulations, whereas acupuncture at LI.4 was used to demonstrate common brain activation patterns after stimulation of different acupoints.

Subject preparation and instructions.—The subjects were blinded about the type, block design, and order of stimulations and were instructed that all stimulations would be endurable. To minimize the effect of anticipation, subjects were instructed that any combination of different or same types of stimulation may be performed in a paradigm (although, for the purpose of group analysis, the stimulation paradigms were performed with a fixed block design in a balanced order). Before performance of the second stimulation paradigm, we determined that each subject's psychophysical state and autonomic function had returned to neutral baseline levels after approximately 20 minutes. Informed consent was obtained from all subjects, and both the acupuncture and functional MR imaging arms of the experiment were approved by the institutional ethics committees at Massachusetts General Hospital (Boston) and Kaohsiung Veterans General Hospital (Taiwan).

Stimulation paradigm design.—The block design for all four stimulation paradigms consistently was B_{120}-A-B_{150}-A-B_{90}, in which two stimulation periods (A, needle manipulation for 60 seconds) were interposed within three rest periods (B_{120}, B_{150}, and B_{90}, no needle present for 120, 150 and 90 seconds, respectively). All stimulation paradigms were performed by one experienced acupuncturist (J.X.).

Experiment 1.—In the first paradigm (real acupuncture at ST.36), a stainless steel acupuncture needle (Lhasa Medical, Accord, Mass) with a diameter of 0.25 mm and a length of 30 mm was inserted to a depth of about 2 cm into acupoint ST.36, which is located four finger breadths below the lower margin of the patella and one finger breadth laterally from the anterior crest of the tibia. The needle was manipulated by twirling approximately 90° and lifting-thrusting approximately 0.6–1.0 cm coordinately in a balanced reinforcing and reducing manner at about 1–2 Hz (24,30).

In the second paradigm (superficial pricking), an acupuncture needle was used to gently prick (approximately 1 mm deep at 1 Hz) the skin at ST.36.

Experiment 2.—In the first paradigm, real acupuncture was performed at acupoint LI.4, which is located at the first dorsal intermetacarpal space with a depth of approximately 1 cm (24,30). Manipulation of the needle was similar to that for ST.36. In the second paradigm (minimal acupuncture), the needle location was chosen at a nonmeridian focus near ST.36 (approximately 2–3 cm distant laterally) on the left leg. The manipulation was performed more lightly than in real acupuncture, with a depth of approximately 5 mm (31,32).

Data Acquisition

Psychophysical and autonomic function assessment.—After completion of each stimulation paradigm, subjects used a 10-point scale to self rate the perceived intensities of pain, the *De-Qi* effect, unpleasantness, and anxiety. A score of 0 indicated no intensity at all, and a score of 10 indicated the strongest imaginable intensity. Heart rate and end-tidal CO_2 level were continuously monitored (Omni-Trak 3100; Invivo Research, Orlando, Fla) throughout the experiments.

MR imaging.—MR imaging was performed with a quadrature head coil and a 1.5-T MR imager (Signa; GE Medical Systems, Milwaukee, Wis) that had been modified for echo-planar imaging (Advanced NMR System; Advanced NMR, Wilmington, Mass). To reduce head motion, subjects were immobilized with foam support cushions and adhesive strips.

Imaging involved the following protocol. First, a sagittal localizer image was obtained with a conventional T1-weighted spoiled gradient-echo sequence (25/5 [repetition time msec/echo time msec]; flip angle, 35°; field of view, 23 cm; matrix, 192 × 256; through-plane resolution, 2.8 mm; 60 sections) to orient, for subsequent acquisitions, 17 contiguous axial sections along the anterior commissure–posterior commissure line and to cover both cerebral hemispheres. This localizer image also was used as the structural image for transformation to Talairach coordinates of the imaging data.

Next, an automated shimming technique was used to optimize B_0 (constant magnetic induction field) homogeneity (33). This was followed by acquisition of a spoiled gradient-echo T1-weighted flow-compensated MR image (170/8; flip angle, 60°; resolution, 1.6 × 1.6 × 7.0 mm; field of view, 20 cm; matrix, 128 × 128), which was obtained primarily to aid in Talairach transformation during data analysis. The third imaging sequence was a T1-weighted echo-planar inversion-recovery sequence (∞/5/1,200 [repetition time/echo time msec/inversion time msec]; resolution, 1.6 × 1.6 × 7.0 mm), which was used to obtain structural images for the construction of preliminary statistical maps (but not Talairach-transformed or averaged maps).

Finally, a gradient-echo T2*-weighted sequence (∞/40; flip angle, 90°; field of view, 20 cm; matrix, 64 × 64 for a voxel resolution of 3.125 × 3.125 × 7.000 mm; 17 contiguous axial sections along the anterior commissure–posterior commissure line and covering both cerebral hemispheres) was performed. This sequence, which is sensitive to signal changes that arise from small changes in blood oxygenation, was used for measurements of brain activation (27). One complete set of 17 sections was obtained repeatedly every 3.5 seconds to obtain 136 time points during 8 minutes.

Autonomic Function and Psychophysical Data Analysis

Autonomic function and psychophysical data (heart rate and end-tidal CO_2 level) were averaged across the two stimulation periods and across the three rest periods separately, to calculate the mean values in the stimulation and rest states, respectively. Heart rates and end-tidal CO_2 levels in the stimulation and rest states for each paradigm were compared by using both the paired Student *t* test and the Wilcoxon signed-rank test to determine whether there were significant stimulation-related changes in autonomic function. The changes induced by means of stimulation were further normalized to percentage changes, as indexed to the mean values of the rest periods.

Multivariate analyses of variance (with four indicator variables for the four types of stimulation and one indicator variable for order effects of stimulation) were used in the analysis of differences among the four psychophysical scores and among heart rate changes associated with the four stimulation paradigms. Multivariate analyses of variance also were used in the analysis of differences among psychophysical scores and heart rate changes between the two true acupuncture paradigms and between the true acupuncture paradigm and the control stimulation paradigm. Comparisons among individual psychophysical score and heart-rate changes were performed with analyses of variance, with a threshold *P* value of less than .003 (ie, type I error rate α = .05/[3 × 5]; Bonferroni correction).

Image Analysis

Motion correction.—The echo-planar imaging data were motion corrected by using a ratio-variance minimization algorithm (called "automatic image registration", or AIR) (34) adapted from Woods et al (35). After motion correction, residual motion was reduced to less than 0.5 mm, and no time-series data evidenced residual motion in the form of cortical rim or ventricular artifacts for either the acupuncture or the control stimulations.

Talairach transformation, normalization, and averaging.—Both morphologic and functional imaging data for each subject were transformed to correspond to the Talairach stereotactic system (36) and were resectioned in coronal orientation over 57 sections with isotropic voxel dimensions of 3.125 × 3.125 × 3.125 mm. If movement was apparent between acquisitions of structural and functional images, the functional data were further fit to the structural data by translating exterior contours.

Talairach-transformed functional data were intensity scaled so that all mean baseline raw MR signal intensities were equal. Group data for each stimulation paradigm were obtained by averaging the Talairach-transformed functional data across nine subjects. The structural imaging data also were obtained by averaging across nine subjects.

Voxel-by-voxel statistical mapping and anatomic localization.—Stimulation-induced changes in functional MR imaging signal intensity were assessed by using nonparametric Kolmogorov-Smirov statistical maps (28,37–39) constructed from these averaged data sets. These maps were used for the comparisons among the two stimulation and three rest periods of each paradigm. Kolmogorov-Smirov maps were constructed after an in-plane Hanning spatial filter was applied that smoothed adjacent voxels. The Kolmogorov-Smirov probability map was converted to a logarithmic color scale and was overlaid on anatomic T1-weighted images of the same location for visual inspection. Kolmogorov-Smirov maps for group results were created with a threshold for significant changes in signal intensity established with a *P* value of less than .00001. Kolmogorov-Smirov maps also were constructed for individuals, to determine the percentage of subjects who showed activation or deactivation (with a threshold of $P < .01$) of the areas noted in the group data. Brain areas with increased signal intensity during stimulation periods were defined as activated areas, and those with decreased signal intensity during stimulation periods were defined as deactivated areas.

The time courses of signal intensity changes were evaluated for each putative activation or deactivation identified on statistical maps derived from averaged data. These signal intensity–versus-time determinations were assessed to ascertain that the changes in signal intensity did not precede stimulus presentation and that the changes specifically followed performance of the stimulation paradigm. All activations and deactivations had to meet these two criteria.

Statistical maps were superimposed on conventional T1-weighted images that also had been transformed into the Talairach domain.

RESULTS

Autonomic Function and Psychophysical Assessments

The autonomic function assessments showed that the average heart rate (± SD) was significantly decreased by means of acupuncture at ST.36 (from 64.4 beats per minute ± 7.3 in the rest periods to 60.5 beats per minute ± 7.8 in the stimulation periods, $P < .001$) and at LI.4 (from 68.1 beats per minute ± 4.8 to 64.2 beats per minute ± 5.3 , $P < .001$). No significant changes were induced by the control stimulations (Fig 1). End-tidal CO_2 level was not significantly changed in any subject.

The analysis of the four psychophysical scores and changes in heart rate indicated no significant order effects ($F_{5,27} = 0.907$, $P = .491$) for the stimulations. Because there were no significant differences between assessments of acupuncture at ST.36 and LI.4 ($F_{5,27} = 0.483$, $P = .786$), we combined the two data sets to represent the results of real acupuncture. We found significant differences between real acupuncture and minimal acupuncture ($F_{5,27} = 14.45$, $P < .001$), as well as between real acupuncture and superficial pricking ($F_{5,27} = 27.15$, $P < .001$). Comparisons among each psychophysical score and change in heart rate showed that real acupuncture resulted in significantly higher degrees of *De-Qi* and a more severe bradycardia response ($P < .001$ for both) than did minimal acupuncture, whereas real acupuncture caused significantly less pain, a higher degree of *De-Qi*, and a more severe bradycardia effect ($P < .001$ for all) than did superficial pricking (Fig 1).

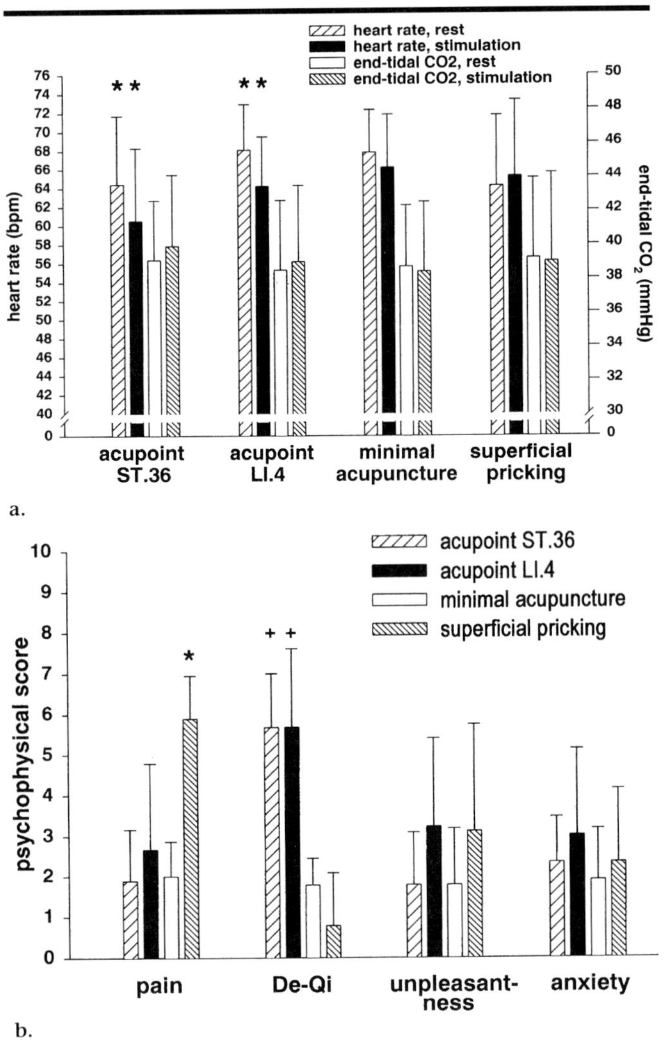

Figure 1. **(a)** Bar graph shows heart rate averaged across nine subjects in the rest and stimulation periods for each stimulation paradigm. *bpm* = beats per minute, * = significant difference ($P < .001$). **(b)** Bar graph shows average psychophysical responses reported by the subjects, who used a score of 0–10 for each variable on the horizontal axis. * = significantly different from other stimulations ($P < .001$), + = significantly different from control stimulations ($P < .001$) but not between two real acupuncture stimulations.

Functional MR Imaging Findings

Group results for functional MR imaging (Figs 2, 3; Table) during acupuncture at ST.36 showed an activation pattern in the hypothalamus and limbic system, that is, activation (signal intensity increased during stimulation as compared with that during rest) in the contralateral hypothalamus and nucleus accumbens. Deactivation (signal intensity decreased during stimulation as compared with that during rest) was noted bilaterally in the anterior cingulate cortex (rostral part, Brodmann area 24b [22]), ipsilaterally in the orbital and basal gyri, contralaterally in the amygdala formation, and bilaterally in the hippocampal complex. In addition, activation occurred in the contralateral primary somatosensory cortex, ipsilateral parietal operculum (Brodmann area 40), and bilateral prefrontal cortex (Brodmann areas 8, 9, and 10). The involvement of the limbic system was replicated with acupuncture at LI.4 in experiment 2; however, the hypothalamus appeared to show more extensive activation bilaterally.

With regard to the control stimulations, minimal acupuncture induced activation over the contralateral supplementary motor area and the anterior cingulate cortex (Brodmann area 32), the contralateral frontal operculum (Brodmann area 44 and primary motor area M1), and the ipsilateral parietal operculum (Brodmann area 40). Superficial pricking induced activation over the primary somatosensory cortex, the thalamus, the anterior cingulate cortex (Brodmann areas 32 and 24′), the contralateral supplementary motor area, the bilateral prefrontal cortex (Brodmann areas 8, 9, and 10), the bilateral frontal operculum (Brodmann area 44 and primary motor area M1), and the bilateral parietal operculum (Brodmann area 40). In addition, there was activation in the ipsilateral lentiform nucleus and the bilateral insula. No area showed a significant decrease in signal intensity (Fig 2, Table).

DISCUSSION

The distinction between the two real acupuncture stimulations and the two control stimulations was clearly reflected in the autonomic function results and psychophysical responses. The bradycardia associated with real acupuncture is a rather characteristic autonomic response that has been widely observed clinically

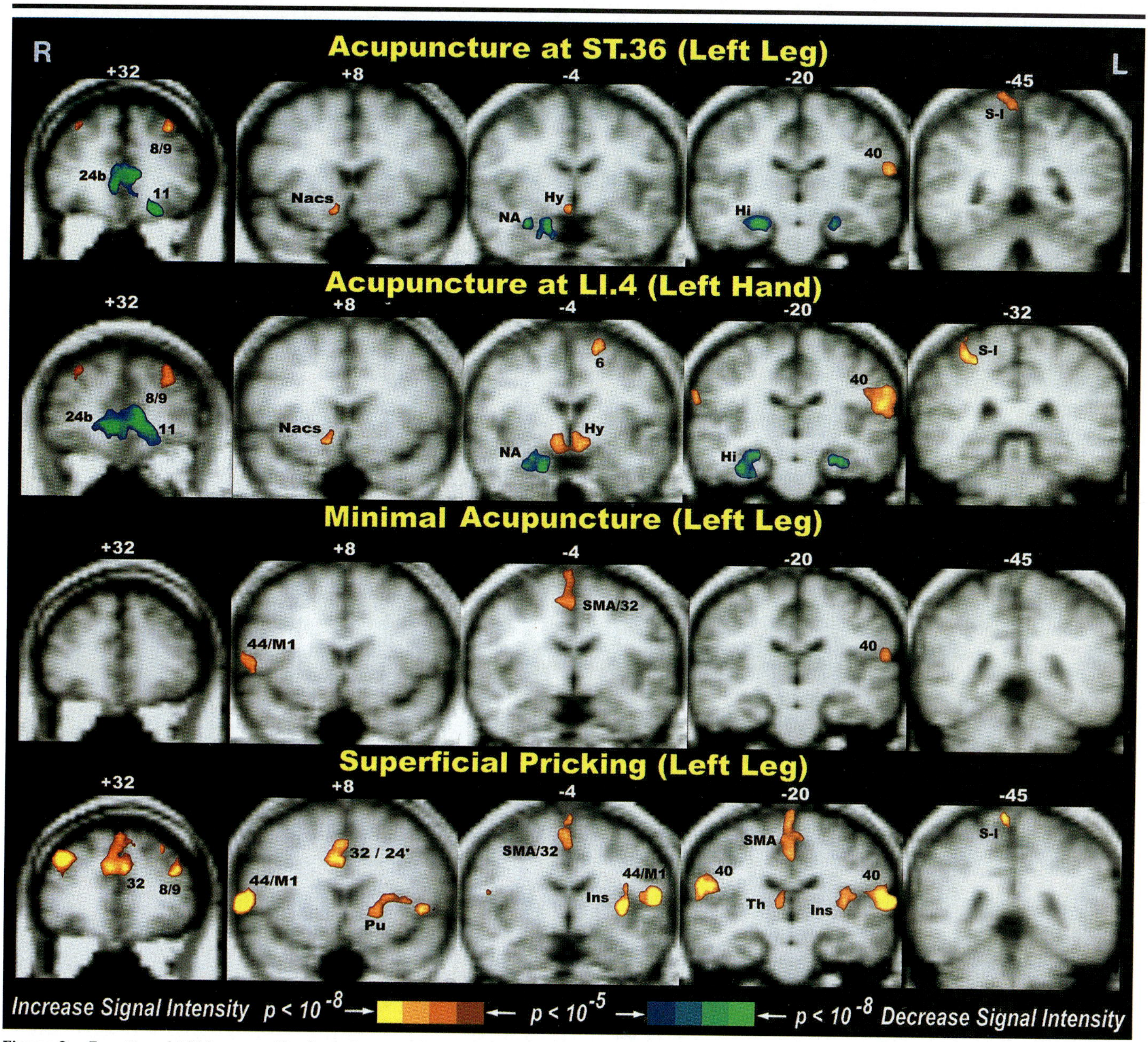

Figure 2. Functional MR images of brain activation show mean results for nine subjects in each stimulation paradigm. Representative color-coded statistical maps derived from data obtained during the four stimulation paradigms (overlaid on morphologic MR images [25/5, 35° flip angle]) show the distribution of foci with significant increases (shown in the spectrum from red to yellow) and decreases (shown in the spectrum from blue to green) in signal intensity, relative to that of the respective rest states. The threshold for a significant change in signal intensity was a *P* value of less than .00001 (Kolmogorov-Smirov method). Numbers above each image indicate the distance in millimeters anterior (+) and posterior (−) to the anterior commissure. Numbers in cortical areas of the images correspond to Brodmann areas. *Hi* = hippocampus, *Hy* = hypothalamus, *Ins* = insula, *M1* = primary motor cortex, *NA* = amygdala, *Nacs* = nucleus accumbens, *Pu* = putamen, *S-I* = primary somatosensory cortex, *SMA* = supplementary motor cortex, *Th* = thalamus.

and experimentally and hypothesized to be triggered by sufficient activation of characteristic acupuncture afferent pathways, concomitant with the state of *De-Qi* (4,24,40). It is unlikely that such bradycardia could cause substantial changes in brain activation patterns. Instead, the bradycardia reinforced the psychophysical assessment results and was supportive of the notion that our subjects achieved the state of *De-Qi* specifically by means of real acupuncture stimulation.

Of note, in the healthy subjects in our study, none of whom had a painful condition, it was difficult to demonstrate an analgesic effect of acupuncture. Furthermore, the clinical effect of acupuncture analgesia usually necessitates longer and multiple stimulation sessions; thus, it is difficult to assess the analgesic effect in an experimental functional MR imaging setting. However, presence of the *De-Qi* state, which is a prerequisite for and often an indicator of a clinical acupuncture effect (2,4,5,24,25), was sufficient to support our hypothesis that functional MR imaging findings indeed reflected the CNS pathways that mediate the acupuncture effect.

The activation of the hypothalamus

and nucleus accumbens by means of acupuncture at both acupoints was consistent with the results from animal experiments and supported the notion that acupuncture afferent pathways engage the structures of the descending antinociceptive system, particularly the hypothalamus (2,4,10,11,14,16,17). The hypothalamus, with the most abundant endorphinergic neurons and long descending projections to the raphe nucleus and periaqueductal gray matter of the mesencephalon, has repeatedly been shown (15–17,41) to be critical for acupuncture analgesia. The nucleus accumbens, with interconnections to the descending pathway from the hypothalamus to the raphe nucleus and periaqueductal gray matter, is another important structure for both opioid- and acupuncture-induced analgesia (14,15,18,41).

An important finding was that the hypothalamus showed a tendency for sustained activation on the MR images obtained after acupuncture (Fig 3). Such sustained activation of the hypothalamus may have a bearing on the long-lasting analgesic effect of acupuncture in the clinical setting (2–4,11,24,42). The finding that acupuncture at LI.4 activated the hypothalamus more extensively than did acupuncture at ST.36 may be in agreement with the clinical observation that acupuncture at the LI.4 acupoint has a stronger analgesic effect.

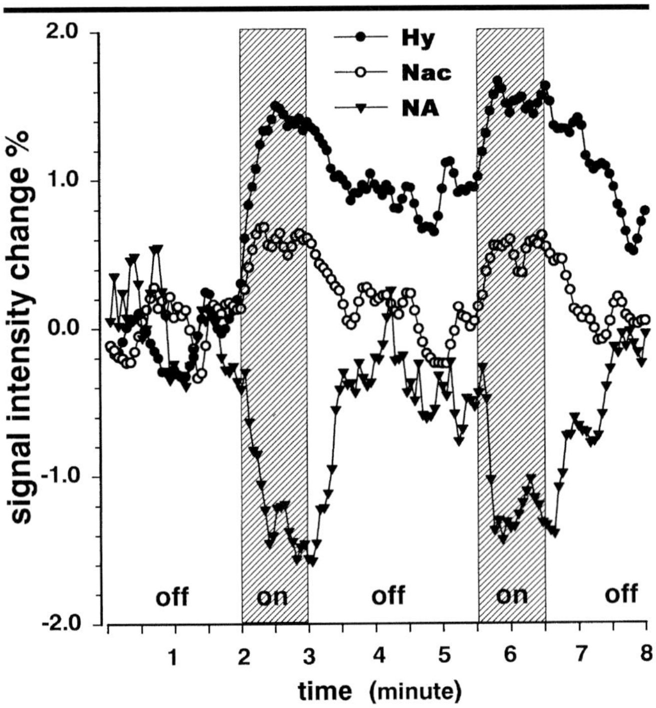

Figure 3. Graph shows the time course of changes in signal intensity (averaged across nine subjects) during acupuncture at ST.36. *Hy* = hypothalamus, *Nac* = nucleus accumbens, *NA* = amygdala. Signal intensity was normalized to the average of that measured at the first rest period and is expressed as percentage change. Note that the signal intensity of the hypothalamus showed prolonged elevation through postacupuncture MR acquisitions. The time courses of signal intensity during acupuncture at LI.4 (not shown) were similar.

Although it has been generally accepted (27) that increases in signal intensity at functional MR imaging indicate neuronal excitation (ie, activation), the physiologic meaning of a decrease in signal intensity awaits further investigation. A plausible explanation is a summed decrease in neuronal activity (ie, deactivation) (43). In the present study, the only areas of deactivation that we observed were in the limbic system during real acupuncture. This finding is noteworthy because it has been suggested (19,20,22) that the limbic system participates in pain perception, particularly the affective-cognitive aspect. Results of animal studies have demonstrated that the amygdala formation has abundant opiate receptors and participates in both opioid analgesia and acupuncture analgesia (18,44). Hippocampal activity can be strongly modulated by means of both pain and acupuncture stimulation (17,45). Furthermore, the rostral part of the anterior cingulate cortex, which has extensive connections to the amygdala and periaqueductal gray matter, is a key modulator of the internal emotional response to pain (22). On the basis of these linkages, we hypothesized that an important mechanism of acupuncture analgesia may be deactivation of limbic areas and attenuation of the affective response to pain as a result of acupuncture stimulation.

We ascribed the discrepancy between the activation pattern associated with real acupuncture and that associated with minimal acupuncture to the notably lower degree of *De-Qi* in minimal acupuncture as rated by the subjects. Minimal acupuncture has recently been recommended as an appropriate control for real acupuncture, because minimal acupuncture minimizes the specific effects of the needle manipulation while maintaining the psychologic effect (31,32). The activation of the supplementary motor cortex, parietal operculum, and frontal operculum in minimal acupuncture may be suggestive of an orientation of attention toward incoming sensory stimulation (46,47). We did not use "sham acupuncture," in which the needle manipulation and depth are identical to those used in real acupuncture, but the manipulations are performed at a nonacupoint. It has been pointed out (3,4,31,32) that sham acupuncture produces a substantial acupuncture effect that overlaps that of real acupuncture, and a huge number of subjects are needed to differentiate the effects of these two types of stimulation. On the other hand, the multiple distributed activations noted at superficial pricking—such as those of the contralateral anterior cingulate cortex (Brodmann area 24′) and thalamus, the ipsilateral lentiform nucleus, and the bilateral insula, frontal operculum (Brodmann area 44 and primary motor area M1), and parietal operculum (Brodmann area 40)—are consistent with activations identified in previous human experimental neuroimaging studies of pain (21,23,47–51). Such activation patterns were consistent with the higher pain scores given by the subjects for superficial pricking relative to those given for the deep-tissue stimulation of acupuncture.

We emphasized the group results in the present study. Given that the hypothalamus and limbic system are close to the skull base, which contains air and bone structures, it is possible that substantial susceptibility artifact (ie, decreased functional MR signal) will be produced, along with an increased potential for a type II

Foci with Significant Change in Signal Intensity between Rest and Stimulation Periods

Region	ST.36 Acupuncture					LI.4 Acupuncture					Minimal Acupuncture					Superficial Pricking				
	Side	Signal Intensity	Coordinates*	P Value†	No. of Subjects‡	Side	Signal Intensity	Coordinates*	P Value†	No. of Subjects‡	Side	Signal Intensity	Coordinates*	P Value†	No. of Subjects‡	Side	Signal Intensity	Coordinates*	P Value†	No. of Subjects‡
Hypothalamus	Right	Increase	−5, −11, +3	$<10^{-7}$	8	Right	Increase	−3, −2, +4	$<10^{-8}$	8										
						Left	Increase	−4, −4, −5	$<10^{-8}$	7										
Nucleus accumbens	Right	Increase	+8, −7, +8	$<10^{-7}$	7	Right	Increase	+10, −4, +10	$<10^{-8}$	7										
Anterior cingulate gyrus (rostral, Brodmann area 24b)	Right	Decrease	+33, +10, +4	$<10^{-9}$	8	Right	Decrease	+35, +10, +4	$<10^{-9}$	8										
	Left	Decrease	+32, +9, −7	$<10^{-10}$	8	Left	Decrease	+33, +8, −4	$<10^{-9}$	8										
Anterior cingulate gyrus (posterior-caudal, Brodmann area 24)							Increase	0, +32, +4	$<10^{-5}$	5						Right	Increase	+8, +34, +3	$<10^{-9}$	9
Anterior cingulate gyrus (Brodmann area 32)											Right	Increase	−3, +45, +4	$<10^{-6}$	7	Right	Increase	+32, +29, +5	$<10^{-10}$	9
																Left	Increase	+30, +26, −6	$<10^{-9}$	9
Amygdala formation	Right	Decrease	−8, −12, +21	$<10^{-9}$	8	Right	Decrease	−4, −13, −20	$<10^{-10}$	8										
Hippocampal complex	Right	Decrease	−20, −12, +28	$<10^{-10}$	9	Right	Decrease	−22, −10, +30	$<10^{-8}$	7										
	Left	Decrease	−24, −13, −25	$<10^{-7}$	7	Left	Decrease	−20, −18, −39	$<10^{-8}$	7										
Thalamus																Right	Increase	−20, +5, +9	$<10^{-6}$	9
Primary somatosensory	Right	Increase	−44, +65, +6	$<10^{-6}$	9	Right	Increase	−33, +60, +35	$<10^{-9}$	9						Right	Increase	−45, +66, +7	$<10^{-9}$	9
Prefrontal (Brodmann areas 8, 9, 10)	Right	Increase	+28, +45, +40	$<10^{-5}$	7	Right	Increase	+30, +44, +39	$<10^{-5}$	7						Right	Increase	+32, +31, +50	$<10^{-11}$	9
	Left	Increase	+32, +43, −33	$<10^{-8}$	7	Left	Increase	+30, +40, −38	$<10^{-6}$	7						Left	Increase	+30, +28, −48	$<10^{-10}$	9
Prefrontal (Brodmann areas 44/M1)											Right	Increase	+7, +19, +57	$<10^{-6}$	6	Right	Increase	+8, +15, +50	$<10^{-11}$	9
																Left	Increase	+0, +20, +12	$<10^{-11}$	9
Prefrontal (Brodmann area 6)						Left	Increase	−6, +61, +21	$<10^{-7}$	8										
Supplementary motor cortex						Right	Increase	−12, +56, +5	$<10^{-5}$	6	Right	Increase	−6, +60, +5	$<10^{-6}$	6	Right	Increase	−16, +58, +4	$<10^{-7}$	9
Insula																Right	Increase	0, +2, +32	$<10^{-6}$	8
																Left	Increase	+10, −4, −37	$<10^{-10}$	9
Lentiform nucleus																Left	Increase	+7, +4, −17	$<10^{-6}$	8
Posterior parietal (inferior, Brodmann area 40)						Right	Increase	−20, +28, +61	$<10^{-7}$	7						Right	Increase	−35, +30, +58	$<10^{-10}$	9
	Left	Increase	−23, +21, −53	$<10^{-7}$	9	Left	Increase	−24, +30, −57	$<10^{-8}$	9	Left	Increase	−21, +20, −54	$<10^{-7}$	6	Left	Increase	−28, +30, −51	$<10^{-11}$	9

Note.—Blank cells indicate areas in which change in signal intensity did not reach the significance threshold (ie, $P < .00001$).
* Data are Talairach coordinates (anterior-posterior, superior-inferior, right-left) of maximal change in signal intensity in terms of group results.
† P values calculated with the Kolmogorov-Smirov method.
‡ Data are number of subjects with significant change in signal intensity in the vicinity of the coordinates for the entire group.

statistical error; therefore, we used group averages in the data analyses to increase the contrast-to-noise ratio (39). On the other hand, the fact that not all subjects showed activation in the foci determined from the group results (Table) may reflect the clinical observation that individual variation is common in the treatment response of acupuncture therapy (2,4,24). Future studies with large groups of patients in which correlations among functional MR imaging findings, psychophysical and autonomic responses, and treatment effectiveness are investigated may provide results that are relevant to this clinical issue.

Although acupuncture analgesia is among the earliest, and so far most advanced, aspects of acupuncture application to be explained in scientific terms, it has been suggested (5) that a proposed mechanism for the acupuncture effect must be able to account for its action in both painful and nonpainful conditions. Given that the hypothalamus and limbic system provide multidimensional integration of neuroendocrinal and autonomic homeostasis (41), our finding that acupuncture activates the hypothalamus and limbic system also may provide a basis for the versatility of acupuncture for use in conditions other than pain disorders, such as management of nausea and vomiting, asthma, and substance addiction (4,5,52,53).

These preliminary results suggest that functional MR imaging is useful for demonstrating brain activation associated with acupuncture stimulation. We also characterized a nervous pathway in the hypothalamus and limbic system that may mediate the *De-Qi* state. Activation of the hypothalamus and nucleus accumbens of the descending antinociceptive system and deactivation of limbic areas, which are associated with pain perception, provide a neurophysiologic mechanism for the analgesic effect of acupuncture. Our findings also provide a basis for future comprehensive investigations of endogenous pain modulation circuits in the human brain.

Acknowledgments: This work is in memory of Hong N. Yang, PhD, (1950–1997), who was a mentor of young investigators in MR research in Taiwan. The authors thank Ping-Hong Lai, MD, for insightful comments; Yi-Hsin Connie Yang, PhD, for consultation on the statistical analyses; Tsung-Lung Yang, MD, for the preparation of illustrations; and Po-Chou Chen, PhD, for computer programming.

References

1. Nathan PW. Acupuncture analgesia. Trends Neurosci 1978; 21–23.
2. Han JS. Neurochemical basis of acupuncture. Annu Rev Pharmacol Toxicol 1982; 22:193–220.
3. Melzack R. Folk medicine and the sensory modulation of pain. In: Wall PD, Melzack R, eds. The textbook of pain. 3rd ed. London, England: Churchill Livingstone, 1994; 1209–1218.
4. Pomeranz B. Scientific basis of acupuncture. In: Stux G, Pomeranz B, eds. Basics of acupuncture. 3rd ed. New York, NY: Springer-Verlag, 1995; 4–60.
5. Filshie J, White A. Medical acupuncture: a Western scientific approach. London, England: Churchill Livingstone, 1998.
6. Eisenberg DM, Kesseler RC, Foster C, Norlock FE, Calkins DR, Delbanco TL. Unconventional medicine in the United States: prevalence, costs and patterns of use. N Engl J Med 1993; 328:246–252.
7. Fisher P, Ward A. Complementary medicine in Europe. Br Med J 1994; 309:107–111.
8. 1993 exploratory grants for alternative medicine: National Institutes of Health guide. Bethesda, Md: National Institutes of Health, 1993.
9. Bowsher D. Mechanisms of acupuncture. In: Filshie J, White A, eds. Medical acupuncture: a Western scientific approach. London, England: Churchill Livingstone, 1998; 69–82.
10. Peets JM, Pomeranz B. CXBK mice deficient in opiate receptors show poor electroacupuncture analgesia. Nature 1978; 273:675–676.
11. Clement-Jones V, McLoughlin L, Tomlin S, Besser GM, Rees LH, Wen HL. Increased beta-endorphin but not met-enkephalin levels in human cerebrospinal fluid after acupuncture for recurrent pain. Lancet 1980; 2:946–949.
12. Kiser RS, Khatami MJ, Gatchel RJ, Huang XY, Bhatia K, Altshuler KZ. Acupuncture relief of chronic pain syndrome correlates with increased plasma met-enkephalin concentrations. Lancet 1983; 2:1394–1396.
13. Ng LKY, Katims JJ, Lee MHM. Acupuncture, a neuromodulation technique for pain control. In: Aronoff GM, ed. Evaluation and treatment of chronic pain. 2nd ed. Baltimore, Md: Williams & Wilkins, 1992.
14. Jin WQ, Zhou ZF, Han JS. Electroacupuncture and morphine analgesia potentiated by bestatin and thiorphan administered to the nucleus accumbens of the rabbit. Brain Res 1986; 380:317–324.
15. Yu LC, Han JS. Involvement of arcuate nucleus of hypothalamus in the descending pathway from nucleus accumbens to periaqueductal gray subserving an antinociceptive effect. Int J Neurosci 1989; 48: 71–78.
16. Wang Q, Mao L, Han JS. The arcuate nucleus of hypothalamus mediates low but not high frequency electroacupuncture in rats. Brain Res 1990; 513:60–66.
17. Takeshige C. The acupuncture point and its connecting central pathway for producing acupuncture analgesia. Brain Res Bull 1993; 30:53–67.
18. Zhou Z, Du M, Wu W, Jiang Y, Han J. Effect of intracerebral microinjection of naloxone on acupuncture- and morphine-analgesia in the rabbit. Sci Sin 1981; 24: 1166–1177.
19. Melzack R, Casey KL. Sensory, motivational and central control determinants of pain. In: Kenshalo DR Jr, ed. The skin senses. Springfield, Ill: Thomas, 1968.
20. Bonica JJ. Basic considerations of pain. In: The management of pain. 2nd ed. Philadelphia, Pa: Lea & Febiger, 1990; 2–208.
21. Hsieh JC, Belfrage M, Stone-Elander S, Hansson P, Ingvar M. Central representation of chronic ongoing neuropathic pain studied by positron emission tomography. Pain 1995; 63:225–236.
22. Devinsky O, Morrell MJ, Vogt BA. Contributions of anterior cingulate cortex to behavior. Brain 1995; 118:279–306.
23. Rainville P, Duncan GH, Price DD, Carrier B, Bushnell C. Pain affect encoded in human anterior cingulate but not somatosensory cortex. Science 1997; 277:968–971.
24. Beijing College of Traditional Chinese Medicine, Shanghai College of Traditional Chinese Medicine, Nanjing College of Traditional Chinese Medicine, Acupuncture Institute of the Academy of Traditional Chinese Medicine. Essentials of Chinese acupuncture. Beijing, People's Republic of China: Foreign Language Press, 1980.
25. Vincent CA, Richardson PH, Black JJ, Pither CE. The significance of needle placement site in acupuncture. J Psychosom Res 1989; 33:489–496.
26. Cho ZH, Chung SC, Jones JP, et al. New findings of the correlation between acupoints and corresponding brain cortices using functional MRI. Proc Natl Acad Sci USA 1998; 95:2670–2673.
27. Kwong KK, Belliveau JW, Chesler DA, et al. Dynamic magnetic resonance imaging of human brain activity during primary sensory stimulation. Proc Natl Acad Sci USA 1992; 89:5675–5679.
28. Cohen MS, Bookheimer SY. Localization of brain function using magnetic resonance imaging. Trends Neurosci 1994; 17:268–277.
29. Wu MT, Xian J, Kwong KK, Yang P, Rosen BR. Central processes of acupuncture assessed by functional MR imaging (abstr). Radiology 1997; 202(2):56A.
30. State Administration of Traditional Chinese Medicine. The location of acupoint: state standard of the People's Republic of China. Beijing, People's Republic of China: Foreign Language Press, 1995.
31. Vincent CA, Lewith G. Placebo controls for acupuncture studies. J R Soc Med 1995; 88:199–202.
32. Lewith GT, Vincent CA. The clinical evaluation of acupuncture. In: Filshie J, White A, eds. Medical acupuncture: a Western scientific approach. London, England: Churchill Livingstone, 1998; 205–224.
33. Reese TG, Davis TL, Weisskoff RM. Automated shimming at 1.5 T using echo planar image frequency maps. JMRI 1995; 5:739–745.
34. Jiang A, Kennedy DN, Baker JR, et al. Motion detection and correction in functional MR imaging. Hum Brain Mapp 1995; 3:1–12.
35. Woods RP, Cherry SR, Mazziotta JC. Rapid automated algorithm for aligning and reslicing PET imaging. J Comput Assist Tomogr 1992; 16:620–633.
36. Talairach J, Tournoux P. Co-planar stereotaxic atlas of the human brain. New York, NY: Thieme Medical, 1988.
37. Stuart A, Ord JK, eds. Kendall's advanced

theory of statistics. New York, NY: Oxford University Press, 1991.
38. Baker JR, Weisskoff RM, Stern CE, et al. Statistical assessment of functional MRI signal change (abstr). In: Book of abstracts: Society of Magnetic Resonance in Medicine 1992. Berkeley, Calif: Society of Magnetic Resonance in Medicine, 1992; 626.
39. Breiter HC, Etcoff NL, Whalen PJ, et al. Response and habituation of the human amygdala during visual processing of facial expression. Neuron 1996; 17:875–887.
40. Nishijo K, Mori H, Yosikawa K, Yazawa K. Decreased heart rate by acupuncture stimulation in humans via facilitation of cardiac vagal activity and suppression of cardiac sympathetic nerve. Neurosci Lett 1997; 227:165–168.
41. Angevine JB, Cotman CW. The limbic system and hypothalamus. In: Principles of neuroanatomy. New York, NY: Oxford University Press, 1981; 253–293.
42. Lewith GT, Machin D. On the evaluation of the clinical effects of acupuncture. Pain 1983; 16:111–127.
43. Le Bihan D, Dohi M. Can fMRI detect decreased neuronal activity? (abstr). In: Proceedings of the Society of Magnetic Resonance in Medicine and the European Society of Magnetic Resonance in Medicine. Berkeley, Calif: Society of Magnetic Resonance in Medicine, 1995; 452.
44. Manning BH, Mayer DJ. The central nucleus of the amygdala contributes to the production of morphine antinociception in the rat tail-flick test. J Neurosci 1995; 15:8199–8213.
45. Khanna S, Sinclair JG. Responses of the CA1 region of the rat hippocampus to a noxious stimulus. Exp Neurol 1992; 117: 28–35.
46. Posner MI, Rothbart MK. Attentional mechanisms and conscious experience. In: Milner AD, Rugg MD, eds. The neuropsychology of consciousness. London, England: Academic Press, 1991; 91–111.
47. Derbyshire SW, Jones AK, Gyulai F, Clark S, Townsend D, Firestone LL. Pain processing during three levels of noxious stimulation produces differential patterns of central activity. Pain 1997; 73:431–445.
48. Coghill RC, Talbot JD, Evans AC, et al. Distributed processing of pain and vibration by the human brain. J Neurosci 1994; 14:4095–4108.
49. Hsieh JC, Stahle-Backdahl M, Hagermark O, Stone-Elander S, Rosenquist G, Ingvar M. Traumatic nociceptive pain activates the hypothalamus and the periaqueductal gray: a positron emission tomography study. Pain 1995; 64:303–314.
50. Hsieh JC, Hannerz J, Ingvar M. Right-lateralized central processing for pain of nitro-glycerine–induced cluster headache. Pain 1996; 67:59–68.
51. Derbyshire SWG, Jones AKP, Devani PFKJ, et al. Cerebral responses to pain in patients with atypical facial pain measured by positron emission tomography. J Neurol Neurosurg Psychiatry 1994; 57:1166–1172.
52. Clement-Jones V, McLoughlin L, Lowry PJ, Besser GM, Rees LH, Wen HL. Acupuncture in heroin addicts: changes in met-enkephalin and beta-endorphin in blood and cerebrospinal fluid. Lancet 1979; 2:380–383.
53. Jobst K, Chen JH, McPherson K, et al. Controlled trial of acupuncture for disabling breathlessness. Lancet 1986; 2:1416–1419.

Interlude

Left Ventricular Mouse

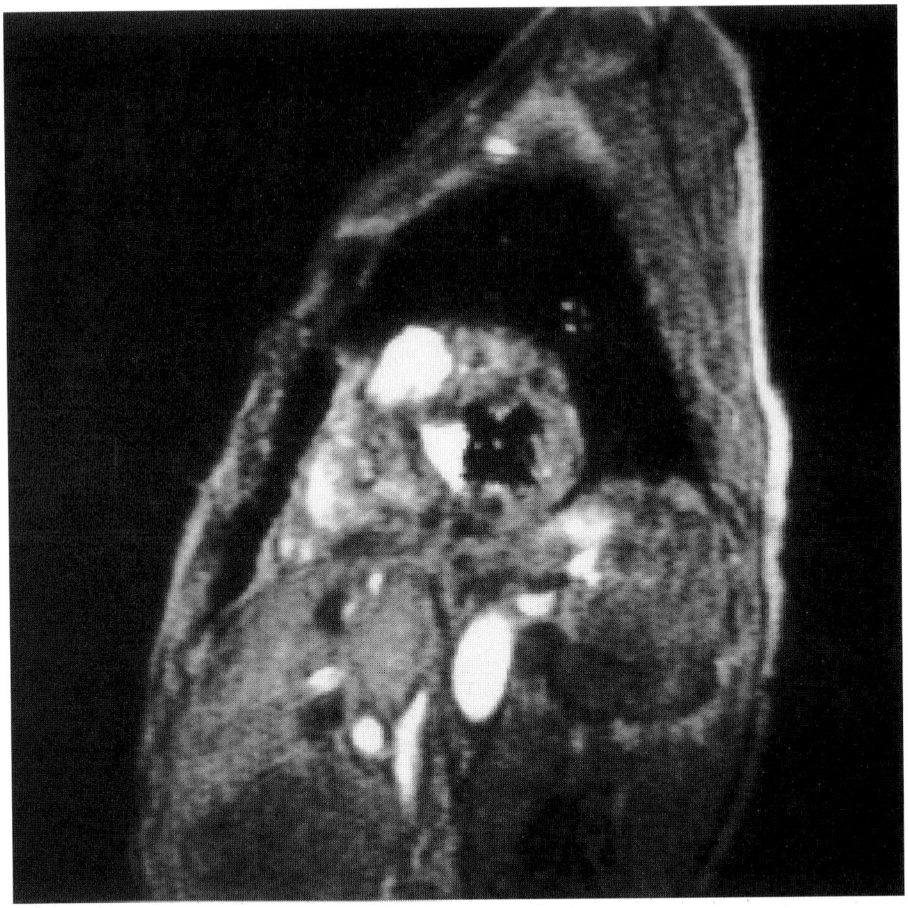

Courtesy of Raad Mohiaddin, MD, PhD, FESC, FRCR, London, United Kingdom

Stereotactic Radiosurgical Pallidotomy and Thalamotomy with the Gamma Knife: MR Imaging Findings with Clinical Correlation—Preliminary Experience[1]

David P. Friedman, MD
H. Warren Goldman, MD, PhD
Adam E. Flanders, MD
Stephen M. Gollomp, MD
Walter J. Curran, Jr, MD

Index terms:
Basal ganglia, MR, 142.121413, 142.12143
Parkinson disease, 142.881, 143.881
Stereotaxis, 142.1267, 143.1267
Thalamus, 143.121413, 143.12143
Therapeutic radiology, technology, 142.1267, 142.1299, 143.1267, 143.1299

Radiology 1999; 212:143–150

Abbreviation:
RF = radio frequency

[1] From the Departments of Radiology (D.P.F., A.E.F.), Neurosurgery, Neurosensory Institute, Wills Eye Hospital (H.W.G.), and Radiation Oncology (W.J.C.), Jefferson Medical College and Thomas Jefferson University Hospital, 132 S 10th St, Suite 1072 Main Building, Philadelphia, PA 19107, and the Department of Neurology, Lankenau Medical Building East, Wynnewood, Pa (S.M.G.). From the 1997 RSNA scientific assembly. Received August 26, 1998; revision requested September 22; final revision received November 16; accepted January 21, 1999. **Address reprint requests to** D.P.F. (e-mail: *friedm11@jeflin.tju.edu*).

PURPOSE: To evaluate the temporal evolution and appearance of a radiosurgical lesion at magnetic resonance (MR) imaging and the clinical response in patients undergoing stereotactic radiosurgical pallidotomy or thalamotomy with the gamma knife.

MATERIALS AND METHODS: Seventeen patients with medically refractory movement disorders underwent stereotactic radiosurgical pallidotomy ($n = 2$) or thalamotomy ($n = 15$). A single dose of 120–140 Gy was administered to a target in the globus pallidus interna or ventralis intermedius thalamic nucleus. Postprocedure gadolinium-enhanced MR imaging and clinical assessment were performed at 1 month and 3 months.

RESULTS: At 3 months, the radiosurgical lesion most commonly ($n = 11$) appeared as a ring-enhancing focus 5 mm or less in diameter surrounded by vasogenic edema that extended less than 7 mm in radius beyond the target. Five patients had ring-enhancing lesions 7 mm or more in diameter; four of these developed symptomatic perilesional edema at 3 ($n = 2$) or 8 ($n = 2$) months after the procedure. Onset of therapeutic effect began approximately 4 weeks after treatment. In the 15 patients with tremor, there was a mean decline of 2.1 on the Tremor Rating Scale.

CONCLUSION: Findings in this pilot study suggest that radiosurgical thalamotomy is a promising treatment for medically refractory tremor. Three-month follow-up MR studies show a ring-enhancing lesion surrounded by a variable amount of vasogenic edema. Visualization of the radiosurgical lesion and the clinical response are delayed compared to that with radio-frequency procedures.

In recent years, there has been increasing interest in the stereotactic neurosurgical treatment (radio-frequency [RF] pallidotomy or thalamotomy) of movement disorders (1–5). This interest has been prompted by recognition of the limitations of pharmacotherapy for Parkinson disease and other movement disorders, improvements in neuroradiologic imaging, and development of more sophisticated stereotactic neurosurgical techniques. Unfortunately, a large minority of patients who could benefit from RF pallidotomy or thalamotomy are poor neurosurgical candidates because of advanced age or coexistent medical conditions (eg, atherosclerotic cardiovascular disease, hypertension, chronic anticoagulant therapy). Moreover, intraparenchymal hemorrhage, which is perhaps the most serious potential catastrophic complication of stereotactic neurosurgery, is more common in elderly patients (particularly among those with one or more of the aforementioned conditions) (1,2).

Stereotactic radiosurgical ablation of the globus pallidus interna (pallidotomy) or ventralis intermedius nucleus of the thalamus (thalamotomy) with the gamma knife

Author contributions:
Guarantor of integrity of entire study, D.P.F.; study concepts, D.P.F., H.W.G.; study design, D.P.F., H.W.G., S.M.G.; definition of intellectual content, D.P.F.; literature research, D.P.F., H.W.G., S.M.G., W.J.C.; clinical studies, D.P.F.; experimental studies, D.P.F.; data acquisition, D.P.F., H.W.G., S.M.G.; data analysis, D.P.F., A.E.F.; statistical analysis, D.P.F.; manuscript preparation and editing, D.P.F.; manuscript review, all authors.

stereotactic radiosurgery unit represents a new treatment for patients with severe movement disorders, particularly those who are poor candidates for stereotactic neurosurgical procedures (6–10). Radiosurgery with the gamma knife is a minimally invasive, closed-head procedure that offers the possibility of safer ablation of the target than is possible with conventional open neurosurgical procedures; in particular, the risk of acute hemorrhage should be totally eliminated. Prior descriptions of these procedures have been mostly limited to very small series or case reports, without systematic follow-up magnetic resonance (MR) imaging (6–10). In this pilot study, we evaluated the temporal evolution and appearance of the radiosurgical lesion at MR imaging and the clinical response in a group of patients undergoing stereotactic radiosurgical pallidotomy or thalamotomy.

MATERIALS AND METHODS

During a 14-month interval (July 1996 through September 1997), 17 patients (seven men, 10 women; age range, 37–84 years; mean age, 69 years) with medically refractory movement disorders underwent stereotactic radiosurgery (Leksell Gamma Knife; Elekta Instruments, Atlanta, Ga). Preprocedure diagnoses included Parkinson disease (n = 5) and benign essential tremor (n = 12). The average duration of Parkinson disease was 12 years and of benign essential tremor was 25 years. Patients usually sought treatment when pharmacotherapy became ineffective or the slowly progressive disability resulting from their movement disorder interfered with activities of daily living (especially feeding, dressing, and handwriting). Three patients with resting tremor due to Parkinson disease and 12 patients with benign essential tremor underwent radiosurgical thalamotomy. Two patients with Parkinson disease and dyskinesia underwent radiosurgical pallidotomy. Informed consent was obtained from each patient prior to the radiosurgical procedure.

The first 10 patients in this study were believed to be poor candidates for stereotactic neurosurgery primarily because of advanced age or cardiovascular disease. After the first 10 patients had been treated, the preference of subsequent patients as to either RF or radiosurgical therapy entered into the decision-making process. One patient, a 37-year-old man, underwent expansion of a preexisting RF lesion. Owing to the proximity of the pallidotomy target to the internal capsule and optic tract, radiosurgical pallidotomy was not performed unless the patient had undergone ipsilateral (n = 1) or contralateral (n = 1) RF pallidotomy, in which stereotactic coordinates had been verified by means of electrophysiologic testing. Because of this restriction, it was more difficult to recruit patients for radiosurgical pallidotomy.

All patients were assessed clinically by a neurologist specializing in movement disorders (S.M.G.). At a minimum, patients were evaluated at baseline and at approximately 1 and 3 months after radiosurgery. In the 15 patients with tremor, the clinical evaluation included a neurologic examination and assignment of a score from the four-point Tremor Rating Scale (11,12): 0, absent; 1, slight, present with action; 2, moderate in amplitude, present with action; 3, moderate in amplitude with posture holding and action; 4, marked in amplitude, interferes with feeding. In addition, the patient assigned a self-assessment subjective score after the procedure: mild, moderate, or substantial improvement. All patients underwent radiosurgery on the side contralateral to their most functionally affected upper extremity.

Prior to radiosurgery, the patient was placed in the MR-compatible four-pin stereotactic frame. The patient was then brought to a 1.5-T superconducting MR imager (Magnetom; Siemens Medical Systems, Iselin, NJ), and imaging was performed with a gadolinium-enhanced T1-weighted inversion-recovery prepared three-dimensional fast spoiled gradient-echo sequence (repetition time msec/echo time msec/inversion time msec = 18.7/5.5/500 with 30° flip angle). Gadopentetate dimeglumine (Magnevist; Berlex Laboratories, Wayne, NJ) was administered at a dose of 0.1 mmol per kilogram of body weight. The inversion-recovery sequence provided excellent differentiation between gray and white matter and readily depicted the anterior and posterior commissures. The MR imaging data were transferred to the plan station of the gamma knife, where a three-axis reconstruction was performed. MR-based stereotactic localization was used in conjunction with the Schaltenbrand and Wahren atlas (13) for target localization.

The boundaries of the globus pallidus interna and the ventralis intermedius nucleus of the thalamus cannot be definitively identified on the basis of MR imaging characteristics. Hence, localization of these structures with stereotactic techniques is critical for optimal placement of the radiosurgical lesion. Stereotactic coordinates are calculated relative to a line connecting, but not including, the anterior and posterior commissures (intercommissural line) (Fig 1a). This line is typically 24–32 mm long (Fig 1b) (1,2).

The principal indication for stereotactic thalamotomy is tremor. The target is the ventralis intermedius nucleus of the thalamus (Fig 1c), which is a subnucleus of the ventral lateral nucleus. The ventral lateral nucleus receives projections from the contralateral cerebellum via the brachium conjunctivum. The ventralis intermedius nucleus is only 3–4 mm in anteroposterior thickness. The location of the target is 7–8 mm anterior to the posterior commissure along the intercommissural line and 11–13 mm lateral and 2 mm superior to the intercommissural line (2,3).

The principal indications for stereotactic pallidotomy are the hypokinetic or hyperkinetic symptoms of Parkinson disease. The target resides within the posteroventral globus pallidus interna (Fig 1c). The posteroventral globus pallidus interna makes up a major part of the thalamocortical circuit of the basal ganglia. Ideally, the lesion should be placed immediately lateral to the internal capsule, just above the optic tract, and immediately posterior to the mamillary bodies. The location of the target is 2–3 mm anterior to the midcommissural point and 18–23 mm lateral and 4–6 mm inferior to the intercommissural line (1,4,5).

After appropriate localization and verification, a single dose of 120–140 Gy was administered with a 4-mm collimator to the target in the globus pallidus interna or ventralis intermedius nucleus by using the cobalt 60 sources of the gamma knife. Treatment time was typically between 45 and 60 minutes. Dexamethasone (10 mg) was administered intravenously immediately preceding application of the stereotactic frame and every 6 hours thereafter for 24 hours. The patient was also observed in the hospital for 24 hours after the procedure.

Routine gadolinium-enhanced MR imaging was performed with a 1.5-T imager in three patients at approximately 1 month after the procedure and in 16 patients at approximately 3 months after the procedure. Five patients underwent additional MR studies after the 3-month examination. Gadopentetate dimeglumine was administered at a dose of 0.1 mmol/kg. The images were assessed by a neuroradiologist (D.P.F.) for size and appearance of the radiosurgical lesion and the degree of surrounding edema (mild, moder-

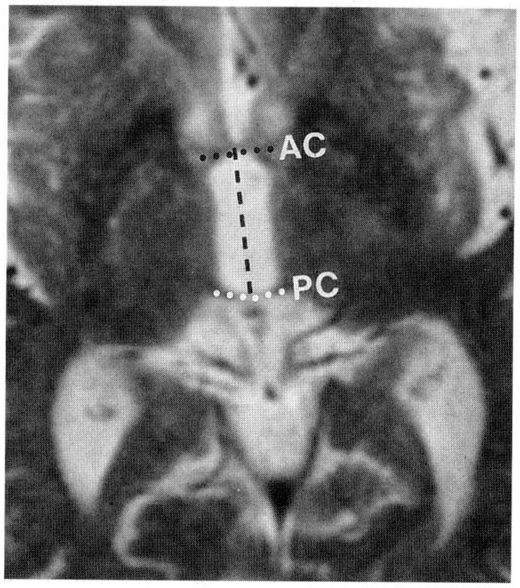

a.

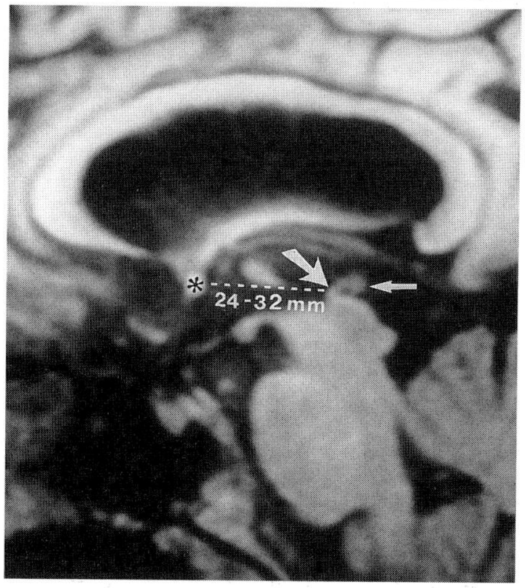

b.

Figure 1. Normal anatomy. **(a)** Axial T2-weighted (2,400/80) MR image shows the anterior commissure (*AC*) (black dots), posterior commissure (*PC*) (white dots), and intercommissural line (dashed line). Stereotactic coordinates are calculated relative to this line. **(b)** Sagittal T1-weighted inversion-recovery prepared three-dimensional fast spoiled gradient-echo (11.7/2.4/500 with 30° flip angle) MR image shows the anterior commissure (*), posterior commissure (thick arrow), and pineal gland (thin arrow). The intercommissural line (dashed line) is typically between 24 and 32 mm long. **(c)** Diagram shows the left thalamus and lentiform nucleus in the axial plane. The target for stereotactic thalamotomy is the ventralis intermedius (*vim*) thalamic nucleus (curved arrow); the ventralis intermedius is a subnucleus of the ventralis lateralis (*VL*) nucleus. The target for stereotactic pallidotomy resides within the posteroventral globus pallidus interna (*Gpi*). *Gpe* = globus pallidus externa, *IC* = internal capsule, *P* = putamen, *va* = ventralis anterior nucleus, *vp* = ventralis posterior nucleus, *v3* = third ventricle.

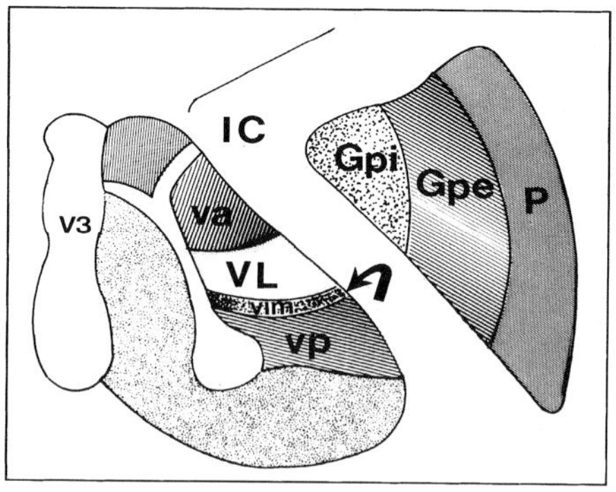

c.

ate, severe). Mild edema was arbitrarily defined as hyperintensity on long repetition time images that extended less than 7 mm in radius beyond the radiosurgical target. Moderate edema was defined as hyperintensity on long repetition time images in asymptomatic patients that extended more than 7 mm in radius beyond the radiosurgical target; for patients who underwent thalamotomy, the edema had to be confined to the thalamus, internal capsule, basal ganglia, or midbrain. Severe edema was defined as hyperintensity on long repetition time images in symptomatic patients that extended into the lobar white matter, beyond the thalamus, internal capsule, basal ganglia, or midbrain.

RESULTS

All patients with tremor experienced amelioration of their symptoms on the side contralateral to the radiosurgical thalamotomy. Onset of therapeutic effect usually began approximately 4 weeks after treatment; peak sustained therapeutic effect occurred 2–4 weeks later. Before treatment, two patients had a score of 2 on the Tremor Rating Scale, 12 had a score of 3, and one had a score of 4. Three months after treatment, three patients had a score of 0, 11 had a score of 1, and one had a score of 2. This resulted in a mean decline in score of 2.1 per patient on the Tremor Rating Scale. All 15 patients with tremor described their improvement subjectively as "substantial." Neurologic examination of the two patients who underwent radiosurgical pallidotomy showed complete resolution (n = 1) or mild improvement (n = 1) of dyskinesia.

The 1-month follow-up MR examination was discontinued after the first three patients showed no discernible change. One patient did not return for any follow-up MR imaging. On the 3-month follow-up studies, the remaining 16 patients had accurate placement of the radiosurgical lesion in the expected location of the globus pallidus interna or ventralis intermedius nucleus (Figs 2, 3). In each patient, the radiosurgical lesion was isointense to hypointense compared with the parenchyma on T1-weighted images and of variable signal intensity (ranging from hypointense to hyperintense) on T2-weighted images. There were no areas of hemorrhage seen to extend beyond the target in any case. In each patient, the radiosurgical lesion showed ring enhancement. The ring was 5 mm or less in diameter in 11 patients (range, 3–5 mm) (Figs 2, 3) and 7 mm or more in diameter in five patients (range, 7–13 mm) (Figs 4, 5). Perilesional edema was rated as mild in 11 patients (Figs 2, 3), moderate in three (Fig 4), and severe in two (Fig 5); the latter two were the patients with ring-enhancing lesions 10 mm or more in diameter. Two of the patients with moderate edema at 3 months after the procedure developed severe edema at approximately 8 months after the procedure (Fig 4); in these patients, the ring-enhancing lesion increased in diameter from 7 to 12 mm and from 9 to 15 mm, respectively.

Nine patients developed recognizable clinical complications. Two patients with essential tremor who underwent radiosurgical thalamotomy developed transient, mild slowing of rapid fine finger movements that resolved without treatment. One patient with Parkinson disease who underwent radiosurgical thalamotomy experienced marked improvement in a resting tremor but developed an action tremor in the same upper extremity. One patient with Parkinson disease who underwent radiosurgical enlargement of prior RF pallidotomy subsequently developed right hemiparesis at 8 months after treatment; an MR study showed a large lacunar infarction in the left corona radiata (Fig 3b). One patient with Parkinson disease and a prior left RF pallidotomy who underwent right radiosurgical pallidotomy developed hypophonia and swallowing difficulties. These are known risks of bilateral procedures. Four patients ultimately developed severe, symptomatic edema (Figs 4, 5) that required treatment with steroids; as stated previously, this was seen at 3 months after the procedure in two patients and at 8 months after the procedure in an additional two patients. However, the extent of hyperintensity on T2-weighted images was disproportionately large compared with the effect on neurologic function in these patients. Of these four patients, two are currently being treated and are improving, one experienced complete resolution of edema-related symptoms, and one developed dysarthria, akinesia, and weakness. A summary of the clinical and radiologic data for each patient is presented in the Table.

DISCUSSION

In patients with medically refractory movement disorders, stereotactic radiosurgery, which is a closed-head procedure, offers the possibility of safer target ablation than does stereotactic neurosurgery, since the risk of acute hemorrhage should be totally eliminated. This technique should also be an acceptable alternative for patients who are poor neurosurgical candidates. Stereotactic radiosurgery, as exemplified by the Leksell Gamma Knife, employs 201 separate, precisely directed sources (^{60}Co) configured to deliver gamma radiation in a hemispheric array to a preselected target. This delivers a biologically lethal dose of radiation to the targeted tissue while sparing adjacent nontargeted tissues. The target is placed at the convergence of the sources of gamma radiation by means of stereotactic guidance (14,15). The gamma knife has an established role in the treatment of cerebral arteriovenous malformations, cerebral metastases, and certain primary intracranial neoplasms, but its role in the treatment of other diseases, including movement disorders, is currently under evaluation.

To our knowledge, there are very few studies in the literature that evaluate the efficacy of stereotactic radiosurgery for movement disorders; most of the studies contain a very small number of patients, and the reported clinical response was variable (6–10). Findings in our pilot study show that radiosurgical thalamotomy with the gamma knife is a promising treatment for patients with medically refractory tremor. In patients with tremor at 3 months after treatment, there was a mean decline in score of 2.1 per patient on the four-point Tremor Rating Scale, and patients were consistently satisfied with their degree of improvement. Indeed, 14 of 15 patients had either complete resolution or only a slight residual tremor at 3 months after treatment. These results are comparable to those seen after RF thalamotomy, in which near or total resolution of tremor occurs in 94%–100% of patients. However, one of the disadvantages of radiosurgical therapy is that there is a delayed clinical response. In this series, the peak sustained clinical response was usually seen approximately 2 months after treatment. A corollary of this limitation is that an inadequate radiosurgical lesion cannot be recognized at the time of treatment; nevertheless, on

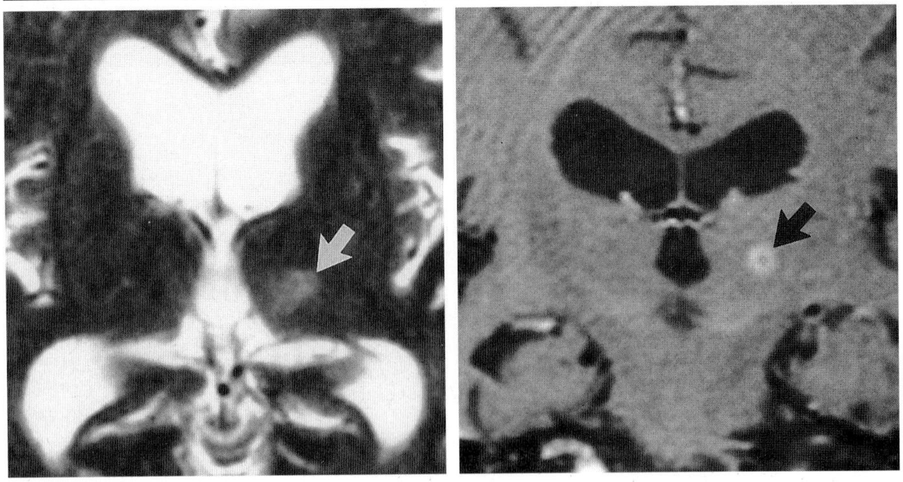

a. b.

Figure 2. Patient 10. Images in an 80-year-old man with a 5-year history of essential tremor. **(a)** Axial T2-weighted (4,000/95) fast spin-echo MR image obtained approximately 3 months after left radiosurgical thalamotomy shows a small focus of hyperintensity (edema) (arrow) in the expected location of the left ventralis intermedius thalamic nucleus. The degree of edema was rated as mild. **(b)** Gadolinium-enhanced coronal T1-weighted (600/12) MR image shows a 5-mm-diameter ring-enhancing lesion (arrow) in the same location. The lesion presumably represents a focus of radiation necrosis. This pattern of edema and enhancement was seen in 11 of 16 patients in this study.

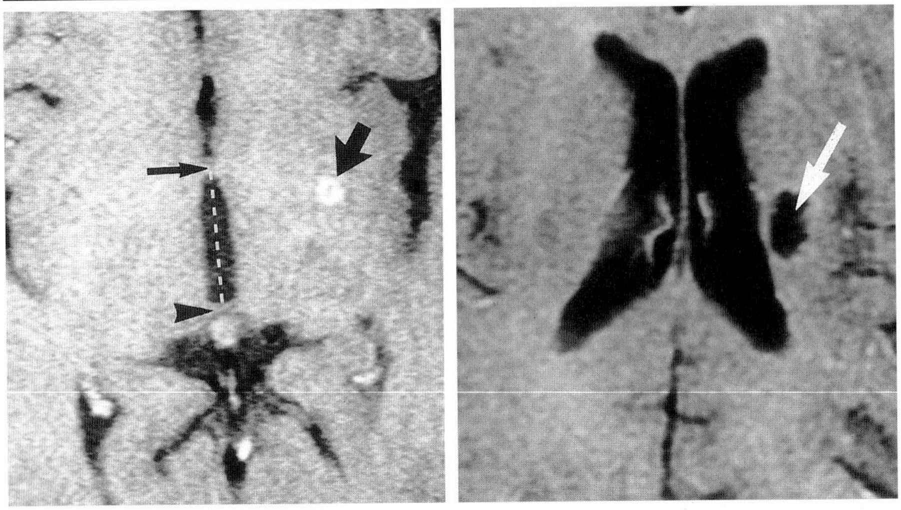

a. b.

Figure 3. Patient 4. Images in a 37-year-old man with an 8-year history of Parkinson disease and severe dyskinesia. The patient had undergone remote left RF pallidotomy. **(a)** Gadolinium-enhanced axial T1-weighted (724/12) MR image obtained approximately 3 months after left radiosurgical pallidotomy shows a 4-mm-diameter ring-enhancing lesion (thick arrow) in the area of the left globus pallidus interna. The lesion placement in this patient was modified from standard placement on the basis of electrophysiologic data from the prior RF procedure. The anterior commissure (thin arrow), posterior commissure (arrowhead), and intercommissural line (dashed line) are identified in this section. **(b)** Gadolinium-enhanced axial T1-weighted (550/12) MR image obtained approximately 8 months after the procedure shows a presumed large lacunar infarction (arrow) in the left corona radiata.

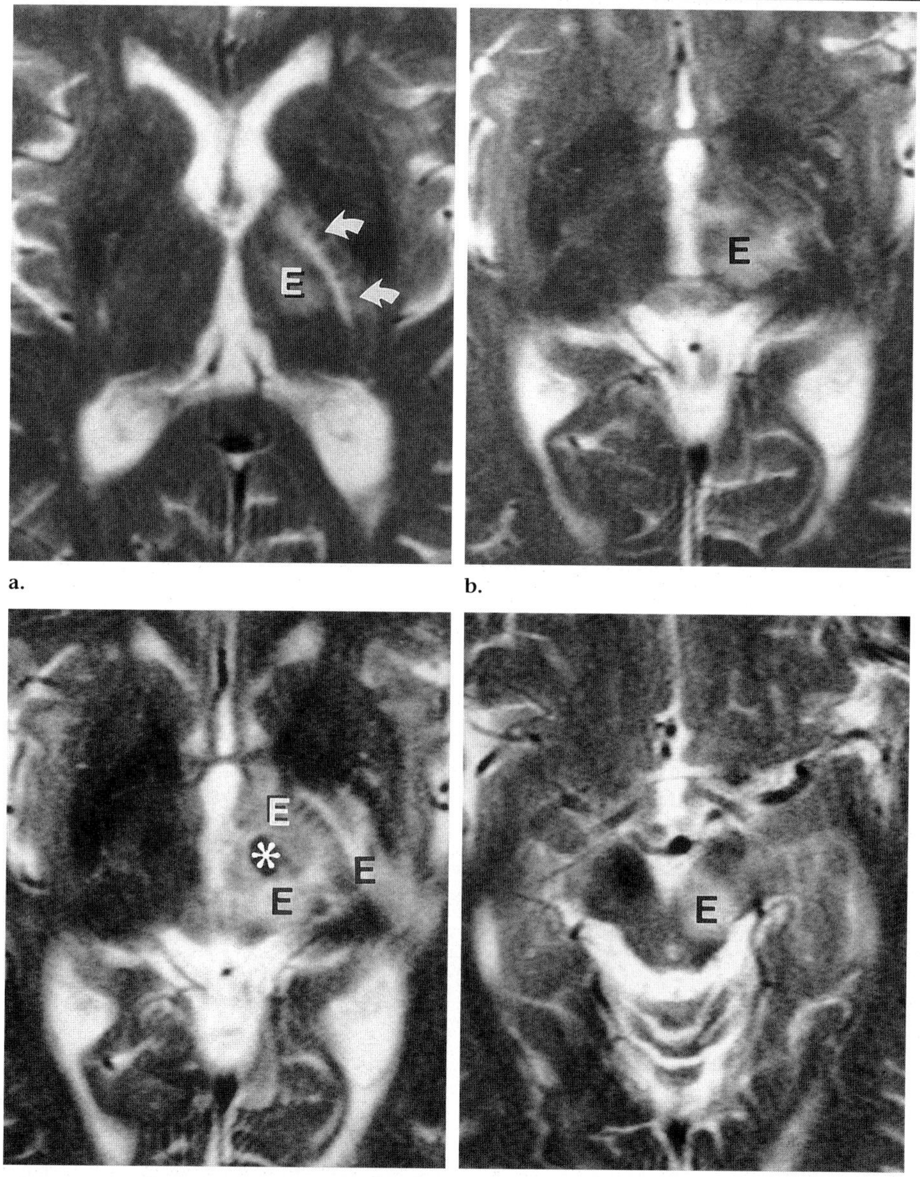

a. b. c. d.

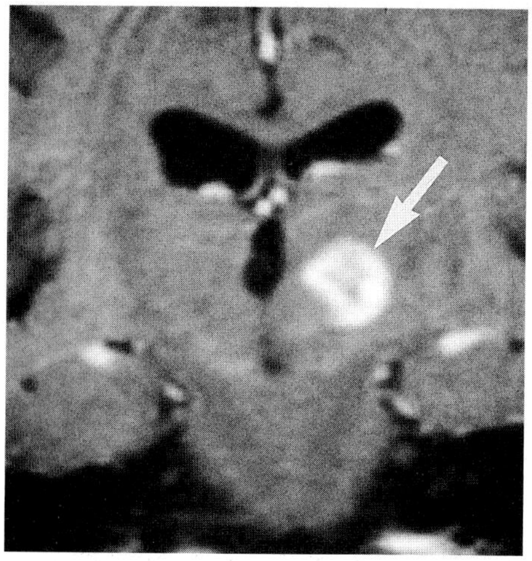

e.

Figure 4. Patient 9. Images in a 69-year-old woman with 13-year history of essential tremor. **(a)** Axial T2-weighted (3,200/105) fast spin-echo MR image obtained approximately 3 months after left radiosurgical thalamotomy shows hyperintense edema (*E*) in the left thalamus. The edema extends to the internal capsule and globus pallidus (curved arrows). The degree of edema was rated as moderate. **(b)** Axial section 7.5 mm caudad to **a** shows more extensive edema (*E*) in the left thalamus. A ring-enhancing lesion (not shown) was 7 mm in diameter. **(c)** Axial T2-weighted (3,200/105) fast spin-echo MR image obtained approximately 8 months after the procedure, to evaluate right-arm weakness and dysmetria, shows progressive edema (*E*) in the left thalamus, basal ganglia, and temporal white matter. The degree of edema was rated as severe. The radiosurgical target (*) is hypointense compared with the parenchyma, suggesting the presence of blood products. **(d)** Axial section 7.5 mm caudad to **c** shows edema (*E*) and swelling in the left midbrain. **(e)** Coronal gadolinium-enhanced T1-weighted (640/12) MR image shows a 12-mm-diameter ring-enhancing lesion (arrow) in the left thalamus.

the basis of findings in this study, this seems to be a theoretic rather than a practical concern. RF therapy offers the possibility of an immediate, maximum clinical response.

In this series, only two patients underwent radiosurgical pallidotomy. Because of the proximity of the internal capsule to the pallidotomy site, this procedure was performed only if the patient had previously undergone ipsilateral or contralateral RF pallidotomy, in which stereotactic coordinates had been verified by means of electrophysiologic testing. In the setting of prior RF pallidotomy, performance of a radiosurgical procedure on the contralateral side assumes symmetry between the two hemispheres; this may or may not be a true assumption, particularly in older patients in whom other diseases (eg, prior infarction) can produce spatial discrepancies between the hemispheres (16,17).

The need for electrophysiologic confirmation of the target location owing to individual anatomic variations has been emphasized in the functional neurosurgery literature for many years (1,2). This confirmation is clearly not obtained in stereotactic radiosurgery, which is a closed-head procedure. As such, this represents a potentially important limitation of this technique. On the other hand, although electrophysiologic monitoring may provide a more precise target, this location is the center for a thermal discharge intended to ablate only a limited but nevertheless variable volume of normal tissue. In practice, if the patient (who is awake during the RF procedure) does not respond appropriately, a larger lesion is made or the device making the lesion is moved (7). In any event, almost all the patients in this series who underwent radiosurgical thalamotomy experienced noticeable amelioration of their tremor. Along with postprocedure MR studies that consistently show the radiosurgical lesion to be included in the expected location of the ventralis intermedius thalamic nucleus, this provides indirect evidence that satisfactory localization of the target can be achieved without electrophysiologic monitoring.

On MR images obtained in the first three patients 1 month after treatment, there was no identifiable lesion; hence, these examinations were discontinued. This normal imaging appearance is in contradistinction to the changes seen on early postoperative (within 24 hours) MR studies obtained in patients who underwent stereotactic RF pallidotomy or thalamotomy; the RF lesion has a "target" appearance on axial T2-weighted images (Fig 5a). This target lesion is composed of three concentric zones of alternating signal intensity. The alternating signal intensity consists of a punctate central area of hyperintensity (coagulum) surrounded by a halo of mild hypointensity (presumably, deoxyhemoglobin) surrounded by a halo of hyperintensity (presumably, edema) (18).

On MR images obtained 3 months after treatment, the most common appearance of the radiosurgical lesion was a small (≤5 mm in diameter) ring-enhancing focus surrounded by a small (<7 mm in radius) halo of edema (Figs 2, 3). Given the dose of radiation used for this procedure, this appearance presumably represents a small focus of radiation necrosis surrounded by radiation-induced vasogenic edema. This appearance was noted in 11 of 16 patients; clinically, none of these patients subsequently developed any neurologic signs or symptoms suggesting either progressive edema or radiation necrosis. Two patients with ring-enhancing lesions 10 mm or more in diameter at 3 months after treatment experienced severe, symptomatic edema requiring treatment with steroids (Fig 5). Moreover, two of three patients with ring-enhancing lesions 7 mm or more in diameter and moderate edema at 3 months after treatment progressed to severe, symptomatic edema at 8 months after treatment; the radiosurgical lesion also enlarged noticeably in these two patients (Fig 4). On the basis of these limited data, patients with moderate edema or a ring-enhancing lesion 7 mm or more in diameter at 3 months after treatment should be considered at risk for developing further radiation necrosis and edema. Careful surveillance of these patients for at least 1 year appears warranted.

Regarding focal radiation injury of the brain with traditional doses and delivery systems, approximately 70% of all cases occur during the first 2 years. Necrosis is the most common clinically recognized form of focal radiation injury (19). Treatment of movement disorders with the gamma knife is different from traditional forms of radiation therapy in that a much higher dose is delivered to the target with the intention of creating a focal injury; moreover, the target is composed of macroscopically normal tissue. In this series, the occurrence of more extensive radiation necrosis or edema appeared to be a random event. The dosages of radiation were comparable in all patients. The unpredictable development of edema following the treatment of tumors and arteriovenous malformation with the gamma knife has already been described (20,21).

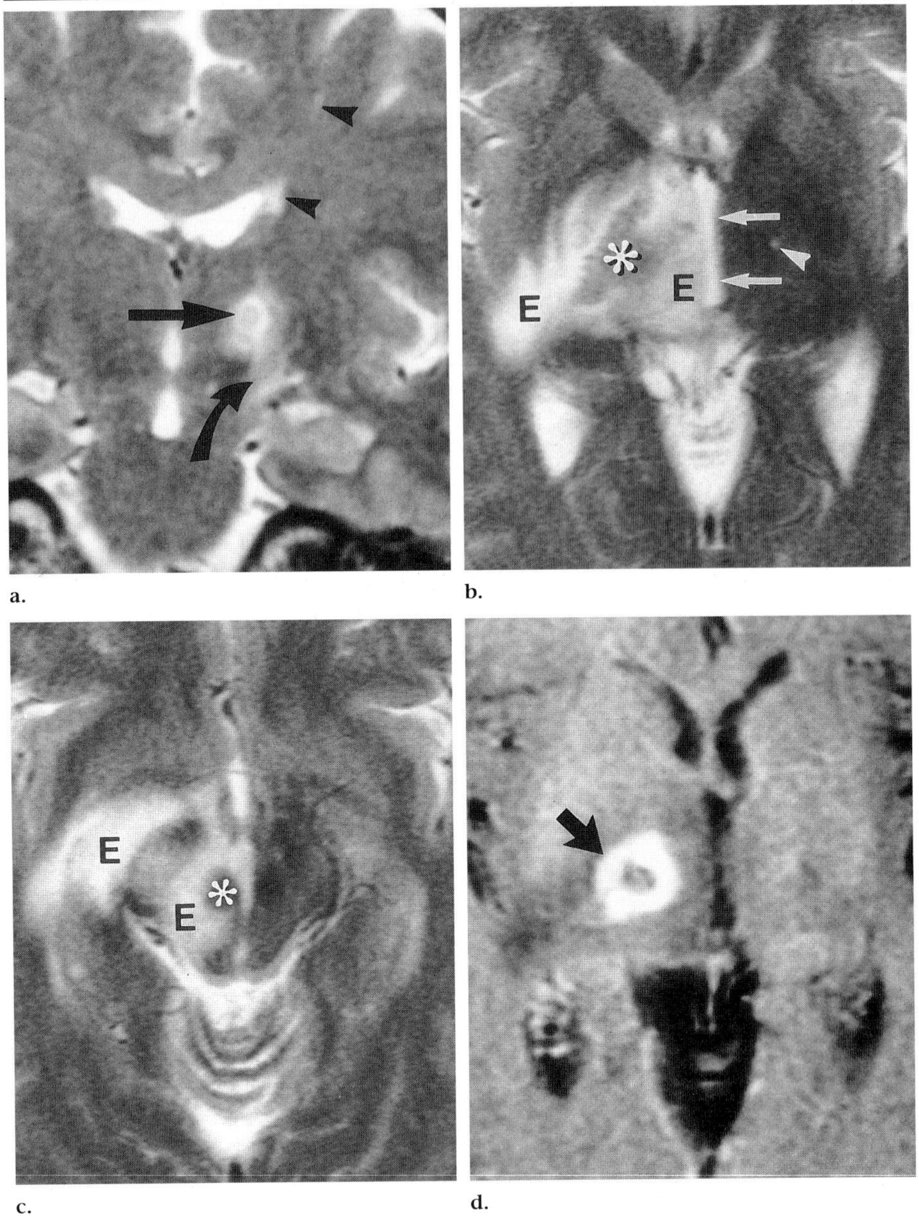

Figure 5. Patient 3. Images in a 50-year-old woman with a 15-year history of Parkinson disease and tremor. **(a)** Coronal T2-weighted (2,400/80) MR image obtained 24 hours after left RF thalamotomy in 1995 shows the characteristic "target" lesion (straight arrow) composed of concentric zones of alternating signal intensity. There is mild hyperintense edema (curved arrow) adjacent to the RF lesion. Faint, discontinuous hyperintensity (arrowheads) is seen along the RF probe tract. **(b)** Axial T2-weighted (2,600/105) fast spin-echo MR image obtained approximately 3 months after right radiosurgical thalamotomy shows the mildly hypointense radiosurgical lesion (*) surrounded by extensive hyperintense edema (*E*). The degree of edema was rated as severe. The third ventricle (arrows) is mildly compressed and displaced to the left. The patient's clinical symptoms included weakness and confusion. The residuum (arrowhead) of the prior RF thalamotomy is identified. **(c)** Axial section 7.5 mm caudad to **b** shows edema (*E*) in the right midbrain and frontotemporal white matter. * = red nucleus. **(d)** Gadolinium-enhanced axial T1-weighted (480/12) MR image shows a 13-mm-diameter ring-enhancing lesion (arrow) in the right thalamus.

Clinical and MR Imaging Findings in 17 Patients Undergoing Stereotactic Radiosurgery for Movement Disorders

Patient No./ Age (y)/Sex	Diagnosis, Duration	Preoperative Evaluation*	Postoperative Evaluation at 3 mo*	Gamma Knife Procedure	MR Findings at 3 mo: Diameter (mm) of Ring-enhancing Lesion	MR Findings at 3 mo: Degree of Vasogenic Edema	MR Findings at 8 mo	Adverse Effects at 3 mo	Comments
1/76/M	Essential tremor, 45 y	Left tremor (score, 3)	Left tremor (score, 2)	Right thalamotomy	≤5	Mild	NP	None	None
2/58/M	Essential tremor, 10 y	Right tremor (score, 3)	Right tremor (score, 1)	Left thalamotomy	10	Severe	NP	Severe edema	Improved with steroid therapy
3/50/F†	Parkinson disease, 15 y	Left tremor (score, 3)	Left tremor (score, 0)	Right thalamotomy	13	Severe	NP	Severe edema	Improved with steroid therapy, but residual deficit
4/37/M‡	Parkinson disease, 8 y	Severe right dyskinesia	Resolved	Left pallidotomy	≤5	Mild	Lacunar infarct, left corona radiata	None	Right hemiparesis at 8 mo
5/81/F	Essential tremor, 5 y	Right tremor (score, 3)	Right tremor (score, 0)	Left thalamotomy	7	Moderate	NP	Right side, transient incoordination	Resolved
6/80/F	Parkinson disease, 8 y	Right tremor (score, 4)	Right tremor (score, 1)	Left thalamotomy	≤5	Mild	NP	Developed mild action tremor	None
7/72/M	Essential tremor, 8 y	Right tremor (score, 3)	Right tremor (score, 1)	Left thalamotomy	≤5	Mild	NP	None	None
8/71/F	Parkinson disease, 10 y	Left tremor (score, 3)	Left tremor (score, 1)	Right thalamotomy	≤5	Mild	NP	None	None
9/69/F	Essential tremor, 13 y	Right tremor (score, 3)	Right tremor (score, 1)	Left thalamotomy	7	Moderate	Severe edema, 12-mm-diameter ring lesion	None	Symptomatic edema at 8 mo
10/80/M	Essential tremor, 5 y	Right tremor (score, 3)	Right tremor (score, 1)	Left thalamotomy	≤5	Mild	NP	None	None
11/61/F§	Parkinson disease, 20 y	Severe left dyskinesia	Mild improvement	Right pallidotomy	NP	NP	NP	None	Subsequently developed hypophonia and swallowing difficulties
12/84/F‖	Essential tremor, 20 y	Right tremor (score, 3)	Right tremor (score, 1)	Left thalamotomy	≤5	Mild	NP	None	None
13/81/F	Essential tremor, 22 y	Left tremor (score, 3)	Left tremor (score, 1)	Right thalamotomy	≤5	Mild	NP	Left side, transient incoordination	Resolved
14/75/M	Essential tremor, 16 y	Right tremor (score, 3)	Right tremor (score, 1)	Left thalamotomy	≤5	Mild	NP	None	None
15/68/F	Essential tremor, 55 y	Right tremor (score, 2)	Right tremor (score, 1)	Left thalamotomy	≤5	Mild	NP	None	None
16/56/M	Essential tremor, 40 y	Right tremor (score, 3)	Right tremor (score, 1)	Left thalamotomy	9	Moderate	Severe edema, 15-mm-diameter ring lesion	None	Symptomatic edema at 8 mo
17/73/F	Essential tremor, 60 y	Left tremor (score, 2)	Left tremor (score, 0)	Left thalamotomy	≤5	Mild	NP	None	None

Note.—NP = not performed.

* Tremor Rating Scale scores: 0, absent; 1, slight, present with action; 2, moderate in amplitude, present with action; 3, moderate in amplitude with posture holding and action; 4, marked in amplitude, interferes with feeding.

† Prior left RF thalamotomy, 10/95.

‡ Prior left RF pallidotomy, 7/95.

§ Prior left RF pallidotomy, 5/96.

‖ Prior right RF thalamotomy, 2/96.

Although all patients in this series with severe edema were symptomatic, the degree of neurologic dysfunction was relatively mild compared with the extent of abnormality on the MR study (22). However, one of these patients ultimately developed fixed neurologic deficits.

One patient in this series (a 37-year-old man with Parkinson disease) who underwent radiosurgical expansion of an RF pallidotomy experienced complete resolution of dyskinesia on the contralateral side; however, he ultimately developed right hemiparesis. MR imaging performed approximately 8 months after treatment showed a large lacunar infarction in the left corona radiata (Fig 3b). It is not known if the prior RF procedure predisposed this young patient in any way to develop this infarction. The relationship between the radiosurgical procedure and the infarction, if any, is also unclear.

The permanent morbidity rate for unilateral RF thalamotomy is approximately 3%. Transient deficits can be seen in 10% of patients. The major morbidity of thalamotomy (hypophonia, dysarthria, dysphasia, memory dysfunction) is usually related to bilateral procedures. Surgical mortality is rare (0.5%–1.0% of cases) and is almost exclusively due to intraoperative hemorrhage (2,3). Although radiosurgical thalamotomy eliminates the risk of procedure-related hemorrhage, on the basis of findings in this series, it exposes a small but important minority of patients to the unpredictable development of symptomatic radiation necrosis and edema.

The improvement in contralateral tremor seen after RF thalamotomy is fairly persistent in approximately two-thirds of patients. Long-term follow-up shows that even 10–15 years after unilateral or bilateral RF thalamotomy, a majority of patients continue to demonstrate improvement from their preoperative baseline (23). Clearly, similar data are not available for radiosurgical thalamotomy. Hence, these data pose both a challenge and an opportunity for this new, minimally invasive technique. Larger studies and longer follow-up of patients will be required to determine if this technique can meet or exceed the performance of RF thalamotomy.

Acknowledgments: The authors thank Karen McGlinn, RN, MS, for gathering the clinical data and the MR images; Stephen Purcell for typing the manuscript; and Ken Goodman and Fred Ross for preparing the illustrations.

References

1. Laitinen LV. Pallidotomy for Parkinson's disease. Neurosurg Clin N Am 1995; 6:105–112.
2. Burchiel KJ. Thalamotomy for movement disorders. Neurosurg Clin N Am 1995; 6:55–71.
3. Fox MW, Ahlskog JE, Kelly PJ. Stereotactic ventrolateralis thalamotomy for medically refractory tremor in post-levodopa era Parkinson's disease. J Neurosurg 1991; 75:723–730.
4. Iacono RP, Shima F, Lonser RR, Kuniyoshi S, Maeda G, Yamada S. The results, indications, and physiology of posteroventral pallidotomy for patients with Parkinson's disease. Neurosurgery 1995; 36:1118–1127.
5. Laitinen LV, Bergenheim AT, Hariz MI. Leksell's posteroventral pallidotomy in the treatment of Parkinson's disease. J Neurosurg 1992; 76:53–61.
6. Rand RW, Jacques DB, Melbye RW, Copcutt BG, Fisher MR, Levenick MN. Gamma knife thalamotomy and pallidotomy in patients with movement disorders: preliminary results. Stereotact Funct Neurosurg 1993; 61(suppl 1):65–92.
7. Friedman JH, Epstein M, Sanes JN, et al. Gamma knife pallidotomy in advanced Parkinson's disease. Ann Neurol 1996; 39: 535–538.
8. Ohye C, Shibazaki T, Hirato M, Inoue H, Andou Y. Gamma thalamotomy for Parkinsonian and other kinds of tremor. Stereotact Funct Neurosurg 1996; 66(suppl 1):333–342.
9. Otsuki T, Jokura H, Takahashi K, et al. Stereotactic gamma thalamotomy with a computerized brain atlas: technical case report. Neurosurgery 1994; 35:764–768.
10. Lindquist C, Steiner L, Hindmarsh T. Gamma knife thalamotomy for tremor: report of two cases. In: Steiner L, ed. Radiosurgery: baseline and trends. New York, NY: Raven, 1992; 237–243.
11. Fahn S, Marsden CD, Calne DB, Goldstein M, eds. Recent developments in Parkinson's disease. Vol 2. Florham Park, NJ: Macmillan Health Care Information, 1987; 153–163.
12. Fahn S, Marsden CD, Calne DB, Goldstein M, eds. Recent developments in Parkinson's disease. Vol 2. Florham Park, NJ: Macmillan Health Care Information, 1987; 293–304.
13. Schaltenbrand G, Wahren W. Atlas for stereotaxy of the human brain. 2nd ed. Stuttgart, Germany: Thieme, 1977.
14. Lunsford LD, Flickinger J, Lindner G, Maitz A. Stereotactic radiosurgery of the brain using the first United States 201 cobalt-60 source gamma knife. Neurosurgery 1989; 24:151–159.
15. Lutz W. Radiation physics for radiosurgery. In: Alexander E, Loeffler JS, Lunsford LD, eds. Radiation physics for radiosurgery. New York, NY: McGraw Hill, 1993; 7–15.
16. Brierly J, Beck E. The significance in human stereotactic brain surgery of individual variations in the diencephalon and globus pallidus. J Neurol Neurosurg Psychiatry 1959; 22:286–298.
17. Kelly PJ, Derome P, Guiot G. Thalamic spatial variability and the surgical results of lesions placed with neurophysiologic control. Surg Neurol 1978; 9:307–315.
18. Friedman DP, Goldman HW, Flanders AE. MR imaging of stereotaxic pallidotomy and thalamotomy. AJR 1997; 169:894–896.
19. Valk PE, Dillon WP. Radiation injury of the brain. AJR 1991; 156:689–706.
20. Pollock BE, Lunsford LD, Kondziolka D, Bissonette DJ, Flickinger FC. Stereotactic radiosurgery for postgeniculate visual pathway arteriovenous malformations. J Neurosurg 1996; 84:437–441.
21. Niemela M, Lim YJ, Soderman M, Jaaskelainen J, Lindquist C. Gamma knife radiosurgery in 11 hemangioblastomas. J Neurosurg 1996; 85:591–596.
22. Goldman HW, Gollomp S, Friedman D. Clinical implications of delayed white matter changes following gamma knife stereotactic radiosurgical thalamotomy. Presented at the 48th Annual Meeting of the Congress of Neurological Surgeons, Seattle, Washington, October 3–8, 1998.
23. Broggi G, Giorgi C, Servello D. Stereotactic neurosurgery in the treatment of tremor. Acta Neurochir Suppl (Wien) 1987; 39:73–76.

Robert L. Williams, MD
Randall L. Beatty, MD
Emanuel Kanal, MD
Jane L. Weissman, MD

Index terms:
Brain, MR, 161.121411, 161.121413, 161.121414, 161.121415
Brain, ventricles, 161.458
Cytomegalovirus, 2245.2066
Eye, diseases, 2245.2066, 2245.241, 2245.892
Eye, MR, 2245.121411, 2245.121413, 2245.121414, 2245.121415
Retina, 2245.892
Silicone, 161.458, 2244.126

Radiology 1999; 212:151–154

[1] From the Departments of Radiology (R.L.W., E.K., J.L.W.), Ophthalmology (R.L.B.), and Otolaryngology (J.L.W.), University of Pittsburgh Medical Center, Rm D132PUH, 200 Lothrop St, Pittsburgh, PA 15213. Received March 26, 1998; revision requested June 24; revision received September 18; accepted December 8. **Address reprint requests to** R.L.W. (e-mail: *williamsrl@radserv.arad.upmc.edu*).

Author contributions:
Guarantor of integrity of entire study, R.L.W.; study concepts and design, R.L.W.; definition of intellectual content, J.L.W.; literature research, R.L.W., R.L.B.; data acquisition and analysis, R.L.W., E.K.; manuscript preparation, R.L.W.; manuscript editing and review, R.L.B., J.L.W., E.K.

MR Imaging of Intraventricular Silicone: Case Report[1]

A 42-year-old man with human immunodeficiency viral infection developed cytomegaloviral retinitis that was complicated by retinal detachment and was treated with an intravitreous injection of silicone. Fifteen months later, magnetic resonance imaging revealed intraocular and intraventricular silicone. Signal intensity characteristics and chemical shifts of silicone in the two locations were identical.

Intraocular silicone is an increasingly common finding on magnetic resonance (MR) studies of the brain due to the high success rate of silicone tamponade in treating retinal detachment (1). Intravitreous silicone maintains retinal attachment, primarily because silicone has a higher surface tension than water has. Small retinal tears are functionally closed, which prevents repeated detachment of the retina (2).

The MR imaging appearance of intraocular silicone oil has been well described (3–6). However, to our knowledge, there are no prior reports of the extension of silicone into the ventricles and of the corresponding MR imaging findings. A mechanism of communication between the vitreous body and the cerebrospinal fluid is proposed for this unusual complication that follows the repair of retinal detachment.

Case Report

A 42-year-old man with a 13-year history of human immunodeficiency viral infection was examined at an ophthalmologic consultation 2 years prior to MR imaging, when he complained of a 1-week history of a decrease in vision in the left eye. At examination, the visual acuity was 20/20 in the right eye and 20/200 in the left eye. Retinal evaluation revealed cytomegaloviral retinitis with cytomegaloviral optic neuritis. Both of these gradually resolved following treatment with intravenous injection of ganciclovir sodium (Cytovene; Hoffmann-La Roche, Nutley, NJ).

Five months later, the cytomegaloviral retinitis recurred, with an associated retinal detachment. The patient was treated with an intravitreous injection of the antiviral agent foscarnet sodium (Foscavir; AstraZeneca, Wayne, Pa). The patient returned in 3 months, at which time his visual acuity had decreased to only light perception. The patient was treated with a second intravitreous injection of foscarnet sodium. To treat the retinal detachment, he underwent an orbiculus ciliaris vitrectomy, an orbiculus ciliaris lensectomy, a gas and fluid exchange, and the injection of 5,000-centistoke-viscosity (50 cm^2/sec) silicone oil.

Intraocular pressure was elevated following the procedure, and medications used to treat glaucoma were administered. Following surgery, visual acuity gradually deteriorated to no light perception. The cytomegalovirus appeared to be completely inactive; only retinal scarring was observed. However, damage to the optic nerve due to glaucoma was considerable and included cupping of the optic disc.

Seven months after retinal detachment surgery, subconjunctival silicone oil was noted during a slit-lamp examination. The patient's health began to deteriorate, and 8 months later, he developed a peripheral neuropathy. Due to the new neurologic deficit, we obtained MR images of the brain and cervical spine.

MR imaging was performed on two occasions over 5 months, with a 1.5-T unit (Signa; GE Medical Systems, Milwaukee, Wis) (Figs 1, 2). Sagittal T1-weighted spin-echo (500–566/14 [repetition time msec/echo time msec], one signal acquired), axial intermediate-weighted fast spin-echo (2,000–2,366/13–39, one signal acquired), axial T2-weighted fat-saturated chemical shift–selective fast spin-echo (2,183–2,500/104–105, one signal acquired), and axial fluid-attenuated inversion-recovery fast spin-echo (9,002–10,002/172–175/2,200 [repetition time msec/echo time msec/inversion time msec], one signal acquired) images were all obtained. A section thickness of 5 mm, an intersection gap of 1 mm, a field of view of 20 × 20 cm, an image matrix of 256 × 160 pixels, and a bandwidth of ±16 kHz (32 kHz) were used.

The condition was clinically stable when repeat imaging was performed 5 months later. MR imaging was performed as described but with an increase in the matrix to 256 × 192 and with a decrease in the bandwidth of 7.82 kHz before and after interchanging the phase- and frequency-encoding directions (Fig 2c, 2d). An axial T1-weighted series (600/12, one signal acquired) was obtained with the fat-saturated chemical shift–selective technique, and intermediate-weighted images (2,000/16, one signal acquired) were also obtained, with the patient prone, after the field of view was increased to 22 × 22 cm.

Silicone in the left globe was hyperintense when compared with normal vitreous on the T1-weighted and fluid-attenuated inversion-recovery images (Fig 1a). Identical signal intensity on the T1-weighted images was seen in the substance in the lateral ventricle (Fig 1b). Silicone was hypointense when compared with vitreous in the globe (Fig 1c) and with the substance in the ventricle (Fig 1d) on the T2-weighted fat-saturated images. On the intermediate-weighted images, the silicone was slightly hyperintense when compared with normal vitreous (Fig 2a). Similar signal intensity was present in the substance in the ventricle, as seen on images obtained with the same sequence (Fig 2b).

A prominent chemical shift artifact was present along the frequency-encoding direction, which changed appropriately as the phase and frequency directions were interchanged (Fig 2c, 2d). Chemical shift artifact between silicone and water and between fat and water increased as the bandwidth decreased. A substance with a small (7-mm-long), oval shape in the left lateral ventricle and a round 1-mm focus in the right lateral ventricle had, on images obtained from all MR sequences, signal intensities and associated artifact that were identical to the signal intensity and associated artifact of the silicone in the globe. Similar signal intensity was also present along the superior aspect of the intracranial optic nerve on the left (Fig 2e). The substance in the ventricle was nondependent and changed in position as the patient's position changed from supine to prone.

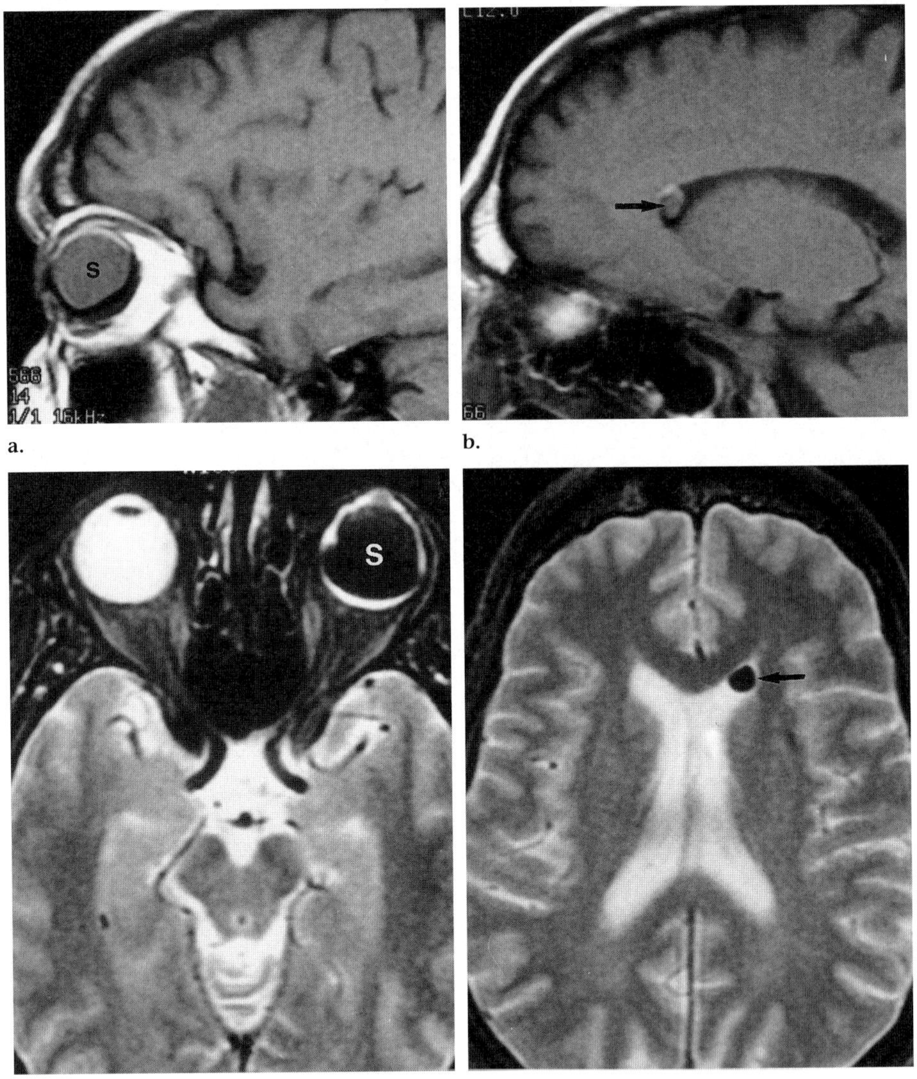

a. b. c. d.

Figure 1. **(a, b)** Sagittal T1-weighted spin-echo MR images (566/14) demonstrate **(a)** intraocular silicone (*S*), which is hyperintense when compared with normal vitreous, and **(b)** intraventricular silicone (arrow), which is hyperintense when compared with cerebrospinal fluid. **(c, d)** Axial T2-weighted fat-saturated fast spin-echo MR images (2,500/104) demonstrate hypointense signal in **(c)** the silicone (*S*) in the left globe and **(d)** the silicone (arrow) in the left lateral ventricle.

On images obtained with fat-saturation techniques, the substance in the lateral ventricles and superior to the optic nerve had signal intensity loss identical to the signal intensity loss of silicone in the globe. The magnitude and direction of the chemical shift artifact also suggested that the substances in the ventricles and in the globe were identical.

We calculated the frequency shift (in Hertz) between the silicone in the left globe, with surrounding water protons, and the substance in the ventricles, with surrounding water protons, on the basis of the known relationship among the amount of shift in the frequency direction (in millimeters), the field of view (in millimeters), and the bandwidth (in Hertz). This was calculated as follows: $FS = (x/FOV) \times BW$, where FS is the frequency shift in Hertz, x is the frequency direction, FOV is the field of view, and BW is the bandwidth.

The magnitude and direction of the chemical shift were identical between the silicone in the globe and the substance in the ventricles. With bandwidths of 32.00 and 7.82 kHz, the displacements in the frequency-encoding direction were 2 and 7 mm, respectively, which corresponded to calculated frequency differences of 273 and 320 Hz, respectively. The calculated frequency shifts are, in each case, within one

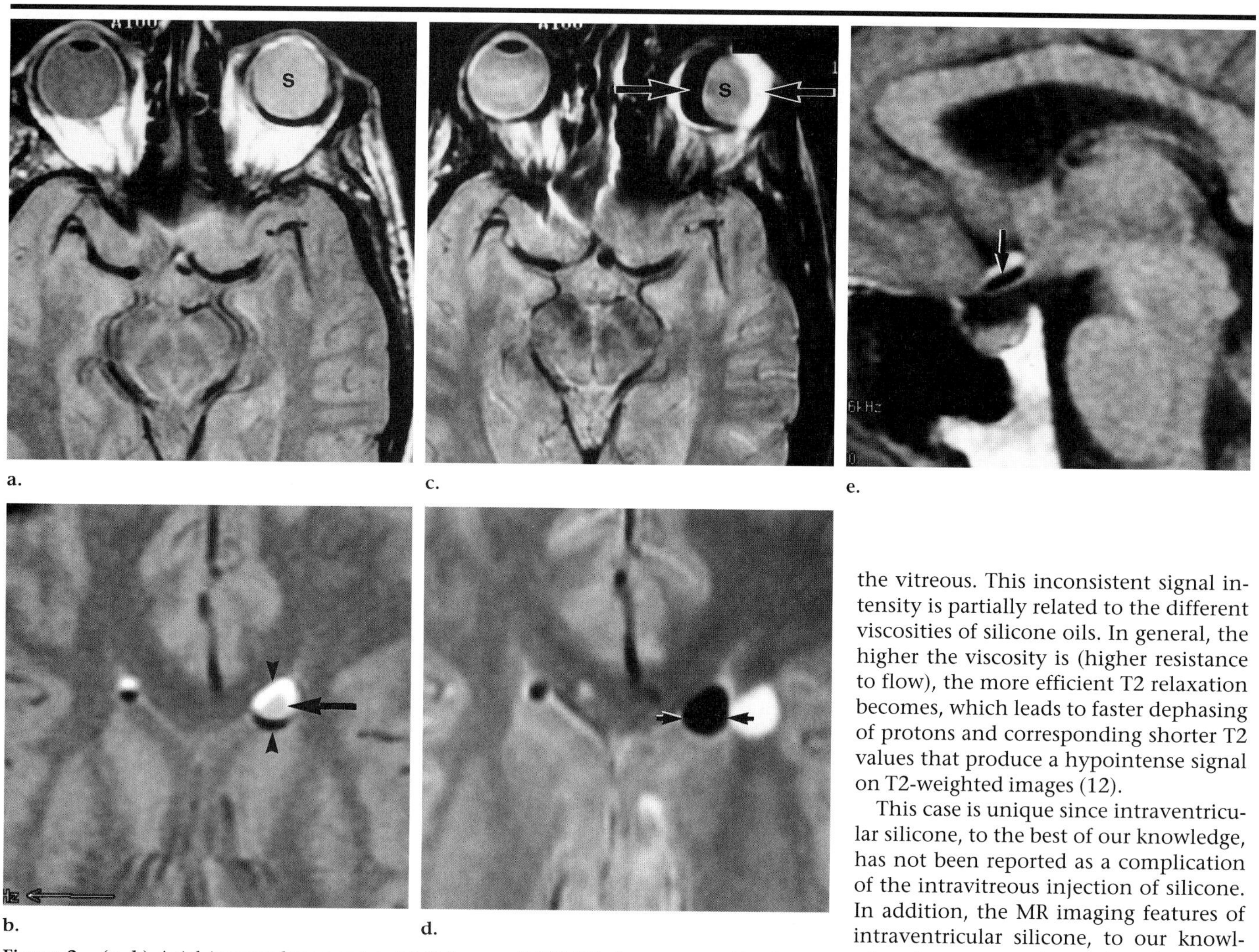

Figure 2. (a, b) Axial intermediate-weighted MR images (2,333/15) demonstrate (a) silicone (*S*) in the left globe, which is slightly hyperintense when compared with normal vitreous, and (b) similar signal intensity (arrow) and chemical shift artifact (arrowheads) in the silicone in the left lateral ventricle. Only chemical shift artifact is seen from the silicone in the right lateral ventricle. (c, d) Axial intermediate-weighted images (2,366/39) obtained with the low bandwidth technique and with interchanged phase and frequency directions show that (c) the hyper- and hypointense bands of signal (arrows) from chemical shift artifact adjacent to the silicone (*S*) in the left globe have changed in direction and are more apparent. (d) The chemical shift artifact at the lateral ventricles is identical to the artifact seen in the globe. The magnitude of the chemical shift (arrows) was measured and was used to calculate the frequency shift in Hertz. (e) Sagittal T1-weighted image (500/14) demonstrates silicone within or adjacent to the intracranial left optic nerve and chiasm (arrow).

frequency column of resolution from the known 290 Hz of shift from the water peak, as seen in some types of silicone (7). The accuracy of this calculation is limited by the bandwidth per pixel and the spatial resolution of the study parameters. These similarities between the material in the globe and the material in the ventricles are compelling evidence that silicone is in the ventricles.

Discussion

Intravitreous silicone oil is injected to provide a mechanical tamponade that maintains retinal attachment following retinal detachment repair. The MR imaging appearance of intraocular silicone oil has been well described (Table). Signal intensity characteristics are variable and depend on the sequence parameters, field strength, and viscosity of silicone oil, as measured in stokes (centimeters squared per second) (6).

Typically, in vivo silicone oil is hyperintense on T1-weighted images, when compared with normal vitreous, and variably is iso-, hypo-, or hyperintense on T2-weighted images, when compared with the vitreous. This inconsistent signal intensity is partially related to the different viscosities of silicone oils. In general, the higher the viscosity is (higher resistance to flow), the more efficient T2 relaxation becomes, which leads to faster dephasing of protons and corresponding shorter T2 values that produce a hypointense signal on T2-weighted images (12).

This case is unique since intraventricular silicone, to the best of our knowledge, has not been reported as a complication of the intravitreous injection of silicone. In addition, the MR imaging features of intraventricular silicone, to our knowledge, have never been described. The pathway that allows the transit of silicone from the vitreous to the cerebrospinal fluid is uncertain. There is no normal anatomic communication between the vitreous and the subarachnoid space (13).

Silicone oil has a propensity to leak through very small openings, such as the 1-mm sclerotomy sites, despite tight suturing of these sites. Silicone may even egress through the entrance and exit sites of the needle during suture placement (14). The presence of silicone in the subconjunctival space is, therefore, not unusual in cases in which the vitreous has been replaced with silicone oil for the treatment of retinal detachment (15). Subconjunctival oil, however, has no access to the subarachnoid space that surrounds the intraorbital optic nerve.

We hypothesize that the silicone may have entered the atrophic optic disc due to the raised intraocular pressure (15,16). The intraneural silicone then coalesced and extended posteriorly, eventually mi-

MR Findings of Intraocular Silicone

Study	MR Field Strength (T)	Silicone Viscosity* (centistoke)	Silicone Signal Intensity† T1-weighted	Intermediate-weighted	T2-weighted	Chemical Shift
Gross et al (8) (6 cases)	1.5	1,000 (10)	Hyperintense	Hyperintense	Hyperintense	Present
Lidov et al (3) (1 case)	0.5	NA	Hyperintense	Isointense	Hypointense	Present
Murray et al (5) (2 cases)	0.35	NA	Hyperintense	Hyperintense	Hyperintense	Present
Manfre et al (9) (7 cases)	0.5	NA	Hyperintense	Hyperintense	Hyperintense	NA
Mathews et al (6) (2 cases)	1.5	5,000 (50)	Hyperintense	Isointense	Hypointense	Present
Girardot et al (4) (1 case)	0.5	1,000 (10)	Hyperintense	Hyperintense	Isointense	Present
Yoshida et al (10) (5 cases)	1.5	1,000 (10)	NA	NA	Hyperintense	Present
Mafee et al (11) (1 case)	1.5	NA	NA	Isointense	Hypointense	Present
Herrick et al (7) (11 cases)	1.5	NA	Hyperintense	Questionably isointense	Questionably isointense	Present

Note.—NA = not available.
* Viscosity in SI units appears in parentheses (1 centistoke = 10^{-2} cm^2/sec).
† When compared with vitreous.

grating into the subarachnoid space that surrounds the optic nerve. Communication of the subarachnoid space that surrounds the optic nerve with the intracranial subarachnoid space would then allow the passage of silicone into the ventricles.

This theory is supported by case reports that demonstrate the extension of intravitreous silicone into the intraorbital optic nerve (15,16). In fact, the potential for the extension of intravitreous silicone into the central nervous system was originally predicted by Shields and Eagle (16). In addition, the clinical histories of patients in whom extravitreous silicone has been identified included severely elevated intraocular pressure (15,16), as seen in our case.

This correlation with severe glaucoma has also been noted in cases of cystic degeneration of the optic nerve. Zimmerman et al (17) theorized that cystic degeneration of the optic nerve is caused by ischemic necrosis of the nerve, which develops secondarily to severe acute glaucoma. The cystic spaces in cystic degeneration were filled with vitreous, which was believed to be "forced into the optic nerve" (17). Similar cystic spaces were filled with silicone in one report (16), a finding that may be present in our case. Damage to the optic nerve due to glaucoma may, therefore, be required to allow oil to enter the optic disc and nerve. Continued elevation of intraocular pressure may also promote extension of silicone through the nerve.

Imaging evidence that supports this theory is present in our case, in which silicone is seen immediately adjacent to the intracranial optic nerve (Fig 2e). This silicone is believed to be intraneural, since the silicone has not changed in position between the two studies. Further imaging evidence is found in another case in which MR imaging demonstrated perfluorocarbon liquid (an intravitreous substance which is also used for mechanical tamponade of retinal detachment) within the intraorbital optic nerve sheath (7). Subarachnoid space involvement confirms our theory that intravitreous substances may enter the perineural subarachnoid space.

In conclusion, MR imaging demonstrated, in a patient who was treated for retinal detachment with intravitreous silicone, intraocular and intraventricular silicone oil, as confirmed by identical signal intensity characteristics and chemical shifts in the two locations. The MR appearance of intraventricular silicone may vary with the field strength, the sequence parameters, and the viscosity of the silicone injected. The proposed pathway for the extension of silicone is through the optic nerve, which migrates into the surrounding subarachnoid space and which communicates with the ventricles. This mechanism may require a necrotic optic nerve and a raised intraocular pressure.

Acknowledgment: We express our appreciation to Karol Rosengarth for assistance with manuscript preparation.

References

1. Regillo CD, Vander JF, Duker JS, Fischer DH, Belmont JB, Kleiner R. Repair of retinitis-related retinal detachments with silicone oil in patients with acquired immunodeficiency syndrome. Am J Ophthalmol 1992; 113:21–27.
2. McCuen BW III, de Juan E Jr, Machemer R. Silicone oil in mitreoretinal surgery. I. Surgical techniques. Retina 1985; 5:189–197.
3. Lidov MW, Maldjian J, Glajchen N, Som PM. MR appearance of intraocular silicone oil. J Comput Assist Tomogr 1994; 18:131–132.
4. Girardot C, Hazebroucq VG, Fery-Lemonnier E, et al. MR imaging and CT of surgical materials currently used in ophthalmology: in vitro and in vivo studies. Radiology 1994; 191:433–439.
5. Murray JG, Gean AD, Barr RM. Intraocular silicone oil for retinal detachment in AIDS: CT and MR appearances. Clin Radiol 1996; 51:415–417.
6. Mathews VP, Elster AD, Barker PB, Buff BL, Haller JA, Greven CM. Intraocular silicone oil: in vitro and in vivo MR and CT characteristics. AJNR 1994; 15:343–347.
7. Herrick RC, Hayman LA, Maturi RK, Diaz-Marchan PJ, Tang RA, Lambert HM. Optimal imaging protocol after intraocular silicone oil tamponade. AJNR 1998; 19:101–108.
8. Gross JG, Hesselink JR, Press GA, Goldbaum MH, Freeman WR. Magnetic resonance imaging in the evaluation of vitreoretinal disease in eyes with intraocular silicone oil. Am J Ophthalmol 1990; 110:366–370.
9. Manfre L, Fabbri G, Avitabile T, Biondi P, Reibaldi A, Pero G. MRI and intraocular tamponade media. Neuroradiology 1993; 35:359–361.
10. Yoshida A, Cheng HM, Kwong KK, Ogasawara H, Garrido L, McMeel JW. Magnetic resonance imaging of intraocular tamponades. Ophthalmic Surg 1991; 22:287–291.
11. Mafee MF, Peyman GA, Grisolano JE, et al. Malignant uveal melanoma and simulating lesions: MR imaging evaluation. Radiology 1986; 160:773–780.
12. Fullerton G. Physiologic basis of magnetic relaxation. In: Stark DD, Bradley WG Jr, eds. Magnetic resonance imaging. 2nd ed. St Louis, Mo: Mosby–Year Book, 1992; 88–108.
13. Garfinkle AM, Danys IR, Nicolle DA, Colohan AR, Brem S. Terson's syndrome: a reversible cause of blindness following subarachnoid hemorrhage. J Neurosurg 1992; 76:766–771.
14. Donahue SP, Friberg TR, Johnson BL. Intraconjunctival cavitary inclusions of silicone oil complicating retinal detachment repair. Am J Ophthalmol 1992; 114:639–640.
15. Ni C, Wang WJ, Albert DM, Schepens CL. Intravitreous silicone injection: histopathologic findings in a human eye after 12 years. Arch Ophthalmol 1983; 101:1399–1401.
16. Shields CL, Eagle RC Jr. Pseudo-Schnabel's cavernous degeneration of the optic nerve secondary to intraocular silicone oil. Arch Ophthalmol 1989; 107:714–717.
17. Zimmerman LE, De Venecia G, Hamasaki DI. Pathology of the optic nerve in experimental acute glaucoma. Invest Ophthalmol 1967; 6:109–125.

Choong R. Kim, MD
Beverly A. Eaton, RT(T)
Kenneth R. Stevens, Jr, MD

Index terms:
Therapeutic radiology, 854.1269
Treatment planning, 854.1269
Uterine neoplasms, therapeutic radiology, 854.1269, 854.32

Radiology 1999; 212:155–158

[1] From the Department of Radiation Oncology, St John Medical Center, 1614 E Kessler Blvd, Longview, WA 98632 (C.R.K., B.A.E.), and the Department of Radiation Oncology, School of Medicine, Oregon Health Sciences University, Portland, Ore (K.R.S.). From the 1996 RSNA scientific assembly. Received October 7, 1997; revision requested December 16; final revision received August 28, 1998; accepted December 15. **Address reprint requests to** C.R.K.

Author contributions:
Guarantors of integrity of entire study, C.R.K., K.R.S.; study concepts, C.R.K.; study design, C.R.K., B.A.E.; definition of intellectual content, C.R.K., K.R.S.; literature research, C.R.K.; clinical studies, C.R.K., B.A.E.; data acquisition, C.R.K., B.A.E.; data analysis, C.R.K.; manuscript preparation, C.R.K., B.A.E.; manuscript editing, B.A.E., K.R.S.; manuscript review, K.R.S.

Localization of the Apex of the Vagina: Implications for Radiation Therapy Planning[1]

PURPOSE: To evaluate (*a*) the displacement of the vaginal apex by a rod during radiation therapy simulation for gynecologic malignancy and (*b*) apical localization with implanted radiopaque markers.

MATERIALS AND METHODS: Metallic markers were implanted in the cervix or vaginal cuff in nine patients with cervical or endometrial carcinoma who underwent irradiation. In all but one patient, radiographs were obtained with and then without the vaginal rod. Displacement of the markers relative to bone landmarks was measured. The total displacement was the square root of the sum of the squares of displacement in each axial direction.

RESULTS: All patients showed displacement of the cervical markers by the vaginal rod (mean total displacement, 1.9 cm; range, 0.6–3.6 cm). The greatest displacement was cephalic (mean, 1.5 cm; range, 0.5–2.4 cm). Anteroposterior displacement occurred in all patients but was not as predictable as cephalic displacement. Displacement was anterior in five of the eight patients, posterior in three patients, and lateral in four patients.

CONCLUSION: Displacement of the vaginal apex and/or cervix with placement of the vaginal rod during simulation was marked in all patients. Use of implanted cervical markers to localize the vaginal apex or the cervix during simulation is more accurate than use of a vaginal rod.

Radiation treatment is widely used as either the primary or a postoperative adjuvant therapy for cervical or endometrial carcinoma. Irradiation options for gynecologic malignancy often involve external-beam radiation therapy of the whole pelvis, with an additional dose to the cervix, apex of the vagina, or vaginal cuff. The boost dose to this area can be delivered by using either a vaginal intracavitary implant or small fields of external-beam irradiation.

The external boost irradiation generally consists of a four-field box technique or bilateral arc rotation with the isocenter at the vaginal apex. Fields are small to avoid an excessive dose to the rectum and bladder. Simulation procedures usually involve placement of a rigid vaginal rod into the vagina to radiographically determine the location of the vaginal cuff or cervix at the tip of the vaginal rod. The isocenter is then set at the tip of the vaginal rod. However, the vagina is flexible and expandable, and the apex or the cervix can easily be displaced by the vaginal rod. This may result in a misapplication of irradiation and an underdosing to the apex of the vagina.

We performed this study to measure and evaluate the displacement of the vaginal apex due to placement of the vaginal rod and to evaluate the implantation of metallic markers in the vaginal apex or cervix for localizing the vaginal apex.

MATERIALS AND METHODS

From April 1993 through February 1996, nine patients with cervical or endometrial carcinoma who underwent radiation treatment and implantation of cervical markers were evaluated. All patients were informed of the risks of the procedure and consented to the

TABLE 1
Patient Characteristics

Patient No./ Age (y)	Location of Carcinoma	FIGO Stage
1/30	Cervix	IB
2/36	Cervix	IB
3/40	Cervix	IB
4/44	Cervix	IB
5/57	Cervix	IIA
6/65	Cervix	IB
7/73	Cervix	IIIB
8/56	Endometrium	IB
9/72	Endometrium	Recurrent

TABLE 2
Displacement of Cervical Markers after Placement of the Vaginal Rod during Simulation

Patient No.	Cephalic Displacement (cm)	Anteroposterior Displacement (cm)	Lateral Displacement (cm)	Total Displacement (cm)
1	1.5	0.7 (anterior)	0	1.7
2	1.0	1.4 (anterior)	0.4 (left)	1.8
3	1.4	NA	0	NA
4	2.4	2.5 (posterior)	1.0 (right)	3.6
5	2.1	0.8 (anterior)	1.0 (left)	2.5
6	1.1	0.6 (posterior)	0.2 (right)	1.3
7	0.5	0.5 (anterior)	0	0.6
8	2.0	0.8 (anterior)	0	2.2
9	1.1	1.0 (posterior)	0	1.5
Mean	1.5	1.0	0.2	1.9

Note.—NA = not available.

TABLE 3
Location of the Tip of the Vaginal Rod Relative to the Cervical Marker

Patient No.	Cephalic Location (cm)	Anteroposterior Location (cm)	Lateral Location (cm)
1	1.0	0.5 (anterior to marker)	1 (right of marker)
2	2.0	2.0 (anterior to marker)	Midline without shift
4	1.5	2.0 (posterior to marker)	1 (left of marker)

placement of the cervical markers. The median age was 56 years (age range, 30–73 years). The patient characteristics are shown in Table 1.

All patients received external-beam irradiation of the whole pelvis (4,500 cGy), which included parametrial and pelvic lymph nodes. Three of the seven patients with cervical cancer received radiation treatment as the primary therapy, with an additional dose administered by using cesium 137 in a Fletcher-Suit applicator. Three patients underwent total abdominal hysterectomy and received postoperative adjuvant external-beam radiation therapy, with an additional dose administered to the vaginal cuff by using 5 × 5-cm fields. One patient with locally advanced cervical carcinoma received palliative radiation treatment for uncontrolled bleeding.

One of the two patients with the endometrial carcinoma received postoperative adjuvant therapy, which included placement of an intracavitary vaginal implant with ^{137}Cs sources by using the vaginal applicator. The other patient with endometrial carcinoma received radiation therapy for recurrence.

All patients had gold markers (Anderson Marker; Best Industries, Springfield, Va) implanted in either the cervix or the vaginal cuff after 4,500-cGy external-beam irradiation of the whole pelvis. Markers were placed at the 5- and 11-o'clock positions. Orthogonal radiographs (Cascade Simulator; Cascade X-ray, Yakima, Wash; with barium [Liquid Polibar Plus, E-Z-Em, Westbury, NY] in the rectum [30–50 mL]) were obtained with and then without the vaginal rod, except in patient 3, in whom a lateral image was not obtained. The location of the markers was referenced to the top of the symphysis pubis and the most anterior tip of S1. The displacement of the markers was measured in the cephalocaudal, anteroposterior, and lateral directions by using simulation radiographs. The total displacement was determined by using the Pythagorean theorem (by determining the square root of the sum of the squares of displacement in each direction).

Computed tomography (CT; CT HiSpeed Advantage, GE Medical Systems, Milwaukee, Wis) was performed with the vaginal rod and then without the vaginal rod in patient 2, who had cervical carcinoma.

RESULTS

All patients showed displacement of the cervical markers by the vaginal rod (Table 2). The mean total displacement was 1.9 cm (range, 0.6–3.6 cm). The most substantial displacement was in the cephalic direction. The mean cephalic shift was 1.5 cm (range, 0.5–2.4 cm). Due to the pressure to keep the rod in place, the length of the vagina increased when the vaginal rod was placed. Figure 1 shows the displacement of the cervical marker in the cephalic direction.

The tip of the vaginal rod was more cephalic than the implanted cervical markers in three patients (Table 3, Fig 1). Their ages were 30, 36, and 44 years. They all had cervical carcinoma, and radiation treatment was the primary treatment. The tip of the vaginal rod was 1–2 cm more cephalic than the original location of the cervical markers. This finding was confirmed with CT in patient 2. The tip of the vaginal rod was 2 cm more cephalic, as shown in Figure 2.

The anterior and posterior displacements of the marker were also noted in all patients (Table 2), but these were not as predictable as cephalic displacement. Five of the eight patients evaluated showed a mean anterior displacement of the implanted markers of 0.8 cm (range, 0.5–1.4 cm). Three patients showed posterior displacement of markers of 0.6, 1.0, and 2.5 cm. The tip of the vaginal rod was 0.5 and 2.0 cm more anterior to the implanted markers in patients 1 and 2, respectively. The tip of the vaginal rod was 2.0 cm more posterior to the markers in patient 4.

Lateral displacement of the implanted markers was not as marked. Only four of the nine patients showed lateral displacement. Two patients showed a shift to the right (0.2 and 1.0 cm), and two patients showed a shift to the left (0.4 and 1.0 cm).

DISCUSSION

Localization of the apex of the vagina during simulation may involve the placement of a vaginal rod. The rod is usually a rigid straight applicator with radiopaque

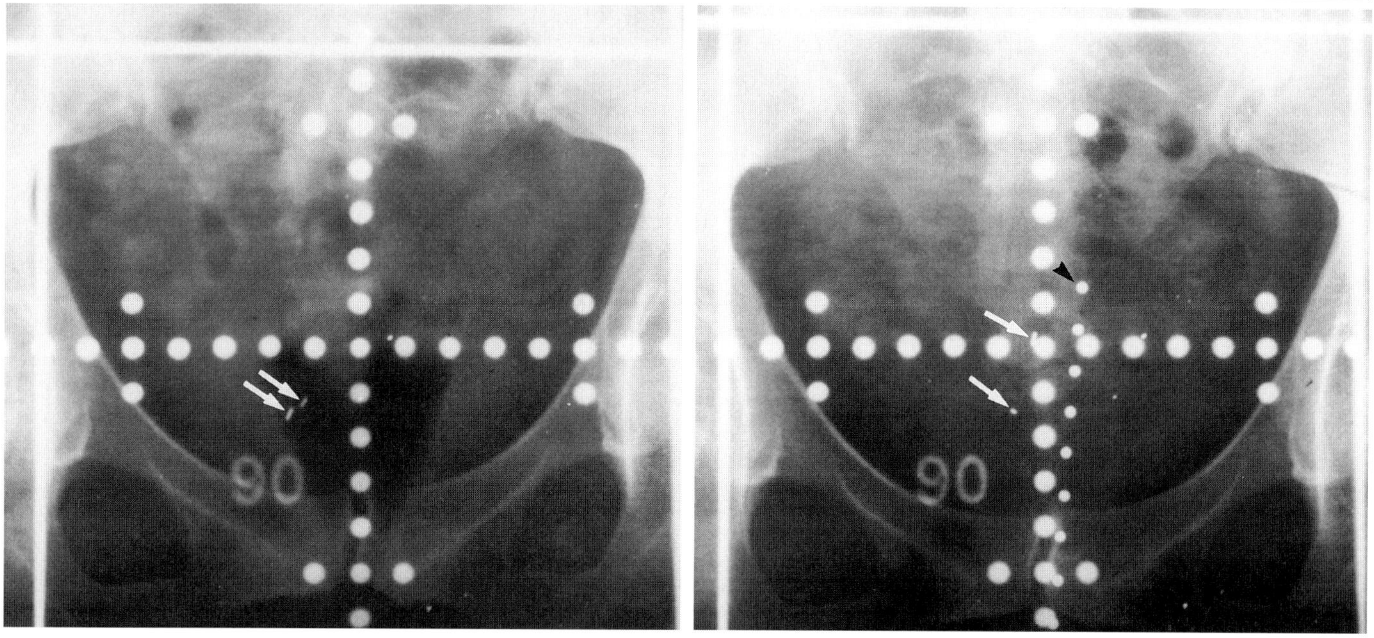

a. b.

Figure 1. Anteroposterior radiographs obtained during simulation **(a)** without and **(b)** with the vaginal rod in place. In **b**, the cervical markers (arrows in **a** and **b**) with the rod in place show the cephalic displacement. The tip of the vaginal rod (arrowhead) is more cephalic than the markers.

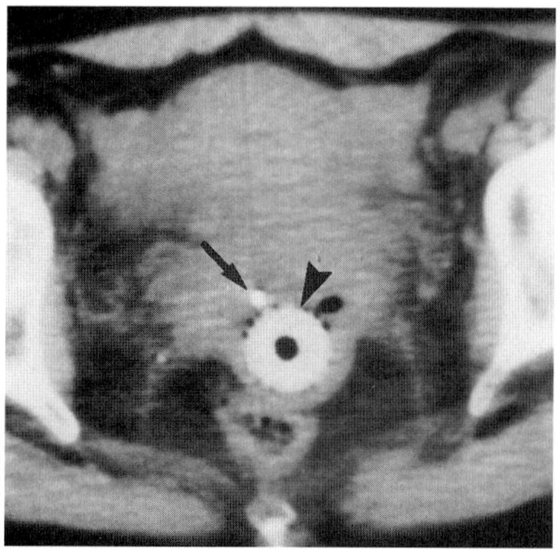

Figure 2. CT scan of the pelvis with the vaginal rod in place. The location of the implanted marker (arrow) is noted in relation to the vaginal rod (arrowhead). The tip of the vaginal rod was 2 cm cephalic to the markers on another image (not shown).

measurement markers. The apex of the vagina is assumed to be at the tip of the rod, and the isocenter is usually set on it during simulation. However, the displacement of the vaginal apex due to the rod during simulation is not recognized.

The vagina is expandable, with great potential to change its length and diameter. Placement of the vaginal rod causes displacement of the vaginal apex.

The tip of the vaginal rod, when it is placed in the vaginal vault during simulation, does not necessarily indicate the location of the cervix. The cervix or vaginal cuff can shift up to 3.6 cm. When the vaginal rod is removed, the apex of the vagina reverts back to its normal position, and the apex of the vagina may be missed with a small field. This becomes clinically important when external irradiation is used to boost a small area in the apex of the vagina.

The change in the location of the apex of the vagina or cervix was previously noted with gynecologic brachytherapy that involves placement of rigid implants. Grigsby et al (1) reported on 40 patients who underwent irradiation and received two intracavitary implants with a Fletcher-Suit tandem and ovoids; these patients had displacement of the reference points between the first Fletcher-Suit implantation and the second implantation. The displacement of the individual reference points ranged from 0 to 2.6 cm. Grigsby et al postulated the change in the anatomy was due to tumor shrinkage and fibrosis. They did not mention the possibility of geometric variation due to the pressure from the vaginal packing and the Fletcher-Suit tandem and ovoids placed during the implantation procedure. Kim et al (2) reported that posterior vaginal packing was responsible for 20% of geographic variation between multiple high-dose-rate applications of brachytherapy for cervical carcinoma.

The shift of other soft and expandable tissues from the position of the body has been reported. Smoron et al (3) observed that the esophagus is not fixed and can shift up to 6 cm anteriorly or posteriorly with a change from supination to pronation. Corn et al (4) reported that the esophagus can shift anteriorly up to 4.2 cm with a change from supination to pronation.

The displacement of a semifixed soft-tissue organ such as the prostate to expansion or contraction of the lumen of the rectum and bladder during simulation in patients with prostate cancer has been reported. Ten Haken et al (5) reported the displacement of the prostate gland was a mean of 0.5 cm (range, 0–2 cm) in 31 of 50 consecutive patients, with the bladder and the rectum naturally filled or emptied. These differences were noted between CT-based treatment plans and simulation radiographs obtained during simulation. Pickett et al (6) demonstrated anterior movement of the prostate on the CT scan when the rectum was filled with barium solution compared with the position when the rectum was empty. The full rectum displaced the prostate anteriorly and superiorly. Beard et al (7) reported that distention of the rectum can change the position of the prostate and the seminal vesicles up to 1.5 to 2.2 cm. The direction of displacement of the prostate or the seminal vesicles could not be predicted in their studies.

Findings of our study demonstrate that the vaginal rod causes displacement of the vaginal apex during the simulation performed to establish the locations of small boost irradiation fields. This may result in a misapplication of irradiation in the treatment due to substantial displacement of the vaginal apex during the simulation. Implanted cervical or vaginal markers are more accurate for localizing the cervix or the apex of the vagina during simulation.

References

1. Grigsby PW, Georgiou A, Williamson JF, Perez CA. Anatomic variation of gynecologic brachytherapy prescription points. Int J Radiat Oncol Biol Phys 1993; 27:725–729.
2. Kim RY, Meyer JT, Plott WE, et al. Major geometric variations between multiple high-dose-rate applications of brachytherapy in cancer of the cervix: frequency and type of variation. Radiology 1995; 195:419–422.
3. Smoron GL, O'Brien CA, Sullivan CA. Tumor localization and treatment technique for cancer of the esophagus. Radiology 1974; 111:735–736.
4. Corn BW, Coia LR, Chu JCH, Hwang CC, Stafford PM, Hanks GE. Significance of prone position in planning treatment for esophagus cancer. Int J Radiat Oncol Biol Phys 1991; 21:1303–1309.
5. Ten Haken RK, Forman JD, Heimberger DK, et al. Treatment planning issues related to prostate movement in response to differential filling of the rectum and bladder. Int J Radiat Oncol Biol Phys 1991; 20:1317–1324.
6. Pickett B, Roach M III, Verhey L, et al. The value of nonuniform margins for six-field conformal irradiation of localized cancer. Int J Radiat Oncol Biol Phys 1995; 32:211–218.
7. Beard CJ, Kijewski P, Bussiere M, et al. Analysis of prostate and seminal vesicle motion: implication for treatment planning. Int J Radiat Oncol Biol Phys 1996: 34:451–458.

Transrectal versus Transvaginal Abscess Drainage: Survey of Patient Tolerance and Effect on Activities of Daily Living[1]

David M. Hovsepian, MD
Joseph R. Steele, MD
Celette Sugg Skinner, PhD
Eric S. Malden, MD

Index terms:
Abscess, drainage, 757.1263, 791.1263, 855.1263
Abscess, US, 857.12986
Interventional procedures, 757.1263, 791.1263, 855.1263
Pelvic organs, abscess, 85.211
Pelvic organs, interventional procedures, 757.1263, 791.1263, 855.1263
Pelvic organs, US, 757.12986, 791.12986, 855.12986

Radiology 1999; 212:159–163

[1] From the Departments of Radiology (D.M.H., J.R.S., C.S.S., E.S.M.) and Surgery (D.M.H., E.S.M.), Washington University Medical Center, Mallinckrodt Institute of Radiology, 510 S Kingshighway Blvd, St Louis, MO 63110. From the 1997 RSNA scientific assembly. Received July 27, 1998; revision requested August 27; revision received October 22; accepted December 21. **Address reprint requests to** D.M.H. (e-mail: *hovsepian@mirlink.wustl.edu*).

Author contributions:
Guarantors of integrity of entire study, D.M.H., J.R.S.; study concepts, D.M.H., J.R.S.; study design, D.M.H., J.R.S., C.S.S.; literature research, D.M.H., J.R.S.; clinical studies, D.M.H., J.R.S.; data acquisition, D.M.H., J.R.S., E.S.M.; data analysis, D.M.H., J.R.S.; statistical analysis, D.M.H.; manuscript preparation, D.M.H., J.R.S.; manuscript editing, D.M.H., J.R.S., C.S.S.; manuscript review, E.S.M.

PURPOSE: To evaluate patient perception of pain related to transrectal and transvaginal drainage and the catheter's effect on activities of daily living.

MATERIALS AND METHODS: From July 1993 to August 1997, 22 male and 40 female patients (mean age, 41 years; age range, 4–80 years) underwent transrectal or transvaginal aspiration or drainage. Fifty-seven drainages were performed. In a follow-up survey, patients were asked to score pain experienced during the procedure and afterward on a scale of 1–10 and to rate the effect of the catheter on their activities of daily living.

RESULTS: Twenty-two patients participated in the telephone survey. For those able to recall the insertion procedure, the mean pain score was 3.2 for transrectal and 5.9 for transvaginal drainage. Mean indwelling catheter pain was 1.6 for transrectal and 4.8 for transvaginal drainage. Pain after removal was 1.4 for transrectal and 2.3 for transvaginal drainage. Only one patient with a transrectal catheter reported severe limitation (bowel movement), with no reports of any serious effect on urinating, bathing, sitting, or walking. Transvaginally placed catheters caused marked limitation in all categories and were more painful than transrectal catheters ($P < .05$).

CONCLUSION: Of the transrectal and transvaginal approaches, transrectal is better tolerated.

The transrectal and transvaginal routes have been increasingly advocated for drainage of deep pelvic abscesses. Many authors (1–7) have described excellent results with few complications. It is known that pelvic surgery has a profound effect on patients, particularly with respect to limitations on personal hygiene, bowel and bladder function, and personal and sexual relations (8,9). Therefore, transrectal and transvaginal catheters have the same potential to be uncomfortable, inconvenient, and awkward.

Despite the claim that transvaginal drainage is well tolerated (2), our impression has been that patients tolerate both the transvaginal catheter insertion procedure and indwelling transvaginal catheters less well than they do the placement of transrectal catheters. The purpose of this study was to evaluate patients' perceptions of transrectal and transvaginal abscess drainage and the effect of the catheter on their activities of daily living. We conducted a telephone interview of patients treated with transrectal or transvaginal catheter drainage at our institution to determine which route may be most appropriate and which subsets of patients may tolerate these approaches.

MATERIALS AND METHODS

Institutional review board approval was granted for a retrospective review of all patient charts and for telephone follow-up of all patients who underwent transrectal or transvaginal catheter drainage during the 48-month period from July 1993 to August 1997. The

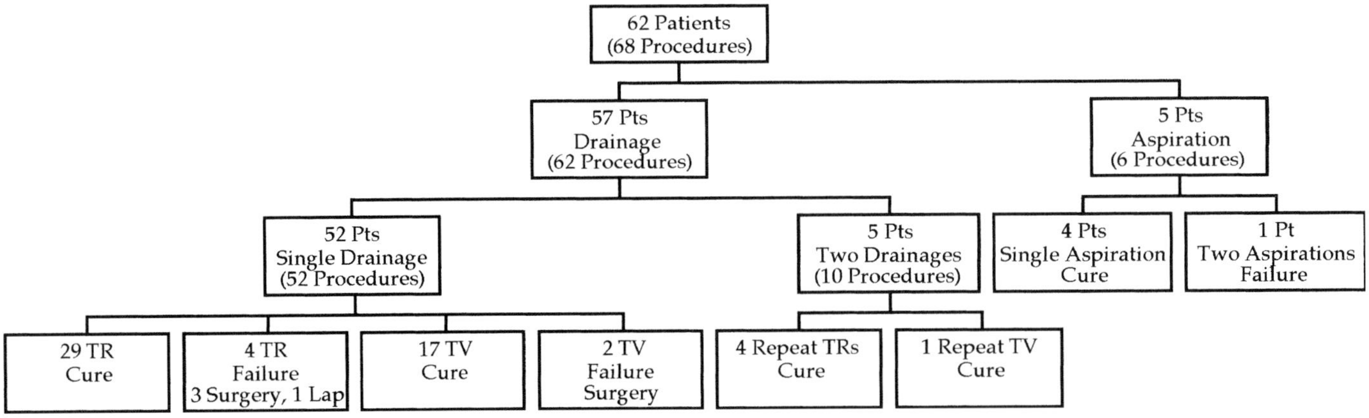

Figure 1. Flowchart shows the distribution of the 68 transrectal (*TR*) and transvaginal (*TV*) procedures among the 62 patients (*Pts*), with the successes and failures for single and multiple procedures indicated. *Lap* = laparoscopic surgery, *Surgery* = open surgery.

study included 62 patients (22 male patients, 40 female patients; age range, 4–84 years; mean age, 40 years; median age, 46 years).

Patients were treated by using the standard ultrasonographically (US) guided techniques that have been described by other authors in detail (2,4). Briefly, only with use of intravenous conscious sedation, access into the pelvic collection was attained by using endoluminal US, with a biopsy guide in most cases (transrectal, $n = 42$; transvaginal, $n = 16$). Fluoroscopy (transvaginal, $n = 6$), transabdominal US guidance (transrectal, $n = 2$), and digital palpation (transrectal, $n = 2$) were used for guidance in the remaining cases. The collections were then opacified with water-soluble contrast material, and the procedures were converted to fluoroscopic control for tract dilation and drainage.

No specific bowel preparation was used prior to transrectal drainage, and no patient received an enema prior to the procedure. No effort was made to sterilize the vaginal canal prior to transvaginal drainage. Collections were not lavaged with saline or povidone iodine, nor were antibiotics administered in the cavity. All patients were receiving antibiotics intravenously prior to drainage, and in most cases antibiotics were continued afterward. Drainage catheters were self-retaining (locking-loop type) and were 8–16 F (median size, 10 F for both transrectal abscess drainage and transvaginal abscess drainage), and all were placed to drain only by means of gravity.

At the request of the institutional review board, patients were first contacted by mail and then by telephone by medically trained research assistants who were not present during the original procedures. After explaining the purpose of the study, the assistants asked the patients for permission to conduct the interview. The 53-question telephone survey was used to gather demographic data; quantify patients' perceived pain or discomfort levels during and after the procedure (on a scale of 1–10); and evaluate the effect of the indwelling catheter on activities of daily living, employment, and sexual activity.

Five specific aspects of activities of daily living were investigated: bathing, bowel movements, urinating, sitting, and walking. The effect on activities of daily living was evaluated both for the time that catheters were in place and also after they were removed. Responses were classified as "very limited," "somewhat limited," or "not limited at all." Patients were also asked to assess whether they thought the informed consent process accurately prepared them for the procedure and the effect that the catheter would have on their activities of daily living.

The data were tabulated and analyzed by using statistical software (Statview; Abacus Concepts, Berkeley, Calif). Comparisons of pain scores were made by using the Student t test or Fisher exact test. Contingency tables were analyzed to determine the relative effect on activities of daily living. A P value less than .05 was considered to indicate a statistically significant difference.

RESULTS

Transrectal or transvaginal aspiration or drainage was performed 68 times in 62 patients, with the intent to place a drainage catheter in each case (Fig 1). The indication for transrectal or transvaginal aspiration or drainage was a fluid collection within the deep pelvis in close proximity to the vagina or rectum, with associated clinical signs and symptoms. In all cases, transperitoneal access was unavailable or deemed risky.

Fifty-seven patients underwent successful insertion of catheters, and five of them required two procedures. The technical success rate for placing a drainage catheter, therefore, was 91%. In six procedures, a catheter could not be placed owing to technical factors—small size ($n = 1$), lack of fluid ($n = 4$), or inability to dilate the tissues ($n = 1$)—and only aspiration was performed. Patients who underwent aspiration only were not included in the catheter effect survey.

Twenty-two (39%) of the 57 patients who had undergone placement of a drainage catheter agreed to participate in the telephone survey: five male patients who underwent transrectal procedures and 17 female patients, seven of whom underwent transrectal procedures and 10 of whom underwent transvaginal procedures. Three patients had undergone two procedures, so 25 questionnaires were completed. The remaining 35 patients were unable to complete the questionnaire process owing to refusal ($n = 2$), death ($n = 3$), lost to follow-up ($n = 18$), failure to return multiple messages ($n = 8$), inability to recall having undergone the procedure ($n = 2$), and serving a jail sentence ($n = 2$).

Transrectal aspiration or transrectal abscess drainage accounted for 46 procedures, with an even distribution of male patients ($n = 23$) and female patients ($n = 23$), and an additional 22 procedures were performed by means of the transvaginal route (Fig 2). Only one patient underwent both transrectal and transvaginal procedures, which were unsuccessful aspiration attempts. Therefore, our clinical

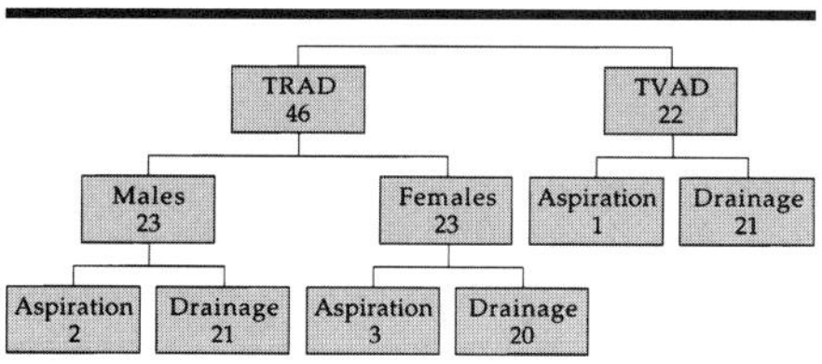

Figure 2. Flowchart shows the distribution of transrectal procedures among male patients and female patients and of transrectal and transvaginal procedures among those who underwent aspiration and those who underwent drainage. *TRAD* = transrectal abscess drainage, *TVAD* = transvaginal abscess drainage.

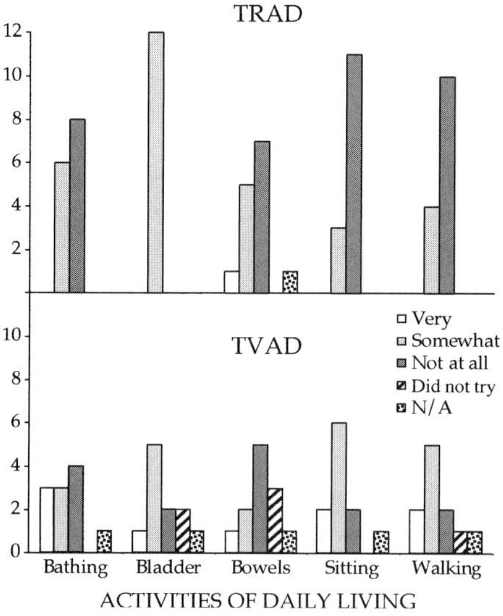

Figure 3. Bar graph shows the effect of both transrectal and transvaginal catheters on the activities of daily living, specifically bathing, bowel and bladder function, sitting, and walking. *N/A* = not applicable, *Somewhat* = somewhat limited, *TRAD* = transrectal abscess drainage, *TVAD* = transvaginal abscess drainage, *Very* = very limited.

success rate, defined as those patients adequately treated with one or more radiologic procedures (drainage or aspiration), was 89% (55 of 62 patients). The mean catheter duration was 5.7 days for transrectal abscess drainage and 6.5 days for transvaginal abscess drainage (mode, 3 days; median, 4 days for both transrectal abscess drainage and transvaginal abscess drainage).

Thirty-seven fluid collections were thought to be abscesses that arose after surgery, 20 were abscesses without a history of recent surgery, six fluid collections developed after gunshot wounds, four resulted from Crohn disease, and one patient had a painful postoperative lymphocele. Forty-two specimens grew a variety of bacteria, with *Escherichia coli* being the most common pathogen (12 cases). Thirteen specimens showed no growth. No specimen could be obtained in two cases; no specimen could be obtained in two repeat drainages; and culture results were not found during chart review in nine cases.

Pain

In our questionnaire, procedural pain was graded on a scale of 1–10, with 10 being the highest. Patients who received a transrectal catheter were sufficiently sedated to be unable recall the procedure during nine (64%) of 14 procedures. Therefore, no pain score was given, and the means reflect only those who recalled the procedure.

Pain-scale measurements were recorded for the insertion of the catheter, the time while the catheter was indwelling, and the period after the catheter was removed. Mean scores (± SD) for transrectal catheters were as follows: insertional pain, 3.2 ± 3.9; indwelling pain, 1.6 ± 1.5; and postremoval pain, 1.4 ± 1.3. There were no differences in the pain scores of men and women undergoing transrectal abscess drainage for these three parameters ($P = .67$, $P = .29$, and $P = .62$, respectively). The patients who underwent transrectal drainage and who recalled the experience rated the pain during insertion as only 3 or less, with only one patient complaining of severe pain with a score of 10. Respondents also reported a similar level of pain while the transrectal catheter was indwelling: 13 of 14 procedures were given a pain score of 4 or less (mean, 1.6 ± 1.5). The one patient who reported a pain score of 10 during catheter insertion complained of a pain score of 6 while it was indwelling. Pain resolved in all patients on catheter removal.

Mean pain scores (± SD) for transvaginal catheters were as follows: insertion, 5.9 ± 3.5; indwelling, 4.8 ± 3.9; and postremoval, 2.3 ± 2.8. In contrast to the relative ease of sedating patients undergoing transrectal abscess drainage to the point that the procedure was not recalled, in four (36%) of 11 cases, patients undergoing transvaginal abscess drainage reported that they did not recall the procedure. In four cases, patients scored the pain of insertion as 5 or greater. Perception of pain with an indwelling catheter was higher for patients with transvaginal catheters; there were five scores for pain of 5 or greater (mean, 4.8 ± 3.9; $P = .01$). Again, all respondents reported that the pain resolved after the transvaginal catheter was removed.

Analysis of women undergoing transvaginal abscess drainage versus transrectal abscess drainage showed higher transvaginal abscess drainage pain scores for all three parameters, but these trends did not approach statistical significance ($P > .99$, $P = .32$, and $P > .99$), mainly owing to the small sample size. This observed trend also applied to the entire patient population; women receiving transvaginal catheters generally experienced greater pain as compared with both male and female patients receiving transrectal catheters, but this observation, too, did not reach statistical significance ($P = .24$).

Effect on Activities of Daily Living

The effects of both transrectal and transvaginal catheters on activities of daily living are summarized in Figure 3. The majority of patients reported that the indwelling transrectal or transvaginal catheter either did not limit or only somewhat limited their activities of daily living. Activities of daily living were limited in only one patient who underwent transrectal drainage, which was in the movement of her bowels.

Transvaginal catheters were generally perceived as more limiting than the transrectal catheters, and some of the differences proved significant. Three patients thought the transvaginal catheter limited their ability to bathe ($P = .11$), walking was very limited in two ($P = .06$), two could not sit comfortably ($P = .01$), the ability to urinate was very limited in one patient ($P = .02$), and another was very limited in moving her bowels ($P = .22$). The limitations that were perceived by patients who received a transvaginal catheter resolved quickly after removal of the catheter, except for two patients: one who required a month to regain normal bowel function and another whose ability to urinate was limited for 2 days after removal of the drainage catheter.

Employment

Eleven of the 22 respondents were employed full time prior to the drainage procedure, two were part-time workers, and one was a student. One full-time worker returned to work while her transvaginal catheter was in place. Seven full-time workers and both part-time workers returned to work within 60 days of catheter removal (mean, 35 days; median, 28 days). Three patients had not returned to work at the time of follow-up. Concurrent illness was often the major influence on hospital course, discharge date, and the time taken before returning to work.

Sexual Function

Twenty-one of the respondents were over the age of 18. Thirteen were sexually active prior to the procedure and agreed to answer questions in this area. Nine transrectal and six transvaginal drains were placed in this subgroup, as two patients underwent two procedures. Of the nine transrectal catheters, three were in patients who were in the hospital the entire time the catheter was in place and there was no opportunity for sexual activity. Three transrectal catheters were associated with no sexual limitation at all, one was said to be somewhat limiting, and in two patients the catheter was thought to be very limiting. Normal sexual function was reported by all patients after the transrectal catheter was removed, except in one male patient who stated that he remained somewhat limited sexually.

Four of the six patients who had transvaginal catheters reported the catheters were very limiting to their sexual activity ($P = .31$). The remaining two patients were in the hospital the entire time and had no opportunity for sexual activity. Three patients reported the return of normal sexual function after removal of the catheter, but the fourth believed she remained somewhat limited at the time of follow-up.

Informed Consent

Twenty-one of the 22 respondents reported that the procedure was explained well to them prior to the initiation of treatment. Patients' expectations of the effect of the procedure and indwelling catheter, however, often differed from what they experienced. Six patients believed that they underestimated the amount of pain that would be involved, and eight thought they were more limited in their activities of daily living than they thought they would be. None stated that this reflected a deficiency in the informed consent process.

DISCUSSION

Advances in endoluminal US are responsible for an increase in the acceptance of the transrectal and transvaginal routes to pelvic drainage by making the procedures safer and easier. The effectiveness of both approaches is now well documented (1–5,10).

The most commonly used alternative to these technically challenging fluid collections is to approach them transgluteally, usually under computed tomographic guidance (11–13). However, transgluteal catheters are often accompanied by prolonged pain and discomfort (11), which may not subside until the catheter is removed. There is also a potential for transgluteal catheter insertion to injure large blood vessels, with resultant severe hemorrhage (14), which has not been reported in any transrectal or transvaginal series, to our knowledge.

Nevertheless, there remains some apprehension on the part of patients, referring physicians, and radiologists regarding use of the transrectal and transvaginal approaches. The reasons for this are uncertain but may include unfamiliarity with the techniques involved or a concern over the amount of pain and discomfort that the patient might experience. Transrectal and transvaginal drains are frequently anticipated by patients as awkward or unusual. Patients who are treated and discharged home in their own care may not express concerns over maintenance of hygiene and other factors. Interventional radiologists have assumed responsibility for the care and follow-up of patients, so it is imperative that they understand the issues involved in patients' acceptance of these types of catheters.

The effect of pelvic surgery, for instance, on body image, quality of life, and activities of daily living has been well described (8,9). We sought to obtain similarly objective data regarding the effect of radiologically placed transrectal and transvaginal catheters on patients and their activities of daily living by rating pain on a linear scale and asking questions about activities of daily living that would elicit discrete, quantifiable responses.

We found that despite a trend for greater pain during the insertion of transvaginal as compared with transrectal catheters (5.9 vs 3.2, $P = .24$), only the pain level while the transvaginal catheters were indwelling proved to be significantly greater (4.8 vs 1.6, $P = .01$). Pain resolved in every case after the catheter was removed.

Transrectal catheters had minimal effect on the patients' activities of daily living, whereas transvaginal catheters appeared to have a greater effect on walking, bathing, and bowel habits, with a significant ($P < .05$) effect on urination and sitting. Describing patients' limitations in general terms (eg, somewhat limited, very limited) does not allow identification of specific problem areas, such as pain on urination versus urinary incontinence. However, the purpose of this study was to determine if there was an overall greater negative effect with the transvaginal approach, and the data support this hypothesis. While we would have preferred to include very specific details, the small number of patients presented here often included too few data points for statistical validation of a number of interesting observations.

Ideally, the issue should be studied prospectively, with inclusion of patients undergoing transgluteal, transabdominal, and transperineal pelvic abscess drainage for comparison of all methods. This would necessitate studying a very large number of patients with close follow-up intervals, because many patients are unable to recall the precise details of distant events. Statistical analysis of specific complaints related to each type of approach would require many times the number of patient responses gathered in this study.

Limited as this study might otherwise be, there were no obvious predictive factors for those patients who would or would not tolerate transvaginal or transrectal drainage. There was no apparent correlation between the size of the catheter, the age of the patient, the duration of the catheter placement, the cause of the collection, the time from catheter removal to the date of the interview, or the physician placing the catheter with the amount of pain experienced or the effect on activities of daily living. Patients thought that they were properly informed, and, therefore, tolerance of the procedure or the effect of the indwelling catheter on activities of daily living is influenced by a variety of factors unrelated to the informed consent process.

In summary, given the increased pain and inconvenience associated with transvaginal drainage catheters, we prefer to use the transrectal approach. However, for female patients who are postmenarchal, we still opt for the transvaginal approach in three clinical settings: when the transrectal approach is no longer available (eg, following abdominoperineal resection), when there has been dehiscence of a vaginal cuff (no transvaginal needle or tract dilation is needed), and in patients with active inflammatory bowel disease.

Prior to pelvic abscess drainage, especially by means of the transvaginal route, patients and referring physicians should be made well aware of the potential for discomfort and severe limitations on activities of daily living.

Acknowledgments: The authors thank Patricia L. Norton, BS, RN, and Patricia M. Suntrup, RT, for administering the patient survey and Roberta L. Yoffie, RT, for helping to coordinate follow-up efforts. We are also grateful to Thomas K. Pilgram, PhD, for his statistical help and advice.

References

1. Kuligowska E, Keller E, Ferrucci JT. Treatment of pelvic abscess: value of one-step sonographically guided transrectal needle aspiration and lavage. AJR 1995; 164:201–206.
2. Feld R, Eschelman DJ, Sagerman JE, Segal S, Hovsepian DM, Sullivan KL. Treatment of pelvic abscess and other fluid collections: efficacy of transvaginal sonographically guided aspiration and drainage. AJR 1994; 163:1141-1145.
3. Nelson AL, Sinow RM, Renslo R, Renslo MJ, Atamdede F. Endovaginal ultrasonographically guided transvaginal drainage for treatment of pelvic abscesses. Am J Obstet Gynecol 1995; 172:1926–1932.
4. Alexander AA, Eschelman DJ, Nazarian LN, Bonn J. Transrectal sonographically guided drainage of deep pelvic abscesses. AJR 1994; 162:1227–1230.
5. vanSonnenberg E, D'Agostino HB, Casola G, Goodacre BW, Sanchez RB, Taylor B. US-guided transvaginal drainage of pelvic abscesses and fluid collections. Radiology 1991; 181:53–56.
6. Bennett JD, Kozak RI, Taylor BM, Jory TA. Deep pelvic abscesses: transrectal drainage with radiologic guidance. Radiology 1992; 185:825–828.
7. Mauro MA, Jacques PF, Mandell VS, Mandel SR. Pelvic abscess drainage by the transrectal catheter approach in men. AJR 1985; 144:477–479.
8. Hawighorst-Knapstein S, Schonfuss G, Hoffmann SO, Knapstein PG. Pelvic exenteration: effects of surgery on quality of life and body image—a prospective longitudinal study. Gynecol Oncol 1997; 66: 495–500.
9. McLeod RS, Fazio VW. Quality of life with the continent ileostomy. World J Surg 1984; 8:90–95.
10. Pereira JK, Chait PG, Miller SF. Deep pelvic abscesses in children: transrectal drainage under radiologic guidance. Radiology 1996; 198:393–396.
11. Butch RJ, Mueller PR, Joseph T, et al. Drainage of pelvic abscess through the greater sciatic foramen. Radiology 1986; 158:487–491.
12. vanSonnenberg E, D'Agostino HB, Casola G, Halasz NA, Sanchez RB, Goodacre BW. Percutaneous abscess drainage: current concepts. Radiology 1991; 181:617–626.
13. Jaques PF, Mauro M. Drainage of pelvic abscesses through the greater sciatic foramen (letter). Radiology 1986; 160:278–279.
14. Malden ES, Picus D. Hemorrhagic complications of transgluteal pelvic abscess drainage: successful percutaneous treatment. JVIR 1992; 3:323–328.

Book Review

Vascular Brachytherapy. 2nd ed.

Edited by Ron Waksman, MD
Armonk, NY: Futura, 1998. ISBN 0-87993-4131.
Hardcover, $149.00; pp 654; 232 figures; tables.

Dr Ron Waksman, director of the Experimental Angioplasty and Vascular Brachytherapy Institute at the Washington Hospital Center, has compiled the only textbook currently available (to our knowledge) that provides a comprehensive overview of vascular brachytherapy. A novel therapeutic application of ionizing radiation, vascular brachytherapy is the placement of radioactive material within coronary or peripheral arteries immediately after balloon angioplasty. The goal of radiation therapy in this setting is to inhibit the intimal hyperplasia that frequently occurs in response to vessel dilatation and negates much of the procedure's beneficial effect by impeding blood flow. In the past, this mechanism of restenosis has invariably frustrated interventional cardiologists. Pharmacologic intervention has been largely unsuccessful, and expansile intraluminal stents have only partially mitigated the problem.

Insofar as vascular brachytherapy emerged as a collaboration among radiation oncologists, cardiologists, interventional radiologists, and vascular surgeons who care for patients with atherosclerotic disease, these specialists form the core of Dr Waksman's target audience. Other interested readers would be medical physicists who develop and monitor vascular brachytherapy devices, as well as scientists who study intracellular molecular events and tissue effects triggered by balloon injury and by ionizing radiation within arteries.

This textbook was developed from the syllabus of the annual course entitled "Cardiovascular Radiation Therapy" directed by Dr Waksman and colleagues at his institution. The material is organized into nine parts that comprise 53 individual chapters. The first three parts contain background information on the pathophysiology of arterial stenosis, basic principles of radiobiology, and fundamentals of brachytherapy dosimetry. Three more parts that summarize numerous preclinical experimental results are followed by a seventh that surveys major clinical studies. The final two parts include additional descriptions of vascular radiation therapy systems currently being investigated, as well as commentary regarding radiation safety issues and pertinent federal regulatory guidelines.

The book is printed on high-quality glossy paper and contains numerous helpful illustrations. This edition is almost twice as large as the previous one, which was published only 3 years ago; the growth is a direct reflection of burgeoning investigational activity at numerous research centers that is expanding the available fund of knowledge about vascular brachytherapy. Overall, Dr Waksman has done a splendid job of cataloguing the established data and ongoing dynamic investigations in a rapidly evolving field of study. Generally highly informative and well written, the book's imperfections ironically stem from the effort to be almost too encyclopedic. There are so many authors and chapters that there is overlap in the material presented. Future editions will be improved if some portions are consolidated into streamlined presentations of the larger common topics, especially for the introductory sections.

A concise review of coronary anatomy and angioplasty techniques would suffice to orient the radiation oncologist and physicist to the cardiac catheterization laboratory. Other readers might find it more useful to have a single background radiobiology chapter briefly synopsizing clonogen survival–based classic radiobiology and highlighting the relevant molecular radiobiology that characterizes important signal transduction pathways triggered by nonlethal doses of ionizing radiation in quiescent and proliferating cells. When the currently active clinical protocols have matured, it will be easier to compose coherent overviews of the results by discussing the nuances that distinguish each trial.

We recommend *Vascular Brachytherapy* as an excellent reference textbook for anyone currently participating in clinical trials or preclinical experimentation in the field. As the indications for vascular brachytherapy crystallize and techniques of administration are refined, the modality will likely become more widely used. Cardiologists, vascular interventional radiologists, and radiation oncologists who are not yet familiar with the topic will find the book to be an ideal starting point for their education about a therapeutic intervention that is potentially beneficial to the many thousands of patients who annually undergo angioplasty for atherosclerotic disease.

Reviewed by Brian D. Kavanagh, MD,
and Douglas W. Arthur, MD

Joseph E. Cox, MD
Caroline Chiles, MD
Christopher M. McManus, MD
Suzanne L. Aquino, MD
Robert H. Choplin, MD[2]

Index terms:
Biopsies, complications, 60.411, 60.732
Computed tomography (CT), guidance, 60.12111
Lung, biopsy, 60.126, 60.732
Pneumothorax, 60.411, 60.732

Radiology 1999; 212:165–168

Abbreviation:
TNAB = transthoracic needle aspiration biopsy

[1] From the Department of Radiology, Wake Forest University School of Medicine, Winston-Salem, NC. Received June 17, 1998; revision requested July 30; revision received September 22; accepted December 16. **Address reprint requests to** J.E.C., 59 MDW/MTRD, 2200 Bergquist Dr, Suite 1, Lackland AFB, TX 78236-5300 (e-mail: *joecox@aol.com*).

[2] Current address: Department of Radiology, Presbyterian Hospital, Philadelphia, Pa.

Author contributions:
Guarantors of integrity of entire study, J.E.C., C.C., C.M.M.; study concepts and design, J.E.C., C.C., C.M.M.; definition of intellectual content, J.E.C.; literature research, J.E.C., C.M.M.; clinical studies, all authors; data acquisition, all authors; data analysis, J.E.C.; statistical analysis, J.E.C.; manuscript preparation, J.E.C.; manuscript editing and review, J.E.C., C.C., R.H.C.

Transthoracic Needle Aspiration Biopsy: Variables That Affect Risk of Pneumothorax[1]

PURPOSE: To analyze the influence of multiple variables on the rate of pneumothorax and chest tube placement associated with transthoracic needle aspiration biopsy of the lung.

MATERIALS AND METHODS: In 346 patients, 331 computed tomographically (CT) guided and 24 fluoroscopically guided lung biopsies were performed. Variables analyzed were lesion size, depth, and location; number of pleural passes; needle size; presence of emphysema; and training level of the person who performed the biopsy.

RESULTS: Pneumothorax occurred at 144 (40.4%) of 356 biopsies, including 139 (42.0%) CT-guided and five (21%) fluoroscopically guided biopsies. Chest tube placement was needed in 25 (17.4%) of 144 cases of pneumothorax (7% of all biopsies). An increased rate of pneumothorax was correlated with smaller lesion size (P = .001) and presence of emphysema (P = .01). Patients with emphysema were three times as likely to require chest tube placement. The pneumothorax rate was 15% (16 of 105) if no aerated lung was traversed and approximately 50% if aerated lung was penetrated. Lesion location, needle size, number of pleural passes, and level of training were not correlated with pneumothorax rate.

CONCLUSION: Smaller lesion size and emphysema are strongly correlated with occurrence of pneumothorax. Pneumothorax was more than three times less frequent if no aerated lung was traversed. After pneumothorax, chest tube placements were related to the presence of emphysema.

Percutaneous transthoracic needle aspiration biopsy (TNAB) of the lung is a well-established method for obtaining pulmonary tissue for pathologic examination (1–6). Accuracy for the diagnosis of benign and malignant diseases is greater than 80% and 90%, respectively (4–6).

Fatal complications due to systemic air embolism, hemorrhage, or pericardial tamponade have been described (3,7–10), but these complications are rare. Other serious complications, such as seeding of malignant cells into the needle track (11), lung torsion (12), and empyema (7), also are rare and should not alter indications for TNAB.

Pneumothorax is, by far, the most frequent complication of the procedure: Reported (2,8,13–23) rates range widely, from 5% to 61%. Most of these data pertain to fluoroscopically guided TNAB. Overall, TNAB performed with computed tomographic (CT) guidance may be associated with a higher frequency of pneumothorax than fluoroscopically guided TNAB, probably because CT requires more time, and the average size of the lesion is smaller. The reported rate of pneumothorax with CT-guided biopsy may also be slightly higher because CT is more sensitive for the detection of pneumothorax. The authors of several investigations (1,13,24) have reported a 22%–45% risk of pneumothorax for CT-guided TNAB. The purpose of this study was to examine the influence of multiple variables on the frequency of pneumothorax and chest tube placement.

MATERIALS AND METHODS

Between January 1993 and June 1997, 356 percutaneous TNABs were performed in 346 patients at our institution. Ten patients underwent biopsy twice, both times with CT guidance. The study population included 226 men and 120 women aged 18–92 years (mean age, 64 years). Of the 356 biopsies, 331 were performed with CT guidance, 24 were performed with fluoroscopy, and the procedure was performed "blindly" (without imaging guidance) in one patient in the intensive care unit.

All procedures were performed by a staff radiologist (J.E.C., C.C., S.L.C., R.H.C.) or by a radiology resident (C.M.M.) with staff supervision, in accordance with the protocol followed by the thoracic radiology section at our institution (North Carolina Baptist Hospital, Winston-Salem). Biopsies were assigned randomly to the resident or staff radiologist who was covering the chest CT service. Informed consent was obtained before each biopsy.

The procedure was performed with the patient in a prone, supine, or lateral decubitus position, depending on the location of the lesion. Conscious sedation was used in anxious patients and on request. Local anesthesia was administered by means of a subcutaneous injection of 1% lidocaine. Coaxial procedures were performed with a 19-gauge outer needle (Greene needle; Cook, Bloomington, Ind) and a 22-gauge inner needle. Biopsy of a peripheral lesion often was performed directly with a 22-gauge needle. If CT guidance was used, axial images were acquired before needle aspiration to document the position of the 19- or 22-gauge needle in the lesion. Nine biopsies were performed with an 18-, 20-, or 21-gauge needle. Pleural effusions, fissures, and bullae were avoided during biopsy if possible. As a general rule, the radiologists would not refuse to perform a biopsy because of emphysema.

The frequency of pneumothorax and chest tube placement was analyzed in relationship to several variables, including lesion location (upper lobe, lower lobe, right middle lobe), lesion size, lesion depth, number of pleural passes, size of the needle used to traverse the pleura, presence of emphysema in lobe in which biopsy was performed, and level of training of person performing the biopsy.

For CT-guided biopsies, images were first acquired at 3- or 5-mm collimation through the lesion by using a CT HiSpeed Advantage scanner (GE Medical Systems, Milwaukee, Wis). Lesion size was determined on the basis of the average lesion diameter in two axial planes. CT scans were available for all fluoroscopically guided biopsies. (Fluoroscopically-guided biopsies generally were performed when the CT scanner was not immediately available.) Lesion depth was the amount of aerated lung traversed from the surface of the pleura to the edge of the lesion. The presence of any type of emphysema in the lobe in which biopsy was performed was determined on the basis of CT results alone. At our institution, thin-section (1-mm-collimation) CT images of the lung are routinely acquired and could be used to evaluate for emphysema in most cases. The level of training (1st- through 4th-year resident or staff physician) of each person performing the procedure was recorded.

A cytotechnologist and resident or staff cytopathologist were present at all biopsies. All specimens obtained were immediately smeared and then stained by the cytotechnologist. The adequacy of the specimen for diagnosis was assessed by the resident pathologist, the staff pathologist, or both. If possible, additional aspirates were obtained when specimens were not sufficient for diagnosis.

After the procedure, patients were placed on a stretcher for 1 hour in the puncture-side-down position, with the supervision of a nurse. Chest radiographs were obtained 1–2 hours after biopsy, with the patient in the erect position. The procedure was complicated by pneumothorax if pneumothorax was seen on either the follow-up CT scan obtained immediately after biopsy or on the chest radiograph obtained 1–2 hours after biopsy. An enlarging or symptomatic pneumothorax was treated with placement of a chest tube. The relationship between pneumothorax and quantitative variables was analyzed by using the Fisher exact test or the χ^2 statistic.

TABLE 1
Correlation of Pneumothorax Rate with Level of Training

Level of Training	No Pneumothorax (n = 209)	Pneumothorax (n = 143)	Total (n = 352)	Pneumothorax Rate (%)
1st-year resident	29	20	49	41
2nd-year resident	76	53	129	41
3rd-year resident	50	40	90	44
4th-year resident	36	18	54	33
Staff physician	18	12	30	40

Note.—Procedure was performed by two physicians in four patients.

TABLE 2
Correlation of Pneumothorax Rate with Number of Pleural Passes

No. of Passes	No Pneumothorax (n = 212)	Pneumothorax (n = 144)	Total (n = 356)	Pneumothorax Rate (%)
1	106	61	167	37
2	45	42	87	48
3	34	22	56	39
4	18	7	25	28
≥5	9	12	21	57

RESULTS

Pneumothorax was seen in 139 (42.0%) of 331 cases of CT-guided TNAB. Pneumothorax was seen in five (21%) of 24 cases of fluoroscopically guided TNAB. Only 24 (6.7%) of 356 biopsies were performed with fluoroscopic guidance. Of the 144 cases of pneumothorax, 25 (17.4%) necessitated chest tube placement.

Table 1 shows the comparison of the frequency of pneumothorax and the level of training of the physician who performed the procedure. No significant difference in pneumothorax rate was found when the procedure was performed by a junior resident (73 [41%] of 178), a senior resident (58 [40%] of 144), or a staff physician (12 [40%] of 30).

No significant correlation was found between lesion location (upper lobe vs lower lobe) and frequency of pneumothorax. Pneumothorax occurred at 87 (40%) of 216 upper lobe biopsies, and at 48 (42%) of 113 lower lobe biopsies. TNAB of 20 right middle lobe lesions resulted in six (30%) pneumothoraces. In the remaining seven patients, the fissure was crossed during biopsy.

Table 2 shows the comparison of the frequency of pneumothorax with the number of passes made across the pleural surface with the needle. No significant

TABLE 3
Correlation of Pneumothorax Rate with Distance from Pleural Surface

Distance from Pleural Surface (cm)	No Pneumothorax (n = 192)	Pneumothorax (n = 144)	Total (n = 356)	Pneumothorax Rate (%)
0	89	16	105	15
>0–1	40	44	84	52
>1–2	29	25	54	46
>2–3	22	25	47	53
>3–4	13	18	31	58
>4–5	13	10	23	43
>5	6	6	12	50

TABLE 4
Correlation of Pneumothorax Rate with Presence of Emphysema as Determined at Thin-Section CT

Emphysema	No Pneumothorax (n = 212)	Pneumothorax (n = 144)	Total (n = 356)	Pneumothorax Rate (%)
Present	68	66	134	49.3
Absent	144	78	222	35.1

TABLE 5
Correlation of Pneumothorax Rate with Lesion Size

Lesion Size (cm)	No Pneumothorax (n = 212)	Pneumothorax (n = 144)	Total (n = 356)	Pneumothorax Rate (%)
0–1	8	15	23	65
>1–2	43	57	100	57
>2–3	75	43	118	36
>3–4	36	19	55	35
>4–5	23	6	29	21
>5	27	4	31	13

correlation between these two variables was found. Pneumothorax occurred in 103 (40.6%) of 254 biopsies performed with two or fewer pleural passes and in 41 (40.2%) of 102 biopsies performed with three or more pleural passes. In addition, no significant difference in the prevalence of pneumothorax was found when comparing one pass with multiple passes ($\chi^2 = 1.71$).

In almost all patients, the pleural surface was traversed with a 19- or 22-gauge needle. The frequency of pneumothorax with the larger (19-gauge) needle (45 [39.1%] of 115) was not significantly different from the frequency with the smaller (22-gauge) needle (91 [39.6%] of 230).

Table 3 shows the comparison of the frequency of pneumothorax with the distance of the lesion from the pleural surface, that is, amount of aerated lung traversed by the needle. A measurement of 0 cm indicates that the lesion contacted the pleural surface, and no aerated lung was traversed during the TNAB. For these peripheral lesions, pneumothorax occurred at only 16 (15%) of 105 biopsies. If any amount of aerated lung was traversed during biopsy, the rate of pneumothorax approximated 50%. The pneumothorax rate did not increase with increasing distance of the lesion from the pleural surface (if peripheral lesions are excluded from consideration).

Table 4 demonstrates the significantly greater frequency of pneumothorax ($\chi^2 = 6.9$, $P < .01$) in patients who had CT evidence of emphysema (usually determined on the basis of thin-section CT findings) in the lobe in which biopsy was performed. In patients in whom biopsy was complicated due to pneumothorax, the frequency of chest tube placement was significantly greater ($\chi^2 = 7.12$, $P < .01$) in those with CT evidence of emphysema (18 [27%] of 66) than in those with no CT evidence of emphysema (seven [9%] of 78).

Table 5 shows the comparison of the frequency of pneumothorax with the size of the lesion in which the biopsy was performed. Smaller lesion size correlated strongly ($P = .001$) with the development of pneumothorax. For lesions 2 cm or smaller, the pneumothorax rate was 58.5% (72 of 123). Biopsy of lesions larger than 2 cm resulted in pneumothorax in 72 (30.9%) of 233 procedures.

DISCUSSION

Prior investigators (13–16,24) have reported that a greater depth of needle penetration from the pleural surface to the edge of the lesion is associated with a higher rate of pneumothorax. Technically, our results support this conclusion, although the data can be somewhat misleading. Most previously published reports (1–3,5–8,13–16,24) included biopsy of peripheral lung lesions in the calculation of pneumothorax rates, even if no aerated lung was traversed. Our data show that in 105 pleural-based lesions in which biopsy was performed (without traversal of aerated lung), the pneumothorax rate was only 15% (16 of 105). However, if any amount of aerated lung was traversed, the pneumothorax rate was approximately 50%, and this rate did not increase with increasing depth of the lesion (Table 3). For example, for lesions at a depth of 0–2 cm (excluding peripheral pleural lesions), the frequency of pneumothorax was 50.0% (69 of 138), as compared with a frequency of 52.2% (59 of 113) for lesions that necessitated needle penetration of more than 2 cm through aerated lung. Our results do not support the findings of Poe et al (14), who reported that increasing depth of needle penetration increased the risk for pneumothorax, even after exclusion of lesions that contacted the pleural surface. Direct comparison of the results of these studies is difficult, however, given that Poe and colleagues performed the biopsies fluoroscopically and with different techniques.

There is some debate in the literature about the correlation between abnormal pulmonary function test results and the risk of development of pneumothorax. Recently, Anderson et al (17) and Kazerooni et al (24) found that pulmonary function test results had no predictive value with regard to the frequency of pneumothorax in their studies of CT-guided TNAB in 93 and 121 patients, respectively. In contrast, both Fish et al (15) and Miller et al (16) found that obstructive lung disease was a factor that affected the pneumothorax rate. In those studies, pneumothorax developed in approximately 45% of patients with an obstructive pulmonary abnormality, as compared with about 20% of patients with normal pulmonary function. Poe et al (14) found a twofold increase in the prevalence of pneumothorax in patients who had greater than 120% of predicted total lung capacity.

In our study, thin-section CT (usually 1–3-mm collimation) was used to determine if emphysema was visible in the lobe in which biopsy was performed. We found a significantly higher ($\chi^2 = 7.45$, $P < .01$) risk of pneumothorax in patients with emphysema (49% vs 35% in those without emphysema) when evaluated as a single independent variable. Also, patients with emphysema in whom a pneumothorax developed required chest tube placement at three times the rate of those with pneumothorax but no CT evidence of emphysema (27% and 9%, respectively).

The increased likelihood of chest tube placement in patients who have obstructive lung disease has previously been demonstrated (15,24,25) and could be due to several factors. Patients with emphysema have decreased pulmonary reserve and are more likely to have a symptomatic pneumothorax. Also, disruption of dilated air spaces may prevent rapid sealing of the air leak (24). Pneumothorax resorbs more slowly in patients with an obstructive pulmonary abnormality (26).

The strong correlation between pneumothorax rate and lesion size is difficult to explain, although this correlation has previously been reported (15,24). It could be argued that larger lesions are more likely to contact the pleural surface and, hence, not require needle passage through aerated lung. However, the correlation of increasing frequency of pneumothorax with decreasing lesion size persists, even if lesions with pleural contact are eliminated from consideration. The pneumothorax rate was 64.2% (68 of 106) for lesions 2 cm or less in size, as compared with 41.4% (60 of 145) for lesions more than 2 cm in size (excluding the 105 lesions in contact with pleura). A possible explanation for this finding is that the up-and-down movement of the needle tip during aspiration biopsy results in more tearing of adjacent lung parenchyma when the lesion is relatively small.

No relationship was found between the number of pleural passes and the pneumothorax rate. Although this lack of association is surprising, other studies (14–16,24) have shown similar results. There also was no correlation between pneumothorax rate and needle size (19-gauge vs 22-gauge) or lesion location (upper lobe vs lower lobe). Of interest, the risk of pneumothorax was nearly identical when TNAB was performed by a junior resident, senior resident, or staff physician, possibly because the factors that influence the pneumothorax rate are not operator dependent.

In conclusion, the only factors that independently altered the risk of pneumothorax were size of the lesion and presence of emphysema. If no aerated lung was traversed during needle penetration, the pneumothorax rate was low. However, the rate of pneumothorax was approximately 50% if any amount of aerated lung was penetrated. The presence of emphysema increased the likelihood that chest tube placement would be necessary.

References

1. Li H, Boiselle PM, Shepard JO, Trotman-Dickenson B, McCloud TC. Diagnostic accuracy and safety of CT-guided percutaneous needle aspiration biopsy of the lung: comparison of small and large pulmonary nodules. AJR 1996; 167:105–109.
2. Harter LP, Moss AA, Goldberg HI, Gross BH. CT-guided fine-needle aspirations for diagnosis of benign and malignant disease. AJR 1983; 140:363–367.
3. Perlmutt LM, Johnston WW, Dunnick NR. Percutaneous transthoracic needle aspiration: a review. AJR 1989; 152:451–455.
4. Stanley JH, Fish GD, Andriole JG, et al. Lung lesions: cytologic diagnosis by fine-needle biopsy. Radiology 1987; 162:389–391.
5. Westcott JL. Percutaneous transthoracic needle biopsy. Radiology 1988; 169:593–601.
6. Khouri NF, Stitik FP, Erozan YS, et al. Transthoracic needle aspiration biopsy of benign and malignant lung lesions. AJR 1985; 144:281–288.
7. Sinner WN. Complications of percutaneous transthoracic needle aspiration biopsy. Acta Radiol 1976; 17:813–828.
8. Herman PG, Hessel SJ. The diagnostic accuracy and complications of closed lung biopsies. Radiology 1977; 125:11–14.
9. Tolly TL, Feldmeier JE, Czcernecki D. Air embolism complicating percutaneous lung biopsy. AJR 1988; 150:555–556.
10. Aberle DR, Gamsu G, Golden JA. Fatal systemic arterial air embolism following lung needle aspiration. Radiology 1987; 165:351–353.
11. Müller NL, Bergin CJ, Miller RR, Ostrow DN. Seeding of malignant cells into the needle track after lung and pleural biopsy. Can Assoc Radiol J 1986; 37:192–194.
12. Graham RJ, Heyd RL, Raval VA, Barrett TF. Lung torsion after percutaneous needle biopsy of lung. AJR 1992; 159:35–37.
13. vanSonnenberg E, Casola G, Ho M, et al. Difficult thoracic lesions: CT-guided biopsy experience in 150 cases. Radiology 1988; 167:457–461.
14. Poe RH, Kallay MC, Wicks CM, Odoroff CL. Predicting risk of pneumothorax in needle biopsy of the lung. Chest 1984; 85:232–235.
15. Fish GD, Stanley JH, Miller KS, Schabel SI, Sutherland SE. Postbiopsy pneumothorax: estimating the risk by chest radiography and pulmonary function tests. AJR 1988; 150:71–74.
16. Miller KS, Fish GB, Stanley JH, Schabel SI. Prediction of pneumothorax rate in percutaneous needle aspiration of the lung. Chest 1988; 93:742–745.
17. Anderson CLV, Crespo JCA, Lie TH. Risk of pneumothorax not increased by obstructive lung disease. Chest 1994; 105:1705–1708.
18. Haramati LB, Austin JHM. Complications after CT-guided needle biopsy through aerated versus nonaerated lung. Radiology 1991; 181:778.
19. Fontana RS, Miller WE, Beabout JW, Payne WS, Harrison EG Jr. Transthoracic needle aspiration of discrete pulmonary lesions: experience in 100 cases. Med Clin North Am 1970; 54:961–971.
20. Coleman R, Driver M, Gishen P. Percutaneous lung biopsy: experiences during the first 54 biopsies. Cardiovasc Intervent Radiol 1982; 5:61–63.
21. Jereb M. The usefulness of needle biopsy in chest lesions of different sizes and locations. Radiology 1980; 134:13–15.
22. Jackson R, Coffin LH, DeMeules JE, Miller DB, Dietrich P, Fairbank J. Percutaneous needle biopsy of pulmonary lesions. Am J Surg 1980; 139:586–590.
23. Gibney RTN, Man GCW, King EG, leRiche J. Aspiration biopsy in the diagnosis of pulmonary disease. Chest 1981; 80:300–303.
24. Kazerooni EA, Lim FT, Mikhail A, Martinez FJ. Risk of pneumothorax in CT-guided transthoracic needle aspiration biopsy of the lung. Radiology 1996; 198:371–375.
25. Perlmutt LM, Braun SD, Newman GE, et al. Transthoracic needle aspiration: use of a small chest tube to treat pneumothorax. AJR 1987; 148:849–851.
26. Dines DE, Clagett OT, Payne WS. Spontaneous pneumothorax in emphysema. Mayo Clin Proc 1970; 45:481–487.

Descending Thoracic Aortic Aneurysm: Thoracic CT Findings after Endovascular Stent-Graft Placement[1]

Toyohiko Sakai, MD
Michael D. Dake, MD
Charles P. Semba, MD
Tetsuhisa Yamada, MD
Akihiko Arakawa, MD
Stephen T. Kee, MD
Nobushige Hayashi, MD
Mahmood K. Razavi, MD
Daniel Y. Sze, MD

Index terms:
Aneurysm, aortic, 563.732, 943.73
Aorta, grafts and prostheses, 563.1269, 943.1268
Aorta, interventional procedures, 563.1269, 943.1268

Radiology 1999; 212:169–174

[1] From the Department of Cardiovascular and Interventional Radiology, Stanford University Medical Center, 300 Pasteur Dr, Suite H3630, Stanford, CA 94305-1056 (T.S., M.D.D., C.P.S., T.Y., A.A., S.T.K., M.K.R., D.Y.S.), and the Department of Radiology, Fukui Medical University School of Medicine, Fukui, Japan (N.H.). Received April 1, 1998; revision requested June 25; revision received September 14; accepted December 16. **Address reprint requests to** M.D.D. (e-mail: *mddake@stanford.edu*).

PURPOSE: To evaluate the usefulness of thoracic computed tomography (CT) after placement of an endovascular stent-graft for the treatment of descending thoracic aortic aneurysm.

MATERIALS AND METHODS: From 1992 to 1996, 85 patients with thoracic aortic aneurysm underwent stent-graft placement. In 63 patients, thoracic CT scans were obtained both before and within 10 days after placement. The CT findings were retrospectively studied, and their clinical effect analyzed. In 20 of 63 patients, long-term follow-up CT findings were also evaluated.

RESULTS: After stent-graft placement in the 63 patients, CT demonstrated an increase in pleural effusion in 46 (73%), periaortic changes in 21 (33%), perigraft leak in 13 (21%), atelectasis in six (10%), mural thrombus within the stent-graft in two (3%), and new aortic dissection in one (2%). The mean maximum diameter of the aneurysm was 58.8 mm before and 60.0 mm after stent-graft insertion. Sixty-two (98%) patients were successfully treated until discharge. Interventional procedures were performed to eliminate the leakage into the aneurysm sac in 10 patients with perigraft flow depicted at CT. Other complications were managed conservatively.

CONCLUSION: Thoracic CT is useful in the treatment of patients after stent-graft insertion for the management of descending thoracic aortic aneurysm.

Endoluminal stent-graft placement is currently being tested as a less invasive alternative than conventional surgery for the treatment of descending thoracic aortic aneurysm. Although long-term evaluation is definitely necessary to determine the efficacy of the stent-grafts in preventing further aneurysmal dilation and rupture, preliminary results suggest the procedure is feasible, safe, and promising with acceptable midterm results (1–6).

In our institution, patients treated with stent-grafts routinely undergo a thoracic computed tomographic (CT) examination before their discharge to evaluate patency of the graft and the possibility of perigraft leak or other complications. Several changes depicted at thoracic CT have been reported after stent-graft insertion, such as an increase in pleural effusion (1), but we believe detailed CT findings after stent-graft placement in the thoracic aorta have not been well described. The purpose of this study was to analyze the findings at thoracic CT after stent-graft insertion in relation to the indication for treatment, aneurysm anatomy, and final outcome and, thus, to clarify the clinical effect of these findings on the treatment of the patients.

MATERIALS AND METHODS

From July 1992 through June 1996, 85 patients with thoracic aortic aneurysm were treated with placement of an endovascular stent-graft. The investigative protocol was approved by the Stanford University Institutional Review Board, and informed consent was obtained in each case. The protocol required that all patients undergo follow-up chest radiography,

Author contributions:
Guarantors of integrity of entire study, T.S., M.D.D.; study concepts and design, T.S.; definition of intellectual content, T.S., M.D.D.; literature research, T.S.; clinical studies, M.D.D., M.K.R., C.P.S., S.T.K., D.Y.S.; data acquisition, T.S., T.Y., A.A.; data analysis, T.S., N.H.; manuscript preparation and editing, T.S., M.D.D.; manuscript review, T.S., N.H., M.D.D.

arteriography, and contrast material–enhanced spiral CT before hospital discharge after stent-graft placement. Among the 85 patients, this study included 63 patients (46 men and 17 women; age range, 35–84 years; mean age, 68.4 years) who underwent thoracic CT both before and within 10 days after the treatment to evaluate acute changes in thoracic CT findings after stent-graft placement. In order to focus on the acute and possibly transient CT changes caused by stent-graft placement, the remaining 22 patients were excluded from this study because they had undergone an additional procedure such as embolization of a perigraft leak with transcatheter deposition of coils before the first CT examination after stent-graft placement ($n = 3$) or follow-up CT was performed more than 10 days after placement ($n = 19$).

The endovascular stent-graft was custom designed for each patient and comprised a stainless steel endoskeleton consisting of modified Z-stents (Cook, Bloomington, Ind) covered with woven polyester graft material (Cooley Veri-Soft; Meadox/Boston Scientific, Watertown, Mass). All procedures were performed in the operating room with general anesthesia. The femoral artery, iliac artery, or abdominal aorta was surgically exposed and a 24-F Teflon sheath and polyethylene dilator were introduced over the guide wire and advanced with fluoroscopic guidance until the sheath was positioned proximal to the aneurysm. Then, the stent-graft was advanced through the Teflon sheath by using a solid pusher and was deployed at the appropriate position by holding the pusher firmly in position and quickly withdrawing the sheath.

CT was performed with a whole-body scanner (Somaton Plus-S, Siemens Medical Systems, Iselin, NJ, or CT HiSpeed Advantage, GE Medical Systems, Milwaukee, Wis) with capability for spiral scanning and three-dimensional reconstruction (7,8). The patient was instructed to hyperventilate and maintain the same degree of inspiration for 30 seconds. After placement of a 20-gauge intravenous catheter into an antecubital vein, a 150-mL bolus of nonionic iodinated contrast media (Isovue 300; Squibb, New Brunswick, NJ) was administered at a flow rate determined to deliver the volume of contrast media in a period of time equivalent to the duration scanning. A delay after the initiation of the contrast media infusion was calculated for each patient on the basis of findings at dynamic scanning performed through the level of interest after injection of a 20-mL bolus of contrast media. After the predetermined delay, spiral scans were obtained with 3-mm collimation at a table speed of 5 or 6 mm/sec (pitch, 1.7 or 2.0), depending on the required volume of interest. The spiral acquisition was reconstructed into axial sections with 5–9-mm collimation every 2–6 mm to achieve at least 33% overlap.

The CT scans were retrospectively interpreted in an independent manner by three experienced radiologists (T.S., T.Y., A.A.). Subsequently, final consensus agreement was achieved regarding the CT findings in each case. Findings on CT scans obtained after stent-graft placement were compared to those evident before placement with special attention to the following features: pleural effusion, atelectasis without massive pleural effusion, periaortic changes, perigraft leak, and other complications related to stent-graft placement. In addition, the maximum diameter of the aneurysm was compared on the CT scans obtained before and after placement. The CT scans were interpreted without knowledge of three-dimensional reconstruction, angiographic, or chest radiographic findings or patient prognosis.

Passive atelectasis associated with massive pleural effusion was commonly observed, but it was excluded from evaluation as a separate pathologic finding because it was not considered a primary process.

Aortic or periaortic changes evident at CT included aortic wall thickening, periaortic effusion, and periaortic atelectasis. Aortic wall thickening was diagnosed when the aortic wall was thicker on the postplacement than on the preplacement CT scans. Periaortic effusion was diagnosed when a fluid collection was observed around only the descending aorta without any other effusion identified on the same image. Periaortic atelectasis was diagnosed when focal atelectasis was noted adjacent to the aorta without atelectasis evident in other areas on the same image. In this study, if these findings existed on a CT scan before stent-graft placement and were unchanged on the postplacement CT images, they were not considered abnormal findings due to the stent-graft placement.

In 20 of the 63 patients, long-term follow-up CT scans (mean, 388 days; range, 6 months to 3.5 years) were also available for evaluation.

RESULTS

Sixty-two (98%) of the 63 patients were successfully treated by means of endovascular stent-graft placement without open surgery. One of the 63 patients died of respiratory failure 21 days after stent-graft insertion (mortality rate, 2%). In this case, CT performed 5 days after the procedure revealed an increase in pleural effusion with no evidence of pneumonia, atelectasis, or perigraft leakage of contrast media into the aneurysm sac. Subsequently, respiratory failure progressed, and prolonged intubation was necessary. This was complicated by pneumonia. Retrospectively, there was no evidence on sequential chest radiographs of a further increase in pleural effusion after the first postplacement CT scan was obtained.

TABLE 1
Summary of Abnormal Thoracic CT Findings after Stent-Graft Placement in 63 Patients

Abnormal Finding	No. of Patients	Frequency (%)
Pleural effusion	46	73
Periaortic changes	21	33
Perigraft leak	13	21
Atelectasis	10	16
Mural thrombus	2	3
Dissection	1	2
Pneumonia	1	2
None	9	14

After stent-graft insertion in the 63 patients, fever (>38°C) was recorded in 23 (37%) and leukocytosis (>11,000/μL [11.0×10^9/L]) in 48 (76%). In general, these findings were self-limited and improved within 7 days in all cases. Blood was cultured in 10 patients. No growth was observed in any culture.

In all 63 patients, CT images after stent-graft deployment were without major artifacts caused by the stent-graft. Minimal artifacts caused by the stent-graft were a relatively common finding on postplacement CT scans, but they did not prohibit interpretation of the images.

CT findings in the 63 patients are summarized in Table 1. The amount of pleural effusion increased in 46 (73%) patients, did not change in 10 (16%), and decreased in seven (11%). In the 46 patients with increased pleural effusion (Fig 1), the amount of pleural effusion increased on both sides of the pleural cavity in 27 (43%), on only the left side in 15 (24%), and on only the right side in four (6%). None of the patients underwent chest tube drainage, and all were treated conservatively. In all cases, a subsequent decrease in pleural effusion was confirmed at chest radiography before discharge. In all 13 patients with long-term follow-up

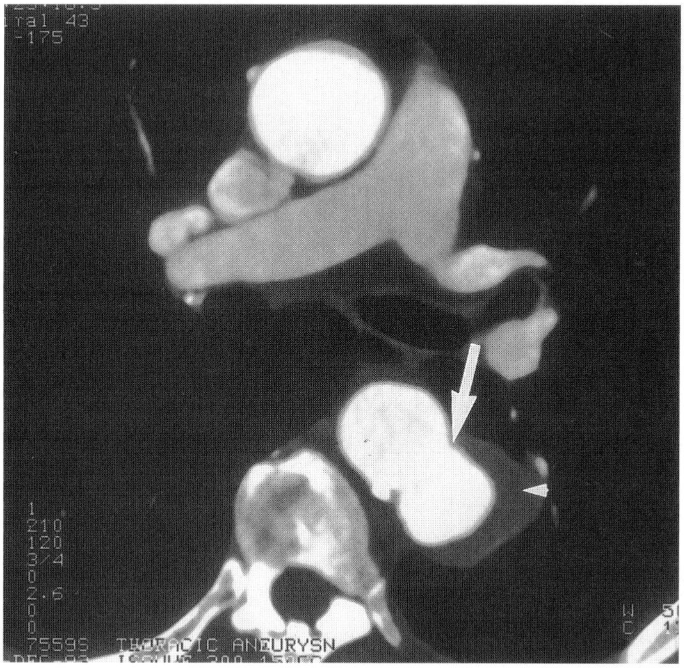

a.

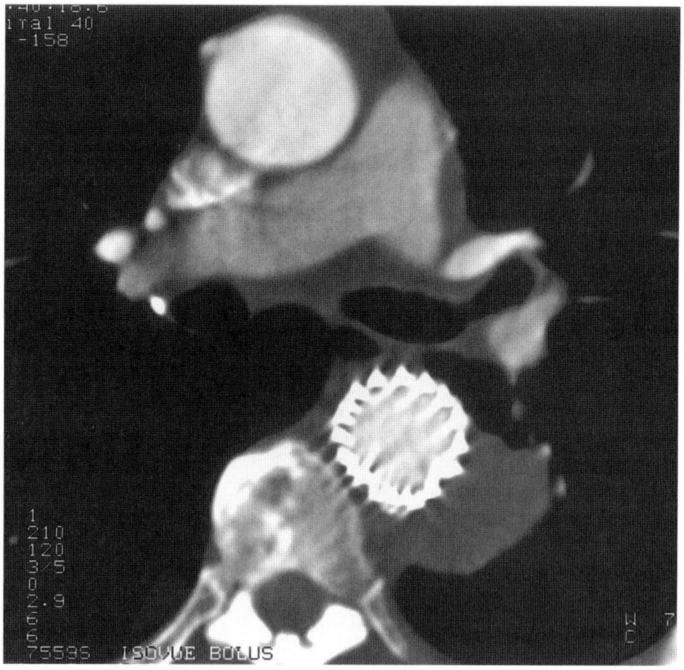

c.

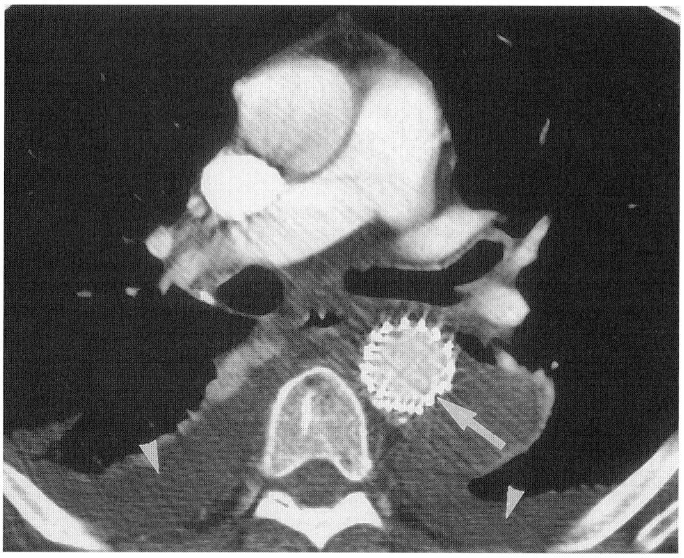

b.

Figure 1. Contrast-enhanced chest CT images depict a saccular aneurysm of the descending thoracic aorta. **(a)** Before stent-graft placement, aneurysm (arrow) has some mural thrombus (arrowhead). **(b)** Two days after placement, the thrombotic aneurysm is depicted, as are the stent-graft (arrow) and bilateral pleural effusions (arrowheads). **(c)** Six months after placement, the pleural effusions are improved.

CT scans, resolution of the effusion was confirmed. Atelectasis without massive pleural effusion was observed in six (10%) patients. Five of the six patients were treated conservatively with medication or nebulizer therapy, and their improvement was confirmed before discharge on the basis of findings at chest radiography, clinical symptoms, or laboratory data. In the remaining patient, a metallic endobronchial stent was placed 18 hours after stent-graft deployment to treat postplacement left-lung atelectasis (Fig 2). Before stent-graft placement in this patient, the left main bronchus had been noted to be severely compressed by the aneurysm. The patient recovered uneventfully after placement of the endobronchial stent, and complete resolution of the atelectasis was depicted at radiography 12 hours after the procedure.

Perigraft leak was observed in 13 (21%) of the 63 patients. These leaks were not detected in the operating room at intraprocedural angiography with a mobile C-arm image intensifier system. Perigraft leaks in 10 of the 13 patients were successfully treated with coil embolization (9) or placement of an additional stent-graft. Resolution of the leak was confirmed at CT in eight of the 10 patients. In the other three patients (5%), the perigraft leak persisted, but further endovascular treatment was not performed because of unsolvable technical problems related to anatomic issues in two patients and refusal by one patient.

Aortic or periaortic changes were observed in 21 (33%) of the 63 patients. These findings included aortic wall thickening in 13, periaortic atelectasis in 15, and periaortic effusion in four. In 20 of the 21 patients, there was no associated back or chest pain. One patient with a periaortic change depicted at CT experienced back pain. Arteriography was performed, and no abnormalities were identified. The patient was observed, and an oral antiinflammatory medication was administered. The back pain disappeared completely, and he was asymptomatic 6 days after stent-graft placement. In 10 of the 21 patients, long-term follow-up CT scans were available for evaluation. In all cases, the abnormal findings disappeared without any specific treatment.

A small amount of mural thrombus lined the stent-graft on postplacement

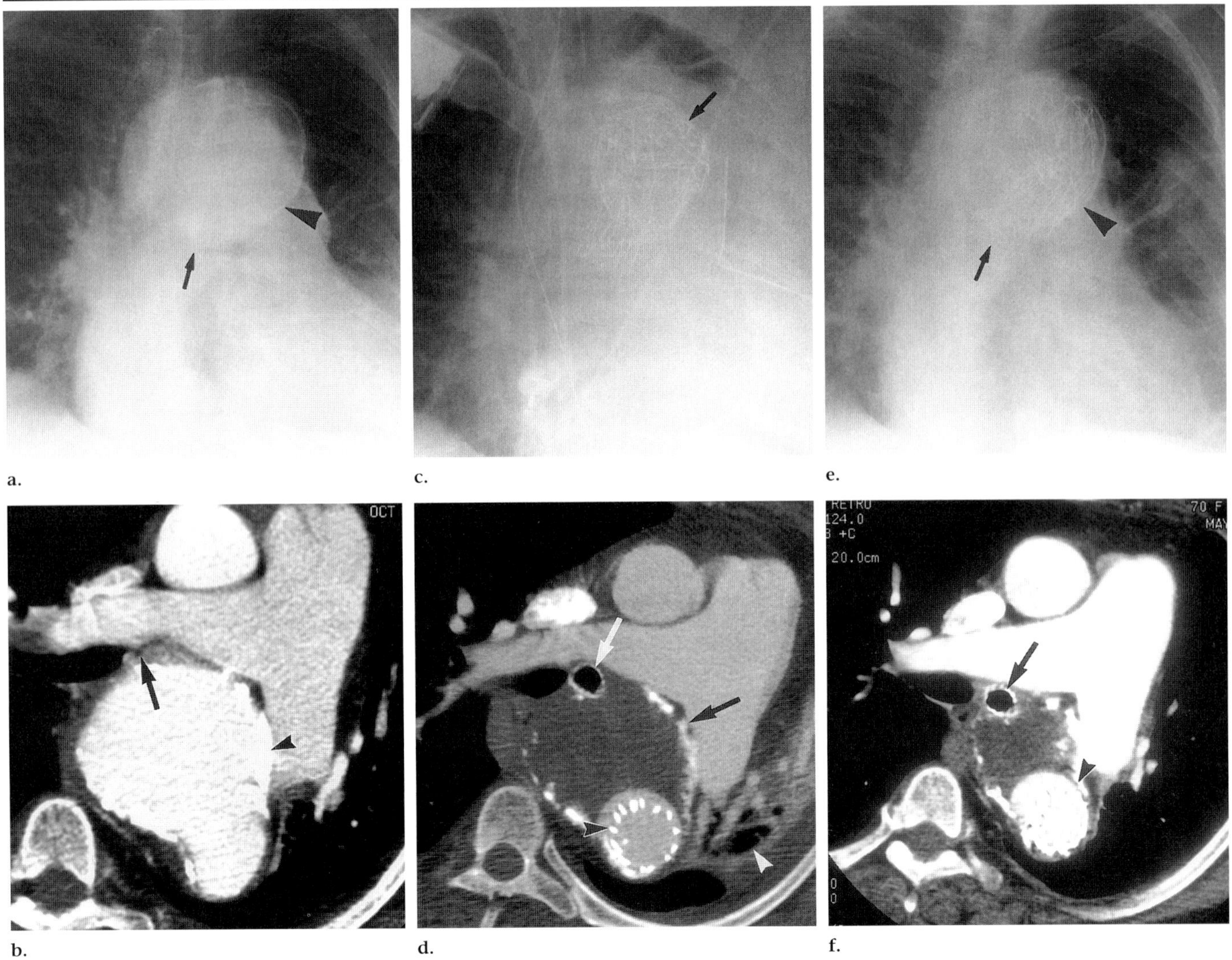

Figure 2. Chronic posttraumatic aneurysm. **(a)** Chest radiograph and **(b)** thoracic CT image obtained before treatment depict a large descending thoracic aortic aneurysm (arrowhead) and narrowing of the left main bronchus (arrow). **(c)** Chest radiograph obtained 12 hours after placement of the stent-graft (arrow) shows complete opacity of the left hemithorax with ipsilateral mediastinal shift consistent with atelectasis. A Palmaz stent (Johnson & Johnson Interventional Systems, Warren, NJ) was placed in the left main bronchus 18 hours after the procedure. **(d)** Chest CT image obtained 5 days after stent-graft placement demonstrates thrombotic aneurysm (black arrow), patent stent-graft (black arrowhead), the Palmaz stent in the left main bronchus (white arrow), and some aeration (white arrowhead) in the collapsed left lung. **(e)** Chest radiograph obtained at 25 days and **(f)** thoracic CT image obtained 6 months after stent-graft placement demonstrate the stent-graft (arrowhead), the Palmaz stent in the left main bronchus (arrow), and resolution of the left-lung atelectasis.

CT scans in two (3%) asymptomatic patients.

Aortic dissection not evident at preprocedural CT was detected in one (2%) patient after stent-graft deployment. In this patient, the dissection was located in the aortic arch and was presumably caused by a retrograde injury from introduction of the stent-graft delivery system. The patient was hemodynamically stable and experienced no back or chest pain. He was treated medically because he was considered a poor surgical risk and was alive without symptoms 36 months after the procedure.

Pneumonia was diagnosed in one patient, who was treated with antibiotics and recovered without sequelae.

The maximum diameter of the aneurysm increased (+3 mm or more) in 18 (29%) of the 63 patients, did not change (from −3 to +3 mm) in 36 (57%), and decreased (−3 mm or more) in nine (14%) (Table 2A). The mean maximum diameter of the aneurysm before stent-graft placement was 58.8 mm and within 10 days after the procedure was 60.0 mm. Among the 13 patients with perigraft leak, the maximum diameter of the aneurysm after stent-graft deployment was larger in two (15%), the same in 10 (77%), and smaller in one (8%) (Table 2A). Among the 50 patients without perigraft leak, the maximum diameter of the aneurysm after stent-graft deployment was larger in 16 (32%), the same in 26 (52%), and smaller in eight (16%) (Table 2A). No interventional procedure was performed in the patients with an aneurysm that enlarged without evidence of perigraft leak. At long-term follow-up CT (mean, 388 days; range, 6 months to 3 years) in 20 patients, the mean maximum diameter of the aneurysm was 59.5 mm before stent-graft placement, 60.8 mm shortly

TABLE 2
Summary of Aneurysm Diameter Changes after Stent-Graft Placement

A: Caliber Changes on CT Scans Obained before and Immediately after Placement (n = 63)

Diameter	Leak	No Leak	Total
Increase	2 (15)	16 (32)	18 (29)
No change	10 (77)	26 (52)	36 (57)
Decrease	1 (8)	8 (16)	9 (14)
Total	13	50	63

B: Caliber Changes on CT Scans Obtained Immediately and Longer than 6 Months after Placement (n = 20)

Diameter	Persistent Leak	Treated Leak	No Leak	Total
Increase	1 (50)	2 (25)	3 (30)	6 (30)
No change	1 (50)	2 (25)	3 (30)	6 (30)
Decrease	0 (0)	4 (50)	4 (40)	8 (40)
Total	2	8	10	20

Note.—A change in aneurysm diameter between two successive CT scans of +3 mm or more is considered an increase, +3 to −3 mm as no change, and −3 mm or more as a decrease. Data are the number of cases. Numbers in parentheses are percentages.

after placement, and 58.7 mm more than 6 months after placement. In a comparison of CT scans obtained shortly after and more than 6 months after stent-graft placement, the diameter of the aneurysm increased in three (30%) of 10 patients with no leak, in two (25%) of eight patients with a treated leak, and in one (50%) of two patients with a persistent leak (Table 2B).

DISCUSSION

Endovascular stent-graft placement is a less invasive technique than conventional surgery for the management of descending thoracic aortic aneurysm. Recent clinical studies have reported acceptable midterm results and findings suggest that stent-graft placement could be a good alternative treatment especially in patients with major surgical risks (2,4–6). Although there is considerable interest in this new therapy, the short-term radiologic changes after stent-graft treatment of thoracic aortic aneurysm and the long-term effects have not been well documented, to our knowledge.

In our study, development of pleural effusion or increase of an existing pleural effusion, either unilateral or bilateral, was a very common finding (73%) after thoracic aortic stent-graft placement. In most cases, it was managed successfully with conservative therapy including appropriate medication. No patient required external drainage with a chest tube. CT was an excellent modality for the detection and follow-up of pleural effusion and could clearly show the response to treatment.

Pneumonia or atelectasis without massive pleural effusion was demonstrated in 10% of our patients. Because most patients had evidence of inflammation such as leukocytosis or high fever immediately after the stent-graft placement, CT was a helpful tool to diagnose pneumonia or atelectasis and to prompt use of medications such as antibiotics or nebulizer therapy. The cause of atelectasis was not clear, but it may be related to general anesthesia. Atelectasis is a recognized complication of endobronchial intubation and mechanical ventilation (10,11). In one patient, a metallic endobronchial stent was placed because the descending thoracic aortic aneurysm was seen at CT to mechanically compress the left main bronchus (Fig 2). CT was useful in this case to determine the choice of treatment for atelectasis because it clearly demonstrated the bronchial stenosis due to external compression by the aneurysm.

Perigraft leak is relatively common and is one of the most disappointing complications of stent-graft treatment of aortic aneurysm because it may lead to failure of the therapy (12–15). Indeed, a perigraft leak with persistent flow in the aneurysm sac is potentially fatal and may cause aneurysm rupture (16). Consequently, it is our policy to detect and aggressively treat a perigraft leak as soon as possible. The initial detection of perigraft leak may occur at angiography in the operating suite immediately after stent-graft deployment. Unfortunately, however, there are several limitations in the operating room to the detection of a perigraft leak. The angiographic equipment we used was a mobile C-arm unit, which does not produce image quality comparable to that achieved with a stationary unit in the radiology suite. The ideal angulation to view the aneurysm and its necks was difficult to obtain because of limitations in C-arm angulation, the surgical table, and the ability of the unit to optimally compensate for the wide range of tissue densities in the chest. Rozenblit et al (12) reported in their series of stent-graft treatment for abdominal aortic aneurysm that CT depicted perigraft leak in four of seven patients whereas angiography in the operating room depicted it in only one.

The effectiveness of selective coil embolization of a perigraft tract for the treatment of perigraft leak was previously reported (9). Once a perigraft leak is detected at CT, our strategy is prompt treatment with coil embolization or placement of an additional stent-graft. In this series, leaks were successfully managed endoluminally before discharge in eight of 13 patients.

A new dissection in the aortic arch and ascending aorta was depicted at CT in one case. In general, the management philosophy for type A dissection is surgical repair, but this patient was treated medically because he was not a surgical candidate.

Aortic or periaortic changes are also relatively common findings and were detected in 33% of our patients. In all cases, the changes were not associated with any clinical symptoms, appeared self-limited, and were completely resolved at long-term follow-up CT without any treatment other than antiinflammatory drugs.

Periaortic changes and increased pleural effusion are commonly encountered, but their causes are unknown. They may represent reactive inflammatory processes because they are frequently associated with elevated fever and leukocytosis. Previously, Sapoval et al (17) reported transient perivascular thickening evident at CT after placement of a stent-graft in the iliac artery. Perivascular soft-tissue changes are also reported at magnetic resonance imaging after insertion of a polyester-covered stent in the femoral, iliac, or subclavian arteries (18,19). In both sheep and swine models, histologic examination shows an infiltration of inflammatory cells adjacent to the polyester 1–4 weeks after stent-graft insertion (20,21). The authors speculate that such inflammatory reactions are responsible for the perivascular changes noted on imaging studies. The polyester graft material, not the stainless steel stent, is considered responsible for the inflammatory reaction (19–25). It may be a foreign-body reaction to polyester (25), or it may be due to the accumulation of proinflammatory substances as part of its processing (19).

A thin focal lining of mural thrombus was rarely encountered at CT after stent-graft placement. In our experience, no specific treatment was required, and there were no instances of clinical symptoms including embolization or progression of the clot on subsequent CT scans.

Change in the diameter of the aneurysm is a finding not well understood. The maximum diameter increased slightly after stent-graft placement in 30% of our patients without evidence of perigraft leak. In 30% of the patients without perigraft leak who underwent long-term follow-up CT, the caliber of the aneurysm further increased compared with its diameter at CT immediately after stent-graft placement. To date, there have been no cases of rupture in this group. In the previous literature of endovascular treatment of abdominal aortic aneurysms (12), it was suggested that any enlargement of the aneurysm after treatment indicates a failure of the procedure. In our experience, however, a slight enlargement of the aneurysm diameter was a common finding after stent-graft placement. The mechanism of change in aneurysm caliber is unknown. If it is not associated with perigraft leak at CT, our current practice is to continue CT observation every 6 months without immediate intervention. Further study is necessary to clarify the real clinical effect and possible mechanism of the changes in aneurysm diameter because our long-term follow-up data include a small number ($n = 20$) of patients with relatively short-term follow-up (mean, 388 days).

In summary, several abnormal findings were detected at thoracic CT after stent-graft insertion for the treatment of descending thoracic aortic aneurysm. Pleural effusion was a common finding (73%) after stent-graft insertion, but it could be managed conservatively without external drainage. Perigraft leak was detected in 21% of our patients, and most of them were successfully treated endoluminally. Atelectasis was observed in 16% of our patients, and most of them could be treated with appropriate medication. Periaortic changes were relatively common (33%), but no treatment was necessary. The other complications were rarely encountered.

In conclusion, thoracic CT is useful in the treatment of patients after stent-graft insertion for management of descending thoracic aortic aneurysm. The clinical importance of changes in the aneurysm diameter after stent-graft placement remains unknown but is an important issue that requires clarification before this therapy can be recommended for general clinical use.

References

1. Dake MD, Miller DC, Semba CP, et al. Transluminal placement of endovascular stent-grafts for the treatment of descending thoracic aortic aneurysms. N Engl J Med 1994; 331:1729–1734.
2. Mitchell RS, Dake MD, Semba CP, et al. Endovascular stent-graft repair of thoracic aortic aneurysms. J Thorac Cardiovasc Surg 1996; 111:1054–1062.
3. Fann JI, Dake MD, Semba CP, et al. Endovascular stent-grafting after arch aneurysm repair using the "elephant trunk." Ann Thorac Surg 1995; 60:1102–1105.
4. Semba CP, Kato N, Kee ST, et al. Acute rupture of the descending thoracic aorta: repair with use of endovascular stent-grafts. JVIR 1997; 8:337–342.
5. Semba CP, Sakai T, Slonim SM, et al. Mycotic aneurysms of the thoracic aorta: repair with use of endovascular stent-grafts. JVIR 1998; 9:33–40.
6. Kato N, Dake MD, Miller DC, et al. Traumatic thoracic aortic aneurysm: treatment with endovascular stent-grafts. Radiology 1997; 205:657–662.
7. Rubin GD. Three-dimensional helical CT angiography. RadioGraphics 1994; 14: 905–912.
8. Rubin GD, Alfrey EJ, Dake MD, et al. Assessment of living renal donors with spiral CT. Radiology 1995; 195:457–462.
9. Kato N, Semba CP, Dake MD. Embolization of perigraft leaks after endovascular stent-graft treatment of aortic aneurysms. JVIR 1996; 7:805–811.
10. Rothen HU, Sporre B, Engberg G, et al. Prevention of atelectasis during general anaesthesia. Lancet 1995; 345:1387–1391.
11. Brismar B, Hedenstierna G, Lundquist H, et al. Pulmonary densities during anesthesia with muscular relaxation: a proposal of atelectasis. Anesthesiology 1985; 62: 422–428.
12. Rozenblit A, Marin ML, Veith FJ, et al. Endovascular repair of abdominal aortic aneurysm: value of postoperative follow-up with helical CT. AJR 1995; 165:1473–1479.
13. Blum U, Langer M, Spillner G, et al. Abdominal aortic aneurysms: preliminary technical and clinical results with transfemoral placement of endovascular self-expanding stent-grafts. Radiology 1996; 198:25–31.
14. Parodi JC. Endovascular repair of abdominal aortic aneurysms and other arterial lesions. J Vasc Surg 1995; 21:549–557.
15. Chuter TAM, Risberg B, Hopkinson BR, et al. Clinical experience with a bifurcated endovascular graft for abdominal aortic aneurysm repair. J Vasc Surg 1996; 24:655–666.
16. Lumsden AB, Allen RC, Chaikof EL, et al. Delayed rupture of aortic aneurysms following endovascular stent grafting. Am J Surg 1995; 170:174–178.
17. Sapoval MR, Gaux JC, Long AL, et al. Transient periprosthetic thickening after covered-stent implantation in the iliac artery. AJR 1995; 164:1271–1273.
18. Link J, Müller-Hülsbeck S, Brossmann J, et al. Perivascular inflammatory reaction after percutaneous placement of covered stents. Cardiovasc Intervent Radiol 1996; 19:345–347.
19. Kellner W, Küffer G, Pfluger T, et al. MR imaging of soft-tissue changes after percutaneous transluminal angioplasty and stent placement. Radiology 1997; 202: 327–331.
20. Schürmann K, Vorwerk D, Bücker A, et al. Perigraft inflammation due to Dacron-covered stent-grafts in sheep iliac arteries: correlation of MR imaging and histopathologic findings. Radiology 1997; 204: 757–763.
21. Link J, Feyerabend B, Grabender M, et al. Dacron-covered stent-grafts for the percutaneous treatment of carotid aneurysms: effectiveness and biocompatibility—experimental study in swine. Radiology 1996; 200:397–401.
22. Rousseau H, Joffre F, Raillat C, et al. Self-expanding endovascular stent in experimental atherosclerosis: work in progress. Radiology 1989; 170:773–778.
23. Vorwerk D, Redha F, Neuerberg J, et al. Neointima formation following arterial placement of self-expanding stents of different radial force: experimental results. Cardiovasc Intervent Radiol 1994; 17: 27–32.
24. Rousseau H, Puel J, Joffre F, et al. Self-expanding endovascular prosthesis: an experimental study. Radiology 1987; 164: 709–714.
25. Vollmar JF, Guldner NW, Mohr W, et al. Perigraft-reaction after implantation of vascular prosthesis: pathogenesis, clinical picture and treatment. Int Angiol 1987; 6:287–293.

Treatment of Hemodialysis-related Central Venous Stenosis or Occlusion: Results of Primary Wallstent Placement and Follow-up in 50 Patients[1]

Patrick Haage, MD
Dierk Vorwerk, MD
Werner Piroth, MD
Karl Schuermann, MD
Rolf W. Guenther, MD

Index terms:
Dialysis, shunts
Veins, grafts and prostheses, 9461.1286, 9462.1286
Veins, innominate, 9461.752
Veins, stenosis or obstruction, 9461.454, 9462.454
Veins, subclavian, 9462.752
Veins, thrombosis, 9461.752, 9462.752
Veins, transluminal angioplasty, 9461.1286, 9462.1286

Radiology 1999; 212:175–180

[1] From the Department of Diagnostic Radiology, University of Technology, Pauwelsstrasse 30, D-52057 Aachen, Germany (P.H., W.P., K.S., R.W.G.) and the Department of Diagnostic and Interventional Radiology, Klinikum Ingolstadt, Germany (D.V.). From the 1998 RSNA scientific assembly. Received July 10, 1998; revision requested August 28; revision received October 2; accepted January 19, 1999. **Address reprint requests to** P.H. (e-mail: *haage@rad.rwth-aachen.de*).

PURPOSE: To analyze the effectiveness of stent placement as the primary treatment for central venous obstruction in patients undergoing hemodialysis.

MATERIAL AND METHODS: Fifty-seven Wallstents were placed in 50 patients with symptomatic shunt dysfunction and arm swelling due to central venous obstruction. Technical success, complication, and patency rates were evaluated.

RESULTS: Stent deployment was successful in all patients, and early rethrombosis (within 1 week) was noted in one patient (2%). Seventy-three episodes of reobstruction occurred and were treated percutaneously with angioplasty alone in 54 cases (74%). Nineteen cases (26%) necessitated additional stent placement. The 3-, 6-, 12-, and 24-month primary patency rates were 92%, 84%, 56%, and 28%, respectively. Cumulative overall stent patency was 97% after 6 and 12 months, 89% after 24 months, and 81% after 36 and 48 months.

CONCLUSION: In the treatment of brachiocephalic and subclavian venous obstruction, stent placement shows excellent technical results and helps preserve vascular access for a substantial period. Multiple repeat interventions are, however, frequently required to maintain patency.

Of the more than 200,000 patients with end-stage renal disease in 1990, at least 85%–90% were treated with hemodialysis at some point during their lifetime (1,2). Investigators with the U.S. Renal Data System have recently reported (3) that hemodialysis access failure is the most frequent cause of hospitalization among patients with end-stage renal disease and accounts for the largest number of hospital days in some centers. Therefore, in patients undergoing hemodialysis, maintenance of vascular access is of essential importance to the patient and his or her physician.

Since Dotter (4) reported early experimental results of stent placement in vessels in 1969, vascular stents have been used to maintain the patency of the vessel after balloon angioplasty. Vascular endoprostheses have achieved excellent results in the arterial system and are a relative recent adjunct in venous applications. Nonsurgical techniques have become a mainstay in the treatment of hemodialysis-related obstruction most frequently encountered in the venous outflow tract of the hemodialysis shunt.

Central venous stenoses or occlusions in patients undergoing hemodialysis are considered to be due to high flow states, in contrast to the low flow normally seen in veins, and occur at sites of turbulence (eg, valves or kinked vessels) (5,6). Injury during or after insertion of a temporary or tunneled dialysis access catheter placed with a jugular and subclavian route has also been recognized as a risk factor for central venous obstruction, with a reported (7) prevalence as high as 40%. The prevalence varies depending on catheter type and access and is especially high for subclavian catheters (7).

In past years, percutaneous intervention in central venous obstruction has consisted of either balloon angioplasty alone (with which modest results were obtained with respect to

Author contributions:
Guarantor of integrity of entire study, P.H.; study concepts and design, P.H., D.V.; definition of intellectual content, P.H., D.V., R.W.G.; literature research, P.H., W.P.; clinical studies, all authors; data acquisition, P.H., W.P.; data analysis, P.H., D.V., W.P.; statistical analysis, P.H., D.V.; manuscript preparation, P.H.; manuscript editing, P.H., D.V.; manuscript review, all authors.

technical outcome and primary patency) (5,6,8–10) or additional stent placement in case of angioplasty failure.

We performed this study to determine the efficacy of stent placement as the primary treatment of brachiocephalic and subclavian vein obstruction in patients undergoing hemodialysis. Herein, we report and provide follow-up data from 50 hemodialysis patients who were initially treated with self-expanding stents after balloon dilation.

MATERIALS AND METHODS

Of 298 patients with a hemodialysis fistula who were referred for angiographic analysis and percutaneous treatment of shunt malfunction between January 1988 and January 1998, 50 had obvious arm swelling and increased venous counterpressure at dialysis. There were 27 men and 23 women aged 40–79 years (mean age, 59.9 years). Before the intervention, informed consent was obtained from all patients. Fifteen patients had a polytetrafluoroethylene implant graft (Gore-Tex; W. L. Gore and Associates, Elkton, Md), and 35 had an autologous arteriovenous fistula. Shunt location was on the right side in 21 patients and on the left side in 29.

Angiographically, an obstruction was situated in the subclavian vein in 35 patients and in the brachiocephalic vein in 15. Of the 35 patients with obstruction in the subclavian vein, 25 (71%) had a high-grade stricture, and 10 (29%) had an occlusion. Of the 15 patients with obstruction in the brachiocephalic vein, 13 (87%) had a severe stenosis, and two (13%) had an occlusion. Well-pronounced collateral veins almost always were present.

A central venous lesion was defined as an indication for primary stent placement due to the reported poor outcome of percutaneous angioplasty alone, partly because of the lack of available high-pressure, large-diameter balloons that fit through the 9-F or smaller sheath recommended for treatment via the dialysis access. A self-expanding metallic stent (Wallstent; Schneider, Bülach, Switzerland) was placed in all patients admitted to our interventional unit with central venous stenosis or occlusion. Stent placement was always performed after conventional balloon dilation, after which most of the obstructed vessels showed considerable residual stenosis despite application of high balloon pressures.

An insufficient result was defined as ongoing compromised shunt flow with persistent collateral veins (if observed) or a residual stenosis of at least 50%. There were three kinked stenoses and six elastic stenoses, all of which immediately collapsed after balloon deflation. The length of the obstruction ranged from less than 1 cm to 9 cm; most were short (mean length ± SD, 2.9 cm ± 1.5). Placement of two overlapping stents was required in seven patients with long stenotic segments.

Before angioplasty and stent deployment, preimplantation angiography with a digital subtraction technique was performed to study the anatomic and pathologic characteristics of the vessel after antegrade venous puncture of a shunt-leading vein or the graft itself with a 20-gauge sheath needle (Abbocath; Abbott, Sligo, Ireland). Intervention was performed with an antegrade approach via the venous outflow tract by using the Seldinger technique. Recanalization usually was attempted with a hydrophilic-coated, steerable, 0.035-inch guide wire (Terumo, Leuven, Belgium) for vessel stenosis and a straight guide wire with a movable core (Cook, Bjaeverskov, Denmark) for occlusion. After safe passage of the obstructed segment, a balloon catheter of adequate diameter, usually 8–10 mm, was advanced into the segment and dilated. Normally, balloons were dilated several times by hand, without pressure monitoring. Inflation time depended on how well the obstruction responded to dilation. In highly resistant lesions, Olbert-type balloons were preferred.

Next, a flexible, self-expanding Wallstent endoprosthesis, which is a tube woven from stainless steel alloy filaments (0.08–0.10-mm diameter), was introduced through a 9-F introducing catheter, which is flexible enough to allow implantation even in kinked vessels. Correction of the Wallstent position for exact placement was done by pulling the partially deployed stent to the affected region. Further technical properties and placement techniques have been described in detail elsewhere (11,12). Stents were dilated with a balloon of suitable size after deployment to ensure as close contact to the venous wall as possible.

Traversal of the lesion and recanalization were always attempted with a brachial approach, except when the shunt vein was severely kinked and too small for a 9-F catheter, which was the case in two patients. In these two patients, the obstruction could not be negotiated with the brachial approach, and dilation was performed with a transfemoral approach followed by stent placement with a

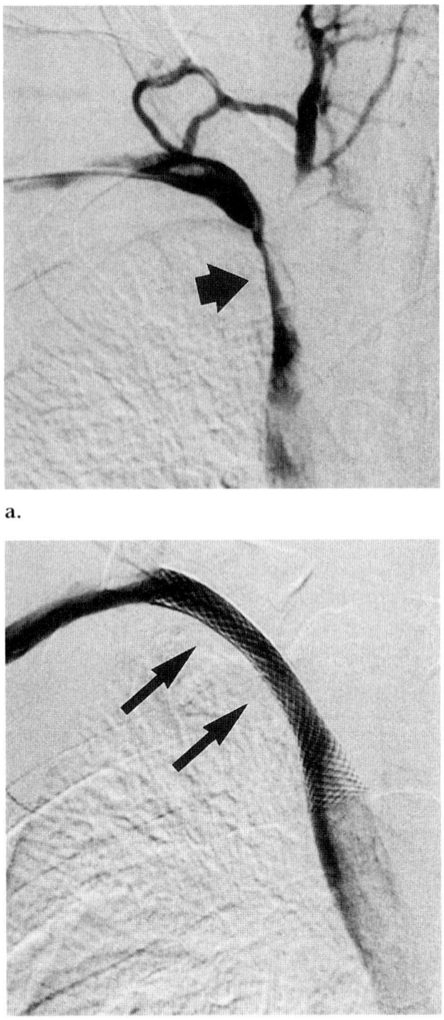

a.

b.

Figure 1. **(a)** Digital subtraction angiogram (frontal view with arm abducted) demonstrates a high-grade stenosis (arrow) of the right brachiocephalic vein draining a Brescia-Cimino fistula. **(b)** Digital subtraction angiogram (frontal view) shows restoration of flow (arrows) and vanishing of collateral vessels after placement of a 14 × 64-mm Wallstent.

transbrachial approach. "Through-and-through" access (13), where the transbrachially placed guide wire is pulled out through the femoral access, was performed in two patients with an extremely rigid and sharply angulated right-sided stenosis of the proximal subclavian vein.

A total of 57 stents were placed. The stent was kept as short as possible but was long enough to bridge the entire lesion with a slight overlap at its proximal and distal ends. The largest possible stent diameter was used and was dependent on lesion site. Size was adapted to the diameter of the adjacent nonobstructed vessel segment. In the 43 patients who required

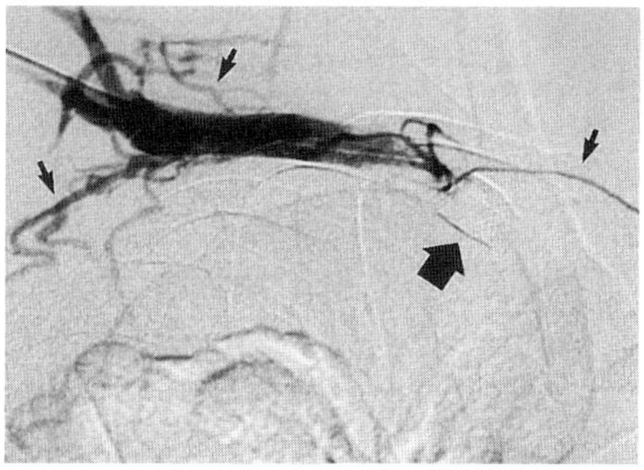

a.

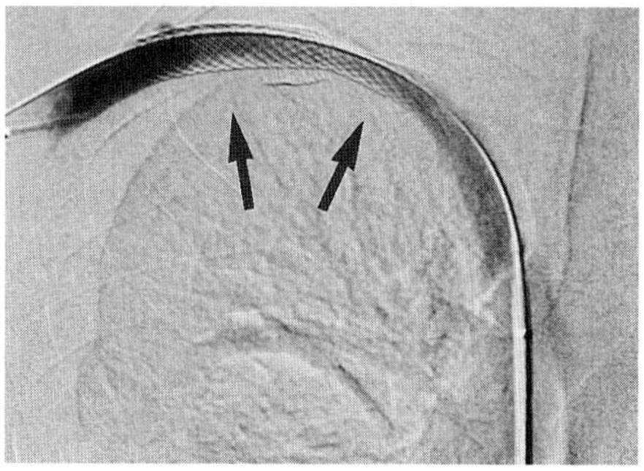

b.

Figure 2. **(a)** Angiogram (oblique view) shows occlusion of the right subclavian vein with pronounced collateral flow (small arrows) in a patient complaining of arm swelling 7 months after deployment of a 12 × 33-mm Wallstent (large arrow). **(b)** Frontal view obtained after percutaneous transluminal angioplasty at the occluded site and subsequent stent placement (arrows) across the originally placed stent shows that full patency has been reestablished.

placement of only one stent, four 10-mm-diameter, 18 12-mm-diameter, 16 14-mm-diameter, and five 16-mm-diameter Wallstents were placed in the obstructed central vein. Two patients were treated with two 12-mm-diameter stents, one with one 12- and one 14-mm-diameter stent, one with two 16-mm-diameter stents, and three with two 14-mm-diameter stents.

Periprocedural anticoagulation was mandatory and was administered intravenously at the beginning of the intervention (5,000 IU heparin). Heparin administration was continued during hemodialysis performed immediately after the end of the procedure via the native or implant shunt or a jugular Shaldon catheter (Vygon, Aachen, Germany).

Outpatient treatment, which was preferred, consisted of subcutaneous injection of 7,500 IU of heparin three times a day for 24 hours. Inpatient treatment consisted of intravenous administration of 1,000 IU of heparin per hour for 24 hours. We recommended that the patients take 100 mg per day of acetylsalicylic acid as a chronic oral medication. No preoperative medication was administered.

Only clinical follow-up was performed, which consisted of monitoring of the dialysis protocols with respect to decreased access flow, decrease in measurement of dialysis dose, deviant urea measurements, and elevation of venous dialysis pressure. Abnormal physical findings (eg, development of arm swelling) were highly suggestive of central venous reobstruction due to stent failure. When abnormal clinical and physiologic parameters were detected, patients were referred to our interventional unit for repeat angiography. If stenosis within the stent with or without the demonstration of collateral veins or stenosis anywhere along the venous outflow tract was found, repeat intervention was indicated. Endoprosthesis shortening that uncovered the lesion was another indication for repeat intervention.

Treatment outcomes were evaluated on the basis of patency of the stent after correction of subclavian or brachiocephalic obstruction.

Primary patency of the Wallstent was diagnosed if there was no evidence of access failure related to restenosis or reocclusion by neointimal hyperplasia or thrombosis within the stent or substantial stent shortening. If shunt failure occurred owing to a condition other than stent obstruction or shortening, the stent was defined as patent. Primary patency ended when repeat intervention was necessary or when the hemodialysis fistula had to be abandoned. The interval between primary stent placement and permanent stent occlusion, including, if feasible, multiple recanalizations, was defined as cumulative stent patency. Primary and cumulative stent patency rates were calculated by means of Kaplan-Meier life-table analysis as follows: $p_{n,n} + 1 = p_n \times p_{n+1}$ and $p_n = 1 - [f_n(n_n - c_n/2)]$, where p is patency, n is the total number of patients at the beginning of an interval, f is the number of failures within the indicated interval, and c is the number of patients censored within the interval.

RESULTS

Fifty primary central venous stent implantation procedures were performed during the 10 years of this study. During that time, more than 800 hemodialysis shunt–associated interventions were performed in our department in 298 patients, for an incidence of primary subclavian and brachiocephalic stent placement of about 6% of all procedures in 17% of patients. The initial deployment of 57 Wallstents was technically successful, with proper positioning in all 50 patients (100%). Insertion of one Wallstent was sufficient to cover the entire lesion in 43 patients; two stents were required for coverage in seven patients (Fig 1). There were no episodes of local bleeding at the catheter site. Venous perforation and disruption did not occur during stent placement. Immediate or delayed central migration of the endoprosthesis was not noted. Also, acute pulmonary hemorrhage or retroperitoneal bleeding during heparin therapy was not reported.

Early rethrombosis within 7 days after initial stent placement occurred in one patient with a right-sided brachiocephalic stent and was treated with hydrodynamic thrombectomy for thrombus fragmentation with a hydrolyser catheter (Cordis, Roden, the Netherlands) followed by balloon angioplasty and deployment of additional overlapping 14-mm-diameter Wallstents proximal to the originally treated lesion and within the originally placed stent. Hypercoagulability and stent shortening were the assumed cause of early thrombosis. Despite documented stent positioning within the obstructed lesion, delayed endoprosthesis shortening toward the distal end occurred 7 months after stent placement in one patient with a brachiocephalic stent and within 3 and 7 months in two patients with a subclavian stent (Fig 2). Complete obstruction had developed in the uncovered segment, and angioplasty and additional successful stent placement were performed with a transbrachial approach in the latter patient and with a transfemoral approach in the other two.

Seventy-three episodes of reobstruction occurred within the observation period. Mean follow-up was 18.4 months ± 15.8 (SD), with the longest follow-up being 55 months. Restenosis or reocclusion within the stent was noted in 61 cases. One patient experienced early thrombosis within the lesion with the stent. Eleven obstruction episodes occurred outside of, but close to, the segment with stent. Stent reobstruction was not observed in 25 patients. An episode of obstruction occurred once in nine patients, twice in five patients, and four times in five patients. Six patients had five to seven stent reobstruction episodes. Wallstent patency rates are summarized in Tables 1 and 2. The mean duration of primary access patency was 10.6 months ± 10.1. The mean primary stent patency period was 11.1 months ± 10.1. The intervals between the first obstruction episode and the second, third, and fourth episodes were not significantly different; these intervals were 7.1 months ± 4.7 between the first and second reobstruction episodes, 5.9 months ± 4.1 between the second and third episodes, and 5.7 months ± 3.8 between the third and fourth episodes. The mean interval between two episodes of restenosis or reocclusion was 6.4 months ± 4.1.

Primary and cumulative Wallstent patency rates determined with life-table analysis are shown in Figure 3. Fifty-four of the 73 repeat interventions consisted of percutaneous angioplasty alone. Stent dilation usually was performed with 10–14-mm-diameter, high-pressure, Olbert-type balloons. In 49 cases, percutaneous revision and passage through the obstruction were easy to perform, in part because the segment was outlined by the Wallstent. In two cases, we failed to cross the occluded segment with the catheter and guide wire, and a femoral approach was used for subsequent successful recanalization. In two patients, segment crossing was not feasible with either the brachial or the femoral approach, and the Wallstent was left occluded. The end points for cumulative stent patency in these two patients were determined after 6 and 29 months. The latter patient had undergone four repeat interventions before permanent stent occlusion, including additional stent placement to retain patency. Both patients had pronounced collateral veins; therefore, the access site of the ipsilateral extremity was not abandoned, and hemodialysis was continued. During dilation of an occluded subclavian stent, one patient experienced extreme chest pain and died of cardiac arrest 2 hours later in the intensive care unit. Pulmonary embolism had been excluded angiographically, and perforation of the right atrium with the guide wire was the probable reason; however, autopsy results did not confirm this (14).

Fourteen patients had at least one reobstruction episode that could not be sufficiently treated with angioplasty alone. A total of 25 stents had to be deployed in addition to the initially placed stent to maintain patency.

In 19 patients, reobstruction occurred within (n = 13) or adjacent to (n = 6) the original lesion. Proximal stent shortening necessitated stent placement in three patients, and additional deployment was necessary because of early rethrombosis within the stent in one patient. Sixteen repeat interventions required one stent per intervention for successful recanalization. To bridge the entire obstruction, we placed two additional stents in three patients and three stents in one patient at one session. A brachial approach was used in 12 of the 16 interventions, and a femoral approach was used in four. Repeat placement of one stent at two sessions due to repeated development of intimal hyperplasia was performed successfully in three patients. The interval between the two obstruction episodes ranged from 5 to 13 months (mean, 10 months).

In each of two patients, a total of three stents were deployed in two repeat intervention sessions. The venogram obtained in the first patient demonstrated thrombosis within the recently placed second stent despite intravenous anticoagulation treatment with 1,000 IU of heparin per hour. Mechanical thrombectomy with the Amplatz thrombectomy device (Microvena, Vadnais Heights, Minn) was performed, followed by placement of two overlapping Wallstents. In the latter patient, two additional stents were placed 11 months after the initial deployment. Repeat dilation was necessary 4 and 9 months after the second stent placement owing to restenosis. One month later, the patient reported to our interventional unit with arm swelling. Angiography showed occlusion of the segment with the stent. Thrombectomy and insertion of yet another stent were necessary because recanalization with a high-pressure angioplasty balloon proved to be unsuccessful.

The 3-, 6-, 12-, and 24-month primary patency rates were 92%, 84%, 56%, and 28%, respectively (Table 1). Overall stent patency was 97% after 6 and 12 months, 89% after 24 months, and 81% after 36 and 48 months (Table 2). In 35 patients, the shunt remained open until the end of the observation period or until the patient's death. The remaining patients were lost to follow-up or underwent renal transplantation.

TABLE 1
Primary Wallstent Patency

Follow-up (mo)	No. of Patients	Patency Rate (%)	Standard Error (%)
3	50	92	4.2
6	26	84	6.7
12	17	56	11.2
24	8	28	11.4

TABLE 2
Cumulative Wallstent Patency

Follow-up (mo)	No. of Patients	Patency Rate (%)	Standard Error (%)
6	50	97	2.5
12	27	97	2.5
24	22	89	8.7
36	12	81	10.8
48	9	81	10.8

Statistical analysis of primary and cumulative stent patency in the patients with 10-, 12-, 14-, and 16-mm-diameter Wallstents showed no statistically significant differences during the observation period. Comparison of primary and cumulative Wallstent patency rates of stents deployed on the right and left side also revealed no significant differences. Furthermore, there were no significant differences in primary and cumulative patency rates when we compared data about initial placement in the brachiocephalic vein with data about initial placement in the subclavian vein.

DISCUSSION

To achieve and improve long-term hemodialysis access function, percutaneous interventional techniques have been widely used in the management of fistula dysfunction. Early detection and treatment of complications is essential to provide adequate care for the patient being treated with hemodialysis. Central venous obstruction is a commonly seen, serious problem in these patients. Clinically, these patients present with arm swelling and occasionally obvious widespread subcutaneous collateral vessels around the shoulder and thoracic aperture. Additional ipsilateral swelling of the face, neck, and breast may develop. Schumacher et al (15) reported a 14% incidence of central venous stenosis and occlusion in their hemodialysis population. Of the patients undergoing hemodialysis in our study who were referred for treatment, 17% had central venous occlusive disease.

Abandonment and removal of the vascular access should be avoided as long as other therapeutic options are available. Surgical bypass procedures with use of polytetrafluoroethylene grafts or the saphenous vein as an initial treatment for central venous obstruction are difficult and seldom performed, because of the substantial morbidity and even mortality rates in these chronically ill patients (16).

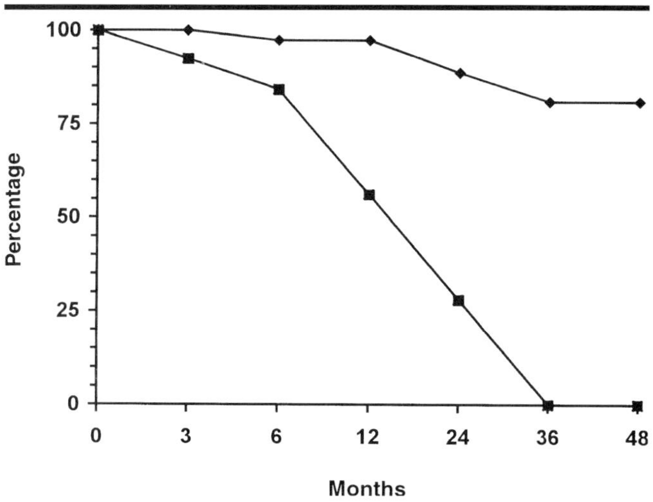

Figure 3. Follow-up findings. Graph shows the primary (■) and cumulative (◆) Wallstent patency rates obtained with life-table analysis.

Authors (17) of earlier reports about surgical reconstruction have described modest results. Only Bhatia et al (18) reported similar success, complication, and patency rates when they retrospectively compared balloon angioplasty results with stent placement and surgical bypass results.

Early clinical applications of percutaneously placed stents were described by Zollikofer et al (19) in 1988. Today, interventional radiologic measures are the primary treatments of choice, and percutaneous transluminal angioplasty has been advocated (5,8,13,20) as an effective, safe, and comparatively inexpensive procedure with a high technical success rate. Central venous obstruction, however, has a tendency to recur earlier than does peripheral venous stenosis after percutaneous transluminal angioplasty (21,22). Severe elastic recoil after balloon dilation in central venous lesions is thought to be the underlying factor for the unsatisfactory long-term results (23). Kinked stenoses due to elongation of veins also respond well to balloon inflation but often collapse immediately after deflation. Kovalik et al (21) reported a 100% recurrence rate with a mean time to recurrence of 2.9 months following percutaneous transluminal angioplasty of elastic stenoses (ie, ≤50% improvement in the diameter of the lesion after angioplasty). In patients with nonelastic stenoses, defined as lesions with more than 50% reconstitution of the vessel lumen after percutaneous transluminal angioplasty, the mean time to recurrence was 7.6 months, with a recurrence rate of 81%. Glanz et al (9) found patency rates of 50% at 6 months, 30% at 1 year, and 0% at 2 years after subclavian vein dilation; their initial success rate was 77%. Beathard (8) reported a 6-month patency rate of 29% and a 1-year patency rate of 0% after percutaneous transluminal angioplasty for central venous stenosis. Better results were reported by Lund et al (24), who reported a patency rate of 26% after a mean follow-up of 7 months after percutaneous transluminal angioplasty.

Because even longer primary and cumulative patency rates are being strived for, additional tools, including stents and, in some instances atherectomy, were sought to achieve this goal. Vascular endoprostheses have been successfully used in the arterial system and consequently were added to the basic therapeutic adjuncts in the treatment of hemodialysis-associated venous obstructions.

Stents are particularly helpful in the treatment of elastic and kinked stenoses. Furthermore, metallic endoprostheses are used for sealing circumscribed perforations and dissections and for reestablishing patency of chronic venous occlusions (25). Quinn et al (10) treated 40 patients with 50 endoluminal prostheses, using the Gianturco stent whenever possible (n = 44). The primary patency rates in their trial were 67%, 11%, and 11% at 2, 6, and 12 months, respectively. Their cumulative 1-year patency rate was 78%. They stated that no conclusions about the role of endovascular stent placement versus balloon angioplasty for the treatment of central venous stenoses and occlusions could be made on the basis of these intermediate patency results. Vesely et al (26) reported primary patency rates of 42% after 6 months and 25% after 1 year. The cumulative patency rate in 20 patients undergoing hemodialysis who were treated with Wallstents was 64% at 6 months, 56% at 12 months, and 22% at 24 months. Kovalik et al (21) reported a mean primary patency duration of 9.8 months in patients with elastic lesions and 4.2 months in patients with nonelastic lesions; they concluded that nonelastic lesions do not respond to intraluminal stent placement in central venous obstruction. Gray et al (27) placed Wallstents in 32 central veins and 24 peripheral veins, with a technical success rate of 96%. The primary patency rate was 46% after 6 months and 20% after 12 months. With repeat interventions, the cumulative patency rate increased to 76% at 6 months and 33% at 12 months (27). Mickley et al (16) implanted 15 Wallstents in 14 patients undergoing hemodialysis. Results of life-table analysis revealed primary patency rates of 70% and 50% after 1 and 2 years, respectively. The cumulative secondary patency rates were 100% and 85% at 12 and 24 months, respectively. Shoenfeld et al (28) reported a primary patency rate of 68% and a cumulative assisted patency rate of 93% at 17-month follow-up. The overall patency rate in their study is similar to that in ours, although the primary patency rates we found were lower (56% at 12 months and 28% at 24 months) and were more comparable to those in the study of Mickley et al (16).

Except for the studies undertaken by Quinn et al (10), Shoenfeld et al (28), and Mickley et al (16), stent deployment was always performed after failed angioplasty or because of recurrent stenosis but not as the initial therapy. This may be a contributing factor in the shorter cumulative patency rates in these studies compared with those for primary stent implantation, including the rates in our study.

With regard to the patency of the central venous stent, there is no evident difference with respect to the type of dialysis graft (ie, the synthetic bridge graft and the autologous arteriovenous graft). It is well known that native fistulas offer superior long-term patency rates. The observation time in patients with an autologous graft might therefore be longer; thus, follow-up data about ipsilateral central venous stent placement may be obtainable over a longer period.

Our results indicate that primary Wallstent placement for central venous obstruction is useful in the salvage and maintenance of hemodialysis access patency. Technical success rates are better than those of balloon angioplasty alone. Repeat intervention for the treatment of reobstruction can often be performed with balloon dilation alone. Twenty-six percent of reobstruction episodes necessitated additional stent placement owing to unsatisfactory results of percutaneous transluminal angioplasty. In all but four cases, the stent was in place and could be traversed and dilated easily, which led to excellent patency rates. Atherectomy has not been used as a primary therapy for central venous obstructions, mainly because of the sharp angles and thin vessel walls in this region. Conversely, atherectomy devices such as the Simpson atherectomy device (Mallinckrodt, St Louis, Mo) are effective tools for debulking neointimal tissue in case of stent reobstruction.

The choice of a suitable endoprosthesis for central veins depends on several factors. The stent should be flexible enough to be used in curved and tortuous vessels. To avoid stent dislocation and central embolization, a self-adjusting stent is advantageous because especially chronic venous occlusions may undergo progressive luminal enlargement after stent placement (14). Also, the size of the delivery system should be moderate. For these reasons, the self-expanding Wallstent is the preferred stent at many institutions, including ours. We believe that stents with available diameters of 10–16 mm should be used for central veins to maintain good stent contact with the adjacent vessel wall.

Bridging of side branches should be avoided whenever possible. Because there is a gradual increase in venous diameter at the planned stent site, we use a Wallstent that matches the size of the larger-diameter central vein. Stent length should be kept as short as possible, covering the entire lesion with a slight overlap. To avoid stent infection, stent placement should be delayed if there are signs of active infection in the patient. We did not administer prophylactic antibiotics during the procedure, and there were no cases of sepsis after deployment, such as were described by Quinn et al (29). There are no data to help prove that periprocedural application of heparin offers a substantial prolongation of acute patency after central venous stent implantation. Anticoagulants, however, have been used by some investigators to reduce chances of early rethrombosis in central venous interventions (9,13) and are recommended at least for the interval between the beginning of the interventional procedure and end of dialysis.

In conclusion, stents evidently do not decrease the likelihood of recurrence in central venous obstructions but prolong patency intervals and allow for easy repeat intervention. Restenosis or reocclusion represent an ongoing process, with no apparent regression over time. The interventional radiologist must be prepared for repeat, sometimes multiple, interventions during the years after stent placement. To minimize intimal hyperplasia, safe stent fixation with an adequate stent size and the maintenance of as small a stent overlap as possible are advisable.

Our results suggest that initial Wallstent deployment is effective in the treatment of central venous stenosis or occlusion and shows improved long-term patency rates as compared with those of other therapeutic modalities (eg, percutaneous balloon angioplasty alone). Continued technical improvements in stent design and thrombolytic devices are necessary to specify definite treatment guidelines. The aim of future stent modifications, such as pharmacologically manipulated stents, biodegradable stents, and radiolabeled stents, will be to prevent restenosis due to intimal hyperplasia. At present, we propose liberal use of stents only in central venous lesions. Early detection and treatment of complications are mandatory to preserve the functionality of the dialysis access graft during a prolonged period.

References

1. U.S. Renal Data System. USRDS 1993 annual data report. Bethesda, Md: National Institute of Diabetes and Digestive and Kidney Disease, National Institutes of Health; 1993.
2. Klein AS, Fair JH. Vascular access. In: Cameron JL, ed. Current surgical therapy. 4th ed. St Louis, Mo: Mosby–Year Book, 1992; 745–758.
3. Mayers JD, Markell MS, Cohen LS, Hong J, Lundin P, Friedman EA. Vascular access for hemodialysis: variables in hospital stay. ASAIO J 1992; 38:113–115.
4. Dotter C. Transluminally-placed coilspring endoarterial tubegrafts: long-term patency in canine popliteal artery. Invest Radiol 1969; 57:5–10.
5. Glanz S, Gordon DH, Butt K, Hong J, Lipkowitz G. The role of percutaneous angioplasty in the management of chronic hemodialysis fistulas. Ann Surg 1987; 206:777–781.
6. Schwab SJ, Quarles LD, Middleton JP, Cohan RH, Saeed M, Dennis VW. Hemodialysis-associated subclavian vein stenosis. Kidney Int 1988; 33:1156–1159.
7. Surrat R, Picus D, Hicks M, et al. The importance of preoperative evaluation of the subclavian vein in dialysis access planning. AJR 1991; 156:623–625.
8. Beathard G. Percutaneous transvenous angioplasty in the treatment of vascular access stenosis. Kidney Int 1992; 42:1390–1397.
9. Glanz S, Gordon D, Lipkowitz G, Butt K, Hong J, Sclafani S. Axillary and subclavian vein stenosis: percutaneous angioplasty. Radiology 1988; 168:371–373.
10. Quinn SF, Schuman ES, Demlow TA, et al. Percutaneous transluminal angioplasty versus endovascular stent placement in the treatment of venous stenoses in patients undergoing hemodialysis: intermediate results. JVIR 1995; 6:851–855.
11. Günther R, Vorwerk D, Bohndorf K, et al. Venous stenosis in dialysis shunts: treatment with self-expanding metallic stents. Radiology 1989; 170:401–405.
12. Vorwerk D, Günther RW, Bohndorf K, Kistler D, Gladziwa U, Sieberth HG. Follow-up results after stent placement in failing arteriovenous shunts: a three-year experiment. Cardiovasc Intervent Radiol 1991; 14:285–289.
13. Ingram TL, Reid SH, Tisnado J, Cho SR, Posner MP. Percutaneous transluminal angioplasty of brachiocephalic vein stenoses in patients with dialysis shunts. Radiology 1988; 166:45–47.
14. Vorwerk D, Günther RW, Mann H, et al. Venous stenosis and occlusion in hemodialysis shunts: follow-up results of stent placement in 65 patients. Radiology 1995; 195:140–146.
15. Schumacher KA, Walker B, Weidenmaier W, Friedrich JM. Shuntferne venöse okklusionen als störungsfaktor bei der hämodialyse. ROFO 1989; 150:198–201.
16. Mickley V, Görich J, Rilinger N, Storck M, Abendroth D. Stenting of central venous stenoses in hemodialysis patients: long-term results. Kidney Int 1997; 51:277–280.
17. Wisselink W, Money SR, Becker MO, et al. Comparison of operative reconstruction and percutaneous balloon dilatation for central venous obstruction. Am J Surg 1993; 166:200–205.
18. Bhatia DS, Money SR, Ochsner JL, et al. Comparison of surgical bypass and percutaneous balloon dilatation with primary stent placement in the treatment of central venous obstruction in the dialysis patient: one-year follow-up. Ann Vasc Surg 1996; 10:452–455.
19. Zollikofer C, Largiader I, Bruhlmann W, Uhlschmid G, Marty A. Endovascular stenting of veins and grafts: preliminary clinical experience. Radiology 1988; 167:707–712.
20. Bohndorf K, Gladziwa U, Kistler D, et al. Rekanalisation von stenosierten oder verschlossenen hämodialyseshunts. ROFO 1993; 158:525–531.
21. Kovalik EC, Newman GE, Suhocki P, Schwab SJ. Correction of central venous stenoses: use of angioplasty and vascular Wallstents. Kidney Int 1994; 45:1177–1181.
22. Newman GE, Davidson CJ, McCann RL, Schwab SJ. Functional restenosis after hemodialysis graft angioplasty (abstr). J Am Soc Nephrol 1991; 2:341.
23. Davisdon CJ, Newman GE, Sheikh KH, Kisslo K, Stack RS, Schwab SJ. Mechanisms of angioplasty in hemodialysis fistula stenoses evaluated by intravascular ultrasound. Kidney Int 1991; 40:91–95.
24. Lund GB, Trerotola SO, Mitchell SE, et al. Central venous angioplasty: an exercise in futility in hemodialysis patients? (abstr). Radiology 1993; 189(P):198.
25. Vorwerk D, Günther RW. Percutaneous interventions in the support of failing hemodialysis fistulae. Semin Intervent Radiol 1994; 11:321–331.
26. Vesely TM, Hovsepian DM, Pilgram TK, Coyne DW, Shenoy S. Upper extremity central venous obstruction in hemodialysis patients: treatment with Wallstents. Radiology 1997; 204:343–348.
27. Gray RJ, Horton KM, Dolmatch BL, et al. Use of Wallstents for hemodialysis access–related venous stenoses and occlusions untreatable with balloon angioplasty. Radiology 1995; 195:479–484.
28. Shoenfeld R, Hermans H, Novick A, et al. Stenting of proximal venous obstructions to maintain hemodialysis access. J Vasc Surg 1994; 19:532–538.
29. Quinn S, Schuman E, Hall L, et al. Venous stenoses in patients who undergo hemodialysis: treatment with self-expandable endovascular stents. Radiology 1992; 183:499–504.

Jeffrey H. Burkhardt, PhD
Jonathan H. Sunshine, PhD

Index terms:
Breast, biopsy, 00.125, 00.1261, 00.1267
Cost-effectiveness

Radiology 1999; 212:181–188

[1] From the Research Department, American College of Radiology, 1891 Preston White Dr, Reston, VA 20191-4397. Received April 3, 1998; revision requested June 29; final revision received November 18; accepted January 7, 1999. Supported in part by National Cancer Institute grant U01CA62462 and in part by the American College of Radiology. **Address reprint requests to** J.H.B.

Author contributions:
Guarantor of integrity of entire study, J.H.B.; study concepts and design, J.H.S.; definition of intellectual content, J.H.S.; literature research, J.H.B.; data acquisition, J.H.B.; data and statistical analyses, J.H.B.; manuscript preparation, J.H.B.; manuscript editing and review, J.H.B., J.H.S.

Core-Needle and Surgical Breast Biopsy: Comparison of Three Methods of Assessing Cost[1]

PURPOSE: To compare and evaluate the measures of costs for core-needle and surgical breast biopsies.

MATERIALS AND METHODS: Three measures of costs were evaluated: (*a*) input resources, (*b*) actual payments, and (*c*) billed charges. A combination of methods were used for data collection from 10 sites enrolled in a large-scale, multiinstitutional, randomized controlled clinical trial.

RESULTS: Input resource cost data (42 core-needle and eight surgical biopsies) were the most difficult to obtain. Actual payments and billed charges data collection (32 core-needle and 44 surgical biopsies) was hampered by the difficulty of obtaining data from all providers involved in the procedures. Average direct input resource costs for surgical biopsy (including needle localization) were almost three times as high as those for core-needle biopsy ($698 vs $243). Actual payments ($2,398 vs $799) and billed charges ($3,764 vs $1,496) for surgical biopsy averaged two and a half to three times higher than those for core biopsy ($P < .001$).

CONCLUSION: There was remarkable consistency in relative costs. Input resource costs were much more difficult to obtain than were either actual payments or billed charges. However, input resource costs present a more reliable indication of the actual costs of a procedure than do the other measures. Given the difficulty in obtaining input resource costs, analyses by using actual payments may be preferred.

Cost has become increasingly important in the evaluation of new medical technologies. In the past, when new medical technologies were evaluated, the determining criterion in most cases was whether the new technology was at least as effective as current technology. Generally, there was no reference to, or consideration of, the cost of performing the procedure. In current evaluations of new medical procedures, however, acceptance is frequently based on procedures that are "effective in terms of increased survival or increased quality of life or both but also that [are] economically sound" (1).

Stereotactic core-needle biopsy has been adopted into widespread use and advocated as a lower cost, less invasive alternative to open excisional biopsy for diagnosing nonpalpable lesions detected by using mammography. This change happened without controlled scientific studies to verify its efficacy (2,3). Hence, the National Cancer Institute sought researchers to conduct a large-scale, multiinstitutional, randomized controlled clinical trial to compare core-needle breast biopsy and fine-needle aspiration with surgical breast biopsy. In its solicitation, the National Cancer Institute also required a cost analysis, which the American College of Radiology performed. This article presents the results of that cost analysis. We compared the costs of core-needle biopsy, with either stereotactic or ultrasonographic (US) guidance, with the costs of needle localization followed by excisional biopsy. (Only surgical biopsies that were preceded by needle localization were included in this analysis, because the National Cancer Institute study is directed at biopsy of nonpalpable lesions. Furthermore, fine-needle aspiration was dropped from the clinical study protocol, so it was omitted from this study also.) When the clinical phase of the research is complete and its results are reported, we hope to combine these cost results with clinical results in a cost-effectiveness analysis.

Because the funding source, the National Cancer Institute, has a high level of interest in costs, we conducted not only an analysis of costs but also applied research into the methodology for studying costs. Health care costs can be measured in three different ways—by evaluating (*a*) costs of input resources, (*b*) actual payments, and (*c*) billed charges.

Data reflecting input resource costs—that is, the actual dollars expended in producing a product or service—are the best cost measures. Unfortunately, in health care studies, these data are rarely used because of the difficulty and expense of obtaining them.

Actual payments—that is, the dollars expended in purchasing a product or service—are a measure of the dollars that become unavailable for purchasing other things in the economy and are widely used in health care cost studies. Actual payments are the direct costs to society for compensating health care providers for performing procedures. These payments include co-payments, deductibles, self payments, and payments by third-party payers. They are another measure that we used in this study.

The third measure of cost that is widely used in health care studies is billed charges, or the dollar amount the consumer is billed for a service or product. Outside of health care, these "list" prices are rarely used in cost analyses, because they do not reflect actual payments, which often are lower. In addition, in health care, billed charges are infrequently paid by insurers or payers, and they may have little relationship to the costs of labor, equipment, and other resource inputs in the procedure or to the actual payments received. Actual payments are often either a discount from billed charges or derived from a payer's fee schedule. In most studies, actual payments or, less satisfactorily, billed charges are used as the measure of costs. We studied all three measures of cost because they each have advantages and disadvantages.

Our study of costs was, given its research nature, designed to answer several questions other than how core-needle biopsy and excisional biopsy compare in cost. Specifically, we also sought to answer the following questions: (*a*) How feasible is it to measure costs by using each of the three measures (input resources, actual payments, and billed charges)? (*b*) What difficulties are encountered? (*c*) How can these difficulties be overcome? (*d*) How similar are the three measures of cost in their findings with regard to the relative costs of the two kinds of biopsy?

MATERIALS AND METHODS

Introduction

The cost analyses described in this study began approximately 12 months after the commencement of the clinical study, in which data accrual began in April 1994. Delaying the start of the cost analyses allowed the clinical process to become routine and the start-up problems to be resolved. We expected this to lead to more consistent and realistic measures of costs, especially for resource input costs.

We used a combination of methods for data collection: We gathered concurrent data for resource cost estimation with time and motion studies, obtained retrospective data on actual payments and billed charges, and distributed questionnaires for estimating patient time. Because of the time and expense of implementing all of these methods, all of them are not typically used in health care research. For this project, however, they were the source of data.

Approximately 22 sites were enrolled in the clinical research project, and the seven facilities that performed the largest number of core-needle biopsies were initially designated for site visits for cost data collection. These sites performed approximately 63% (945 of 1,508) of the core-needle biopsies during the first 2 years of the study. Because surgical biopsies were relatively uncommon, we also visited three additional facilities to obtain data on larger numbers of surgical biopsies. Overall, 10 sites received site visits. Although institutional review board approval and informed consent were required at each site participating in the overall study, not all sites needed these approvals for the site visits and patient questionnaires associated with this economic analysis.

Input Resource Costs

Five components were included in our measurement of input resources: (*a*) labor time of physicians, nurses, technologists, and other health care workers; (*b*) supplies; (*c*) equipment; (*d*) facilities (room time); and (*e*) patient time. Data on the first four input components were collected during on-site visits, and data on patient time were obtained from answers to a separate patient questionnaire.

Data on the labor component of the resource inputs were collected during on-site time and motion studies. Information about the quantity and cost of supplies, equipment, and facilities was also obtained during this visit, when possible. Patient questionnaires with self-addressed stamped envelopes were distributed during each visit and given to approximately 10 consecutive patients who would be undergoing core-needle biopsy and 10 consecutive patients who would be undergoing surgical biopsy.

Labor.—The labor cost of the health care providers involved in the procedures was expected to be the largest portion of the total cost of each procedure, so the greatest effort was devoted to obtaining information on this input. In the time and motion studies, an observer was located in an unobtrusive location outside the procedure room to record the times the patient and each provider entered and exited the room. To maintain consistency in the collection of the time and motion data, one observer (J.H.B.) performed all site visits.

Generally, when a physician was not in the procedure room, even during an ongoing procedure, his or her time was not attributed to the procedure. This is because physicians would often interpret images from other studies or observe other patients while waiting for a patient to be positioned or film to be developed. Technologist time was treated differently and generally allocated to the procedure, even when the technologist had left the procedure room. Technologists rarely treated more than one patient at a time, but they would perform multiple tasks for the ongoing procedure, such as processing film, hanging film for the radiologist, and preparing or cleaning the procedure room.

Many of the facilities in the study were academic institutions. Consequently, residents and fellows were frequently included in the procedures for teaching purposes. Their time was treated the same as that of other physicians, and a national average income for residents was used (4).

The dollar value per minute of the provider time was calculated from the national average hourly salary or annual income for each type of provider. Published national averages (4–6) rather than site-specific salaries and incomes were used to eliminate the variation due solely to differences in salaries and incomes between sites, practice types, or regions of the country. We estimated the vacation and other fringe benefit costs at 22% of salary (American Hospital Association Trend Analysis Group, personal communication, May 1997).

Supplies.—We asked managers at each site to provide a list, with prices, of supplies used for each procedure. Supply costs for core-needle biopsy, including both stereotactic and US-guided procedures, were received from six sites and averaged, as were the supply costs from the two sites that provided information on needle localization supplies. Costs from one surgical site provided the basis for the data used to estimate the surgical biopsy supply costs.

Equipment.—Information on the prices of equipment used for needle localizations and core biopsies was obtained from three radiology department managers and equipment manufacturer representatives. Data on the prices of equipment used in surgery suites and recovery rooms and on actual patient load statistics were collected from one surgery department manager. This formed the basis for the surgical biopsy equipment cost component. By using (*a*) the price information, (*b*) an expected equipment useful life of 5 years for both core-needle and excisional biopsy equipment, and (*c*) an estimated annual cost for capital and maintenance of 5% each, we calculated the cost of equipment per procedure while operating the equipment at 100% of capacity (ie, full capacity). Full capacity was defined as the capacity of equipment used 8 hours per day, 5 days per week, and 52 weeks per year. On the basis of estimates from the time and motion studies, eight core-needle biopsies or five surgical biopsies per 8-hour day would be performed in a facility (room) functioning at full capacity.

Facility.—Facility (procedure room) costs were calculated by multiplying the estimated cost per minute by the average time per procedure. The average time expended per procedure was collected during the time and motion studies by recording the time that a room was devoted to the actual procedure. This included room set-up time, procedure time, and room cleanup time after the procedure. Per-minute costs were calculated by estimating the average room size, construction costs (Paul Durance, Huron Systems, Ann Arbor, Mich, personal communication, May 1997), capital costs, and maintenance costs for radiology rooms, surgical suites, and preoperative/recovery rooms. From these estimates, the cost per minute for operating the rooms at full capacity was used to compute the facility cost per procedure for the radiology, surgery, and preoperative/recovery rooms.

Patient time.—The cost of the patient's time in undergoing and recovering from the biopsy procedure was the fifth component of the input resource costs. Questionnaires, on which patients were asked how many days (or hours if less than 1 day) it took before she was able to resume usual daily activities after the biopsy, were left with personnel in the radiology department during each site visit. These were to be distributed to 10 consecutive core-needle biopsy patients and 10 consecutive needle localization patients who would be undergoing surgical biopsy. The cost in patient time was calculated by using the 1994 median earnings published by the U.S. Bureau of the Census for year-round, full-time female workers (7).

Indirect and overhead costs.—In hospital accounting systems, adding in indirect and overhead costs is an entire discipline in itself, is unavoidably arbitrary in some of its allocations, and has been heavily criticized. Therefore, we ignored all indirect and overhead costs when we calculated input resource costs. For example, we counted only the purchase price of supplies, ignoring the internal warehousing costs and the labor costs of moving the supplies from bulk cartons to the procedure/operating rooms. For labor costs, we assumed that physicians and other health care personnel have no "down time" between procedures and spend no time before or after procedures communicating with colleagues or patients. Similar omissions for other categories of cost were also made. Because of the omission of indirect and overhead costs, the absolute amounts in our input resource cost analysis are low, but the ratios should be relatively sound.

Sensitivity Analyses for Input Resource Costs

Not all core-needle and surgical biopsies are performed under the same conditions. Variation occurs in equipment (US vs stereotactic guidance), facilities (free-standing breast clinic vs hospital, minor surgery facility vs surgical suite), supplies (vacuum-assisted biopsy probes vs long-throw, core-biopsy needles), and facility operating workloads. Therefore, we performed sensitivity analyses by changing various assumptions to see what difference they would make with regard to input resource costs. For one, we calculated the effect of using vacuum-assisted biopsy probes rather than long-throw biopsy needles. Two of the six sites from which we obtained supply cost data used vacuum-assisted biopsy probes for stereotactic breast biopsies rather than the less expensive long-throw, core-biopsy needles.

Second, we explored the costs per procedure of a facility functioning at the actual operating level of one of the sites in the study (67% and 64% of capacity for excisional biopsy and core-needle biopsy, respectively) rather than at the assumed 100% of capacity. This is equivalent to performing 3.4 surgical biopsies daily instead of five at full capacity and to performing 5.2 core-needle biopsies out of a possible eight per day.

Third, because many of the patients involved in this study were either retired or full-time homemakers, we computed the effect of eliminating the cost of patient time. Some authorities take the view that the cost assigned to patient time should be the patients' actual wages. If so, a cost of $0 would be assigned to the time of retirees and full-time homemakers.

Actual Payments and Billed Charges

Although actual payments and billed charges are two different ways of measuring costs, in this study, the method of obtaining information about them was the same, so they are reported together. One of the difficulties in obtaining accurate payment and charge information from available data sets such as Part B Medicare Annual Data files or commercial claims sources is the Physicians' Current Procedural Terminology coding system. Prior to 1994, the costs of the two biopsy procedures—that is, fine-needle aspiration and core-needle breast biopsy—could be submitted to third-party payers for payment by using the same Current Procedural Terminology code. Furthermore, there were multiple ways to code core-needle biopsy, so obtaining payment and charge data from Part B of the Medicare annual data files or commercial sources was unreliable.

Because preexisting claims databases could not be used owing to coding inconsistencies, patient encounter logs were reviewed during site visits to obtain the names of approximately 20 patients who had actually undergone core-needle breast biopsy and 20 who were documented to have undergone excisional breast biopsy. We then requested that hospital departments and physicians' billing offices provide us with the total billed charges and total actual payments from all payers for the approxi-

TABLE 2
Input Resource Costs: Labor

Provider	Biopsies in Which This Provider Was Involved (%)*		Average No. of Provider Minutes per Procedure*†		Average Hourly Wage or Annual Income ($)‡	Average Provider Cost per Procedure ($)#	
	Core-Needle	Surgical	Core-Needle	Surgical		Core-Needle	Surgical
Radiology technologist	100	100	56	48	16.51/hr§	15	13
Registered nurse	60	100	44	174	23.07/hr§	17	67
Nurse anesthetist	0	25	NA	85	41.02/hr§	NA	58
Medical assistant	21	88	39	51	19.85/hr§	13	17
Resident	2	75	19	107	41,102/yr‖	6	35
Radiologist	100	100	24	19	237,400/yr¶	46	36
Anesthesiologist	0	88	NA	52	218,100/yr¶	NA	91
Surgeon	0	100	NA	72	240,000/yr¶	NA	138

Note.—NA = not available.
* Source.—ACR time and motion study, 1995.
† Average number of minutes when provider is involved in the procedure.
‡ Includes fringe benefits.
§ Source.—reference 4.
‖ Source.—reference 6.
¶ Source.—reference 5.
\# Data are average provider cost when provider is involved in the procedure. Total average provider cost was $76 for core-needle biopsy versus $392 for surgical biopsy.

TABLE 1
Average Input Resource Costs

Component	Core-Needle Biopsy Costs ($)	Surgical Biopsy Costs ($)
Provider time	76	392
Supplies	66	93
Equipment	25	57
Facility (room)	2	8
Patient time	74	148
Total average cost	243	698

TABLE 3
Input Resource Costs: Supplies

Institution	Core-Needle Biopsy Costs ($)		Needle Localization and Surgical Biopsy Costs ($)		
	Stereotactic	US	Stereotactic	US	Surgery
B	51.20	NA	33.80	NA	NA
C	24.43	NA	NA	NA	NA
E	185.71*	41.21	58.12	37.94	49.58
F	142.00*	33.00	NA	NA	NA
G	32.40	56.16	NA	NA	NA
H	25.17	NA	NA	NA	NA
Overall average	66.00		43.00		50.00

Note.—Data are average costs. NA = not available.
* Only vacuum-assisted biopsy probes were used for stereotactic procedures at these sites.

mately 20 patients in each biopsy group who we identified from the patient encounter logs. Each patient had undergone the procedure at least 6 months previously, so providers would have had sufficient time to receive essentially all the payments.

Billed charges and actual payments can differ systematically among sites. For example, they may be systematically higher in high-cost cities. Avoiding this source of variation requires analysis in addition to that of the overall averages we present. To eliminate this variation, we compared actual payments and billed charges separately at each of the two institutions that provided data on patients who had undergone multiple core-needle biopsies and on those who had undergone multiple excisional biopsies.

RESULTS

Data Obtained

Ten sites were visited during the data collection phase of this study. We were able to observe 42 core-needle biopsies and eight surgical biopsies during the site visits, which encompassed approximately 40 observer work days (not counting travel time). These numbers indicate the rate at which a site visitor could expect to generate data in a geographically dispersed, multicenter trial.

Approximately 160 questionnaires were left at the sites to be distributed to patients. Sixty-two surveys were returned, and 44 were usable for analysis. The others were unusable, primarily because the type of procedure was not indicated.

Three of the 10 sites visited were able to provide complete billed charges and actual payments data both on patients who had undergone core-needle biopsy and on those who had undergone surgical biopsy. One of these three sites reported data on only one patient who had undergone surgical biopsy and on seventeen patients who had undergone core-needle biopsy. A fourth site provided data only on patients who had undergone surgical biopsy. In total, we obtained complete actual payments and billed charges data on 32 core-needle biopsy and 44 surgical biopsy cases.

Difficulties in Data Collection

Collecting cost data in all three ways was both time-consuming and expensive. Despite the expenditure of approximately 40 observer days in the field and additional time at the office, data were obtained on a relatively small number of cases. Many pitfalls and problems were encountered as data—on input resource costs, actual payments, and billed charges—were being collected for this

TABLE 4
Input Resource Costs: Equipment

Variable	Core-Needle Biopsy	Needle Localization and Surgical Biopsy
Maximum number of procedures per day	8	5
Assumed capacity (%)	100	100
No. of days per year	260	260
No. of procedures per year	2,080	1,300
Surgical equipment cost ($)	NA	120,750
Radiology equipment cost ($)	172,500	125,000
Useful life of equipment (y)	5	5
Cost of capital (%)	5	5
Maintenance cost (%)	5	5
Cost per procedure ($)	25	57

Note.—Data are average values. NA = not available.

project. Some were related to the willingness of contacts to provide data, whereas others stemmed from the availability of the data we needed.

Due to the time necessary to perform time and motion studies for each procedure, considerably fewer surgical biopsies than core-needle biopsies were observed during site visits. If appointments were fully scheduled in a day (which they rarely were), four to six core biopsies, which lasted about an hour, could be studied. However, only one surgical biopsy could be observed in a day, because it usually required 5-6 hours of elapsed time (for needle localization plus surgical biopsy). At one site, because of unusual circumstances, no surgical or core biopsies were performed during the entire site visit, precluding the obtaining of any data for the time and motion study.

Because input resource measurements included those in both radiologic procedures and surgical procedures, approval from radiology departments and surgery departments was necessary to observe the providers during the time and motion studies. Even with surgery department approval, some surgeons were still unwilling to allow the American College of Radiology staff member to be outside the operating room to record provider time.

It was difficult to obtain detailed cost information about supplies, particularly those for surgery, because our contacts with surgical personnel were more indirect. Normally, surgery departments would refer us to the medical supply department for data on prices paid for supplies, and the supply departments did not spend the time to collect the data that we needed. As a result, we were unable to perform statistical comparisons of the supply data.

Billing systems presented problems in data collection. Frequently, there were separate billing offices with separate computer systems for hospital and physician charges, and there often was no interaction between these systems. One site had separate billing systems for the radiology department, surgery department, radiology professional services, and surgery professional services. This made it necessary for us to navigate between numerous administrative units, frequently unsuccessfully, to collect data from all sources of billed charges from and actual payments to providers (including radiologists, surgeons, anesthesiologists, hospitals, and pathologists) for patient procedures.

Actual payments and billed charges for all providers were requested during data collection. Two of the sites provided actual payments and billed charges data with Current Procedural Terminology code detail, so it was obvious that all providers, including pathologists, were represented. However, the small sample size in our study, especially for surgical biopsies, introduced a possible response bias, because some sites that were supposed to provide data did not. Our comparison of core-needle and surgical biopsy costs at individual institutions that provided data on both types of biopsy addresses this response bias issue. The findings indicate that this was not a problem.

Input Resource Costs

Data on each component of input resource costs in a baseline case are shown in Table 1. The total average input resource cost for surgical biopsy was almost three times as high as that for core-needle biopsy ($698 vs $243). Moreover, for every component, surgical biopsy appeared to have a higher average cost than did core-needle biopsy. The difference was real and statistically significant ($P < .001$) for the components for which a statistical comparison was possible—provider time, facilities, and patient time. (Because only one site reported the cost of surgical supplies and equipment, we could not compute an SD and thus could not perform a statistical comparison of the average supply or equipment costs of the two types of breast biopsy.)

Provider time was the largest component of cost for surgical biopsy (Tables 1 and 2). At an average cost of $392, it constituted more than half of the total cost. No other component composed more than 25% of the cost. For core-needle biopsy, provider time (average cost, $76), supplies (average cost, $66), and patient time (average cost, $74) each made up about 30% of the procedural cost (Table 1).

The average cost of supplies for core-needle biopsy ($66) appeared to be lower than the average combined cost of supplies for needle localization and surgical biopsy ($93) (Tables 1 and 3). We were unable to statistically compare the supply costs, because we had surgical supply data based on only one observation. The average equipment cost for surgical biopsy ($57) appeared to be considerably higher than that for core-needle biopsy ($25) (Tables 1 and 4), but again, we were unable to statistically compare these costs because we had only one observation in which to obtain surgical equipment data.

Facility (room) costs composed a minimal portion of the total cost for each procedure. On average, they constituted $2 of the total cost for core-needle biopsy and $8 of that for surgical biopsy (Tables 1 and 5).

The cost of the patient's time during biopsy and recovery was a major factor in the cost of both types of biopsy (Tables 1 and 6). Among the patients who returned the questionnaire, the 23 who underwent core-needle biopsy were able to perform their usual activities after an average of 24 hours, whereas the 21 who underwent surgical biopsy were able to perform their usual activities after an average of 48 hours. These times were converted into 8-hour workdays (24 and 48 hours constituting 1 and 2 workdays, respectively). At $10.68 per hour, this added an average of $74 to the cost of core-needle breast biopsy and an average of $148 to the cost of surgical breast biopsy (Tables 1 and 6).

Sensitivity Analyses for Input Resource Costs

The results of sensitivity analyses of input resource costs showed the magnitude of differences in the total cost of biopsies under the various assumptions. We report the results of three different sensitivity analyses: use of vacuum-assisted biopsy probes versus long-throw biopsy needles, operation at actual versus full capacity, and elimination of patient time costs.

Institutions differed in the supplies used for core-needle biopsy. As Table 7 shows, the estimated average cost for core-needle biopsy with a long-throw needle was $215, and that for core-needle biopsy with a vacuum-assisted probe was $341. The cost of excisional biopsy was unaffected.

When we assumed that the facility, equipment, and providers functioned at capacities of about 67% (excisional biopsy) and 64% (core-needle biopsy), which were the actual operating levels at one of the sites in the study, the average cost of both types of biopsy was greater. The average cost of excisional biopsy was $925, and that for core-needle biopsy was $299. When patient time was omitted, the average costs of excisional and core-needle biopsies were $550 and $169, respectively. With all variants and assumptions, the average cost of excisional biopsy was two to three and a half times higher than that of core-needle biopsy.

TABLE 5
Input Resource Costs: Facility (Room)

Variable	Core-Needle Biopsy	Needle Localization and Surgical Biopsy: Radiography	Preoperative Care and Recovery	Surgery
Room size (sq ft)	225	225	80	300
Construction cost per square foot ($)	200	200	200	200
Useful life of facility (y)	30	30	30	30
Cost of capital (%)	5	5	5	5
Maintenance cost (%)	2	2	2	2
Cost per year ($)	4,650	4,650	1,653	6,200
Minutes per year	124,800	124,800	124,800	124,800
Assumed capacity (%)	100	100	100	100
Cost per minute ($)	0.0373	0.0373	0.0132	0.0497
Minutes per procedure	58	79	115	64
Cost per procedure ($)	2	3	2	3
Average total cost ($)	2		8	

Source.—Paul Durance, Huron Systems, personal communication, May 1997. Data are average values.

Actual Payments

The comparison of actual payments for surgical biopsy and core-needle biopsy is shown in the Figure. For all institutions combined, the average actual payment for surgical biopsy preceded by needle localization ($2,398) was three times as high as that for core-needle biopsy ($799) ($P < .001$). At the two institutions that provided information on more than one excisional biopsy patient and on more than one core-needle biopsy patient, the actual payments for the former group were at least two and a half times as high as those for the latter patients ($P < .01$).

Billed Charges

The Figure also shows the difference between billed charges for surgical biopsy and those for core-needle biopsy. For all institutions combined, billed charges were two and a half times as high as those for surgical biopsy; the average cost for surgical biopsy was $3,764, and that for core-needle biopsy was $1,496 ($P < .001$). For both institutions that provided information on more than one surgical biopsy patient and on more than one core-needle biopsy patient, the billed charges were at least two and a half times as high ($P < .01$).

DISCUSSION

We calculated the costs of core-needle and surgical breast biopsy in three different ways. Two of the measures, actual payments and billed charges, are commonly used in cost studies. We calculated a third measure, input resource cost, which more accurately reflects the actual dollars expended in producing the procedures. By comparing the three measures, we sought to determine (*a*) the feasibility of measuring costs in each of the three ways, (*b*) the difficulties encountered in data collection, (*c*) the methods needed to overcome those difficulties, and (*d*) the similarity, or disparity, in the three measures of relative cost for the two types of biopsy.

TABLE 6
Input Resource Costs: Patient Time

Biopsy	No. of Observations	Average Work Hours Lost	Average Cost ($)
Core-needle	23	6.9	74
Surgical	21	13.9	148

Source.—U.S. Bureau of the Census. The 1994 median hourly earnings for year-round, full-time female workers was $10.68.

Interpretation of Findings

Our principal finding about relative costs—that the billed charges, actual payments, and resource inputs of surgical breast biopsy were greater than those for core-needle biopsy—was no surprise. However, the magnitude of the difference has not been well documented previously in the literature. The difference between core-needle biopsy and surgical biopsy in our baseline case input resource cost analysis was almost three-fold. In all the sensitivity analyses, the costs for surgical breast biopsy were also between two and three and a half times as high as those for core-needle biopsy. The difference in billed charges and payments for the two types of biopsy also was almost threefold.

In all three measures, surgical breast biopsy is approximately two and a half to three times as costly as core-needle biopsy. This suggests that actual payments or billed charges may be reasonable measures for estimating relative costs, even though they both inconsistently reflect true costs and billed charges are an overestimation of costs. It may not be necessary to spend the time and money collecting input cost data, as we did, if the goal is to compare the relative savings of one procedure over another in percentages. However, measuring actual input resource costs, as we did, seems necessary to confirm findings about billed charges or actual payments, because the charges and payments may be arbitrary.

The purpose of this article is not to calculate the effect of altering the choice of breast biopsy on total health spending in the United States. However, one must consider that the difference in cost (as measured by payments) for the approximately one million breast biopsies performed in the United States annually (8) would be about $1.6 billion.

In reality, savings of $1.6 billion should not be expected. Core-needle biopsy may not be appropriate for all patients. It is, however, less invasive and less costly than surgical biopsy. If its diagnostic accuracy is adequate to replace surgical biopsy

TABLE 7
Average Costs Based on Sensitivity Analyses

Baseline Case	Cost Components: Provider Time	Supplies	Equipment	Facilities	Patient Time	Total Average Cost
Full capacity						
Surgical biopsy	392	93	57	8	148	698
Core-needle biopsy	76	66	25	2	74	243
With different needles						
Surgical biopsy	392	93	57	8	148	698
Core-needle biopsy with long-throw needles	76	38	25	2	74	215
Core-needle biopsy with vacuum-assisted probes	76	164	25	2	74	341
Actual capacity*						
Surgical biopsy	588	93	84	12	148	925
Core-needle biopsy	117	66	39	3	74	299
Excluding patient time						
Surgical biopsy	392	93	57	8	0	550
Core-needle biopsy	76	66	25	2	0	169

Note.—All data are average costs in dollars.
* Average costs based on the assumption that the facility, equipment, and providers are functioning at a capacity of 67%.

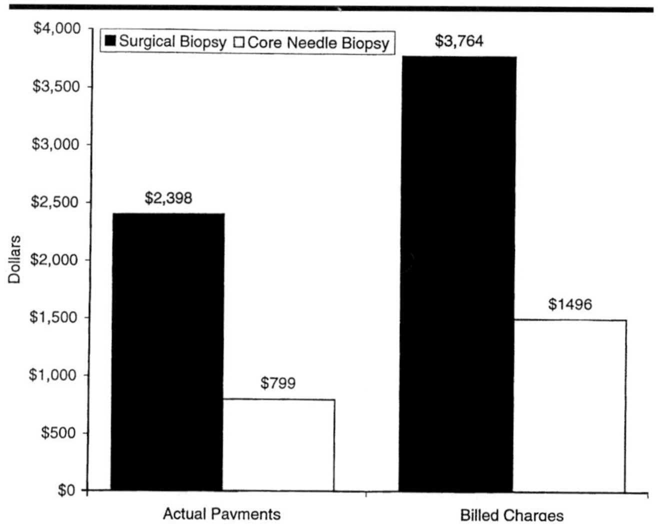

Graph shows a comparison of actual payments and billed charges for surgical and core-needle biopsies.

in most cases, then, as occurred when laparoscopic cholecystectomy replaced surgical cholecystectomy (9,10), core-needle biopsy will be performed at a lower threshold of suspicion than will surgical biopsy. This means that some of the health spending reduction that would be achieved by a simple one-for-one replacement will not occur. Instead, some of the potential reduction will be spent to achieve better care as women who previously did not undergo biopsy because it was too expensive or too invasive gain from undergoing this diagnostic procedure.

Data for use in cost studies are available in several different forms. For our study, we used three different ways of measuring costs and found remarkable consistency in relative costs. Given the difficulty of obtaining resource input cost data—including the necessity of time and motion studies because the needed information is not otherwise available—analyses with actual payments may be preferred; however, this must be recognized as a less reliable method.

Strengths and Limitations of the Study

As with any study, our study has both strengths and limitations. The principal strength of our study is that cost was measured in a variety of ways. When we calculated costs in terms of input resource costs, actual payments, and billed charges, we found remarkable consistency in relative costs among the measures: Surgical biopsy, including needle localization, was uniformly two and a half to three times more expensive than core-needle biopsy. Having three different measures of cost adds strength to the results: If the findings are in agreement with one another, as ours were, they lend credence to the observed relationships. Furthermore, Hillner et al (2), by using cost-to-charge ratios specific to their institution, found a similar consistency in ratios of surgical biopsy and core-needle biopsy costs in their study.

Liberman et al (11) and Lee et al (12) used a different approach in computing costs for their economic models. They based their estimates on the Current Procedural Terminology codes that are commonly used for submitting charges to Medicare for stereotactic core-needle breast biopsy and surgical breast biopsy. Although this is a readily obtainable source for developing estimates, the inconsistency in coding among providers, which prompted the American College of Radiology to issue coding guidelines for core-needle breast biopsy, make this an inaccurate representation of the actual charges for both procedures. Furthermore, actual Medicare charges or payments are not accurate representations of the costs of procedures. Compared with the measures used and reported in this study, these easily accessible cost data methods have the disadvantage of being less reliable.

Although actual payments and billed charges are more easily accessible than are input resource costs, limiting our research to these two measures would have eroded the validity of our findings. The calculated costs obtained from the time and motion studies give strength to the observed relationships and ratios.

As demonstrated in each of the three referenced cost studies (2,11,12), modeling is a popular method used in cost studies. If correct assumptions are made, modeling can be a feasible alternative to the more time-consuming and expensive direct study that we performed. However, as we have described, assumptions often are seriously problematic.

At some facilities, core-needle breast biopsies were so widely accepted by all physicians that surgical breast biopsies were rarely performed. Therefore, it was impossible to observe excisional biopsies for the time and motion studies or to collect actual payments and billed charges data on surgical biopsies. This is an aspect of the "moving target" problem that is frequent in fields such as radiology where technology changes rapidly.

In spite of making additional site visits to increase the number of surgical biopsies observed in the time and motion studies, we faced a possible response bias due to the small number of observations. Our comparison of core-needle and surgical biopsy costs at individual institutions, which provided data on both procedures, addressed this response bias issue. The findings of this comparison indicate that it was not a problem.

Most of the institutions involved in the study were academic facilities and had residents and/or fellows either participating in or performing the procedures. Consequently, the times for both core-needle biopsy and surgical biopsy may be higher than are those normally found in the nonacademic community.

Because the study was conducted only at sites that participated in the clinical research study, there was further potential for bias in the results. Specifically, a common problem in observing patients involved in a study is that procedures take longer when a protocol is followed. In our research, only a portion of the core-needle biopsy patients observed for this project were "protocol patients," and none of the surgical biopsy patients were protocol patients. We did not limit our selection of patients to observe for the time and motion studies to only those enrolled in the clinical study. Rather, we chose all patients who were undergoing core-needle breast biopsy during the week of the site visit. This may have introduced some protocol-based bias in the length of time to perform the procedure, because one-third of the core-needle patients observed were enrolled in the clinical study.

On the other hand, our method may have reduced selection bias, because all patients were observed. In any case, the bias would be against core-needle biopsy, because following a protocol (presumably) lengthened the time to perform some core-needle biopsies, whereas the time for none of the surgical biopsies was lengthened by following a protocol. Thus, the differences in input resource costs between surgical biopsy and core-needle biopsy may be even larger than those we observed.

We calculated costs in three different ways—in terms of input resource costs, actual payments, and billed charges–and found remarkable consistency in relative costs among the measures, with surgical biopsy, including needle localization, uniformly costing two and a half to three times as much as core-needle biopsy. Input resource cost data were much more labor-intensive and difficult to obtain than were either actual payments or billed charges data. However, input resource costs present a more reliable indication of the actual cost of a procedure than do the other measures. Given the difficulty in obtaining resource input costs, analyses with actual payments may be preferred.

Acknowledgments: We thank the members of the executive team of the Radiological Diagnostic Oncology Group V of the American College of Radiology. Barbara J. McNeil, MD, Laurie Fajardo, MD, Etta Pisano, MD, W. J. Frable, MD, and Cynthia Olson were particularly helpful in this economic analysis. Their comments and insights aided in the development of the study and greatly enhanced the quality of this article.

References

1. Hunink MG. Cost-effectiveness research in radiology. Acad Radiol 1996; 3(suppl 1): 13–16.
2. Hillner BE, Bear HD, Fajardo LL. Estimating the cost-effectiveness of stereotaxic biopsy for nonpalpable breast abnormalities: a decision analysis model. Acad Radiol 1996; 3:351–360.
3. Fajardo LL. Cost-effectiveness of stereotaxic breast core needle biopsy. Acad Radiol 1996; 3(suppl 1):21–23.
4. Hospital & Healthcare Compensation Service. Hospital salary survey report 1994-95. Oakland, NJ: Hospital & Healthcare Compensation Service, 1994.
5. American Medical Association. Physician marketplace statistics 1995. Chicago, Ill: American Medical Association, 1995.
6. Hospital & Healthcare Compensation Service. Physician salary survey report 1995. Oakland, NJ: Hospital & Healthcare Compensation Service, 1995.
7. US Bureau of the Census. Current population reports, series P60-189: income, poverty, and valuation of noncash benefits. Washington, DC: Government Printing Office, 1996.
8. Nields MW. Cost-effectiveness of image-guided core-needle biopsy versus surgery in diagnosing breast cancer. Acad Radiol 1996; 3(suppl 1):138–140.
9. Escarce JJ, Chen W, Schwartz JS. Falling cholecystectomy thresholds since the introduction of laparoscopic cholecystectomy. JAMA 1995; 273:1581–1585.
10. Nenner RP, Imperato PJ, Rosenberg C, Ronberg E. Increased cholecystectomy rates among Medicare patients after the introduction of laparoscopic cholecystectomy. J Community Health 1994; 19:409–415.
11. Liberman L, Fahs MC, Dershaw DD, et al. Impact of stereotaxic core breast biopsy on cost of diagnosis. Radiology 1995; 195:633–637.
12. Lee CH, Egglin TK, Philpotts L, Mainiero MB, Tocino I. Cost-effectiveness of stereotactic core-needle biopsy: analysis by means of mammographic findings. Radiology 1997; 202:849–854.

Follow-up of Breast Lesions Diagnosed as Benign with Stereotactic Core-Needle Biopsy: Frequency of Mammographic Change and False-Negative Rate[1]

Carol H. Lee, MD
Liane E. Philpotts, MD
Laura J. Horvath, MD
Irena Tocino, MD

Index terms:
Breast, biopsy, 00.1267
Breast neoplasms, diagnosis, 00.1267
Breast radiography, utilization

Radiology 1999; 212:189–194

Abbreviation:
SCNB = stereotactic core-needle biopsy

[1] From the Department of Diagnostic Radiology, Yale University School of Medicine, 333 Cedar St, New Haven, CT 06520. From the 1997 RSNA scientific assembly. Received August 11, 1998; revision requested September 25; revision received November 10; accepted January 11, 1999. **Address reprint requests to** C.H.L.

PURPOSE: To determine how often lesions diagnosed as benign with stereotactic core-needle biopsy (SCNB) change at follow-up mammography and to determine the optimal follow-up strategy and the delayed false-negative rate.

MATERIALS AND METHODS: From July 1992 through December 1995, 355 of 540 cases (66%) in which SCNB yielded benign results were managed with follow-up mammography. Mammographic follow-up was available for 298 of these cases (84%). Follow-up mammography reports were reviewed. When a change was reported, pre- and postbiopsy mammograms, pathology reports, and results of subsequent mammographic follow-up were reviewed.

RESULTS: Mammographic change occurred in 21 of 298 cases (7%) at intervals of 6–55 months (mean, 20 months). Change occurred after initial mammographic stability in 10 of 21 cases. Repeat biopsy was performed in 18 of 21 cases. Malignancy was diagnosed in two cases: one mass that changed at 6 months and one case of microcalcifications that changed at 24 months. This represented a delayed false-negative rate of 2% (two of 105 malignancies among 540 biopsies).

CONCLUSION: A small percentage of cases diagnosed as benign with SCNB will change on follow-up mammograms, which may necessitate repeat biopsy. These results suggest that 6-month follow-up for cases that yield nonspecific benign results at SCNB and yearly screening mammography for cases with specific benign results is a reasonable management strategy.

Stereotactic core-needle biopsy (SCNB) is now widely used as an alternative to open surgical biopsy for the evaluation of nonpalpable breast lesions (1). Findings of initial studies in which SCNB was immediately followed by open surgical biopsy indicate a high degree of concordance between the results obtained with the two procedures (2–5). However, to our knowledge, long-term follow-up information in patients who have undergone SCNB with benign results and who have not subsequently undergone open surgical biopsy have, until recently, been limited (6–8).

In addition, unlike in excisional biopsy, the aim of SCNB is to sample rather than completely remove the mammographic abnormality. Therefore, the potential exists for the lesion to change during follow-up, which at times prompts repeat biopsy. Follow-up mammograms are necessary to determine the stability of the remaining lesion in those cases in which SCNB yields benign histologic findings. The optimal mammographic follow-up strategy for these cases is yet to be determined, to our knowledge. The best strategy would balance the need for detecting false-negative cases as soon as possible against the inconvenience and added cost of short-interval follow-up examinations. The reported follow-up protocol for cases with benign results of SCNB varies, with some

Author contributions:
Guarantor of integrity of entire study, C.H.L.; study concepts, C.H.L., I.T.; study design, C.H.L.; definition of intellectual content, C.H.L.; literature research, C.H.L.; clinical studies, C.H.L., L.E.P., L.J.H., I.T.; experimental studies, C.H.L., L.E.P., L.J.H., I.T.; data analysis, C.H.L.; statistical analysis, C.H.L.; manuscript preparation, C.H.L.; manuscript editing, C.H.L., L.E.P., L.J.H., I.T.; manuscript review, L.E.P., L.J.H., I.T.

TABLE 1
Masses That Changed by Follow-up Mammography

Case No.	SCNB Histologic Results	Timing of Change (mo)	Change	Management	Biopsy or Follow-up Result
1	Fibroadenoma	12	Increase from 1.5 to 2.0 cm	Excisional biopsy	Fibroadenoma with atypia
2	Fibroadenoma	18	Increase from 1.2 to 1.7 cm	Excisional biopsy	Fibroadenoma
3	Fibroadenoma	18	Palpable, increase from 2.0 to 3.0 cm	Excisional biopsy	Fibroadenoma
4	Fibroadenoma	19	Increase from 1.2 to 1.8 cm	Mammographic follow-up	Decrease to 1.5 cm at 36 mo
5	Fibroadenoma	18	Increase from 1.9 to 2.3 cm	Excisional biopsy	Fibroadenoma
6	Fibroadenoma	6	Increase from 2.5 to 2.9 cm	Excisional biopsy	Fibroadenoma
7	Fibroadenoma	24	Increase from 0.8 to 1.3 cm	Excisional biopsy	Nonspecific benign result
8	Nonspecific benign result	20	Increase from 0.5 to 0.7 cm	Excisional biopsy	Nonspecific benign result
9	Nonspecific benign result	6	Increase from 1.1 to 1.2 cm, spiculated margins	Excisional biopsy	Invasive ductal carcinoma

recommending short-interval follow-up for all such cases (6) and others recommending 12-month follow-up for all cases (9) or 6-month follow-up for some cases with benign results and 12-month follow-up for others (10).

The purpose of this study was to determine how often lesions diagnosed as benign with SCNB change at follow-up mammography, which type of lesion is likely to change, and when the change occurs in these lesions. This information should help determine the optimum management strategy for cases with benign results of SCNB and help determine the delayed false-negative rate among these cases.

MATERIALS AND METHODS

All cases in which SCNB was performed at our facility during the 41 months from July 1992 through December 1995 for which benign results were obtained and for which the management recommendation was follow-up mammography were tracked to determine outcome. Biopsy was performed with a dedicated prone stereotactic table (Stereoguide; LoRad, Danbury, Conn) by using an automated biopsy device (Biopty; Bard Urological, Covington, Ga) and a 14-gauge needle (Biopty-Cut; Bard Urological). The technique of SCNB as performed at our facility has been previously described (10). The mean number of passes was six for all cases, with a mean of five for masses or seven for calcifications.

During the study, 540 SCNB procedures were performed at our facility in 472 patients. The patients were aged 31–84 years, with a mean age of 54 years. In 367 of the 540 biopsies (68%), benign histologic results were obtained for which the management recommendation was either short-interval or routine yearly mammographic follow-up. In 12 of these cases, the patient underwent further surgery despite the recommendation for mammographic follow-up. In five cases, this was done because of the patient's and/or the referring physician's unwillingness to accept the results of the SCNB. In another four cases, the lesion was excised along with a second lesion in proximity in the same breast, which was excised because of a diagnosis of atypical hyperplasia or because an insufficient sample was obtained at SCNB. In three cases, the lesion was removed when a malignancy elsewhere in the same breast was excised. Of the remaining 355 biopsies, 298 (84%) have mammographic follow-up information available.

Follow-up information was obtained through May 1998 from computerized mammography records at our facility, from outside facilities, from the referring physician, or from the patient herself. Follow-up examination was performed at our institution in 231 of the 298 cases (78%). In the remaining 67 cases (22%), follow-up mammograms were obtained at a number of outside facilities.

A substantial change in the mammographic appearance was defined as an increase in size for masses or an increase in number for calcifications and/or a more suspicious morphology for both masses and calcifications. In cases in which a substantial change was reported, the original and follow-up mammograms were obtained and independently reviewed by one of the authors (C.H.L.) for the initial mammographic finding, the type and magnitude of change, and the interval between the SCNB and the mammographic change. Lesion size was recorded as the greatest diameter among the three dimensions. The histologic results of tissue obtained at the time of initial SCNB and subsequent biopsy were noted.

At our facility, short-interval follow-up mammography is usually recommended despite lesions in which a nonspecific benign result concordant with the mammographic impression is obtained. Our short-interval follow-up protocol consists of a unilateral mammographic examination at 6 months, then bilateral diagnostic mammographic examinations at 12 and 24 months. If stability is documented at these examinations, the patient is advised to resume routine yearly screening at 36 months. When the lesion that is being followed up consists of calcifications, magnification views are usually obtained. When SCNB yields a specific benign result that is concordant with the mammographic finding, the management recommendation is usually screening mammography at 1 year. Immediate biopsy is recommended for benign results when atypical hyperplasia, lobular carcinoma in situ, radial scar, or insufficient material is obtained or when there is a perceived discrepancy between the mammographic impression and the histologic result or when the pathologist recommends that more tissue be obtained for a definitive diagnosis.

Histologic results considered to be nonspecific benign findings include fibrocystic changes, apocrine metaplasia, benign breast tissue, and fibrous breast tissue. Specific benign diagnoses include fibroadenoma, lymph node, and cyst. The categories of specific and nonspecific benign findings serve as general guidelines for management decisions, and the final recommendations are made after consideration of the histologic, mammographic, and clinical features of each case. Therefore, occasionally, when a nonspecific benign result is obtained but the level of suspicion based on the mammographic finding is low, a 12-month follow-up examination might be recommended.

Patients in whom no mammographic follow-up or less than 12 months of mammographic follow-up was obtainable were cross-referenced with the Connecticut Tu-

TABLE 2
Calcifications That Changed by Follow-up Mammography

Case No.	SCNB Histologic Results	Timing of Change (mo)	Management	Biopsy or Follow-up Result
1	Fibroadenoma	24	Excisional biopsy	Fibroadenoma
2	Fibroadenoma	17	Mammographic follow-up	No change at 30 months
3	Fibroadenoma	33	Repeat SCNB	Fibroadenoma
4	Nonspecific benign result	55	Excisional biopsy	Nonspecific benign result
5	Sclerosing adenosis	12	Excisional biopsy	Sclerosing adenosis
6	Nonspecific benign result	21	Excisional biopsy	Papilloma
7	Nonspecific benign result	18	Excisional biopsy	Fibroadenoma
8	Nonspecific benign result	36	Repeat SCNB	Nonspecific benign result
9	Nonspecific benign result	13	Mammographic follow-up	No change at 24 months
10	Nonspecific benign result	12	Excisional biopsy	Papilloma
11	Nonspecific benign result	12	Excisional biopsy	Atypical lobular hyperplasia
12	Nonspecific benign result	24	Excisional biopsy	Ductal carcinoma in situ with microinvasion

mor Registry (Connecticut Department of Public Health, Hartford) to attempt to identify possible cases of breast cancer that may have been diagnosed subsequent to the SCNB. The total number of malignancies diagnosed in all patients who underwent SCNB during the study was determined to calculate the false-negative rate. The Student *t* test was used to compare differences in the timing of change of masses and of calcifications.

RESULTS

Of the 298 cases in this series for which mammographic follow-up findings are available, 179 (60%) manifested mammographically as masses, 106 (36%) manifested as calcifications, and 13 (4%) manifested as masses with associated calcifications. Nonspecific benign results were obtained at SCNB in 192 cases (64%), fibroadenoma was found in 85 (29%), and other specific benign results were found in 21 (7%). The management recommendation was for short-interval follow-up mammography in 180 (60%) and for yearly screening mammography in 118 (40%).

For the 298 cases, the duration of mammographic follow-up was 5–65 months, with a mean of 33 months. Mammographic follow-up of 22 months or longer or histologic results of repeat biopsy were available for 253 cases (85%). Of the 45 cases with less than 22 months of follow-up, 25 were masses, 19 were calcifications, and one was a mass with calcifications. Seven of these had follow-up of 5–11 months, 20 had follow-up of 12–17 months, and the remaining 18 had follow-up of 18–21 months. Among the 180 cases in which short-interval mammography was recommended, mammography was performed in 110 (61%) within 9 months of the SCNB procedure. Among the 118 cases in which follow-up mammography at 12 months was recommended, mammography was performed in 69 (58%) within 15 months of the biopsy. In 169 (57%) of the 298 cases, at the time this article was written, either 3 years of mammographic follow-up had been completed or the recommended follow-up was being complied with.

Twenty-one (7%) of the 298 cases showed a substantial change on follow-up mammograms. These included 12 cases of calcifications, which represented 11% of all of the cases of calcifications for which follow-up information was available, and nine masses, which represented 5% of the masses in this series. Details of these 21 cases are presented in Tables 1 and 2. The ages of the women in whom the lesions changed ranged from 31 to 74 years, with a mean age of 48 years. The mammographic change in all of the cases of calcifications was an increase in the number of calcifications. None of the cases with an increased number of calcifications showed a more suspicious morphology. All of the masses that changed increased in size, with the amount of increase ranging from 1 to 10 mm and a mean change of 4.7 mm. One mass became palpable and increased in size at 18 months. One mass increased only minimally in size but became more spiculated.

In 10 of the 21 (48%) cases that changed, the histologic diagnosis of the sample obtained at SCNB was fibroadenoma. These 10 cases constitute 12% of all fibroadenomas diagnosed with SCNB in this series. The 10 patients with these 10 cases were aged 33–74 years, with a mean age of 46 years. Five of the 10 patients were younger than 40 years, and an additional three were younger than 50 years. Eight of the 10 were premenopausal. One of the two postmenopausal patients was receiving hormone replacement therapy. The mammographic finding in this patient was an enlarging mass. The second postmenopausal woman was not receiving estrogen, but the only finding on her mammogram was calcifications that increased in number. Of the remaining 11 cases that changed during follow-up, 10 had nonspecific benign histologic results of SCNB and one had a papilloma.

In 18 of the 21 cases that changed, repeat biopsy was performed. The correlation between SCNB histologic results and the repeat biopsy results in these cases is detailed in Table 3. Representative cases are shown in Figures 1 and 2. In two cases, repeat SCNB was performed and again yielded benign results. In both these cases, continued mammographic stability has been documented for 9 and 15 months at the time this article was written.

Excisional biopsy was performed in the remaining 16 cases. Two of the cases that changed were found to be malignant with repeat biopsy. The first case was a lobulated mass in a 48-year-old woman that had yielded a nonspecific benign diagnosis with SCNB. At the 6-month mammographic follow-up examination, the mass appeared only minimally increased in size, but the margins were more irregular. Excisional biopsy results showed a 1.2-cm invasive ductal carcinoma. Axillary lymph nodes in this patient were negative. The second case that had malignant repeat biopsy results manifested mammographically as calcifications. This case is illustrated in Figure 3.

The remaining 16 cases in which repeat biopsy was performed were benign. In three of the 21 cases that changed, continued mammographic surveillance rather than repeat biopsy was elected by the patient and/or her referring physician. In the first case, which manifested as calcifications at mammography and which had a nonspecific benign diagnosis, no further increase was shown after an additional 11 months of follow-up, for a total follow-up of 24 months. In the second case, which also manifested as calcifications, a fibroadenoma was diagnosed with SCNB, and there was no further increase in the number of calcifications after an additional 13 months of follow-up, for a total follow-up of 30 months. In the third case, a mass was diagnosed as a fibroadenoma at core biopsy. It had enlarged at 19 months but had decreased in size at 36 months of follow-up.

The interval between the SCNB and mammographic change for the 21 cases was 6–55 months, with a mean of 20 months. The time of the first mammographic follow-up examination for the 21 cases ranged from 5 to 29 months, with a mean of 13 months. Ten of the 21 cases showed either a decrease in the size of the mass or in the number of calcifications or no change on the first follow-up mammogram but an increase on a subsequent mammogram. The time in which masses changed was 6–24 months, with a mean of 16 months. The time in which calcifications changed was 12–55 months, with a mean of 23 months. This difference was not statistically significant (P = .129). None of the cases manifesting as calcifications changed before 12 months, including the one false-negative case. Of the nine masses, two changed at 6 months, including the false-negative case. The second mass that changed at 6 months was a cellular fibroadenoma, which was diagnosed with SCNB. In this case, a 6-month follow-up examination was recommended despite the specific benign result because of the cellularity of the lesion. None of the masses changed after 24 months.

Cross-reference with the Connecticut Tumor Registry did not reveal any cases of breast carcinoma diagnosed among the 64 women in our series for whom no mammographic follow-up or less than 12 months of follow-up information was available. Of the 540 SCNB procedures performed during the study, 105 (19%) revealed malignancy. Ninety-two of these cancers were diagnosed initially with SCNB. Thirteen were diagnosed with excisional biopsy immediately following the SCNB procedure because of insufficient sampling (three cases) or a high-risk lesion such as atypical hyperplasia (10 cases). The other two cases were those described in this report in which the diagnosis was made after a mammographic change at 6 and 24 months. If only these two cases are considered to be delayed false-negative cases, the delayed false-negative rate for our series was 2% (two of 105).

TABLE 3
Histologic Results at SCNB and Repeat Biopsy for Lesions That Changed

No. of Cases (n = 18)	Mammographic Findings	SCNB Histologic Results	Repeat Biopsy Histologic Results
5	Mass	Fibroadenoma	Fibroadenoma
1	Mass	Fibroadenoma	Nonspecific benign result
1	Mass	Nonspecific benign result	Nonspecific benign result
1	Mass	Nonspecific benign result	Invasive ductal carcinoma
3	Calcifications	Nonspecific benign result	Nonspecific benign result
2	Calcifications	Fibroadenoma	Fibroadenoma
2	Calcifications	Nonspecific benign result	Papilloma
1	Calcifications	Nonspecific benign result	Fibroadenoma
1	Calcifications	Nonspecific benign result	Atypical lobular hyperplasia
1	Calcifications	Nonspecific benign result	Ductal carcinoma in situ with microinvasion

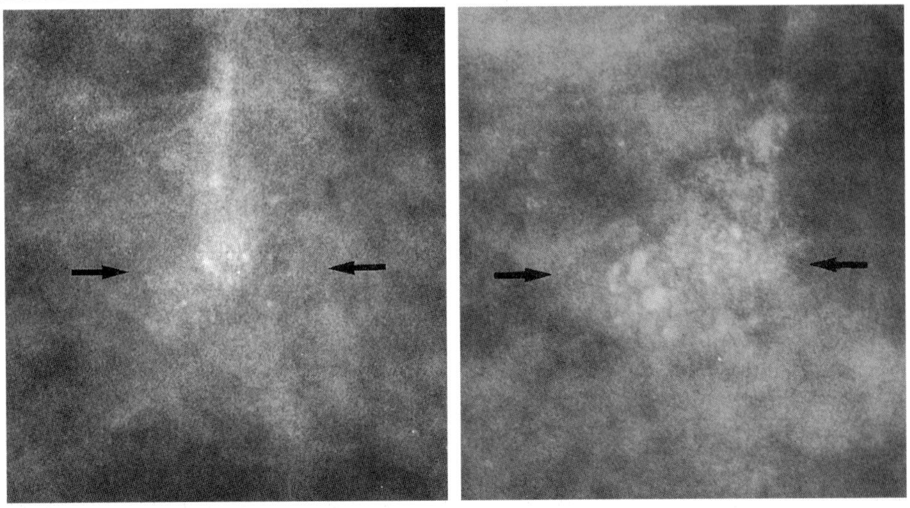

a. b.

Figure 1. Increase in the number of calcifications. **(a)** Magnification craniocaudal view from a mammogram in a 47-year-old woman shows clustered pleomorphic microcalcifications (arrows). SCNB histologic analysis revealed fibrocystic change and ductal hyperplasia, with no evidence of malignancy. Microcalcifications were seen in nonproliferative lobules. **(b)** Magnification craniocaudal view from the same area on a mammogram obtained 36 months after the original SCNB shows an increase in the number of microcalcifications (arrows). Repeat SCNB yielded blunt ductal adenosis with microcalcifications.

DISCUSSION

Among the 298 cases in this series that yielded benign results and for which the management recommendation was follow-up mammography, 21 (7%) changed on subsequent mammograms and repeat biopsy was performed in 18 (6%). These results are similar to those recently reported by Jackman et al (8). In their series, 26 (9%) of 295 lesions that had yielded benign results of SCNB showed progression at mammographic follow-up. In their series, 12% of calcifications and 5% of masses showed progression, which is also similar to our findings of substantial change in 11% of calcifications and 5% of masses.

A large percentage of the lesions that changed in our series (48%) were determined with histologic SCNB findings to be fibroadenomas. When a previously diagnosed fibroadenoma increases in size, the possibility that it actually represents a phyllodes tumor or that a malignancy is present within or adjacent to the fibroadenoma must be considered (11,12). However, these entities are relatively rare, whereas growth of fibroadenomas has been well described (13–15). Meyer et al (14) reported mammographically documented growth in 22 of 254 fibroadenomas (9%) that were subsequently excised, and, in another series (15),

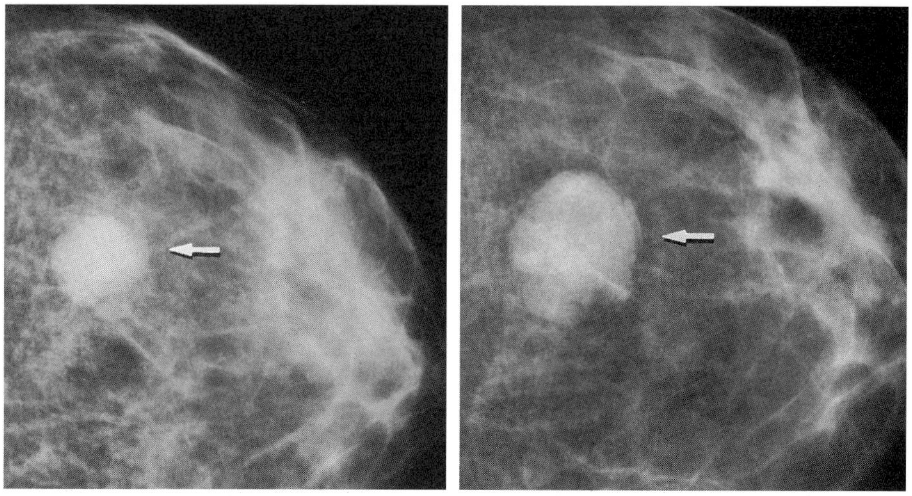

a. b.

Figure 2. Increase in the size of a mass. **(a)** Left craniocaudal mammogram shows a lobulated, 2-cm mass (arrow) in a 36-year-old woman. The mass was not palpable and was diagnosed as a fibroadenoma with SCNB. **(b)** Left craniocaudal mammogram obtained at 18 months after the biopsy shows that the mass (arrow), which was clinically palpable, has increased to 3 cm. Excisional biopsy revealed a fibroadenoma with no evidence of malignancy.

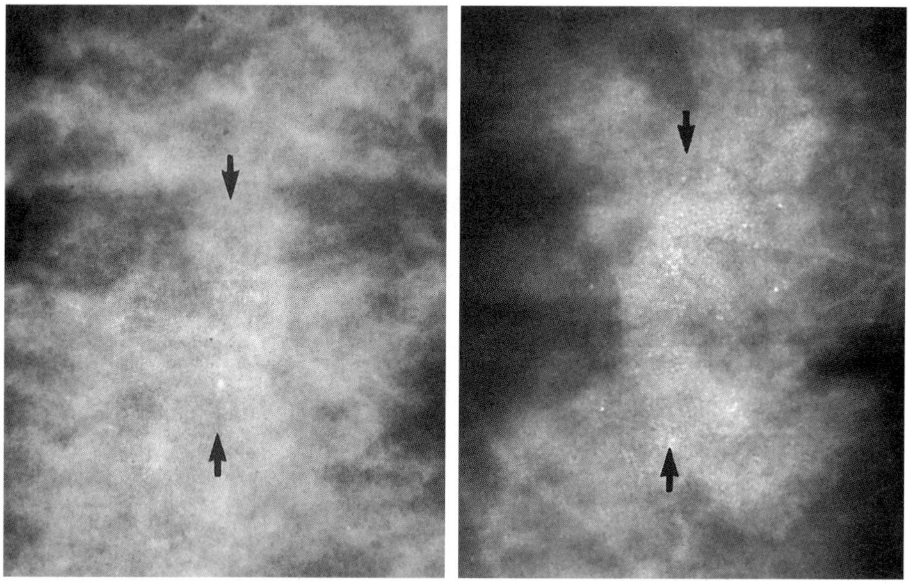

a. b.

Figure 3. False-negative case. **(a)** Magnification craniocaudal mammogram in a 45-year-old woman shows calcifications (arrows) in the right breast, which had nonspecific benign SCNB histologic results. Retrieval of calcifications was documented with radiography of specimens, and calcifications were seen on the histologic slides. On the first follow-up mammogram in this patient, which was obtained 11 months after SCNB, the number of calcifications at the biopsy site was decreased. **(b)** Magnification craniocaudal mammogram obtained at the 24-month follow-up examination, however, shows that calcifications (arrows) at the site are increased in number. Excisional biopsy revealed ductal carcinoma in situ with microinvasion.

four of 279 (1%) clinically palpable fibroadenomas increased in size and were subsequently excised.

Malignancy has not been diagnosed among our cases of fibroadenomas that changed, although one was found at excision to be associated with atypia within the fibroadenoma. Our series was too small to definitively conclude that repeat biopsy is unnecessary for lesions diagnosed as fibroadenomas with SCNB that have changed by follow-up mammography. However, findings in these cases suggest that continued short-interval mammographic follow-up may be a reasonable alternative to repeat biopsy in premenopausal women. Another alternative to excisional biopsy or continued mammographic surveillance for these women might be repeat SCNB with an 11-gauge vacuum-assisted device. Further studies are needed to determine if this is a valid management strategy.

Change on a follow-up mammogram occurred at 6 months in two cases manifesting mammographically as masses, including one of the false-negative cases. None of the cases of calcifications that were followed up showed an increase before 12 months, including the one false-negative case that was seen mammographically as calcifications. Three cases of calcifications changed after 24 months of follow-up, whereas none of the masses did. The difference in the mean time of change for masses and calcifications was not statistically significant.

Our results suggest that recommending 6-month follow-up mammography is a prudent course of action for noncalcified masses when nonspecific benign results are obtained with SCNB. Because the difference in the time of change for masses and calcifications was not significantly different, the recommendation in cases of calcifications that yield nonspecific benign results should probably also be 6-month follow-up mammography, despite the fact that none of the calcification cases in our series changed prior to 12 months.

Since none of the masses in our series changed after 24 months, our results suggest that women with masses who undergo short-interval follow-up can undergo yearly screening after 24 months of stability has been documented. The interval before routine yearly screening mammography can be recommended may need to be longer for calcifications, which usually require magnification views to be adequately followed up.

Our results show that stability or an actual decrease in size or number on the initial follow-up mammogram does not necessarily exclude change at a subsequent examination, nor does it exclude the presence of malignancy. In 11 (52%) of the 21 cases that changed in our series, the first postbiopsy mammogram showed stability, but change was found on a subsequent follow-up mammogram. This occurred in one of the false-negative cases that manifested as calcifications. The calcifications were actually decreased in number on the first follow-up mammogram obtained at 12 months but were increased in number at 24 months. This emphasizes the importance of continued follow-up of lesions diagnosed as benign with SCNB, particularly those that manifest mammographically as calcifications.

While the false-negative rate of SCNB as determined by means of correlation with immediate surgical excision has been evaluated by several investigators, reports of false-negative cases detected after mammographic follow-up rather than immediate surgery (the delayed false-negative rate) have, until recently, been limited (6–8,16,17). In a study (7) of 84 cases with benign SCNB results followed up clinically and mammographically for a mean of 24 months, no delayed false-negative cases were found.

In a multiinstitutional study, Parker et al (6) reported on 2,429 cases with at least 6 months of mammographic follow-up. Of these, 2,402 cases showed no change, 27 showed change at follow-up, and five malignancies were diagnosed. In addition, Parker et al (16) also reported an additional four cancers detected among their cases after an additional year of follow-up. The total length of follow-up was not specified in this report.

Fajardo (17) reported on three cases of malignancy diagnosed among a total of 400 cases, 271 of which were followed up mammographically for 2 years after a benign SCNB diagnosis. These false-negative cases were discovered at 6, 8, and 13 months after SCNB. It is difficult to precisely determine the false-negative rate in this report, as the total number of cancers diagnosed in the group was not explicitly given. In the series of Jackman et al (8), two of the 26 lesions that showed mammographic progression at follow-up were malignant at repeat biopsy. One was a mass that showed progression at 18 months and proved to be a stage I invasive ductal carcinoma, and the second was a cluster of calcifications that increased at 6 months and was diagnosed as ductal carcinoma in situ at repeat biopsy. Their delayed false-negative rate was 1.2% (two of 161 carcinomas).

We had a delayed false-negative rate of 2%. It is possible that additional malignancies have occurred among cases in our series for which no follow-up information is available. This is thought to be unlikely, however, given that no such cases have been identified by means of cross-reference with the Connecticut Tumor Registry. Malignancy may yet be diagnosed in those five cases in which repeat SCNB or continued mammographic follow-up examination rather than excisional biopsy was performed after mammographic change. However, this is thought to be unlikely given that continued mammographic stability has been documented in these cases. It is also possible that additional malignancies will eventually be identified among the 44 cases in our series with less than 22 months of follow-up.

Comparing the delayed false-negative rate for SCNB with that for excisional biopsy of nonpalpable breast lesions is problematic in that, in most series of needle-localized lesions in which excision is performed, unsuccessful excision rates are reported rather than actual false-negative rates based on long-term follow-up of cases in which unsuccessful excisional biopsy has been performed.

Jackman and Marzoni (18) recently reviewed this literature extensively. Misses at the time of excisional biopsy are often apparent on the radiograph of the specimen, and many patients in whom misses occur will undergo immediate repeat excision (19). However, radiographs of specimens are not always obtained and do not always reliably indicate if a lesion, particularly a noncalcified mass, has indeed been excised (20). It is likely that the delayed false-negative rate for needle-localized excisional biopsy, although very low, is not zero.

In the cases in our series, biopsy was performed with the 14-gauge automated biopsy device and a mean of only six passes per case. With the vacuum-assisted biopsy device, more tissue is usually removed (21), and it is possible that the optimal mammographic follow-up protocol for cases in which SCNB is performed with this technique will be different from that for cases in which biopsy is performed with the automated biopsy gun. Long-term follow-up studies are needed to determine this and to determine if the use of the vacuum-assisted device will decrease the delayed false-negative rate (22).

In conclusion, we found that 7% of cases that yielded benign results of SCNB had changed by follow-up mammography which prompted repeat biopsy in 6%. This was particularly likely in young women in whom a fibroadenoma was diagnosed with SCNB findings. The change did not necessarily occur on the first posttreatment mammogram and tended to occur later with calcifications rather than with masses, although the difference was not statistically significant. We found a 2% delayed false-negative rate after a mean of 33 months of mammographic follow-up. On the basis of our results, we believe that 6-month follow-up mammography for cases with nonspecific benign diagnoses and routine yearly screening mammography for cases with specific benign histologic results is a reasonable management strategy. Because the mammographic change sometimes occurred after the first follow-up examination, patients and referring physicians need to be aware of the importance of continued mammographic follow-up after a benign diagnosis is obtained with SCNB.

Acknowledgment: We thank Robert C. Lange, PhD, for his assistance in data analysis.

References

1. March DE, Raslavicus A, Coughlin BF, Klein SV, Makari-Judson G. Use of breast core biopsy in the United States: results of a national survey. AJR 1997; 169:697–701.
2. Parker SH, Lovin JD, Jobe WE, et al. Stereotactic breast biopsy with a biopsy gun. Radiology 1990; 176:741–747.
3. Dronkers DJ. Stereotaxic core biopsy of breast lesions. Radiology 1992; 183:631–634.
4. Elvecrog EL, Lechner MC, Nelson MT. Nonpalpable breast lesions: correlation of stereotaxic large-core needle biopsy and surgical biopsy results. Radiology 1993; 188:453–455.
5. Gisvold JJ, Goellner JR, Grant CS, et al. Breast biopsy: a comparative study of stereotaxically guided core and excisional techniques. AJR 1994; 162:815–820.
6. Parker SH, Burbank F, Jackman RJ, et al. Percutaneous large-core breast biopsy: a multi-institutional study. Radiology 1994; 193:359–364.
7. Head JF, Haynes AE, Elliott MC, Elliott RL. Stereotaxic localization and core needle biopsy of nonpalpable breast lesions: two-year follow-up of a prospective study. Am Surg 1996; 62:1018–1023.
8. Jackman RJ, Nowels KW, Rodriguez-Soto J, Marzoni FA, Finklestein SI, Shepard MJ. Stereotactic, automated, large-core needle biopsy of nonpalpable breast lesions: false-negative and histologic underestimation rates after long-term follow-up. Radiology 1999; 210:799–805.
9. Liberman L, Fahs MC, Dershaw DD, et al. Impact of stereotaxic core breast biopsy on cost of diagnosis. Radiology 1995; 195:633–637.
10. Mainiero MB, Philpotts LE, Lee CH, Lange RC, Carter D, Tocino I. Stereotaxic core needle biopsy of breast microcalcifications: correlation of target accuracy and diagnosis with lesion size. Radiology 1996; 198:665–669.
11. Dershaw DD, Morris EA, Liberman L, Abramson AF. Nondiagnostic stereotaxic core breast biopsy: results of rebiopsy. Radiology 1996; 198:323–325.
12. Pick PW, Iossifides IA. Occurrence of breast carcinoma within a fibroadenoma. Arch Pathol Lab Med 1984; 108:590–594.
13. Dixon JM. Cystic disease and fibroadenoma of the breast: natural history and relation to breast cancer risk. Br Med Bull 1991; 47:258–271.
14. Meyer JE, Frenna TH, Polger M, Sonnenfeld MR, Shaffer K. Enlarging occult fibroadenoma. Radiology 1992; 183:639–641.
15. Cant PJ, Madden MV, Coleman MG, Dent DM. Non-operative management of breast masses diagnosed as fibroadenoma. Br J Surg 1995; 82:792–794.
16. Parker SH, Burbank F, Jackman RJ, et al. Response to "Caution on core." Radiology 1994; 193:326–327.
17. Fajardo LL. Cost and efficacy trade-offs of stereotaxic core biopsy versus surgical biopsy of nonpalpable breast lesions (abstr). Radiology 1995; 197(P):203.
18. Jackman RJ, Marzoni FA. Needle-localized breast biopsy: why do we fail? Radiology 1997; 204:677–684.
19. Kopans DB. Caution on core. Radiology 1994; 193:325–326.
20. Hasselgren PO, Hummel RP, Georgian-Smith D, Fieler M. Breast biopsy with needle localization: accuracy of specimen x-ray and management of missed lesions. Surgery 1993; 114:836–842.
21. Burbank F, Parker S, Fogarty T. Stereotactic breast biopsy: improved tissue harvesting with the Mammotome. Am Surg 1996; 62:738–744.
22. Jackman RJ, Marzoni FA Jr, Nowels KW. Percutaneous removal of benign mammographic lesions: comparison of automated large-core and directional vacuum-assisted stereotactic biopsy techniques. AJR 1998; 171:1325–1330.

Chandu Karadi, PhD
Christopher F. Beaulieu, MD, PhD
R. Brooke Jeffrey, Jr, MD
David S. Paik, MS
Sandy Napel, PhD

Index terms:
Computed tomography (CT), image display and recording, 75.12115, 75.12117
Computed tomography (CT), three-dimensional, 75.12117
Computers, simulation
Colon, CT, 75.12111, 75.12115, 75.12117
Colon, neoplasms, 75.3119

Radiology 1999; 212:195–201

Abbreviations:
ROC = receiver operating characteristic
2D = two-dimensional
3D = three-dimensional

[1] From the Departments of Medicine (C.K., D.S.P.) and Radiology (C.F.B., R.B.J., S.N.), Stanford University School of Medicine, Lucas MRS Center P-268, Stanford, CA 94305-5488. Received July 20, 1998; revision requested September 24; revision received November 18; accepted January 11, 1999. Supported in part by National Institutes of Health grants 1R01 CA72023, 1P41 RR09784-01, and LM 07033, the Packard Foundation (Los Altos, Calif), the Lucas Foundation (Menlo Park, Calif), and the Phil N. Allen Trust (Menlo Park, Calif). C.F.B. is a 1997 RSNA Scholar. C.K. is a 1998 GENDEX/RSNA Medical Student/Scholar Assistant. **Address reprint requests to** S.N. (e-mail: *snapel@stanford.edu*).

See also the article by Beaulieu et al (pp 203–212) in this issue.

Author contributions:
Guarantors of integrity of entire study, C.F.B., S.N.; study concepts and design, C.F.B., C.K.; definition of intellectual content, C.F.B., C.K., S.N.; literature research, C.F.B., C.K.; experimental studies, C.F.B., R.B.J., C.K.; data acquisition, D.S.P., C.K.; data analysis, C.K., C.F.B.; statistical analysis, C.F.B., C.K.; manuscript preparation, C.K., C.F.B., S.N.; manuscript editing, R.B.J., D.S.P.; manuscript review, all authors.

Display Modes for CT Colonography

Part I. Synthesis and Insertion of Polyps into Patient CT Data[1]

PURPOSE: To develop and validate a method for the insertion of digitally synthesized polyps into computed tomographic (CT) images of the human colon for use as ground truth for evaluation of virtual colonoscopy.

MATERIALS AND METHODS: Spiral CT simulator software was used to generate 10 synthetic polyps in various configurations. Additional software was developed to insert these polyps into volume CT scans. Ten polyps in eight patients were selected for comparison. Three radiologists evaluated whether two-dimensional (2D) CT images and three-dimensional (3D) volume-rendered CT images showed synthetic or real polyps.

RESULTS: Edge-response profiles and noise of simulated polyps matched those of native polyps. Frequency distributions of reviewers' responses were not significantly different for synthetic versus real polyps in either 3D or 2D images. Responses were clustered around the response of "unsure" if lesions were real or synthetic. Receiver operating characteristic curves had areas of 0.54 (95% CI = 0.39, 0.68) for 3D and 0.39 (95% CI = 0.25, 0.53) for 2D images, which were not significantly different from random guessing (P = .70 and .28 for 3D and 2D images, respectively).

CONCLUSION: Synthetic polyps were indistinguishable from real polyps. This method can be used to generate ground truth experimental data for comparison of CT colonographic display and detection methods.

Computed tomographic (CT) colonography, also known as virtual colonoscopy, is a promising technique for detection of colonic polyps. Initial results (1) have indicated that the majority of clinically important lesions can be detected; however, there is a wide variety of data review methods ("display modes"), and the most accurate and efficient means of interpreting the acquired CT data has yet to be determined.

Thus far, most investigators (2–5) have used a combination of two-dimensional (2D) and three-dimensional (3D) display modes. When 2D and 3D modes are used together in an unblinded fashion, it is difficult or impossible to establish accurately the relative diagnostic contribution of each mode. The authors of one initial study (2) suggested that 3D display added incremental value over 2D display alone, by increasing the sensitivity for lesion detection. However, more recent data (6,7) suggest that 2D display of "source" axial CT images alone may be sufficiently sensitive for lesion detection.

Several 3D display methods have been used (8–12), and more are under development. These approaches differ from one another not only in terms of the way the images are presented but also in their relative computational complexity and efficiency of viewing. Thus, an important remaining issue in the development of CT colonography for application to screening populations is to determine an efficient yet accurate means of reviewing the acquired image data for the detection of colonic polyps.

To optimize these display tools, a large number of data sets with known true polyps are needed. Typically, one compares CT colonographic images with fiberoptic colonoscopic images, the current reference standard, in the same patients. There are a number of difficulties with this approach. In screening populations, few patients have lesions in the clinically relevant size range of larger than 1 cm in diameter (1). In addition, fiberoptic colonoscopy is less than perfect, in part because the instrument fails to reach the cecum 5%–10% of the time (13). The colon also "telescopes" during the procedure, which makes precise reconciliation of CT findings with fiberoptic colonoscopic findings difficult. Last, because only a small number of lesions are available, radiologists may be able to recall specific lesions seen with different display modes according to shape or local surroundings and, hence, bias results.

A reference standard better than that available with fiberoptic colonoscopy and a large collection of polyps are needed for rigorous evaluation and optimization of CT colonography. The purpose of our study was to develop and validate a method for the generation and insertion of digitally synthesized polyps into CT images of the human colon for use as ground truth in evaluations of virtual colonoscopy. In this article, we describe and evaluate our method, which allows generation of realistic polyps of various sizes and shapes that can be placed anywhere inside a patient's CT-imaged colon. This high degree of control over polyp characteristics allows the generation of multiple phantom CT data sets, which can then be used for systematic evaluation of the trade-offs among the many display techniques currently under investigation for CT colonography. Such an approach can help determine which display method, if any, will prove to be a feasible clinical tool.

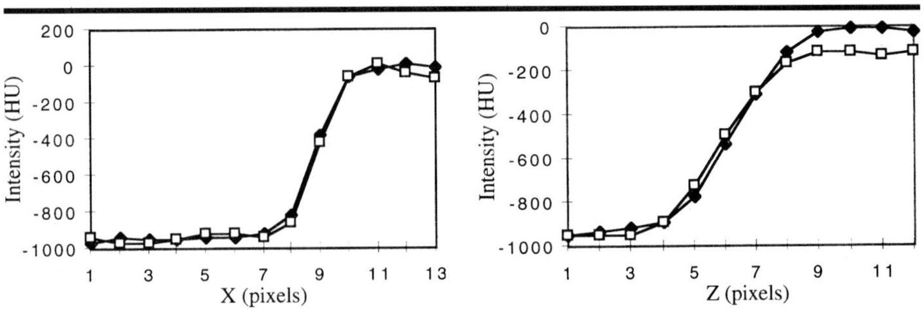

a. b.

Figure 1. Graphs show **(a)** in-plane and **(b)** longitudinal profiles of CT intensity of a synthetic polyp (◆) and the edge of patient's colon (□) as a function of pixel location (*X* in **a**, *Z* in **b**). As one moves from the lumen (air attenuation, −1,000 HU) to the polyp or colonic wall (soft-tissue attenuation, approximately 50 HU), the slope of the line describing the change in attenuation is determined by either in-plane or through-plane partial volume averaging. By matching the input parameters of the CT simulator with those of the base data, closely matched profiles can be obtained.

MATERIALS AND METHODS

Our study involved three phases: (*a*) collection of CT image data in patients undergoing CT colonography, (*b*) synthesis and insertion of polyps into one of the patient data sets, and (*c*) a validation study to compare the synthetic polyps with real lesions.

CT Colonographic Acquisition

For this study, we selected CT colonographic data sets obtained in eight patients (five men, three women; mean age, 56 years; age range, 30–75 years); the data sets were part of a separate ongoing clinical trial (4), approved by our institutional review board, to compare CT colonography and fiberoptic colonoscopy. In all participants, previous sigmoidoscopic results were positive, and the participants had been referred for fiberoptic colonoscopy.

Prior to CT, patients underwent standard precolonoscopy cleansing with a solution of polyethylene glycol and electrolytes (GoLYTELY; Braintree Laboratories, Braintree, Mass). After informed consent had been obtained, CT was performed (CT HiSpeed Advantage scanner; GE Medical Systems, Milwaukee, Wis) at 120 kVp, 200 mA, 3-mm collimation, and 6 mm/sec table speed (pitch, 2.0). The patient was in the supine position, and air insufflation of the colon was performed. Patients were instructed to hold their breath as long as comfortably possible, with quiet breathing, if necessary, during the later part of the study, which covered the pelvic region. CT scanning extended from the dome of the diaphragm to the pubic symphysis, with a total acquisition time of 60 seconds.

Scans were reconstructed at 1-mm intervals with a display field of view of 36–40 cm by using the manufacturer's standard soft-tissue reconstruction algorithm. All images were reconstructed with a 512 × 512 matrix, which resulted in an in-plane pixel size of 0.625–0.703 mm. Reconstructed image data sets were transferred to the Stanford University Department of Radiology 3D Medical Imaging Laboratory.

A positive CT finding for at least one polyp was obtained in each of the eight patients included in this study, and the CT finding was directly correlated with a positive finding at fiberoptic colonoscopy. We selected imaging data from one of the eight patients (a 60-year-old man), hereafter referred to as the "base" data set, for synthetic polyp insertion. For comparison, we chose 10 regions that contained a single true polyp from the data sets obtained in the other seven patients. These 10 polyps were sessile, with various shapes and sizes between 8 and 13 mm.

CT Simulator Parameters

Parameter	Value
Source-to-isocenter distance (mm)	630
Source-to-detector distance (mm)	1,099.3
Height and width of source (mm)	1.2
No. of detectors	852
Height of detector (mm)	3
Width of detector (mm)	1.139
Collimation width (mm)	3
Table speed (mm/sec)	6
Projections per gantry rotation	1,000
Reconstruction algorithm	Helical extrapolative
Reconstruction grid	32 × 32
Field of view (mm)	22.5
In-plane pixel size (mm)	0.703 × 0.703
Reconstruction interval (mm)	1

Creation of Phantom Data

All software was implemented on workstations (O2; Silicon Graphics, Mountain View, Calif) equipped with an R10000 processor and 256 Mbyte of main memory. All volume rendering was performed by using VoxelView software (version 2.5.4; Vital Images, Minneapolis, Minn).

Polyp synthesis.—To create the synthetic polyps, we used a software spiral CT simulator. This simulator allows one to define the shape of an object with geometric primitives and generates projection data and CT reconstructions by using configurable scanner geometry, acquisition parameters, and reconstruction

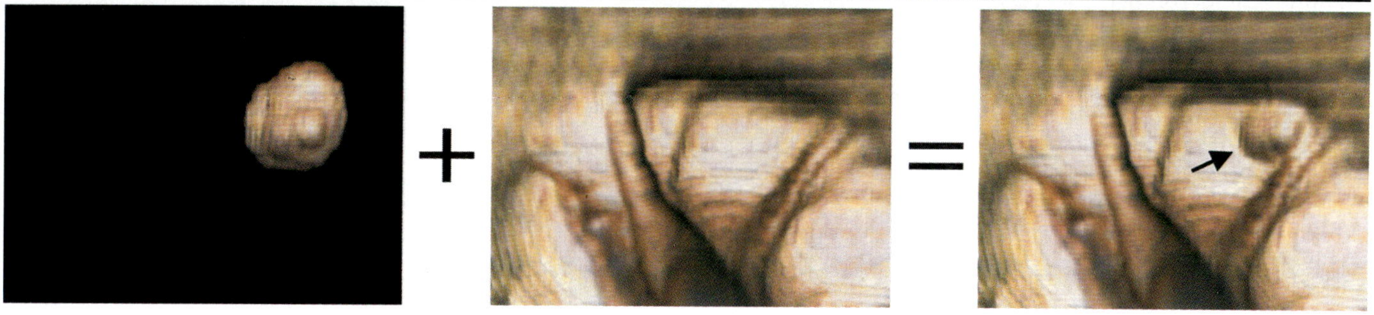

a. b. c.

Figure 2. Three volume-rendered images illustrate creation of phantom data. **(a)** A synthetic free-standing polyp is inserted, or composited (+), into **(b)** polyp-free patient colon data, which results (=) in **(c)** a new colon data set with a polyp (arrow). These images are 2D renderings of the component parts **a** and **b** and the result **c**.

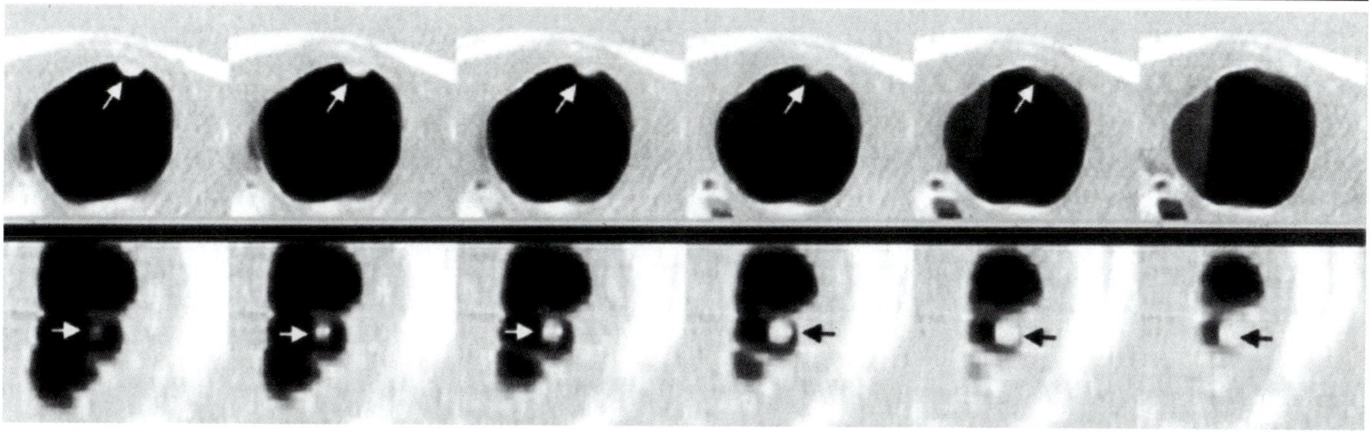

Figure 3. Top: Axial CT sections separated by 1-mm increments through a 10-mm synthetic spherical polyp (arrow). Bottom: Coronal CT sections separated by 0.7-mm increments through the same 10-mm synthetic polyp (arrow).

parameters. We configured the simulator parameters to match those of the CT scanner used to acquire the patient data (Table). Because polyps are small, however, we needed to simulate only those projections that covered a small field of view (22.5 mm) and to reconstruct the images with a 32 × 32 matrix. The resultant in-plane pixel size (0.703 × 0.703 mm) matched that of the base data set we chose for synthetic polyp insertion. In addition, the simulator allowed specification of the variance of a Poisson noise source to be added to the detector measurements, thereby correlating the noise in the reconstructed images in a manner similar to that in reconstructions obtained with actual CT scanners. We adjusted the Poisson noise variance empirically, so that the SDs in regions of interest in the polyps were in the same range as similar measurements made in soft tissue in the base data (approximately 15–25 HU).

To synthesize a polyp, the user defines the CT attenuation value and shape of the polyp. Polyp attenuation was assigned to that of soft tissue. Measurements of attenuation in native polyps ranged from −100 to +70 HU, depending on the size of the lesion and the amount of partial volume averaging with adjacent air. For simulation, a starting attenuation of 0 HU was used. This value was modified by 25–50 HU, as necessary, to match the final attenuation profile with that of real lesions or the air–colonic wall interface.

The shape of each polyp was defined by using a combination of geometric primitives, such as ellipsoids, cylinders, and cones. By using combinations of such primitives, lesions of nearly any shape could be constructed, the simplest being a single sphere. Lesions with a cylindric base and a hemispheric cap were constructed by simulating scans of an object represented by the union of a cylinder and a sphere. Nodular, grossly hemispheric lesions were constructed by simulating scans of an object represented by the union of one large sphere (approximately 10 mm in diameter) and multiple smaller spheres (2–3 mm in diameter) arranged around the surface of the large sphere. We simulated the CT scans of each user-defined polyp and reconstructed 30 cross sections (to cover 30 mm) through each lesion.

Each voxel in the reconstructed volume contained a 16-bit integer value that corresponded to the CT intensity (in Hounsfield units) of the scanned polyp. The polyp was inserted into the patient's colon data by using the algorithm described in the next paragraph.

Polyp insertion.—We developed a software package that allows the user to insert a synthetic polyp into a volume CT study. The key features of the insertion algorithm are that it allows (*a*) smooth insertion of the synthetic polyp into patient data and (*b*) maintenance of the partial volume effects and noise in the synthetic polyp and original patient data. The insertion algorithm operates on a voxel-by-voxel basis by using either direct voxel replacement or nonlinear addition with no spatial averaging.

To understand the insertion algorithm, consider a fixed location in the original patient data with a voxel CT intensity I_P. At the corresponding location in the synthetic polyp data set, there will be a voxel

CT intensity I_S. The insertion algorithm combines I_P and I_S into a final voxel intensity I_F. There are two cases to consider, depending on whether the patient voxel definitely lies inside soft tissue. When $I_P > 0.95 \times I_A$, where I_A is the average CT intensity of the tissue surrounding the air-filled lumen, we can be fairly certain that the voxel lies within tissue; in this case, we set $I_F = I_P$. When $I_P \leq 0.95 \times I_A$, we assume that the voxel is fully or partially in the air-filled lumen; in this case we set $I_F = I_S + I_P - I_S \times I_P/I_A$.

This method, known as compositing, is commonly used in computer graphics for smoothly blending two images together (14). Note that when I_S and I_P are small, I_F is approximately equal to the sum of I_S and I_P. When I_S and/or I_P is nearly equal to I_A, I_F is saturated at the expected value I_A. This saturation, though, leads to a substantial reduction in the noise in those voxels for which both I_S and I_P are large. We therefore compensated for this effect by adding spatially correlated noise weighted by the factor $[2 - (1 - I_P/I_A)^2 - (1 - I_S/I_A)^2]^{1/2}$. Note that when I_S and I_P are small, the weight is small, and little noise is added. The compensation increases, however, as I_S and I_P approach I_A. The correlated noise source was created by simulating a large spherical object with the CT simulator.

Quantification of polyp edge profiles and comparison with features of the base CT data were performed by using software (NIH IMAGE; National Institutes of Health. Available at: *http://rsb.info.nih.gov/nih-image/*. Accessed January 10, 1998.) and various models of Macintosh desktop computers (Apple Computers, Cupertino, Calif). Profiles of image intensity versus pixel number were generated in both the in-plane and the through-plane directions. Through-plane intensity profiles were generated from sagittal or coronal reformatted images created with VOXELVIEW. Note that the intensity profile obtained at the traversal from air to soft tissue, such as that encountered at the normal colonic wall, should be analogous to the profile obtained at the traversal from air to a polyp with soft-tissue attenuation. Intensity profiles with which synthetic lesions were compared with features of the native colon were inspected visually, and iterative adjustments were made in the simulation parameters to minimize observed differences between the profiles.

To determine how the polyp synthesis and insertion techniques work in a simple case, consider a 10-mm spherical polyp that was generated as described earlier.

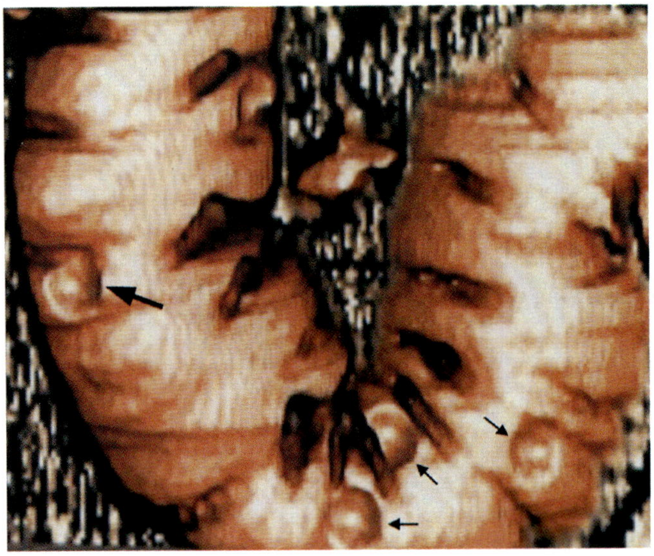

Figure 4. A 3D volume-rendered view of four 10-mm polyps (arrows), including the polyp (large arrow) shown in Figure 3, placed in patient colon data.

Figure 1 shows representative in-plane and longitudinal profiles for the air-tissue interfaces in both a patient colon and a synthetic polyp. This particular polyp required 30 seconds of computation time to be generated. (More complex shapes may take up to 2 minutes.) One can clearly see that the profiles of the air-tissue and air-polyp interfaces agreed well in both the in-plane and the longitudinal directions, with the 10%–90% transition occurring over 2.1 pixels (1.5 mm) in-plane, and 3.7 pixels (3.7 mm) longitudinally. These results show that partial volume effects can be accurately simulated with our system, and the same degree of edge blurring in synthetic lesions as in native tissue-air interfaces in the base colon data can be provided. This modeling is necessary to eliminate spurious visual cues such as overly sharp edges when viewing simulated lesions in polyp detection trials.

Once the polyp is simulated, it can be inserted into the colon by using the previously described algorithm. Figure 2 illustrates the process of creation and insertion of synthetic polyps with three volume-rendered images: a synthetic polyp consisting of four intersecting ellipsoids (Fig 2a), the region of the colon chosen for polyp insertion (Fig 2b), and the same region after polyp insertion (Fig 2c). Figure 3 demonstrates the result of this process with axial and coronal CT images. The top panel shows a series of axial CT sections at 1-mm increments through a 10-mm polyp. From left to right, one sees the appearance of the haustral fold as it smoothly blends into the polyp. The bottom panel in Figure 3 shows a series of coronal sections through the same polyp. From left to right (in 0.7-mm increments), the polyp appearance changes from fully detached in the air space to smoothly embedded in the tissue.

Figure 4 shows a 3D volume-rendered view of four 10-mm-diameter polyps. The specific polyp we have been discussing is shown on the left side, next to a haustral fold. There are three other 10-mm polyps on the lower right side to show that polyps may be inserted in a variety of locations.

Validation Study

To validate our method of polyp creation and insertion, we performed a study to determine if radiologists experienced with CT colonography and trained in 3D visualization methods and standard 2D axial CT could distinguish real polyps from synthetic polyps. Ten synthetic polyps were generated and inserted into polyp-free sections of the base colon data by using the previously described algorithms. The polyps were sessile and were 8–13 mm in diameter.

We generated 3D virtual endoscopic volume-rendered images of the synthetic polyps and the real polyps by using VOXELVIEW. The color, opacity, and lighting settings for all polyps were similar to those reported by McFarland et al (12). We saved 2D color images of the renderings, each annotated with a black caret that clearly identified each polyp.

In addition to the 3D volume-rendered images, standard gray-scale 2D axial CT

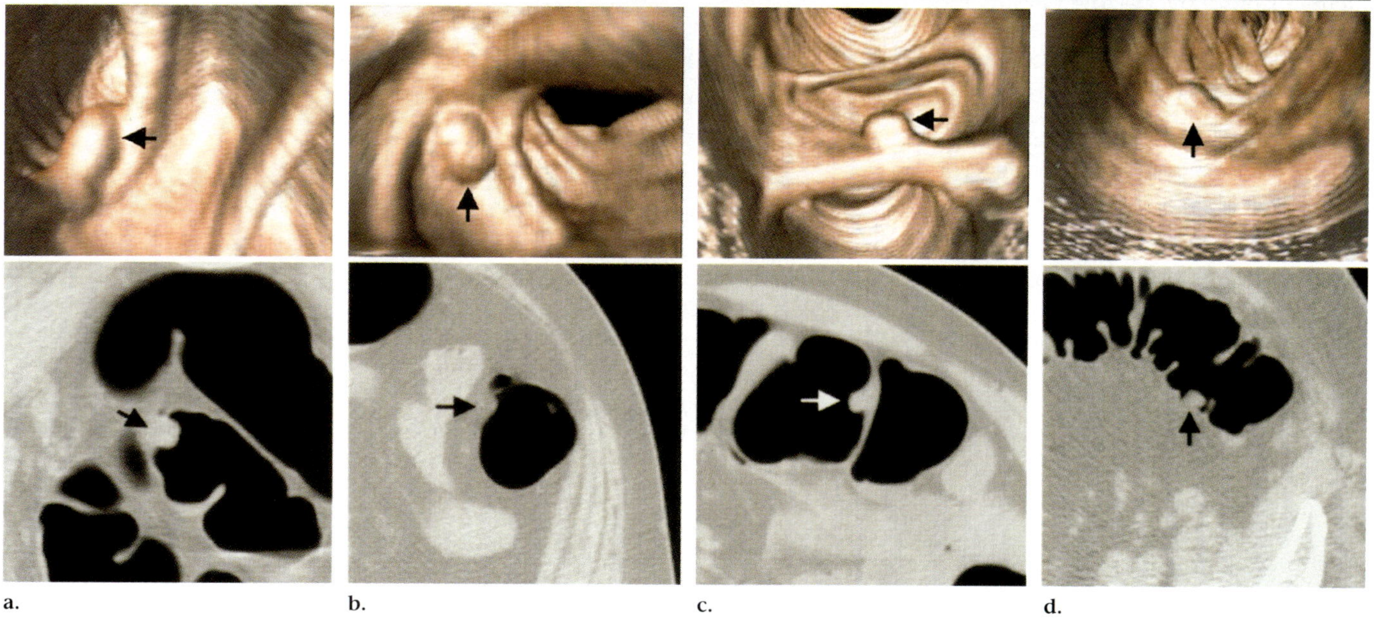

Figure 5. Paired 3D volume-rendered images (top) and 2D axial CT sections (bottom). **(a, c)** Real polyp (arrow). **(b, d)** Synthetic polyp (arrow).

images of each polyp were obtained. The level and window settings were −200 and 800 HU, respectively. In addition, each image was magnified by a factor of three to render it more visible. Each gray-scale image was then annotated with a black caret to identify the polyp.

The 40 images (20 volume-rendered and 20 axial CT images) were then incorporated onto a single World Wide Web page. All images were stored in Joint Photographic Experts Group, or JPEG, format, with the quality factor set to the highest level (ie, with minimal compression). We arranged the 3D and 2D images of the 40 polyps on the page in random order.

Three radiologists (including R.B.J.) were asked to independently score each image by using the following World Wide Web–based interface. Next to each image was a series of five "radio buttons." Button 1 was for rating a lesion as definitely synthetic; button 2, for rating a lesion as possibly synthetic; button 3, for a rating of unsure if synthetic or real; button 4, for rating a lesion as possibly real; and button 5, for rating a lesion as definitely real. Only one button could be toggled for each image. The readers were not told the number of real and synthetic polyps. They were told only that there was a mixture of real and synthetic polyps and that there was no correlation between the 2D axial sections and the 3D volume-rendered images. Each reader was asked to spend approximately 20 seconds studying each image, but no time limit was imposed.

Results for each reader were analyzed as frequency distributions that represented the number of responses in each of the five categories. The frequency histograms for individual readers were not significantly different from each other, so we pooled the results to maximize the statistical power of the observations and as a convenient means of data summary.

Two analyses were performed with the results to test for differences between real and synthetic polyps. First, the frequency distributions for real and synthetic polyps were compared against each another for each of the 3D and 2D display modes. The Wilcoxon rank sum test was used, which is appropriate for ordinal data without the need to assume an underlying normal distribution, with a P value of .05 or less indicative of a significant difference (15).

Second, receiver operating characteristic (ROC) curve analysis was performed by using the program ROCKIT (version 0.9B [beta]; Metz CE, Chicago, Ill). In this analysis, the input data were pairs of values that represented each category along the spectrum from "definitely synthetic" to "definitely real" and its corresponding response frequency for the pooled readers' results. By varying the definition of a true-positive response across the categories, pairs of ROC operating points that represented true-positive observations (sensitivity) versus false-positive observations (1 − specificity) were generated. Mathematically fitted ROC curves were compared against an ROC curve that represented random guesses about which polyps were real and which were synthetic. (This "random guess" curve is a diagonal line, and the area under the curve, or A_z value, is 0.5). The A_z values, 95% CIs, SDs of A_z values, and P values for ROC curve comparison were generated by the ROCKIT program.

RESULTS

Figure 5 shows paired 3D volume-rendered and axial CT views of four representative polyps (two real and two synthetic) used in the study. Figure 6a shows the distribution of reviewers' scores for the 3D volume-rendered images, and Figure 6b shows the distribution of scores for the 2D axial CT sections. In both cases, the distributions were summed for the three reviewers. Note that if the reviewers could readily distinguish between definitely synthetic (score = 1) and definitely real (score = 5) polyps, one would expect the scores to cluster around the values of 1 and 5.

For the 3D volume-rendered images (Fig 6a), the histograms representing real and synthetic lesions overlapped substantially, with most scores clustered around a score of 3 (unsure), which suggests that the reviewers could not readily differentiate between real and synthetic lesions. For real lesions, the median and modal scores were both 4, whereas for the synthetic lesions, the median and modal scores were both 3. The Wilcoxon rank sum test for significant differences between the histograms yielded a P value of .56.

For the 2D axial CT display (Fig 6b), there also was considerable overlap between the frequency distributions. For real lesions, the median and modal scores were 3 and 2, respectively, whereas for the synthetic polyps, the median and modal scores were both 3. The test for statistically significant differences between real and synthetic polyps yielded a P value of .11, which again was indicative of no difference. Note that although no significant differences between the two distributions were detected, there was a tendency with 2D axial CT sections for readers to interpret real lesions as synthetic.

By using ROC curve analysis, we evaluated whether the readers performed significantly better than would be expected from random guessing. Figure 7 shows ROC curves that depict the true-positive fraction (sensitivity) as a function of the false-positive fraction (1 − specificity). An observed ROC curve that is positioned above and to the left of the diagonal line that represents random guessing would be suggestive of the ability to distinguish real from synthetic lesions. For 3D displays, the ROC curve closely paralleled that of random guessing, with an A_z value of 0.54 (SD = 0.08; 95% CI = 0.39, 0.68). The test for significant differences between this curve and random guessing yielded a P value of .70, or no significant difference. For 2D axial CT, the ROC curve tended to be positioned below the level expected for random guessing, with an A_z value of 0.39 (SD = 0.07; 95% CI = 0.25, 0.53). The test for significant differences between this curve and random guessing yielded a P value of .28, or no significant difference.

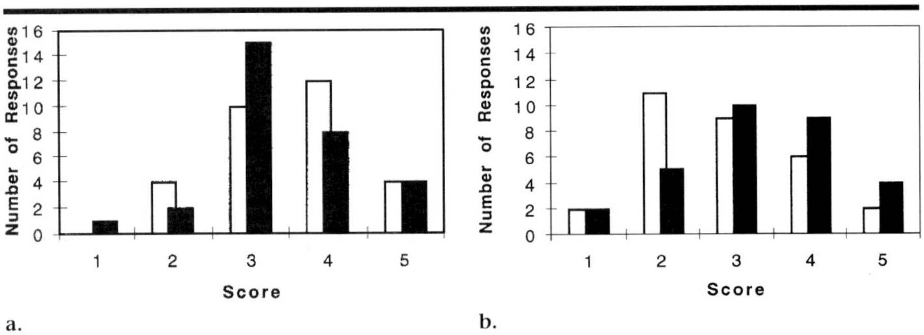

Figure 6. Histograms show distribution of scores, summed over all reviewers, for real (white bars) and synthetic (black bars) polyps on **(a)** 3D volume-rendered images and **(b)** 2D axial CT sections. Scores could range from 1, for a "definitely synthetic" polyp, to 5, for a "definitely real" polyp. If readers could definitively distinguish synthetic from real lesions, responses should cluster around scores of 1 and 5, respectively. Instead, responses for both real and synthetic lesions were clustered around a score of 3, for "unsure" whether the polyp was real or synthetic.

DISCUSSION

Creation of well-defined phantom colon data sets is a useful first step in the systematic evaluation and optimization of different 3D display tools for virtual colonoscopy. Generation of realistic phantom data sets is challenging for a number of reasons.

To create synthetic polyps that appear to be composed of real tissue, the synthetic polyps must have the correct partial volume effects. Mismatched partial volume effects can lead to artifacts on both 2D axial sections and 3D volume-rendered images; these artifacts can cause the synthetic polyps to appear conspicuously "computer generated" rather than resemble real tissue. Thus, we chose to create polyps with a CT simulator to match the partial volume effects in synthetic polyps with those in real tissue.

A second important factor is that the noise in the synthetic polyp must match the noise in the tissue. The CT simulator permits addition of noise to the simulated projections, thereby resulting in synthetic polyps that have noise fluctuations with SD and spatial correlation parameters similar to those seen in tissue.

Another important factor is that the polyps must have a realistic shape. Naturally occurring sessile polyps come in a variety of types, such as marble, mountain, clam shell, and carpet (16). To our knowledge, the frequency of occurrence of specific polyp types in any given patient population has not been reported. Nevertheless, our technique provides the flexibility to generate almost any type of shape by using a combination of ellipsoids, cones, and cylinders.

To validate that the polyps we generated had a realistic appearance, we performed a study to determine if radiologists could distinguish synthetic from real polyps. Because the artifacts seen on 3D images may not be the same as those seen on 2D images, we performed separate evaluations for 3D volume-rendered images and 2D axial sections (Fig 6). Whether we analyzed the results to detect for significant differences between the histograms of radiologists' scores for real and synthetic lesions or the ROC curves to compare observer performance with the hypothetical case of random guessing, we did not detect statistically significant differences between real and synthetic lesions. In fact, there was a tendency (nonsignificant) for readers to interpret real lesions as synthetic on 2D axial CT sections (Fig 6b), a factor that resulted in the ROC curve for the 2D display to be positioned somewhat below the curve for random guessing (Fig 7).

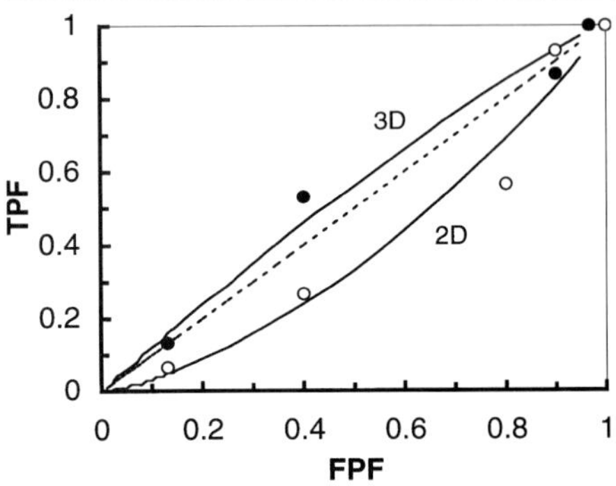

Figure 7. ROC curves for the three radiologist observers (pooled results). The observers attempted to distinguish real from synthetic lesions on 3D volume-rendered images (●) and 2D axial CT sections (○). If the readers had been able to distinguish real from synthetic lesions, the ROC curves for 3D and/or 2D images would be positioned above and to the left of the curve that represents random guessing (dashed line). Instead, the observed ROC curves were not significantly different from random guessing. *FPF* = false-positive fraction, *TPF* = true-positive fraction.

Precisely what visual features of lesions were underlying these trends is unknown; however, a bias toward interpretation of real lesions as synthetic is the opposite of would be expected if the readers could truly identify synthetic lesions. This provides some reassurance that our methods for creation and insertion of synthetic lesions are sound. On the basis of results from the validation study, we conclude that the synthetic lesions mimic real lesions closely enough to be used as a model system for tests of display modes in virtual colonoscopy.

Other groups have developed different methods to construct colonic polyp phantoms. One technique involves the use of a pig colon (17), in which polyps are formed by "puckering" the mucosa with suture material. A limitation of this method is that the haustral folds in a pig colon are different from those in a human colon, and human colonic polyps are often located on or behind a fold. Also, a limited number of polyps may be formed in a single specimen, and the precision and range of shapes available are limited. The use of ex vivo specimens also makes it difficult to mimic the overall complexity involved in a study of the entire human colon.

Another phantom-generation method involves direct copying of voxels from images of patient tissue and insertion of those voxels near the imaged colonic surface (2). However, this method cannot be used to achieve partial volume effects at the edge of the simulated polyp that are the same as those in the nearby colonic wall, and the spatial discontinuity in attenuation at the edge of the "pasted" polyp may render it more visible than a real polyp, thereby biasing the results for display and/or detection methods.

Our approach is most closely related to that reported by Seltzer et al (18), who analytically calculated the partial volume effects for spherical lung nodules and volume averaged the analytic models on a voxel grid matched to patient CT scans of the lungs. In the lung, extension of these methods to other than spherical shapes is not necessary, and the problem of insertion of synthetic nodules at the edge of a structure with comparable attenuation was not addressed. Finally, we note that an important feature of our technique is that any number of user-defined polyps can be placed into patient data at random locations; when used in evaluation of display and detection methods, review of these data sets closely mimics the overall complexity and tedium of review of actual patient studies.

One limitation of our method was that the creation of different polyp shapes is more an art than an exact science. Each polyp was designed by hand, one at a time, with random asymmetries. Because polyps should not be identical, this process had to be repeated for each new polyp. A more systematic approach would be to prepare a library of basic polyp shapes from which the user could choose. The user could then further specify the size and orientation of the polyp. The program would generate a list of ellipsoids, cones, and cylinders that would constitute the polyp. In addition, the program could make small random modifications to the shape so that each polyp is unique.

Another potential limitation of our study was our use of one base data set obtained in a single patient, rather than several data sets from different patients, for insertion of synthetic polyps. However, because the geometry of even a single colon varies considerably over its length and because we inserted lesions at numerous locations in the colon, the only variability one would expect among patient data sets would result from differences in scanning parameters and image noise levels. Note that in the early stages of this work and later in subsequent studies, we did use imaging studies obtained in several patients as base data. Our experience suggests that as long as individual variations in pixel dimensions and image noise are considered, the simulation and insertion process appears to be valid.

A final limitation of our study was that although we could not demonstrate a significant difference between observations of real and synthetic lesions, this result does not explicitly prove that simulated lesions are identical to real lesions. This lack of a difference was largely a result of the relatively small number of real lesions with which the synthetic lesions could be compared. It is no coincidence that this paucity of real lesions provided much of the motivation for the development of synthetic lesions in the first place. In the context of the current work, we can conclude that the synthetic lesions did not contain notably "artificial" features that allowed their differentiation from real lesions. From this, one can make the assumption, albeit untested, that the conspicuity of synthetic lesions should be similar to that of real lesions. Given these limitations, we believe that our results are sufficiently sound to begin application of the phantom system to initial trials in which the display modes are compared (19).

In summary, our polyp synthesis and insertion method allows the generation of a variety of realistic colonic polyps that could not be distinguished from real lesions by experienced observers and, therefore, can facilitate the comparison of display techniques. The fine control over polyp shape, size, and location will facilitate the development and optimization of the many display tools currently under investigation for CT colonography.

Acknowledgments: The authors are grateful to Carl R. Crawford, MD, (Analogic, Peabody, Mass) for providing the core of the CT simulator software; Roger Y. Shifrin, MD, and Elizabeth G. McFarland, MD, for review of the CT data; and Laura Logan, RT, for assistance in the 3D Medical Imaging Laboratory. The authors also thank Silicon Graphics (Mountain View, Calif).

References

1. Hara AK, Johnson CD, Reed JE, et al. Detection of colorectal polyps with CT colography: initial assessment of sensitivity and specificity. Radiology 1997; 205:59–65.
2. Hara AK, Johnson CD, Reed JE, Ehman RL, Ilstrup DM. Colorectal polyp detection with CT colography: two versus three-dimensional techniques. Radiology 1996; 200:49–54.
3. Hopper KD, Naus MS, Khandelwal M, Wise SW, Iyriboz TA, Weaver JS. CT colonoscopy used as a routine screening procedure (abstr). Radiology 1997; 205(P):721.
4. Beaulieu CF, Jeffrey RB, Paik DS, Slosberg EA, Young HA, Napel S. Three-dimensional computed tomography colonography (3DCTC): initial clinical experience with 3 mm collimation and perspective volume rendering (abstr). Radiology 1997; 205(P):196.
5. Fenlon HM, Ferrucci JT. Virtual colonoscopy: what will the issues be? AJR 1997; 169:453–458.
6. Hara AK, Johnson CD, Reed JE. CT colography (CTC) for clinical use: a new method to reduce evaluation time (abstr). Radiology 1997; 205(P):718.
7. Dachman AH, Kuniyoshi JK, Boyle CM, et al. Interactive CT colonography with three-dimensional problem solving for detection of colonic polyps. AJR 1998; 171:989–995.
8. Lorensen WE, Jolesz FA, Kikinis R. The exploration of cross-sectional data with a virtual endoscope. In: Satava RM, Morgan K, Sieburg HB, et al, eds. Interactive technology and the new paradigm for health care: Medicine Meets Virtual Reality III proceedings. Amsterdam, the Netherlands: IOS, 1995; 221–230.
9. Rubin GD, Beaulieu CF, Argiro V, et al. Perspective volume rendering of CT and MR images: applications for endoscopic imaging. Radiology 1996; 199:321–330.
10. Paik DS, Beaulieu CF, Jeffrey RB, Rubin GD, Napel S. Automated flight path planning for virtual endoscopy. Med Phys 1998; 25:629–639.
11. Vining DJ, Shifrin RY, Grishaw EK, Liu K, Gelfand DW. Virtual colonoscopy (abstr). Radiology 1994; 193(P):446.
12. McFarland EG, Brink JA, Loh J, et al. Visualization of colorectal polyps with spiral CT colography: evaluation of processing parameters with perspective volume rendering. Radiology 1997; 205:701–707.
13. Waye JD, Bashkoff E. Total colonoscopy: is it always possible? Gastrointest Endosc 1991; 37:152–154.
14. Foley JD, vanDam A, Feiner SK, Hughes JF. Computer graphics, principles and practice. 2nd ed. New York, NY: Addison-Wesley, 1992.
15. Rosner B. Nonparametric methods. In: Fundamentals of biostatistics. Boston, Mass: Duxbury, 1986; 288–293.
16. O'Brien M, Winawer SJ, Waye JD. Colorectal polyps. In: Winawer SJ, Kurtz RC, eds. Gastrointestinal cancer. New York, NY: Gower Medical, 1992; 3.1–3.41.
17. Dachman AH, Lieberman J, Osnis RB, et al. Small simulated polyps in pig colon: sensitivity of CT virtual colography. Radiology 1997; 203:427–430.
18. Seltzer SE, Judy PF, Adams DF, et al. Spiral CT of the chest: comparison of cine and film-based viewing. Radiology 1995; 197:73–78.
19. Beaulieu CF, Jeffrey RB Jr, Karadi C, Paik DS, Napel S. Display modes for CT colonography. II. Blinded comparison of axial CT and virtual endoscopic and panoramic endoscopic volume-rendered studies. Radiology 1999; 212:203–212.

Book Review

PACS: Basic Principles and Applications

H. K. Huang, DSc
New York, NY: Wiley-Liss, 1999. ISBN 0-471-25393-6.
Softcover, $89.95; pp 556; 259 figures; tables.

The evolution of electronic systems to manage, display, communicate, and archive digital radiologic images gradually evolved so that by the mid-1980s university radiology departments developed functional systems. Dr H. K. Huang was one of the pioneers who developed such a system. His informatics laboratory and graduate program joined the talents of informatics scientists, medical practitioners, and representatives of industry. He related his experience in *PACS: Picture Archiving and Communication Systems in Biomedical Imaging* (New York, NY: Wiley-VCH, 1996), which is devoted to the training of medical informatics scientists and physicists. *PACS: Basic Principles and Applications* is an exciting new book that provides a basic understanding of imaging technology and presents the advances made since publication of Dr Huang's previous book. Part of this evolution came from the union of the picture archiving and communication system (PACS) with the hospital information system (HIS) and the rest of the enterprise system related to patient records.

Dr Huang has had the unusual opportunity to build PACS for two major universities: the University of California, Los Angeles, and the University of California, San Francisco. His experience is reflected in this book. The success of large PACS projects and the availability of practical working systems from industry widens the audience for which this book is intended. All health care workers who would use, order, or pay for these systems must understand their design and function, as well as their potential for streamlining the management of radiologic images. That group includes radiologists, radiology residents, technologists, student technologists, health care planners, administrators, and those in industry who are involved with PACS. This book provides an excellent approach to understanding the basics, as well as the latest about PACS.

After the introduction, the following topics are discussed: imaging basics, projection radiography digitization, digital radiography, sectional imaging, image acquisition, communication and networking, telemedicine and teleradiology, pitfalls and bottlenecks, and future developments and research. In the rapidly developing specialty of digital imaging terminology, acronyms spring up like weeds. A list of these terms is provided just before the foreword. A distinctive feature in the introduction is a diagram of the organization of the book that shows the interrelationship of the topics and chapters.

This is an excellent book that fulfills vital needs at a time when the technology has reached a level of development that requires medical planners to determine when digital imaging equipment is to be acquired. This book should help make that decision easier. The style of writing is clear and concise. Some sections are the same as in Dr Huang's previous book in that they refer to basics that have not changed. Whether one reads the book straight through or refers to various sections, the system of organization is simple and easy to follow. The paper is acid free, and the printing is easy to read. The diagrams and graphs are excellent.

PACS: Basic Principles and Applications is useful and will fill a gap in this rapidly changing and evolving field. Since there are few textbooks on PACS, it will provide the latest information, particularly for those in training. I strongly recommend it.

Reviewed by Jack I. Eisenman, MD

Display Modes for CT Colonography

Part II. Blinded Comparison of Axial CT and Virtual Endoscopic and Panoramic Endoscopic Volume-rendered Studies[1]

Christopher F. Beaulieu, MD, PhD
R. Brooke Jeffrey, Jr, MD
Chandu Karadi, PhD
David S. Paik, MS
Sandy Napel, PhD

Index terms:
Computed tomography (CT), image display and recording, 75.12115, 75.12117
Computed tomography (CT), three-dimensional, 75.12117
Computers, simulation
Colon, CT, 75.12111, 75.12115, 75.12117
Colon, neoplasms, 75.3119

Radiology 1999; 212:203–212

Abbreviations:
2D = two-dimensional
3D = three-dimensional

[1] From the Department of Radiology, Rm S-056, 300 Pasteur Dr, Stanford University School of Medicine, Stanford, CA 94305.

Received July 20, 1998; revision requested September 24; revision received November 18; accepted January 11, 1999. Supported in part by National Institutes of Health grants 1R01 CA72023, 1P41 RR09784-01, LM 07033; the Society for Computed Body Tomography and Magnetic Resonance; the Packard Foundation; the Lucas Foundation; and the Phil N. Allen Trust. C.F.B. is a 1997 RSNA Scholar. C.K. is a 1998 GENDEX/RSNA Medical Student/Scholar Assistant. **Address reprint requests to** C.F.B. (e-mail: *cfb@s-word.stanford.edu*).

See also the article by Karadi et al (pp 195–201) in this issue.

Author contributions:
Guarantor of integrity of entire study, C.F.B.; study concepts, C.F.B., C.K., S.N.; study design, C.F.B., R.B.J., S.N.; definition of intellectual content, C.F.B., S.N.; literature research, C.F.B., C.K.; experimental studies, D.S.P., C.F.B., R.B.J., C.K.; data acquisition, C.F.B., R.B.J., C.K.; data analysis, C.F.B., C.K.; statistical analysis, C.F.B.; manuscript preparation, C.F.B.; manuscript editing and review, all authors.

PURPOSE: To determine the sensitivity of radiologist observers for detecting colonic polyps by using three different data review (display) modes for computed tomographic (CT) colonography, or "virtual colonoscopy."

MATERIALS AND METHODS: CT colonographic data in a patient with a normal colon were used as base data for insertion of digitally synthesized polyps. Forty such polyps (3.5, 5, 7, and 10 mm in diameter) were randomly inserted in four copies of the base data. Axial CT studies, volume-rendered virtual endoscopic movies, and studies from a three-dimensional mode termed "panoramic endoscopy" were reviewed blindly and independently by two radiologists.

RESULTS: Detection improved with increasing polyp size. Trends in sensitivity were dependent on whether all inserted lesions or only visible lesions were considered, because modes differed in how completely the colonic surface was depicted. For both reviewers and all polyps 7 mm or larger, panoramic endoscopy resulted in significantly greater sensitivity (90%) than did virtual endoscopy (68%, $P = .014$). For visible lesions only, the sensitivities were 85%, 81%, and 60% for one reader and 65%, 62%, and 28% for the other for virtual endoscopy, panoramic endoscopy, and axial CT, respectively. Three-dimensional displays were more sensitive than two-dimensional displays ($P < .05$).

CONCLUSION: The sensitivity of panoramic endoscopy is higher than that of virtual endoscopy, because the former displays more of the colonic surface. Higher sensitivities for three-dimensional displays may justify the additional computation and review time.

Virtual colonoscopy, or computed tomographic (CT) colonography, is a rapidly evolving field. CT colonography involves spiral CT of the cleansed colon to help detect polyps and masses (1–3). Images of lesions in the clinically relevant size range of 1 cm in diameter and larger are reliably captured in the scan data as long as there is adequate distention of a clean colon (4,5).

A major obstacle to the implementation of CT colonography in routine clinical practice, however, is the need to view an enormous amount of imaging data, which often includes 200–350 axial sections for a supine study and may be double that if imaging is also performed with the patient in the prone position. There is continuing debate (6–10) about whether review of two-dimensional (2D) axial CT sections alone is adequate or whether some form of three-dimensional (3D) display is necessary to increase polyp detection to the highest level. In early studies, differentiation of the relative contributions of 2D and 3D viewing strategies was difficult, because both strategies were most often used together (3). Complicating this issue is the fact that 2D and 3D viewing or display modes are being developed at an increasing rate. To determine the most efficient method of image review for CT colonography and to validate new methods, the efficacy of each display mode must be rigorously determined under controlled conditions.

To establish a "ground-truth" model for the testing of CT colonographic display modes, we developed methods for electronic insertion of polyps into CT colonographic data obtained in patients enrolled in a clinical trial (11). The realism of the synthetic polyps has been validated in a blinded trial in which radiologists experienced with CT colonography reviewed sets of axial CT sections and 3D endoscopic volume renderings of synthetic lesions and true lesions. The reviewers were unable to distinguish synthetic lesions from true lesions (11).

In this report, we describe our initial experience with the synthetic polyp model system to independently evaluate three display modes for CT colonography. Experimental data sets that contained sets of synthetic polyps were generated and reviewed by radiologists in axial CT mode, virtual endoscopic mode with forward- and reverse-viewing fly-through volume-rendered movies, and panoramic endoscopic mode, a recently developed 3D rendering method for depiction of the topography of the inner colonic surface as a flattened structure. Our purpose was to determine the sensitivity of radiologist observers for the detection of colonic polyps with each of these data review (display) modes.

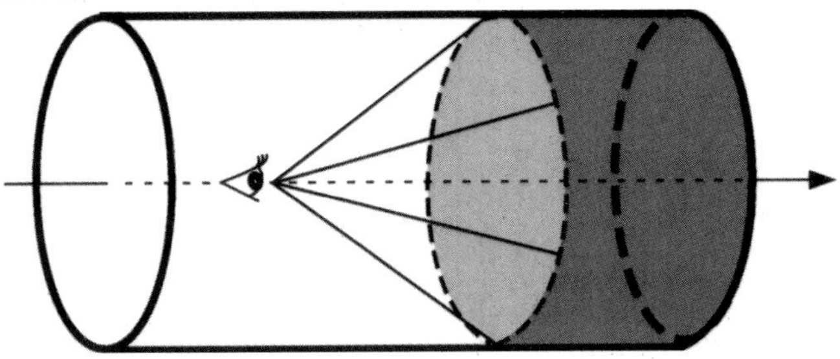

Figure 1. Schematic of virtual endoscopy. The colon is represented by a cylinder, and the position of the virtual camera is shown by the eye. The straight dashed line shows the preplanned path through the center of the colon. By orienting the camera parallel to the path, the part of the colon depicted by the shaded area is visualized. Reverse viewing is achieved by means of 180° rotation of the camera.

MATERIALS AND METHODS

Case Generation

Four identical copies of a control, or "base," data set were generated from a CT colonographic study in a 60-year-old man in whom no polyps were seen at colonoscopy but who, incidentally, had a 2-cm-diameter lipoma of the hepatic flexure. CT data obtained in this patient were used in the polyp-validation phase of this and another current study (11). The patient was enrolled in a clinical CT colonography trial that had been approved by the investigational review board of the university.

Colonic cleansing was performed with a solution of polyethylene glycol and electrolytes (GoLYTELY; Braintree Laboratories, Braintree, Mass). After informed consent was obtained, air insufflation of the colon was performed, followed by CT with the patient in the supine position. A CT HiSpeed Advantage scanner (GE Medical Systems, Milwaukee, Wis) was used, with the following parameters: 120 kVp, 240 mA, 3-mm collimation, and 6 mm/sec table speed (pitch of 2.0). Scans were reconstructed at 1.0-mm intervals with a display field-of-view of 36 cm by using the manufacturer's standard reconstruction algorithm. There was essentially no retained water or fecal material present on the CT colonographic study. Reconstructed CT images of this patient's colon were used for each of the four test cases. In this way, identical "background" colonic morphology was provided for each case, and the only differences between cases were in the locations and sizes of inserted polyps.

Polyps with a simulated diameter of 3.5, 5, 7, or 10 mm were created as spherical objects by using a software CT simulator initially developed elsewhere and modified in our laboratory. The polyp diameters were chosen to represent approximate factor-of-two differences in cross-sectional area between the size categories: If the cross-sectional area is equal to πr^2, where r is the radius, and the diameter is 10 mm, then the cross-sectional area is 78.5 mm^2; if the diameter is 7 mm, the area is 38.5 mm^2; if the diameter is 5 mm, the area 19.6 mm^2; and if the diameter is 3.5 mm, the area is 9.6 mm^2.

The polyps were inserted along the inner aspect of the colonic wall according to methods described in detail elsewhere (11). Insertion locations were randomly selected in the subvolume of data that represented the colonic surface as follows: First, a random point along a path describing the centerline of the colon was chosen (12). Second, a random radial ray was cast from the path point to the nearby colonic surface, and the intersection of the ray with the wall represented the insertion point. When added to the base data, the initially spherical synthetic polyps became hemispheric, and approximately half their diameter protruded into the lumen. The portion of the polyp that overlapped the colonic wall itself or adjacent abdominal fat did not alter the attenuation or noise in the base CT data, owing to the use of nonlinear compositing methods. These methods also allowed the addition of polyps to thin haustral folds, with the resultant lesion protruding from only one side of the mucosal surface of the fold. Although we did not quantitatively assess the depth of insertion, we did inspect each polyp by using axial and focused virtual endoscopic views to verify that the lesions were indeed visible as protrusions from the colonic surface.

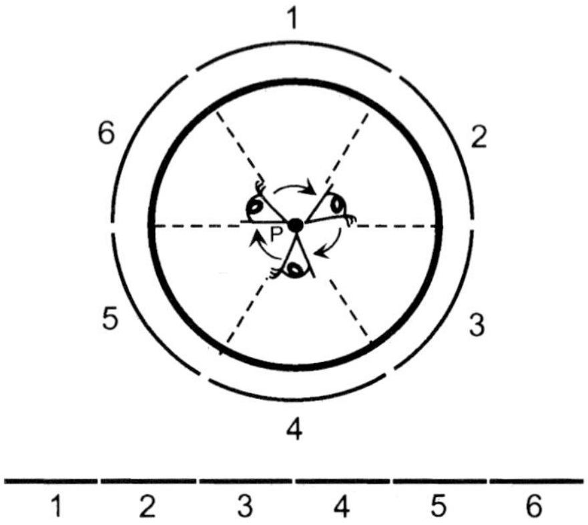

Figure 2. Two-dimensional schematic of panoramic endoscopy. A cross-section through the colon is represented by the continuous inner circle, and the path (●, *P*) is in the center of this circle. The virtual camera, indicated by the eyes, is oriented perpendicular to the path. The virtual camera captures one-sixth of the circumference of the colon at each position (dashed lines, *1–6*), with a 60° camera field of view. An image panel for that camera position and orientation is generated, as indicated by the interrupted outer circle (*1–6*). Contiguous panels displaying the colonic circumference are generated by rotating the camera in 60° increments around the path (arrows). Once generated, the six image panels are displayed side-by-side as an elongated, flattened view of the inner colonic lining. Subsequent panoramic endoscopic views are generated by moving along the path in 3-mm increments and repeating panoramic rendering.

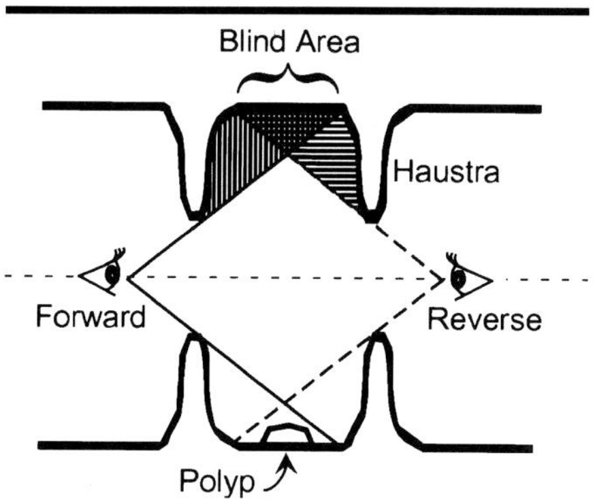

Figure 3. Schematic shows blind areas at virtual endoscopy. This longitudinal cross section of the colon contains normal haustral folds, with diagrams for forward- and reverse-viewing virtual endoscopic cameras with a 60° camera field of view. Blind, or nonvisible, areas occur for both viewing directions when the camera is oriented parallel to the path (thin dashed line), because the outer margins of the camera's visual cone (solid lines for forward viewing, thick dashed lines for reverse viewing) do not capture areas obscured by haustral folds. Blind areas for forward viewing are indicated by vertical stripes; those for reverse viewing, by horizontal stripes. While bidirectional virtual endoscopic movies help reduce the amount of blind area, a polyp such as that shown at the bottom of the diagram may not be visible, because the virtual camera never "captures" the lesion in an image frame. The exact amount of the colonic surface that cannot be visualized is a function of a complex relationship between camera field of view, the convention chosen for the viewing direction (instantaneously tangent to the path or looking toward the furthest visible path point), the amount of gross colonic curvature, the diameter of the colon, the spacing between haustral folds, and the degree to which haustra project into the lumen.

A total of 40 synthetic polyps were added to the four copies of the base data by randomly distributing lesions according to size category and location. Specifically, 10 lesions were added to each of two copies of the base data, nine were added to one copy, and 11 were added to the fourth copy. No changes in lesion location had to be made because of retained fluid in the base data, and lesions that were randomly assigned to be inserted on a haustral fold were not moved. In addition to these experimental data sets, we created "answer" data sets by adding 10-mm-diameter synthetic lesions with high attenuation (1,000 HU) to four additional copies of the base data. The answer lesions were inserted at exactly the same locations as the experimental synthetic lesions and were used by the study coordinator (C.K.) in the data analysis phase (described subsequently). These data were not available to the radiologist reviewers during the blinded portion of the study.

Three-dimensional Rendering

Rendering and image review were performed with Infinite Reality or O2 workstations (Silicon Graphics, Mountain View, Calif) equipped with 256–384 Mbyte of random access memory. Rendering engine software (Voxel View, version 2.5.1; Vital Images, Minneapolis, Minn) was used for 3D volume renderings and for review of axial CT sections in stack, or cine, mode. Central-path–planning software (12,13) that we developed was used for segmentation of the air-containing colon and generation of a central flight path that was used to create key-frame animations with the rendering engine, similar to the process described by Rubin et al (14).

Forward- and reverse-viewing volume-rendered endoscopic movies were created by using a 60° camera field of view. A diagram of the geometry involved is shown in Figure 1. Volume rendering parameters were similar to those being used by groups (14–17) using these techniques for virtual colonoscopy. These parameters include specification of opacity tables to render air transparent, application of a color table to render the colon in a pinkish hue, and application of a lighting model to simulate the reflectiveness of the inner colonic lining. Volume rendering parameters were kept fixed throughout the study. For each forward- or reverse-viewing movie, an image frame was created every 3 mm along the central path of the colon, which resulted in generation of 400 frames for each movie.

Overall, data preprocessing and rendering for virtual endoscopic movies required approximately 1 hour per case. Although this precomputation process constrained the readers' visualization to only those parts of the colonic surface within the viewing frustum of the virtual camera, it also ensured identical image content for both readers. As technology progresses, truly interactive, nearly real-time volume-rendering systems will become available. With such systems, a reader should be able to navigate efficiently through the colon without being constrained by a predefined visualization direction. At the same time, differences between readers in navigation skills will then become an additional variable that could affect detection sensitivity. It is thus owing to a combination of system limitations and a desire for experimental control that we used precomputed animations as opposed to interactive volume rendering. In future studies, this constraint will be relaxed.

The third display mode we tested was a recently developed mode termed "panoramic endoscopy." The geometry for this mode is illustrated in Figure 2. The central path through the colon was used as the location of a 60°–field-of-view virtual camera, with the camera viewing direction perpendicular to the local direction of the path. The camera was rotated around the path in 60° increments, which generated six image panels. When these image panels were displayed side by side, they depicted a panoramic view of the colonic wall around the current location. Sequential panoramic frames were generated by moving the camera location along the path in 3-mm increments, with 360° (six by 60°) panoramic rendering at each point. The overall number of panoramic frames per case (400 frames) was designed to be similar to the number of images reviewed in an axial CT study and in the forward- and reverse-viewing endoscopic movies. Typically, preprocessing and rendering of the movies for panoramic endoscopy took 1½ hours per case.

Review

Training images were provided to the radiologists before the study to illustrate the appearance of each polyp size as it would appear on studies obtained with each of the rendering modes. The reviewers were very experienced with visualization issues involved in CT colonography. During the formal study, two radiologists (C.F.B., R.B.J.) reviewed the four test cases independently. Although more readers would have been ideal and will be incorporated in the future, we wanted to maintain a similar level of experience between the readers and did not have access to other similarly trained individuals at the time of data collection. The reviewers were aware that digital lesions of the sizes described had been added to four copies of the same base data, but they did not know the exact number or size distribution of lesions that would be presented in each case.

Each case was reviewed and scored for each of the three display modes: axial CT, virtual endoscopy, and panoramic endoscopy. Sets of axial images or animations for each case were randomized and presented to the reviewers on separate days. For example, during a given session, a reviewer might score axial CT sections from case 1, virtual endoscopic mode animations from case 2, and panoramic endoscopic mode animations from case 3. This mixing of modes and cases was performed to remove the ability to correlate findings from one display mode with those from another and to minimize case memory. Cases were reviewed during 1 month, with approximately 1 week between review sessions.

Axial CT images were viewed in a cine, or stack, mode on the workstation, with an image size of approximately 5 × 6 inches. All images were reviewed at window and level settings of 800 and −100 HU, respectively. Reviewers were allowed to adjust interactively the window and level settings, but they typically did not modify the settings. For each test data set, a total of 355 axial CT sections were reviewed.

Virtual endoscopic movies were reviewed by using MOVIEPLAYER software (Silicon Graphics) to interactively play animations to represent forward- and reverse-viewing movies. Reviewers could move forward or backward along the path of the colon but could not adjust rendering parameters or the viewing direction in these precomputed frames.

Panoramic endoscopic movies were reviewed similarly by using a customized MOVIEPLAYER interface. As with the virtual endoscopic mode, reviewers could move forward or backward along the path of the colon but could not otherwise adjust rendering parameters or viewing direction.

For each case and display mode, the reviewers recorded the spatial coordinates of each possible lesion and the review time. Estimates of lesion size were not solicited, because the study was designed to evaluate detection sensitivity and not necessarily lesion classification.

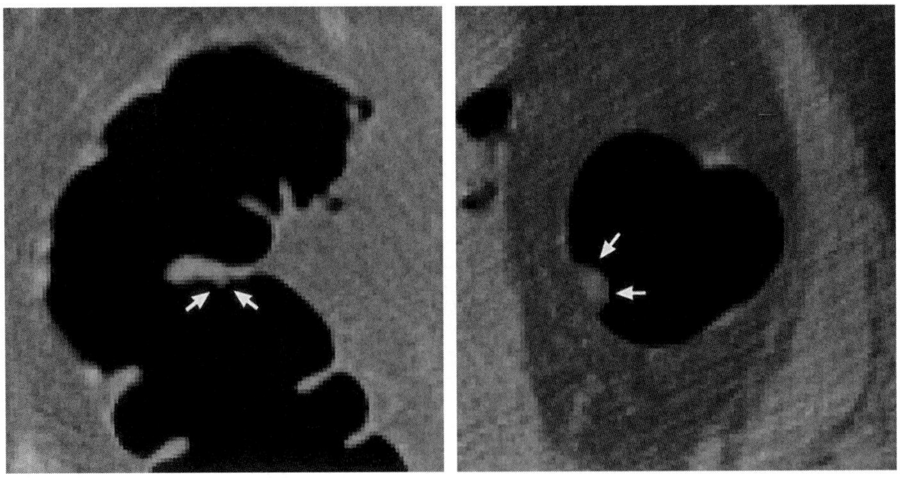

a. b.

Figure 4. Axial CT display mode. **(a)** Magnified view shows a 3.5-mm digitally synthesized polyp (arrows) inserted along a haustral fold. **(b)** Magnified view shows a 10-mm digitally synthesized polyp (arrows) inserted along the colonic wall. The radiologist observers viewed full-scan field-of-view studies, on which the lesions were less conspicuous than they are on these images. A total of 355 axial sections were reviewed in stack, or cine, mode at a graphics workstation. Note that the compositing process with the base data did not create artifacts or variations in image noise that could present additional, unrealistic stimuli to the observers.

Analysis

The study coordinator was required to reconcile each reviewer's findings against truth on the bases of a thorough familiarity with the base data and knowledge of the exact spatial locations of inserted synthetic polyps. For axial CT study review, accurate identification of which synthetic lesions were detected and which were overlooked was relatively straightforward, because pixel coordinates for a reviewer's true-positive observations typically matched the insertion locations within a 2–3-pixel radius.

Reconciliation of the reviewers' results with the truth for the 3D modes was more challenging because the exact location and appearance of a synthetic lesion transformed from a 2D to a 3D representation was not necessarily intuitive. On a 3D image, one would expect that an inserted synthetic lesion should perturb the experimental image relative to a 3D image of the base data as generated from identical virtual-camera viewpoint and viewing directions.

For most of the 7- and 10-mm synthetic lesions, perturbations from matched 3D renderings of the base data were obvious. For some of the larger lesions and for many of the smaller lesions, however, precisely what had changed between the base and experimental 3D data sets was not immediately apparent, so further analysis was necessary. For this, we used the answer data sets, as described earlier, which contained 10-mm, high-attenuation synthetic lesions that were location-matched with the experimental polyps. By comparing 3D renderings of the answer data with identical renderings of the base data, we could determine precisely where a colonic surface perturbation would be expected on a matched rendering of the experimental data.

Once the exact 3D location was identified, a direct comparison of the experimental 3D image was made with the base 3D image to determine whether the experimental lesion was adequately represented to the reviewer in the precomputed animations. This process was very important for data analysis reasons, because for the 3D modes, not all of the inserted lesions were actually visible to the reviewers, owing to geometric or optical considerations involved in generation of the renderings. In the current implementation of the virtual endoscopic mode in particular, forward- and reverse-viewing movies created with a 60° camera field of view and the camera oriented toward the furthest visible point along the central path do not display the entirety of the colonic lining, as illustrated in Figure 3.

Results for the two reviewers were analyzed separately to compare trends in detection sensitivity and to evaluate interobserver variability. When interobserver variability was not statistically significant, combined results from the readers were computed. Sensitivity for polyp detection was calculated in two ways. The first method yielded sensitivity on the basis of all of the polyps inserted in the base data set for each viewing mode. The second method allowed compensation for failed detection due to inserted lesions that did not substantially change the appearance of the colon from that in the base data, that is, for lesions that were not actually visible on studies generated with one or more of the display modes.

Statistical analysis involved pairwise comparisons of sensitivity levels between display modes or between reviewers. When comparing modes, the statistical

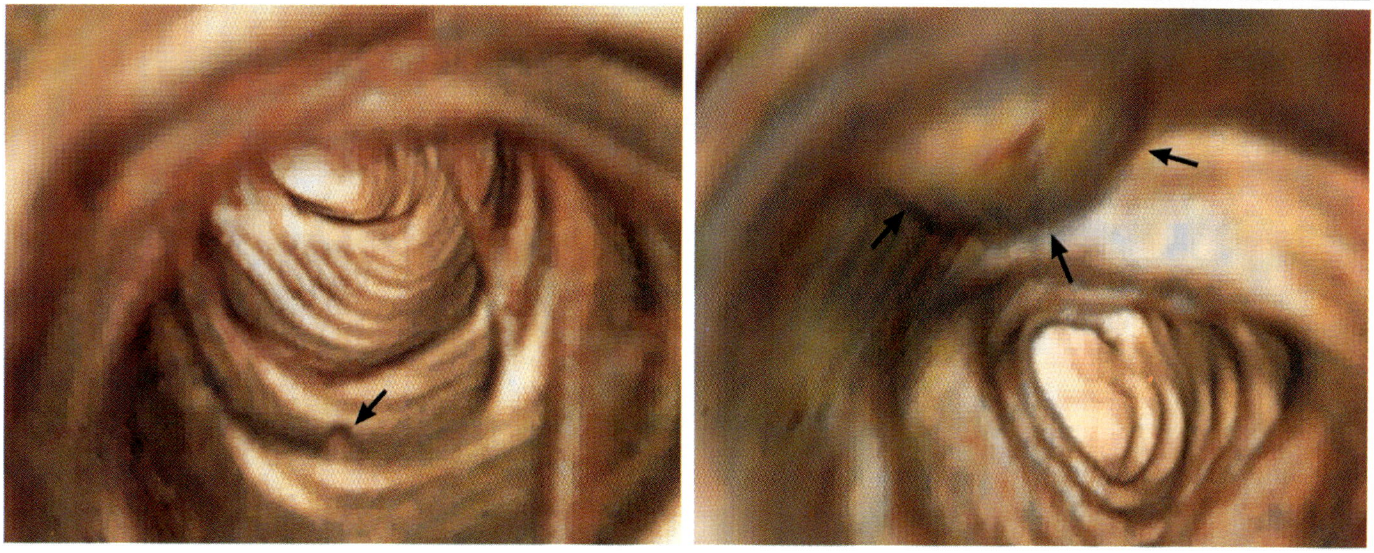

a. b.

Figure 5. Virtual endoscopy display mode. Volume-rendered virtual endoscopic images of **(a)** a 3.5-mm polyp (arrow) and **(b)** a 10-mm polyp (arrows). The observers viewed animations consisting of approximately 400 image frames, of which **a** and **b** are examples, for both forward- and reverse-viewing endoscopic movies, and results obtained with both viewing directions were combined to determine the detection sensitivity.

power was, in some instances, increased by pooling observations across all polyp sizes or by pooling results obtained for the larger (7- and 10-mm) lesions. We have explicitly identified calculations based on such combinations. Because the sample sizes were relatively small, the most appropriate statistical model was one in which estimates of binomial proportions are used (18). Significant differences were obtained when the *P* value was less than or equal to .05.

Examples of Display Modes

Examples of the synthetic lesions used in the visualization trials are shown in Figures 4–6. Figure 4 shows axial CT scans of 3.5-mm and 10-mm synthetic polyps. In Figure 4a, a 3.5-mm lesion was randomly inserted on a haustral fold; in Figure 4b, a 10-mm lesion was inserted along the colonic wall. These magnified views illustrate the individual lesions but do not demonstrate that the reviewers' task was to identify such lesions within the context of the full field-of-view study of 355 CT sections. Figure 5 shows examples of virtual endoscopic images of 3.5-mm and 10-mm polyps. In this display mode, the reviewer's task was to identify polypoid lesions and to differentiate them from normal haustral folds. Figure 6 shows examples of 3.5- and 10-mm polyps on panoramic endoscopic images. As with the virtual endoscopic mode, the readers' task was to identify polypoid lesions and to differentiate them from haustral folds in the base data.

For the 3D modes, identical computer graphics rendering parameters were used for opacity mapping and color and lighting encoding. The principle difference between the 3D modes was the viewing orientation of the virtual camera, as shown schematically in Figures 1 and 2.

RESULTS

Detection of Inserted Lesions

Results of blinded, randomized reviews of axial CT, virtual endoscopic, and panoramic endoscopic studies are shown in Figures 7 and 8. Table 1 summarizes the sensitivity results when lesions were pooled across all sizes.

Figure 7 shows the results when the number of polyps that can possibly be detected matches the number of polyps that were inserted (10 of each size, total of 40 lesions). This analysis permits us to draw conclusions about the sensitivity of each mode as influenced by visual presentation of the data—2D or 3D—as well as by the "visibility coverage" of the colonic surface with the different modes.

Figure 7a shows the detection sensitivity for reader 1 as a function of polyp size. A general trend of increasing detection sensitivity with increasing lesion size was present for each display mode. For the 3.5-, 5-, and 7-mm lesions, the following trend was observed: Sensitivity of panoramic endoscopy was greater than that of axial CT, which was greater than that of virtual endoscopy. Within each size category, differences between display modes were not statistically significant. For 10-mm lesions, the trend was as follows: Sensitivity of panoramic endoscopy was greater than that of virtual endoscopy, which was greater than that of axial CT. When we pooled results obtained with lesions of all sizes (Table 1) and tested for differences between the various pairs of display modes (eg, axial CT vs virtual endoscopy, virtual endoscopy vs panoramic endoscopy), there was no statistically significant difference in sensitivity between the three modes.

Analogous results for reader 2 are shown in Figure 7b. For detection sensitivity for reader 2, the trend was as follows: Sensitivity of panoramic endoscopy was greater than that of virtual endoscopy, which was greater than that of axial CT. When we pooled results across lesion sizes, the panoramic endoscopic and virtual endoscopic modes were significantly more sensitive than axial CT (P = .007 and .002, respectively), but the sensitivity of panoramic endoscopy was not significantly different from that of virtual endoscopy (P = .34).

Comparison of Figure 7a with Figure 7b and the pooled results in Table 1 shows that there were differences in sensitivity between the two reviewers despite identical image content and display methods for the test cases. When display modes were considered separately but results with polyps of all diameters were pooled (Table 1), the sensitivity of axial CT for reader 1 (60%) was significantly higher than that for reader 2 (28%; $P = .001$).

Interobserver differences were not significant when results obtained with the virtual endoscopic mode (55% vs 42% for reader 1 and reader 2, respectively; $P = .26$) or the panoramic endoscopic mode (75% vs 58%; $P = .10$) were compared. Overall, reader 1 detected 76 (63%) and reader 2 detected 51 (43%) of 120 lesions, for a significant difference owing to the discrepancy in sensitivity with the axial CT mode ($P = .002$).

Because of interobserver variability with axial CT scans, results for the two readers could not be combined for this mode. The two readers' results could, however, be combined for virtual endoscopy and panoramic endoscopy. This yielded a sensitivity of 66% (53 of 80 lesions) for panoramic endoscopy and 49% (39 of 80 lesions) for virtual endoscopy (Table 1). Although this result was statistically significant ($P = .025$), the overall sensitivity of 66% was not impressive. However, these results were obtained by pooling lesions of all sizes. By pooling results only from the lesions in the "clinically relevant" size categories of 7 and 10 mm (see Fig 7), the readers in combination detected 90% (36 of 40) of lesions at panoramic endoscopy and 68% (27 of 40) at virtual endoscopy, which was a statistically significant difference ($P = .014$).

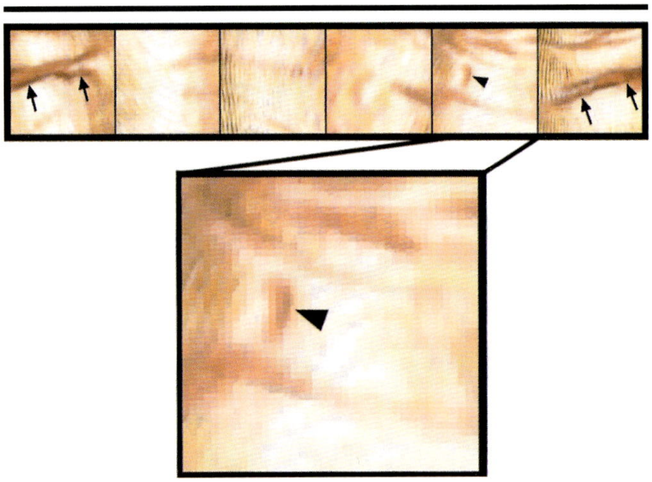

a.

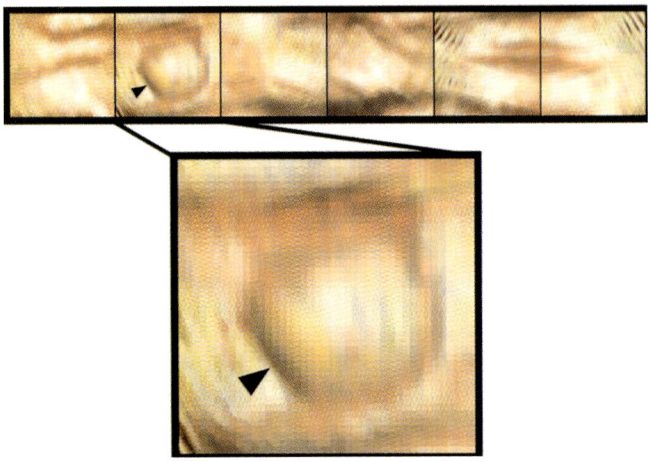

b.

Figure 6. Panoramic endoscopy display mode. **(a)** Top: Elongated panoramic display. Bottom: Magnified view of the fifth panel from the panoramic display. A 3.5-mm synthetic polyp (arrowhead) can be seen in the fifth panel of the panoramic display and in the magnified view. The six panels represent the 360° display of the local colonic wall. Portions of a normal haustral fold (arrows) are seen in the first and sixth panels of the panoramic display. **(b)** Top: Elongated panoramic display. Bottom: Magnified view of the second panel from the panoramic display. A 10-mm synthetic polyp (arrowhead) is located in the second panel of the panoramic display. The observers viewed a total of 400 sequential panoramic frames for each experimental data set.

Detection of Visible Lesions

As already described, the results shown in Figure 7 include influences on the readers due to different modes of data presentation and to "colonic surface coverage" with the 3D display modes. For each mode, the specific lesions that created a substantial perturbation in the base data were explicitly determined by means of careful comparison by the study coordinator of the experimental, base, and answer data sets. Table 2 shows the actual number of visible lesions for each display mode. Whereas all 40 inserted polyps were visible as distinct differences from the base data on axial CT studies, 26 inserted polyps were truly visible at virtual endoscopy, and 37 were visible at panoramic endoscopy.

The geometry of the virtual camera, which led to the decreased visibility in the virtual endoscopic mode, is shown in Figure 3. For the panoramic mode, the specific reason for the "invisibility" of three of the smaller lesions (Table 2) was not clear. It is possible that the lesions were distorted by means of rendering artifacts near the edges of the panels or were made inconspicuous due to the orientation of the polyps with respect to the simulated light source.

Figure 8 illustrates the detection sensitivities of the different display modes for each reader when only the visible lesions were considered as potential observations. Table 3 summarizes the pooled sensitivity results for these visible lesions. By considering polyps of all sizes pooled together, the sensitivity of reader 1 (Fig 8a, Table 3) was essentially the same for virtual endoscopy (85%) and panoramic endoscopy (81%, $P = .72$). Both virtual endoscopy and panoramic endoscopy were significantly more sensitive than axial CT (60%) for the entire range of polyp sizes ($P = .03$ for both virtual endoscopy vs axial CT and panoramic endoscopy vs axial CT). Figure 8b shows analogous results for reader 2. As for reader 1, virtual endoscopy and panoramic endoscopy, with sensitivities of 65% and 62%, respectively, were significantly more sensitive than axial CT, which had a sensitivity of 28% (virtual endoscopy vs axial CT, $P < .001$; panoramic endoscopy vs axial CT, $P = .001$).

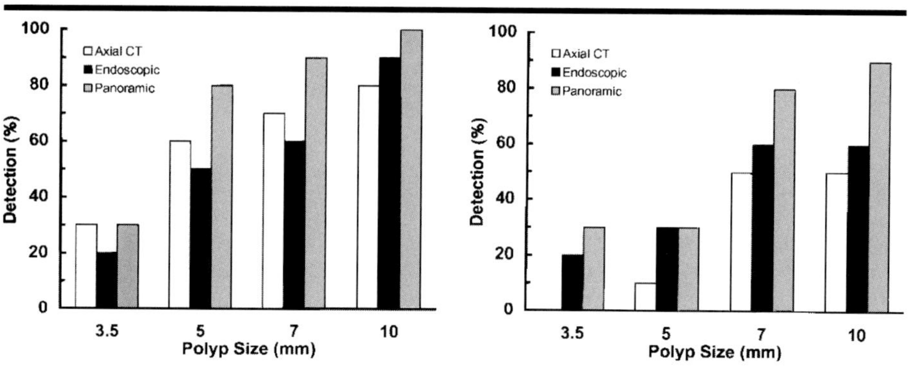

a. b.

Figure 7. Bar graphs show detection sensitivity as a function of polyp size and display mode for **(a)** reader 1 and **(b)** reader 2. A total of 10 polyps of each size were potentially detectable in the four experimental data sets. Note that for both readers, detection increased as polyp size increased. There were significant interobserver differences in detection with the axial CT mode.

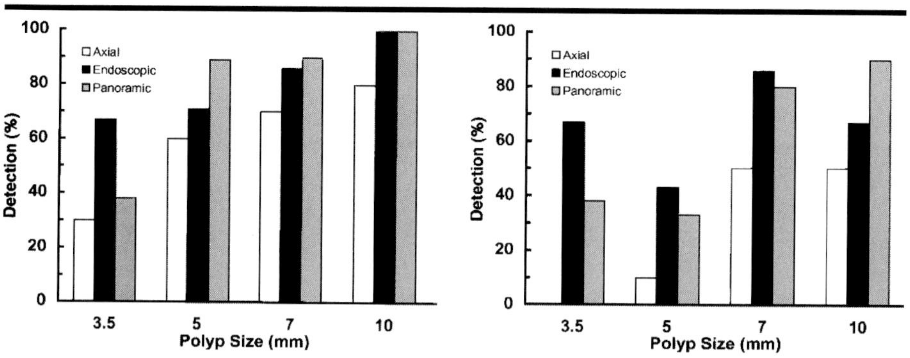

a. b.

Figure 8. Bar graphs show detection sensitivity as a function of polyp size after correction for lesion visibility for **(a)** reader 1 and **(b)** reader 2. The number of potentially detectable polyps is given in Table 2. Because inserted but invisible lesions on renderings from a particular display mode were excluded from this analysis, detection sensitivity was higher than that for all inserted lesions (see Fig 7). Trends toward a higher degree of detection for smaller lesions are present, especially for the 3D modes.

TABLE 1
Detection Sensitivity for Inserted Polyps

Reader	Axial CT	Virtual Endoscopy	Panoramic Endoscopy
1	24/40 (60)	22/40 (55)	30/40 (75)
2	11/40 (28)	17/40 (42)	23/40 (58)
Both 1 and 2	Not calculated*	39/80 (49)	53/80 (66)†

Note.—Data are the number of polyps of all sizes detected/total number of polyps inserted in the base data. Number in parentheses is the percentage.
* Sensitivity not calculated due to high interobserver variability.
† Sensitivity at panoramic endoscopy was significantly higher than that at virtual endoscopy ($P = .025$).

In contrast to the significantly higher sensitivity of panoramic endoscopy when all inserted lesions were considered, the correction for lesion visibility removed this advantage, such that the sensitivities of virtual endoscopy and panoramic endoscopy were not significantly different ($P = .6$; Table 3). In the detection of small (3.5- and 5-mm) polyps by reader 2 (Fig 8b), there was a notable trend toward higher sensitivity for virtual endoscopy and panoramic endoscopy than for axial CT, although the difference was not significant ($P > .05$).

TABLE 2
Influence of Imaging Mode on Visibility of Inserted Polyps

Polyp Size (mm)	Axial CT	Virtual Endoscopy	Panoramic Endoscopy
3.5	10	3	8
5.0	10	7	9
7.0	10	7	10
10.0	10	9	10
Total	40	26	37

Note.—Data are the number of polyps.

Review Time

Average case review times are given in Table 4. In general, the 3D studies took longer to review than did the axial CT studies. Mean review times were as follows: for axial CT studies, 8 minutes; for virtual endoscopic studies, 12.5 minutes; and for panoramic endoscopic studies, 13.2 minutes.

DISCUSSION

In CT colonography, important issues remain unsettled in many areas, including optimal methods of bowel cleansing, data acquisition, image rendering, and diagnostic interpretation (1,2,7,9,16,19,20). The latter issues—rendering and interpretation—are particularly challenging, because the sheer volume of imaging data is enormous compared with that of typical clinical studies. CT colonography also involves a different type of diagnostic interpretation: that of searching for polypoid lesions along the wall of an air-inflated, distended colon. Such issues have stimulated interest in the study of a variety of 2D and 3D display modes (6–8,14,17).

To date, there have not been rigorous trials in which different display modes of CT colonography were compared, to our knowledge. In most series (3,15,16), results from a combination of 2D and 3D display modes were compared with results from fiberoptic colonoscopy. When 2D and 3D modes are used together, it is difficult to establish independently the relative diagnostic contribution of each. Although results from initial investigations (7) suggested that 3D studies added incremental value over 2D studies, the authors of recent reports (6,8) have suggested that 2D studies alone may be sufficiently sensitive for initial data screening.

Whether a 2D, a 3D, or a hybrid approach will be the best initial screening method for CT colonographic data is important, because the effort involved in generating images for review is markedly different for 2D versus 3D modes. It ultimately will be crucial to determine if the extra effort required to produce 3D views is justified by the improved detection sensitivity.

A major confounding issue in clinical series is related to the reconciliation of CT colonographic results with those of the reference standard of fiberoptic colonoscopy. Operator dependence and inaccuracy in unique identification of neighboring lesions make reports of lesion-to-lesion correspondence between detection at CT colonography and detection at fiberoptic colonoscopy an educated guess, at best (21,22). Also limiting is the fact that relatively few clinically important lesions (≥1 cm in diameter) are detected in screening patient populations. In one study (3), only 15 lesions in this size range were identified in 70 patients, and in another study (8), only six lesions with a diameter larger than 8 mm were found in 44 patients.

In this report, we have described systematic work designed to elucidate the most sensitive methods for initial review of CT colonographic data. By using a system of synthetic polyps inserted into CT data obtained in a patient, we have a ground-truth model with which we were able to exercise control over many potentially confounding experimental variables. Our motivation for developing such a model was similar to that of Seltzer and colleagues (23), who used synthetic pulmonary nodules to study display modes for chest CT.

In blinded trials, we assessed the sensitivity of two radiologists at review of studies obtained with axial CT, virtual endoscopy, and a recently developed display mode termed panoramic endoscopy. When all inserted synthetic lesions were considered, the results of reader 1 followed the trend of sensitivity of panoramic endoscopy greater than that of axial CT, which was greater than that of virtual endoscopy, without significant differences between the modes. For reader 2, the trend was of sensitivity of panoramic endoscopy greater than that of virtual endoscopy, which was greater than that of axial CT; for reader 2, the 3D modes resulted in significantly better sensitivity than did the 2D mode.

Differences in sensitivity trends for the two observers are largely explained in terms of different performances with axial CT studies: The sensitivity for reader 1 was significantly greater than that for reader 2 (Fig 7). We believe this finding highlights one of the major challenges with regard to interpretation of CT colonographic studies as a stack of axial sections as compared with interpretation of 3D studies, namely, that of directing the radiologist's attention to an area of interest. In an axial CT study, any given image may contain multiple colonic cross sections, so a systematic search of the colon is necessary to prevent overlooking lesions. Also, the relative size of polyps in a display can be very small as compared with the overall diameter of the abdomen (6). The relatively complex visual search required for axial CT scans is in contrast to that for 3D displays, in which the observer's visible scene is typically constrained to a specific segment of the colon. In the latter circumstance, even relatively subtle lesions may be detectable, as suggested by the trend toward improved detection of small (3.5- and 5-mm) lesions by reader 2 (Fig 8b).

When we asked how the review of axial sections was approached by each of our readers, reader 1 indicated that he traced the colon systematically, whereas reader 2 used a section-by-section approach, attempting to detect lesions on all sections of colon visible on a particular CT image. Given similar amounts of CT colonographic interpretation experience, these different search patterns for axial CT studies may account for the interobserver variability we encountered.

By analyzing the results as a function of all lesions inserted in the base data (Fig 7), we attempted to model a clinical CT colonographic study, in which polyps are distributed relatively uniformly along the colonic mucosa, without necessarily a tendency toward location either on or between haustral folds. (More general tendencies toward a larger number of distal vs proximal colonic lesions do occur but on a larger spatial scale [24].)

With 3D virtual endoscopy, it often is assumed that all of the colonic surface is presented for visualization and thus detection. In reality, polyps located around corners or behind haustral folds may not be within the visible portion of the colon, which makes detection of such polyps impossible (Fig 3). The combination of results from forward- and reverse-viewing directions helps minimize this problem but does not ensure 100% coverage (25). In the current study, the virtual endoscopic mode demonstrated 26 of the 40 (65%) inserted lesions, whereas 37 (92%) lesions were visible on panoramic endoscopic studies (Table 2). These findings help explain why detection sensitivity was significantly higher with panoramic endoscopy (66%) than with virtual endoscopy (49%) when results from the two readers were combined across all lesion sizes (Table 1). Moreover, the absolute sensitivity of panoramic endoscopy for lesions in the 7-and 10-mm categories (90%) was statistically higher than that of virtual endoscopy (68%).

On the basis of these results, we infer that virtual endoscopy as currently implemented has an upper limit in terms of sensitivity for polyp detection, because not all of the colonic surface is presented to the reader. As technology advances to the point that interactive or real-time volume rendering becomes possible, the sensitivity of virtual endoscopy could improve, because an observer would be able to move the virtual camera at will in the attempt to maximize surface display.

By analyzing the detection results only for the lesions that were potentially visible in the renderings shown to the reviewers, we compensated for variations in colonic surface visibility between display modes. We found that the sensitivity trends for the two readers were similar (Fig 8), with no significant differences between panoramic endoscopy and virtual endoscopy. This suggests that the 3D modes depicted individual lesions equally well, despite differences in image appearance due to orientation of the virtual camera. However, the sensitivities of the 3D modes significantly exceeded that of 2D axial CT for both reviewers (Table 3). This suggests that presentation of the imaging data in a 3D format provided important visual cues that made polyp detection easier than that with 2D data.

The concept that the 3D modes effectively constrain the reader's visual field and direct a start-to-finish search through the colon was alluded to earlier. Another contribution to the improved effectiveness of 3D display may be that haustral folds are depicted as they appear in their natural state, which allowed quick identification of the folds as normal structures. The apparent limitations of 2D review alone might be surmountable with training or improvements in image display that help guide the observer through the colon. In addition, augmentation of axial images with coronal, sagittal, or multiplanar reformations could help improve detection at the expense of some additional review time.

Our study has several limitations. A first limitation was our use of synthetic polyps rather than true lesions. This provided maximal control over the variables of lesion size, shape, and location (11).

TABLE 3
Detection Sensitivity for Visible Polyps

Reader	Axial CT	Virtual Endoscopy	Panoramic Endoscopy
1	24/40 (60)	22/26 (85)	30/37 (81)
2	11/40 (28)	17/26 (65)	23/37 (62)
Both 1 and 2	Not calculated*	39/52 (75)	53/74 (72)†

Note.—Data are the number of polyps of all sizes detected/total number of polyps visible in the base data. Number in parentheses is the percentage.
* Sensitivity not calculated due to high interobserver variability.
† In this analysis, there was no difference between sensitivities for panoramic and virtual endoscopy ($P = .63$).

TABLE 4
Mean Review Times for the Imaging Modes and the Four Experimental Data Sets

Reader	Axial CT (min)	Virtual Endoscopy (min)	Panoramic Endoscopy (min)
1	7	12.0	15.0
2	9	13.0	11.5
Mean of both readers	8	12.5	13.2

Although we believe that these simulated lesions accurately model the primary visual cues of native polyps, it is difficult to control for all facets of visual perception that could affect lesion detection.

A second limitation was the use of a single patient's colon for the base data. One could argue that expert reviewers seeing the same colon 12 times would recognize its features. However, because the appearance of the colon varied substantially between the three display modes we tested, the reviewers saw similar colons on only four occasions, so this source of case memory was less of an influence than might be expected. We recognize, however, that each patient has unique colonic curvatures and haustral fold morphology and variable amounts of retained fluid that will affect lesion detection. For this basic trial, which focused on relative performances with display modes, however, we believed that the benefits of a single well-cleansed colon outweighed the disadvantages. The primary advantage was that the background morphology was identical between experimental cases; thus, results from the four cases could be combined without concern about the introduction of a confounding variable.

A third limitation was that we inserted a relatively large number of lesions (nine to 11) in each experimental data set—more lesions than would be expected in a clinical case. Because this was a direct comparison between display modes, this issue probably is less important than it would be in clinical trials, where a "needle-in-a-haystack" search must be performed for what might be one clinically important polyp. In such a setting, reviewer fatigue likely will affect detection sensitivity.

Fourth, we used only spherical simulated lesions, which became hemispheric when composited with the base data. From a practical standpoint, insertion of spherical lesions is easier than insertion of asymmetric lesions, which might require a defined orientation with respect to the colonic wall. From a theoretic standpoint, we did not want to introduce shape features as an additional visual detection cue.

Finally, it is reasonable to question the value of studying each of the modes in a completely blinded fashion. To achieve rigorous, independent results, the rationale behind this design is obvious. In practice, however, a combination of 2D and 3D display modes will likely be needed to achieve not only the sensitivity but also the specificity necessary for clinical CT colonography (2,9,10,19). Lesion specificity, which is concerned with whether a detected polypoid structure represents a true polyp, a focus of retained stool, or a normal structure such as the ileocecal valve, is a critical issue for the overall success of CT colonography but was not the focus of the current study. Future investigators should also systematically address the effect of false-positive observations among different display modes, which could influence patient care with CT colonography.

Ultimately, what we expect is that an initial rapid screening of the imaging data in either a 3D or a 2D mode will be performed to identify areas of concern; then, supplementary images of the area will be created to aid in further analysis of the suggestive areas and decisions about whether the patient should be referred for fiberoptic colonoscopy. Although the current results are suggestive of an incremental value associated with 3D display for initial lesion detection, these results must be considered in the context of our specialized display methods and relatively limited sample sizes. We intend that this work will serve as a useful conceptual framework for future studies in which visualization issues will be systematically addressed.

In summary, we applied a ground-truth model system in initial evaluations of display modes for CT colonography. For 2D axial CT, detection sensitivity differed significantly between the two reviewers, a finding that may be related to different search patterns used during review. When we controlled for true lesion visibility, both reviewers achieved significantly higher detection sensitivity with the 3D modes of virtual endoscopy and panoramic endoscopy than with axial CT, which suggests that 3D images contained visual cues that made lesion detection easier, although review of 3D images was more time-consuming. On a lesion-by-lesion basis, reviewers performed similarly with both virtual endoscopic and panoramic endoscopic modes. However, for all inserted lesions, our panoramic rendering technique significantly increased the sensitivity for polyp detection above that of a display mode in which a conventional virtual camera is used, by increasing the percentage of displayed surface area. Thus, when comparing different display modes, one must recognize that detection sensitivity can be substantially limited because of geometric and optical constraints on the virtual camera, factors that, a priori, limit colonic surface depiction. Such factors could affect polyp detection at clinical CT colonography.

Acknowledgments: The authors are grateful to Carl R. Crawford, MD, (Analogic, Peabody, Mass) for providing the core of the CT simulator software and Laura Logan, RT, for assistance at the Stanford University 3D Medical Imaging Laboratory. The authors also thank Silicon Graphics (Mountain View, Calif).

References

1. Vining DJ, Shifrin RY, Grishaw EK, Liu K, Gelfand DW. Virtual colonoscopy (abstr). Radiology 1994; 193(P):446.
2. Vining D. Virtual colonoscopy. Gastrointest Endosc Clin N Am 1997; 7:285–291.
3. Hara AK, Johnson CD, Reed JE, et al. Detection of colorectal polyps with CT colography: initial assessment of sensitivity and specificity. Radiology 1997; 205:59–65.

4. Dachman AH, Lieberman J, Osnis RB, et al. Small simulated polyps in pig colon: sensitivity of CT virtual colography. Radiology 1997; 203:427–430.
5. Beaulieu CF, Napel S, Daniel BL, et al. Detection of colonic polyps in a phantom model: implications for virtual colonoscopy data acquisition. J Comput Assist Tomogr 1998; 22:656–663.
6. Hara AK, Johnson CD, Reed JE. CT colography (CTC) for clinical use: a new method to reduce evaluation time (abstr). Radiology 1997; 205(P):718.
7. Hara AK, Johnson CD, Reed JE, Ehman RL, Ilstrup DM. Colorectal polyp detection with CT colography: two- versus three-dimensional techniques. Radiology 1996; 200:49–54.
8. Dachman AH, Kuniyoshi JK, Boyle CM, et al. Interactive CT colonography with three-dimensional problem solving for detection of colonic polyps. AJR 1998; 171: 989–995.
9. Fenlon HM, Ferrucci JT. Virtual colonoscopy: what will the issues be? AJR 1997; 169:453–458.
10. Royster AP, Fenlon HM, Clarke PD, Nunes DP, Ferrucci JT. CT colonoscopy of colorectal neoplasms: two-dimensional and three-dimensional virtual-reality techniques with colonoscopic correlation. AJR 1997; 169:1237–1242.
11. Karadi C, Beaulieu CF, Jeffrey RB Jr, Paik DS, Napel S. Display modes for CT colonography. I. Synthesis and insertion of polyps into patient CT data. Radiology 1999; 212:195–201.
12. Paik DS, Beaulieu CF, Jeffrey RB, Rubin GD, Napel S. Automated flight-path planning for virtual endoscopy. Med Phys 1998; 25:629–639.
13. McFarland EG, Wang G, Brink JA, Balfe DM, Heiken JP, Vannier MW. Spiral computed tomographic colonography: determination of the central axis and digital unraveling of the colon. Acad Radiol 1997; 4:367–373.
14. Rubin GD, Beaulieu CF, Argiro V, et al. Perspective volume rendering of CT and MR images: applications for endoscopic imaging. Radiology 1996; 199:321–330.
15. Beaulieu C, Jeffrey R, Paik D, Slosberg E, Young H, Napel S. Three-dimensional computed tomography colonography (3DCTC): initial clinical experience with 3 mm collimation and perspective volume rendering (abstr). Radiology 1997; 205(P):196.
16. Hopper KD, Naus MS, Khandelwal M, Wise SW, Iyriboz TA, Weaver JS. CT colonoscopy used as a routine screening procedure (abstr). Radiology 1997; 205(P):721.
17. McFarland EG, Brink JA, Loh J, et al. Visualization of colorectal polyps with spiral CT colography: evaluation of processing parameters with perspective volume rendering. Radiology 1997; 205:701–707.
18. Daniel WW. Hypothesis testing. In: Biostatistics: a foundation for analysis in the health sciences. 7th ed. New York, NY: Wiley, 1999; 252–254.
19. Kay CL, Evangelou HA. A review of the technical and clinical aspects of virtual endoscopy. Endoscopy 1996; 28:768–775.
20. Vining DJ. Virtual endoscopy: is it reality? (editorial). Radiology 1996; 200:30–31.
21. Rex DK, Cutler CS, Lemmel GT, Rahmani EY, et al. Colonoscopic miss rates of adenomas determined by back-to-back colonoscopies. Gastroenterology 1997; 112:24–28.
22. Haseman JH, Lemmel GT, Rahmani EY, Rex DK. Failure of colonoscopy to detect colorectal cancer: evaluation of 47 cases in 20 hospitals. Gastrointest Endosc 1997; 45:451–455.
23. Seltzer SE, Judy PF, Adams DF, et al. Spiral CT of the chest: comparison of cine and film-based viewing. Radiology 1995; 197: 73–78.
24. O'Brien MJ, Winawer SJ, Zauber AG, et al. The National Polyp Study: patient and polyp characteristics associated with high-grade dysplasia in colorectal adenomas. Gastroenterology 1990; 98:371–379.
25. Paik DS, Beaulieu CF, Jeffrey RB, Napel S. Virtual colonoscopy visualization modes using cylindrical and planar map projections: technique and evaluation (abstr). Radiology 1998; 209(P):429.

Pancreatic Carcinoma versus Chronic Pancreatitis: Dynamic MR Imaging[1]

Pamela T. Johnson, MD
Eric K. Outwater, MD

Index terms:
Pancreas, MR, 77.121411, 77.121412, 77.121415, 77.12143
Pancreas, neoplasms, 77.321
Pancreatitis, 77.291

Radiology 1999; 212:213–218

Abbreviations:
GRE = gradient echo
SE = spin echo

[1] From the Department of Radiology, Thomas Jefferson University Hospital, 132 S 11th St, 7th Floor Main Bldg, Philadelphia, PA 19107. From the 1997 RSNA scientific assembly. Received May 21, 1998; revision requested July 14; revision received October 9; accepted December 16. **Address reprint requests to** P.T.J. (e-mail: *johnson5@jeflin.tju.edu*).

Author contributions:
Guarantor of integrity of entire study, P.T.J.; study concepts and design, P.T.J., E.K.O.; definition of intellectual content, P.T.J., E.K.O.; literature research, P.T.J.; clinical studies, P.T.J., E.K.O.; data acquisition and analysis, P.T.J., E.K.O.; statistical analysis, P.T.J., E.K.O.; manuscript preparation, P.T.J.; manuscript editing, P.T.J., E.K.O.

PURPOSE: To determine if dynamic gadolinium-enhanced magnetic resonance (MR) imaging can distinguish chronic pancreatitis from pancreatic carcinoma.

MATERIALS AND METHODS: A retrospective review of MR and pathology examination findings was performed for 24 patients with pancreatic ductal adenocarcinoma and seven with chronic pancreatitis who underwent dynamic gadolinium-enhanced breath-hold spoiled gradient-echo imaging. Arterial, portal, and delayed phase images were obtained after injection of gadopentatate dimeglumine. The MR images of 14 patients without clinical evidence of pancreatic disease were also reviewed as controls. Signal intensity (SI) was measured on the precontrast (pre) and gadolinium-enhanced (post) images of the area of the pancreas sampled at biopsy and of the nontumorous pancreas. Percentage enhancement was defined as $SI_{pre}/SI_{post} \times 100$.

RESULTS: Normal pancreas showed rapid enhancement that peaked in the arterial or portal phase. For both diseases, T1-weighted images showed hypointense masses with progressive enhancement (differences were significant [$P < .05$] on only delayed fat-saturated images). Differences in enhancement between either disease state and normal pancreas were significant for at least one phase. Nontumorous pancreas in patients with carcinoma showed gradual enhancement that was significantly different from that of normal pancreas.

CONCLUSION: Chronic pancreatitis and pancreatic carcinoma show abnormal pancreatic enhancement, but the two were not distinguished on the basis of degree and time of enhancement.

Advances in technology for magnetic resonance (MR) imaging and computed tomography (CT) have improved the ability to detect pancreatic carcinoma (1–4). Findings in several studies have suggested that MR imaging may be superior to CT in pancreatic lesion detection and preoperative staging (5,6). However, chronic pancreatitis remains difficult to distinguish from pancreatic carcinoma on the basis of imaging criteria because both demonstrate low signal intensity on T1-weighted images and are associated with ductal obstruction (7,8).

A recent study compared images of the pancreas obtained with dynamic gadolinium-enhanced fast multiplanar spoiled gradient-echo (GRE), T1- and T2-weighted spin-echo (SE), and gadolinium-enhanced T1-weighted SE sequences. Dynamic gadolinium-enhanced multiplanar fast spoiled GRE images were found to result in more accurate and specific diagnoses of pathologic conditions in the pancreas (2). The purpose of this study was to determine if the contrast enhancement pattern on dynamic gadolinium-enhanced multiplanar fast spoiled GRE images of the pancreas could distinguish masses due to chronic pancreatitis from those due to pancreatic carcinoma.

MATERIALS AND METHODS

A computer search identified 145 MR imaging examinations performed between 1992 and 1996 at our institution in which a pancreatic mass was detected. In 43 patients, pathologic confirmation of the diagnosis was obtained by means of ultrasonography (US)-guided biopsy, intraoperative biopsy, or resection of the pancreatic mass. Twelve of these 43 patients were excluded because the original MR imaging archive could not be retrieved, no intravenous contrast material was administered, an inadequate arterial bolus was used, the MR imaging protocol varied from the standard dynamic breath-hold fast multiplanar spoiled GRE sequence, or the mass could not be defined and measured when the image was reviewed. Of the remaining 31 patients, 24 (13 men and 11 women; age range, 52–77 years; mean age, 66 years) had pancreatic carcinoma and seven (five men and two women; age range, 46–66 years; mean age, 55 years) had chronic pancreatitis.

The diagnosis of pancreatic carcinoma was confirmed at surgical excision of the mass by means of a Whipple procedure in seven of the 24 patients. Intraoperative biopsy was performed in 12 patients with unresectable tumors. The remaining five patients underwent US-guided fine-needle aspiration (n = 4) or core biopsy (n = 1); their tumors were deemed unresectable at preoperative imaging.

In the seven patients with the diagnosis of chronic pancreatitis, the pathologic correlation was obtained by means of US-guided fine-needle aspiration (n = 2), surgical resection of the mass (n = 1), or intraoperative biopsy (n = 4). Two of the patients who underwent intraoperative biopsy also underwent fine-needle aspiration or pancreatic duct brushing. Findings at follow-up (range, 3–17 months) MR imaging, CT, or endoscopic retrograde cholangiopancreatography confirmed no change in two patients. Two patients underwent follow-up MR imaging that depicted enlargement of the mass, but no further biopsies were performed. Three patients did not undergo follow-up imaging.

Fourteen patients who underwent dynamic imaging of the liver for indications unrelated to pancreatic disease served as control subjects. Their examinations were performed to evaluate hemangioma, fatty liver, or parenchymal liver disease.

All examinations were performed on a 1.5-T system (GE Medical Systems, Milwaukee, Wis). The following parameters were used in the multiplanar fast spoiled GRE sequence: repetition time msec/echo time msec, 100–170/1.3–2.9; flip angle, 90°; matrix, 256 × 128 to 256 × 192; one signal acquired; section thickness, 7–9 mm; gap, 1–2 mm; field of view, 24–38 cm. Gadopentatate dimeglumine (Magnevist; Berlex Laboratories, Wayne, NJ) was administered (0.1 mmol/L per kilogram of body weight) intravenously at approximately 2 mL/sec by means of hand injection followed by a 20-mL saline solution flush. Imaging was initiated after 10 mL of the flush had been infused.

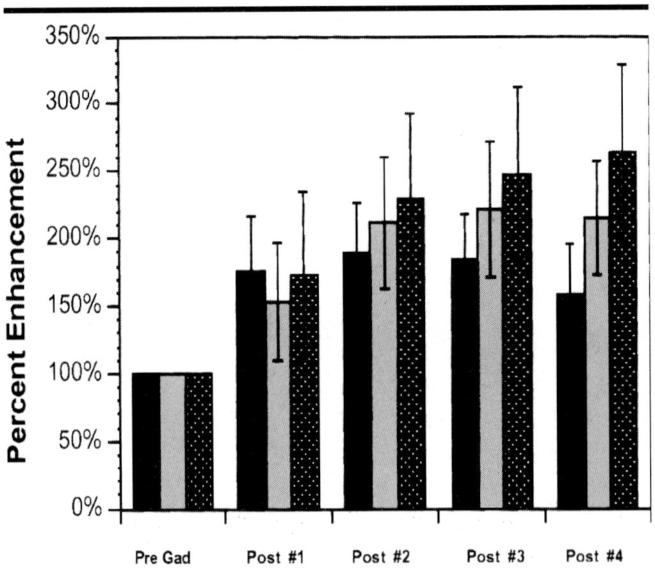

Figure 1. Bar graph depicts mean percentage enhancement after injection of gadopentatate dimeglumine for normal pancreas in control subjects (black bars), chronic pancreatitis (gray bars), and pancreatic cancer (dotted black bars). Error bars represent mean plus or minus SD. The series represents the percentage enhancement before injection of gadopentatate dimeglumine (*Pre Gad*) and after injection in the arterial (*Post #1*), portal venous (*Post #2*), parenchymal- (*Post #3*), or delayed (*Post #4*) phases. In the normal pancreas, the percentage enhancement peaks in the arterial dominant or portal venous phase. Pancreatic carcinoma and chronic pancreatitis demonstrate more gradual enhancement.

Imaging was performed with four breath-hold gadolinium-enhanced sequences in most patients. These sequences correlated approximately with arterial dominant (n = 45), portal venous (n = 45), parenchymal (n = 38), and delayed (n = 42) phases of contrast enhancement. Eight patients with pancreatic cancer underwent imaging with only three gadolinium-enhanced sequences (only one delayed sequence was performed). Five of the eight patients did not undergo imaging with the third gadolinium-enhanced sequence, and three did not undergo imaging with the final delayed fat-saturated sequence. All seven of the patients with chronic pancreatitis underwent imaging with all four sequences.

During review of each case, an adequate bolus was confirmed on the basis of the presence of a moiré pattern in the spleen, absence of hepatic vein contrast enhancement, and corticomedullary differentiation of the kidneys. On the basis of these criteria, two patients were excluded because of an inadequate bolus. The final delayed fat-saturated sequence usually required two breath holds.

The original MR imaging data were loaded onto a workstation (Cannon; Sun Microsystems, Palo Alto, Calif) by means of software (RATIONAL IMAGING; Intuitive Software, West Hills, Calif). Each study was reviewed with the pathology report and US-guided biopsy report or intraoperative note to confirm the location of the mass sampled at biopsy. In the patients with pancreatic carcinoma or chronic pancreatitis, the largest possible region of interest was drawn when the signal intensity of the mass or the nontumorous pancreas was measured proximal to tumor. In the control subjects, region-of-interest measurements were obtained from the pancreatic head and body or tail. The signal intensity was measured on the precontrast and gadolinium-enhanced multiplanar fast spoiled GRE images (n = 31). All regions of interest were placed by one author (P.T.J.).

Percentage enhancement values for the pancreatic mass, nontumorous pancreas, and normal pancreas were calculated by dividing the gadolinium-enhanced signal intensity by the precontrast signal intensity and multiplying by 100. A Student two-tailed t test was performed to com-

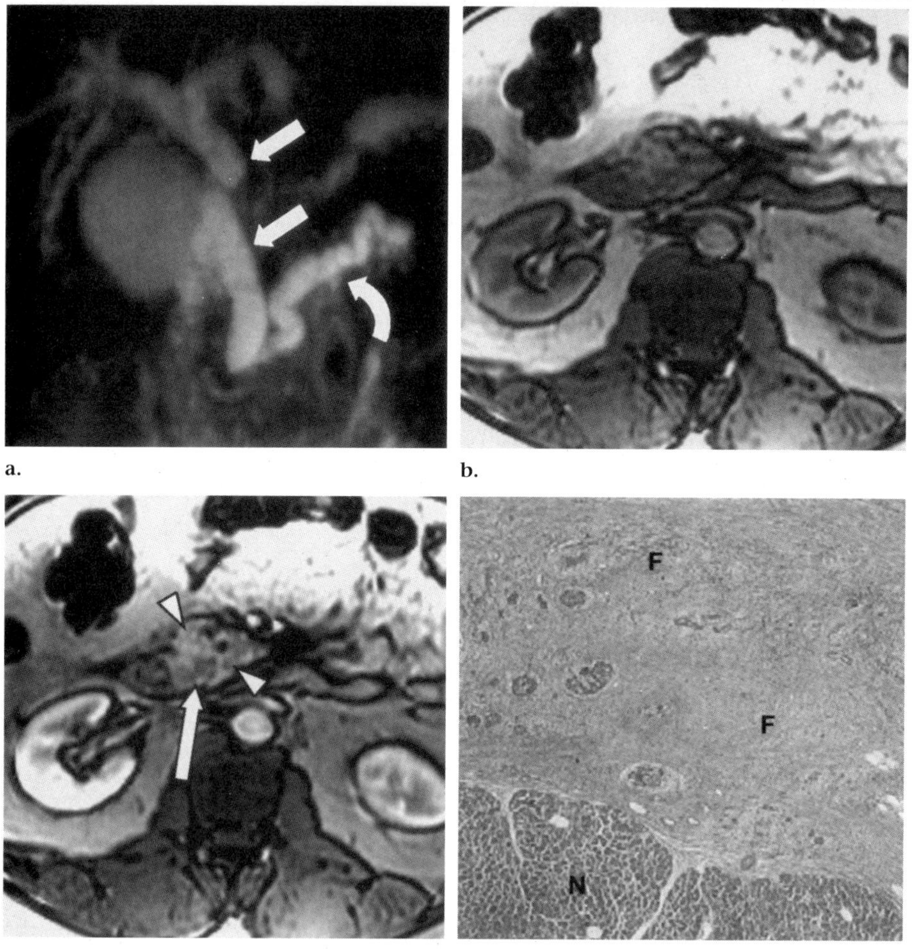

Figure 2. Contrast enhancement of pancreatic carcinoma. **(a)** Reconstructed MR cholangiogram (1,2000/255) depicts distal obstruction of the common bile duct (straight arrows) and pancreatic duct (curved arrow) with ductal dilatation due to a pancreatic adenocarcinoma near the ampulla. **(b, c)** T1-weighted GRE images (155/2.2) were obtained **(b)** before injection of gadopentatate dimeglumine and **(c)** during the arterial phase of contrast enhancement. In **c**, enhancement of the tumor (arrow) is less than that of normal pancreatic parenchyma (arrowheads). **(d)** Photomicrograph shows extensive fibrosis (*F*) throughout the tumor, which borders normal pancreatic parenchyma (*N*).

pare the percentage enhancement of carcinoma, nontumorous pancreas proximal to tumor, chronic pancreatitis, and normal pancreas.

RESULTS

The normal pancreas enhanced rapidly after infusion of gadopentatate dimeglumine and remained enhanced on the portal venous and first delayed images (Fig 1). The percentage enhancement of the normal pancreatic head peaked on the arterial dominant or portal venous phase images. The percentage enhancement of the pancreatic body did not differ significantly from that of the head.

Twenty-four of the patients had biopsy-proved pancreatic carcinoma (mean transverse diameter, 3.2 cm ± 1.2). Seventeen masses were located in the pancreatic head, two in the uncinate process, and five in the pancreatic body. After infusion of gadopentatate dimeglumine, these masses showed gradual progressive enhancement (Fig 2). The percentage enhancement was statistically different from normal on the second (P = .015), third (P = .001), and delayed fat-saturated (P < .001) gadolinium-enhanced images (Fig 1).

Seven masses were pathologically proved chronic pancreatitis (mean transverse diameter, 3.3 cm ± 1.7). All seven were located in the pancreatic head. After infusion of gadopentatate dimeglumine, these masses showed a more gradual enhancement compared with that of the normal pancreas (Fig 3), with peak enhancement on the third gadolinium-enhanced series (Fig 1). The percentage enhancement was statistically different from normal on the delayed fat-saturated gadolinium-enhanced images (P = .01).

The pattern of gradual enhancement of chronic pancreatitis and cancer was similar. However, a statistically significant difference was detected between the two pathologic conditions when the percentage enhancement was compared on the delayed fat-saturated images (P = .04). Considerable overlap was noted when peak percentage enhancement was compared between masses due to chronic pancreatitis or pancreatic cancer. Of the seven masses due to chronic pancreatitis, peak percentage enhancement occurred during the portal venous phase in one, parenchymal phase in four, and delayed phase in two. Of the 24 masses due to pancreatic carcinoma, peak percentage enhancement occurred during the portal venous phase in five, parenchymal phase in four, and delayed phase in 15.

In the setting of a pancreatic head carcinoma, the nontumorous pancreatic body or tail (n = 19) showed gradual progressive enhancement after administration of gadopentatate dimeglumine that peaked on the delayed fat-saturated images (Fig 4). The percentage enhancement of the body or tail was significantly different from that of the normal pancreatic body on the portal venous phase (P = .003), parenchymal (P = .005), and delayed fat-saturated (P < .001) gadolinium-enhanced images. The nontumorous body and tail demonstrated a decreased precontrast signal intensity (Fig 5), which accounted in part for the differences in percentage enhancement.

DISCUSSION

The ability to detect and stage pancreatic carcinoma has improved owing to advances in MR imaging and CT technology. Findings in comparative studies suggest that fast MR imaging sequences may be superior to helical CT for preoperative tumor detection and determination of tumor extension (4,6). Administration of antiperistaltic agents and imaging with fast breath-hold sequences have resulted in images with less motion artifact. Use of faster sequences has also facilitated dynamic gadolinium-enhanced imaging of the pancreas during multiple phases of contrast enhancement. Data continue to emerge about which dynamic sequences are optimal for lesion detection (9).

In many studies, CT has been used in an attempt to distinguish chronic pancreatitis from pancreatic carcinoma. Karawasa et al (10) evaluated the pancreatic duct caliber and contour and found that smooth or beaded dilatations of the duct are more common with an obstructing neoplasm. Chronic pancreatitis more frequently results in an irregularly dilated duct, often with intraductal calcification. Additionally, they found a statistically significant difference in the ratio of duct caliber to pancreatic gland width, which is higher in patients with cancer (10). Megibow et al (11) originally described thickening of the celiac artery or superior mesenteric artery as specific for carcinoma. However, more recent work by Baker (8) and Shulte et al (12) demonstrates that acute and chronic inflammatory processes can result in infiltration of the fat around the superior mesenteric artery and encasement of the vessel by a mass or periarterial adenopathy. Recognizing that periarterial findings are nonspecific, Elmas et al (13) measured the diameter of the superior mesenteric artery and vein in patients with chronic pancreatitis or pancreatic carcinoma. They found that the artery enlarges in the setting of cancer, and carcinoma should be suspected if the artery-to-vein ratio is greater than 1.0.

As MR imaging techniques improve, findings in comparative studies reveal potentially higher diagnostic accuracy compared to that with other modalities in the evaluation of pancreatic disease (3,5). The study by Semelka et al (3) compared MR imaging with CT and revealed significantly diminished delayed contrast enhancement at MR imaging in chronic pancreatitis compared to nonnecrotic acute pancreatitis or normal pancreas. The more recent work by Gohde et al (2) compared a dynamic gadolinium-enhanced multiplanar fast spoiled GRE sequence to T1- and T2-weighted SE sequences and a gadolinium-enhanced T1-weighted SE sequence with fat saturation. The multiplanar fast spoiled GRE sequence has higher sensitivity, specificity, and accuracy for detection of pancreatic disease and yields images of higher quality with better delineation of pancreatic anatomy.

In several studies, MR imaging was used in an attempt to distinguish pancreatic diseases. Jenkins et al (14) found that there is no statistically significant difference in T1 and T2 between chronic pancreatitis and pancreatic carcinoma, although the relaxation times for cancer differed from normal findings in control subjects. More recently, Sittek et al (15) used fast multiplanar MR imaging to demonstrate that chronic pancreatitis and cancer enhance differently from normal pancreas or unaffected pancreatic parenchyma in patients with a mass. Semelka et al (3) compared calcific versus noncalcific chronic pancreatitis imaged with fast GRE and fat-suppressed SE sequences. Percentage contrast enhancement is significantly different between the two groups (16).

The promising work in CT and MR imaging combined with the higher diagnostic accuracy of the dynamic multiplanar fast spoiled GRE sequence prompted us to compare the dynamic multiplanar MR characteristics of chronic pancreatitis with those of pancreatic carcinoma. Both pathologic entities resulted in gradual progressive enhancement of the involved pancreatic parenchyma that would be difficult to distinguish subjectively. Although there was a significant difference in percentage enhancement between the two diseases with the delayed fat-saturated sequence, the amount of overlap would preclude distinguishing the two subjectively on this basis.

Evaluation of the histology of chronic pancreatitis and carcinoma reveals abundant fibrosis in both pathologic conditions (Figs 2, 3), which likely accounts for their similar imaging appearance. Additionally, the pancreas proximal to an obstructing mass may undergo atrophy and fibrosis that lead to an altered pattern of enhancement when compared to that of normal pancreatic parenchyma. Interestingly, this pattern of gradual enhancement in the nontumorous body of a

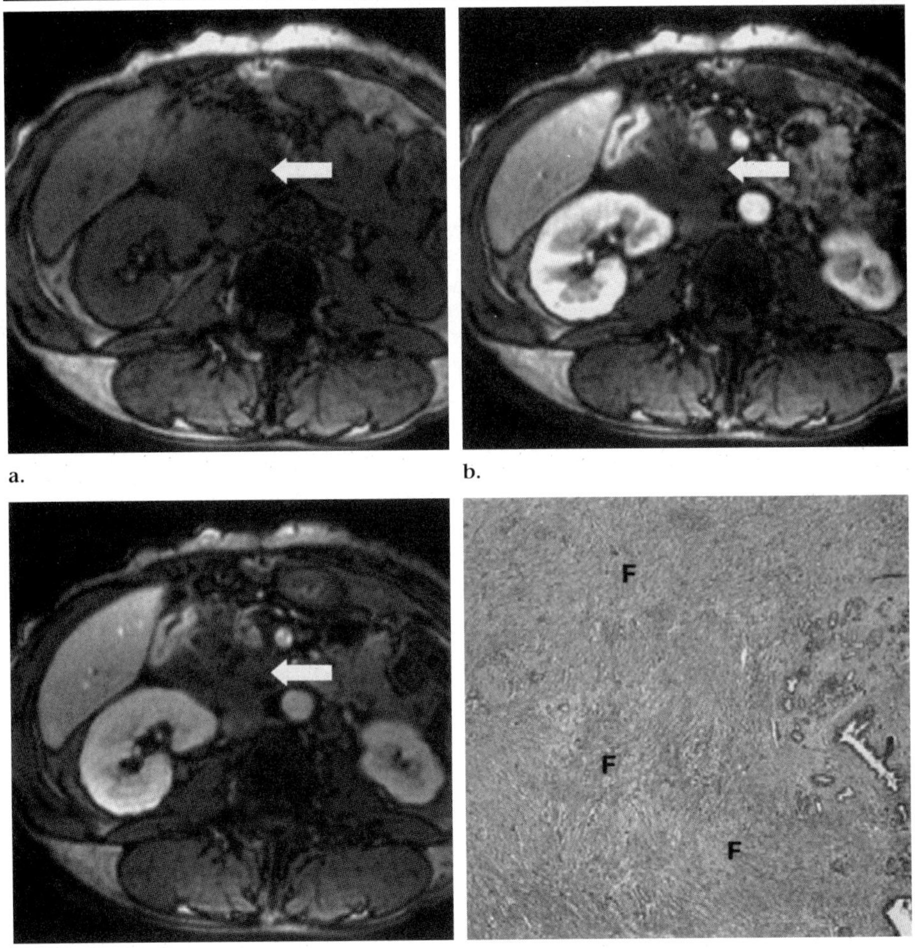

a. b. c. d.

Figure 3. Contrast enhancement of chronic pancreatitis. **(a–c)** T1-weighted GRE images (140/2.5) were obtained **(a)** before injection of gadopentatate dimeglumine and during the **(b)** arterial and **(c)** portal venous phases of contrast enhancement. **b** and **c** depict only slight enhancement of the pancreatic head mass (arrow). **(d)** Photomicrograph shows extensive fibrosis (*F*) throughout the chronic pancreatitis.

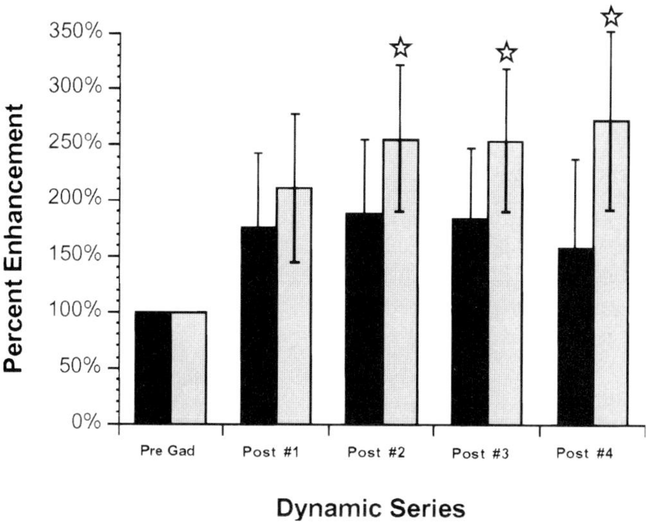

Figure 4. Bar graph depicts mean percentage enhancement after injection of gadopentatate dimeglumine in the normal pancreas of control patients (black bars) and nontumorous portion of the pancreas in patients with pancreatic carcinoma (gray bars). The series represents the percentage enhancement before injection of gadopentatate dimeglumine (*Pre Gad*) and after injection during the arterial (*Post #1*), portal venous (*Post #2*), parenchymal (*Post #3*), and delayed (*Post #4*) phases. The nontumorous pancreas demonstrates gradually increasing enhancement over time that is significantly different from that of normal pancreas (☆ = $P < .005$) and peaks on the delayed fat-saturated image (*Post #4*). Error bars represent mean plus or minus SD.

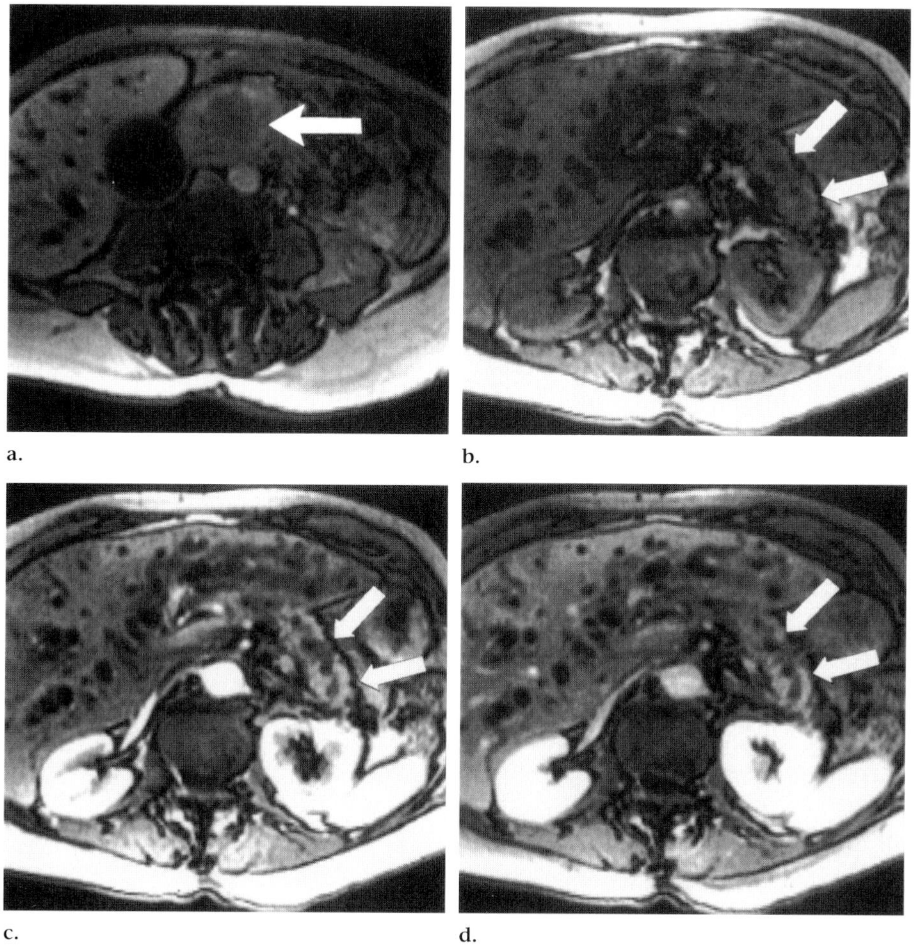

Figure 5. Enhancement of chronic pancreatitis due to obstructing pancreatic head carcinoma. **(a)** Gadolinium-enhanced T1-weighted GRE image shows the pancreatic carcinoma (arrow) in the head of the pancreas. **(b–d)** In the same patient, T1-weighted GRE images (115/2.2) of the pancreatic body and tail obtained **(b)** before injection of gadopentatate dimeglumine and after injection during the **(c)** arterial and **(d)** portal venous phases of enhancement. Enhancement of the pancreatic parenchyma (arrows) is lower than that of the normal pancreas. In **c**, the dilated pancreatic duct appears as a beaded low-signal-intensity structure in the parenchyma of the body and tail.

pancreas with a pancreatic head mass was more similar to the enhancement of the cancer itself than to that of chronic pancreatitis. This may be due to the lack of inflammation that accompanies typical chronic pancreatitis.

In conclusion, masses due to pancreatic carcinoma and chronic pancreatitis show a pattern of contrast enhancement after dynamic infusion of gadopentatate dimeglumine that is altered compared to that of normal pancreas. The similar gradual pattern of enhancement and overlap in peak enhancement preclude distinction of the two entities on the basis of gadolinium-enhanced MR findings. Further work must address other dynamic MR imaging features that may help distinguish the two pathologic entities.

References

1. Semelka RC, Ascher SM. MR imaging of the pancreas. Radiology 1993; 188:593–602.
2. Gohde SC, Toth J, Krestin GP, Debatin JF. Dynamic contrast-enhanced FMPSPGR of the pancreas: impact on diagnostic performance. AJR 1997; 168:689–696.
3. Semelka RC, Kroeker MA, Shoenut JP, Kroeker R, Yaffe CS, Micflikier AB. Pancreatic disease: prospective comparison of CT, ERCP, and 1.5-T MR imaging with dynamic gadolinium enhancement and fat suppression. Radiology 1991; 181:785–791.
4. Gabata T, Masui S, Kadoya M, et al. Small pancreatic adenocarcinomas: efficacy of MR imaging with fat suppression and gadolinium enhancement. Radiology 1994; 193:683–688.
5. Vellet AD, Romano W, Bach DB, Passi RB, Taves DH, Munk PL. Adenocarcinoma of the pancreatic ducts: comparative evaluation with CT and MR imaging at 1.5 T. Radiology 1992; 183:87–95.
6. Ichikawa T, Haradome H, Hachiya J, et al. Pancreatic ductal adenocarcinoma: preoperative assessment with helical CT versus dynamic MR imaging. Radiology 1997; 202:655–662.
7. DelMaschio A, Vanzulli A, Sironi S, et al. Pancreatic cancer versus chronic pancreatitis: diagnosis with Ca 19-9 assessment, US, CT, and CT-guided fine-needle biopsy. Radiology 1991; 178:95–99.
8. Baker ME. Pancreatic adenocarcinoma: are there pathognomonic changes in the fat surrounding the superior mesenteric artery? Radiology 1991; 180:613–614.

9. Lu DS, Vedantham S, Krasny RM, Kadell B, Berger WL, Reber HA. Two-phase helical CT for pancreatic tumors: pancreatic versus hepatic phase enhancement of tumor, pancreas, and vascular structures. Radiology 1996; 199:697–701.
10. Karawasa E, Goldberg HI, Moss AA, Federle MP, London SS. CT pancreatogram in carcinoma of the pancreas and chronic pancreatitis. Radiology 1983; 148:489–493.
11. Megibow AJ, Bosniak MA, Ambos MA, Beranbaum ER. Thickening of the celiac axis and/or superior mesenteric artery: a sign of pancreatic carcinoma on computed tomography. Radiology 1981; 141: 449–453.
12. Shulte SH, Baron RL, Freeny PC, Patten RM, Gorell HA, Maclin ML. Root of the superior mesenteric artery in pancreatitis and pancreatic carcinoma: evaluation with CT. Radiology 1991; 180:659–662.
13. Elmas N, Yorulmaz I, Oran I, Oyar O, Ozutemiz O, Ozer H. A new criterion in differentiation of pancreatitis and pancreatic carcinoma: artery-to-vein ratio using the superior mesenteric vessels. Abdom Imaging 1996; 21:331–333.
14. Jenkins JP, Braganza JM, Hickey DS, Isherwood I, Machin M. Quantitative tissue characterisation in pancreatic disease using magnetic resonance imaging. Br J Radiol 1987; 60:333–341.
15. Sittek H, Heuck AF, Folsing C, Gieseke J, Reiser M. Static and dynamic MR tomography of the pancreas: contrast media kinetics of the normal pancreatic parenchyma in pancreatic carcinoma and chronic pancreatitis. ROFO 1995; 162: 396–403.
16. Semelka RC, Shoenut JP, Kroeker MA, Micflikier AB. Chronic pancreatitis: MR imaging features before and after administration of gadopentatate dimeglumine. JMRI 1993; 3:79–82.

Pancreatic CT Imaging: Effects of Different Injection Rates and Doses of Contrast Material[1]

Tonsok Kim, MD
Takamichi Murakami, MD, PhD
Satoru Takahashi, MD
Atsuya Okada, MD
Masatoshi Hori, MD
Yoshifumi Narumi, MD, PhD
Hironobu Nakamura, MD, PhD

Index terms:
Computed tomography (CT), contrast enhancement, 770.12112, 770.12119
Pancreas, CT, 770.12112, 770.12119
Pancreas, neoplasms, 770.32

Radiology 1999; 212:219–225

[1] From the Department of Radiology, Osaka University Medical School, 2-2 Yamadaoka, Suita City, Osaka 565-0871, Japan. From the 1997 RSNA scientific assembly. Received June 17, 1998; revision requested July 30; revision received September 22; accepted December 15. **Address reprint requests to** T.K. (e-mail: *kim@radiol.med.osakau.ac.jp*).

PURPOSE: To assess the effects of the intravenous injection rate and dose of contrast material on pancreatic computed tomography (CT).

MATERIALS AND METHODS: A total of 126 patients were divided at random into four groups with different injection rates and doses. Groups 1 and 2 underwent injection of 2 mL per kilogram of body weight of 300 mg of iodine per milliliter of contrast material, and groups 3 and 4 underwent injection of 1.5 mL/kg. The injection rate was 5 mL/sec for groups 1 and 3 and 3 mL/sec for groups 2 and 4. Single-level serial CT scanning was performed at the level of the pancreatic head, and the pancreatic enhancement value was calculated.

RESULTS: The maximum pancreatic enhancement value was 99 HU ± 18 (mean ± SD) for group 1, 90 HU ± 18 for group 2, 86 HU ± 15 for group 3, and 74 HU ± 13 for group 4. There were significant differences in the maximum pancreatic enhancement value between groups 1 and 2 ($P = .045$), between groups 3 and 4 ($P = .001$), between groups 1 and 3 ($P = .016$), and between groups 2 and 4 ($P = .001$).

CONCLUSION: Both a higher dose and a faster injection rate increased the maximum pancreatic enhancement value.

Helical computed tomography (CT) reduces the scanning time and allows for imaging of the abdomen during the optimal phase after intravenous injection of a bolus of contrast material (1). Helical CT is widely used for multiphase imaging of the entire liver (2,3). Several groups of investigators (4–9) have reported the effects of various intravenous contrast material injection techniques on hepatic enhancement, and these effects are now well known. Helical CT is also used for examination of the pancreas (10–16). However, our search of the literature revealed only a few reports (17,18) in which the effects of intravenous contrast material injection techniques on pancreatic enhancement have been evaluated.

One of the most common goals of pancreatic CT examination with use of contrast material is diagnosis of pancreatic ductal adenocarcinoma. Pancreatic adenocarcinomas are hypovascular (19), and theoretically, therefore, the greatest conspicuity of these tumors should be achieved when the pancreatic parenchyma is highly enhanced. Visualization of both the major peripancreatic arteries and portal venous system are also required for adequate staging of the tumor.

In this study, we evaluated the effects of different injection rates and doses of contrast material on pancreatic CT imaging through analysis of the enhancement of the pancreatic parenchyma, aorta, and superior mesenteric vein to identify the optimal injection technique.

MATERIALS AND METHODS

This study was performed in a prospective fashion. Consecutive patients who had malignancies and who were referred for abdominal CT examination to evaluate liver metastasis were considered for this study. In our institution, portal venous phase CT

Author contributions:
Guarantors of integrity of entire study, T.K., T.M., Y.N., H.N.; study concepts and design, T.K., T.M.; definition of intellectual content, T.K., T.M.; literature research, T.K.; clinical studies, T.K., S.T., A.O., M.H.; data acquisition and analysis, T.K.; statistical analysis, T.K.; manuscript preparation, T.K.; manuscript editing, T.K., T.M.; manuscript review, Y.N., H.N.

scanning of the liver is routinely performed for the evaluation of liver metastasis. Patients with one or more of the following diseases or conditions that could affect arterial and venous flow of the pancreas and mesentery were excluded: poor general condition; early postoperative phase; extensive tumor involvement of the liver, pancreas, or mesentery; cirrhosis; portal venous thrombosis; compression or invasion of arteries or veins around the pancreas; ascites; and cardiovascular disease.

We explained to the patients the purpose of this study, and we explained that radiation levels would be slightly increased, that the added radiation level would be about equal to that of several sections of our routine abdominal CT, and that the study would not interfere with the patients' clinical examinations. The patients who did not agree to this study were excluded, and all the patients included in this study gave informed consent. This study adhered to the Declaration of Helsinki principles (20). Patients in whom a 19-gauge plastic cannula could not be placed in an antecubital vein at the time of the CT examination were also excluded from this study.

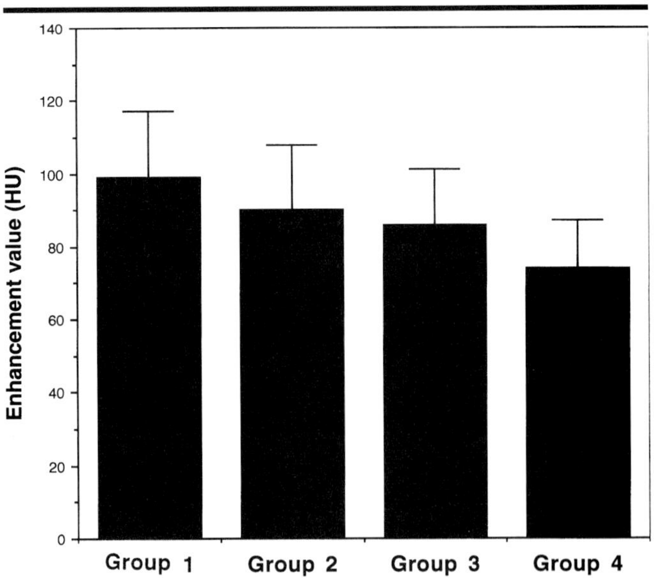

Figure 1. Bar graph shows the mean maximum enhancement value of the pancreas for the four groups. Error bars show SDs. Group 1 underwent injection with a dose of 2 mL/kg at a rate of 5 mL/sec, group 2 underwent injection with 2 mL/kg at 3 mL/sec, group 3 underwent injection with 1.5 mL/kg at 5 mL/sec, and group 4 underwent injection with 1.5 mL/kg at 3 mL/sec. The mean maximum enhancement value of the pancreas was greatest for group 1 and was greater for the groups with the higher dose.

Ultimately, 126 patients (63 women, 63 men; age range, 21–88 years; mean age, 56 years; weight range, 30–80 kg; mean weight, 55 kg) who met all the criteria for inclusion were entered into this study. The patients were divided at random into four groups with different monophasic intravenous injection protocols for the contrast material. In this study, two different injection rates (faster rate: 5 mL/sec and slower rate: 3 mL/sec) and two different doses (higher dose: 2 mL/kg and lower dose: 1.5 mL/kg) were adopted. For the contrast material, 300 mg of iodine per milliliter of nonionic contrast material (iomeprol; Iomeron; Eisai, Tokyo, Japan) was used. Group 1 (29 patients) underwent injection of a dose of 2 mL per kilogram of body weight at a rate of 5 mL/sec, group 2 (30 patients) underwent injection of a dose of 2 mL/kg at 3 mL/sec, group 3 (32 patients) underwent injection of a dose of 1.5 mL/kg at 5 mL/sec, and group 4 (35 patients) underwent injection of a dose of 1.5 mL/kg at 3 mL/sec.

The patients were examined after fasting for at least 4 hours. All CT scanning was performed with a HiSpeed Advantage scanner (GE Medical Systems, Milwaukee, Wis). Several nonenhanced CT images covering the pancreas were obtained in the form of contiguous 10-mm sections. These nonenhanced images were used to establish a single reference level, namely the section that included the pancreatic head and the superior mesenteric vein and that was caudal to the confluence of the splenic and the superior mesenteric veins. Single-level serial CT images were obtained at this level during a single breath hold every 2 seconds from 22 seconds until 60 seconds after the initiation of contrast material injection with an automatic injector (Autoenhance A50; Nemotokyorindo, Tokyo, Japan) through a 19-gauge plastic cannula placed in an antecubital vein.

Single-level serial CT scanning was performed with a 1-second scanning time, a 1-second interscan delay, 10-mm sections, an 80-mA electric current, and 140 kV. The electric current used for this study was reduced to 80 mA, although a 240-mA current is used for routine CT imaging in our institution. This method of repeated single-level CT sections at reduced milliamperage is used routinely in the commercial packages that monitor CT enhancement to optimize timing of scans relative to a bolus administration of contrast material (21). After this single-level scanning, CT scanning of the liver during the portal venous phase, as routinely performed in our hospital, was initiated 70 seconds after the start of the injection of contrast material. This study involved a minimal increase in radiation levels and did not interfere with clinical examinations.

Quantitative data acquisition was followed by measurement in Hounsfield units of the resultant attenuation values of the pancreatic head and aorta by using a circular region-of-interest cursor placed on the images by one author (T.K.) before and every 2 seconds from 22 seconds until 60 seconds after the initiation of injection of contrast material for a total of 21 images. Every attempt was made to align the regions of interest on all the images and to maintain a constant region-of-interest area of at least 1 cm^2 in the pancreatic head and aorta. Care also was taken to exclude vessels and ductal structures from the region of interest in the pancreatic head.

The enhancement value at each time point was calculated for each of the patients as the difference in attenuation value (in Hounsfield units) between the nonenhanced and the contrast material–enhanced images for the pancreatic parenchyma and aorta.

The maximum enhancement values of the pancreatic parenchyma within 60 seconds after the injection of contrast material were determined for each patient. If the enhancement value of the pancreas did not show a peak within 60 seconds after the initiation of injection and was still increasing at 60 seconds, the maximum enhancement value of the pancreas was regarded as the enhancement value

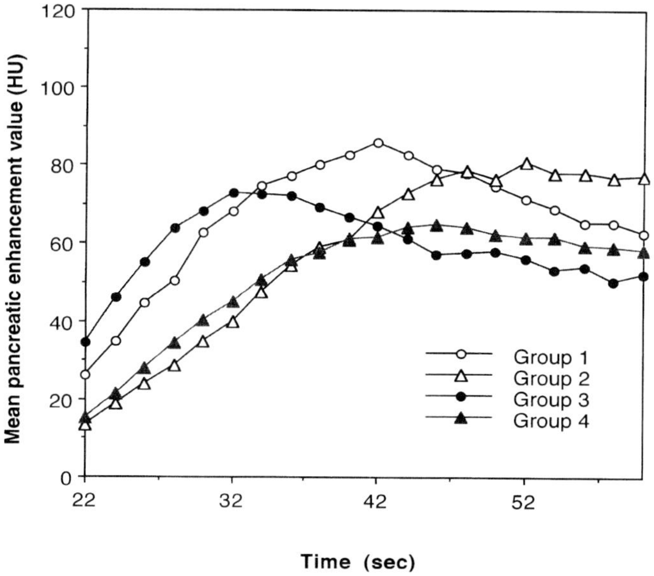

Figure 2. Graph shows the mean enhancement value of the pancreas at each of the time points after the injection of contrast material. The mean enhancement values of the pancreas for patients in groups 1 and 3, who underwent the same higher injection rate, nearly overlapped in the early period and so did those for the patients in groups 2 and 4, who underwent the same slower injection rate.

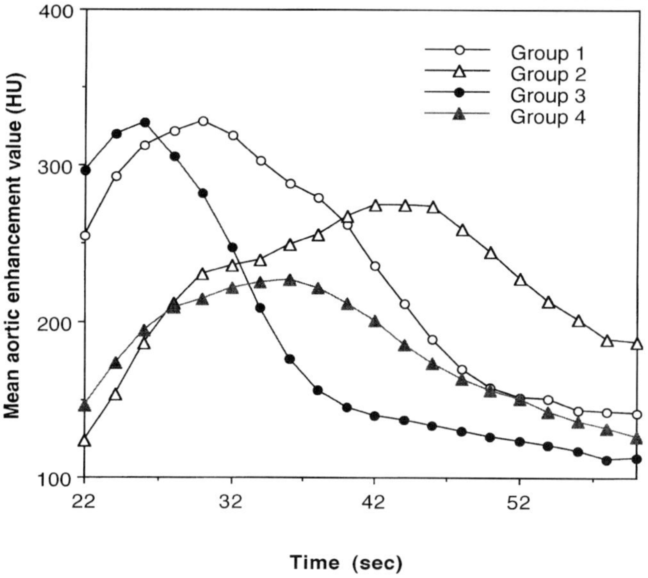

Figure 3. Graph shows the mean enhancement value of the aorta at each of the time points after the injection of contrast material. The mean enhancement value of the aorta for the groups with the faster injection rate increased more rapidly than that for the groups with the slower injection rate, and it decreased more rapidly after the peak.

at 60 seconds. Maximum enhancement values of the pancreas for the four groups were then compared statistically. An overall test was performed with the Kruskal-Wallis test. When the differences in ratings among the four groups were statistically significant, the Mann-Whitney *U* test was used to compare the data for the groups. A two-tailed *P* value less than .05 was considered statistically significant.

The mean enhancement values of the pancreas and the aorta at each time point for each group were calculated and plotted on graphs to show the enhancement patterns of the pancreas and the aorta according to the different injection protocols. From these graphs, the time point when the mean enhancement value of the pancreas reached 50 HU was obtained for each group, and this time point was defined as the average onset of the pancreatic phase during which the pancreatic parenchyma was optimally enhanced (10,11). The time points when the mean enhancement values of the pancreas and the aorta reached their maximum were also obtained for each group.

Two authors (T.K., T.M.) evaluated by consensus the enhancement of the superior mesenteric vein on the images obtained with single-level serial scanning. The time when the superior mesenteric vein was completely opacified without defects caused by the mixing of contrast material and blood was determined for each patient.

RESULTS

The patients' ages were 54 years ± 18 (mean ± SD) in group 1, 57 years ± 15 in group 2, 56 years ± 14 in groups 3, and 58 years ± 14 in group 4. The patients' mean body weights were 56 kg ± 10 in group 1, 56 kg ± 10 in group 2, 56 kg ± 10 in group 3, and 55 kg ± 10 in group 4. There was no significant difference in age or body weight between the four groups. The amount of contrast material administered was 66–140 mL (mean, 112 mL) for group 1, 70–160 mL (mean, 112 mL) for group 2, 54–114 mL (mean, 81 mL) for group 3, and 45–105 mL (mean, 83 mL) for group 4. The mean time used to inject the contrast material was 22 seconds for group 1, 37 seconds for group 2, 16 seconds for group 3, and 28 seconds group 4.

The enhancement value of the pancreas reached its maximum within 60 seconds after the start of injection in all patients, except for four patients in group 2 and two patients in group 4. The maximum enhancement value of the pancreas was 99 HU ± 18 for group 1, 90 HU ± 18 for group 2, 86 HU ± 15 for group 3, and 74 HU ± 13 for group 4 (Fig 1). The resultant *P* values of statistical comparison of the maximum enhancement values were .045 between groups 1 and 2, .016 between groups 1 and 3, less than .001 between groups 1 and 4, .67 between groups 2 and 3, .001 between groups 2 and 4, and .001 between groups 3 and 4. There were significant differences between all groups except for between groups 2 and 3. The maximum enhancement value of the pancreas for group 1, in which the patients underwent injection with the higher dose at the faster rate, was greater than for the other groups.

Figure 2 shows the mean enhancement values of the pancreas at the different time points after the injection of contrast material. The time until the point when the mean enhancement value of the pancreas reached 50 HU, which was defined as the average onset of the pancreatic phase, was 28 seconds for group 1, 36 seconds for group 2, 26 seconds for group 3, and 34 seconds for group 4. The time until the average onset of the pancreatic phase was nearly identical for the groups with the same injection rates and was shorter for the groups with the faster injection rate. The time point when the mean enhancement value of the pancreas reached its maximum was 42 seconds for group 1, 52 seconds for group 2, 32 seconds for group 3, and 46 seconds for group 4. To reach the maximum mean enhancement of the pancreas, less time was needed for the group with the shorter contrast material injection time.

Figure 3 shows the mean enhancement values of the aorta at each of the time

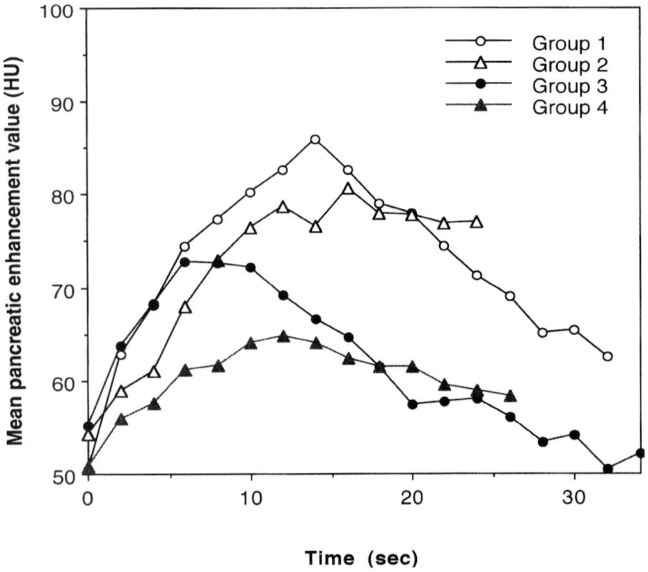

Figure 4. Graph shows the mean enhancement values of the pancreas by group after the average onset of the pancreatic phase. The time point of 0 seconds represents the average onset of the pancreatic phase. The pancreatic enhancement was maintained more constantly at a high level during the pancreatic phase in the groups with the higher dose than in those with the lower dose.

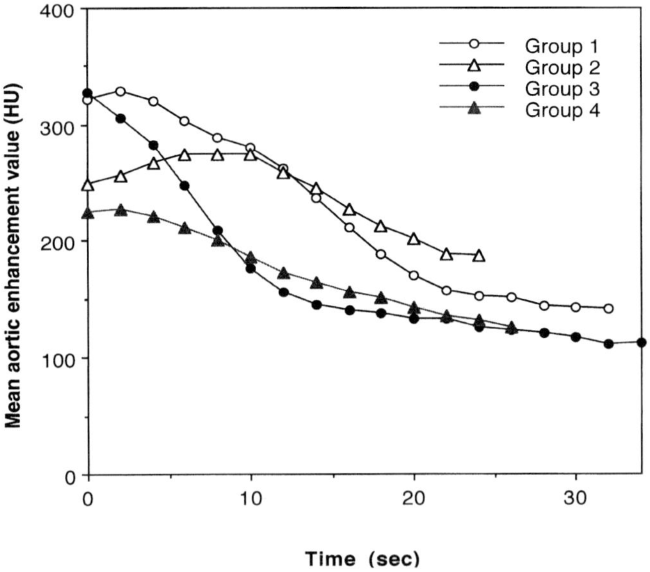

Figure 5. Graph shows the mean enhancement values of the aorta by group after the average onset of the pancreatic phase. The time point of 0 seconds represents the average onset of the pancreatic phase. In the groups with an injection rate of 5 mL/sec, aortic enhancement decreased relatively rapidly in the later part of the pancreatic phase. In the groups with an injection rate of 3 mL/sec, constant aortic enhancement was attained throughout the pancreatic phase, although the actual maximum enhancement values were lower.

points after the injection of contrast material. The time point when the mean enhancement value of the aorta reached its maximum was 30 seconds for group 1, 44 seconds for group 2, 26 seconds for group 3, and 36 seconds for group 4. The mean enhancement value of the aorta reached its maximum 2 seconds after the average onset of the pancreatic phase in group 1, 8 seconds in group 2, 0 seconds in group 3, and 2 seconds in group 4.

Figures 4 and 5 show the mean enhancement values of the pancreas and the aorta, respectively, for each group for the period after the average onset of the pancreatic phase. The mean enhancement value of the pancreas was maintained at a high level for a longer period after the average onset of the pancreatic phase in the groups with the higher dose (Fig 4). The mean enhancement value of the aorta almost decreased in groups 1, 3, and 4 throughout this interval, while it reached its maximum approximately at the midpoint of the interval in group 2. The mean enhancement value of the aorta was maintained at a high level for a longer period in the groups with the higher dose. A comparison between the groups with the same dose (groups 1 and 2 and groups 3 and 4) showed that while aortic enhancement was higher for the groups with the faster injection rate in the earlier part of the interval, it was higher for the groups with the slower injection rate in the later part, and it was maintained more constantly at a high level in the groups with the slower injection rate (Fig 5).

Complete opacification of the superior mesenteric vein without defects caused by the mixing of contrast material and blood could not be attained by 60 seconds after the injection in three patients of group 1, nine patients of group 2, and eight patients of group 3 (Figs 6–9). The mean time for the superior mesenteric vein to be completely opacified in the patients in whom complete opacification was seen within 60 seconds was 47 seconds for group 1, 51 seconds for group 2, 47 seconds for group 3, and 49 seconds for group 4.

DISCUSSION

Contrast-enhanced CT is the dominant imaging modality used for the diagnosis and staging of pancreatic ductal adenocarcinoma. The efficacy of helical CT for the diagnosis of pancreatic adenocarcinoma has been reported by several groups of investigators (10–14). Contrast material injection techniques have varied in previous studies. The dose range was 120–150 mL of nonionic contrast material at 300 mg of iodine per milliliter, which was injected intravenously at rates ranging between 1.5 and 5 mL/sec, and the time delay between the start of the injection and the start of scanning was 25–70 seconds (10–13). These differences in injection rates, doses of contrast material, and the scanning delay times appear to indicate that the techniques have not been optimized yet.

The pancreatic phase was defined by Lu et al (10) as the period during which the pancreatic parenchyma is most markedly enhanced, and the pancreatic phase in their study was 40–70 seconds after the infusion of 150 mL of contrast material at a rate of 3 mL/sec. For our study, we defined the time point when the mean enhancement value of the pancreas reaches 50 HU as the average onset of the pancreatic phase. A clinically valid definition of the start and end of a phase, such as the hepatic arterial phase, the hepatic portal venous phase, and the pancreatic phase, is difficult to obtain.

The results of our study revealed that the time until the average onset of the pancreatic phase was nearly identical for the groups with the same injection rate, which indicates that this period depends on the injection rate. The results of our study also support the definition of Lu et

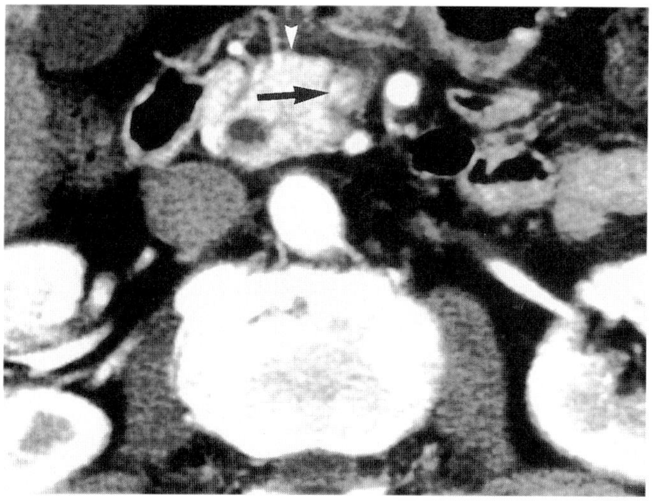

Figure 6. CT image of the abdomen obtained 36 seconds after the initiation of injection of 110 mL of contrast material at a rate of 5 mL/sec in a 73-year-old man with a body weight of 55 kg in group 1. The enhancement value of the pancreas (arrowhead) is at its maximum and registered 115 HU at this time point. The superior mesenteric vein (arrow) is not completely opacified yet.

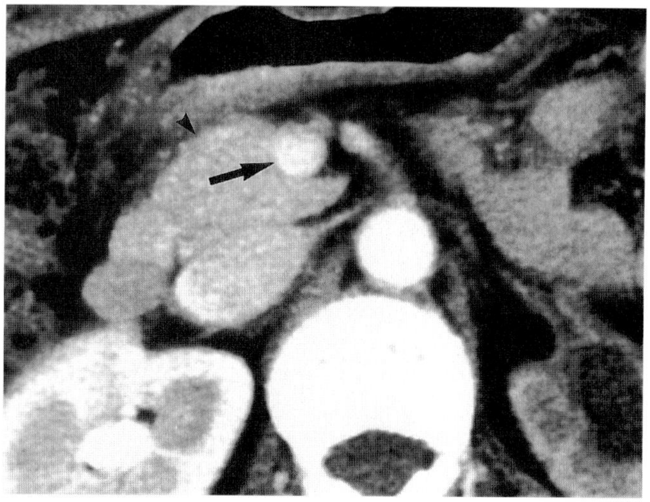

Figure 7. CT image of the abdomen obtained 52 seconds after the initiation of injection of 112 mL of contrast material at a rate of 3 mL/sec in a 45-year-old woman with a body weight of 56 kg in group 2. The enhancement value of the pancreas (arrowhead) is at its maximum and registered 89 HU at this time point. The superior mesenteric vein (arrow) is completely opacified.

al (10) of the start of the pancreatic phase when the injection rate is 3 mL/sec, because the average time of onset of the pancreatic phase was 34–36 seconds after the start of injection in our groups with an injection rate of 3 mL/sec. However, the corresponding onset occurred 26–28 seconds after the start of injection in our groups with an injection rate of 5 mL/sec. Therefore, the pancreatic phase starts earlier when the injection rate is faster. It has been reported that the faster rate of injection decreases the time during which pancreatic enhancement is high (18). In addition, our study results showed that the duration of the pancreatic phase depended on the dose of contrast material because the mean pancreatic enhancement was maintained at a high level for a longer period in the groups with the higher dose.

Keogan et al (14) reported that "arterial phase" scans obtained 20–40 seconds after the injection of contrast material at a rate of 4 mL/sec, and obtained in addition to "venous phase" scans acquired 70–100 seconds after injection, did not improve the detection of pancreatic malignancies. Graf et al (16) also reported that the conspicuity of pancreatic adenocarcinomas was substantially greater on the "portal phase" CT scan started 60 seconds after the start of injection of 160 mL of contrast material at a rate of 4 mL/sec than on the "arterial-phase" CT scan started 18 seconds after the start of injection. However, Lu et al (10) reported that the mean tumor-pancreatic contrast was significantly greater during the "pancreatic phase" (40–70 seconds after the infusion of contrast material at a rate of 3 mL/sec) than during the "hepatic phase" (70–100 seconds after infusion). Our study results suggest that the arterial phase scan in the studies by Keogan et al (14) and Graf et al (16) started before the pancreatic parenchyma began to be greatly enhanced and that the pancreatic phase scan in the study by Lu et al (10) started after such notable enhancement.

Pancreatic ductal adenocarcinomas are hypovascular (19), and theoretically, therefore, the greatest conspicuity of these tumors should be achieved when the pancreatic parenchyma is greatly enhanced. Although, to our knowledge, there have been no reports comparing the efficacy of arterial phase imaging with that of pancreatic phase imaging for the detection of pancreatic adenocarcinoma, we hypothesize that pancreatic phase imaging is more effective for attaining the greatest conspicuity of hypovascular pancreatic adenocarcinoma.

Bonaldi et al (18) reported that a faster injection rate did not increase the maximum pancreatic enhancement. Our study results do not support the conclusion of Bonaldi et al because our results show that the faster injection rate of 5 mL/sec substantially increased the maximum enhancement value of the pancreas above that of the slower injection rate of 3 mL/sec for both the higher dose (2 mL/kg) and the lower dose (1.5 mL/kg) groups. The lower dose in our study was the same as the dose used by Bonaldi et al, and a comparison of the results of the groups in their study and of the lower dose groups in our study shows that the maximum enhancement value of the pancreas was 71 HU ± 15 for a rate of 6 mL/sec and 72 HU ± 17 for a rate of 2 mL/sec in the study of Bonaldi et al, and 86 HU ± 15 for a rate of 5 mL/sec and 74 HU ± 13 for a rate of 3 mL/sec in our study. The maximum enhancement values of the pancreas for the slower rates (2 mL/sec and 3 mL/sec) in the two studies were thus almost identical, but those for the faster rates (6 mL/sec and 5 mL/sec) were quite different.

Bonaldi et al (18) started CT scanning 30 seconds after the start of contrast material injection, while we started 20 seconds after the start of contrast material injection. In our study, moreover, the time point when the mean enhancement value of the pancreas reached its maximum was 32 seconds for the group of patients who underwent an injection of 1.5 mL/kg at a rate of 5 mL/sec. As a result of comparing the results of Bonaldi et al with ours, we presume that CT scanning could have been started after the actual peak pancreatic enhancement in some patients in the study by Bonaldi et al and that therefore they may have underestimated the maximum enhancement value of the pancreas for a rate of 6 mL/sec.

To our knowledge, there have been no reports to evaluate the effects of different doses of contrast material injection on pancreatic CT imaging. Our study results

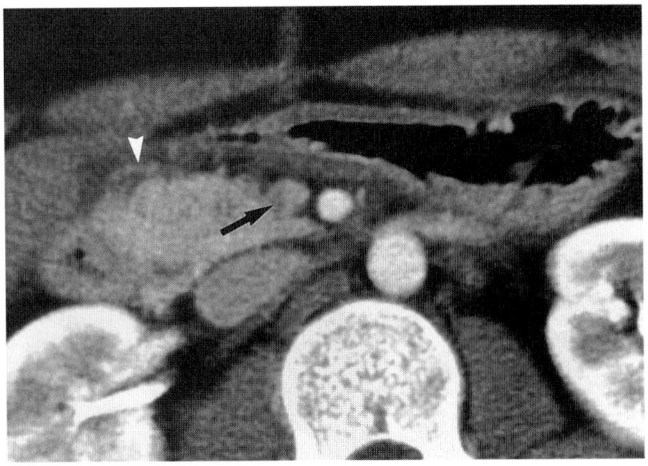

Figure 8. CT image of the abdomen obtained 50 seconds after the initiation of injection of 105 mL of contrast material at a rate of 5 mL/sec in a 25-year-old man with a body weight of 70 kg in group 3. The enhancement value of the pancreas (arrowhead) is at its maximum and registered 86 HU at this time point. The superior mesenteric vein (arrow) is not completely opacified yet.

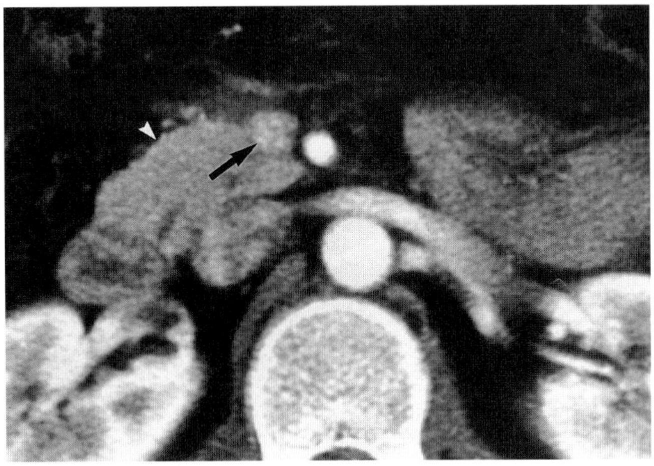

Figure 9. CT image of the abdomen obtained 56 seconds after the initiation of injection of 105 mL of contrast material at a rate of 3 mL/sec in a 36-year-old man with a body weight of 70 kg in group 4. The enhancement value of the pancreas (arrowhead) is at its maximum and registered 86 HU at this time point. The superior mesenteric vein (arrow) is not completely opacified yet.

clearly showed that a higher dose substantially increases the maximum pancreatic enhancement. Both a higher dose and a faster rate for the injection of contrast material thus appear to increase the maximum pancreatic enhancement. A higher dose results in both greater pancreatic enhancement and more constant maintenance of high pancreatic and arterial enhancement during the pancreatic phase. A faster injection rate also results in greater pancreatic enhancement. However, if the dose is reduced, a faster injection rate may decrease the duration of high pancreatic and arterial enhancement in the pancreatic phase.

Of the four injection protocols evaluated in this study, an injection of a dose of 2 mL/kg at a rate of 5 mL/sec achieved the greatest maximum enhancement value of the pancreas, but this injection did not produce constant maintenance of high arterial enhancement throughout the pancreatic phase. Such high arterial enhancement was maintained most constantly with the injection of a dose of 2 mL/kg at a rate of 3 mL/sec.

For staging of pancreatic adenocarcinomas, evaluation of arterial involvement is required. For this purpose, high arterial enhancement should be maintained constantly throughout the pancreatic phase. The dose of 2 mL/kg used as the higher dose in this study is the same as the usual clinical dose. When injected at a rate of 5 mL/sec, however, this dose is not enough to maintain constantly high arterial enhancement throughout the pancreatic phase. We therefore think that the arterial structures can be evaluated better if a dose of more than 2 mL/kg is injected at a rate of 5 mL/sec for the diagnosis of pancreatic adenocarcinoma, unless a patient has renal dysfunction. If intravenous access is poor and a higher injection rate cannot be achieved in some patients, increasing the dose of contrast material may result in an increase in pancreatic enhancement.

The involvement of veins, including the superior mesenteric vein, should also be evaluated for the staging of pancreatic adenocarcinomas. Lu et al (10) reported that substantially greater enhancement in all vessels, including the superior mesenteric vein, was attained during the pancreatic phase rather than the hepatic phase. However, our study results showed that complete opacification of the superior mesenteric vein without defects caused by the mixing of contrast material and blood could not be attained consistently throughout the pancreatic phase. And if the superior mesenteric vein is not completely opacified with contrast material, venous involvement by pancreatic adenocarcinomas cannot be precisely evaluated. Therefore, our study results indicate that second-phase imaging performed after the pancreatic phase is needed for the evaluation of venous involvement, regardless of injection technique. Portal venous phase imaging is usually performed as the second-phase imaging (10–17). Portal venous phase imaging is necessary not only for the detection of hypovascular liver metastases from pancreatic adenocarcinomas but also for the precise evaluation of the venous involvement of pancreatic adenocarcinomas.

In summary, our study results indicate that the average time until the onset of the pancreatic phase depends on the injection rate. A higher dose results in both greater pancreatic enhancement and more constant maintenance of high pancreatic and arterial enhancement during the pancreatic phase. A faster injection rate also results in greater pancreatic enhancement. However, if the dose of contrast material is reduced, a faster injection rate may decrease the duration of high pancreatic and arterial enhancement in the pancreatic phase. Our study results lead us to hypothesize that pancreatic phase and portal venous phase helical CT scans with the injection of contrast material at a higher dose and at a faster rate can provide better results for the detection and staging of pancreatic adenocarcinoma. Further clinical study in patients with pancreatic adenocarcinoma is needed to prove this hypothesis.

References

1. Zeman RK, Fox SH, Silverman PM, et al. Helical (spiral) CT of the abdomen. AJR 1993; 160:719–725.
2. Hollett MD, Jeffrey RB Jr, Nino-Murcia M, Jorgensen MJ, Harris DP. Dual-phase helical CT of the liver: value of arterial phase scans in the detection of small malignant hepatic neoplasms. AJR 1995; 164:879–884.
3. Baron RL, Oliver JH, Dodd GD III, Nalesnik M, Holbert BL, Carr B. Hepatocellular carcinoma: evaluation with biphasic, contrast-enhanced, helical CT. Radiology 1996; 199:505–511.

4. Baron RL. Understanding and optimizing use of contrast material for CT of the liver. AJR 1994; 163:323–331.
5. Silverman PM, O'Malley J, Tefft MC, Cooper C, Zeman RK. Conspicuity of hepatic metastases on helical CT: effect of different time delays between contrast administration and scanning. AJR 1995; 164:619–623.
6. Garcia PA, Bonaldi VM, Bret PM, Liang L, Reinhold C, Atri M. Effect of rate of contrast medium injection on hepatic enhancement at CT. Radiology 1996; 199:185–189.
7. Foley WD, Hoffmann RG, Quiroz FA, Kahan CE, Perret RS. Hepatic helical CT: contrast material injection protocol. Radiology 1994; 192:367–371.
8. Heiken JP, Brink JA, McClennan BL, Sagel SS, Crowe TM, Gaines MV. Dynamic incremental CT: effect of volume and concentration of contrast material and patient weight on hepatic enhancement. Radiology 1995; 195:353–357.
9. Chambers TP, Baron RL, Lush RM. Hepatic CT enhancement. Radiology 1994; 193:513–522.
10. Lu DSK, Vedantham S, Krasny RM, Kadell B, Berger WL, Reber HA. Two-phase helical CT for pancreatic tumors: pancreatic versus hepatic phase enhancement of tumor, pancreas, and vascular structures. Radiology 1996; 199:697–701.
11. Lu DS, Reber HA, Krasny RM, Kadell BM, Sayre J. Local staging of pancreatic cancer: criteria for unresectability of major vessels as revealed by pancreatic-phase, thin-section helical CT. AJR 1997; 168:1439–1443.
12. Zeman RK, Cooper C, Zeiberg AS, et al. TNM staging of pancreatic carcinoma using helical CT. AJR 1997; 169:459–464.
13. Bluemke DA, Cameron JL, Hruban RH, et al. Potentially resectable pancreatic adenocarcinoma: spiral CT assessment with surgical and pathologic correlation. Radiology 1995; 197:381–385.
14. Keogan MT, McDermott VG, Paulson EK, et al. Pancreatic malignancy: effect of dual-phase helical CT in tumor detection and vascular opacification. Radiology 1997; 205:513–518.
15. Van Hoe L, Gryspeerdt S, Marchal G, Baert AL, Mertens L. Helical CT for the preoperative localization of islet cell tumors of the pancreas: value of arterial and parenchymal phase images. AJR 1995; 165:1437–1439.
16. Graf O, Boland GW, Warshaw AL, Fernandez-del-Castillo C, Hahn PF, Mueller PR. Arterial versus portal venous helical CT for revealing pancreatic adenocarcinoma: conspicuity of tumor and critical vascular anatomy. AJR 1997; 169:119–123.
17. Hollett MD, Jorgensen MJ, Jeffrey RB Jr. Quantitative evaluation of pancreatic enhancement during dual-phase helical CT. Radiology 1995; 195:359–361.
18. Bonaldi VM, Bret PM, Atri M, Garcia P, Reinhold C. Comparison of two injection protocols using helical and dynamic acquisitions in CT examinations of the pancreas. AJR 1996; 167:49–55.
19. Megibow AJ. Pancreatic adenocarcinoma: designing the examination to evaluate the clinical questions. Radiology 1992; 183:297–303.
20. 41st World Medical Assembly. Declaration of Helsinki: recommendations guiding physicians in biomedical research involving human subjects. Bull Pan Am Health Organ 1990; 24:606–609.
21. Silverman PM, Roberts S, Tefft MC, et al. Helical CT of the liver: clinical application of an automated computer technique, SmartPrep, for obtaining images with optimal contrast enhancement. AJR 1995; 165:73–78.

Interlude

Before Biopsy: A Worried Hepatocellular Carcinoma

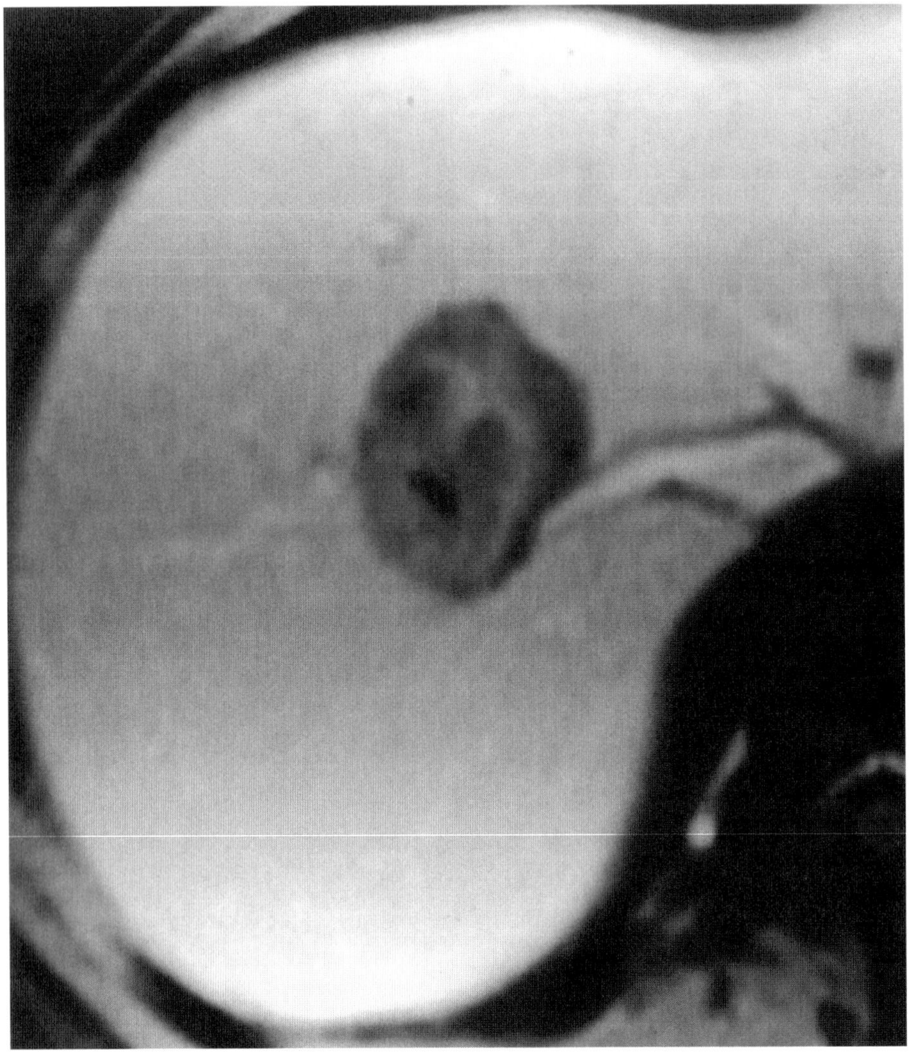

Gadolinium-enhanced fat-suppressed T1-weighted fast low-angle shot magnetic resonance image (165/2, 60° flip angle) shows hepatocellular carcinoma (biopsy proved) with focal fatty change.

Courtesy of Declan G. Sheppard, FRCR, Dundee, United Kingdom

Hepatic Iron Concentration: Noninvasive Estimation by Means of MR Imaging Techniques[1]

Herbert L. Bonkovsky, MD
Richard B. Rubin, MD[2]
Edward E. Cable, PhD[3]
Ashley Davidoff, MD
Tammo H. Pels Rijcken, MD[4]
David D. Stark, MD[5]

Index terms:
Hemochromatosis, 761.659
Iron
Liver, biopsy, 761.1261
Liver, diseases, 761.659
Liver, iron content, 761.659
Magnetic resonance (MR), comparative studies, 761.121411, 761.121412

Radiology 1999; 212:227–234

Abbreviations:
GRE = gradient-recalled echo
ln = natural logarithm
SNR = signal-to-noise ratio

[1] From the Dept of Medicine, Div of Digestive Disease and Nutrition (H.L.B., R.B.R., E.E.C.), Dept of Radiology (A.D., T.H.P.R., D.D.S.), and Center for Study of Disorders of Iron and Porphyrin Metabolism (H.L.B., R.B.R., E.E.C.), University of Massachusetts Medical School and University of Massachusetts Memorial Health Care, Rm S6-737, 55 Lake Ave North, Worcester, MA 01655. Received Feb 20, 1998; revision requested Apr 27; revision received Sep 8; accepted Dec 17. H.L.B. supported in part by the Magnetic Resonance Imaging Center of Central Massachusetts and by a grant from the National Institutes of Health (DK 38825). **Address reprint requests to** H.L.B. (e-mail: *Herbert.Bonkovsky@ummhc.org*).

The opinions expressed in this paper are those of the authors; they do not necessarily reflect the official views of the National Institutes of Health.

[2] Current address: Port Jefferson, NY.

[3] Current address: Dept of Microbiology and Immunology, Penn State College of Medicine, Hershey, Pa.

[4] Current address: Dept of Radiology, Onze Lieve Vrouwe Gasthuis, Amsterdam, the Netherlands.

[5] Current address: Dept of Radiology, University of Nebraska Medical Center, Omaha, Neb.

Author contributions:
Guarantor of integrity of entire study, H.L.B.; study concepts, H.L.B., A.D., D.D.S.; study design, H.L.B., E.E.C., R.B.R.; definition of intellectual content, all authors; literature research, T.H.P.R., H.L.B., R.B.R., E.E.C.; clinical studies, T.H.P.R., H.L.B., R.B.R., A.D.; experimental studies, T.H.P.R., H.L.B., D.D.S.; data acquisition, T.H.P.R., H.L.B., R.B.R., A.D., D.D.S.; data analysis, T.H.P.R., H.L.B., R.B.R., E.E.C.; statistical analysis, H.L.B., R.B.R., E.E.C.; manuscript preparation, H.L.B., R.B.R., E.E.C., A.D., D.D.S.; manuscript editing, H.L.B., A.D., D.D.S.; manuscript review, H.L.B., R.B.R., A.D., D.D.S.

PURPOSE: To identify a magnetic resonance (MR) imaging method sufficiently sensitive and specific in the estimation of hepatic iron content to obviate liver biopsy.

MATERIALS AND METHODS: Thirty-eight patients underwent percutaneous needle biopsy of the liver with chemical measurement of the hepatic iron concentration and hepatic MR imaging with several spin-echo and gradient-recalled-echo (GRE) techniques. Correlations between MR imaging parameters and the hepatic iron concentration were determined.

RESULTS: Inverse curvilinear relationships were noted between several MR parameters and hepatic iron concentrations. GRE sequences with short repetition and echo times were more accurate and precise than spin-echo sequences for the estimation of hepatic iron concentration. A GRE sequence with a repetition time of 18 msec, an echo time of 5 msec, and a flip angle of 10° showed close correlation between the hepatic iron concentration and the natural logarithm of the ratio of the signal intensity of liver to the SD of background noise ($r = -0.94$) and low coefficient of variation (12%).

CONCLUSION: MR imaging with these parameters is a rapid, noninvasive, and accurate modality for estimation of hepatic iron concentration; it is sufficiently accurate and precise to obviate liver biopsy for the purpose of measuring hepatic iron concentration.

Hereditary *HLA*-linked hemochromatosis is an autosomal recessive condition characterized by excessive intestinal absorption of iron, which leads to deposition of the metal in the liver, heart, pancreas, and other organs. Timely diagnosis of hereditary hemochromatosis and treatment with phlebotomy can prevent this organ damage (1). Mutations in the *HFE* gene are responsible for the common form of *HLA*-linked hereditary hemochromatosis that occurs with high prevalence among non-Jewish whites of northern European origin (2,3). DNA-based tests for the two mutations that have been linked to the hemochromatosis phenotype (nucleotide *G745A*, amino acid *C282Y*, and nucleotide *C187G*, amino acid *H63D*) are now available at our (University of Massachusetts Memorial Health Care) and other centers; these tests have helped to establish definitive diagnosis, particularly in patients and their families with the classic form of hereditary hemochromatosis.

However, in the United States only about 80%–85% of patients with the hemochromatotic phenotype have these mutations in the *HFE* gene, and their prevalence is even lower in other geographic regions (4–7). In addition, an appreciable number of subjects who are homozygous abnormal, especially women, do not express the iron overload phenotype (8). Then too, there are clearly other types of hereditary hemochromatosis (eg, those occurring in black Africans or Melanesians), in which causative mutations occur in other still unidentified genes (9).

Because the liver is the principal organ responsible for the storage and detoxification of iron, and also the first and foremost organ damaged by heavy iron overload, the standard for the diagnosis of hemochromatosis is liver biopsy with determination of the hepatic iron index value (10). This index is defined as the hepatic iron concentration, expressed as micromoles of iron per gram of dry liver, divided by the age of the patient in years. Liver biopsy, however, is invasive and may be associated with complications. Furthermore, the variability in measured hepatic iron concentrations in small liver samples from patients with cirrhosis may be considerable (11,12).

To avoid liver biopsy, attempts have been made to devise noninvasive means of estimating the hepatic iron concentration. A dedicated device to measure magnetic susceptibilities, the superconducting quantum interference device, is highly sensitive for the detection of iron but is not widely available (13). Although computed tomography demonstrates an increase in the attenuation of the liver in hepatic iron overload, it is relatively insensitive to mild degrees of increased hepatic iron, especially if there is associated fatty change in the liver (14). Magnetic resonance (MR) imaging has been considered a promising noninvasive modality to estimate hepatic iron concentration (15–17). An increase in hepatic iron concentration decreases the T2 relaxation time, which decreases the liver's signal intensity and makes the liver appear dark on typical MR images.

Standard MR imaging sequences, known as spin-echo sequences, have been shown to be sensitive, but not specific, for distinguishing mild from marked degrees of iron excess (18). Newer gradient-recalled-echo (GRE) sequences, which are more sensitive to the field inhomogeneities induced by paramagnetic substances such as iron, have shown more promise (15,19) but have not been widely used to study hemochromatosis. The present study was undertaken to develop a rapid, cost-effective, accurate test to estimate hepatic iron concentration without the need for performance of percutaneous needle biopsy of the liver.

TABLE 1
Final Diagnoses and Laboratory Characteristics of Study Patients

Final Diagnosis	No. of Patients (*N* = 38)	Transferrin Saturation (%)	Ferritin (ng/mL)*	Bilirubin (mg/dL)*	Alk Phos (U/L)	AST (U/L)	ALT (U/L)	HIC (µg/g dry liver)*
HHC	15	88	492	1.1	98	44	68	8,520
Viral hepatitis	16	55	291	0.9	103	51	72	2,000
Alcoholic liver disease	5	48	251	0.8	99	56	31	1,860
Steatohepatitis	2	48	541	1.0	114	62	63	889
Normal range	NA	20–50	15–218	0.3–1.2	30–115	10–40	10–40	300–1,200

Note.—Data are mean values. Alk Phos = alkaline phosphatase, ALT = alanine aminotransferase, AST = aspartate aminotransferase, HHC = hereditary homozygous hemochromatosis, HIC = hepatic iron concentration, NA = not applicable.

* To convert ferritin levels to SI units (µg/L), multiply by 1. To convert bilirubin levels to SI units (µmol/L), multiply by 17.1. To convert HIC to SI units (µmol), divide by 55.85.

TABLE 2
MR Imaging Sequences Tested

Method	Repetition Time (msec)	Echo Time (msec)	Flip Angle (degree)	*r* Value*
Spin echo	600	17	90	−0.61
Spin echo	2,000	80	90	−0.55
Spin echo	2,000	12	90	−0.53
GRE	18	5	10	−0.94
GRE	18	5	70	−0.92
GRE	39	30	10	−0.74
GRE	39	30	70	−0.68
GRE	120	5	10	−0.59
GRE	120	5	70	−0.61

* The *r* value refers to the correlation of ln (SNR) and hepatic iron concentration.

MATERIALS AND METHODS

Patients

We examined 38 patients (30 men, eight women; age range, 28–68 years; median age, 44 years) who were referred for evaluation of hepatic iron overload on the basis of clinical criteria or because of an increased serum ferritin or transferrin saturation. The study protocol and informed consent form were approved by the Committee for Protection of Human Subjects in Research of the University of Massachusetts Medical School. Each patient gave written informed consent to participate in the study.

On the basis of a synthesis of the clinical history, hepatic iron index value, and serum study and hepatic histologic findings, final diagnoses were made. As shown in Table 1, 15 patients had hereditary hemochromatosis, 16 had chronic viral hepatitis, five had alcoholic liver disease, and two had steatohepatitis. Each patient in the study underwent both percutaneous needle biopsy of the liver with chemical measurement of the hepatic iron concentration and MR imaging. The two studies were carried out within 1 month of one another. Patients did not receive iron removal therapy during the interval between the two tests.

Patients confirmed to have hereditary hemochromatosis were advised to begin vigorous programs of therapeutic phlebotomy. Evaluation of first-degree relatives was also recommended. All patients were initially examined prior to 1996, when the *HFE* gene was identified (2). Therefore, a diagnosis of hemochromatosis was made based on traditional criteria. We were able to obtain *HFE* mutational analysis in one of the patients with hereditary hemochromatosis in our study. This confirmed that the patient is homozygous for the *C282Y* mutation.

Liver Biopsy

Biopsy of the right lobe of the liver was performed with a 16-gauge Klatskin-modified Menghini needle (Becton-Dickinson, Rutherford, NJ) by using the intercostal, percutaneous approach. Biopsies were performed through the eighth right intercostal space at the midaxillary line. The majority of the specimen was placed in Carnoy solution or 10% buffered formaldehyde saline, processed routinely, embedded in paraffin, and sectioned. The embedded sections were stained with hematoxylin-eosin, Masson trichrome, and Perls stains. Another portion of the biopsy specimen was dried, weighed, ashed, and submitted to measurement of the hepatic iron concentration by a colorimetric procedure (20).

MR Imaging Procedures

Within 1 month of the time of liver biopsy, all patients underwent MR imag-

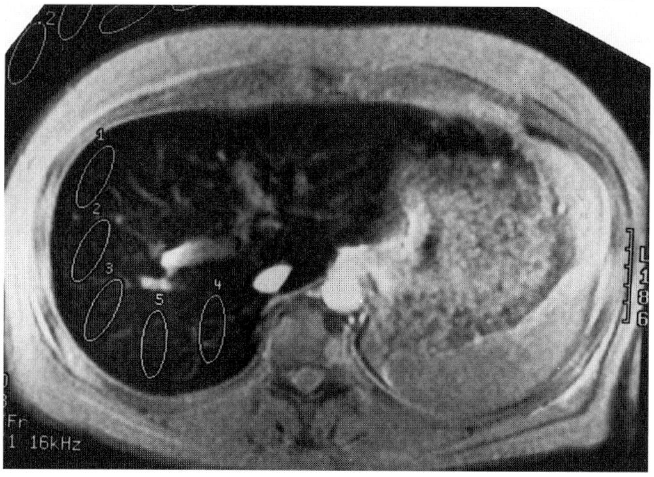

Figure 1. Transverse GRE MR image (18/5, 10° flip angle) obtained in a 52-year-old man with genetic homozygous hemochromatosis who underwent breath-hold imaging shows operator-defined regions of interest used in this study. Note the markedly decreased signal intensity of the liver compared with that of structures such as the paraspinous muscles and the spleen. Representative regions of interest are outlined on the liver and background air.

ing with a unit (Signa; GE Medical Systems, Milwaukee, Wis) operating at a field strength of 1.5 T. In all but five patients, the MR study was performed prior to the biopsy. The following sequences were used for all patients (Table 2): Spin-echo sequence 600/17 (repetition time msec/echo time msec), 2,000/80, and 2,000/12; GRE sequence (18/5) with flip angles of 10° and 70°; GRE sequence (39/30) with flip angles of 10° and 70°; and GRE sequence (120/5) with flip angles of 10° and 70°. These sequences were selected by performing pilot experiments, which tested machine limits in various combinations of repetition time, echo time, and flip angle. Sequences outside these limits showed no improvement or substantial degradation of signal-to-noise ratios (SNRs) per unit of time. The GRE sequences (18/5) were performed with the patients holding their breath at the end of inspiration. A single 2-cm section was chosen that included both the liver and the spleen. The examinations were performed with two signals acquired, and the matrix was held constant at 256 × 128 pixels. One patient also was examined with a fast spin-echo (6,000/117) sequence (see Results).

Signal intensities were measured in operator-defined regions of interest in 2-cm-thick sections. Hepatic regions of interest were chosen to avoid major vascular structures. Regions of interest were drawn to contain at least 50 pixels. In initial studies, regions of interest were also drawn on paraspinous muscle, spleen, fat, and the air just anterior to the torso of the patient. The latter were drawn on the same transverse sections as those used for measuring hepatic intensities and in the phase-encoding direction of the data acquisition process (to minimize noise arising from motion artifacts).

In general, five regions of interest each were drawn on each liver and five on the air above the patient and other tissues. From these, mean values for signal intensities were obtained (Fig 1). The regions of interest included the region of the right lobe of the liver on which biopsy was performed. Ratios were calculated by dividing the mean signal intensity of the liver by that of the SD of the mean of the signal intensity of the overlying air, or noise, or the mean signal intensities of the other tissues (21). Initial plots of these ratios as functions of hepatic iron concentration revealed curvilinear relationships. Therefore, natural logarithms (ln) of the ratios were calculated. Plots of the ln of the ratios versus hepatic iron concentration were linear and inverse and were thus used in subsequent analysis. The coefficient of variation for the ln of the ratios was calculated as the SD of this parameter divided by its mean value multiplied by 100 to convert it to a percentage.

Statistical Analysis

All of the data were entered into computer files that contained an identifying code number for each patient to ensure confidentiality. Scatterplots were obtained and were inspected for linearity and closeness of fit. The correlation between hepatic iron concentration and ln (mean signal intensity of liver/SD of air) or (mean signal intensity of liver/mean signal intensity of other tissue) was determined by using linear regression analysis with the assistance of statistical software (JMP 3.0.2; SAS Institute, Cary, NC). Statistical significance was assessed with the Wilcoxon rank sum test and the Spearman rank correlation coefficient. A P value less than .05 was considered to indicate a statistically significant difference.

RESULTS

Clinical and Routine Laboratory Findings in Patients Examined

Table 1 summarizes the final diagnoses and laboratory findings in the 38 patients examined. Most patients with hereditary hemochromatosis had normal or nearly normal serum liver chemistries (serum bilirubin, alkaline phosphatase, aspartate aminotransferase, and alanine aminotransferase levels). Liver chemistries of patients with alcoholic liver disease or chronic viral hepatitis were slightly more abnormal than those of patients with hereditary hemochromatosis. As expected, most patients with hereditary hemochromatosis had strikingly abnormal serum transferrin saturations and serum ferritins with a markedly elevated mean transferrin saturation of 88%. Many patients with chronic viral hepatitis also had elevations of serum transferrin saturations.

Hepatic iron concentrations were highest in patients with untreated hereditary hemochromatosis (mean, 8,520 μg [153 μmol] of iron per gram of dry liver). The mean hepatic iron concentration was only mildly elevated in patients with chronic viral hepatitis or alcoholic liver disease (mean values, 2,000 μg [35.8 μmol]/g dry liver and 1,860 μg [33.3 μmol]/g dry liver, respectively). Hepatic iron concentration values were normal in the two patients with steatohepatitis.

Preliminary MR Imaging Studies

In preliminary studies, regions of interest were drawn on the liver, as well as on the fat, spleen, paraspinous muscles, and air overlying the patient in the same transverse section (Fig 1). Regions of interest on the fat were difficult to draw in a standardized manner because of variations in body habitus of the patients. The coefficient of variation for the determination of the signal intensity of fat in an individual patient was usually greater than 30%. In contrast, the SD of pixel signal intensities of the overlying air, or noise, was easily measured in a standard manner in all patients and was not affected by body habitus. This SD was reproducible. Because variances were consistently lower when hepatic signal intensities were normalized to the overlying air, or noise, for routine use, the signal intensity ratio of the liver to that of this SD was used in all subsequent studies.

MR Imaging Characteristics of Patients in the Study

The GRE sequences, sensitive as they are to minute fluctuations in the local magnetic field, generally tended to perform better than the standard MR imaging sequences. An inverse linear correlation was noted with all MR imaging sequences between hepatic iron concentration and ln (SNR). The closest inverse linear correlation between hepatic iron concentration and ln (SNR) was with the GRE sequence (18/5) with a flip angle of 10° ($r = -0.94$, $P < .001$) (Table 2).

A scatterplot of hepatic iron concentration versus ln (SNR) in our optimal MR imaging sequence of GRE (18/5) with a flip angle of 10° is depicted in Figure 2. The straight line shows the least-squares best-fit of the data, and the curved lines indicate 95% confidence limits. No patient with ln (SNR) greater than 3.2 had hepatic iron concentration greater than three times the upper limit of normal (3,600 µg [64.5 µmol]/g dry liver). At levels of mild to moderate hepatic iron overload (2,500–7,500 µg [44.8–134 µmol]/g dry liver, $n = 8$), our optimal GRE sequence performed well in that a close inverse linear relationship between hepatic iron concentration and ln (SNR) was observed within this range. With this optimal GRE sequence (18/5, 10° flip angle), the determination of ln (SNR) was highly reproducible at hepatic iron concentration less than 10,000 µg (179 µmol)/g dry liver, with a coefficient of variation of only 8%–13%.

In cases of heavy hepatic iron overload (hepatic iron concentration greater than 10,000 µg [179 µmol]/g dry liver, $n = 7$), MR imaging estimation of hepatic iron concentration was somewhat less precise. At this level of heavy iron overload, the absolute signal intensities of the livers studied were low and differed little from one another, even with our optimal GRE sequence. The coefficient of variation for determination of ln (SNR) in this range of iron concentrations was 13%–20%. For the entire data set, the coefficient of variation was 12%.

Figure 1 depicts an MR image of a man with *HLA*-linked hemochromatosis. A striking feature of this image is the markedly diminished signal intensity of the liver in comparison with surrounding structures such as the spleen and paraspinous muscles.

An example of the benefits of short GRE images with breath-hold techniques is shown in Figure 3. The conventional T2-weighted image (2,000/80) shows a dark liver. However, in this relatively long, non–breath-hold sequence, motion artifact from respiration contributes to appreciable background noise and degradation of contrast between liver and paraspinous muscle (Fig 3a). With more recently developed fast spin-echo T2-weighted images (6,000/117), data are rapidly acquired, and motion artifact is decreased. However, the difference between liver and muscle has been virtually eliminated because of the heavy T2 weighting (Fig 3b). In contrast, our optimal GRE sequence provides excellent contrast and limited motion artifact (Fig 3c).

The ability of the optimal GRE sequence to distinguish moderate hepatic iron overload from normal hepatic iron concentrations is shown in Figure 4. Note the clear difference in appearance of the livers and compare these images with those in Figures 1 and 3.

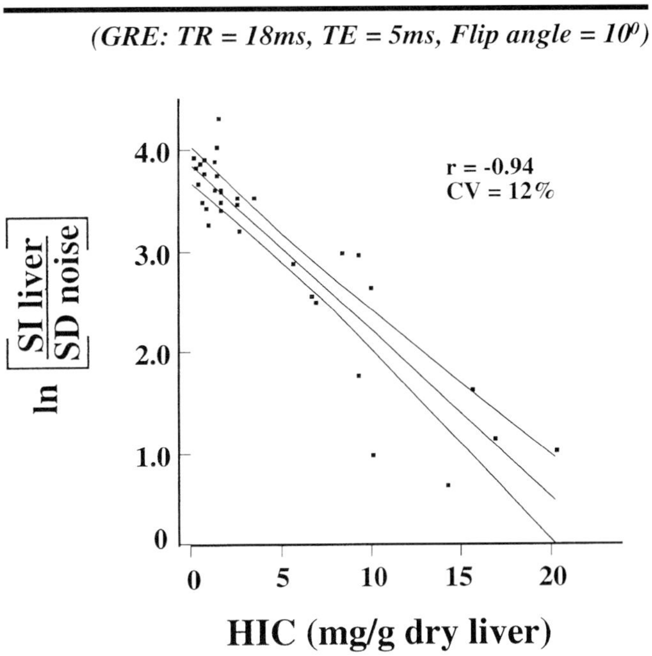

Figure 2. Scatterplot of the hepatic iron concentration versus the ln of the ratio of the signal intensity (*SI*) of the liver to the SD of the background air, or noise (SNR). Note the inverse linear relation between the variables ($r = -0.94$, $P < .001$). The curved lines indicate 95% CIs. *CV* = coefficient of variation, *HIC* = hepatic iron concentration, *ms* = milliseconds, *TE* = echo time, *TR* = repetition time.

DISCUSSION

The physical basis of the use of MR imaging for estimation of hepatic iron concentration is the well-known but still incompletely understood effect of iron on the T2, or transverse relaxation time (22,23). However, comparison of absolute signal intensities from one MR imaging unit to another is unreliable because of substantial intermachine variation. The ratio of signal intensities of the liver and another structure on the same image gives a more reliable estimate of the hepatic iron concentration.

We found that, with all of the MR imaging sequences studied, there was an inverse linear correlation between the hepatic iron concentration and the ln (SNR). Standard sequences performed less well than the newer GRE sequences (Table 2, Figs 3, 4), which is in agreement with other recent results (19). As recently noted by Stark (15), the inherent sensitivity of GRE sequences to paramagnetic sub-

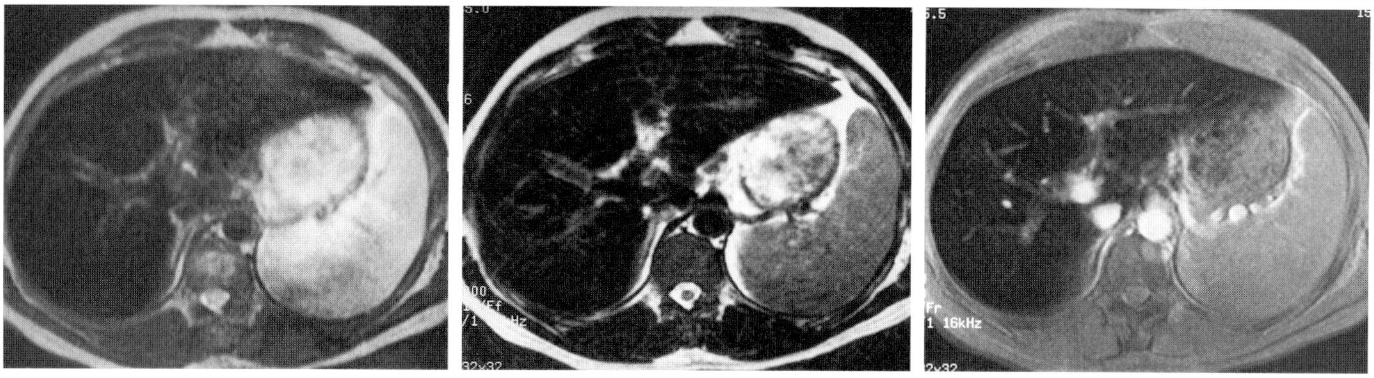

a. b. c.

Figure 3. Transverse MR images obtained by using conventional T2-weighted MR sequences and the optimal GRE sequence used in this study. (a) Conventional T2-weighted sequence (2,000/80) performed in a 58-year-old man with iron overload (hepatic iron concentration = 15,630 µg [280 µmol]/g dry liver). Although the liver shows lower signal intensity than that of the paraspinous muscle, there is considerable motion artifact in the background, which causes image degradation. (b) Heavily T2-weighted fast spin-echo sequence (6,000/117) performed in the same patient and in which motion artifact has been limited, but the contrast difference between the muscle and liver is virtually eliminated because of the heavy T2 weighting. (c) GRE image (18/5, 10° flip angle) obtained in the same patient. Note the much improved contrast and limited motion artifact. This proved to be the optimal sequence in this study.

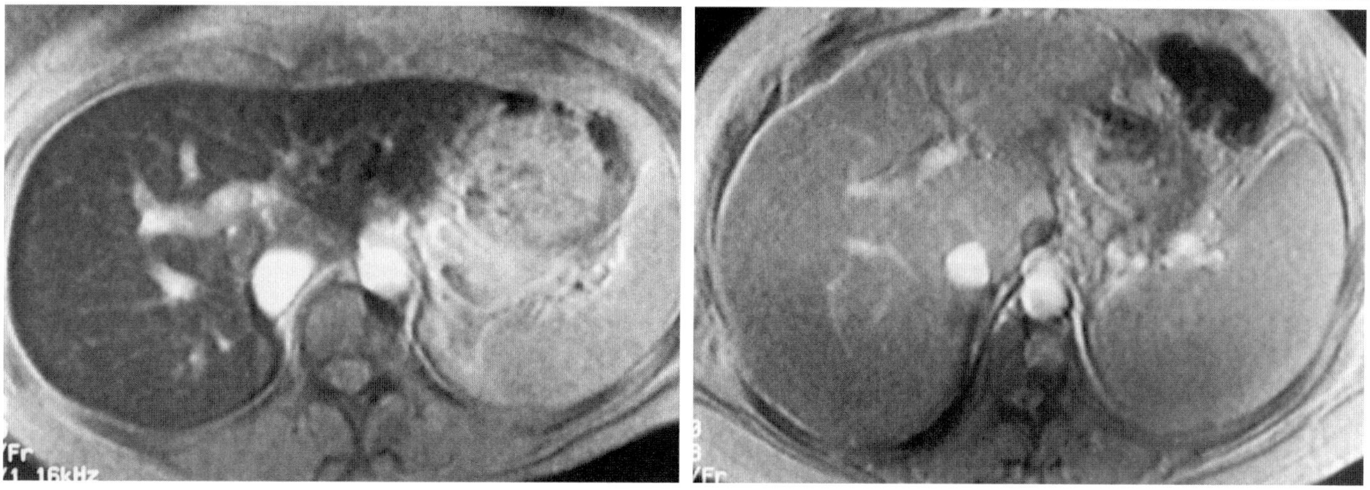

a. b.

Figure 4. Transverse MR images obtained with the optimal GRE sequence used in this study shows (a) iron overload and (b) normal hepatic iron concentrations. (a) GRE image (18/5, 10° flip angle) obtained in a 38-year-old woman with homozygous hereditary hemochromatosis whose hepatic iron concentration was 5,640 µg (101 µmol)/g dry liver (4.7-fold above the upper limit of normal). This is the typical MR appearance of hepatic iron overload. (b) GRE image (18/5, 10° flip angle) obtained in a 50-year-old man with a normal hepatic iron concentration (880 µg [15.8 µmol]/g dry liver). The liver in **a** shows less signal intensity than that in **b**.

stances is consistent with the superior performance of the GRE sequences in this study. Another major advantage of the GRE sequences is that, unlike the standard sequences that take 10 minutes to perform, they can be performed in a matter of seconds.

Of the various GRE sequences studied, the GRE sequence with the shortest repetition and echo times performed the best. This is probably because data acquisition was of sufficiently short duration that the patients were able to comfortably hold their breath during the sequence, thus minimizing motion artifact and other sources of noise. Noise has been noted previously to be a major problem in quantitative MR imaging (24).

From analysis of the scatterplot of hepatic iron concentration versus ln (SNR) with our optimal GRE sequence (Fig 2), we were able to establish a retrospective arbitrary threshold at ln (SNR) of 3.2; no patient with ln (SNR) greater than 3.2 had hepatic iron concentration greater than three times the upper limit of normal (3,600 µg [64.5 µmol]/g dry liver). The value of such a threshold for the clinician is that it allows one, by using only 19 seconds of imager time, to exclude clinically important hepatic iron overload in an individual patient.

For completion of data acquisition with this optimal sequence, the total facility time, including turnover time between patients, was approximately 15 minutes. At the current rate of charge for imager time in the United States of $800 per hour, the charge for this test might be only about $200, which is far less than the charges for liver biopsy and measurement of hepatic iron concentration at our

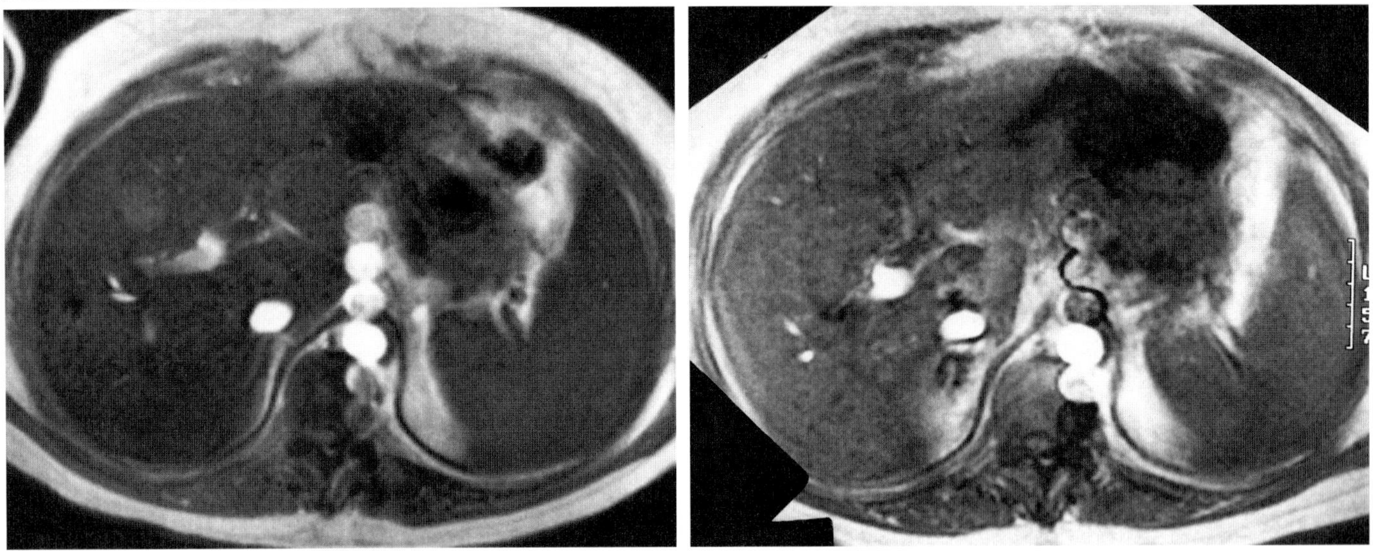

a. b.

Figure 5. Transverse MR images obtained to follow the progress of iron removal. A 54-year-old man with chronic hepatitis B and thalassemia intermedia was treated with phlebotomy to ameliorate his viral hepatitis and secondary iron overload (28). Interferon alfa-2b had been administered previously without clinical or biochemical improvement. **(a)** MR image obtained with our optimal method (GRE sequence; 18/5, 10° flip angle) prior to therapeutic phlebotomy; note the decreased signal intensity of the liver compared with that of the paraspinous muscle and spleen. The estimated hepatic iron concentration was 17,500 µg (313 µmol)/g dry liver. **(b)** MR image obtained with our optimal method (GRE sequence; 18/5, 10° flip angle) after iron depletion was achieved by removal of more than 15 L of blood; note that the signal intensity of the liver is now similar to that of the paraspinous muscle and spleen. The estimated hepatic iron concentration was 300 µg (5.37 µmol)/g dry liver; the hepatic iron concentration measured chemically in a portion of a biopsy specimen obtained around the same time was 270 µg (4.83 µmol)/g dry liver. Clinical aspects of the patient have been described (29).

and most other centers. At our center (University of Massachusetts Memorial Health Care), for example, typical charges for liver biopsy with quantitative hepatic iron concentration measurement are as follows: The short-stay facilities charge is $170, the hepatologist's fee for performing biopsy is $330, the fee for processing the specimen is $237, the pathologist's fee for interpretation of biopsy results is $220, the fee for hepatic iron concentration measurement is $146, and the total is $1,103. The average actual reimbursement to our clinical system and group practice is considerably lower because of discounts negotiated with third-party insurers. In addition, because the MR imaging procedure is noninvasive, it is more comfortable than liver biopsy for many patients, although some who are claustrophobic are unable to lie in the MR imaging machine, even for 15 minutes.

Chemical measurement of hepatic iron concentration is accurate and precise when adequate samples are assayed under ideal conditions (25). However, errors occur in standard practice, probably owing to inadequate specimen sizes, contamination, or laboratory error. Then, too, the variability of hepatic iron concentration estimation in cirrhotic livers is substantial, with coefficients of variation as high as 30%–40% (11,12). With respect to the concern of possible sampling error, MR imaging has an advantage in that the entire liver is visualized, and several truly representative regions of interest can be selected and results averaged among them (Fig 1). For example, in our study the mean coefficient of variation for the determination of ln (SNR) was only 12%, and the coefficients of variation for patients with cirrhosis in our study were not different from those without cirrhosis.

Another potential advantage of MR imaging over liver biopsy is that, due to the excellent visualization of the liver, important additional information may be obtained. In this study, for example, an operable hepatocellular carcinoma was found in one patient, and unanticipated hepatic lesions were discovered in another.

Because of the inability of MR imaging to show hepatic histopathology, liver biopsy retains its importance in the assessment of hepatic fibrosis and inflammation. As a rule, we continue to recommend liver biopsy in all patients with palpable livers, increased serum aminotransferase, or serum ferritin levels greater than 1,000 ng/mL (1,000 µg/L). Biopsy results that show fibrosis or cirrhosis provide important prognostic information and suggest the need to evaluate the severity of portal hypertension and the need for close follow-up for development of hepatocellular carcinoma. However, our results establish that MR imaging is useful to exclude iron overload in patients in whom there is only a low to moderate suspicion of the disease (eg, in a sibling of a person known to have hemochromatosis with normal or only mildly elevated iron study results).

MR imaging can also be useful in patients who adamantly refuse liver biopsy or those with decompensated liver disease and severe coagulopathy, in whom needle biopsies pose increased risks (eg, heavy drinkers with elevated liver chemistries, prothrombin times, and serum ferritin levels or transferrin saturations). Another potential role for quantitative MR imaging is to follow patients noninvasively through the course of phlebotomy or chelation therapy for primary or secondary hemochromatosis. Such uses for quantitative hepatic MR imaging have already been described (26,27). Figure 5 shows the usefulness of MR imaging in following up a patient during the course of phlebotomy therapy.

Several previous investigators focused on the liver-to-paraspinous muscle intensity ratio as the most convenient way to normalize hepatic intensity. For example,

Kaltwasser et al (16) used spin-echo sequences to determine the correlation between the hepatic iron concentration and the signal intensity ratio of liver to paraspinous muscle and found a correlation coefficient of −0.91. Hernandez et al (30) studied the relationship between the hepatic iron concentration and the ratio of signal intensities between the liver and paraspinous muscle and found a moderately good relationship ($r = -0.77$).

Bonkovsky et al (18) used a heavily T2-weighted spin-echo MR imaging sequence to examine 48 patients with abnormal iron parameters and found a correlation coefficient of −0.8 between the hepatic iron concentration and the signal intensity ratio of liver to paraspinous muscle. However, the 95% CIs still were thought to be too wide for this MR imaging method to be practical clinically. In addition, the spin-echo MR imaging sequences showed a lack of specificity. Figure 3 provides an example of the limitations of standard T2-weighted spin-echo or fast spin-echo sequences compared with rapid GRE sequences.

In agreement with the findings of an earlier pilot study (31), the results of this study showed that the ratio of signal intensities of liver to overlying air, or noise, had a closer relationship to the hepatic iron concentration values than the ratio of signal intensities of liver to that of fat, muscle, or spleen (Table 2). Our results are also in accord with those of Gandon et al (19) who also found the GRE sequences more sensitive than the standard sequences. Our results differ, however, in that Gandon et al (19) found that the liver-to-fat signal intensity ratios generally correlated more closely with hepatic iron concentration values than did the liver-to-air ratios. We speculate that the reason we found the liver-to-air ratios more precise is because of the artifactual variability of subcutaneous fat on MR images, which is related to variations in body habitus, radio frequency, and the positioning of the magnet.

Because higher magnetic field strengths provide larger magnetization gradients, higher signal contrasts can be achieved with 1.5-T than with 0.5-T magnets (24). Therefore, our 1.5-T unit, theoretically, is better suited for quantitation of hepatic iron concentration than the 0.5-T unit used by Gandon et al (19). The magnetization of ferritin itself is proportional to the strength of the ambient magnetic field (32), and previous studies (33) have suggested that higher magnetic field strength increases transverse relaxation. Thus, higher field strength imaging systems are more sensitive and accurate for the estimation of hepatic iron concentration in the range of clinical interest.

With regard to future directions and developments, the most challenging problem is finding a way to standardize noninvasive estimation of hepatic iron concentrations from one MR imaging facility to another. Measurements of signal intensity may vary from one machine to another, even if the machines are of the same type. Therefore, other investigators will need to calibrate their MR imaging machines against chemical measurements, as was done in this study. Ideally, phantoms that could be used to establish standard curves for iron measurements by means of MR imaging instruments would be developed, thus obviating the use of human subjects for machine calibration. Such phantoms would have to be stable, durable, and available at a reasonable cost and in sufficient quantity such that they would be generally available.

In summary, this study demonstrates that rapid GRE MR imaging at high magnetic field strength is a sensitive, accurate, and noninvasive modality for the estimation of hepatic iron concentration and for ruling out clinically important hepatic iron overload (ie, greater than three times the upper limit of normal). Because of the greater sensitivity and reduced random variability of results obtained with GRE sequences, such methods are preferred. Indeed, the variability of results with such noninvasive methods applied to cirrhotic livers appears to be less than that of traditional direct chemical measurements performed on small portions of biopsy specimens. Furthermore, they should be less costly than liver biopsy with direct measurement of hepatic iron concentration, although liver biopsy retains an important place in evaluation and management because of the other information it can uniquely provide.

Acknowledgments: We thank the technical and professional staffs of the Magnetic Resonance Center of Central Massachusetts for their help in carrying out this study and Rebecca Jordan for typing the manuscript. We thank Otto Gildemeister, PhD, for help with preparation of Figure 2.

References

1. Niederau C, Fisher R, Sonnenberg A, et al. Survival and causes of death in cirrhotic patients with primary hemochromatosis. N Engl J Med 1985; 313:1256–1262.
2. Feder JN, Gnirke A, Thomas W, et al. A novel MHC class I-like gene is mutated in patients with hereditary hemochromatosis. Nat Genet 1996; 13:399–408.
3. Beutler E, Gelbart R, West C, et al. Mutation analysis in hereditary hemochromatosis. Blood Cells Mol Dis 1996; 22:187–194.
4. Merryweather-Clarke AT, Pointon HH, Shearman JP, Robson KJH. Global prevalence of putative hemochromatosis mutations. J Med Genet 1997; 34:275–278.
5. Carella M, D'Ambrosio L, Totaro A, et al. Mutation analysis of the *HLA-H* gene in Italian hemochromatosis patients. Am J Hum Genet 1997; 60:828–832.
6. Chang JG, Liu TC, Lin SF. Rapid diagnosis of the *HLA-H* gene *Cys 282 Tyr* mutation in hemochromatosis by polymerase chain reaction: a very rare mutation in the Chinese population. Blood 1997; 89:3492–3493.
7. Beckman LE, Saha N, Spitsyn V, Van Landeghem G, Beckman L. Ethnic differences in the *HFE* codon 282 (*Cys/Tyr*) polymorphism. Hum Hered 1997; 47:263–267.
8. Crawford DH, Jazwinska EC, Cullen LM, Powell LW. Expression of *HLA*-linked hemochromatosis in subjects homozygous or heterozygous for the *C282Y* mutation. Gastroenterology 1998; 114:1003–1008.
9. Moyo VM, Mandishona E, Hasstedt SJ, et al. Evidence of genetic transmission in African iron overload. Blood 1998; 91:1076–1082.
10. Barry M. Liver iron concentration, stainable iron and total body storage iron. Gut 1974; 15:411–415.
11. Villeneuve JP, Bilodeau M, Lepage R, et al. Variability in hepatic iron concentration measurement from needle-biopsy specimens. J Hepatol 1996; 25:172–177.
12. Bronner MP, Kowdley KV, Carlson TH, et al. Intraorgan variability of hepatic iron concentration with hepatitis C (abstr). Hepatology 1995; 22:276A.
13. Brittenham GM. Noninvasive methods for the early detection of hereditary hemochromatosis. Ann N Y Acad Sci 1988; 526:199–208.
14. Howard JM, Ghent CN, Carey LS, et al. Diagnostic efficacy of hepatic computed tomography in the detection of body iron overload. Gastroenterology 1983; 84:209–215.
15. Stark DD. Hepatic iron overload: paramagnetic pathology (editorial). Radiology 1991; 179:333–335.
16. Kaltwasser JP, Gottschalk R, Schalk KP, et al. Noninvasive quantitation of liver iron overload by magnetic resonance imaging. Br J Haematol 1990; 74:360–363.
17. Villari N, Caramella D, Lippi A, et al. Assessment of liver iron overload in thalassemic patients by MR imaging. Acta Radiol 1992; 33:347–350.
18. Bonkovsky HL, Slaker DP, Bills EB, Wolf DC. Usefulness and limitations of laboratory and hepatic imaging studies in iron-storage disease. Gastroenterology 1990; 99:1079–1091.
19. Gandon Y, Guyader D, Heautot JF, et al. Hemochromatosis: diagnosis and quantification of liver iron with gradient-echo MR imaging. Radiology 1994; 193:533–538.
20. Barry M. Determination of chelated iron in the liver. Clin Pathol 1968; 21:166–168.
21. Stark DD, Hendrick RE, Hahn PF, Ferrucci JT Jr. Motion artifact reduction with fast spin-echo imaging. Radiology 1987; 164:183–191.
22. Stark DD, Moseley ME, Bacon BR, et al.

Magnetic resonance imaging and spectroscopy of hepatic iron overload. Radiology 1985; 154:137–142.
23. Josephson L, Lewis J, Jacobs B, Hahn PF, Stark DD. The effects of iron oxides on proton relaxivity. Magn Reson Imaging 1988; 6:647–653.
24. Henkelman RM. Measurement of signal intensities in the presence of noise in MR imaging. Med Phys 1985; 12:232–233.
25. Overmoyer BA, McLaren CE, Brittenham GM. Uniformity of liver density and nonheme (storage) iron distribution. Arch Pathol Lab Med 1987; 111:549–555.
26. Jensen PD, Jensen FT, Christensen T, et al. Evaluation of transfusional iron overload before and during iron chelation by magnetic resonance imaging of the liver and determination of serum ferritin in adult non-thalassemic patients. Br J Haematol 1995; 89:880–889.
27. Chan PC, Liu P, Cronin C, et al. The use of nuclear magnetic resonance imaging in monitoring total body iron in hemodialysis patients with hemosiderosis treated with erythropoietin and phlebotomy. Am J Kidney Dis 1992; 19:484–489.
28. Bonkovsky HL, Banner BF, Rothman AL. Iron and viral hepatitis. Hepatology 1997; 25:759–768.
29. Rubin RB, Barton AL, Banner BF, Bonkovsky HL. Iron and chronic viral hepatitis: emerging evidence for an important interaction. Dig Dis 1995; 13:223–238.
30. Hernandez RJ, Sarnaik SA, Lande I, et al. MR evaluation of liver iron overload. J Comput Assist Tomogr 1988; 12:91–94.
31. Pels Rijcken TH, Rubin RB, Davidoff A, et al. Are liver biopsies necessary in the evaluation of liver iron overload? (abstr). Am J Radiol 1994; 21:149A.
32. Koenig SH, Brown RD, Gibson JF, Ward RJ, Peters TJ. Relaxometry of ferritin solutions and the influence of Fe^{3+} core ions. Magn Reson Med 1986; 3:755–767.
33. Gillis P, Koenig SH. Transverse relaxation of solvent protons induced by magnetized spheres: application to ferritin, erythrocytes, and magnetite. Magn Reson Med 1987; 5:323–345.

Hepatocellular Carcinoma: Association with Increased Iron Deposition in the Cirrhotic Liver at MR Imaging[1]

Katsuyoshi Ito, MD
Donald G. Mitchell, MD
Toshifumi Gabata, MD
Hie-Won L. Hann, MD
Pyo N. Kim, MD
Takeshi Fujita, MD
Hitomi Awaya, MD
Kazumitsu Honjo, MD
Naofumi Matsunaga, MD

Index terms:
Hepatitis, 761.291
Liver, cirrhosis, 761.794
Liver, iron content, 761.659
Liver, MR, 761.121411, 761.121412, 761.121415, 761.12143
Liver, nodules, 761.3198
Liver, regeneration, 761.3198
Liver neoplasms, diagnosis, 761.121411, 761.121412, 761.121415, 761.12143, 761.323

Radiology 1999; 212:235–240

Abbreviations:
GRE = gradient echo
HCC = hepatocellular carcinoma
SE = spin echo

[1] From the Department of Radiology, Thomas Jefferson University Hospital, 132 S 10th St, 1096 Main Bldg, Philadelphia, PA 19107 (K.I., D.G.M., T.G., P.N.K.); the Department of Radiology, Kanazawa University School of Medicine, Kanazawa, Japan (T.G.); the Department of Medicine, Jefferson Medical College, Philadelphia, Pa (H.W.L.H.); and the Department of Radiology, Yamaguchi University School of Medicine, Yamaguchi, Japan (T.F., H.A., K.H., N.M.). Received June 30, 1998; revision requested August 5; revision received September 29; accepted January 19, 1999. **Address reprint requests to** D.G.M. (e-mail: *Donald.Mitchell@mail.tju.edu*).

Author contributions:
Guarantors of integrity of entire study, K.I., D.G.M.; study concepts, K.I., D.G.M., H.W.L.H.; study design, K.I.; definition of intellectual content, K.I.; literature research, K.I., P.N.K.; clinical studies, D.G.M., H.W.L.H., T.F., H.A., K.H., N.M.; data acquisition, K.I., D.G.M., T.G.; data analysis, K.I., D.G.M.; statistical analysis, K.I.; manuscript preparation, K.I.; manuscript editing, D.G.M.; manuscript review, D.G.M., T.G., H.W.L.H.

PURPOSE: To determine whether the frequency of hepatocellular carcinoma (HCC) in patients with cirrhosis is affected by hepatic iron deposition as detected with magnetic resonance (MR) imaging.

MATERIALS AND METHODS: In a retrospective search of MR imaging and histopathology records, 196 patients with histopathologically proved cirrhosis and with (n = 80) or without (n = 116) HCC who underwent T2-weighted conventional or fast spin-echo and gradient-echo (GRE) (echo time ≥ 6.0 msec) imaging were identified. MR images were qualitatively and quantitatively evaluated for diffuse hepatic iron deposition and siderotic regenerative nodules to assess their correlation with the presence of HCC.

RESULTS: Hepatic parenchymal iron deposition was seen in 79 (40%) patients, and iron deposition in regenerative nodules was seen in 71 (36%) at MR imaging. The mean signal intensity ratio of GRE images in patients with hepatic iron deposition was significantly lower than that in patients without it (P < .001). The frequency of HCC in patients with iron deposition in regenerative nodules (52% [37 of 71 patients]) was significantly higher (P = .015) than that in patients without iron in regenerative nodules (34% [43 of 125 patients]).

CONCLUSION: The occurrence of HCC may be associated causally with iron deposition in regenerative nodules in patients with cirrhosis. MR imaging can enable detection of iron deposition in regenerative nodules as a possible risk factor for the development of HCC.

Patients with high iron levels have been noted to have an increased risk of developing cancers. An increased probability of developing hepatocellular carcinoma (HCC) has been reported in patients with idiopathic hemochromatosis (1,2) and in patients with viral hepatitis and with persistently elevated serum ferritin levels (3).

Magnetic resonance (MR) imaging is an effective modality for evaluating patients with cirrhosis because of its capability to depict HCC and dysplastic nodules and to help assess the severity of cirrhosis (4–7). An additional advantage of MR imaging is its ability to help assess hepatic iron overload qualitatively and quantitatively in patients with cirrhosis or patients at risk for cirrhosis as well as in patients with β-thalassemia major and hemochromatosis (8–11). Thus, MR imaging may play a role in the assessment of hepatic iron deposition as a possible risk factor for the development of HCC in patients with cirrhosis. To our knowledge, however, this potential role has not been evaluated. The purpose of our study was to determine whether the frequency of HCC in patients with cirrhosis is affected by hepatic iron deposition as detected at MR imaging.

MATERIALS AND METHODS

Patient Population

Liver MR records and clinical MR requests from June 1994 to December 1997 obtained from Yamaguchi University (Japan) and Thomas Jefferson University Hospital (Philadel-

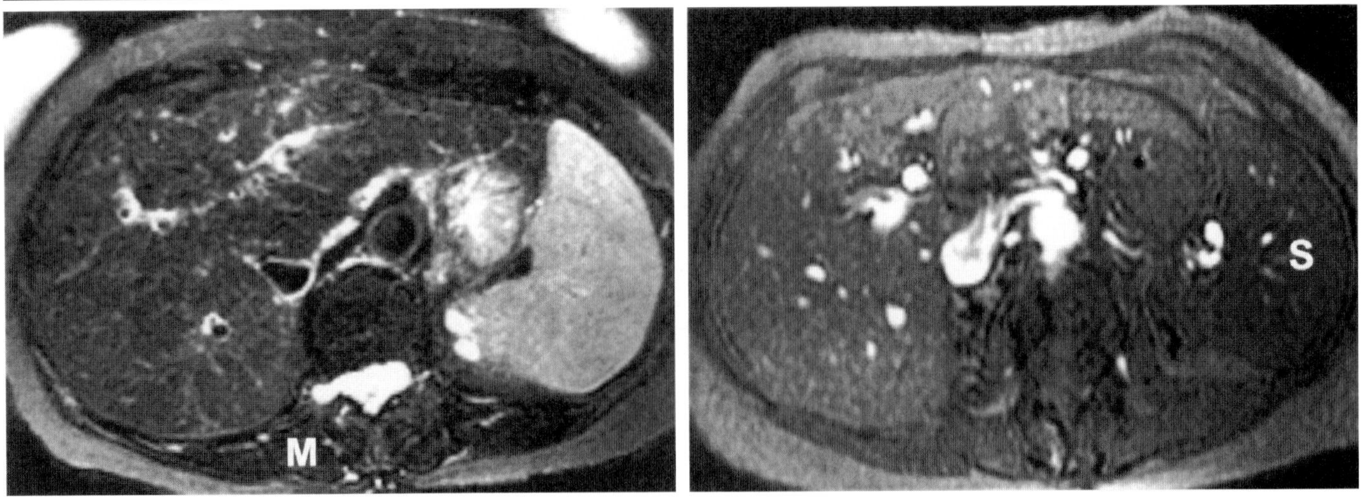

a. b.

Figure 1. Cirrhosis without hepatic iron deposition in an 84-year-old woman. **(a)** Axial T2-weighted fast SE image (6,000/144) demonstrates normal liver signal intensity, which is higher than the signal intensity of the skeletal muscle (*M*). **(b)** Axial GRE image (32/8.7, 45° flip angle) shows normal liver signal intensity, which is higher than that of the spleen (*S*) and the skeletal muscle, consistent with no hepatic iron deposition.

phia, Pa) were searched and then cross-referenced to the histopathology records to identify patients with histopathologically proved cirrhosis. The criteria for inclusion of patients in this study were that (*a*) diagnoses of cirrhosis and HCC (if present) were confirmed by means of histopathologic examination, and (*b*) for the purpose of analysis of hepatic iron deposition, both T2-weighted spin-echo (SE) or fast SE sequences and gradient-echo (GRE) sequences with an echo time 6.0 msec or greater were performed as a part of our routine abdominal MR examination.

Patients were excluded if (*a*) they had genetic hemochromatosis or Wilson disease, (*b*) MR images were degenerated by metallic artifacts due to surgical clips, (*c*) diffuse HCC was present throughout the liver, (*d*) MR studies could not be recovered from digital archive media, or (*e*) a hypervascular focal mass strongly suggestive of HCC but without histopathologic confirmation was identified on a contrast material–enhanced dynamic study. We included the last criterion to avoid having these cases categorized in the patient group without HCC, and 24 patients were excluded from this study on this basis. Consequently, this study population comprised 196 patients with cirrhosis and with HCC (n = 80) or without HCC (n = 116).

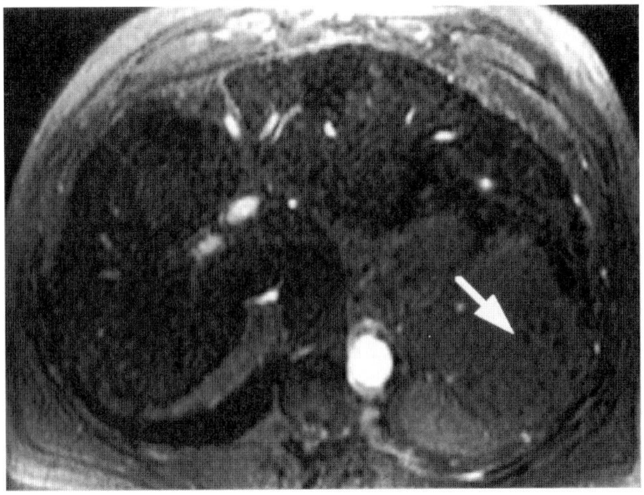

Figure 2. Cirrhosis with hepatic parenchymal iron deposition in a 59-year-old man. Axial GRE image (33/8.7, 45° flip angle) shows the liver with low signal intensity compared with the skeletal muscle. Siderotic nodules (arrow) are present in the spleen.

These patients had been referred for MR imaging for evaluation of the severity of cirrhosis and portal hypertension, for the preoperative evaluation of liver transplantation, or for the screening or further examination of hepatic lesions that were suspected with other imaging modalities. There were 121 men and 75 women (age range, 22–84 years; mean age, 53.2 years) with cirrhosis caused by viral infection (hepatitis B [n = 32], C [n = 93], or B and C [n = 10]), alcohol abuse (n = 19), and α_1-antitrypsin deficiency (n = 3); primary biliary cirrhosis (n = 6) and cryptogenic cirrhosis (n = 9); and undetermined causes of cirrhosis owing to insufficient clinical data (n = 24). Cirrhosis was histopathologically confirmed by means of percutaneous liver biopsy in 126 patients, liver transplantation in 27, transjugular liver biopsy in 20, surgical resection in 17, and autopsy in six. The diagnosis of HCC was proved at histopathologic examination in all 80 patients by means of percutaneous liver biopsy (n = 52), surgical resection (n = 17), liver transplantation (n = 9), and autopsy (n = 2).

MR Imaging Technique

MR imaging was performed with a 1.5-T unit (Signa, GE Medical Systems, Milwaukee, Wis; Magnetom H-15 or Vision, Siemens, Erlangen, Germany) with the use of either a whole-body coil (n = 41) or a phased-array torso coil (n = 155). Because

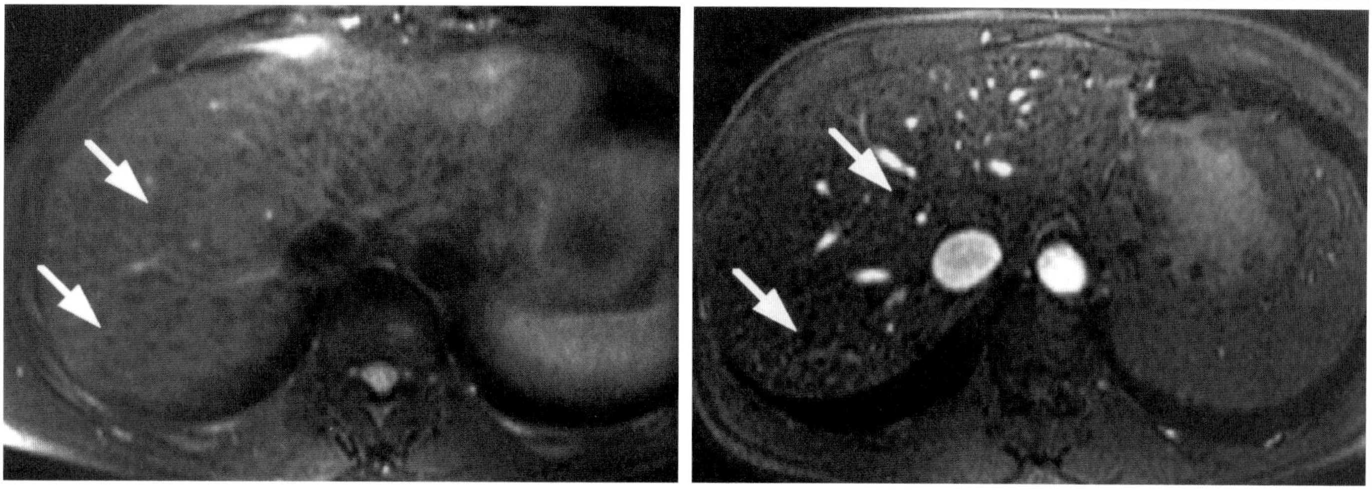

a.   b.

Figure 3. Cirrhosis with iron deposition in hepatic regenerative nodules in a 54-year-old man. **(a)** Axial T2-weighted SE image (2,000/50) demonstrates small low-intensity nodules (arrows) in the liver. **(b)** Axial GRE image (33/8.7, 45° flip angle) clearly shows multiple low-intensity nodules (arrows) in the liver, which are consistent with siderotic regenerative nodules.

TABLE 1
Comparison of Signal Intensity Ratios in Patients with and Patients without Hepatic Iron Deposition and in Patients with and Patients without HCC

	Iron in Regenerative Nodules			Iron in Liver Parenchyma			HCC		
Sequence	Positive* (n = 71)	Negative* (n = 125)	P Value†	Positive* (n = 79)	Negative* (n = 117)	P Value†	Positive* (n = 80)	Negative* (n = 116)	P Value†
T2-weighted SE	1.33 ± 1.00	1.54 ± 0.81	NS	0.97 ± 0.32	1.85 ± 0.97	<.001	1.38 ± 0.75	1.52 ± 0.86	NS
GRE	0.82 ± 0.39	1.13 ± 0.45	<.001	0.76 ± 0.29	1.25 ± 0.42	<.001	0.97 ± 0.32	1.06 ± 0.48	NS

* Data are the mean signal intensity ratios ± SD.
† NS = not significant.

the purpose of our study was to assess hepatic iron deposition, T2-weighted SE or fast SE images and GRE images (echo time ≥ 6.0 msec) were reviewed in all patients. These sequences have been relatively sensitive to the paramagnetic effects of hepatic iron among the MR images obtained at our routine abdominal examination.

Previous reports (9,10,12) showed a statistically significant correlation between the hepatic iron concentration revealed at MR imaging with T2-weighted or T2*-weighted sequences and the hepatic iron concentration value measured at biopsy, and they indicated that MR imaging with these sequences can be used to accurately quantify the amount of hepatic iron. T2-weighted imaging included conventional SE (1,500–3,000/50–100 [repetition time msec/echo time msec]), respiratory-triggered fast SE (3,000–7,500/91–144 [effective echo time]) with or without fat suppression, or breath-hold fast SE (2,500–4,200/70–138 [effective echo time]) sequences.

GRE images were obtained with a repetition time of 22–150 msec, an echo time of 6.0–9.9 msec, and a flip angle of 20°–60°. In addition, in-phase GRE (80–210/4.2, 90° flip angle), contrast-enhanced GRE (80–170/2.2–4.8, 70°–90° flip angle), and phase-contrast GRE (30–39/9.9, 30° flip angle) images with or without contrast enhancement were also reviewed as supplemental sequences, if available, although GRE images with shorter echo times generally are less sensitive in the detection of hepatic iron compared with T2-weighted SE and GRE (echo time ≥ 6.0 msec) sequences.

Contrast-enhanced GRE images were obtained after the administration of 0.1 mmol of gadopentetate dimeglumine (Magnevist, Berlex Laboratory, Wayne, NJ, or Japan-Schering, Osaka, Japan) per kilogram of body weight, but these images were not used to evaluate hepatic iron. Other imaging parameters included a 256 or 512 × 128–256 imaging matrix, usually with use of a rectangular field of view to reduce the number of phase-encoding views, and a 5–10-mm section thickness with a section gap of 2 mm or less.

Image Interpretation

MR images of each patient were evaluated on a computer monitor (SPARC 20; Sun Microsystems, Palo Alto, Calif). Three representative images per sequence obtained at different levels (eg, upper, middle, and lower level) of the liver were given to the readers (K.I., D.G.M., T.G.). Consequently, the total image number was six to 15 per patient—in most patients, nine or 12 images. The images in which HCC was seen were not included because knowledge of the presence of HCC might bias the readers' evaluation for hepatic iron deposition. Thus, the readers were blinded with regard to the presence of HCC in each patient during their reading. The images obtained in patients with HCC or without HCC were intermixed randomly and presented to the readers.

MR images were qualitatively evaluated for (*a*) hepatic parenchymal iron deposition and (*b*) iron deposition in regenerative nodules to assess the correlation with the presence of HCC. Hepatic parenchymal iron deposition was considered present when the signal intensity of the liver diffusely decreased and was scored with use of the following four-point severity scale: "0" was defined as absent if the signal intensity of the liver was greater than that of skeletal muscle; "1," as mild if the signal intensity of the liver was equal to or slightly less than that of skeletal muscle; "2," as moderate if the signal intensity of the liver was moderately less than that of skeletal muscle; and "3," as severe if the signal intensity of the liver was markedly less than that of skeletal muscle. We used skeletal muscle as a reference tissue according to the findings of prior studies (10,11,13) because iron tends not to accumulate in skeletal muscle in patients with iron overload. Iron deposition in regenerative nodules was scored "0" for absent, "1" for probably present, and "2" for definitely present. Siderotic regenerative nodules were defined as small nodules with low signal intensity compared with surrounding hepatic parenchyma on GRE images (14,15).

Images were reviewed retrospectively and independently by three radiologists (K.I., D.G.M., T.G.) experienced in the interpretation of MR images of the liver. When there was disagreement in their opinions regarding the absence or presence of hepatic iron deposition, a majority opinion was used as the final decision. When hepatic iron deposition was determined to be present, a mean score of the three observers' readings was used for further analysis.

For the quantitative evaluation, region-of-interest analysis of the images was performed by a single observer (K.I.). Region-of-interest measurements were made of the liver and the right paraspinous muscles by using the T2-weighted SE and GRE (echo time ≥ 6.0 msec) images; the same location on the images was used for the measurements. Signal intensities were measured on the posterior part of the right hepatic lobe adjacent to the right paraspinous muscles because the signal intensity of the central portion of the liver often decreased on MR images obtained with a phased-array torso coil. Vessels were excluded from the region of interest as much as possible. The liver-to-muscle signal intensity ratio was calculated from region-of-interest measurements. The signal intensity ratio was defined as the signal intensity of the liver divided by the signal intensity of the paraspinous muscle.

TABLE 2
Frequency of HCC in Patients with and Patients without Hepatic Iron Deposition

HCC	Iron in Regenerative Nodules: Positive (*n* = 71)	Iron in Regenerative Nodules: Negative (*n* = 125)	Iron in Liver Parenchyma: Positive (*n* = 79)	Iron in Liver Parenchyma: Negative (*n* = 117)
Positive (*n* = 80)	37	43	32	48
Negative (*n* = 116)	34	82	47	69

Note.—Data are the number of patients.

Statistical Analysis

The χ^2 test was used to compare the difference of the frequency of HCC between the patients with and the patients without hepatic iron deposition. Comparisons of the signal intensity ratios were performed with an unpaired two-tailed Student *t* test between subgroups with and subgroups without hepatic iron deposition or between those with and those without HCC. Data were presented as the mean ± SD. A *P* value of less than .05 was considered to indicate a statistically significant difference. To assess interobserver variability in the reading, κ values were calculated for the three readers (16). The level of agreement was defined as follows: no agreement, κ < 0; poor agreement, κ = 0.01–0.40; good agreement, κ = 0.41–0.75; and excellent agreement, κ = 0.76–1.00.

RESULTS

In the analysis of interobserver variability for the three readers, the κ values for MR imaging findings showed good agreement (0.50–0.72).

At visual inspection, the signal intensity of the liver was equal to or less than that of skeletal muscle in 79 (40%) of the 196 patients, which indicates the presence of hepatic parenchymal iron deposition (Figs 1, 2). The mean visual score in these patients was 1.22 ± 0.67. Iron deposition in regenerative nodules was seen in 71 (36%) of the 196 patients, with a mean visual score of 1.42 ± 0.50 (Fig 3). Iron deposition in both the hepatic parenchyma and regenerative nodules was seen in 43 (22%) of the 196 patients. In the quantitative analysis, the 79 patients with visible hepatic parenchymal iron deposition had significantly lower mean signal intensity ratios than did the 117 patients without it on both T2-weighted SE (0.97 ± 0.32 vs 1.85 ± 0.97, *P* < .001) and GRE images (0.76 ± 0.29 vs 1.25 ± 0.42, *P* < .001). The 71 patients with siderotic regenerative nodules on GRE images had significantly lower mean signal intensity ratios than did the 125 patients without them (0.82 ± 0.39 vs 1.13 ± 0.45, *P* < .001). There was no significant difference in the mean signal intensity ratio between the 80 patients with HCC and the 116 patients without HCC (Table 1).

The difference in the frequency of HCC between patients with and patients without hepatic iron deposition is shown in Table 2. HCC was seen in 32 (41%) of the 79 patients with visible hepatic parenchymal iron deposition and was seen in 48 (41%) of the 117 patients without it (no significant difference). The frequency of HCC in patients with siderotic regenerative nodules was higher (52% [37 of 71 patients]) than that in patients without siderotic regenerative nodules (34% [43 of 125 patients]; *P* = .015) (Fig 4).

Among patients with siderotic regenerative nodules (*n* = 71), differences in the signal intensity ratio were compared between subgroups with HCC (*n* = 37) and those without HCC (*n* = 34) to determine whether the prevalence of HCC is associated with the severity of hepatic iron deposition (Table 3). There was no significant difference in the signal intensity ratio between subgroups with HCC and those without HCC.

DISCUSSION

Because iron can accumulate diffusely within the hepatic parenchyma or focally within regenerative nodules in patients with cirrhosis, we evaluated MR images of these two findings in association with the presence of HCC. In this study, hepatic parenchymal iron deposition was visible in 79 (40%) patients, with a mean score of 1.22 ± 0.67 in the qualitative analysis. The mean signal intensity ratio in these 79 patients was significantly lower than that in 117 patients without visible he-

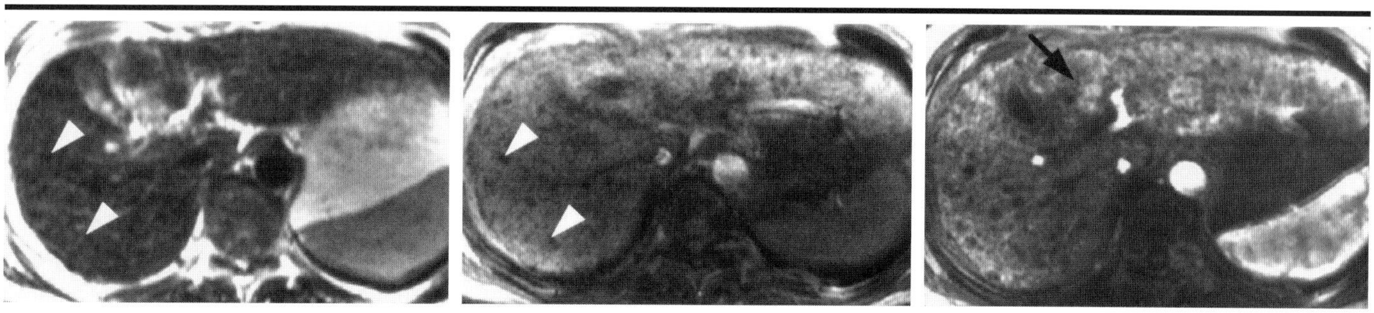

a. b. c.

Figure 4. Cirrhosis with HCC and iron deposition in hepatic regenerative nodules in a 68-year-old man. **(a)** Axial T2-weighted fast SE image (2,500/99) and **(b)** axial GRE image (150/6, 60° flip angle) show multiple siderotic regenerative nodules (arrowheads) with low signal intensity. **(c)** Axial arterial-phase contrast-enhanced dynamic GRE image (150/6, 60° flip angle) demonstrates HCC as a nodule (arrow) with early enhancement.

TABLE 3
Comparison of Signal Intensity Ratios in Subgroups with HCC and Subgroups without HCC among Patients with Iron Deposition in Regenerative Nodules

	Positive for Iron in Regenerative Nodules (n = 71)		
Sequence	HCC Positive (n = 37)*	HCC Negative (n = 34)*	P Value†
T2-weighted SE	1.34 ± 0.95	1.33 ± 1.05	NS
GRE	0.79 ± 0.34	0.84 ± 0.41	NS

* Data are the mean signal intensity ratios ± SD.
† NS = not significant.

patic parenchymal iron deposition, which indicates that visual inspection was correlated with quantitative analysis for diffuse iron accumulation and confirms that mild hepatic siderosis is common in cirrhosis (12). Ludwig et al (17) have shown a similar frequency (32.4% [145 of 447]) of mild hemosiderosis in cirrhosis on the basis of analysis of tissue iron of specimens obtained at orthotopic liver transplantation.

Siderotic regenerative nodules are seen frequently in cirrhotic livers at MR imaging (14,15). In the current study, iron deposition in regenerative nodules was seen in 71 (36%) patients at visual inspection. The mean signal intensity ratio in these 71 patients was significantly lower than that in 125 patients without siderotic regenerative nodules on GRE images, probably owing to the inclusion of microscopic siderotic nodules within measured regions.

Our methodology did not include histopathologic proof that decreased signal intensity is caused by hepatic iron deposition. However, similar imaging techniques have been used to detect hepatic iron overload and siderotic regenerative nodules, and results have been confirmed with quantitative histopathologic measurements (9,10,15). Because of little attention to hepatic iron deposition in many histopathology reports, limited availability of histopathologic specimens, and the small number of iron stains and quantitative tissue iron studies of hepatic specimens, direct correlation between findings in MR studies and at histopathologic examination regarding the degree and distribution of hepatic iron deposition was difficult and was not performed in this study.

Excessive tissue iron is potentially toxic and mutagenic and can lead to malignant transformation, and the liver is especially vulnerable (18). Authors of prior reports (19–21) have shown an association between HCC and the histopathologic findings of hepatic iron excess, and they have indicated that hepatic iron overload is a risk factor for developing HCC, even in the absence of genetic hemochromatosis. In the current study, the frequency of HCC in patients with siderotic regenerative nodules visible on MR images was significantly higher than that in patients without iron in regenerative nodules.

Our results suggest that the occurrence of HCC may be causally related to iron concentration within regenerative nodules that are large enough to be visible on MR images and that MR imaging can depict these siderotic regenerative nodules as a marker of HCC development. However, depiction of these siderotic regenerative nodules is not a mandatory process leading to the development of HCC, because there were some patients with HCC but without visible siderotic regenerative nodules. In our analysis of subgroups (n = 71) with visible iron deposition in regenerative nodules (Table 3), there was no significant difference in the signal intensity ratio between patients with HCC (n = 37) and those without HCC (n = 34). Therefore, it seems that the severity of diffuse hepatic parenchymal iron deposition is unlikely to affect the prevalence of HCC among patients with visible siderotic regenerative nodules.

Prior reports offer two explanations as to how increased hepatic iron may contribute to hepatocarcinogenesis. One possible direct mechanism is that free cellular iron may induce mutations by generating reactive oxygen species. A number of DNA changes are produced by reactive oxygen species (22). An indirect possibility is that excess hepatic iron may facilitate the persistence of chronic hepatitis B and C viral infections, both of which are major risk factors for the development of HCC (21).

Histopathologic observations further support a role for iron-accumulative regenerative nodules in carcinogenesis. Authors of previous reports (23–25) have described the emergence of hyperplastic or malignant foci with atypical hepatocytes within large regenerative nodules, which suggests incipient neoplastic hepatocellular lesions. In one autopsy series (26), the frequency of hyperplastic foci within large regenerative nodules in patients with cirrhosis was higher in patients with iron-accumulative nodules versus those without iron-accumulative nodules (57% [20 of 35] vs 31% [20 of 64]). Iron concentration within regenerative nodules may expose hyperplastic or dysplastic foci to the tumor-stimulating effects of iron. Malignant foci within iron-accumulative regenerative nodules can show a nodule-within-nodule appearance on MR images (27) because these malignant foci do not contain iron (28). Therefore, MR imaging may be used to follow up patients with cirrhosis with iron-accumulative regenerative nodules for the early detection of malignant foci.

It is unclear why a subset of regenerative nodules in some patients with cirrhosis tends to accumulate iron. Because hepatocellular iron uptake is largely mediated by transferrin receptor proteins (29), these proteins may be abnormal in iron-accumulative regenerative nodules. The iron in regenerative nodules has been shown to disappear with the development of iron deficiency anemia (30), which suggests that iron deposition in regenerative nodules can be reversible and that the intralesional iron is metabolically available for redistribution for hematopoiesis. Therefore, phlebotomy may reduce iron deposition in regenerative nodules and potentially decrease the risk of HCC. MR imaging could help evaluate the changes of iron in regenerative nodules during the clinical course as well as after phlebotomy.

Our study has some limitations. First, the MR imaging parameters and sequences differed between patients. Recent technical improvements have allowed the use of more efficient pulse sequences, including fast SE and GRE imaging with a short echo time. Fast SE sequences are less sensitive than conventional SE sequences to magnetic field heterogeneities because of the use of repeated 180° refocusing pulses, which probably results in overlooking mild hepatic iron overload. GRE sequences with an echo time longer than 15 msec are considered preferable for detecting slight hepatic iron (12). More standardized pulse sequences optimized for iron sensitivity may have resulted in the detection of more cases of mild hepatic iron deposition. However, it was not practical to include these less efficient sequences in the current routine abdominal protocol.

Second, we could not exclude the possibility of small HCCs, if they were not seen on the images, being categorized in the group of patients without HCC. It is not possible to reliably exclude this possibility without histopathologic investigation of the whole hepatic specimen. However, these limitations do not reduce the validity of the correlation we observed between visible siderotic regenerative nodules and the frequency of HCC.

In conclusion, the occurrence of HCC may be associated causally with iron deposition in large regenerative nodules in patients with cirrhosis, and MR imaging is a useful modality for assessing iron deposition in these regenerative nodules as a possible risk factor for the development of HCC.

References

1. Bradbear RA, Bain C, Siskind V, et al. Cohort study of internal malignancy in genetic hemochromatosis and other chronic non-alcoholic liver diseases. J Natl Cancer Inst 1985; 75:81–84.
2. Niederau C, Fischer R, Sonnenberg A, Stremmel W, Trampisch HJ, Strohmeyer G. Survival and causes of death in cirrhotic and in non-cirrhotic patients with primary hemochromatosis. N Engl J Med 1985; 313:1256–1262.
3. Hann HWL, Kim CY, London WT, Blumberg BS. Increased serum ferritin in chronic liver disease: a risk factor for primary hepatocellular carcinoma. Int J Cancer 1989; 43:376–379.
4. Matsui M, Kadoya M, Kameyama T, et al. Adenomatous hyperplastic nodules in the cirrhotic liver: differentiation from hepatocellular carcinoma with MR imaging. Radiology 1989; 173:123–126.
5. Ito K, Choji T, Nakada T, Nakanishi T, Kurokawa F, Okita K. Multislice dynamic MRI of hepatic tumors. J Comput Assist Tomogr 1993; 17:390–396.
6. Yamashita Y, Mitsuzaki K, Yi T, et al. Small hepatocellular carcinoma in patients with chronic liver damage: prospective comparison of detection with dynamic MR imaging and helical CT of the whole liver. Radiology 1996; 200:79–84.
7. Ito K, Mitchell DG, Hann HWL, Outwater EK, Kim Y. Compensated cirrhosis due to viral hepatitis: using MR imaging to predict clinical progression. AJR 1997; 169: 801–805.
8. Gomori JM, Horev G, Tamary H, et al. Hepatic iron overload: quantitative MR imaging. Radiology 1991; 179:367–369.
9. Gandon Y, Guyader D, Heautot JF, et al. Hemochromatosis: diagnosis and quantification of liver iron with gradient-echo MR imaging. Radiology 1994; 193:533–538.
10. Ernst O, Sergent G, Bonvarlet P, Canva-Delcambre V, Paris JC, L'Hermine C. Hepatic iron overload: diagnosis and quantification with MR imaging. AJR 1997; 168: 1205–1208.
11. Siegelman ES, Mitchell DG, Outwater E, Munoz SJ, Rubin R. Idiopathic hemochromatosis: MR imaging findings in cirrhotic and precirrhotic patients. Radiology 1993; 188:637–641.
12. Siegelman ES, Mitchell DG, Semelka RC. Abdominal iron deposition: metabolism, MR findings, and clinical importance. Radiology 1996; 199:13–22.
13. Siegelman ES, Mitchell DG, Rubin R, et al. Parenchymal versus reticuloendothelial iron overload in the liver: distinction with MR imaging. Radiology 1991; 179:361–366.
14. Ohtomo K, Itai Y, Ohtomo Y, Shiga J, Iio M. Regenerating nodules of liver cirrhosis: MR imaging with pathologic correlation. AJR 1990; 154:505–507.
15. Murakami T, Kuroda C, Marukawa T, et al. Regenerating nodules in hepatic cirrhosis: MR findings with pathologic correlation. AJR 1990; 155:1227–1231.
16. Fleiss JL. Statistical methods for rates and proportions. 2nd ed. New York, NY: Wiley, 1973; 211–236.
17. Ludwig J, Hashimoto E, Porayko MK, Moyer TP, Baldus WP. Hemosiderosis in cirrhosis: a study of 447 native livers. Gastroenterology 1997; 112:882–888.
18. Bonkovsky HL. Iron and the liver. Am J Med Sci 1991; 301:32–43.
19. Zhou X, Detolla L, Custer RP, London WT. Iron, ferritin, hepatitis B surface and core antigens in the livers of Chinese patients with hepatocellular carcinoma. Cancer 1987; 59:1430–1437.
20. Turlin B, Juguet F, Moirand R, et al. Increased liver iron stores in patients with hepatocellular carcinoma developed on a noncirrhotic liver. Hepatology 1995; 22: 446–450.
21. Mandishona E, MacPhail AP, Gordeuk VR, et al. Dietary iron overload as a risk factor for hepatocellular carcinoma in Black Africans. Hepatology 1998; 27:1563–1566.
22. Meneghini R. Iron homeostasis, oxidative stress, and DNA damage. Free Radic Biol Med 1997; 23:783–792.
23. Arakawa M, Kage M, Sugihara S, Nakashima T, Suenaga M, Okuda S. Emergence of malignant lesions within an adenomatous hyperplastic nodule in a cirrhotic liver: observations in five cases. Gastroenterology 1986; 91:198–208.
24. Furuya K, Nakamura M, Yamamoto Y, Togei K, Otsuka H. Macroregenerative nodule of the liver: a clinicopathological study of 345 autopsy cases of chronic liver disease. Cancer 1988; 61:99–105.
25. Terada T, Nakanuma Y. Iron-negative foci in siderotic macroregenerative nodules in human cirrhotic liver. Arch Pathol Lab Med 1989; 113:916–920.
26. Terada T, Nakanuma Y. Survey of iron-accumulative macroregenerative nodules in cirrhotic livers. Hepatology 1989; 10: 851–854.
27. Mitchell DG, Rubin R, Siegelman ES, Burk DL Jr, Rifkin MD. Hepatocellular carcinoma within siderotic regenerative nodules: appearance as a nodule within a nodule on MR images. Radiology 1991; 178:101–103.
28. Terada T, Kadoya M, Nakanuma Y, Matsui O. Iron-accumulating adenomatous hyperplastic nodule with malignant foci in the cirrhotic liver: histopathologic, quantitative iron, and magnetic resonance imaging in vitro studies. Cancer 1990; 65: 1994–2000.
29. Bomford AB, Munro HN. Transferrin and its receptor: their roles in cell function. Hepatology 1985; 5:870–875.
30. Murakami T, Nakamura H, Kuroda C, et al. Siderotic nodules in hepatic cirrhosis disappearing after biliary hemorrhage: MR imaging. J Comput Assist Tomogr 1991; 15:1039–1041.

Young H. Kim, MD
Hyo K. Lim, MD
Joon K. Han, MD
Byung I. Choi, MD
Yong I. Kim, MD
Won J. Lee, MD
Seung H. Kim, MD

Index terms:
Gastritis, 72.202, 72.291
Lymphoma, 72.34
Lymphoma, diagnosis, 72.123, 72.1261
Peptic ulcer, 72.25
Stomach, biopsy, 72.123, 72.1261

Radiology 1999; 212:241–248

Abbreviations:
GI = gastrointestinal
MALT = mucosa-associated lymphoid tissue

[1] From the Department of Radiology, Samsung Medical Center, College of Medicine, Sungkyunkwan University, 50 Ilwon-dong, Kangnam-ku, Seoul 135-710, Korea (H.K.L., W.J.L., S.H.K.), and the Departments of Radiology (Y.H.K., J.K.H., B.I.C.) and Pathology (Y.I.K.), Seoul National University Hospital, Korea. From the 1997 RSNA scientific assembly. Received April 20, 1998; revision requested July 2; revision received August 19; accepted November 20. **Address reprint requests to** H.K.L.

Low-Grade Gastric Mucosa-associated Lymphoid Tissue Lymphoma: Correlation of Radiographic and Pathologic Findings[1]

PURPOSE: To describe upper gastrointestinal (GI) examination findings of low-grade gastric mucosa-associated lymphoid tissue (MALT) lymphoma and to correlate them with pathologic examination findings.

MATERIALS AND METHODS: A retrospective review of upper GI examinations was performed in 25 patients with proved low-grade gastric MALT lymphomas. Upper GI examinations were reviewed for common findings and most probable diagnosis, and these findings were correlated with pathologic findings in resected specimens in 15 patients.

RESULTS: The common findings at upper GI examination included mucosal nodularity (n = 13), ulcer (n = 12), rugal thickening (n = 6), mass (n = 4), and enlarged areae gastricae (n = 2). The most probable diagnoses were early gastric carcinoma (n = 7), advanced gastric carcinoma (n = 6), gastritis (n = 9), and lymphoma (n = 3). Of 17 lesions found on resected specimens, six ulcers and two masses were not depicted at barium study. Disorganized convergent rugae projecting to multiple points and vague ulcer margins were present in four and seven lesions, respectively. Multiple ulcers were seen in two patients.

CONCLUSION: Although the common radiographic and pathologic findings observed in low-grade gastric MALT lymphomas were similar to those of gastric carcinomas or gastritis, disorganized convergent rugae, vague ulcer margins, and multiplicity of lesions may be helpful in differentiating them from gastric carcinomas or gastritis.

The gastrointestinal (GI) tract, particularly the stomach, is the most common primary site of extranodal lymphoma. However, primary gastric lymphoma is uncommon and constitutes only 2%–5% of malignant gastric lesions (1,2). Most gastric lymphomas are of B-cell lineage (3). Among them, most primary low-grade B-cell lymphomas of the stomach have long been known as "pseudolymphomas" or "lymphoreticular hyperplasia" because of the presence of reactive follicles and mixed inflammatory cell infiltration at histopathologic examination and because of the favorable prognosis (4,5). However, recent immunohistochemical studies (6,7) have shown that most pseudolymphomas are monoclonal B-cell proliferations and that the majority of these B cells are considered to originate from mucosa-associated lymphoid tissue (MALT). These B cells have the same cytologic and immunophenotypic characteristics as the B cells that are normally found around the mantle zones of Peyer patches (8–10). Therefore, these low-grade B-cell lymphomas, which have the morphologic features of MALT with the high-grade lesions that may evolve from them, are known as MALT lymphoma (11–13).

There have been some reports (14–16) describing the radiographic findings of pseudolymphoma and gastric MALT lymphoma (17–20). Suekane et al (18) stated that friable mucosa and ulcers simulating early gastric carcinoma were frequent findings in low-grade gastric MALT lymphoma. Yoo et al (20) reported that round nodularity was the most common finding at double-contrast barium study. To our knowledge, however, there has been no

Author contributions:
Guarantors of integrity of entire study, H.K.L., Y.H.K.; study concepts and design, H.K.L., J.K.H.; definition of intellectual content, H.K.L.; literature research, Y.H.K.; clinical studies, W.J.L., H.K.L., J.K.H., B.I.C.; data acquisition, S.H.K., Y.H.K.; data analysis, Y.H.K., Y.I.K.; manuscript preparation, Y.H.K.; manuscript editing, H.K.L.; manuscript review, B.I.C., H.K.L.

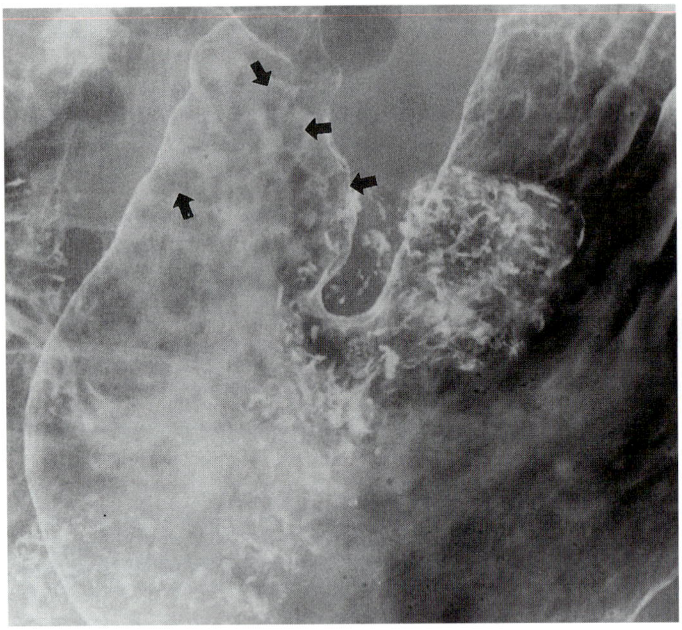

a.

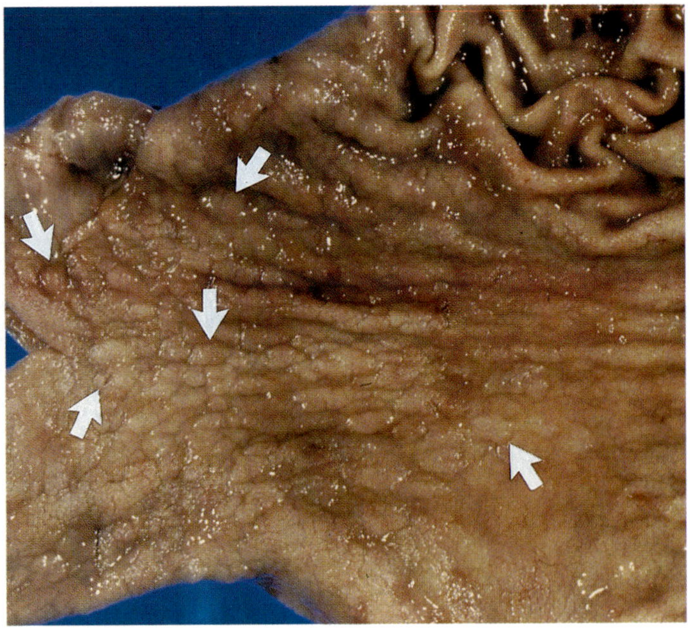

b.

Figure 1. Low-grade gastric MALT lymphoma with diffuse mucosal nodularity in a 60-year-old woman. **(a)** Spot radiograph of upper GI examination shows diffuse nodules of varying sizes (arrows) in the gastric antrum. **(b)** Magnification photograph (original magnification ×2) of the resected specimen shows diffuse nodularities (arrows) in the gastric antrum. At histopathologic examination, low-grade MALT lymphoma was found in the mucosa of the entire gastric antrum (not shown).

prior report describing the radiologic-pathologic correlation of this entity in the English-language radiology literature.

The purpose of this study was to evaluate the findings of double-contrast upper GI examinations in 25 patients with histopathologically proved low-grade gastric MALT lymphoma and to correlate them with pathologic findings.

MATERIALS AND METHODS

A review of the pathologic and radiologic databases during a 5-year period (1993–1997) revealed 121 consecutive patients with gastric lymphomas at our institutions. Among them were 25 patients (16 women, nine men; age range, 24–75 years; mean age, 32 years) with low-grade gastric MALT lymphomas histopathologically proved at endoscopic biopsy. Twenty of these patients underwent either total ($n = 12$) or subtotal ($n = 8$) gastrectomy. The presence of *Helicobacter pylori* infection was histopathologically confirmed in 23 patients by means of endoscopic biopsy, and the remaining two patients had a history of treatment for gastritis or peptic ulcer.

All patients underwent double-contrast upper GI examinations that were adequate for the analysis of the lesions. All upper GI examinations were performed within 2 weeks (mean, 5 days) of endoscopy. The upper GI examination was performed to evaluate the extent of the lesions in patients ($n = 20$) who were scheduled to undergo surgery. The surgeons at our institutions wanted the barium study before surgery to help them decide what type of surgery to perform. The barium study in the remaining five patients treated with antibiotics or chemotherapy was requested as a baseline study for follow-up. We used intramuscular injection of 20 mg of scopolamine butylbromide (Buscopan; Boehringer Ingelheim Korea, Seoul, Korea) as a hypotonic agent and oral administration of 200–250 mL of 140% wt/vol barium suspension (Solotop-HD; Taejoon Pharm, Kyungkido, Korea). Oral administration of an effervescent agent was used for adequate gastric distention. Under fluoroscopic observation, multiple spot radiographs were obtained after adequate mucosal coating.

The findings at upper GI examination were reviewed independently at each institution by four radiologists (Y.H.K., H.K.L., J.K.H., W.J.L.). This retrospective review was performed without knowledge of the endoscopic and pathologic findings but with knowledge of the final diagnosis of low-grade gastric MALT lymphoma. Final interpretations were made by consensus. The radiologic signs evaluated were the pattern of areae gastricae, presence of ulcer, mass formation, mucosal nodularity, and rugal thickening. The extent of the lesions was categorized as being in the antrum, body, or fundus.

TABLE 1
Findings at Upper GI Examination in 25 Patients with Low-Grade Gastric MALT Lymphoma

Radiographic Findings	No. of Patients
Mucosal nodularity	13 (52)
Ulcer (either shallow or deep)	12 (48)
Fold thickening	6 (24)
Mass	4 (16)
Single	1 (4)
Multiple	3 (12)
Enlarged areae gastricae	2 (8)
Two or more findings	15 (60)

Note.—Data in parentheses are percentages.

Of 20 patients who underwent surgical resection, the pathologic specimens were available in 15 patients. The pathologic specimens were reviewed by one experienced pathologist (Y.I.K.) for the extent and morphologic features of the lesions. The depth of invasion and involvement of lymph nodes were also determined at histopathologic examination. Although

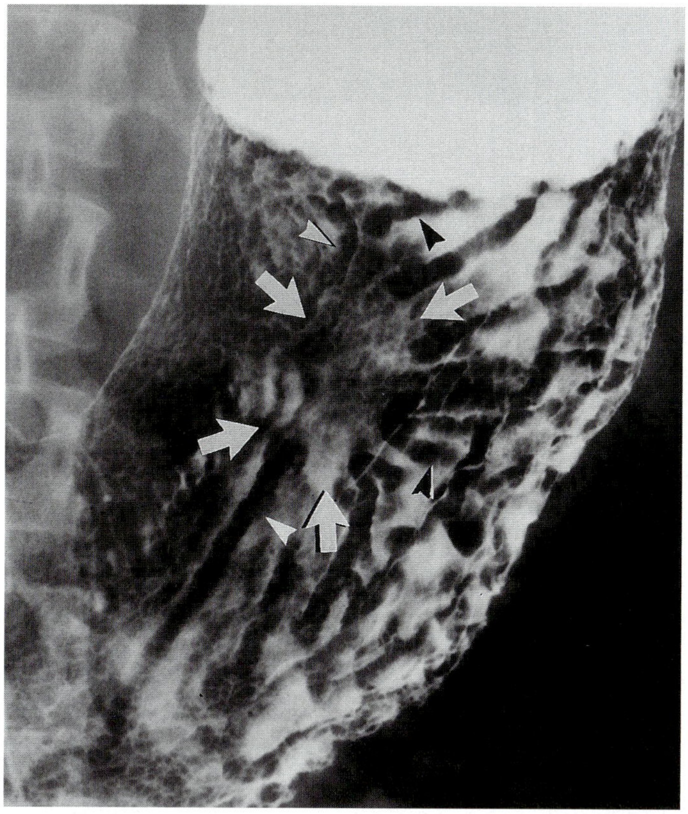

a.

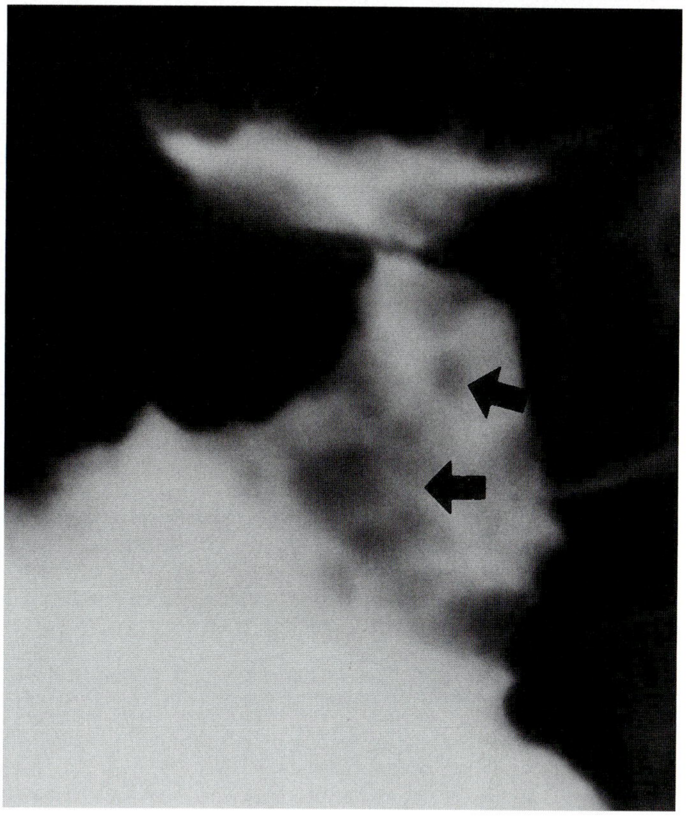

b.

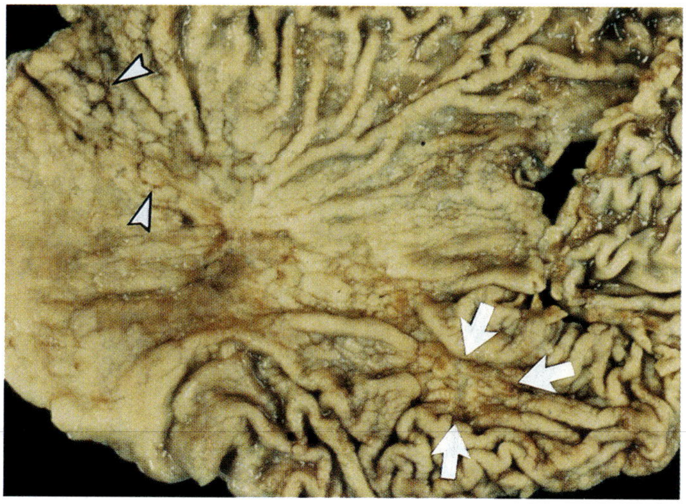

c.

Figure 2. Low-grade gastric MALT lymphoma with ulcer in a 33-year-old woman. **(a)** Spot radiograph of upper GI examination shows a large shallow ulcer (arrows) with vague margins in the posterior wall of the gastric body. Note the convergent rugae (arrowheads) that project to multiple points. **(b)** Compression radiograph of the distal antrum shows multiple nodules (arrows) of varying sizes. **(c)** Photograph of the resected specimen shows a shallow ulcer (arrows) with convergence of the surrounding rugae in the posterior wall of the gastric body. Note the associated mucosal nodularities (arrowheads) in the antrum. At histopathologic examination, both lesions had low-grade MALT lymphoma (not shown).

detailed histopathologic mapping of the whole resected specimen was not performed, the pathologist tried to evaluate the histopathologic features of all visible lesions. We then correlated the findings of double-contrast upper GI examinations with those of pathologic examinations, and we reviewed the clinical indications for endoscopy and the clinical staging of the disease.

RESULTS

Clinical Findings

The clinical indications for endoscopy in 25 patients included abdominal discomfort in 16 (64%), dyspepsia in four (16%), abdominal pain in three (12%), and GI bleeding in two (8%) patients. Five patients (20%) had anemia at laboratory examination.

On the basis of records of clinical, surgical, and histopathologic examinations, the Ann Arbor staging scheme was applied in all 25 patients. Of these, 23 patients had stage IE, and two had stage IIE.

Of 25 patients, five underwent administration of antibiotics for eradication of *H pylori*. Complete remission was defined as resolution of clinical evidence of disease and of endoscopic lesions, with negative biopsy specimen findings and absence of extragastric localization. Partial remission was defined as improvement of clinical symptoms and endoscopic lesions with a decrease in tumoral infiltration. Complete remission was attained in one patient, and partial remission was attained in four. Three of four patients with partial remission underwent surgical resection, and the remaining one underwent chemotherapy. Seventeen pa-

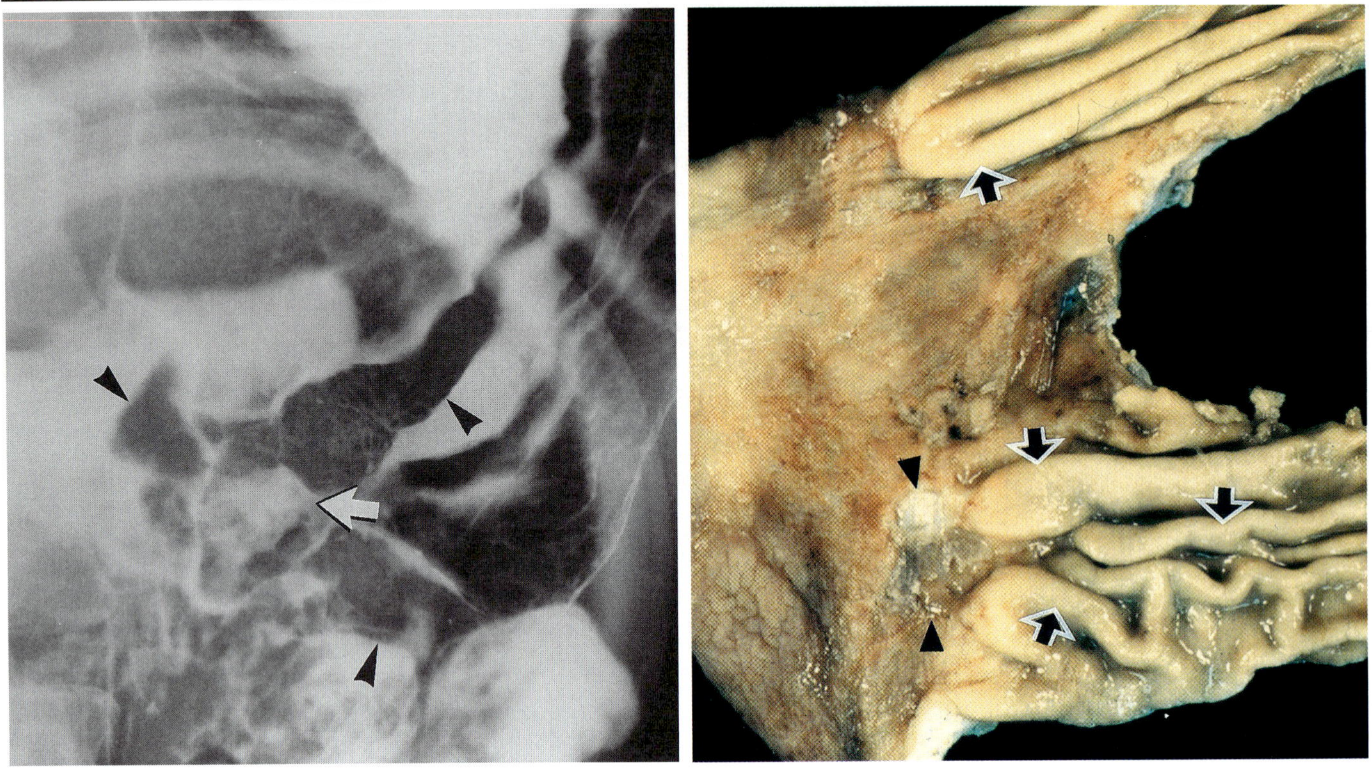

a. b.

Figure 3. Low-grade gastric MALT lymphoma with rugal thickening in a 34-year-old woman. **(a)** Compression spot radiograph of the gastric body shows marked rugal thickening (arrowheads). A large deep ulcer (arrow) is associated. **(b)** Photograph of the resected specimen shows thickened rugae (arrows) that converge to a deep ulcer (arrowheads) in the gastric body. At histopathologic examination, low-grade MALT lymphoma was found in both the thickened rugae and the ulcer.

tients underwent curative surgical resection without preoperative medical therapy. Three patients were lost to follow-up after endoscopy and upper GI examination. Two patients received adjunctive radiation therapy, and one patient received adjunctive chemotherapy owing to the involvement of regional lymph nodes (n = 2) and resection margins (n = 1).

There were no surgical deaths in the current study, but two patients had early perioperative complications: leakage from gastrojejunostomy site (n = 1) and wound infection (n = 1). During follow-up, one patient experienced postoperative adhesive ileus, which was resolved with conservative treatment. The remaining 17 patients had no peri- or postoperative complications. All 25 patients are alive with disease in complete remission after follow-up (range, 6–70 months; mean, 38.1 months).

Findings at Upper GI Examination

All 25 patients with low-grade MALT lymphoma showed abnormal findings at upper GI examination. Of these patients, nine had lesions in the antrum, seven had lesions in the body, seven had lesions in the antrum and body, one had lesions in the fundus, and the remaining one had lesions in the body and fundus. Thus, 16 patients (64%) had involvement of the gastric antrum.

The findings observed at upper GI examination are summarized in Table 1. Mucosal nodularity, found in 13 patients (52%), was the most common finding (Fig 1). These nodules were distinct in margin and round or oval in shape. The nodules were variable in size (less than 1 cm in greatest diameter) and were located in the antrum (n = 6), antrum and body (n = 5), fundus (n = 1), and nearly the whole stomach (n = 1). Thus, 12 patients (92%) had nodularity in the gastric antrum.

The next common finding, seen in 12 patients (48%), was ulcers (either shallow or deep) similar in appearance to gastric carcinoma (Fig 2). The ulcers were of varying size, were either shallow or deep, and were mostly indistinct in margin. Of 12 patients with ulcers, two had two ulcers, and nine had mucosal convergence around the ulcer. These ulcers were located in the antrum (n = 6) and body (n = 6). The other findings included rugal thickening (n = 6) (Fig 3), single or multiple mass formation (n = 4) (Fig 4), and diffusely enlarged areae gastricae (n = 2) (Fig 5). Fifteen patients (60%) had two or more findings.

After an analysis of the upper GI examinations, we tried to make the most probable diagnosis based on upper GI findings. The diagnosis of gastric carcinoma was made in 13 patients (52%) owing to ulcers, masses, and rugal convergence. Among 13 patients, seven had morphologic features similar to those of early gastric carcinoma (Fig 2), and the remaining six demonstrated findings mimicking advanced gastric carcinoma (Fig 3). In nine patients (36%), gastritis was diagnosed on the basis of nodularity, coarse areae gastricae, rugal thickening, and erosive lesions (Figs 1, 3, 5). In three patients (12%), malignant lymphoma was diagnosed on the basis of single or multiple polypoid lesions and rugal thickening (Fig 4).

Pathologic Findings and Radiographic-Pathologic Correlation

In the pathologic specimens of 15 patients, 17 discrete abnormalities were

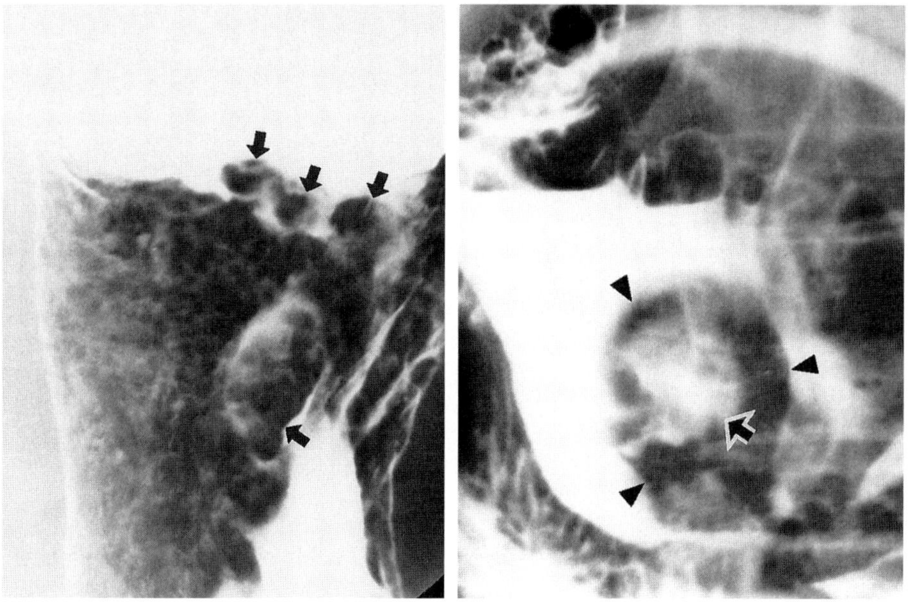

a. b.

Figure 4. Low-grade gastric MALT lymphoma with a mass. **(a)** Spot radiograph of upper GI examination shows multiple well-circumscribed masses (arrows) in the gastric body in a 40-year-old man. **(b)** Compression spot radiograph of the gastric antrum in an 80-year-old man shows a single well-demarcated mass (arrowheads) with a central ulcer (arrow).

found. Three patients had two discrete lesions. One patient had no definite focal abnormality on the specimen. Nine lesions involved the antrum, six involved the body, and two involved the gastric angle. The correlation of the pathologic and radiographic findings in 15 patients is summarized in Table 2.

On pathologic specimens, the morphologic features of these lesions resembled the morphologic features of gastric carcinomas. Nine lesions (60%) had shallow ulcers with convergent rugae (Fig 2). Shallow ulcers with surrounding or internal nodularity were demonstrated in three lesions. Three lesions demonstrated focal masses that mimicked elevated early gastric carcinoma. Two lesions had deep ulcers with convergent rugae and mimicked advanced gastric carcinoma (Fig 3). Of all 17 lesions, 14 abnormalities in 12 patients were shallow or deep ulcers with convergent rugae. Seven lesions had vague ulcer margins, and four of these had disorganized convergent rugae that projected to multiple points (Fig 2). Multiple ulcers were seen in two patients.

At histopathologic examination, all lesions invaded only the submucosal layer. One patient with no definite focal abnormality at pathologic examination demonstrated disseminated tumor cell infiltration along the mucosa and submucosa from antrum to fundus. Regional lymph node dissection was performed in all patients who underwent surgical resection. Two of 20 patients had involvement of regional lymph nodes. The resection margin was involved by tumor cells in two patients. All ulcers and focal masses demonstrated at double-contrast upper GI examinations and in pathologic specimens had tumor cells.

Mucosal nodularity, enlarged areae gastricae, and thickened rugae had involvement of MALT lymphoma in some areas and *H pylori* gastritis in other areas. It was almost impossible to distinguish MALT lymphoma from *H pylori* gastritis in each of these lesions demonstrated at double-contrast upper GI examination. *H pylori* gastritis of varying degrees coexisted with low-grade MALT lymphoma in all cases.

Of 17 lesions found at pathologic examination, only nine lesions in eight patients were detected at upper GI examination. Six shallow ulcers and two masses were not depicted at double-contrast upper GI examination. However, six shallow ulcers, two deep ulcers, and one focal mass seen at upper GI examination correlated well with the lesions seen in the resected specimens in terms of morphology.

DISCUSSION

MALT lymphoma is characterized as a distinctive type of lymphoma that manifests as localized disease and, in general, has a favorable prognosis (21). The characteristic histologic finding in MALT lymphoma is a diffuse cellular infiltrate of small centrocyte-like cells that may invade the epithelial lining of glands or crypts and form lymphoepithelial lesions (9,11). Although the stomach is the most common site of extranodal lymphoma, including MALT lymphoma, there is normally no lymphoid tissue in the gastric mucosa.

The paradox of lymphomas arising in the stomach has been explained by the observation of MALT in the stomach in response to infections by *H pylori* and by the presence of this organism in more than 90% of gastric MALT lymphomas (22–25). In some cases, low-grade MALT lymphomas have regressed with eradication of *H pylori* (26). In our study, 23 (92%) of 25 patients had histopathologic evidence of *H pylori* infection. This finding correlates well with findings of previous reports (24–26) and supports the suggestion that *H pylori* infection acts as a predisposing factor in the development of gastric MALT lymphoma.

In our study, the mean age of the patients was 32 years, and a female predominance of 16:9 was noted. These results did not match with the findings of previous reports (5,6,8,9,13,17,18,27,28) of MALT lymphoma or pseudolymphomas. In previous reports (5,6,8,9, 13,17,18, 27,28), the mean age was 50-60 years, and an equal sex ratio or slight male predominance was noted. Although it is difficult to explain the exact cause of the younger age of patients and of female predominance our study, the small number of patients included or selection bias may contribute to these differences. Another possible explanation for the younger age would be in practice pattern. In our country, gastric carcinoma is a common malignancy, and gastroscopy is a routine procedure in patients with GI symptoms. Widespread and early use of endoscopy, even in young patients, may enable early diagnosis.

Low-grade MALT lymphoma manifests at an early stage and has a good prognosis (9,27–29). All 25 patients had Ann Arbor stage IE (n = 23) or IIE (n = 2) and remained alive during a mean follow-up of 38.1 months in our study. The stage of primary gastric lymphoma was one of the most important prognostic factors. Other prognostic factors are tumor location, tumor size, depth of invasion, grade of tumor, and involvement of regional lymph nodes (29–33). Manifestation at an early stage, the superficial nature of

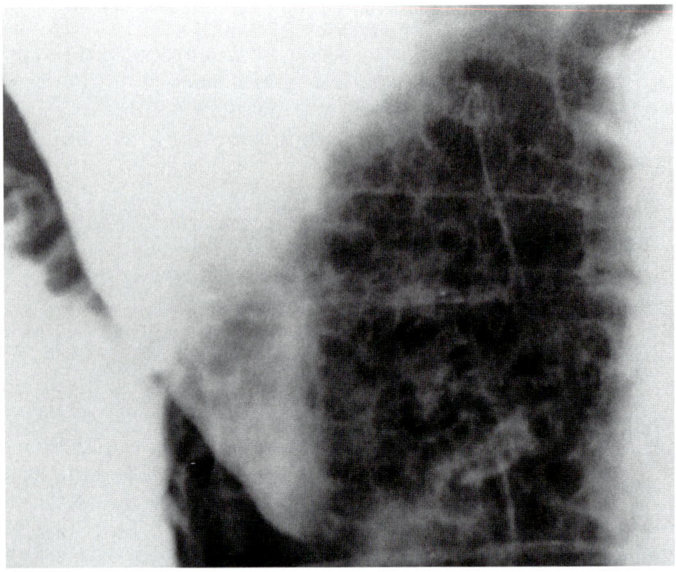

a.

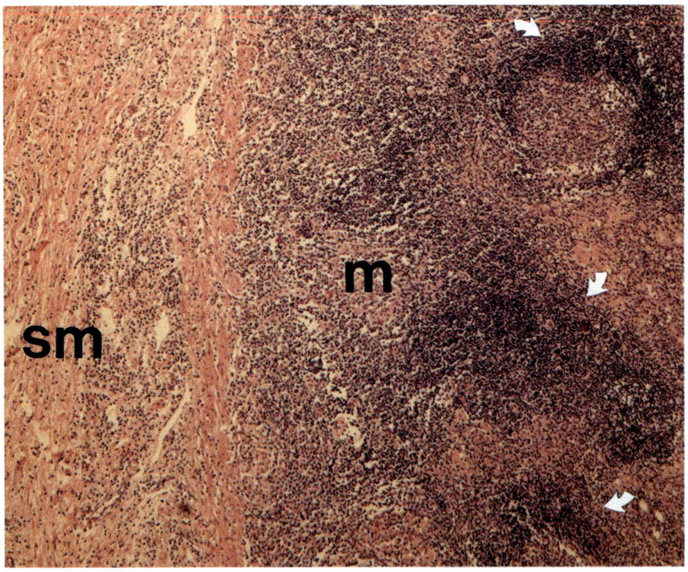

b.

Figure 5. Low-grade gastric MALT lymphoma with enlarged areae gastricae in a 75-year-old man. **(a)** Compression spot radiograph of the gastric body and antrum shows diffuse enlargement of the areae gastricae with a coarse pattern. **(b)** Photomicrograph (hematoxylin-eosin stain; original magnification, ×100) of the resected specimen shows tumor cells (arrows) in the mucosal layer. The tumor cells are diffusely distributed throughout the gastric body and antrum. On the pathologic specimen, no focal lesion was found (not shown). *m* = mucosa, *sm* = submucosa.

the lesions (confined to submucosa), and the infrequent involvement of regional lymph nodes indicate a good prognosis for the patients in our study.

The strategy for treatment of low-grade MALT lymphoma remains somewhat controversial. Some investigators (29,32,33) reported that adequate staging and long-term survival were attained with radical gastrectomy, with or without adjuvant treatment, in patients with low-grade MALT lymphoma. However, other nonsurgical treatments, such as chemotherapy or eradication of *H pylori*, also were recommended (26,34). In the patients in our study, radical gastrectomy, with or without adjuvant therapy, was performed in 20 patients. All these patients have been alive with disease in complete remission until now. Although direct comparison would be difficult because of the small number of patients who underwent nonsurgical treatment, surgical resection can be an appropriate treatment of low-grade MALT lymphoma, especially in the case of failure of antibiotics or in institutes that have skilled surgeons. The effects of nonsurgical treatment, especially eradication of *H pylori*, should be evaluated in further studies.

Gastric lymphomas are demonstrated on barium studies by a spectrum of findings, including thickened rugae, submucosal masses, centrally ulcerated (bull's-eye or target) lesions, polypoid lesions, nodules, and ulcers. There have been some reports in which radiographic findings of gastric MALT lymphomas have been described in the Japanese-language (17,18) and English-language literature (19,20). According to one Japanese report (18) in which 20 patients with low-grade gastric MALT lymphoma were analyzed, the largest group of patients with this disease, to our knowledge, friable mucosa and shallow ulcers mimicking early gastric carcinoma were frequent findings at upper GI examination. At endoscopy, the lesions affected the body and the antrum and consisted of an irregular and large ulcer with raised edges and erosions, small nodules, and localized or diffuse rugal thickening (28). Our study results are similar to those of the study by Suekane et al (18).

Perez and Dorfman (14) reported radiologic findings of pseudolymphoma, including tumor mass with ulceration, infiltrating constrictive lesions associated with ulceration, solitary well-defined ulcer craters, and enlarged gastric rugae. Other authors (15,16) described radiographic and pathologic findings of pseudolymphoma. They described radiologic findings such as ulcerating masses, submucosal masses, enlarged gastric rugae, and benign-appearing ulcers. At pathologic examination, ulcers were shown in all cases, and about half demonstrated multiple lesions. Considering that the majority of pseudolymphomas originated from MALT, our findings of low-grade MALT lymphoma are comparable to those of pseudolymphoma. However, multiple lesions were less frequent in our study (20%) than were pseudolymphomas.

TABLE 2
Correlation of Radiographic and Pathologic Findings in 15 Patients

Morphologic Features	Number of Lesions Detected at Upper GI Examination (*n* = 9)	Number of Lesions Detected at Pathologic Examination (*n* = 17)
Shallow ulcer	4	9
Shallow ulcer with nodularity	2	3
Mass	1	3
Deep ulcer	2	2

Early gastric lymphoma was defined as lymphoma invasion limited to the mucosa or the submucosa of the stomach wall, regardless of the presence of lymph node metastases (35). These tumors usually manifested as localized smooth enlargement of the rugae, poorly defined shallow ulcers, or well-defined deep ulcers. The ulcers usually were associated with mucosal convergence, enlargement of the rugae, and smooth marginal elevation. Multiple lesions were noted in 40%–50% of cases (30,35). Kitamura et al (30) reported that five of 10 early gastric lymphomas had pathologic features of MALT lymphoma.

In our study, the depth of invasion of all tumors was limited to the submucosa, and only two patients had regional lymph node metastases. On the basis of depth of invasion, the MALT lymphomas in our study can be classified as early gastric lymphoma. The findings obtained from our analysis of the upper GI examinations and pathologic examinations are similar to those of early gastric lymphoma, which frequently exhibits enlarged rugae, either shallow or deep ulcers, and multiplicity of lesions.

In our study, low-grade MALT lymphomas were confused with gastric carcinoma (especially early gastric carcinoma), gastritis, and lymphoma at double-contrast upper GI examination and pathologic examination. Compared with the findings of previous reports of MALT lymphoma (28), pseudolymphoma (14–16), and early gastric lymphoma (35), our results are not surprising. Chiles and Platz (15) reported that pseudolymphomas and early gastric lymphomas were usually diagnosed as gastric carcinomas or benign ulcers. Differentiation from gastric carcinoma was the most frequent diagnostic problem (30,35). Carcinoma that originates in the mucosa produces mucosal destruction and desmoplastic changes in the submucosa. In gastric carcinoma of the ulcerative type, these pathologic changes usually manifest as well-defined, irregular, shallow ulcers with abrupt disruption of the normal mucosa and often manifest as a striking convergence of the rugae. In contrast, early lymphoma that arises from the lymphatic tissue in the deeper layer mainly produces submucosal tumor growth, and desmoplastic reaction is rare. Therefore, smooth enlarged rugae with slight convergence indicating the submucosal nature of early lymphoma and poorly defined ulceration indicating poor desmoplastic reaction were findings suggestive of early lymphoma (35).

Kitamura et al (30) reported a higher prevalence of multifocal lesions in early gastric lymphoma than in gastric carcinoma. In our study, four (29%) of 14 ulcers had disorganized convergent rugae projecting to multiple points, and seven (50%) had vague ulcer margins. Two patients (14%) had multiple ulcers. Our results and the findings of previous reports (30,35) suggest that disorganized convergent rugae, vague ulcer margins, and multiple lesions may be useful in differentiating low-grade gastric MALT lymphoma from gastric carcinoma, especially the ulcerative type.

In some reports (36–38), *H pylori* gastritis manifested as thickened, nodular rugae in the gastric antrum and enlarged areae gastricae. Mucosal nodularity was the most frequent finding at upper GI examination in our study, so low-grade MALT lymphoma can mimic *H pylori* gastritis. Although all low-grade gastric MALT lymphomas did not have ulcers, the presence of ulcers may play a useful role in the differentiation of the two diseases. However, low-grade gastric MALT lymphoma manifesting as nodularity or thickened rugae alone is difficult to differentiate from *H pylori* gastritis on the basis of findings at upper GI examination.

Although we could not perform detailed histopathologic mapping of the entire gastrectomy specimen, all abnormal areas demonstrated at upper GI examination had involvement of MALT lymphoma with a background of diffuse gastritis. Hoshida et al (29) reported that multiple superficial spreading (slightly elevated lesions or thickened rugae), restricted invasion within the submucosa, and manifestation at an early stage were characteristic features of low-grade MALT lymphoma. In other reports (9,30) of MALT lymphoma and early gastric lymphoma, superficial spreading lesions were noted as frequent findings. Considering the superficial spreading nature of low-grade MALT lymphoma, the mucosal nodularity, enlarged areae gastricae, and thickened rugae seen at upper GI examination in our study could be represented by infiltration of MALT lymphoma.

When upper GI examination findings were correlated with pathologic examination findings, six shallow ulcers and two focal elevated lesions were missed at upper GI examination. Of the missed shallow ulcers, four were interpreted as normal, and two were interpreted as mucosal nodularity. Two cases of missed focal elevated lesions were interpreted as rugal thickening and mucosal nodularity. The inadequate upper GI examination, shallow nature of the lesions, and nonspecific findings, such as mucosal nodularity and rugal thickening that are commonly seen in *H pylori* gastritis, may contribute to the low detection rate of main lesions at upper GI examination.

In conclusion, low-grade gastric MALT lymphomas manifested as mucosal nodularity, either shallow or deep ulcers, and rugal thickening at upper GI examination and showed similar findings to those of gastric carcinoma and *H pylori* gastritis. Disorganized convergent rugae, vague ulcer margins, and multiple lesions may be helpful in differentiating low-grade gastric MALT lymphomas from gastric carcinomas.

References

1. Freemen C, Berg JW, Cutler SJ. Occurrence and prognosis of extranodal lymphomas. Cancer 1972; 29:252–260.
2. Aozasa K, Tsujimoto M, Inoue A, et al. Primary gastrointestinal lymphoma. Oncology 1985; 42:97–103.
3. Grody WW, Magidson JG, Weiss LM, Hu E, Warnke RA, Lewin KJ. Gastrointestinal lymphomas: immunohistochemical studies on the cell of origin. Am J Surg Pathol 1985; 9:328–337.
4. Jacobs DS. Primary gastric malignant lymphoma and pseudolymphoma. Am J Clin Pathol 1963; 40:379–394.
5. Tokunaga O, Watanabe T, Morimatsu M. Pseudolymphoma of the stomach: a clinicopathologic study of 15 cases. Cancer 1987; 59:1320–1327.
6. Eimoto T, Futami K, Naito H, Takeshita M, Kikuchi M. Gastric pseudolymphoma with monotypic cytoplasmic immuno-globulin. Cancer 1985; 55:788–793.
7. Spencer J, Diss T, Isaacson PG. Primary B cell gastric lymphoma: a genotypic analysis. Am J Pathol 1989; 135:557–564.
8. Moore I, Wright DH. Primary gastric lymphoma: a tumor of mucosa-associated lymphoid tissue—a histological and immunohistochemical study of 36 cases. Histopathology 1984; 8:1025–1039.
9. Isaacson PG, Spencer J, Finn T. Primary B-cell gastric lymphoma. Hum Pathol 1986; 17:72–82.
10. Abbondanzo SL, Sobin LH. Gastric pseudolymphoma: a retrospective morphologic and immunophenotypic study of 97 cases. Cancer 1997; 79:1656–1663.
11. Isaacson PG, Wright DH. Extranodal malignant lymphoma arising form mucosa-associated lymphoid tissue. Cancer 1984; 53:2515–2524.
12. Isaacson PG, Spencer J. Malignant lymphoma of mucosa-associated lymphoid tissue. Histopathology 1987; 11:445–462.
13. Chan JK, Ng CS, Isaacson PG. Relationship between high-grade lymphoma and low-grade B-cell mucosa-associated lymphoid tissue lymphoma (MALToma) of the stomach. Am J Pathol 1990; 136:1153–1164.
14. Perez CA, Dorfman RF. Benign lymphoid hyperplasia of the stomach and duodenum. Radiology 1966; 87:505–510.
15. Chiles JT, Platz CE. The radiographic manifestations of pseudolymphoma of the stomach. Radiology 1975; 116:551–556.
16. Martel W, Abell MR, Allan TNK. Lymphoreticular hyperplasia of the stomach (pseudolymphoma). AJR 1976; 127:261–265.
17. Baba Y. Image diagnosis of gastric malignant lymphoma and its mimicking lesions-focused on the low-grade malignant lymphoma (MALT lymphoma). Stomach Intestine 1996; 31:41–58. [Japanese]
18. Suekane H, Iida M, Nakamura S, et al. Differential diagnosis between so-called reactive lymphoid hyperplasia (RLH) and mucosa-associated lymphoid tissue (MALT) lymphomas in the stomach: studies on radiographic, endoscopic, and endosonographic findings. Stomach Intestine 1996; 31:59–73. [Japanese]
19. Levine MS, Elmas N, Furth EE, Rubesin SE, Goldwein MI. *Helicobacter pylori* and gastric MALT lymphoma. AJR 1996; 166: 85–86.

20. Yoo CC, Levine MS, Furth EE, et al. Gastric mucosa-associated lymphoid tissue lymphoma: radiologic findings in six patients. Radiology 1998; 208:239–243.
21. Harris NL. Low-grade B-cell lymphoma of mucosa-associated lymphoid tissue and monocytoid B-cell lymphoma: related entities that are distinct from other low-grade B-cell lymphomas (editorial). Arch Pathol Lab Med 1993; 117:771–775.
22. Wyatt JI, Rathbone BJ. Immune response of the gastric mucosa to *Campylobacter pylori*. Scand J Gastroenterol 1988; 142(suppl): 44–49.
23. Stolte M, Eidt S. Lymphoid follicles in the antral mucosa: immune response to *Campylobacter pylori*. J Clin Pathol 1989; 42: 1269–1271.
24. Wotherspoon AC, Ortiz-Hidalgo C, Falzon MR, Isaacson PG. *Helicobacter pylori*-associated gastritis and primary B-cell gastric lymphoma. Lancet 1991; 338:1175–1176.
25. Stolte M. *Helicobacter pylori* and gastric MALT-lymphoma. Lancet 1992; 339:745–746.
26. Wotherspoon AC, Doglioni C, Diss TC, et al. Regression of primary low-grade B-cell gastric lymphoma of mucosa-associated lymphoid tissue after eradication of *Helicobacter pylori*. Lancet 1993; 342:575–577.
27. Castrillo JM, Montalban C, Obeso G, Piris MA, Rivas MC. Gastric B-cell mucosa associated lymphoid tissue lymphoma: a clinicopathological study in 56 patients. Gut 1992; 33:1307–1311.
28. Blazquez M, Haioun C, Chaumette MT, et al. Low grade B cell mucosa associated lymphoid tissue lymphoma of the stomach: clinical and endoscopic features, treatment, and outcome. Gut 1992; 33: 1621–1625.
29. Hoshida Y, Kusakabe H, Furukawa H, et al. Reassessment of gastric lymphoma in light of the concept of mucosa-associated lymphoid tissue lymphoma. Cancer 1997; 80: 1151–1159.
30. Kitamura K, Yamaguchi T, Okamoto K, et al. Early gastric lymphoma: a clinicopathologic study of ten patients, literature review, and comparison with early gastric adenocarcinoma. Cancer 1996; 77:850–857.
31. Azab MB, Henry-Amar M, Rougier P, et al. Prognostic factors in primary gastrointestinal non-Hodgkin's lymphoma. Cancer 1989; 64:1208–1217.
32. Papachristodoulou A, Misiakos E, Kouraklis G, Androulaki A, Gogas J. Surgical treatment of gastrointestinal B-cell mucosa-associated lymphoid tissue lymphomas. South Med J 1997; 90:723–728.
33. Kodera Y, Yamamura Y, Nakamura S, et al. The role of radical gastrectomy with systematic lymphadenectomy for the diagnosis and treatment of primary gastric lymphoma. Ann Surg 1998; 227:45–50.
34. Hammel P, Haioun C, Chaumette MT, et al. Efficacy of single-agent chemotherapy in low-grade B-cell mucosa-associated lymphoid tissue lymphoma with prominent gastric expression. J Clin Oncol 1995; 13:2524–2529.
35. Sato T, Sakai Y, Ishiguro S, Furukawa H. Radiologic manifestations of early gastric lymphoma. AJR 1986; 146:513–517.
36. Morrison S, Dahms BB, Hoffenberg E, Czinn SJ. Enlarged gastric folds in association with *Campylobacter pylori* gastritis. Radiology 1989; 171:819–821.
37. Sohn J, Levine MS, Furth EE, et al. *Helicobacter pylori* gastritis: radiographic findings. Radiology 1995; 195:763–767.
38. Levine MS, Rubesin SE. The *Helicobacter pylori* revolution: radiologic perspective. Radiology 1995; 195:593–596.

MR Cholangiography in the Evaluation of Neonatal Cholestasis[1]

Twei-Shiun Jaw, MD
Yu-Ting Kuo, MD
Gin-Chung Liu, MD
Shaou-Hsium Chen, MD
Chien-Kuo Wang, MD

Index terms:
Bile ducts, abnormalities, 768.1434
Bile ducts, MR, 768.121411, 768.121413, 768.121415, 768.121416
Bile ducts, radionuclide studies, 768.12172
Gallbladder, 762.1434
Infants, 762.1434

Radiology 1999; 212:249–256

Abbreviations:
IR = inversion recovery
MIP = maximum intensity projection
SE = spin echo
2D = two-dimensional
3D = three-dimensional

[1] From the Departments of Radiology (T.S.J., Y.T.K., G.C.L., C.K.W.) and Pediatric Surgery (S.H.C.), Kaohsiung Medical College, 100 Shih-Chuan First Rd, Kaohsiung 807, Taiwan, Republic of China. From the 1997 RSNA scientific assembly. Received April 29, 1998; revision requested June 16; final revision received December 15; accepted January 19, 1999. **Address reprint requests to** T.S.J. (e-mail: *m810101@cc.kmc.edu.tw*).

PURPOSE: To evaluate the usefulness of magnetic resonance (MR) cholangiography in excluding biliary atresia as the cause of neonatal cholestasis.

MATERIALS AND METHODS: MR cholangiography was performed on 10 control and 16 jaundiced neonates and infants aged 3 days to 5 months. Diagnosis of biliary atresia (n = 6) was confirmed with surgery and liver biopsy, with or without surgical cholangiography. Diagnosis of neonatal hepatitis (n = 9) was confirmed with clinical follow-up until jaundice resolved. In one infant, paucity of intrahepatic ducts was diagnosed at liver biopsy. MR cholangiography was performed with respiratory-triggered, heavily T2-weighted turbo spin-echo and optional inversion-recovery turbo spin-echo sequences. Diagnosis of biliary atresia was based on nonvisualization of either the common bile duct or common hepatic duct. Cholescintigraphy with technetium 99m disofenin was performed in all 16 jaundiced patients.

RESULTS: In the 10 controls, the nine patients with neonatal hepatitis, and the one infant with paucity of intrahepatic ducts, MR cholangiography clearly depicted the gallbladder and common hepatic and common bile ducts. MR cholangiography was 100% accurate in excluding biliary atresia as the cause of neonatal cholestasis, while ^{99m}Tc disofenin cholescintigraphic findings were false-positive in four of 10 patients with nonobstructive cholestasis.

CONCLUSION: MR cholangiography can be used to depict the major biliary structures of neonates and small infants and to exclude biliary atresia as the cause of neonatal cholestasis by allowing visualization of the biliary tract.

Prompt and accurate differentiation of biliary atresia from other causes of neonatal cholestasis is of great clinical importance because patients with biliary atresia must undergo surgery as soon as possible to have a better surgical outcome (1,2). Until now, cholescintigraphy has been thought to be the most sensitive modality (97%–100%) to distinguish biliary atresia from other causes of neonatal cholestasis, but the specificity of cholescintigraphy varies from 67% to 93%, depending on the technetium 99m–labeled radiopharmaceutical agent used (3–6). Recently, magnetic resonance (MR) cholangiography has been used to demonstrate the normal biliary tree in neonates and infants (7,8). We speculate that MR cholangiography may replace diagnostic laparotomy and surgical cholangiography in jaundiced neonates in whom no bowel excretion is seen on cholescintigrams. The purpose of this study was to evaluate the usefulness of MR cholangiography in excluding biliary atresia as the cause of neonatal cholestasis.

MATERIALS AND METHODS

Patients

Using MR cholangiography, we prospectively evaluated the bile duct anatomy of 26 neonates and infants, aged 3 days to 5 months. Ten neonates and infants were nonjaundiced control subjects who were undergoing MR imaging of the brain, and 16 neonates and infants had jaundice. The study protocols had been approved by our institutional review boards. Informed consent to perform MR cholangiography was obtained from the parents.

The control group included seven male and three female neonates and infants, aged 3

Author contributions:
Guarantor of integrity of entire study, T.S.J.; study concepts, T.S.J.; study design, T.S.J., Y.T.K.; definition of intellectual content, T.S.J.; literature research, T.S.J., Y.T.K.; clinical studies, T.S.J., S.H.C.; data acquisition, T.S.J., Y.T.K.; data analysis, T.S.J., Y.T.K., C.K.W., G.C.L.; statistical analysis, T.S.J.; manuscript preparation, T.S.J.; manuscript editing, T.S.J., G.C.L.; manuscript review, G.C.L.

Clinical Data, Imaging Findings, and Final Diagnoses in 16 Patients with Neonatal Cholestasis

Patient No./Age (d)/Sex	Serum Bilirubin Level (mg/dL)		GGT Level (U/L)	Scintigraphic Findings*		MR Cholangiographic Findings*				Proof	Final Diagnosis
	Total	Direct		GB	Bowel	GB Length (cm)	CBD	CHD	IHD		
1/32/M	5.7	4.8	129	−	−	0.9	−	−	−	Laparotomy, Kasai operation, biopsy	Biliary atresia (type A)
2/47/F	6.6	5.3	955	−	−	0.8	−	−	−	Laparotomy, Kasai operation, biopsy, died (6 mo)	Biliary atresia (type A)
3/57/F	9.5	5.6	282	−	−	2.1	−	−	±	Laparotomy, Kasai operation, biopsy	Biliary atresia (type A)
4/41/M	7.1	5.2	196	−	−	1.0	−	−	−	Laparotomy, Kasai operation, OPC, biopsy	Biliary atresia (type B)
5/57/M	6.9	5.2	665	−	−	1.4	−	−	−	Laparotomy, Kasai operation, OPC, biopsy	Biliary atresia (type B)
6/23/M	6.8	4.5	532	−	−	1.2	−	Cystic	±	Laparotomy, choledochojejunostomy (29 d), OPC, Kasai operation (40 d), biopsy	Biliary atresia (type C)
7/32/F	11.3	9.9	78	−	−	2.9	+	+	−	Biopsy Died at 3½ mo	Paucity of IHD
8/49/M	6.7	5.1	129	1 h	4 h	1.4	+	+	+	Jaundice-free by 3 mo	Neonatal hepatitis
9/65/M	4.5	3.3	102	2 h	1 h	3.2	+	+	+	Jaundice-free by 2½ mo	Neonatal hepatitis
10/48/M	6.4	3.2	97	−	−	3.0	+	+	+	Jaundice-free by 4 mo	Neonatal hepatitis
11/64/F	9.0	6.1	50	−	5 h	2.4	+	+	+	Jaundice-free by 5 mo	Neonatal hepatitis
12/46/F	6.0	4.7	20	−	−	3.0	+	+	+	Jaundice-free by 3 mo	Neonatal hepatitis
13/15/M	12.2	9.2	174	−	4 h	2.8	+	+	+	Jaundice-free by 2 mo	Neonatal hepatitis
14/43/M	6.5	2.7	91	−	4 h	3.6	+	+	+	Jaundice-free by 3 mo	Neonatal hepatitis
15/62/M	9.3	6.8	158	−	−	2.2	+	+	+	Biopsy Jaundice-free by 6 mo	Neonatal hepatitis
16/48/M	4.5	2.5	30	1 h	1 h	4.5	+	+	+	Jaundice-free by 2½ mo	Neonatal hepatitis

Note.—CBD = common bile duct, CHD = common hepatic duct, GB = gallbladder, GGT = γ-glutamyltransferase, IHD = intrahepatic ducts, OPC = operative cholangiography.
* − = invisible, + = visible, ± = incompletely visible.

days to 5 months (mean age, 106 days). Sixteen consecutive neonates and infants who had neonatal cholestatic jaundice were included in this prospective study. They included 11 male and five female neonates and infants, aged 15–65 days (mean age, 46 days). Clinically, these patients had clay-colored stool and prolonged conjugated hyperbilirubinemia that occurred within the first 2 months of life (9). Prolonged conjugated hyperbilirubinemia was defined as a total serum bilirubin level of more than 3.0 mg/dL (51 µmol/L), with the direct form more than 40% of the total (normal values, 0.2–1.0 mg/dL [3.4–17 µmol/L] and 0–0.2 mg/dL [0–3.4 µmol/L], respectively). Most of the jaundiced patients also had an increased serum γ-glutamyltransferase level (normal values, 3–30 U/L) (Table).

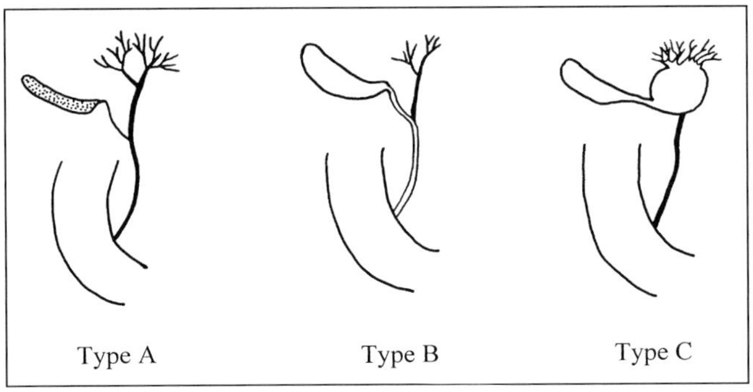

Figure 1. Drawing shows the three types of biliary atresia. Type A (n = 3) has complete fibrous obliteration of the entire extrahepatic bile duct. Type B (n = 2) shows a patent but extremely hypoplastic common bile duct with atretic hepatic ducts. Type C (n = 1) has a cystic dilatation of the common hepatic duct with an atretic common bile duct.

In the six patients with biliary atresia, the findings were confirmed at laparotomy; three underwent surgical cholangiography. Surgical cholangiography was not performed in the other three patients with biliary atresia because only fibrotic remnants of ducts were found at surgery. Of the six patients with biliary atresia, three had complete fibrous obliteration of the extrahepatic bile duct (type A), two had a patent but extremely thin common bile duct with atretic hepatic ducts (type B), and one had a cyst at the hilum of the liver with an atretic common bile duct (type C) (Fig 1) (Table) (10). All patients with biliary atresia underwent a Kasai operation (hepatoportoenterostomy).

Liver aspiration biopsy was performed in eight patients, including six patients with biliary atresia, one patient with neonatal hepatitis, and the one patient with paucity of intrahepatic ducts. Liver biopsy was not performed in the remaining eight patients with neonatal hepatitis; in six patients, liver biopsy was not performed because biliary atresia could be excluded by the presence of bowel activity on cholescintigrams, and for two patients, the parents refused biopsy.

The findings from liver biopsy revealed

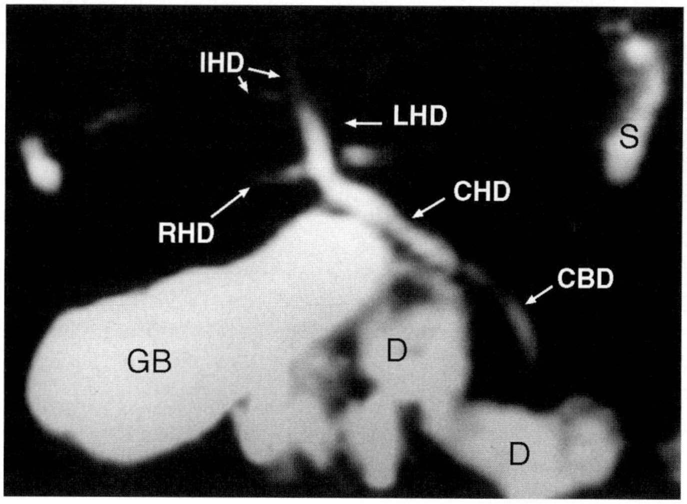

a.

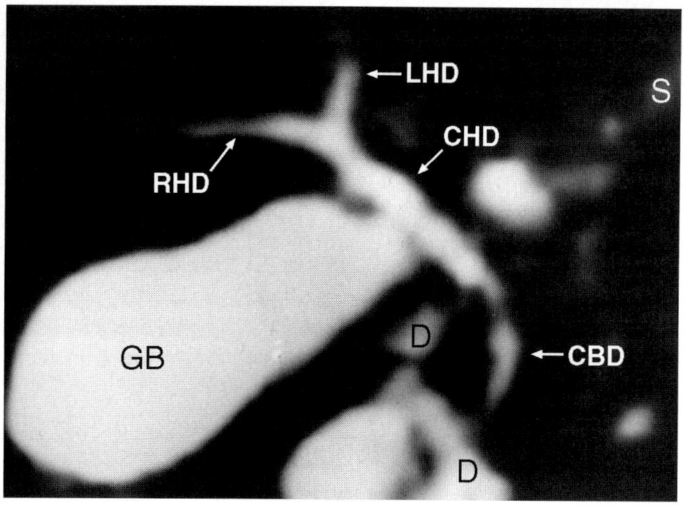

b.

Figure 2. MR cholangiograms in a 3-month-old nonjaundiced male infant. *S* = stomach, *D* = duodenum. **(a)** T2-weighted turbo SE image (3,000/700 [effective]) with 2D acquisition by using an MIP algorithm clearly depicts the gallbladder (*GB*), common bile duct (*CBD*), common hepatic duct (*CHD*), right and left hepatic ducts (*RHD, LHD*), and the second-order intrahepatic ducts (*IHD*). **(b)** T2-weighted IR turbo SE image (7,000/1,000 [effective]/50) with 3D acquisition by using an MIP algorithm shows the biliary structures up to the right and left hepatic ducts (*RHD, LHD*). The second-order intrahepatic duct is not visible. *CBD* = common bile duct, *CHD* = common hepatic duct, *GB* = gallbladder.

that four patients with biliary atresia showed typical histopathologic features, with bile duct proliferation, bile plugs, and periportal fibrosis. In the other two patients with biliary atresia, the findings from biopsy showed giant cell transformation and canalicular and cellular bile stasis, without definite bile duct proliferation or periportal fibrosis. In one patient with neonatal hepatitis, the findings from biopsy showed giant cell transformation, inflammatory cell infiltration, and lobular disorganization. The results of liver biopsy in the patient with paucity of intrahepatic ducts showed no interlobular bile duct in several portal areas.

In the nine patients with idiopathic neonatal hepatitis, the diagnosis was verified by the patient's recovery from jaundice and the normalization of laboratory values during the clinical follow-up period. The duration of follow-up was 3–12 months. In the patient with paucity of intrahepatic ducts, azotemia and imaging findings of infantile polycystic kidney disease were noted in addition to the cholestasis.

Imaging

All patients had fasted for at least 3 hours before the MR examination and were sedated with rectal administration of secobarbital (5–10 mg per kilogram of body weight) or with oral or rectal administration of chloral hydrate (50 mg/kg). MR examination was performed with a 1.5-T magnet (Gyroscan ACS-NT; Philips Medical Systems, Best, the Netherlands). A flexible surface coil (E1; rectangular and measuring 16 × 13.5 cm) was wrapped around the upper portion of the abdomen of the neonates and infants.

MR imaging sequences included a coronal T2-weighted, spectral presaturation with inversion recovery (IR), turbo spin-echo (SE) sequence (1,650/80 [repetition time msec/effective echo time msec]) with an echo train length of 14; an axial T2-weighted, turbo SE sequence (1,650/100 [effective]) with an echo train length of 18; and an axial T1-weighted turbo gradient-echo sequence (15/5; flip angle, 25°). MR cholangiography was performed with a two-dimensional (2D), non–breath-hold, respiratory-triggered, heavily T2-weighted, fat-suppressed, turbo SE sequence (3,000/700 [effective]) with an echo train length of 128. Coronal source images were obtained with a 2-mm section thickness and a 1-mm overlap. The number of signals acquired was six. We used a 195 × 256 matrix. In addition, a three-dimensional (3D) IR turbo SE sequence (7,000/1,000 [effective]/50 [repetition time msec/effective echo time msec/inversion time msec]) with an echo train length of 116 was also used in five control subjects, six neonates and infants with biliary atresia, and one infant with paucity of intrahepatic ducts. The number of signals acquired was two.

The 2D or 3D acquisition images were reformatted by using a standard maximum intensity projection (MIP) algorithm to create a rotating display. Imaging time for MR cholangiography varied from 6 minutes 11 seconds to 12 minutes 36 seconds. The total imaging time ranged from 20 to 30 minutes.

Cholescintigraphy with ^{99m}Tc disofenin was also performed with a gamma camera scanner (GCA 602A; Toshiba, Nasu, Japan) in all 16 patients within a week of MR examination. Phenobarbital (5 mg/kg/d) was given to each patient for at least 5 days before scintigraphic examination. The neonates and infants had fasted for 3 hours before the examination. Cholescintigraphy was performed with intravenous administration of ^{99m}Tc disofenin in a dose of 0.25 mCi/kg (9.25 MBq/kg). Sequential anterior scintigrams of the abdomen were obtained at 1, 5, 15, and 30 minutes after injection and at 1, 2, 4, and 6 hours. Delayed images were obtained at 24 hours if there was still no visualization of bowel activity by 6 hours (11). The hepatic uptake of radiotracer, the depiction of the gallbladder, and the presence of activity in the bowel were observed on the serial scans within 6 hours and on a 24-hour–delay scan.

Image Analysis

All MR images were interpreted independently by three radiologists (Y.T.K., C.K.W., G.C.L.) who were experienced in abdominal MR imaging and were blinded to the clinical history and the results of

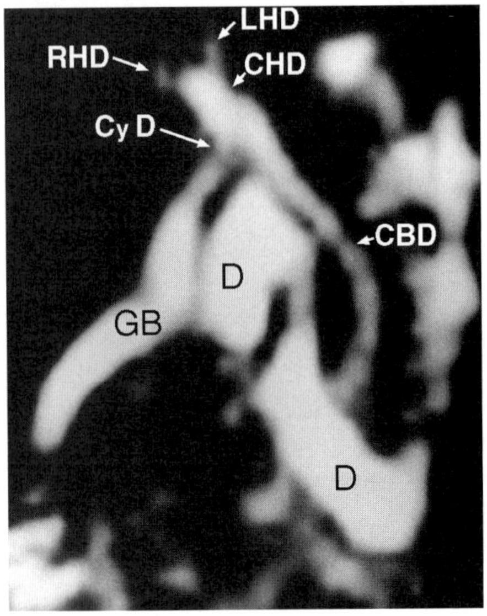

Figure 3. MR cholangiogram in a 3-day-old nonjaundiced male neonate. T2-weighted turbo SE image (3,000/700 [effective]) in steep oblique projection shows the gallbladder (*GB*), cystic duct (*CyD*), common bile duct (*CBD*), common hepatic duct (*CHD*), and right and left hepatic ducts (*RHD, LHD*), but the second-order intrahepatic ducts are not shown. *D* = duodenum.

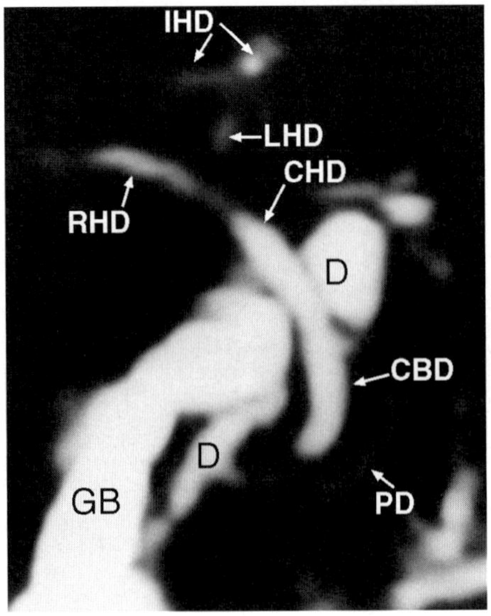

Figure 4. MR cholangiogram in a 46-day-old female infant with neonatal hepatitis. T2-weighted turbo SE image (3,000/700 [effective]) obtained from frontal projection shows clearly visible gallbladder (*GB*), common bile duct (*CBD*), common hepatic duct (*CHD*), and right and left hepatic ducts (*RHD, LHD*) and faintly visible second-order intrahepatic ducts (*IHD*). The pancreatic duct (*PD*) is also seen. *D* = duodenum.

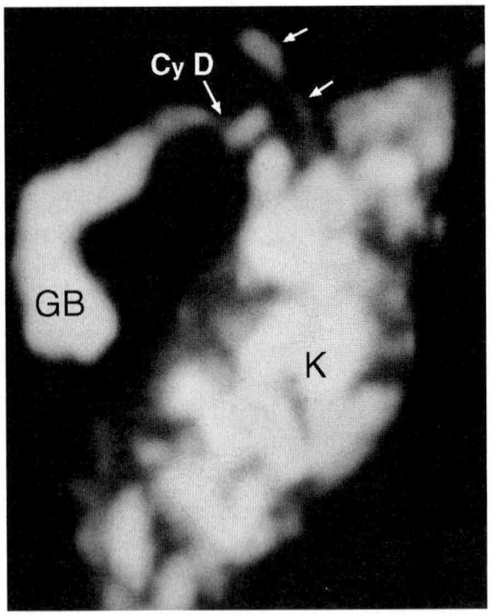

Figure 5. MR cholangiogram in a 32-day-old female infant with paucity of intrahepatic ducts and infantile polycystic kidney disease. T2-weighted turbo SE image (3,000/700 [effective]) obtained with steep oblique coronal projection depicts the gallbladder (*GB*), cystic duct (*Cy D*), and extrahepatic bile duct (arrows). Also seen is the enlarged right kidney (*K*) with small hyperintense cystic lesions.

other tests of the patients. The conspicuity or visibility of the common bile duct, common hepatic duct, gallbladder, cystic duct, and intrahepatic ducts was evaluated on the basis of the source and MIP-reformatted images. Discrepancies among observers were resolved by consensus.

For the patients with neonatal cholestasis, biliary atresia was excluded if there was visualization of a normal extrahepatic biliary system at MR cholangiography. In the patients with biliary atresia, MR findings were correlated with those found at surgery. The studies of the 10 control patients, who underwent MR imaging only, were interpreted in the same manner as those for the 16 jaundiced patients. The cholescintigraphic studies were interpreted in the same fashion as the MR images. The interpretation of the MR images and cholescintigraphic studies was separated by 1–2 weeks to prevent recall of the findings, and the patient order in which those two types of studies were interpreted was different.

Statistical Analysis

The McNemar exact test was used to compare the visibility of intrahepatic ducts between 2D turbo SE and 3D IR turbo SE images in five control pairs. The Student *t* test was used to evaluate the statistically significant difference in the mean gallbladder size between patients with neonatal hepatitis and those with biliary atresia. The Fisher exact test was used to test the significance of a small gallbladder on the MR cholangiogram in the differentiation of biliary atresia from other causes of neonatal cholestasis. A P value of less than .05 was considered to indicate a statistically significant difference.

RESULTS

The gallbladder, common bile duct, common hepatic duct, and right and left hepatic ducts were visible in all 10 nonjaundiced neonates and infants, while the cystic duct was visible in six of the 10 nonjaundiced control subjects. The second-order intrahepatic ducts were visualized in only five control subjects (50%). The caliber of the common bile duct ranged from 2.0 to 3.5 mm (mean ± SD, 2.6 mm ± 0.5). The gallbladder was 2.2–4.6 cm in length (mean ± SD, 3.3 cm ± 0.9). In addition to 2D turbo SE images, 3D IR turbo SE images were also obtained in five of the 10 control neonates and infants. The 2D turbo SE images tended to depict more secondary branches of the intrahepatic ducts than did the 3D IR turbo SE images in these five control subjects, although the difference was not statistically significant (three of five vs one of five; McNemar exact test, P = .5) (Fig 2). An example of duct visibility in a 3-day-old control neonate is illustrated in Figure 3.

The Table lists the clinical data, various imaging findings, and the final diagnoses in the 16 patients with neonatal cholestasis. In the nine patients with neonatal hepatitis, the gallbladder, common bile duct, common hepatic duct, and right and left hepatic ducts were clearly depicted at MR cholangiography (Fig 4). The cystic duct was visible in five of the nine patients with neonatal hepatitis. In the infant with paucity of intrahepatic ducts, cholescintigraphy with ^{99m}Tc disofenin did not allow visualization of the gallbladder or of bowel activity, with retention of tracer in the liver up to 24 hours. However, MR cholangiography depicted the gallbladder, cystic duct, common bile duct, and common hepatic duct, and the hepatic ducts were faintly visible (Fig 5). The 3D IR turbo SE images were slightly inferior to the 2D turbo SE images in the depiction of the hepatic ducts in this patient.

In the six patients with surgically confirmed biliary atresia, no MR cholangio-

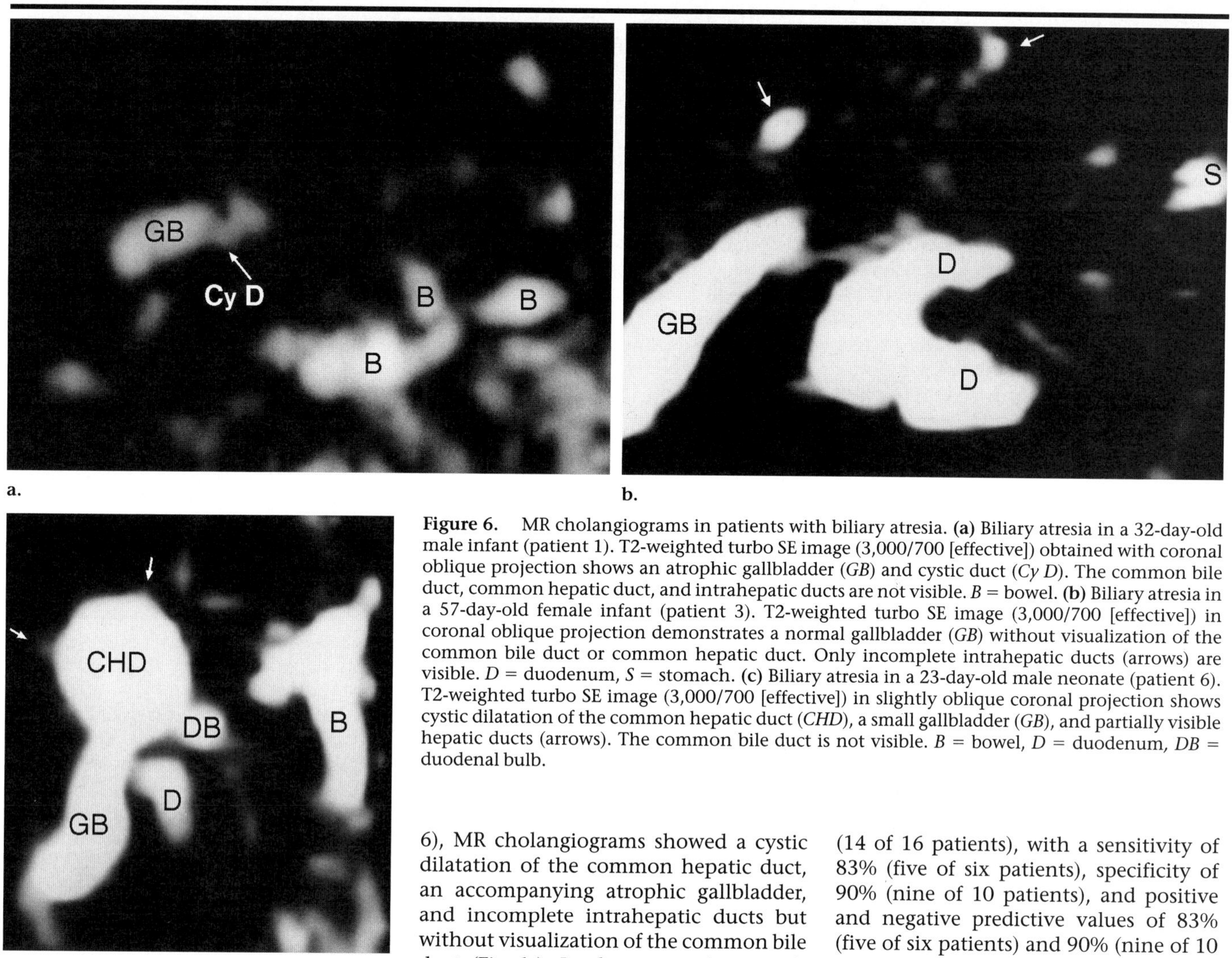

a. b. c.

Figure 6. MR cholangiograms in patients with biliary atresia. **(a)** Biliary atresia in a 32-day-old male infant (patient 1). T2-weighted turbo SE image (3,000/700 [effective]) obtained with coronal oblique projection shows an atrophic gallbladder (*GB*) and cystic duct (*Cy D*). The common bile duct, common hepatic duct, and intrahepatic ducts are not visible. *B* = bowel. **(b)** Biliary atresia in a 57-day-old female infant (patient 3). T2-weighted turbo SE image (3,000/700 [effective]) in coronal oblique projection demonstrates a normal gallbladder (*GB*) without visualization of the common bile duct or common hepatic duct. Only incomplete intrahepatic ducts (arrows) are visible. *D* = duodenum, *S* = stomach. **(c)** Biliary atresia in a 23-day-old male neonate (patient 6). T2-weighted turbo SE image (3,000/700 [effective]) in slightly oblique coronal projection shows cystic dilatation of the common hepatic duct (*CHD*), a small gallbladder (*GB*), and partially visible hepatic ducts (arrows). The common bile duct is not visible. *B* = bowel, *D* = duodenum, *DB* = duodenal bulb.

gram showed a visible common bile duct (Fig 6). The common hepatic duct was not depicted in five of these six patients and was cystic in another patient. The intrahepatic ducts were not visible at all in four of the six patients with biliary atresia and were only partially visible in two patients. All of the six patients but one had a small gallbladder, which was defined as less than 1.5 cm in length (12). The cystic duct was depicted in four of the six patients with biliary atresia. No obvious difference in duct conspicuity could be noted between the 2D turbo SE images and the 3D IR turbo SE images because the extrahepatic and intrahepatic ducts were not depicted in most of these patients.

Patients with type A and type B biliary atresia had similar MR cholangiographic findings; that is, both groups had an invisible extrahepatic bile duct. In the patient with type C biliary atresia (patient 6), MR cholangiograms showed a cystic dilatation of the common hepatic duct, an accompanying atrophic gallbladder, and incomplete intrahepatic ducts but without visualization of the common bile duct (Fig 6c). In the two patients with type B biliary atresia, MR cholangiography failed to depict the extremely hypoplastic common bile duct, which was visible at surgical cholangiography with a caliber of less than 0.5 mm. On the basis of nonvisualization of the entire extrahepatic biliary tree, the authors were consistently correct in predicting biliary atresia as the cause of the jaundice.

The neonates and infants with neonatal hepatitis had gallbladders ranging from 1.4 to 4.5 cm in length (mean ± SD, 2.9 cm ± 0.9), while the gallbladders in the neonates and infants with biliary atresia were 0.8–2.1 cm in length (mean ± SD, 1.2 cm ± 0.4) (Student *t* test, $t = 4.33$, $P < .001$). MR cholangiography showed small gallbladders in all patients with biliary atresia except one and showed a small gallbladder in only one of the 10 patients without biliary atresia (Fisher exact probability test, $P < .001$). Thus, a small gallbladder could be considered highly suggestive but not diagnostic of biliary atresia. The diagnostic accuracy was 88% (14 of 16 patients), with a sensitivity of 83% (five of six patients), specificity of 90% (nine of 10 patients), and positive and negative predictive values of 83% (five of six patients) and 90% (nine of 10 patients), respectively.

Periportal fibrosis, as defined by the presence of increased T2 signal intensity on the T2-weighted conventional MR images, was seen in four of the six patients with biliary atresia (Fig 7) and in none of the nonjaundiced cohort and none of the patients with nonobstructive cholestasis. However, periportal thickening was hardly appreciable on MIP-reformatted MR cholangiographic images.

The findings from cholescintigraphy with ^{99m}Tc disofenin in all of the neonates and infants with biliary atresia were nonvisualization of the gallbladder and of bowel activity by 24 hours. In the group of patients with neonatal hepatitis, the images showed both the gallbladder and bowel activity in three patients and showed bowel activity alone in three patients. In the remaining three patients with neonatal hepatitis, as well as the infant with paucity of intrahepatic ducts, neither the gallbladder nor bowel activity by 24 hours was visible. For the diagnosis of biliary atresia, the sensitivity was 100% (six of six patients), but the specificity was only 60% (six of 10 patients). The accuracy was 75% (12 of 16 patients), and the positive predictive value was 60% (six of 10 patients).

DISCUSSION

This preliminary study shows that MR cholangiography in small infants can provide images of such diagnostic quality that the common bile and common hepatic ducts can be depicted clearly.

With these images, biliary atresia can be definitely excluded if the entire extrahepatic bile duct is visualized on the MR cholangiograms. If no complete extrahepatic bile duct can be visualized, especially when accompanied by an atrophic gallbladder, biliary atresia is suggested.

Biliary atresia and neonatal hepatitis are the two major causes of cholestatic jaundice in neonates and young infants (13). Biliary atresia was theorized to result from destructive inflammatory processes, leading to progressive fibrosis and obliteration of the extrahepatic bile duct (1). Patients with biliary atresia require an early surgical intervention, at best before 2 months of age (14). Many tests have been used to evaluate cholestasis in infants; however, none has proved infallible (9). A percutaneous liver biopsy has an extremely variable diagnostic accuracy of 60%–96.8% (9,13,15,16). Imaging studies, including ultrasonography, hepatobiliary scintigraphy, and endoscopic retrograde cholangiopancreatography, have been used to exclude biliary atresia as the cause of neonatal cholestasis (3–6,17–20). Use of endoscopic retrograde cholangiopancreatography to view the biliary tree presents a challenge in infants because of the lumen-to-tube ratio (21). Although laparotomy with surgical cholangiography can provide a direct and definite diagnosis, it is undesirable if alternative techniques are available.

MR cholangiography has developed rapidly over the past few years. Promising results in adult biliary disorders have been well documented in the literature (22–24). The feasibility and preliminary applications of MR cholangiography in neonates and infants have been mentioned in two recent articles (7,8). In our study, with the use of a non–breath-hold, respiratory-triggered, heavily T2-weighted, fat-suppressed, turbo SE technique, the main biliary structures were depicted in all control neonates and infants younger than 5 months of age. The second-order intrahepatic ducts could be visualized in half of the control group. This reflected that the resolution and quality of MR cholangiograms could ensure a clinical application for neonates and small infants.

The technique we used had several advantages: (*a*) higher signal-to-noise and contrast-to-noise ratios, which allow the use of thin sections, even for 2D imaging, and (*b*) diminished sensitivity to both motion artifact and slow flow (24). These advantages are mandatory for imaging neonates or small infants who have small-caliber biliary ducts and unavoidable motion. In addition, the respiratory-triggering technique allowed a non–breath-hold examination, which made imaging a baby possible.

These non–breath-hold fast SE techniques rely on an increase in signal acquisition (up to six signals acquired) to increase the signal-to-noise ratio and to compensate for signal losses caused by motion (25,26). The increase in the number of signals acquired, however, results in a long acquisition time, which should be minimized by choosing an adequate echo train length. Applying a surface coil instead of a body coil increases the signal-to-noise ratio and, therefore, improves visualization of small nondilated ducts (27). The addition of a fat-saturation technique has also improved the conspicuity of bile ducts from the surrounding intraabdominal fat while decreasing the motion artifacts associated with hyperintense subcutaneous fat (24).

In our control group, the 3D IR turbo SE images were slightly inferior to the 2D turbo SE images, especially in depicting the intrahepatic ducts. In the jaundiced cohort, 3D IR turbo SE imaging was performed only in the six patients with biliary atresia and the infant with paucity of intrahepatic ducts. Because none or only a few bile ducts were depicted in these patients, it is hard to compare these two sequences in the jaundiced group. In general, 3D IR turbo SE images proved to be slightly inferior in quality compared with the 2D turbo SE images. The increased motion artifacts caused by thin sections, the limitation of the number of signals acquired, and the long acquisition time degrade the visualization of the small-caliber intrahepatic ducts in small infants imaged with 3D IR turbo SE sequences. Because of the relatively higher quality and the shorter imaging time, we recommend 2D turbo SE sequences for MR cholangiographic study in small infants.

In this study, the extrahepatic bile ducts were visualized well in the nine patients with neonatal hepatitis and the infant with paucity of intrahepatic ducts. Biliary atresia was thereby excluded, and an unnecessary laparotomy was avoided in the four patients who had no evidence of hepatobiliary excretion at cholescintigraphy.

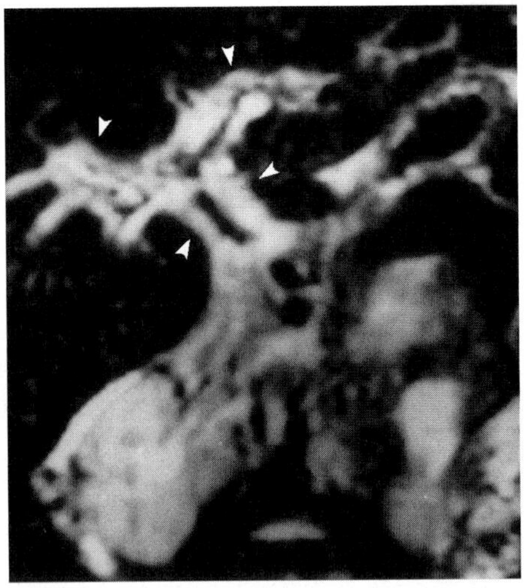

Figure 7. MR cholangiogram in a 47-day-old female infant with biliary atresia (patient 2). Paracoronal T2-weighted, spectral presaturation with IR, turbo SE (1,650/80 [effective]) image shows marked periportal thickening (arrowheads).

MR cholangiograms of all of the six patients with biliary atresia did not show the extrahepatic bile duct, except for one patient with cystic dilatation of the common hepatic duct. In the two patients with type B biliary atresia, a patent but very thin common bile duct with an atretic common hepatic duct was disclosed with surgical cholangiography. The lack of adequate water content in the hypoplastic common bile duct and its extremely small caliber (<0.5 mm) made it unable to be visualized on MR cholangiograms. Nevertheless, this did not affect the diagnosis of biliary atresia from a clinical point of view, nor did it have an influence on the choice of surgical procedures or the predicted outcome. In four patients with biliary atresia, MR cholangiograms also did not show the intrahepatic ducts. This was consistent with the surgical and histopathologic findings on the sections through the porta hepatis, which showed only a fibrous cord of the common hepatic duct and prominent fibrotic tissues with small bile ductules without normal structures of hepatic ducts.

Guibaud et al (7) have reported a false-positive diagnosis of biliary atresia in an infant with sclerosing cholangitis, in whom MR cholangiography did not depict the extrahepatic bile duct because of the small caliber of the ducts. Someday, with further improvements in the imaging resolution of MR cholangiography, visualization might be possible in cases such as that of the previous patient with sclerosing cholangitis and hypoplastic common bile ducts in type B biliary atresia. At such time, a reference to the normal caliber of the common bile duct (mean, 2.6 mm ± 0.5; range, 2.0–3.5 mm) will be necessary.

Guibaud et al (7) described periportal thickening on MR cholangiograms in all three of their patients with biliary atresia. Hyperintense periportal thickening was also found on T2-weighted MR images in our four patients with biliary atresia. However, periportal thickening was hardly appreciable on heavily T2-weighted MIP MR cholangiograms. The use of too heavily T2-weighted sequences and the MIP algorithm may suppress the signal intensity of periportal fibrosis.

Periportal thickening corresponded to the histologic findings of expansion of the portal tract by varying amounts of fibrosis, bile duct proliferation, and mixed inflammatory infiltrates (28). In the two patients with biliary atresia without MR findings of periportal thickening, no periportal fibrosis was noted at histopathologic examination of the specimen from liver biopsy. No periportal thickening was seen in our patients with nonobstructive cholestasis. This could be caused by the fact that progression of periportal fibrosis in intrahepatic cholestasis is not as prominent as that encountered in biliary atresia (29). Therefore, periportal thickening could also be a useful MR finding of biliary atresia. Larger prospective studies are required to determine the accuracy of periportal thickening in the diagnosis of biliary atresia.

In this prospective study of consecutive neonates and infants with neonatal cholestasis, the diagnostic accuracy of MR cholangiography was 100% (16 of 16 patients), while the accuracy of cholescintigraphy with ^{99m}Tc disofenin for the diagnosis of biliary atresia was only 75%, with a specificity of only 60%. The results of our scintigraphic studies are consistent with those from previous reports, which have revealed excellent sensitivity but low specificity in depicting biliary atresia (3–5). The liver uptake and excretion of the ^{99m}Tc-labeled radiopharmaceuticals are affected by the serum bilirubin levels and hepatic function of the patients (30). Therefore, several other causes of neonatal cholestasis may produce findings on cholescintigrams similar to those of biliary atresia (ie, lack of visualization of the gallbladder and of bowel activity, with retention of tracer in the liver by 24 hours), decreasing the specificity of the findings.

Guibaud et al stated, "The conditions that mimic biliary atresia on scintigraphy will also mimic biliary atresia on MR cholangiography" (7, p 30). However, in the present study, MR cholangiography depicted the extrahepatic bile ducts in three patients with neonatal hepatitis and in the infant with paucity of intrahepatic ducts, all of whom showed neither the gallbladder nor bowel activity at cholescintigraphy. Unlike cholescintigraphy, MR cholangiography is not limited by serum bilirubin levels or the hepatic function of the patients.

MR cholangiography depicts fluid in the bile duct, rather than only bile. In healthy individuals, mucus-producing glands located in the deep layers of the extrahepatic bile ducts connect with the lumen by long ducts and secrete white viscous secretions (31). Although bile secretion is retarded in severe intrahepatic cholestasis, this white viscous secretion, together with that of the neck glands of the gallbladder, might contribute to the visualization of the extrahepatic bile ducts with MR cholangiography.

Several major drawbacks still need to be addressed. The spatial resolution and signal-to-noise ratio need to be improved. There are problems of motion induced by respiration, by bowel peristalsis, or especially by inadequate sedation, which is also the major cause of a failed examination. Appropriate sedation is mandatory. The presence of fluid within the regional gastrointestinal tract may obscure the bile ducts, although some fluid in the duodenum can serve as a good anatomic landmark. Adequate fasting or administration of negative contrast agents may reduce this bowel interference.

In conclusion, MR cholangiography can be used to depict the major biliary structures of neonates and small infants, and it can be used to accurately exclude biliary atresia as the cause of neonatal cholestasis by allowing visualization of the biliary tract. Further efforts are needed in improving the image resolution and in obtaining more clinical experience to investigate the accuracy of MR cholangiography in excluding biliary atresia.

References

1. Balistreri WF, Grand R, Hoofnagle JH, et al. Biliary atresia: current concepts and research directions—summary of a symposium. Hepatology 1996; 6:1682–1692.
2. Ohi R, Hanamatsu M, Mochizuki I, Chiba T, Kasai M. Progress in the treatment of biliary atresia. World J Surg 1985; 9:285–293.
3. Gerhold JB, Klingensmith WC, Kuni CC, et al. Diagnosis of biliary atresia with radionuclide hepatobiliary imaging. Radiology 1983; 146:499–504.
4. Kirks DR, Coleman RE, Filstron HC, Rosenberg ER, Merten DF. An imaging approach to persistent neonatal jaundice. AJR 1984; 142:461–466.
5. Cox KL, Stadalnik RC, McGahan JP, Sanders K, Cannon RA, Ruebner BH. Hepatobiliary scintigraphy with technetium-99m disofenin in the evaluation of neonatal cholestasis. J Pediatr Gastroenterol Nutr 1987; 6:885–891.
6. Ben-Hain S, Seabold JE, Kao SCS, Johnson J, Tran D, Brown BP. Utility of Tc-99m mebrofenin scintigraphy in the assessment of infantile jaundice. Clin Nucl Med 1995; 20:153–163.
7. Guibaud L, Lachaud A, Touraine R, et al. MR cholangiography in neonates and infants: feasibility and preliminary applications. AJR 1998; 170:27–31.
8. Miyazaki T, Yamashita Y, Tang Y, Tsuchigame T, Takahashi M, Sera Y. Single-shot MR cholangiopancreatography of neonates, infants, and young children. AJR 1998; 170:33–37.
9. Lai MW, Chang MH, Hsu SH, et al. Differential diagnosis of extrahepatic biliary atresia from neonatal hepatitis: a prospective study. J Pediatr Gastroenterol Nutr 1994; 18:121–127.
10. Karrer FM, Raffensperger JG. Biliary atresia. In: Raffensperger JG, ed. Swenson's pediatric surgery. 5th ed. Norwalk, Conn: Appleton & Lange, 1990; 650.
11. Nadel HR. Hepatobiliary scintigraphy in children. Semin Nucl Med 1996; 26:25–42.
12. McGahan JP, Phillips HE, Cox KL. Sonography of the normal pediatric gallbladder and biliary tract. Radiology 1982; 144: 873–875.
13. Mowat AP, Psacharopoulos HT, Williams R. Extrahepatic biliary atresia versus neonatal hepatitis: review of 137 prospectively investigated infants. Arch Dis Child 1976; 51:763–770.
14. Kasai M. Treatment of biliary atresia with special reference to hepatic portoenterostomy and its modifications. Prog Pediatr Surg 1974; 6:5–52.
15. Manolaki AG, Larcher VF, Mowat AP, Barrett JJ, Portmann B, Howard ER. The prelaparotomy diagnosis of extrahepatic biliary atresia. Arch Dis Child 1983; 58: 591–594.
16. Brough AJ, Bernstein J. Conjugated hyperbilirubinemia in early infancy: a reassessment of liver biopsy. Hum Pathol 1974; 3:507–516.
17. Abramson SJ, Treves S, Teele RL. The infant with possible biliary atresia: evaluation by ultrasound and nuclear medicine. Pediatr Radiol 1982; 12:1–5.
18. Ikeda S, Sera Y, Akagi M. Serial ultrasonic examination to differentiate biliary atresia from neonatal hepatitis: special reference to change in size of the gallbladder. Eur J Pediatr 1989; 148:396–400.
19. Gurlrud M, Jaen D, Mendoza S, Plaz J, Torres P. ERCP in the diagnosis of extra-

hepatic biliary atresia. Gastrointest Endosc 1991; 37:522–526.
20. Ohnuma N, Takahasi H, Tanabe M, Yoshida H, Iwai J. The role of ERCP in biliary atresia. Gastrointest Endosc 1997; 45:365–370.
21. Shirai Z, Toriya H, Maeshiro K, Ikeda S. The usefulness of endoscopic retrograde cholangiopancreatography in infants and small children. Am J Gastroenterol 1993; 88:536–541.
22. Laurent G, Bret PM, Reinhold C, Atri M, Barkun AN. Bile duct obstruction and choledocholithiasis: diagnosis with MR cholangiography. Radiology 1995; 197:109–115.
23. Chan YI, Chan ACW, Lam WWM, et al. Choledocholithiasis: comparison of MR cholangiography and endoscopic retrograde cholangiography. Radiology 1996; 200:85–89.
24. Reinhold C, Bret PM. Current status of MR cholangiopancreatography. AJR 1996; 166:1285–1295.
25. Macaulay SE, Schulte SJ, Sekijima JH, et al. Evaluation of a non–breath-hold MR cholangiography technique. Radiology 1995; 196:227–232.
26. Reinhold C, Bret PM, Guibaud L, Barkun ANG. MR cholangiopancreatography: potential clinical applications. RadioGraphics 1996; 16:309–320.
27. Takehara T, Ichijo K, Tooyama N, et al. Breath-hold MR cholangiopancreatography with a long-echo-train fast spin-echo sequence and a surface coil in chronic pancreatitis. Radiology 1994; 192:73–78.
28. Park WH, Kim SP, Park KK, Choi SD, Lee HJ, Kwon KY. Electron microscopic study of the liver with biliary atresia and neonatal hepatitis. J Pediatr Surg 1996; 31:367–374.
29. Shirahase I, Ooshima A, Tanaka K, et al. The slow progression of hepatic fibrosis in intrahepatic cholestasis as compared with extrahepatic biliary atresia. Eur J Pediatr Surg 1995; 5:77–81.
30. Chervu LR, Nunn AD, Loberg MD. Radiopharmaceuticals for hepatobiliary imaging. Semin Nucl Med 1982; 9:5–17.
31. Netter FH, Popper H, Cliffton EE. Normal anatomy of the liver, biliary tract and pancreas. In: Oppenheimer E, ed. The CIBA collection of medical illustrations. Vol 3, Digestive system. Part III. Liver, biliary tract and pancreas. 2nd ed. Summit, NJ: CIBA, 1979; 22.

Autoimmune Lymphoproliferative Syndrome: A Syndrome Associated with Inherited Genetic Defects That Impair Lymphocytic Apoptosis—CT and US Features[1]

Nilo A. Avila, MD
Andrew J. Dwyer, MD
Janet K. Dale, RN, MPH
Uri A. Lopatin, BA
Michael C. Sneller, MD
Elaine S. Jaffe, MD
Jennifer M. Puck, MD
Stephen E. Straus, MD

Index terms:
Autoimmune lymphoproliferative syndrome, 99.39
Familial conditions
Lymphatic system, CT, 99.12911, 99.12912
Lymphatic system, diseases, 99.822
Lymphatic system, US, 99.12983, 99.12984

Radiology 1999; 212:257–263

Abbreviation:
ALPS = autoimmune lymphoproliferative syndrome

[1] From the Diagnostic Radiology Department, Warren Grant Magnuson Clinical Center, National Institutes of Health, Bldg 10, Rm 1C660, 10 Center Dr, MSC 1182, Bethesda, MD 20892-1182 (N.A.A., A.J.D.); the Laboratories of Clinical Investigation (J.K.D., U.A.L., S.E.S.) and Immunoregulation (M.C.S), National Institute of Allergy and Infectious Diseases, Bethesda, Md; the Laboratory of Pathology, National Cancer Institute, Bethesda, Md (E.S.J.); and the National Human Genome Research Institute, Bethesda, Md (J.M.P.).

Received July 6, 1998; revision requested August 27; final revision received October 26; accepted January 19, 1999.

Address reprint requests to N.A.A. (e-mail: *navila@nih.gov*).

Author contributions:
Guarantor of integrity of entire study, N.A.A.; study concepts, S.E.S., N.A.A.; study design, N.A.A.; literature research, S.E.S., N.A.A.; clinical studies, M.C.S., E.S.J., J.K.D., S.E.S.; experimental studies, J.M.P.; data acquisition, J.K.D., U.A.L.; data analysis, N.A.A., U.A.L.; manuscript preparation, A.J.D., N.A.A., S.E.S.; manuscript editing and review, all authors.

PURPOSE: To describe the imaging findings in patients with autoimmune lymphoproliferative syndrome (ALPS) and to relate the findings to the clinical and genetic features of this recently recognized syndrome.

MATERIALS AND METHODS: Retrospective or prospective reviews of the computed tomographic (CT) and ultrasonographic (US) studies and the clinical features in 19 consecutive patients with ALPS were performed.

RESULTS: Most patients presented in the 1st year of life with symptoms of adenopathy and hepatosplenomegaly. At the time of presentation to the institution, 12 patients had already undergone splenectomy, and 14 patients had developed autoimmune disorders. All patients had multifocal adenopathy, which was massive in some patients; 14 of 15 patients who underwent CT of the chest had an enlarged thymus, and all six patients who retained their spleens and who underwent imaging had splenomegaly. Ten of 18 patients who underwent liver imaging had hepatomegaly. The adenopathy at US was hyper- and/or isoechoic relative to the liver and thyroid and was enhanced at CT in some patients. All patients had defective lymphocytic apoptosis, or programmed cell death, which was due to specific Fas (*APT1* [*TNFRSF6*]) mutations in 15 patients.

CONCLUSION: Patients with ALPS demonstrate nonspecific but often dramatic imaging findings of lymphoproliferative disorders, such as adenopathy, splenomegaly, thymic enlargement, and hepatomegaly. The stability of the clinical findings over months to years and the pattern of lymph node echogenicity may suggest the diagnosis of ALPS.

Apoptosis, or programmed cell death, maintains immune homeostasis by limiting lymphocytic accumulation and by minimizing reactions against self-antigens (1,2). Findings of recent studies have shown that defective lymphocytic apoptosis caused by specific genetic mutations manifests as a human disorder termed the autoimmune lymphoproliferative syndrome (ALPS) (3–6). ALPS manifests in early childhood. The defining clinical features of ALPS are chronic, diffuse, nonmalignant lymphadenopathy and splenomegaly of occasionally massive proportions. Autoimmune diseases, which include autoantibody-mediated hemolytic anemia and thrombocytopenia, manifest in most patients.

Splenectomy is commonly required to control the cytopenia caused by hypersplenism and acutely aggravated by these autoimmune phenomena. There is an expansion of a usually rare (<1%) population of double-negative ($CD4^-CD8^-$) T cells that expresses the $\alpha\beta$ T-cell receptor and of defective lymphocytic apoptosis in vitro (7,8). In most patients with

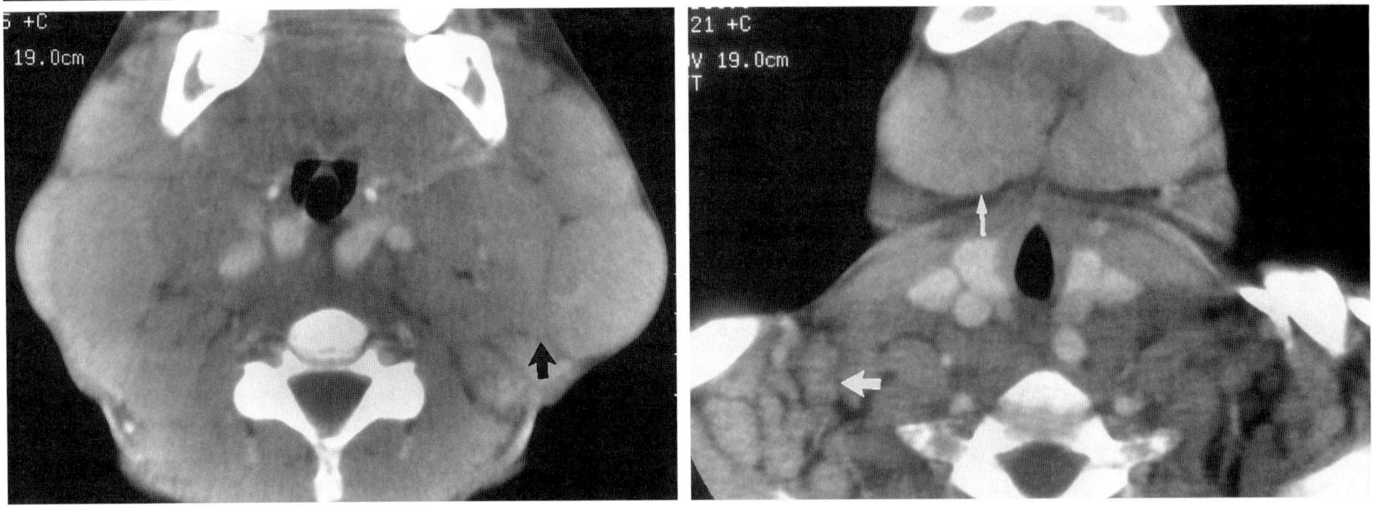

a. b.

Figure 1. CT images of the neck in a 4-year-old patient with ALPS. **(a)** Axial section at the level of the mandible shows extensive cervical adenopathy (arrow). **(b)** Axial section at the base of the neck shows extensive supraclavicular adenopathy (large arrow) and submental adenopathy (small arrow).

ALPS, functional mutations can be identified in the gene *APT1* (*TNFRSF6*), which encodes Fas, one of the key apoptosis-signaling proteins (3,4,6,9,10).

We conducted radiologic examinations in 19 consecutive patients with ALPS to relate the imaging findings to the clinical and genetic features of this syndrome and to determine whether the imaging findings might aid in diagnostic evaluation of ALPS.

MATERIALS AND METHODS

We performed retrospective or prospective reviews of the imaging studies in 19 consecutive patients with ALPS who presented to our institution, Warren Grant Magnuson Clinical Center, National Institutes of Health, Bethesda, Md, during their evaluations for ALPS and its complications. Six patients were examined at our institution before we developed the computed tomographic (CT) imaging protocol outlined in Materials and Methods; the imaging studies in these patients were reviewed retrospectively. Thirteen patients were examined prospectively after the initiation of the CT protocol outlined in Materials and Methods. All patients or parents of patients under 18 years of age consented in writing for the study of ALPS under internal review board–approved (National Institute of Allergy and Infectious Diseases, Bethesda, Md) protocols.

All imaging studies were reviewed by one radiologist (N.A.A.), who was blinded to the clinical and laboratory findings but who was aware of the diagnosis of ALPS. As patient schedules permitted, patients underwent CT of the neck ($n = 12$), chest ($n = 15$), abdomen ($n = 15$), or thymus ($n = 15$) by using a Highlite Advantage scanner (GE Medical Systems, Milwaukee, Wis). The CT images of the neck and thymus were obtained with 5-mm collimation, whereas the images of the chest and abdomen were obtained with 10-mm collimation. Thirteen of the 15 patients who underwent CT did so after intravenously receiving nonionic contrast material (iopamidol [Isovue 300]; Bracco Diagnostics, Princeton, NJ); two patients reported having allergic reactions in the

TABLE 1
Clinical and Demographic Data for Patients with ALPS

Patient No.*	Sex	Age (y)†	Adenopathy‡ (scale 0–4+)	Splenomegaly	Hepatomegaly	Autoimmune Disease: AIHA	ITP	AIN	GN	GB	PBC
1§	M	0.3	3+	Yes	Yes	No	Yes	No	No	No	No
2§	F	1.5	4+	Yes	Yes	No	Yes	No	Yes	No	Yes
3§	M	5.0	2+	Yes	No	Yes	Yes	Yes	No	No	No
4§	M	2.0	3+	Yes	Yes	No	No	No	No	No	No
5§	M	0.2	4+	Yes	No	Yes	Yes	Yes	No	No	No
6§	F	0.3	4+	Yes	Yes	Yes	No	No	No	No	No
11	F	0.8	4+	Yes	Yes	Yes	No	No	No	No	No
14§	F	0.8	4+	Yes	Yes	Yes	No	No	No	No	No
17§	F	0.3	4+	Yes	Yes	Yes	No	Yes	No	No	No
20§	F	3.0	2+	Yes	Yes	No	No	No	No	Yes	No
23	F	0.1	1+	Yes	No	Yes	No	Yes	No	No	No
27	M	5.0	2+	Yes	No	No	No	No	No	No	No
30	M	1.0	1+	Yes	No	Yes	Yes	Yes	Yes	No	No
30A	F	7.0	1+	Yes	No	No	No	No	No	No	No
31	F	0.8	1+	Yes	Yes	Yes	Yes	No	No	No	No
31A	F	0.0	1+	Yes	No	No	No	No	No	No	No
31B	F	4.0	1+	Yes	No	No	No	No	No	No	No
31C	F	2.0	1+	Yes	Yes	No	Yes	Yes	No	No	No
35	M	0.5	2+	Yes	No	Yes	No	No	No	No	No

Note.—AIHA = autoimmune hemolytic anemia, AIN = autoimmune neutropenia, GB = Gullian-Barré syndrome, GN = glomerulonephritis, ITP = idiopathic thrombocytopenic purpura, PBC = primary biliary cirrhosis.

* A, B, C = parents or siblings of the proband.

† Age at which ALPS was first documented.

‡ 1+ = multiple chains of detectable but <1.0-cm lymphnodes, 2+ = multiple chains of 1–2-cm nodes, 3+ = multiple chains visible without palpation, 4+ = massive adenopathy that distorted normal anatomic landmarks.

§ Previously published data (6).

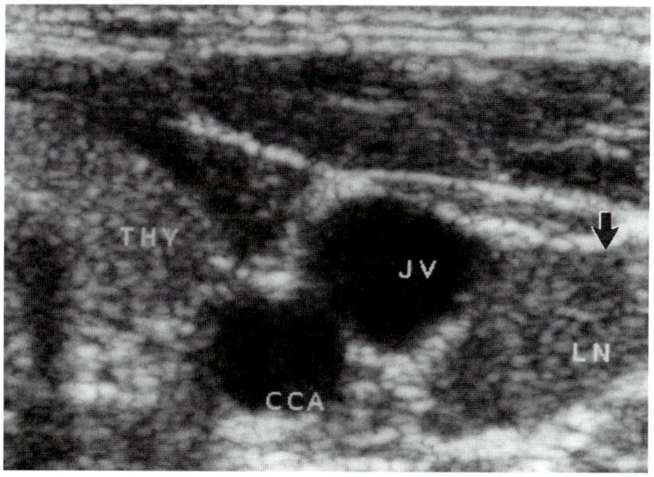

Figure 2. Transverse gray-scale US image of the neck in a 16-year-old patient with ALPS shows an enlarged lymph node (arrow) with echogenicity similar to that of the thyroid gland. *CCA* = common carotid artery, *JV* = jugular vein, *LN* = lymph node, *THY* = thyroid.

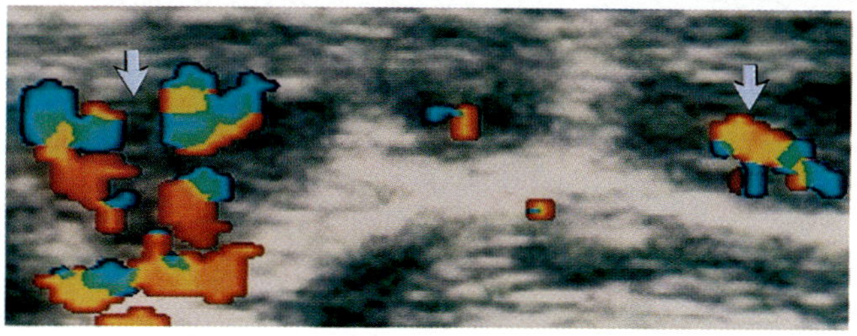

Figure 3. Transverse color Doppler US image of the submental region in a 10-year-old patient with ALPS shows moderate vascularity (arrows) within the submental lymph nodes.

past and did not receive intravenous contrast material.

CT findings were documented as follows: Lymph nodes were characterized according to size, site, and presence of enhancement. The thymus was measured in maximal craniocaudal, anteroposterior, and transverse dimensions; thymic thickness (the largest dimension perpendicular to the long axis of the thymus) was also measured and was compared with standards that were previously published (11). The maximal craniocaudal dimensions of the liver and spleen, when they had not been surgically removed, were recorded.

Eight patients underwent abdominal ultrasonography (US) that was performed with either a model 128 or a model 128 XP unit (Acuson, Mountain View, Calif); from the US images, the presence and echogenicity of abdominal lymphadenopathy were recorded. Five patients underwent gray-scale and color Doppler US of the submental lymph nodes; the size, echogenicity, and presence of internal vascularity of the nodes were recorded.

The patients' clinical charts were reviewed (by J.K.D. and U.A.L.). Pertinent clinical, genetic, and demographic data were recorded. The clinical and genetic features of ALPS in nine patients had been previously reported by Sneller et al (6).

RESULTS

Nineteen patients were examined; 12 were female patients, and seven were male patients. The age at which the patients first presented with symptoms of adenopathy or splenomegaly ranged from birth to 5 years; a majority of the patients ($n = 10$) presented before their first birthday. At the time of referral to our institution, the patients had a median age of 10 years (age range, 1–39 years). Thus, they had had clinical evidence of marked lymphoproliferation for a median of 7.2 years (range, 0.7–37.0 years).

Of the 19 patients, seven had persistent splenomegaly that was determined at clinical examination, and 12 patients had already undergone splenectomy, 10 patients had hepatomegaly, and 14 patients had documented autoimmune disorders (Table 1). All patients met the criteria for ALPS by virtue of their chronic lymphoproliferation, increased double-negative T-cell percentages, and defective lymphocytic apoptosis in vitro.

Fifteen patients had defined mutations in the gene encoding Fas. These mutations occur throughout the gene but cluster with the gene region that codes for the cytoplasmic death–signaling domain. Four patients were presumed to have had unrecognized defects in other genes that regulate apoptosis (6).

Cervical Lymph Nodes

CT images of the neck showed submental lymph nodes (which ranged from 1.0 to 4.0 cm in maximal diameter for the largest lymph node in each patient) and cervical lymph nodes (which ranged from 1.0 to 3.0 cm in maximal diameter) in all 12 of the patients who underwent CT of the neck (Fig 1). Enhancement of the submental nodes was seen in two patients, and enhancement of the cervical nodes was seen in five patients. All five patients who underwent US of the submental lymph nodes showed enlarged submental and cervical lymph nodes that were either isoechoic or slightly less echogenic than was the thyroid gland and that were either minimally or moderately vascular at color Doppler evaluation (Figs 2, 3).

Histologic findings of cervical lymph node biopsy specimens typically showed florid, reactive follicular hyperplasia and paracortical expansion, with immunoblasts, plasma cells, and a markedly expanded $CD3^+CD4^-CD8^-$ subset of T cells (Fig 4).

Chest and Abdominal Lymph Nodes

CT images of the chest and abdomen obtained in 15 patients showed lymph nodes in the following sites: axillary, in 15 patients, often with multiple lymph nodes that ranged in size from 0.9 to 3.8 cm; mediastinal, in 12 patients (size range, 0.5–5.0 cm); periportal, in three patients (size range, 1.8–4.0 cm); retroperitoneal, in 12 patients (size range, 0.8–3.0 cm); mesenteric, in 10 patients (size range, 0.8–3.0 cm); pelvic, in four patients (size range, 1.5–2.0 cm); and inguinal, in 10 patients (size range, 0.6–1.8 cm). Lymph nodes in the following anatomic locations showed CT enhancement: axillary, in 10 patients; retroperitoneal, in two patients; mesenteric, in one patient; and inguinal, in nine patients (Fig 5).

US of the abdomen revealed lymph nodes in seven of the eight patients who underwent abdominal US; in all seven patients, the lymph nodes were isoechoic when compared with the liver and were periportal in seven patients and retroperitoneal in four patients. One of the seven patients also had some periportal lymph nodes that were hyperechoic relative to the liver parenchyma (Fig 6).

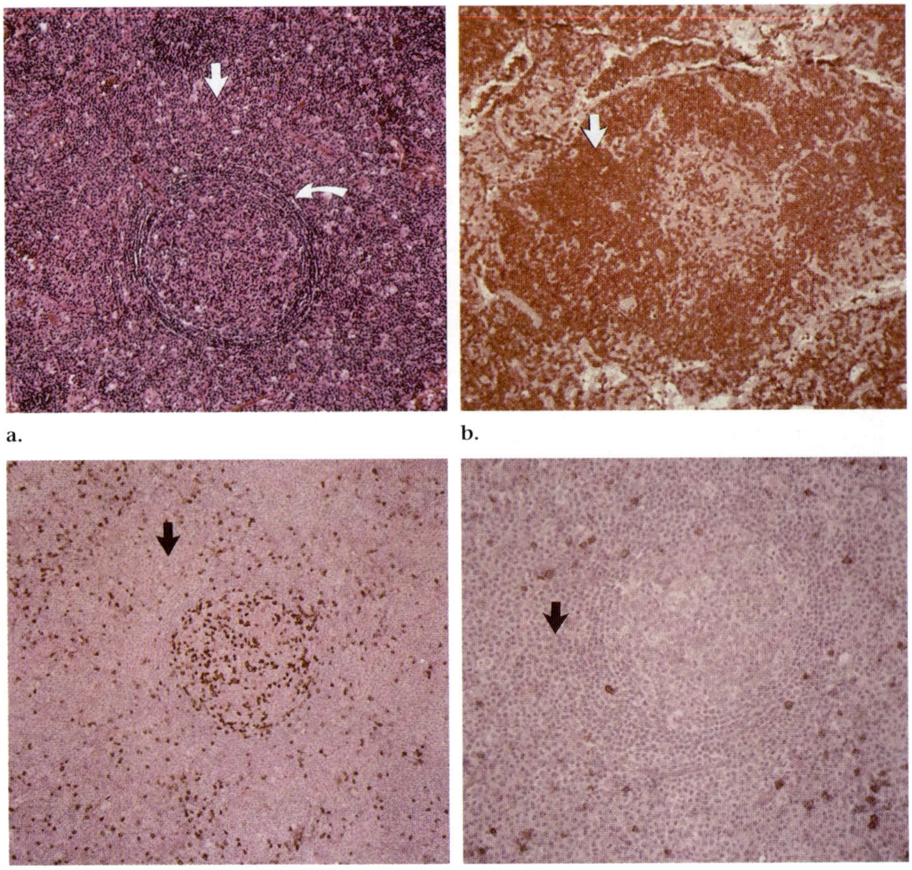

a. b. c. d.

Figure 4. Histologic results from a cervical lymph node biopsy in a patient with ALPS shows florid reactive hyperplasia and a markedly expanded $CD3^+CD4^-CD8^-$ subset of T cells. **(a)** Photomicrograph obtained with hematoxylin-eosin staining shows preservation of the lymph node architecture (curved arrow), marked reactive follicular hyperplasia, and paracortical expansion (straight arrow), with immunoblasts and plasma cells. **(b–d)** Photomicrographs obtained following staining of lymph node sections for **(b)** CD3, **(c)** CD4, and **(d)** CD8 show extensive accumulation of T cells (arrow) in the paracortical region. The absence of staining for **(c)** CD4 or **(d)** CD8 in the lymph node photomicrographs shows that most $CD3^+$ cells are $CD4^-$ and $CD8^-$. (In **a–d**, original magnification, ×100.)

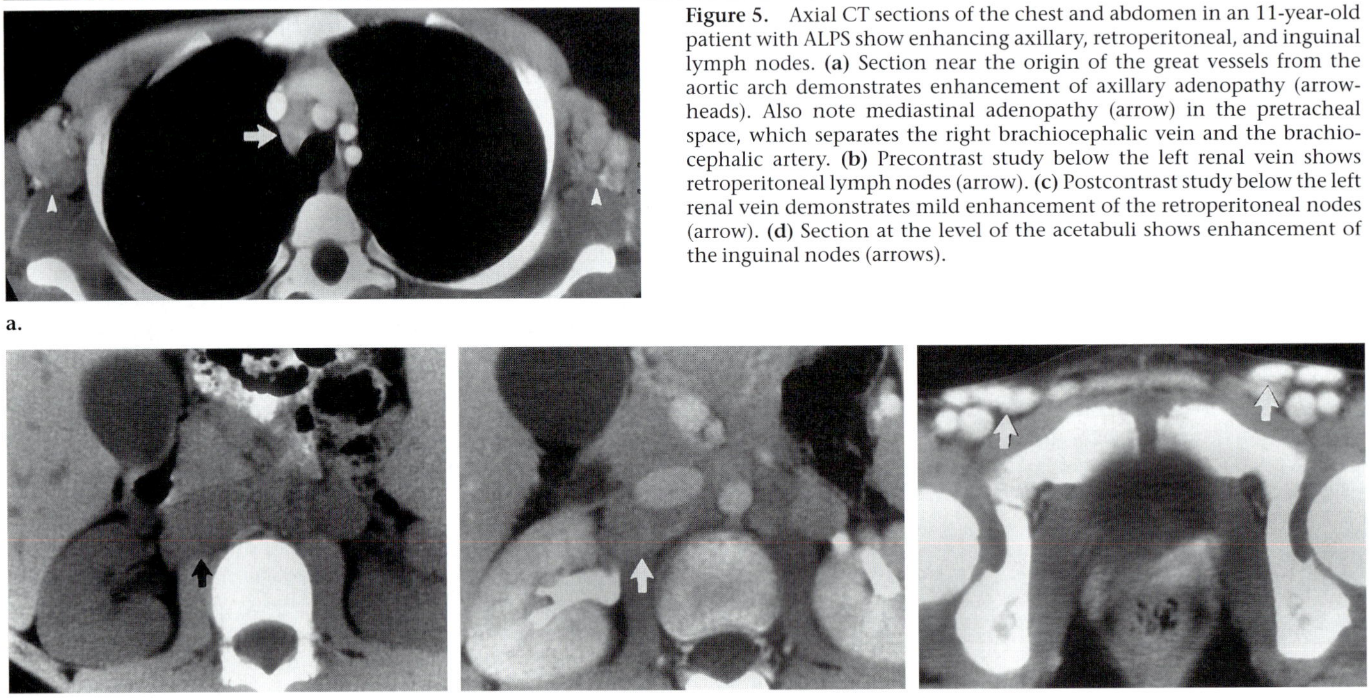

a. b. c. d.

Figure 5. Axial CT sections of the chest and abdomen in an 11-year-old patient with ALPS show enhancing axillary, retroperitoneal, and inguinal lymph nodes. **(a)** Section near the origin of the great vessels from the aortic arch demonstrates enhancement of axillary adenopathy (arrowheads). Also note mediastinal adenopathy (arrow) in the pretracheal space, which separates the right brachiocephalic vein and the brachiocephalic artery. **(b)** Precontrast study below the left renal vein shows retroperitoneal lymph nodes (arrow). **(c)** Postcontrast study below the left renal vein demonstrates mild enhancement of the retroperitoneal nodes (arrow). **(d)** Section at the level of the acetabuli shows enhancement of the inguinal nodes (arrows).

Thymic Enlargement

The thymus was enlarged in 14 of the 15 patients who underwent CT of the chest. The thymus thickness was above the normal, published, age-related standards (11), and the thymic attenuation was similar to the attenuation of muscle in these 14 patients. The thymus was diffusely enlarged and preserved a triangular shape in seven of these patients, had lobulated contours in two patients, and had a multinodular appearance in the other five patients (Figs 7, 8). Patient 17, a 20-year-old woman, had almost complete fatty replacement of the thymus, with a few remaining nodular areas that measured less than 0.5 cm in maximal diameter.

Liver

Ten of the 19 patients had hepatomegaly at clinical examination (Table 1). Eighteen patients underwent imaging of the liver; 15 underwent only CT, and three underwent only US (Table 2). The maximal craniocaudal dimension of the liver was measured (Table 2). Ten of the 18 patients who had undergone liver imaging had imaging proof of hepatomegaly, according to the published age-adjusted standards (12). No focal liver lesions were found.

Spleen

All 19 patients had splenomegaly detected at clinical examination or by determining medical history (Table 1). Eighteen patients underwent imaging of the spleen; 15 patients underwent only CT, and three patients underwent only US (Table 2). Twelve of the 18 patients had undergone splenectomy. The spleen was diffusely enlarged in all six patients who had not undergone splenectomy. No focal splenic lesions were identified.

Indications for splenectomy included the following: hypersplenism, severe hemolytic anemia, refractory thrombocytopenia, and suspicion of lymphoma. Histologic examination of the splenic specimens showed lymphoid hyperplasia of the white pulp with histologic features similar to those of the involved lymph nodes, that is, expansion of the white pulp with reactive follicles.

DISCUSSION

ALPS is a disorder of lymphocytic apoptosis that results in splenomegaly, adenopathy, and autoimmune phenomena. The syndrome manifests in early childhood, often with massive splenomegaly and chronic lymphadenopathy. This prompts consideration of several lymphoproliferative disorders, including infectious diseases and malignant lymphoma, before the histologic, cellular, genetic, and immunologic features of ALPS allow its definitive diagnosis.

Our results suggest that the US and CT features of the adenopathy may help in the distinction of ALPS from other lymphoproliferative processes, including malignant lymphoma. First, the adenopathy and splenomegaly may persist with only moderate alterations in size for many

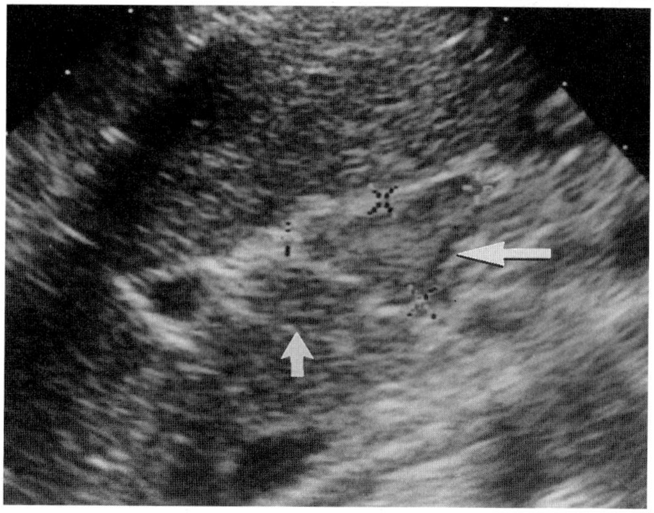

Figure 6. Longitudinal US image of periportal adenopathy in a 9-year-old patient with ALPS shows lymph nodes that are isoechoic (short arrow) and hyperechoic (long arrow) relative to the liver. (Crosshairs indicate location of calipers.)

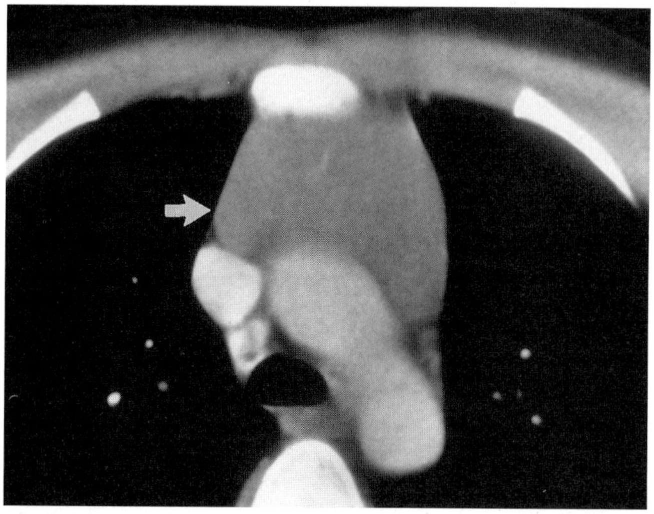

Figure 7. Axial CT image at the level of the anterior mediastinum in a 4-year-old patient with ALPS demonstrates a diffusely enlarged thymus (arrow).

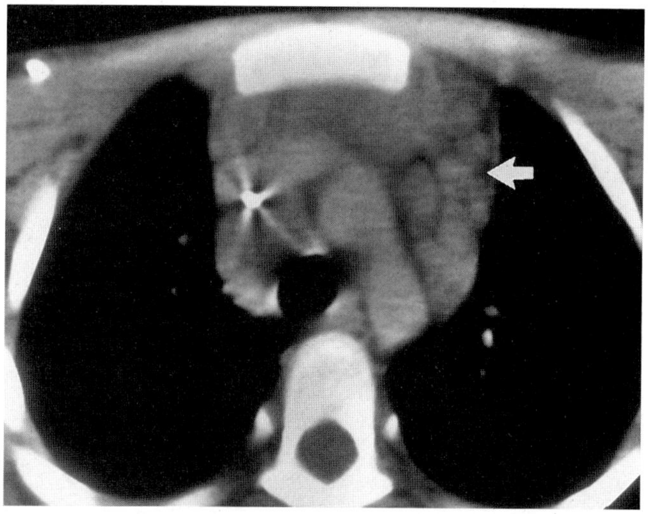

Figure 8. Axial CT image at the level of the anterior mediastinum in a 9-year-old patient with ALPS demonstrates an enlarged thymus (arrow) with a multinodular appearance.

TABLE 2
Imaging Findings in Patients with ALPS

Patient No.*	Age (y)[†]	Lymph Nodes (cm): Submental	Cervical	Axillary	Mediastinal	Periportal	Retro-peritoneal	Mesenteric	Pelvic	Inguinal	Craniocaudal Diameter (cm): Liver	Spleen	Thymus: Shape[‡]	Thickness (cm)	Miscellaneous CT and US Findings
1	6	NA	NA	NA	NA	2.0[§]	1.5[§]	NA	NA	NA	12[§]	Removed	NA	NA	US: periportal and retroperitoneal nodes isoechoic to liver
2	10	NA	NA	2.2	3.0	None	2.2	1.0	2.0	1.8	14	Removed	3.0 × 4.0 × 5.0, triangular	1.8	CT: axillary nodes with necrotic centers US: periportal nodes isoechoic to liver, submental nodes isoechoic to thyroid, increased vascularity
3	10	NA	NA	NA	NA	1.5[§]	NA	NA	NA	NA	16[§]	Removed	NA	NA	US: periportal and retroperitoneal nodes isoechoic to liver
4	9	NA	NA	NA	NA	2.2[§]	1.8[§]	1.5[§]	NA	NA	15[§]	14[§]	NA	NA	US: periportal and retroperitoneal nodes isoechoic and hyperechoic to liver
5	6	NA	NA	1.0	0.6	None	1.2	1.0	None	0.8	16	Removed	3.0 × 2.5 × 2.0, triangular	1.4	CT: enhancing axillary nodes
6	1	NA	NA	NA	NA	NA	NA	NA	NA	NA	NA	NA	NA	NA	. . .
11	4	4.0	3.0	2.2	5.0	4.0	2.5	2.0	2.0	1.5	17	Removed	3.5 × 4.0 × 3.5, lobulated	4.0	CT: enhancing cervical and inguinal nodes US: periportal and retroperitoneal nodes isoechoic to liver
14	8	2.0	1.5	1.8	1.0	1.8	1.8	1.5	1.5	1.0	14	Removed	2.8 × 2.5 × 3.0, triangular	1.5	CT: enhancing inguinal nodes
17	20	2.5	1.0	3.0	1.0	None	1.5	None	None	1.0	17	Removed	0.5-cm nodules, fat replaced	NA	CT: enhancing axillary and inguinal nodes US: submental nodes less echogenic than thyroid, mild vascularity
20	13	2.0	2.0	3.0	1.5	None	2.0	1.5	1.5	None	25	23	3.2 × 2.8 × 4.0, multinodular	1.6	CT: enhancing axillary and cervical nodes US: submental nodes less echogenic than thyroid, mild vascularity
23	9	1.0	1.5	1.6	3.0	None	None	None	None	None	15	14	4.0 × 5.0 × 3.0, multinodular	3.0	CT: enhancing cervical, axillary, and inguinal nodes
27	8	NA	NA	1.8	1.2	None	1.2	3.0	None	1.5	15	Removed	5.0 × 6.0 × 5.0, multinodular	2.5	CT: enhancing axillary, mesenteric, and inguinal nodes US: abdominal nodes isoechoic to liver
30	8	2.0	1.6	3.8	None	None	None	1.0	None	1.5	14	Removed	5.0 × 4.8 × 7.0, lobulated	3.2	CT: enhancing axillary and inguinal nodes US: periportal nodes isoechoic to liver
30A	12	1.0	1.2	1.2	None	None	0.8	0.8	None	0.6	14	14	3.5 × 3.0 × 5.0, triangular	2.0	. . .
31	16	1.0	1.5	2.0	1.5	4.0	None	None	None	None	22	Removed	4.5 × 6.2 × 7.0, multinodular	2.8	CT: enhancing axillary and inguinal nodes US: submental nodes less echogenic than thyroid, mild vascularity
31A	11	1.8	1.6	1.0	0.9	None	1.0	0.8	None	None	16	20	3.8 × 2.1 × 3.5, triangular	1.5	CT: enhancing submental and cervical nodes
31B	14	1.0	1.2	1.5	0.5	None	2.0	1.2	None	1.8	20	Removed	2.2 × 3.2 × 4.0, triangular	1.8	CT: enhancing cervical, axillary, retroperitoneal, and inguinal nodes
31C	39	1.2	1.0	0.9	None	None	1.2	None	None	None	20	Removed	4.2 × 4.0 × 8.0, multinodular	2.0	CT: enhancing submental and axillary nodes US: submental nodes less echogenic than thyroid, avascular
35	11	2.0	1.0	3.0	1.5	None	3.0	None	None	1.0	15	19	5.0 × 3.0 × 4.0, triangular	1.2	CT: enhancing axillary, retroperitoneal, and inguinal nodes

Note.—All lymph node sizes are the greatest diameter for the largest lymph node found in a given anatomic area. NA = This anatomic area was not imaged.

* A, B, C = parents or siblings of the proband.

† Age at the time of the imaging examination.

‡ Anteroposterior × transverse × craniocaudal.

§ US finding. No CT was performed of this area.

years. In the present series, which to our knowledge is the largest series of patients with ALPS reported to date, the median duration of lymphoproliferation at the time of imaging was 7.2 years. Although we have just begun a longitudinal evaluation of these patients, their medical histories, including their requirement of splenectomy years to decades earlier, verify the chronicity of the condition. Our initial impression suggests that, if anything, the adenopathy becomes relatively less prominent after childhood.

Second, in seven of eight patients who underwent US, the abdominal adenopathy was isoechoic or hyperechoic relative to the liver and was distinct from the adenopathy of malignant lymphoma, which is usually hypoechoic (13). Of less use in the differential diagnosis is that in all 13 patients who underwent contrast-enhanced CT, some of the lymph nodes enhanced (this has been previously described in patients with Castleman disease, tuberculosis, or reactive hyperplasia), which suggests an infectious or reactive cause. However, the same finding has also been reported in some patients with neoplasms, such as lymphoma and melanoma (14,15).

The radiologic similarities between the adenopathy in ALPS and the adenopathy in more conventional reactive and infectious processes parallel the histologic findings. In ALPS, the histologic features of the lymph nodes resemble those of viral lymphadenitis, except for the conspicuous absence of histiocytes normally seen to contain apoptotic debris. The lymph node architecture is preserved. There is florid follicular hyperplasia and paracortical expansion by a mixed infiltrate that includes $CD3^{+}CD4^{-}CD8^{-}$ T cells (5,6). This combination of follicular hyperplasia and paracortical expansion, with $CD4^{-}$ and $CD8^{-}$ T cells that express the $\alpha\beta$ T-cell receptor in the lymph nodes and spleen, appears unique to ALPS and, hence, constitutes a virtually certain pathognomonic histologic feature.

There is insufficient long-term clinical follow-up of patients with ALPS to predict their ultimate outcome. Most patients with ALPS experience autoimmune complications—commonly hemolytic anemia and thrombocytopenia—although autoimmune neutropenia, glomerulonephritis, autoimmune hepatitis, and Guillain-Barré syndrome have been seen. Most patients eventually require splenectomy, usually for hypersplenism, severe hemolytic anemia, or refractory thrombocytopenia.

Some patients have developed postsplenectomy sepsis with encapsulated bacteria, including *Streptococcus pneumoniae* and *Haemophilus influenzae*. There is, however, no other recognized predisposition to infections in patients with ALPS. Although adenopathy may be massive, the lymphoproliferative aspect of ALPS per se does not affect vital organ function. Whether patients with ALPS are predisposed to malignancy remains to be proved, but isolated cases have been confirmed in extended studies of ALPS kindreds (3,6).

Apoptosis is a crucial cellular mechanism that normally limits lymphocytic accumulation and the potential for some aberrant clones that can react against self-antigens to persist (1,2). In ALPS, lymphocytic apoptosis is disrupted by heritable defects in genes that regulate it. This disruption results in the accumulation in lymphoid organs of mature, activated $CD4^{-}$ and $CD8^{-}$ lymphocytes that have escaped apoptosis. These lymphocytes, together with additional reactive cells, produce the microscopically massive follicular hyperplasia and/or paracortical expansion and the macroscopic adenopathy, splenomegaly, and hepatomegaly that are characteristic of ALPS.

Similarly, the autoimmune phenomena can be explained by the faulty apoptosis of T and B cells, the failure to eliminate mature T cells with receptors that recognize self-antigens, the excess of helper T cells for self-reactive B cells, the excess of B cells with self-reactive potential, the excessive release of cytokines that induce lymphocytes to exhibit autoimmune phenomena, or by a combination of these mechanisms (16).

The clinical and immunologic features in patients with ALPS resembled those of mice with mutations that impair lymphocytic apoptosis. This observation provided the first clue to the factors involved in the cause of ALPS (5). The demonstration that most ALPS patients have alterations in Fas, the same gene product that is abnormal in a strain of mice with a similar disorder, established the nature of ALPS (3,4).

It is apparent that not all patients with ALPS have Fas mutations. Mutations in other apoptosis genes are being sought. Our recent study of one large family revealed the pattern of inheritance of the mutation and its variable clinical consequences (17). Of 11 family members in four generations with the identical Fas mutation and with defective lymphocytic apoptosis in vitro, three members were entirely asymptomatic, five members had one or more features of ALPS, and three members had the full-blown syndrome.

Patients with autoimmune lymphoproliferative syndrome demonstrate nonspecific imaging findings of lymphoproliferative disorders (adenopathy, splenomegaly, thymic enlargement, and hepatomegaly); the stability of the clinical findings over months to years and the pattern of lymph node echogenicity may suggest the diagnosis. Imaging examinations have various roles in managing ALPS: (*a*) providing accurate measures of organ involvement, (*b*) depicting lymphoproliferation that can elude clinical examination, (*c*) and helping to rule out other unanticipated or complicating conditions.

References

1. Lenardo MJ. Fas and the art of lymphocyte maintenance. J Exp Med 1996; 183:721–724.
2. Lenardo MJ. Interleukin-2 programs mouse alpha beta T lymphocytes for apoptosis. Nature 1991; 353:858–861.
3. Fisher GH, Rosenberg FJ, Straus SE, et al. Dominant interfering Fas gene mutations impair apoptosis in a human autoimmune lymphoproliferative syndrome. Cell 1995; 81: 935–946.
4. Rieux-Leucat F, Le Deist F, Hivroz C, et al. Mutations in Fas associated with human lymphoproliferative syndrome and autoimmunity. Science 1995; 268:1347–1349.
5. Sneller MC, Straus SE, Jaffe ES, et al. A novel lymphoproliferative/autoimmune syndrome resembling murine lpr/gld disease. J Clin Invest 1992; 90:334–341.
6. Sneller MC, Wang J, Dale JK, et al. Clinical, immunologic, and genetic features of an autoimmune lymphoproliferative syndrome associated with abnormal lymphocyte apoptosis. Blood 1997; 89:1341–1348.
7. Shivakumar S, Tsokos G, Datta S. T cell receptor alpha/beta expressing double negative (CD4-/CD8-) and CD4+ T helper cells in humans augment the production of pathogenic anti-DNA autoantibodies associated with lupus nephritis. J Immunol 1989; 43: 103–112.
8. de la Hera A, Toribio ML, Marquez C, Martinez C. Interleukin 2 promotes growth and cytolytic activity in human T3+4-8- thymocytes. Proc Natl Acad Sci USA 1985; 82:6268–6271.
9. Drappa J, Vaishnaw AK, Sullivan KE, et al. Fas gene mutations in the Canale-Smith syndrome, an inherited lymphoproliferative disorder associated with autoimmunity. N Engl J Med 1996; 335:1643–1649.
10. Bettinardi A, Brugnoni D, Quiros-Roldan E, et al. Missense mutations in the Fas gene resulting in autoimmune lymphoproliferative syndrome: a molecular and immunological analysis. Blood 1997; 89:902–909.
11. Baron RL, Lee JKT, Sagel SS, Peterson RR. Computed tomography of the normal thymus. Radiology 1982; 142:121–125.
12. Keats TE, Lusted LB. Determination of liver size in infancy and childhood. In: Keats TE, Lusted LB. Atlas of roentgenographic measurement. 5th ed. Chicago, Ill: Year Book Medical, 1985; 323–328.
13. Nyman R, Rehn S, Glimelius B, et al. Magnetic resonance imaging, chest radiography, computed tomography and ultrasonography in malignant lymphoma. Acta Radiol 1987; 28:253–262.
14. Pombo F, Rodriguez E, Caruncho MV, Villalva C, Crespo C. CT attenuation values and enhancing characteristics of thoracoabdominal lymphomatous adenopathies. J Comput Assist Tomogr 1994; 18:59–62.
15. Shirkhoda A, Albin J. Malignant melanoma: correlating abdominal and pelvic CT with clinical staging. Radiology 1987; 165:75–78.
16. Fuss IJ, Strober W, Dale JK, et al. Characteristic T helper 2 T cell cytokine abnormalities in autoimmune lymphoproliferative syndrome, a syndrome marked by defective apoptosis and humoral autoimmunity. J Immunol 1997; 158:1912–1918.
17. Infante AJ, Britton HA, DeNapoli T, et al. The clinical spectrum in a large kindred with autoimmune lymphoproliferative syndrome caused by a Fas mutation that impairs lymphocyte apoptosis. J Pediatr 1998; 133:629–633.

Interlude

An Egg-ceptional Dissection of the Ascending Aorta

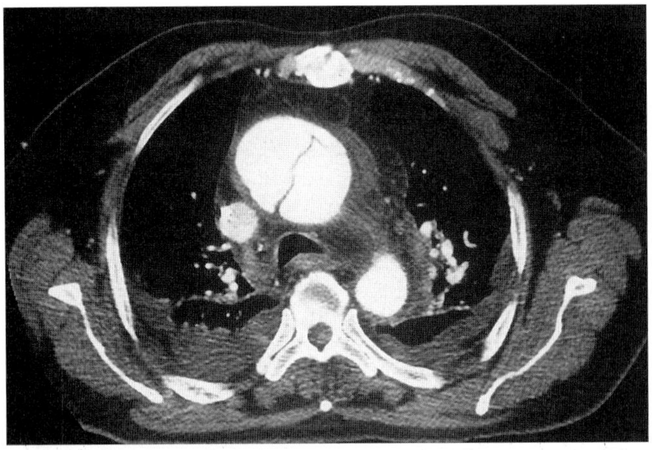

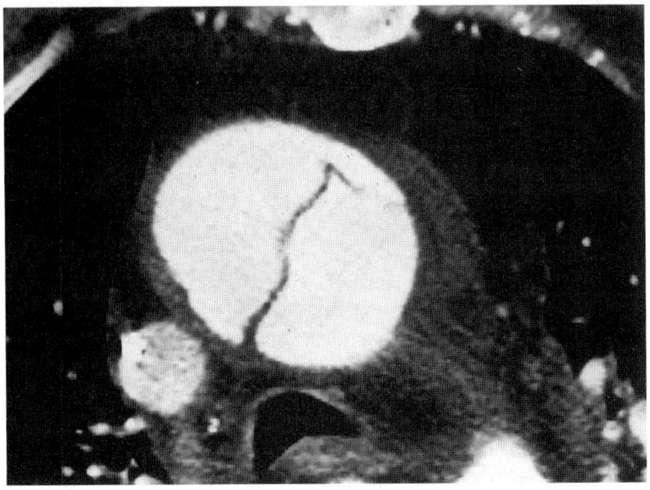

Courtesy of Uri Rimon, MD, and Tali Jonas, MD, Tel-Hashomer, Israel

MR Colonography: Optimized Enema Composition[1]

Wolfgang Luboldt, MD
Johannes M. Frohlich, PhD
Nicole Schneider, MD
Dominik Weishaupt, MD
Franziska Landolt, MSc
Jorg F. Debatin, MD

Index terms:
Colon, MR, 75.121412, 75.121419, 75.12143
Gadolinium
Iron
Magnetic resonance (MR), contrast agents, 75.121412, 75.121419, 75.12143
Magnetic resonance (MR), contrast enhancement, 75.12143
Manganese

Radiology 1999; 212:265–269

Abbreviations:
CNR = contrast-to-noise ratio
GRE = gradient-recalled echo
SE = spin echo
SI = signal intensity
2D = two-dimensional
3D = three-dimensional

[1] From the Institute of Diagnostic Radiology, University Hospital Zurich, Ramistrasse 100, CH-8091 Zurich, Switzerland. Received May 27, 1998; revision requested August 5; revision received September 10; accepted December 16. Supported in part by German Research Foundation stipend Lu 687/1-1. **Address reprint requests to** J.F.D. (e-mail: *debatin@drnr.usz.ch*).

Author contributions:
Guarantor of integrity of entire study, J.F.D.; study concepts, J.F.D., W.L., J.M.F.; study design, W.L.; definition of intellectual content, J.F.D., W.L., J.M.F.; literature research, W.L., N.S., F.L., D.W.; experimental studies, W.L., N.S., F.L.; data acquisition, W.L., N.S., D.W.; data analysis, D.W.; statistical analysis, D.W., N.S.; manuscript preparation and editing, W.L., J.F.D., D.W.; manuscript review, J.F.D., D.W., J.M.F.

Manganese chloride, iron glycerophosphate, and cellulose additive were assessed as base materials for use in a T1-shortening single contrast enema for magnetic resonance (MR) colonography. Contrast-to-noise ratios (CNRs) were compared to those with the standard 10 mmol/L gadolinium–based enema. On T1-weighted three-dimensional gradient-recalled-echo images, CNRs with the iron glycerophosphate enema exceeded those with the manganese- and gadolinium-based enemas. Use of an additive of 0.8% wt/wt cellulose was found to be practicable as it increased viscosity sufficiently without altering CNR. The gadolinium-based enema can be replaced with an iron glycerophosphate enema to render MR colonography less costly.

Magnetic resonance (MR) colonography combines the application of a rectal enema containing paramagnetic contrast agent with breath-hold, T1-weighted, high-spatial-resolution, three-dimensional (3D) imaging and heavily T2-weighted, two-dimensional (2D), single-shot, spin-echo (SE) imaging (1). Beyond being biocompatible, the enema used at MR colonography needs to fulfill MR signal intensity (SI) and mechanical requirements. For reconstruction of endoscopic views, the enema should be homogeneously bright on T1-weighted, 3D, gradient-recalled-echo (GRE) images and homogeneously dark on T2-weighted images for better depiction of pathologic conditions contained within the colonic wall. In addition, the enema needs to homogeneously fill and distend the colon. These mechanical properties are mainly dependent on the viscosity of the enema.

Presently, an enema with 10 mmol of gadopentetate dimeglumine (Magnevist; Berlex Laboratories, Wayne, NJ) per liter of water is used for MR colonography. Although it fulfills the SI requirements, the low viscosity induces backflow into the small bowel, which complicates subsequent analysis and reduces colonic distention. More important however, the enema has a volume of up to 2,000 mL and thus requires use of as much as 40 mL of a 0.5 mol/L paramagnetic contrast agent formulation. The associated cost is high, which negatively effects consideration of MR colonography as a screening alternative for colonic polyps.

The purpose of this study was to identify a less costly, more viscous enema with SI characteristics similar to those with the 10 mmol/L gadopentetate dimeglumine and water enema currently employed.

Materials and Methods

MR Imaging

All imaging was performed on a 1.5-T system (Signa Acuspot; GE Medical Systems, Milwaukee, Wis). To ensure a sufficiently large field of view to cover the entire colon, the body coil was used for signal transmission and reception. Two sequences were employed: 3D spoiled GRE (repetition time msec/echo time msec = 4.7/2, 45° flip angle, 0.5 signals acquired, 62.5-kHz bandwidth, 382 × 192 matrix, 40 × 40-cm field of view, 2.4-mm section thickness) and 2D single-shot fast SE (65-msec echo time, 31.3-kHz bandwidth, 256 × 192 matrix, 40 × 40-cm field of view, 6-mm section thickness).

Assessment of New Contrast Media

Two agents—manganese chloride and iron glycerophosphate—were assessed as possible replacements for gadopentetate dimeglumine. Water-based dilution series with each agent and with gadopentetate dimeglumine were imaged with the 3D spoiled GRE and 2D single-shot fast SE sequences. In addition, a water-dilution series with iron glycerophosphate and 600 mg of manganese chloride was imaged to determine possible synergistic effects with the two substances. On the basis of SI data acquired on 3D spoiled GRE images, the concentration with which the maximum SI was achieved was determined with a finely incremented dilution series. SI-concentration curves were obtained for each of the four evaluated contrast media.

The contrast media that provided the maximum contrast-to-noise ratio (CNR) on the 3D spoiled GRE images was used at the optimum concentration to fill the colon of three anesthetized pigs. The experiments were conducted in accordance with state regulations governing animal experiments. The colon was imaged with both the 3D spoiled GRE and 2D single-shot fast SE sequences. To determine CNR, SI characteristics of the contrast agent–filled colonic lumen were evaluated relative to the colonic wall and surrounding structures. Additionally, three colonic specimens exposed to the enema were obtained for histologic examination of iron uptake with Prussian blue staining.

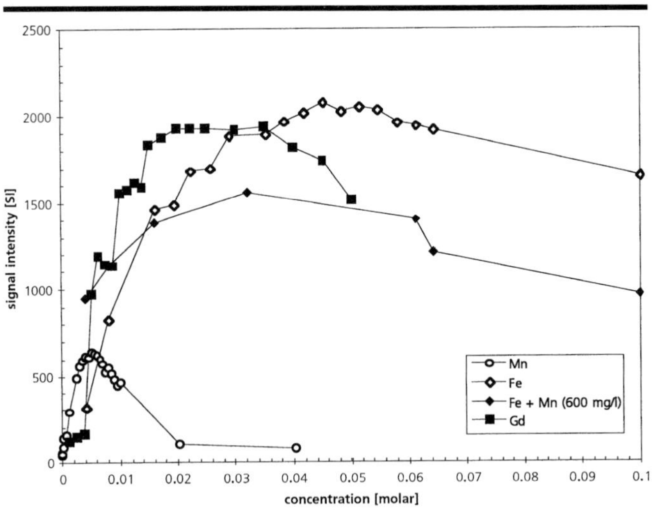

Figure 1. For T1-weighted 3D spoiled GRE images, graph plots SIs relative to dilution series of manganese chloride (*Mn*), iron glycerophosphate (*Fe*), manganese chloride and iron glycerophosphate [*Fe + Mn (600 mg/l)*], or gadopentetate dimeglumine (*Gd*). In all cases, an initial SI increase is followed by an eventual SI decrease. This appearance reflects the rising T2-shortening effect of these substances as their concentration is increased. The highest maximum was measured with iron glycerophosphate.

Optimization of Enema Viscosity

Cellulose was added to enhance the mechanical properties of the enema by increasing its viscosity. In an initial step, the maximum additive of cellulose was determined that allowed passage of the mixture through the enema tip at 1.5 m of hydrostatic pressure. With this maximum cellulose concentration as a baseline, the enema viscosity was titrated for MR colonography by means of progressive dilution with water until complete colonic filling at 1.5-m hydrostatic pressure was possible.

Dilution experiments were performed in six patients (four men and two women; age range, 53–72 years; mean age, 61 years) undergoing MR colonography in a larger study designed to determine the diagnostic performance of MR colonography in the detection of colonic masses. This study had been approved by the local ethics committee, and written informed consent was obtained from all patients. The patients had undergone colonic preparation for subsequent conventional colonoscopy. Colonic filling was monitored with a non–section-selective 2D spoiled GRE acquisition collecting one image every second. The acquired images permitted assessment of colonic distention and reflux into the small bowel.

To determine the influence on SI characteristics of the cellulose additive in its previously optimized concentration, the gadopentetate dimeglumine and iron glycerophosphate dilution series were repeated with and without the cellulose additive, with the 3D spoiled GRE sequence. The ratio of the resultant SIs with and SIs without cellulose ($SI_{with}/SI_{without}$) were plotted against the concentrations of gadopentetate dimeglumine and iron glycerophosphate. The paired Student *t* test was used to assess statistically significant differences in the collected data sets.

Results

On the T1-weighted 3D spoiled GRE images, both manganese chloride and iron glycerophosphate resulted in an initial concentration-dependent increase in SI followed by an eventual decrease in SI as T2-shortening effects began to dominate T1 effects with increased concentrations (Fig 1). The highest SI was achieved with the iron glycerophosphate and water solution at a concentration of 45 mmol/L, which corresponds to an iron load of 28 g/L. Manganese chloride solutions were associated with lower SI values. Maximum SI was observed with a concentration of 5 mmol/L, which corresponds to a manganese load of 1 g/L. The combination of manganese chloride and iron glycerophosphate showed a synergistic effect as evidenced by SI values that exceeded those with only iron glycerophosphate up to a concentration of 15 mmol/L of iron glycerophosphate (Fig 1). Beyond 15 mmol/L, iron glycerophosphate provided SI values higher than the combination of iron glycerophosphate and manganese chloride. Results with the gadopentetate dimeglumine dilution series revealed a maximum SI at a concentration of 23 mmol/L. The maximum gadopentetate dimeglumine value (SI, 1,932) exceeded values with manganese chloride (SI, 640) but remained lower than the maximum value with iron glycerophosphate (SI, 2,078).

In pigs, the 45 mmol/L iron glycerophosphate solution provided homogeneously high SI within the colonic lumen on the T1-weighted 3D spoiled GRE images (Fig 2a), which permitted reconstruction of virtual endoscopic images. The mean for CNRs of the colonic lumen relative to surrounding structures was 48 ± 5 (SD). On T2-weighted 2D single-shot fast SE images, the colonic lumen was homogeneously dark, which permitted easy delineation of the hyperintense colonic wall (Fig 2b). The means for CNRs of the colonic wall relative to the colonic lumen or surrounding structures were 21 ± 3 and 10 ± 4, respectively. Histologic analysis of the colonic specimen revealed no evidence of iron uptake into the colonic mucosal cells.

The cellulose additive beyond 2% wt/wt precluded passage through the enema tip. To ensure easy filling of the entire colon under in vivo conditions, the cellulose additive was lowered to 0.8% wt/wt

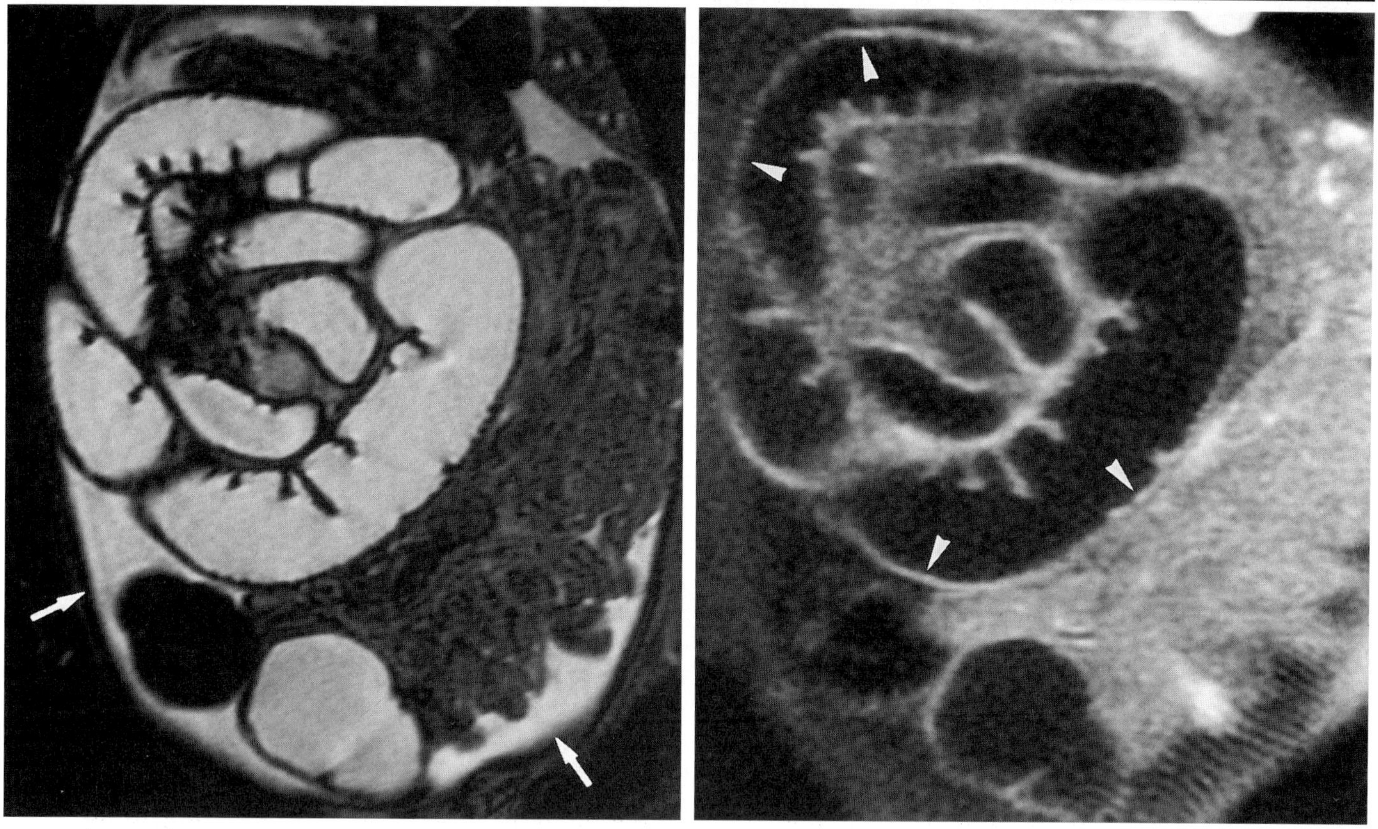

a. b.

Figure 2. Coronal **(a)** 3D spoiled GRE and **(b)** 2D single-shot fast SE images of the colon after rectal administration of a highly concentrated (28 g/L) iron glycerophosphate enema to a pig. The colonic lumen is bright in **a**. Even at this high concentration, iron glycerophosphate caused no artifacts. Since the colon of the pig was artificially perforated, the T1-shortening iron glycerophosphate can also be identified within the peritoneal cavity (arrows in **a**). In **b**, the colonic lumen is dark. Having inherently high SI on T2-weighted images, the colonic wall (arrowheads) is clearly delineated from the colonic lumen and surrounding structures.

(Fig 3). At this concentration, there was no reflux noted in any of the six patients. The addition of cellulose at this concentration had no effect on the SI characteristics on 3D spoiled GRE images for either the gadopentetate dimeglumine or iron glycerophosphate dilution series (Fig 4). The paired Student t test revealed no statistically significant differences in SI ($P > .5$).

Discussion

The potential benefits of colonic polyp screening are well documented (2). Recently, we reported promising results with MR colonography (3). Although the cost of MR colonography depends on the content of the enema, its performance depends on the intraluminal SI and distention of the colon. The cost of MR colonography has been rather high, which predominantly reflects the use of as much as 40 mL of gadopentetate dimeglumine as the contrast agent for the enema. Findings in this study demonstrate that the enema can be optimized to dramatically lower the overall cost of an MR colonographic examination.

Presently, the amount of gadopentetate dimeglumine required for optimum contrast on both T1-weighted 3D spoiled GRE and T2-weighted 2D single-shot fast SE images represents a cost factor that would preclude use of MR colonography for screening purposes. Since the contrast agent is administered rectally and not intravenously, there is a considerably wider latitude regarding tolerance and safety of agents. We evaluated two considerably less expensive agents with known T1- and T2-shortening effects as possible alternatives to gadopentetate dimeglumine: manganese chloride and iron glycerophosphate. Manganese was chosen as it is the substance responsible for the T1-shortening effects inherent in blueberry juice (4). Manganese chloride provided a maximum SI (SI, 640) that was 41% of that achieved with gadopentetate dimeglumine (SI, 1,560) at the 10 mmol/L concentration (Fig 1). This cannot be considered sufficient for MR colonography.

Subsequently, iron was tested in its most tolerable form as iron glycerophosphate (5). SI values achieved with iron glycerophosphate were far higher than those associated with manganese chloride and even exceeded those with gadopentetate dimeglumine (Fig 1). Maximum SI values were seen at a concentration of 45 mmol/L, which corresponds to an iron load of 28 g/L. In an attempt to lower the concentration of iron glycerophosphate, manganese chloride was added. The amount of manganese chloride added corresponded to the concentration associated with 87% (SI, 558) of the maximum SI increase in the manganese chloride dilution series (SI, 640). Indeed, the addition of manganese chloride to iron glycerophosphate resulted in higher SI values at lower concentrations. At higher concentrations, the combination reached a maximum SI value of 75% (SI, 1,560) of the maximum SI achieved with iron glycerophosphate alone (SI, 2,078) (Fig 1).

The in vivo imaging characteristics of iron glycerophosphate are favorable for MR colonography. At a concentration of 45 mmol/L, the enema was displayed as homogeneously bright on T1-weighted 3D spoiled GRE images and totally dark on T2-weighted 2D single-shot fast SE images (Fig 2). The visual impressions are corroborated by the high CNRs. In contrast to superparamagnetic iron oxide, which requires matching with diamagnetic barium sulfate particles to avoid susceptibility artifacts (6,7), images obtained with iron glycerophosphate depicted no artifacts up to the tested concentration of 45 mmol/L (Fig 2).

Iron glycerophosphate appears to be a safe agent. In fact, it has been used in high doses without relevant side effects in pediatric populations (8). It is poorly absorbed when administered orally (9,10). Although conclusive data are not available, it is not likely to cause any side effect if administered rectally. As was also confirmed in our study, there is no measurable resorption of this physiologic iron compound in the colon (11). It is conceivable, however, that iron could be resorbed if reflux occurs far into the proximal small bowel. Even if such an extensive reflux were to occur, the transient nature of the iron present in the small bowel would obviate any serious imbalance in iron metabolism. As an additional safeguard, iron could be embedded in macromolecules (iron-dextran, iron-cellulose) that are not resorbed. In this manner, the potential toxicity would be reduced as the viscosity increased.

Similar to double contrast barium enema examination (12,13), accurate assessment of the colonic lumen with MR colonography mandates adequate colonic distention (3). Beyond the administration of antiperistaltic, distention is dependent on the viscosity of the enema. Currently, the enema used at MR colonography consists mainly of water, which results in quick passage of enema fluid through the ileocecal valve into the small bowel in a vast majority of patients. Increases in viscosity must, however, be balanced against the need for easy and fast filling of the colon, particularly in view of limitations regarding usable hydrostatic pressure. Although results of in vitro experiments identified a 2% wt/wt cellulose additive as maximum, results of in vivo evaluations in six patients demonstrated a cellulose additive beyond 0.8% wt/wt to be impracticable. At this concentration, there was no reflux of contrast material into the small bowel and, consequently, distention was good (Fig 3). Results of in vitro experiments showed that the addition of cellulose to the enema did not have any measurable effect on SIs on 3D spoiled GRE images (Fig 4).

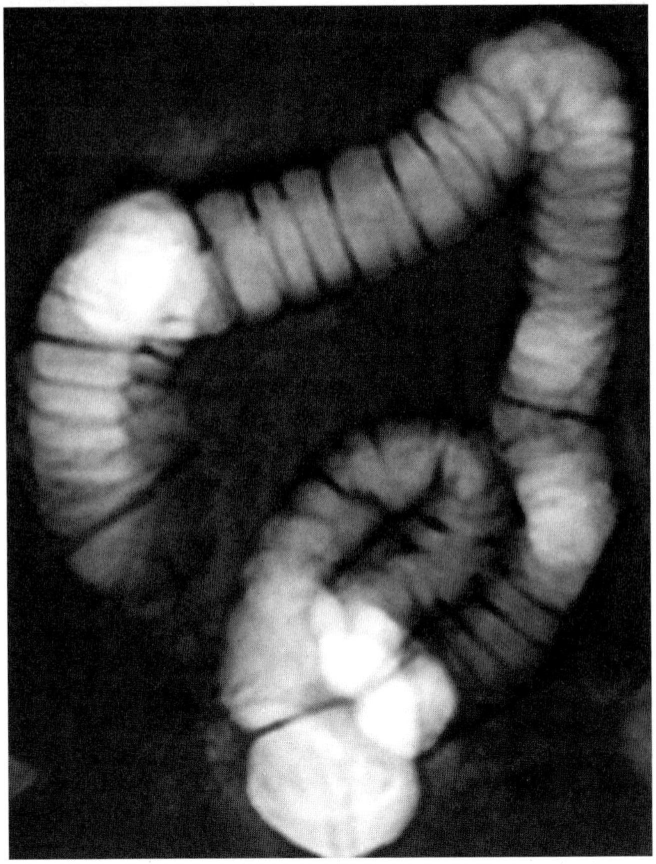

Figure 3. MR image of colonic filling permits assessment of colonic distention and reflux into the small bowel. The additive of cellulose prevented reflux of contrast agent into the small bowel in all six patients and resulted in good colonic distention.

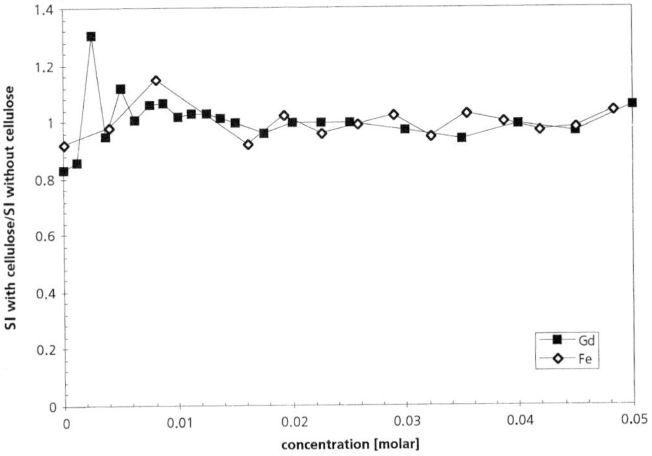

Figure 4. For T1-weighted 3D spoiled GRE images, graph plots the ratio of SIs obtained with and SIs obtained without the addition of 0.8% wt/wt cellulose depending on the concentration of gadopentetate dimeglumine (*Gd*) or iron glycerophosphate (*Fe*). Cellulose had no measurable influence on SIs.

Iron glycerophosphate seems to be a feasible alternative to gadopentetate dimeglumine as a contrast enema in MR colonography. Before any clinical use, more safety data need to be collected (eg, by means of radiolabeling techniques with the radioactive isotope iron-59 instead of iron-56 [14]). A relative price difference of a factor of approximately 25 in conjunction with slightly better SI characteristics makes this a worthwhile endeavor. Even though MR colonography may become less expensive with the use of iron glycerophosphate, a cost analysis of MR colonography compared with other modalities, such as barium enema examination or colonoscopy, will need to be performed.

References

1. Luboldt W, Bauerfeind P, Steiner P, Fried M, Krestin GP, Debatin JF. Preliminary assessment of three-dimensional magnetic resonance imaging for various colonic disorders. Lancet 1997; 349:1288–1291.
2. Winawer SJ, Zauber AG, Ho MN, et al. Prevention of colorectal cancer by colonoscopic polypectomy: the National Polyp Study Workgroup. N Engl J Med 1993; 329:1977–1981.
3. Luboldt W, Steiner P, Bauerfeind P, Pelkonen P, Debatin JF. Detection of mass lesions with MR colonography: preliminary report. Radiology 1998; 207:59–65.
4. Hiraishi K, Narabayashi I, Fujita O, et al. Blueberry juice: preliminary evaluation as an oral contrast agent in gastrointestinal MR imaging. Radiology 1995; 194:119–123.
5. Layrisse M, Martinez Torres C, Divo MR, Jaffe W, Torres Suarez JE. Iron absorption from skim milk enriched with iron glycerophosphate (letter). Arch Latinoam Nutr 1973; 23:145–150.
6. Liebig T, Stoupis C, Ros PR, Ballinger JR, Briggs RW. A potentially artifact-free oral contrast agent for gastrointestinal MRI. Magn Reson Med 1993; 30:646–649.
7. Briggs RW, Wu Z, Mladinich CR, et al. In vivo animal tests of an artifact-free contrast agent for gastrointestinal MRI. Magn Reson Imaging 1997; 15:559–566.
8. Pobedinskaia VN. Use of large doses of iron glycerophosphate in the therapy and prevention of allergic diseases in children. Vopr Okhr Materin Det 1976; 21:61. [Russian]
9. Hallberg L, Solvell L, Brise H. Search for substances promoting the absorption of iron: studies on absorption and side-effects. Acta Med Scand Suppl 1966; 459:11–21.
10. Anghileri LJ, Cordova Martinez A, Maincent P, Robert J. In vivo behaviour of low molecular weight iron complexes. Eur J Drug Metab Pharmacokinet 1991; 16:203–206.
11. Lombard M, Chua E, O'Toole P. Regulation of intestinal non-haem iron absorption. Gut 1997; 40:435–439.
12. Goei R, Nix M, Kessels AH, Ten Tusscher MP. Use of antispasmodic drugs in double contrast barium enema examination: glucagon or buscopan? Clin Radiol 1995; 50:553–557.
13. Rubesin SE, Furth EE, Rose D, Levine MS, Laufer I. The effects of distention of the colon during air-contrast barium enema on colonic morphology: anatomic correlation. AJR 1995; 164:1387–1389.
14. Chouly C, Pouliquen D, Lucet I, Jeune JJ, Jallet P. Development of superparamagnetic nanoparticles for MRI: effect of particle size, charge and surface nature on biodistribution. J Microencapsul 1996; 13:245–255.

Haim Azhari, DSc
Didi Sazbon, MSc

Index terms:
Breast, US, 00.12989
Computed tomography (CT), ultrasound (US)
Ultrasound, experimental studies, 00.12989
Ultrasound computed tomography (US/CT), 00.12989

Radiology 1999; 212:270–275

Abbreviation:
3D = three-dimensional

[1] From the Department of Biomedical Engineering, Technion, Israel Institute of Technology, Haifa 32000, Israel. Received September 15, 1997; revision requested November 24; final revision received November 20, 1998; accepted January 15, 1999. Supported in part by the Israel Science Foundation (grant Z-953/93), the Technion Vice Provost for Research Fund (J. Tal Equipment and Research Fund 130-304), the Irving and Adele Rosenberg Foundation, and the Israel Cancer Association (grants 960023-B and 972025-B). **Address reprint requests to** H.A. (e-mail: *haim@biomed.technion.ac.il*).

Volumetric Imaging with Ultrasonic Spiral CT[1]

To examine the feasibility of implementing spiral computed tomography (CT) in ultrasonic imaging as a potential method for breast screening, an algorithm for x-ray spiral CT was applied to ultrasonic waves on a specially built ultrasonic tomographic system. Three-dimensional reconstructions of various phantoms were obtained. Spiral ultrasonic CT is feasible, and it may have clinical merit as a breast imaging method.

Breast cancer is a major cause of mortality in women. Current statistics indicate that one in eight women (12.5%) may be affected by breast cancer in their lifetimes (1). Mammography is currently the accepted screening tool for breast imaging. However, mammography has some major disadvantages. It has been proved ineffective as an imaging modality for women with dense breasts and undesirable in young women (ultrasonography is the preferred modality in these cases [2,3]), has limited tissue characterization capability, and provides only two-dimensional projections of the breast. Furthermore, mammography involves hazardous ionizing radiation, which renders this method undesirable for mass screening and frequent follow-up.

Ultrasonic imaging, in comparison, is considered safe; is suitable for women in any age group; enables tissue characterization on the basis of a variety of parameters such as backscatter, attenuation, and speed of sound (3–6); depicts tissue morphology; and is a relatively cost-effective modality. Currently, pulse-echo imaging (B scan) is the most widely applied ultrasonic technique, but its ability to discriminate between solid masses is limited (7). Ultrasonic computed tomography (CT) has been suggested as an alternative imaging technique that provides better tissue characterization (8,9), but the large number of projections required to obtain a high-spatial-resolution image requires use of large (and costly) transducer arrays or results in a long acquisition time.

Spiral CT is a relatively new approach implemented in modern x-ray imaging (10–12). With spiral CT, a continuous scan is obtained of a volume of interest, which provides the data for a three-dimensional (3D) reconstruction of the studied object. Spiral CT provides information for a much more detailed 3D reconstruction of the object and is more efficient than is conventional CT performed with the same scanning parameters. On the basis of its 3D nature, spiral CT can provide longitudinal and arbitrarily oriented cross sections in addition to the axial images commonly obtained with conventional CT.

The objective of this study was to examine the feasibility of implementing spiral CT in ultrasonic imaging as a potential method for 3D breast imaging.

Materials and Methods

Ultrasonic CT

Ultrasonic CT images are commonly reconstructed from the detected acoustic waves passing through an insonified object (forming its acoustic projections) by means of a backprojection process. Projections of the object are acquired from various directions around it to constitute its Radon transform. By using the relation between the Fourier transform of the projection and the two-dimensional Fourier transform of the object (by means of the slice theorem [13]), the measured projections are used to obtain the Fourier domain of the object. The image of the object can be reconstructed by using the inverse Fourier transform of these data. With ultrasonic CT, tomograms can be obtained that depict the acoustic attenuation coefficients or the local refraction index, defined as 1/wave velocity. By ignoring diffraction effects, a relatively simple model is implied for ultrasonic CT. The ultrasonic wave propagation paths in soft tissues are assumed to be approximately along straight lines (8,14). Hence,

Author contributions:
Guarantor of integrity of entire study, H.A.; study concepts and design, H.A.; definition of intellectual content, H.A.; literature research, D.S.; experimental studies, H.A., D.S.; data acquisition and analysis, D.S.; manuscript preparation and editing, H.A., D.S.; manuscript review, H.A.

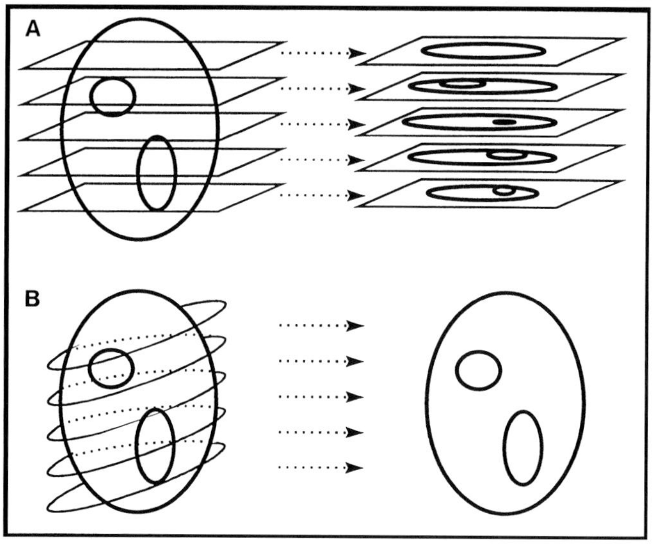

Figure 1. Schematic illustrates *A*, conventional 3D reconstruction versus *B*, volumetric spiral reconstruction. A set of parallel cross sections is provided in *A*, whereas a single data set (volumetric) is obtained in *B*. Note that small objects located between two consecutive scanned planes may disappear in *A*.

images can be reconstructed in a manner similar to that with x-ray CT by applying the filtered backprojection algorithm (14). (A more accurate model that accounts for diffraction effects would require a computationally more intensive algorithm [15]). Consequently, the following relations can be implemented.

Refraction index projections can be estimated by measuring the time of flight of the ultrasonic wave through the object by using the following line integral (along each ray) (8):

$$\int_{\text{ray}} N_r(x,y)\,\mathrm{d}s = T_{\text{rec}} - T_{\text{trans}}, \quad (1)$$

where N_r is the refraction index, T_{trans} is the transmission time, and T_{rec} is the receiving time.

Attenuation coefficient projections can be estimated by measuring the amplitude of the through transmitted ultrasonic wave. In this case, the following line integral is used (8):

$$\int_{\text{ray}} \mu_0(x,y)\,\mathrm{d}s = -\ln(A_{\text{rec}}/A_{\text{trans}}), \quad (2)$$

where μ_0 is the equivalent attenuation coefficient (ie, ignoring dependency on the frequency), A_{trans} is the transmitted wave amplitude, and A_{rec} is the received wave amplitude. In this study, we chose to focus on attenuation imaging alone. Tomograms, obtained with ultrasonic CT based on Equation (1), have been published previously (14,16).

Spiral CT

Spiral CT provides volumetric information from the object. Unlike conventional CT, which scans the object section by section (Fig 1a), spiral CT scans the entire object along a spiral path (Fig 1b). Accordingly, if the helical pitch (defined as the axial displacement of the detectors per revolution) is properly selected, spiral CT contains information from all regions of the object. Consequently, small abnormal regions located between two consecutive planes, which may disappear in the 3D reconstruction obtained with conventional CT, are likely to be detected with spiral CT. Naturally, this also depends on other scanning parameters (ie, section thickness [which is fixed by the collimator], the number of sampled rays, the number of projections acquired, and the quality of the reconstruction algorithm used).

Spiral CT is also more efficient than conventional CT in the sense that it can provide a much larger number of sections within a given scanning time. Scanning time is determined by the time required to acquire a single projection (Δt) multiplied by the number of projections (N_P) required to reconstruct the object. Given a total scanning time (T) as a constraint, the number of available projections is determined by $N_P = T/(\Delta t)$. If the number of projections used to reconstruct a single section is N_1, conventional CT can yield only N_P/N_1 sections, whereas spiral CT can yield $N_P - (2 \cdot N_1)$ sections. For example, if the total number of projections acquired is 640 and $N_1 = 64$, conventional CT can produce only 10 sections whereas spiral CT can produce as many as 512 sections.

With ultrasonic CT, no hazardous radiation is involved. Therefore, total acquisition time is not limited by dose factors but merely by the patient's comfort. The time required to acquire a single ultrasonic projection (Δt) is determined mainly by engineering factors (data storage and mechanical movements). The physical limitation here is almost negligible (ultrasonic travel time through 200-mm-thick tissue is about 0.13 msec). Thus, a projection of 128 rays, for example, will require about 17 msec plus the time required for the hardware to sample and store the data. (With modern hardware and array transducers, an acquisition rate of more than 10 projections per second can be achieved.)

Object reconstruction from spiral CT data can be achieved by using alternative approaches. In this study, linear interpolation of the projection data into a set of parallel planes (17,18) was used. The interpolation method is described in detail in the Appendix. Basically with this method, the spiral CT data set is first resampled into a set of many planar Radon transforms by using the interpolation algorithm. Then, by applying a conventional backprojection algorithm to each Radon transform, a set of parallel cross sections is generated. Consequently, the number of planes reconstructed is substantially larger than the number obtained by conventional CT with the same scanning parameters. This leads to a much more detailed 3D reconstruction of the object. However, the penalty for that procedure is an increase in the section sensitivity profile (ie, the effective section width is increased [19–22]). It should be noted that the section sensitivity profile depends strongly on the helical pitch used (ie, a smaller pitch will provide a narrower effective section width and vice versa). Nevertheless, with a smaller pitch, a larger number of windings will be required to cover the object, which leads to an increase in the total scanning time.

Spiral Ultrasonic CT Experimental System

The experimental system used to implement spiral CT to ultrasonic waves comprises a water bath with a specially built computer-controlled mechanism that can produce spatial motion with 3 *df* [x, z, θ] for a pair of 5-MHz focused transducers

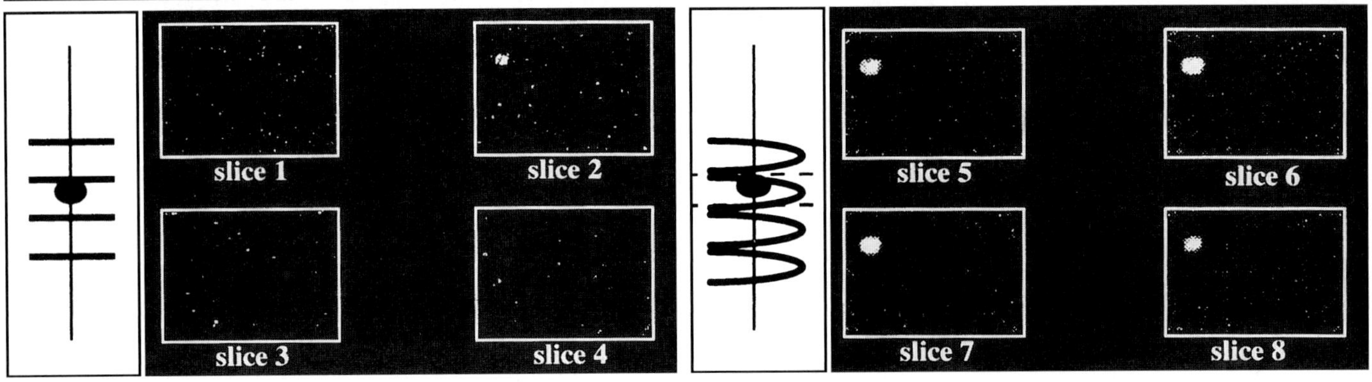

a. b.

Figure 2. Plasticine spherical target. **(a)** Conventional 3D scan depicts four sections (*slice 1–4*) 10 mm apart (schematically illustrated on the left). Only the second section (*slice 2*) depicts a cross-sectional image of the upper part of the sphere. Note that the sphere would have been undetected with a slight change in section position. **(b)** Spiral CT scan was obtained with four spirals and 10-mm pitch (schematically illustrated on the left). The four sections (*slice 5–8*) depict cross sections located between the two dashed lines in the schematic and passing through the sphere. In this case, the spiral reconstruction consists of 16 sections.

(Panametrics; Waltham, Mass). Section thickness is determined on the basis of the diameter of the acoustic beam generated by the transducers. We estimated it to be about 5 mm in this case. The system can scan a cylindric volume defined by the user (up to 20 cm in diameter and 30 cm high) located in the center of the water bath. The system can currently acquire a 15-cm-long projection with 600 rays in 10 seconds. The helical pitch, defined as the axial displacement of the ultrasonic transducers per revolution, can be set arbitrarily by the user (0–300 mm per revolution).

A pulser receiver (model 5800; Panametrics) was used to transmit and receive the ultrasonic waves. A two-channel 20-MHz analog-to-digital converter (model R2000; Rapid Systems, Seattle, Wash) was used to digitally store the detected waves. For image reconstruction, the peak-to-peak amplitude of each wave was registered. The system was controlled with a 66-MHz computer (PC/486; Fox Computers, Taiwan). Codes for data acquisition, image reconstruction, and image display were written in our laboratory by using a C++ compiler (Borland International, Scotts Valley, Calif).

Objects Tested and Protocols Used

Three objects were used to evaluate spiral ultrasonic CT performance.

Plasticine spherical target.—A 7-mm-diameter plasticine sphere (Cope 4516; PanArt, Jerusalem, Palestine) was used to simulate a single tissue target and allow comparison of conventional ultrasonic CT with spiral ultrasonic CT. The sphere was positioned within the scanner water tank. It was positioned in the water tank by using a very thin wire (about 0.2-mm diameter), which was too thin to be detected by the system (the corresponding ultrasonic wavelength in water is about 0.3 mm). Scout acoustic attenuation projections based on Equation (2) were acquired for general orientation. With use of these scout projections, the coordinates of the desired imaging windows (ie, minimum and maximum spatial coordinates of the scanned volume) were set manually.

Tomographic images of the sphere were initially obtained by using reconstructions of four conventional ultrasonic CT sections with a resolution of 128 × 128 pixels. Each pixel was 1 × 1 mm. A 10-mm distance between sections was used. (This distance was used to ensure the sphere was detected in only one section of the conventional ultrasonic CT scan.) Next, the same sphere was reconstructed with use of a spiral ultrasonic CT scan with four spiral windings and a 10-mm pitch. The corresponding cross sections were also reconstructed with a resolution of 128 × 128 pixels. In-plane resolution was again 1 × 1 mm.

On the ultrasonic attenuation tomograms, brighter gray levels indicated higher attenuation. Thus, because the ultrasonic attenuation coefficient of plasticine is higher than that of the background (ie, water), the sphere appeared as a bright spot on a relatively dark background. The sphere was detected within the tomographic reconstructions by two observers (H.A., D.S.) on the basis of consensus. The sphere was easily detected (Fig 2). Because we merely compared the two methods for detection, no tests of reproducibility were performed.

Egg phantom.—A hard-boiled egg was positioned within a condom. An egg was chosen because its acoustic properties are close to that of tissue and its internal geometry is known. The hard-boiled egg was positioned approximately at the center of the water tank of the scanner (by using the condom for suspension). By acquiring scout projections, the coordinates of the desired imaging window were set manually. A 3D reconstruction of the egg at 128 × 128 × 128-voxel resolution was obtained from a spiral ultrasonic CT scan with eight spiral windings and a 10-mm pitch. Voxel size ($\Delta x \Delta y \Delta z$) was 1.00 × 1.00 × 0.62 mm. Again the images were analyzed by consensus. The purpose of this study was merely to validate that the reconstructions produced with spiral ultrasonic CT matched the expected cross sections of the hard-boiled egg. Hence, no tests of reproducibility were performed.

Breast phantom.—The breast biopsy phantom (model BB-1; ATS Laboratories, Bridgeport, Conn) mimics the appearance, size, and acoustic properties of the human breast. The phantom contains eight target structures embedded randomly throughout. The target structures are similar to abnormal tissue and are 5–10 mm in diameter. The phantom was imaged with spiral ultrasonic CT with 16 spiral windings and 5-mm pitch. A 128 × 128 × 64-voxel reconstruction of the phantom was obtained. Voxel size ($\Delta x \Delta y \Delta z$) was 1.40 × 1.40 × 1.25 mm.

Abnormal tissue–mimicking targets were characterized in the tomograms with

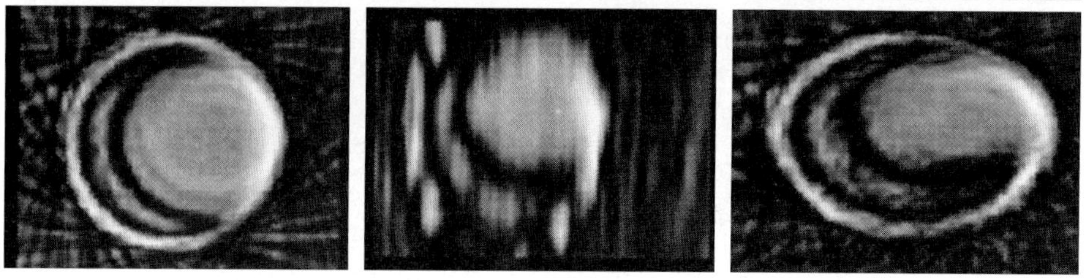

a. b. c.

Figure 3. Hard-boiled egg phantom. Spiral reconstructions obtained with eight spiral windings and 10-mm pitch depict the following cross-sectional views: **(a)** axial, **(b)** longitudinal, and **(c)** oblique (tilted 35° relative to the axial plane).

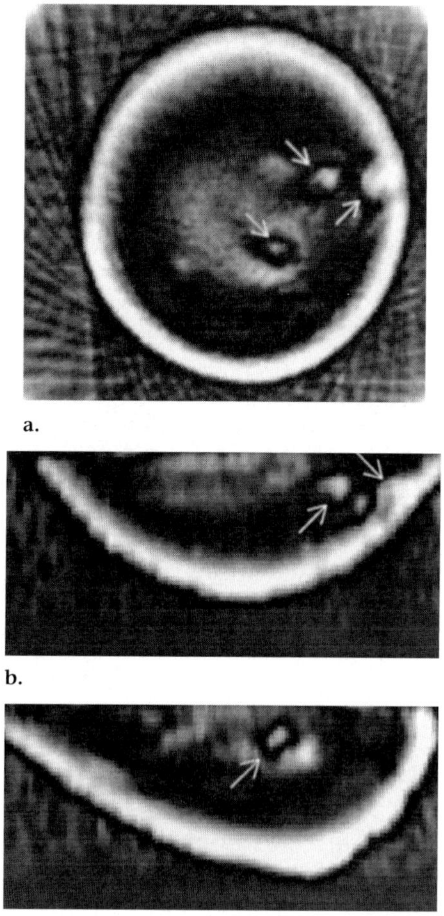

a. b. c.

Figure 4. Breast biopsy phantom. Spiral reconstructions, obtained with 16 spirals and 5-mm pitch, consist of 128 × 128 × 64 voxels of 1.4 × 1.4 × 1.25 mm. Abnormal tissue targets (arrows) are clearly visible. **(a)** Coronal cross section 10 (of 64). **(b)** Axial cross section 56 (of 128). **(c)** Sagittal cross section 80 (of 128).

relatively higher attenuation coefficients (ie, high gray level) and a dark corona (presumably a diffraction effect). The same two observers detected the targets by consensus. For validation, the phantom was also scanned manually by a third observer with a conventional ultrasonic scanner (Synergy-B; Diasonics, Israel) with a 3.5-MHz transducer in the B-scan mode.

Reproducibility of Data Acquisition

The reproducibility of the system in acquiring the data required for image reconstruction was also evaluated. The system was given a reset command and the transducers moved to their home position. Then the system was ordered to acquire a single acoustic projection of the breast phantom with coordinates arbitrarily set by the user. The acquired data were stored on the computer disk. The procedure (ie, a reset command followed by an acquisition command) was repeated several times. Finally, the correlation coefficients between 10 pairs of these acoustic projections (acquired from the same location of the breast phantom) were calculated by using a library function (MATLAB; Math Works, Natick, Mass). A high correlation coefficient indicates high reproducibility.

Results

Spiral Ultrasonic CT versus Conventional Ultrasonic CT

Plasticine spherical target.—The cross sections of the plasticine sphere obtained with conventional ultrasonic CT are displayed in Figure 2a. Note that the second section was deliberately positioned to obtain a cross-sectional image of the upper part of the sphere; clearly, the sphere would not have been detected if the section position were changed slightly. On the other hand, spiral ultrasonic CT scans the entire volume, which can produce a large number of cross sections. The number of cross sections reconstructed in this case was arbitrarily set at 16. Four reconstructed cross sections passing through the sphere (covering the slab marked by the dashed lines in the schematic) are depicted in Figure 2b. Note that the sphere is clearly depicted.

Hard-boiled egg phantom.—Axial, longitudinal, and oblique (35° relative to the axial plane) cross sections of the hard-boiled egg obtained from the reconstructed spiral ultrasonic CT data are depicted in Figure 3. As can be noted, the structure of the egg is clearly visible in all the cross-sectional images. However, the longitudinal cross section is blurred and inferior in quality relative to the axial cross section. This may be attributed to the large helical pitch chosen.

Breast biopsy phantom.—The abnormal tissue–mimicking targets were clearly depicted on the spiral ultrasonic CT reconstruction of the breast phantom. Coronal, axial, and sagittal cross-sectional images of the volumetric reconstruction depicting the abnormal tissue targets are given in Figure 4. The general orientations of the targets depicted in Figure 4 were confirmed with an independent B-scan study. On the basis of its volumetric nature, spiral ultrasonic CT allowed production of a 3D object that can be displayed in various modes. To further demonstrate the volumetric nature of the reconstruction, the boundaries of the breast phantom were semiautomatically traced, and a 3D computer rendering (Fig 5) was obtained. The breast phantom was virtually cut about 10 mm from its base to enable a look inside at its lesions. Furthermore, it should be noted that with use of a dynamic computer display mode, it is also possible to move virtually through the imaged breast and study its internal structure more closely.

Reproducibility of Data Acquisition

Correlation coefficients were calculated between 10 pairs of acoustic projections acquired in the same location of the breast phantom on different scans. The mean correlation coefficient was 0.9976 (range, 0.9972–0.9980), indicating high reproducibility for data acquisition.

Discussion

The feasibility of imaging with spiral ultrasonic CT was verified in this study. The ability to obtain 3D reconstructions of selected objects by measuring the through transmitted acoustic waves with spiral ultrasonic CT was demonstrated experimentally. This method may provide an additional imaging tool to the practicing radiologist.

Spiral ultrasonic CT offers several advantages. The first stems from the inherent properties of the ultrasonic modality, which is considered hazardless and relatively cost-effective. This implies applicability to mass screening and potential use in clinics and hospitals.

The second advantage is derived from the information provided by the ultrasonic CT images. Although the commonly used pulse-echo techniques have been very useful in depicting breast cysts (1,2), their ability to differentiate solid masses is limited (2). On the other hand, analyses based on speed of sound (23,24) and acoustic attenuation have demonstrated clinical potential (eg, Scherzinger et al [25] achieved approximately 90% sensitivity and specificity in depicting breast cancer with ultrasonic CT).

In addition, spiral ultrasonic CT offers the main advantage provided by x-ray spiral CT, which is a volumetric coverage of the object with an efficient scan. Volumetric imaging also offers better diagnostic potential over conventional two-dimensional imaging. This property was demonstrated in our study for the spherical target and the egg and breast phantoms. As shown in Figure 2, spiral ultrasonic CT depicted the spherical target that conventional ultrasonic CT may have missed. Furthermore, the 3D reconstructions obtained for the egg and breast phantoms enabled the display of arbitrarily oriented cross sections, as depicted in Figures 3 and 4, respectively. In addition, by using a dynamic display, the diagnostic physician could virtually move through the object and locate the lesions. Finally, with the 3D display of the breast (Fig 5), the surgeon could obtain a more realistic orientation and possibly design a better surgical intervention.

However, spiral ultrasonic CT also has several disadvantages that should be noted. Owing to the facts that through transmission is required and ultrasonic waves can barely penetrate the bones and the lungs, spiral ultrasonic CT is limited almost exclusively to the breast. Moreover, axillary regions of the breast or regions very proximal to the ribs cannot be imaged with this technique. Hence, spiral ultrasonic CT must be coupled with the standard pulse-echo technique. In addition, the major disadvantage of x-ray spiral CT also applies here. As a result of the interpolation between data acquired at different heights (relative to the spiral axis), the effective section profile is substantially increased (twice the spiral pitch [19–21]). Consequently, if the spiral pitch is large, notable blurring may occur along the longitudinal direction. This was demonstrated on the longitudinal cross-sectional images obtained in the egg (Fig 3). Optimization between the desired section sensitivity profile and the width of the pitch might give better results for a given imaged object.

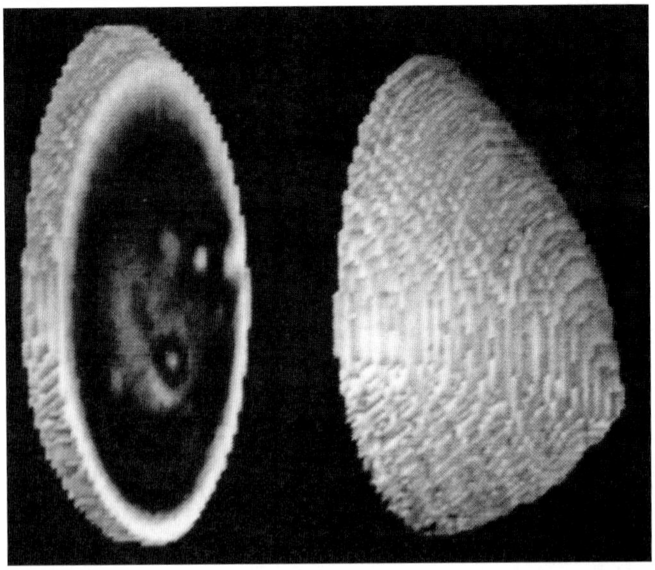

Figure 5. Breast biopsy phantom. On the 3D computer rendering, the phantom was virtually cut about 10 mm from its base to enable a look inside at its lesions. This type of presentation may provide a better orientation to the physician and may help plan more effective surgical procedures.

In addition, several limitations of the present study should be pointed out. For computational simplicity, we ignored diffraction effects. This assumption is not entirely valid. A more accurate model should also account for diffraction effects. An algorithm that accounts for diffraction effects, such as the filtered back-propagation algorithm suggested by Devaney (15), might produce more accurate reconstructions. However, this algorithm is computationally much more intensive. Furthermore, Schreiman et al (26) have already demonstrated that clinically valuable images of the breast can be obtained with ultrasonic CT by means of a straight line model. As the objective of this study was merely to demonstrate feasibility, we chose to implement the simpler model.

A second simplification was to ignore the dependency of the attenuation coefficient on the frequency. A more accurate approach would be to apply spectral analysis to the signals. Alternatively, one can assume a linear relation between the attenuation coefficients and the frequency and can implement one of the methods reviewed by Kak and Slaney (14).

Finally, it should be pointed out that although attenuation tomograms were obtained in this study, with a slight modification (ie, measuring time of flight instead of wave amplitude), tomograms depicting speed of sound distribution may be produced. This acoustic parameter (ie, speed of sound) has been shown to provide valuable clinical information (23,24).

In conclusion, findings in this study demonstrate that spiral ultrasonic CT is feasible. This imaging method may find clinical application as a breast screening tool.

Appendix

The interpolation method applied in this study is based on the method presented by Bresler and Skrabacz (17) and Ruimi (18). With this approach, the spiral data set in the projection domain is first converted (resampled) by means of interpolation into a set of planar Radon transforms. Then, application of a conventional two-dimensional reconstruction algorithm to each plane yields a set of parallel cross sections.

In spiral CT, the position, z, along the spiral axis and the angle, θ_P, at which the projection is acquired, are linearly related by

$$\theta(z) = \theta_P = (2\pi \cdot z/D) \bmod 2\pi,$$

where D is the spiral pitch.

To resample the spiral projections into a set of parallel Radon planes, the z value of each desired plane is first set. By using this relation, three consecutive projections (previous [prev], current [cur], and next) are selected that were acquired at different heights (z values) but correspond to the same angle. Then, the weighted average of these projections is calculated by

$$P(\theta) = w_{\text{prev}} \cdot P_{\text{prev}}(\theta) + w_{\text{cur}} \cdot P_{\text{cur}}(\theta) + w_{\text{next}} \cdot P_{\text{next}}(\theta).$$

The weights, w, for $0 \le \theta \le \theta_P$ are given by

$$\begin{cases} w_{\text{prev}}(\theta) = 0 \\ w_{\text{cur}}(\theta) = 1 + [(\theta - \theta_P)/2\pi] \\ w_{\text{next}}(\theta) = -[(\theta - \theta_P)/2\pi], \end{cases}$$

and for $\theta_P \le \theta \le 2\pi$ are given by

$$\begin{cases} w_{\text{prev}}(\theta) = [(\theta - \theta_P)/2\pi] \\ w_{\text{cur}}(\theta) = 1 - [(\theta - \theta_P)/2\pi] \\ w_{\text{next}}(\theta) = 0. \end{cases}$$

The resultant vector $\boldsymbol{P}(\theta)$ is the new resampled projection at angle θ. The procedure is repeated to cover all θ values from 0 to π, and the filtered backprojection is applied to reconstruct the corresponding section (at the desired height z).

References

1. Cardenosa G. Breast imaging companion. 2nd ed. Philadelphia, Pa: Lippincott-Raven, 1997.
2. Jokich PM, Monticciolo DL, Adler YT. Breast ultrasonography. Radiol Clin North Am 1992; 30:993–1009.
3. Vilaro MM, Kurtz AB, Needleman L, et al. Hand-held and automated sonomammography: clinical role relative to x-ray mammography. Ultrasound Med 1989; 8:95–100.
4. Greenleaf JF, Johnson SA, Lee SL, Herman GT, Wood EH. Algebraic reconstruction of spatial distributions of acoustic absorption within tissue from their two-dimensional acoustic projections. In: Green PS, ed. Acoustical holography. New York, NY: Plenum, 1974; 5:966–972.
5. Glover GH, Sharp JC. Reconstruction of ultrasound propagation speed distributions in soft tissue: time-of-flight tomography. IEEE Trans Sonics Ultrasonics 1977; 24:229–234.
6. Richard AR. Three-dimensional biomedical imaging. In: Robinson BS, Greenleaf JF, eds. Computerized ultrasound tomography. Boca Raton, Fla: CRC, 1985; 2:57–78.
7. Jackson VP. The role of US in breast imaging. Radiology 1990; 177:305–311.
8. Greenleaf JF, Bahn RC. Clinical imaging with transmissive ultrasonic computerized tomography. IEEE Trans Biomed Eng 1981; 28:177–185.
9. Greenleaf JF, Ylitalo J, Gisvold JJ. Ultrasonic computed tomography breast examination. IEEE Eng Med Biol 1987; 27: 27–32.
10. Kalender WA, Vock P, Seissler W. Spiral CT scanning for fast and continuous volume data acquisition: advances in CT. Heidelberg, Germany: Springer-Verlag, 1990; 55–64.
11. Heiken JP, Brink JA, Vannier MW. Spiral (helical) CT. Radiology 1993; 189:647–656.
12. Kalender WA. Technical foundations of spiral CT. Semin Ultrasound CT MRI 1994; 15:81–89.
13. Parker JA. Image reconstruction in radiology. Boca Raton, Fla: CRC,1991.
14. Kak AC, Slaney M. Principles of computerized tomographic imaging. New York, NY: Institute of Electrical and Electronic Engineers, 1987.
15. Devaney AJ. A filtered backpropagation algorithm for diffraction tomography. Ultrason Imaging 1982; 5:336–350.
16. Azhari H, Stolarski S. Hybrid ultrasonic computed tomography. Comput Biomed Res 1997; 30:35–48.
17. Bresler Y, Skrabacz CJ. Optimal interpolation in helical scan 3D computerized tomography. IEEE Int Conf Acoust Speech Signal Process 1989; 3:1427–1425.
18. Ruimi D. Study of computed tomography with simultaneous patient translation on a multiple slice scanner. Dissertation. Department of Biomedical Engineering, Tel Aviv University, Israel, 1994.
19. Kalender WA, Polacin A. Physical performance characteristics of spiral CT scanning. Med Phys 1991; 18:910–915.
20. Polacin A, Kalender WA, Marchal G. Evaluation of section sensitivity profiles and image noise in spiral CT. Radiology 1992; 185:29–35.
21. Wang G, Vannier MW. Helical CT image noise: analytical results. Med Phys 1993; 20:1635–1640.
22. Wang G, Vannier MW. Longitudinal resolution in volumetric x-ray computerized tomography: analytical comparison between conventional and helical computerized tomography. Med Phys 1994; 21: 429–433.
23. Richter K, Heywang-Kobrunner SH. Sonographic differentiation of benign from malignant breast lesions: value of indirect measurement of ultrasound velocity. AJR 1995; 165:825–831.
24. Edmonds PD, Mortensen CL, Hill JR, et al. Ultrasound tissue characterization of breast biopsy specimens. Ultrason Imaging 1991; 13:162–185.
25. Scherzinger AL, Belgam RA, Carson PL, et al. Assessment of ultrasonic computed tomography in symptomatic breast patients by discriminant analysis. Ultrasound Med Biol 1989; 15:21–28.
26. Schreiman JS, Gisvold JJ, Greenleaf JF, Bahn RC. Ultrasound computed tomography of the breast. Radiology 1984; 150: 523–530.

Emanuele Neri, MD
Davide Caramella, MD
Fabio Falaschi, MD
Paola Sbragia, MD
Claudio Vignali, MD
Edoardo Laiolo, MD
Adriano Viviani, MD
Carlo Bartolozzi, MD

Virtual CT Intravascular Endoscopy of the Aorta: Pierced Surface and Floating Shape Thresholding Artifacts[1]

Index terms:
Aorta, CT, 56.12115, 56.12116, 56.12117
Aortography, virtual, 56.12117
Computed tomography (CT), image display and recording, 56.12116, 56.12117
Computed tomography (CT), three-dimensional, 56.12117

Radiology 1999; 212:276–279

[1] From the Department of Oncology, Diagnostic and Interventional Radiology, University of Pisa, Via Roma 67, I-56100 Pisa, Italy. Received December 15, 1997; revision requested March 2, 1998; final revision received November 6; accepted January 19, 1999. **Address reprint requests to** E.N. (e-mail: *neri@do.med.unipi.it*).

Author contributions:
Guarantors of integrity of entire study, E.N., D.C., C.B.; study concepts, E.N., D.C., C.B.; study design, E.N., D.C.; definition of intellectual content, E.N., D.C.; literature research, E.L., A.V.; clinical studies, E.N., D.C., F.F., P.S., C.V.; data acquisition, E.N., D.C., F.F., P.S., C.V.; data analysis, E.N.; statistical analysis, E.N.; manuscript preparation, E.N., D.C.; manuscript editing and review, E.N., D.C., C.B.

Two types of artifacts may appear in virtual computed tomographic endoscopic views of the aorta rendered at different threshold levels: pierced surface and floating shape artifacts. A positive correlation was found between mean attenuation of the aorta and the threshold levels at which these artifacts appeared. The correlation was statistically significant ($0.71 \leq r \leq 0.86$) for floating shape. An artifact-free threshold range can be predicted on the basis of aortic enhancement.

Virtual computed tomographic (CT) endoscopy, an imaging technique performed by means of internal rendering of CT and magnetic resonance (MR) data sets, has been used to create endoscopic views of the bronchial tree (1–5), colon (6,7), vessels (8–12), ear (13,14), and biliary (15,16) and urinary (17) tracts.

Two virtual CT endoscopic techniques have been developed on the basis of surface and volume rendering. With volume rendering, a continuous attenuation table is applied that allows individual voxels to be visualized with variable transparency. With surface rendering, image data are segmented on the basis of two levels of attenuation—low threshold and high threshold—that allow rendering of the voxels within that range. The operation results in a binary data set. As a result of correct segmentation with surface rendering, virtual CT intravascular endoscopy generates smoothed internal walls of a vessel with an empty lumen, which is assumed to be the normal pattern (8–12).

The segmentation threshold required to generate surface models influences the quality of endoscopic views. Furthermore, as reported in recent experiences with MR data sets, incorrect segmentation causes the appearance of artifacts on the rendered images (9). These artifacts, defined as "floating shape," were interpreted as dark voxels mistakenly rendered as distinct objects within the lumen because the selected attenuation range did not include them.

Herein, we describe a different type of artifact, which consists of voxels mistakenly not rendered in the reconstructed image. Thus, the presence of a hole is simulated in the vessel wall. We called this a "pierced surface" artifact.

Since spiral CT data sets require a preliminary threshold-based segmentation, our purpose was to study the presence and pattern of artifacts arising from this kind of segmentation. We also sought to determine any correlation between the threshold levels at which artifacts can be observed and the contrast enhancement achieved inside the aorta.

Materials and Methods

We retrospectively reviewed the imaging data sets obtained at spiral CT (HiSpeed Advantage; GE Medical Systems, Milwaukee, Wis) in 45 patients (22 men and 23 women; age range, 25–76 years; mean age, 63 years) who underwent evaluation of the abdominal (29 cases) or thoracic (16 cases) aorta. All patients underwent scanning with the same acquisition protocol. The abdominal aorta was scanned in the cephalocaudal direction during a single breath hold starting just above the superior mesenteric artery (beam collimation, 3 mm; pitch, 1; table incremental speed, 3 mm/sec; tube rotation, 1 second; tube current, 250–280 mA with 120 kVp; field of view, 30–35 cm). Acquisition time was 25–30 seconds, and the total scanning length was 75–90 mm. The thoracic aorta was scanned in the cephalocaudal direction during a single breath hold from the aortic arch to the diaphragm (beam collimation, 5 mm; pitch, 1.0–1.5; table incremental speed, 5.0–7.5 mm/sec; tube views of surface-rendered anatomic structures. Segmentation is performed by using low and high thresholds. With this method, all the voxels excluded from the selected range of Hounsfield units are considered by the system as not belonging to the object, and, subsequently, they are not rendered. To generate the surface from the segmented voxel, the software uses the marching cube algorithm. With this approach, the voxels of the volume edges are transformed into a smooth surface of triangles or patches (18).

Virtual CT intravascular endoscopic perspectives are created by simulating the conic view of fiberoptic endoscopy, and the field of view can range from 15° to 60°.

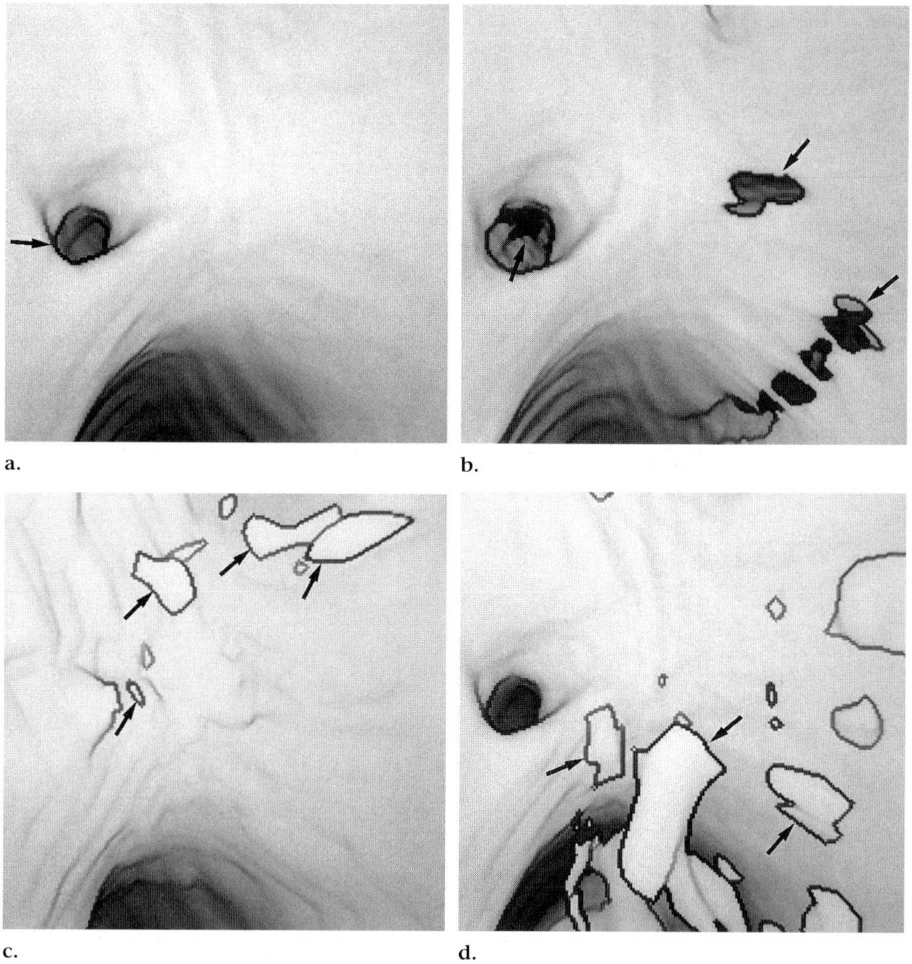

Figure 1. Virtual CT intravascular endoscopic images of the abdominal aorta show the internal surface at the level of the ostium (arrow in **a**) of the right renal artery. **(a)** Field of view, 60°; low threshold, 200 HU; high threshold, 500 HU. No artifacts are visible. **(b)** Low threshold, 120 HU; high threshold, 500 HU. The low-threshold pierced surface artifacts appear as holes through the aortic and renal artery walls (right arrows and left arrow, respectively). **(c)** Low threshold, 240 HU; high threshold, 500 HU. The low-threshold floating shape artifacts (arrows) appear inside the aortic lumen. The threshold level excludes the ostium of the right renal artery from the rendered data set. **(d)** Low threshold, 200 HU; high threshold, 350 HU. Low-threshold pierced surface and floating shape artifacts are not present. The ostium of the right renal artery is visible, but high-threshold floating shape artifacts (arrows) are visible inside the lumen.

current, 250–280 mA with 120 kVp; field of view, 30–35 cm).

In all cases, a volume of 150 mL of iohexol (300 mg of iodine per milliliter) (Omnipaque 300; Nycomed Imaging, Oslo, Norway) was administered with a power injector (MCT/MCT Plus; Medrad, Indianola, Pa) via the antecubital vein with a flow rate of 3 mL/sec. To select the scanning delay, the circulation time was determined by means of a dynamic scanning test with use of a semiautomatic bolus tracking program (SMARTPREP; GE Medical Systems). To measure the aortic peak, a circularly shaped region of interest was traced within the aortic lumen at the level of the arch in the thorax or the renal arteries in the abdomen. To avoid artifacts in the three-dimensional model, no oral contrast agent was administered.

All axial images were reconstructed with 180° linear interpolation at 1-mm spacing by using a standard reconstruction algorithm. Spatial resolution of sections was $512 \times 512 \times 12$ bits (384 kbytes of memory). The total number of images reconstructed for each study ranged between 75 and 90 images (28.0–33.8 Mbytes).

Image Processing and Display

Spiral CT data sets were surface rendered by using software (NAVIGATOR; GE Medical Systems) on a workstation (SunSparc 20; Sun Microsystems, Mountain View, Calif). The software allows users to display internal

Image Analysis

Three radiologists (C.V. and others) independently reviewed the virtual CT intravascular endoscopic images created from inside the aorta at the level of the renal arteries or aortic arch. These images simulated visualization of renal artery ostia, including the tract of the aorta 3 cm above and below the ostia (abdominal aorta), or of all epiaortic branch ostia (thoracic aorta). The observers were required to determine if the artifacts appeared as a result of manipulating the low- and high-threshold levels during rendering. In particular, a floating shape artifact was defined as data that should not have been present within the lumen that were mistakenly rendered. A pierced surface artifact was defined as parietal voxel data that were mistakenly not rendered, thus simulating a hole.

For this determination, the low and high thresholds were progressively changed, in steps of 10 HU, from 0 to 500 HU and from 500 to 0 HU, respectively, to detect alterations in the aortic internal surface and the presence of floating shape inside the lumen. Agreement was considered to occur when at least two observers agreed concerning the threshold level at which artifacts started to appear. Agreement was considered a difference of 1–10 HU and disagreement a difference of more than 10 HU.

All evaluations were performed at the workstation, and no time limits were imposed.

Statistical Analysis

To evaluate aortic enhancement on axial images, a histogram was originated from data in a circularly shaped region of interest within the aorta at the level of the renal arteries (abdominal aorta) or aortic arch (thoracic aorta). Maximum, minimum, and mean attenuation values were calculated directly with the software.

Data series were processed with software (STATVIEW; Abacus Concepts, Berkeley, Calif). Mean attenuation values were calculated for low and high thresholds of artifact

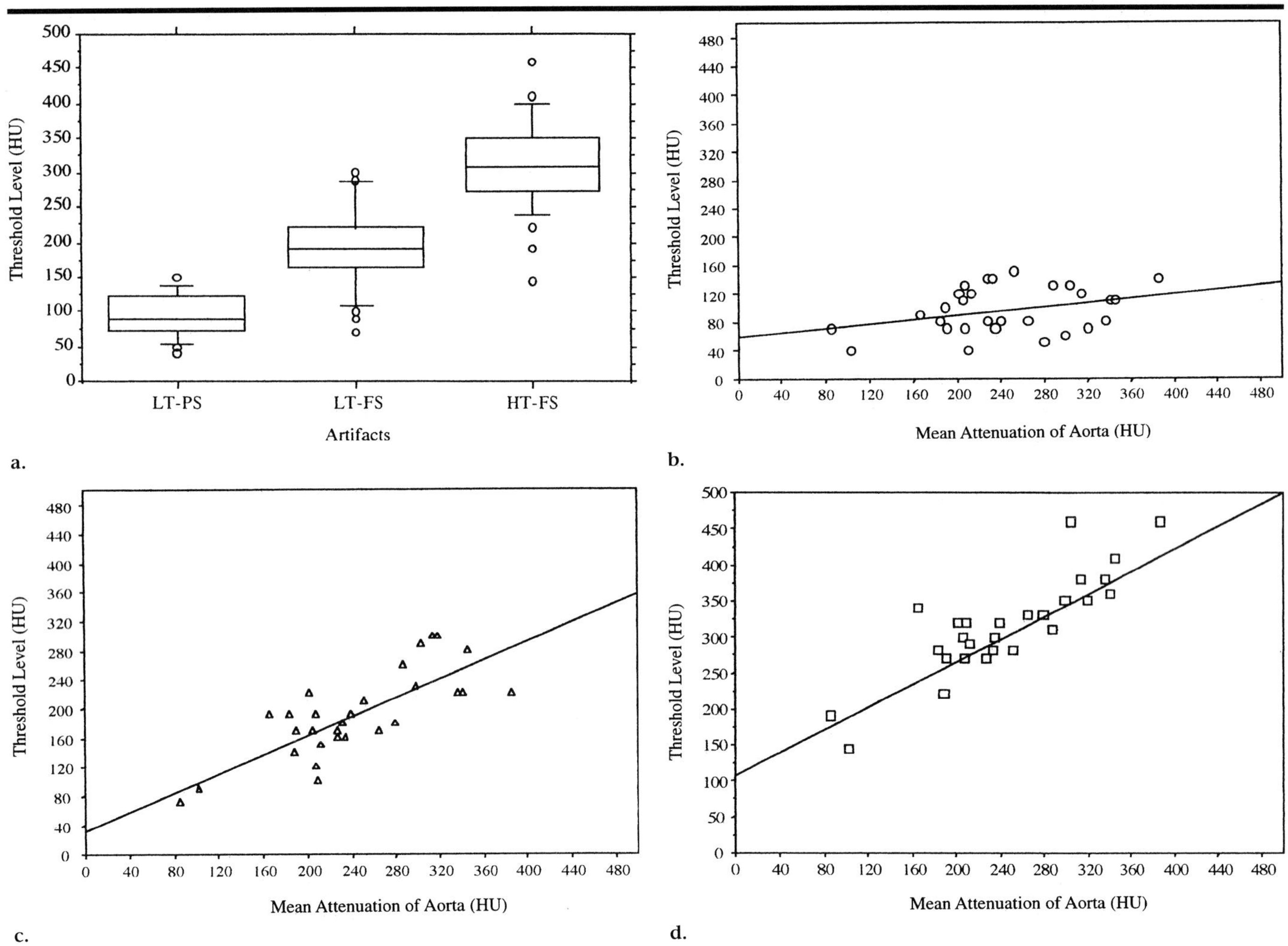

Figure 2. Artifacts observed at virtual CT intravascular endoscopy in the abdominal aorta. **(a)** Box plots compare threshold levels for low-threshold pierced surface (*LT-PS*) artifacts (range, 40–150 HU; mean, 95.862 ± 32.129), low-threshold floating shape (*LT-FS*) artifacts (range, 70–300 HU; mean, 191.034 ± 59.121), and high-threshold floating shape (*HT-FS*) artifacts (range, 145–460 HU; mean, 312.241 ± 69.018). Upper and lower margins of box plots represent the 75th and 25th percentiles, respectively. The median is the line bisecting the box. Error bars represent SD. ○ = outliers. **(b)** Linear regression analysis shows a not statistically significant correlation between mean attenuation value and low-threshold pierced surface artifact ($r = 0.325$, $P = .086$). **(c)** Scattergram shows a positive and good ($r > 0.7$) correlation between mean attenuation and low-threshold floating shape artifacts ($r = 0.77$, $P = .001$). **(d)** Scattergram shows the same correlation between mean attenuation and high-threshold floating shape artifacts ($r = 0.86$, $P = .001$).

appearance and for the geometric mean, maximum, minimum, and SD. The ranges were calculated between maximum and minimum values and between low and high thresholds.

Linear regression analysis was performed to investigate the correlation between the mean attenuation value and the low or high thresholds at which artifacts appeared. A correlation coefficient (*r*) greater than 0.7 was considered indicative of good correlation. A *P* value less than .05 (95% CI) was considered indicative of a statistically significant difference.

Results

The scanning delay for the thoracic aorta ranged between 17 and 27 seconds (22.1 seconds ± 3.3 [mean ± SD]; range, 10 seconds) and for the abdominal aorta, between 18 and 32 seconds (23.1 seconds ± 4.5; range, 14 seconds). The mean attenuation inside the thoracic aorta ranged between 73 and 420 HU (280.3 HU ± 63.5; range, 347 HU) and for the abdominal aorta, between 86 and 387 HU (243.6 HU ± 70.4; range, 301 HU). Intraluminal contrast was heterogeneous. All histograms showed a Gaussian distribution, with the majority of voxels grouped in the center of the curve, close to the mean attenuation value.

Virtual CT intravascular endoscopic images of the aorta showed a smoothed internal surface with an empty lumen (Fig 1a). At specific attenuation values, variations in the low and high thresholds influenced the rendering pattern and determined the appearance of the two types of artifacts. Agreement between observers was reached in 91% (41 of 45) of the cases. In the remaining 9% (four cases), disagreement was due to the adoption of different conic fields of view. However, correction of the field of view allowed complete agreement.

The first type of artifact—pierced surface—appeared after variations in the low threshold. This artifact caused the pierced appearance of the internal surface of the vessels, with scattered holes visible at any viewing angle (Fig 1b).

The second type of artifact—floating shape—appeared inside the lumen after variations in both the low and high thresholds (Fig 1c, 1d).

Linear regression analysis was performed to correlate mean attenuation with the appearance of artifacts. For floating shape artifacts on abdominal aorta studies, a positive and statistically significant correlation ($r > 0.7$) was found between mean attenuation and both the low ($r = 0.77$, $P = .001$) and high ($r = 0.86$, $P = .001$) thresholds. For pierced surface artifacts on abdominal aorta studies, a positive correlation was found between mean attenuation and the low threshold, but the correlation was not statistically significant ($r = 0.325$, $P = .086$) (Fig 2).

For floating shape artifacts on thoracic aorta studies, a positive and statistically significant correlation was found between mean attenuation and both the low ($r = 0.71$, $P = .001$) and high ($r = 0.78$, $P = .001$) thresholds. For pierced surface artifacts on thoracic aorta studies, a positive correlation was found between mean attenuation and the low threshold, but the correlation was not statistically significant ($r = 0.43$, $P = .072$).

Discussion

Rendering artifacts have been described in a previous article (9) concerning virtual intravascular endoscopy with MR angiographic data sets. Those authors described the floating shape as low-signal-intensity voxels mistakenly rendered as distinct objects within the lumen. These artifacts were the result of flow turbulence detected at MR angiography.

A similar hypothesis can be made for virtual intravascular endoscopy with CT angiographic data sets. In fact, we may expect that the inhomogeneity of attenuation values of enhanced blood is the cause of the appearance of floating shape. In our study, the threshold levels at which floating shape started to appear showed a positive and statistically significant correlation with aortic enhancement. This proves that if the mean attenuation of the aorta increases, the threshold values at which low- and high-threshold floating shape artifacts start to be observed also increase.

Conversely, to our knowledge, pierced surface artifacts have not been previously reported. We believe that these artifacts are caused by inherent difficulties in separating the hyperattenuating voxels at the periphery of the lumen from surrounding structures by means of this thresholding technique. Consequently, these voxels are not rendered, and holes through the surface of the aorta are simulated. Additional causes that may be involved in the generation of pierced surface artifacts are the existence of peripheral flow turbulences, irregularities of vascular walls, and the vicinity of the wall to hyperattenuating structures such as the renal vein, superior vena cava, or vertebral bodies.

Contrast enhancement of the aorta is the most important factor that enables determination of the threshold levels at which artifacts start to be observed. In our study, we demonstrated that the threshold levels at which low- and high-threshold floating shape started to appear increased with mean attenuation. In contrast, the threshold levels for low-threshold pierced surface artifacts increased with the mean attenuation of the aorta, although the correlation did not reach statistical significance. By comparing the slopes of the regression lines shown in the graphs concerning the appearance of the low-threshold pierced surface (Fig 2b), low-threshold floating shape (Fig 2c), and high-threshold floating shape (Fig 2d) artifacts, we can appreciate that the artifact-free threshold range is larger for higher mean attenuation of the aorta. This observation suggests that the degree of aortic attenuation is an important factor in the performance of high-quality virtual CT intravascular endoscopy. In turn, aortic attenuation depends on the type of contrast medium, the flow rate, the correct selection of the scanning delay, and the possibility of performing the examination during a single breath hold. In some situations, however, use of the guidelines described herein is not entirely feasible, such as in emergency patients (no time for a circulation time test, reduced respiratory capacity), in patients with difficult venous access (flow rate must be reduced to less than 3 mL/sec), and in patients with pathologic conditions in the aorta that are capable of creating flow turbulence (stenosis, aneurysm, rupture). We did not investigate any of these difficult cases, but we suspect that the correlation between mean attenuation and threshold levels of artifacts might be altered in these situations. Another issue to be considered concerns variations in the attenuation of blood at different levels in the aorta. This stresses the importance of choosing the appropriate scanning delay to obtain an optimal distribution of the contrast material at the selected aortic tract.

In conclusion, knowledge about segmentation pitfalls can help avoid the appearance of artifacts on virtual CT intravascular endoscopic images, thus preventing wrong interpretations of endoluminal findings. We believe that floating shape and pierced surface artifacts have a negative effect on the diagnostic performance of virtual CT intravascular endoscopy, and more studies are needed to investigate the clinical implications of these artifacts. However, the artifacts described herein are probably related to our threshold-based selection of voxels. In the future, it must be ascertained whether the appearance of artifacts can be prevented by using more sophisticated segmentation methods.

References

1. Vining DJ, Shifrin RY, Haponik EF, Liu K, Choplin RH. Virtual bronchoscopy (abstr). Radiology 1994; 193(P):261.
2. Rubin GD, Beaulieu CF, Argiro V, et al. Perspective volume rendering of CT and MR images: applications for endoscopic imaging. Radiology 1996; 199:321–330.
3. Lacrosse M, Trigaux JP, Van Beers BE, Weynants P. 3D spiral CT of the tracheobronchial tree. J Comput Assist Tomogr 1995; 19:341–347.
4. Buthiau D, Antoine E, Piette JC, Nizri D, Baldeyrou P, Khayat D. Virtual tracheobronchial endoscopy: educational and diagnostic value. Surg Radiol Anat 1996; 18:125–131.
5. Rodenwaldt J, Kopka L, Roedel R, Grabbe E. Three-dimensional surface imaging of the larynx and trachea by spiral CT: virtual endoscopy. ROFO 1996; 165:80–83.
6. Hara AK, Johnson CD, Reed JE, Lehman RL, Ilstrup DM. Colorectal polyp detection with CT colography: two- versus three-dimensional techniques—work in progress. Radiology 1996; 200:49–54.
7. Luboldt W, Steiner P, Bauerfeind P, Plelkonen P, Debatin JF. Detection of mass lesions with MR colonography: preliminary report. Radiology 1998; 207:59–65.
8. Davis CP, Ladd ME, Gohde SC, Pfammatter T, Fass L, Debatin JF. Virtual intravascular endoscopy in the renal arteries: a new way of observing 3-D-MIR angiography data sets. ROFO 1996; 165:257–263.
9. Davis CP, Ladd ME, Romanowski BJ, Wildermuth S, Knoplioch JF, Debatin JF. Human aorta: preliminary results with virtual endoscopy based on three-dimensional MR imaging data sets. Radiology 1996; 199:37–40.
10. Kimura F, Shen Y, Date S, Mochizuki T. Thoracic aortic aneurysm and aortic dissection: new endoscopic mode for three-dimensional CT display of the aorta. Radiology 1996; 198:573–578.
11. Hayashi H, Kobayashi H, Kumazaki T, Goto Y. Virtual CT endoscopy "cruising eye view": development and clinical applications. Nippon Igaku Hoshasen Gakkai Zasshi 1996; 56:135–136.
12. Bartolozzi C, Neri E, Caramella D. CT in vascular pathologies. Eur Radiol 1998; 8:679–684.
13. Neri E, Battolla L, Bartolozzi C, et al. Virtual human otoscopy of spiral CT data sets (abstr). Radiology 1997; 205(P):695.
14. Frankenthaler RP. Virtual otoscopy. Otolaryngol Clin North Am 1998; 31:383–392.
15. Dubno B, Luboldt WW, Schmidt M, McKinnon GC, Krestin GP, Debatin JF. Virtual endoscopy in MR-cholangiopancreaticography (MRCP) (abstr). Radiology 1997; 205(P):197.
16. Neri E, Boraschi P, Braccini G, Caramella D, Perri G, Bartolozzi C. MR virtual endoscopy of the pancreaticobiliary tract. Magn Reson Imaging 1999; 17:59–67.
17. Frank R, Stenzl A, Frede T, et al. Three-dimensional computed tomography of the reconstructed lower urinary tract: technique and findings. Eur Radiol 1998; 8:657–663.
18. Lorensen WE, Cline H. Marching cubes: a high resolution 3D surface construction algorithm. Comput Graphics 1987; 21:163–169.

John A. Kaufman, MD
Stuart C. Geller, MD
Hasan Bazari, MD
Arthur C. Waltman, MD

Index terms:
Angiography, contrast media, 566.1245, 80.1248, 982.1245
Venae cavae, angiography, 566.1245, 80.1248, 982.1245
Venography, 566.1245, 80.1248, 982.1245

Radiology 1999; 212:280–284

Abbreviations:
IVC = inferior vena cava
DOTA = tetraazacyclododecane-tetraacetic acid
DSA = digital subtraction angiography
SVC = superior vena cava

[1] From the Division of Vascular Radiology (J.A.K., S.C.G., A.C.W.) and the Department of Medicine, Division of Nephrology (H.B.), Harvard Medical School, Massachusetts General Hospital, GRB 290, 55 Fruit St, Boston, MA 02114. Received April 30, 1998; revision requested July 6; revision received August 18; accepted December 15. **Address reprint requests to** J.A.K. (e-mail: *kaufmanfamily@sprintmail.com*).

Author contributions:
Guarantor of integrity of entire study, J.A.K.; study concepts and design, J.A.K.; definition of intellectual content, all authors; literature research, J.A.K.; clinical studies, all authors; data acquisition, J.A.K.; data analysis, all authors; statistical analysis, J.A.K.; manuscript preparation and editing, J.A.K.; manuscript review, all authors.

Gadolinium-based Contrast Agents as an Alternative at Vena Cavography in Patients with Renal Insufficiency—Early Experience[1]

The authors reviewed results of digital subtraction vena cavography with a gadolinium-based contrast agent in 14 patients with serum creatinine levels greater than or equal to 1.5 mg/dL (133 µmol/L). All cavograms were diagnostic. In 11 patients, there was no impairment of renal function. In three patients, a rise in serum creatinine level of greater than or equal to 0.5 mg/dL (44 µmol/L) was attributable to concurrent medical problems. Gadolinium-based contrast agents may be suitable for digital subtraction vena cavography in patients with renal insufficiency.

Invasive imaging of the vena cava is usually performed with iodinated contrast agents. In patients with renal insufficiency (serum creatinine level, ≥1.5 mg/dL [133 µmol/L]), an alternative contrast agent with a low risk of contrast agent–induced acute renal failure would be desirable. Gaseous CO_2, which has no nephrotoxicity, has been used as a contrast agent for inferior vena cavography (1,2). Care must be exercised when preparing CO_2 for injection, as it indistinguishable from room air. Injection rates are difficult to control because CO_2 must be injected by hand unless a power injector is available. Invasive imaging of the vena cava without any contrast agent is possible with intravascular ultrasonography, but this requires use of specialized equipment (3). A simple to use, readily available alternative contrast agent for procedures in the vena cava would be useful.

In several case reports, the application of gadolinium-based magnetic resonance (MR) imaging contrast agents for digital subtraction angiography (DSA) has been described (4–6). These contrast agents appear to have little clinical nephrotoxicity (4–8). In this study, we used gadolinium-based contrast agents for diagnostic and interventional procedures in the vena cava. To our knowledge, this application of gadolinium-based contrast agents has not been reported previously.

Materials and Methods

From July 1996 through March 1998, 14 patients (six men, eight women; age range, 37–86 years; mean age, 66 years ± 17 [SD]) with serum creatinine levels greater than or equal to 1.5 mg/dL (133 µmol/L) underwent invasive catheter-based procedures in the vena cava (inferior vena cava [IVC] in 13 patients and superior vena cava [SVC] in one) performed with gadolinium-based contrast agents (gadodiamide, Omniscan, Nycomed, Princeton, NJ, or gadopentetate dimeglumine, Magnevist, Berlex Laboratories, Wayne, NJ) alone (n = 12) or in conjunction with CO_2 (n = 2). The procedures were IVC filter placement in 10 patients, thrombolysis of the IVC in one, and diagnostic studies in three (Table). All filter placements were in patients with documented thromboembolic disease and either contraindications to or failed anticoagulation therapy. During the same time, no patients with elevated serum creatinine levels underwent cavography with CO_2 alone. The gadolinium-based contrast agent used was based on availability in the angiography suite.

In our institution, gadolinium-based contrast agents are routinely used alone or in conjunction with CO_2 as alternative contrast agents for DSA in nonpregnant, nonlactating adult (older than 18 years) patients with a serum creatinine level

Patient Data

Patient No./ Sex/Age (y)	Procedure	Serum Creatinine Level (mg/dL)*	Coexistent Conditions
1/M/77	IVC filter placement	1.8	Multiple trauma
2/F/74	IVC filter placement	2.1	Congestive heart failure, urinary tract infection, renal artery stenosis
3/F/76	IVC filter placement	1.7	Urinary tract infection
4/F/76	IVC filter placement	1.6	Postoperative sepsis, disseminated intravascular coagulation
5/F/86	IVC filter placement	2.1	Multiple trauma
6/F/65	IVC filter placement	3.2	Wegener granulomatosis, multiple organ system failure
7/M/41	IVC filter placement	1.9	Human immunodeficiency virus, sepsis, compartment syndrome
8/M/80	IVC filter placement	2.1	Gastrointestinal bleeding, pneumonia
9/F/59	IVC filter placement	4.3	Pancreatic carcinoma
10/M/82	IVC filter placement	3.4	Chronic obstructive uropathy
11/M/37	Inferior vena cavography	4.5	Liver and kidney transplant
12/F/74	Inferior vena cavography	3.3	Stroke, patent foramen ovale
13/M/49	IVC thrombolysis	4.5	Liver transplant
14/F/45	Superior vena cavography	2.1	SVC stenosis

*Conversion factor, ×88.4 μmol/L.

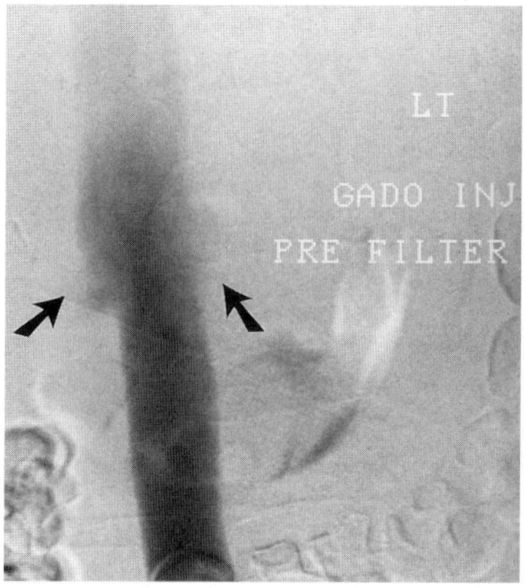

a.

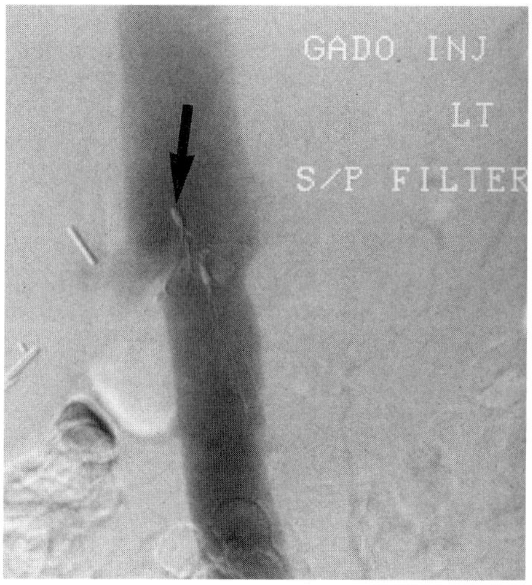

b.

Figure 1. Patient 5. IVC filter placement in an 86-year-old woman with deep venous thrombosis and a closed head injury, with use of diluted gadodiamide (*GADO INJ*) as a contrast agent. *LT* = left. **(a)** Digital subtraction inferior vena cavogram was obtained prior to (*PRE FILTER*) filter placement after injection of gadodiamide diluted 2:1 with normal saline solution at a rate of 15 mL/sec for 2 seconds through a 5-F pigtail catheter positioned at the confluence of the iliac veins. Contrast agent density is adequate. The renal veins (arrows) are readily identified. **(b)** Digital subtraction inferior vena cavogram was obtained through the filter delivery sheath with the same contrast agent and injection rates after placement (*S/P FILTER*) of the filter (arrow).

greater than or equal to 1.5 mg/dL (133 μmol/L) when it is anticipated that only a limited volume of contrast agent will be necessary. The maximum dose of gadolinium-based contrast agent never exceeds 0.4 mmol per kilogram of body weight (0.8 mL/kg), or 60 mL. These are the same guidelines observed in our clinical practice of MR angiography, during which a gadolinium-based contrast agent is injected into a peripheral vein. This dose of gadolinium-based contrast agent for venous injection is not considered investigational in our institution, and thus institutional review board approval was not required.

Written informed consent was obtained prior to all procedures. In 13 patients, a common femoral vein approach was used to place a 5.0–7.1-F pigtail catheter (Cook, Bloomington, Ind) in the infrarenal IVC. The SVC study was performed by injecting the contrast agent through an existing chest port. In 12 cases, gadodiamide (0.3–0.4 mmol/kg) was diluted 2:1 with normal saline solution, usually resulting in 60–80-mL total volume (Fig 1). In two cases, undiluted contrast agent (gadodiamide or gadopentetate dimeglumine) was used (Fig 2). In all cases, the majority of the contrast agent was loaded into a power injector, with approximately 10 mL reserved for test injections by hand. After the operator was satisfied with the position of the catheter, digital subtraction cavography (large focal spot, 70–80 kV) was performed with power injection of 15–20 mL of contrast agent for 1–2 seconds, with acquisition at a rate of 2–6 frames per second. When IVC filters were placed, a completion cavogram was obtained through the filter introducer sheath with use of a similar rate and volume of contrast agent and the same digital subtraction technique.

When CO_2 was used, aliquots of 20–40 mL were injected by hand with use of techniques described previously (1,2). In patient 13, CO_2 was used in conjunction with gadolinium-based contrast agent because multiple injections were performed during catheter positioning. CO_2 was also used in patient 7 because the serum creatinine level was rising acutely, and there seemed to be little advantage to use of a gadolinium-based contrast agent. However, the CO_2 inferior vena cavogram was considered inadequate for planning filter placement, and gadolinium-based contrast agent was then used to obtain a satisfactory study.

During the procedures, all patients underwent monitoring of vital signs, cardiac rhythm, and oxygen saturation, according to routine departmental protocols. The serum creatinine level was measured at 24 and 48 hours after the procedure in all patients, also according to routine protocol for angiography in patients with an abnormal serum creatinine level. Acute renal failure was defined as a rise in serum creatinine level of greater than or equal to 0.5 mg/dL (44 μmol/L) within 48 hours before or after the procedure (9).

Patient charts were reviewed for clinical evidence of acute renal failure (decreased or absent urine output, elevation of serum creatinine level, need for dialysis) within 48 hours before or after the procedure. Concurrent medical and surgical conditions were also recorded.

Results

The mean serum creatinine level the day of the procedure was 2.8 mg/dL ± 1.1

(248 μmol/L ± 97). Patient 13 underwent vena cavography on three successive days during a thrombolysis procedure (total volume of gadodiamide, 130 mL). His data were excluded from the calculation of averages. For the remaining 13 patients, the average serum creatinine level at 48 hours after the procedure was 2.8 mg/dL ± 1.3 (248 μmol/L ± 115). The average volume of gadolinium-based contrast agent was 45 mL ± 11. There were no anaphylactic or other adverse reactions to the gadolinium-based contrast agent.

In eight patients, the serum creatinine level decreased an average of 0.3 mg/dL ± 0.3 (26 μmol/L ± 26) after the procedure. The serum creatinine level increased in six patients at 48 hours, including patient 13. In patients 5, 6, and 11, the rise in creatinine level was less than or equal to 0.3 mg/dL (26 μmol/L). This was not considered evidence of contrast agent–induced renal failure.

A rise in serum creatinine level greater than or equal to 0.5 mg/dL (44 μmol/L) occurred in three patients but was attributed to causes other than the contrast agent in all cases. In patient 2, the rise in creatinine level was 0.5 mg/dL (44 μmol/L). This patient had a history of congestive heart failure, coronary artery disease, a single kidney with a severe proximal renal artery stenosis, and past episodes of azotemia with aggressive diuresis. She was in congestive heart failure with a urinary tract infection and was undergoing aggressive diuresis at the time of the IVC filter placement. In the 24 hours prior to the filter placement, her serum creatinine level had risen slightly. The aggressive diuresis continued following filter placement. The nephrology service evaluated the patient on multiple occasions during her admission and attributed her rise in creatinine level to intravascular volume depletion due to diuresis.

Patient 7 had a rise in creatinine level of 1.3 mg/dL (115 μmol/L) at 48 hours. This immunocompromised patient previously had a normal serum creatinine level. On the day of IVC filter placement, he presented with hypotension, sepsis, phlegmasia cerulea dolens that required emergent surgical intervention, myoglobinuria, and elevated serum creatinine level of 1.9 mg/dL (168 μmol/L). The IVC filter was placed with use of both CO_2 and gadodiamide. The patient remained vasopressor dependent, developed progressive multiple organ system failure, and died after 7 days. His renal failure was considered to be related to hypotension and myoglobinuria.

Patient 13 presented with anuria and IVC thrombosis. The patient had an underlying chronic right renal vein thrombosis that had occurred after liver transplantation. In the 48 hours preceding thrombolysis, his creatinine level had risen from 1.9 to 4.5 mg/dL (from 168 to 398 μmol/L). At the time of initiation of thrombolysis, he was found to have thrombosis of the IVC to the level of the hepatic veins with obstruction of both renal veins. He was studied on three successive days during catheter-directed thrombolysis, each time with CO_2 and 40–50 mL of gadodiamide. At 48 hours after initiation of thrombolysis, he began to urinate, but his creatinine level had risen to 5.5 mg/dL (486 μmol/L). On the third day (at the time his last gadodiamide-enhanced cavogram was obtained), his serum creatinine level decreased to 5.0 mg/dL (442 μmol/L). At 48 hours after acquisition of his last cavogram, his creatinine level further decreased to 4.1 mg/dL (362 μmol/L). His creatinine level returned to baseline over the following week. The nephrology service attributed his rise in creatinine level to mechanical obstruction of the renal veins by thrombus, which was not relieved until the second day of thrombolysis.

In patients 7 and 13, the two patients in whom both CO_2 and gadodiamide were used, the CO_2 was injected first. Gadodiamide was then used because the angiographer performing the study determined that the CO_2 images were unsatisfactory (Fig 2). All gadolinium-enhanced cavograms were considered diagnostic and of satisfactory quality to allow planning of interventions at the time of the procedure. Specifically, the IVC could be evaluated from the level of the confluence of the iliac veins to the diaphragmatic hiatus, allowing identification of the renal veins and, in one case, intraluminal thrombus. There were no instances in which the operator decided to switch to iodinated contrast agents in order to obtain a satisfactory study.

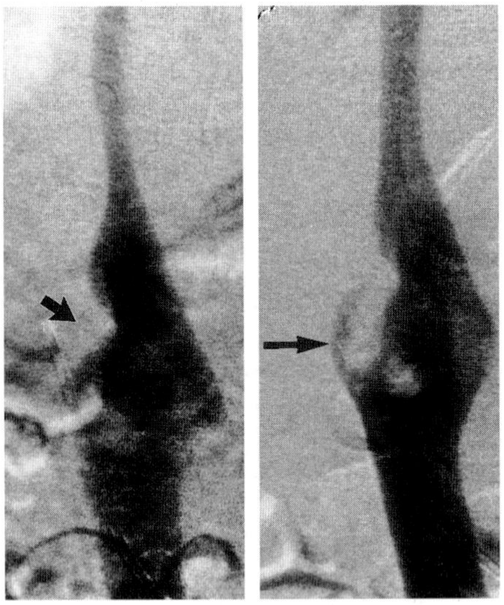

a. b.

Figure 2. Patient 13. IVC thrombolysis in a 49-year-old man with IVC thrombosis. **(a)** Digital subtraction inferior vena cavogram was obtained at 48 hours after thrombolysis by means of hand injection of 40 mL of CO_2 through a 5-F pigtail catheter. A poorly defined mural filling defect (arrow) is depicted in the region of the right renal vein orifice. **(b)** Repeat digital subtraction inferior vena cavogram through the same catheter was obtained with undiluted gadodiamide at 20 mL/sec for 2 seconds. The residual thrombus (arrow) in the region of the right renal vein (a posterior structure) is better defined with the gadodiamide, which mixes with blood rather than displacing it. Note the apparent difference in caliber of the suprarenal IVC when compared with **a** as a result of anterior layering of CO_2.

Discussion

Catheter-based imaging and interventions in the vena cava are an important part of radiologic practice. Iodinated contrast agents are suitable for the majority of patients with normal renal function who require invasive procedures in the vena cava. Patients with renal insufficiency, however, are at increased risk of contrast agent–induced acute renal failure following angiography with iodinated contrast agents (9,10). The risk of contrast agent–induced acute renal failure is difficult to predict, as it varies on the basis of patient profile, type of iodinated contrast agent, and definition of renal failure. With use of the definitions and guidelines proposed by Solomon et al (9), the incidence of contrast agent–induced acute renal failure is 11% in patients with a baseline creatinine level greater than or equal to 1.5 mg/dL (133 μmol/L) who undergo cardiac catheterization. To our knowledge, there are no studies of contrast agent–induced renal failure following cavography with iodinated contrast agents. An alternative contrast agent that permits invasive imaging of the vena cava without the risk of nephrotoxicity would be useful for this subset of patients.

Gadolinium-based contrast agents were developed for and are primarily used in MR imaging (11). These contrast agents have an excellent safety profile in patients with renal insufficiency (7,8,12). Although decreased creatinine clearance has been observed in isolated ischemic rat nephrons after perfusion with gadolinium tetraazacyclododecanetetraacetic acid (DOTA) (13), other studies have shown no change or slight increase in glomerular filtration rate with high doses (0.5–0.6 mmol/kg) of Gd-DOTA in isolated rat kidneys and in vivo in dogs (14,15). To our knowledge, the explanation for the lack of nephrotoxicity of gadolinium-based contrast agents is not known. In this series, 11 of 14 patients experienced either a decrease in serum creatinine level or an elevation that was less than 0.5 mg/dL (44 μmol/L) at 48 hours after their procedure.

The three patients in this series who experienced an elevation in serum creatinine level of greater than or equal to 0.5 mg/dL (44 μmol/L) at 48 hours after cavography with gadodiamide had other explanations for their renal failure. These cases underscore the important point that the use of a gadolinium-based contrast agent will not halt or reverse ongoing acute renal failure or overcome other causes of renal dysfunction. Furthermore, these cases reflect the observational nature of this series. The presence of ongoing acute decompensation of renal function did not preclude the use of gadolinium-based contrast agent in these patients, although we currently avoid use of gadolinium-based contrast agent in such cases because there seems to be little benefit in terms of renal function.

Use of gadolinium-based contrast agents is not entirely without risk. Adverse reactions, including true anaphylaxis, are rare but do occur (16). Fortunately, cross sensitivity in patients with prior anaphylaxis to iodinated contrast agents does not appear to be a problem (16). In one study of patients with a baseline serum creatinine level greater than or equal to 2.0 mg/dL (177 μmol/L) who received 0.1 mmol/kg of gadopentetate dimeglumine intravenously for brain MR imaging, the overall adverse reaction rate was 3.6% within 72 hours of injection (8). None of the events was considered serious or life threatening. The patients in the current series tolerated the injections of gadolinium-based contrast agent without incident.

Theoretically, gadolinium-based contrast agents should work well as a radiologic contrast agent. The k edge of gadolinium-based contrast agents is 52 and exceeds that of iodine, which is 33. In vitro experimental findings have shown that above a mean 72 kVp ± 6, image contrast is better with gadolinium-based contrast agents than with iodinated agents (17). Below this kilovolt peak setting, iodine provides image contrast superior to that with gadolinium-based contrast agents (17). Quinn and co-workers (18) determined in a tissue phantom that at equimolar concentrations, gadopentetate dimeglumine caused 250% greater attenuation than did iopromide (Ultravist 370; Berlex Laboratories) in a CT scanner at 120 kV, 250 mA, with 5-mm section thickness, and a 2.5-second exposure. They found that 90 mL of gadopentetate dimeglumine (47 mmol, equal to 10 times the U. S. Food and Drug Administration approved dose) injected intravenously provided satisfactory enhancement of the circle of Willis.

Despite the theoretically favorable x-ray imaging properties of gadolinium-based contrast agent, the actual vascular enhancement observed during DSA is weaker than that observed with iodinated contrast agents. This is due to the relatively low concentration of gadolinium in currently available MR imaging contrast agents. In one study, the density of gadopentetate dimeglumine diluted 50% with normal saline solution was found to be equivalent to that of a solution of 40 mg of iodine per milliliter at 80 kVp (5). The typical iodine content of contrast agents used for DSA is 200–300 mg of iodine per milliliter (19).

The low density of current gadolinium-based contrast agents presents a dilemma when used for DSA. Ideally, the contrast agent should not be diluted, to maximize its density during imaging (6). However, the maximum dose of gadodiamide approved by the U. S. Food and Drug Administration is 0.3 mmol/kg, or 0.6 mL/kg (manufacturer's recommendation, Nycomed, Princeton, NJ). The maximum approved dose of gadopentetate dimeglumine is only 0.1 mmol/kg, or 0.2 mL/kg (manufacturer's recommendation, Berlex Laboratories, Wayne, NJ). Therefore, dilution is usually necessary in most cases in order to achieve a contrast agent volume that is sufficient for cavography without vastly exceeding the approved dosages. We were unwilling to exceed a dose of 0.4 mmol/kg (0.8 mL/kg) because of a lack of published safety data.

The choice of definition of contrast agent–induced renal failure has a major effect on any study in which this entity is examined (10,20). Some authors have advocated use of a percentage change instead of or in addition to an absolute rise in serum creatinine level, as well as extension of the period of observation to 72 hours (10,20). We chose the definition of a rise in serum creatinine level greater than or equal to 0.5 mg/dL (44 μmol/L) at 48 hours as this is among the criteria for contrast agent–induced acute renal failure used by the nephrology service in our hospital.

In most situations, CO_2 gas is an inexpensive, safe alternative contrast agent for DSA studies. The actual cost of the volume of CO_2 used for most angiographic applications is pennies (1,21). The limitations associated with CO_2-enhanced venography include the need to temporarily displace all of the blood in the IVC with a large volume of gas for accurate imaging (Fig 2) and lack of readily available CO_2 power injectors for controlled administration of the contrast agent (21). Venous administration of large volumes of CO_2 to a patient in the supine position can, rarely, result in trapping of the gas in the anterior pulmonary artery outflow tract, with obstruction of blood flow ("vapor lock") and cardiovascular compromise (22). Furthermore, cavography with CO_2 may be contraindicated in patients with intracardiac or intrapulmonary right-to-left shunts. Ehrman et al (22) noted seizures in two patients and loss of consciousness in a third patient in whom reflux of CO_2 occurred into the arterial circulation during imaging of upper extremity hemodialysis fistulas.

Gadolinium-based contrast agents can be used in any patient (with the exception of patients who are pregnant or lactating or experienced anaphylaxis after exposure to gadolinium) for diagnostic and interventional procedures in the vena cava without the need for specialized equipment. Owing to the expense of the gadolinium-based contrast agents (purchase price of $70–$100 per 20-mL vial) and the limited volumes that can be used, they are most suitable for patients with contraindications to conventional contrast agents such as renal insufficiency. Gadolinium-based contrast agents may be of special utility for venographic studies in patients with renal insufficiency and known or suspected right-to-left shunts.

The risk factors for contrast agent–induced acute renal failure in patients with renal insufficiency include contrast agent type, patient hydration, diabetes, site of injection, prior episodes of contrast agent–induced renal failure, and the volume of contrast agent used (23). A safe threshold volume of iodinated contrast agent that can be used without risk of contrast agent–induced renal failure in these patients has not been determined. Similarly, the minimal volume of iodinated contrast agent required for cavography has not been established. In our institution, we regularly inject 30–40 mL of contrast agent per cavogram and obtain both a pre- and postplacement cavogram when placing an IVC filter. The typical total volume of contrast agent, including test injections by hand to confirm catheter placement, ranges from 70 to 100 mL for an IVC filter placement. The purchase price of 100 mL of nonionic contrast agent varies greatly by region and manufacturer, but it is currently approximately $45 at our institution.

This article is a description of our initial limited experience with gadolinium-based contrast agents in vena cavography. A multiinstitutional, prospective, randomized comparative study with either CO_2 or a conventional iodinated contrast agent is required to fully evaluate this application of gadolinium-based contrast agents. Inclusion of only those patients with stable renal insufficiency would simplify data analysis and interpretation.

Gadolinium-based contrast agents have been described as alternative contrast agents at DSA in case reports by several authors (4–6). Findings in this small series suggest that gadolinium-based contrast agents are suitable as an alternative at digital subtraction vena cavography in patients with renal insufficiency, particularly when a limited volume of contrast agent is needed.

References

1. Kerns SR, Hawkins IF Jr. Carbon dioxide digital subtraction angiography: expanding applications and technical evolution. AJR 1995; 164:735–741.
2. Sullivan KL, Bonn J, Shapiro MJ, Gardiner GA. Venography with carbon dioxide as a contrast agent. Cardiovasc Intervent Radiol 1995; 18:141–145.
3. McCowan TC, Ferris EJ, Carver DK. Inferior vena caval filter thrombi: evaluation with intravascular US. Radiology 1990; 177:783–788.
4. Kinno Y, Odagiri K, Andoh K, Itoh Y, Tarao K. Gadopentetate dimeglumine as an alternative contrast material for use in angiography. AJR 1993; 160:1293–1294.
5. Kaufman JA, Geller SC, Waltman AC. Renal insufficiency: gadopentetate dimeglumine as a radiographic contrast agent during peripheral vascular interventional procedures. Radiology 1996; 198:579–581.
6. Matchett WJ, McFarland DR, Russell DK, Sailors DM, Moursi MM. Azotemia: gadopentetate dimeglumine as a contrast agent at digital subtraction angiography. Radiology 1996; 201:569–571.
7. Prince MR, Arnoldus C, Frisoli JK. Nephrotoxicity of high-dose gadolinium compared with iodinated contrast. JMRI 1996; 5:162–166.
8. Aresenault TM, King BF, Marsh JW Jr, et al. Systemic gadolinium toxicity in patients with renal insufficiency and renal failure: retrospective analysis of an initial experience. Mayo Clin Proc 1996; 71:1150–1154.
9. Solomon R, Werner C, Mann D, D'Elia J, Silva P. Effects of saline, mannitol, and furosemide on acute decreases in renal function induced by radiocontrast agents. N Engl J Med 1994; 331:1416–1420.
10. Lautin EM, Freeman NJ, Schoenfeld AH, et al. Radiocontrast-associated renal dysfunction: incidence and risk factors. AJR 1991; 157:49–58.
11. Brasch RC. Introduction to the gadolinium class. J Comput Assist Tomogr 1993; 17(suppl):19–23.
12. Haustein J, Niendorf HP, Krestin G, et al. Renal tolerance of gadolinium-DTPA/dimeglumine in patients with chronic renal failure. Invest Radiol 1992; 27:352–354.
13. Brillet G, Dubois M, Beaufils H, Bourbouze R, Deray G. Renal tolerance of gadolinium-DOTA and gadolinium-DTPA in rats. Invest Radiol 1994; 29:352–354.
14. Katzberg RW, Sahler LG, Duda SW, et al. Renal handling and physiologic effects of the paramagnetic contrast medium Gd-DOTA. Invest Radiol 1990; 25:714–719.
15. Brown PWG, Haylor JL, Morcos SK, El Nahas AM. The functional effects of gadolinium-DTPA on the isolated perfused rat kidney. Eur J Radiol 1993; 16:85–89.
16. Murphy KJ, Brunberg JA, Cohan RH. Adverse reactions to gadolinium contrast media: a review of 36 cases. AJR 1996; 167:847–849.
17. Cardinal HN, Holdsworth DW, Drangova M, Hobbs BB, Fenster A. Experimental and theoretical x-ray imaging performance: comparison of iodine and lanthanide contrast agents. Med Phys 1993; 20:15–31.
18. Quinn AD, O'Hare NJ, Wallis FJ, Wilson GF. Gd-DTPA: an alternative contrast medium for CT. J Comput Assist Tomogr 1994; 18:634–636.
19. Bettman MA. Angiographic contrast media. In: Kandarpa K, Aruny JE, eds. Handbook of interventional radiologic procedures. 2nd ed. Boston, Mass: Little Brown, 1996; 313–317.
20. Rudnick MR, Berns JS, Cohen RM, Goldfarb S. Nephrotoxic risks of renal angiography: contrast media-associated nephrotoxicity and atheroembolism—a critical review. Am J Kidney Dis 1994; 24:713–727.
21. Caridi JG, Hawkins IF. CO_2 digital subtraction angiography: potential complications and their prevention. JVIR 1997; 8:383–391.
22. Ehrman KO, Taber TE, Gaylord GM, Brown PB, Hage JP. Comparison of diagnostic accuracy with carbon dioxide versus iodinated contrast material in the imaging of hemodialysis access fistulas. JVIR 1994; 5:771–775.
23. Bettmann MA. Physiologic effects and systemic reactions. In: Baum S, ed. Abram's angiography. Boston, Mass: Little Brown, 1997; 22–37.

Yoshimi Anzai, MD
Satoshi Minoshima, MD, PhD
Gregory T. Wolf, MD
Richard L. Wahl, MD

Index terms:
Head and neck neoplasms, diagnosis, 20.30
Head and neck neoplasms, emission CT (ECT), 20.12163

Radiology 1999; 212:285–290

Abbreviations:
FDG = 2-[fluorine-18]fluoro-2-deoxy-D-glucose
PCA = principal components analysis
SUV = standardized uptake value

[1] From the Departments of Radiology (Y.A., R.L.W.), Internal Medicine (Nuclear Medicine) (S.M., R.L.W.), and Otolaryngology and Head and Neck Surgery (G.T.W.), the University of Michigan Medical Center, B1G505 University Hospital, 1500 E Medical Center Dr, Ann Arbor, MI 48109-0028. From the 1996 RSNA scientific assembly. Received April 1, 1998; revision requested June 25; revision received October 2; accepted December 16. Supported in part by National Institutes of Health grants CA 52880, MO1RR 00042, CA 53172, and CA 56731, and the High Technology funding initiative of the University of Michigan Medical Center and Clinical Research Center. **Address reprint requests to** R.L.W. (e-mail: *rwahl@umich.edu*).

Author contributions:
Guarantors of integrity of entire study, Y.A., R.L.W.; study concepts, Y.A., S.M., R.L.W.; study design, Y.A., R.L.W.; definition of intellectual content, Y.A., R.L.W.; literature research, Y.A., R.L.W.; clinical studies, R.L.W., G.T.W.; data acquisition, R.L.W., G.T.W.; data analysis, Y.A., S.M.; statistical analysis, Y.A., S.M.; manuscript preparation, all authors; manuscript editing, Y.A., S.M., R.L.W.; manuscript review, R.L.W., G.T.W.

Head and Neck Cancer: Detection of Recurrence with Three-dimensional Principal Components Analysis at Dynamic FDG PET[1]

Fully automated principal components analysis (PCA) was applied to dynamic 2-[fluorine-18]fluoro-2-deoxy-D-glucose (FDG) positron emission tomographic (PET) images obtained in 15 patients with previously treated head and neck cancer. PCA with time-activity curves incorporated kinetic information about FDG uptake, which improved tissue characterization on FDG PET images. The combination of standardized uptake value and PCA image sets likely will improve the reliability of tumor detection in head and neck cancers.

Imaging with 2-[fluorine-18]fluoro-2-deoxy-D-glucose (FDG) positron emission tomography (PET) has been shown to be a valuable technique in tumors to detect and stage various malignant neoplasms (1–5). Extracranial head and neck cancer is also reported to be FDG avid, and FDG PET permits detection of head and neck cancers that might not be diagnosed with computed tomography (CT) or magnetic resonance (MR) imaging (6–8). The work-up for newly diagnosed head and neck cancers includes CT or MR imaging in conjunction with thorough clinical examination, which is sufficient in most cases. In contrast, early diagnosis of recurrent head and neck cancer following radiation therapy or surgery is diagnostically challenging. The presence of edema in the mucosal surface and the distortion of anatomic fascial planes secondary to prior surgery or radiation therapy make differentiation of recurrent tumors from post-therapeutic changes difficult if not impossible. FDG PET plays an important role in the diagnosis of such recurrent head and neck cancers (6,8–12). Diagnostic accuracy with FDG PET has been reported as better than that with MR imaging in patients with clinically suspected recurrent head and neck cancers (12).

Accurate interpretation of FDG PET images of the head and neck, however, is not necessarily straightforward. On FDG PET images typically obtained at 50–70 minutes after radiotracer injection, physiologic FDG uptake can be seen in lymphoid tissue, nasal mucosa, or salivary gland. Radioactivity in large vessels may mimic focal tumor uptake especially at earlier imaging times. Muscle uptake may be substantial in certain cases (13). Postirradiation or surgical changes may increase FDG uptake in the soft tissue, which may not be easily distinguished from uptake associated with tumor recurrence. Such physiologic FDG uptake in the head and neck can be asymmetric, particularly postoperatively, simulating a pathologic condition at FDG PET. These findings suggest that information other than the static distribution of FDG activity after tracer injection is necessary to improve accuracy of FDG PET image interpretation.

On the basis of findings in autoradiographic studies, it has been speculated that time courses of FDG uptake may have valuable information in the distinction of neoplastic from nonneoplastic tissue activities (14). FDG uptake within a tumor gradually increases over time after intravenous administration of the radioisotope. Nonneoplastic cellular activities have been shown to have a different kinetic behavior of FDG uptake from that of neoplastic tissues. Intravascular FDG activity initially increases following injection and rapidly diminishes thereafter. Thus, examination of time courses of FDG uptake may give us additional insight to distinguish tumor versus nontumor tissues on FDG PET images.

Principal components analysis (PCA) is a multivariate correlation analysis (15) that explains algebraically a variance-covariance structure of observed data sets with a few linear combinations of original variables. When applied to dynamic FDG PET image sets, PCA finds clusters of pixels that have similar kinetic behavior of FDG uptake and summarizes them into a component. This method was applied previously in dynamic FDG PET of the liver in two dimensions (16).

PCA of dynamic FDG PET images was chosen to be explored in this study for two reasons. First, tumor tissues are heterogeneous, and conventional compartment models may not describe tumor FDG uptake adequately. This requires more complex modeling that does not guarantee the validity of the model among different tumors (17). Model-independent, data-driven analysis such as PCA may have an advantage in this regard. Second, results of PCA can be easily depicted as parametric images, which are suitable for visual interpretation of FDG PET image data.

The aim of this study was to explore the use of PCA to detect recurrent head and neck cancers. Our underlying hypothesis was that use of FDG kinetics as side information or as an alternative to a static FDG distribution image would improve the accuracy of FDG PET in the distinction of tumor from nontumor tissues in the head and neck. In this initial study, fully automated PCA was implemented in three dimensions, and resultant parametric image sets were interpreted in comparison with conventional standardized uptake value (SUV) image sets.

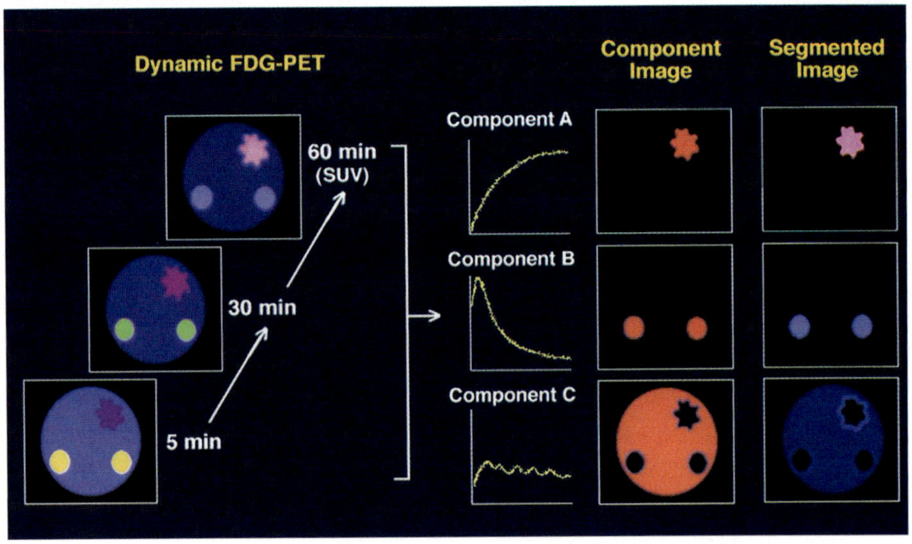

Figure 1. Schematic of PCA and its application to dynamic FDG PET in this study.

Materials and Methods

Patients

Dynamic FDG PET data for 15 patients (14 men and one women; age range, 33–80 years; mean age, 63 years) were drawn from an ongoing study of FDG PET to diagnose recurrent head and neck cancers. Only patients with pathologic confirmation of tumor recurrence (at either surgery or biopsy) or those with nonrecurrent tumor after clinical follow-up of longer than 6 months were included. No patients satisfying these criteria were excluded from the study unless they could not complete FDG PET or substantial body motion occurred during imaging. All patients had been treated for primary tumors with surgery, radiation therapy, or chemotherapy and had clinical signs or symptoms suspicious for tumor recurrence in the head and neck. Twelve patients had squamous cell carcinoma, and one each had melanoma, adenoid cystic carcinoma, and small cell carcinoma. Primary sites of cancers were the larynx (n = 8), oropharynx (n = 1), hypopharynx (n = 1), parotid gland (n = 1), skin over the lower neck (n = 1), temporal bone (n = 1), or oral cavity (n = 1), or the primary site was unknown (n = 1). Previous treatment was both radiation therapy and surgery in seven patients, surgery alone in four, and radiation therapy alone in four. Two patients were also treated with chemotherapy. The minimum time from the last prior therapy until the imaging study was 2 months (mean, 26.4 months; range, 2–108 months).

The study was conducted with the approval of the institutional review board, with the radiopharmaceutical FDG (in-house production) administered under conditions of an investigational new drug application on file with the U. S. Food and Drug Administration. Written informed consent was obtained from all patients.

Dynamic FDG PET

Dynamic FDG PET was performed with two scanners (CTI/Siemens, Knoxville, Tenn): an Ecat Exact 921 scanner in nine patients and an Ecat 931/08–12 scanner in six patients. All patients underwent FDG PET after at least 4 hours of fasting. Transmission scanning for attenuation correction was performed before emission scanning with a germanium 68 ring source. Transmission and emission images were obtained between the level of the external auditory canal and the thoracic inlet depending on clinical symptoms suspected for tumor recurrence. After intravenous administration of 370 MBq (10 mCi) of FDG, dynamic image sets were obtained between 0 and 60 minutes after injection.

To examine PCA in various imaging protocols, image data obtained with different dynamic imaging protocols were tested. In four patients, six 10-minute frames were obtained (total, six frames). In eight patients, six 10-second frames, three 20-second frames, two 90-second frames, one 5-minute frame, and five 10-minute frames were obtained (total, 17 frames). In one patient, six 10-second frames, three 20-second frames, two 90-second frames, five 5-minute frames, and three 10-minute frames were obtained (total, 19 frames). In two patients, 12 10-second frames, three 20-second frames, two 60-second frames, five 5-minute frames, and three 10-minute frames were obtained (total, 25 frames).

Images were reconstructed with a Hanning filter (cutoff frequency, 0.3 cycles per projection element), resulting in approximately 12-mm full width at half maximum in-plane resolution. The reconstructed voxel size for the Ecat 931 scanner was 4.69 mm in plane with 6.75-mm section thickness and for the Ecat Exact scanner was 4.22 mm in plane with 3.375-mm section thickness.

PCA Method

In PCA, a three-dimensional dynamic image data set was rearranged first in a data matrix ($n \times p$, where n is the number

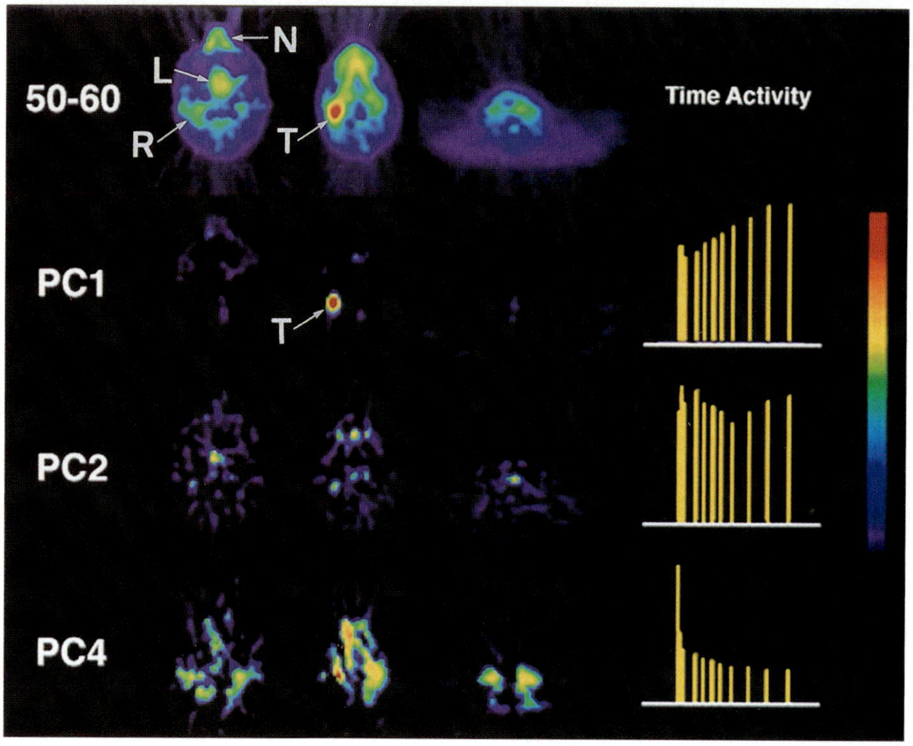

Figure 2. PCA (*PC1, PC2, PC4*) in a patient with small cell carcinoma of the larynx, which was previously treated with irradiation and chemotherapy, who presented with a right-side neck mass. SUV image set (*50–60* [minutes]) shows moderate FDG uptake in the nasal mucosa (*N*) and lymphoid tissue in the oropharynx (*L*) and postirradiation changes in the neck (*R*) and some intravascular activities. Tumor uptake (*T*) is also identifiable on the right side of the neck. Principal component image sets revealed focal tumor uptake with markedly suppressed physiologic soft-tissue uptake in the first component (*PC1*). Vascular activities are separated in the fourth component (*PC4*). The second component (*PC2*) represents other noise variances.

of dynamic frames and p is the number of pixels within a frame). Pixels within a single dynamic frame were rearranged into a single column of the data matrix from the rightmost anterior pixel to the leftmost posterior pixel of the body and then from the top to the bottom sections. A variance-covariance matrix was derived from the data matrix and then standardized to a correlation matrix ($p \times p$). PCA was used to solve eigenvalue-eigenvector pairs from the correlation matrix. This mathematic operation is described elsewhere (15). One practical difficulty was to manipulate a large correlation matrix on a workstation with a limited amount of memory and computational power since the number of pixels within a single frame p is typically greater than 5×10^5. To overcome this problem, the data matrix was transformed and transposed to a $p \times n$ matrix to allow subsequent calculation of eigenvalue-eigenvector pairs in a correlation matrix $n \times n$ (18,19). Initial estimates of principal components were then rotated to a simpler structure by means of a Varimax rotation method (20). Resultant principal component image sets consisted of elements of rotated eigenvectors, and the number of principal components was no greater than n, the number of dynamic frames.

Pixel values in resultant PCA image sets represented correlation coefficients with latent principal components, with the maximum value of 1 being most significantly correlated with the component. For each principal component, each frame of the dynamic image set was segmented with a given PCA image set by means of multiplication. A time-activity curve for each principal component was then calculated by averaging radioactivity within pixels with the highest 1% of correlation coefficients in the PCA image matrix. Along with the time-activity curves for principal components, segmented FDG image sets of the last dynamic frame (50–60 minutes after injection) in each PCA image set were used for image interpretation (hereafter, "PCA image sets") (Fig 1). The last dynamic frame was also used to create an SUV image set (21).

These algorithms were implemented on a workstation (Sparc Station 2; Sun Microsystems, Mountain View, Calif) by means of a standard C language. A dynamic FDG PET image set was processed in approximately 3–8 minutes, depending on the number of sections and frames.

PCA and SUV Image Evaluation

Time-activity curves and PCA image sets were evaluated by consensus of a head and neck radiologist (Y.A.) and a nuclear medicine physician (S.M.) along with clinical information including locations of primary cancers, previous treatment, presenting symptoms, and pathology results. SUV image sets were also available at the time of interpretation of PCA image sets, which was performed in two steps. First, time-activity curves of principal components were reviewed in each patient. According to the previous knowledge of FDG accumulation in viable tumors (14,22,23), components with gradually increasing FDG uptake over time or gradually increasing FDG uptake followed by a relatively stable phase were considered to be tumor or tumorlike components, respectively. PCA image sets corresponding to such time-activity curves were considered tumor PCA image sets, and they were inspected visually to localize tumor or tumorlike activities. Tumor PCA image sets were compared with an SUV image set obtained in the same patient.

To compare distinction of tumor activities from physiologic nontumor activities, structures that were visible on tumor PCA image sets and SUV image sets were examined. In this comparison, activities suspicious for or similar to tumor uptake were defined first on PCA and SUV image sets. These activities were then localized to specific structures on CT or MR images or to locations of tumor recurrence confirmed pathologically. In addition, tumor-to-background contrast ratios (CR) were calculated for both tumor PCA and SUV image sets by means of the following equation: $CR = |\text{tumor activity} - \text{background activity}| \div (\text{tumor activity} + \text{background activity})$. Background activity was measured at neck structures contralateral to tumors. By definition, the minimum and maximum contrasts were 0 and 1, respectively. A nonparametric sign test was used to assess differences in contrast ratios on PCA versus SUV image sets.

Results

Identification of Tumor Components

Twelve of 15 patients were found to have recurrent tumors that were confirmed at biopsy or surgery. The average SUV for all 12 tumors was 6.22. Three patients with negative biopsy results had clinical follow-up for more than 6 months without clinical evidence of tumor recurrence, and their cases are considered negative for tumor involvement.

Inspection of time-activity curves of principal components revealed 10 patients with tumor (n = 8) or tumorlike (n = 2) components (Figs 2, 3). PCA failed to detect a tumor component in one patient with adenoid cystic carcinoma of the parotid gland (Fig 4). One recurrent tumor that was not detected with an SUV image set was also not differentiated with PCA from physiologic soft-tissue activities. In contrast, no tumor component was detected in three patients who had no recurrent tumors. When the diagnostic accuracy of PCA was calculated on the basis of identification of tumor components on a patient-by-patient basis, the sensitivity and specificity, respectively, were 83% (10 of 12 patients with tumor recurrence) and 100% (no tumor component detected in three patients without recurrence).

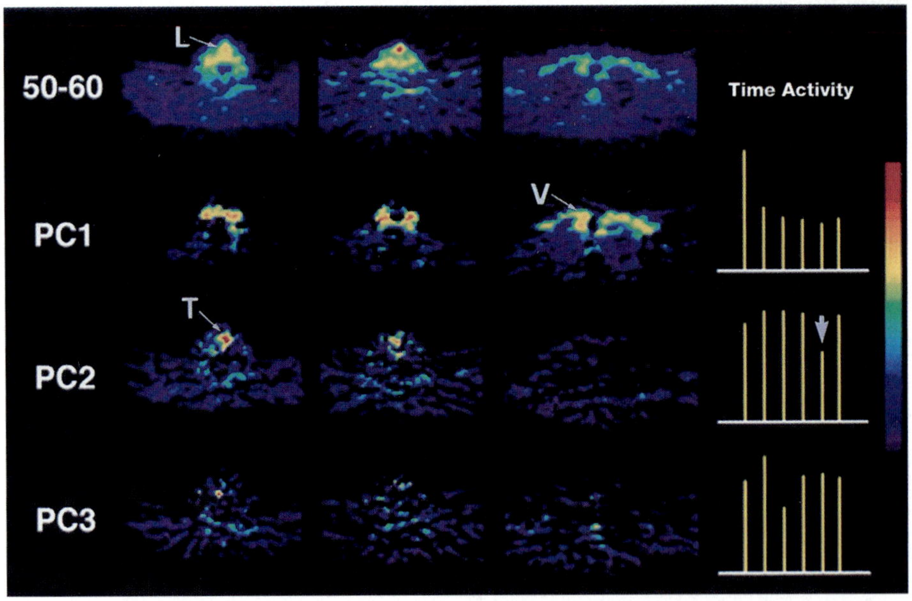

Figure 3. PCA (*PC1–PC3*) in a patient with laryngeal cancer, which had been treated with irradiation, who presented with sore throat and hoarseness. SUV image (*50–60* [minutes]) shows diffuse mildly increased FDG uptake in the previously irradiated larynx (*L*), but the tumor is not conspicuous. The first component (*PC1*) is the vascular component (*V*). The second component (*PC2*) is the tumor component, which corresponds to a focus of recurrent laryngeal tumor (*T*) in the true vocal cord that extends into the anterior commissure. This tumor component image clearly separates tumor from residual FDG uptake in the postirradiation changes. In the time-activity curve, there is a small dip (arrow) that most likely relates to noise or patient motion. The third component (*PC3*) represents residual noises without apparent physiologic correlates.

Structures Depicted on Tumor PCA and SUV Image Sets

Visual inspection of PCA image sets corresponding to tumor components typically revealed discrete areas of tumor uptake corresponding to a biopsy- or surgically proved recurrent tumor (Figs 2, 3). Physiologic soft-tissue activity was suppressed substantially on tumor PCA image sets, which improved tumor-to-background contrast.

The number of identifiable physiologic soft-tissue activities on SUV image sets was reduced markedly on tumor PCA image sets with minimal loss of tumor detectability (Table). Particularly, vascular activities were suppressed completely from tumor components. Other physiologic activities such as lymphoid tissues and postirradiation or surgical changes were suppressed on tumor PCA image sets, but suppression was not complete compared to that of the vascular structures.

Tumor-to-Background Contrast Ratios on PCA and SUV Image Sets

Tumor-to-background contrast ratios were significantly improved on tumor PCA image sets. They were 0.48 ± 0.14 (mean ± SD) on SUV image sets and 0.79 ± 0.21 on tumor PCA images (sign test, $P < .001$). In five of 12 patients with recurrent tumor, background activity in the neck contralateral to tumors was nearly negligible at visual inspection of images (Figs 2, 3).

Discussion

Findings in this initial study demonstrate the feasibility of pixel-by-pixel, three-dimensional PCA applied to dynamic FDG PET studies in the head and neck regions. The analysis is able to cluster pixels with a similar kinetic behavior and generate multiple time-activity curves for physiologic interpretation. By using this approach, tumor activities can be separated from other background activities that can be confounded in the interpretation of FDG PET images, particularly in postoperative patients with asymmetrically distorted anatomy of the head and neck. As shown in Results, vascular-related and other physiologic activities such as mucosal activities were well suppressed on tumor PCA images, and PCA improved tumor-to-background ratios compared with those on conventional SUV images. We found that this analysis substantially increased the lesion conspicuity on PET images and also helped correlation with anatomic images when necessary.

The analysis of tumor FDG PET data by means of kinetic information has been explored previously. Compartmental analysis is one of the common approaches to estimate tumor biochemical parameters. However, a difficulty with this approach is "compartmental" modeling of tumor tissues, as they may be highly heterogeneous and their compartments potentially cannot be determined precisely in human subjects. The PCA is at the opposite end of the spectrum in that it does not rely on modeling; instead, it explores variance structures of observed data. Because of its exploratory nature and pixel-by-pixel approach, the current method does not require prospective placement of regions of interest, which obviates biases potentially introduced by observers. PCA distinguishes different kinetic components contributing to the same image pixel (such as blood flow vs metabolism of the tumor), and the magnitudes of contribution of different components are summarized into different component image sets. This type of parametric imaging cannot be achieved with region-of-interest analysis on conventional SUV image sets. However, resultant component image sets can be analyzed subsequently by placing regions of interest to obtain quan-

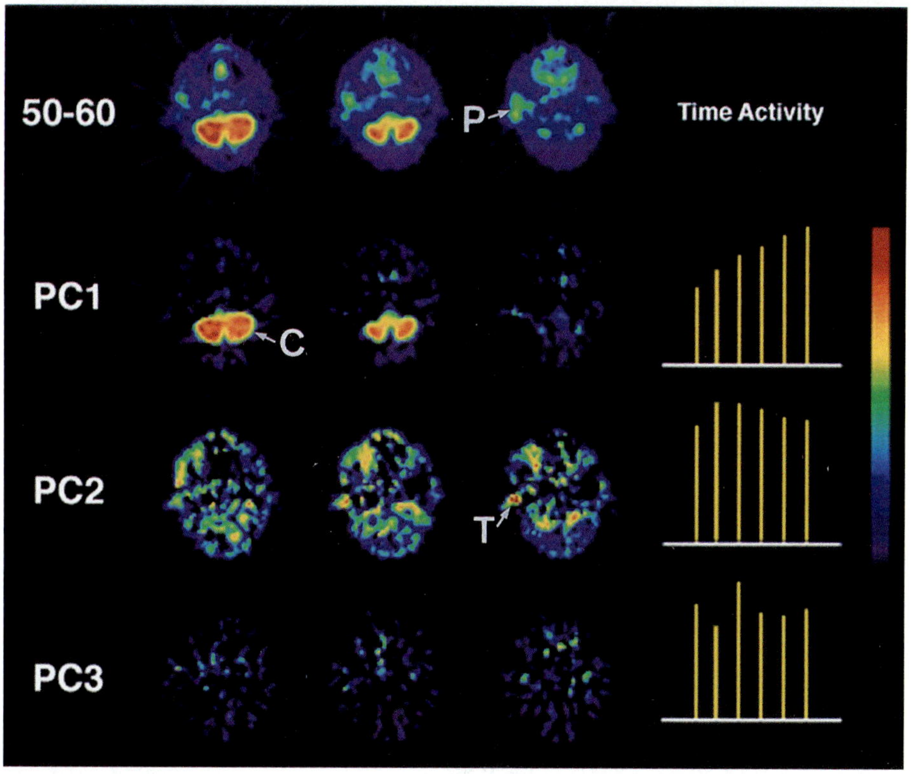

Figure 4. PCA (*PC1–PC3*) in a patient with adenoid cystic carcinoma of the right cheek and parotid gland that had been partially resected. The patient presented with swelling of the right cheek. SUV image (*50–60* [minutes]) shows very mild radiotracer uptake in the right parotid gland (*P*). The first component image (*PC1*) shows gradual increase in FDG uptake, which is expected to be tumor component, corresponding to the cerebellum (*C*). Tumor (*T*) was classified into the second component image (*PC2*), which shows initial increase followed by gradual decrease in FDG uptake. At PCA, this tumor was not detected in the component of increasing activity (*PC1*) because the kinetic behavior of this particular tumor was similar to that of residual soft tissue. The third component (*PC3*) represents residual noises without apparent physiologic correlates.

titative indexes (such as estimations of contrast ratios in this study). Thus, these two approaches can be used complementarily.

Other parametric imaging techniques such as influx imaging require either sequential arterial sampling to estimate an input function of radiotracer or manual placement of regions of interest within a vascular structure (2). The former technique is invasive and may not be necessarily suitable for routine clinical use. The latter technique is suitable for thoracic neoplasms, and the drawing of regions of interest in the major vascular structures in the chest, such as aorta, is relatively straightforward. In contrast, accurate placement of a region of interest within the carotid artery in the neck can be difficult on FDG PET images. PCA is, again, advantageous in this regard since it does not require either input function or manual placement of regions of interest in the vascular structures. In addition, PCA can be used in preprocessing of dynamic images to segment vascular components, which can be used subsequently to estimate input function on dynamic images. The use of PCA for preprocessing of dynamic PET images is still under investigation. The vascular structures can be discriminated from tumor uptake by simply comparing an early postinjection FDG PET image with a standard plateau-phase image. PCA not only distinguished vascular structures but also identified different physiologic components on the basis of a variance-covariance matrix of observed data. One noticeable advantage of PCA is suppression of the background random noise component, which results in improved signal-to-noise ratios for tumors.

The application of pixel-by-pixel PCA to PET is a relatively new field. Pedersen and colleagues (16) applied the technique to abdominal tumors in two dimensions (on a single PET section) to distinguish tumor activity from nontumor background activities. A similar technique was also applied to PET brain activation data to elucidate patterns of intercorrelation of regional brain functions (24). The method to deal with a large variance-covariance matrix for PET images in the PCA was investigated by Friston and colleagues (25) for PET brain activation studies by means of an iterative algorithm. We implemented a faster and more accurate analytic algorithm (18) to process large three-dimensional volumetric dynamic PET images on a common workstation. Compared with analysis of a single section (16), inclusion of the whole image data set improves the stability of separating kinetically intercorrelated pixels in the head and neck region such as vascular components. Execution time for the algorithm was not measured systematically in the current study, but the analysis was completed in 3–8 minutes depending on the number of frames and sections of dynamic PET studies. This suggests a potential routine application of such computationally extensive analysis to clinical FDG PET studies in conjunction with evaluation of conventional SUV images.

Certain limitations exist in PCA analysis. The capability of PCA to detect tumors is governed by kinetic behaviors of FDG in tumor and nontumor soft-tissue structures. For example, the cerebral cortex has FDG kinetics similar to those of tumors, and it can be clustered in the same component, although such structures can be distinguished easily by means of correlative anatomic imaging. In addition, the analysis itself does not give the physiologic importance of each component. Thus, side information such as a time-activity curve for the component or correlative anatomic imaging is essential when results of PCA analysis are interpreted. In the current implementation, a time-activity curve for each component was generated automatically by the algorithm. This was found to be extremely useful because observers could screen the results by using time-activity curves to determine if components suspicious for tumors were seen in the observed data set. PCA and any other kinetic analysis are sensitive to patient motion during dynamic imaging, which may be improved by employing a frame-to-frame image registration algorithm.

Several dynamic imaging protocols were tested empirically in this study. The maximum number of components is equal to the number of frames (ie, a 17-frame study provided 17 components). Component image sets with large eigenvalues were displayed first in the current implementation. The first few component image sets often contained tumors. The last several components often indicated noise components. However, in a patient with a small tumor seen on a dynamic PET study covering the large field of the upper mediastinum and the neck, the tumor component was identified in the sixth component. We did not observe definite correlation between the number of frames acquired during dynamic imaging and the detectability of tumors with PCA, although this evaluation is still not complete because of insufficient experience with different imaging protocols. The greater the number of frames, the more detailed an analysis could be performed. The optimal or minimal number of frames necessary for accurate PCA analysis at dynamic PET must be established in further investigations.

In conclusion, we demonstrated the feasibility of pixel-by-pixel, three-dimensional PCA application to dynamic FDG PET tumor imaging. PCA incorporates kinetic information about FDG uptake in parametric image display and interpretation, improving tissue characterization on FDG PET images. Findings in this study demonstrate improved distinction of tumors in the head and neck regions with PCA images as compared to that with conventional SUV images. Implementation of the method permits an acceptable execution time for a routine analysis. A prospective evaluation of PCA versus static FDG imaging will be of considerable interest, as well as the application of the PCA method to tumors located in other areas of the body.

Structures Seen on SUV and Tumor PCA Image Sets in 12 Patients with Recurrent Tumor

Structure	SUV	Tumor Principal Component	Percentage Improvement*
Tumor	11	10	
Vascular structures	7	0	100 (7 of 7)
Salivary gland	8	2	75 (6 of 8)
Lymphoid tissue	11	5	55 (6 of 11)
Nasal mucosa	9	3	67 (6 of 9)
Muscle	2	1	50 (1 of 2)
Areas of prior surgery and radiation therapy	3	1	67 (2 of 3)

Note.—Numbers are the number of structures.
* (SUV − tumor principal component)/SUV × 100. Cerebral uptake is not included since it is not consistently imaged.

Acknowledgments: The authors thank cyclotron operators and PET radiochemists at our institution for the production of radiopharmaceuticals and PET technologists for the skillful acquisition of images.

References

1. Gritters LS, Francis IR, Zasadny KR, Wahl RL. Initial assessment of positron emission tomography using 2-fluorine-18-fluoro-2-deoxy-D-glucose in the imaging of malignant melanoma. J Nucl Med 1993; 34:1420–1427.
2. Newman JS, Francis IR, Kaminski MS, Wahl RL. Imaging of lymphoma with PET with 2-[F-18]-fluoro-2-deoxy-D-glucose: correlation with CT. Radiology 1994; 190: 111–116.
3. Wahl RL, Cody RL, Hutchins GD, Mudgett EE. Primary and metastatic breast carcinoma: initial clinical evaluation with PET with the radiolabeled glucose analogue 2-[F-18]-fluoro-2-deoxy-D-glucose. Radiology 1991; 179:765–770.
4. Wahl RL, Quint LE, Greenough RL, Meyer CR, White RI, Orringer MB. Staging of mediastinal non–small cell lung cancer with FDG PET, CT, and fusion images: preliminary prospective evaluation. Radiology 1994; 191:371–377.
5. Strauss LG, Clorius JH, Schlag P, et al. Recurrence of colorectal tumors: PET evaluation. Radiology 1989; 170:329–332.
6. Jabour BA, Choi Y, Hoh CK, et al. Extracranial head and neck: PET imaging with 2-[F-18]fluoro-2-deoxy-D-glucose and MR imaging correlation. Radiology 1993; 186: 27–35.
7. Minn H, Joensuu H, Ahonen A, Klemi P. Fluorodeoxyglucose imaging: a method to assess the proliferative activity of human cancer in vivo—comparison with DNA flow cytometry in head and neck tumors. Cancer 1988; 61:1776–1781.
8. Rege S, Maass A, Chaiken L, et al. Use of positron emission tomography with fluorodeoxyglucose in patients with extracranial head and neck cancers. Cancer 1994; 73:3047–3058.
9. Greven KM, Williams DW III, Keyes JW Jr, et al. Positron emission tomography of patients with head and neck carcinoma before and after high dose irradiation. Cancer 1994; 74:1355–1359.
10. Haberkorn U, Strauss LG, Dimitrakopoulou A, et al. Fluorodeoxyglucose imaging of advanced head and neck cancer after chemotherapy. J Nucl Med 1993; 34: 12–17.
11. Lapela M, Grenman R, Kurki T, et al. Head and neck cancer: detection of recurrence with PET and 2-[F-18]fluoro-2-deoxy-D-glucose. Radiology 1995; 197:205–211.
12. Anzai Y, Carroll WR, Quint DJ, et al. Recurrence of head and neck cancer after surgery or irradiation: prospective comparison of 2-deoxy-2-[F-18]fluoro-D-glucose PET and MR imaging diagnoses. Radiology 1996; 200:135–141.
13. Kostakoglu U, Wong JC, Barringston SF, Cronin BF, Dynes AM, Maisey MN. Speech-related visualization of laryngeal muscles with fluorine-18-FDG. J Nucl Med 1996; 37:1771–1773.
14. Kubota R, Kutoba K, Yamada S, Tada M, Ido T, Takahashi N. Microautoradiographic study for the differentiation of intratumoral macrophages, granulation tissues and cancer cells by the dynamics of fluorine-18-fluorodeoxyglucose uptake. J Nucl Med 1994; 35:104–112.
15. Johnson RA, Wichern DW. Principal components. In: Johnson RA, ed. Applied multivariate statistical analysis. Englewood Cliffs, NJ: Prentice Hall, 1992; 356–395.
16. Pedersen F, Bergstrom M, Bengtsson E, Langstrom B. Principal component analysis of dynamic positron emission tomography images. Eur J Nucl Med 1994; 21: 1285–1292.
17. Wu HM, Huang SC, Choi Y, Hoh CK, Hawkins RA. A modeling method to improve quantitation of fluorodeoxyglucose uptake in heterogeneous tumor tissue. J Nucl Med 1995; 36:297–306.
18. Minoshima S, Koeppe RA. Fast and accurate numerical method for principal components analysis dealing with large image data sets. Kaku Igaku 1996; 33:431–434.
19. Reyment RA, Jöreskog KG. Basic structure of a matrix and the Eckart-Young theorem. In: Ramond RA. Applied factor analysis in the natural sciences. Cambridge, Mass: Cambridge University Press, 1996; 62–66.
20. Harris RJ. Rotation of principal components. In: Harris RJ. A primer of multivariate statistics. Orlando, Fla: Academic Press, 1985; 264–297.
21. Zasadny KR, Wahl RL. Standardized uptake values of normal tissues at PET with 2-[fluorine-18]-fluoro-2-deoxy-D-glucose: variations with body weight and a method for correction. Radiology 1993; 189:847–850.
22. Wahl RL, Zasadny K, Helvie M, Hutchins GD, Weber B, Cody R. Metabolic monitoring of breast cancer chemohormonotherapy using positron emission tomography: initial evaluation. J Clin Oncol 1993; 11:2101–2111.
23. Zasadny KR, Wahl RL. Enhanced FDG PET tumor imaging with correlation-coefficient filtered influx-constant images. J Nucl Med 1996; 37:371–374.
24. Yap JT, Cooper M, Chen CT, Cunningham VJ. Generation of parametric images using factor analysis of dynamic PET. In: Myers R, Cunningham V, Bailey D, Jones T, eds. Quantification of brain function using PET. San Diego, Calif: Academic Press, 1996; 292–296.
25. Friston KJ, Frith CD, Liddle PF, Frackowiak RS. Functional connectivity: the principal-component analysis of large (PET) data sets. J Cereb Blood Flow Metab 1993; 13:5–14.

Letters to the Editor

Can Inversion-Recovery Gradient- and Spin-Echo T2-weighted MR Imaging Be an Alternative to Fast Spin-Echo Imaging with Fat Suppression?

From:
Masayuki Kanematsu, MD, and Hiroaki Hoshi, MD
Department of Radiology, Gifu University School of Medicine
40 Tsukasamachi, Gifu 500-8705, Japan

Editor:
Dr Pijl and colleagues are to be congratulated for their splendid article on T2-weighted MR imaging of the liver in the November 1998 issue of *Radiology* (1). In the article, they concluded that the respiratory-triggered inversion-recovery gradient- and spin-echo (IR GRASE) sequence is a fast alternative to the respiratory-triggered fast spin-echo (SE) sequence in the evaluation of suspected liver metastases. Their results showed that the mean contrast-to-noise ratio for metastases, the tumor sensitivity, and the diagnostic accuracy determined with receiver operating characteristic analysis were somewhat greater with IR GRASE than with the fast SE sequence. We especially mention three merits of the IR GRASE sequence evaluated by Dr Pijl and colleagues: homogeneous fat suppression, suppressed signal intensity from hepatic vasculature, and shortened acquisition time due to acceleration of k-space data filling. We also believe that all these merits contributed to tumor detection and clinical usefulness.

However, we still emphasize one of the limitations of Dr Pijl and colleagues' study as described in their article: no use of the chemical-shift-selective fat-suppression technique with the respiratory-triggered fast SE sequence. As findings of a previous study (2) have suggested its usefulness, we also grant that use of the fat-suppression technique greatly increases the detection of focal hepatic lesions. First, the liver parenchyma turns darker with fat suppression than without fat suppression, because physiologically existing lipid in the liver is suppressed, which leads to better tumor-to-liver contrast. Second, fast SE imaging with a phased-array multicoil produces a prominent high signal intensity of the abdominal wall adjacent to the coils because of the high signal intensity from fat and the near-field effect. This causes serious ghosting artifacts over the liver, which may obscure the focal hepatic lesions. However, use of a chemical-shift-selective fat-suppression pulse can decrease such ghosting artifacts, leading to improved lesion detectability.

We have attested to the advantage of using fat suppression with respiratory-triggered T2-weighted fast SE imaging to detect focal hepatic lesions in previous studies (3,4). With regard to acquisition time, in our most recent study (4), we imaged the patients in 4–6 minutes (identical to the acquisition time with IR GRASE imaging in the study of Dr Pijl and colleagues) with a fat-suppressed respiratory-triggered fast SE sequence with 256 phase-encoding steps, an echo train length of eight to 18, and four signals acquired. However, this shorter acquisition time was enabled by a shorter interecho space (11 msec) with our enhanced gradient system with echo-planar capability when a wider receiver bandwidth (±62 kHz) was used. In conclusion, we confirmed a substantial increase in malignant tumor detectability by using fat suppression with the respiratory-triggered fast SE sequence.

We thank Dr Pijl and colleagues again for their dedicated study, and we respectfully expect their continued evaluation of the usefulness of the IR GRASE sequence compared with the fat-suppressed fast SE sequence in the detection of focal hepatic lesions.

References
1. Pijl MEJ, Wasser MNJM, van Meerten ELvP, et al. Comparison of inversion-recovery gradient- and spin-echo and fast spin-echo techniques in the detection and characterization of liver lesions. Radiology 1998; 209:427–434.
2. Schwartz LH, Seltzer SE, Tempany CMC, et al. Prospective comparison of T2-weighted fast spin-echo, with and without fat suppression, and conventional spin-echo pulse sequences in the upper abdomen. Radiology 1993; 189:411–416.
3. Kanematsu M, Hoshi H, Murakami T, et al. Focal hepatic lesion detection: comparison of four T2-weighted MR imaging pulse sequences. Radiology 1998; 206:167–175.
4. Kanematsu M, Hoshi H, Itoh K, et al. Focal hepatic lesion detection: comparison of four fat-suppressed T2-weighted MR imaging pulse sequences. Radiology 1999; 211:363–371.

Dr Wasser and colleagues respond:

We thank Drs Kanematsu and Hoshi for their comments. As we stated in our article (1), we did not compare our IR GRASE sequence with a fat-suppressed T2-weighted fast SE sequence. At the time of our study, fat-suppressed fast SE was not considered to be substantially better than T2-weighted fast SE without fat saturation. Moreover, the addition of fat saturation would have greatly lengthened our T2-weighted sequence, and one aim of our study was to accelerate T2-weighted imaging.

The sequence described by Drs Kanematsu and Hoshi combines a T2-weighted fast SE acquisition with fat suppression and therefore may be equivalent to our IR GRASE sequence, although the actual T2 contrast weighting may be different. It would be interesting to compare their sequence with IR GRASE in a prospective randomized study.

Reference
1. Pijl MEJ, Wasser MNJM, van Meerten ELvP, et al. Comparison of inversion-recovery gradient- and spin-echo and fast spin-echo techniques in the detection and characterization of liver lesions. Radiology 1998; 209:427–434.

Martin N. J. M. Wasser, MD, Milan E. J. Pijl, MD, Els L. van Persijn van Meerten, MD, Jan-Willem C. Gratama, MD, and Johan L. Bloem, MD
Department of Radiology, C2-S, Leiden University Medical Center Albinusdreef 2, 2333 AA Leiden, the Netherlands

Audience Preference for Scientific Presentation Method

From:
Edward I. Bluth, MD,* and Kent Nash, PhD†
Department of Radiology, Ochsner Clinic and Alton Ochsner Medical Foundation
1514 Jefferson Highway, New Orleans, LA 70121*
Nash & Associates, West Chicago, Ill†

Editor:

At a recent RSNA refresher course, as the result of adverse circumstances one of five speakers was unable to attend at the last minute. These five speakers had made the same presentations the previous year, which were videotaped. Since two of the presentations were given with traditional slides, two were given with computer-generated slides, and the presentation by the speaker who was unable to attend was videotaped, we used this opportunity to poll course attendees regarding their preference for the type of scientific presentation. The attendees were asked to rate their preference for the presentation method separately from giving their opinions regarding scientific quality. The presentations were rated on a 1–5 scale, with 5 indicating the most preferred (excellent) method. The responses were compared by using a two-sample test of proportions.

Approximately 180 course attendees responded. Overall, 82% (145/178) rated traditional slides as excellent or very good, compared with 87% (156/180) for computer-generated slides and 32% (56/174) for the videotaped presentation. By combining the excellent and very good ratings, differences were found to be significant for traditional slides versus videotapes and for computer-generated slides versus videotapes at the 5% level of significance ($P < .05$). The test failed to reject the null hypothesis, and there was no difference at the 5% level of significance in the percentage of respondents who rated computer-generated slides and traditional slides as excellent or very good.

The audience members who responded to the survey preferred live presentation with the use of either traditional or computer-generated slides compared with videotapes. Most written responses criticized the videotaped presentation because audience members were unable to ask questions and request the presenter to further define points that they did not understand. Several attendees found the computer-generated slides distracting because of the motion activity related to adding words. In fact, some found it distracting to see information coming from the left or the right side of the slide. Others found this type of presentation more lively and said that it "kept them awake." Attendees criticized the "fumbling around" that was required to hook up the computers for computer-generated slides when the presenters changed. In addition, several attendees preferred the double-projection format of traditional slides compared with the single-projection format of computer-generated slides.

In summary, and perhaps most important, attendees at the RSNA scientific assembly who were polled preferred in-person presentations with either traditional or computer-generated slides.

Abstracts of Current Literature

Thorax

Usefulness of D-Dimer, Blood Gas, and Respiratory Rate Measurements for Excluding Pulmonary Embolism. Paul Egermayer, G. Ian Town, John G. Turner, et al. *Thorax* 1998; 53:830–834. (G.I.T., Canterbury Respiratory Research Group, Christchurch School of Medicine, PO Box 4345, Christchurch, New Zealand)

Background: A study was undertaken to assess the usefulness of the SimpliRED D-dimer test, arterial oxygen tension, and respiratory rate measurement for excluding pulmonary embolism (PE) and venous thromboembolism (VTE). *Methods:* Lung scans were performed in 517 consecutive medical inpatients with suspected acute PE over a one year period. Predetermined end points for objectively diagnosed PE in order of precedence were (1) a post mortem diagnosis, (2) a positive pulmonary angiogram, (3) a high probability ventilation perfusion lung scan when the pretest probability was also high, and (4) the unanimous opinion of an adjudication committee. Deep vein thrombosis (DVT) was diagnosed by standard ultrasound and venography. *Results:* A total of 40 cases of PE and 37 cases of DVT were objectively diagnosed. The predictive value of a negative SimpliRED test for excluding objectively diagnosed PE was 0.99 (error rate 2/249), that of Pa_{O_2} of ≥80 mm Hg (10.7 kPa) was 0.97 (error rate 5/160), and that of a respiratory rate of ≤20/min was 0.95 (error rate 14/308). The best combination of findings for excluding PE was a negative SimpliRED test and Pa_{O_2} ≥80 mm Hg, which gave a predictive value of 1.0 (error rate 0/93). The predictive value of a negative SimpliRED test for excluding VTE was 0.98 (error rate 5/249). *Conclusions:* All three of these observations are helpful in excluding PE. When any two parameters were normal, PE was very unlikely. In patients with a negative SimpliRED test and Pa_{O_2} of ≥80 mm Hg a lung scan is usually unnecessary. Application of this approach for triage in the preliminary assessment of suspected PE could lead to a reduced rate of false positive diagnoses and considerable resource savings.
Authors' Abstract

Reason for selecting abstract:
• Important clinical information
Selected by *David L. Spizarny, MD*
Henry Ford Hospital, Detroit, Mich

Genitourinary System

Ablation of Renal Tumors in a Rabbit Model with Interstitial Saline-augmented Radiofrequency Energy: Preliminary Report of a New Technology. Thomas J. Polascik, Ulrike Hamper, Benjamin R. Lee, et al. *Urology* 1999; 53: 465–472. (T.J.P., Division of Urologic Surgery, Duke University Medical Center, Durham, NC 27710)

Objectives: To evaluate the efficacy of interstitial saline radiofrequency energy for reproducibly ablating nonmalignant (control) and malignant (the VX-2 tumor) renal tissue in a rabbit model, and to determine the ability of conventional gray-scale and power sonography to image the tumor and ablative process in real time before, during, and after treatment. *Methods:* The VX-2 tumor was implanted beneath the renal capsule in 18 rabbit kidneys. Twelve days after implantation, 50 W of 500-kHz radiofrequency energy was delivered into the surgically externalized renal tumor and contralateral control kidney for 30 or 45-second treatment intervals using an interstitial saline-augmented radiofrequency probe (the virtual electrode). Localization of the tumor and response to treatment were imaged with gray-scale and power Doppler ultrasonography. The effect of radiofrequency and extent of the destructive process on benign and malignant renal tissue were evaluated histologically. *Results:* Mean tumor size was 1.3 × 0.7 cm. Both 30 and 45-second treatment intervals provided marked tissue/tumor ablation. Gross anatomic and histologic analysis showed time-dependent ablated lesions averaging 1.4 ± 0.3 × 1.0 ± 0.3 cm (30-second treatment) and 1.8 ± 0.4 × 1.5 ± 0.3 cm (45-second treatment), with clear demarcation of the surrounding parenchyma. Conventional gray-scale sonography allowed visualization of the ablative process, and power Doppler ultrasound demonstrated changes in the vascular pattern of the tumor both before and after ablation. No immediate treatment-related complications were observed. *Conclusions:* These preliminary studies in a rabbit model demonstrate the feasibility of using the interstitial saline-augmented electrode to ablate small renal tumors and the ability to simultaneously visualize the ablative process using real-time ultrasonography. This technology may have the potential to treat small renal tumors in a minimally invasive manner in the clinical setting.
Authors' Abstract

Reason for selecting abstract:
• New renal tumor ablation technique
Selected by *Stanford M. Goldman, MD*
University of Texas, Houston

Positron Emission Tomography in the Clinical Staging of Patients with Stage I and II Testicular Germ Cell Tumors. Peter Albers, Hans Bender, Hasan Yilmaz, et al. *Urology* 1999; 53:808–811. (P.A., Department of Urology, Bonn University, Bonn D-53105, Germany)

Objectives: To evaluate the accuracy of fluorodeoxyglucose positron emission tomography (PET) compared with computed tomography (CT) staging in patients with Stage I and II testicular germ cell tumors (GCTs). *Methods:* From January 1995 to July 1997, in 37 patients with clinical Stage (CS) I (n = 25) and CS II (n = 12) GCT (24 nonseminomas, 13 seminomas), PET and CT were compared in the initial staging. After PET, the patients with nonseminomatous GCT were staged surgically by retroperitoneal lymph node dissection and the patients with seminomatous GCT were followed up clinically. *Results:* Correct staging by PET was achieved in 34 of 37 patients compared with correct CT staging in 29 of 37 patients. Of 10 metastatic lesions, 7 and 4 were detected by PET and CT, respectively. PET did not show false-positive signals. PET was unable to detect vital cancer with a maximal diameter less than 0.5 cm or teratoma at any size. *Conclusions:* PET was useful for detecting viable tumor in lesions that are visible on CT scan and, thus, it may omit false-positive CS II lesions. However, PET was not able to identify mature teratoma. In this study, PET did not improve the staging in patients with CS I tumor.
Authors' Abstract

Reason for selecting abstract:
• Informational article on the future use of PET
Selected by *Stanford M. Goldman, MD*
University of Texas, Houston

Ultrasound-guided Needle Aspiration in Prostatic Abscess. Argimiro Collado, Juan Palou, Javier García-Penit, et al. *Urology* 1999; 53:548–552. (J.P., Department of Urology, Universidad Autónoma de Barcelona, Fundació Puigvert, c/Cartagena 340-350, Barcelona 08025, Spain)

Objectives: To review the clinical presentation of prostatic abscess and to assess the usefulness of ultrasound-guided needle aspiration as a treatment option for this condition. *Methods:* Between October 1984 and November 1997, prostatic abscess was diagnosed in 31 patients. The average age was 60 years (range 29 to 79). Prostate ultrasound was performed using either a hypogastric or transrectal approach. Initial therapy included ultrasound-guided needle aspiration in 24 (77.4%), transurethral resection of prostate (TURP) in 5 (16.1%), or conservative management with antibiotic therapy. During follow-up, ultrasound examinations and urine cultures were performed on an outpatient basis. *Results:* Past medical history most often included previous urinary infection (15 patients, 48%) and bladder outlet obstruction (13 patients, 42%). Sixty-one percent of patients presented with irritative voiding symptoms at the time of diagnosis. Ultrasound-guided needle aspiration resolved 83.3% of cases; 2 patients needed a second procedure. Three patients required TURP for drainage and 2 to remove an obstruction after abscess resolution. *Conclusions:* A high degree of suspicion is needed to diagnose prostatic abscess clinically. Transrectal ultrasound is necessary for the differential diagnosis. Transrectal ultrasound-guided needle aspiration is a technically simple and effective therapeutic procedure with no morbidity and, in case of failure, may be repeated or a drainage TURP may be undertaken.
Authors' Abstract

Reason for selecting abstract:
• Excellent alternative to surgery
Selected by *Stanford M. Goldman, MD*
University of Texas, Houston

Yield and Efficacy of Biopty Gun Testis Needle Biopsy. Allen F. Morey, Michael F. MacDonald, Thomas A. Rozanski, et al. *Urology* 1999; 53:604–607. (A.F.M., Urology Service, Department of Surgery, Brooke Army Medical Center, MCHE-SDU, Bldg 3600, Rm 225-5, 3851 Roger Brooke Dr, Fort Sam Houston, TX 78234)

Objectives: To assess whether a preliminary skin incision enhances diagnostic yield of percutaneous testis biopsy and to further evaluate the clinical efficacy of this procedure. *Methods:* A total of 45 men (67 testes) underwent testicular biopsy with two passes of a Biopty gun spring-loaded needle. Twenty-seven biopsies were performed without a preliminary skin incision (group 1), and 40 were performed after a small scrotal incision (group 2). In 56 testes, needle biopsy histopathologic diagnosis was compared with that of open biopsy or orchiectomy specimens from the same patient. Needle and surgical specimens were fixed in Bouin's solution and sent separately for independent, blinded, histologic interpretation. *Results:* Complications of the procedure were negligible. In all 67 needle biopsies, specimen quality was adequate for histopathologic interpretation. The mean number of seminiferous tubules obtained from needle biopsy was 28% higher among patients having a preliminary skin incision (25.9) compared with those without (18.7, $P = 0.023$). Correlation between needle and open histopathologic diagnosis was excellent (55 of 56, 98%). *Conclusions:* A preliminary skin incision made before needle biopsy increases the diagnostic yield of percutaneous testis biopsy. Percutaneous testis biopsy using the Biopty gun needle provides equal diagnostic information when compared with open testis biopsy or orchiectomy specimens. The concomitant reduction in morbidity and cost make this an attractive diagnostic procedure.
Authors' Abstract

Reason for selecting abstract:

- Procedure that may replace testicular removal

Selected by *Stanford M. Goldman, MD*
University of Texas, Houston

Cardiovascular System

Prevalence and Risk Factors of Carotid Plaque in Women with Systemic Lupus Erythematosus. Susan Manzi, Faith Selzer, Kim Sutton-Tyrrell, et al. *Arthritis Rheum* 1999; 42:51–60. (S.M., University of Pittsburgh School of Medicine, Liliane Kaufman Bldg, 3471 5th Ave, Suite 502, Pittsburgh, PA 15312)

Objective: To determine the prevalence of carotid atherosclerosis and associated risk factors in women with systemic lupus erythematosus (SLE). *Methods:* Carotid plaque and intima-media wall thickness (IMT) were measured by B-mode ultrasound in women with SLE. Risk factors associated with carotid plaque and IMT were determined at the time of the ultrasound scan and included traditional cardiovascular risk factors, SLE-specific variables, and inflammation markers. *Results:* The 175 women with SLE were predominantly white (87%), with a mean age of 44.9 years (SD 11.5). Twenty-six women (15%) had a previous arterial event (10 coronary [myocardial infarction or angina], 11 cerebrovascular [stroke or transient ischemic attack], and 5 both). The mean ± SD IMT was 0.71 ± 0.14 mm, and 70 women (40%) had focal plaque. Variables significantly associated with focal plaque ($P < 0.05$) included age, duration of lupus, systolic, diastolic, and pulse pressure, body mass index, menopausal status, levels of total and low-density lipoprotein (LDL) cholesterol, fibrinogen and C-reactive protein levels, SLE-related disease damage according to the Systemic Lupus International Collaborating Clinics (SLICC) damage index (modified to exclude cardiovascular parameters), and disease activity as determined by the Systemic Lupus Activity Measure. Women with longer duration of prednisone use and a higher cumulative dose of prednisone as well as those with prior coronary events were more likely to have plaque. In logistic regression models, independent determinants of plaque ($P < 0.05$) were older age, higher systolic blood pressure, higher levels of LDL cholesterol, prolonged treatment with prednisone, and a previous coronary event. Older age, a previous coronary event, and elevated systolic blood pressure were independently associated with increased severity of plaque ($P < 0.01$). Older age, elevated pulse pressure, a previous coronary event, and a higher SLICC disease damage score were independently related to increased IMT ($P < 0.05$). *Conclusion:* B-mode ultrasound provides a useful noninvasive technique to assess atherosclerosis in women with SLE who are at high risk for cardiovascular disease. Potentially modifiable risk factors were found to be associated with the vascular disease detected using this method.
Authors' Abstract

Reason for selecting abstract:

- Use of ultrasonography in complications associated with lupus erythematosus

Selected by *David J. Sartoris, MD*
Veterans Affairs Medical Center, San Diego, Calif

An Algorithm for Noninvasive Identification of Angiographic Three-Vessel and/or Left Main Coronary Artery Disease in Symptomatic Patients on the Basis of Cardiac Risk and Electron-Beam Computed Tomographic Calcium Scores. Axel Schmermund, Kent R. Bailey, John A. Rumberger, et al. *J Am Coll Cardiol* 1999; 33:444–452. (From the Division of Cardiovascular Diseases and Internal Medicine, Mayo Clinic and Foundation, Rochester, Minn)

Objectives: We sought to model an algorithm for noninvasive identification of angiographically obstructive three-vessel and/or left main disease based on conventional cardiac risk assessment and site and extent of coronary calcium determined by electron-beam computed tomography (EBCT). *Background:* Such an algorithm would greatly facilitate clinical triage in symptomatic patients with no previous diagnosis of coronary artery disease (CAD). *Methods:* We examined 291 patients with suspected, but not previously diagnosed, CAD who underwent coronary angiography for clinical indications. Cardiac risk factors were determined as defined by the National Cholesterol Education Program. An EBCT scan was performed in all patients, and a coronary calcium score (Agatston method) was computed. Total per-patient calcium scores and separate scores for the major coronary arteries were generated. These scores were also analyzed for localization of coronary calcium in the more distal versus proximal tomographic sections. These parameters and the risk factors were considered for the model described in the following section. *Results:* Sixty-eight patients (23%) had angiographic three-vessel and/or left main CAD. Multiple logistic regression analysis determined male sex, presence of diabetes and left anterior descending (LAD) and circumflex (LCx) coronary calcium scores, independent from more distal calcium localization, as independent predictors for identification of three-vessel and/or left main CAD. Based on this four variable model, a simple noninvasive index (NI) was constructed as the following: $\log_e$(LAD score) + $\log_e$(LCx score) + 2[if diabetic] + 3[if male]. Receiver operating characteristic curve analysis for this NI yielded an area under the curve of 0.88 ± 0.03 ($p < 0.0001$) for separating patients with, versus without, angiographic three-vessel and/or left main CAD. Various NI cutpoints demonstrated sensitivities from 87–97% and specificities from 46–74%. The NI values >14 increased the probability of angiographic three-vessel and/or left main CAD from 23% (pretest) to 65–100% (posttest), and NI values <10 increased the probability of no three-vessel and/or left main CAD from 77% (pretest) to 95–100% (posttest). *Conclusions:* On the basis of a simple algorithm ("noninvasive index"), EBCT calcium scanning in conjunction with risk factor analysis can rule in or rule out angiographically severe disease, i.e., three-vessel and/or left main CAD, in symptomatic patients.
Authors' Abstract

Reason for selecting abstract:

- Efficacy algorithm for EBCT

Selected by *Robert M. Steiner, MD*
New York Methodist Hospital–Weill Medical College of Cornell University, New York, NY

Assessment of Myocardial Viability by Dobutamine Echocardiography, Positron Emission Tomography and Thallium-201 SPECT: Correlation with Histopathology in Explanted Hearts. Helmut Baumgartner, Gerold Porenta, Yuk-Kong Lau, et al. *J Am Coll Cardiol* 1998; 32:1701–1708. (H.B., Department of Cardiology, Vienna General Hospital, University of Vienna, Währinger Gürtel 18-20, A-1090 Vienna, Austria)

Objectives: We examined the relationship among viability assessment by dobutamine echocardiography (DE), positron emission tomography (PET) and thallium-201 single-photon emission computed tomography (Tl-SPECT) to the degree of fibrosis. *Background:* DE, PET and Tl-SPECT have been shown to be sensitive in identifying viability of asynergic myocardium. However, PET and Tl-SPECT indi-

cated viability in a significant percentage of segments without dobutamine response or functional improvement after revascularization. *Methods:* Twelve patients with coronary artery disease and severely reduced left ventricular function (EF 14.5 ± 5.2%) were studied with DE prior to cardiac transplantation: 5 had additional PET and 7 had Tl-SPECT studies. Results of the three techniques were compared to histologic findings of the explanted hearts. *Results:* Segments with >75% viable myocytes by histology were determined to be viable in 78%, 89% and 87% by DE, PET and Tl-SPECT; those with 50–75% viable myocytes in 71%, 50% and 87%, respectively. Segments with 25–50% viable myocytes showed response to dobutamine in only 15%, but were viable in 60% by PET and 82% by Tl-SPECT. Segments with <25% viable myocytes responded to dobutamine in 19%; however, PET and Tl-SPECT demonstrated viability in 33% and 38%, respectively. Discrepant segments without dobutamine response but viability by PET and SPECT had significantly more viable myocytes by pathology than did those classified in agreement to be nonviable but had significantly less viable myocytes than those classified in agreement to be viable (p < .001). *Conclusions:* These findings suggest that contractile reserve as evidenced by a positive dobutamine response requires at least 50% viable myocytes in a given segment whereas scintigraphic methods also identify segments with less viable myocytes. Thus, the methods may provide complementary information: Nuclear techniques appear to be highly sensitive for the detection of myocardial viability, and negative tests make it highly unlikely that a significant number of viable myocytes are present in a given segment. Conversely, dobutamine echo may be particularly useful for predicting recovery of systolic function after revascularization.
Authors' Abstract

Reasons for selecting abstract:
- Imaging modality comparison
- Indications for PET

Selected by *Robert M. Steiner, MD*
New York Methodist Hospital–Weill Medical College of Cornell University, New York, NY

Significance of Rest Technetium-99m Sestamibi Imaging for the Prediction of Improvement of Left Ventricular Dysfunction after Q Wave Myocardial Infarction: Importance of Infarct Location Adjusted Thresholds. Christian A. Schneider, Eberhard Voth, Sybille Gawlich, et al. *J Am Coll Cardiol* 1998; 32:648–654. (C.A.S., Klinik III für Innere Medizin, Universität zu Köln, Joseph-Stelzmann-Strasse 9, 50934 Cologne, Germany)

Objective: The value of rest technetium-99m (Tc-99m) sestamibi scintigraphy under oral nitrate medication to predict myocardial viability was examined in patients with chronic infarcts. *Background:* The value of rest Tc-99m sestamibi to predict viability in infarct regions has not been fully established because significant underestimation of viability, especially in the inferior myocardial wall, has been reported. *Methods:* Forty patients with Q wave myocardial infarction underwent Tc-99m sestamibi single-photon emission computed tomography under nitrate medication before revascularization of the infarct-related artery. Wall motion was quantified from paired angiograms before and 4 months after revascularization. Tracer uptake was quantified in the central infarct region identified on the angiogram. *Results:* The average Tc-99m sestamibi uptake in the central infarct region of patients with anterior infarcts and improvement of left ventricular function was significantly higher (68 ± 12%, mean ± SD) than in patients without improvement of function (40 ± 14%, p < 0.02). The average Tc-99m sestamibi uptake in the central infarct region of patients with improvement of function and inferior infarcts was significantly lower (43 ± 7%) than in patients with anterior infarcts (68 ± 12%, p < 0.003), but was significantly higher than in patients with inferior infarction and no improvement of function (31 ± 7%, p < 0.02). Using an infarct location adjusted optimal threshold (50% for anterior infarcts, 35% for inferior infarcts), Tc-99m sestamibi had a positive predictive value of 90% and a negative predictive value of 91% for improvement of left ventricular function. *Conclusion:* Quantitative rest Tc-99m sestamibi scintigraphy after oral nitrates reliably predicts improvement of left ventricular function after revascularization if infarct location adjusted thresholds are used.
Authors' Abstract

Reasons for selecting abstract:
- Indications for nuclear cardiac imaging
- Cardiac pathophysiology

Selected by *Robert M. Steiner, MD*
New York Methodist Hospital–Weill Medical College of Cornell University, New York, NY

Musculoskeletal System

The Bath Ankylosing Spondylitis Radiology Index (BASRI): A New, Validated Approach to Disease Assessment. Kirsten MacKay, Christopher Mack, Sinead Brophy, et al. *Arthritis Rheum* 1998; 41:2263–2270. (Andrei Calin, Royal National Hospital for Rheumatic Diseases, Upper Borough Walls, Bath BA1 1RL, United Kingdom)

Objective: To develop a reproducible and simple radiologic scoring system for the spine in patients with ankylosing spondylitis (AS): the Bath Ankylosing Spondylitis Radiology Index for the spine (BASRI-s). *Methods:* Radiographs of 470 patients with AS were scored using the New York criteria for the sacroiliac joints and, similarly, grading the lumbar and cervical spine on a scale of 0–4 (for normal, suspicious, mild, moderate, and severe). These 3 scores were added together to produce the BASRI-s score (scored 2–12). Radiographs of 188 patients were used to test reproducibility. Blinded radiographs of 89 non-AS patients were included, randomly, to assess disease specificity. Sensitivity to change was assessed using 177 radiographs from 58 AS patients. *Results:* Intra- and interobserver variation showed 75–86% and 73–79% complete agreement at all sites, respectively. Specificities of 0.83–0.89 suggested that the lumbar and cervical spine BASRI scores were disease specific. Sensitivity to change became apparent at 2 years ($P < 0.001$). Using a lateral view *and* an anteroposterior view of the lumbar spine was more sensitive than using a lateral view alone. Grading a set of radiographs (sacroiliac joints, lumbar spine, and cervical spine) took 30 seconds. *Conclusion:* BASRI is a reliable method for grading radiographic changes in patients with AS. It is disease specific, sensitive to change, valid, simple, and rapid to perform.
Authors' Abstract

Reason for selecting abstract:
- Method to grade ankylosing spondylitis

Selected by *David J. Sartoris, MD*
Veterans Affairs Medical Center, San Diego, Calif

Grip Strength and the Risk of Developing Radiographic Hand Osteoarthritis: Results from the Framingham Study. Christine E. Chaisson, Yuqing Zhang, Leena Sharma, et al. *Arthritis Rheum* 1999; 42:33–38. (C.E.C., Boston University Arthritis Center, Boston University School of Medicine, 715 Albany St, A-203, Boston, MA 02118)

Objective: In knees, quadriceps strength may protect against osteoarthritis (OA). Muscle activity is a major determinant of forces at the hand joints, and grip is a common task during which high muscle forces are sustained, especially at the proximal hand joints (metacarpophalangeal [MCP] joints and thumb base). This longitudinal study of radiographic hand OA examined the association between incident OA at different hand joints and maximal grip strength. *Methods:* Four hand joint groups were studied: distal interphalangeal (DIP), proximal interphalangeal (PIP), MCP, and the base of the thumb (carpometacarpal and scaphotrapezial combined). Subjects were members of the Framingham OA Study who had a baseline radiograph in 1967–1969 and a followup radiograph in 1992–1993 (mean followup 24 years) and had no prevalent radiographic OA in any hand joint at baseline. Incident disease was defined as development of OA defined as a modified Kellgren/Lawrence grade of ≥2. Grip strength was measured in kilograms by dynamometer in 1958–1961 and again in 1960–1963, and the 2 measures were averaged and divided into sex-specific tertiles. Joint-based analysis was performed by adjusting for age, physical activity, and occupational category using the lowest grip strength tertile as the referent. *Results:* Baseline and followup radiographs were obtained from 746 subjects. Of these, 453 subjects with no prevalent OA at baseline were eligible for analysis. In men, higher maximal grip strength was associated with an increased risk of OA in the PIP (highest tertile odds ratio [OR] 2.8 compared with lowest tertile, 95% confidence interval [95% CI] 1.2–6.7), MCP (highest tertile OR 2.9, 95% CI 1.1–7.4), and thumb base joints (highest tertile OR 2.8, 95% CI 1.1–7.4). In women, there was increased risk of OA in the MCP joints (highest tertile OR 2.7, 95% CI 1.1–6.4). *Conclusion:* Men with high maximal grip strength are at

increased risk for the development of OA in the PIP, MCP, and thumb base joints, and women, in the MCP joints. No association was found between maximal grip strength and incident OA in the DIP joints of men or women.
Authors' Abstract
Reason for selecting abstract:
- Factor relating to risk of developing osteoarthritis

Selected by *David J. Sartoris, MD*
Veterans Affairs Medical Center, San Diego, Calif

The Impact of Hemiparalysis on the Expression of Osteoarthritis. Rafael Segal, Eliezer Avrahami, Ela Lebdinski, et al. *Arthritis Rheum* 1998; 41:2249–2256. (Dan Caspi, Rheumatology Day Care Unit, Tel Aviv Medical Center, 6 Weizman St, Tel Aviv 64239, Israel)

Objective: Primary generalized osteoarthritis (OA), the most prevalent joint disease, is usually symmetric. Sporadic case reports mention decreased OA manifestations in limbs in which there are neurologic deficits, but no systematic research has been published. The aim of the present study was to examine these observations in a planned and controlled survey in a group of patients with OA. *Methods:* Seventy-five geriatric patients with a history of stroke and hemiparalysis were studied clinically and radiographically (hand radiographs; graded according to a modified Altman method) for the presence and the degree of OA in the hands. Detailed clinical and radiologic scores were calculated for each hand. Demographic, occupational, and neurologic data were collected. Patients with other joint or neurologic conditions were excluded. A group of 55 elderly patients without stroke were similarly studied (controls). Scores in the paralyzed hand were compared with those in the nonparalyzed hand in the stroke patients and subgroups (by Student's paired *t*-test and Wilcoxon test). Scores in the dominant hands were compared with those in the nondominant hands in stroke patients and control subjects (by Student's paired *t*-test and Mann-Whitney test). Correlation between the degree of neurologic damage and OA asymmetry (Pearson's correlation coefficient) was also sought. *Results:* Paralyzed hands showed significantly fewer OA changes than nonparalyzed hands, both clinically and radiologically. This trend, accentuated in patients with more severe paralysis, disappeared in those with mild residual paresis. Asymmetry of OA was more pronounced in patients with flaccid, compared with spastic, paralysis. The degree of paralysis and loss of muscle strength correlated with the degree of OA asymmetry. Women had significantly higher OA scores than men. In the control group, dominant hands had higher OA scores, but this finding was concealed among hemiparalyzed patients. Lifetime gross occupational load and present grip strength did not correlate with the degree of OA. *Conclusion:* In elderly patients, hemiparalysis reduces ipsilateral hand expression of OA, while OA is accentuated (or increased) in the dominant hand of patients without paralysis. This first systematic study confirms the findings of previous case reports and lends support to the role of biomechanical factors in the development of OA.
Authors' Abstract
Reason for selecting abstract:
- Causative factor for osteoarthritis

Selected by *David J. Sartoris, MD*
Veterans Affairs Medical Center, San Diego, Calif

Incidence and Risk Factors for Radiographic Knee Osteoarthritis in Middle-aged Women: The Chingford Study. Deborah J. Hart, David V. Doyle, Tim D. Spector. *Arthritis Rheum* 1999; 42:17–24. (D.J.H., Twin Research and Osteoporosis Unit, St Thomas' Hospital, Lambeth Palace Rd, London SE1 7EH, United Kingdom)

Objective: To examine the natural history, role of risk factors, and incidence of knee osteoarthritis (OA) in a prospective study of women from a population cohort. *Methods:* Women from the Chingford Study who had been recruited in 1989 were followed up with knee radiographs 4 years later. A total of 715 paired radiographs (71% of the original sample) were graded for osteophytes and 644 for joint space narrowing (JSN). Women whose radiographs had been graded as 0 in 1989 and as ≥14 years later were classified as having incident disease. Incident cases were compared with controls for associations with a number of risk factors. *Results:* Eighty-one women (12.6%) developed JSN of the knee, equating to an incidence of 3.1% per year. No clear risk factors for JSN were identified. Reproducibility of measures of joint space is poor, however, leading to inaccuracy of definition. Incident knee osteophytes developed in 95 women (13.3%), equating to an incidence of 3.3% per year. Compared with controls, women with incident knee osteophytes were older, heavier, and had more hand OA and knee symptoms. Women in the top tertile of obesity (body mass index >26.4) had a significantly increased risk of incident knee osteophytes (odds ratio [OR] 2.38, 95% confidence interval [95% CI] 1.29–4.39). Incident knee osteophytes increased by 20% per 5-year age increase. A nonsignificant protective effect for incident knee osteophytes was seen with current estrogen replacement therapy (ERT) (OR 0.41, 95% CI 0.12–1.42). No effect was associated with smoking, physical activity, hysterectomy, or previous knee injury. *Conclusion:* Obesity and aging are associated with a high risk of new knee OA developing in women. Evidence of a protective effect of ERT was seen. No clear association was found for incident JSN, suggesting that different etiologic mechanisms are operating or that standard radiographs are an inaccurate measure of incident narrowing.
Authors' Abstract
Reason for selecting abstract:
- Risk factors for osteoarthritis

Selected by *David J. Sartoris, MD*
Veterans Affairs Medical Center, San Diego, Calif

Neurosciences

Discrepancy between Regional Cerebral Blood Flow and Glucose Metabolism of the Brain in Systemic Lupus Erythematosus Patients with Normal Brain Magnetic Resonance Imaging Findings. Chia-Hung Kao, Yung-Jen Ho, Jung-Liang Lan, et al. *Arthritis Rheum* 1999; 42:61–68. (C.H.K., Department of Nuclear Medicine, Taichung Veterans General Hospital, 160 Taichung Harbor Rd, Section 3, Taichung 40705, Taiwan, Republic of China)

Objective: In this study, 2 updated brain-imaging modalities, technetium-99m hexamethylpropylene amine oxime–single-photon–emission computed tomography (HMPAO-SPECT) and fluorine-18 2-fluoro-2-deoxy-D-glucose-positron emission tomography (FDG-PET), were used to simultaneously detect regional cerebral blood flow (rCBF) and glucose metabolism of the brain in patients with systemic lupus erythematosus (SLE). *Methods:* Twenty-five female SLE patients, ages 25–40 years, were enrolled in this study and assigned to 1 of 2 groups. Group 1 consisted of 13 patients with neuropsychiatric manifestations (7 had major and 6 had minor manifestations). Group 2 consisted of 12 patients without neuropsychiatric manifestations. Serum levels of anticardiolipin antibodies (aCL) and anti-ribosomal P antibodies (anti-P) were measured. All patients had normal brain magnetic resonance imaging (MRI) findings. Ten healthy female volunteers also underwent brain MRI, HMPAO-SPECT, and FDG-PET for comparison. *Results:* ^{99m}Tc-HMPAO-SPECT revealed hypoperfusion lesions in 11 (44%) of 25 SLE patients, including 9 (69%) of the 13 patients in group 1, 7 (100%) of the 7 patients with major manifestations, 2 (33%) of the 6 patients with minor manifestations, and 2 (17%) of the 12 patients in group 2. Parietal lobes were the areas most commonly involved. FDG-PET revealed hypometabolism in 7 (54%) of the group 1 patients, 6 (86%) of the 7 patients with major manifestations, and 1 (17%) of the 6 patients with minor manifestations. Temporal lobes were the most commonly involved areas. However, no significant hypometabolism brain lesions were found in group 2 patients. All of the 4 patients with headaches and dizziness or headaches alone had normal findings on HMPAO-SPECT and FDG-PET. Nine (36%) of the 25 patients were positive for aCL. However, the presence of aCL was not related to neuropsychiatric manifestations or to HMPAO-SPECT or FDG-PET findings. Five (20%) of the 25 patients had anti-P antibodies and psychosis/depression. *Conclusion:* In patients with normal brain MRI findings, decreases in glucose metabolism coupled with decreases in rCBF are associated with serious neuropsychiatric SLE (NPSLE) presentations, while normal glucose metabolism with decreases in rCBF may be found in SLE patients with or without NPSLE.
Authors' Abstract
Reason for selecting abstract:
- Importance of glucose metabolism in lupus erythematosus

Selected by *David J. Sartoris, MD*
Veterans Affairs Medical Center, San Diego, Calif

Classified Services

POLICY

As a service to its readers, *Radiology* accepts classified advertising, and every effort is made to ensure that the ads are relevant to the practice of radiology. Acceptable categories include positions available, positions sought, fellowships, announcements of post-graduate courses or symposia, practices for sale, medical facilities for rent or sale, used radiologic equipment and apparatus for sale, medical employment bureau advertising, academic posts to be filled, available posts for interns and residents, and malpractice insurance. We retain the right to refuse any advertisement considered not relevant, and respondents are advised to investigate each offer since we cannot assume responsibility for the offers or claims of advertisers.

RATES (per month, per insertion)

Line ads in *Radiology* (no agency commission)

50 words or less $100.00

51–100 words $145.00

Each word over 100—$1.00 per word.

Box Number—$30.00 additional per each insertion (this service is optional).

TERMS

Payment must accompany order.* Make checks payable to **Radiological Society of North America.** We accept American Express, VISA, Mastercard, and Diners Club for classified ads. Call for details. Send payment to:

RSNA, Radiology Classified Ad Department
Accounts Payable, 820 Jorie Boulevard
Oak Brook, IL 60523-2251 USA.

*Purchase Order Numbers are accepted with prior approval.

Please mark each issue:

❒ Jan ❒ Feb ❒ Mar ❒ Apr ❒ May ❒ June
❒ July ❒ Aug ❒ Sept ❒ Oct ❒ Nov ❒ Dec

Send invoice and tearsheet to:

____

____

____

____

Advertisers who cancel ads will not receive refunds.

DEADLINE

Copy must be received by the **20th of the second month preceding issue**. Please submit copy typed and double-spaced. Initials or abbreviations equal one word. Telephone numbers with area code equal one word.

CLASSIFIED DISPLAY ADVERTISING

Black and white frequency rates are based on the total number of insertions used within a 12-month period from date of first insertion.

Ad Space	Size	1X	6X	12X
1 page	7" x 9-1/2"	$2350	2270	2190
2/3 pg vert	4-1/2" x 9-1/2"	$2000	1930	1860
1/2 pg horzt	7" x 4-1/2"	$1550	1490	1430
1/2 pg vert	3-3/8" x 9-1/2"	$1550	1490	1430
1/2 pg island	4-1/4" x 7-1/2"	$1550	1490	1430
1/3 pg vert	2-1/4" x 9-1/2"	$1100	1050	1000
1/3 pg square	4-1/2" x 4-1/2"	$1100	1050	1000
1/4 page	3-3/8" x 4-1/2"	$ 900	860	820
1/6 page	2-1/4" x 4-1/2"	$ 650	630	610
1/9 page	2-1/4" x 3"	$ 450	430	410

Preferred materials are composite negatives, right-reading, emulsion side down. (Conversion materials such as positive film, repro proofs, and camera-ready artworks are acceptable; there may be an additional charge.)

Customer supplied negative: cost as noted
Customer supplied copy to be set and ad prepared: add 20%

Call Production Department for additional information.
Address for correspondence, insertion orders, copy, proofs, box number, and payment:

***Radiology* Advertising Production Office**
820 Jorie Boulevard
Oak Brook, IL 60523-2251

To respond to a box number ad, send your CV and/or any other information to the above address; on the front of the envelope, please indicate the appropriate box number.

For further information:
Carissa Muccianti, *Advertising Coordinator*
630.571.7817
630.571.7837 (fax)

Positions Available

THE DEPARTMENT OF RADIOLOGY AT THE UNIVERSITY OF ALABAMA AT BIRMINGHAM—Is actively recruiting an interventional radiologist. The section of Vascular and Interventional Radiology provides services for 1,100-beds at the University and Verteran's Administration Hospitals and performs over 5,500 procedures per year. Currently there are three full-time faculty members. Facilities include a Siemens Multistar TOP and two Philips angio suites currently under construction. Applicants must be Board certified in diagnostic radiology, have a CAQ in vascular and interventional radiology (or eligible for a CAQ), and eligible for licensure in the state of Alabama. Duties include medical student and resident teaching, radiology service and clinical research. Academic rank and tenure status will depend upon qualifications and experience. Interested candidates should submit their CV to Robert J. Stanley, MD, Department of Radiology, University of Alabama at Birmingham, AL 35233. The University of Alabama at Birmingham is an affirmative action/equal opportunity employer.

THE UNIVERSITY OF KENTUCKY—Is seeking a full-time, tenured line, open rank academic thoracic radiologist. Must be Board eligible; certification preferred. Duties would also include interpretation of film for evaluation of occupational lung disease. Responsibilities include patient care, medical student and resident teaching, and regularly scheduled interdepartment conferences. Opportunity to pursue clinical research. Please mail or fax letter of interest and curriculum vitae to James C. Reed, MD, Chairman, Department of Radiology, HX304, UK Medical Center, Lexington, KY 40536-0084; fax 606-257-6014. UK is an equal opportunity employer.

ASHEVILLE, NC— A board certified radiologist is needed to help with night, weekend day, and holiday call coverage of 21 person group practice in major refereral center. Partnership track available with excellent time off and benefits package in beautiful mountain vacation area. Send CV to Ms. Sue Spivey, P.O. Box 2959, Ashe-ville, NC 28802

CROSS-SECTIONAL IMAGER (CT, ULTRASOUND AND MRI)—Northeastern PA partnership track position. Interventional skills a definite plus. Eight man group currently provides complete range of services for a busy community hospital, two MRI imaging centers, and a private office practice. Generous salary and outstanding benefit package. Flexible timetable, but can start immediately. Reply to Radiological Group, Inc, c/o J.F. Sauchak, Business Manager, 327 N Washington Ave, Suite 400, Scranton, PA 18503; telephone 717-346-7501; fax 717-344-3858.

MUSCULOSKELETAL AND EMERGENCY RADIOLOGIST—The Department of Radiology at the University of Rochester Medical Center has a faculty position available in musculoskeletal and emergency radiology. Clinical services at Strong Memorial Hospital perform 200,000 diagnostic examinations per year. State-of-the-art facilities are available in all modalities. The emergency department is a level one trauma center and the musculoskeletal unit performs 5,000 radiological examinations per year. Fellowship training is preferred but not required. Send cover letter and CV to Arvin E. Robinson, MD, Chair, Department of Radiology, University of Rochester Medical Center, Box 648, 601 Elmwood Ave, Rochester, NY 14642 or fax to 716-756-8290. Deadline for applications is March 1, 1999. The University of Rochester is an equal opportunity employer.

NEURORADIOLOGIST/MRI/INTERVENTIONALIST—NE PA, partnership track position. Eight member group seeking neuroradiologist (or equivalent expertise) with neurological and musculoskeletal MRI skills, and strong interventional background. Group currently provides complete range of services for a community hospital, MRI imaging center and a private office practice. Generous salary and outstanding benefit package. Flexible timetable, but can start immediately. Reply to Radiological Group, Inc, c/o J.F. Sauchak, Business Manager, 327 N Washington Ave, Suite 400, Scranton, PA 18503; telephone 717-346-7501.

ABERDEEN, SD—Excellent opportunity for Board certified diagnostic radiologist to join a group of five well-established radiologists. Must be seasoned in all aspects of radiology. Strong interest in musculoskeletal preferred but not necessary. Minimal angio/interventional procedures required. This beautiful regional medical center is located in a crime free, family-oriented community. Excellent salary, benefits, paid vacation and CME allowance. Contact Robin Lorber, EMSA, 1-800-422-3672 ext 7397; fax 954-424-3270. EEO/AA/M/F.

RADIOLOGISTS (ALL TYPES)—Kendall and Davis has numerous radiology openings nationwide. For a detailed description of these positions, check out our website at *www.KENDALLandDAVIS.com*, or if you prefer, call Judi Phillips at 800-950-1551 or fax your CV to 314-843-2262. Sorry, no J-1 positions available.

THE UNIVERSITY OF TENNESSEE, MEMPHIS—Is actively recruiting for a radiologist specializing in cross-sectional imaging. The Radiology Department provides services for 1,600 adult and pediatric beds in an urban medical center which includes the Regional Medical Center at Memphis and its Level I trauma center, the tertiary UT/Bowld Hospital and its active renal, liver and pancreas transplant service, the Memphis VA Medical Center, the LeBonheur Children's Hospital and the Jude Cancer Research Institute. Applicants must be Board certified or eligible in diagnostic radiology, fellowship trained in body imaging and eligible for licensure in the state of Tennessee. Sub-specialty training is preferable but not required. Appointment will be at the Assistant to Associate level depending upon experience and qualifications. Interested applicants should respond with a letter of interest, current curriculum vitae and the names and addresses of three references to Robert E. Gold, MD, Chair, Department of Radiology, The University of Tennessee, Memphis, 800 Madison Ave, Memphis, TN 38163. The University of Tennessee is an equal opportunity/affirmative action/Title IX/Section 504/ADA employer.

NIGHT RADIOLOGISTS—Bay Imaging Consultants Medical Group, Inc, a large San Francisco Bay area private practice radiology group with multiple outpatient and hospital sites, is seeking night radiologists for the night rotation. The night rotation is comprised of 12-hour rotations from 7:00pm to 7:00am. Must be Board certified. Competitive salary. Start date as soon as possible. Please submit your CV, a cover letter and the names of three references to Human Resources, 175 Lennon Ln, Suite 100, Walnut Creek, CA 94598. EOE.

EXPERIENCED BOARD CERTIFIED DIAGNOSTIC RADIOLOGIST—Join 15 radiologists in a highly successful group covering multiple hospitals and OP facilities. High volume practice includes all aspects of general radiology. Specific interest in body MR, US, and nuclear medicine preferred. Partnership tract includes excellent compensation/benefit package including paid vacation, malpractice & health insurance pension with CME and moving allowance. Very progressive medical community located 90 miles from Dallas in East Texas. Send CV to Larry Smith, Practice Administrator, Tyler Radiology Assoc, 1407 S Fleishel, Suite 301, Tyler, TX 75701 or fax to 903-593-0559.

DIAGNOSTIC RADIOLOGIST—With stable five person group in Duluth, MN. Candidate must be proficient in all aspects of diagnostic imaging, routine angiography and interventional procedures. Fellowship training strongly preferred. Position leads to partnership. Apply to Calvin C. Loken, MD, 924 E Superior St, Suite 109, Duluth, MN 55802.

VASCULAR/INTERVENTIONAL RADIOLOGIST—The Department of Radiology at Saint Louis University Health Sciences Center is seeking an ABR eligible or certified, fellowship trained vascular/interventional radiologist for a full-time, faculty position open in July, 1999. The rapidly expanding practice has a case load including diagnostic angiography (including pulmonary angiography), angioplasty, central venous access, thrombolysis, embolization, IVC Filter placement, biliary and uroradiology, TIPS, percutaneous biopsy and percutaneous gastrostomy. A broad range of teaching and research opportunities is available. Appointment is anticipated at the Assistant Professor level. For information, contact Thomas Bocchini, MD, Chief, Section of Interventional Radiology, Department of Radiology, Saint Louis University Health Sciences Center, 3635 Vista at Grand Boulevard, St. Louis, MO 63110-0250. Phone 314-268-5784; fax 314-268-5116. Saint Louis University Health Sciences Center is an equal opportunity employer M/F/D/V.

RADIOLOGY, SALEM, OR—Northwest Permanente, PC, a physician managed, multispecialty group serving the members of Kaiser Permanente in the northwest division, has an excellent opportunity beginning in 1999 for a BC/BE radiologist to join two radiologists at our medical facilities in Salem, OR capital city. Located 45 miles South of Portland, our Salem 40-physician multispecialty group currently offers professional services to 43,000 plan members in the area. Our need is for a general radiologist whose skills include CT, US, fluoroscopy and mammography. Northwest Permanente has a total of 32 radiologists at our clinics and affiliated hospitals in the Portland metropolitan area and Salem providing quality care to over 430,000 plan members in Oregon and Washington. Ours is a collegial and stimulating practice in one of the most successful managed care programs in the country. In addition to a lifestyle inherent to the beautiful Pacific Northwest, we offer a predictable work schedule, and a competitive salary and benefit package which includes professional liability coverage, a comprehensive pension program, sabbatical leave and more. For additional information please forward CV to R.A. Clark, Director, Physician Resources, Northwest Permanente, PC, 500 NE Mult-nomah, Suite 100, Portland, OR 97232-2099. EOE.

PEDIATRIC RADIOLOGIST—The University of Mississippi Medical Center is actively seeking a fellowship-trained pediatric radiologist. Candidates must be certified by the American Board of Radiology and must have or be eligible to sit for the certificate of added qualification in pediatric radiology. Letters of interest and CV should be addressed to Dr Brent Harrison, Professor and Chairman, Department of Radiology, The University of Mississippi Medical Center, 2500 North State St, Jackson, MS 39216. EOE, M/F/D/V.

NAVAJO INDIAN HEALTH SERVICE—Wanted! Full time radiologist for Navajo Indian Health Hospitals: Shiprock, NM, Gallup, NM, Chinle, AZ and Tuba City, AZ, serving the Navajo nation. Modalities include general radiology US, CT, mammography, ultrasound and mobile MRI. Teleradiology services available. Government benefits. Live within driving distance of the Grand Canyon, Mesa Verde, Monument Valley & canyon lands of southern Utah. Send CV to Jim Jones, Acting Director/Recruitment, PO Box 9020, Window Rock, AZ 86515, fax 520-871-5868 or call 520-871-5880. An equal opportunity employer. Preference in filling positions given to qualified Native Americans in accordance with the Indian Preference Act. US citizenship required. Not a J-1 visa sponsor.

RADIA MEDICAL IMAGING—A 36+ member progressive radiology practice serving the Seattle area and extending East and North is seeking Board certified radiologists. Candidates with fellowship training are preferred. Radia serves five hospitals, one large multi-specialty clinic and various outpatient sites. Implementation of 24-hour emergency services coverage via a teleradiology network and elevated exam volumes have increased a need for radiologists. Positions open include: general "nighthawk" radiologist with cross-sectional imaging expertise, women's imager with expertise in breast and pelvic imaging, nuclear medicine, and neuroradiologist. If you are interested in working in a high quality, progressive practice and living in an environment that allows access to a multitude of metropolitan and outdoor recreational activities, please forward your CV to Physician Recruitment Committee, c/o Cheryl West, Radia Medical Imaging, Inc, 728 134th St SW 120, Everett, WA, 98204; fax 425-297-6250, e-mail *cwest@radiax.com.*

PRICE, UTAH—Small group practice on beautiful Colorado plateau seeks ABR certified/eligible general radiologist. Fellowship preferred but not required. All modalities except angiography. Southeastern Utah Radiology PC, PO Box 255, Price, Utah 84501, fax 435-613-0345, or e-mail *psheya@castlenet.com.*

RADIOLOGISTS-WISCONSIN—LaSalle Clinic, a 190-plus physician multi-specialty group with 27 locations in northeast Wisconsin, is recruiting two BE/BC radiologists to join their five physician radiology team. Successful candidates will perform the full gamut of diagnostic and interventional radiology services. Neuroradiology fellowship desirable for one position. Industry-leading salary and benefits package. Enjoy diverse social and cultural activities. Live and practice in a safe, comfortable family environment and benefit from a growing local economy and nationally acclaimed educational systems. For more information, contact LaSalle Clinic Medical Staffing, PO Box 8005, Menasha, WI 54952-8005; phone 800-722-9989, e-mail *cfielkow@affinityhealth.org, http://www.lasalleclinic.com*

A 130-BED COMMUNITY HOSPITAL IN NORTH CAROLINA—Seeks two Board certified or Board eligible radiologists (requires one with an interventional fellowship). Scenic, family-oriented community offers year-round activities, close proximity to mountains and beaches. Competitive salary, paid malpractice, excellent fringe benefits. Please forward confidential CV to Box R-106.

GEORGIA—Immediate opening for Board certified radiologist to join a six-member group expanding to seven due to practice growth. Group covers three hospitals and a brand new 5200 sq ft outpatient imaging center with state-of-the-art equipment, including Acuson Sequoia Ultrasound, three Helical CT scanners, ADAC variable head nuclear medicine camera and GE Horizon 1.5 Tesla MRI. Position is a partnership track with excellent benefits and salary, located 90 minutes south of Atlanta. Please send CV to Scott M. Stephen, MD, 748 F North Houston Rd, Warner Robins, GA 31093 or fax to 912-922-6116. For further information, call Kim at 912-922-5214.

GREATER CINCINNATI AREA—General radiologist needed to join strong, progressive 22-member group. Special interest in nuclear medicine, body imaging and/or mammography would be helpful. Nonvascular interventional skills required. This is a partnership track position. Please send CV to Mr Joe Roesel, PO Box 17630, 170 Barnwood Dr, Edgewood, KY 41017; fax 606-344-1117; e-mail *Dlubbers @msn.com*

TIFTON, GEORGIA—A three-man radiology group in South Georgia seeks general radiologist with special interest/training in MR or interventional radiology. Partnership track position to begin July 2000. Generous time off. Two hours to Atlantic or Gulf. Send CV to Dr Kelley P. Douglas, Tifton Radiology, PC, 1495 Kennedy Rd, Tifton, GA 31794 or fax to 912-386-4495.

VERMONT—Community hospital practice in lovely rolling hills of southern Vermont has an opening for full-time general diagnostic (BC/BE) radiologist. Department features all modalities including up-to-date digital fluoro, spiral CT, new US units and mobile MRI. Exceptionally vibrant community with active music, theater, dance. Outdoor sports virtually out your back door. Competitive salary leading to full partnership in one year. Please reply to Peter D. Gibbons, MD, Brattleboro Memorial Hospital, 17 Belmont Ave, Brattleboro, VT 05301. (E-mail *gbbn@sover.net*)

DIAGNOSTIC RADIOLOGIST—The Department of Radiology at Wayne State University and the Detroit Medical Center has an immediate opening for a Board certified radiologist with significant experience or with fellowship training in cross sectional imaging. The department offers an extremely competitive compensation package as well as an opportunity to actively participate in its teaching and research programs. Interested candidates should send a current curriculum vitae and introductory letter to Lawrence P. Davis, MD, FACR, Associate Chair, Department of Radiology DRH 3L8, 4201 St. Antoine, Detroit, MI 48201. Telephone 313-745-8585, fax 313-577-8600, *ldavis @med.wayne.edu*. Equal opportunity employer.

WESTERN NORTH CAROLINA—Diagnostic radiologist needed to practice and live in Brevard, NC, a beautiful college town in the Smoky Mountains located 30 miles from Asheville. Individuals should have skills and interest in all phases of diagnostic radiology, including CT, NM, US, mammography and basic interventional/special procedures. This is a partnership track position within a 24-physician practice based in Asheville which will provide subspecialty backup, vacation coverage and after hours teleradiology. The individual selected for this position will rotate through the Asheville practice on a regular basis. Please contact Sue Spivey, PO Box 2959, Asheville, NC 28802.

RADIOLOGY OPENING—Growing practice in Dallas/Fort Worth area seeks well trained, Board certified, personable radiologist, fellowship-trained in neuroradiology, to join our group as we practice quality radiology and enjoy a great lifestyle in a suburban practice. The ideal candidate will be CAQ eligible or certified in neuroradiology, but comfortable with a wide range of modalities, including interventional. Partnership track position. Contact Greg Naugher, MD, Family Radiology, 1614 Scripture, Suite 2, Denton, TX 76201-3892.

BREAST IMAGING RADIOLOGIST—The Department of Radiology at Wayne State University and the Detroit Medical Center has an immediate opening for a Board certified radiologist with fellowship training in mammography. The position requires expertise in mammography, breast ultrasound and interventional breast procedures. The department offers an extremely competitive compensation package as well as an opportunity to actively participate in its teaching and research programs. Interested candidates should send a current curriculum vitae and introductory letter to Lawrence P. Davis, MD, FACR, Associate Chair, Department of Radiology DRH 3L8, 4201 St. Antoine, Detroit, MI 48201. Telephone 313-745-8585, fax 313-577-8600, *ldavis @med.wayne.edu*. Equal opportunity employer.

DIRECTOR OF BREAST IMAGING—Suburban LA hospital seeks breast imager to direct large breast imaging center affiliated with a 400-bed in-patient facility. Has screening, diagnostic mammography services, ultrasound, ABBI, mammotome, and access to MRI. Must be Board certified in radiology and capable of performing other routine radiographic studies. Please reply to Box R-107.

VASCULAR/INTERVENTIONAL RADIOLOGIST—Seeking a fellowship-trained vascular/interventional radiologist competent in vascular access and magnetic resonance angiography to join three interventionalists. The position is a partnership position with a private practice group consisting of 22 diagnostic radiologists and four radiation oncologists. The group serves two tertiary care hopitals -total of 900 beds- and a regional VA hospital. Sioux Falls is a referral center for eastern South Dakota, northwestern Iowa and southwestern Minnesota. Approximately 1800 interventional procedures are performed annually. Medical X-Ray Center offers an excellent salary and benefits package. For more information, see our website at *www.medx-ray.com*. Please forward CVs to Sandy Fox, Medical X-Ray Center, 1417 S Minnesota Ave, Sioux Falls, SD 57105; fax 605-373-0718, e-mail *sfox @medx-ray.com*.

CARDIOVASCULAR/INTERVENTIONALIST—The SUNY Health Science Center at Syracuse Department of Radiology has immediate openings for full-time academic cardiovascular/interventional radiologists, one of whom will be the director of the Division of CVI Radiology. The division performs 3800 procedures per year plus an additional 750-800 cases per year at the Syracuse Veterans Administration Medical Center. Fellowship training and ABR certification in diagnostic radiology is required. CAQ in interventional radiology is highly desirable. Responsibilities include teaching, research publication and patient care. The division is staffed by nine dedicated CVI technologists, ten CVI nurses, two radiology residents and one fellow participating in our ACGME-accredited fellowship program. Excellent equipment, work environment, support personnel and research facilities are available. The level of faculty appointment and salary will depend upon the applicant's experience and academic productivity. The SUNY Health Science Center is a 380-bed tertiary care academic health care center in Syracuse, New York, a short drive from the Adirondack Mountains and Lake Ontario. Applicants should respond with a letter of interest and copy of their current CV to John F. Cardella, MD, Chairman, Department of Radiology, SUNY Health Science Center, 750 East Adams St, Syracuse, NY 13210 or *cardellj@mailbox .hscsyr.edu*. SUNY Health Science Center is a smoke-free campus, an equal opportunity/affirmative action employer, and encourages minority and female applicants to apply.

THE DEPARTMENT OF REGIONAL RADIOLOGY AT THE CLEVELAND CLINIC FOUNDATION—Cleveland, Ohio, is in the process of recruiting ABR certified general diagnostic radiologists to practice in community hospitals and ambulatory care facilities, which are part of the Cleveland Clinic Health System. The department consists of 20 staff radiologists servicing four community hospitals and seven ambulatory care facilities/surgi centers. Approximately 278,000 examinations were performed at the sites in 1998. The hospital departments and outpatient facilities are fully networked (imaging and RIS) with the Cleveland Clinic Foundation main campus radiology department, which is staffed by 48 subspecialty radiologists. If this opportunity is appealing to you, please contact Gregory P. Borkowski, MD, FACR, Chairman, Regional Radiology Practice, The Cleveland Clinic Foundation, Department of Radiology, Hb-6, 9500 Euclid Ave, Cleveland, OH 44195; phone 216-444-6625, fax 216-445-4432, e-mail *borkowg @cesmtp.ccf.org*.

PRIVATE PRACTICE OPPORTUNITY IN OLYMPIA, WA—Immediate opening for a Board certified general radiologist with additional experience and fellowship training. The practice is in a rapidly expanding medical community and covers a 340-bed referral hospital, two small community hospitals, an outpatient imaging office, and a large multi-specialty clinic. Intention of long-term partnership is necessary. Contact Jim Bonifield, MD, at 3417 Ensign Rd NE, Olympia, WA 98506-5075. Telephone 360-493-4602, or fax 360-493-4603.

EXPERIENCED BODY MR RADIOLOGIST—Wayne State University Department of Radiology seeks an experienced body MR radiologist for section chief and medical director of the MR Center. Responsibilities include teaching, research, patient care and administration of a center which has three state-of-the-art whole body magnets, one of which is dedicated to research, and a 4.7T animal imager. The center currently performs 10,500 studies per year. There is an active interdisciplinary research program in both MRI and MRS with full-time physicists, biochemists and graduate students. Send inquiries with CV to Renate Soulen, MD, MR Center, Harper Hospital, 3990 John R St, Detroit, MI 48201, e-mail *rsoulen@med.wayne.edu*. Wayne State University is an equal opportunity/affirmative action employer.

EVENING/WEEKEND DIAGNOSTIC RADIOLOGISTS—Midwest group seeking Board certified (eligible) individuals to rotate coverage. General, CT, US, nuclear medicine skills needed. Basic angio helpful. Salaried positions; 810-412-9944, ask for Judi.

MINNESOTA: BUSY MINNESOTA RADIOLOGY PRACTICE—Dakota Clinic, a 175-physician-owned multispecialty clinic based in Fargo, North Dakota, is seeking a BE/BC radiologist for our Thief River Falls, Minnesota division for the summer of 2000. Located in northwest Minnesota, this 16-physician group is looking to replace its retiring radiologist with an eager individual proficient in general, CT, MRI and nuclear radiology. Enjoy a new 50,000 square foot state-of-the-art clinic and modern hospital. We offer a competitive salary and benefits package with stockholdership available after two years. Thief River Falls, the home of Arctic Cat snowmobiles, is a growing community of 9,000 with a service area of 45,000. This family-oriented community offers excellent schools, low crime, hunting, fishing and easy access to Minnesota lakes. To learn more about this opportunity, mail, fax or e-mail your CV to Dick Reis, Physician Recruitment Manager, Dakota Clinic Ltd, 1702 S University Dr, Fargo, ND 58103. Fax 701-280-3229, e-mail *dreis@dakcl.com*, toll-free number 1-800-882-7310. Dakota Clinic: *www.dakotaclinic.com*.

INTERVENTIONAL RADIOLOGIST—Needed to replace retiring partner in expanding 22-person quality private practice. Multiple hospitals and clinics will see 2300 or more cases of all types this year including transplant work. You will join three other interventionalists who have good working relationship with vascular surgeons and others. This is the senior radiology practice in Iowa. Desirable urban location. Please respond to Jeffrey H. Watters, MD, Radiology PC, 1221 Pleasant, Ste 150, Des Moines, IA 50309. 515-979-4419.

NEURORADIOLOGIST—The University of Michigan at Ann Arbor is seeking an academic neuroradiologist. Call or e-mail Dr. Gebarski for details at 734-936-4484; *gebarski@umich.edu*.

VISITING FACULTY POSITION IN CLINICAL CT RESEARCH—The Department of Radiology at Indiana University School of Medicine has a research position for a radiologist with clinical research interest in multi-slice spiral CT. The researcher will help design and carry out clinical research studies in collaboration with faculty subspecialty radiologists in thoracic, abdominal, musculoskeletal and neuroradiology and write manuscripts for publication in peer-reviewed journals. There is excellent supporting infrastructure including research nurses, technologists, secretaries, statisticians, PACS, workstations, graphics/photographic equipment, and information systems. Rank and salary will be commensurate with experience and qualifications. Interested applicants should send their curriculum vitae to Dr Kenyon Kopecky, Department of Radiology, Indiana University Hospital Room 0279, 550 N University Blvd, Indianapolis, IN 46202-5253 or e-mail *kkopecky @iupui.edu*. Indiana University is an EO/AA employer.

CENTRAL MASSACHUSETTS—Group of nine seeking fellowship-trained or experienced radiologist with cross sectional or neuro expertise. Busy practice with expanding CT and MRI volume. Basic angiography skills a plus. Competitive salary and partnership track. Contact Dr Mark Sykes, 33 Oak Ave, Worcester, MA 01605. 508-753-8151, fax 508-752-2759.

GENERAL RADIOLOGIST—Progressive radiology group located in Southwest seeks Board certified, fellowship-trained general radiologist for partnership track position. Should be competent in all modalities. Excellent lifestyle, salary and benefits. Reply to Box R-108.

NEURORADIOLOGIST POSITION—The Medical College of Wisconsin is recruiting a neuroradiologist to its six-person neuroradiology section. The position offers excellent academic opportunity, in particular the use of fMRI and MR spectroscopy. Imaging facilities include three state-of-the-art CT scanners with helical capabilities and a Light Speed QX\i GE CT scanner; three MR scanners (Signa plus Horizon LX) and access to an experimental 3.0T imager; three up-to-date angiographic suites with state-of-the-art digital biplane capabilities. Staffing includes six neuroradiologists with excellent academic credentials and specialized areas of expertise. The clinical rotations are equalized and the staff functions as a team. Send letters of application and CV to David Daniels, MD, Chief of Neuroradiology, 9200 W Wisconsin Ave, Milwaukee, WI 53226; or via e-mail *ddaniels@mcw.edu* or fax 414-259-9290; or phone 414-259-3122. The Medical College of Wisconsin is an affirmative action/ equal opportunity employer.

NEURO-INTERVENTIONALIST POSITION—The Medical College of Wisconsin is recruiting a neuro-interventionalist to its six-person neuroradiology section. The neuro-interventionalist should be prepared to build a neuro-interventional program, and must have completed a neuro-interventional fellowship. The position offers excellent academic opportunity, in particular the use of fMRI and MR spectroscopy in planning and monitoring interventional procedures. Imaging facilities include three state-of-the-art CT scanners with helical capabilities; three Signa MR scanners and access to an experimental 3.0T imager; three up-to-date angiographic suites with state-of-the-art digital biplane capabilities. Staffing includes six neuroradiologists with excellent academic credentials and specialized areas of expertise. Send letters of application and CV to David Daniels, MD, Chief of Neuroradiology, 9200 W Wisconsin Ave, Milwaukee, WI 53226; or via e-mail *ddaniels@mcw.edu* or fax 414-259-9290; or phone 414-259-3122. The Medical College of Wisconsin is an affirmative action/ equal opportunity employer.

WANTED: BOARD CERTIFIED RADIOLOGISTS IN NE PENNSYLVANIA—Radiological Consultants, Inc, has a demand for several radiologists secondary to both retiring members as well as an expanding service area. We are group of 17 radiologists in northeast Pennsylvania covering two hospitals in Scranton, one hospital in Wilkes Barre, one hospital in Nanticoke, as well as an MRI center which houses two 1.5 Tesla magnets as well as an open 0.3 Tesla magnet. We are currently targeting fellowship trained or an equivalent experienced radiologist. Competitive salary and benefits are being offered for this excellent opportunity. Reply to Radiological Consultants, Inc, c/o John J. Culliney, MD, 751 Keystone Industrial Park, Dunmore, PA 18512. Phone 717-346-8272 or fax CV to 717-346-4872.

MAMMOGRAPHER IN CENTRAL JERSEY—Group of five hospital-based private practice radiologists seeking fellowship trained mammographer for new state-of-the-art women's center including stereotactic biopsy. Partnership opportunity. Please contact Dr. McManus, 732-886-4445.

GENERAL RADIOLOGIST—Board certified general radiologist for non-partnership track position with highly desirable large southwestern diagnostic radiology practice. Must be competent in all modalities. Competitive salary and benefits. Reply to Box R-105.

MAMMOGRAPHER—The Elizabeth Wende Breast Clinic in Rochester, New York, under the direction of Dr Wende Logan-Young, is seeking a radiologist specializing in mammography. Candidates must be Board certified in radiology and must have completed a fellowship in mammography, breast ultrasonography and interventional breast procedures. Excellent patient and staff rapport a must. Initial salary and benefits, leading to partnership. Send inquiries/CVs to Theresa Wade, The Elizabeth Wende Breast Clinic, 1351 Mt Hope Ave, Rochester, NY 14620; phone 716-442-8054, fax 716-442-1837.

EXCELLENT PARTNERSHIP OPPORTUNITY IN LOUISIANA!—Growing, dynamic radiology group of nine is seeking two new partners to begin in June 2000. Group covers four hospitals performing 180k exams per year. Practice is located in northwest Louisiana in a beautiful community of 200k. Applicant should be Board certified and fellowship trained in interventional radiology or body imaging. Applicant should be competent in all areas of radiology. Please send your CV to J. Paul Price, MD, 939 Delaware St, Shreveport, LA 71106. Or via e-mail *Magnethead @msn.com*.

BOARD-CERTIFIED RADIOLOGIST (MR/ NEURO IMAGING)—An established outpatient radiology practice in Kansas City, MO, is seeking a full-time radiologist skilled in all modalities, with special interest/expertise in neuro MR. This fast-paced practice performs in excess of 150,000 outpatient exams/year. The 10-member group is independent from any hospital, and owns and operates five imaging locations. State-of-the-art equipment is used at all sites. An ability to communicate and interact effectively with patients, colleagues and staff is essential. No evenings, holidays, Sundays, or call. Competitive salary and benefits. Please forward CV and cover letter to Michelle Watzig, Practice Coordinator, Diagnostic Imaging Center, 6724 Troost, #900, Kansas City, MO 64131.

NEURORADIOLOGY—We are a rapidly expanding, not-for-profit, multi-specialty group practice located in South Florida. We are recruiting a neuroradiologist who is committed to excellence in patient care, with an interest in clincial investigation and education. The candidate should have strong clinical and academic skills. Prior post-graduate experience is desirable. Fort Lauderdale offers an ideal climate, excellent schools, a diverse culture, and is a great place to raise a family. Please contact the office of Professional Staff Affairs, 3000 W Cypress Creek Rd, Ft Lauderdale, FL 333309; fax 954-978-7416.

GOSHEN, IN—Full-time position available beginning on July 12, 1999 for general radiologist in hospital-based three-person group. The position includes MRI, angio/intervention, mammography, CT, US, NM and general diagnostics. Partnership track. 1/3 year off. Good support from the hospital administration and board. Full benefits package available. For more information, contact John F. Maesaka, MD, at e-mail *john_anne.maesaka @ibm.net*, fax 219-533-2413, phone 219-535-2604, or send CV to John F. Maesaka, Dept of Radiology, Goshen General Hospital, 200 High Park, Goshen, IN 46526.

VASCULAR/INTERVENTIONAL—The University of Texas M.D. Anderson Cancer Center at Houston has an immediate opening for a full-time vascular and interventional radiologist. Applicants should be fellowship trained and ABR certified. The vascular and interventional section performs all non-coronary and non-neurologic vascular diagnostic and interventional procedures as well as the full range of non-vascular intervention. Applicants must be committed to patient care, teaching and research. Academic rank is dependent on qualifications. Interested candidates should submit a CV to Marshall E. Hicks, MD, UTMDACC, Diagnostic Radiology Box 57, 1515 Holcombe Blvd, Houston, TX 77030, Telephone 713-792-8295; fax 713-792-4098. U.T.M.D. Anderson Cancer Center is an equal opportunity employer. Women and minority candidates are encouraged to apply. Smoke-free environment.

THE UNIVERSITY OF CINCINNATI, DEPARTMENT OF RADIOLOGY—Seeks qualified candidates for non-tenure track positions at the assistant or associate professor level, rank commensurate with experience. Opportunities are available for physicians with subspecialty interest in one or more of the following areas: general body imaging, abdominal, thoracic, breast imaging, body MRI, and angio/interventional. Fellowship training is preferred but not required. Must be ABR/AOBR certified and have, or be eligible for, an Ohio medical license. Applicants should be interested in pursuing a combined academic/clinical career. Responsibilities include clinical patient care and teaching/supervision of residents, fellows and students. Participation in basic and clinical research is supported. Letters of inquiry and CV should be forwarded to Ms Shira Karns, Radiology Business Office, 2600 Euclid Ave, Cincinnati, OH 45219. The University of Cincinnati is an AA/EOE/ADA employer. Women, minorities, persons with disabilities, Vietnam era and disabled veterans are encouraged to apply. UC is a smoke-free work environment.

PEORIA RADIOLOGY ASSOCIATES, PC—Is currently recruiting two general radiologists for one of our satellite institutions. This represents a unique career opportunity to join a large private subspecialty radiology group with close university affiliation. This is a partnership track offer. Peoria Radiology Associates, PC, is a 25-person, highly subspecialized group that has an active teaching program including radiology residents and fellowships in neuroradiology, breast imaging and interventional radiology. There is an excellent compensation and benefit package. Clinical responsibilities include all areas of medical imaging, including MRI and possibly some interventional radiology. All inquiries will be held confidential. Please indicate whether you wish to be contacted at home or at work. Please reply with CV to Kay Springer, Peoria Radiology Associates, PC, 530 NE Glen Oak Ave, Peoria, IL 61637, or fax 309-655-2951.

THE UNIVERSITY OF KENTUCKY MEDICAL CENTER—Is offering an unusual opportunity for an individual whose expertise and interest include adult and pediatric plain film, GI/GU, CT, ultrasound, nuclear medicine and mammography. Candidate must be certified by the American Board of Radiology. The opportunity presented is to live in a small, scenic, historical college town approximately 40 miles southeast of Lexington, be part of the University of Kentucky Department of Diagnostic Radiology faculty with regular participation in the teaching of residents and medical students. The position includes UK hospital privileges, as well as the local community hospital with an enlarged, newly renovated department, excellent equipment and technical staff. This opportunity offers UK benefits and open academic rank based on qualifications. If this unusual opportunity appeals to you, please send or fax your letter of interest and CV to James C. Reed, MD, Chairman, Department of Diagnostic Radiology, A110 KY Clinic, Lexington, KY 40536-0284; fax 606-257-6014. Position available immediately. The University of Kentucky is an equal opportunity employer.

MUSCULOSKELETAL RADIOLOGY STAFF POSITION—Available at the Cleveland Clinic Foundation. An opportunity exists for a Board-certified, fellowship-trained musculoskeletal radiologist to join a diverse, dynamic group of colleagues at one of the leading health care centers in the country. Our section works closely with the departments of orthopedics, rheumatology and endocrinology. Academic interests are encouraged. The section provides full musculoskeletal diagnostic and interventional services. Teaching within the department and in other departments is expected. The section performs over 100,000 studies per year in an atmosphere of cutting-edge technology. For further information or to forward your resume, please contact: Bradford J. Richmond, MD, Desk A-21, Cleveland Clinic Foundation, 9500 Euclid Ave, Cleveland, OH 44195; 216-444-3931.

INTERVENTIONAL RADIOLOGIST—Radia Medical Imaging, the Pacific Northwest's largest private practice group, is seeking a fellowship-trained, CAQ interventionalist, experience preferred. Progressive busy practice with full interventional service includes complex vascular interventions, fibroid embolizations, venous access, GI and GU interventions, intracranial thrombolysis, MRA and CTA. Growth in volumes necessitates an additional interventionalist at our downtown location. The Seattle area is consistently rated as one of the top areas of the country to live and work, with an abundance of outdoor recreation, a progressive metropolitan area and a robust economy. Please forward your CV to: Mark Churchill, Radia Medical Imaging, 728-134th Street SW, Suite 120, Everett, WA 98204. Fax: 425-297-6250 or e-mail to: *mchurchill @radlax.com*

DYNAMIC RADIOLOGY GROUP—In beautiful Pacific NW seeking a generalist with specialty expertise. 380+-bed, level II trauma center. Partnership track. Great community; affordable living; close to skiing, fishing, boating, wilderness. Qualified applicants please send CV to Ronald J. Cocchiarella, MD, 801 W 5th Ave, #205, Spokane, WA 99204 or fax 509-747-1180.

SEATTLE—Five-member group seeks ABR-certified diagnostic radiologist for partnership track position. MRI, mammography, and/or interventional skills with fellowship training is desirable, but must be comfortable with all modalities. Both hospital- and outpatient-based practice with adjoining facilities in a growing community hospital. The hospital includes new Siemens angio suite and spiral CT. Outpatient practice has busy US, MRI, and mammography service. Competitive compensation package and partnership offered after 1 year. Flexible start date. Please send CV to Peter A. Ory, MD, Southwest Medical Imaging, 16259 Sylvester Road SW, Seattle, WA 98166. Phone: 206-248-8900, Fax: 206-248-8000

GENERAL DIAGNOSTIC RADIOLOGIST—Position available immediately for BC/BE general diagnostic radiologist skilled in CT, US, MRI and mammography. We are a 14-member radiology group in southern central Pennsylvania with hospital and private office practices. Telephone 717-652-5840, x130. Fax 717-652-2165, Attention: Paul DeLoia, Jr.

A LARGE MULTI-SPECIALTY PRIVATE RADIOLOGY GROUP—On Long Island seeks an ABR-certified radiologist with specialty credentials in breast imaging. Expertise in all aspects of diagnostic and interventional breast imaging (mammography, breast ultrasound, ultrasound-guided fine needle and core biopsies, stereotaxic biopsy, galactography, needle localization and breast MRI) is required. Familiarity with OB-GYN and general ultrasound procedures, barium and plain film work, and bone densitometry is preferred. Competitive salary and benefits. Please address inquiries and accompanying CVs to Melinda J. Staiger, MD, Director of Breast Imaging, South Shore Radiologists, PC, 759 Montauk Hwy, West Islip, NY 11795.

MAINE, DIAGNOSTIC RADIOLOGY—Private practice opportunity with full partnership after 1-year. Mammography, nuclear, MRI, CT, ultrasound. Join a successful B/C radiologist in a practice that does 30,000 annual exams. Live in a family-safe riverside community close to Maine's best ski resort and a beautiful lake region. Affiliate with a strong 90-bed community hospital. Escape traffic and gated communities. For more information, contact Lianne Harris, New England Health Search, 63 Forest Ave, Orono, ME 04473. Telephone 207-866-5680. Fax 207-866-5696.

RADIOLOGIST—The Department of Veterans Affairs Medical Center, Fayetteville, Arkansas is seeking a Board certified radiologist, US citizen preferred. The position offers excellent benefits, liberal vacation, sick and educational leave, competitive salary with tenure incentives. No malpractice insurance required. The medical center is a 51-bed general medical and surgical facility providing acute health care for both inpatient and outpatient services. Fayetteville is located in beautiful Northwest Arkansas with abundant outdoor and community activities. Information on Fayetteville area available at *www.fayettevillear.com*. Inquiries should be addressed to Mark Enderle, Chief of Staff, VA Medical Center, 1100 N College, Fayetteville, AR 72703 or 501-444-5050. Equal opportunity employer.

DIAGNOSTIC RADIOLOGY/BEAUTIFUL NORTH GEORGIA—Major lake community of 10,000, one hour North of Atlanta, near major university and North Georgia Mountains. Staff positions available to cover 150-bed facilities. Imaging services include MRI, CT, ultrasound, nuclear medicine and mammography. Direct contract with the hospital system, offering competitive salary, production incentive and benefit package including retirement plan. Call David King (King Search, Inc) at 800-990-0780, 770-886-0780 or fax 770-886-9522. Send CV to King Search & Consulting, Inc, 1380 Zephyr Ct, Cumming, GA 30041, *Kingsearch@msn.com*.

DIAGNOSTIC RADIOLOGIST—Immediate opportunity for Board certified radiologist. Primary responsibilities include MR, CT, mammography, ultrasound and general diagnostics. Skills in routine angiography and additional training in cross-sectional imaging would be beneficial. Hospital is located in the Northwest suburbs of Chicago. Please fax CV to Dr Edwin Willgress, Good Shepherd Hospital, Barrington, IL 60010 at 847-842-4472.

NEURORADIOLOGIST—Radiology practice is seeking a Board certified, fellowship-trained radiologist for a full-time position. A strong background in neuroangiography, myelography, CT and MRI is required. Applicants should possess skills in general radiology, including fluoroscopy and ultrasound. Basic body angio skills are required. This is a dynamic group practice located

A CENTURY OF RESEARCH & EDUCATION
RSNA 1999

1999 RSNA REFRESHER COURSE ENROLLMENT, SCIENTIFIC PROGRAM, ADVANCE REGISTRATION AND HOUSING

85th Scientific Assembly and Annual Meeting
November 28 – December 3, 1999

McCormick Place
Chicago, Illinois

Physics program in joint sponsorship with the American Association of Physicists in Medicine

RSNA Radiological Society of North America Founded in 1915

American Association of Physicists in Medicine

WELCOME

MESSAGE TO ATTENDEES

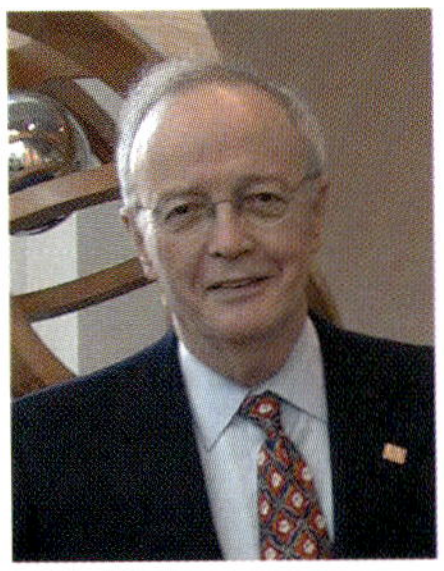

On behalf of the Board of Directors, I invite you to attend the 85th Scientific Assembly and Annual Meeting of the Radiological Society of North America. This year we celebrate a century of research and education—a century marked by rapid progress in radiology, from the Curies' 1903 Nobel Prize for the discovery of radium to the modern-day use of functional imaging techniques. The ultimate aim of our research is the improvement of patient care.

The rapid progression of our profession has created new challenges and opportunities for us in communication. The 1999 RSNA meeting will feature a dramatic demonstration of how we can share information in the Integrated Healthcare Enterprise.

Paralleling our profession's growth, the RSNA Scientific Assembly and Annual Meeting has grown from a 2-day meeting in 1915 at the Hotel Sherman, Chicago, with 30 of the RSNA's 62 members from 17 states in attendance, to a 6-day meeting that consumes the McCormick Place Complex and the city of Chicago with its attendance of nearly 60,000 representing more than 100 countries.

Again this year, you will have access to the latest radiologic research and unprecedented educational opportunities through scientific papers, refresher courses, scientific and *info*RAD exhibits, technical exhibits, demonstrations, workshops, and symposia. But most of all, you will have a chance to meet and exchange ideas with radiology professionals from around the world.

As we reflect on the tremendous progress of the past 100 years, we are reminded of our charge for the 21st Century—to break new ground in radiologic practice, technology, and most important, patient care. I look forward to seeing you at this year's Annual Meeting.

Seymour H. Levitt

Seymour H. Levitt, MD
President

TABLE OF CONTENTS

President's letter	*IFC*
Introduction	*01*
Scientific highlights	*03*
Meeting at-a-glance	*08*
Hotel listings	*26-28*
Registration instructions	*29*
Advance registration and housing form	*30-31*

RSNA link

If you're an Internet user, RSNA gives RSNA/AAPM members and non-member physicians the opportunity to register for the Annual Meeting online. Simply connect to RSNA Link and fill out the on-screen advance registration form.

For up-to-the-minute information about RSNA 1999 and a wealth of other radiologic information, visit RSNA's Web site.

www.rsna.org

The RSNA takes great pride in the range of educational opportunities and the advancements in research and technology that make the RSNA Scientific Assembly and Annual Meeting the premier radiology event in the field. This year, RSNA celebrates a century of research and education—a century marked by rapid progress and brilliant discoveries.

The rapid progress in radiologic science and technology in the past 100 years has had a dramatic impact on the educational opportunities that help radiologists enhance patient care.

ENGAGE IN A CENTURY OF RESEARCH AND EDUCATION

The exchange of scientific information is one of the reasons radiologic professionals from around the world regard the RSNA Scientific Assembly and Annual Meeting as the most important educational event in the field. Professional attendees—nearly 25,000—arrive each year ready to study and to learn.

Radiology professionals have come to expect an impressive array of lectures, courses, orations, symposia, panel discussions, poster sessions, paper presentations, and workshops. For RSNA, education is the focal point of the meeting. This is also true for most of our attendees. The educational programs are designed so that all radiologic professionals can benefit from attending the Annual Meeting (See the RSNA 1999 Scientific Program Highlights section on page 3 for detailed information.)

PROFESSIONAL AND SUBSPECIALTY DISTRIBUTION

Radiologic Specialty

Diagnostic Radiology	3,914
Vascular and Interventional	971
Neuroradiology	948
Magnetic Resonance	913
Radiation / Physics	652
Breast / Mammography	569
Computed Tomography (Body Imaging)	566
Ultrasound	487
Nuclear Medicine	460
Musculoskeletal Radiology	441
Radiation Oncology	337
Pediatric Radiology	370
Chest Radiology	287
Gastrointestinal Radiology	252
Cardiac Radiology	184
Head & Neck	94
Genitourinary Radiology	93
Radiobiology	45
Health Policy & Practice	43
Unspecified	552
Total Radiologists	**12,178**

Healthcare Professionals

Radiologists	12,178
Radiology Support Personnel / Hospital Staff	5,759
Residents	1,472
Students (Medical & Associated Sciences)	1,136
Physicists	1,054
Technical & *info*RAD VIP Guests	881
Hospital Executives	406
Consultants	356
Commercial R & D Personnel	564
Other Physicians	252
Medical Service Organization	166
Student Members	24
Total Healthcare Professionals	**24,248**

The demographic information provided here was collected from the RSNA '98 Scientific Assembly and Annual Meeting.

CONTINUING MEDICAL EDUCATION CREDIT AVAILABLE

The Radiological Society of North America is accredited by the Accreditation Council for Continuing Medical Education to sponsor continuing medical education for physicians.

The RSNA designates this continuing medical education activity for a maximum of 61 hours of Category 1 credit toward the AMA Physician's Recognition Award. Each physician should claim only those hours of credit that he or she actually spends in the educational activity.

This educational activity is approved to grant Medical Physics Continuing Education Credit (MPCEC) by the Commission on the Accreditation of Medical Physics Education Programs (CAMPEP).

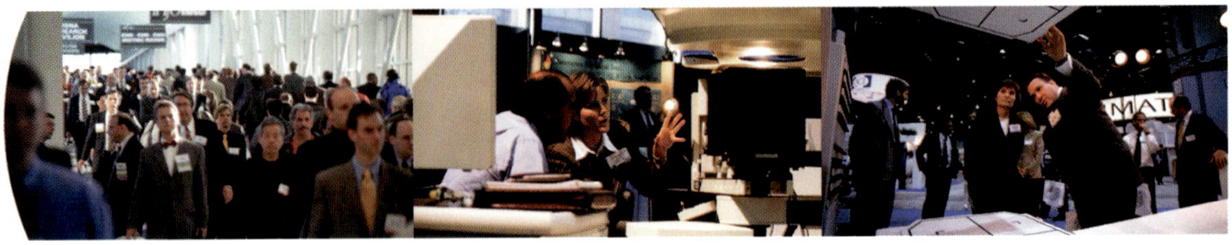

RSNA 1999 LEARNING OBJECTIVES

RSNA has developed a set of learning objectives that serve as guidelines for selecting the educational content of the meeting. RSNA 1999 attendees will be able to:

- Learn about the results of new research
- Review basic knowledge and skills
- Understand the state of the art
- Assess the latest in radiologic equipment and services
- Exchange ideas in radiologic science and technology
- Study on their own at scientific and *info*RAD exhibits

SUBSPECIALTIES UNDER THE RSNA "UMBRELLA"

This peer-reviewed scientific program features the most highly respected academicians addressing topics and concerns of specific interest to you and your practice. If you are involved in any of the following areas, you are certain to benefit by attending and participating in RSNA 1999:

- Breast Imaging
- Cardiovascular
- Chest
- Computed Tomography
- Diagnostic Radiology
- Gastrointestinal
- Genitourinary
- Health Policy & Practice
- Interventional
- Magnetic Resonance
- Musculoskeletal
- Neuroradiology/Head & Neck
- Nuclear Medicine
- Pediatric Radiology
- Physics
- Radiation Oncology
- Radiobiology
- Ultrasound

HOW TO GET THE MOST OUT OF YOUR EDUCATIONAL EXPERIENCE

Since there is so much to see and accomplish during the week, the RSNA provides attendees with several resources to help them spend their time at the Annual Meeting wisely and efficiently.

The official Scientific Program is improved each year in order to help you plan your time at the Annual Meeting. The program includes learning objectives for plenary sessions, refresher courses, scientific and *info*RAD exhibits and abstracts for scientific papers. All the meeting has to offer—from paper presentations to plenary sessions—is outlined for attendees in this publication, available in print in October and at the RSNA Web site (www.rsna.org) in early November.

The *Walk Through the Week* brochures that are available at the meeting also help you plan your time by breaking down the scientific program into 21 subspecialty areas. *Walk Through the Week* brochures are categorical listings of all the scientific sessions, refresher courses, and exhibits within a particular subspecialty—from administration to ultrasound.

The Buyer's Guide to Radiologic Products and Services, formerly *On Display,* lists all of the technical exhibitors, identifies all of their products and services, and gives diagrams of all the exhibit halls. This publication allows you to identify the exhibits that might offer information especially useful to you. *The Buyer's Guide to Radiologic Products and Services* is available to attendees onsite at the Annual Meeting in print and at the RSNA Web site in November.

Important Note:
An even simpler way to enhance your RSNA 1999 experience is to utilize RSNA's Web site, RSNA *Link* (www.rsna.org), to plan your schedule of participation at various sessions, symposia, workshops, and courses. RSNA *Link* has available all meeting and program information at the touch of your fingertips. The *Scientific Program* and *The Buyer's Guide to Radiologic Products and Services* are both available online in November through RSNA *Link*, which offers electronic searching.

WHO WILL ATTEND RSNA 1999

The RSNA Annual Meeting is well represented by all categories of medical and health care professionals involved in the science and practice of radiology:

- Radiologists (all subspecialties)
- Physicists
- Radiology residents
- Physicians impacted by radiology
- Healthcare professionals
  - *Radiologic technologists*
  - *Engineers*
  - *Radiology department administrators*
  - *Nurses*
  - *Educators*
  - *Computer analysts*
  - *Radiology facility architects*
  - *Government employees*
  - *Network managers*
  - *Systems operators*
  - *Telemedicine/communication specialists*
  - *Facility managers*
- Hospital/healthcare executives
  - *CEOs, CFOs, CIOs*
  - *Vice presidents*
  - *Corporate purchasing executives*
  - *Medical service organizations*
  - *Chief administrators*
  - *Senior executives*
  - *Purchasing agents*

OPPORTUNITIES TO BUILD PROFESSIONAL RELATIONSHIPS

The RSNA Annual Meeting is the largest medical meeting in the world. Radiology professionals from around the world—25,000 of them—gathering together each year under one roof for a week creates a very exciting and inspiring atmosphere. This "community" of your peers engaged in exchanging ideas, sharing knowledge, and networking is a professional advantage you won't want to miss. This is your chance to hear a distinguished radiologist give a lecture, to learn side-by-side with radiology professionals from around the world, to hear first-hand the latest advances in your subspecialty, and to catch up on news from your colleagues.

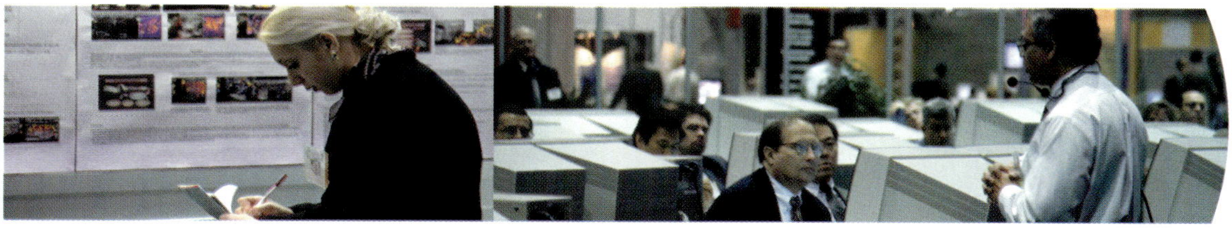

RSNA 1999 SCIENTIFIC PROGRAM HIGHLIGHTS

The educational opportunities at the Annual Meeting are as broadly based as the science of radiology itself. The quality of the information presented, however, is of paramount importance to the RSNA. Each paper, course, and exhibit is carefully scrutinized and hand-picked by an RSNA committee dedicated to high standards of excellence. Following is a listing of the major 1999 scientific program components:

Scientific Sessions — Choose from 200 sessions featuring more than 1,600 scientific papers and presentations representing 14 radiologic subspecialties.

Refresher Courses — Increase not only your knowledge but also your Category 1 CME credits by attending any of the 275 refresher courses. Courses include 32 limited-attendance workshops (16 "How-to" and 16 "Hands-on" Workshops) that feature intensive demonstration, discussion, and expanded Q&A opportunities.

Scientific Exhibits — Experience more than 1,000 scientific exhibits, ranging from backlit displays to fully interactive computer-assisted demonstrations. RSNA's scientific exhibits highlight the latest, most important research from the finest minds in radiology. All scientific exhibits offer an opportunity to earn Category 2 CME credit; selected exhibits are available for Category 1 credit.

infoRAD — *info*RAD provides a dynamic learning experience featuring hands-on computer-assisted self-instruction, Web-based applications, clinical software, virtual reality, and Integrating the Healthcare Enterprise exhibits. All *info*RAD exhibits allow you to earn Category 2 CME credit. Also, special 1-1/2 hour tutorials provide opportunities to obtain Category 1 credit. (For more information about *info*RAD, please see below.)

THE RSNA IS CONNECTED TO THE FUTURE

Getting your hands on the future is what the RSNA Annual Meeting is all about. This is where thousands of radiology professionals will gather to explore all the new technological developments that will surely impact our future.

Practical demonstrations and hands-on learning

*info*RAD is a section within the RSNA Annual Meeting devoted exclusively to hands-on computer learning. Teleradiology and telemedicine applications are presented in practical, realistic settings that give attendees hands-on exposure to the latest in high-speed network technology and services.

In the *info*RAD exhibit area, more than 150 educational and 10 commercial exhibits showcase computer-aided instruction, computer-based literature searches, computer workstations for radiologists, Internet instruction, and new electronic technology in radiologic education and information management. Designed to provide a laboratory-like learning environment, *info*RAD offers attendees the opportunity to interact one-on-one with exhibitors who will train professionals on the latest system upgrades.

Hands-on Computer Workshops: Basic Training for Radiologists

Again this year, RSNA is giving attendees an opportunity to participate in Hands-on Computer Workshops. Conducted by commercial leaders in the industry, computer workshops provide attendees with first-hand experience with the latest products available in the field.

Workshops provide radiology professionals first-hand experience in:

- Training on state-of-the-art computer equipment
- New techniques used for computer-assisted diagnosis
- Integrating computers into radiology practice
- Picture Archiving and Communications Systems (PACS)
- Radiology Information Systems (RIS)

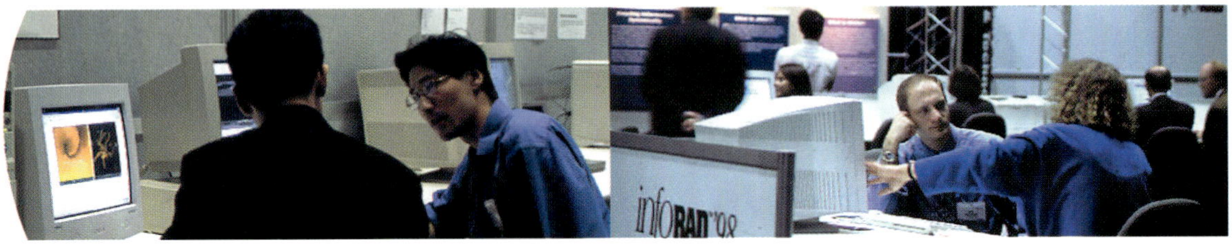

Integrating the Healthcare Enterprise

IHE Vendor Demonstration

RSNA 1999 will mark the first demonstration in the IHE initiative, a new phase in the Society's efforts to encourage integration of information systems across the healthcare enterprise. For several years RSNA has advocated adoption of the Digital Imaging and Communications in Medicine (DICOM) standard, which has revolutionized the practice of radiology. This year, the first of a planned series of IHE demonstrations will showcase the progress made under this new initiative, sponsored jointly by RSNA and the Healthcare Information and Management Systems Society (HIMSS). Vendors of imaging modalities, PACS systems, radiological information systems and hospital/clinical information systems will demonstrate their ability to exchange messages in an open environment based on existing standards such as DICOM and HL7. The range of capabilities to be demonstrated will broaden with each succeeding year of the initiative.

Participation in the IHE demonstration includes a series of technical workshops leading up to an interoperability trial, or "Connect-a-thon," as well as the demonstration at RSNA 1999 and a companion demonstration at HIMSS 2000. Participation is open to all qualified vendors. Further information can be found at RSNA's Web site, RSNA *Link*, www.rsna.org/IHE.

IHE Symposium

To coincide with the IHE demonstration, RSNA will present the inaugural IHE Symposium, to be held December 1-3, 1999 (Wed.- Fri.). This "Meeting within the RSNA Meeting" offers a full slate of tutorials, workshops, papers, lectures, and discussion groups addressing topics related to the integration of information systems in healthcare. In addition to interested physicians and radiological professionals, the IHE Symposium is expected to attract delivery network and hospital executives, healthcare information managers, medical informatics researchers, systems developers and vendors, and representatives of other interested sectors of the healthcare industry.

RSNAnet

RSNA 1999 attendees will be able to interface with the future, thanks to a complex computer network—the most intricate of any medical meeting in the world—installed throughout McCormick Place. Called RSNAnet, this high-speed network enables attendees to experience advanced telecommunications technology and applications as they would in an actual hospital setting. Participating exhibitors will demonstrate DICOM compliance by exchanging medical information from booth to booth, exhibit hall to exhibit hall, building to building, or around the world via the Internet.

WHAT'S NEW AT RSNA 1999

RSNA 1999 will emphasize practical applications to your specialty more than ever before. Some examples:

- *Special Course in Pediatric Radiology*
- *Categorical Course in Diagnostic Radiology: Body MR*
- *Two Categorical Courses in Diagnostic Radiology Physics: "Electronic Radiology Practice–Technical and Practical" and "Physical Aspects of Breast Imaging–Current and Future Considerations"*
- *One new minicourse: Body CT*

THE VALUE OF MEMBERSHIP

As an RSNA member, you're entitled to a number of privileges that make attending the Society's Annual Meeting easier and more convenient.

- Advance enrollment in refresher courses
- Early meeting and hotel registration privileges
- Complimentary registration (a $390 value)

REGISTER ONLINE (WWW.RSNA.ORG)

RSNA*link* RSNA offers the convenience of registering for the Annual Meeting online.

RSNA/AAPM members and non-member physicians simply connect to RSNA's Web site at **www.rsna.org** and fill out the on-screen advance registration form. We will confirm your registration via e-mail, fax, or mail.

Also, a special online feature within RSNA *Link* helps you plan your schedule of participation at various sessions, symposia, workshops, and courses.

For up-to-the-minute information about RSNA 1999 and a wealth of other timely information, visit **www.rsna.org**.

The IHE Symposium at RSNA 1999 is the first in a series of annual meetings designed to address the major changes in the organization and delivery of healthcare and the information technology needed to support those changes. The theme of the inaugural symposium is "Architecting Cost Effective, High Quality, Patient-Centered Care for the New Millennium."

The meetings are intended to provide a forum for discussion of new health enterprises, economic and cost-effective considerations, the role of the Internet, the impact of consumer activism, an expanded focus on health and wellness, and software and hardware strategies needed to provide information infrastructure for healthcare systems of the future.

THE IHE SYMPOSIUM: MEETING WITHIN RSNA 1999.

The recent increase in the number of non-radiology healthcare professionals, healthcare executives, information technology professionals, and vendors who attend the RSNA meeting has prompted the Society to establish the IHE symposium. The meetings will be held concurrently with the RSNA meeting capitalize on the synergies of focus, participation, and facilities.

The 1999 IHE symposium will feature keynote lectures; presentations of clinical scenarios highlighting the importance of integration; scientific papers, case studies and panel discussions.

Intended audiences of the meetings are physicians; CEOs and other healthcare executives for HMOs, healthcare delivery networks, teaching hospitals and healthcare chains; CIOs, academic medical informatics specialists; and representatives of various healthcare industries.

Topics for the 1999 meeting include:

- Strategies for Integration
- Web-Based EMR
- Security and Confidentiality
- The IHE Connectivity Initiative
- Patient-Centered Computing/ Consumer Health/Healthcare Education
- Healthcare Intranets
- Image Integration
- Component-based Technologies
- Computer-aided Decision Support Clinical Guidelines
- Telemedicine
- Internet Tools and Services
- Standards and Vocabulary
- Forces for Healthcare Integration, Drivers, Priorities

Wednesday and Thursday's schedules will include plenary sessions from 1:00 – 2:15 p.m., featuring "Developing and Managing Network Environments for the Enterprise," and "Industry Experience with Enterprise Integration."

Sessions will be featured in three separate tracks, including **Track 91:** Management Oriented, **Track 92:** Clinically Oriented and **Track 93:** Technical, In-depth.

The IHE Symposium at RSNA 1999 complements the IHE Demonstration of vendor interoperability. This is a demonstration to showcase integrated systems prototypes emphasizing component-based building block approaches, and standards-based interfaces. The IHE Demonstration is the result of an initiative jointly sponsored by RSNA and the Healthcare Information and Management Systems Society (HIMSS).

1999 Honarary Members

1:00 pm Monday

Nina Einhorn, MD. PhD
Stockholm, Sweden

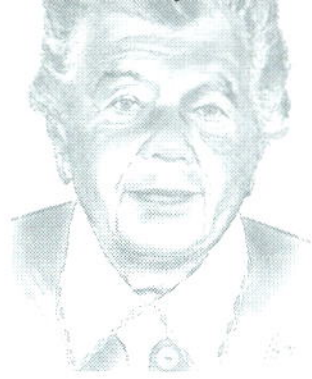

Ulrik Ringborg, MD
Stockholm, Sweden

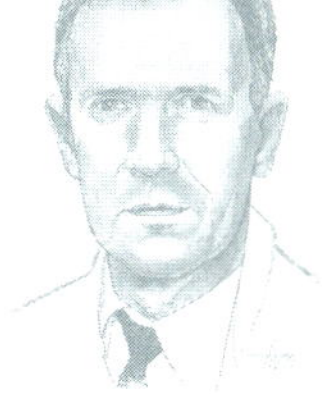

Rolf Sauer, MD
Erlangen, Germany

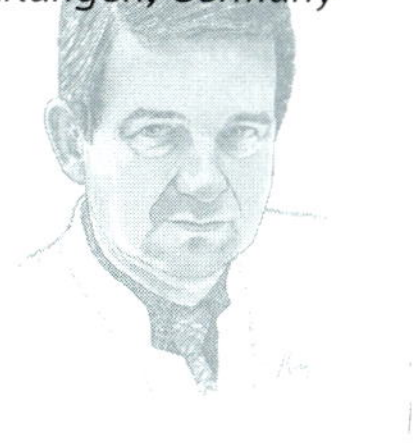

1999 Gold Medalists

1:00 pm Tuesday

Malcolm A. Bagshaw, MD
Stanford, CA

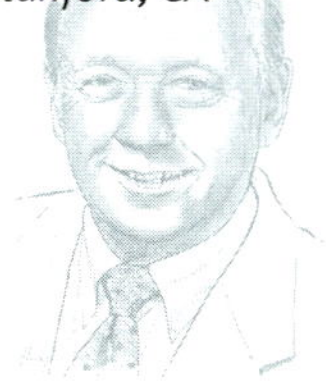

Jerzy Einhorn, MD, PhD
Stockholm, Sweden

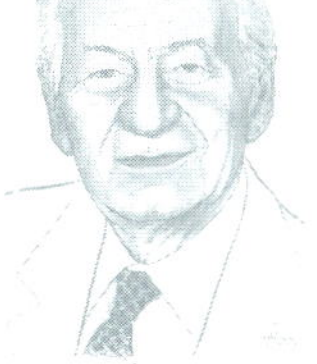

O. Wayne Houser, MD
Rochester, MN

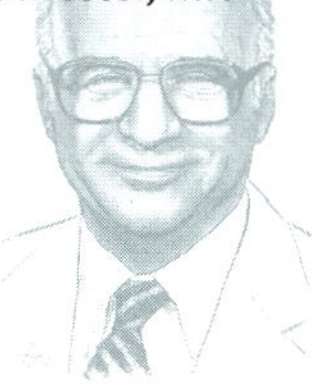

Eugene P. Pendergrass New Horizons Lecture

1:00 pm Monday

"Imaging Cancer in the New Millennium: Form Follows Function"
Richard Wahl, MD
Ann Arbor, MI

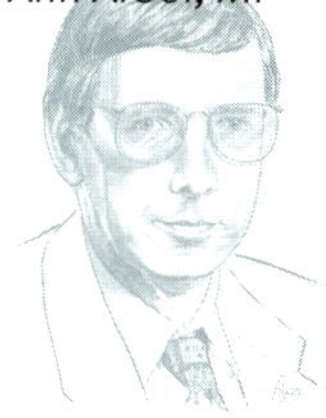

Annual Oration in Diagnostic Radiology

1:00 pm Tuesday

"Ultrasound: Advances in Contrast Agents and 3D Imaging"
Barry B. Goldberg, MD
Philadelphia, PA

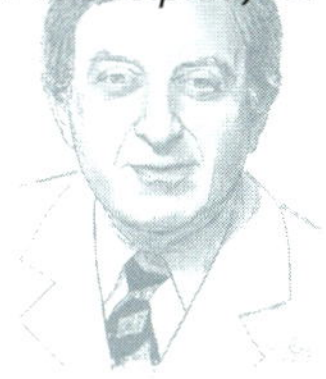

Annual Oration in Radiation Oncology

1:00 pm Wednesday

"Radiation Therapy in Early Stage Breast Cancer: Biologic and Clinical Rationale"
Lars E. Rutqvist, MD, PhD
Stockholm, Sweden

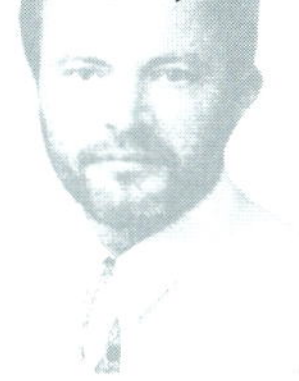

Special Focus Sessions

4:00 - 5:30 pm Tuesday

"CT Screening for Lung Cancer: Results and Critical Issues," *moderated by Claudia I. Henschke, MD, PhD*

"Current Clinical Applications of PET Imaging in the Oncology Patient, " *moderated by Edward Patz, Jr., MD*

"Evidence-based Radiology," *moderated by Harald O. Solberg, MD*

"Computer-aided Mammographic Diagnosis: Are Computers Telling Us Something We Should Know?" *moderated by Carl J. Vyborny, MD, PhD*

"Sonography of the Shoulder and Musculoskeletal System: Can You/Should You Do It?" *moderated by William Middleton, MD*

"Liver Tumor Ablation with Image Guidance" *moderated by Robert L. Bree, MD, MHSA*

"Compliance, Documentation, and How to Avoid Fraud in Your Practice," *moderated by Robert Zeman, MD*

"Screening Mammography: A World View," *moderated by Linda Warren, MD*

4:15 - 5:45 pm Thursday

"Role of Imaging in Epilepsy Surgery: Present and Future," *moderated by Clifford Jack, Jr, MD*

"Tuberculosis from Head to Toe," *moderated by Melissa L. Rosado de Christenson, MD*

"Battle for Supremacy in Abdominal Imaging: Helical CT versus MR Imaging," *moderated by Joseph K. T. Lee, MD*

"When Appendicitis is Suspected in Children," *moderated by Carlos Sivit, MD*

"Physician-Patient Relationships," *moderated by Wilbur Smith, Jr., MD*

"Mouse Genomics and Phenotypic Imaging," *moderated by R. Nick Bryan, MD, PhD*

"Update on the Activities of the American College of Radiology Imaging Network (ACRIN)" *moderated by Bruce J. Hillman, MD*

1999 MEETING SCHEDULE

Times: 8:30 AM, 9:00, 9:30, 10:00, 10:30, 11:00, 11:30, 12:00 NOON, 12:30 PM, 1:00, 1:30, 2:00, 2:30, 3:00, 3:30, 4:00, 4:30, 5:00, 5:30, 6:00

Saturday

10:15 – 4:00
Associated Sciences Workshop; "New Realities in Radiology: Multidisciplinary Strategies for Compliance"

1:00 – 5:00
AAPM/RSNA Physics Tutorial for Residents: "Fluoroscopy"
Beth A. Schueler, PhD

2:00 – 5:00
AAPM/RSNA Basic Tutorial on Equipment Selection: "MR Imaging"
Ronald R. Price, PhD

3:00 – 4:30
AAPM/RSNA Basic Physics Lecture for the Radiologic Technologist: "Digital Imaging: What You Need to Know Now and What You Need to Know Next"
Gerald A. White, Jr, MS

Sunday

8:30 – 10:15
President's Address "Impact of Changes in the Health Care System on Patient Care, Research, and Education"
Seymour Levitt, MD,

Oncologic Imaging, "What the Oncologist Wants to Know about Diagnostic Imaging"
Samuel Hellman, MD

"Advances in Oncologic Imaging: The Diagnostic Radiologist's Perspective"
Hedvig Hricak, MD, PhD

10:15 – 10:35
Business Session

10:45 – 12:15
Scientific Sessions

12:15–1:30
Lunch

Visit Exhibits

1:30 – 3:00
Refresher Courses (100s)

Workshops (100s)

3:30 – 5:15
Research and Education Foundation Awards

Image Interpretation Session
N.Reed Dunnick, MD

Monday

8:30 – 10:00
Refresher Courses (200s)

Workshops (200s)

10:30 – 12:00
Scientific Sessions

12:00 – 1:00
Lunch

Visit Exhibits

1:00 – 2:00
Eugene P. Pendergrass New Horizons Lecture, "Imaging Cancer in the New Millennium: Form Follows Function"
Richard Wahl, MD

2:30 – 3:30
Scientific Sessions

4:00 – 5:30
Refresher Courses (300s)

Workshops (300s)

Tuesday

8:30 – 10:00
Refresher Courses (400s)

Workshops (400s)

10:15 – 10:35
Business Session

10:30 – 12:00
Scientific Sessions

12:00 – 1:00
Lunch

Visit Exhibits

1:00 – 2:00
Annual Oration in Diagnostic Radiology, "Ultrasound: Advances in Contrast Agents and 3D Imaging"
Barry Goldberg, MD

2:30 – 3:30
Scientific Sessions

4:00 – 5:30
Special Focus Sessions

Wednesday

8:30 – 10:00
Refresher Courses (500s)

Workshops (500s)

10:30 – 12:00
Scientific Sessions

12:00 – 1:00
Lunch

Visit Exhibits

1:00 – 2:00
Scientific Exhibit Awards

Annual Oration in Radiation Oncology, "Radiation Therapy in Early Stage Breast Cancer: Biologic and Clinical Rationale"
Lars E. Rutqvist, MD

2:30 – 3:30
Scientific Sessions

4:00 – 5:30
Oncodiagnosis Panel, "Diagnosis and Multidisciplinary Approach for Lung Cancer"
Ritsuko Komaki, MD

Thursday

8:30 – 10:00
Refresher Courses (6c

Workshops (600s)

10:30 – 12:00
Scientific Sessions

12:00 – 1:00
Lunch

Visit Exhibits

1:00 – 2:15
RSNA/AAPM Sympos
"Spiral CT, 10 Years in
David R. Pickens, PhL

Inauguration of 2000 Board of Directors

AAPM Leadership Introduction

2:30 – 4:00
Refresher Courses (7

Workshops (700s)

4:15 – 5:45
Special Focus Sessio

This is an abbreviated schedule of the week's events. All programs are presented in English.

Plenary Sessions · Refresher Courses & Workshops · Scientific Sessions · IHE Workshops

Friday	Wednesday	Thursday	Friday
– 10:00 esher Courses (800s) kshops (800s)		8:30 – 10:00 691. *Healthcare intranets* 692. *The electronic medical record as an integration tool* 693. *Designing reliable high performance networks*	8:30 – 10:00 891. *Standards, architectures, organization initiatives* 892. *Clinical guidelines* 893. *Strategic integration of IT*
o – 12:00 ntific Sessions		10:30 – 12:00 R91. *Strategies for integration* R92. *Multimedia and image integration* R93. *Developing and managing an enterprise Web site*	10:30 – 12:00 U91. The IHE initiative U92. *Security, confidentiality, privacy update* U93. *Building the infrastructure*
– 12:30 n / Visit *info*RAD and ntific Exhibits		12:00 – 1:00 Lunch Visit Exhibits	
– 3:00 y Imaging Symposium, orithmic Controversies" *Gottschalk, MD*	1:00 – 2:15 N01. Industry Experience with Enterprise Integration	1:00 – 2:15 S01. Developing and Managing Network Enviornments for the Enterprise	
	2:30 – 3:30 P91. *Integration: Drivers, Trends* P92. *Telemedicine as a strategic tool* P93. *Standards activities*	2:30 – 3:30 791. *Internet tools and resources* 792. *Relationship building* 793. *Net-based technologies in health care*	
	4:00 – 5:30 Q91. *Priorities for integration: CIO perspective* Q92. *Consumer-focus, outreach, patient-centered care* Q93. *Data warehousing, data mining, analysis*	4:00 – 5:30 T91. *National-level integration initiatives* T92. *Computer-aided decision support* T93. *Integration paradigms*	

REGISTRATION

On-site Registration

Hours at McCormick Place for physicians, technologists, and related professionals

Saturday, November 27	12:00 pm – 6:00 pm
Sunday – Thursday, November 28 – December 2	7:00 am – 6:00 pm
Friday, December 3	7:00 am – 1:00 pm

Students

Medical students and students in the associated sciences with proper identification may register at no charge in the General Registration area.

Accompanying Family Members

Register and purchase tour tickets, if desired, at either of two locations:

McCormick Place South, Tours and Activities Desk:

Saturday, November 27	12:00 pm – 6:00 pm
Sunday, November 28	7:00 am – 6:00 pm
Monday – Thursday, November 29 – December 2	7:00 am – 4:00 pm

Palmer House Hotel, Monroe Ballroom:

Saturday – Thursday, November 27 – December 2	8:30 am – 6:00 pm

EXHIBIT HOURS

Technical Exhibits

Sunday – Thursday, November 28 – December 2	10:00 am – 6:00 pm

Scientific Exhibit

Sunday, November 28	8:00 am – 6:00 pm
Monday – Thursday, November 29 – December 2	7:00 am – 10:00 pm
Friday, December 3	7:00 am – 12:30 pm

IHE/infoRAD Exhibits

Sunday – Thursday, November 28 – December 2	8:00 am – 5:00 pm
Friday, December 3	8:00 am – 12:30 pm

infoRAD Classroom Tutorial Enrollment

Seating is limited to 50 people. See information below for number of Category 1 credits earned for each course. If the *info*RAD course that you choose runs concurrently with a selected refresher course, and both are available, please indicate on the Course Enrollment Form your course preference - the *info*RAD course or the refresher course.

The Internet and Its Medical Information/Education Resources

This tutorial is a basic introduction to the Internet and its medical information and education resources. Internet's client server architecture and the varied ways it can be accessed are described. The configuration and use of Web browsers to display multimedia information are discussed. Medical information and education resources that are on the Internet are surveyed and the Internet's future directions are reviewed. The tutorial is intended for clinicians and academic clinicians who are interested in knowing more about how the Internet works and/or the varied medically related resources that are available. At the conclusion of the tutorial, participants should be able to configure and use their Web browser to access multimedia information sources on the Internet.

Objectives:

1. Understand NLM's High Performance Computing and Communication initiatives and the information available on *The Learning Center* for Interactive Technology Web server.

2. To obtain more in-depth, hands on experience with the Internet and some of its information resources.

Day	*Time*	*Course No.*	*Credits*
Monday	3:30pm – 5:00pm	010	1.5
Tuesday	10:30am – 12:00pm	011	1.5
	1:30pm – 3:00pm	012	1.5
Wednesday	8:30am – 10:00am	013*	1.5
	10:30am – 12:00pm	014	1.5
	1:30pm – 3:00pm	015	1.5
Thursday	10:30am – 12:00pm	016	1.5
	1:30pm – 3:00pm	017*	1.5

**(Courses in red run concurrently with refresher courses.)*

RSNA Research and Education Resources

This 90-minute talk and tutorial provides information on the research and educational opportunities offered through several programs of The RSNA Research and Education Foundation and The RSNA Education Center. Discussion will cover the contents of these resources, how to access them over the RSNA Web site and how to link to other resources such as the RSNA Office of Research Development Database of Funding Opportunities. In addition, ways and means of obtaining Continuing Medical Education (CME) from the RSNA Scientific Assembly and from the two RSNA educational journals, *RadioGraphics* and *EJ*, will be discussed along with other means of obtaining CME in the radiological sciences.

Day	*Time*	*Course No.*	*Credits*
Sunday	10:30am – 12:00pm	020	1.5
Thursday	3:30pm – 5:00pm	021*	1.5

**(Courses in red run concurrently with refresher courses.)*

infoRAD Workstation Classroom Enrollment

Seating is limited to 75 people. See information below for number of Category 1 credits earned for each course.

"Hands-On Workshop: Radiology and Clinical Information Integration"

Note: This workshop will be repeated 3 times during the meeting, in identical presentation. This is NOT a sequential course of 3 sessions. If you do not have prior experience with a PACS workstation, it is strongly suggested that you enroll in one of the basic workstation refresher courses (153, 253, 453, or 653) as a prerequisite.

The objective of this workshop is to demonstrate how intranet and internet technology can enhance patient care by bi-directional exchange of information between radiology and other clinical (enterprise) systems. Ability to switch from PACS to RIS or HIS windows at a radiologist's workstation will be demonstrated, including web-enabled interaction between these systems such that patient focus is communicated between the systems.

Central to the demonstration is the concept of worklists of patients and studies. Bi-directional modality worklist is a new important addition to the DICOM standard for downloading worklists and appropriate demographic information directly into the imaging device for the RIS. Interaction between the systems enables the radiologist to obtain clinical information from the HIS for scheduled CT exams, such as lab data, to select exam protocols and convey them to the technologist. Radiologist access to clinical information such as history and physical, laboratory data and physician notes (including speech recognition), and radiology procedure requests will be demonstrated.

Furthermore, radiologists at a PACS workstation will have access to other medical image data such as endoscopy. RIS worklists can trigger sequential presentation of unread cases, along with appropriate comparison studies.

Ability to push image and report information via Web/email techniques to referring clinicians will be demonstrated, including stat reports with return receipt.

General clinician access to radiology reports and images through Web techniques will also be demonstrated, including access to preliminary reports (notes or digitized speech). Ability to retrieve historical studies from PACS through a Web browser will be included.

Finally, digital radiology consultation and conferencing as well as digital teaching file technology will be demonstrated.

Objectives:

How intranet and internet technology can enhance patient care by the seamless exchange of information between radiology and other clinical systems.

Day	*Time*	*Course No.*	*Credits*
Tuesday	2:30pm – 4:00pm	030	1.5
Wednesday	2:30pm – 4:00pm	031	1.5
Thursday	10:30am – 12:00pm	032	1.5

***info*RAD tutorial and presentation learning objectives are to enable the attendee to:**

1. Assess new computer technologies for research, education, and practice.
2. Operate computer-aided instruction programs.
3. Operate computer-aided diagnostic programs and assess their own role in practice.
4. Appreciate the options for connectivity in radiology through PACS, workstations, and Internet.
5. Make use of the Internet for research, education, and practice.

*info*RAD Guided Tours Schedule

Tours are limited to 90 people per hour.

Note: No CME credit is given for the info*RAD guided tour.*

Guided tours will be scheduled on the days and times indicated below. Authors are present at the exhibits between 10:00am and 2:00pm. Pre-registration is required. Make your selections on the Course Enrollment Form under the *info*RAD Guided Tours section. Tours will be approximately 30 to 45 minutes long.

Sunday

Time	*Tour No.*
9:00am	050
10:00am	051
11:00am	052
12:00pm	053
1:00pm	054
2:00pm	055
3:00pm	056

Monday

Time	*Tour No.*
9:00am	057
10:00am	058
11:00am	059
12:00pm	060
1:00pm	061
2:00pm	062
3:00pm	063

Tuesday

Time	*Tour No.*
9:00am	064
10:00am	065
11:00am	066
12:00pm	067
1:00pm	068
2:00pm	069
3:00pm	070

Wednesday

Time	*Tour No.*
9:00am	071
10:00am	072
11:00am	073
12:00pm	074
1:00pm	075
2:00pm	076
3:00pm	077

Thursday

Time	*Tour No.*
9:00am	078
10:00am	079
11:00am	080
12:00pm	081
1:00pm	082
2:00pm	083
3:00pm	084

Friday

Time	*Tour No.*
9:00am	085
10:00am	086

Hands-on Computer Workshops:
Basic Training for Radiologists

Again this year, RSNA is giving attendees an opportunity to gain valuable insight into the use of computers in radiology from experts in the field. Commercial leaders in the industry have reserved classroom space near the IHE/*info*RAD exhibit area to conduct classes on their respective proprietary computer systems.The classrooms will hold 30 participants for each session; preregistration is advised.

The Hands-on Computer Workshops at RSNA 1999 are designed to give radiology professionals first-hand experience in:

- Training on state-of-the-art computer equipment
- Integrating computers into radiology practice
- Radiology Information Systems (RIS)
- Picture Archiving and Communications Systems (PACS)
- New techniques used for computer-assisted diagnosis

Remember: *Attendance is limited, reserve space now.*

While workshop reservations are made through the RSNA, the workshops are not offered for CME credit.

AGFA Medical, AGFA Corporation

Course	*S*	*M*	*T*	*W*	*T*	*F*
Integrated Voice Recognition & PACS 9:00 – 10:00 am	BA10	BA20	BA30	BA40	BA50	BA60
Seamless RIS/PACS Integration and The Electronic Patient Record 10:15 – 11:15 am	BA11	BA21	BA31	BA41	BA51	BA61
Implications of DIN-PACS on Commercial PACS 11:30 – 12:30 pm	BA12	BA22	BA32	BA42	BA52	BA62
Image Processing Paradigms and Their Effect on Computed Radiography Images 12:45 – 1:45 pm	BA13	BA23	BA33	BA43	BA53	—
Integrated Voice Recognition and PACS 2:00 – 3:00 pm	BA14	BA24	BA34	BA44	BA54	—
Seamless RIS/PACS Integration and The Electronic Patient Record 3:15 – 4:15 pm	BA15	BA25	BA35	BA45	BA55	—

ISG Technologies, Inc.

Course	*S*	*M*	*T*	*W*	*T*	*F*
Workflow 9:30 - 10:30 am	BD10	BD20	BD30	BD40	BD50	—
Value Added Radiology 11:00 am - 12:00 pm	BD11	BD21	BD31	BD41	BD51	—
On Demand Imaging 2:00 - 3:00 pm	BD12	BD22	BD32	BD42	BD52	—

Siemens Medical Systems, Inc

Course	*S*	*M*	*T*	*W*	*T*	*F*
The Integrated Radiology PACS 8:30 - 10:00 am	BB10	BB20	BB30	BB40	BB50	—
Enterprise PACS 10:00 - 11:30 am	BB11	BB21	BB31	BB41	BB51	—
The Integrated Radiology PACS 1:00 - 2:30 pm	BB12	BB22	BB32	BB42	BB52	—
Enterprise PACS 3:00 - 4:30 pm	BB13	BB23	BB33	BB43	BB53	—

Vital Images, Inc

Course	*S*	*M*	*T*	*W*	*T*	*F*
Fast, Simple 3-D Imaging for Routine CT & MR Applications 8:30 – 9:30 am	BC10	BC20	BC30	BC40	BC50	BC60
Fast, Simple 3-D Imaging for Routine CT & MR Applications 10:00 – 11:00 am	BC11	BC21	BC31	BC41	BC51	BC61
Fast, Simple 3-D Imaging for Routine CT & MR Applications 11:30 – 12:30 pm	BC12	BC22	BC32	BC42	BC52	—
Fast, Simple 3-D Imaging for Routine CT & MR Applications 2:00 – 3:00 pm	BC13	BC23	BC33	BC43	BC53	—
Fast, Simple 3-D Imaging for Routine CT & MR Applications 3:30 – 4:30 pm	BC14	BC24	BC34	BC44	BC54	—

Categorical Course

A series of eight courses covering a subject, accompanied by a syllabus. The topic is coordinated with at least one other organization. The Categorical Courses and their directors are:

_02*
Categorical Course in Diagnostic Radiology: Body MR
Shirley M. McCarthy, MD, PhD Director
Caroline Reinhold, MD Co-director
William E. Palmer, MD Co-director

_23**
Categorical Course in Diagnostic Radiology Physics: Electronic Radiology Practice—Technical and Practical
Nicholas J. Hangiandreou, PhD Co-director
Jeremy W. R. Young, MD Co-director
Richard L. Morin, PhD Co-director

_25***
Categorical Course in Diagnostic Radiology Physics: Physical Aspects of Breast Imaging—Current and Future Considerations
Arthur G. Haus, Co-director
Martin J. Yaffe, PhD Co-director

Special Course

A series of eight courses encompassing an entire topic area organized solely by the RSNA; a syllabus is produced. The Special Course and the director is:

_13+
Special Course in Pediatric Radiology: Current Concepts in Body Imaging at the Millennium
Marilyn J. Siegel, MD Director

Minicourse

A series of four courses covering a topic area organized solely by the RSNA; no syllabus is produced.

"How-to"

A course with limited audience permitting the attendee the opportunity for intimate exchange with the faculty.

"Hands-on"

A course with limited audience permitting the attendee the opportunity to utilize medical equipment and/or devices.

The Refresher Courses Learning Objectives are to enable the attendees to:

1. Identify basic anatomic, pathologic, and physiological principles as they apply to specific disease processes, organ-based diagnostic imaging, or radiation oncology.
2. Describe the physics of particular imaging and therapeutic modalities for improving quality while reducing patient risk and/or expense.
3. Analyze current and future imaging and therapeutic techniques with respect to protocol development, patient management, algorithms, and cost/efficiency.
4. Assess the influence of socioeconomic issues on current and future practice patterns.
5. Learn indications and contradictions for and techniques of specific image-guided procedures.

Refresher Course, Workshops, and IHE Enrollment

Act promptly. Attendance at each session is limited to the room seating capacity. Enrollment requests will be honored in the order of receipt. Registrants enrolling in a complete Categorical Course, Mini-course or Special Course will be given priority over registrants requesting a single session within a course.

Each refresher course and workshop is approved for 1-1/2 hours of Category 1 credit.

Refresher courses, workshops, and IHE are grouped according to the last two digits:

Chest 01
Categorical Course in Diagnostic Radiology: Body MR 02
Cardiovascular 03
Musculoskeletal 04
Neuroradiology 05
Head and Neck 06
Genitourinary 07
Emergency Radiology 08
Gastrointestinal 09
Ultrasound 10
Nuclear Medicine 11
CT 12
Special Course in Pediatric Radiology: Current Concepts in Body Imaging at the Millennium 13
Interventional 14
Breast Imaging 15
Miscellaneous . . . . . 16, 17 and 29
Oncologic Imaging 18
Radiation Oncology . . . . . 19 and 20
Physics . . . . . 21, 22 and 28
Categorical Course in Diagnostic Radiology Physics: Electronic Radiology Practice—Technical and Practical 23
Associated Sciences 24
Categorical Course in Diagnostic Radiology Physics: Physical Aspects of Breast Imaging—Current and Future Considerations 25
Computers 26
Health Policy and Practice 27
Minicourses: Women's Health in Imaging/New Developments in Body CT Scanning 30
"How-to" Workshops . . . . . 50 and 51
"Hands-on" Workshops . . . . . 52 and 53
IHE: Management 91
IHE: Clinical 92
IHE: Technical 93

Sunday, November 28, 1999
1:30 pm to 3:00 pm
Courses 101–130 14
Workshops 150–153 15

Monday, November 29, 1999
8:30 am to 10:00 am
Courses 201–230 15
Workshops 250–253 16

4:00 pm to 5:30 pm
Courses 301–330 16
Workshops 350–353 17

Tuesday, November 30, 1999
8:30 am to 10:00 am
Courses 401–430 18
Workshops 450–453 19

Wednesday, December 1, 1999
8:30 am to 10:00 am
Courses 501–530 19
Workshops 550–553 20

Thursday, December 2, 1999
8:30 am to 10:00 am
Courses 601–630 20
Workshops 650–653 22
IHE 691–693 22

2:30 pm to 4:00 pm
Courses 701–730 22
Workshops 750–753 23
IHE 791–793 23

Friday, December 3, 1999
8:30 am to 10:00 am
Courses 801–830 23
Workshops 850–853 24
IHE 891–893 24

Sunday, November 28, 1999
1:30 pm to 3:00 pm

101
Imaging of the Airways
David P. Naidich, MD
Philippe A. Grenier, MD

102
Categorical Course in Diagnostic Radiology: Body MR*
A. Chest
Warren B. Gefter, MD
B. Breast
Susan G. Orel, MD
C. Interventional MR Imaging: Abdominal Applications
Stuart G. Silverman, MD

103
MR Imaging of Congenital Heart Disease
Charles B. Higgins, MD
Albert De Roos, MD

104
Imaging of Sports-related Injuries: An Overview
Thomas L. Pope, Jr, MD
Coordinator
Leon Lenchik, MD
Arthur H. Newberg, MD

105
Acute Cerebral Ischemia: Physiologic Imaging and Image-guided Therapy
Richard E. Latchaw, MD
R. Gil Gonzalez, MD, PhD
William T. Yuh, MD, MSEE

106
Technique and Pitfalls: How to Avoid Misdiagnosis in Head and Neck Imaging
A. Techniques in Head and Neck Imaging
Daniel W. Williams III, MD
B. Pitfalls
Lawrence E. Ginsberg, MD

107
Adrenal Imaging: Current Concepts
Michael J. Lee, MD
Giles W. Boland, MD
William W. Mayo-Smith, MD
Richard B. Noto, MD

108
Head Trauma and Nontraumatic Central Nervous System Emergencies
A. Head Trauma
James G. Smirniotopoulos, MD
B. Nontraumatic Central Nervous System Emergencies
James M. Provenzale, MD

109
Colorectal Cancer Screening and Diagnosis: Back to the Future
C. Daniel Johnson, MD
G. Scott Gazelle, MD, MPH
Harvey M. Goldstein, MD

110
Practical Tips in US: Pelvis
A. Ovarian Masses: What to Look for
Roy A. Filly, MD
B. The Uterus
Beverly G. Coleman, MD

111
Practical Cardiovascular Nuclear Medicine
Jack A. Ziffer, MD, PhD
Moderator
Naomi P. Alazraki, MD

112
CT of the Liver: Principles and Practice
Michael P. Federle, MD
Erik K. Paulson, MD

113
Special Course in Pediatric Radiology: Current Concepts in Body Imaging at the Millennium—Techniques in Pediatric Body Imaging+
A. Sedation in Noninvasive CT and MR Imaging
George S. Bisset III, MD
B. Helical CT in the Pediatric Abdomen: Techniques and Applications
Donald P. Frush, MD
C. Helical CT in the Pediatric Chest: Techniques and Applications
Sandra S. Kramer, MD

114
Interventional Radiology in Esophageal and Gastrointestinal Strictures and Fistulas
Andreas N. Adam, MD
Christoph L. Zollikofer, MD

115
Percutaneous Breast Biopsy
A. US Guidance
W. Phil Evans, MD
B. Stereotactic Guidance
D. David Dershaw, MD

116
What to Order When
Ronald L. Eisenberg, MD, JD
William P. Dillon, MD
Charles E. Putman, MD
N. Reed Dunnick, MD
Alexander R. Margulis, MD

117
Summary of the International Working Group on Breast MR Imaging
Steven E. Harms, MD
Debra M. Ikeda, MD
Nola Michiko Hylton, PhD
Mitchell D. Schnall, MD, PhD
Suzanne Klimberg, MD

118
Imaging Lymphoma
A. Thorax
Herman I. Libshitz, MD
B. Abdomen and Pelvis
Janet E. Husband, MD

119
Gastrointestinal Tract Malignancies
A. Radiation Treatment of Gastrointestinal Tract Malignancies
Tyvin A. Rich, MD
B. Management of Cancer of the Esophagus
Jaffer A. Ajani, MD

120
Tumor Biology and Mechanism of Cell Death
A. Apoptosis: Role in Tumor Growth and Tumor Therapy with Radiation and Other Cytotoxic Agents
Luka Milas, MD, PhD
B. Molecular Biology of Breast Cancer
Thomas A. Buchholz, MD

121
High-Frequency X-ray Generator Basics
Wlad T. Sobol, PhD

122
Stereotactic Radiation Treatment Approaches and Devices
J. Daniel Bourland, PhD

123
Categorical Course in Diagnostic Radiology Physics: Electronic Radiology Practice—Technical and Practical: The Importance of Electronic Practice**
A. A CEO's Perspective
Leo F. Black, MD

A CENTURY OF RESEARCH & EDUCATION
RSNA 1999

sunday

monday

tuesday

RSNA 1999 Weekly Planner

Detach and plan your week at RSNA with ease

wednesday

thursday

friday

RSNA® | Radiological Society of North America Founded in 1915

18 **Oncologic Imaging**	**118** Imaging Lymphoma	**218** Primary Intrathoracic and Malignant Tumors	**318** Imaging of the Surgically Altered Breast	**418** Pancreatic Neop
19 and 20 **Radiation Oncology**	**119** Gastrointestinal Tract Malignancies **120** Tumor Biology and Mechanism of Cell Death	**219** Management of Regionally Localized, High-Risk Prostate Cancer **220** Radioprotectors	**319** Stereotactic Radiosurgery for Central Nervous System Tumors **320** Radiation Therapy for Prostate Cancer: Dose Escalation with 3D Conformal Radiation Therapy	**419** Lung Cancer **420** Combined Surge Therapy for Adva Cancers
21, 22 and 28 **Physics**	**121** High-Frequency X-ray Generator Basics **122** Stereotactic Radiation Treatment Approaches and Devices **128** Physics: Imaging in Radiation Therapy	**221** How to Run with the PACS **222** Multileaf Collimators and Dynamic Wedges **228** Physics: Imaging in Radiation Therapy	**321** US Artifacts **322** Physics of Intravascular Brachytherapy **328** Physics: Imaging in Radiation Therapy	**421** The Physicist an Technologist **422** SPECT and Coinci **428** Physics: Imaging Therapy
23 **Categorical Course in Diagnostic Radiology Physics: Electronic Radiology Practice — Technical and Practical**	**123** The Importance of Electronic Practice	**223** PACS for the Electronically Challenged	**323** Real Life Electronic Practice – An Interview with Trench Dwellers	**423** Electronic Image Technical Aspect
24 **Associated Sciences**	**124** Organizational Culture and Health System Change	**224** Asset Management for High-Technology Systems	**324** Economic Implications of Regulatory Change	**424** Managing a Mul Network
25 **Categorical Course in Diagnostic Radiology Physics: Physical Aspects of Breast Imaging — Current and Future Considerations**	**125** Categorical Course in Diagnostic Radiology Physics: Physical Aspects of Breast Imaging—Current and Future Considerations	**225** Categorical Course in Diagnostic Radiology Physics: Physical Aspects of Breast Imaging—Current and Future Considerations	**325** Categorical Course in Diagnostic Radiology Physics: Physical Aspects of Breast Imaging—Current and Future Considerations	**425** Categorical Cour Radiology Physic of Breast Imagin Future Considera
26 **Computers**	**126** PACS and Radiology Informatics: Making the Business Argument for PACS	**226** PACS and Radiology Informatics: Update on PACS Technology and Infrastructure	**326** PACS and Radiology Informatics: Getting from Here to There—"Change Management" in PACS	**426** PACS and Radiol Writing the PACS Proposal and Op Vendor Relation
27 **Health Policy and Practice**	**127** Entrepreneurship and Marketing for Radiologists	**227** Coding and Billing Tips to Optimize Revenue	**327** Turf Battles in Radiology: How to Fight Them and Win!	**427** Management Ch Academic and C Radiology Depa to Meet Them
30 **Minicourses: Women's Health in Imaging — New Developments in Body CT Scanning**	**130** Minicourse: Women's Health in Imaging	**230** Minicourse: Women's Health in Imaging after Menopause	**330** Minicourse: Women's Health in Imaging before Menopause	**430** Minicourse: Wo Imaging-Advanc
50 and 51 **"How-to" Workshops**	**150** Hysterosalpingography and Selective Salpingography **151** Managing Complications of Central Venous Access	**250** Carotid Stent Placement **251** Dialysis Graft Thrombectomy and Thrombolysis	**350** Percutaneous CT-guided Biopsy of the Spine **351** How to Prepare and Deliver Electronic Presentations	**450** Strategies for O the Vascular Sys **451** Lymph Node Ma
52 and 53 **"Hands-on" Workshops**	**152** Real-Time Interventional Ultrasound **153** How to Use a PACS Workstation: Basic	**252** Musculoskeletal US **253** How to Use a PACS Workstation: Basic	**352** Interventional Breast Procedures **353** How to Use a PACS Workstation: Advanced	**452** Venous Access **453** How to Use a P Basic
91, 92 and 93 **Integrating the Healthcare Enterprise**				

s: CT and MR	**518** Evaluation of Hepatic Metastatic Disease: CT, MR, and US	**618** Gynecologic Malignancies: Imaging Evaluation and Follow-up	**718** PET Scanning in Oncology	**818** Primary Bone Tumor and Limb-sparing Surgery: Imaging Evaluation and Follow-up
nd Radiation d Head and Neck	**519** Lymphoma **520** Radiation: The Two-edged Sword—Risk Factors and Protection	**619** Management of Non-CNS Pediatric Tumors **620** Brachytherapy for Gynecologic Cancer	**719** Radiation Therapy in Cervical Cancer **720** Breast Cancer	**819** Management of Soft-Tissue Sarcoma **820** Prostate Brachytherapy
Mammography e Imaging Basics Radiation	**521** Technical Aspects of Interventional Fluoroscopic Systems **522** RSO Basics **528** Physics: Imaging in Radiation Therapy	**621** Fundamentals of Flat Panel X-ray Detector Physics **622** Medical Physics Practice Basics **628** Physics: Imaging in Radiation Therapy	**721** MR Accreditation Physics **722** Digital Radiographic Image Quality and System Optimization **728** Physics: Imaging in Radiation Therapy	**821** Radiation Shielding **822** Basic MR Imaging QC **828** Physics: Imaging in Radiation Therapy
uisition—	**523** Electronic Image Acquisition—Practice Aspects	**623** Electronic Image Infrastructure	**723** Electronic Image Interpretation	**823** Electronic Image Distribution
Radiology	**524** Current Challenges in Radiology and Planning and Design	**624** Specialized Accreditations: A Cost of Doing Business	**724** Multidisciplinary Standards for the New Millennium	**824** Marketing Radiology: Getting the Message out
Diagnostic hysical Aspects urrent and s	**525** Categorical Course in Diagnostic Radiology Physics: Physical Aspects of Breast Imaging—Current and Future Considerations	**625** Categorical Course in Diagnostic Radiology Physics: Physical Aspects of Breast Imaging—Current and Future Considerations	**725** Categorical Course in Diagnostic Radiology Physics: Physical Aspects of Breast Imaging—Current and Future Considerations	**825** Categorical Course in Diagnostic Radiology Physics: Physical Aspects of Breast Imaging—Current and Future Considerations
nformatics: uest for zing the User-	**526** PACS and Radiology Informatics: Getting the Message Out—Update on Voice Recognition, Structured Reporting, and Value Innovation	**626** PACS and Radiology Informatics: Practical and Operational Issues in PACS	**726** PACS and Radiology Informatics: Decision Support	**826** PACS and Radiology Informatics: Challenges and Strategies for Enterprise Radiology Informatics
ges Facing unity Hospital nts and How	**527** Risk Management in Radiology: How to Stay Out of Trouble with the Courts	**627** Negotiating a Managed Care Contract	**727** New Ways to Organize Radiology Practices: Physician Practice Management Companies, Networks, and Mergers—Are They the Wave of the Future?	**827** How to Measure Productivity in Your Radiology Department
s Health in Breast Imaging	**530** Minicourse: New Developments in Body CT Scanning - New Developments in Abdominal CT	**630** Minicourse: New Developments in Body CT Scanning - 3D CT Angiography and Virtual Imaging	**730** Minicourse: New Developments in Body CT Scanning - New Developments in Chest CT	**830** Minicourse: New Developments in Body CT Scanning - High-Resolution CT of the Chest
zing Spiral CT of g	**550** Sympathetic Blockades for Pain Management: Radiologic and Medical Strategies for Pain Management **551** Thrombolytic Therapy in Venous Disease	**650** Nonbiopsy Spine Procedures **651** Fetal Imaging with US and MR Imaging: How We Do It	**750** MR Imaging of the Abdomen: How We Do It **751** MR Imaging in Sports Medicine	**850** Radiologic Evaluation of the Solitary Pulmonary Nodule **851** FDA Regulation of Medical Devices: Practical Approaches to Everyday Problems
Vorkstation:	**552** Venous Thrombosis: Doppler Sonography **553** How to Use a PACS Workstation: Advanced	**652** Freehand Invasive Sonography for the Breast **653** How to Use a PACS Workstation: Basic	**752** Techniques of Freehand Invasive Sonography **753** How to Use a PACS Workstation: Advanced	**852** Techniques of Invasive Sonography **853** How to Use a PACS Workstation: Advanced
		691 Healthcare Intranets: How to Develop and Support an Intranetl What Functions it Should have, Successful Approaches **692** The Electronic Medical Record as an Integration Tool: Strategies for Accessing, Coordinating, and Updating the EMR Across a Network **693** Designing Reliable High Performance Networks: Network Design Issues and Approaches: Also Generation Internet	**791** Internet Tools and Resources: Content, Tools, Services, Consortia For Health Care Networks **792** Relationship Building: Issues Facing PCP's Patients in a Network, and How Info Systems Can Support These Needs **793** Net-based Technologies in Health Care: A Focus on Java, CORBA, DCOM, XML	**891** Standards, Architectures, Organization Initiatives: A Standard Road Map, How the Effort Interacts **892** Clinical Guidelines: Roles for Clinical Guidelines in Workstation Design, Referral Management, and Workflow Optimization **893** Strategic Integration of IT: Selecting Priorities, Developing a Plan, Engaging the Participants, Managing the Process

REFRESHER COURSE PLAN OF PRESENTATION

	Sunday, November 28 1:30pm – 3:00pm	Monday, November 29 8:30am – 10:00am	Monday, November 29 4:00pm – 5:30pm	Tuesday, Nov 8:30am – 10:
01 Chest	101 Imaging of the Airways	201 The Diagnosis of Pulmonary Embolism: A Rational Approach to Familiar Tests and New Technologies	301 Differential Diagnosis of Mediastinal Masses	401 High-Resolution Parenchyma: A
02 Categorical Course in Diagnostic Radiology: Body MR	102 Categorical Course in Diagnostic Radiology: Body MR	202 Categorical Course in Diagnostic Radiology: Body MR	302 Categorical Course in Diagnostic Radiology: Body MR	402 Categorical Cou Radiology: Body
03 Cardiovascular	103 MR Imaging of Congenital Heart Disease	203 Three-dimensional Contrast MR Angiography	303 Practical Cardiac MR Imaging: Principles, Pearls, and Protocols for Success	403 Assessment of L Function and Via Role of MR Imag and Nuclear Car
04 Musculoskeletal	104 Imaging of Sports-related Injuries: An Overview	204 Imaging Enigmas of the Hip	304 MR Imaging of Athletic Injuries of the Knee	404 Interventional M Radiology
05 Neuroradiology	105 Acute Cerebral Ischemia: Physiologic Imaging and Image-guided Therapy	205 The New WHO Classification of Brain Tumors: Imaging Correlations	305 Spinal Imaging: Dealing with Back Pain	405 Congenital and Abnormalities
06 Head and Neck	106 Technique and Pitfalls: How to Avoid Misdiagnosis in Head and Neck Imaging	206 The Sinonasal Cavities and the Ostiomeatal Complex	306 Advanced Concepts in Head and Neck Cancer	406 The Temporal Bo
07 Genitourinary	107 Adrenal Imaging: Current Concepts	207 Pelvic Prolapse: The New Way to Image	307 Genitourinary Tract Imaging in Pregnant and Postpartum Patients	407 US of the Genito and Controversi
08 Emergency Radiology	108 Head Trauma and Nontraumatic Central Nervous System Emergencies	208 Imaging Chest Trauma	308 Helical CT of Nontraumatic Abdominal Emergencies	408 Helical CT and U Trauma
09 Gastrointestinal	109 Colorectal Cancer Screening and Diagnosis: Back to the Future	209 Minimally Invasive Treatment of Malignant Hepatic Tumors	309 Imaging of the Acute Abdomen	409 Radiology of the Curve to the Oth
10 Ultrasound	110 Practical Tips in US: Pelvis	210 Practical Tips in US: Obstetrics	310 Practical Tips in US: Breast	410 Practical Tips in
11 Nuclear Medicine	111 Practical Cardiovascular Nuclear Medicine	211 Advances in Nuclear Oncology	311 Musculoskeletal Nuclear Imaging	411 Infection Imagin
12 CT	112 CT of the Liver: Principles and Practice	212 Advances and Controversies in CT and MR of the Genitourinary Tract	312 Three-dimensional CT Imaging: Principles, Techniques, and Clinical Applications	412 The Acute Abdo
13 Special Course in Pediatric Radiology: Current Concepts in Body Imaging at the Millennium	113 Techniques in Pediatric Body Imaging	213 Imaging the Pediatric Chest: Current Applications	313 MR Imaging of Congenital Cardiovascular Disease	413 CT and MR Imag Disorders: Curre
14 Interventional	114 Interventional Radiology in Esophageal and Gastrointestinal Strictures and Fistulas	214 Stent-Grafts of the Aorta and Peripheral Vessels	314 Transjugular Intrahepatic Portosystemic Shunts: From Patient Selection to Surveillance and Revision	414 Endovascular Ma Vein and Pulmor
15 Breast Imaging	115 Percutaneous Breast Biopsy	215 Correlating Pathology of Benign and Malignant Breast Lesions with Mammography and US	315 Reducing False-Positive Mammogram Interpretations	415 Strategies to Re Mammographic Problems, Soluti Studies
16, 17 and 29 Miscellaneous	116 What to Order When 117 Summary of the International Working Group on Breast MR Imaging 129 Technology Assessment in Radiology: Part I-Basic Principles of Testing: Diagnostic Accuracy and Decision-making in Radiology	216 Imaging the Hot Zone: What Every Radiologist Should Know about Emerging Infectious Diseases and Food-borne Illnesses 217 American College of Radiology Standards and Accreditation Programs: Major Issues and Update 1999 229 Technology Assessment in Radiology: Part II-Outcomes and Cost-Effectiveness Research	316 Current Activities of the Residency Review Committee and the American Board of Radiology in Regard to Diagnostic Radiology 317 AIDS Imaging: A Critical Clinical Approach 329 Transplants: Use of US	416 "Getting Your W Editors and Auth 417 Preserving Your Share: Malpracti and Antitrust 429 Do Not Resuscita Complying with in the Radiology

er 30 n	Wednesday, December 1 8:30am – 10:00am	Thursday, December 2 8:30am – 10:00am	Thursday, December 2 2:30pm – 4:00pm	Friday, December 3 8:30am – 10:00am
f the Lung ical Approach	**501** Optimization of Spiral CT of the Thorax	**601** Chest Infections: Typical Presentations, Complications, and Management	**701** Digital Chest Radiography: Techniques and Clinical Applications	**801** Lung Cancer: Role of Diagnostic Imaging
n Diagnostic	**502** Categorical Course in Diagnostic Radiology: Body MR	**602** Categorical Course in Diagnostic Radiology: Body MR	**702** Categorical Course in Diagnostic Radiology: Body MR	**802** Categorical Course in Diagnostic Radiology: Body MR
entricular y: The Emerging Relative to Echo gy	**503** Noninvasive Vascular Imaging: Applications of CT and MR Angiography	**603** Coronary Artery Disease Assessed with MR and CT: At Which Shop to Stop	**703** Thoracic Aortic Disease: New Concepts in Diagnosis and Intervention	**803** Perfusion and Function in Nuclear Cardiology: Explanation of Techniques and How to Use Them
loskeletal	**504** MR Imaging of the Shoulder: Glenohumeral Joint Instability	**604** MR Imaging of the Ankle and Foot	**704** Imaging of Ligaments, Capsules, and Tendons of the Wrist and Hand	**804** A Systematic Approach to Imaging of Musculoskeletal Tumors
lopment	**505** MR Nerve Imaging: Neuroimaging of the Peripheral Nervous System to Include the Brachial and Sacral Plexuses	**605** Neurologic Interventions: Endovascular Treatment of Acute Cerebral Ischemia	**705** Functional Brain Mapping	**805** New MR Techniques for Neurologic Disease
	506 The Orbit and Optic Pathways	**606** Oncologic Overview of Head and Neck Malignancy	**706** Pediatric Ear, Nose, and Throat	**806** Skull Base and Craniovertebral Junction: Normal Anatomy, Congenital and Acquired Lesions, including Trauma
ary Tract: Update	**507** Genitourinary Imaging 1999: When to Use Intravenous Pyelography, US, CT, and MR	**607** Problematic Renal Masses: What You Need to Know	**707** MR Imaging in Gynecology	**807** Classic Signs in Uroradiology
Abdominal	**508** Imaging of Vertebral Trauma	**608** Imaging Upper-Extremity Trauma with Plain Films, CT, and MR	**708** Imaging Lower-Extremity Trauma with Plain Films, CT, and MR	**808** Pediatric Emergencies of the Chest, Abdomen, and Pelvis
nach: From One	**509** Imaging of Diffuse Liver Disease: Practical Approach	**609** A Trio of Small-Bowel Diseases: Ischemia, Malabsorption, and Obstruction	**709** Radiologic Evaluation of Pharyngeal and Anorectal Disorders: From One End to the Other	**809** Abdominal MR Imaging: Myth versus Reality
Doppler	**510** Practical Tips in US: Small Parts	**610** Practical Tips in US: Liver	**710** Practical Tips in US: Obstetrics	**810** Practical Tips in US: Abdomen
date	**511** Scintimammography, Lymphoscintigraphy, and Sentinel Node Imaging	**611** Perfusion Brain Imaging	**711** Optimal Imaging Modalities for Disorders of the Hepatobiliary Tree, Infection, and Gastrointestinal Bleeding	**811** Clinical PET Imaging
CT Evaluation	**512** Spiral (Helical) CT: Principles and Clinical Applications	**612** CT of the Small Bowel and Colon: Principles, Techniques, and Applications	**712** Helical CT of the Kidneys: New Concepts in Tumor Detection and Differentiation, CT Angiography, Renal Infection, and Stone Detection	**812** Cutting-Edge Technologies in CT Scanning: Multidetector Helical CT and Virtual Imaging
n Abdominal pplications	**513** Imaging in Oncology: Diagnosis and Treatment-related Issues	**613** MR Imaging of Extremities: Marrow and Soft Tissues	**713** Imaging of Extremities: Cartilage and Bone	**813** Interventional Radiology: Pediatric Considerations
ement of Deep Thrombosis	**514** Gynecologic Embolotherapy	**614** Current Trends in Dialysis Access Placement and Management	**714** Renal and Carotid Disease: Current Trends in Noninvasive Evaluation and Endovascular Therapy	**814** Abdominal Interventions: New Insights into Routine and Difficult Case Management
False-Negative rpretation: and Case	**515** Effect of Tumor Biology on Breast Cancer Detection	**615** Characterizing, Categorizing, and Managing	**715** Evaluation of the Breast after Surgery	**815** The Assessment of Screening Mammography Programs
ublished": ell All cal Market Managed Care, DNR) Orders: nced Directives artment	**516** Extramural and Intramural Opportunities through the National Institutes of Health **529** Antecedents of Osteoporosis	**616** Malignant Neoplasia: A Primer of Primaries **629** Bone Densitometry in Osteoporosis	**716** Clinical PACS: Eight Years of Experience in Vienna **729** PACS: Its Impact on Facility Design	**829** Strategic Thinking in Radiology

	Sunday, November 28		Monday, November 29		Tuesday, November 30	
8:00am						
8:30am						
9:00am		050 *info*RAD Guided Tours Schedule		057 *info*RAD Guided Tours Schedule		064 *info*RAD Gu Tours Schec
9:30am						
10:00am		051 *info*RAD Guided Tours Schedule		058 *info*RAD Guided Tours Schedule		065 *info*RAD Gu Tours Schec
10:30am	020 RSNA Research and Education Resources				011 The Internet and its Medical Information/ Education Resources	
11:00am		052 *info*RAD Guided Tours Schedule		059 *info*RAD Guided Tours Schedule		066 *info*RAD Gu Tours Schec
11:30am						
12:00onn		053 *info*RAD Guided Tours Schedule		060 *info*RAD Guided Tours Schedule		067 *info*RAD Gu Tours Schec
12:30pm						
1:00pm		054 *info*RAD Guided Tours Schedule		061 *info*RAD Guided Tours Schedule		068 *info*RAD Gu Tours Schec
1:30pm					012 The Internet and Its Medical Information/ Education Resources	
2:00pm		055 *info*RAD Guided Tours Schedule		062 *info*RAD Guided Tours Schedule		069 *info*RAD Gu Tours Schec
2:30pm					030 *"Hands-On Workshop:" Radiology and Clinical Information Integration*	
3:00pm		056 *info*RAD Guided Tours Schedule		063 *info*RAD Guided Tours Schedule		070 *info*RAD Gu Tours Schec
3:30pm			010 The Internet and its Medical Information/ Education Resources			
4:00pm						
4:30pm						
5:00pm						

***info*RAD tutorial and presentation learning objectives are to enable the attendee to:**

1. Assess new computer technologies for research, education, and practice.
2. Operate computer-aided instruction programs.
3. Operate computer-aided diagnostic programs and assess their role in practice.
4. Appreciate the options for connectivity in radiology through PACS, workstations, and Internet.
5. Make use of the Internet for research, education, and practice.

Wednesday, December 1		Thursday, December 2		Friday, December 3	
013 The Internet and its Medical Information/ Education Resources					
	071 *info*RAD Guided Tours Schedule		078 *info*RAD Guided Tours Schedule		085 *info*RAD Guided Tours Schedule
	072 *info*RAD Guided Tours Schedule		079 *info*RAD Guided Tours Schedule		086 *info*RAD Guided Tours Schedule
014 The Internet and its Medical Information/ Education Resources		016 The Internet and its Medical Information/ Education Resources; 032 *"Hands-On Workshop:" Radiology and Clinical*			
	073 *info*RAD Guided Tours Schedule		080 *info*RAD Guided Tours Schedule		
	074 *info*RAD Guided Tours Schedule		081 *info*RAD Guided Tours Schedule		
	075 *info*RAD Guided Tours Schedule		082 *info*RAD Guided Tours Schedule		
015 The Internet and its Medical Information/ Education Resources		017 The Internet and its Medical Information/ Education Resources			
	076 *info*RAD Guided Tours Schedule		083 *info*RAD Guided Tours Schedule		
031 *"Hands-On Workshop:"*	077 *info*RAD Guided Tours Schedule		084 *info*RAD Guided Tours Schedule		
		021 RSNA Research and Education Resources			

IHE SYMPOSIUM: PROPOSED SESSIONS AND SPEAKERS

91: *Management oriented*	92: *Clinically oriented*	93: *Technical, in-depth*

Wednesday, December 1

Plenary 1:00–2:15 pm

N01. Industry Experience with Enterprise Integration

Scientific Session 2:30–3:30 pm

91: Management oriented	92: Clinically oriented	93: Technical, in-depth
P91. *Integration: drivers, trends* Forces at work, key factors pushing toward integration	**P92.** *Telemedicine as a strategic tool* Applications, economics, legal issues, and experience to identify key settings for telemedicine	**P93.** *Standards activities* Detailed discussion of alternative approaches and how they relate

Scientific Session 4:00–5:30 pm

91: Management oriented	92: Clinically oriented	93: Technical, in-depth
Q91. *Priorities for integration: CIO perspective* Examining the range of possibilities and narrowing the focus	**Q92.** *Consumer-focus, outreach, patient-centered care* Demands, needs of patients & public, and how they are driving IDNs; successful approaches	**Q92.** *Data warehousing, data mining, analysis* Methodologies for data discovery from large databases, and for providing institutional information support

Evening Reception

Thursday, December 2

Scientific Session 8:30–10:00 am

91: Management oriented	92: Clinically oriented	93: Technical, in-depth
691. *Healthcare intranets* How to develop and support an intranet; what functions it should have, successful approaches	**692.** *The electronic medical record as an integration tool* Strategies for accessing, coordinating, and updating the EMR across a network	**693.** *Designing reliable high performance networks* Network design issues and approaches, also Next Generation Internet

Scientific Session 10:30–12:00 pm

91: Management oriented	92: Clinically oriented	93: Technical, in-depth
R91. *Strategies for integration* Examples, demos of integration approaches; Partners, CareWeb, BJC, Regenstrieff, Columbia	**R92.** *Multimedia and image integration* Feasibility and desirability of distributing clinical images, as part of the EMR, and for consultation, successful approaches	**R93.** *Developing and managing an enterprise Web site* Issues and approaches

Lunch and exhibits/tour

Plenary 1:00–2:15 pm

S01. Developing and Managing Network Environments for the Enterprise

Scientific Session 2:30–3:30 pm

91: Management oriented	92: Clinically oriented	93: Technical, in-depth
791. *Internet tools & resources* Content, tools, services, consortia for health care networks	**792.** *Relationship building* How networked enterprises can enhance communications between patients and providers	**793.** *Net-based technologies in healthcare* A focus on Java, COBRA, DCOM, XML

Scientific Session 4:00–5:30 pm

91: Management oriented	92: Clinically oriented	93: Technical, in-depth
T91. *National-level integration initiatives* Management and organizational approaches to integrating diverse systems	**T92.** *Computer-aided decision support* Achieving the benefits of integration through data mining, data analysis, and decision aids	**T93.** *Integration paradigms* Client-server and internet-based architectures

Friday, December 3

Scientific Session 8:30–10:00 am

91: Management oriented	92: Clinically oriented	93: Technical, in-depth
891. *Standards, architectures, organization initiatives* A standards road map, how the efforts interact	**892.** *Clinical guidelines* Roles for clinical guidelines in workstation design, referral management, and workflow optimization	**893.** *Strategic integration of IT* Selecting priorities, developing a plan, engaging the participants, managing the process

Scientific Session 10:30–12:00pm

91: Management oriented	92: Clinically oriented	93: Technical, in-depth
U91. *The IHE initiative* Goals, vendor, health enterprise, perspectives, future plans	**U92.** *Security, confidentiality, privacy update* Tradeoffs, issues for meeting the needs without making the system unwieldy	**U93.** *Building the infrastructure* Technology for integrating distribution systems

B. A Radiologist's Perspective
Edward V. Staab, MD

C. A Clinician's Perspective
Eric G. Tangalos, MD

124

Organizational Culture and Health System Change

Sponsored by the Associated Sciences Consortium
Paula Maramonte, MEd, RT(R) (AERS) Coordinator
Cornelius J. Rater, MD (AERS)
Harry J. Granito, MS (RBMA)
Susan K. Snyder, BS, EdD (ASRT)

125

Categorical Course in Diagnostic Radiology Physics: Physical Aspects of Breast Imaging—Current and Future Considerations***

A. Radiology of Minimal Breast Cancer
Laszlo Tabar, MD

B. Epidemiology of Breast Cancer
Robert A. Smith, PhD

126

PACS and Radiology Informatics: Making the Business Argument for PACS

Paul J. Chang, MD Moderator
Sean O'Rourke
Bruce I. Reiner, MD
Eliot L. Siegel, MD
Philip A. Templeton, MD

127

Entrepreneurship and Marketing for Radiologists

Elias A. Zerhouni, MD
Derace L. Schaffer, MD

128

Physics: Imaging in Radiation Therapy

Arthur L. Boyer, PhD Director

A. State of the Art in Medical Imaging
John D. Hazle, PhD

B. Imaging for Conformal Therapy and Intensity-modulated Radiation Therapy
Arthur L. Boyer, PhD

129

Technology Assessment in Radiology: Part I-Basic Principles of Testing: Diagnostic Accuracy and Decision-making in Radiology

William C. Black, MD
Curtis P. Langlotz, MD, PhD

130

Minicourse: Women's Health in Imaging

Ellen B. Mendelson, MD Director

A. Bone Density Evaluation
Donald M. Bachman, MD

B. Vascular Disease in Women
Harvey L. Neiman, MD

C. Interventional Procedures
Eric vanSonnenberg, MD

150

Hysterosalpingography and Selective Salpingography ("How-to" Workshop)

Amy S. Thurmond, MD
Lindsay S. Machan, MD
Antoine J. Maubon, MD
Jean-Pierre Rouanet, MD
David M. Hovsepian, MD
Arl V. Moore, Jr, MD
Ronald J. Zagoria, MD
James C. Bass, MD

151

Managing Complications of Central Venous Access ("How-to" Workshop)

George G. Hartnell, MD
Philip D. Orons, DO
Anthony F. Watkinson, MD
Clement J. Grassi, MD
James F. Benenati, MD

152

Real-Time Interventional Ultrasound ("Hands-on" Workshop)

Mark B. Saker, MD
Carolyn K. Donaldson, MD
David M. Ayoub, MD
Michael C. Brunner, MD
Meri E. Chen, MD
Horacio B. D'Agostino, MD
Janice J. Dieschbourg, MD
Gregory S. Foster, DO
Angelo N. Makris, MD
Terence A. Matalon, MD
Virginia McDonald, MD
Albert A. Nemcek, Jr, MD
Myra I. Rapoport, MD
Bruce Silver, MD
Robert I. Silvers, MD

153

How to Use a PACS Workstation: Basic ("Hands-on" Workshop)

David E. Avrin, MD, PhD Co-moderator
Janice C. Honeyman, PhD Co-moderator
Katherine P. Andriole, PhD Co-moderator
Keith J. Dreyer, MD, PhD Co-moderator

Monday, November 29, 1999 8:30 am to 10:00 am

201

The Diagnosis of Pulmonary Embolism: A Rational Approach to Familiar Tests and New Technologies

Jeffrey R. Galvin, MD
Martine J. Remy-Jardin, MD, PhD

202

Categorical Course in Diagnostic Radiology: Body MR*

A. Liver
Donald G. Mitchell, MD

B. Hepatobiliary System and Pancreas
Matthew A. Barish, MD

C. Adrenal Glands and Kidneys
Peter L. Choyke, MD

203

Three-dimensional Contrast MR Angiography

Thomas M. Grist, MD
Martin R. Prince, MD, PhD
Jorg F. Debatin, MD

204

Imaging Enigmas of the Hip

B. J. Manaster, MD, PhD Coordinator
Carol L. Andrews, MD
Cheryl A. Petersilge, MD

205

The New WHO Classification of Brain Tumors: Imaging Correlations

James G. Smirniotopoulos, MD
Carolyn C. Meltzer, MD

206

The Sinonasal Cavities and the Ostiomeatal Complex

A. The Ostiomeatal Complex
Vijay M. Rao, MD

B. Inflammatory Disease and Neoplasms
Patricia A. Hudgins, MD

207

Pelvic Prolapse: The New Way to Image

Amy S. Thurmond, MD
Antoine J. Maubon, MD
Zoran L. Barbaric, MD
Jean-Pierre Rouanet, MD

208

Imaging Chest Trauma

Steven L. Primack, MD
Stuart E. Mirvis, MD

209

Minimally Invasive Treatment of Malignant Hepatic Tumors

Gerald D. Dodd III, MD
William R. Lees, MBBS
Fred T. Lee, Jr, MD

210

Practical Tips in US: Obstetrics

A. Premenopausal Bleeding
Edward A. Lyons, MD

B. First Trimester
Donald S. Emerson, MD

C. Third Trimester
Michael L. Manco-Johnson, MD

211

Advances in Nuclear Oncology

Alan Waxman, MD Moderator
Robert E. Henkin, MD
Jonathan M. Links, PhD

212

Advances and Controversies in CT and MR of the Genitourinary Tract

Melvyn T. Korobkin, MD
Janet E. Husband, MD
Cary L. Siegel, MD

213

Special Course in Pediatric Radiology: Current Concepts in Body Imaging at the Millennium—Imaging the Pediatric Chest: Current Applications+

A. CT and MR Imaging of Mediastinal Masses
Beverley Newman, MD

B. High-Resolution CT of Pediatric Parenchymal Disorders
Jerald P. Kuhn, MD

C. CT of Acute Lung Disease: Infection and Trauma
Lane F. Donnelly, MD

214
Stent-Grafts of the Aorta and Peripheral Vessels

Curtis W. Bakal, MD
Stuart C. Geller, MD
James F. Benenati, MD

215
Correlating Pathology of Benign and Malignant Breast Lesions with Mammography and US
Gilda Cardenosa, MD
G. W. Eklund, MD

216
Imaging the Hot Zone: What Every Radiologist Should Know about Emerging Infectious Diseases and Food-borne Illnesses

Sponsored by the RSNA Committee on International Relations and Education
Anne G. Osborn, MD
C. J. Peters, MD
Loren H. Ketai, MD

217
American College of Radiology Standards and Accreditation Programs: Major Issues and Update 1999

In conjunction with the American College of Radiology
E. Stephen Amis, Jr, MD Moderator
D. David Dershaw, MD
Stephen R. Baker, MD
Robert K. Zeman, MD

218
Primary Intrathoracic and Malignant Tumors

A. Missed Lung Cancer at Radiography: What Can Be Done?
John H. Austin, MD

B. Diagnosis, Work-up, and Staging of Lung Cancer
Robert D. Pugatch, MD

C. Role of PET Scanning in the Diagnosis, Staging, and Follow-up of Lung Cancer
Steven M. Larson, MD

219
Management of Regionally Localized, High-Risk Prostate Cancer

Alan Pollack, MD, PhD

220
Radioprotectors

Scott P. Tannehill, MD

221
How to Run with the PACS

Katherine P. Andriole, PhD

222
Multileaf Collimators and Dynamic Wedges

Jatinder R. Palta, PhD
Chihray Liu, PhD

223
Categorical Course in Diagnostic Radiology Physics: Electronic Radiology Practice—Technical and Practical: PACS for the Electronically Challenged**

Nicholas J. Hangiandreou, PhD
Richard L. Morin, PhD

224
Asset Management for High-Technology Systems

Sponsored by the Associated Sciences Consortium
Chester T. Szerlag, MBA (SROA) Coordinator
Tim Guertin (SROA)
Sheila M. Sferrella (AHRA)
Dennis A. Bair, RT(R)(CV) (AVIR)

225
Categorical Course in Diagnostic Radiology Physics: Physical Aspects of Breast Imaging—Current and Future Considerations***

A. X-ray Equipment Considerations
Gary T. Barnes, PhD

B. Screen-Film-processing Considerations
Arthur G. Haus

226
PACS and Radiology Informatics: Update on PACS Technology and Infrastructure

Paul J. Chang, MD Moderator
Fred W. Prior, PhD
G. Michael LaChance
Sridhar B. Seshadri, MSEE, MBA
Douglas M. Tucker, PhD

227
Coding and Billing Tips to Optimize Revenue

Walt Blackham
Joy Pratt

228
Physics: Imaging in Radiation Therapy

Arthur L. Boyer, PhD Director
A. Standards for Radiation Therapy Image Communication
Bruce H. Curran, PhD

B. Coordinate Systems in Radiation Oncology
George Starkschall, PhD

229
Technology Assessment in Radiology: Part II-Outcomes and Cost-Effectiveness Research

Bruce J. Hillman, MD
Maria G. Hunink, MD, PhD

230
Minicourse: Women's Health in Imaging after Menopause

Ellen B. Mendelson, MD Director
A. Effects of Tamoxifen and Hormone Replacement Therapy
Marcela Bohm-Velez, MD

B. CT Staging of Pelvic Neoplasms
Elliot K. Fishman, MD

C. Staging of Endometrial Carcinoma with Use of Appropriateness Criteria
Hedvig Hricak, MD, PhD

250
Carotid Stent Placement ("How-to" Workshop)

Donald E. Schwarten, MD

251
Dialysis Graft Thrombectomy and Thrombolysis ("How-to" Workshop)

Scott O. Trerotola, MD
Matthew S. Johnson, MD
Karim Valji, MD

252
Musculoskeletal US ("Hands-on" Workshop)

Marnix T. Van Holsbeeck, MD Moderator
J. Antonio Bouffard, MD
Etienne Cardinal, MD
David P. Fessell, MD
Ghyiath Habra, MD
Joseph H. Introcaso, MD
Jon A. Jacobson, MD
Doohi Lee, MD
William D. Middleton, MD
Matthieu J. Rutten, MD
Glenn M. Strome, MD
Joseph G. Craig, MD

253
How to Use a PACS Workstation: Basic ("Hands-on" Workshop)

David E. Avrin, MD, PhD Co-moderator
Janice C. Honeyman, PhD Co-moderator
Katherine P. Andriole, PhD Co-moderator
Keith J. Dreyer, MD, PhD Co-moderator

Monday, November 29, 1999 4:00 pm to 5:30 pm

301
Differential Diagnosis of Mediastinal Masses

Melissa L. Rosado de Christenson, MD
Ella A. Kazerooni, MD

302
Categorical Course in Diagnostic Radiology: Body MR*

A. Female Pelvis: Benign Disease
Caroline Reinhold, MD

B. Female Pelvis: Malignant Disease
Susan M. Ascher, MD

C. Male Pelvis
Hedvig Hricak, MD, PhD

303
Practical Cardiac MR Imaging: Principles, Pearls, and Protocols for Success

Vivian S. Lee, MD, PhD
David A. Bluemke, MD, PhD

304
MR Imaging of Athletic Injuries of the Knee

Arthur A. De Smet, MD Coordinator
Michael J. Tuite, MD

305
Spinal Imaging: Dealing with Back Pain

Jeffrey S. Ross, MD
Michael T. Modic, MD
Michael N. Brant-Zawadzki, MD

306
Advanced Concepts in Head and Neck Cancer

A. Imaging Considerations
Anthony A. Mancuso, MD

B. Nodes
Peter M. Som, MD

307
Genitourinary Tract Imaging in Pregnant and Postpartum Patients

Deborah Levine, MD
Michelle M. McNicholas, MD

308
Helical CT of Nontraumatic Abdominal Emergencies

A. Helical CT of Appendicitis and Diverticulitis
Patrick M. Rao, MD

B. Helical CT of Bowel Obstruction
Michael P. Federle, MD

C. Helical CT of Urinary Tract Stones: Leave No Stone Unseen
Robert C. Smith, MD

309
Imaging of the Acute Abdomen

Bernard A. Birnbaum, MD
Julien B. Puylaert, MD, PhD
Kyunghee C. Cho, MD

310
Practical Tips in US: Breast

A. Breast US
A. Thomas Stavros, MD

B. Breast Fine-Needle Aspiration Biopsy
Paula B. Gordon, MD

C. Breast Core Biopsy
Steve H. Parker, MD

311
Musculoskeletal Nuclear Imaging

Manuel L. Brown, MD
Moderator
Lawrence E. Holder, MD

312
Three-dimensional CT Imaging: Principles, Techniques, and Clinical Applications

Geoffrey D. Rubin, MD
Elliot K. Fishman, MD

313
Special Course in Pediatric Radiology: Current Concepts in Body Imaging at the Millennium—MR Imaging of Congenital Cardiovascular Disease+

A. Cardiovascular MR Imaging Techniques
Kerry M. Link, MD

B. Cardiac Applications
Fernando R. Gutierrez, MD

C. Evaluation of the Great Vessels
Ramiro J. Hernandez, MS, MD

314
Transjugular Intrahepatic Portosystemic Shunts: From Patient Selection to Surveillance and Revision

Charles A. Owens, MD
Jeanne M. LaBerge, MD
Ziv J. Haskal, MD

315
Reducing False-Positive Mammogram Interpretations

A. Mammography Screening: Reducing the Recall Rate
Edward A. Sickles, MD

B. Problem-solving Imaging: Reducing the Benign Tissue Diagnosis Rate
Debra M. Ikeda, MD

316
Current Activities of the Residency Review Committee and the American Board of Radiology in Regard to Diagnostic Radiology

In Conjunction with the Residency Review Committee and the American Board of Radiology

A. Current Activities of the Residency Review Committee
Albert A. Moss, MD
Judith S. Armbruster, PhD

B. Current Activities of the American Board of Radiology
William J. Casarella, MD
M. Paul Capp, MD

317
AIDS Imaging: A Critical Clinical Approach

Jacques W.A.J. Reeders, MD, PhD

318
Imaging of the Surgically Altered Breast

A. Mammography of the Postconservation Breast
D. David Dershaw, MD

B. Mammography of the Augmented Breast
R. James Brenner, MD, JD

C. MR Imaging after Conservation and Augmentation
Susan G. Orel, MD

319
Stereotactic Radiosurgery for Central Nervous System Tumors

Shiao Y. Woo, MBBS

320
Radiation Therapy for Prostate Cancer: Dose Escalation with 3D Conformal Radiation Therapy

Jeff M. Michalski, MD

321
US Artifacts

Lance V. Hefner, MS
Donovan M. Bakalyar, PhD
Beatrice L. Madrazo, MD
Frederick W. Kremkau, PhD

322
Physics of Intravascular Brachytherapy

Charles W. Coffey II, PhD
Dennis M. Duggan, PhD

323
Categorical Course in Diagnostic Radiology Physics: Electronic Radiology Practice—Technical and Practical: Real Life Electronic Practice—An Interview with Trench Dwellers**

Byrn Williamson, Jr, MD
Jeremy W. R. Young, MD
Eliot L. Siegel, MD
Thomas H. Berquist, MD

324
Economic Implications of Regulatory Change

Sponsored by the Associated Sciences Consortium
DuVonne Campbell (ASRT)
Coordinator
Cherrill Farnsworth (AHRA)
Sherry Makely, PhD (ASRT, SNM)
Donna L. Wright, EdD, RT(R) (AERS)

325
Categorical Course in Diagnostic Radiology Physics: Physical Aspects of Breast Imaging—Current and Future Considerations***

A. Optimizing Mammography Technique Factors
R. Edward Hendrick, PhD

B. Radiation Dose in Mammography
Lawrence N. Rothenberg, PhD

C. Risk, Benefit, and Controversies in Mammographic Screening
Stephen A. Feig, MD

326
PACS and Radiology Informatics: Getting from Here to There—"Change Management" in PACS

Janice C. Honeyman, PhD
Moderator
Patrice M. Bret, MD
Trevor D. Cradduck, PhD
Loretta L. Hanwell, MPA (AHRA)

327
Turf Battles in Radiology: How to Fight Them and Win!

David C. Levin, MD
Robert L. Bree, MD
Vijay M. Rao, MD
Harvey L. Neiman, MD

328
Physics: Imaging in Radiation Therapy

Arthur L. Boyer, PhD
Director

A. Three-dimensional Data Derived from Spiral CT
Willi A. Kalender, PhD

B. CT Numbers and Electron Density
Frank E. Zink, PhD

329
Transplants: Use of US

Brian Gorman, MBBCh

330
Minicourse: Women's Health in Imaging before Menopause

Ellen B. Mendelson, MD
Director

A. Infertility
Amy S. Thurmond, MD

B. Sonography of Pelvic Masses and Its Impact on Patient Management
Arthur C. Fleischer, MD

C. Managing Breast Masses in Young, Lactating, or Pregnant Women
Ellen B. Mendelson, MD

350
Percutaneous CT-guided Biopsy of the Spine ("How-to" Workshop)

Glen K. Geremia, MD
William M. Greenlee, MD
Anne M. Dowd, MD
Subba Raju, MD
David B. Granato, MD
Tae Woo Kim, MD
Calvin H. Flowers, MD
Richard T. Falter, Jr, MD
Todd R. Brack, DO
Douglas S. Fenton, MD

351
How to Prepare and Deliver Electronic Presentations ("How-to" Workshop)

Robert J. Pizzutiello, Jr, MS
Brent H. Adler, MD
Franklin N. Tessler, MD

352
Interventional Breast Procedures ("Hands-on" Workshop)

W. Phil Evans, MD
Frederick Ronald Margolin, MD
Carl J. D'Orsi, MD
Michele R. Miles, MD
Bruno D. Fornage, MD
Handel E. Reynolds, MD
Laura Liberman, MD
Etta D. Pisano, MD
Eva Rubin, MD
Elsie Levin, MD

353
How to Use a PACS Workstation: Advanced ("Hands-on" Workshop)

David E. Avrin, MD, PhD Co-moderator
Janice C. Honeyman, PhD Co-moderator
Katherine P. Andriole, PhD Co-moderator
Keith J. Dreyer, MD, PhD Co-moderator

Tuesday, November 30, 1999 8:30 am to 10:00 am

401
High-Resolution CT of the Lung Parenchyma: A Practical Approach
W. Richard Webb, MD
Nestor L. Muller, MD, PhD

402
Categorical Course in Diagnostic Radiology: Body MR*

A. Cardiac
Andre J. Duerinckx, MD, PhD

B. Aorta
Neil M. Rofsky, MD

C. Renal and Mesenteric MR Angiography
Martin R. Prince, MD, PhD

D. Peripheral Vasculature
James F. Meaney, MD

403
Assessment of Left Ventricular Function and Viability: The Emerging Role of MR Imaging Relative to Echo and Nuclear Cardiology

Kerry M. Link, MD
Thomas Wallhaus, MD

404
Interventional Musculoskeletal Radiology
Phoebe A. Kaplan, MD Coordinator
Robert G. Dussault, MD
Jean-Denis Laredo, MD

405
Congenital and Development Abnormalities

A. Dorsal and Ventral Neural Tube Defects
Marvin D. Nelson, Jr, MD

B. Migrational and Proliferative Disorders
Thomas P. Naidich, MD

C. Neurocutaneous Syndromes
James G. Smirniotopoulos, MD

406
The Temporal Bone

A. Anatomy, Congenital Abnormalities, and the Anatomy and Pathology of the Facial Nerve
Mahmood F. Mafee, MD

B. Inflammatory Disease, Sensorineural Hearing Deficit, and the Neurovascular Compartments
Joel D. Swartz, MD

407
US of the Genitourinary Tract: Update and Controversies

Matthew D. Rifkin, MD
Franklin N. Tessler, MD
Mitchell E. Tublin, MD
Neil T. Wolfman, MD

408
Helical CT and US of Abdominal Trauma

A. Helical CT of Abdominal Trauma
Diego B. Nunez, Jr, MD
Robert A. Novelline, MD

B. US of Abdominal Trauma
Kimberley L. McKenney, MD

409
Radiology of the Stomach: From One Curve to the Other

Marc S. Levine, MD
Richard M. Gore, MD
Frank H. Miller, MD

410
Practical Tips in US: Doppler

A. Lower Extremity Deep Venous Thrombosis: Doppler
John J. Cronan, MD

B. Carotid: Doppler
Joseph F. Polak, MD, MPH

C. Abdomen: Doppler
Laurence Needleman, MD

411
Infection Imaging Update

Donald S. Schauwecker, PhD, MD Moderator
Ethan M. Braunstein, MD
Christopher J. Palestro, MD

412
The Acute Abdomen: CT Evaluation

Jay P. Heiken, MD
Bruce A. Urban, MD

413
Special Course in Pediatric Radiology: Current Concepts in Body Imaging at the Millennium—CT and MR Imaging in Abdominal Disorders: Current Applications+

A. Blunt Abdominal Trauma: Imaging and Outcome
George A. Taylor, MD

B. CT in Nontraumatic Gastrointestinal Diseases
Carlos J. Sivit, MD

C. MR Imaging and MR Angiography in the Pediatric Abdomen
Peter J. Strouse, MD

414
Endovascular Management of Deep Vein and Pulmonary Thrombosis

Charles P. Semba, MD
Mahmood K. Razavi, MD

415
Strategies to Reduce False-Negative Mammographic Interpretation: Problems, Solutions, and Case Studies

Lawrence W. Bassett, MD
Valerie P. Jackson, MD
R. James Brenner, MD, JD

416
"Getting Your Work Published": Editors and Authors Tell All

In Conjunction with the American Association for Women Radiologists
Melissa L. Rosado de Christenson, MD Moderator
Anthony V. Proto, MD
William W. Olmsted, MD
Laurens V. Ackerman, MD, PhD
B. J. Manaster, MD, PhD
Wendy R.K. Smoker, MD

417
Preserving Your Medical Market Share: Malpractice, Managed Care, and Antitrust

Sponsored by the RSNA Medical Legal Committee
Leonard Berlin, MD
Harry Zibners, MD, JD
John J. Smith, MD, JD
Ronald L. Eisenberg, MD, JD

418
Pancreatic Neoplasms: CT and MR

Chusilp Charnsangavej, MD
Richard C. Semelka, MD

419
Lung Cancer

A. Management of Small Cell Lung Cancer
Ritsuko U. Komaki, MD

B. Three-dimensional Conformal Treatment for Lung Cancer
Bahman Emami, MD

420
Combined Surgery and Radiation Therapy for Advanced Head and Neck Cancers

Louis G. Portugal, MD
Adam S. Garden, MD

421
The Physicist and the Mammography Technologist

Robert J. Pizzutiello, Jr, MS
Debra H. Deibel, RT(R)M
Rita W. Heinlein, RT(R)(M)

422
SPECT and Coincidence Imaging Basics
Mark T. Madsen, PhD
James A. Patton, PhD

423
Categorical Course in Diagnostic Radiology Physics: Electronic Radiology Practice—Technical and Practical: Electronic Image Acquisition—Technical Aspects**

A. Computed and Digital Radiography
Katherine P. Andriole, PhD

B. Digitization: Film and Video
Jon H. Trueblood, PhD

C. Modality Interfacing via DICOM
Steven C. Horii, MD

424
Managing a Multisite Radiology Network

Sponsored by the Associated Sciences Consortium
Kathryn J. Canny, (RBMA) Coordinator
Larry A. Ranahan, MBA (RBMA) Moderator
Charles Deschamps RT(R)(MR) (SMRT)
Scott Seberg, MS (RBMA)
Chester T. Szerlag, MBA (RBMA)

425
Categorical Course in Diagnostic Radiology Physics: Physical Aspects of Breast Imaging—Current and Future Considerations***

A. Mammography Quality Standards Act
John L. McCrohan, MS

B. Changes in the 1999 ACR Quality Control Manual
Priscilla F. Butler, MS

C. Quality Mammography in a Managed Care Environment
Ronald F. Bernardi, BA, RT(R)

426
PACS and Radiology Informatics: Writing the PACS Request for Proposal and Optimizing the User-Vendor Relationship

Eliot L. Siegel, MD Moderator
Paul J. Chang, MD
Robert Cooke
Sean O'Rourke
Donald R. Peters, MD
Philip A. Templeton, MD

427
Management Challenges Facing Academic and Community Hospital Radiology Departments and How to Meet Them

Steven E. Seltzer, MD
William R. Poller, MD

428
Physics: Imaging and Radiation Therapy

Arthur L. Boyer, PhD Director
A. Active Matrix Flat-Panel Imagers for Electronic Portal Imager
Arthur L. Boyer, PhD

B. Real-Time Imaging for Patient Position Alignment
Martin Murphy, PhD

429
Do Not Resuscitate (DNR) Orders: Complying with Advanced Directives in the Radiology Department

Sponsored by the RSNA Ethics Committee
Franklin Earnest IV, MD
Heather J. Ohrt, MD
Donald M. Bachman, MD

430
Minicourse: Women's Health in Imaging-Advances in Breast Imaging

Ellen B. Mendelson, MD Director
A. MR Imaging
Mitchell D. Schnall, MD, PhD

B. Scintimammography and Sentinel Node Imaging
Iraj Khalkhali, MD

C. US in Local Staging of Breast Cancer and in Guiding New Interventional Procedures
Bruno D. Fornage, MD

450
Strategies for Optimizing Spiral CT of the Vascular System ("How-to" Workshop)

Geoffrey D. Rubin, MD
Mathias Prokop, MD

451
Lymph Node Mapping ("How-to" Workshop)

Deepak G. Bedi, MD
Kelly K. Hunt, MD
Ebrahim S. Delpassand, MD
Gary J. Whitman, MD

452
Venous Access ("Hands-on" Workshop)

Robert D. Lyon, MD
James C. Andrews, MD
John F. Cardella, MD
Peter G. Chait, MD
Howard B. Chrisman, MD
John David Lane, MD
Mark L. Lukens, MD
Matthew A. Mauro, MD
Philip C. Pieters, MD
Joseph A. Ronsivalle, DO
Melvin Rosenblatt, MD

453
How to Use a PACS Workstation: Basic ("Hands-on" Workshop)

David E. Avrin, MD, PhD Co-moderator
Janice C. Honeyman, PhD Co-moderator
Katherine P. Andriole, PhD Co-moderator
Keith J. Dreyer, MD, PhD Co-moderator

Wednesday, December 01, 1999 8:30 am to 10:00 am

501
Optimization of Spiral CT of the Thorax

Ann N. Leung, MD
Jeffrey S. Klein, MD

502
Categorical Course in Diagnostic Radiology: Body MR*

A. Bone Marrow
Harry K. Genant, MD

B. Osseous Tumors
Leanne L. Seeger, MD

C. Soft-Tissue Masses: A Systematic Approach to MR Evaluation
Mark J. Kransdorf, MD

503
Noninvasive Vascular Imaging: Applications of CT and MR Angiography

Geoffrey D. Rubin, MD
Jorg F. Debatin, MD

504
MR Imaging of the Shoulder: Glenohumeral Joint Instability

A. Normal Anatomy, Anatomic Variations, and Pathologic Anatomy
Donald L. Resnick, MD

B. Bankart and Bankart Variation Lesions: MR Arthrography
Phillip F. Tirman, MD

C. Glenoid Labral Articular Disruptions (GLAD) and Superior Labrum Anterior and Posterior (SLAP) Lesions: MR Arthrography
Javier Beltran, MD

D. Glenohumeral Joint Instability: Noncontrast MR Imaging
Mahvash Rafii, MD

505
MR Nerve Imaging: Neuroimaging of the Peripheral Nervous System to Include the Brachial and Sacral Plexuses

Brian C. Bowen, MD, PhD
Kenneth R. Maravilla, MD

506
The Orbit and Optic Pathways

A. The Pediatric Orbit
Patricia C. Davis, MD

B. The Adult
Jane L. Weissman, MD

507
Genitourinary Imaging 1999: When to Use Intravenous Pyelography, US, CT, and MR

Ronald J. Zagoria, MD
Philip J. Kenney, MD
Evan S. Siegelman, MD

508
Imaging of Vertebral Trauma

A. Radiography: The ABCs
Richard H. Daffner, MD

B. Helical CT
James T. Rhea, MD

C. MR Imaging
Andrew L. Goldberg, MD

509
Imaging of Diffuse Liver Disease: Practical Approach

Pablo R. Ros, MD
Richard L. Baron, MD
Christoph D. Becker, MD

510
Practical Tips in US: Small Parts

A. What's New?
Peter L. Cooperberg, MD

B. Shoulder
Thomas C. Winter III, MD

C. Other Musculoskeletal US
William D. Middleton, MD

511
Scintimammography, Lymphoscintigraphy, and Sentinel Node Imaging

Naomi P. Alazraki, MD
Patrick J. Peller, MD

512
Spiral (Helical) CT: Principles and Clinical Applications

Robert K. Zeman, MD
Paul M. Silverman, MD
Janet E. Kuhlman, MD

513
Special Course in Pediatric Radiology: Current Concepts in Body Imaging at the Millennium—Imaging in Oncology: Diagnosis and Treatment-related Issues+

A. Wilms Tumor
Nancy S. Rosen, MD

B. Neuroblastoma
Sara J. Abramson, MD

C. Malignant Bone Tumors
Barry D. Fletcher, MD

514
Gynecologic Embolotherapy

Richard D. Shlansky-Goldberg, MD
Lindsay S. Machan, MD
Scott C. Goodwin, MD

515
Effect of Tumor Biology on Breast Cancer Detection

A. Breast Cancer Growth Rates
Eva Rubin, MD

B. Effect of Tumor Biology on Breast Cancer Detection
Daniel B. Kopans, MD

C. Missed Cancers, Interval Studies, and Maximizing Screening Techniques
Carl J. D'Orsi, MD

516
Extramural and Intramural Opportunities through the National Institutes of Health

Lee A. Rosen, PhD
Daniel Carl Sullivan, MD
R. Nick Bryan, MD, PhD

518
Evaluation of Hepatic Metastatic Disease: CT, MR, and US

A. CT
James H. Oliver III, MD

B. MR
Marc J. Fenstermacher, MD

C. US
Laurence Needleman, MD

519
Lymphoma

A. Expanding Role of Radiation Therapy for Malignant Lymphoma
James D. Cox, MD

B. Management of Hodgkin Disease
Chul S. Ha, MD

520
Radiation: The Two-edged Sword—Risk Factors and Protection

Eric J. Hall, DPhil, DSc

521
Technical Aspects of Interventional Fluoroscopic Systems

Stephen Balter, PhD

522
RSO Basics

Jean M. St Germain, MS
Kenneth Miller, MS

523
Categorical Course in Diagnostic Radiology Physics: Electronic Radiology Practice—Technical and Practical: Electronic Image Acquisition—Practice Aspects**

A. Mechanisms for RIS Interfaces
Janice C. Honeyman, PhD

B. Imaging Workflow
Richard Olinger, RT(R)

C. Examination Quality Control
Lisa L. Jorgenson, RT(R)

524
Current Challenges in Radiology and Planning and Design

Sponsored by the Associated Sciences Consortium
Morris A. Stein (AIA-AAH) Coordinator
Bill Rostenberg (AIA-AAH)
Jerry W. Froelich, MD (AIA-AAH)
Eliot L. Siegel, MD (AIA-AAH)

525
Categorical Course in Diagnostic Radiology Physics: Physical Aspects of Breast Imaging—Current and Future Considerations***

A. Stereotactic Breast Biopsy: Clinical Overview
Jean R. Paquelet, MD

B. Stereotactic Imaging: Physical Considerations
R. Edward Hendrick, PhD

C. Medical Physics Surveys and Accreditation of Stereotactic Breast Biopsy Units
Robert J. Pizzutiello, Jr, MS

526
PACS and Radiology Informatics: Getting the Message Out—Update on Voice Recognition, Structured Reporting, and Value Innovation

Paul J. Chang, MD Moderator
W. Dean Bidgood, Jr, MD, MS
Peter K. Kijewski, PhD
Donald F. Schomer, MD

527
Risk Management in Radiology: How to Stay Out of Trouble with the Courts

Leonard Berlin, MD

528
Physics: Imaging in Radiation Therapy

Arthur L. Boyer, PhD Director

A. Volume Rendering
Charles Pelizzari, ME

B. CT Simulation
Bruce H. Curran, ME

529
Antecedents of Osteoporosis

In Conjunction with the American Association for Women Radiologists
M. Ines Boechat, MD Moderator
Dorothy Nelson, PhD
Sharmila Majumdar, PhD
Vicente Gilsanz, MD, PhD

530
Minicourse: New Developments in Body CT Scanning - New Developments in Abdominal CT

Elliot K. Fishman, MD Co-director
Nestor L. Muller, MD, PhD Co-director

A. Multislice CT Scanning: A New Imaging Paradigm
W. Dennis Foley, MD

B. Multiphase Imaging of the Liver
Michael P. Federle, MD

C. Multiphase Imaging of the Pancreas
R. Brooke Jeffrey, Jr, MD

550
Sympathetic Blockades for Pain Management: Radiologic and Medical Strategies for Pain Management ("How-to" Workshop)

Wade H. Wong, DO
Mark S. Wallace, MD
Scott Magnuson, MD

551
Thrombolytic Therapy in Venous Disease ("How-to" Workshop)

Haraldur Bjarnason, MD
Charles P. Semba, MD

552
Venous Thrombosis: Doppler Sonography ("Hands-on" Workshop)

Lynwood W. Hammers, DO
Leslie M. Scoutt, MD
Janis M. Brown, MD
Janis G. Letourneau, MD
Thomas R. Beidle, MD
Deborah J. Rubens, MD

553
How to Use a PACS Workstation: Advanced ("Hands-on"Workshop)

David E. Avrin, MD, PhD Co-moderator
Janice C. Honeyman, PhD Co-moderator
Katherine P. Andriole, PhD Co-moderator
Keith J. Dreyer, MD, PhD Co-moderator

Thursday, December 02, 1999
8:30 am to 10:00 am

601
Chest Infections: Typical Presentations, Complications, and Management

Georgeann McGuinness, MD
H. Page McAdams, MD

602
Categorical Course in Diagnostic Radiology: Body MR*

A. Hip
Robert D. Boutin, MD

B. Ankle
Hollis G. Potter, MD

C. Wrist: Ligaments and Triangular Fibrocartilage Complex
Donald L. Resnick, MD

603
Coronary Artery Disease Assessed with MR and CT: At Which Shop to Stop

A. MR Assessment
Roderic I. Pettigrew, MD, PhD

B. CT Assessment
William Stanford, MD

604
MR Imaging of the Ankle and Foot

Zehava S. Rosenberg, MD Coordinator
Javier Beltran, MD

605
Neurologic Interventions: Endovascular Treatment of Acute Cerebral Ischemia

Thomas A. Tomsick, MD
Charles A. Jungreis, MD

606
Oncologic Overview of Head and Neck Malignancy

A. Larynx and Hypopharynx
Hugh D. Curtin, MD

B. Nasopharynx and Oropharynx
Laurie A. Loevner, MD

607
Problematic Renal Masses: What You Need to Know

David S. Hartman, MD
Peter L. Choyke, MD

608
Imaging Upper-Extremity Trauma with Plain Films, CT, and MR

Louis A. Gilula, MD Moderator
A. Shoulder Injuries
David A. Rubin, MD
B. Elbow Injuries
O. Clark West, MD
C. Wrist and Hand Injuries
William G. Totty, MD

609
A Trio of Small-Bowel Diseases: Ischemia, Malabsorption, and Obstruction

Francis J. Scholz, MD
Ellen L. Wolf, MD
David H. Frager, MD

610
Practical Tips in US: Liver

A. Sonography of Liver Lesions: Benefits of Contrast Agents and Pulse Inversion Imaging
Stephanie R. Wilson, MD
B. Sonographically Guided Biopsy
Rendon C. Nelson, MD
C. Sonographically Guided Ablation
J. W. Charboneau, MD

611
Perfusion Brain Imaging

Masanori Ichise, MD Moderator
Ronald L. Van Heertum, MD
Michael Devous, Sr, MD

612
CT of the Small Bowel and Colon: Principles, Techniques, and Applications

Richard M. Gore, MD
Elizabeth G. McFarland, MD
Karen M. Horton, MD

613
Special Course in Pediatric Radiology: Current Concepts in Body Imaging at the Millennium—MR Imaging of Extremities: Marrow and Soft Tissues+

A. Musculoskeletal Techniques
Carol E. Barnewolt, MD
B. Bone Marrow: Normal and Variants
Marilyn J. Siegel, MD
C. Soft-Tissue Masses
James S. Meyer, MD
D. Vascular Malformations
Patricia E. Burrows, MD

614
Current Trends in Dialysis Access Placement and Management

A. Hemodialysis Catheters: Go with the Flow
Scott O. Trerotola, MD
B. Screening and Prophylactic Angioplasty in Hemodialysis Grafts
Himanshu Shah, MD
C. Placement and Repositioning of Peritoneal Dialysis Catheters
Scott J. Savader, MD

615
Characterizing, Categorizing, and Managing

A. Calcifications in the Breast
Stephen A. Feig, MD
B. Breast Masses
Laura Liberman, MD

616
Malignant Neoplasia: A Primer of Primaries

Melissa L. Rosado de Christenson, MD
Gregory N. Bender, MD
Mark D. Murphey, MD
Paula J. Woodward, MD
Kelly K. Koeller, MD

618
Gynecologic Malignancies: Imaging Evaluation and Follow-up

A. Cervix
Susan M. Ascher, MD
B. Corpus Uterus
Caroline Reinhold, MD
C. Adnexa
Eric K. Outwater, MD

619
Management of Non-CNS Pediatric Tumors

Paula J. Schomberg, MD
Kevin J. Murray, MD

620
Brachytherapy for Gynecologic Cancer

Beth A. Erickson, MD
Michael T. Gillin, PhD

621
Fundamentals of Flat Panel X-ray Detector Physics

John A. Rowlands, PhD
John Yorkston, PhD

622
Medical Physics Practice Basics

Kenneth N. Vanek, PhD
Robert J. Pizzutiello, Jr, MS

623
Categorical Course in Diagnostic Radiology Physics: Electronic Radiology Practice—Technical and Practical: Electronic Image Infrastructure**

A. Networks
Robert Cooke
B. Compression of Medical Images
Bradley J. Erickson, MD, PhD
C. Archives
Robert Cecil, PhD

624
Specialized Accreditations: A Cost of Doing Business

Sponsored by the Associated Sciences Consortium
Luann J. Culbreth, MEd, RT(R) (SMRT) Moderator
John Kovelski, RT(R) (SMRT)
Karol Handrahan, RT(R) (SMRT)
Sandra Katanick, RN, RVT (SDMS)
Ronald F. Bernardi, BA, RT(R) (AHRA)

625
Categorical Course in Diagnostic Radiology Physics: Physical Aspects of Breast Imaging—Current and Future Considerations***

A. Digital Mammography: Technical Aspects
Martin J. Yaffe, PhD
B. Clinical Aspects
Etta D. Pisano, MD
C. Future Directions for Breast Imaging
Daniel B. Kopans, MD

626
PACS and Radiology Informatics: Practical and Operational Issues in PACS

Paul J. Chang, MD Moderator
Janice C. Honeyman, PhD
Steven C. Horii, MD
Eliot L. Siegel, MD
Charles E. Willis, PhD

627
Negotiating a Managed Care Contract

Fred Gaschen, MBA
David C. Levin, MD
Jeffrey Oxendine, MBA

628
Physics: Imaging in Radiation Therapy

Arthur L. Boyer, PhD Director
A. Use of MR Imaging Data for Treatment Planning
Marc L. Kessler, PhD
B. Subjective Target Volume and Normal Structure Segmentation
Mary M. Austin-Seymour, MD

629
Bone Densitometry in Osteoporosis

Leon Lenchik, MD
Bradford J. Richmond, MD

630
Minicourse: New Developments in Body CT Scanning - 3D CT Angiography and Virtual Imaging

Elliot K. Fishman, MD Co-director
Nestor L. Muller, MD, PhD Co-director
A. Principles and Applications of 3D CT Angiography
Elliot K. Fishman, MD
B. CT Angiography: Imaging the Aorta and Kidneys
Patricia A. Smith, MD
C. Virtual Imaging: Concepts and Applications in the Abdomen
Geoffrey D. Rubin, MD

650
Nonbiopsy Spine Procedures (“How-to” Workshop)

Robert A. Koenigsberg, DO
Eric A. Brandser, MD
Orlando Ortiz, MD, MBA
Michelle S. Barr, MD

651
Fetal Imaging with US and MR Imaging: How We Do It ("How-to" Workshop)

Deborah Levine, MD
Vickie A. Feldstein, MD

652
Freehand Invasive Sonography for the Breast ("Hands-on" Workshop)

Alda F. Cossi, MD
Dianne Georgian-Smith, MD
James J. Roebker, MD
Handel E. Reynolds, MD
Lauren I. McCurdy, MD
Michael P. McNamara, Jr, MD
Gary J. Whitman, MD
Judy S. Blebea, MD
Sally H. Bass, MD
Linda N. Michelson, MD
Alice S. Rim, MD
Paula B. Gordon, MD
Ann T. Rolfs, MD

653
How to Use a PACS Workstation: Basic ("Hands-on" Workshop)

David E. Avrin, MD, PhD
Co-moderator
Janice C. Honeyman, PhD
Co-moderator
Katherine P. Andriole, PhD
Co-moderator
Keith J. Dreyer, MD, PhD
Co-moderator

Integrating the Healthcare Enterprise

691
Healthcare Intranets: How to Develop and Support an Intranet: What Functions it Should have, Successful Approaches

692
The Electronic Medical Record as an Integration Tool: Strategies for Accessing, Coordinating, and Updating the EMR Across a Network

693
Designing Reliable High Performance Networks: Network Design Issues and Approaches—Also Next Generation Internet

Thursday, December 02, 1999 2:30 pm to 4:00 pm

701
Digital Chest Radiography: Techniques and Clinical Applications

Denise R. Aberle, MD
Stuart S. Sagel, MD

702
Categorical Course in Diagnostic Radiology: Body MR*

A. Knee: Menisci
Phoebe A. Kaplan, MD
B. Knee: Ligaments
Clyde A. Helms, MD
C. Knee: Cartilage
Thomas R. McCauley, MD

703
Thoracic Aortic Disease: New Concepts in Diagnosis and Intervention

Richard D. White, MD
Bart L. Dolmatch, MD

704
Imaging of Ligaments, Capsules, and Tendons of the Wrist and Hand

Louis A. Gilula, MD
Coordinator
Marnix T. Van Holsbeeck, MD
David A. Rubin, MD

705
Functional Brain Mapping

Vincent P. Mathews, MD
R. Nick Bryan, MD, PhD
Joseph T. Lurito, MD, PhD
John L. Ulmer, MD

706
Pediatric Ear, Nose, and Throat

A. Pediatric Neck Masses
Larissa T. Bilaniuk, MD
B. Pediatric Sinus, Inflammation
Bernadette L. Koch, MD

707
MR Imaging in Gynecology

A. Benign Disease of the Uterus
Shirley M. McCarthy, MD, PhD
B. Uterine Cancer
Juergen E. Scheidler, MD
C. Ovarian Cancer: Lesion Characterization and Staging
Hedvig Hricak, MD, PhD

708
Imaging Lower-Extremity Trauma with Plain Films, CT, and MR

A. Hip Injuries
Joseph S. Yu, MD
B. Knee Injuries
Lee F. Rogers, MD
C. Foot and Ankle Injuries
Eric A. Brandser, MD

709
Radiologic Evaluation of Pharyngeal and Anorectal Disorders: From One End to the Other

Stephen E. Rubesin, MD
Bronwyn Jones, MD
Frederick M. Kelvin, MD

710
Practical Tips in US: Obstetrics

A. Fetal Anomalies: Skeletal Thorax
Peter W. Callen, MD
B. Fetal Anomalies II: Chromosomal Markers
Beryl R. Benacerraf, MD
C. Fetal Anomalies III: The Heart
Douglas L. Brown, MD

711
Optimal Imaging Modalities for Disorders of the Hepatobiliary Tree, Infection, and Gastrointestinal Bleeding

Darlene Fink-Bennett, MD

712
Helical CT of the Kidneys: New Concepts in Tumor Detection and Differentiation, CT Angiography, Renal Infection, and Stone Detection

Bernard A. Birnbaum, MD
Patricia A. Smith, MD
Stanford M. Goldman, MD

713
Special Course in Pediatric Radiology: Current Concepts in Body Imaging at the Millennium—Imaging of Extremities: Cartilage and Bone+

A. MR Imaging of Musculoskeletal Trauma
Diego Jaramillo, MD
B. MR Imaging of Infectious and Inflammatory Disorders
Michel E. Azouz, MD
C. Helical CT Applications in Musculoskeletal Disorders
Tal Laor, MD

714
Renal and Carotid Disease: Current Trends in Noninvasive Evaluation and Endovascular Therapy

Alan H. Matsumoto, MD
Klaus D. Hagspiel, MD
David F. Kallmes, MD
Klaus D. Mathias, MD

715
Evaluation of the Breast after Surgery

A. Mammography and US in Follow-up of the Breast Cancer Patient
Ellen B. Mendelson, MD
B. MR Imaging in the Postsurgical Breast
Gillian M. Newstead, MD

716
Clinical PACS: Eight Years of Experience in Vienna

Walter F. Hruby, MD

718
PET Scanning in Oncology

A. Head and Neck
R. Edward Coleman, MD
B. Chest
George Segall, MD
C. Abdomen and Pelvis
Peter E. Valk, MD

719
Radiation Therapy in Cervical Cancer

Nina A. Mayr, MD

720
Breast Cancer

A. Radiation Therapy Management of Noninvasive and Early-Stage Invasive Carcinoma of the Breast
Robert R. Kuske, MD
B. Management of Locally Advanced Breast Cancer
Eric A. Strom, MD

721
MR Accreditation Physics

Geof Clarke, PhD
R. Edward Hendrick, PhD
L. K. Hedges, PhD

722
Digital Radiographic Image Quality and System Optimization

Perry Sprawls, Jr, PhD

723
Categorical Course in Diagnostic Radiology Physics: Electronic Radiology Practice—Technical and Practical: Electronic Image Interpretation**

A. Workstation Design
Alan H. Rowberg, MD

B. Workstation Function
Kenneth M. Spicer, MD, PhD

C. Radiologist Workflow
David W. Piraino, MD

724
Multidisciplinary Standards for the New Millennium

Sponsored by the Associated Sciences Consortium
Susan S. Weiss, CNMT (SNM-TS) Moderator
William R. Poller, MD (SNM-TS)
Michael R. Bloyd, RT(R), BSN (ASRT)
Sue M. Smith, RT(R)(CV)(M), FAVIR (AVIR)

725
Categorical Course in Diagnostic Radiology Physics: Physical Aspects of Breast Imaging—Current and Future Considerations***

A. Computer-aided Diagnosis in Breast Imaging
Maryellen L. Giger, PhD

B. Telemammography: Technical Aspects
H. K. Huang, DSc

C. Computer-aided Diagnosis and Telemammography: Clinical Perspective
Edward A. Sickles, MD

726
PACS and Radiology Informatics: Decision Support

Charles E. Kahn, Jr, MD Moderator
Kevin W. McEnery, MD
John Eng, MD

727
New Ways to Organize Radiology Practices: Physician Practice Management Companies, Networks, and Mergers—Are They the Wave of the Future?

Lawrence R. Muroff, MD
Thomas Fortner
Michael L. Sherman, MD

728
Physics: Imaging in Radiation Therapy

Arthur L. Boyer, PhD Director

A. Objective Gross Target Volume and Normal Structure Segmentation
Daniel Fritsch, PhD

B. Imaging in Stereotactic Treatment Planning
Frank Bova, PhD

729
PACS: Its Impact on Facility Design

Bill Rostenberg (AIA-AAH)
Morris A. Stein (AIA-AAH)
Edward V. Staab, MD

730
Minicourse: New Developments in Body CT Scanning - New Developments in Chest CT

Elliot K. Fishman, MD Co-director
Nestor L. Muller, MD, PhD Co-director

A. Advanced Visualization of the Thoracic Aorta
Charles S. White, MD

B. Advanced Visualization of the Pulmonary Vessels
Martine J. Remy-Jardin, MD, PhD

C. Advanced Visualization of the Airways
David P. Naidich, MD

750
MR Imaging of the Abdomen: How We Do It ("How-to" Workshop)

Evan S. Siegelman, MD
Russell N. Low, MD
Thomas K. Helmberger, MD

751
MR Imaging in Sports Medicine ("How-to" Workshop)

David W. Stoller, MD Moderator
J. Bruce Kneeland, MD
Antoni Capdevila, MD

752
Techniques of Freehand Invasive Sonography ("Hands-on" Workshop)

Brian D. Coley, MD
William E. Shiels II, DO
Robert D. Lyon, MD
John David Lane, MD
Neil D. Johnson, MD
H. Theodore Harcke, Jr, MD
Alda F. Cossi, MD
Clark L. Searle, MD
Russell B. Midkiff, MD
Stephen C. O'Connor, MD
Peter G. Chait, MD
James S. Donaldson, MD

753
How to Use a PACS Workstation: Advanced ("Hands-on" Workshop)

David E. Avrin, MD, PhD Co-moderator
Janice C. Honeyman, PhD Co-moderator
Katherine P. Andriole, PhD Co-moderator
Keith J. Dreyer, MD, PhD Co-moderator

Integrating the Healthcare Enterprise

791
Internet Tools and Resources: Content, Tools, Services, Consortia For Health Care Networks

792
Relationship Building: Issues Facing PCP's Patients in a Network, and How Info Systems Can Support These Needs

793
Net-based Technologies in Health Care: A Focus on Java, CORBA, DCOM, XML

Friday, December 03, 1999
8:30 am to 10:00 am

801
Lung Cancer: Role of Diagnostic Imaging

Edward F. Patz, Jr, MD
Ann N. Leung, MD

802
Categorical Course in Diagnostic Radiology: Body MR*

A. Shoulder: Techniques and Anatomy
Mini N. Pathria, MD

B. Shoulder: Rotator Cuff
Lynne S. Steinbach, MD

C. Shoulder: Labrum and Instability
William E. Palmer, MD

803
Perfusion and Function in Nuclear Cardiology: Explanation of Techniques and How to Use Them

E. Gordon DePuey, MD
Jack A. Ziffer, MD, PhD
Raymond Taillefer, MD

804
A Systematic Approach to Imaging of Musculoskeletal Tumors

Mark D. Murphey, MD
Murali Sundaram, MD

805
New MR Techniques for Neurologic Disease

Allen D. Elster, MD
John L. Ulmer, MD
A. Gregory Sorensen, MD

806
Skull Base and Craniovertebral Junction: Normal Anatomy, Congenital and Acquired Lesions, including Trauma

Wendy R.K. Smoker, MD

807
Classic Signs in Uroradiology

Raymond B. Dyer, MD
Christopher M. McManus, MD

808
Pediatric Emergencies of the Chest, Abdomen, and Pelvis

A. Pediatric Airway and Chest Emergencies
Janet L. Strife, MD

B. Emergency Abdominal Conditions in Children
Carlo Buonomo, MD

C. Emergency Scrotal and Gynecologic Conditions in Children
Brian D. Coley, MD

809
Abdominal MR Imaging: Myth versus Reality

Herbert Y. Kressel, MD
Richard C. Semelka, MD
Bernd K. Hamm III, MD

810
Practical Tips in US: Abdomen

A. The Peritoneal Space
Anthony E. Hanbidge, MB

B. US in Appendicitis
Julien B. Puylaert, MD, PhD

C. Focused Abdominal Sonography for Trauma (FAST) by Radiologists
John P. McGahan, MD

811
Clinical PET Imaging

R. Edward Coleman, MD Co-moderator
Richard L. Wahl, MD Co-moderator
R. Edward Coleman, MD
Richard L. Wahl, MD

812
Cutting-Edge Technologies in CT Scanning: Multidetector Helical CT and Virtual Imaging

Rendon C. Nelson, MD
Christopher F. Beaulieu, MD, PhD

813
Special Course in Pediatric Radiology: Current Concepts in Body Imaging at the Millennium—Interventional Radiology: Pediatric Considerations+

A. Chest Interventions
James S. Donaldson, MD

B. Abdominal Drainage and Biopsy Interventions
Fredric A. Hoffer, MD

C. Retroperitoneal Interventions
Douglas C. Redd, MD

814
Abdominal Interventions: New Insights into Routine and Difficult Case Management

Peter R. Mueller, MD
Eric vanSonnenberg, MD

815
The Assessment of Screening Mammography Programs

A. The Mammography Audit
Michael N. Linver, MD

B. Cost-Effectiveness Analysis of Mammographic Screening
Karen K. Lindfors, MD

818
Primary Bone Tumor and Limb-sparing Surgery: Imaging Evaluation and Follow-up

A. Preoperative Evaluation
B. J. Manaster, MD, PhD

B. Postoperative Appearance after Limb Salvage Surgery
Kevin W. McEnery, MD

819
Management of Soft-Tissue Sarcoma

Beatriz E. Amendola, MD

820
Prostate Brachytherapy

Peter D. Grimm, DO

821
Radiation Shielding

Douglas J. Simpkin, PhD

822
Basic MR Imaging QC

Joel P. Felmlee, PhD

823
Categorical Course in Diagnostic Radiology Physics: Electronic Radiology Practice—Technical and Practical: Electronic Image Distribution**

A. Hospital and Clinic Strategies
Michael M. Abiri, MD

B. Remote Site Strategies
Keith J. Dreyer, MD, PhD
Amit Mehta, MD

C. Legal Issues
Charles K. Showalter, MS

824
Marketing Radiology: Getting the Message out

Sponsored by the Associated Sciences Consortium
Ronald F. Bernardi, BA, RT(R) (AHRA) Moderator
Cherrill Farnsworth (AHRA)
Michael R. Favreau (AHRA)

825
Categorical Course in Diagnostic Radiology Physics: Physical Aspects of Breast Imaging—Current and Future Considerations***

A. Role of MR Imaging in Breast Imaging
Gillian M. Newstead, MD

B. Role of US in Breast Imaging
Ellen B. Mendelson, MD

C. Breast Imaging Based on Viscoelastic Properties
Donald B. Plewes, PhD

826
PACS and Radiology Informatics: Challenges and Strategies for Enterprise Radiology Informatics

Paul J. Chang, MD Moderator
John A. Carrino, MD
John Eng, MD
Ramin Khorasani, MD

827
How to Measure Productivity in Your Radiology Department

Carl E. Ravin, MD
Michael T. Nelson, MD
Douglas M. Cassel, MD

828
Physics: Imaging in Radiation Therapy

Arthur L. Boyer, PhD Director

A. Film Systems for Radiation Therapy Imaging
Arthur G. Haus

B. Three-dimensional Dosimetry with Gels and MR Imaging
Lars E. Olsson, PhD

829
Strategic Thinking in Radiology

Ronald B. Schilling, PhD
Edward V. Staab, MD

830
Minicourse: New Developments in Body CT Scanning - High-Resolution CT of the Chest

Elliot K. Fishman, MD Co-director
Nestor L. Muller, MD, PhD Co-director

A. Interstitial Lung Disease
W. Richard Webb, MD

B. Obstructive Lung Disease
Nestor L. Muller, MD, PhD

C. Acute Lung Disease
Georgeann McGuinness, MD

850
Radiologic Evaluation of the Solitary Pulmonary Nodule ("How-to" Workshop)

Paul L. Molina, MD
Phillip M. Boiselle, MD
John E. Connolly, Jr, MD

851
FDA Regulation of Medical Devices: Practical Approaches to Everyday Problems ("How-to" Workshop)

John J. Smith, MD, JD
Susan Alpert, MD, PhD
Bruce Beauchemin
Anne C. Roberts, MD

852
Techniques of Invasive Sonography ("Hands-on" Workshop)

William E. Shiels II, DO
Mark J. Hogan, MD
Robert D. Lyon, MD
John David Lane, MD
H. Theodore Harcke, Jr, MD
Alda F. Cossi, MD
Dianne Georgian-Smith, MD
Clark L. Searle, MD
Russell B. Midkiff, MD
Stephen C. O'Connor, MD
Peter G. Chait, MD
James W. Murakami, MD

853
How to Use a PACS Workstation: Advanced ("Hands-on" Workshop)

David E. Avrin, MD, PhD Co-moderator
Janice C. Honeyman, PhD Co-moderator
Katherine P. Andriole, PhD Co-moderator
Keith J. Dreyer, MD, PhD Co-moderator

Integrating the Healthcare Enterprise

891
Standards, Architectures, Organization Initiatives: A Standards Road Map, How the Efforts Interact

892
Clinical Guidelines: Roles for Clinical Guidelines in Workstation Design, Referral Management, and Workflow Optimization

893
Strategic Integration of IT: Selecting Priorities, Developing a Plan, Engaging the Participants, Managing the Process

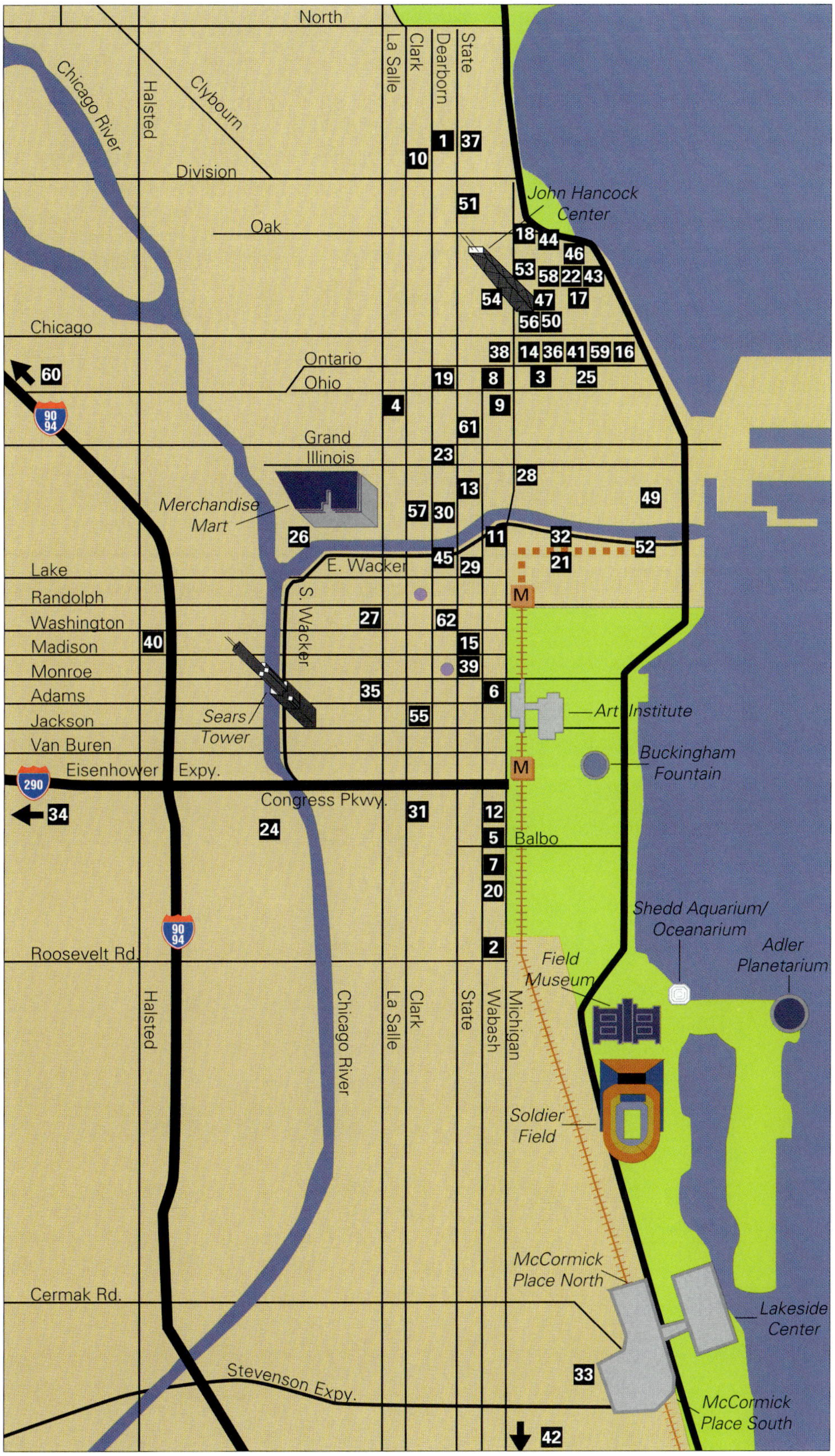

(MAP NOT TO SCALE)

*Special Notes: Rates do not include 14.9% (subject to change) Chicago hotel tax.

A service fee has been included in your room rate to defray the cost of housing, registration, and transportation services.

Hotel No. 34 is at Ashland and Harrison;

Hotel No. 60 is in the suburb of Rosemont.

Shuttle bus service will be provided as indicated in hotel profile.

● = Downtown CTA Stations
········ = CTA Rapid Transit line from O'Hare
M = Metra Electric

The information provided below is based on single occupancy. Type of bed (king, double, twin) may be requested but cannot be confirmed until check-in. For triple and quad rate information please contact I.T.S. at (847) 940-2155.

A first and last night room deposit totaling $300 is required when a hotel is requested.

Please note: To uphold the professional and educational standards of the RSNA Meeting, children under 16 years of age are not permitted in the exhibit halls or sessions. Child care is available. See the back cover of this brochure for details. Your hotel may also provide child care services. Please check the Hotel Profile for the child care icon or call your hotel to determine if child care services are available.

HOTEL	SINGLE	DOUBLE	SUITE	AMENITIES
1 Ambassador West	$135	$155	$325+	
2 Best Western Grant Park Hotel	$115	$115	$169+	
3 Best Western Inn of Chicago	$126	$136	$210+	
4 Best Western River North Hotel	$107	$107	$209+	
5 Blackstone	$99	$109	$159+	
6 Chicago Athletic Association**	$143	$154	$187+	
7 Hilton and Towers — Chicago	$175	$197	$473+	
Hilton Towers	$226	$247		
8 Chicago's Lenox Suites Hotel (AS)				
Standard Studio	$115	$125	$155+	
Deluxe Double/Double		$150		
9 Chicago Marriott Downtown	$152	$152	$545+	
10 Claridge Hotel	$130	$155	$185+	
11 Clarion Executive Plaza Hotel	$139	$157	$275+	
12 Congress Plaza Hotel	$105	$115	$350+	
13 Courtyard By Marriott/Chicago Downtown	$146	$146	$209	
14 Crowne Plaza Allerton	$195	$220	$350	
Deluxe	$205	$230		
15 Crowne Plaza Silversmith	$195	$220	$289	
16 Days Inn Lake Shore Drive	$116	$126	$299+	
17 Doubletree Guest Suites (AS)	$196	$218		
18 Drake Hotel	$213	$234	$350+	
19 Embassy Suites Hotel (AS)	$200	$220		
20 Essex Inn	$113	$123	$150+	

** *Charges an 18% non-member surcharge instead of the 14.9% city hotel tax.*

Legend

= On Premises Parking
= On-site Business Center
= Laundry/Valet Service
= Lounge
= Handicap Accessible
= Dataport
= Room Service
= Lounge with Music
= No Smoking Policy Rooms/Floors
= Fitness Room
= 24-Hour Room Service
= Shuttle Bus
= Child Care
= Pool
= Restaurant/Cafe
= Metra Service

AS = All Suites

HOTEL	SINGLE	DOUBLE	SUITE	AMENITIES
21 Fairmont Hotel	$201	$224	$411+	
22 Four Seasons Hotel	$322	$343		
Executive Suites	$358	$379		
23 Hampton Inn & Suites	$149	$159		
Studio Suites	$169	$179	$209+	
24 Holiday Inn and Suites	$135	$155	$199	
25 Holiday Inn Chicago City Centre Hotel	$144	$157	$350	
26 Holiday Inn Mart Plaza	$135	$148		
27 Hotel Allegro Chicago	$177	$177	$375	
28 Hotel Inter-Continental Chicago				
Superior Rooms North Tower	$159	$179	$475+	
Deluxe Rooms South Tower	$214	$234		
29 Hotel Monaco	$205	$205	$320	
30 House of Blues	$200	$200	$280+	
31 Hyatt on Printers Row	$168	$193	$550+	
32 Hyatt Regency Chicago	$166	$166	$565+	
Regency Club	$201	$236		
33 Hyatt Regency McCormick Place	$187	$204	$395+	
34 Hyatt at University Village	$147	$158	$325+	
35 Midland Hotel	$176	$176	$450	
Executive Level	$216	$216		
36 Motel 6 Chicago	$101	$101		
37 Omni Ambassador East	$195	$215	$265+	
38 Omni Chicago Hotel (AS)	$214	$234	$385+	
39 Palmer House Hilton	$168	$188		
Palmer House Hilton Towers	$213	$233	$465+	

Housing changes, cancellations, and early departures.

Prior to October 29, 1999 mail or fax arrival/departure date changes and room cancellations for full deposit refunds to I.T.S./RSNA 1999.

After November 8, 1999 direct all arrival/departure date changes and room cancellations to the hotel.

Changes to reservations

After October 29, 1999 changes to reservations are subject to availability and rate.

Changes made after October 29, 1999 and/or up to seven days prior to date of arrival that result in a reduction of total room nights stayed will incur a $50 fee by the hotel.

Changes in arrival and departure dates less than one week prior to arrival that result in a reduction of nights stayed may be considered cancellations by the hotel and may result in forfeiture of partial or all deposits paid.

Failure to check-in at the hotel on your scheduled arrival day will result in forfeiture of your reservations and hotel deposit. The hotel will accommodate you on a space available basis.

Early departure will result in the hotel's retaining the fee for one night's room plus tax or the last night room deposit of $150, whichever is less.

Room cancellations

Reservations cancelled after October 29, 1999, and/or up to seven days prior to date of arrival will incur a $50 cancellation fee.

Cancellations received less than seven days prior to date of arrival will result in forfeiture of full $300 deposit.

When cancelling your room reservation directly with the hotel, please note the date and time of your call, with whom you spoke, and make sure to obtain a cancellation number.

HOTEL	SINGLE	DOUBLE	SUITE	AMENITIES
40 Quality Inn Chicago Downtown	$103	$111	$135+	
41 Radisson Hotel and Suites Chicago	$151	$167	$202+	
42 Ramada Inn Lake Shore	$97	$97	$150	
43 Raphael Chicago	$199	$199		
44 Regal Knickerbocker Hotel	$192	$202	$285	
45 Renaissance Chicago Hotel	$207	$227	$390+	
Renaissance Club Level	$257	$277		
46 Residence Inn by Marriott (AS)	$151	$151	$208+	
47 Ritz-Carlton Chicago	$322	$343		
Executive Suite	$358	$379		
49 Sheraton Chicago Hotel	$166	$166		
Club	$208	$228		
Towers	$226	$246		
50 Summerfield Suites Hotel Chicago (AS)				
Studio	$205	$205		
Parlor	$215	$215		
One Bedroom	$225	$225		
51 Sutton Place Hotel	$220	$245		
52 Swissótel Chicago	$176	$187	$395+	
53 Talbott Hotel	$160	$180	$275+	
54 Tremont Hotel	$215	$215		
55 Union League Club**	$163	$163		
56 Westin Michigan Ave	$175	$195		
Towers	$205	$225		
57 Westin River North Chicago	$207	$227	$490+	
Skyline	$227			
58 Whitehall Hotel	$219	$219	$571+	
59 Wyndham Hotel and Suites	$205	$225		
60 Holiday Inn O'Hare (transportation is not provided)	$135	$135		
61 Homewood Suites (AS)	$169	$169		
62 Hotel Burnham	$190	$190		

*** Charges an 18% non-member surcharge instead of the 14.9% city hotel tax.*

Legend

P = On Premises Parking
= Handicap Accessible
= No Smoking Policy Rooms/Floors
= Child Care
AS = All Suites
= On-site Business Center
= Dataport
= Fitness Room
= Pool
= Laundry/Valet Service
= Room Service
= 24-Hour Room Service
= Restaurant/Cafe
= Lounge
= Lounge with Music
= Shuttle Bus
= Metra Service

IMPORTANT!

Please read this information before completing the registration form.

ADVANCE REGISTRATION & HOUSING DEADLINES:

Non-North American

October 1, 1999

North American

October 29, 1999

HOW TO REGISTER

By telephone

(If no verification is required)

- Completed registration form
- Air travel information
- Registration fee and first and last night room deposit
- Credit card number and expiration date (AMEX, Diners, Discover, MasterCard, VISA)
- **Call I.T.S./RSNA 1999 at (800) 650-7018**
- **Outside U.S. and Canada, call (847) 940-2155**
- **Hours: 8:00am–5:30pm CST**

By fax

(Payment must be made by credit card)

- Completed registration form
- Verification letter or business card (if applicable)
- Registration fee and first and last night room deposit
- Credit card number and expiration date
- **Fax I.T.S./RSNA 1999 at (800)521-6017**
- **Outside U.S. and Canada, fax (847) 940-2386**

By Internet

Register online at www.rsna.org

(for RSNA/AAPM members and non-member physicians)

- Credit card number and expiration date must be provided

By mail

(Include the following)

- Completed registration form
- Verification letter or business card (if applicable)
- Registration fee and first and last night room deposit
- Check or money order made payable to RSNA 1999 in U.S. funds and drawn on a U.S. bank, or
- Credit card number and expiration date, or
- Wire transfer in U.S. funds (Call I.T.S. (847) 940-2155 for instructions)

Please Note: Registration will not be processed without payment

A confirmation will be sent by email, fax, or mail for each registration processed and every time a change is made. Allow seven days for receipt of confirmation and if not received please contact I.T.S./RSNA 1999

- (800) 650-7018 (U.S.)
- (847) 940-2155 (Outside U.S. & Canada)
- Email: RSNA@ITVLSVC.com
- Fax: (800) 521-6017 (U.S.)
- Fax: (847) 940-2386 (Outside U.S. & Canada)

SPECIAL REGISTRATION / HOUSING NOTES

If, at RSNA 1999, you need aid or services as identified under the Americans With Disabilities Act, call RSNA (630) 571-7846 before October 29, 1999.

ADVANCE REGISTRATION AND HOUSING (FORM 1)

RSNA

Advance Registration Deadline:

Non-North American registrations must be received by October 1, 1999

North American registrations must be received by October 29, 1999

FOR RSNA OFFICE USE	
CO#	Deposit

Please check one: ☐ Attending RSNA only ☐ Attending RSNA & IHE ☐ Attending IHE only

Name / address information (Place peel-off address label over areas 1, 2, & 3 if all information is correct.)

PLACE LABEL IN THIS AREA

1 ______ LAST NAME/FAMILY NAME

______ FIRST NAME/GIVEN NAME DEGREE TITLE

2 ______ ADDRESS TO WHICH MATERIALS SHOULD BE SENT

Address is: ☐ Home ☐ Office

______ CITY / STATE / ZIP / COUNTRY

( ) ______ PHONE (COUNTRY & CITY CODE IF APPLICABLE)

( ) ______ FAX (COUNTRY & CITY CODE IF APPLICABLE)

3 ______ NAME OF INSTITUTION / OFFICE / HOSPITAL

______ EMAIL ADDRESS

4 ______ NAME AS IT SHOULD APPEAR ON BADGE IF DIFFERENT THAN ABOVE

5 **Classification Code** ______ 6 **Subspecialty Code** ______
(IMPORTANT! WRITE ONE NUMBER AND LETTER IN EACH SPACE. SEE LISTINGS IN INSTRUCTIONS)

7 Classification Codes 22, 23, 24, 30, or 31 must attach a business card or verification letter (25 and 26 must attach both), or your registration will not be processed.

☐ Check box if you are a contributor to the R&E Fund

☐ Check box if you are a *Radiology* subscriber

☐ Check box if this is your first RSNA Meeting

☐ Boxed Lunch for Associated Sciences $11.50

Accompanying spouse/family member(s) ______
SPOUSE/FAMILY MEMBER WILL RECEIVE A COMPLIMENTARY BADGE. CHILDREN UNDER THE AGE OF 16 WILL NOT BE ADMITTED TO THE RSNA ANNUAL MEETING.

Badge classification is subject to RSNA approval.

Hotel reservation

8 I do not require a hotel reservation because I am: ☐ staying at a local residence ☐ sharing a room reserved by ______

To contact me, I have reservations at (hotel) ______
THIS INFORMATION IS IMPORTANT FOR ENTRY IN THE REGISTRATION LOCATOR/MESSAGE CENTER SYSTEM.

9 ______ 1ST CHOICE HOTEL # & NAME ______ 2ND CHOICE HOTEL # & NAME ______ 3RD CHOICE HOTEL # & NAME

$______ ROOM RATE DESIRED ☐ single (1 BED) ☐ double (2 PERSONS/1 BED) ☐ twin (2 PERSONS/2 BEDS) ☐ suite ☐ smoking ☐ non-smoking

10 Person(s) Sharing My Room ______ (OTHER THAN SPOUSE/FAMILY WRITTEN IN ABOVE)

11 Arrival Day/Date ______ Departure Day/Date ______

12 Hotel choice based primarily on: ☐ rate ☐ location ☐ a particular hotel

☐ other consideration ______

Please Note: Hotel rooms become very limited after August 1. Please check one of the boxes below:

☐ **If no rooms are available in the downtown hotels, please do not assign me a room in a suburban or airport hotel. I will try to book a room on my own.**

☐ **If no rooms are available in the downtown hotels, I am willing to be assigned a suburban or airport hotel.**

Room cancellations and early departures

Reservations cancelled after October 29, 1999 and / or up to seven days prior to date of arrival will incur a $50 cancellation fee.
Cancellations received less than seven days prior to date of arrival will result in forfeiture of full $300 deposit.
Early departure will result in the hotel's retaining the fee for one night's room plus tax or the last night room deposit of $150, whichever is less.

☐ ♿ **Please check here if under the Americans with Disabilities Act you may require special accommodations or services in order to attend. You will be contacted by RSNA.**

Payment information *(for all registrants)*

Registration fee (see page 34) $______

Hotel reservation deposit enclosed ($300 deposit for first and last night must accompany this form.) $ 300.00

Check # ______
(PAYABLE TO RSNA 1999)

Total Payment Enclosed (U.S. Funds Only) $______

Credit card information

☐ American Express
☐ Diners Club
☐ Discover
☐ MasterCard
☐ VISA

______ CARD NUMBER

______ NAME AS IT APPEARS ON CARD

______ SIGNATURE (REQUIRED) ______ / ______ EXPIRES (MONTH/YEAR)

If registering by mail, send your completed form to:

RSNA
108 Wilmot Road, Suite 400
Deerfield, IL 60015-0825, USA

Telephone
1(800) 650-7018 (U.S.)
1(847) 940-2155 (Outside U.S. & Canada)

Fax
1(800) 521-6017 (U.S.)
1(847) 940-2386 (Outside U.S. & Canada)

Note: *Requests for courses and tutorials will not be accepted by telephone. If you have faxed your course or tutorial requests,* ***do not*** *mail this form.*

Email
rsna@itvlsvc.com

COURSE ENROLLMENT (FORM 2)

RSNA

Advance Registration Deadline:

Non-North American registrations must be received by October 1, 1999

North American registrations must be received by October 29, 1999

FOR RSNA OFFICE USE	
CO#	Deposit

Important: You MUST be registered for the RSNA Annual Meeting in order to register for courses. You may mail or FAX this form. We are sorry, but course enrollment cannot be handled by telephone. Follow these steps to register for courses:

If you have previously registered for RSNA 1999:

- Complete your name and Registration I.D. # as it appears in the upper right hand section of your RSNA 1999 confirmation. Mail or FAX this form.

If you have not registered for RSNA 1999:

Or

- And plan to register by phone, ask for your Registration I.D. #. Fill in your name, city and state, and Registration I.D. #. Mail or FAX this form.
- Mail or FAX your registration form and course enrollment form together. Your Registration I.D. # will be assigned upon receipt of your registration.

Please check one: ☐ Attending RSNA only ☐ Attending RSNA & IHE ☐ Attending IHE only

Please complete the following, type or print (RSNA Members–do not use your address label on this form):

LAST NAME/FAMILY NAME FIRST NAME/GIVEN NAME DEGREE

IF ALREADY REGISTERED, YOUR REGISTRATION I.D.#

ADDRESS

( ) PHONE (COUNTRY & CITY CODE IF APPLICABLE)

CITY / STATE / ZIP

( ) FAX (COUNTRY & CITY CODE IF APPLICABLE)

COUNTRY

EMAIL

Refresher Course, Workshop, and IHE Enrollment (1 ½ Hours Category 1 Credit)

After reviewing the Refresher Course Plan of Presentation on pages 14-24, complete the numbers on this form to indicate your choices. Each course has a three digit number. The first digit is printed on the form; please fill in the remaining two digits.

Time Period	*1st Choice*	*2nd Choice*	*3rd Choice*	*Time Period*	*1st Choice*	*2nd Choice*	*3rd Choice*
Sunday, November 28, 1:30 pm	1 __ __	1 __ __	1 __ __	Wednesday, December 1, 8:30 am	5 __ __	5 __ __	5 __ __
Monday, November 29, 8:30 am	2 __ __	2 __ __	2 __ __	Thursday, December 2, 8:30 am	6 __ __	6 __ __	6 __ __
Monday, November 29, 4:00 pm	3 __ __	3 __ __	3 __ __	Thursday, December 2, 2:30 pm	7 __ __	7 __ __	7 __ __
Tuesday, November 30, 8:30 am	4 __ __	4 __ __	4 __ __	Friday, December 3, 8:30 am	8 __ __	8 __ __	8 __ __

*info*RAD Course Enrollment (Category 1 Credit)

After reviewing the *info*RAD Plan of Presentation on pages 10-11, complete the numbers on this form to indicate your choices. Each course has a three digit number. The first digit is printed on the form; please fill in the remaining two digits. If your *info*RAD choice runs concurrently with a refresher course, and both are available, check the box to indicate your preference—*info*RAD course or refresher course.

	1st Choice	*2nd Choice*	*3rd Choice*	*Course Preference (check one box only)*
The Internet and Its Medical Information/ Education Resources	0 __ __	0 __ __	0 __ __	☐ *info*RAD Course ☐ Refresher Course
RSNA Research and Education Resources	0 __ __	0 __ __	0 __ __	
Hands-On Workshop: Radiology and Clinical Information Integration	0 __ __	0 __ __	0 __ __	

*info*RAD Guided Tour Selection

1st Choice	*2nd Choice*	*3rd Choice*
0 __ __	0 __ __	0 __ __

*info*RAD Hands-on Computer Workshops: Basic Training for Radiologists

After reviewing the Workshops on page 12, complete the numbers on this form to indicate your choices.

B __ __ __	B __ __ __	B __ __ __	B __ __ __
B __ __ __	B __ __ __	B __ __ __	B __ __ __

If registering by mail, send your completed form to:

RSNA
108 Wilmot Road, Suite 400
Deerfield, IL 60015-0825, USA

Telephone
1(800) 650-7018 (U.S.)
1(847) 940-2155 (Outside U.S. & Canada)

Fax
1(800) 521-6017 (U.S.)
1(847) 940-2386 (Outside U.S. & Canada)

Note: *Requests for courses and tutorials will not be accepted by telephone. If you have faxed your course or tutorial requests,* ***do not*** *mail this form.*

Email
rsna@itvlsvc.com

Follow these numbered instructions carefully to complete the Advance Registration & Housing Form

(1-4) Complete the appropriate information

(5) Classification Code Section

Select your classification code from the following categories and the appropriate letter code (23a, 24b, etc.), which describes your primary occupation.

Physicians – no verification letter required

11 RSNA Member (No Fee)
- **a** radiologist
- **b** physicist
- **c** dentist
- **d** veterinarian
- **e** computer scientist
- **f** electrical engineer

12 RSNA Member-In-Training (No Fee)

13 Non-Member Refresher Course Instructor, Paper Presenter, Scientific or Electronic Education (*info*RAD) Exhibitor (No Fee)

14 Non-Member Radiologist ($390 Fee)

15 Non-Member Resident/Trainee ($100 Fee)

16 Other Physician ($390 Fee)

17 RSNA Medical Student Member

Medical Physicists

21 AAPM Member (No Fee)

22 Non-Member Physicist ($390 Fee – *letter of verification or business card required*)

Healthcare Professional – *Employed in a hospital/medical care/university or research facility/ corporate healthcare provider*

23 Radiology Support Personnel or other Hospital Staff ($100 Fee – *letter of verification or business card required*)
- **a** technologist
- **b** engineer
- **c** radiology business manager
- **d** radiology department administrator
- **e** nurse
- **f** radiology educator
- **g** computer scientist
- **h** architect
- **i** government employee
- **j** network manager
- **k** systems operator
- **l** telemedicine/ communications specialist
- **m** facility manager

24 Hospital Executive (Individuals directly employed by a healthcare institution, network, or corporate healthcare provider; $390 Fee – *letter of verification or business card required*)
- **a** hospital administrator
- **b** purchasing agent
- **c** corporate purchasing executive
- **d** CEO
- **e** CFO
- **f** CIO
- **g** Legal (in-house counsel)

Research & Development – *Those registering under categories 25 and 26 must be R&D personnel of a company currently involved in radiologic research and development.*

25 Commercial research and development personnel, employee of RSNA 1999 technical exhibitor ($390 Fee – *letter of verification and business card required*).

26 Physicist or other personnel involved in commercial research and development directly related to the field of radiology, and employee of any non-exhibiting company at RSNA 1999 ($390 Fee – *letter of verification and business card required*)

Medical Service Organization – *Qualified individuals employed in a non-hospital based environment providing radiology support services. This includes departmental management; purchasing; staffing; imaging and therapy services.*

30 MSO employee ($390 Fee – *letter of verification or business card required*)

Healthcare Consultant – *Currently under contract to radiologic health care provider including hospitals, free-standing clinics, corporate healthcare providers, or networks*

31 Consultant ($390 Fee – *letter of verification from healthcare provider required*)
- **a** computer analyst
- **b** investment broker or banker
- **c** purchasing consultant
- **d** attorney
- **e** financial analyst
- **f** architectural designer

Badge classification is subject to RSNA approval.

LETTERS OF VERIFICATION

For categories requiring a letter of verification or business card (22, 23, 24, 25, 26, 30, or 31):

- The letter of verification must be on letterhead from the employer and state the objective of attending the RSNA Annual Meeting.
- The business card must include the registrant's name, title, employer name, complete address, and telephone number.
- Those registrations requiring verification will not be processed unless a letter or business card is received with the registration form.

(6) Subspecialty Code Section

If your classification code is 11, 12, 13, 14, 21, or 22, select one subspecialty code from the following.

Breast/Mammography	54
Cardiovascular	45
Chest	55
Computed Tomography (Body Imaging)	53
Diagnostic Radiology	41
Gastrointestinal	57
Genitourinary	58
Head and Neck	50
Health Policy & Practice	59
Interventional	51
Magnetic Resonance	52
Musculoskeletal	56
Neuroradiology	46
Nuclear Medicine	42
Pediatric Radiology	44
Physics	47
Radiation Oncology	49
Radiobiology	48
Ultrasound	43

(7) Follow Instructions on Form

HOTEL RESERVATIONS

(8-12) Follow instructions on form and complete the Hotel Reservation section to request your housing through the RSNA. Hotel reservations through the RSNA 1999 registration system are only available to registered RSNA attendees. The hotels listed on pages 26–28 have reserved blocks of rooms for RSNA registrants at reduced rates. Hotels will not accept direct reservations for rooms until after November 9, when remaining rooms (if any) from the RSNA block will be released back to the hotel. RSNA hotel rates are subject to change for reservations made directly with the hotel.

If your hotel selections are no longer available, we will be able to serve you better if you indicate which is the most important...the cost of your room, the location of your hotel, being in one particular hotel, or other considerations as noted on the form.

Please remember hotel reservations are made on a first-come, first-served basis. Hotels fill up quickly, so the sooner you register, the better your chance of booking the hotel of your choice.

Professional attendees may not request housing through technical exhibiting companies.

PROFESSIONAL REGISTRANTS, REGISTER PROMPTLY

Requests are processed on a first-come, first-served basis. Registration materials (including badges) will be mailed the second week of November.

STUDENTS

Students (technical, medical, and nursing) register at Onsite Registration. No fee is required for students with proper identification.

TO REGISTER AFTER THE ADVANCE REGISTRATION DEADLINES

Advance registration forms will be accepted at I.T.S./RSNA through October 29. After this date, individuals will be required to register onsite.

Registration forms will be available onsite for registrants to complete. Identification and verification will be required at the credentials desk along with the completed registration form and will follow the same rules as in the advance process.

Non-physician healthcare professionals who are employed in a hospital/medical care/university/research facility or by a corporate healthcare provider are required to present a letter of verification or business card. The letter of verification should be on letterhead from the employer and state the objective in attending the RSNA Annual Meeting. The business card should include the registrant's name and title, employer's name, complete address, and telephone number.

Additional credentials may be required from time to time in order to maintain the quality of attendance verification.

If you are unable to register in advance, on-site registration takes place at McCormick Place, South Building, beginning Saturday, November 27, noon to 6:00 pm. Sunday–Thursday, November 28–December 2, 7:00 am to 6:00 pm. Friday, December 3, registration hours are 7:00 am to 1:00 pm (shortest registration lines are on Saturday).

Non-North American registrations received after October 1 may pick up advance registration materials at McCormick Place, Registration, Desk A, beginning Saturday, November 27.

REGISTRATION CANCELLATION

Registration cancellations must be in writing to I.T.S./RSNA 1999. A $25.00 fee will be charged for cancellations received by October 29. After that date, there are no registration refunds.

HOUSING CHANGE, CANCELLATION, AND EARLY DEPARTURES

Prior to October 29, 1999 mail or fax all arrival/departure date changes, and room cancellations for full deposit refunds to I.T.S./RSNA 1999.

After November 8, 1999 direct all arrival/departure date changes, and room cancellations to the hotel.

CHANGES TO RESERVATIONS

After October 29, 1999 changes to reservations are subject to availability and rate.

Changes made after October 29, 1999 and/or up to seven days prior to date of arrival that result in a reduction of total room nights stayed will incur a $50 fee by the hotel.

Changes in arrival and departure dates less than one week prior to arrival that result in a reduction of nights stayed, may be considered cancellations by the hotel and may result in forfeiture of partial or all deposits paid.

Failure to check-in at the hotel on your scheduled arrival day will result in forfeiture of your reservations and hotel deposit. The hotel will accommodate you on a space available basis.

Early departure will result in the hotel's retaining the fee for one night's room plus tax or the last night room deposit of $150, whichever is less.

ROOM CANCELLATIONS

Reservations cancelled after October 29, 1999 and/or up to seven days prior to date of arrival will incur a $50 cancellation fee.

Cancellations received less than seven days prior to date of arrival will result in forfeiture of full $300 deposit.

When cancelling your room reservation directly with the hotel, please note the date and time of your call, with whom you spoke, and make sure to obtain a cancellation number.

REGISTRATION FEES AT-A-GLANCE

RSNA Member	No Fee
RSNA Member-In-Training	No Fee
Non-Member Refresher Course Instructor, Paper Presenter, Scientific or Electronic Education (*info*RAD) Exhibitor	No Fee
Non-Member Radiologist	$390.00
Non-Member Resident/Trainee	$100.00
Other Physician	$390.00
RSNA Medical Student Member	No Fee
AAPM Member	No Fee
Non-Member Physicist*	$390.00
Radiology Support Personnel*	$100.00
Hospital Executive*	$390.00
Commercial Research and Development Personnel* *(Physicist or other personnel involved in commercial research and development directly related to the field of radiology and employee of any non-exhibiting company at RSNA 1999)*	$390.00
Commercial Research & Development Personnel* *(non-exhibitor at RSNA 1999)*	$390.00
Medical Service Organizations*	$390.00
Healthcare Consultant*	$390.00

Letter of verification or business card required.

Air Fare Discounts

RSNA now offers its attendees two ways to save on air fare. Both United Airlines and Delta Air Lines offer discounts from 5% – 10% or take advantage of the area pricing / zone fares.

Area Pricing / Zone Fares – No Saturday night stay over required, two day minimum stay, air fare does not fluctuate, and is fully refundable (less service fee). Additional restrictions may apply.

You can call I.T.S. (International Travel Service) at 1-800-621-1083 and use your credit card to purchase your discounted tickets, which will then be mailed directly to you.

If you prefer to use your personal travel agent or call the airlines directly, simply refer to the RSNA ID Numbers: United Airlines 544XE or Delta Air Lines 121523A.

UNITED AIRLINES

1-800-521-4041
Monday–Sunday 7:00 a.m.–12:00 Midnight EST
ID Number: **544XE**

UNITED AIRLINES AREA PRICING

Cost for a round trip coach class ticket to Chicago, Illinois (Area 4)

Area 1	DC / MA / MD / PA / VA	$402.00
Area 2	CT / DE / ME / NH / NJ / NY / RI / VT / WV / CANADA - ON	$402.00
Area 3	AL / FL / GA / MS / NC / SC / TN/ SAN JUAN PR	$410.00
Area 4	IA / IL / IN / KS / KY / MI / MN / MO / NE / OH / WI	$352.00
Area 5	AR/ LA/ NM/ OK/ TX	$372.00
Area 6	CO/ MT/ ND/ SD/ UT/ WY	$410.00
Area 7	ID / OR / WA / CANADA - AB / BC	$478.00
Area 8	AZ / CA / NV	$457.00
Area 9	AK	$504.00

DELTA

1-800-241-6760
Monday - Friday 7:30 a.m.–11:00 p.m. EST
Weekends 8:30 a.m.–11:00 p.m. EST
ID Number: **121523A**

DELTA AIR LINES ZONE FARES

Cost for a round trip coach class ticket to Chicago, Illinois (Area D)

Area A	FL / GA / AL / MS / TN / SC / NC	$390.00
Area B	ME / NH / VT / RI / MA / CT / NY / NJ / PA / DE / DC / MD / WV/	$383.00
Area C	NM / OK / AR / TX / LA	$354.00
Area D	MN / WI / MI / NE / IA / IL / IN / OH / KY / MO / KS	$335.00
Area E	ID / MT / ND / SD / WY/ UT/ CO	$390.00
Area F	WA / OR / CA / NV/ AZ	$445.00

International Travel Packages

The most economical way to make arrangements for travel to RSNA is to work directly with I.T.S. and your preferred air carrier. For individuals from Europe, Middle East, Asia,Central and South America, interested in an all inclusive RSNA Meeting Travel Package, please contact ESA Voyages and ESA North America for details:

Individuals from Europe, and the Middle East please contact:
ESA Voyages
32 rue De La Boétie
75008 Paris, France
phone: 33 1 53 53 01 35
fax: 33 1 53 53 01 45

ygrandjean@esavoyages.com
www.esavoyages.fr

Individuals from Asia and Central and South America please contact:
ESA North America
27 East Monroe, Suite 900
Chicago, Illinois, 60603
phone: (312) 917-4947
fax: (312) 917-4946

moconnell@esanorthamerica.com
www.esanorthamerica.com

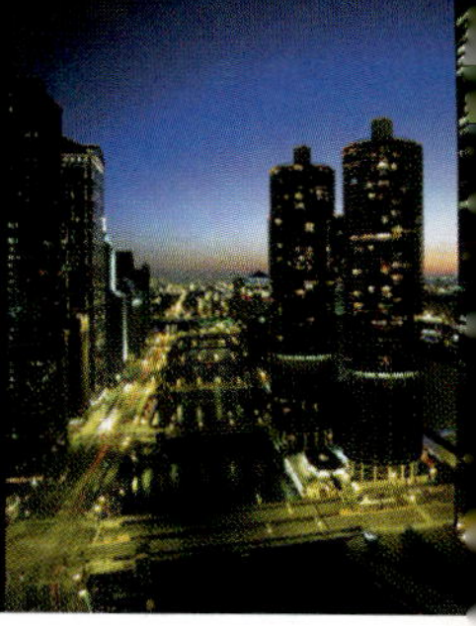

RSNA 1999 CONVENTION CAMP REGISTRATION FORM

Advance Registration Deadline: November 18, 1999

FOR RSNA OFFICE USE	
CO#	Deposit

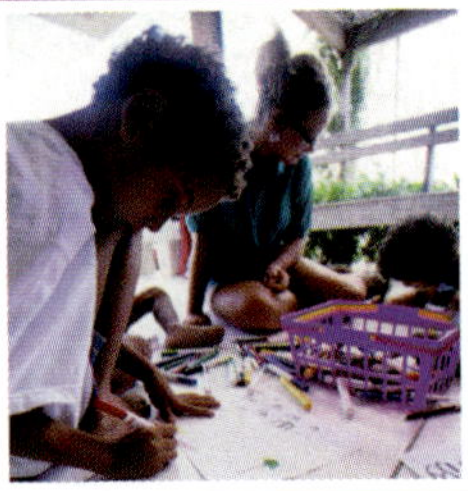

Camp RSNA childcare is open to children ages 6 months – 12 years.

A one-time $25.00 per child non-refundable registration fee is required for both advance and on-site registration. November 18th is the deadline for advance registration; after the date, registration is subject to availability and increased prices. For further information regarding the Childcare Center, please call ACCENT on Children's Arrangements, Inc. at (504)524-1227.

Rates: Children 6 – 30 months. $12.00 per hour (A three consecutive hour minimum)
Children 31 months – 12 years. $10.00 per hour(A three consecutive hour minimum)

CHILD'S NAME ____ AGE ____ SEX ____ BIRTHDATE ____

CHILD'S NAME ____ AGE ____ SEX ____ BIRTHDATE ____

CHILD'S NAME ____ AGE ____ SEX ____ BIRTHDATE ____

☐ Check here if your child has needs under the Americans with Disabilities Act. We will contact you.

The Child(ren) named above will be released ONLY to the person(s) signing this application.

FATHER / GUARDIAN FULL NAME ____ SIGNATURE ____

MOTHER / GUARDIAN FULL NAME ____ SIGNATURE ____

ADDRESS ____ ( ) DAYTIME TELEPHONE ____ ( ) FAX ____

CITY ____ STATE/PROVINCE ____ ZIP/POSTAL CODE COUNTRY ____ INTERNET/E-MAIL ADDRESS ____

Payment method (makes checks payable to ACCENT on Children's Arrangements, Inc.)
Check: Number ____

Credit Card Information: ☐ MasterCard ☐ VISA

CARD NUMBER ____ EXPIRES ____

NAME AS IT APPEARS ON CARD ____ SIGNATURE ____

Special Note: Parents must provide their own transportation to McCormick Place.RSNA does not allow children under the age of 16 on the RSNA Shuttles.
Registration confirmation will be sent upon receipt of this form.

Meals are not included in the registration. Those planning to enroll children in the Center over meal times may order meals on this Registration form. We will assume your child will attend during the hours registered. If your schedule changes we need **as much** notice as possible. You will receive a refund for a cancellation received in writing to ACCENT offices by **November 18, 1999**. You will receive no refund for a cancellation made after that time. "No shows" receive no refund. This policy is to ensure proper staffing, which is in the best interest of your child. ACCENT reserves the right to substitute programs of same/greater value, or cancel programs based on enrollment.

DATE	DROP-OFF TIME	PICK-UP TIME	NO. OF HOURS	NO. OF CHILDREN	LUNCHES @ $12	TOTAL (ADV. RATE)
Sunday, November 28, 1999 7:00 am – 7:30am, Parents Open House						
Sunday, November 28, 1999 7:30 am – 6:00 pm, Hello Chicago						
Monday, November 29, 1999 7:30 am – 6:00 pm, Windy City Wonders						
Tuesday, November 30, 1999 7:30 am – 6:00 pm, Chicago Cubs						
Wednesday, December 1, 1999 7:30 am – 6:00 pm, Lake Michigan Magic						
Thursday, December 2, 1999 7:30 am – 6:00 pm, Animal Encounter						
Friday, December 3, 1999 7:30 am – 3:00 pm, Holiday Season						
NON-REFUNDABLE ONE-TIME REGISTRATION FEE $25 PER CHILD					x $25	
				TOTAL		

November 18th is the deadline for Advance Registration. After this date, registration is subject to availability and increased prices.

Mail completed form to: **RSNA/ACCENT Convention Camp**
938 Lafayette St., Suite 201
New Orleans, LA 70113
Phone (504) 524-1226 Fax (504) 524-1229

RSNA

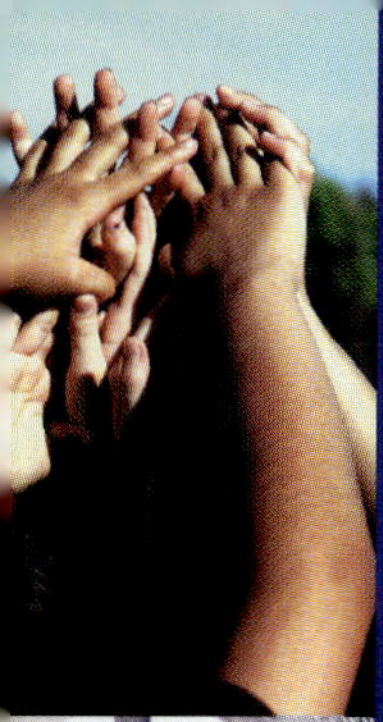
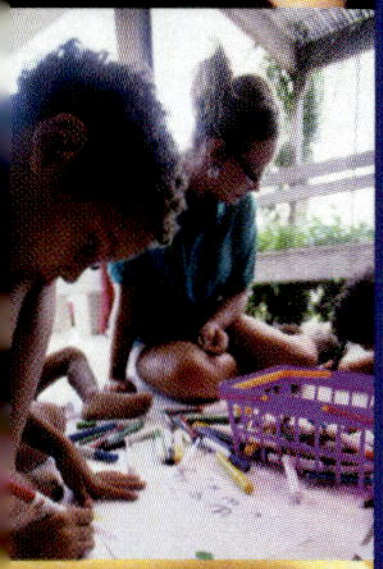
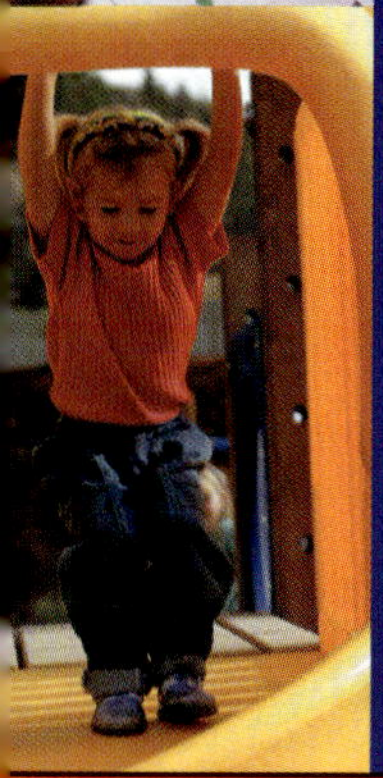

Hey Moms and Dads!

This year there's a solution for what to do with the children while you go to the meeting.

ACCENT on Children's Arrangements, Inc., has planned a great child's activity center for the RSNA attendees' children. ACCENT is a nationally recognized professional child care company organized to provide onsite children's activities in a nurturing, safe, educational environment. The Center will be located in the McCormick Place Complex. Daily activity themes such as Lake Michigan Magic and Chicago Cubs will reinforce the children's experiences of Chicago. With arts and crafts activities, active games and special guests, ACCENT's Convention Camp is sure to be great fun for all ages. All of ACCENT's counselors are fun-loving professionals who will care for and love your children.

ACCENT provides exceptional caregiver to child ratio: 1:2 for children ages 6 – 30 months, 1:4 ages 30 months to 4 years, 1:6 ages 4 – 6 years, and 1:8 ages 6 –12 years. For further information, call (504) 524-1227. We look forward to seeing you and your child in Chicago!

Dates child care is available: November 28 – December 3, 1999

Hands-on Computer Workshops:
Basic Training for Radiologists

Again this year, RSNA is pleased to offer a unique opportunity for meeting attendees to gain valuable insight into the use of computers in radiology from experts in the field.

Commercial leaders in the industry will conduct computer classes designed to give radiology professionals first-hand experience in:

- Using state-of-the-art computer equipment
- Integrating computers into radiology practice
- Radiology Information Systems (RIS)
- Picture Archiving and Communications Systems (PACS)
- New techniques used for computer-assisted diagnosis

Workshops will be held Sunday through Friday during the Annual Meeting in an area adjacent to the infoRAD area in the Lakeside Center, McCormick Place. Registration information can be found on page 12 of this brochure.

Remember: Attendance is limited, reserve space now.

While workshop reservations are made through the RSNA, they do not offer CME credit.

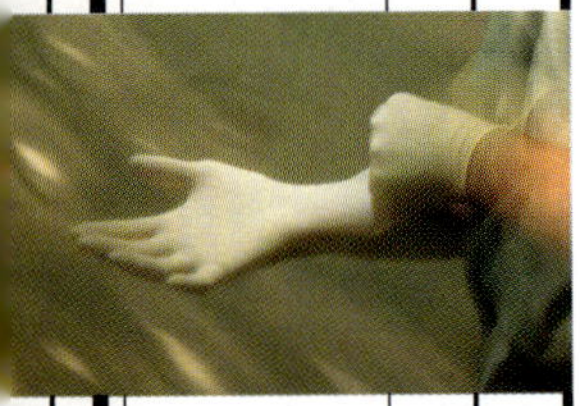

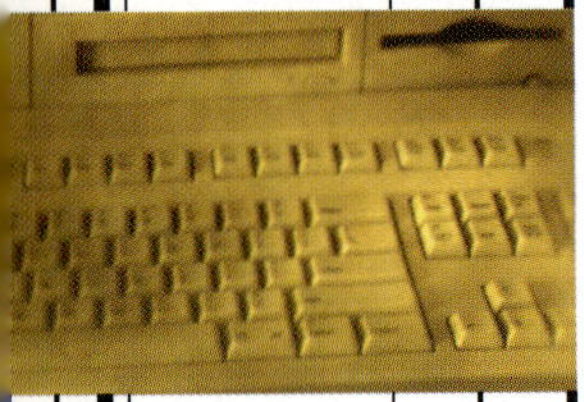

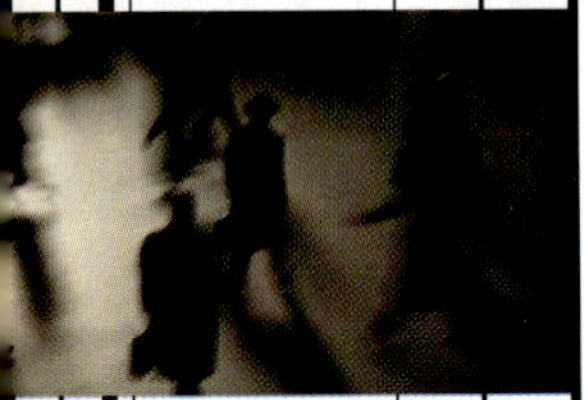

IHE Symposium: Integrating the Healthcare Enterprise

Architecting Cost Effective, High Quality, Patient-centered Care for the New Millennium

Introducing a new phase in RSNA's efforts to encourage the integration of information systems across the healthcare enterprise.

Audience:

- Physician
- CIOs
- CEOs
- other healthcare executives
- academic medical informatics specialists
- representatives of various healthcare industries.

Learn about:

- new healthcare enterprises
- economic and cost-effectiveness considerations
- the role of the Internet
- the impact of consumer activism
- the expanded focus on health and wellness
- software and hardware strategies.

"Bootcamp" for developers and commercial exhibitors on:

- components software tools
- information resources
- development environments
- applications
- services
- other related capabilities.

SEE INSIDE FOR DETAILS

Sponsored by RSNA and Healthcare Information and Management Systems Society (HIMS

RSNA 1999
108 Wilmot Road, Suite 400
Deerfield, IL 60015-0825, USA

Forwarding and Address Correction Requested

FUTURE RSNA ANNUAL MEETING DATES:

November 26 – December 1, 2000, Chicago
November 25 – November 30, 2001, Chicago
December 1 – December 6, 2002, Chicago
November 30 – December 5, 2003, Chicago
November 28 – December 3, 2004, Chicago

IMPORTANT!

ADVANCE REGISTRATION MATERIAL

INTERVENTIONAL RADIOLOGIST—Bay Imaging Consultants Medical Group, Inc, a large San Francisco Bay area private practice radiology group with multiple outpatient and hospital sites, is seeking a fellowship-trained inter-ventional radiologist with experience in all general radiology modalities, as well as experience and interest in mammographic procedures. Must be Board certified. Partnership track. Competitive salary. Start date is around July 1999 or later. Please submit your CV, a cover letter and the names of three references to Human Resources, Attn: Jill Carley, 175 Lennon Lane, Suite 100, Walnut Creek, CA 94598. EOE.

SOUTH FLORIDA—Immediate openings. Desirable private practice with two hospitals in need of fellowship-trained MRI radiologist, fellowship-trained interventional radiologist, and fellowship-trained pediatric radiologist. The successful candidates must be willing to do general radiology as well. Excellent positions for excellent individuals. Please fax CVs to 561-488-8347.

NONINVASIVE CARDIOVASCULAR IMAGER—The Department of Radiology, Cleveland Clinic Foundation, is seeking an ABR-certified imager with expertise in noninvasive cardiovascular imaging (MRI and CT) to become a member of the Section of Cardiovascular Imaging, which supports the efforts of the active Heart Center (over 4,600 open-heart surgical procedures/year). Clinical noninvasive cardiovascular imaging activities include MRI (over 900 patients/year) and helical CT with gated sub-second acquisition capabilities (over 500 patients/year) for acquired or congenital diseases of the heart and great vessels. This work and related clinical and basic research activities are supported by three Siemens MRI systems (one Symphony-Sonata, two Visions) and four Siemens Helical CT systems. Direct all correspondence to Richard D. White, MD (Head, Section of Cardiovascular Imaging), Division of Radiology: Hb-6, Cleveland Clinic Foundation, 9500 Euclid Ave, Cleveland, OH 44195, 216-444-2740.

CALIFORNIA CENTRAL COAST—Partnership track radiology position in challenging practice; 65-bed hospital three-man practice with new CT, MRI, and ultrasound and mammo equipment. Must be highly skilled in all modalities. No catheter angiography. Family oriented community of 40,000 plus. Please send inquiries and CV to David McAninch, MD, 1111 E Ocean Ave, Suite 2, Lompoc, CA 93436; fax 805-735-8540.

SALT LAKE CITY RADIOLOGY GROUP—Seeks Board certified radiologist, fellowship training desirable to join established five-member group starting immediately. Practice includes all modalities including angio/interventional. Send CV to Jonathan Naatz, MD, Valley Radiology, 632 W 7250 South, Midvale, UT 84047 or fax to 801-561-5520.

GENERAL RADIOLOGIST—Beautiful coastal community in central eastern Florida is seeking a radiologist with fellowship training preferably in MRI or musculoskeletal radiology. Partnership track position with excellent benefits. Send CV or contact Peter Joyce, MD, Vero Radiology Associates, Vero Beach, FL; 561-567-1942, fax 561-562-1505.

BOARD-CERTIFIED RADIOLOGIST—Wanted for hospital-based New Hampshire radiology practice (54 miles north of Boston). Must be competent in CT, US, MRI, mammography, and general radiology. Fellowship trained individual preferred. Generous salaried position. A 3-yr partnership track. For further information, contact G. Eric Geslien, MD, Department of Diagnostic Imaging, Exeter Hospital, PO Box 790, Exeter, NH 03833 or e-mail *RGESLIEN@EHR.ORG* or fax 603-778-6707.

NUCLEAR RADIOLOGY—The Penn State Geisinger Health System is currently seeking a fellowship trained and licensed nuclear radiologist to join the Geisinger Medical Center in Danville, PA. The practice will combine general and nuclear radiology. Background and experience in nuclear medicine, MRI, CT, ultrasound and general diagnostic radiology is preferred. Call coverage is on a rotational basis with 12 other diagnostic radiologists. The position will include both clinical and teaching responsibilities in a 458-bed tertiary care hospital and level 1 trauma center with its own radiology program. Geisinger Medical Center supports a 40-county area throughout northeastern and central Pennsylvania. We offer a competitive salary and excellent benefit package. For additional information regarding this opportunity please contact Kurt

Scott, Penn State Geisinger Health System, Department of Professional Staffing and Credentialing (RAD-CT), 100 N Academy Ave, Danville, PA 17822-1528; phone 800-845-7112. CVs can be faxed to 800-622-2515. EOE, M/F/H/V.

RADIOLOGIST—Community hospital, 180 beds, near shore resorts in Delaware, seeks radiologist fellowship-trained in cross-sectional imaging or interventional radiology to join three-man group. Partnership track, a competitive salary, benefits and vacation. Contact E.J.Goldstein, MD, 8 Lexington Dr, Milford DE 19963, phone after 6 pm 302 424-0613, e-mail *egoldstein@mmh .bayhealth.org.*

THE UNIVERSITY OF MISSISSIPPI MEDICAL CENTER—Department of Radiology is seeking an additional mammographer. The University of Mississippi Medical Center is among the fastest growing academic medical centers in the United States. The equipment is state-of-the-art. There is an opportunity to perform breast procedures on the General Electric interventional magnet. This magnet is one of 11 in the world. Salary is commensurate with training, experience and productivity. Interested parties should contact Dr Brent Harrison, Department of Radiology, 2500 N State St, Jackson, MS 39216, 601-984-2515, *RBHARRISON@email.MSN.com.* EOE, M/F/D/V.

NUCLEAR MEDICINE—Progressive subspecialized large private practice radiology group is seeking individual fellowship-trained in nuclear medicine. The practice is affiliated with a medical school and residency program, thereby offering the benefits of both private practice and the pursuit of academic interests. Position will include eventual directorship of nuclear medicine department. The practice is located on the Atlantic coastline with a mild climate and all water sports available. Interested persons should send a CV or contact Stephen Carr, MD, Director of Recruiting, Medical Center Radiologists, 6330 N Center Dr, Bldg 13, Ste 220, Norfolk, VA 23502; 757-466-0089 or fax 757-466-8017.

MUSCULOSKELETAL RADIOLOGIST—Progressive subspecialized large private practice radiology group is seeking individual with subspecialty training in musculoskeletal MR. The practice is affiliated with a medical school and residency program, thereby offering the benefits of both private practice and the pursuit of academic interests. The practice is located in coastal Virginia with a mild climate and many recreational activities available with the Chesapeake Bay and Atlantic Ocean nearby. Interested persons should send a CV or contact Stephen Carr, MD, Director of Recruiting, Medical Center Radiologists, 6330 N Center Dr, Bldg 13, Ste 220, Norfolk, VA 23502; 757-466-0089 or fax 757-466-8017.

GENERAL RADIOLOGIST—Progressive subspecialized large private practice radiology group is seeking a qualified body imaging radiologist comfortable with all modalities of diagnostic radiology except angiography and interventional. The practice is affiliated with a medical school and residency program, thereby offering the benefits of both private practice and the pursuit of academic interests. The practice is located on the Atlantic coastline with a mild climate and all water sports available. Interested persons should send a CV or contact Stephen Carr, MD, Director of Recruiting, Medical Center Radiologists, 6330 N Center Dr, Bldg 13, Ste 220, Norfolk, VA 23502; 757-466-0089 or fax 757-466-8017.

INTERVENTIONAL RADIOLOGIST—Progressive subspecialized large private practice radiology group is seeking an interventional radiologist. The practice is affiliated with a medical school and residency program, thereby offering the benefits of both private practice and the pursuit of academic interests. The practice is located in coastal Virginia with a mild climate and many recreational activities available with the Chesapeake Bay and Atlantic Ocean nearby. Interested persons should send a CV or contact Stephen Carr, MD, Director of Recruiting, Medical Center Radiologists, 6330 N Center Dr, Bldg 13, Ste 220, Norfolk, VA 23502; 757-466-0089 or fax 757-466-8017.

MRI STAFF POSITION—The MRI Section at the University of Pennsylvania is seeking applicants for a faculty position at the assistant professor rank in the area of MRI. Applicants should have fellowship training in MRI and clinical experience with body and musculoskeletal MRI. Experience in clinical research is desired. Clinical responsibilities will be split between body and musculoskeletal MRI. Applications should include a curriculum vitae, a statement of research interests, and the names and addresses of three references. Applications should be sent to Mitchell D. Schnall, MD, PhD, MRI Section, Department of Radiology, Hospital of the University of Pennsylvania, 3400 Spruce St, Philadelphia, PA 19104. The University of Pennsylvania is an equal opportunity/affirmative action employer. Qualified female and minority candidates are encouraged to apply.

MAMMOGRAPHY AND BODY IMAGING POSITIONS-FLORIDA—Watson Clinic, LLP, is a 175-physician multispecialty group seeking two radiologists. Join 14 radiologists in this fully diversified practice which includes MRI, CT, mammography, DEXA, GI/IVP, US and interventional work and a 660-bed tertiary care hospital two blocks south of the clinic. One position available to join one other in mammography. Ability to perform stereotactic needle biopsies required. Additional practice opportunity available in CT body imaging. We offer early partnership, salary guarantee with production incentive, excellent benefits package and paid malpractice insurance. Located between Tampa and Orlando, Lakeland offers a secure family environment with abundant recreational opportunities. Interested candidates should please send a CV to Professional Services, Watson Clinic LLP, 1600 Lakeland Hills Blvd, Lakeland, FL 33804; 800-854-7786, fax 941-680-7951.

LAKE MICHIGAN SHORELINE COMMUNITY—Progressive six-member practice seeks Board-certified, preferably fellowship-trained radiologist for partnership track. Busy, rapidly expanding practice, with all modalities, including MRI and angiography/interventional. Candidate would be expected to cover all modalities. Generous compensation, benefit and vacation package. Community is in western Michigan, which offers low cost of living and abundant recreational activities, amongst other perks. Please reply to Box R-109.

INTERVENTIONAL RADIOLOGIST-NORTHWEST INDIANA—Board certified general diagnostic radiologist, fellowship trained in angio/interventional radiology with competency in all modalities needed to join a multi-specialty group of 12 radiologists serving three area hospitals and eight clinic locations. Competitive benefits and compensation. Contact and/or send a CV to James M. Forde, MD, 825 E Lincolnway, Valparaiso, IN 46383; telephone 219-464-4891, fax 219-465-0193.

RADIOLOGIST/ASSOCIATE PROFESSOR—Medical University of South Carolina Radiology Department: Opening for Board-certified or equivalent radiologist with GI and computed tomography experience, also teaching, research in academic environment. Includes appointment to College of Medicine as associate professor. Send CV by July 31, 1999 to Jeremy Young, MD, Professor and Chairman, c/o Melanie Jackson, MUSC Radiology Department, 169 Ashley Ave, PO Box 250322, Charleston, SC 29425. Women and minorities encouraged to apply.

NEURORADIOLOGIST—For university practice in Massachusetts. Includes a university appointment and involves clinical duties at the University Hospital in an associated private practice with teaching of residents and fellows. Fellowship required, CAQ preferred. Interest or experience in advanced MRI techniques helpful. Contact Edward H. Smith, Chairman, Department of Radiology, phone 508-856-3252, fax 508-856-4669. EOE.

The Department of Diagnostic Imaging at Temple University School of Medicine is recruiting board-certified faculty to participate in our clinical, research and teaching programs in:

NEURORADIOLOGY - Assistant Professor. Interest and training in Interventional Neuroradiology preferred.

THORACIC RADIOLOGY - Assistant Professor. To participate in all aspects of chest imaging, including PET.

AVAILABLE EQUIPMENT - Fully digital format using an AGFA network; two 1.5 GE Sigma MRI scanners upgraded to an LX Platform; two Picker spiral CT scanners; two Voxel-Q work stations for three-dimensional imaging and virtual endoscopy; a third CT scan, a PET scanner and open MRI scanner to be installed; seven ultrasound scanners; CVIS system for endo-luminal and vascular ultrasound; two Philips and one Siemens PSA rooms. GE PET scanner being installed.

Send current CV and cover letter to: **Robert A. Gatenby, M.D., Professor and Chairperson, Department of Diagnostic Imaging, Temple University School of Medicine, 3401 N. Broad Street, Philadelphia, PA 19140.** Temple University School of Medicine is an Affirmative Action/Equal Opportunity Employer and strongly encourages women and minorities to apply.

STATE UNIVERSITY OF NEW YORK AT STONY BROOK—Has unexpected opening in our diagnostic radiology residency program at both junior and senior levels to begin July 1, 1999. We are a 504-bed tertiary care referral center and Level I trauma center. State-of-the-art equipment and 24 full-time subspecialty-trained faculty members dedicated to resident teaching provide a sound educational experience. Interested applicants, send curriculum vitae and references to Kathleen Finzel, MD, Program Director, Department of Radiology, SUNY- Stony Brook, Stony Brook, NY 11794-8460, or fax 516-444-7538.

FACULTY POSITION IN US AND CT, THOMAS JEFFERSON UNIVERSITY HOSPITAL—The Department of Radiology at Thomas Jefferson University Hospital in Philadelphia seeks a junior faculty member to join its very large practice in US and body CT. Jefferson performs 35,000 US exams of all types and 12,000 body CT exams per year on state-of-the-art equipment. The department has seven cross sectional imaging fellows per year, as well as 24 residents. We offer an abundance of interesting clinical and teaching material, numerous opportunities for research, and an excellent infrastructure to support clinical and research activities. Individuals just completing fellowship or scheduled to complete one in June 2000 are encouraged to apply. The position is available immediately but the start date can be delayed until July 2000 if necessary. Interested candidates should contact Barry B. Goldberg, MD, Director, Division of Diagnostic Ultrasound, Thomas Jefferson University Hospital, Philadelphia, PA 19107. Phone 215-955-6227, fax 215-955-8549.

ASSISTANT/ASSOCIATE PROFESSOR—Full-time faculty position available September 1, 1999. The Department of Radiology at the University of Wisconsin Medical School, Madison, is seeking a fellowship-trained radiologist with experience in women's imaging with additional skills in abdominal radiology. Duties include medical student and resident teaching, radiology service and clinical research. Candidates must be Board certified in diagnostic radiology. Cover letter and resume should be made in application to Patrick Turski, MD, Professor and Chairman, Department of Radiology, E3/311, Clinical Science Center, 600 Highland Ave, Madison, WI 53792-3252. Unless confidentiality is requested in writing, information regarding the applicants must be released upon request. Finalists cannot be guaranteed confidentiality. An equal opportunity/affirmative action employer.

BREAST IMAGING RADIOLOGIST—A 16-member group in North Florida seeking fellowship-trained mammographer or candidate with special interest in mammography for partnership position. Strong general radiology skills required. Please reply to B.L. Storm, MD, PO Box 12219, Tallahassee, FL 32317-2219; office telephone 850-942-4497, fax 850-942-1610.

NEURORADIOLOGY FACULTY POSITION—The Division of Neuroradiology in the Department of Radiology at Emory University School of Medicine, Atlanta, GA, is offering a full-time faculty position as assistant or associate professor in neuroradiology, to begin July 1, 1999. Candidates should be Board-certified radiologists who have completed a fellowship, preferably 2 years, in an accredited neuroradiology program, and who are CAQ certified or eligible. A strong background and interest in academic radiology, cerebral angiography, myelography, CT, MR and MR angiography are required. Academic interest in functional MR is preferable. The neuroradiology division is extremely well balanced with expertise in pediatric neuroradiology, head and neck radiology, interventional neuroradiology and functional imaging. Equipment includes seven high field MRI units, including DWI, PWI, fMRI and MR spectroscopy (an MR research center, to include a 3T magnet, will be in place soon), seven CT scanners and three neuroangiographic suites. Interdepartmental conferences and research collaboration are conducted with neurology, neurosurgery, orthopedic surgery and otolaryngology. Applications will be accepted until position is filled. For more information, please contact Patricia A. Hudgins, MD, Director, Neuroradiology, Department of Radiology/B-115, Emory University School of Medicine, 1364 Clifton Rd, NE, Atlanta, GA 30322; phone 404-712-4583, fax 404-712-7957.

Geisinger Medical Center
Danville, PA

Nuclear Radiology

The **Penn State Geisinger Health System** is currently seeking a fellowship trained and licensed nuclear radiologist to join the Geisinger Medical Center in Danville, PA. The practice will combine general and nuclear radiology. Background and experience in nuclear medicine, MRI, CT, ultrasound and general diagnostic radiology is preferred. Call coverage is on a rotational basis with 12 other diagnostic radiologists. The position will include both clinical and teaching responsibilities in a 458-bed tertiary care hospital and level 1 trauma center with its own radiology program. Geisinger Medical Center supports a 40 county area throughout northeastern and central Pennsylvania. We offer a competitive salary and excellent benefits package. For additional information, please contact:

Kurt Scott, Professional Staffing and Credentialing (RAD-DK)
Penn State Geisinger Health System
100 N. Academy Avenue
Danville, PA 17822-1528
Phone: 800-845-7112 Fax: 800-622-2515

PennState Geisinger
Health System
THE POWER OF HEALTH

E.O.E.
M/F/H/V

CHIEF OF RADIOLOGY

NEW YORK MEDICAL COLLEGE

New York Medical College seeks a dynamic Radiologist to lead the Department of Radiology at its academic affiliate, Metropolitan Hospital Center, a 494-bed Health and Hospitals Corporation acute care facility on the Upper East Side of Manhattan.

The successful candidate will have extensive clinical and administrative experience and qualify for academic appointment at the level of Associate Professor or Professor of Radiology at New York Medical College.

Candidates should submit current CV to:

Catherine Hinterbuchner, M.D.
Chairman, Search Committee
Code: RJ
New York Medical College
Metropolitan Hospital Center
Department of Rehabilitation Medicine
1901 First Avenue
Room 327
New York, NY 10029
Fax: (212) 423-6326

New York Medical College is an AA/EOE.

THE DEPARTMENT OF RADIOLOGY AT STANFORD UNIVERSITY SCHOOL OF MEDICINE—Invites applications from qualified individuals for 2 years of research training in brain imaging. We are actively recruiting for 1999 and 2000 postdoctoral trainee positions. This is an NIH-funded program in advanced techniques in cancer imaging with opportunities for brain and central nervous system imaging research using MR imaging and MR spectroscopy (using 1.5T, 2.0T and 3.0T), CT (using conventional, ultrafast and electron beam scanners) and ultrasound. Preceptors drawn from both the radiology and electrical engineering departments include Gary H. Glover, PhD, Scott W. Atlas, MD, Michael Mosley, PhD, Sandy Napel, PhD, Dwight Nishimura, PhD, and Norbert J. Pelc, ScD. The ideal candidates will be either MDs who have completed at least 2 years in an approved radiology residency program, or PhDs in an imaging-related field from an approved doctoral program within 4 years of acceptance to this training program. For candidates who have completed radiology residency training, the fellowship includes 6 months of clinical neuroradiology under the direction of Scott W. Atlas, MD, in addition to 18 months of neuroimaging research. The Stanford University Medical School is committed to increasing representation of women and members of minority groups and encourage all qualified candidates to apply. In accordance with NIH regulations, applicants must be citizens, permanent residents, or naturalized citizens of the United States. Applicants should send a curriculum vitae, a statement about interest in the program and research career goals, and letters from three referees to Ms Donna Cronister, Training Program Administrator, Department of Radiology, Stanford University, Lucas Center for Magnetic Resonance Spectroscopy and Imaging, Mail Code 5488, Room P-260, Stanford, CA 94305-5488.

LINDE HEALTHCARE—(*www.Lindehc.com*) Has openings for radiologist interested in locum tenens. Work in an environment catered to your lifestyle. Want to work full-time locums, pick up extra hours, or explore positions leading to permanent placement? Linde HealthCare provides competitive pay, malpractice, travel and lodging, while maintaining a high level of confidentiality. Call us @ 800-588-4343, fax your CV to 314-843-2262, or send it to *Info@lindehc.com.*

MUSCULOSKELETAL RADIOLOGIST—A 16-member group in North Florida seeking BC/BE MSK radiologist with strong general radiology skills for partnership position. Please reply to B.L. Storm, MD, PO Box 12219, Tallahassee, FL 32317-2219; office telephone 850-942-4497, fax 850-942-1610.

BODY IMAGING RADIOLOGIST—A 16-member group in North Florida seeking fellowship-trained candidate for partnership position. Candidate should be skilled in body MRI and basic GI interventions. Please reply to B.L. Storm, MD, PO Box 12219, Tallahassee, FL 32317-2219; office telephone 850-942-4497; fax 850-942-1610

THE DEPARTMENT OF RADIOLOGY AT STANFORD UNIVERSITY SCHOOL OF MEDICINE—Invites applications from qualified individuals for 2 years of research training in advanced techniques in cancer imaging. We are currently recruiting for 1999 and 2000 postdoctoral trainee positions. This is an NIH-funded program with opportunities for research in magnetic resonance imaging and spectroscopy (using 1.5T, 2.0T and 3.0T), CT (using conventional, ultrafast and electron beam scanners) and ultrasound. The program is intended for trainees to develop expertise in cancer-related imaging research. Preceptors drawn from the radiology and electrical engineering departments are Gary M. Glazer, MD, Gary H. Glover, PhD, Robert J. Herfkens, MD, R. Brooke Jeffrey, MD, King Li, MD, Michael Moseley, PhD, Sandy Napel, PhD, Dwight Nishimura, PhD, Norbert J. Pelc, ScD, and F. Graham Sommer, MD. The ideal candidates will be individuals who have received an MD in an imaging-related field or a PhD equivalent degree from an approved doctoral program within 4 years of acceptance to this training program. MD candidates must have completed at least 2 years in an approved radiology residency program. The Stanford University Medical School is committed to increasing representation of women and members of minority groups and encourages all qualified candidates to apply. In accordance with NIH regulations, applicants must be citizens, permanent residents or naturalized citizens of the United States. Applicants should send a curriculum vitae, a statement about interest in the program and research career goals, and letters from three referees to Ms Donna Cronister, Training Program Administrator, Department of Radiology, Stanford University, Lucas Center for Magnetic Resonance Spectroscopy and Imaging, Mail Code 5488, Room P-260, Stanford, CA 94305-5488. Application deadline for 1999 appointments is July 15, 1999. Notification of acceptance into the program will occur within 4 months of deadline date.

DIAGNOSTIC RADIOLOGY-MOBILE, AL—Growing Gulf Coast community (300,000+ metro area) with abundant recreational opportunities has an expanding radiology practice that needs an additional partnership track radiologist to cover all diagnostic areas: MR, US, NM, mammo, general diagnostic, angio and basic interventional. Broad referral base at hospital and adjacent outpatient center. Position available immediately. Very generous salary, benefit and vacation package. Send letter and CV to Ann Bradley, 6576 Airport Blvd, #C-2, Mobile, AL 36608.

WOMEN'S IMAGING RADIOLOGIST—Fairfax Radiology Consultants is a large subspecialized radiology group in the northern Virginia suburbs of Washington, DC. We are seeking an individual, experienced or fellowship-trained in women's imaging modalities, to join our growing women's imaging practice. This is a unique opportunity to join a subspecialized private practice that includes a complete breast imaging center and a free-standing ultrasound imaging center as well as several multi-modality imaging centers that perform a large percentage of women's imaging. Direct inquiries and CVs to Roberta Illy, Human Resources Director, PO Box 3650, Merrifield, VA 22116; phone 703-698-4444, fax 703-698-4451. EOE.

ANGIO-INTERVENTIONAL/GENERAL RADIOLOGIST—Private practice of five, with four outpatient clinics and a new 230-bed active community hospital seeking general radiologist with angio/interventional capability. Excellent pay, liberal benefits, minimal call. Position to be filled immediately. Fax resume to 313-581-3000.

DIRECTOR OF INTERVENTIONAL RADIOLOGY—The Department of Radiology at the University of Iowa College of Medicine is seeking a director of Interventional Radiology. We are accepting applications for a full-time faculty position with open rank. As one of the largest teaching hospitals in the country, the University of Iowa Hospitals and Clinics provide a high volume of diverse and complex interventional radiology cases. Excellent clinical facilities, interdepartmental and core research laboratories, animal imaging facilities, and an engineering center experienced in custom stent/filter device design and fabrication are available. Applicants must be Board certified by the American Board of Radiology or equivalent and possess the Certificate of Added Qualification (CAQ) in interventional radiology. Applicants must have experience in vascular and non-vascular interventional radiology. Strong evidence of clinical productivity, scholarly works and prior administrative experience are desirable. Salary is commensurate with experience. Women and members of minority groups are strongly encouraged to apply. Send applications to George El-Khoury, MD, University of Iowa Hospitals and Clinics, 200 Hawkins Dr, Iowa City, IA 52242. The University of Iowa is an affirmative action/equal opportunity employer.

FELLOWSHIP-TRAINED RADIOLOGISTS—Premier radiology group in Illinois seeks radiologists with body imaging, musculoskeletal or interventional training and experience. We offer top earning potential, excellent benefits and partnership track. If you are looking for a successful collegial practice environment located in a safe, family-oriented community, contact Kathy Jordan at 1-800-765-3055; fax 314-726-3009. e-mail *kjordan@cejka.com.* ID# 6074RA. Visit our website at *www.cejka.com.*

MAMMOGRAPHER WANTED—Come live in the beautiful oceanside community of Cape Cod, MA. We are a 10-member, well-established group of radiologists providing care for Cape Cod hospital and three private offices. Seeking an individual with extensive training/interest in mammography and breast biopsies for full-time partnership track position. Duties include mostly mammography and breast biopsies, but also include CT/US, fluoroscopy and plain film readings. Send curriculum vitae to Dr Gordon K. Kanzer, MD, Cape Cod Radiology Associates and Women's Imaging Center, 66 Lewis Bay Rd, Hyannis, MA 02601. Telephone 508-775-3515, fax 508-778-9381.

INTERVENTIONAL RADIOLOGIST—An experienced, fellowship-trained vascular/interventional radiologist is sought to join the radiology department of a 930-bed teaching hospital in suburban Detroit. Opportunities are available for teaching and research. There is a large residency program as well as positions for two fellows each in accredited fellowships in vascular/interventional and neuroradiology. The candidate must have experience in a broad range of diagnostic and therapeutic interventional procedures. Board certification is required as well as being interventional CAQ certified or eligible. An interest in non-invasive vascular imaging is also desirable. Reply to Kenneth Matasar, MD, FACR, Chairman, Diagnostic Radiology, William Beaumont Hospital, 3601 West 13 Mile Road, Royal Oak, MI 48073. Fax 248-551-5490.

GENERAL RADIOLOGIST, LAS VEGAS, NV—Expanding, stable and progressive 13-member outpatient practice is seeking two BC fellowship-trained radiologists for two excellent partnership track positions in one of the fastest growing cities in the United States. The practice runs three of the largest state-of-the-art imaging centers in the nation and includes six MRIs, four CT scanners, two angio suites, nuclear medicine, mammography and US. Strong general radiology skills needed (no interventional skills required). Interest in mammography would be beneficial for one position, but not required. These positions currently involve no call and no angio coverage. Positions are available immediately, but start date is flexible to summer of 2000. Please send CV to Dr Chang, 2950 S Maryland Pkwy, Las Vegas, NV 89109.

THE DEPARTMENT OF RADIOLOGY AT THE UNIVERSITY OF PITTSBURGH SCHOOL OF MEDICINE—Is recruiting for the position of an interventional radiologist. The incumbent will provide clinical service at a UPMC-affiliated community hospital and, potentially, UPMC Presbyterian, and serve on the faculty of the University of Pittsburgh School of Medicine. This is a non-tenure clinical position with an expected hiring date in the summer of 1999. Salary and rank are dependent on qualifications and experience. The position requires Board certification with an interventional fellowship required. The physician should be licensed (or eligible for licensure) to practice medicine in the Commonwealth of Pennsylvania. Clinical research opportunities are available to interested candidates. Interested candidates should submit a curriculum vitae to Barry McCook, MD, Assistant Professor of Radiology, UPMC, Department of Radiology, 200 Lothrop St, Pittsburgh, PA 15213-2582. The University of Pittsburgh is an affirmative action/equal opportunity employer.

BC RADIOLOGIST—The Fallon Clinic, a 250-member multispecialty group practice seeks BC radiologist to provide high quality care to our patients. Join a dedicated outpatient department committed to excellence. Additional training or special interest in mammography, ultrasound and spiral CT are desirable. We are affiliated with a major teaching hospital and have been serving the community for over 70 years. Enjoy life in scenic and culturally rich New England. We offer an excellent salary and benefits package. For confidential inquiry, please contact Physician Services at 508-795-1157 or mail CV to Physician Services, 100 Central St, Worcester, MA 01698. Fax 508-793-0909; e-mail *omd@fallon-clinic.com.* EOE.

METRO ST. LOUIS—Well established, large private practice group continuing to expand is recruiting two new radiologists for partnership track. Candidate should be ABR-certified; fellowship training is highly desirable. Our new radiologists would be expected to make an impact by continuing to develop new imaging approaches and state-of-the-art techniques for our hospital and outpatient practice. We currently staff three busy suburban hospitals and own and operate three additional free-standing imaging centers. Salary and benefits are very competitive. For more information, contact Darryl Zuckerman, MD, Department of Radiology, St. Joseph Health Center, 300 First Capitol Dr, St. Charles, MO 63301; phone 314-947-5444, fax 314-947-9860.

BREAST IMAGING POSITION—The Department of Radiology at the University of Pennsylvania Medical Center is seeking an additional faculty member with academic experience or fellowship training in breast imaging. The breast imaging section provides a full range of breast imaging modalities, including mammography, ultrasound, MRI and full-field digital mammography. The rich research program allows collaboration within radiology as well as other departments. Clinical services are performed at the Hospital of the University of Pennsylvania and affiliated locations. Responsibilities of the position include clinical, teaching and research activities. Appointments to the university will be at the assistant or associate professor level in the full-time clinician educator track, non-tenure, depending on qualifications. Interested applicants should send a curriculum vitae to Emily F. Conant, MD, Chief of Breast Imaging, Department of Radiology, 1 Silverstein Bldg, 3400 Spruce St, Philadelphia, PA 19104. The University of Pennsylvania Medical Center is an affirmative action/equal opportunity employer. Minority and women candidates are encouraged to apply.

SEATTLE POSITION AVAILABLE—Move to Seattle and the beautiful Pacific Northwest. Growing private practice in a desirable Seattle suburb seeks thirteenth full-time radiologist. Inpatient/outpatient setting with a 250-bed multispecialty hospital and several imaging centers. Individual sought with experience and skills in neuro and musculoskeletal MRI. Presently two magnets (including Siemen's Vision 1.5T with Echo Planer Imaging), third installation planned. Would also participate in other general radiology rotations and equal call. Partnership track, competitive benefits and salary. Please direct inquiries to Steve Sperling, MD, Overlake Hospital Medical Center, 1035 116th Ave NE, Bellevue, WA 98004; 425-688-5537.

MUSCULOSKELETAL/BODY IMAGER-SILVER SPRING, MD—A 14-person subspecialty-oriented, Washington, DC, suburban radiology practice has immediate opening for partnership-track position for Board-certified candidate with fellowship training in musculoskeletal or body MRI. Candidate must also be competent in all aspects of diagnostic imaging. Group has both hospital and outpatient MRI systems (GE Echo Speed, GE Signa and Toshiba Opart). Please reply to R.W. Zimmerman, MD, Diagnostic Medical Imaging, PA, 1500 Forest Glen Rd, Silver Spring, MD 20910. Fax 301-681-7609, e-mail *zimmeRo @holycrosshealth.org.*

RADIOLOGY OPPORTUNITIES—Watson Clinic LLP is a 175-physician multispecialty group seeking two radiologists. Join 14 radiologists in this fully diversified practice which includes MRI, CT, mammogram, DEXA, GI/IVP, U/S and interventional work at a 660-bed tertiary care hospital two blocks south of the clinic. One position available to join one other in mammography. Ability to perform stereotactic needle biopsies required. Additional practice opportunity available in CT/body imaging. We offer early partnership, salary guarantee with production incentive, excellent benefits package and paid malpractice insurance. Please send a CV to Professional Services, Watson Clinic, LLP, 1600 Lakeland Hills Blvd, Lakeland, FL 33804; phone 800-854-7786, fax 941-680-7951.

BODY CROSS-SECTIONAL IMAGING RADIOLOGIST—The Department of Radiology at the University of Rochester Medical Center has a faculty position available in body cross-sectional imaging (CT, US, MRI). Clinical services at Strong Memorial Hospital perform 200,000 diagnostic examinations per year. State-of-the-art facilities are available in all modalities. The emergency department is a level I trauma center and hospital services include active organ transplant and oncologic programs. Fellowship training is required. Send cover letter and CV to Arvin E. Robinson, MD, Chair, Department of Radiology, University of Rochester Medical Center, Box 648, 601 Elmwood Ave, Rochester, NY 14642 or fax to 716-756-8290. Deadline for applications is December 1, 1999. The University of Rochester is an equal opportunity employer.

CHIEF OF NEURORADIOLOGY—The Department of Radiology at the University of Chicago is seeking candidates for the position of Chief of Neuroradiology. The university has exceptionally active clinical and research programs in neurosurgery, neurology, radiation oncology and ENT that collaborate intensively with neuroradiology. The section provides a full range of imaging and interventional services, utilizing state-of-the-art 1.5T MRI scanners, spiral CT units and angiography suites in both inpatient and outpatient facilities. A 3T MRI unit that will be dedicated to neuroscience research (especially fMRI and MRS) will be installed in winter/spring 2000. Our ideal candidate will have an outstanding academic record in neuroradiology research. In addition, this individual will have the ability to lead a very busy clinical service and to supervise the teaching of both residents and neuroradiology fellows. A CAQ in neuroradiology is highly desirable and eligibility for licensure in Illinois is a prerequisite. An appointment will be made at the level of professor or associate professor. The University of Chicago is located 10 minutes from the heart of downtown Chicago along the shores of Lake Michigan. Interested parties should send a letter and a CV to the Search Committee c/o David N. Levin, MD, PhD, Department of Radiology, The University of Chicago, 5841 S Maryland Ave, Chicago, IL 60637; phone 773-702-6511, fax 773-702-1161, *dlevin@uchicago.edu*. The University of Chicago is an equal opportunity/affirmative action employer.

THE UCLA DEPARTMENT OF RADIOLOGICAL SCIENCES—Is seeking a full-time faculty member in the rank of assistant or associate professor-in-residence. Clinical responsibilities will include shared coverage of diagnostic neuroradiology inpatient and outpatient facilities, cerebral angiography, myelography, discography and image-guided biopsies. The candidate will supervise and teach neuroradiology fellows and residents in diagnostic radiology. Strong research interest with experience in MR techniques, including MRI, spectroscopy, interventional MR and/or diffusion/perfusion desirable. The position requires excellent clinical skills, teaching ability and experience in clinical or basic research. The candidate must be Board certified in diagnostic radiology and CAQ certified in neuroradiology. Please send CV and names of five professional references to Richard Steckel, MD, Chairman, Department of Radiological Sciences, UCLA School of Medicine, Los Angeles, CA 90095-1721. The University of California is an EO/AA employer.

MEDICAL PHYSICS FACULTY POSITION-RADIOLOGICAL SCIENCES—The graduate program in radiological sciences at the University of Texas Health Sciences Center at San Antonio is seeking a medical physicist specializing in diagnostic imaging to serve as a core faculty member in the continuing development of the medical physics graduate program. The program is one of nine certified medical physics graduate programs in North America certified by CAMPEP (see web site for details: *http://radscience.uthscsa.edu/*). The successful candidate will join a multidisciplinary faculty of 46. He/she will be responsible for teaching portions of two diagnostic physics courses (Fundamentals of Diagnostic Physics and Physics of Nuclear Imaging). In addition, the new junior faculty member will be expected to actively develop an independent research program

RADIOLOGIST

www.lahey.org

Lahey Clinic is seeking a board-certified Radiologist with special interest in ultrasound. The ultrasound section supports a busy liver transplant service. We are seeking an individual familiar with intraoperative and laproscopic ultrasound. Responsibilities include clinical work in abdominal and general ultrasound, GYN (primarily infertility and gynecologic oncology), prostate (including biopsy), endorectal and endoanal, small parts, breast (including interventional procedures) and non-invasive vascular imaging (performed in our ICAVL accredited vascular laboratory). Additional work in general radiology including plain film, CT, fluoroscopy and mammography can be expected. The practice includes an active residency program and medical student teaching.

Lahey Clinic Medical Center is a large, non-profit, physician-directed, multi-specialty group practice in a 249-bed hospital with a trauma center and outpatient clinics in virtually all subspecialties, located 30 minutes northwest of Boston in Burlington, MA. We are a large, non-profit, physician-directed multi-specialty group practice with 300 physicians and a growing network of community-based primary and specialty care in Eastern and Central Massachusetts.

Salary is commensurate with experience and qualifications. Interested applicants should send curriculum vitae to: ***Richard A. Baker, M.D., Chairman, Department of Diagnostic Radiology, Lahey Clinic, 41 Mall Road, Burlington, MA 01805****. For further information contact* ***Alda F. Cossi, M.D., at (781) 744-8170, Fax: (781) 744-5232*** *or e-mail* ***Alda.F.Cossi@lahey.org***

An Equal Opportunity/Affirmative Action Employer.

Lahey CLINIC

in one of the existing imaging laboratories or clinics. Collaboration with existing projects in interventional cardiovascular imaging, nuclear imaging pharmacology, interventional tumor ablation, functional imaging- MRI and PET and/ or electronic imaging is encouraged. Imaging equipment for research is available in both research and clinical settings. Candidates must have a doctoral degree in medical physics, physics, biomedical engineering or other appropriate physical science. Experience with nuclear imaging, MR and electronic imaging methodologist is highly desirable. This position carries a tenure-track academic appointment in the Department of Radiology. Salary and academic rank commensurate with qualifications. Send curriculum vitae and references to Medical Physics Faculty Recruitment, c/o Gary D. Fullerton, PhD, Professor and Chief, Radiological Sciences Division, University of Texas HSCSA, 7703 Floyd Curl Dr, San Antonio, TX 78284-7800. The University of Texas HSCSA is an equal opportunity/affirmative action employer.

DIAGNOSTIC RADIOLOGIST NEEDED in GROWING MW CITY

18 physician radiology group, income potential in the top 5%, 13 weeks vacation/CME, partnership opportunity. Premier radiology group seeks a BC/BE radiologist to join a rapidly expanding practice. Full range of diagnostic radiology services with state-of-the-art equipment, including high field and open M.R.I units, DEXA, and teleradiology. Join 18 BC colleagues providing expertise in all areas of radiology. A fellowship in one of the following areas is required: Neuroradiology Interventional, Neurointerventional or Mammography.

Call Barb Kennington, 1-800-765-3055
ID#: 6574RA, Fax: 314-726-3009
E-mail: bkenning@cejka.com
Visit our website: www.cejka.com

STAFF RELIEF, INC.
Continuity in Radiology

OPPORTUNITIES PERMANENT & LOCUM TENENS

Staff Relief, Inc., has immediate openings for Radiologists nationwide. Must be Board Certified or Board eligible. If you are interested in locum tenens or permanent placement fax your CV to 713-956-6847 or e-mail to Misty@StaffRelief.com

New Positions Added Daily

If you are seeking a Radiologist please call 1-800-996-7828. We have many Board Certified, Fellowship trained radiologists available for locum tenens and permanent opportunities.

NEURORADIOLOGY FACULTY POSITION—The Neuroradiology/Interventional Neuroradiology Division of the Department of Radiology at the University of Vermont/Fletcher Allen Health Care is recruiting a new faculty member in diagnostic neuroradiology at the assistant professor level. The candidate must be Board certified in diagnostic radiology with completion of a minimum of 1 year of training in neuroradiology in an ACGME-accredited program and be CAQ certified or eligible. The candidate must be familiar with all aspects of neuroimaging, including CT, MRI/MRA, CT angiography, myelography and angiography. Candidates with some experience and a strong interest in functional MRI will be preferred. Occasional staffing of interventional neuroradiology will be required, as will be participation in teaching of residents and fellows. Imaging facilities include three recent GE helical CT scanners, one GE 1.5T MRI scanner and another one currently being installed with perfusion/diffusion imaging and spectroscopy capability, two standard angiography suites and a soon-to-be installed state-of-the-art biplane neurointerventional angiography suite. The candidate will be expected to participate in research in collaboration with other neuroscience services. Eligibility for Vermont medical licensure is required. Women and minority candidates are encouraged to apply. The deadline for receipt of applications is Tuesday, August 31, 1999. Interested applicants should forward their CV to and contact Lotfi Hacein-Bey, MD, Director, Diagnostic and Interventional Radiology, University of Vermont College of Medicine, FAHC-Patrick 107, 111 Colchester Ave, Burlington, VT 05401. Telephone 802-656-3592, fax 802-656-4822, e-mail *Lotfi.Hacein-Bey@vtmednet.org*. Fletcher Allen Health Care and the University of Vermont are equal opportunity/affirmative action employers.

WEST TEXAS-EXCELLENT RADIOLOGY OPPORTUNITY—Midland is a community of approximately 100,000 people in West Texas with a surrounding area of 150,000. Seven radiologists at two hospitals seek additional radiology support and expertise. We currently have three MR scanners, three helical CT scanners and two modern angio suites. There is an outpatient imaging facility and an established women's imaging center which includes on-site ultrasound and a stereotactic breast biopsy system. The women's imaging center, ultrasound practice and one MR scanner are ACR certified. We seek a body imaging fellowship-trained individual with a desire to complement our busy US/CT/MR practice and expand the mammography program. A second fellowship-trained interventionalist to assist with an established interventional radiology practice is also required. The group will consider a salaried or part-time position with no call responsibilities for an individual interested in mammography only. These are 2-year to partnership track positions with eight weeks vacation. Midland is a safe and clean community. There are good private schools, many church groups, warm climate and traffic is never a problem. There is a new, convenient airport with commercial jet service to anywhere in the country. Please contact us or forward your CV to Marlon D. Hughes, MD, 4 Dunblane, Midland, TX 79707, phone 915-685-1580 (work), 915-694-3150 (home), *mdhughesmd@msn.com*.

DEPARTMENT OF VETERANS AFFAIRS MEDICAL CENTER, ST. LOUIS, MO—Is seeking a part-time Board-certified diagnostic radiologist. The medical center is a 300-bed, dual division, tertiary care hospital with large outpatient department. Skills in general radiography, ultrasound, CT, neuroradiology and MRI with some angiography and interventional experience are desired. The VAMC offers good working conditions, competitive salary and excellent benefits in a moderately sized metropolitan area. Interested candidates should send CV to VAMC, Attn: Nancy Lauermann (O5JB), #1 Jefferson Barracks Dr, St. Louis, MO 63125. Phone 314-894-6620. EOE.

THE NEURORADIOLOGY SECTION AT THE UNIVERSITY OF ALABAMA AT BIRMINGHAM—Is recruiting two Board-certified neuroradiologists (CAQ certified) to join four neuroradiologists. Coverage for UAB Hospital, VAH and Kirklin Clinic includes 24,000 procedures annually, teaching house staff and research. The radiology department in the medical center has 4 GE CT/I helical scanners, and 4 MRI scanners: two GE Signa 1.5T, one Siemens Expert 1T and one GE Signa 1T; and one biplane Siemens Neurostar angiography room. Contact Dr Robert Stanley, Department of Radiology, University of Alabama at Birmingham, Birmingham, AL 35233; phone 205-934-9577, fax 205-934-8110. UAB is an equal opportunity employer.

RADIOLOGIST—Excellent opportunity awaits you to serve our nation's veterans at the VA Medical Center in Alexandria, LA. Board-certified/eligible. Special pay incentives. Generous federal employees benefits. EOE. Contact Lillian Cavin, MD, at 318-473-0010 x 2329.

RADIOLOGIST, PORTLAND, OR—Our well-established eight-member group has an immediate opening for a Board-certified radiologist with additional training in body imaging or interventional radiology. Other fellowship training considered. We anticipate the position to lead to partnership in 2 to 3 years. We practice at a major central city hospital with a large pediatric program and a Level I trauma center. Salary and benefits are competitive. Send CV to Blaine Kozak, MD, or fax to 503-413-2554. Call 503-413-4032 or e-mail *bkozak@lhs.org*.

SEEKING A BOARD CERTIFIED RADIOLOGIST—To join a progressive multi-hospital group practice in beautiful western Maryland. All modalities including '98 GE Horizon 1.5T MRI and Digital Siemens Angio Suite. Interventional training or experience preferred. Excellent compensation toward partnership. Contact Jong Kim, MD, Sacred Heart Hospital, Radiology Department, 900 Seton Dr, Cumberland, MD 21502, phone 301-723-5133.

FELLOWSHIP-TRAINED MUSCULOSKELETAL RADIOLOGIST—Sought for progressive, high-quality practice in the Pacific Northwest. Radia Medical Imaging is a 40+ radiologist group in the Seattle/Everett area which staffs several hospital systems and one multispecialty clinic. Our focus is on subspecialty practice. We also own and operate a series of well-established outpatient offices. The Seattle area is consistently rated as one of the top areas of the country to live and work, with an abundance of outdoor recreation, a progressive metropolitan area and a robust economy. If you are seeking an equitable group focused on the future, forward your CV to Mark Churchill, Radia Medical Imaging, 728 134th St SW, Ste #120, Everett, WA 98204. Fax 425-297-6250 or e-mail *mchurchill@radiax.com*. For more information on our practice, visit our website at *www.radiax.com*.

NUCLEAR MEDICINE—Portland, OR. Northwest Permanente, PC, a physician-managed multispecialty group serving over 440,000 members of Kaiser Permanente in the Northwest has an excellent opportunity in the Portland area for a radiologist, Board-certified or eligible in nuclear medicine. Our program in Oregon and Washington offers a collegial and professionally stimulating environment in one of the most successful managed care systems in the country, plus a quality lifestyle in the Northwest. In addition, we provide a competitive salary and benefit package which includes a generous retirement program, sabbatical leave, professional liability coverage and more. Please forward CV to N.M. Clark, Director, Professional Resources, Northwest Permanente, PC, 500 NE Multnomah, Ste 100, Portland, OR 97232-2099. EOE.

NEURORADIOLOGIST/ASSISTANT PROFESSOR—Medical University of South Carolina Radiology Department: Opening for fellowship-trained neuroradiologist beginning Fall 1999, to complete group of three neuro faculty, one neuro fellow. There are four CT scanners (two multi-slice) and four up-to-date MRI scanners; 22 full-time radiologists, 26 residents and four fellows; includes College of Medicine appointment as assistant professor. Submit CV by August 30, 1999 to Jeremy W.R. Young, MD, Professor and Chairman, c/o Melanie Jackson, MUSC Radiology Department, 169 Ashley Ave, PO Box 250322, Charleston, SC 29425. Women and minorities encouraged to apply.

NEURORADIOLOGIST—The Veterans Affairs Pittsburgh Healthcare System seeks to add a neuroradiologist to its eight-physician imaging group at a state-of-the-art tertiary referral center affiliated with the University of Pittsburgh. Board certification, fellowship training and CAQ certification or eligibility required. Position entails about two-thirds neuro (angio and imaging), one-third general radiology, and teaching opportunities with house staff and students. Located in Pittsburgh's culturally rich East End. Flexible start date. Please reply with CV to Frank Allen Mino, MD, Radiology (132X-U), VA Pittsburgh Healthcare System, University Dr, Pittsburgh, PA 15240; fax 412-688-6856, e-mail *fmino26702@aol.com*. EOE.

VA SIERRA NEVADA HEALTH CARE SYSTEM, RENO, NV—Is actively recruiting for a full-time Board-certified radiologist with interventional and/or MRI skills. Reno is located in the foothills of the Sierra Nevada mountains and offers a wide variety of outdoor sports, recreational and cultural activities. Nevada has no state income tax. Interested and qualified candidates are requested to send their CV to Human Resources Management Service (05), VA SNHCS, 1000 Locust St, Reno, NV 89520 or fax 775-328-1754. For further questions, please call Beth Rottmann, Human Resources Management Service, at 775-328-1252 or Dr James Hecker, Acting Chief, Diagnostic Imaging Service, at 775-328-1444. Equal opportunity employer.

RADIOLOGY—The University of Wisconsin Medical School has a full-time faculty position available as of July 1, 1999, for an assistant professor in musculoskeletal radiology. Applicants must be Board certified and fellowship training in musculoskeletal radiology preferred. The musculoskeletal section has six faculty members and two fellows in a subspecialty practice, which includes musculoskeletal plain film examinations, extremity and spine CT and MR imaging, spine and joint injections and extremity ultrasound. The institution has three spiral CT scanners and four 1.5T GE MR magnets with one of the mag-

Paediatric Diagnostic Imaging & Paediatric Neuro-Imaging

CLINICIAN SCIENTISTS

The Hospital for Sick Children, affiliated with the University of Toronto in Canada, is one of the largest paediatric teaching hospitals in the world. It serves as a tertiary referral centre for Canada, and accepts worldwide referrals. The Department of Diagnostic Imaging is one of the world's busiest paediatric radiology departments, performing approximately 110,000 studies per year. It has strong subspecialty programs in Cardiac and Interventional Radiology, and Neuroradiology.

A health care, teaching, and research centre dedicated exclusively to children; affiliated with the University of Toronto.

The Department of Diagnostic Imaging at the Hospital for Sick Children has immediate openings for a Clinician Scientist in Body Imaging and a Clinician Scientist in Neuro-Imaging. Recent acquisition of state-of-the-art MR imaging technology, PACS, and planned installation of Magnetoencephalography (MEG) later this year will provide an exciting work environment.

Candidates should have experience in developing and managing a clinical and research program with proven research experience. The Diagnostic Imaging role will require technical and academic excellence in Ultrasound, Body MR, Digital imaging or interest in another subspecialty along with completion of a fellowship in Paediatric Radiology. The Diagnostic Neuro-Imaging position calls for technical and academic achievements in MRI, especially functional MRI or MEG, as well as completion of a fellowship in Neuroradiology. All candidates may be required to complete radiology certification examinations in Canada (FRCP). Salary and benefits are competitive.

Applicants should submit their curriculum vitae, along with three references, by July 31, 1999, to: **Paul Babyn, M.D., Department of Diagnostic Imaging, The Hospital for Sick Children, 555 University Avenue, Toronto, Ontario, M5G 1X8 Canada** *The University of Toronto encourages applications from qualified women and men, members of visible minorities, aboriginal peoples and persons with disabilities. In accordance with Canadian immigration requirements, this advertisement is directed firstly to Canadian citizens and permanent residents.*

University of Toronto

THE HOSPITAL FOR SICK CHILDREN

nets dedicated to extremity and spine imaging by the section. Spine and sports medicine are particular strengths of the institution. Cover letter and resume should be made in application to Patrick Turski, MD, Professor and Chairman, Department of Radiology E3/311, Clinical Science Center, 600 Highland Ave, Madison, WI 53792-3252. Unless confidentiality is requested in writing, information regarding the applicants must be released upon request. Finalists cannot be guaranteed confidentiality. An equal opportunity/affirmative action employer.

THE SECTION OF NEURORADIOLOGY IN THE DEPARTMENT OF RADIOLOGY AT THE CLEVELAND CLINIC FOUNDATION—Is offering 2 full-time staff positions due to rapid growth of their practice. Candidates should be Board-certified radiologists who have completed a fellowship, preferably two years, in an accredited neuroradiology program, and who are CAQ certified or eligible. A strong background in academic radiology, cerebral angiography, myelography, CT, MR and MR angiography is required. (Clinical interest in functional MR is particularly valuable.) The neuroradiology section provides a well-balanced team atmosphere with existing expertise in pediatric neuroradiology, interventional neuroradiology and three PhD level staff physicists and two (PhD and masters level) biostatisticians. A research center with a large commitment to vascular disease is available for basic investigations in interventional neuroradiology; clinical research protocols for all facets of neurointervention are already in place. Applications will be accepted until positions are filled. For more information, please contact Thomas J. Masaryk, MD, Section Head, Neuroradiology, Department of Radiology, Hb-6, 9500 Euclid Ave, Cleveland, OH 44195; e-mail *masaryk@ccisd2.ccf.org*. Equal opportunity/affirmative action employer.

FACULTY POSITIONS—In abdominal, pediatric, pediatric interventional, neurointerventional and thoracic radiology. The Department of Radiology at Indiana University School of Medicine is pleased to announce the availability of tenure track faculty positions. Candidates must be Board certified in diagnostic radiology and have fellowship training. Responsibilities will include clinical care, teaching and research. Salary and academic rank will be commensurate with experience and qualifications. Interested applicants should send their curriculum vitae to Dr Mervyn Cohen, Chairman, Department of Radiology, Indiana University Hospital Room 0663, 550 N University Blvd, Indianapolis, IN 46202-5253; or e-mail *jamriley@iupui.edu*. Indiana University is an equal opportunity/affirmative action employer.

RADIOLOGIST-OPENINGS IN NORTH CAROLINA, SOUTH CAROLINA AND NEW MEXICO—Community-based outpatient imaging centers need BC radiologists for state-of-the-art imaging centers; one facility is a full-service center, the others are MRI and CT. Monday through Friday, no call and no weekends, excellent compensation and benefits. Send CV to HR Manager, 3295 River Exchange Dr, Ste 270, Norcross, GA 30092, fax CV to 770-300-0429, or, for immediate information, call Mark Rooney at 800-849-3713.

Positions Sought

BOARD CERTIFIED—Experienced radiologist with recent formal MRI training and full year of imaging fellowship desires partnership in west, northwest, or southwest United States. Basic interventional. Voice: 310-454-3363.

LOOKING—For PGY II or III position in diagnostic radiology starting July 1, 1999. Please call 617-720-2711.

Fellowships

THE DEPARTMENT OF RADIOLOGY OF THE BRIGHAM AND WOMEN'S HOSPITAL-HARVARD MEDICAL SCHOOL—Offers 1 or 2-year fellowship positions in the following areas: 1) cardiovascular and interventional, 2) neuroradiology, 3) abdominal, 4) abdominal interventional, 5) magnetic resonance, 6) women's imaging, 7) oncoradiology, 8) chest, 9) bone, 10) nuclear medicine, 11) computer science, 12) mammography, 13) EW. For more information please send curriculum vitae specifying your area of interest to Steven E. Seltzer, MD, Chairman, Department of Radiology, Brigham and Women's Hospital, 75 Francis St, Boston, MA 02115. Harvard Medical School and Brigham and Women's Hospital are equal opportunity, affirmative action employers.

INDIANA UNIVERSITY SCHOOL OF MEDICINE FELLOWSHIPS—The Department of Radiology at Indiana University in Indianapolis offers fellowships in abdominal imaging, breast imaging, chest imaging, musculoskeletal imaging, neuroradiology, nuclear medicine, pediatric radiology, and vascular and interventional radiology. Indiana has a 40-member teaching faculty, state-of-the-art equipment, a large clinical practice (over 400,000 patient examinations per year), and active research. For more information please visit our web site at *www.indyrad.iupui.edu*. Must obtain license to practice medicine in the state of Indiana. Grant (award) type/term/amount: competitive; 1-2-years. Department funding, contact Kathie Pedersen, Indiana University Hospital 0279, 550 N University Blvd, Indianapolis, IN 46202-5253; telephone 317-274-1840, fax 317-274-1848, e-mail *kmpeders@iupui.edu*. Deadlines: n.a. Key words: abdominal imaging, breast imaging, chest imaging, musculoskeletal imaging, neuroradiology, nuclear medicine, pediatric radiology, vascular and interventional radiology. Award amount key: n.a. Links: go to RFP/A.

FELLOWSHIPS AT THE UNIVERSITY OF ROCHESTER SCHOOL OF MEDICINE—The Department of Radiology at the University of Rochester Medical Center has openings for fellowships in pediatric radiology, body imaging, neuroradiology, angiography and interventional radiology, and musculoskeletal radiology for July 2000. Strong Memorial Hospital is a tertiary care teaching facility performing 195,000 radiologic procedures/year in a single location. Please direct your inquiry and send your curriculum vitae to Arvin E. Robinson, MD, Chair, Department of Radiology, Box 648, University of Rochester Medical Center, Rochester, NY 14642-8648; phone 716-275-2733. The University of Rochester is an equal opportunity employer.

NEURORADIOLOGY FELLOWSHIP POSITION FOR JULY 2000—A 1 or 2-year neuroradiology fellowship accredited by the ACGME. Training includes all aspects of neuroradiology, head and neck radiology and participation in interventional neuroradiology procedures. A one-month elective away is offered in pediatric neuroradiology or interventional for those in the 2nd-year. The hospital has state-of-the-art equipment: 1) three helical GE CT scanners, 2) two GE 1.5T Signa MR scanners, echospeed on one scanner and plans to upgrade to echospeed on the other, and 3) new biplane Toshiba neuroangio-graphy unit. The outpatient center has an echospeed 1.5T Signa MR scanner with plans for addition of another MR scanner and helical CT scanner. There are five full-time neuroradiology, three PhD physicists and three visiting research faculty. The neuroradiology section conducts many research projects, including those in functional MRI. Research facilities include small and large animal surgical suites, chemistry, physiology, and physics laboratories. In addition, a 2.0T, 30cm bore MRI animal scanner is available in the NMR Medical Center Laboratory. Direct inquiries to Henry Wang, MD, PhD, Department of Radiology, University of Rochester Medical Center, 601 Elmwood Ave, Box 648, Rochester, NY 14642; phone 716-273-4133, fax 716-473-4861, e-mail *henry_wang@urmc.rochester.edu*. The University of Rochester is an equal opportunity employer.

MEMORIAL SLOAN-KETTERING CANCER CENTER, DEPARTMENT OF RADIOLOGY—Offers fellowship positions. Body imaging (1-year, 5 positions) fellowship provides extensive experience in body CT, body MRI and ultrasound, including imaging of chest/abdomen/pelvis/extremities in adult and pediatric patients. State-of-the-art equipment includes six CT scanners, three 1.5T MRI scanners, and six ultrasound units. Director: David Panicek, MD. Breast imaging (six months, plus six months of body imaging; 5 positions) provides comprehensive training in all aspects of breast diagnosis (mammography, sonography, MRI, screening and diagnosis) and intervention (including ultrasound and stereotactic biopsy). Director: David Dershaw, MD. Other fellowships include nuclear medicine (2-years; contact Steven Larson, MD, at MSKCC), and combined New York Presbyterian/MSKCC fellowships in neuroradiology (2-years; contact Michael Deck, MD, at NYP) and vascular/interventional radiology (1-year; contact Thomas Sos, MD, at NYP). Excellent opportunities for research exist at this Cornell University Medical College affiliate, with competitive salary and benefits. Request brochure and application from David Panicek, MD, Department of Radiology, Memorial Sloan-Kettering Cancer Center, 1275 York Avenue, New York, NY 10021; e-mail *panicekd@mskcc.org*. *http://www.mskcc.org*. An equal opportunity employer.

MAYO CLINIC—The Mayo Clinic, Department of Radiology, Rochester, MN, has an unanticipated opening for a fellowship beginning June

26, 1999. There is the potential for a fellowship position in the following areas: nuclear medicine, thoracic imaging and musculoskeletal imaging. Address correspondence to Thomas E. Hartman, MD, Department of Radiology, Mayo Clinic, Rochester, MN, 55095.

MAYO CLINIC—The Mayo Clinic, Department of Radiology, Rochester, MN, has unanticipated openings for fellowships beginning July 1, 2000. There is the potential for fellowship positions in the following areas: angiography/interventional radiology, nuclear medicine, abdominal imaging, thoracic imaging and musculoskeletal imaging. Address correspondence to Thomas E. Hartman, MD, Department of Radiology, Mayo Clinic, Rochester, MN 55905.

NEURORADIOLOGY FELLOWSHIP—Mallinckrodt Institute of Radiology has an unexpected opening for a fellowship position starting July 1, 2000, with clinical, research and teaching duties. This ACGME accredited program is staffed by 10 sub-specialized neuroradiologists who cover both adult and pediatric hospitals. Applicant must be Board certified and must have completed their residency in radiology by starting date. Interested candidates may contact Daniel K. Kido, MD, Neuroradiology Section, Mallinckrodt Institute of Radiology, Washington University School of Medicine, 510 S Kings Highway Blvd, St. Louis, MO 63110; phone 314-362-5950, fax 314-362-4886.

NEURORADIOLOGY FELLOWSHIP, UNIVERSITY OF MICHIGAN—Due to expansion of our program, the University of Michigan at Ann Arbor is opening two new neuroradiology fellowship positions. One position each is available starting July 1999 and July 2000. For more information, please contact Dr. Gebarski at 734-936-4484. (*gebarski@umich.edu)*

A 6-MONTH OPEN MRI FELLOWSHIP - SAN FRANCISCO BAY AREA—Potential to join radiology group after fellowship. Currently three radiologists reading for three open magnets; soon to expand to five open magnets. Competitive pay and benefits. Please fax CV to 510-784-1142 attn Peter Rothschild, MD.

BODY IMAGING FELLOWSHIP—University of Vermont/Fletcher Allen Health Care, Burlington, VT. One-year fellowship position in body imaging available at University of Vermont commencing July 2000. The fellowship program is based at Fletcher Allen Health Care, a 500-bed tertiary-care teaching hospital offering the full range of medical and surgical specialty care and a Comprehensive Cancer Center (as designated by NCI). The fellowship has excellent exposure to all facets of imaging including body CT, ultrasound (including obstetric, pediatric, and vascular ultrasound), and body and musculoskeletal MRI. Extensive experience in CT and ultrasound-guided interventional procedures is also part of the training. Equipment includes three GE Hi-Speed helical CT scanners, two state-of-the-art GE MR units, eight US rooms with GE or Acuson equipment, and PACS/3D workstations. The Medical Center offers a collegial environment, and Burlington is truly one of the best small cities in the United States. FACH is an equal opportunity/affirmative action employer. Please address all inquiries to: Robert K. Zeman, MD, Professor and Chairman, Dept of Radiology, Fletcher Allen Health Care, MCHV Campus-Patrick 113, 111 Colchester Ave, Burlington, VT 05401; 802-656-3592.

BODY AND BREAST IMAGING FELLOWSHIPS—William Beaumont Hospital has seven positions for body imaging fellowships beginning July 2000. Two of these positions are combined body imaging/mammography. The duration of fellowship is 1 year and includes training and extensive experience in sectional body imaging and vascular ultrasound. The combined mammography fellowship would include 6 months of breast imaging. Participation in ongoing programs of research and publication are encouraged. The division has eight radiologists and three physicists devoted to body imaging, as well as physics of CT/ultrasound and MRI. Equipment available includes five spiral CT scanners, three Vision MRI units and 10 state-of-the-art ultrasound. Applicants must be Board eligible with strong recommendation. An interview is required. Please contact Ali Shirkhoda, MD, Department of Diagnostic Radiology, William Beaumont Hospital, Royal Oak, MI 48073. You may check the website at *www.beaumont.edu* or call 248-551-1001 for the application.

THORACIC IMAGING FELLOWSHIP, UNIVERSITY OF MIAMI—The Department of Radiology, University of Miami School of Medicine, Miami, FL, offers a 1-year fellowship in comprehensive thoracic imaging to begin July 1, 2000. The department is based at Jackson Memorial Hospital, a 1600-bed primary and tertiary care center with outstanding clinical opportunities. Facilities include a new outpatient center (opened 1998) with state-of-the-art equipment, a dedicated breast health center, and an MR research magnet. Rotations in breast imaging may be incorporated into the fellowship experience. Research participation is actively encouraged. Interested candidates should contact Joel Fishman, MD, PhD, Department of Radiology, Jackson Memorial Hospital, West Wing 279, 1611 NW 12th Ave, Miami, FL 33136 (*jfishman@mednet.med.miami.edu*)

NONINVASIVE CARDIOVASCULAR IMAGING FELLOWSHIP-CLEVELAND CLINIC FOUNDATION—The Section of Cardiovascular Imaging (Division of Radiology) announces a 1-year noninvasive cardiovascular imaging fellowship position for 1999 (July 1, 1999 - June 30, 2000) to interested and qualified BC/BE radiologists. This fellowship emphasizes integrated diagnostic imaging of acquired and congenital diseases of the heart and thoracic vasculature using noninvasive tomographic techniques (MRI and helical CT with gated sub-second acquisition capabilities). Extensive exposure to cardiovascular MRI (over 900 cases/year) is included. Direct all correspondence to Richard D. White, MD, (Head, Section of Cardiovascular Imaging), Division of Radiology: Hb-6, Cleveland Clinic Foundation, 9500 Euclid Ave, Cleveland, OH 44195, 216-444-2740.

THE UNIVERSITY OF MASSACHUSETTS MEDICAL CENTER—Offers fellowship positions in neuroradiology, vascular/interventional and body imaging/MRI. The University of Massachusetts includes a medical school and a 388-bed hospital and trauma center located 40 miles west of Boston. The radiology department performs approximately 200,000 exams per year. State-of-the-art equipment includes two vascular/interventional, two CT and two 1.5Tesla MRI units. The positions include teaching of medical students and residents with opportunities for research and conference attendance. The neuroradiology and vascular/interventional fellowships are approved by ACGME. For information, contact John Knorr, DO, for neuroradiology, Ducksoo Kim, MD, for vascular/interventional, and Ashley Davidoff, MD, for body imaging at University of Massachusetts Medical Center, Department of Radiology, 55 Lake Ave N, Worcester, MA 01655; 508-856-2215.

NEURORADIOLOGY FELLOWSHIP POSITION—The Department of Radiology, Section of Neuroradiology, Emory University School of Medicine has an opening for a 2nd-year fellowship position beginning July 1, 1999. The fellowship year will consist of both clinical and research opportunities in general neuroradiology, pediatric neuroradiology, ENT and interventional neuroradiology. Equipment includes seven high field MRI units, including DWI, PWI, fMRI and MR spectroscopy, seven CT scanners and three neuroangiographic suites. Interdepartmental conferences and research collaboration are conducted with neurology, neurosurgery and otolaryngology. Contact Patricia A. Hudgins, MD, Director, Neuroradiology, Emory University School of Medicine, Department of Radiology/Neuroradiology, 1364 Clifton Rd NE, Atlanta, GA 30322; phone 404-712-4583. Emory University is an equal opportunity/affirmative action employer.

BODY IMAGING—The Department of Radiology, University of Iowa Hospitals and Clinics, Iowa City, IA, offers a 1-year fellowship in body imaging. We currently are accepting applications for July 2000 and July 2001. The Division of Diagnostic Radiology consists of 50 attending staff, including the Body Imaging Section, consisting of eight staff physicians. Their primary interest is adult body imaging: GI and GU fluoroscopy and contrast studies, CT, US, MRI, mammography, and image-guided biopsy and drainage. Candidates have protected time for research/academic activities and gain experience using our state-of-the-art scanners. Experience in anorectal, laparoscopic and endo-sonographic ultrasound procedures are provided. Candidates must have completed an accredited diagnostic radiology residency program and be certified or eligible for certification by the American Board of Radiology. Women and members of minority groups are encouraged to apply. Interested applicants should respond to Bruce P. Brown, MD, Department of Radiology, The University of Iowa Hospitals and Clinics, 200 Hawkins Drive, Iowa City, IA 52242. The University of Iowa is an affirmative action/equal opportunity employer.

VASCULAR AND INTERVENTIONAL RADIOLOGY—The Department of Radiology of the University of Pennsylvania Medical Center (HUP) has an unexpected opening in its six-fellow ACGME-accredited program starting July 1, 2000. Fellows perform the entire spectrum of vascular and interventional procedures, including arteriography, arterial interventions, biliary procedures, interventional GU and GI, and a wide variety of dialysis and venous access procedures. State-of-the-art interventions such as aortic stent grafts, TIPS, uterine fibroid embolization and chemoembolization are integral to our practice, as are CTA and MRA. Typically, there are two residents, two medical students and a vascular access PA on the service at HUP. We also utilize the Children's Hospital of Philadelphia, the Veterans Medical Center of Philadelphia, and the Presbyterian Hospital (a part of the UPMC) for training and clinical practice. Currently, we have three angio rooms at HUP, soon to be four rooms. Research is encouraged with specific allotted time and ample lab facilities. Contact David B. Freiman, MD, or Gwen Gilbert at Interventional Radiology, 1 Silverstein, 3400 Spruce St, Philadelphia, PA 19104 or 215-662-6839 or -3040.

BODY IMAGING FELLOWSHIP-JULY 1, 2000—The University of Colorado Health Sciences Center, Denver, CO, has an unexpected fellowship opening in body imaging commencing July 2000. The 1-year program has a total of four body imaging fellows who rotate through University Hospital in MRI, CT and ultrasound (including fetal ultrasound at the Prenatal Diagnosis Center on campus), and at the Denver Veterans' Administration Hospital. The program provides extensive training in all aspects of body cross sectional imaging and considerable experience in interventional procedures guided by ultrasound and CT. State-of-the-art ultrasound, CT and MRI equipment are available at all practice sites. Address inquiries to Dr Scott Evans, Department of Radiology, University of Colorado Health Sciences Center, Box C277, 4200 E 9th Ave, Denver, CO 80262. Telephone 303-372-6195, fax 303-372-6626.

THE DEPARTMENT OF RADIOLOGY AT GEORGETOWN UNIVERSITY—Seeks candidates for fellowships in musculoskeletal imaging, to begin in both 1999 and 2000. The fellow will participate in resident teaching, interdisciplinary conferences, and the clinical MRI service. There are excellent opportunities and resources for clinical musculoskeletal and MRI research. Contact Lawrence Yao, MD, MRI, 2nd flr CCC Bldg, Georgetown University Medical Center, 3800 Reservoir Rd NW, Washington, DC 20007. e-mail *yaol@gunet.georgetown.edu*, fax 202-784-3862, phone 202-784-5469.

Practices for Sale

EXCELLENT INCOME OPPORTUNITY—Radiology practice for sale in central California. Excellent location across from district hospital. Mammography, diagnostic imaging, MRI, CT and ultrasound. Terms available to qualified buyer. Call 970-259-3822 or mail letters of interest to PO Box 932, Sunset Beach, CA 90742.

Practices Wanted

BOARD-CERTIFIED RADIOLOGIST—Interested in purchasing a practice. Open to all areas for the right opportunity; prefer West Coast. Confidentiality a must. Please reply to Box R-110.

Radiology Business Information

Radiology, a monthly journal devoted to clinical radiology and allied sciences, is owned and published by

The Radiological Society of North America, Inc (RSNA)
820 Jorie Boulevard
Oak Brook, IL 60523-2251 USA
(630) 571-2670 • FAX (630) 571-7837
RSNA Link *http://www.rsna.org*

Delmar J. Stauffer, *Executive Director and Business Manager for Publications*

■ JOURNAL BUSINESS

Send new manuscripts to the address given in the Publication Information for Authors.

Correspondence concerning accepted or published material should be addressed to

Anthony V. Proto, MD–Editor, *Radiology*
Radiology Editorial Office • 1001 East Broad Street
Suite 310 • Richmond, VA 23219
(804) 644-5667 FAX (804) 644-5672
e-mail: *proto@rsna.org*

■ COPYRIGHT AND PERMISSIONS

■ PHOTOCOPYING

Authorization to photocopy items for internal or personal use, or the internal or personal use of specific clients and educators, is granted by RSNA, provided that the appropriate fee is paid directly to Copyright Clearance Center, Inc (CCC), 222 Rosewood Dr, Danvers, MA 01923 (phone 978-750-8400; FAX 978-750-4744).

Consent for photocopying does not extend to copying for general distribution, resale, or advertising and promotional purposes, or for creating new collective works. Permission for the latter categories may be sought by writing to the Permissions Coordinator, RSNA Publications, Oak Brook, IL (address above).

■ SUBSCRIPTION INFORMATION

The nonmember subscription rate for the USA is $215.00 per year; for outside USA, $260.00 (includes postage). (Air freight is available; rates are furnished on request.) Residents who are members of the RSNA may subscribe to **both** *Radiology* and *RadioGraphics* for a special rate of $80.00 (for North American addresses; residents from outside North America, add $60.00 for postage). Single copies are $25.00 (air freight, $11.00). Orders for subscriptions, remittances, and questions about subscriptions should be sent to

RSNA Subscriptions Department
820 Jorie Boulevard
Oak Brook, IL 60523-2251 USA
(630) 571-7873
FAX (630) 571-7837
e-mail: *subscrib@rsna.org*

■ CHANGE OF ADDRESS

The Post Office will not forward your journal to a new address. To avoid missing any issues, you must notify us of a change in address. At least 5 weeks before you move, please send (*a*) your **new address,** with zip code, and (*b*) your **current mailing label** with your old address to the address above.

■ MISSING ISSUES AND BACK COPIES

Claims for copies lost in the mail are allowed within 90 days of issue. Claims are not allowed for issues lost as a result of insufficient notice of change of address. To replace a missing issue or order a back copy contact RSNA Subscriptions Department at the address above. Back copies cost $25.00 (air freight, $11.00).

■ REPRINTS

The first footnote on the first page of each *Radiology* article contains the name and address of the author who answers requests for reprints. For reprint orders of 100 or more, contact

(continued)

The page containing advertising information (Advertisers' Index) may be located by consulting the Departments section in the Table of Contents.

RSNA DEPARTMENT TELEPHONE NUMBERS

Accounting	(630) 571-7812
Advertising	(630) 571-7817
Copyrights and Permissions	(630) 571-7829
Executive	(630) 571-7866
Learning Center	(630) 368-3753
Meetings	(630) 571-7850
Membership	(630) 571-7873
Office of Research	(630) 368-3756
Permissions	(630) 571-7829
Program	(630) 571-7874
Research and Education Foundation	(630) 571-7816
Reprints	(610) 250-7244
Subscriptions	(630) 571-7873
Syllabus sales	(800) 272-2920
Main telephone	(630) 571-2670
FAX	(630) 571-7837

Radiology Reprints
1991 Northampton St
Easton, PA 18042-3189 USA
(610) 250-7244

For reprints of advertisements, contact the Advertising Production Manager (address under Advertising).

■ MICROFORM

Radiology is available in microfilm and microfiche from

University Microforms International
300 N Zeeb Road
Ann Arbor, MI 48106 USA
(800) 521-3044

■ INDEXES

Radiology is included in the *RSNA Index to Imaging Literature,* a 3-year cumulative subject and author index of *Radiology* and 41 radiologic journals, available for $35.00 per copy (air freight, $11.00). Subscribers to the Journal receive the index free of charge. *Radiology* is indexed in *Current Contents/Clinical Medicine,* available from the Institute for Scientific Information, and *Index Medicus,* available from the National Library of Medicine.

■ BOOK REVIEWERS AND BOOKS FOR REVIEW

Any person who would like to help in reviewing books for *Radiology* should contact

Richard A. Szucs, MD, Book Review Editor
Radiology Editorial Office
1001 E Broad St
Suite 310
Richmond, VA 23219

Publishers wishing to have books reviewed should send them to the same address.

■ PUBLISHERS' ROW

As a service to readers and colleagues in medical publishing, *Radiology* publishes a list of current imaging publications of interest to radiologists and allied scientists. Complete addresses and phone numbers of participating publishers are included. Publishers' Row is featured quarterly, in the March, June, September, and December issues. For information on publishing a list, contact Nancy Osborne at RSNA Publications at the Oak Brook address.

■ ADVERTISING

The advertising policy appears on the Advertisers' Index of each issue. Questions about advertising and billing, advertising contracts, and insertion orders and requests for media kits should be addressed to

James F. Drew, *Director of Advertising*
RSNA Publications
820 Jorie Boulevard
Oak Brook, IL 60523-2251 USA
(630) 571-7819
FAX (630) 571-7837

Questions about advertising production should be addressed to:

Pat Hollingsworth, *Advertising Production Manager*
RSNA Advertising Department
820 Jorie Boulevard
Oak Brook, IL 60523-2251 USA
(630) 571-7818
FAX (630) 571-7837

■ CLASSIFIED ADVERTISING

As a service to readers, *Radiology* accepts classified advertising, and every effort is made to ensure that the ads are relevant to the practice of radiology. For more details on the classified advertising policy and procedures, see the Classified Advertising section in each issue (consult the Departments section in the Table of Contents for page number) or contact the Advertising Production Manager (address under Advertising).

CHANGE OF ADDRESS FORM

Please allow 90 days for change to take effect

Name: ____________________

Previous Address

Address: ____________________

____

____

City/State/Zip: ____________________

New Address

Address: ____________________

____

____

City/State/Zip: ____________________

Mail to:
RSNA Subscriptions Department • 820 Jorie Boulevard • Oak Brook, IL 60523-2251 USA **FAX:** (630) 571-7837

RSNA®

RSNA Executive Offices • 820 Jorie Boulevard
Oak Brook, IL 60523 • (630) 571-2670

Bulletin Board

July 1999

✓ **RSNA Plans IHE Year 1 Symposium at Annual Meeting**

✓ **RSNA '99-A Smoke Free Meeting**

✓ **1999 Camp RSNA**

■ The RSNA has announced it will sponsor an inaugural 3-day slate of presentations on healthcare information systems integration from December 1-3, 1999. The IHE Year 1 Symposium will be held as a "Meeting within RSNA '99". The Symposium program coincides with the IHE Year 1 Demonstration. Together, these events represent a major evolution in the focus on medical information technology at the RSNA annual meeting. The Symposium will offer a full slate of tutorials, workshops, papers, lectures, and discussion groups addressing topics related to the integration of information systems in healthcare. The Year 1 Symposium and Year 1 Demonstration will be held alongside *info*Rad, in the Lakeside Center of McCormick Place.

■ Attendees will be glad to see the promotion of RSNA '99 as a smoke-free meeting. While no-smoking regulations have existed in the past, they were difficult to enforce due to the sheer size of the meeting. This year, the only smoking areas will be outside of the building and the no-smoking regulation will be strictly enforced. RSNA asks that exhibitors and attendees alike help enforce the no-smoking rule by directing persons who wish to smoke outside the building. These areas will be clearly marked for ease of use.

■ For the second year, ACCENT on Children's Arrangements, Inc, has planned a great activity center for the RSNA attendees' children—Camp RSNA. ACCENT is a nationally recognized professional child care company organized to provide onsite children's activities in a nurturing, safe, educational environment. Camp RSNA will be located in the McCormick Place Complex. Daily activity themes have been planned, as well as arts and crafts activities, active games, and special guests. Camp RSNA is sure to be great fun for all ages and will be available from November 28 to December 3, 1999. Space is limited so you'll want to register early. For details, please call ACCENT on Children's Arrangements at 504 524-1226 or e-mail inquiries to Production@accentoca.com.

■ The following is a list of applicants for RSNA membership, published as provided by the bylaws of the Society. Society members are asked to review these names. Should a member have a question concerning the eligibility of an applicant, within 30 days of the publication of this list, the member should request that the applicant's membership be withheld pending investigation and reconsideration by the Membership and Credentials Board. Please mark your signed letter of protest "Confidential" and address it to Secretary-Treasurer, RSNA, 820 Jorie Blvd, Oak Brook, IL 60523. Please note that listed here are only the locations in which the prospective members reside and the counselors for those areas.

ARIZONA
Counselor: Pamela J. Lund, MD
Todd A. Steinberg, MD, Scottsdale

ARKANSAS
Counselor: Thomas W. Koonce, MD
Cheryl L. Green, MD, Little Rock

CALIFORNIA
Counselors: Deborah S. Ablin, MD
Kenneth W. Chin, MD
Nancy A. Ellerbroek, MD
Gary R. Hansen, MD
Eric W. Olcott, MD
Dolores H. Pretorius, MD
Osman M. Ratib, MD, PhD, Los Angeles
Robert E. Lundahl, MD, San Francisco
Michael P. Norton, MD, Carmichael

KANSAS
Counselor: Peter E. Schloesser, MD
Debbie A. Desilet-Dobbs, MD, Wichita

LOUISIANA
Counselor: David R. Hunter, MD
Pensinee Tontiplaphol, MD, Metairie

MASSACHUSETTS
Counselor: Robert H. Cleveland, MD
Claudia S. Reynders, MD, Hamilton

MINNESOTA
Counselor: David H. Stephens, MD
Mark S. Collins, MD, Rochester

MISSISSIPPI
Counselor: Margaret T. Hatten, MD
Jani L. Purvis, MD, Brookhaven

MISSOURI
Counselors: David P. Diemer, MD
G. David Dixon, MD
James R. Farkas, MD, Sedalia

NEW YORK
Counselors: Mario A. Grosso, MD
David M. Panicek, MD
Arthur J. Segal, MD
Stuart G. Katz, MD, Center Moriches

PENNSYLVANIA
Counselors: Nilima Dash, MD
Kathryn A. Evers, MD
John E. Madewell, MD
Bruce C. Turner, MD, PhD, Philadelphia

TEXAS
Counselors: Karl A. Glastad, MD
Chandra S. Katragadda, MD
Timothy W. Lillick, MD
Christine A. Keesling, MD, San Antonio
Jacque R. Wettlaufer, MD, San Antonio

VERMONT
Counselor: Howard J. Mindell, MD
Roshan Sivagnanam, MD, Rutland

MEXICO
Counselors: Jose H. Arredondo, MD
Manuel A. Cabal, MD
Jose M. Cardoso, MD
Miguel A. Carrillo, MD
Ramon R. Ponte, MD
Francisco J. Reynaga-Garcia, MD
Oscar Perez Rocha, MD, Guadalajara
Gerardo L. Villegas, Jr, MD, Mexico

CANADA

ALBERTA
Counselor: Thomas E. Ackerman, MD
Lee S. Paskar, MD, Edmonton

NOVA SCOTIA
Counselor: Robert A. Vandorpe, MD
Allister J. McGowan, MD, Tide Head

CORRESPONDING
Manuel M. Arboleda, MD, Philippines
Miguel Blanco, MD, Spain
Shira H. De Bie, MD, Netherlands
Bernard P. Duparc, MD, France
Stephen J. Esler, MBBS, Australia
Peter E. Goodwin, MD, Australia
Jan-Willem C. Gratama, MD, Netherlands
Stephane Guth, MD, France
Loi M. Hoang, MD, Vietnam
Volker W. Hoffmann, MD, Germany
Paul A. Hulse, MD, United Kingdom
Ian Levin, MBChB, South Africa
Jianhai Li, MS, Peoples Republic of China
Claes G. Lonnroth, MD, Norway
Yukino Machida, MD, Japan
Mariano Magallanes, MD,Argentina
Chrit T. Moonen, PhD, France
Bruno Morgan, MD,United Kingdom
Tito L. Mundim, MD,Brazil
Shuichi Murashima, MD,Japan
Xiwen Nan, MD, Peoples Republic of China
Norihisa Nitta, MD,Japan
Benu Pankaj, MBBS, MD,India
Jeong Mi Park, MD, South Korea
Horst N. Schaefer, PhD, Germany
Alexandra Seybold-Epting, MD, Germany
Ajai K. Sharma, MBBS, MD,India
Jorge M. Sibina, MD, Peru
Masaki Takahashi, MD, Japan
Francisco M. Tardaguila, MD, Spain
Orlando Valls, MD, DSc, Cuba
Henrique Vilaca-Ramos, MD, Portugal
Louwerens D. Vos, MD, Netherlands

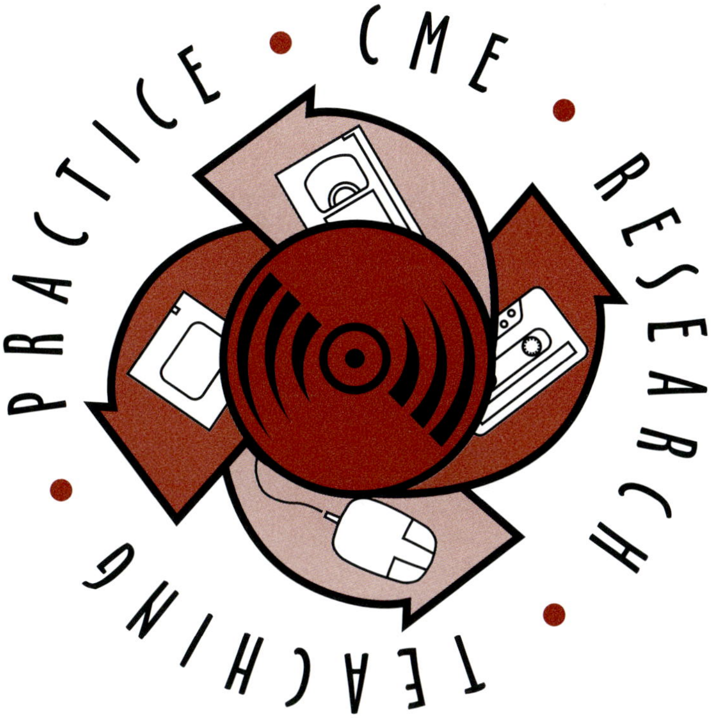

Thoracic

Learning Center Resources

July 1999

RSNA® | Radiological Society of North America
Founded in 1915

Featured Topics

- **Venous Duplex Ultrasound and Thrombolysis in Venous and Pulmonary Occlusive Disease**
- **Digital Chest Radiography: Techniques and Clinical Applications**
- **Diagnosis, Work-up, and Staging of Lung Cancer**
- **Thoracic Manifestations of AIDS**

New Service

The entire 1998–1999 Learning Center Resources Catalog is now available on the RSNA *Link*, the Web site of the Radiological Society of North America, on the Internet.

You can reach us through the World Wide Web (WWW) by entering the uniform resource locator: http://www.rsna.org

We invite you to browse through the catalog, search for specific courses of interest, then simply order via our fax or 800 phone number.

Detach and store for your future use.

The following 21 Thoracic titles are now available in the Learning Center Resources Library. All videotapes are available for purchase or rental (U.S., Canada, and Mexico). All video programs may be purchased in NTSC, PAL, and SECAM television standards. Slides and audiotapes are available for purchase only.

For more information, call or fax the RSNA Learning Center Resources at the numbers listed on the order form. To order by mail, use the form on the back.

NEW!

Venous Duplex Ultrasound and Thrombolysis in Venous and Pulmonary Occlusive Disease *RSP 694*

Steven C. Rose, MD
Charles P. Semba, MD

Venous Duplex Ultrasound

Steven C. Rose, MD

This presentation reviews the use of duplex US for diagnosis of lower-extremity acute deep venous thrombosis and chronic venous insufficiency, and upper-extremity central venous occlusive disease. *Learning objectives:* (1) To understand the role of duplex US for diagnosis of venous disease given specific common clinical presentations. (2) To learn the contributions made by each of the family of duplex techniques and the significance of specific diagnostic findings.

Thrombolysis in Venous and Pulmonary Occlusive Disease

Charles P. Semba, MD

This presentation reviews current management strategies for deep vein thrombosis (DVT) and pulmonary emboli, including use of low-molecular-weight heparin and thrombolytic therapy. The pathophysiology and techniques for endovascular treatment of upper- and lower-extremity DVT, including superior vena cava syndrome, and life-threatening pulmonary emboli are discussed. The role of adjunctive angioplasty, stents, and mechanical thrombectomy devices and the indication for temporary vena caval filters are also reviewed. *Learning objective:* To understand the indications, risks, and benefits of endovascular therapy versus standard anticoagulation in treating symptomatic DVT and pulmonary emboli. *(C.P.S. is a scientific consultant to Abbott Laboratories, Abbott Park, Ill.)*

VHS *M$140, N$160*

Not available in slide/audiotape

NEW!

Digital Chest Radiography: Techniques and Clinical Applications *RSP 715*

Denise R. Aberle, MD
Stuart S. Sagel, MD

This program covers the techniques for acquisition of digital chest radiographic images and their pragmatic use in everyday clinical practice. These methods currently are equivalent or superior diagnostically to the best screen-film combinations. Digital techniques allow the capture and ultimate display of all the disparate densities in the lungs and mediastinum. Chest radiographic images may be acquired digitally by using (1) photostimulable phosphor plates or (2) direct sensors (amorphous selenium or silicon). With storage phosphor imaging, there is no need for significant modification of current radiographic equipment. The density of the final image is set independently of the original exposure level, obviating repeat radiographs when phototiming is not available, as with bedside chest radiography. It also enables reliable and excellent images of nonstandard projections (eg, lateral and decubitus views). Either a video monitor or laser film can be used as the viewing medium. Networking of digital image data allows rapid simultaneous viewing of images at multiple sites, enhancing timely patient care. Direct digital radiography sensors have greater quantum efficiency than the storage phosphor plates and do not require stimulation for image readout, thus eliminating a source of image noise. *Learning objective:* To become familiar with the newer digital chest radiographic techniques, including their advantages and limitations.

125 slides/2 audiotapes *M$205, N$225*
VHS *M$205, N$225*

M/N = Member/Nonmember prices
To order call (800) 272-2920 or FAX (630) 990-9958
(Outside U.S., phone (630) 990-9941)

Clinical Applications and Utility of High-Resolution CT in Lung Disease *(1993)* *RSP 430*
W. Richard Webb, MD
Nestor L. Müller, MD, PhD
Stephen J. Swensen, MD

181 slides/2 audiotapes M$205, N$225
VHS M$205, N$225

Imaging and Staging of Masses in the Chest *(1993)* *RSP 438*
Colleen J. Bergin, MD, ChB
Herrman I. Libshitz, MD
Philip Costello, MD

215 slides/2 audiotapes M$205, N$225
VHS M$205, N$225

Clinical Applications of Chest CT: A Critical Appraisal of Conventional, High Resolution, and Spiral CT *(1994)* *RSP 456*
Janet E. Kuhlman, MD
Elias A. Zerhouni, MD

VHS M$205, N$225
Not available in slide/audiotape

Looking Anew at Pulmonary Pattern Recognition: "Splitters" and "Lumpers" *(1994)* *RSP 457*
David S. Feign, MD
James C. Reed, MD

VHS M$205, N$225
Not available in slide/audiotape

Acute Pulmonary Embolism: Diagnostic and Therapeutic Considerations *(1995)* *RSP 480*
Alan H. Matsumoto, MD

71 slides/audiotape M$140, N$160
VHS M$140, N$160

Helical and Electron-Beam Imaging of the Thorax: Clinical Applications *(1995)* *RSP 481*
Patrick F. Sheedy II, MD
David P. Naidich, MD

VHS M$205, N$225
Not available in slide/audiotape

Radiology of the Critically Ill Patient in the Intensive Care Unit *(1995)* *RSP 482*
Irena Tocino, MD

VHS M$205, N$225
Not available in slide/audiotape

Radiologic Critical Care: Clinically Focused *(1995)* *RSP 483*
Daniel A. Henry, MD

VHS M$140, N$160
Not available in slide/audiotape

Embolization and Interventional Thoracic Procedures *(1995)* *RSP 484*
John R Haaga, MD
George G. Hartnell, FRCR, FACC

VHS M$205, N$225
Not available in slide/audiotape

Mycobacterial and Fungal Diseases in the Chest in Normal and Immunocompromised Patients *(1995)* *RSP 485*
Helen T. Winer-Muram, MD
Sanford A. Rubin, MD

VHS M$205, N$225
Not available in slide/audiotape

Diagnosis and Treatment of Pulmonary Embolism *(1996)* *RSP 527*
Rolf W. Gunther, MD

56 Slides/audiotape M$140, N$160
VHS M$140 N$160

Nonvascular Thoracic Interventional Procedures *(1996)* *RSP 528*
Gerhard B. Adam, MD

48 Slides/audiotape M$140, N$160
VHS M$140, N$160

Blunt Chest Trauma: Pulmonary Contusions and Traumatic Diaphragmatic Rupture *(1996)* *RSP 529*
Charles F. Mueller, MD

114 Slides/audiotape M$140, N$160
VHS M$140, N$160

Blunt Chest Trauma: Extrapleural Air and Acute Traumatic Aortic Injury *(1996)* *RSP 530*
John H. Harris, Jr, MD, DSc

104 Slides/audiotape M$140, N$160
VHS M$140, N$160

Thoracic Venous Anatomy *(1996)* *RSP 531*
Marvin H. Chasen, MD

VHS M$140, N$160
Not available in slide/audiotape

High-Resolution CT of the Lung Parenchyma: A Practical Approach *(1996)* *RSP 532*
W. Richard Webb, MD
Nestor L. Müller, MD, PhD

VHS M$205, N$225
Not available in slide/audiotape

Interventional Thoracic Radiology *(1996)* *RSP 581*
Curtis A. Lewis, MD

102 Slides/audiotape M$140, N$160
VHS M$140, N$160

Diagnosis, Work-up, and Staging of Lung Cancer *(1997)* *RSP 593*
Robert D. Pugatch, MD

61 Slides/audiotape M$140, N$160
VHS M$140, N$160

Thoracic Manifestations of AIDS *(1997)* *RSP 595*
Georgeann McGuinness, MD
Philip C. Goodman, MD

129 Slides/audiotape M$205, N$225
VHS M$205, N$225

Place Stamp Here

TO: RSNA LEARNING CENTER RESOURCES
PO BOX 5316
OAK BROOK, IL 60522-5316
USA

FOLD HERE

PRACTICE • CME • RESEARCH • TEACHING

Order Form

You may mail or fax this form. To fax your order, dial 630-990-9958. Please print.

☐ *RSNA Member* ☐ *Nonmember*

NAME ______________ RSNA MEMBER # (REQUIRED FOR MEMBER PRICING) ______________

ADDRESS ______________

CITY ______________ STATE/COUNTRY ______________ ZIP ______________

PHONE ______________ FAX ______________

Order Information (for purchase and rentals)

Course Number	*Showing Date (Rental Only)*	*Format (Purchase Only)*	*Price*

FOLD HERE

Check one:

☐ *Rental*

☐ *Purchase*

Subtotal ______

Shipping & Handling ______

Total ______

Shipping Information

United States

1 program = $7

2 – 3 programs = $10

4 – 6 programs = $20

7 programs and up = $30

Rental

No charge for shipping to renter. Renter is responsible for return shipping charges.

Outside United States

1 program = $10

Each additional program = $5

All orders from outside the U.S. must be prepaid, either by MasterCard, VISA, AMEX or Diners Club or a check in U.S. dollars, drawn on a U.S. bank.

Payment Information

☐ Payment by check

☐ Payment by credit card: ☐ VISA ☐ MasterCard ☐ AMEX ☐ Diners Club

CARD NUMBER ______________

SIGNATURE ______________ EXP. DATE ______________

For faster service, phone (800) 272-2920 or fax (630) 990-9958 (Outside U.S., phone (630) 990-9941).

TEAR HERE

Foto-Comm Corporation is the distributor of RSNA Learning Center Resources.

RAD 7.99

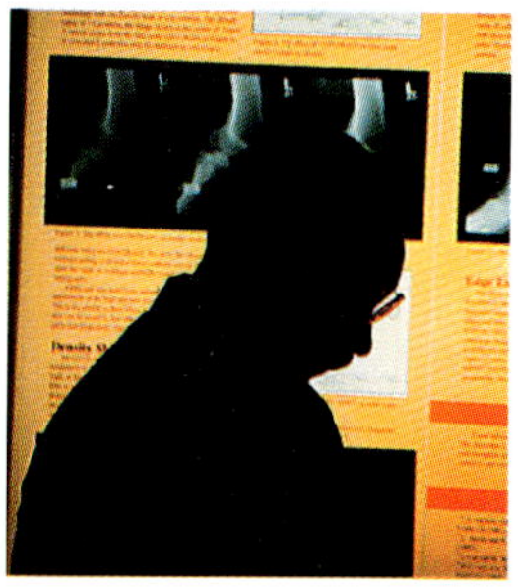

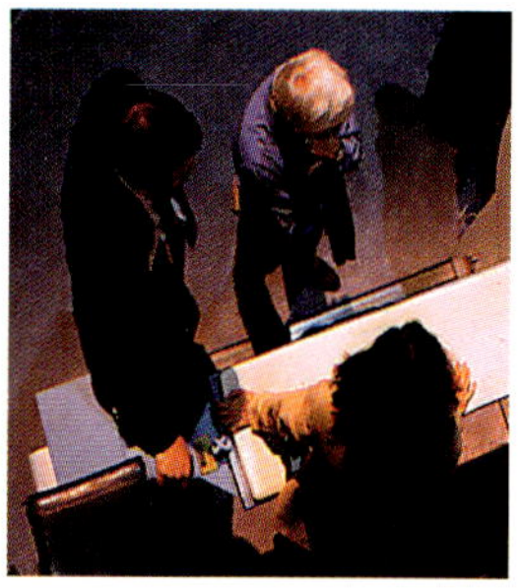

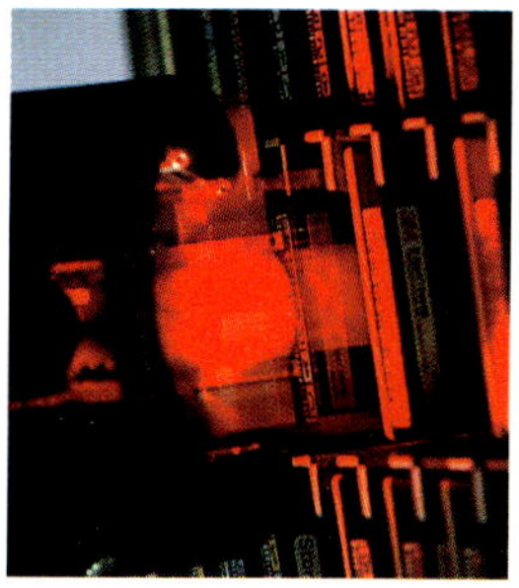

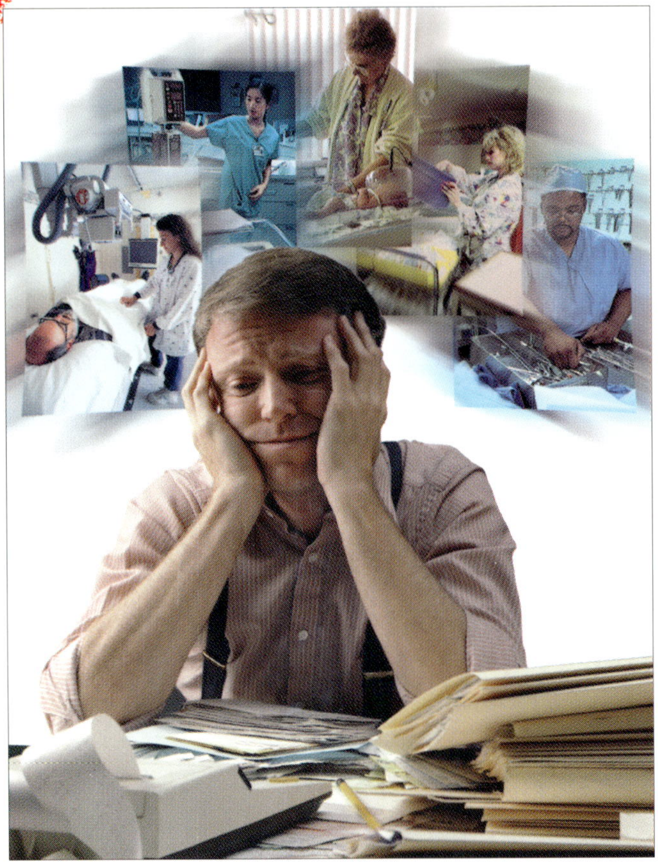

August 1999
Volume 212 • Number 2
RADLAX 212 (2) 297–604

Radiology

From the Editor | 297
Special Communication | 298
Perspectives | 301
Editorial | 305
State of the Art | 307
Neuroradiology | 325
Diagnosis Please:Case 17 | 357
Case 13 Answer | 359
Vascular and Interventional Radiology | 365
Genitourinary Imaging | 395
Special Report | 401
Emergency Radiology | 423
Gastrointestinal Imaging | 431
Experimental Studies | 459
Ultrasonography | 493
Nuclear Medicine | 499
Pediatric Imaging | 515
Musculoskeletal Imaging | 527
Signs in Imaging | 541
Breast Imaging | 543
Computer Applications | 551
Thoracic Imaging | 561
Cardiac Imaging | 573
Technical Developments | 579
Letters to the Editor | 601

THE RADIOLOGICAL SOCIETY OF NORTH AMERICA

RSNA® **85th Scientific Assembly and Annual Meeting**
Chicago, November 28–December 3, 1999

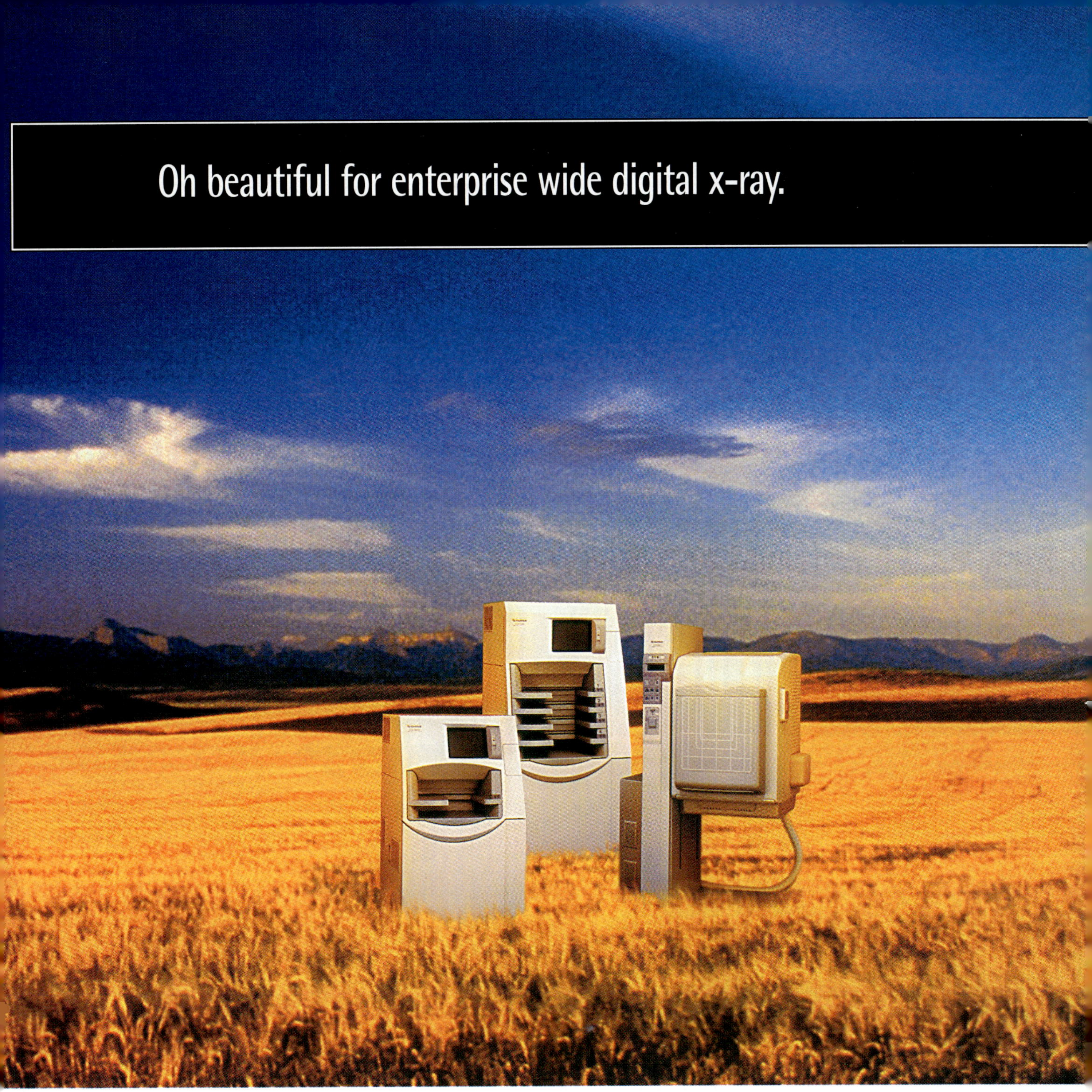
Oh beautiful for enterprise wide digital x-ray.

A CENTURY OF RESEARCH & EDUCATION RSNA 1999

Radiological Society of North America
85th Scientific Assembly and Annual Meeting
November 28–December 3, 1999
McCormick Place, Chicago

New Realities in Radiology: Multidisciplinary Strategies for Compliance

Associated Sciences Program at RSNA 1999

Workshop: Saturday, Nov. 27, 1999 10:15 am - 4:00 pm, McCormick Place South

Refresher Courses: Sunday, Nov. 28, through Friday, Dec 3, 1999

Credits: 5 hours

Welcome and Introduction
10:15 am
Samuel L. Hissong, MD, Chair, Associated Sciences Consortium and Committee
JoAnn Belanger, RN, CRN, Coordinator, Associated Sciences Consortium

Keynote Presentation
10:30 am - 11:50 am
Compliance, Audits and Radiology: The Art of Survival (AHRA)
Karol Handrahan RT(R)

Break
11:50 am - 12:10 pm

Special Luncheon Program
12:10 - 1:20 pm
Uncle Sam Strikes Back: Medicine in the Enforcement Age (RBMA)
Tom Hoffman

Break
1:20 - 1:30 pm

Panel Presentation
1:30 - 4:00 pm
(Break 2:45 pm - 3:00 pm)
Practicum (SROA)
Andrew Woods, Esq.
Gadi Weinreich, Esq.
Bruce Freid, Esq.

AAPM/RSNA Basic Physics Lecture for the Radiologic Technologists: Digital Imaging: What You Need to Know Now and What You Need to Know Next
Organized by
Gerald A. White, Jr., MS
3:00 - 4:30 pm
1½ hours credit

Refresher Courses

(Each Refresher Course is approved for 1½ hours credit)

Sunday RC 124
Organizational Culture and Health System Change
Sponsored by the Associated Sciences Consortium
Paula Maramonte, MEd, RT(R) (AERS) Coordinator
Cornelius J. Rater, MD (AERS)
Harry J. Granito, MS (RBMA)
Susan K. Snyder, BS, EdD (ASRT)

Monday RC 224
Asset Management for High-Technology Systems
Sponsored by the Associated Sciences Consortium
Chester T. Szerlag, MBA (SROA) Coordinator
Tim Guertin (SROA)
Sheila M. Sferrella (AHRA)
Dennis A. Bair, RT(R)(CV) (AVIR)

Monday RC 324
Economic Implications of Regulatory Change
Sponsored by the Associated Sciences Consortium
DuVonne Campbell (ASRT) Coordinator
Cherrill Farnsworth (AHRA)
Sherry Makely, PhD (ASRT, SNM)
Donna L. Wright, EdD, RT(R) (AERS)

Tuesday RC 424
Managing a Multisite Radiology Network
Sponsored by the Associated Sciences Consortium
Kathryn J. Canny, (RBMA) Coordinator
Larry A. Ranahan, MBA (RBMA) Moderator
Charles Deschamps RT(R)(MR) (SMRT)
Scott Seberg, MS (RBMA)
Chester T. Szerlag, MBA (RBMA)

Wednesday RC 524
Current Challenges in Radiology and Planning and Design
Sponsored by the Associated Sciences Consortium
Morris A. Stein (AIA-AAH) Coordinator
Bill Rostenberg (AIA-AAH)
Jerry W. Froelich, MD (AIA-AAH)
Eliot L. Siegel, MD (AIA-AAH)

Thursday RC 624
Specialized Accreditations: A Cost of Doing Business
Sponsored by the Associated Sciences Consortium
Luann J. Culbreth, MEd, RT(R) (SMRT) Moderator
John Kovelski, RT(R) (SMRT)
Karol Handrahan, RT(R) (SMRT)
Sandra Katanick, RN, RVT (SDMS)
Ronald F. Bernardi, BA, RT(R) (AHRA)

Thursday RC 724
Multidisciplinary Standards for the New Millennium
Sponsored by the Associated Sciences Consortium
Susan S. Weiss, CNMT (SNM-TS) Moderator
William R. Poller, MD (SNM-TS)
Michael R. Bloyd, RT(R), BSN (ASRT)
Sue M. Smith, RT(R)(CV)(M), FAVIR (AVIR)

Friday RC 824
Marketing Radiology: Getting the Message Out
Sponsored by the Associated Sciences Consortium
Ronald F. Bernardi, BA, RT(R) (AHRA) Moderator
Cherrill Farnsworth (AHRA)
Michael R. Favreau (AHRA)

Registration Information

Advance registration for the RSNA Scientific Assembly ends October 29. Onsite registration begins at 12:00 noon on Saturday, November 27, at McCormick Place. RSNA shuttle bus service to McCormick Place will be available beginning at 10:00 am on Saturday. Advance registration is not required for the Saturday workshop; however, to receive continuing education credit you must register.

Advance registration information appears in the July issue of *Radiology*. Brochures are also available from your association or from the RSNA, 820 Jorie Boulevard, Oak Brook, IL 60523-1860. Phone: 630/571-7852.

Registration for the RSNA Scientific Assembly includes registration for the Associated Sciences Workshop. A box lunch will be available for purchase to facilitate your attendance at the workshop. These lunches must be purchased with your advance registration for the RSNA Meeting. **If you wish to purchase a box lunch, please check the appropriate box on the RSNA Advance Registration form and enclose your $11.50 payment.**

If you would like a copy of the published Associated Sciences Proceedings, please call 630/571-7874.

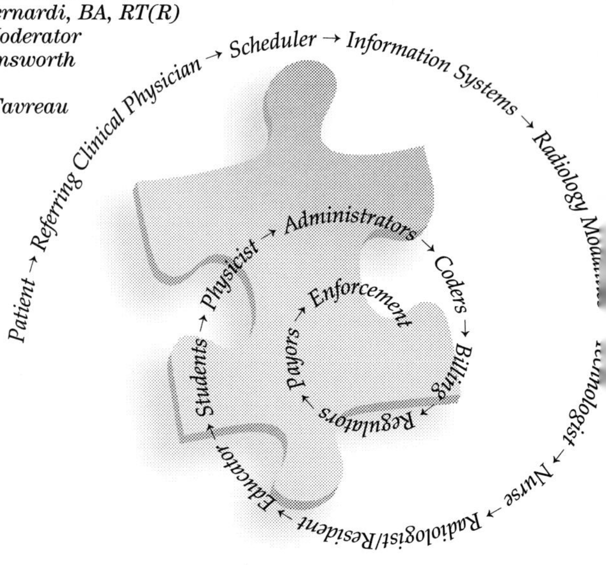

Sponsoring Organizations

- American Healthcare Radiology Administrators (AHRA)
- American Institute of Architects — Academy on Architecture for Health (AIA-AAH)
- American Radiological Nurses Association (ARNA)
- American Society of Radiologic Technologists (ASRT)
- Association of Educators in Radiological Sciences, Inc. (AERS)
- Association of Vascular and Interventional Radiographers (AVIR)
- Radiology Business Management Association (RBMA)
- Society for Radiation Oncology Administrators (SROA)
- Society of Diagnostic Medical Sonographers (SDMS)
- Section for Magnetic Resonance Technologists (SMRT-ISMRM)
- Society of Nuclear Medicine — Technologists Section (SNM-TS)

RSNA® Radiological Society of North America Founded in 1915

820 Jorie Boulevard
Oak Brook, Illinois 60523-1860
630/571-2670 FAX: 630/571-7837
www.rsna.org

Associated Sciences

Radiology

August 1999
Volume 212
Number 2

RSNA®
A monthly journal devoted to clinical radiology and allied sciences, owned and published by THE RADIOLOGICAL SOCIETY OF NORTH AMERICA, INC.
http://www.rsna.org

August 1999
Volume 212 • Number 2

Radiology

A monthly journal devoted to clinical radiology and allied sciences, owned and published by the Radiological Society of North America, Inc.

RSNA

From the Editor

297 *Radiology* 1999: Left-Hand Pages
Anthony V. Proto

Special Communication

298 The Radiological Society of North America 85th Scientific Assembly and Annual Meeting, Sunday, November 28 to Friday, December 3, 1999 McCormick Place, Chicago, Illinois
Seymour H. Levitt

Perspectives

301 The Future of Medicine and Radiology: Part I
Richard M. Friedenberg
Within the next 10 years, clinicians will have to collaborate with a variety of independent and semiindependent practitioners loosely categorized as nonphysician clinicians.

Editorial

305 Old Problems, New Techniques: The Interventional Radiologist and the Lacrimal Apparatus
Jane L. Weissman
The inclination to address epiphora, and other clinical problems, by modifying the existing techniques of interventional radiology is ingenious and important.

State of the Art

307 Imaging of Acute Cerebral Ischemia
Norman J. Beauchamp, Jr, Peter B. Barker, Paul Y. Wang, and Peter C. M. vanZijl
This State of the Art describes the central role of the radiologist and neuroimaging in the diagnosis and subsequent management of acute cerebral ischemia.

Neuroradiology

325 Hyperacute Stroke: Ultrafast MR Imaging to Triage Patients prior to Therapy
Jeffrey L. Sunshine, Robert W. Tarr, Charles F. Lanzieri, Dennis M. D. Landis, Warren R. Selman, and Jonathan S. Lewin
Diffusion- and perfusion-weighted MR imaging can be performed within the time constraints of an acute stroke protocol and provide valuable data to guide critical patient triage and therapeutic decisions.

333 **Acute Cerebral Infarction: Quantification of Spin-Density and T2 Shine-through Phenomena on Diffusion-weighted MR Images**
Jonathan H. Burdette, Allen D. Elster, and Peter E. Ricci
With use of current gradient strengths with *b* values of 1,000 sec/mm^2, T2 (and to a lesser degree spin-density) shine-through effects account for a substantial component of the total MR signal intensity observed on diffusion-weighted images of subacute cerebral infarction, especially beyond 3–4 days.

340 **Moyamoya Disease: Evaluation with Diffusion-weighted and Perfusion Echo-planar MR Imaging**
Ichiro Yamada, Yoshiro Himeno, Tsukasa Nagaoka, Hideaki Akimoto, Yoshiharu Matsushima, Toshihiko Kuroiwa, and Hitoshi Shibuya
Diffusion-weighted and perfusion echo-planar MR imaging are useful methods for evaluating cerebral ischemia in patients with moyamoya disease.

348 **Long-term Angiographic Follow-up of 169 Intracranial Berry Aneurysms Occluded with Detachable Coils**
Christophe Cognard, Alain Weill, Laurent Spelle, Michel Piotin, Lina Castaings, Alain Rey, and Jacques Moret
Despite total occlusion obtained in 148 cases, recurrences were observed in 20 aneurysms (14%).

Diagnosis Please

357 **Case 17**
Noriko Salamon-Murayama, Eric J. Russell, and Barry M. Rabin

359 **Case 13: Polyarteritis Nodosa—Systemic Necrotizing Vasculitis with Involvement of Hepatic and Superior Mesenteric Arteries**
Klaus D. Hagspiel, J. Fritz Angle, David J. Spinosa, and Alan H. Matsumoto
The sensitivity and specificity of angiography in polyarteritis nodosa have been reported to be 89% and 90%, respectively, with a positive predictive value of 55% and a negative predictive value of 98%.

Vascular and Interventional Radiology

365 **Dacryoliths: Nonsurgical Fluoroscopically Guided Treatment during Dacryocystoplasty**
Kai E. Wilhelm, Ulrich Hofer, Hans J. Textor, Thorsten Böker, Holger M. Strunk, and Hans H. Schild
The interventional radiologic procedure we describe should be considered as an alternative to dacryocystorhinostomy in the treatment of dacryolithiasis, and dacryocystorhinostomy can be used in case of failure.

371 **Iliofemoral Arterial Occlusive Disease: Contrast-enhanced MR Angiography for Preinterventional Evaluation and Follow-up after Stent Placement**
Johann Link, Johann C. Steffens, Joachim Brossmann, Joachim Graessner, Stephanie Hackethal, and Martin Heller
Contrast-enhanced MR angiography can enable highly accurate diagnosis of occlusion and stenosis greater than 50% in the iliac and femoral arteries; the patency of stents can be determined, but restenoses within stents may not be detected.

378 **Outcome and Cost Comparison of Percutaneous Transluminal Renal Angioplasty, Renal Arterial Stent Placement, and Renal Arterial Bypass Grafting**
Feiyu Xue, Michael A. Bettmann, David R. Langdon, and Wayne A. Wivell
In our study population, percutaneous transluminal renal angioplasty, percutaneous transluminal stent placement of renal arteries, and renal arterial bypass grafting (RABG) had similar success rates and were equally efficacious for treatment of renovascular hypertension; however, the two percutaneous treatments cost substantially less than RABG.

385 **Secondary Postpartum Hemorrhage: Treatment with Selective Arterial Embolization**
Jean-Pierre Pelage, Philippe Soyer, Danielle Repiquet, Denis Herbreteau, Olivier Le Dref, Emmanuel Houdart, Denis Jacob, Mourad Kardache, Patrick Schurando, Jean-Bernard Truc, and Roland Rymer
Even though retention of gestational products and endometritis are the most frequent causes of secondary postpartum bleeding, angiographic exploration often demonstrates a bleeding artery that is related to previously unsuspected genital tract lesions.

Continued—

Radiology is published monthly by the Radiological Society of North America, Inc, 820 Jorie Boulevard, Oak Brook, IL 60523-2251 (ISSN 0033-8419). Printed in USA. Periodical class postage paid at Oak Brook, Ill, and additional mailing offices. The nonmember subscription rate for the USA is $215.00 per year; for all other countries, $260.00 (includes postage). Information about subscription rates for residents is available on request. (Air freight is available; rates are furnished on request.) Single copies are $25.00 ($36.00 to a non-U.S. address). Notice of missing issues or change of address (include old mailing label and new address) should be sent to RSNA Subscriptions Department, 820 Jorie Boulevard, Oak Brook, IL 60523-2251. Inquiries via e-mail should be directed to *subscrib@rsna.org.* POSTMASTER: Send address correction "changes" to: *Radiology,* RSNA, 820 Jorie Boulevard, Oak Brook, IL 60523-2251.

Claims for copies lost in the mail are allowed within 90 days of the date of issue. Claims are not allowed for issues lost as a result of insufficient notice of change of address.

Membership in the Radiological Society of North America is by formal application. Membership information should be secured from the Executive Director, the Radiological Society of North America, Inc, 820 Jorie Boulevard, Oak Brook, IL 60523-2251. Dues are payable annually in January. In accordance with U.S. postal regulations, $107.50 of active membership dues is allocated to a subscription to *Radiology*.

390 **Postoperative Pelvic Lymphocele: Treatment with Simple Percutaneous Catheter Drainage**
Jae-Kyu Kim, Yong-Yeon Jeong, Yun-Hyeon Kim, Young-Chul Kim, Heoung-Keun Kang, and Ho-Sun Choi
Percutaneous catheter drainage without sclerotherapy is a simple and effective therapeutic method that results in a high success rate in the treatment of a symptomatic lymphocele after radical pelvic lymphadenectomy performed because of uterine malignancy.

Genitourinary Imaging

395 **Role of MR Imaging in the Selection of Patients with Early Cervical Carcinoma for Fertility-preserving Surgery: Initial Experience**
P. Delia Peppercorn, Arjun R. Jeyarajah, Robert Woolas, John H. Shepherd, David H. Oram, Ian J. Jacobs, Peter Armstrong, David Lowe, and Rodney H. Reznek
MR imaging can be used to accurately predict cervical tumor confined to the cervix, which enables patients with early disease who wish to attempt to preserve their fertility to be offered trachelectomy and laparoscopic lymphadenectomy with the understanding that further treatment occasionally may be required.

Special Report

401 **Ovarian Cancer: Comparison of Observer Performance for Four Methods of Interpreting CT Scans**
Patrick J. Fultz, Christina V. Jacobs, W. Jackson Hall, Ronald Gottlieb, Deborah Rubens, Saara M. S. Totterman, Steven Meyers, Cynthia Angel, Giuseppe Del Priore, David P. Warshal, Kelly H. Zou, and David E. Shapiro
Certain interpretative methods, such as the integration of independent readings to form a noninteractive replicated reading, may be helpful for improving observer performance for experienced readers.

411 **TIPS for Prevention of Recurrent Bleeding in Patients with Cirrhosis: Meta-analysis of Randomized Clinical Trials**
Angelo Luca, Gennaro D'Amico, Roberto La Galla, Massimo Midiri, Alberto Morabito, and Luigi Pagliaro
The results of this meta-analysis show that in patients with cirrhosis and previous variceal bleeding, transjugular intrahepatic portosystemic shunt creation is more effective than endoscopic therapy with or without propranolol administration for the prevention of recurrent bleeding but significantly increases the risk of encephalopathy and does not affect survival.

Emergency Radiology

423 **Hemoperitoneum as the Sole Indicator of Abdominal Visceral Injuries: A Potential Limitation of Screening Abdominal US for Trauma**
Kathirkamanathan Shanmuganathan, Stuart E. Mirvis, Caroline D. Sherbourne, William C. Chiu, and Aurelio Rodriguez
Thirty-four percent of patients with abdominal visceral injury following blunt abdominal trauma had no hemoperitoneum at admission, but CT reliably depicted injuries that did not have associated hemoperitoneum.

Gastrointestinal Imaging

431 **Extravasation Detection Accessory: Clinical Evaluation in 500 Patients**
Bernard A. Birnbaum, Rendon C. Nelson, Judith L. Chezmar, and Seth N. Glick
The extravasation detection accessory evaluated in this study demonstrated a sensitivity of 100% (95% CI: 51%, 100%) and a specificity of 98% (95% CI: 96%, 99%) in the detection of clinically important extravasation.

439 **Recurrent Gallbladder Carcinoma along Laparoscopic Cholecystectomy Port Tracks: CT Demonstration**
Corinne B. Winston, June W. Chen, Yuman Fong, Lawrence H. Schwartz, and David M. Panicek
Gallbladder carcinoma can recur in laparoscopic port tracks even if surgical resection of the port sites is performed at subsequent hepatic resection for attempted cure.

445 **Local Extension of Pancreatic Carcinoma: Assessment with Thin-Section Helical CT versus with Breath-hold Fast MR Imaging—ROC Analysis**
Taiji Nishiharu, Yasuyuki Yamashita, Yasuko Abe, Katsuhiko Mitsuzaki, Tadatoshi Tsuchigame, Yoshiharu Nakayama, and Mutsumasa Takahashi
Compared with MR imaging, thin-section CT may have more useful applications in the diagnostic imaging of pancreatic tumor.

453 **Fecal Incontinence: Endoanal US versus Endoanal MR Imaging**
Elena Rociu, Jaap Stoker, Marinus J. C. Eijkemans, W. Ruud Schouten, and Johan S. Laméris
In the current study, the use of endoanal MR imaging findings was superior to the use of endoanal US findings with regard to decisions about the optimal therapy.

Continued—

Experimental Studies

459 **Effects of Superparamagnetic Iron Oxide on Radiofrequency–induced Temperature Distribution: In Vitro Measurements in Polyacrylamide Phantoms and in Vivo Results in a Rabbit Liver Model**
Elmar M. Merkle, S. Nahum Goldberg, Daniel T. Boll, Ajit Shankaranarayanan, Travis Boaz, Gretta H. Jacobs, Michael Wendt, and Jonathan S. Lewin
Our in vitro data suggest that local temperatures can be increased in tissues surrounding a radio-frequency electrode when ablation is performed in the presence of superparamagnetic iron oxide particles.

467 **Infarcted Myocardium in Pigs: MR Imaging Enhanced with Slow-Interstitial-Diffusion Gadolinium Compound P760**
Lucia J. M. Kroft, Joost Doornbos, Rob J. van der Geest, Soraya Benderbous, and Albert de Roos
P760 is a newly designed extracellular contrast agent with improvements over conventional extracellular contrast agents for MR myocardial perfusion imaging.

475 **Delayed Vascular Injury after Single High-Dose Irradiation in the Rat Brain: Histologic, Immunohistochemical, and Angiographic Studies**
Marc W. Münter, Christian P. Karger, Wolfgang Reith, H. Michael Schneider, Peter Peschke, and Jürgen Debus
Vascular changes seem to be major factors that contribute to radiation-induced late effects.

483 **Stent Placement versus Percutaneous Transluminal Angioplasty of Human Carotid Arteries in Cadavers in Situ: Distal Embolization and Findings at Intravascular US, MR Imaging, and Histopathologic Analysis**
Hannu I. Manninen, Heikki T. Räsänen, Ritva L. Vanninen, Pauli Vainio, Mikko Hippeläinen, and Veli-Matti Kosma
Distal embolization was common during both percutaneous transluminal angioplasty and stent placement in situ in the carotid arteries of cadavers, and there was no substantial difference in the severity of distal embolization between the treatments.

Ultrasonography

493 **Assessment of Stenosis: Implications of Variability of Doppler Measurements in Normal-appearing Carotid Arteries**
Vivian S. Lee, Barbara S. Hertzberg, Mark A. Kliewer, and Barbara A. Carroll
We have demonstrated a statistically significant variability in peak systolic velocity and end diastolic velocity along the course of the common carotid artery in patients without visible US evidence of disease.

Nuclear Medicine

499 **Count-based PET Method for Predicting Ischemic Stroke in Patients with Symptomatic Carotid Arterial Occlusion**
Colin P. Derdeyn, Tom O. Videen, Nicholas R. Simmons, Kent D. Yundt, Susanne M. Fritsch, Robert L. Grubb, Jr, and William J. Powers
In this retrospective analysis of St Louis Carotid Occlusion Study data, we have demonstrated that the count-based measurement of oxygen extraction fraction can be used to identify patients at increased risk of ischemic stroke with accuracy similar to that of the quantitative method.

507 **Pediatric Inflammatory Bowel Disease: Assessment with Scintigraphy with ^{99m}Tc White Blood Cells**
Martin Charron, Fernando J. del Rosario, and Samuel A. Kocoshis
In this study, we found high accuracy for scintigraphy with technetium 99m white blood cells in the evaluation of inflammation in children with inflammatory bowel disease.

Pediatric Imaging

515 **Splenic Injury Diagnosed with CT: US Follow-up and Healing Rate in Children and Adolescents**
Kathleen H. Emery, Diane S. Babcock, Andrea S. Borgman, and Victor F. Garcia
There is a clear relationship between the severity of blunt splenic injury in children and adolescents and the time course to US-documented healing; this information may be used to tailor the timing of follow-up imaging.

Continued—

519 **Legg-Calvé-Perthes Disease: MR Imaging Evaluation during Manual Positioning of the Hip—Comparison with Conventional Arthrography**
Diego Jaramillo, Tamara A. Galen, Carl S. Winalski, James DiCanzio, David Zurakowski, Robert V. Mulkern, Patricia A. McDougall, Olga L. Villegas-Medina, Ferenc A. Jolesz, and James R. Kasser
Our data show that MR imaging with use of manual positioning of the hip in an open-configuration magnet system in children with Legg-Calvé-Perthes disease is comparable to conventional arthrography for overall assessment of femoroacetabular relationships (containment and congruency) and detection of hinge abduction.

Musculoskeletal Imaging

527 **Idiopathic Bone Marrow Edema Lesions of the Femoral Head: Predictive Value of MR Imaging Findings**
Bruno C. Vande Berg, Jacques J. Malghem, Frederic E. Lecouvet, Jacques Jamart, and Baudouin E. Maldague
Results from the current study of idiopathic femoral head lesions that show the bone marrow edema pattern at MR imaging demonstrate that precise analysis of the subchondral marrow changes depicted on T2-weighted or contrast-enhanced T1-weighted images helps differentiate irreversible lesions from transient lesions.

537 **Is a Subset of Wrist Ganglia the Sequela of Internal Derangements of the Wrist Joint? MR Imaging Findings**
Khaled I. El-Noueam, Mark E. Schweitzer, Roberto Blasbalg, Aly A. Farahat, Randall W. Culp, Lee A. Osterman, and Amaar Malik
A subset of paraarticular cysts around the wrist may be the sequela of internal derangements.

Signs in Imaging

541 **The Double-Line Sign**
John V. Zurlo
The double-line sign is seen with avascular necrosis (osteonecrosis) on MR images.

Breast Imaging

543 **Breast MR Imaging in Patients with Axillary Node Metastases and Unknown Primary Malignancy**
Susan G. Orel, Susan P. Weinstein, Mitchell D. Schnall, Carol A. Reynolds, Lynn M. Schuchter, Douglas L. Fraker, and Lawrence J. Solin
In this patient population, MR imaging offers potential not only for the detection of a primary ipsilateral breast cancer but also for staging, which may be used to guide treatment planning.

Computer Applications

551 **Breast Cancer: Computer Simulation Method for Estimating Optimal Intervals for Screening**
James S. Michaelson, Elkan Halpern, and Daniel B. Kopans
We developed a computer simulation model of breast cancer growth and spread, and the results of our model suggest that an increase in the frequency of breast cancer screening could lead to substantial reductions in the incidence of metastatic disease and, thus, in the breast cancer death rate.

Thoracic Imaging

561 **Small Pulmonary Nodules: Evaluation with Repeat CT—Preliminary Experience**
David F. Yankelevitz, Rajiv Gupta, Binsheng Zhao, and Claudia I. Henschke
We present one such approach [to observing a nodule], in which we established the usefulness of early repeat CT by demonstrating that growth in a nodule can be reliably detected with repeat CT performed within a clinically acceptable interval.

567 **Lymphocytic Interstitial Pneumonia: Thin-Section CT Findings in 22 Patients**
Takeshi Johkoh, Nestor L. Müller, Heather A. Pickford, Thomas E. Hartman, Kazuya Ichikado, Masanori Akira, Osamu Honda, and Hironobu Nakamura
Lymphocytic interstitial pneumonia is characterized by the presence of ground-glass attenuation, poorly defined centrilobular nodules, and thickening of perilymphatic interstitium.

Continued—

Cardiac Imaging

573 **Composite Graft Replacement of the Ascending Aorta: Leakage Detection with Gadolinium-enhanced MR Imaging**
Rossella Fattori, Benedetta Descovich, Paola Bertaccini, Francesca Celletti, Ilaria Caldarera, Angelo Pierangeli, and Giampaolo Gavelli
MR imaging helped define the morphologic characteristics of the prosthetic graft and the anastomotic sites.

Technical Developments

579 **Submillimeter Three-dimensional Coronary MR Angiography with Real-time Navigator Correction: Comparison of Navigator Locations**
Matthias Stuber, René M. Botnar, Peter G. Danias, Kraig V. Kissinger, and Warren J. Manning
The proximal and middle portions of the left and right native coronary artery system can be reliably depicted with both cardiac and diaphragmatic navigator locations, but the diaphragmatic navigator was objectively found to be superior for distal right coronary artery visualization and left anterior descending artery sharpness.

588 **Lungs in Infants and Young Children: Improved Thin-Section CT with a Noninvasive Controlled-Ventilation Technique—Initial Experience**
Frederick R. Long, Robert G. Castile, Alan S. Brody, Mark J. Hogan, Robert L. Flucke, David A. Filbrun, and Karen S. McCoy
By applying physiologic responses to augmented ventilation, motion-free thin-section CT images of the chest can be acquired noninvasively in the sedated infant or young child at both full lung inflation and deflation.

594 **Bowel Lesions: Percutaneous US-guided 18-gauge Needle Biopsy—Preliminary Experience**
Gareth R. Tudor, Peter M. Rodgers, and Kevin P. West
We found that a diagnostic biopsy can be safely performed percutaneously with an 18-gauge biopsy needle to obtain a satisfactory sample for histologic examination in patients with bowel-wall lesions discovered at US.

598 **Thoracic Duct: Visualization at Nonenhanced MR Lymphography—Initial Experience**
Sanshin Hayashi and Mitsue Miyazaki
MR lymphography with a short echo spacing, three-dimensional, half-Fourier, fast spin-echo sequence can be used to visualize the thoracic duct without use of a contrast agent.

Letters to the Editor

601 **MR Angiography in Acute Pulmonary Embolism**
Mathias Goyen

601 **Reply**
Ashu Gupta and Christopher K. Frazer

601 **CT Reinterpretation**
Thomas J. White, Jr

602 **Reply**
Marc J. Gollub, David M. Panicek, Ariadne M. Bach, and Ronald A. Castellino

Book Reviews

300 **Neuroradiology Companion: Methods, Guidelines, and Imaging Fundamentals. 2nd ed.**
422 **Intraoperative, Laparoscopic, and Endoluminal Ultrasound**
550 **Radiation Protection Dosimetry: A Radical Reappraisal**

Interludes

358 **Swaggering Aorta**
400 **Intestinal Worm**
514 **Patient with a Frog in His Throat**

Departments

603 **Abstracts of Current Literature**
16A **Advertisers' Index**
19A **Announcements and Books, Audiovisual Materials, and Software Received**
2A **Associated Sciences Workshop 1999**
43A **Classified Services**
27A **Continuing Medical Education**
36A **Copyright and Certifications Agreement**
37A **Publication Information for Authors**
31A ***Radiology* Business Information**
41A ***Radiology* Manuscript Categorization Terms**
61A **RSNA Bulletin Board**
15A **RSNA Quick Reference**

RSNA Radiological Society of North America
Founded in 1915

820 Jorie Boulevard
Oak Brook, Illinois 60523-2251
630/571-2670
FAX: 630/571-7837

Quick Reference

RSNA PURPOSE

The purpose of the Radiological Society of North America is to promote and develop the highest standards of radiology and related sciences through education and research. The Society seeks to provide radiologists and allied health scientists with educational programs and materials of the highest quality, and to constantly improve the content and value of these educational activities. The Society seeks to foster closer fellowship among all radiologists and greater cooperation among radiologists and members of other branches of medicine and allied health care professionals.

RSNA OFFICERS FOR 1999

President, **Seymour H. Levitt, MD,** Minneapolis, MN

President-Elect, **C. Douglas Maynard, MD,** Winston-Salem, NC

First Vice-President, **William M. Thompson, MD,** Minneapolis, MN

Second Vice-President, **J. Frank Wilson, MD,** Milwaukee, WI

Third Vice-President, **Stephen Balter, PhD,** New York, NY

Secretary-Treasurer, **David H. Hussey, MD,** Iowa City, IA

Historian, **William R. Eyler, MD,** Beverly Hills, MI

RSNA BOARD OF DIRECTORS FOR 1999

Jerry P. Petasnick, MD, Chairman of the Board, Chicago, IL

David H. Hussey, MD, Secretary-Treasurer, Iowa City, IA

Brian C. Lentle, MD, Liaison for Education, Vancouver, BC

R. Nick Bryan, MD, PhD, Liaison for Publications and Educational Materials, Bethesda, MD

Peggy J. Fritzsche, MD, Liaison for Communications and Corporate Relations, Riverside, CA

Robert R. Hattery, MD, Liaison Designate for Publications and Educational Materials, Rochester, MN

Seymour H. Levitt, MD, President, Minneapolis, MN

C. Douglas Maynard, MD, President-Elect, Winston-Salem, NC

Delmar J. Stauffer, Executive Director

RSNA IMPORTANT TELEPHONE NUMBERS

MAIN TELEPHONE	(630) 571-2670	MEMBERSHIP	(630) 571-7873 e-mail: membersh@rsna.org
FAX	(630) 571-7837	RESEARCH DEVELOPMENT	(630) 368-3756
ACCOUNTING	(630) 571-7812	PROGRAM SERVICES	(630) 571-7874
EXECUTIVE	(630) 571-7866	RESEARCH & EDUCATION FOUNDATION	(630) 571-7816
LEARNING CENTER	(630) 368-3753	ADVERTISING	(630) 571-7817
MARKETING COMMUNICATIONS	(630) 571-7830	CLASSIFIED ADVERTISING	(630) 571-7817
MEETINGS	(630) 571-7850	RSNA LINK	http://www.rsna.org
PERMISSIONS	(630) 571-7829	SUBSCRIPTIONS	(630) 571-7873 e-mail: subscrib@rsna.org

RSNA MEETING DATES AND LOCATIONS

1999 November 28 to December 3
McCormick Place, Chicago

2000 November 26 to December 1
McCormick Place, Chicago

2001 November 25 to November 30
McCormick Place, Chicago

RSNA YEAR-AT-A-GLANCE

September 15, 1999
Third Seed Grant Deadline

September 17–19, 1999
RSNA Board of Directors Meeting

October 1, 1999
Deadline for Non–North American Advance Registration for RSNA Scientific Assembly

October 29, 1999
Deadline for North American Advance Registration for RSNA Scientific Assembly

November 28 to December 3, 1999
RSNA 85th Scientific Assembly and Annual Meeting

January 1, 2000
Call for Scientific Papers, Scientific Exhibits, and *info*RAD Exhibits

January 8, 2000
Deadline for Receipt of all RSNA R&E Foundation Grant Materials

January 15, 2000
First Seed Grant Deadline

February 18–20, 2000
RSNA Board of Directors Meeting

March 1, 2000
Roentgen Centennial Fellow "Preliminary Letter of Interest" Deadline

April 12–13, 2000
R&E Foundation Trustee Meeting

April 15, 2000
Deadline for Submission of Scientific Paper, Scientific Exhibit, and *info*RAD Applications

May 1, 2000
Deadline for Receipt of Editorial Fellowship Applications

May 15, 2000
Second Seed Grant Deadline

June 8–10, 2000
RSNA Board of Directors Meeting

July 1, 2000
Deadline for Receipt of Derek Harwood-Nash Fellowship Application

July 1, 2000
Deadline for Receipt of International Visiting Scholar Application

Advertisers' Index

RSNA Advertising Policy

According to the advertising policy of the Radiological Society of North America, the information describing radiological equipment, products, and services offered by vendors in their advertisements should be ethical, educational, professional, of value in furthering the radiologic evaluation and treatment of patients and furthering the education of the radiologists and allied scientists. The guidelines below should be followed for advertising in RSNA journals.

- All advertising must be directed to radiologic diagnosis, therapy, research, communication and/or to the professional and managerial roles of radiologists and allied scientists. Advertising material should be consistent with the highest standards of professionalism.
- RSNA reserves the right to reject copy which, in its opinion, is not in good taste, is unprofessional, or is inappropriate for a radiology publication, or offers products or services not in the best interest of the patient or the Society. Advertisements that are constructed to resemble the journal's editorial pages will not be accepted in that form.
- Acceptance of advertising does not mean endorsement by RSNA of the products or services advertised, the advertisers, or the claims made.

For media kits and questions about advertising ONLY, contact:

Jim Drew, *Director of Advertising*
RSNA Publications
820 Jorie Boulevard
Oak Brook, IL 60523-2251
(630) 571-2670
FAX (630) 571-7837

For all other RSNA department telephone numbers, see "RSNA Quick Reference"; consult "Departments" in the Table of Contents for page.

American College of Radiology 30A

Bioscan 19A

C.B. Fleet 11A
Catholic Medical Centers 55A

Daniel & Yeager 45A
Diversified Diagnostic Products, Inc 29A, 35A

Franciscan Skemp Healthcare 49A
Fuji Medical Systems IFC–1A

Gammex RMI 9A
GE Medical Systems OBC

Hewlett-Packard 22A–23A, 25A

Interim Physicians 49A

J & C Nationwide 55A

Kaiser Permanente 51A

Locum Medical Group 53A

National University Hospital Singapore 51A

Philips Medical Systems 13A

RadioGraphics 20A
Radiology 34A
RADX 21A
RSNA Associated Sciences 2A
RSNA International Programs 24A
RSNA Learning Center 474, 63A–66A
RSNA *Link* 526
RSNA Membership 26A
RSNA ORD 536
RSNA Resident Membership 17A–18A
RSNA Scientific Assembly and Annual Meeting IBC, 578

Saint Joseph Hospital/Creighton University 57A
Siemens Medical Systems, Inc 7A
Staff Relief, Inc 57A
Staten Island University Hospital 19A

Texas Tech University School of Medicine 47A
Toshiba 4A

U.S. Army Reserve 30A

Vista Staffing Solutions 47A

Which society offers radiology residents the best in radiology at **no charge?**

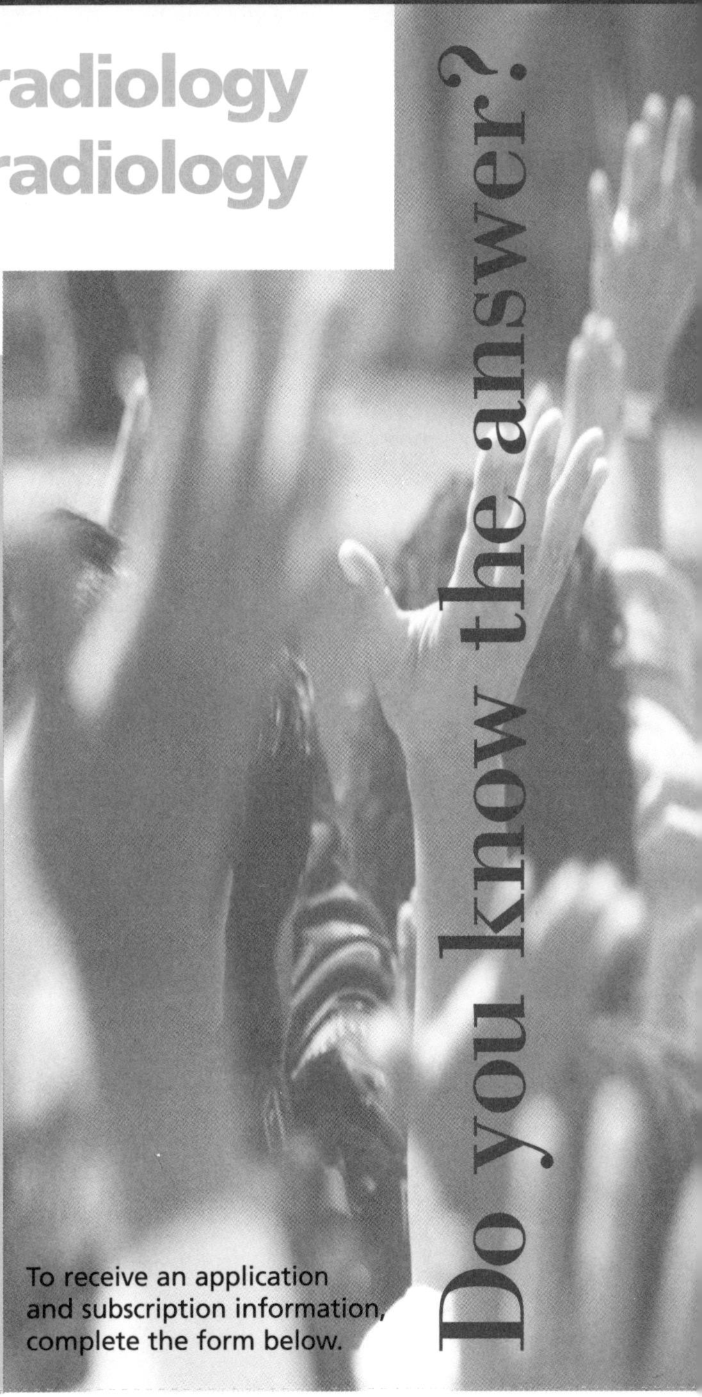

The Radiological Society of North America welcomes radiology residents worldwide by extending **free membership.**

That's right. As a radiology resident actively engaged in a radiological training program, you can benefit from the wealth of educational opportunities available through RSNA:

- **Free admission** to the largest medical meeting in the world—the RSNA Scientific Assembly and Annual Meeting.
- **A highly subsidized subscription rate** of $80 for both RSNA journals–a $325 value.
  Outside North America add $60 for postage.

  Radiology The leading peer-reviewed journal in the field, featuring the latest research in all subspecialties.

  RadioGraphics The peer-reviewed teaching journal investigating the latest news about informatics technology, and featuring scientific exhibits presented during RSNA's Annual Meeting.

You also have the opportunity to learn from and network with the best medical professionals in radiology—RSNA members.

Membership Reply Form

❑ Yes! I would like to receive an application for free membership.

Name

Address (If indicating an institution, please include institution name and department.)

City State Country Zip/Postal Code

Here are the Facts about RSNA

RSNA Scientific Assembly and Annual Meeting

The largest medical meeting in the world.

Professional Attendees	24,248
Technical Exhibits	628
Scientific Exhibits	1,094
Scientific Papers	1,636
Refresher Courses	276
Scientific Sessions	192

Based on 1998 meeting data.

Radiology

The premier peer-reviewed journal in the field of radiology.

296 pages per issue, including:

- Original research
- State-of-the-art reviews
- Editorials
- Abstracts of current literature

More than 600 articles are published annually.

RadioGraphics

The only peer-reviewed journal devoted to scientific exhibits, evolving technology, and continuing education.

- Scientific exhibits from the Scientific Assembly and Annual Meeting
- High-quality, detailed radiologic images
- Opportunity to earn category 1 CME credits*
- Latest in *info*RAD technology
- Imaging and Therapeutic Technology

*Does not apply to residents.

RSNA current membership totals 30,310. The following is a breakdown by status:

Active	17,706
Associate	1,310
Resident/Fellows	4,528
Retired	3,203
Emeritus	8
Corresponding	3,506
Honorary	49

RSNA®
Radiological Society of North America
Founded in 1915
820 Jorie Boulevard
Oak Brook, IL 60523-2251
630/571-2670 FAX: 630/571-7837
www.rsna.org

NO POSTAGE NECESSARY IF MAILED IN THE UNITED STATES

BUSINESS REPLY MAIL
FIRST-CLASS MAIL PERMIT NO. 65 OAK BROOK IL

POSTAGE WILL BE PAID BY ADDRESSEE

RADIOLOGICAL SOCIETY OF NORTH AMERICA
820 JORIE BOULEVARD
OAK BROOK IL 60523-0114

free
membership for residents

Announcements and Books, Audiovisual Materials, and Software Received

Announcements

2nd International Pelvic Floor Imaging Symposium

The Nicolaes Tulp Institute of the University of Amsterdam Academic Medical Centre is sponsoring the 2nd International Pelvic Floor Imaging Symposium on November 5–6, 1999, at the University of Amsterdam, the Netherlands. This symposium is intended for radiologists, urologists, gynecologists, surgeons, gastroenterologists. Organizing committee: Bartram, Rociu, Stoker. For further information, contact the Nicolaes Tulp Institute, University of Amsterdam Academic Medical Centre, Meibergdreef 9, Postbus 23213, 1100 DS Amsterdam, the Netherlands; telephone 31 20 566 8585; fax 31 20 696 3228; e-mail *m.verweij@amc.uva.nl.*

MET 2000

"MET 2000," the International Congress on Multidisciplinary Endovascular Therapy, will be held on January 12–15, 2000, in Rome, Italy. Program director: Rossi. Co-directors: Katzen, Lammer, Odink, Simonetti, Zollikofer. For further information, contact Plinio Rossi, MD, Istituto di Radiologia, Università degli Studi di Roma "La Sapienza," Viale Regina Elena 324, 00161 Rome, Italy; telephone 39 06 446 8587; fax 39 06 445 5602; e-mail *rossi@uniroma1.it; http://www.MET2000.org.*

Books, Audiovisual Materials, and Software Received

Radiology carries a complete listing of all books, CD-ROMs, and other material received by the Radiological Society of North America. If the material is later reviewed, the reviews of books will be printed in *Radiology* and the reviews of CD-ROMs and electronic material will appear in *RadioGraphics*.

Send publications for review to Richard A. Szucs, MD, Book Review Editor, *Radiology* Editorial Office, 1001 E Broad St, Suite 310, Richmond, VA 23219.

Doppler Tissue Imaging Echocardiography. M. A. Garcia-Fernandez, J. Zamorano, J. Azevedo. Hardcover, $98.00; 167 pp, 94 illustrations. ISBN: 84-486-0187-4. New York, NY: McGraw-Hill, 1999.

Lymphatic Drainage of the Skin and Breast: Locating the Sentinel Nodes. Roger F. Uren, John F. Thompson, Robert B. Howman-Giles. Hardcover, $80.00; 196 pp, 76 illustrations. ISBN: 90-5702-410-1. Amsterdam, the Netherlands: Harwood Academic Publishers, 1999.

Practical Radiation Protection and Applied Radiobiology. 2nd ed. Steven B. Dowd, EdD, RT(R), Elwin R. Tilson, EdD, RT(R). Softcover, $34.95; 368 pp, 124 illustrations. ISBN: 0-7216-7523-9. Philadelphia, Pa: Saunders, 1999.

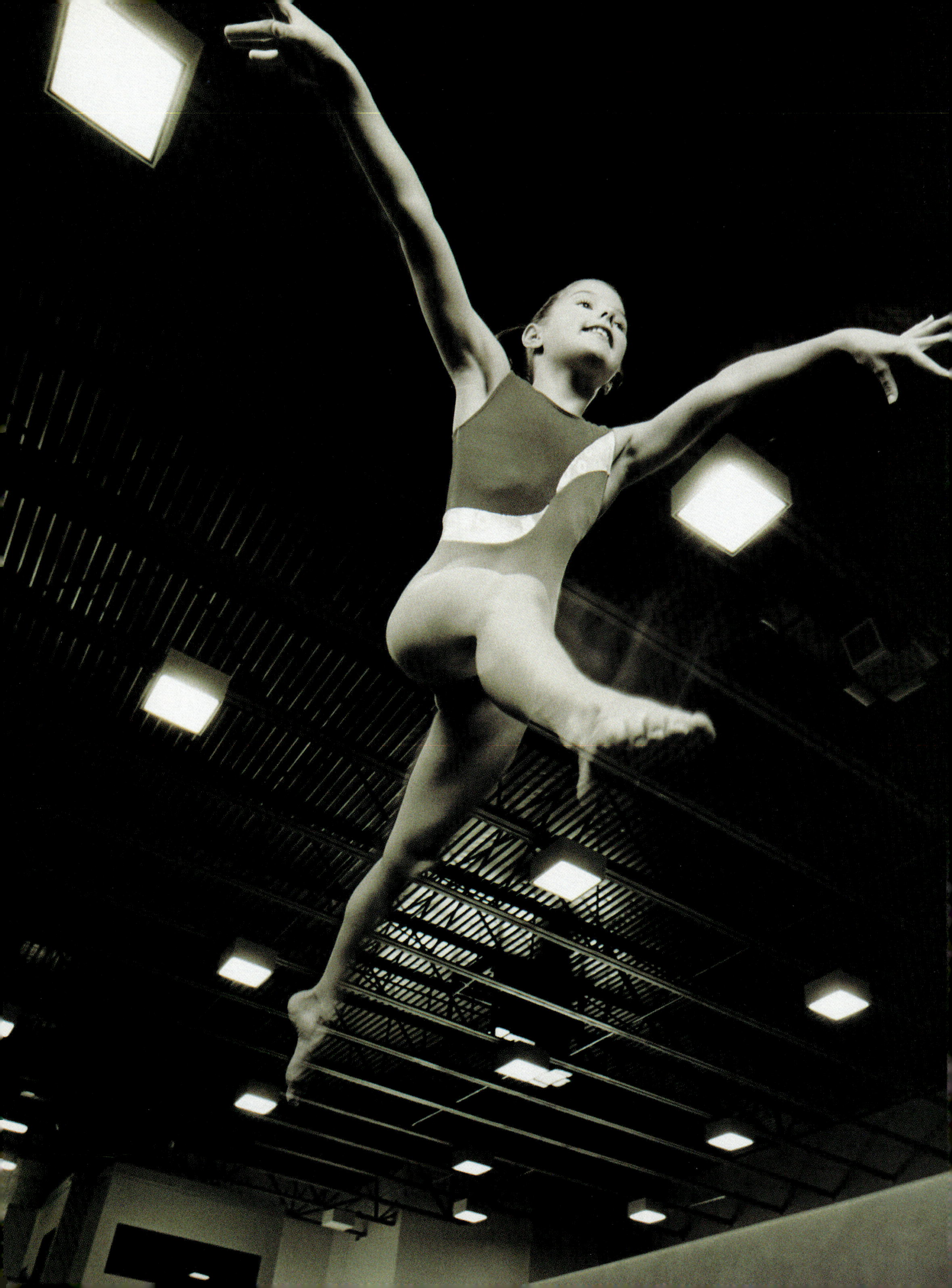

RSNA® International Programs

RSNA International Visiting Professor Program

RSNA is looking for dynamic, experienced radiology teachers interested in enhancing radiologic education in countries outside North America. Teach and travel in countries such as Chile, Ecuador, India, Jordan, Kenya, Malaysia and elsewhere.

Interested applicants willing to devote their time to teach oversees should contact the Committee on International Relations and Education for more information and an application form.

THE DEADLINE IS AUGUST 31, 1999

The RSNA Derek Harwood–Nash R&E Foundation International Fellowship

The RSNA is looking for promising scholars from outside North America who are embarking on a career in academic radiology, who wish to study at a North American institution.

Interested scholars whose educational goals would best be met by a course of study at a North American institution should contact the Committee on International Relations and Education for more information and an application form.

RSNA International Visiting Scholar Program

RSNA is looking for exceptional radiology educators from emerging nations interested in attending the RSNA Scientific Assembly and Annual Meeting to bring first-hand perspectives on the needs and status of radiology education in their nations. The program is intended for scholars who could not otherwise afford to attend the Scientific Assembly and Annual Meeting.

Interested scholars should contact the Committee on International Relations and Education for more information and an application form.

Anne G. Osborn, MD, Chairman
Committee on International Relations and Education

RSNA
820 Jorie Boulevard
Oak Brook, IL 60523-2251

(630) 590-7727 phone
(630) 571-7837 fax
e-mail: ranesbot@rsna.org

RSNA® INTERNATIONAL PROGRAMS

RSNA®
Founded 1915

Radiological Society of North America
820 Jorie Boulevard • Oak Brook, Illinois • 60523-2251
630.590.7727 phone • 630.571.7837 fax

Continuing Medical Education

Notices of continuing medical education programs will be accepted for publication in *Radiology* and *RadioGraphics* (*a*) if the program is directly relevant to radiologic imaging, practice, and oncology; and (*b*) if the course originates directly from and is organized by the radiology department of a medical school or medical center accredited for radiology residency training and approved to offer bona fide CME credit, or a radiologic organization that is a member of the Intersociety Commission of the American College of Radiology and approved to offer bona fide CME credit. Announcements of CME programs that do not meet these criteria will not be published. The RSNA assumes no responsibility for the content of CME programs appearing here.

Notices must include (*a*) the title of the course or meeting, (*b*) date and location, (*c*) listing of faculty, (*d*) fees, (*e*) number of category 1 credits available, (*f*) accredited sponsor of CME course, and (*g*) contact for further information. Notices should be submitted at least 4 months before the date of the meeting.

The opportunity to purchase classified and display ad space is also available.

Address announcements to Julie Pietryla, RSNA Publications, 820 Jorie Blvd, Oak Brook, IL 60523-2251.

Continuing medical education programs are listed according to diagnostic discipline; interdisciplinary programs are grouped under the predominant or first-listed specialty.

Diagnostic Imaging

Foot, Ankle and Knee Advanced Imaging Symposium

A "Foot, Ankle and Knee Advanced Imaging Symposium," sponsored by the Departments of Radiology and Continuing Medical Education, Thomas Jefferson Medical College, will take place on October 9–10, 1999, at Thomas Jefferson University, Philadelphia, Pa. This course is designed for radiologists, orthopedists, and podiatrists who wish to update their skills in the diagnosis and management of foot and ankle disorders. At the conclusion of the course, participants should be able to (*a*) identify normal and abnormal anatomic structures with multiple imaging modalities and (*b*) assess clinical and diagnostic findings to determine the most appropriate medical and surgical treatment. Course directors: Karasick, Schweitzer. Fee: $350; 13.5 hours of category 1 credit will be available. For further information, contact the Education Office, Department of Radiology, Thomas Jefferson University, 132 S 10th St, 780C Main, Philadelphia, PA 19107; telephone (888) 390-5051 or (215) 955-8533; fax (215) 923-9452; e-mail *JUREI@jeflin.tju.edu; http://jeffline.tju.edu/ultrasound.*

23rd Annual Cancer Symposium

The "23rd Annual Cancer Symposium for Physicians," sponsored by the Stevens Cancer Center, Scripps Memorial Hospitals, will be held on October 14–16, 1999, at the Hyatt Regency La Jolla, San Diego, Calif. This course is designed for clinicians involved in the treatment of patients with malignant or hematologic diseases. The purpose is to update the professional on current research and therapy issues in the fields of oncology and hematology. Topics include postmastectomy radiation therapy, radiotherapeutic approaches for localized cancer, and cisplatin-based chemoradiation for cervical cancer. In addition, the 19th Annual Cancer Symposium for Nurses will run concurrently with the physicians symposium. Program chair: Bernstein. Fee: $425 until September 10, $450 thereafter ($215 [$240] for fellows and residents); 16.5 hours of category 1 credit will be available. For further information, contact Ruthanne Crawford, Stevens Cancer Center, Scripps Memorial Hospitals, 9888 Genesee Ave, La Jolla, CA 92037; telephone (619) 626-6756; fax (619) 626-6793; e-mail *racrawford @chw.edu.*

General Radiology and Breast Imaging Review

The Department of Diagnostic Radiology, University of Kentucky College of Medicine, is sponsoring a "General Radiology and Breast Imaging Review" on October 16–17, 1999, at the Embassy Suites, Lexington, Ky. This course is designed to update radiologists on current diagnostic techniques in general radiology, particularly breast imaging, through didactic lectures, panel discussions, and question and answer sessions. Guest faculty: Bird, Cardenosa. Fee: $300 ($150 for residents; $100 for technologists and health care professionals); 9.5 hours of category 1 credit will be available. For further information, contact Brandy Daniels, conference coordinator, Department of Continuing Medical Education, University of Kentucky, L007 Kentucky Clinic, Lexington, KY 40536-0284; telephone (606) 323-5174; fax (606) 323-2008.

Cardiovascular Imaging 1999

The North American Society for Cardiac Imaging (NASCI) will hold its 27th annual meeting and scientific sessions, "Cardiovascular Imaging 1999," on November 6, 1999, in Atlanta, Ga. The program has been designed for radiologists, cardiologists, physicists, and other scientists who are interested in new developments and the clinical use of magnetic resonance (MR) and computed tomography (CT) for cardiovascular imaging. Topics include fast CT for coronary calcium, plaque characterization, interventional cardiovascular MR imaging, and cardiac function/perfusion. Chairmen: Duerinckx, Stillman. Fee: $60 ($30 for NASCI members); 5 hours of category 1 credit will be available. For further information, contact Joan Oefner, CAE, North American Society for Cardiac Imaging, 156 S Spruce Ave, Suite 207A, South San Francisco, CA 94080-4556; telephone (650) 876-0790; fax (650) 876-0791; e-mail *info@nasci .org; http://www.nasci.org.*

Breast Imaging

Mammography in the Diagnosis and Treatment of Breast Diseases

The Baylor College of Medicine and the Houston Radiological Society are co-sponsoring a course entitled "Imaging Perspective VI: Mammography in the Diagnosis and Treatment of Breast Diseases III" on October 9–10, 1999, at the Baylor College of Medicine, Houston, Tex. At the conclusion of this symposium, participants will be able to explain and discuss (*a*) the mammographic findings characteristic of benign and malignant breast disorders, (*b*) the mammographic changes resulting from surgery and radiation therapy, (*c*) how to implement a multidisciplinary approach to the diagnosis and treatment of breast cancer, and (*d*) the techniques used to perform optimal mammographic imaging. Directors: Fahr, Huynh, Shetty, Whitman. Fee: $300 until September 1, $375 thereafter ($125 [$175] for technologists; $75 [$90] for residents and fellows); 16 hours of category 1 credit will be available. For further information, contact Carol J. Soroka, conference coordinator, Office of Continuing Medical Education, Baylor College of Medicine, 1 Baylor Plaza, Suite S-104, Houston, TX 77030; telephone (800) 914-3709 or (713) 798-5602; fax (713) 798-7955; e-mail *cme@bcm.tmc.edu; http://www.bcm.tmc.edu/cme/.*

Computed Tomography

Spiral CT: Applications and Techniques

The Department of Radiology of Duke University Medical Center is sponsoring "Spiral CT: Applications and Techniques,"

Continued

a course to be held on October 4–8, 1999, at the Breakers, West Palm Beach, Fla. This course is designed to update radiologists on practical knowledge of spiral computed tomography including multislice scanning and fluoroscopy, as well as on the evolution of new techniques, faster scanners, and broad applications. Faculty: Donnelly, Enterline, Gray, McAdams, Nelson, Paulson. Fee: $650 until September 3, $700 thereafter; 21.75 hours of category 1 credit will be available. For further information, contact Debbie Sykes, Department of Radiology, Duke University Medical Center, Box 3808, Durham, NC 27710; telephone (919) 684-7228; e-mail *sykes010@mc.duke.edu.*

Interventional Radiology

Interventional/Vascular Radiology Course

The Department of Medical Imaging, University of Toronto, is sponsoring the "6th Annual Interventional/Vascular Radiology Course" on November 4–6, 1999, at the Sunnybrook and Women's College Health Sciences Centre, Toronto, Canada. This course is designed for practicing interventionalists, as well as residents and fellows pursuing careers in angiography and interventional radiology. The course features live video presentation of 15–20 interventional cases performed by University of Toronto faculty, broadcast simultaneously from two state-of-the-art angiographic suites. Directors: Common, Saibil. Guest speakers: Dake, Katzen, Machan. Fee: $300 until October 1, $350 thereafter ($200 [$230] for residents and nurses); 12.5 hours of category 1 credit will be available. For further information, contact Andrew Common, MD, Department of Medical Imaging, St Michael's Hospital, 30 Bond St, Toronto, Ontario, Canada M5B 1W8; telephone (416) 864-5690; fax (416) 864-5380; e-mail *commona@smh.toronto.on.ca; http://www.utoronto.ca/imaging/vir_course .htm.*

Magnetic Resonance

Current Concepts of Magnetic Resonance

"Current Concepts of Magnetic Resonance," a course sponsored by the Department of Radiology, Stanford University School of Medicine, will take place on October 10–14, 1999, at the Monterey Plaza Hotel, Monterey, Calif. This course is intended for practicing radiologists with an interest in the fundamental techniques and clinical applications of magnetic resonance (MR) imaging. Topics include image formation and contrast manipulation mechanisms, gradient echo methods, vascular imaging, and image artifacts. Faculty: Atlas, Beaulieu, Butts, Daniel, Glover, Herfkens, Lane, Li, Marks, Moseley, Napel, Pelc, Sommer, Spielman. Fee: $750 until September 10, $800 thereafter ($400 [$450] for trainees; $500 [$550] for Stanford alumni and military personnel); 30.6 hours of category 1 credit will be available. For further information, contact Donna Cronister, Department of Radiology, Stanford University Medical Center, Lucas MRS Center, 300 Pasteur Dr, Stanford, CA 94305-5488; telephone (650) 723-8205; fax (650) 723-5795; *http://www-radiology .stanford.edu/education/Monterey .html.*

Neuroradiology

Computed Tomography and Magnetic Resonance Imaging of the Brain, Head, Neck and Spine

The "26th Annual Course on Computed Tomography and Magnetic Resonance Imaging of the Brain, Head, Neck and Spine," sponsored by the Department of Diagnostic Radiology, Rush-Presbyterian-St Luke's Medical Center, will be held on November 4–5, 1999, at the Palmer House Hilton Hotel, Chicago, Ill. The course will provide instruction in the performance, interpretation, and comparison of selected computed tomographic (CT) and magnetic resonance (MR) examinations of the brain, head, neck, and spine. It is recommended that registrants have previous knowledge of the basic physical principles of CT and MR imaging, as these topics will be addressed only insofar as they pertain to particular clinical situations. Guest faculty: Ball, Castillo, Hasso, Haughton, Osborn, Ramsey, Russell, Tanenbaum, Thulborn. Local faculty: Colton, Geremia, Huckman. Fee: $495 ($395 for persons in training); 15 hours of category 1 credit will be available. For further information, contact Michael S. Huckman, MD, Department of Diagnostic Radiology, Rush-Presbyterian-St Luke's Medical Center, 1653 W Congress Pkwy, Chicago, IL 60612; telephone (312) 942-5781; fax (312) 942-2114; e-mail *mhuckman@rush.edu.*

Neuroradiology in Nevis

"Neuroradiology in Nevis," a course sponsored by the University of Pennsylvania Medical Center, will take place on November 17–20, 1999, at the Four Seasons Hotel, Nevis, British West Indies. This course will provide a thorough review of magnetic resonance (MR), computed tomography, and angiography as they pertain to the evaluation of diseases of the brain, head and neck, spine, and cerebral vasculature. The latest technical developments, including functional MR imaging, perfusion-diffusion imaging, and interventional angiographic procedures, will be discussed. Course director: Grossman. Fee: $750; 20 hours of category 1 credit will be available. For further information, contact Janice Ford Benner, Department of Radiology, University of Pennsylvania Medical Center, 3400 Spruce St, 1 Silverstein Bldg, Philadelphia, PA 19104; telephone (215) 662-6904; fax (215) 349-5925.

Ultrasonography

Radiology '99: Ultrasound/MRI/Mammography

The Department of Radiology, University of Minnesota, is sponsoring its 62nd annual course, entitled "Radiology '99: Ultrasound/MRI/Mammography," on September 16–18, 1999, at the Radisson Hotel Metrodome, Minneapolis, Minn. Participants will learn to evaluate abdominal disorders appropriately, use diverse imaging techniques in the evaluation of thoracic disorders, and use ultrasonography in the evaluation of selected disorders. Course directors: Engeler, Everson, Thompson, Trenkner, Truwit. Guest faculty: D'Orsi, Filly, Kucharczyk. Fee: $395 ($295 for residents and military personnel); 16.5 hours of category 1 credit will be available. For further information, contact the Office of Continuing Medical Education, University of Minnesota, 615 Washington Ave SE, Suite 107, Minneapolis, MN 55414; telephone (800) 776-8636 or (612) 626-7600; fax (612) 626-7766; *http://www .med.umn.edu/cme/.*

Diagnostic Ultrasound in Gynecology and Obstetrics and Abdomen

The Department of Radiology and Radiological Science, Johns Hopkins University School of Medicine, is sponsoring the

Continued

Continuing Medical Education

"28th Annual Diagnostic Ultrasound in Gynecology and Obstetrics and Abdomen" course on September 17–19, 1999, at the Renaissance Harborplace Hotel, Baltimore, Md. Fee: not available; category 1 accreditation pending. For further information, contact the conference coordinator, Office of Continuing Medical Education, Johns Hopkins University School of Medicine, 720 Rutland Ave, Turner 20, Baltimore, MD 21205-2195; telephone (410) 955-2959; fax (410) 955-0807; e-mail *cmenet @jhmi.edu; http://www.med.jhu.edu/cme.*

Society of Radiologists in Ultrasound

The 9th Annual Meeting and Postgraduate Educational Course of the Society of Radiologists in Ultrasound (SRU), co-sponsored by the American College of Radiology and the SRU, will be held on October 8–10, 1999, at the Sheraton Chicago Hotel and Towers, Chicago, Ill. This year's course is entitled "Advances in Sonography," during which attendees will participate in discussion of current issues pertaining to the practice of ultrasonography. Topics include turf issues, computer applications, compliance with federal regulations for billing and coding, fraud and abuse, and practice accreditation. Program chair: Hertzberg. Fee: $500 for physician nonmembers, $250 for SRU members ($200 for sonographers and technologists); 20.5 hours of category 1 credit will be available. For further information, contact the Society of Radiologists in Ultrasound, 1891 Preston White Dr, Reston, VA 20191; telephone (703) 729-3353; fax (703) 262-9313; *http://www.sru.org.*

Radiology Business Information

Radiology, a monthly journal devoted to clinical radiology and allied sciences, is owned and published by

The Radiological Society of North America, Inc (RSNA)
820 Jorie Boulevard
Oak Brook, IL 60523-2251 USA
(630) 571-2670 • FAX (630) 571-7837
RSNA Link *http://www.rsna.org*

Delmar J. Stauffer, *Executive Director and Business Manager for Publications*

■ JOURNAL BUSINESS

Send new manuscripts to the address given in the Publication Information for Authors.

Correspondence concerning accepted or published material should be addressed to

Anthony V. Proto, MD–Editor, *Radiology*
Radiology Editorial Office • 1001 East Broad Street
Suite 310 • Richmond, VA 23219
(804) 644-5667 FAX (804) 644-5672
e-mail: *proto@rsna.org*

■ COPYRIGHT AND PERMISSIONS

■ PHOTOCOPYING

Authorization to photocopy items for internal or personal use, or the internal or personal use of specific clients and educators, is granted by RSNA, provided that the appropriate fee is paid directly to Copyright Clearance Center, Inc (CCC), 222 Rosewood Dr, Danvers, MA 01923 (phone 978-750-8400; FAX 978-750-4744).

Consent for photocopying does not extend to copying for general distribution, resale, or advertising and promotional purposes, or for creating new collective works. Permission for the latter categories may be sought by writing to the Permissions Coordinator, RSNA Publications, Oak Brook, IL (address above).

■ SUBSCRIPTION INFORMATION

The nonmember subscription rate for the USA is $215.00 per year; for outside USA, $260.00 (includes postage). (Air freight is available; rates are furnished on request.) Residents who are members of the RSNA may subscribe to **both** *Radiology* and *RadioGraphics* for a special rate of $80.00 (for North American addresses; residents from outside North America, add $60.00 for postage). Single copies are $25.00 (air freight, $11.00). Orders for subscriptions, remittances, and questions about subscriptions should be sent to

RSNA Subscriptions Department
820 Jorie Boulevard
Oak Brook, IL 60523-2251 USA
(630) 571-7873
FAX (630) 571-7837
e-mail: *subscrib@rsna.org*

The page containing advertising information (Advertisers' Index) may be located by consulting the Departments section in the Table of Contents.

■ CHANGE OF ADDRESS

The Post Office will not forward your journal to a new address. To avoid missing any issues, you must notify us of a change in address. At least 5 weeks before you move, please send (*a*) your **new address**, with zip code, and (*b*) your **current mailing label** with your old address to the address above.

■ MISSING ISSUES AND BACK COPIES

Claims for copies lost in the mail are allowed within 90 days of issue. Claims are not allowed for issues lost as a result of insufficient notice of change of address. To replace a missing issue or order a back copy contact RSNA Subscriptions Department at the address above. Back copies cost $25.00 (air freight, $11.00).

■ REPRINTS

The first footnote on the first page of each *Radiology* article contains the name and address of the author who answers requests for reprints. For reprint orders of 100 or more, contact

(continued)

RSNA DEPARTMENT TELEPHONE NUMBERS

Accounting	(630) 571-7812
Advertising	(630) 571-7817
Copyrights and Permissions	(630) 571-7829
Executive	(630) 571-7866
Learning Center	(630) 368-3753
Meetings	(630) 571-7850
Membership	(630) 571-7873
Office of Research	(630) 368-3756
Permissions	(630) 571-7829
Program	(630) 571-7874
Research and Education Foundation	(630) 571-7816
Reprints	(610) 250-7244
Subscriptions	(630) 571-7873
Syllabus sales	(800) 272-2920
Main telephone	(630) 571-2670
FAX	(630) 571-7837

Radiology Reprints
1991 Northampton St
Easton, PA 18042-3189 USA
(610) 250-7244

For reprints of advertisements, contact the Advertising Production Manager (address under Advertising).

■ MICROFORM

Radiology is available in microfilm and microfiche from

University Microforms International
300 N Zeeb Road
Ann Arbor, MI 48106 USA
(800) 521-3044

■ INDEXES

Radiology is included in the *RSNA Index to Imaging Literature,* a 3-year cumulative subject and author index of *Radiology* and 41 radiologic journals, available for $35.00 per copy (air freight, $11.00). Subscribers to the Journal receive the index free of charge. *Radiology* is indexed in *Current Contents/Clinical Medicine,* available from the Institute for Scientific Information, and *Index Medicus,* available from the National Library of Medicine.

■ BOOK REVIEWERS AND BOOKS FOR REVIEW

Any person who would like to help in reviewing books for *Radiology* should contact

Richard A. Szucs, MD, Book Review Editor
Radiology Editorial Office
1001 E Broad St
Suite 310
Richmond, VA 23219

Publishers wishing to have books reviewed should send them to the same address.

■ PUBLISHERS' ROW

As a service to readers and colleagues in medical publishing, *Radiology* publishes a list of current imaging publications of interest to radiologists and allied scientists. Complete addresses and phone numbers of participating publishers are included. Publishers' Row is featured quarterly, in the March, June, September, and December issues. For information on publishing a list, contact Nancy Osborne at RSNA Publications at the Oak Brook address.

■ ADVERTISING

The advertising policy appears on the Advertisers' Index of each issue. Questions about advertising and billing, advertising contracts, and insertion orders and requests for media kits should be addressed to

James F. Drew, *Director of Advertising*
RSNA Publications
820 Jorie Boulevard
Oak Brook, IL 60523-2251 USA
(630) 571-7819
FAX (630) 571-7837

Questions about advertising production should be addressed to:

Pat Hollingsworth, *Advertising Production Manager*
RSNA Advertising Department
820 Jorie Boulevard
Oak Brook, IL 60523-2251 USA
(630) 571-7818
FAX (630) 571-7837

■ CLASSIFIED ADVERTISING

As a service to readers, *Radiology* accepts classified advertising, and every effort is made to ensure that the ads are relevant to the practice of radiology. For more details on the classified advertising policy and procedures, see the Classified Advertising section in each issue (consult the Departments section in the Table of Contents for page number) or contact the Advertising Production Manager (address under Advertising).

CHANGE OF ADDRESS FORM

Please allow 90 days for change to take effect

Name: ______________________________

Previous Address

Address: ______________________________
____
____
City/State/Zip: ______________________________

New Address

Address: ______________________________
____
____
City/State/Zip: ______________________________

Mail to:
RSNA Subscriptions Department • 820 Jorie Boulevard • Oak Brook, IL 60523-2251 USA **FAX:** (630) 571-7837

Transfer of Copyright and Certifications Agreement

Manuscript No. (for Editorial Office use only)____________________

Complete copyright to the article entitled:

____

____

is hereby transferred to the Radiological Society of North America (for **U.S. government employees:** to the extent transferable), effective if and when the article is accepted for publication in ***Radiology,*** printed or electronic format. In the case of authors who are officers or employees of the U.S. government, the Radiological Society of North America recognizes that works prepared by them as part of their official government duties are in the public domain.

Authors reserve the following rights:

A. Other than copyright, all proprietary rights including patent rights relating to the subject matter of the article.
B. The license for personal use in lectures, lecture notes, and exhibits.

Please return this form as soon as possible. The signed statement **must** be received by the Editor **before** the manuscript can be processed for publication.

A. All authors certify that this material or similar material has not been and will not be submitted by them or by colleagues in their institution to any other publication prior to its appearance in ***Radiology.***

B. All authors certify that they have read the Publication Information for Authors found in the most recently published issue of ***Radiology*** at the time the manuscript is submitted. They further certify their compliance with the various requirements found therein.

C. All authors certify that they have submitted all required permissions and that all required statements have been inserted in the text where appropriate.

D. All authors certify that all individuals who have participated sufficiently in the conception and design of this work, in the analysis of the data, and in the writing of the manuscript have been listed as authors. All authors further certify that they have read the final version of the manuscript and approve it for submission for publication.

E. All authors certify that the Editor may correspond with the designated *corresponding author* regarding acceptance, rejection, revision of the manuscript and that the corresponding author is responsible for informing all other authors of the same.

F. All authors certify that responses, revisions received by the Editor from the designated *corresponding author* will be treated as if from all authors and that the corresponding author is responsible for informing all other authors of the same.

G. All authors certify that: **(must check one)**

- ❐ they have no direct or indirect financial interest in the products under investigation or subject matter discussed in this manuscript, or
- ❐ one or more (please name) authors do have a direct or indirect financial interest in the products under investigation or subject matter discussed in this manuscript. A separate statement is attached that details this proprietary interest, and the authors hereby grant permission to publish this information or an appropriate summary thereof with the manuscript if the manuscript is published.

TO BE SIGNED BY ALL AUTHORS:

Name (print) (First) ____________________ Signature ____________________

Name (print) ____________________ Signature ____________________

Name (print) ____________________ Signature ____________________

Name (print) ____________________ Signature ____________________

Name (print) ____________________ Signature ____________________

Name (print) ____________________ Signature ____________________

Use additional page if necessary.

This signed form (a photocopy is acceptable) must be submitted with all proffered works.

Radiology Publication Information for Authors

Radiology is published under the supervision of the Board of Directors of the Radiological Society of North America, Inc, which appoints the Editor who selects all material submitted for publication, including advertisements. No responsibility is accepted by the Board of Directors or the appointed Editor for the opinions expressed by the contributors. Please note that the instructions below are in accord with the *Uniform Requirements for Manuscripts Submitted to Biomedical Journals* (*Annals of Internal Medicine* 1997; 126:36-47). Although *Radiology* will receive material prepared and submitted according to these instructions, the right is reserved to introduce any changes necessary to make the contributions conform to the individual editorial standards of this Journal.

Full manuscripts should be addressed to:
Anthony V. Proto, MD—Editor, *Radiology*
Radiology Manuscripts • RSNA Publications
820 Jorie Boulevard • Oak Brook, IL 60523-2251 USA
FAX (630) 571-7837

All other submissions and correspondence concerning accepted or published material should be addressed to:
Anthony V. Proto, MD—Editor, *Radiology*
Radiology Editorial Office • 1001 East Broad Street
Suite 310 • Richmond, VA 23219
(804) 644-5667 FAX (804) 644-5672
e-mail: *proto@rsna.org*

Inquiries about manuscript status and preparation, as well as letters to the editor, can be directed to *radiolog@ rsna.org*

The page containing advertising information (Advertisers' Index) may be located by consulting the Departments section in the Table of Contents.

■ TRANSFER OF COPYRIGHT AND CERTIFICATIONS AGREEMENT

Please send the copyright and certifications agreement with the initial submission of all proffered works. This may be accomplished by using a copy of the form that appears in this issue. **All** authors of any single composition must sign this agreement. In the case of officers or employees of the U.S. government, the Society recognizes that works prepared as part of their official government duties are in the public domain, but they must still sign the copyright and certifications agreement.

■ FINANCIAL INTEREST

Authors must describe any direct or indirect financial interest they may have in the subject matter of a submitted manuscript, and they must authorize the Society to publish this financial disclosure with the article if deemed appropriate. The Society's Financial Disclosure policy is as follows:

"Each author shall describe (*a*) any direct financial interest that author has in the subject matter discussed in the submitted manuscript, and (*b*) any affiliation or financial involvement that author has with or in any organization having a direct financial interest in the subject matter discussed in the submitted manuscript. Such information will be held in the confidence of the journal Editor during the review process. If necessary, in the Editor's view, this information may be shared with reviewers after discussion between the Editor and author. The submission of a manuscript to *Radiology* grants permission for RSNA to publish the financial information described above, or an appropriate summary thereof, with the manuscript if the manuscript is accepted for publication."

■ MANUSCRIPT PREPARATION

Original writings will be accepted only with the understanding that they are contributed solely to *Radiology*. Manuscripts should be typewritten and **double-spaced (all pages)** on only one side of the paper with at least 3-cm margins. Each manuscript component should begin on a **new page** in this order: title pages, abstract, text, acknowledgments, references, tables (each on a separate page), and captions for illustrations. The title pages and abstract page should not be numbered. Sequential numbering should begin with the text. To ensure anonymity in the review process, authors' names should appear on only the full title page; names of authors or the institution should **not** be given in the text or on the illustrations. **Three copies** of the manuscript and three complete sets of mounted illustrations should be submitted. The author should retain a complete copy of the manuscript, since accepted manuscripts will not be returned and only the illustrations of rejected manuscripts will be returned. All manuscripts are acknowledged; please allow 2-3 weeks from the time you mailed the manuscript for receipt of an acknowledgment.

■ TITLE PAGES, AUTHOR CONTRIBUTIONS

Full Title Page: This page should include the title of the manuscript, the first and last names, middle initials, and degrees of all authors, the name and street address (not a postal box) of the institution from which the work originated, the telephone number, the FAX or Telex number, and the e-mail address (if available) of the **corresponding author**, and information concerning grants. The address for reprint requests should include

(continued)

the **complete** name, street address (not a postal box), and zip code. It is important to indicate on this title page whether your paper has been presented at an RSNA meeting (please give year) or has been accepted for presentation at a future meeting.

Abbreviated Title Page: This page should include only the title of the manuscript so as to allow for anonymity during the review process.

Author Contributions: Authors are required to identify their manuscript contributions, for which they are responsible. The author(s) responsible for the integrity of the entire study should also be identified. Please list the following phrases on a separate page, to follow the "*Abbreviated Title Page*," and beside each indicate the name(s) of the author(s) to whom these phrases apply:

- guarantor of integrity of entire study
- study concepts
- study design
- definition of intellectual content
- literature research
- clinical studies
- experimental studies
- data acquisition
- data analysis
- statistical analysis
- manuscript preparation
- manuscript editing
- manuscript review

For those phrases that do not apply, please list them and so indicate.

■ ABSTRACT, KEY WORDS, CATEGORIZATION TERMS, AND SUMMARY STATEMENT

An abstract of 200 words or less must be submitted with each manuscript of a major paper. The abstract must be divided into four paragraphs with the following headings.

PURPOSE: State the hypothesis being tested or the procedure being evaluated.

MATERIALS AND METHODS: Briefly state what was done and what materials were used, including number of subjects. Also include the methods used to assess the data and to control bias.

RESULTS: Provide the findings of the study, including indicators of statistical significance. Include actual numbers, as well as percentages.

CONCLUSION: Summarize in one or two sentences the conclusion made on the basis of the findings.

Below the abstract, please list three to six key words as derived from the terms used in the most recent 3-year *RSNA Index to Imaging Literature*. Also, on the Manuscript Categorization Terms form provided at the end of these instructions, please select as many terms as are appropriate for your manuscript. It is important that you comply with this request, since the terms you select are utilized to match your manuscript with the appropriate reviewers.

On the reverse side of the Manuscript Categorization Terms form, the *author should reproduce from the text the one statement that best conveys or summarizes the message of the study*.

An abstract of 60 words or less must be submitted for each case report or Technical Developments paper. The abstract must state (*a*) what was done, (*b*) what was found, and (*c*) what was concluded.

■ TEXT

The text of observational and experimental studies is arranged in sections with the headings Introduction, Materials and Methods, Results, and Discussion. Lengthy papers may need subheadings within some sections to clarify their content, especially within the Results and Discussion sections.

Introduction: Clearly state the hypothesis or purpose of the study. Give only strictly pertinent references, and do not review the literature extensively.

Materials and Methods: Describe clearly the number and selection of the subjects studied (patients or experimental animals, including controls). Identify the methods, instrumentation (manufacturer's name and address in parentheses), and procedures in sufficient detail to allow other workers to reproduce the results. To ensure anonymity in the review process, do **not** include the name of the institution where the work was performed, either within the text or at the top of each manuscript page. Give references to established methods, including statistical methods that have been published but are not well known; describe new or substantially modified methods and give reasons for using these techniques. Include numbers of observations and the statistical significance of the findings when appropriate. Detailed statistical analyses, mathematical derivations, and the like should be presented in one or more appendixes.

Results: Present the results in logical sequence in the text, along with tables, and illustrations. Do not repeat in the text all the data in the tables and/or illustrations; summarize only important observations.

Discussion: Emphasize the new and important aspects of the study and conclusions that follow from them. Do not repeat in detail the data given in the Results section. Include in the Discussion the implications of the findings and their limitations, in particular with reference to the use of modified methods, statistical or otherwise. Relate the observations to other relevant studies. Link the conclusions with the goals of the study, but avoid unqualified statements and conclusions not supported completely by the data. Avoid claiming priority and alluding to work that has not been completed. State new hypotheses when warranted, but clearly label them as such. Recommendations, when appropriate, may be included.

For experimental studies, please describe the potential importance of your conclusions as they relate to future practical applications. Please identify this paragraph with the title "Practical Application(s)."

■ ACKNOWLEDGMENTS

List here those who have contributed substantially to the work reported in the manuscript, such as editorial and writing assistance, but who are not authors of the study. Authors are expected to obtain written permission of those acknowledged, and to submit the same, as readers might interpret that those acknowledged agree with the data and conclusions of the study.

■ REFERENCES

Number references consecutively in the order in which they are first mentioned. The abbreviations used for periodicals cited in the references should follow the style of *Index Medicus*. For journal articles, list surnames and initials of all authors when six or less, such as:

1. Stuart MJ, Elrad H, Graeber JE, Hakanson DO, Sunderji SG, Barvinchak MK. Increased synthesis of prostaglandin endoperoxides and platelet hyperfunction in infants of mothers with diabetes mellitus. J Lab Clin Med 1979; 94:12–26.

When seven or more authors are listed, only the first three names need to be identified, followed by "et al," such as:

1. Hibbard CT, Campbell S, Sabbagha RE, et al. Demonstration of tissue interfaces within the body by ultrasonic echo sounding. Br J Radiol 1961; 34:539–549.

Abstracts, editorials, and letters to the Editor should be noted as such. In the case of books, the authors of a chapter, title of the chapter, editor(s), title of the book, edition, city, publisher, year, and specific pages must be provided.

1. Brown M, Gray L. Indications for hematology. In: Wintrobe MM, ed. Clinical hematology. 3rd ed. Philadelphia, Pa: Lea & Febiger, 1975; 1146–1167.

It is the responsibility of the author(s) to ensure that all references are listed accurately.

■ TABLES

Tables should be numbered in Arabic numerals and should have a title. All abbreviations used in the table should be explained in a footnote.

Tables should be presented in the style used in recent issues of the Journal. No vertical lines or shading should be included. Avoid excessive use of horizontal lines within the table.

■ CAPTIONS FOR ILLUSTRATIONS

A caption must be supplied for each illustration, including drawings and graphs. It should not duplicate text material and should follow the style used in recent issues of the Journal. All captions should appear collectively on one or more pages separate from the text, and each caption should also appear below the corresponding illustration. It is essential that the caption describes all labels placed on the print of an illustration.

■ ILLUSTRATIONS

Illustrations should be limited to those required to show the essential features described in the manuscript. Space constraints prevent us from publishing redundant or excessive illustrations. Unretouched glossy prints no larger than 12.7 × 17.8 cm (5 × 7 inches) are desirable. Prints to be combined into one array, such as posteroanterior and lateral views, should be the same height or the same width to facilitate reproduction. They should correspond in appearance to the tonal relations of the original radiograph (ie, showing the bones white on a dark background, with the patient's right to the observer's left; computed tomograms and MR images should employ the "view from below"). If an image has been enhanced electronically, explain the alterations that have been made and send an original image along with the enhanced one. Drawings and charts should be rendered professionally in India ink on white paper. In computer-generated artwork, shading should be done in continuous tones (ie, solid black, solid gray, solid white): **Do not use dotted shadings.**

Since the size of the illustration printed in the Journal is typically smaller than that submitted by the author(s), it is essential that each submitted illustration show only the area(s) of interest with enough surrounding area for orientation puposes (e.g., to illustrate a cavity at the right lung apex, show only that area with enough surrounding area for orientation, rather than the entire chest).

All illustrations must be numbered and the top indicated on the back. For protection against loss or damage, each illustration should then be neatly attached to paper (one illustration per page), and the number and top should be reindicated on this page. For attachment, **avoid using glue, staples, or corner mounts.** Because it holds the illustration securely to the page without damage, we recommend Scotch Removable Magic Tape (3M, St Paul, Minn). **Please** do not add letters or numbers to the **face** of the illustration to identify the figure (such as 1A or 1B).

Arrows and other labels should be placed only on the final print, should be of professional quality, and should be **removable**. Professional artist service for such items is available to authors without charge. The desired additions may simply be indicated on tissue or a transparent overlay attached securely to the print.

Illustrations of accepted manuscripts become the property of the RSNA and will be stored for 2 years after publication. Illustrations will be returned only upon receipt of a written request from the corresponding author. We suggest that authors make and keep a set of illustrations in addition to the three sets submitted to the Journal.

■ UNITS AND ABBREVIATIONS

Radiation measurements and laboratory values should be given in the *International System of Units (SI)* (resources: SI Units in Radiation Protection and Measurements, NCRP Report no. 82 [August 1985]; "Now Read This: The SI Units Are Here," *JAMA* 1986; 255:2329–2339). Abbreviations should be spelled out when first used in the text, such as "cerebrospinal fluid (CSF)." Laboratory slang, clinical jargon, and uncommon abbreviations should be avoided.

■ INFORMED CONSENT

Manuscripts reporting the results of experimental studies on human subjects must include a statement in Materials and Methods to the effect that informed consent was obtained after the nature of the procedure(s) had been fully explained. In addition, a statement affirming approval of the appropriate institutional review board is required. If a review board does not exist, then the Declaration of Helsinki principles should be followed and a statement affirming the same should be made (41st World Medical Assembly. Declaration of Helsinki: recommendations guiding physicians in biomedical research involving human subjects. Bull Pan Am Health Organ 1990; 24: 606-609).

The maintenance and care of experimental animals to provide humane treatment and to ensure reliable results are described in the National Institutes of Health guidelines for use of laboratory animals. Authors must affirm compliance with these guidelines or approval of the appropriate institutional review board in the Materials and Methods section.

■ RIGHTS AND PERMISSIONS

Written permission (we require a copy) must be granted by the publisher and author to reproduce any previously published figures, including permission to reproduce in both print and electronic formats; any such material must be clearly noted and its source given in the manuscript. A signed letter of permission must be included with your manuscript for any individual who might be identified due to written descriptions, photographs (masking the eyes in photographs is not sufficient protection of anonymity), or otherwise. Informed consent, which requires that the individual be shown the manuscript, should be affirmed in the Materials and Methods section.

If reference is made in the text to personal communication (oral or written) as a source of information, a signed statement of permission is required from each such source.

■ AUTHOR RESPONSIBILITY

Authors must be certain that no manuscript on the same or similar material has been or will be submitted to another journal by themselves or others at their institution before their work appears in *Radiology*. The submission by authors of similar material to advertising media must be indicated at the time *Radiology* receives the manuscript.

■ ELECTRONIC SUBMISSION OF ACCEPTED MANUSCRIPTS

Text File: Manuscripts that have been accepted for publication must be submitted on computer disk (required for text, desirable for illustrations). Submit text on a $3^1/_2$-inch diskette prepared in WordPerfect or Microsoft Word format for Windows or Macintosh. A hard copy should accompany the diskette and should match the diskette file exactly. The diskette should be labeled with its assigned manuscript number, the first author's last name, the word processing program used, and the file name.

The entire article should be submitted as a single text file, with the elements in the standard order: title pages, abstract, text, acknowledgments, references, tables, captions. *Do not embed illustrations.* Only the final version of the article should be on the submitted disk. Keep the text file as free from formatting codes as possible: Do not use boldface, italic, underlining, strange fonts, codes for centering, unnecessary line spacing, etc. Use the default settings of the word-processing program; especially do not use right-justified margins. Use tabs to indent at the beginnings of paragraphs, and insert only one space after end punctuation marks. Use hard returns only at the ends of paragraphs or between sections of the manuscript; do not insert them mid-paragraph. Do not insert tabs in references; use only one hard return at the end of each reference.

Illustrations File: Although not required, submission of illustrations on $3^1/_2$-inch disk, ZIP disk, or CD is acceptable. All image files should be in PC tif or eps format. Do not sumbit images in bitmap, jpeg, or gif format. *Do not embed images in the text file.*

For black and white images, we require that they be submitted in PC tif or PC eps format with a dot range of 5% Highlight to 95% Shadow and resolution of 500 dpi. Four-color images should also be PC tif or PC eps format with a maximum of 280% total tonal density and resolution of 300 dpi. Note that when your RGB files are converted to CYMK, there will be less color due to conversion. Images should be supplied as close as possible to print size: $2^1/_4$ inches wide for one column, $3^1/_4$ inches wide for $1^1/_2$ columns, $4^5/_8$ inches wide for two columns.

Each image file should be named, and with the diskette or cartridge the following should be provided: a hard-copy inventory with specific information on the image, two sets of proofs obtained at 800–1,800 dpi, and one set of proofs obtained with a laser printer to be used as a reference set.

■ BOOK REVIEWERS

Any person who would like to help in reviewing books for *Radiology* should contact

Richard A. Szucs, MD, Book Review Editor
Radiology Editorial Office
1001 E Broad St
Suite 310
Richmond, VA 23219

■ BOOKS FOR REVIEW

Publishers wishing to have books reviewed should send them to the address above.

✔ Checklist of Requirements:

- ❒ 1. Send 3 copies of manuscript and 3 copies of illustrations.
- ❒ 2. Mount each illustration on a separate page, $8^1/_2 \times 11$ inches. Indicate figure number and top.
- ❒ 3. Double space all parts of manuscript.
- ❒ 4. Send copyright and certifications agreement with signatures of all authors.
- ❒ 5. Send institutional affiliation for each author and corresponding author's name, address, phone number, FAX or Telex number, and e-mail address.
- ❒ 6. Send a **brief** abstract: 200 words or less for regular articles, 60 words or less for case reports and Technical Developments papers.
- ❒ 7. Give SI units for radiation measurements and laboratory values.
- ❒ 8. Send copy of letter of permission to reprint any figure that was published previously or for any other reasons as noted in the instructions found above.
- ❒ 9. Send a completed copy of the Manuscript Categorization Terms form. Please remember to reproduce from the text the one statement that best conveys or summarizes the message of your study.

Radiology Manuscript Categorization Terms

Please PRINT your name: ______________________________

Please print the title of your manuscript ______________________________

____

For each section, please categorize your manuscript by checking off **as many terms as are appropriate.**

Modalities/Techniques

___ Absorptiometry/ Bone Densitometry
___ Angiography
___ Arthrography
___ Conventional Radiography
___ CT
___ CT-Angiography
___ CT-Electron Beam
___ CT-High Resolution
___ CT-Spiral
___ Dacryocystography
___ Defecography
___ Digital Radiography
___ Echocardiography
___ Fluoroscopy
___ Hysterosalpingography
___ Image Manipulation/ Reconstruction
___ Lymphography
___ MR-Angiography
___ MR-Diffusion/Perfusion
___ MR-Functional Imaging
___ MR-Imaging
___ MR-Spectroscopy
___ Neural Networks
___ PACS
___ PET
___ Radionuclide Studies
___ Sialography
___ SPECT
___ Ultrasound
___ Ultrasound-Color Doppler
___ Ultrasound-Doppler
___ Ultrasound-Power Doppler
___ Ultrasound-Spectral Doppler

Procedures

___ Angioplasty
___ Angioscopy
___ Balloon Insertions
___ Biopsy/Drainage
___ Dilation
___ Embolization
___ Endoscopy
___ Filter Insertions
___ Interventional Other ______________
___ Intraoperative
___ Laser
___ Lithotripsy
___ Localization
___ Myelography
___ Percutaneous
___ Radiation Therapy/Oncology
___ Radionuclide Therapy
___ Shunts
___ Stents
___ Thrombolysis

Areas/Systems

___ Abdomen
___ Biliary
___ Breast
___ Cardiac
___ CNS
___ Ear/Nose/Throat
___ Genital/Reproductive
___ GI
___ Head/Neck
___ Hematologic
___ Lymphatic
___ Muscular
___ Nervous-Peripheral
___ Skeletal-Appendicular
___ Skeletal-Axial
___ Soft Tissues/Skin
___ Thorax
___ Urinary
___ Vascular

Structures

___ Adrenal
___ Ankle
___ Anus
___ Aorta
___ Appendix
___ Arteries
___ Bile Ducts
___ Bladder
___ Brain/Brain Stem
___ Breast
___ Cervix
___ Diaphragm
___ Duodenum
___ Ear
___ Elbow
___ Esophagus
___ Extremities
___ Eye
___ Face
___ Fallopian Tubes
___ Foot
___ Gallbladder
___ Hand
___ Heart
___ Hip
___ Jaw
___ Joints
___ Kidney
___ Knee
___ Lacrimal Glands
___ Large Bowel
___ Larynx
___ Ligaments
___ Liver
___ Long Bones
___ Lung
___ Marrow
___ Mediastinum
___ Meninges
___ Mesentery
___ Omentum
___ Orbit
___ Ovaries
___ Pancreas
___ Paranasal Sinuses
___ Parathyroid
___ Pelvis
___ Pelvocalyceal
___ Penis
___ Pericardium
___ Peritoneum
___ Pharynx
___ Pineal
___ Pituitary
___ Pleura
___ Prostate
___ Pylorus
___ Rectum
___ Retina
___ Retroperitoneum
___ Ribs
___ Salivary Glands
___ Scrotum
___ Shoulder
___ Skull
___ Small Bowel
___ Spinal Cord
___ Spine-Cervical
___ Spine-Lumbar

Continued

Structures, continued

___ Spine-Sacrum/Coccyx
___ Spine-Thoracic
___ Spleen
___ Stomach
___ Tendons
___ Testes
___ Thymus
___ Thyroid
___ Tongue
___ Tracheobronchial Tree
___ Ureters
___ Urethra
___ Uterus
___ Vagina
___ Valves
___ Veins
___ Vena Cava
___ Wrist

Topics

___ Abscess
___ Acceptance Testing
___ Acute
___ Adults
___ AIDS
___ Anatomy
___ Aneurysms
___ Animal Investigations
___ Arteriosclerosis
___ Arthritides
___ Artifacts
___ Atelectasis
___ Athletic Injuries
___ AVM
___ Axilla
___ Biological Effects
___ Biostatistics
___ Blood
___ Calcifications/Calculi
___ Cardiac Assist Devices
___ Catheters
___ Cavitation
___ Cerebral Palsy
___ Chemistry
___ Chronic Obstructive Airways Disease
___ Cirrhosis
___ Comparative Studies
___ Complications
___ Computer Applications-3D
___ Computer Applications-Teleradiology
___ Computer Applications-Virtual Imaging
___ Computer Applications-Other___________
___ Congenital
___ Connective Tissue Disorders
___ Contrast Agents-Intravenous
___ Contrast Agents-Oral
___ Cost-effectiveness
___ CSF
___ Cysts
___ Dementia
___ Demineralization-Bone
___ Dilatation
___ Dissection
___ Diverticula
___ Dosimetry
___ Drugs/Reactions
___ Dysplasias
___ Eating Disorders
___ ECMO
___ Edema
___ Education
___ Efficacy Studies
___ Embolism
___ Endocrine Disorders
___ Equipment
___ Ethics
___ Experimental Investigations
___ Fetus
___ Fistula
___ Foreign Bodies
___ Forensics
___ Genetic Defects
___ Grafts
___ Health Policy and Practice
___ Hemangioma
___ Hematologic Diseases
___ Hemodynamics/Flow Dynamics
___ Hemorrhage
___ Hernia
___ History
___ Hyperplasia/Hypertrophy
___ Hypertension
___ Imaging Sequences
___ Infection
___ Inflammation
___ Instrumentation
___ Ischemia/Infarction
___ Laboratory Tests
___ Leukemia
___ Lymphoma
___ Medicolegal Issues
___ Metabolic Disorders
___ Metastases
___ Monoclonal Antibodies
___ Motility
___ Neoplasms-Primary
___ Normal Variants
___ Observer Performance
___ Obstetrics
___ Obstruction/Occlusion
___ Occupational/Environmental Hazards
___ Outcomes Analysis
___ Parasites
___ Pathology
___ Pediatric Population-Adolescents
___ Pediatric Population-Children
___ Pediatric Population-Infants
___ Pediatric Population-Neonates
___ Physics
___ Physiological Studies
___ Pregnancy
___ Prostheses
___ QA/QC
___ Radiation Effects
___ Radiation Safety
___ Radiobiology
___ Safety
___ Screening
___ Sedation
___ Seizure Disorders
___ Socioeconomic Issues
___ Speech Disorders
___ Staging
___ Statistics
___ Surgery
___ Technical Aspects
___ Technology Assessments
___ Tissue Characterization
___ Transplantation
___ Trauma
___ Treatment Effects
___ Tropical Diseases
___ Varices
___ Volvulus

Please reproduce here the **one sentence** from the text that best conveys or summarizes the message of your study.

____

____

Please provide author initials by appropriate author contribution category.

________ Guarantor of integrity of entire study
________ Study concepts
________ Study design
________ Definition of intellectual content
________ Literature research
________ Clinical studies
________ Experimental studies
________ Data acquisition
________ Data analysis
________ Statistical analysis
________ Manuscript preparation
________ Manuscript editing
________ Manuscript review

This form *must be* included with your manuscript submission.

Anthony V. Proto, MD

Radiology 1999: Left-Hand Pages

For the past several years, *Radiology* has maintained a policy of beginning each article within a given section on a right-hand page. A positive feature of this policy has been the convenience provided for the reader who wishes to remove articles from a given issue—no overlap with the last page of the prior article or the first page of the subsequent article. The negative feature of this policy, however, has been the accumulation of some 12–20 potentially blank left-hand pages per issue of the Journal. Rather than leave these pages blank, we have used them for a variety of items such as Interludes, Book Reviews, and others (1).

An exception to our left-hand page policy has been the Technical Developments section. In the past, articles in this section might begin not only on a left-hand page but also in the middle of a page. As of the January 1998 issue, my first as Editor, we continued the policy of beginning articles within the Technical Developments section on left-hand pages, if necessary, but not in the middle of a given page. We have received no negative feedback of this use of left-hand pages.

A number of items have prompted me to reconsider our left-hand page policy: (*a*) Publication space in our Journal is highly sought by authors from within and outside North America; (*b*) our number of submissions has not decreased but, in fact, has increased slightly; (*c*) the availability of the *Radiology* Online Edition has prompted some to no longer remove articles from the Journal in view of their ready availability electronically, thereby saving personal storage space; (*d*) we continue to amass a wealth of important material that deserves dissemination to our readers in as timely a fashion as possible; and (*e*) some highly respected nonimaging journals begin articles on left-hand pages. In view of the foregoing, we have implemented use of left-hand pages to begin articles within the given sections of the Journal. Some of you no doubt noticed this change that began in part with the June 1999 issue and is now fully implemented in the August 1999 issue. At this time, we have no plans to change our policy of beginning the first article in each section on a right-hand page. Thus, some left-hand pages will remain and will be used as in the past.

Radiology seeks to publish the best of the submissions it receives regarding imaging, imaging-related, radiation oncology, and medical physics research that is conducted worldwide and to offer, at the same time, information that is of practical value to its readers. Using left-hand pages in this new manner will help us achieve our goal by providing a more efficient use of the Journal pages. We trust our readers will agree that any inconvenience this new policy will create for them is minor in light of the benefit of improved use of space.

Index terms:
Editorials
Radiology (journal)

Radiology 1999; 212:297

Reference

1. Proto AV. *Radiology*—1998 and the future. Radiology 1998; 206:1–2.

Seymour H. Levitt, MD
President, Radiological Society of North America

The Radiological Society of North America 85th Scientific Assembly and Annual Meeting Sunday, November 28 to Friday, December 3, 1999 McCormick Place, Chicago, Illinois[1]

Just as our knowledge and technology have evolved and improved over the decades, so have the offerings of the RSNA Scientific Assembly and Annual Meeting. The 85th Annual Meeting celebrates "A Century of Research and Education," from the birth of radiology to today's cutting-edge diagnostic imaging and therapeutic technology. The 1999 Scientific Program is dedicated to the memory of Dr Juan A. Del-Regato in honor of his contributions to radiology, and especially to radiation oncology.

As in the past, attendees have a vast array of educational opportunities, through scientific papers, refresher courses, scientific and *info*RAD exhibits, technical exhibits, demonstrations, workshops, and symposia. In keeping with our tradition of growth and enhancement of our Annual Meeting, this year's event places special emphasis on integrating information systems in healthcare with our "Meeting within the RSNA Meeting"—the Integrating the Healthcare Enterprise (IHE) Symposium.

The IHE Symposium, with the theme, "Architecting Cost-effective, High-Quality, Patient-centered Care for the New Millennium," will run concurrently with the RSNA Meeting and include keynote lectures; presentations of clinical scenarios, scientific papers, case studies; and panel discussions. Attendees can register for IHE Symposium sessions only or can incorporate a selection of these sessions into their overall program.

More than 25,000 of your peers will convene this year to benefit from the impressive assemblage of more than 1,700 scientific papers, 200 scientific sessions, 275 refresher courses, 1,000 scientific and *info*RAD exhibits, and 700 technical exhibits, in addition to the many demonstrations, workshops, and symposia.

The **Opening Session**, beginning at 8:30 AM on Sunday, November 28, will feature "Oncologic Imaging, What the Oncologist Wants to Know about Diagnostic Imaging," moderated by Samuel Hellman, MD, and "Advances in Oncologic Imaging: The Diagnostic Radiologist's Perspective," moderated by Hedvig Hricak, MD, PhD. These presentations will be preceded by my Presidential Address, "Impact of Changes in the Health Care System on Patient Care, Research and Education."

On Sunday afternoon, beginning at 3:30, C. Douglas Maynard, MD, chairman of the Board of Trustees of the **RSNA Research and Education Foundation**, will announce the RSNA Roentgen Centennial Fellow for 1999 and present other Foundation news. The always popular **Sunday Image Interpretation Session**, moderated this year by N. Reed Dunnick, MD, will follow Dr Maynard's announcements.

On Monday afternoon at 1:00, RSNA recognizes Nina Einhorn, MD, PhD, and Ulrik Ringborg, MD, both of Stockholm, Sweden, and Rolf Sauer, MD, of Erlangen, Germany, for the contributions they have made to radiology, by awarding them **Honorary Membership** in the Society. Following that presentation, Richard Wahl, MD, will present the **Eugene P. Pendergrass New Horizons Lecture**, "Imaging Cancer in the New Millennium: Form Follows Function."

Tuesday afternoon's activities include a 1:00 PM plenary session, which begins with the presentation of the 1999 **RSNA Gold Medals** to Malcolm A. Bagshaw, MD, of Stanford, Calif; Jerzy Einhorn, MD, PhD, of Stockholm, Sweden; and O. Wayne Houser, MD, of Rochester, Minn. The presentation will be followed by the **Annual Oration in Diagnostic Radiology**, featuring Barry B. Goldberg, MD. He will speak on "Ultrasound: Advances in Contrast Agents and 3D Imaging."

Special Focus Sessions will be presented on Tuesday and Thursday. The eight sessions offered at 4:00 PM on Tuesday are "CT Screening for Lung Cancer: Results and Critical Issues," moderated by Claudia I. Henschke, MD, PhD; "Current Clinical Applications of PET Imaging in the Oncology Patient," by Edward Patz, Jr, MD; "Evidence-based Radiology," by Harald O. Solberg, MD; "Computer-aided Mammographic Diagnosis: Are Computers Telling Us Something We Should Know?" by Carl J. Vyborny, MD, PhD; "Sonography of the Shoulder and

Index term:
Radiological Society of North America, 85th scientific assembly and annual meeting

Radiology 1999; 212:298–299

[1] In accordance with the bylaws of the Radiological Society of North America (section 6.12), the Board of Directors has appointed a Committee on Nominations. In 1999, the Committee on Nominations consists of C. Douglas Maynard, MD, Chairman, Winston-Salem, NC; David B. Fraser, MD, Halifax, NS; and Richard L. Morin, PhD, Jacksonville, FL. Suggestions for nominations should be addressed to the Chairman.

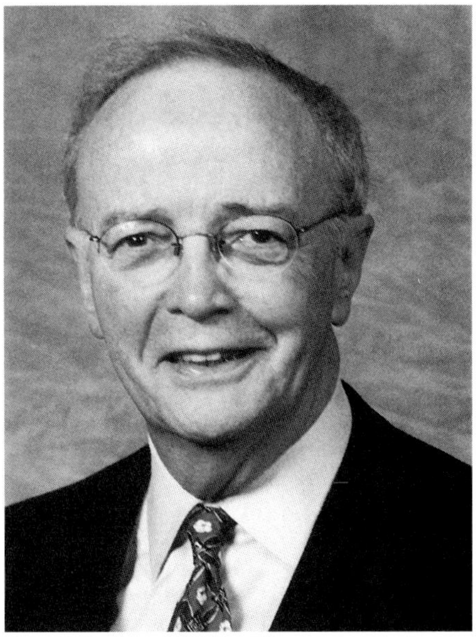

Seymour H. Levitt, MD, President

Musculoskeletal System: Can You/Should You Do It?" by William Middleton, MD; "Liver Tumor Ablation with Image Guidance," by Robert L. Bree, MD, MHSA; "Compliance, Documentation, and How to Avoid Fraud in Your Practice," by Robert Zeman, MD; and "Screening Mammography: A World View," by Linda Warren, MD.

Wednesday's highlights include a 1:00 PM plenary session beginning with the announcement of the **Scientific Exhibit Awards**. After the awards presentation, Lars E. Rutqvist, MD, will deliver the **Annual Oration in Radiation Oncology** on "Radiation Therapy in Early-Stage Breast Cancer: Biologic and Clinical Rationale." At 4:00 PM on Wednesday, Ritsuko Komaki, MD, will moderate the **Oncodiagnosis Panel**, which will discuss "Diagnosis and Multidisciplinary Approach for Lung Cancer."

At 1:00 Thursday afternoon, the **RSNA/AAPM Symposium** will focus on "Spiral CT, 10 Years In," moderated by David R. Pickens, PhD. The inauguration of the 2000 RSNA Board of Directors and introduction of the 1999 AAPM officers and council chairs will follow.

Thursday's seven **Special Focus Session** topics, held at 4:15 PM, are "Role of Imaging in Epilepsy Surgery: Present and Future," moderated by Clifford Jack, Jr, MD; "Tuberculosis from Head to Toe," by Melissa L. Rosado de Christenson, MD; "Battle for Supremacy in Abdominal Imaging: Helical CT versus MR Imaging," moderated by Joseph K. T. Lee, MD; "When Appendicitis is Suspected in Children," by Carlos Sivit, MD; "Physician-Patient Relationships," by Wilbur Smith, Jr, MD; "Mouse Genomics and Phenotypic Imaging," by R. Nick Bryan, MD, PhD; and "Update on the Activities of the American College of Radiology Imaging Network (ACRIN)," by Bruce J. Hillman, MD.

The final plenary session, on December 3, features the **Friday Imaging Symposium**, at 12:30 PM. The symposium topic is "Algorithmic Controversies" and will be moderated by Alex Gottschalk, MD.

The **Refresher Course Program** is a focal part of the meeting. Conducted throughout the week, it features more than 275 courses, including 32 limited-attendance workshops. Three Categorical Courses, one Special Course, and two minicourses will be featured in the Refresher Course program.

The **Categorical Course in Diagnostic Radiology** will focus on body magnetic resonance imaging and is being directed by Shirley M. McCarthy, MD, PhD, Caroline Reinhold, MD, and William E. Palmer, MD. There are two **Categorical Courses in Physics**. The first features "Electronic Radiology Practice: Technical and Practical" directed by Nicolas J. Hangiandreou, PhD, Jeremy W. R. Young, MD, and Richard L. Morin, PhD. The second features "Physical Aspects of Breast Imaging: Current and Future Considerations," directed by Arthur G. Haus, and Martin J. Yaffe, PhD.

The **Special Course** topic is "Pediatric Radiology: Current Concepts in Body Imaging at the Millennium," directed by Marilyn J. Siegel, MD. Minicourse subjects include "Women's Health in Imaging" and "New Developments in Body CT Scanning." Syllabi for the Categorical Courses and the Special Course will be available for purchase at the meeting.

The weeklong event also includes *info*RAD, which features hands-on computer-assisted self-instruction, Web-based applications, clinical software, virtual reality, and Integrating the Healthcare Enterprise exhibits.

Prior to the official opening of the RSNA Scientific Assembly and Annual Meeting, the Associated Sciences Consortium will conduct its **Associated Sciences Workshop**, beginning at 10:15 AM on Saturday, November 27. The theme of the workshop will be "New Realities in Radiology: Multidisciplinary Strategies for Compliance."

Three joint AAPM/RSNA physics presentations are also scheduled for Saturday afternoon. The **AAPM/RSNA Physics Tutorial for Residents**, "Fluoroscopy," organized by Beth A. Schueler, PhD, will be held from 1:00 to 5:00 PM. The **AAPM/RSNA Basic Tutorial on Equipment Selection**, featuring "MR Imaging," with Ronald R. Price, PhD, is scheduled from 2:00 to 5:00 PM. Gerald A. White, Jr, MS, will deliver the **AAPM/RSNA Basic Physics Lecture for the Radiologic Technologist**, "Digital Imaging: What You Need to Know Now and What You Need to Know Next," from 3:00 to 4:30 PM.

The scientific assembly continues to be successful through the untiring efforts of more than 2,000 volunteer committee members. I especially thank the Program Committee, directed by Theresa C. McLoud, MD; the Refresher Course Committee, guided by Glenn S. Forbes, MD; the Scientific Exhibits Committee, chaired by Steven K. Teplick, MD; the Technical Exhibits Committee, headed by Alan E. Oestreich, MD; the Audiovisual Services Committee, directed by Susan A. Stafford, MD; and the Associated Sciences Committee, led by Samuel L. Hissong, MD.

The Program Subcommittee chairs are responsible for selecting the papers and organizing the sessions in their respective disciplines. They are to be commended for the magnitude of work they do and for the excellent results of their efforts. The subcommittee chairs are Kerry M. Link, MD, Cardiovascular Radiology; Lawrence R. Goodman, MD, Chest Radiology; Pablo R. Ros, MD, Gastrointestinal Radiology; Carl J. D'Orsi, MD, General Radiology/Breast Imaging; Stanford M. Goldman, MD, Genitourinary Radiology; Robert L. Bree, MD, Health Services, Policy and Research; Mark D. Murphey, MD, Musculoskeletal Radiology; Allan J. Fox, MD, Neuroradiology/Head and Neck; Gary L. Dillehay, MD, Nuclear Medicine; Joanna J. Seibert, MD, Pediatric Radiology; James A. Seibert, PhD, Physics; Nora A. Janjan, MD, Radiation Oncology and Radiobiology; and Gerald Dodd III, MD, Ultrasound. I thank each subcommittee chair and member for their hard work and dedication.

Equally important to learning and networking is the chance for meeting new colleagues and reacquainting with old friends from around the country, as well as from nations around the world.

This year's Annual Meeting promises a wealth of excitement and educational exchange. Please join us for RSNA 1999.

I'll see you in November at Chicago's McCormick Place.

Book Review

Neuroradiology Companion: Methods, Guidelines, and Imaging Fundamentals. 2nd ed.

Mauricio Castillo, MD
Philadelphia, Pa: Lippincott-Raven, 1998. ISBN 0-7817-1695-0. Softcover, $59.95; pp 384; 239 figures.

This is the second edition of this compact book, whose purpose is to help trainees during their rotations in neuroradiology. It is a single-authored work by the chief of the neuroradiology section at the University of North Carolina Hospital. Since this is an outgrowth of the resident handbook used at the author's institution, it contains a section on protocols and guidelines and another on images with pearls of wisdom. The former section provides practical techniques for caring for the patient and acquiring optimal images. The latter section is a compendium of clinical images with itemized comments about each illustrated disease process.

The format of the second edition is identical to that of the first. However, changes have been made to this edition. Imaging protocols have been updated to reflect the author's current practice. One notable difference is the preference for spiral technique in most computed tomographic (CT) protocols. The angiographic guidelines have been altered in consideration of the change from cut-film to digital subtraction technology. The section on the Wada protocol has been removed, as have the Society of Cardiovascular and Interventional Radiology criteria on indications for cerebral angiography. The techniques for magnetic resonance (MR) imaging are based on those used with Siemens equipment, but no manufacturer-specific acronyms are used. Parenthetically, there are no included protocols for MR imaging of the temporomandibular joints or the brachial plexus.

The section on medications for reactions to contrast media now includes a paragraph on medication given to prevent reactions. The author's suggestions that contrast material reactions are due to allergies and that there is an "iodine allergy" are misleading. It would be more accurate to state that contrast medium reactions are idiosyncratic events and to point out that pretreatment is not foolproof; severe reactions may still occur. Furthermore, the patient with generalized allergies does not always require pretreatment; however, pretreatment of patients who have had documented contrast medium reactions is advisable.

The small section on sedation in the original edition has been expanded to five full pages. The chapter entitled "What Study to Order" has also been revised to include advances in MR imaging in the interval since the previous edition. The entire chapter called "Dictations" has been eliminated, although the reason for this editorial decision is not explained. The section entitled "Imaging Fundamentals" is updated, and most of its images are new. The new edition also adds a chapter on degenerative brain disorders.

This book is not written in narrative style. It contains lists, illustrations, and tables. The lists are clear and the illustrations are very good, considering that they are no more than one-quarter page in size. The bibliography is modern, and there is an index to assist in searching for a topic.

This book is meant to be a guide for radiology residents and neuroradiology fellows. As such, it may be useful given the following caveats. Imaging protocols vary by institution because of differences in equipment. The type of study to order also changes depending on the availability of equipment. The key facts about images and diseases may be a sufficient starting point, but they are not a substitute for intensive and continuous academic inquiry. Trainees must be aware that seeing "typical" images is not a substitute for learning the logical and thorough application of pathophysiologic and imaging principles to the analysis and interpretation of images.

Most radiology house officers should find this manual welcome on call; it would be even more practical if it could be reduced to the size of a laboratory coat pocket. It is not exorbitantly priced for its size. It could be published as a CD-ROM. Future editions could include tables and examples of normal myelination and illustrations of spinal fracture instability, a diagram of the normal cerebral circulation at CT and angiography, and a description of tumor staging by area for head and neck cancers.

This book will likely be of only some interest to most neuroradiology fellows, who will be buying more comprehensive works. It may be of interest to physicians in allied fields such as neurology or neurosurgery who seek quick, concise protocols to incorporate into their own practices. Practicing radiologists may find the protocols and guidelines useful to compare with their own.

Reviewed by David S. Martin, MD

Richard M. Friedenberg, MD

The Future of Medicine and Radiology: Part I[1]

What has happened in medicine over the past several years is history. History is recorded, so one must be careful that one's statements relating to the past are accurate. Efforts to anticipate the future are ubiquitous. The predictor must be cautious—the only thing that is certain is that the future will be different from the present. It is fairly safe to predict the changes that will occur in the next 4 or 5 years—history has shown that over a short time, the changes usually will relate to the past, a variation of the previous 5 years. This is not true for predictions about changes 10–20 years in the future. In the science of futurology, one cannot use simple extrapolation for long-term predictions. Therefore, long-term forecasts must be conditional forecasts. For example, if the Democrats control the U.S. Congress for the majority of the next 20 years, the future practice of medicine may be different than that which would occur if the Republicans maintain control of Congress. Future changes, in other words, are conditional upon other events that are themselves difficult to predict.

One nice thing about predicting the future is that nobody can say that you are wrong—and if, in the future, it turns out that you were wrong, by that time nobody remembers what you said.

Joseph Goldstein, MD, chair of the Department of Molecular Genetics at the University of Texas Southwestern Medical Center in Dallas stated that the three major factors that have transformed our lives in the past century are "McDonald's, the microchip, and the discovery of the genetic code" (1). Obviously, he did not consider it from the viewpoint of physicians, who might have included managed health care in the list of factors that transformed our lives.

In this article, which is the first of two parts, I discuss the changes that have occurred in the practice of medicine and attempt to predict what will evolve in the future; in part II, I will discuss the changes that have occurred in the practice of radiology and my outlook for the future. In radiology, we are intermediaries, and as such we are directly affected by what happens to the rest of medicine (2).

The drastic changes that have occurred in medicine over the past 10 years actually started in 1929, 70 years ago, in Elk City, Oklahoma, where the first medical cooperative was established to provide medical care through prepaid insurance. In the 1930s and 1940s, several large managed health care organizations were formed, including the Ross-Loos Medical Clinic (Calif) in 1929, the Kaiser-Permanente Medical Care Program (Calif) in 1939, the Health Insurance Plan of New York in 1947, and the Group Health Cooperative of Puget Sound (Wash) in 1947 (3).

In 1970, a Minneapolis (Minn) physician by the name of Paul Ellwood, Jr, MD, coined the term health maintenance organization, or HMO, as an alternative to the fee-for-service system. You may not have known that, in 1971, President Nixon, in his health message to Congress, embraced the HMO concept and proposed legislation to allow Medicare participants to join such organizations. Congress passed the Health Maintenance Organization Act of 1973, which provided incentive grants for the establishment of HMOs. From 1970 until approximately 1980, enrollment of patients in HMOs increased from 3 million to 13 million participants (4). In 1985, enrollment was approximately 19 million, and, by 1998, enrollment was estimated to be over 150 million.

Three major stimuli for the development of managed health care were, first, the rapid rise in the cost of health care for workers, which had become a large part of industry's budget, and, second, the government's concern about rising health care costs in the United States, which had increased from $250 million in 1980 to about $1 trillion in 1995. Health care was consuming about 14% of the gross national product (5). The third and precipitating factor was the failure of President Clinton's health care proposals in 1993, after which the government backed off from involvement in structuring of the health care system and left the field wide open to business entrepreneurs. By 1995, HMO enrollment in the United States had grown to 56 million participants, and HMOs were now a powerful force in American medicine (4).

I believe that, in the late 1980s and early 1990s, we physicians made a fundamental mistake. We were so busy trying to protect the fee-for-service system that we were not major players in the establishment of managed health care policy. We forgot that our prime purpose should be as advocates for patients, and, as such, we should have had a major say in the methods of managed health care. Instead, we became recipients of the rules established by the entrepreneurs, which, in many cases, were slanted more toward profit than patient care. Managed health care became too much involved with management and too little involved with the problems of patient care. Profit-oriented

Index terms:
Perspectives
Radiology and radiologists, socioeconomic issues

Radiology 1999; 212:301–304

[1] From the Department of Radiological Sciences, UCI Medical Center, University of California, Irvine, 101 The City Dr, Orange, CA 92868-3298. Received March 16, 1999; accepted May 21. **Address reprint requests to** the author (e-mail: *rmfriede@uci.edu*).

chief executive officers drove down costs, often sacrificing quality in the process. In California, we have experienced the growth of managed health care to the point where unrestricted fee for service is almost extinct. In California, approximately 25% of the population is uninsured. Of the remaining 75%, 49% are participants in HMOs; 22%, in preferred provider organizations (PPOs); 5%, in point-of-service plans, (an HMO hybrid); 21%, in Medicare/Medi-Cal; and approximately 3%, in indemnity fee-for-service plans (6).

Managed health care is deeply rooted in California, which in many ways was the birthplace of modern managed health care. In California, HMOs became the prevalent form of managed health care. Outside of California, PPO plans, which are, in effect, controlled fee-for-service plans, are more popular than the more restrictive HMO plans. To cope with patient demands and physician complaints, HMOs were forced to expand their services, which increased their costs. In 1993 and 1994, approximately 90% of HMOs reported a profit or surplus (4). In 1995, that number declined to 60% and today is probably less than 50%. Stock prices of managed care companies have decreased dramatically over the past 3 years. In 1996 alone, HMO stocks as a group decreased by 22%. The answer for HMOs was to raise rates. Kaiser-Permanente last year increased its rates by up to 14%; increases of 8%–10% were common, and further increases will probably occur this year.

The main base of HMO support is corporate America, because of the lower insurance costs. However, even this may change if there is further public discontent with the restrictions imposed by HMOs. Recently, new Medicare legislation has allowed Medicare beneficiaries to enroll in PPOs, as well as HMOs, and this may stimulate additional PPO growth.

It is interesting to note that when Medicare and Medicaid were created in 1965, politicians were concerned about health care, not costs. In 1965, the budget office projected that the cost in 1990 of Medicare Part A (the hospital insurance portion of Medicare) would be $9 billion. The actual amount in 1990 was $66.9 billion, which shows the difficulty in projecting ahead (7). The percentage of gross national product accounted for by health care costs was 5.1% in 1960 and 13.6% in 1990; in 2030, these percentages are projected to be 37% with indemnity health care and 14% with managed health care (7). The indemnity costs are obviously overinflated, and the managed health care costs are underestimated. Such overinflated estimates have stimulated support for managed health care.

TABLE 1
Nonphysician Clinicians

Traditional	Complementary	Specialty Discipline
Nurse practitioner	Chiropractor	Podiatrist
Certified nurse midwife	Naturopath	Optometrist
Physician assistant	Acupuncturist	Nurse anesthetist
	Herbal medicine practitioner	Clinical nurse specialist

Source.—Reference 9.

Richard Lamm, former governor of Colorado, recently described the clash of ethics between the medical profession and public policy makers (8). This is the clash between those who are patient advocates and believe in a 1:1 ratio between physician and patient and those who believe that the new medicine is related to the overall public interest, which is referred to as the "1:*n* ratio." Changes in the perception of health care can be summarized as follows: From 1940 to 1960, the main concern was with whether the physician was nice and caring, and the physician-to-patient ratio was 1:1; from 1960 to 1990, the concern was with the physician's use of the latest technology, and the ratio was still 1:1; in 2000 and beyond, the concern will be with health care as measured with population-based methods, and the ratio will be 1:*n*.

I believe physicians will find it difficult to abandon the concept of the 1:1 relationship. For those of us who have been practicing medicine for 15 years or longer, the concept of sacrificing the individual patient's welfare for the greater good of the community seems like heresy. Unfortunately, Governor Lamm is correct. The time when we would do whatever is necessary to diagnose disease and to treat the individual patient has disappeared. Whether we like it or not, "spare no cost" medicine is gone. No society can continue to fund an open-ended system. As Governor Lamm pointed out, the health care system can no more do everything beneficial for the individual patient than the educational system can do everything beneficial for the individual student. In the future, tax money and corporate payments will be to benefit the health of the people as a whole, while individuals with problems beyond the standards will have to use their own funds. If society does not want health care distributed in this manner, it should not make health care a responsibility of public policy.

The solution to the problems as described by Governor Lamm is not easy. Although health care is heavily influenced by social problems such as provision of food, sanitation, shelter, work, family, and attention to other problems such as smoking, when and if we solve these problems health care costs will not necessarily be reduced. More individuals will attain an older age, but other illnesses will then consume the dollars saved by preventive medicine in the early years. In fact, as we solve problems that allow individuals to attain an older age, we may well be increasing health care costs over the long run.

Physician mores have changed. Physicians are beginning to be much more selective in the diagnostic work-up and treatment of their patients. They realize the benefits of a public policy that is directed at preventive medicine. They are shocked by the knowledge that there are 40 million or more people without health insurance. But decisions to solve such problems are policy decisions, which have become very politicized. Physicians are not the ones who should decide that every patient over 75 years of age with metastatic carcinoma or every newborn with a serious congenital abnormality should not be treated. These are decisions for public policy makers and they cannot make these decisions without consultation with older patients and parents—this is why such decisions are politically very difficult.

Within the next 10 years, clinicians will have to collaborate with a variety of independent and semiindependent practitioners loosely categorized as nonphysician clinicians (9) (Table 1). Most nonphysician clinicians have 4–6 years of training after high school. The responsibility for regulation of nonphysician clinicians resides with the individual state. Most states permit nurse practitioners and physicians' assistants to perform physical examinations and conduct diagnostic examinations within their area of expertise, and many states allow them to prescribe drugs (Table 2). There may be a requirement for

TABLE 2
State Licensure and Autonomy

Practitioner	Practice Recognized by State	Practitioners Licensed	Independent Practice Licensed
Nurse practitioner	50	35	21
Physician assistant	50	31	0

Note.—Data are number of states.

the involvement of a supervising physician, but this is frequently intermittent and at a distance. The Balanced Budget Act of 1997 expanded Medicare reimbursement directly to nurse practitioners and physicians' assistants and removed requirements for physician involvement. Since their reimbursement rates are substantially less than those of physicians, the use of nonphysician clinicians becomes an attractive means of cost control.

I think it is safe to assume that the number of physicians' assistants and nurse practitioners will more than double in the next 10–15 years and that their ability to practice independently will increase. This will probably decrease the need for physicians. In one poll (10) conducted in Washington, DC, 52% of patients reported that they were willing to see a nurse practitioner rather than a physician for primary care.

Chapman (11), from Leeds, England, wrote that a shortage of radiologists in many radiology departments has encouraged the development of a trend of radiographers performing as nonphysician clinicians. This started with ultrasonography, where it soon became evident that the skill of the radiographer frequently surpassed that of the supervising physician. First, the radiographer dictated provisional reports, supervised by the physician. These reports were considered to be comparable to those of the physician, so the radiographer then dictated final reports directly. Next, radiographers started to perform gastrointestinal fluoroscopy; to inject contrast material; to report results of intravenous pyelography, computed tomography, and magnetic resonance imaging with loose physician supervision; and, finally, to report results of emergency room examinations. Results of a survey (11) in one London (England) hospital that involved 12,000 emergency room reports by nonphysician clinicians showed that trained radiographers had a sensitivity of 96% and a specificity of 99%. Again, this is a substantial cost saving and may lead to a new category of nonphysician clinician in radiology.

What do I think will happen to the practice of medicine over the next 10 years? Much of this will depend on how our political establishment deals with current problems.

1. I believe that managed care will continue to mutate in response to both physician and patient demands. Although these demands will raise costs, politicians will accede to them. Managed health care will have to establish a more patient-centered rather than profit-centered profile. The public will insist on this.

2. I believe that the needs of approximately 42 million uninsured individuals, with an increase of about 1 million per year, must and will be addressed, because this has become a major political problem.

3. I believe that alternative medicine will be encouraged by public policy planners and will continue to grow over the next several years.

4. I do not believe that we will have universal health insurance, but I believe that, in response to public demand, we will have a layered insurance scheme more expensive than today's managed health care system but less costly than our previous fee-for-service system. Layered insurance will allow the patient to select the depth of coverage desired within the managed care program—for a price. This will, in effect, remove the distinctions between the various types of managed health care organizations such as HMOs and PPOs.

a) For those individuals who are currently uninsured and those using Medicaid, the government will subsidize HMO care under a basic health care plan. The government will attempt to ensure that private HMOs accept these patients, but this will be difficult, and the government may be forced to establish its own HMO, which, in effect, will be an extension of Medicaid. The responsibility for administration of this may be at the state level. I believe there will be enough physicians available to staff such a plan.

b) Those individuals who work for corporate America will have access to multitiered HMO and PPO plans. These might be termed "focused care," where the individual selects the desired level of care. Options would include pharmacy, second opinions, ability to see a health care professional outside of the plan, and so forth. There will be copayment for coverage available to those who opt for more sophisticated plans. The cost to corporations to provide even the basic plan will be higher than it is today. I believe that the majority of these patients will select PPO plans.

c) For the more affluent, there will be restricted fee for service. Patients will be able to have a wide choice of physicians who will accept a predetermined fee. There will be a small group of consultants who will not accept any plan and will require private payment of a larger fee.

We should realize that whatever happens to the management of health care will not rid society of medical care problems. There will be continuing flux between managers, patients, and physicians, which will continue to modify the organization and administration of health care. My predictions are based on a moderate continuation of economic growth, with a political balance between liberals and conservatives. Extremes of prosperity or depressed earnings or total control by liberals (advocates of universal health care) or conservatives (advocates of market-driven health care) may affect the balance.

How will physicians be reimbursed? Reimbursement will continue as it does today—capitation, regulated fee for service, or salary. If, in the future, Congress has a liberal orientation, compensation may primarily be through salary and capitation. I believe that it is more likely that regulated fee for service, similar to the PPO structure of today, will be the major form of compensation for most physicians. Small practice groups will disappear—the practice of medicine will be dominated by large group practices affiliated with managed health care organizations. The tendency will be to reimburse support physicians (formerly hospital-based physicians) by means of capitation or salary. Most radiologists will fall into this category. The total income of physicians will continue to decrease over time, as it has in California, although physicians as a group will still earn a reasonable income.

As physicians become more frustrated with the loss of control with regard to patients, reduced fees, and an increased "hassle factor," unions will see an opportunity to organize physicians. The Service

Employees International Union has pledged to spend $1 million per year to recruit physicians (12). Currently, about 6% of doctors are already union members, and the number is increasing. Organizers have said they will first concentrate on California, Florida, and Washington, where unions already have strength. Although the American Medical Association has stated that strikes are contrary to physicians' ethical codes, the unions would not rule out the possibility of strikes. If physician unhappiness in managed health care continues, we may see substantial union activity in the next few years.

There is a separate and serious problem for academic institutions. Because their costs are higher, HMOs do not readily send patients to teaching hospitals. To attract HMO patients, academic centers must match the fees paid to private groups. This means that academic centers must have other means of support to maintain their programs. In 1994, a bill was introduced in Congress to create an academic health center trust fund (7). This was to be financed by a 1.5% tax on health care premiums with an additional 0.25% tax added on for research support. It was calculated that over $17 billion would be collected over 5 years. Unfortunately, the bill did not pass Congress. Senator Moynihan introduced a similar bill in 1997 to establish a medical education trust fund that would have received about $13.5 billion from general funds over 6 years (7). This bill never reached the Senate floor. There is no question that outside support will be needed if we are to maintain the quality of our academic institutions. If an added tax bill does not generate support, I believe that Congress may appropriate $2–3 billion per year from general funds and that this money will be channeled to academic institutions.

As a postscript, in my next Perspective I will present my views on the future of the practice of radiology. Many readers will have different views concerning the future of medicine and radiology. I invite you to send your views to me.

References

1. Harris ED Jr. Dartmouth Medical School bicentennial symposium: great issues for medicine in the twenty-first century—a consideration of the ethical and social issues arising out of advances in the biomedical sciences. Pharos 1998; 61:26–33.
2. Friedenberg RM. The radiologist: a middleman (person) of medicine. Radiology 1994; 190(1):49A–51A.
3. Friedenberg RM. A compendium of managed care: past, present, and hints of the future: part I. Radiology 1998; 208:289–292.
4. Hamer R, VanAntwerp S. Study results show decline in HMO operating margins. Healthc Financ Manage 1997; 51:78–80, 82, 84.
5. Thompson JC. Seedcorn: impact of managed care on medical education and research. Ann Surg 1996; 223:453–463.
6. Insurance Policy Committee of University of California, Berkeley, and UCLA. Bulletin of State Health Insurance Committee of California. Sacramento, Calif: State Health Insurance Committee of California, 1998.
7. Moynihan DP. On the commodification of medicine. Acad Med 1998; 73:453–459.
8. Lamm RD. The coming clash: patient advocates vs the public interests. Pharos 1998; 61:18–20.
9. Cooper RA, Henderson T, Dietrich CL. Roles of nonphysician clinicians as autonomous providers of patient care. JAMA 1998; 280:795–802.
10. Oransky I, Varma JK. Nonphysician clinicians and the future of medicine (editorial). JAMA 1997; 277:1090.
11. Chapman AH. Changing work patterns. Lancet 1997; 350:581–583.
12. Bernstein S, Cleeland N, Riccardi N. Salaried doctors are courted by labor union. Los Angeles Times 1999; March 2:1.

Jane L. Weissman, MD

Old Problems, New Techniques: The Interventional Radiologist and the Lacrimal Apparatus[1]

Therapeutic interventions joined the diagnostic radiology armamentarium in 1964 (1). Remarkable new vistas opened immediately. Since the first reported angioplasty (1), radiologists have been augmenting and refining their ability to accomplish, without surgery or general anesthesia, procedures that previously required both (2,3). The article by Wilhelm et al (4) in the current issue of *Radiology* provides one more example of an ingenious nonsurgical approach to a problem previously deemed exclusively surgical.

External dacryocystorhinostomy is the traditional option to treat lacrimal sac stones (dacryolithiasis), nasolacrimal duct obstruction, and the resultant epiphora (tearing). Dacryocystorhinostomy, the surgical placement of a stent between the lacrimal sac and the nasal cavity, usually requires general anesthesia and always leaves a cutaneous scar (5,6). Other surgical options include endonasal (endoscopic) dacryocystorhinostomy and laser dacryocystorhinostomy (5).

In an elegant nonsurgical procedure, Wilhelm and colleagues crushed dacryoliths with a balloon-tipped catheter, then flushed the fragments out of the nasolacrimal duct into the nose (4). The procedure was performed with fluoroscopic observation. Some patients required intravenous sedation, but no patients required general anesthesia, and the procedure left no visible scars.

Nonsurgical fluoroscopically guided treatment of dacryoliths is the youngest child in a family of interventional radiologic procedures addressing partial and complete obstruction of the lacrimal apparatus. Hanafee and Dayton (7) dilated the nasolacrimal duct with a probe and fluoroscopic guidance in 1978. Radiologists soon were using balloons to dilate the nasolacrimal duct (8–11) and placing metal (12), plastic (13), and polyurethane (14–16) stents in the duct. Ophthalmologists jumped on the balloon bandwagon (17,18). Despite cautionary notes sounded (in this journal) by an ophthalmologist warning radiologists against instrumentation of the lacrimal sac and canaliculi (6), this journal subsequently reported successful balloon dilation of the lacrimal sac by radiologists (19). Radiologists also used balloons to dilate the lacrimal canaliculi (20,21) and placed a lacrimal canaliculus stent (22).

How important is this work? Epiphora occurs in two settings: a normal, patent lacrimal apparatus overwhelmed by a sudden flow of tears (as in crying), and a partially or completely obstructed system unable to drain a normal volume of tears. The latter brings patients to medical attention. Epiphora is a troubling problem but not a debilitating one. It is considered a common ophthalmologic problem but accounts for less than 5% of office visits (4,23).

In the United States, epiphora has not achieved the epidemic proportions or ramifications of cardiovascular disease. I conducted an informal survey of head and neck radiologists practicing in the United States and identified only one radiologist who had dilated a nasolacrimal duct. Yet to consider the utility of interventional radiology in the lacrimal apparatus solely from the perspective of patient numbers or the severity of the affliction does a disservice to this procedure and to the entire field of interventional radiology.

The inclination to design, attempt, and refine a nonsurgical solution to any clinical problem is the basis of the field of interventional radiology. After Dotter and Judkins' groundbreaking report (1), the newfound ability to treat atherosclerotic disease from within (the endovascular approach) rather than from without (surgery) fired the imaginations of radiologists. Reports of "minimally invasive procedures" (3) to treat vascular and, subsequently, nonvascular disease soon began to appear.

Today, the interventional radiology suite has replaced the operating room as the venue for a wide array of therapeutic procedures. The blood supply to aneurysms, vascular malformations, varicoceles, vascular tumors, and vessels damaged by tumor, trauma, or irradiation can be therapeutically interrupted with polyvinyl alcohol particles, gelatin sponge, glue, collagen, coils, and balloons (24–28). The patency of thrombosed vessels can be reestablished with urokinase or

Index terms:
Catheters and catheterization, 223.1263
Editorials
Fluoroscopy, 223.11
Lacrimal gland and duct, 223.1492, 223.818
Lacrimal gland and duct, interventional procedures, 223.1262, 223.1263, 223.1267, 223.1295
Lacrimal gland and duct, radiography, 223.11, 223.1295

Radiology 1999; 212:305–306

[1] From the Department of Radiology, University of Pittsburgh Medical Center, Rm PUH D-132, 200 Lothrop Street, Pittsburgh, PA 15213. Received April 8, 1998; accepted April 16. **Address reprint requests to** the author. (e-mail: *weissmanjl@radserv.arad.upmc.edu*).

See also the article by Wilhelm et al (pp 365–370) in this issue.

tissue plasminogen activator (29), as well as an array of investigational drugs and thrombectomy catheters. Angioplasty preserves or widens a lumen compromised by atherosclerosis, spasm, or irradiation (3). Balloons reestablish, and stents maintain, the patency of blood vessels, ducts (lacrimal, biliary), and hollow viscera (esophagus, bronchus, ureter) (3,30–34). Percutaneous injections obliterate or reduce vascular malformations (35); percutaneous catheters address renal and other obstructions (33). All of these procedures rely on fluoroscopy, and most are quicker, easier (for both the patient and the physician), and less invasive than existing surgical alternatives. In the era of managed care and cost containment, a less invasive procedure that is followed by a more rapid recovery has wide appeal.

The field of interventional radiology is large and continues to grow. The development of new techniques refines and advances the specialty. Applying established techniques to newly identified problems, as Wilhelm and colleagues (4) have done, is yet another way to advance the forefronts of interventional radiology and to provide evidence of the field's vitality.

To the patients affected, epiphora is not a minor problem, and these patients are no less deserving of state-of-the-art medical care because their numbers are small. The inclination to address epiphora, and other clinical problems, by modifying the existing techniques of interventional radiology is ingenious and important. Publication of this work encourages and rewards the authors and, I hope, encourages and inspires others.

Acknowledgment: The author is grateful to Sabrina L. Jennings for her good-natured and skillful manuscript preparation.

References

1. Dotter CT, Judkins MP. Transluminal treatment of arteriosclerotic obstruction: description of a new technic and a preliminary report of its application. Circulation 1964; 30:654–670.
2. Kinney TB. Radiologic history exhibit: Charles T. Dotter—a pioneering interventional radiologist. RadioGraphics 1996; 16:697–707.
3. Vogelzang RL. Future directions in vascular and interventional radiology research. Radiology 1998; 209:17–18.
4. Wilhelm KE, Hofer U, Textor HJ, Böker T, Strunk HM, Schild HH. Dacryoliths: nonsurgical fluoroscopically guided treatment during dacryocystoplasty. Radiology 1999; 212:365–370.
5. Shun-Shin GA, Thurairajan G. External dacryocystorhinostomy: an end of an era? Br J Ophthalmol 1997; 81:716–717.
6. Glatt HJ. Dacryocystoplasty: an oculoplastic surgeon's perspective (letter). Radiology 1991; 180:289–290.
7. Hanafee WN, Dayton GO Jr. Dilatation of the nasolacrimal duct under radiographic control. Radiology 1978; 127:813–815.
8. Munk PL, Lin DTC, Morris DC. Epiphora: treatment by means of dacryocystoplasty with balloon dilation of the nasolacrimal drainage apparatus. Radiology 1990; 177: 687–690.
9. McCullough KM. Naso-lacrimal duct balloon dilatation. Clin Radiol 1994; 49:787–790.
10. Janssen AG, Mansour K, Krabbe GJ, van der Veen S, Helder AH. Dacryocystoplasty: treatment of epiphora by means of balloon dilation of the obstructed nasolacrimal duct system. Radiology 1994; 193: 453–456.
11. Berkefeld J, Kirchner J, Müller HM, Fries U, Kollath J. Balloon dacryocystoplasty: indications and contraindications. Radiology 1997; 205:785–790.
12. Song HY, Ahn HS, Park CK, Kwon SH, Kim CS, Choi KC. Complete obstruction of the nasolacrimal system. II. Treatment with expandable metallic stents. Radiology 1993; 186:372–376.
13. Song HY, Jin YH, Kim JH, Sung KB, Han YM, Cho NC. Nasolacrimal duct obstruction treated nonsurgically with the use of plastic stents. Radiology 1994; 190:535–539.
14. Song HY, Jin YH, Kim JH, et al. Nonsurgical placement of a nasolacrimal polyurethane stent. Radiology 1995; 194:233–237.
15. Song HY, Jin YH, Lee HK, Sung KB. Nonoperative management of dacryolithiasis. JVIR 1995; 6:647–650.
16. Pulido-Duque JM, Reyes R, Carreira JM, et al. Treatment of complete and partial obstruction of the nasolacrimal system with polyurethane stents: initial experience. Cardiovasc Intervent Radiol 1998; 21:41–44.
17. Becker BB, Berry FD. Balloon catheter dilatation in lacrimal surgery. Ophthalmic Surg 1989; 20:193–198.
18. Robinson R, Turner N, Brettle P, Chell PB, Chavda SV, Murray PI. The treatment of epiphora with balloon dacryocystoplasty. Eye 1993; 7:687–690.
19. Lee JM, Song HY, Han YM, et al. Balloon dacryocystoplasty: results in the treatment of complete and partial obstructions of the nasolacrimal system. Radiology 1994; 192:503–508.
20. Ilgit ET, Yuksel D, Unal M, Akpek S, Isik S, Hasanreisoglu B. Transluminal balloon dilatation of the lacrimal drainage system for the treatment of epiphora. AJR 1995; 165:1517–1524.
21. Song HY, Lee CO, Park S, et al. Lacrimal canalicular obstructions: safety and effectiveness of balloon dilation. JVIR 1996; 7:929–934.
22. Song HY, Lee CO, Park S, et al. Lacrimal canaliculus obstruction: nonsurgical treatment with a newly designed polyurethane stent. Radiology 1996; 199:280–282.
23. Song HY, Jin YH, Kim JH, et al. Nonsurgical placement of a nasolacrimal polyurethane stent: long-term effectiveness. Radiology 1996; 200:759–763.
24. Berenstein A, Russell E. Gelatin sponge in therapeutic neuroradiology: a subject review. Radiology 1981; 141:105–112.
25. Picard L, Bracard S, Lehericy S, et al. Endovascular occlusion of intracranial aneurysms of the posterior circulation: comparison of balloons, free coils and detachable coils in 38 patients. Neuroradiology 1996; 38(suppl 1):S133–141.
26. Bavinzski G, Killer M, Ferraz-Leite H, Gruber A, Gross CE, Richling B. Endovascular therapy of idiopathic cavernous aneurysms over 11 years. AJNR 1998; 19:559–565.
27. Coley SC, Jackson JE. Endovascular occlusion with a new mechanical detachable coil. AJR 1998; 171:1075–1079.
28. Chaloupka JC, Putman CM, Citardi MJ, Ross DA, Sasaki CT. Endovascular therapy for the carotid blowout syndrome in head and neck surgical patients: diagnosis and managerial considerations. AJNR 1996; 17:843–852.
29. Fisher M, Bobousslavsky J. Further evolution toward effective therapy for acute ischemic stroke. JAMA 1998; 279:1298–1303.
30. McNicholas MM, Gibney RG, MacErlaine DP. Radiologically guided balloon dilatation of obstructing gastrointestinal strictures. Abdom Imaging 1994; 19:102–107.
31. Huynh PT, de Lange EE, Shaffer HA Jr. Symptomatic webs of the upper esophagus: treatment with fluoroscopically guided balloon dilation. Radiology 1995; 196:789–792.
32. Song HY, Park SI, Do YS, et al. Expandable metallic stent placement in patients with benign esophageal strictures: results of long-term follow-up. Radiology 1997; 203: 131–136.
33. Dunnick NR, Illescas FF, Mitchell S, Cohan RH, Saeed M. Interventional uroradiology. Invest Radiol 1989; 24:831–841.
34. Boguth L, Tatalovic S, Antonucci F, Heer M, Sulser H, Zollikofer CL. Malignant biliary obstruction: clinical and histopathologic correlation after treatment with self-expanding metal prostheses. Radiology 1994; 192:669–674.
35. Casasco A, Herbreteau D, Houdart E, et al. Devascularization of craniofacial tumors by percutaneous tumor puncture. AJNR 1994; 15:1233–1239.

Imaging of Acute Cerebral Ischemia[1]

Norman J. Beauchamp, Jr, MD
Peter B. Barker, DPhil
Paul Y. Wang, MD
Peter C. M. vanZijl, PhD

Index terms:
Brain, infarction, 10.781
Brain, ischemia, 10.781
Cerebral blood vessels, CT, 174.1211
Cerebral blood vessels, flow dynamics, 174.76
Cerebral blood vessels, MR, 174.12141, 174.12142, 174.12145
State-of-art reviews

Radiology 1999; 212:307–324

Abbreviations:
ADC = apparent diffusion coefficient
CSF = cerebrospinal fluid
ECASS = European Cooperative Acute Stroke Study
FLAIR = fluid-attenuated inversion recovery
GRE = gradient-recalled echo
MCA = middle cerebral artery
NAA = *N*-acetylaspartate
NINDS = National Institute for Neurological Diseases and Stroke
rt-PA = recombinant tissue plasminogen activator
SE = spin echo

[1] From the Morgan H. Russell Department of Radiology, Division of Neuroradiology, the Johns Hopkins Hospital, 600 N Wolfe St, Baltimore, MD 21287. Received April 16, 1998; revision requested June 24; final revision received January 13, 1999; accepted March 16. **Address reprint requests to** N.J.B. (e-mail: *nbeauch@welchlink.welch.jhu.edu*).

Until recently, there was no efficacious treatment for acute cerebral ischemia. As a result, the role of neuroimaging and the radiologist was peripheral in the diagnosis and management of this disease. The demonstration of efficacy using thrombolysis has redefined this role, with the success of intervention becoming increasingly dependent on timely imaging and accurate interpretation. The potential benefits of intervention have only begun to be realized. In this State-of-the-Art review of imaging of acute stroke, the role of imaging in the current and future management of stroke is presented. The role of computed tomography is emphasized in that it is currently the most utilized technique, and its value has been demonstrated in prospective clinical trials. Magnetic resonance techniques are equally emphasized in that they have the potential to provide a single modality evaluation of tissue viability and vessel patency in an increasingly rapid evaluation.

Stroke is an injury to the central nervous system that is characteristically abrupt in onset and due to a vascular insult. The term is reflective of damage to the brain secondary to ischemia or hemorrhage. It is the number three cause of mortality and the number one cause of disability in adults in the United States. Strokes are ischemic approximately 80% of the time, and until recently, there was no available beneficial intervention (1,2). In 1995, the published results of the National Institute for Neurological Diseases and Stroke (NINDS) recombinant tissue plasminogen activator (rt-PA) trial represented the first demonstration of efficacious treatment for acute cerebral ischemia (3). This has redefined the role of the radiologist and neuroimaging from peripheral to central in the management of acute cerebral ischemia. This State of the Art describes the central role of the radiologist and neuroimaging in the diagnosis and subsequent management of acute cerebral ischemia.

HISTORY OF STROKE IMAGING

The requirements of stroke imaging are reflective of available treatment options. Before the demonstration of an efficacious intervention, management was largely supportive. Of greatest importance was not the detection of manifest ischemic changes, but the detection of processes such as infection or tumor for which interventions were available. Once processes requiring emergent intervention such as infection and tumor were excluded, supportive measures were instituted, including the prevention of additional thrombus formation with use of anticoagulation. It was well accepted that in the absence of detecting the aforementioned processes, deficits lasting less than 24 hours were due to transient ischemic attacks. Neurologic deficits persisting beyond 24 hours were attributed to infarction. Imaging confirmation of manifest infarction was not needed.

The demonstrated efficacy of the intravenously administered thrombolytic, alteplase ([rt-PA] Activase; Genentech, South San Francisco, Calif), has redefined the requirements for neuroimaging. Optimal management now requires delineation of infarction prior to intervention. This requirement is best understood in the context of the role of thrombolytics for cerebral ischemia and the pathophysiology of cerebral ischemia.

THROMBOLYSIS

Prompt reestablishment of flow with lysis of an occlusive thrombus is the goal of thrombolysis. This is in contrast to anticoagulation, in which new clot formation is

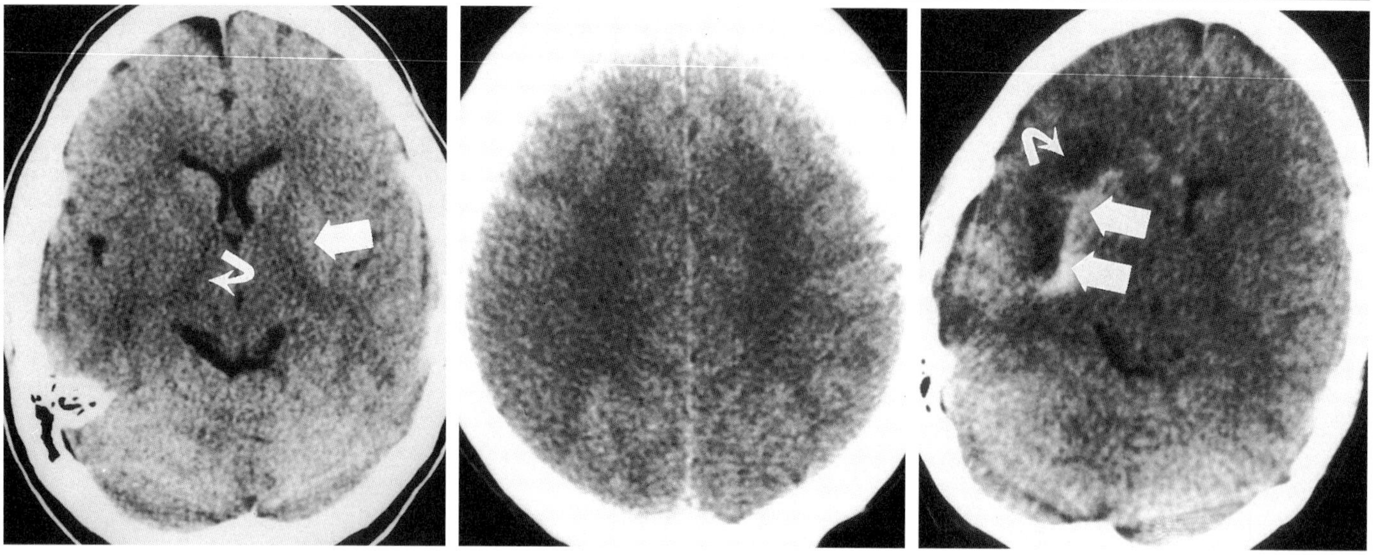

a. b. c.

Figure 1. Left-sided hemiparesis in a 45-year-old man. **(a)** Axial CT scan of the head obtained 6 hours after onset of symptoms. Curved arrow denotes medial demarcation of the posterior limb of the right internal capsule. Note that the lateral margin of the right internal capsule is poorly defined due to decreased attenuation in the structure that makes up the lateral border—the lentiform nucleus. Compare this to the normal left internal capsule and left lentiform nucleus (straight arrow). **(b)** Axial CT scan of the head obtained superior to **a**. There is global decrease in gray matter–white matter differentiation in the right cerebral hemisphere that corresponds to the MCA distribution. **(c)** Axial CT scan of the head was obtained on hospital day 3 and demonstrates an area of increased attenuation (straight arrows) that corresponds to hemorrhage into a region of infarction. The nonhemorrhagic areas of infarction are seen as hypoattenuating (curved arrow).

minimized. These agents convert the proenzyme plasminogen to the active enzyme in thrombin lysis, plasmin. Thrombolysis can be performed by using streptokinase, urokinase, or rt-PA. rt-PA is the most specific of the three agents. It is fibrin specific, activating only thrombin-bound plasminogen. For this reason, it has the most favorable therapeutic index of the three thrombolytic agents.

After thrombolysis was initially proposed in 1958, its acceptability was limited by the inability to differentiate cerebral ischemia from primary intraparenchymal hematoma, the latter a contraindication to thrombolysis (4). Enthusiasm was renewed in the 1990s because of the wide availability of computed tomographic (CT) scanners and the demonstration of efficacy of thrombolytics in the treatment of myocardial ischemia (5,6). This resulted in the performance of numerous clinical trials (3,7–10). Of these, two intravenous rt-PA clinical trials have been of particular importance in defining the current approach to treating cerebral ischemia—the NINDS trials (3) and the European Cooperative Acute Stroke Study (ECASS) (7).

The NINDS trial was the first trial to demonstrate efficacy in the use of the thrombolytics for the treatment of cerebral ischemia (3). The protocol was based on a 3-hour treatment window from the time of ictus to the administration of rt-PA. A CT scan was obtained, and the detection of intracerebral thrombosis was an exclusion criterion. Although no short-term benefits were demonstrated, patients in the treatment group achieved improved stroke scale ratings as compared with those in the placebo group at 3 months. This resulted in approval by the U.S. Food and Drug Administration of rt-PA in June of 1996 and the widespread implementation of acute stroke teams across North America.

The ECASS trial allowed a longer treatment window of 6 hours (7). This time-window prolongation increased the likelihood of manifest infarction at the time of reestablishing flow and thus the risk of reperfusion hemorrhage. In an attempt to avoid reperfusion hemorrhage, a CT scan was obtained to exclude patients with extensive infarction. Patients were excluded if on-site interpretation detected infarction in greater than 33% of the middle cerebral artery (MCA) distribution. Unfortunately, the ECASS group failed to demonstrate efficacy in the intention to treat group. Notably, in addition to the on-site interpretation, CT scans were later reviewed by the ECASS CT review panel. The panel determined that "misinterpretation" by the on-site readers resulted in inappropriate entrance into the trial of 52 individuals (7). By excluding this subgroup of protocol violators, efficacy was demonstrable.

The need for subgroup analysis led to skepticism about the efficacy of thrombolysis beyond 3 hours, which is reflected in the aforementioned approval of a 3-hour treatment window and the relative lack of enthusiasm in the European Community toward implementing thrombolysis. Despite this, the design and outcome of the ECASS trial has had a major effect on defining the optimal approach to stroke intervention in that it has redefined the role for neuroimaging in acute stroke. In this study, CT was used to detect the presence of infarction as opposed to its prior role of excluding other processes such as hemorrhage, tumor, or infection. The ECASS trial also "suggested," based on subgroup analysis, that with neuroimaging it is possible to extend the treatment window beyond 3 hours. This is of great relevance in that on the basis of estimates from the International Stroke Trial, only 4% of acute stroke patients presenting to the hospital are able to arrive within 3 hours (11). Extending the treatment window to 6 hours would make intervention available to approximately 16% of acute stroke patients (11,12).

Finally, this trial demonstrates that "in practice" the early CT changes of infarction are subtle. For example, in 11% of the patients in the ECASS trial, initial

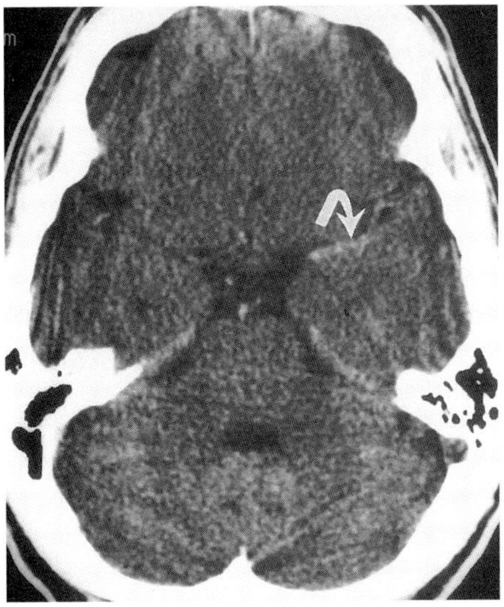

Figure 2. Acute onset of aphasia and right hemiparesis in a 27-year-old man. Axial CT scan of the head obtained 3 hours after onset of symptoms demonstrates a "hyperdense MCA sign" (curved arrow). Note that the vessel is of higher attenuation than that of the contralateral MCA.

interpretation did not detect the presence of infarcts seen on post hoc review. Thus, although enabling of efficacy when the treatment window is less than 3 hours, CT is not the optimal technique for delineating the presence or absence of infarction in the acute period. This "insensitivity" becomes even more important in considering extension of the treatment window beyond 3 hours when the likelihood of infarcted tissue being present and risks of posttreatment hemorrhage are greater.

NEWLY DEFINED ROLE OF CT

CT detection of extended infarction is a recommended exclusion criterion based on the American Heart Association Thrombolysis Practice Advisory Guidelines (13). It is now incumbent on all radiologists to be familiar with the CT evaluation of acute stroke. The sensitivity of CT in the detection of the early changes of infarction is related to the underlying principles of image acquisition. CT images are obtained by projection of a high-kilovoltage collimated beam through the brain. Beam attenuation is due to absorption proportional to the linear attenuation coefficient of the materials through which it passes. The relatively high-kilovoltage x rays used in CT result in linear attenuation primarily due to tissue density. Differentiation of adjacent tissues such as gray matter and white matter depends on perceivable differences in electron density; detection of a pathologic condition requires a perceivable change in electron density.

Fluid redistribution characterizes cerebral ischemia and imparts the changes in electron density detectable with CT. Maintenance of a normal cell volume involves the double-Donnan-equilibrium between electrolytes and fluid exchange between the extra- and intracellular spaces (14,15). This requires a continuous supply of energy to the membrane pumps necessary in maintaining normal intra- and extracellular electrolyte concentration gradients and fluid distribution. With the interruption of blood flow, these energy needs are no longer met, resulting in cytotoxic edema, which is defined as cellular injury with influx of fluid in the intracellular space without an increase in vascular permeability (16).

Neurons are the most sensitive cell to ischemia. These cells are located in gray matter. Initially more dense than the white matter, gray matter becomes increasingly less dense with an increase in water content. The normal gray matter–white matter differentiation that characterizes the normal CT scan progressively declines and results in three of the CT signs of acute cerebral infarction: (*a*) blurring of the clarity of the internal capsule, (*b*) loss of distinctness of the insular ribbon cortex, and (*c*) loss of differentiation between the cortical gray matter and the subjacent white matter (Fig 1) (17,18). In addition to the attenuation changes, morphologic changes occur due to the accumulation of intracellular fluid causing swelling of the cortical gyri. This results in effacement of the spaces demarcated by the gyral infoldings (sulci), known as "sulcal effacement" (19). This is demonstrated prior to the appearance of hypoattenuation. Although these findings become prominent over time, detectable alterations in attenuation are not present at the time of ictus (20).

The "hyperdense MCA sign" is secondary to an embolus lodged in the MCA (Fig 2). This results in increased attenuation in the first segment of the MCA that can be seen at the time of ictus (21). Angiographic correlation has demonstrated a corresponding thrombus, and it is most common with cortical and large deep MCA infarcts. This sign is associated with worse patient outcomes. To avoid misinterpretation of atherosclerotic disease calcifying the MCA and mimicking a thrombus, the following "hyperdense MCA sign" inclusion criteria are important: (*a*) The abnormal vessel should be of higher x-ray attenuation than that of the contralateral MCA and the basilar artery and (*b*) intravenous contrast material has not been administered. A similar "hyperdense" vessel sign has been described for the basilar artery. Whereas prominence of the parenchymal changes associated with vascular occlusion are a contraindication to thrombolysis, the "hyperdense MCA sign" signifies a vascular occlusion and a need for intervention when detected within the treatment window.

As stated above, the ability to exclude intraparenchymal hemorrhage is central to the appropriate treatment of stroke patients. CT has demonstrated nearly 100% sensitivity for the detection of intraparenchymal hemorrhage, except for in very anemic patients with isoattenuating hematomas (hematocrit less than 20%) (13,22). Conspicuity of hemorrhage is based on the differentiation of the attenuation of hemorrhage from that of gray and white matter. Gray matter and white matter have lower attenuation, approximately 39 and 32 HU, respectively (23). Because of the presence of hemoglobin, recent hemorrhage has an attenuation of 56–76 HU and is thus detectable.

Administration of contrast material may be helpful in delineating infarcts in the subacute period when there may be obscuration of the infarct by "fogging" (24). Fogging was described by Becker et al (25) in 1979 as the phenomenon of an area of previously hypoattenuating infarction evolving to a state of isoattenuation between days 14 and 21 after infarction; this occurrence was believed to be secondary to small petechial hemorrhages or infiltration of the infarcted tissue with macrophages (25). Although difficult to see on a nonenhanced study, the area of infarction intensely enhances at the periphery.

Conversely, despite histologic breakdown of the blood-brain barrier beginning on the day of infarction, contrast enhancement is not generally seen during the first 3 days. Further, there is a theoretical concern about intravenous contrast material causing further parenchymal injury in the presence of a disrupted blood-brain barrier (26). Finally, intravenous contrast material has not been demonstrated to increase the detectability of ischemic changes within the first 24 hours (27). Therefore, it is not recommended in the acute evaluation of stroke.

In summary, nonenhanced head CT has a clearly defined role in the current management of acute stroke (Table). A CT scan for the exclusion of hemorrhage is a listed requirement in the package insert for alteplase. Also, in the practice guidelines for the imaging of acute stroke, the Stroke Council of the American Heart Association recommends an initial CT scan (13). It has enabled the implementation of the first efficacious treatment of ischemia. CT is appealing as an imaging study in that it is widely available, can be performed quickly and safely on critically ill patients, and is relatively inexpensive. Further, its utility has been proved in large-scale clinical trials.

Algorithm for Determining the Appropriateness of Administration of rt-PA in Patients Presenting within 3 Hours of Ictus

Grade of Stroke	CT Findings	Recommendation*
0	Normal	None
1	Possible early signs of infarction†: vague blurring of gray matter–white matter boundaries, slight attenuation of the insular ribbon, slight indistinctness of basal ganglia gray matter, suggestion of crowding sulci	May still give rt-PA depending on the neurologist's judgment
2	Subtle but definite signs of early infarction: same as for grade 1 except findings are distinct	Likely will not treat
3	Prominent signs of early infarction: mass effect (ie, ventricular effacement, subfalcine or uncal herniation), clearly demonstrated hypoattenuation	Contraindication to treatment

Source.—Based on recommendations by the American Heart Association (13) and experience from the NINDS (3) and ECASS (7) trials.

* Current recommendations for administration of rt-PA require presentation to the hospital within 3 hours and no CT signs of hemorrhage or extensive infarction.

† In the ECASS trial, the major early signs of infarction included diffuse swelling of the affected hemisphere and effacement of the cerebral sulci in more than 33% of the MCA territory.

LIMITATIONS OF CT IN STROKE INTERVENTION

The current approach to evaluation and treatment of cerebral ischemia with thrombolytics demands further optimization. An analysis of rt-PA thrombolysis estimated that on the basis of the current approach to thrombolysis, there is a 12% chance of an improved outcome at 3 months (28). However, there is also a concomitant 3% increased risk of intracranial hemorrhage. Reperfusion into areas of infarction is associated with an increased risk of hemorrhage (28). As previously noted, in the ECASS study, trained investigators did not detect these "subtle but present changes" in approximately 11% of the patients. von Kummer et al (29) demonstrated that in the first 6 hours after onset of ischemia, 31% of CT scans may be misinterpreted (Fig 3). Although CT may show findings of infarction as early as 3–6 hours after ictus, up to 60% of CT scans are normal in the first few hours after ischemic insult. Thus, despite some reports of high sensitivity in the acute period, it is still accepted that its overall sensitivity is relatively poor (30,31).

A more sensitive method for detecting areas of infarction may lead to improved patient selection for thrombolytic therapy. In the setting of presentation for acute stroke within 3 hours of ictus, a CT scan is typically normal. Aside from the "hyperdense MCA sign," the current approach to selection of a patient as an appropriate candidate for thrombolysis is based on the absence of signs of infarction. For example, a patient presenting with stroke symptoms but a negative CT scan is deemed to be a good candidate for rt-PA. Unfortunately, with this approach, the diagnosis of cerebral ischemic infarction is assigned incorrectly in as many as 20% of these patients (32). Further, analysis of subjects in studies that used similar selection criteria demonstrated that up to 20% of patients will have a negative angiogram, possibly due to early spontaneous lysis of clot (33).

Another 10%–20% had arterial dissections, occlusions sites not readily susceptible to thrombolysis, or minor branch occlusions that without intervention have a favorable natural outcome (33). The lack of sensitivity and specificity in the diagnosis of stroke limits the attainable benefit. Therefore, although CT has proved to be of tremendous benefit, other modalities such as magnetic resonance (MR) imaging may provide an opportunity to further improvements in patient care (12).

CONVENTIONAL MR IMAGING FOR INCREASED SENSITIVITY IN DETECTION OF ACUTE STROKE

Earlier detection of areas of infarction is possible with MR imaging. MR imaging involves placing a patient in an applied external magnetic field. Because of the precessional properties of certain nuclei with an odd molecular mass or odd charge, the most abundant of which is hydrogen, the nuclei will act as small magnets that align with the magnetic field. With the use of applied radiofrequency pulses and receiver coils, it is possible to generate and detect different signals from tissue based on the number of protons per unit volume (ie, spin density) of different substances. MR imaging takes advantage of the fact that water protons have different biophysical relaxation properties, described by times T1 and T2, depending on the microscopic environment of the water protons. Acute cerebral ischemia is characterized by changes in electrolyte and water balance that result in alterations in this environment. These differences can be exploited to increase contrast, and as a result MR imaging is extremely sensitive in the detection of acute infarction.

Acute infarcts are more visible on MR images than on CT scans, with over 80% of MR images positive in the 1st day compared to 60% of CT scans (19). MR imaging is particularly superior in the detection of stroke in the posterior fossa where CT is limited due to beam-hardening artifact from the adjacent skull base. Lacunar infarcts and small cortical strokes are also seen with higher conspicuity (19).

The earliest MR changes are loss of normal intravascular flow voids, morphologic swelling of the gray matter, and increased signal intensity on the T2-weighted and intermediated–weighted (3,000/30 [repetition time msec/echo time msec]) images [Editor's note: The convention of *Radiology* is to term this sequence intermediate weighted although it has also been termed proton-density weighted]. There is normally a loss of intraarterial signal with standard spin-echo (SE) sequences, referred to as a "flow void," due to precessional phase changes induced by blood flow. In low- or no-flow states, there is a loss of the "flow void" such that signal intensity is demonstrated in the

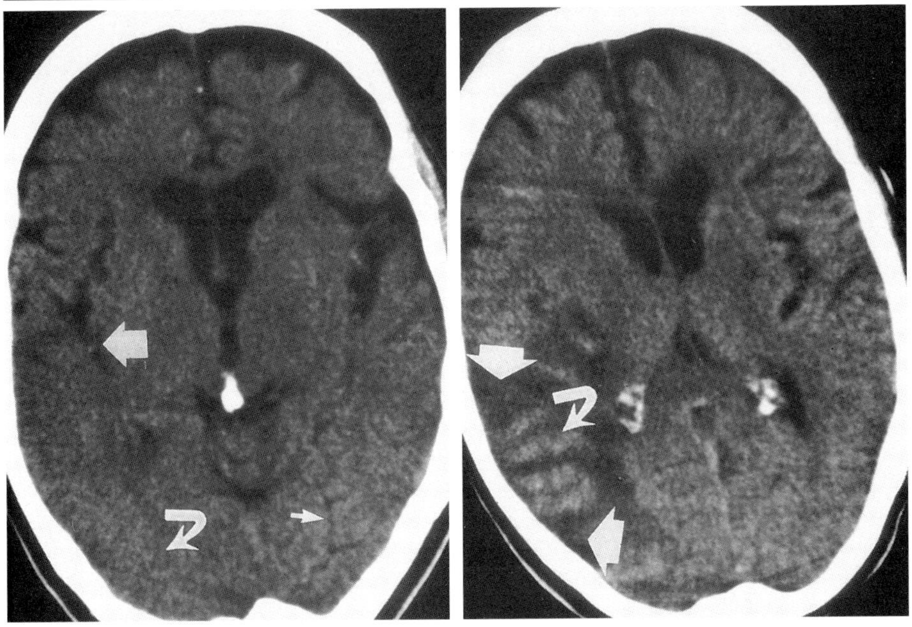

a. b.

Figure 3. Left hemiparesis upon awakening in a 56-year-old man. **(a)** Axial CT scan of the head obtained 2 hours after the patient awakened demonstrates subtle loss of demarcation of the posterior aspect of the insular ribbon (large straight arrow) and sulcal effacement (curved arrow). Compare the loss of the sulci on the right (curved arrow) to the normal sulci on the left (small straight arrow). Interpretation at the time of scanning did not detect these findings. **(b)** Axial CT scan of the head obtained 3 days after presentation demonstrates progression to infarction (straight arrows) and some petechial hemorrhage seen as areas of increased attenuation (curved arrow).

involved vessel (19). Similar to the "hyperdense MCA sign" in CT, absence of flow in involved vessels can be seen immediately after occlusion.

The morphologic changes at MR imaging relate to cellular swelling. These have been shown to appear before the T2 signal changes, although these changes are very subtle. More easily detected are the signal intensity changes that result from an increase in intracellular fluid. These can be detected on both the T2-weighted images or on the intermediated-weighted images with the T1-weighted signal intensity changes the least sensitive for detection of stroke. The changes on the intermediate-weighted changes are often more conspicuous than those on the T2-weighted images, particularly in strokes involving the cortical gray matter (19). The earliest signal intensity changes usually involve the gray matter, with the white matter typically appearing normal in the first 24 hours.

Intermediate-weighted images are also superior for detection of lesions near a ventricle or subarachnoid space. This is because the presence of cerebrospinal fluid (CSF) can make it difficult to identify the lesions on the T2-weighted images given that both CSF and infarcted tissue may have similar signal intensities. CSF is isointense to gray matter, and thus areas of abnormal hyperintensity can be detected. Similarly, intermediate-weighted images enable differentiation of lacunar infarcts from perivascular spaces: the former hyperintense and the latter isointense to CSF.

Intravenous contrast material can provide additional information. Vascular enhancement can be seen in cortical infarcts up to 75% of the time (34). This is believed to be due to slow flow in the region of the infarction. Meningeal enhancement can also be seen acutely in approximately 33% of patients, possibly due to meningeal inflammation (34). Both types of enhancement resolve toward the end of the 1st week. This can potentially delineate the acuteness of a lesion in patients demonstrating more that one area of infarction. In general, however, it is not necessary to administer contrast material to assess the enhancement characteristics of an ischemic lesion. As will be discussed subsequently, the acuteness of a lesion can be adequately determined by using MR diffusion imaging. Administration of contrast material is typically reserved for those instances in which MR perfusion imaging is performed.

New MR techniques are now available to generate images with T2 weighting in less time. A fast SE sequence enables the acquisition of T2-weighted images in a fraction of the time required to obtain similar conventional SE images(roughly four to 16 times faster). This is made possible by acquiring multiple lines in k space per repetition time, TR (number of lines acquired equal to the echo train length). In conventional SE imaging, only one line of k space is acquired per repetition time. Whereas the time of acquisition of an SE image is number of signals acquired (NSA) $\times$ TR $\times$ the number of phase encoding steps (N_{phase}), time of acquisition in fast SE imaging is (NSA $\times$ TR $\times$ N_{phase})/ETL, where ETL is the echo train length. For example, with an echo train length of 8, a fast SE evaluation of equal resolution could be performed as much as eight times faster. This is of particular value in evaluating patients with acute stroke for which prompt diagnosis and institution of therapy portends the greatest likelihood of tissue salvage. Other benefits include reduced flow artifacts due to even echo rephasing, a result of the symmetric sequence design within a repetition time cycle (35). This may increase the conspicuity of posterior fossa lesions where flow-related artifacts can be particularly problematic (36). Further, the ability to rapidly acquire the images enables timely performance of high-spatial-resolution T2-weighted imaging and limits patient motion artifact. Although the information obtained is similar with equivalent detectability of large lesions, the detection of small lesions is decreased (37). This may be due to the image blurring that occurs in the phase direction due to unequal echo delays in the echo train (38). Further, true proton-density–weighted images are not as reliably obtained, limiting the ability to differentiate perivascular spaces from lacunar infarcts.

Lesion conspicuity can be further optimized by using an inversion-recovery sequence in which an initial 180° radio-frequency pulse is followed at an inversion time by a 90° radio-frequency pulse. The latter converts the partially recovered longitudinal magnetization to transverse magnetization, at which point it is detected (39). For a given T1 relaxation time, an inversion time can be used that will result in zero transverse magnetization. A fluid-attenuated inversion-recovery (FLAIR) sequence using an inversion time approximating the null point of CSF (2,200 msec) combined with a long echo time to obtain T2 weighting suppresses

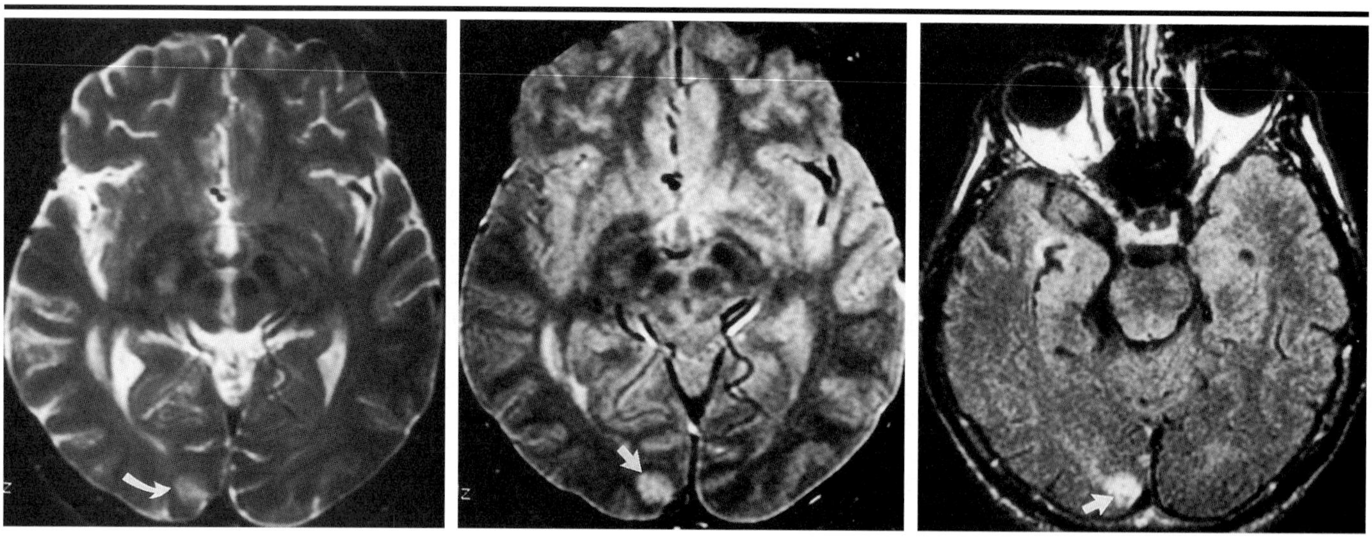

a. b. c.

Figure 4. Left hemianopsia in a 67-year-old woman. MR imaging was performed 12 hours after onset of symptoms. **(a)** Axial T2-weighted MR image (3,000/100 [repetition time msec/echo time msec], 5-mm section thickness, 256 × 192 matrix) demonstrates a subtle area of hyperintensity (arrow) in the right occipital lobe. Proximity to the adjacent CSF obscures this area of infarction. **(b)** Axial intermediate-weighted image (3,000/25, 5-mm section thickness, 256 × 192 matrix) demonstrates the area of hyperintensity (arrow) with increased conspicuity because the CSF signal was isointense to gray matter. **(c)** Axial FLAIR MR image (10,002/104/2,200 [repetition time msec/echo time msec/inversion time msec], 5-mm section thickness, 256 × 192 matrix) demonstrates the area of hyperintensity (arrow) with optimal conspicuity due to nulling of signal from CSF.

the signal from CSF while maintaining the hyperintensity associated with pathologic processes (40). This leads to reduced artifacts due to CSF flow and volume averaging and results in excellent conspicuity of both small and large lesions (41). FLAIR is superior to fast SE T2-weighted and intermediate-weighted images in the evaluation of cerebrovascular disease, with lacunar and cortical infarcts more conspicuous (Fig 4) (42).

Initial clinical implementation of FLAIR was limited because the required inversion time resulted in a relatively inefficient sequence, with the time to evaluate the brain on the order of 12 minutes. Thus, despite the increased conspicuity of abnormalities, the trade-off in time did not warrant the benefits, particularly since an intermediate-weighted image yields similar information. Recently, it became possible to combine the enhanced conspicuity of FLAIR with the speed of fast imaging techniques (43). Modified fast FLAIR and fast SE FLAIR can reduce imaging time to 2–5 minutes (44). As a result, it is now possible to obtain T2-weighted images with high conspicuity (due to CSF suppression) in a short period of time.

MR Exclusion of Intraparenchymal Hemorrhage

As previously mentioned, exclusion of intraparenchymal hemorrhage is central to the evaluation of acute stroke. Conventional SE techniques are highly sensitive for the detection of subacute and chronic hemorrhage. Deoxyhemoglobin, methemoglobin, and hemosiderin are the breakdown products of hemoglobin (45). These substances are paramagnetic and with retraction, into a fibrin clot, they cause a marked alteration in relaxation properties (46). In the hyperacute stages of hemorrhage in which there has been minimal conversion of oxyhemoglobin to breakdown products and no mature clot formation, conventional MR sequences are less sensitive. This has caused reluctance to rely on MR as the primary imaging modality in acute stroke due to concerns of false-negative results.

Conventional SE imaging techniques have a lower sensitivity for the detection of blood products due to an applied 180° radio-frequency phase refocusing pulse. Fast SE techniques have an even lower sensitivity. However, gradient-recalled-echo (GRE) imaging employs a reversal of the readout gradient, without a refocusing radio-frequency pulse, resulting in high sensitivity to magnetic field inhomogeneity induced by the presence of the paramagnetic breakdown products of blood. As a result, GRE images are particularly sensitive in the detection of acute intraparenchymal hemorrhage (45) (Fig 5). When conventional SE sequences are supplemented with GRE hemosiderin-sensitive sequences, the earlier stages of hemorrhage can be diagnosed equally well with MR imaging and CT (45,47). The criteria for the presence of hemorrhage on MR images are increased signal intensity on the T1-weighted images, decreased signal intensity on the T2-weighted images, and/or decreased signal intensity on the GRE images when the signal intensity is compared to that of white matter. In the hyperacute stage, the central area of hemorrhage will appear somewhat similar to CSF, but there is often a subtle halo of hypointensity on GRE images.

Conventional SE and fast SE MR images are also insensitive to the presence of acute subarachnoid hemorrhage. However, FLAIR images have been shown to be highly sensitive in the detection of acute, subacute, and chronic subarachnoid hemorrhage (48,49). Despite this, many radiologists and most clinicians remain more "confident" using CT as the imaging tool for the diagnosis of subarachnoid hemorrhage. Willingness to rely on MR imaging as a primary diagnostic tool in the evaluation of stroke will be benefited by more first-hand experience with the reliability of MR imaging in the detection of intraparenchymal and subarachnoid hemorrhage.

Assessing Large-Vessel Patency

As discussed earlier, approximately 20% of patients presenting with symptoms of acute cerebral ischemia do not have an

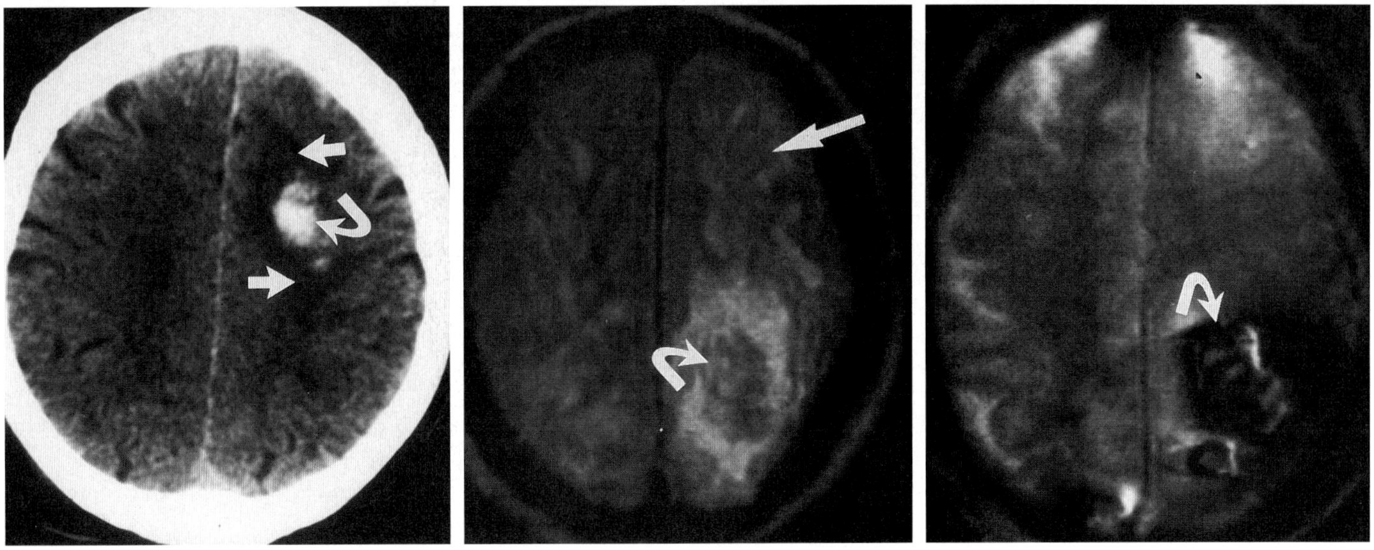

a. b. c.

Figure 5. Acute onset of right hemiparesis and aphasia in a 52-year-old man. CT scan was obtained 4 hours after onset of symptoms and demonstrated a left frontoparietal intraparenchymal hematoma. MR images were obtained 7 hours after onset of symptoms. **(a)** Axial CT scan of the head demonstrates a central area of increased attenuation (curved arrow) compatible with a hemorrhage. Peripherally, there is surrounding edema manifested as decreased attenuation (straight arrows). **(b)** Axial intermediate-weighted MR image (3,000/25, 5-mm section thickness, 256 × 192 matrix) demonstrates diffuse hyperintensity in the left frontoparietal lobe (straight arrow). There is a more focal area posteriorly that is heterogeneous (curved arrow). **(c)** Axial GRE image (3,000/25, 23° flip angle, 5-mm section thickness, 256 × 192 matrix) demonstrates marked hypointensity (curved arrow) compatible with a hematoma. This demonstrates the increased sensitivity of GRE images for the detection of intraparenchymal hemorrhage.

angiographically demonstrable vascular occlusion. An additional 10%–20% have small-vessel occlusions or dissections for which thrombolysis is unlikely to be of benefit. Thus, in addition to demonstrating areas of infarction, it is equally important to demonstrate that there is a vascular lesion that is amenable to thrombolysis.

MR angiography enables the noninvasive evaluation of vascular patency. Images can be generated on which flow within the vessel is increased in signal intensity (bright blood) or on which the lumen is depicted as decreased in signal intensity (black blood); the former is the more commonly used technique. Time of flight is the most frequently used bright-blood MR angiographic technique. Key issues in MR angiography are optimizing intravascular signal intensity and maximizing suppression of stationary spins. Time of flight applies a GRE sequence, enabling the use of a shorter echo time and repetition time than those of SE imaging, important in minimizing signal loss due to intravascular intravoxel phase dispersion and optimizing suppression of stationary tissue, respectively. For evaluating the intracranial circulation, a volumetric (three-dimensional) acquisition is optimal, enabling thinner voxels, which limits intravoxel phase dispersion and the associated artifactual signal loss in the region of stenoses. In time-of-flight MR angiography, background suppression is particularly important. Magnetization transfer and manipulation of echo time such that fat and water are out of phase yield improved background suppression. Additionally, increasing the flip angle in the direction of flow minimizes saturation effects, which optimizes intravascular signal recovery in the more distal vessels. Loss of phase coherence limits usefulness in small peripheral vessels by preventing generation of an intravascular signal. However, an image similar to a conventional arteriogram can be reconstructed from the intravascular signals that is sensitive to large vessel occlusion or narrowing in the internal carotid, vertebral, basilar, and first and second segments of the anterior, middle, and posterior cerebral arteries. Although the value of MR angiography has yet to be shown in a large-scale clinical trial, the need for differentiating which patients have lesions amenable to thrombolysis seems clear given the potential risks of treatment (Fig 6).

Extending the Treatment Window beyond 3 Hours

Thus, the use of conventional MR imaging provides many benefits over CT in the use of thrombolytics within 3 hours of ictus. It has increased sensitivity to the presence of infarction, equivalent sensitivity for the detection of intraparenchymal hemorrhage, and facilitates assessment of large-vessel patency. However, even with conventional MR imaging, areas of infarction are often not demonstrated in the first 6 hours. Thus, despite the increased sensitivity of MR imaging for the detection of infarction, it is still inadequate to extend the treatment window beyond 3 hours. Methods more sensitive to the early changes of infarction are needed to avoid reperfusion of areas of infarction and risk of hemorrhage. Expanding the therapeutic window will require techniques that are not only sensitive to the presence of infarction, but also capable of delineating areas at risk for infarction. This may now be possible with advanced MR imaging techniques.

TREATABLE TISSUE BEYOND 3 HOURS: THE PENUMBRA

Compared to other tissues such as muscle, the brain has little capacity to store energy. In zero-flow states (complete ischemia), the available energy will maintain cell viability for approximately 2–3 minutes. More often, ischemia is incomplete, with the area of greatest compromise located centrally with a large area of surrounding tissue at risk but remaining viable. The central region in which cell death will occur generally corresponds to a region in which energy supply is insufficient to maintain membrane pumps leading to loss of the membrane potential. The surrounding at-risk area can have detectably abnormal evoked potentials but has not undergone cell depolarization. This area is referred to as the *penumbra* (50,51).

The progression of acute stroke is a common occurrence. The mechanisms for progression of infarct are multiple, including cerebral edema, hemorrhagic transformation, poor collateral flow, low blood pressure, or increased blood glucose levels. Animal and human studies (19,52) have documented both reversal of ischemia and progression of ischemic tissue to infarction over periods as long as 36 hours. In a study by Castillo et al (52), 34% of patients demonstrated such progression with a drop in their Canadian Stroke Scale score of 1 or more over 48 hours. Bryan et al (19) demonstrated that at least one-third of MR imaging studies showed that stroke areas increased in size after 24 hours. This suggests that there is salvageable tissue beyond the currently accepted 3-hour therapeutic window.

ADVANCED MR IMAGING TECHNIQUES FOR BETTER DEFINITION OF STROKE

The imaging requirements for extending the treatment window are delineation of areas of infarction and risk of infarction, evaluation of large-vessel patency, and exclusion of nonischemic causes of symptom onset. Conventional CT combined with CT angiography and CT perfusion imaging has promise due to its accessibility and ability to demonstrate areas of hemorrhage, large-vessel occlusions, and regions of hypoperfusion (52a). However, it remains somewhat limited by its current low sensitivity for delineating irreversibly injured tissue in the hyperacute period. Numerous other imaging techniques can contribute in assessing individual parameters, but few are both comprehensive and expeditious. These include xenon-enhanced CT, positron emission tomography (PET), single photon emission CT, and transcranial Doppler ultrasonography. For example, whereas PET provides important quantitative information related to blood flow and oxygen extraction, current limitations in anatomic de-

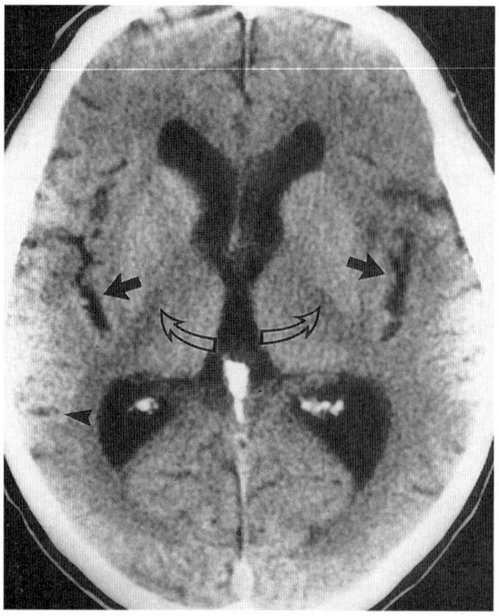

a.

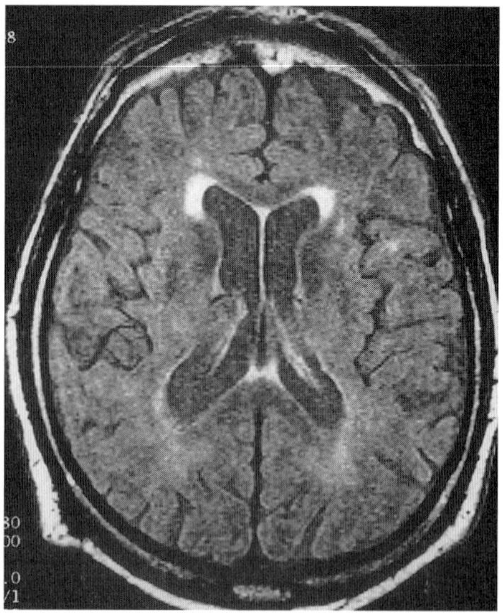

b.

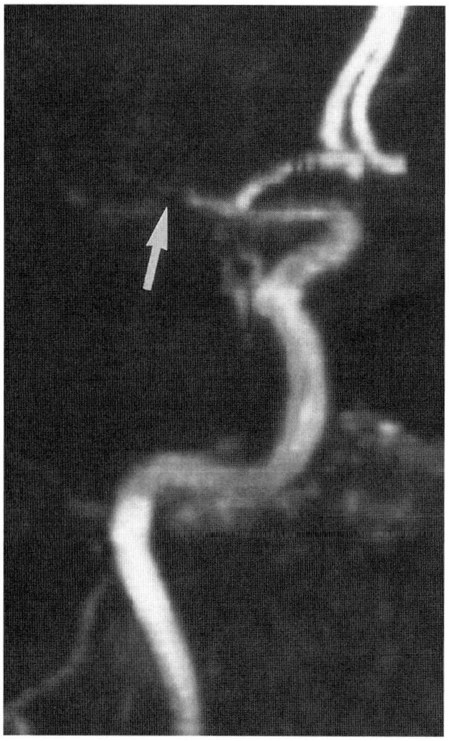

c.

Figure 6. Acute onset of left-sided hemiparesis in a 43-year-old woman with hypertension. CT was performed 4 hours after onset of symptoms. MR imaging was performed 12 hours after onset of symptoms. **(a)** Axial CT scan of the head was interpreted as normal. Note that the insular ribbons (straight arrows), the gray matter–white matter differentiation (arrowhead), and the internal capsules (curved arrows) are normal. **(b)** Axial FLAIR MR image(10,002/104/2,200, 5-mm section thickness, 256 × 192 matrix) demonstrates no evidence of a right hemispheric infarction. **(c)** Three-dimensional time-of-flight MR angiogram (53/4.1, 1.1-mm section thickness, 512 × 192 matrix) demonstrates occlusion (arrow) of the right MCA, potentially amenable to thrombolysis.

lineation (and accessibility) have hampered its routine use in accessing stroke patients (53). Conversely, MR imaging generally has higher spatial resolution than other tomographic techniques (similar to that of CT), enabling anatomic, physiologic, and metabolic analysis in a single examination. Therefore, rather than presenting the wide array of available imaging techniques, in reviewing the state of the art for acute stroke imaging, emphasis is focused on the potential of advanced MR imaging techniques to provide the information relevant to the treatment of cerebral ischemia in a time-efficient and comprehensive fashion. Three newer techniques hold great promise for increasing the sensitivity of detecting infarction and demarcating the area at risk and are reviewed in detail. These techniques include MR diffusion imaging, MR perfusion imaging, and proton MR spectroscopic imaging.

MR Diffusion Imaging

The effects of molecular self-diffusion on the amplitude of SE MR signals was recognized early in the development of nuclear MR spectroscopy (54), and the equations and pulsed field gradient methods published by Stejskal and Tanner (55) in 1965 form the basis of modern diffusion-weighted MR imaging (56). In 1990, Moseley et al (57) demonstrated in an animal stroke model that the apparent

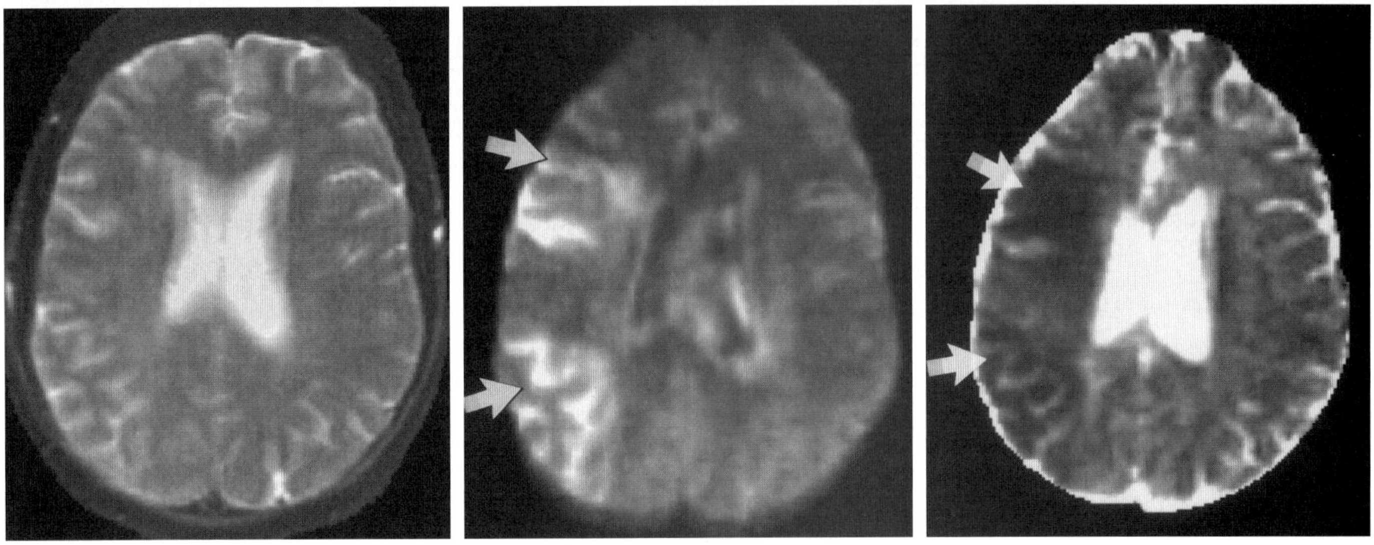

a. b. c.

Figure 7. Acute onset of left-sided hemiparesis in a 72-year-old man. MR images were obtained 4 hours after ictus. **(a)** Axial T2-weighted image (3,000/100, 5-mm section thickness, 256 × 192 matrix) demonstrates no evidence of abnormality. **(b)** Axial, single-shot echo-planar diffusion-weighted image (5,000/126, 5-mm section thickness, 128 × 128) demonstrates two areas of hyperintensity (arrows) in the right MCA distribution. This finding is compatible with an acute infarct. **(c)** Axial, pure diffusion D_{av} MR image (5,000/126, 5-mm section thickness, 128 × 128 matrix) demonstrates decreased signal intensity (arrows) in the right MCA distribution. The areas of decreased ADC (hypointensity) correspond to an acute infarct.

diffusion coefficient (ADC) decreased by approximately 30%–50% within 30 minutes after onset of focal ischemia. This change occurs while other MR image types such as T2- or intermediate-weighted images remain normal (Fig 7) (57,58). It is now well demonstrated that the majority of the diffusion changes coincide with the membrane depolarization due to Na^+,K^+-ATPase pump failure (59–61), and this can be measured instantaneously by using MR imaging (58,62). This coincides with water redistribution between intra- and interstitial space upon energy failure, although the exact physical mechanism for the changes in diffusion-weighted imaging is still a point of discussion (63–67). Although many mechanisms have been proposed, it is generally believed that the most likely cause of the decrease in ADC values is the redistribution of water from the interstitial to the (diffusion-restricted) intracellular space, as the energy-dependent Na^+,K^+-ATPase pumps fail (ie, the initiation of cytotoxic edema) (63,65,68–70). Of note is that there is also ample proof that the explanation based on a high interstitial and low intracellular diffusion constant is somewhat of an oversimplification. Further experimental data are needed to support the interstitial diffusion values that underlie this assumption.

The flow threshold for large ADC reduction (eg, 50%–80% of control values) appears to be in the 15–20 mL/100 g per minute range, (71) similar to the threshold for electrical failure and symptom onset, while small (10%) reductions may be seen below 30 mL/100 g per minute (72). In focal ischemia, the degree of ADC reduction has been reported to depend on both the anatomic location and the duration of ischemia (73–75). Provided that the duration of ischemia is short enough, reperfusion leads to a restoration of normal ADC and energy metabolism (62). If ischemia is prolonged, ADC may not recover fully, depending on the length of ischemia and the value of the ADC immediately before reperfusion (75,76). In one study of fixed ischemic duration (45 minutes), only ischemic tissue with a change in ADC of less than 0.25×10^{-3} mm^2/sec recovered (did not infarct) after reperfusion (77). In studies of human stroke, areas of reduced ADC have almost inevitably progressed to infarction presumably because most of the images are obtained several hours, or even days, after stroke onset (78,79). However, it is generally accepted that a single measure of ADC alone cannot distinguish reversible from irreversible ischemic damage; both the duration of ischemia (which often cannot readily be determined in human stroke) and the reduction in ADC determine reversibility (80,81).

Therefore, there have been attempts to associate diffusion-weighted imaging with other imaging parameters (such as T2), which, when used in combination, may better stage stroke progression (58,82). This was first performed in a permanent MCA occlusion model in the rat; after the initial ADC drop, by 12 hours, as vasogenic edema begins to accumulate, the T2 begins to increase (this stage of stroke is particularly conspicuous on diffusion-weighted images, which, because of limited gradient strength on clinical imagers, are both diffusion- and T2-weighted in most cases) (83). As ischemia continues, the ADC begins to return to normal (12–24 hours in this model) and eventually becomes elevated (24–48 hours) as necrosis occurs. Various combinations of ADC and T2 ("signatures") were identified, which corresponded to the different histopathologic conditions of evolving infarction. The same behavior has also been observed in human stroke, although the time scale appears to be different, with several groups finding a slower recovery and increase in ADC (after several days) compared to that in the animal studies (84,85). However, this has been somewhat controversial and may be partly technique dependent.

Although diffusion-weighted imaging can help identify stroke location, therefore, it is questionable if it alone can differentiate reversible from irreversible ischemic injury. However, the ability to positively diagnose stroke from an imaging perspective is extremely valuable for initiating stroke therapy (86). Diffusion-weighted imaging has also been shown to enable differentiation of acute from nonacute infarcts (87), to help predict outcome (88,89), and to facilitate correlation with final infarct size, although final infarcts were larger than abnormalities at diffusion-weighted imaging seen at 6, 12, or 24 hours (78). It was suggested that enlargement of the area of infarction was likely to occur if the area of perfusion deficit was larger than the area of diffusion abnormality (90). We and others also found that acute perfusion abnormalities tend to be larger than final infarct size (88,91,92). While the exact time scale for ADC reversal is still debated, the ability of diffusion-weighted imaging to distinguish an acute from a chronic lesion is of great clinical interest (93). In addition, it was found possible to predict which strokes would improve versus those that would not on the basis of the diffusion-weighted image: In one report of 40 patients, only four had no detectable abnormality on diffusion-weighted images; in all four of these patients, the neurologic deficit subsequently resolved (90). However, there have been isolated reports of patients with negative diffusion-weighted imaging studies who subsequently developed infarction (94).

For all of these reasons, diffusion-weighted imaging is becoming an essential stroke imaging modality, but diffusion-weighted imaging of the human brain also poses numerous technical challenges. Perhaps the most difficult problem is the elimination of motion artifacts on the heavily diffusion-weighted images. Large phase errors can occur during application of the diffusion gradients as the result of macroscopic sample motion. Various different approaches have been tried to address this problem. One approach is to image as rapidly as possible in order to minimize potential motion. If the image can be recorded in a single shot, for instance by using echo-planar imaging, every line of k space has the same phase error, so no image artifacts are present after Fourier transformation and magnitude calculation (90). Other rapid imaging techniques, such as gradient- and spin-echo (GRASE) or fast low-angle shot (FLASH), may also be used (95,96). An alternative approach is to measure, and correct for, the phase error on each line of k space, by recording a second, non–phase-encoded echo (called a "navigator" echo) (97). This approach allows diffusion imaging to be performed with conventional SE sequences, which are generally less demanding on MR instrumentation and have better signal-to-noise ratio and fewer susceptibility artifacts than those of single-shot imaging sequences. However, adequate correction with navigator echoes is only possible for relatively simple, small amplitude motions, and this approach is less favorable than fast imaging methods, particularly for noncompliant patients, and/or when multiple *b* values and gradient directions are required. As a result, echo-planar diffusion is the most practical and commonly used method for stroke imaging (79).

Another technical issue regards the directional dependence of the ADC. While the ADC in liquids is isotropic, in biological samples the motion of water molecules is partially restricted, resulting in different diffusivities in different directions (anisotropy). Mathematically, diffusion therefore has to be described as a tensor, and the signal attenuation in diffusion-weighted imaging will depend on the direction and amplitude of the applied gradients, which is proportional to the proton gyromagnetic ratio, the gradient length, and the diffusion time, with the time between the (start of) two gradients in the diffusion experiment, and x, y, and z are the orthogonal directions defined by the scanner magnetic field gradients.

In the brain, ADC anisotropy is particularly evident in white matter, due to the greater diffusivity of water parallel (as opposed to perpendicular) to the axonal fibers. This property can potentially be exploited to noninvasively map brain fiber tracts and directions (70), and to study the processes of myelination (98) and demyelinating diseases (99). However, in the context of stroke imaging, diffusion anisotropy is largely an added complication: If only a single diffusion-gradient direction is used (as in the case of most early studies of human stroke), hyperintensity is often observed in the densely myelinated corticospinal tracts, corpus callosum, or other white matter regions, which may be difficult to distinguish from reductions in ADC due to ischemia. This important problem can be avoided by using certain combinations of these ADCs that are not orientation-dependent, such as the so-called trace of the diffusion tensor (100). Trace imaging is a more reliable method for measuring changes in ADCs and may avoid interpretation errors due to the intrinsic anisotropy of the brain (81,100).

With appropriate pulse sequence design, the orientation-independent trace or average value of the diffusion constant, D_{av}, can be measured, which provides nearly uniform diffusion-weighted images in normal brain (90,100). Normal D_{av} values are approximately 3.2×10^{-5} cm^2/sec for CSF and 0.8×10^{-5} cm^2/sec for human brain parenchyma (101). Gray matter may have a slightly higher (by approximately 10%) D_{av} than that of white matter, although it is difficult to measure cortical gray matter regions of interest that are completely free from CSF contamination. Trace images can be constructed either by measuring D_{xx}, D_{yy}, and D_{zz} in separate experiments, or by using sequences that give isotropic diffusion-weighting in a single shot (102). Each approach has its own advantages and disadvantages: The single-shot trace methods are fast and are not subject to errors due to head motion (or different eddy-current artifacts) between different sequences. However, they are more demanding on gradient strength, and with typical currently available gradient sets, maximum *b* values are rather low using acceptable echo times (eg, on our current GE Medical Systems unit [Milwaukee, Wis] with "echo-speed" gradients, $G_{max} = 2.2$ G/cm, with an echo time approximately 126 msec, b_{max} approximately 550 sec/mm^2) (103,104). Ideally, *b* values in the range of 1,000–1,500 sec/mm^2 have been shown to give optimal contrast for stroke diffusion-weighted imaging studies (105). Individual measurements of D_{xx}, D_{yy}, and D_{zz}, as well as applying gradient combinations in the xy, xz, and yz directions, allow the full diffusion tensor to be determined, and to calculate indexes of diffusion anisotropy, which may also change in ischemia (106). Higher *b* values can be obtained for better contrast, but at the expense of increased imaging time compared to that of the single-shot trace methods. A minor advantage of the single-shot trace sequence, but nevertheless an important one in the clinical environment, is that less offline processing is required to view orientation-independent images. Newer imagers with "scalable" gradient driver hardware can produce gradient strengths of up to 4 G/cm, which should enable single-shot imaging with adequate *b*-value weighting (104).

MR Perfusion Imaging

MR imaging of cerebral perfusion can be performed by injecting a bolus of gadopentetate dimeglumine (107). In normal brain, the paramagnetic contrast agent gadopentetate dimeglumine remains enclosed within the cerebral vasculature; this shortens the longitudinal re-

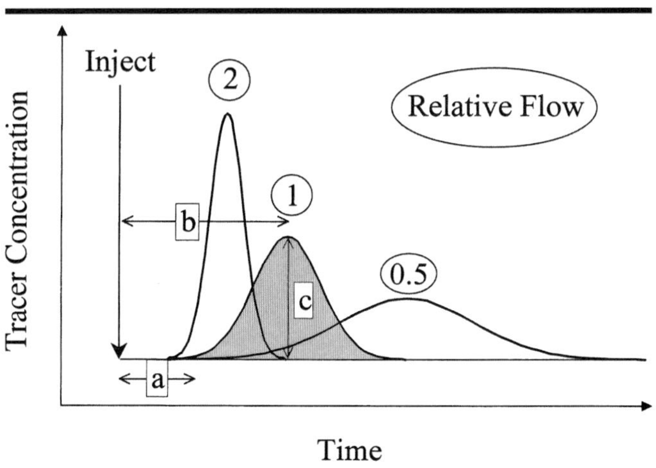

Figure 8. Simulated gamma-variate functions at constant blood volume for three different relative blood flows. The shaded gamma variant function depicts the values of interest including time to peak (*b*) and peak height (*c*). The bolus delay (*a*) is also depicted. The shaded area is proportional to regional cerebral blood volume.

laxation time (T1) of blood, which causes a paramagnetic frequency shift within the vessel, and creates local magnetic field inhomogeneities in surrounding tissues, which shorten the transverse relaxation time constant T2* (108–113). Under certain conditions, each one of these effects is linearly proportional to the concentration of the tracer (contrast agent) within the image pixel. Therefore, by using the theory of tracer kinetics, rapid MR images acquired during the first pass of the contrast agent through the brain can be analyzed to produce images of relative regional cerebral blood volume rCBV (114). If an estimate of the arterial input function is available, the mean transit time MTT, and regional cerebral blood flow rCBF can also be estimated (rCBF = rCBV/MTT) (115,116). In lesions where the blood-brain barrier is disrupted, the latter part of the signal intensity–time curve can also be analyzed to give an index of relative blood-brain barrier permeability (117), although in most patients with acute stroke this may be expected to be small.

The theory of calculating regional cerebral blood flow from data sets of this type is complicated and too involved to be repeated here (116,118). A number of assumptions are required in order to perform the calculation, including such factors as estimation of capillary hematocrit, the assumption that the change in R2* ($\Delta R2^* = -\ln[S/S_0]/\mathrm{TE}$) signal intensity changes follows the same dependency in the microvasculature and major vessels, and the difficulty of performing the appropriate mathematical deconvolution on rather coarsely digitized and noisy data. In some experiments, the input function may not be available, and it is debatable as to where the input function should be determined in stroke patients with occluded major vessels. For these reasons, all MR perfusion studies of human stroke to date have used relative measures of regional cerebral blood volume or other, nonquantitative perfusion-related parameters.

Theoretically, the distribution of an intravenously administered bolus leaving the heart-lung system should follow a gamma-variate function (119). Cerebral blood volume is proportional to the area under the curve; it can be seen that several simple parameters are easily measured and sensitive to changes in blood flow: peak signal intensity changes, time to peak, and width at half height (Fig 8). Each of these parameters is loosely proportional (or inversely proportional) to blood flow. Since, from PET studies, regional cerebral blood volume is known to be relatively nonspecific in stroke (120), these alternative, hemodynamic, flow-related parameters may be more sensitive for detection of abnormalities. PET has shown that cerebral blood volume may be unchanged, increased (as the result of compensatory vasodilatation), or decreased (as the result of collapse and/or occlusion of the ischemic vasculature) in cerebrovascular disease. Blood flow, however, is always reduced unless reperfusion and hyperemia have occurred. We found that arrival time (ie, time to peak) maps were much more sensitive than cerebral blood volume maps in detecting abnormalities in acute stroke, and this has also been the experience of others (92,121). In patients with occluded vessels, bolus arrival times were substantially longer than in contralateral hemispheres with patent vessels. Increased arrival times could be due to two reasons: (*a*) blood flow may be decreased, with increased mean transit times (at constant blood volume), or (*b*) the flow may be collateral or contralateral, with the result that the bolus has to traverse a longer path in order to reach the ischemic region. It is also possible that both mechanisms are involved. This delineation is benefited by assessing for large-vessel occlusion with MR angiography.

Relative, as opposed to absolute, indexes of blood flow (and blood volume) can therefore be useful in acute stroke. It has been shown that MR perfusion imaging can be used to detect early ischemic changes in patients with acute stroke, with much higher sensitivity than that of conventional MR imaging (122). Decreases in apparent blood volume were correlated with the presence of major vessel occlusion as demonstrated with MR angiography and were predictive of poor clinical outcome (122,123). Recently, there have also been reports of perfusion deficits that were not associated with either diffusion-weighted imaging or conventional MR imaging abnormalities, which subsequently proceeded to infarction by the time of the follow-up images (94,124). Presumably, these represent lesions in which the blood flow was in an intermediate region—below the threshold for electrical failure (symptom onset), but above the threshold for cytotoxic edema and reduced ADC. These cases highlight the need for both perfusion and diffusion MR imaging in acute stroke. It has also been reported that the area of perfusion abnormality often exceeds the area of diffusion abnormality, and that this mismatch may represent the ischemic penumbra (Fig 9) (50,78). In support of this, follow-up images in these patients usually depicted larger regions of infarction than seen on (acute) diffusion-weighted images, although not as large as the initial perfusion deficit. Perfusion imaging, alone, therefore, may overestimate areas of final infarction, most likely because it is presently not yet possible to identify a critical flow threshold on the nonquantitative images. In these studies, focal perfusion deficits were identified on cerebral blood volume or mean transit time maps, which were different from the surrounding tissue or contralateral hemisphere. Comparison of perfusion parameters to the contralateral hemisphere is perhaps the easiest way to currently interpret MR perfusion parameters, but should be done with caution since blood flow may not be normal in the contralateral hemisphere for several possible reasons including the occurrence of bilateral atherosclerotic disease, remote effects of the stroke, or old contralateral lesions (125–127).

Perfusion MR imaging with a bolus of gadopentetate dimeglumine requires rapid, susceptibility weighted MR imaging in order to adequately sample the first pass of the bolus through the brain. A temporal resolution of at least one image frame every 2 seconds is preferable. Early studies used single-section conventional GRE imaging (128). However, for stroke, multisection imaging with full brain coverage is desirable; this can only be achieved with rapid, single-shot imaging sequences such as echo-planar imaging "BURST" (ie, frequency shift burst of radio-frequency pulses) or rapid spiral imaging (129–132). We have recently been using a GRE spiral sequence that allows up to 18 sections to be recorded per second (133).

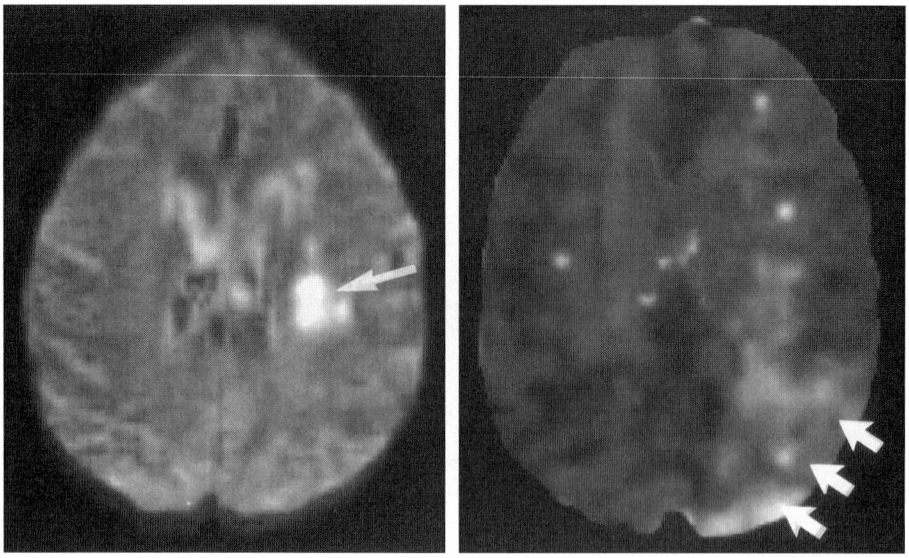

a. b.

Figure 9. Right hemiparesis in a 37-year-old man. MR imaging was performed 8 hours after ictus. **(a)** Axial diffusion-weighted image (5,000/126, 5-mm section thickness, 128 × 128) demonstrates a focal area of hyperintensity (arrow) in the left corona radiata and centrum semiovale. This lesion is too focal to explain the patient's symptom complex. **(b)** Axial echo-planar perfusion MR image (5,000/50, 5-mm section thickness, 128 × 128 matrix) is scaled such that hyperintensity corresponds to delayed time to peak. Note that the area of delayed arrival time (arrows) is larger than the diffusion abnormality. The area of demonstrated abnormality better corresponds to the patient's deficits. This appearance corresponds to the theoretic model of the penumbra.

MR Spectroscopic Imaging

Proton MR spectra of the brain enable detection of resonances that are relevant in the evaluation of patients with cerebral ischemia: lactate at 1.33 parts per million (ppm) and *N*-acetylaspartate (NAA) at 2.02 ppm. Lactate is not present in sufficiently high concentrations to measure in the brain under normal conditions. NAA is normally present and is found only in neurons or axons in mature brain (134,135).

Numerous studies (136,139,141) of animal models have indicated the ability of proton MR spectroscopy to depict acute cerebral ischemia on the basis of increased levels of lactate. In a model of carotid artery occlusion (136–138), it was found that lactate elevation occurred once the blood flow decreased below 20 mL/100 g per minute, similar to the threshold at which (in a number of species) electrical activity ceases (51,72,136–138). In global ischemia (ie, cardiac arrest), the elevation of lactate is rapid (immediately detectable after the onset of ischemia) and reaches a plateau in approximately 10 minutes (59,139). Both the rate of production and final concentration are proportional to the preischemic blood glucose levels, typically reaching about 12 mM in normoglycemic animals (140). Lactate is also detected immediately after the onset of focal and/or incomplete ischemia (141–143). Reperfusion after a short period of ischemia leads to restoration of normal metabolism with low levels of lactate, while longer periods of ischemia may lead to persistent lactic acidosis (144).

NAA decreases after the onset of either global or focal ischemia. In two different studies, there was a 10% decrease immediately after the induction of global ischemia, after which NAA decreased more slowly over a period of hours, with a 50% decrease by about 6 hours (142,145). Note that this has been observed both with MR spectroscopy and with conventional biochemical analysis (141). The decrease in NAA over a period of hours after the onset of ischemia is a critical finding. It appears to be one of the few MR parameters that changes over this period of time and offers the possibility of being able to stage the stroke progression over the critical first few hours. Since lactate and NAA reductions have been shown to correlate with loss of neurons and neuronal function in animal models, it is also tempting (but currently unproved) to speculate that the NAA level may be related to the surviving neuronal population within the ischemic lesion (146,147).

Generally, there is a consensus that elevated lactate levels are observed in the acute stage of human stroke, which can be used to delineate ischemic tissue. After the initial increase in the acute stage, there is usually a slow decline (148,149). However, lactate may remain elevated for extended periods of time (days to weeks), either because of ongoing anaerobic glycolysis, the inability to remove or metabolize lactate after it has been produced, or possibly from the glycolytic metabolism of macrophages in the late subacute or early chronic stages of stroke (150,151).

As discussed above, NAA seems to decrease slowly over a period of hours after stroke onset; by the time tissue has completely infarcted, NAA is either dramatically reduced or completely absent. It is postulated that in acute stroke, tissue that has high lactate, no conventional MR imaging abnormalities, and normal or only slightly reduced NAA levels in the first few hours after stroke onset may represent ischemic tissue at risk of infarction (152,153). This tissue could represent the "penumbra" (Fig 10). We hypothesize that identification of such regions may, in the future, be one of the criteria for initiating thrombolytic therapy (12).

Stroke progression is related not only to residual blood flow but also to the duration of decreased blood flow (51, 154,155). A limitation in the evaluation of patients with acute stroke is that during the acute stages of stroke, most MR

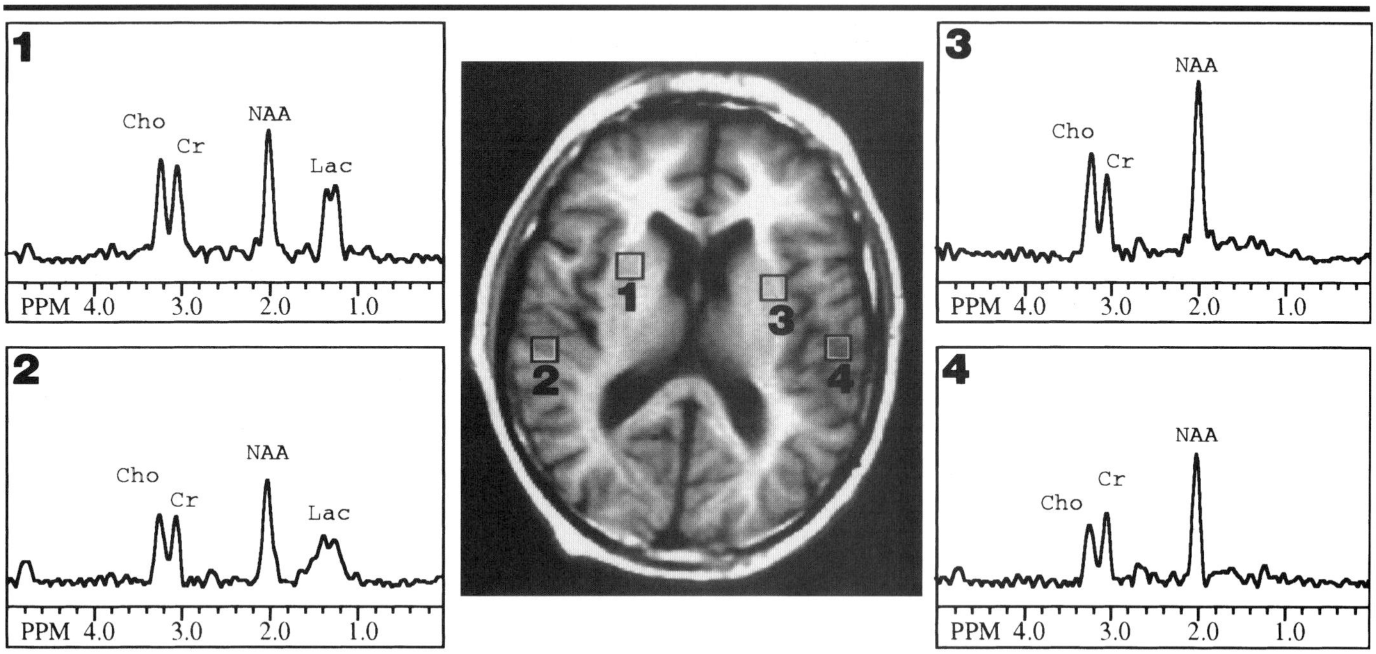

a.

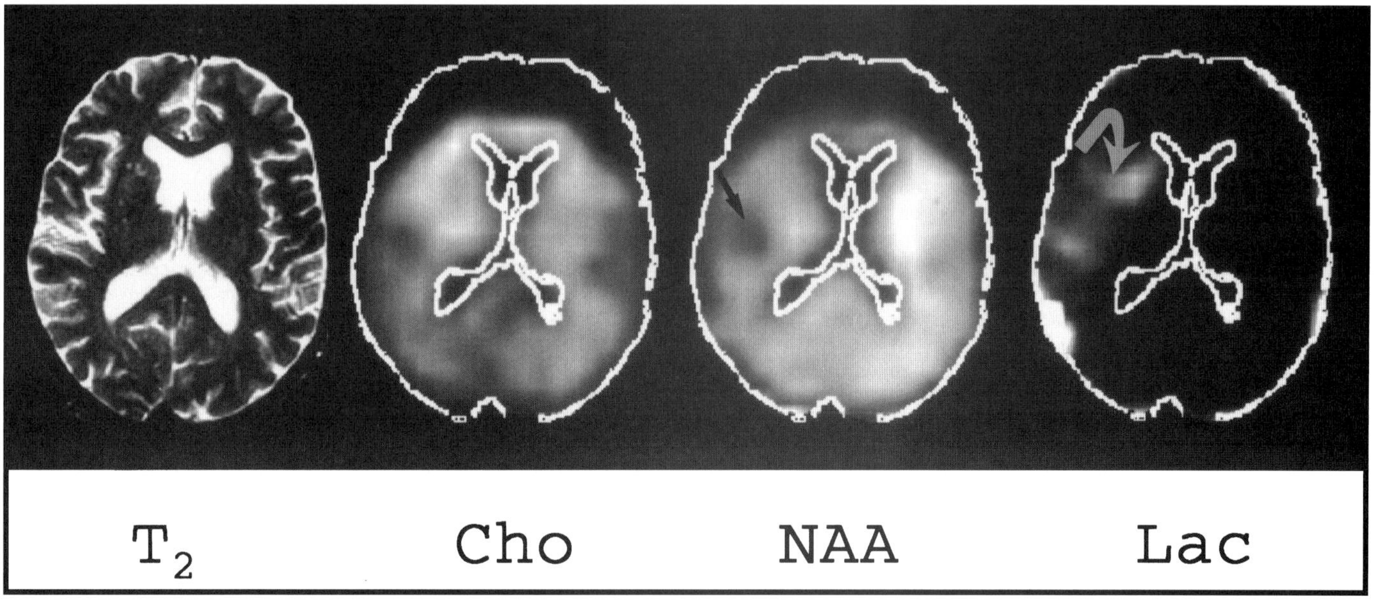

b.

Figure 10. Dense left-sided hemiparesis, severe dysarthria, and a central seventh nerve palsy in a 56-year-old man. Conventional T2-weighted MR image obtained 24 hours after ictus (image labeled T_2 in **b**) demonstrated no areas of hyperintensity. MR angiogram (not shown) demonstrated an occlusion or high-grade stenosis of the right MCA. Multisection two-dimensional proton spectroscopic axial images (2,300/272, 15-mm section thickness, 32 × 32 matrix) (not shown) were also obtained at this time. *Cho* = choline, *Cr* = creatine and phosphocreatine, *Lac* = lactate, *PPM* = parts per million. **(a)** Spectra obtained from four regions in the brain show areas of NAA and lactate abnormality on the right (zones labeled *1* and *2*). Conversely, the spectra obtained from the left cerebral hemisphere (zones labeled *3* and *4*) are normal. Note the absence of a lactate peak in the left hemisphere. **(b)** Metabolite axial MR images (2,300/272, 15-mm section thickness, 32 × 32 matrix) demonstrate an area of NAA decrease (straight arrow) with surrounding lactate elevation (curved arrow). In the area of NAA decrease and highest lactate levels, there was progression to infarction. This appearance corresponds to the theoretic model of the penumbra.

imaging parameters do not appear to change. Specifically, conventional T2-weighted images do not show changes until fairly late after stroke onset. Moreover, perfusion deficits and decreased diffusion, although immediately detectable, may remain static for a considerable period of time. For example, a decreased ADC gives no indication of the duration of ischemia. Conversely, rates of NAA loss and lactate increase appear to be blood flow dependent (154). Therefore, a metabolic-based measure of stroke progression may be more useful than either isolated measures of time after onset or cerebral blood flow in characterizing the ischemic state.

The earliest studies of human stroke

used single-voxel methodologies, such as spatially resolved spectroscopy (SPARS) or stimulated echo acquisition mode (STEAM) (156,157). A major drawback of single-voxel and one-dimensional MR spectroscopic imaging methodologies, however, is that they provide no (or little) information regarding the spatial extent or heterogeneity of the abnormalities, and also require prior knowledge of the stroke location for correct voxel placement. Therefore, two- or three-dimensional MR spectroscopic imaging methods that map metabolite levels over wider regions of the brain are required. Because of the good efficiency of the spectroscopic imaging data acquisition, multidimensional MR spectroscopic imaging data can be obtained with higher spatial resolution than single voxel studies. Early attempts used single-section two-dimensional MR spectroscopic imaging, and more recently we have used a multisection two-dimensional MR spectroscopic imaging method (158–160). This technique allows complete mapping of supratentorial metabolite levels in a 30-minute imaging time, with a nominal spatial resolution of less than 1 cm^3.

It is clear that spectroscopy provides unique and relevant information to the characterization of acute cerebral ischemia, potentially demarcating the penumbra. However, it is important to recognize the limited spatial resolution of the MR spectroscopic imaging data sets (approximately 1 cm^3), and appreciate that intervoxel signal contamination can occur between adjacent voxels (160). Therefore, a voxel of normal brain that lies immediately adjacent to a lactate-containing infarct could easily be mistaken as "tissue at risk," since it will have a normal MR imaging appearance but may appear to contain some lactate signal that actually originates from the adjacent voxel. The spatial resolution is largely signal-to-noise ratio limited, and it does not appear likely to be greatly improved in the near future; clearly, proton MR spectroscopic imaging will not enable detection of lacunar or small infarcts (<1 cm^3). The higher spatial resolution of diffusion and perfusion MR imaging is definitely an advantage is this regard. Further, the implementation of MR spectroscopic imaging is hampered by the limited coverage, and lengthy imaging times (approximately 30 minutes). Whole-brain multisection MR spectroscopic imaging may be possible in the future if enough sections can be interleaved into a single repetition time period. Imaging time reductions are definitely feasible and have already been demonstrated by using either multiecho sequences analogous to fast SE or rapid acquisition with relaxation enhancement (or RARE) sequences or by using proton echo-planar spectroscopic imaging (or PEPSI) (161–163). These fast methods of spatial encoding allow imaging times to be reduced from 30 minutes to under 10 minutes without sacrificing too much sensitivity or resolution. For instance, excellent-quality spectroscopic images were recently demonstrated by using the proton echo-planar spectroscopic imaging sequence with an 8-minute imaging time (163).

OPTIMAL MR IMAGING EVALUATION OF CEREBRAL ISCHEMIA

A comprehensive evaluation of cerebral ischemia is possible with advanced MR techniques. Diffusion techniques provide early delineation of the extent of tissue that is likely to proceed to infarction. Perfusion and spectroscopy aid in delineating the area at risk of infarction, and MR angiography can help determine if there is a thrombus amenable to lysis. GRE sequences enable exclusion of intraparenchymal hemorrhage. Although it can be agreed on that a T2-weighted sequence should be obtained, opinions vary as to whether this should be done by using a FLAIR, fast SE, or conventional SE sequence; we currently use the conventional SE sequence.

This combination of examinations should enable optimal patient selection and minimization of risk of intervention. Further, in delineating the ischemic penumbra, it may also be possible to extend the therapeutic window beyond 3 hours. However, it is important to realize that despite the great promise of MR, only CT has proved beneficial in large-scale prospective trials (3,7). Demonstration of the potential advantages of MR will require further investigation including incorporation into prospective large-scale studies and further clinical validation of its ability to delineate the ischemic penumbra.

HORIZONS IN ADVANCED MR TECHNIQUES

Finally, MR imaging is an ever-expanding source of methodologies, and it is reasonable to expect that several new techniques will become available in the future. Some of these methods are now already being applied in functional MR imaging, such as blood-flow techniques based on arterial spin labeling and the so-called blood oxygen level dependent, or BOLD, approach based on hemoglobin-related magnetic susceptibility changes in and around the blood vessels (130,164–171). Assuming intravascular origin of the blood oxygen level dependent SE effect, it was recently shown that the absolute T2 of blood in perfused tissue is directly related to the tissue oxygen extraction ratio, which is the ratio of oxygen consumption and oxygen delivery (172). Because initial stages of ischemia are characterized by reduced blood flow but maintained oxygen metabolism, one would expect a reduction in the oxygen extraction ratio as has been shown with PET. This should then lead to a reduction in T2, which was recently demonstrated to occur (173). This also explains the origin of T2* and T2 effects found in initial ischemia in animals in recent years (174–176). However, this effect may reverse if oxygen metabolism becomes impaired, and care has to be taken in its interpretation. In addition, these effects are small (a few percentage points) and will not be obvious on T2-weighted images; thus, they have to be carefully measured by using absolute T2 approaches. These effects reduce even more when using multiple SE sequences. Preliminary results on another potentially important new approach were recently reported at a conference, namely, imaging of the so-called spin-lock relaxation rate T1r, which was able to separate reversible from irreversible ischemia in a rat model (173).

Lastly, there has recently been renewed interest in sodium imaging for stroke, which was successfully demonstrated in the clinical setting at 3 T (177). However, just as for phosphorus spectroscopy, this approach is hampered by limited clinical availability. In addition, sodium changes are expected to occur upon membrane depolarization, similar to the major part of the diffusion signal changes, and may be only an early indicator of irreversible damage.

SUMMARY

The state of the art for imaging acute cerebral ischemia has dramatically changed following the demonstration of efficacy of rt-PA. Neuroimaging now occupies a central role in patient care with prompt performance and interpretation of the initial CT study critical to successful intervention. It has been of proved benefit in guiding therapy in prospective clinical trials. Current limitations of CT in this role are a relative lack of sensitivity for the detection of early ischemia and low specificity in determining appropriateness for intervention with thrombolysis. MR imaging has tremendous potential to contribute to stroke management on the basis of a high sensitivity for detection of areas of infarction and the ability to evaluate large-vessel patency and perfusion characteristics. Continued investigation is needed to determine its ability to delineate the penumbra and to affect patient outcome.

References

1. Bryan RN. Imaging of acute stroke. Radiology 1990; 177:615–616.
2. Goldstein M. Decade of the brain: National Institute of Neurological Disorders and Stroke (editorial). Neurosurgery 1993; 32:297.
3. National Institute of Neurological Disease and Stroke rt-PA Study Group. Tissue plasminogen activator for acute ischemic stroke. N Engl J Med 1995; 355: 1581–1587.
4. Sussman BJ, Fitch TS. Thrombolysis with fibrinolysis in cerebral arterial occlusion. JAMA 1958; 167:1705–1709.
5. Wardlaw JM, Warlow CP. Thrombolysis in acute ischemic stroke: does it work? Stroke 1992; 23:1826–1829.
6. Levy DE, Brott TG, Haley EC, et al. Factors related to intracranial hematoma formation in patients receiving tissue-type plasminogen activator for acute ischemic stroke. Stroke 1994; 25:291–297.
7. Hacke W, Kaste M, Fieschi C, et al for the ECASS Study Group. Intravenous thrombolysis with recombinant tissue plasminogen activator for acute hemispheric stroke: the European Cooperative Acute Stroke Study. JAMA 1995; 274:1017–1025.
8. Multicenter Acute Stroke Trial-Italy (MAST-I) Group. Randomized controlled trial of streptokinase, aspirin, and combination of both in treatment of acute ischemic stroke. Lancet 1995; 346:1509–1514.
9. The Multicenter Acute Stroke Trial-Europe Study Group. Thrombolytic therapy with streptokinase in acute ischemic stroke. N Engl J Med 1996; 335:145–150.
10. Donnan GA, Davis SM, Chambers B, et al. Streptokinase for acute ischemic stroke with relationship to time of administration. JAMA 1996; 276:961–966.
11. International Stroke Trial Pilot Study Collaborative Group. Study design of the international stroke trial (IST), baseline data and outcome in 984 randomized patients in the pilot study. J Neurol Neurosurg Psychiatry 1996; 60:371–376.
12. Beauchamp NJ, Bryan RN. Acute cerebral ischemia: a pathophysiologic review and radiologic perspective. AJR 1998; 171: 73–84.
13. Culebras A, Kase CS, Masdeu JC. Practice guidelines for the use of imaging in transient ischemic attacks and acute stroke: a report of the Stroke Council, American Heart Association. Stroke 1997; 28:1480–1497.
14. Macknight ADC, Leaf A. Regulation of cellular volume. Physiol Rev 1977; 37: 510–573.
15. Baethmann A, Staub F. Cellular edema. In: Welch KMA, Caplan LR, Reis DJ, Siesjo BK, Weir B, eds. Primer on cerebrovascular diseases. San Diego, Calif: Academic Press, 1997; 153–156.
16. Klatzo I. Neuropathological aspects of brain edema. J Neuropathol Exp Neurol 1967; 26:1–14.
17. Truwit CL, Barkovich AJ, Gean-Martin A, Hibrin N, Norman D. Loss of the insular ribbon: another sign of CT infarction. Radiology 1990; 176:801–806.
18. Tomura N, Uemura K, Inugami A, Fujita H, Higano S, Shishida F. Early CT finding in cerebral infarction: obscuration of the lentiform nucleus. Radiology 1988; 168: 463–467.
19. Bryan RN, Levy LM, Whitlow WD, Killian JM, Preziosi TJ, Rosario JA. Diagnosis of acute cerebral infarction: comparison of CT and MR imaging. AJNR 1991; 12:611–620.
20. von Kummer R, Meyding-Lamade U, Forsting M, et al. Sensitivity and prognostic value of early CT in occlusion of the middle cerebral artery trunk. AJNR 1994; 15:9–15.
21. Leys D, Pruvo JP, Godefroy O, Rondepierre P, Leclerc X. Prevalence and significance of hyperdense middle cerebral artery in acute stroke. Stroke 1992; 23:317–324.
22. New PFJ, Aronow S. Attenuation measurements of whole blood and blood fractions in computed tomography. Radiology 1976; 121:635–640.
23. Arimitsu I, DiChiro G, Brooks RA, Smith PB. White-gray matter differentiation in computed tomography. J Comput Assist Tomogr 1977; 1:437–442.
24. Wing SD, Norman D, Polock JA, Newton TH. Contrast enhancement of cerebral infarcts in computed tomography. Radiology 1976; 121:89–92.
25. Becker H, Desch H, Hacker H, Pencz A. CT fogging effect with ischemic cerebral infarcts. Neuroradiology 1979; 18:185–192.
26. Kendall BE, Pullicino P. Intravascular contrast injection in ischaemic lesions. II. Effect on prognosis. Neuroradiology 1980; 19:241–243.
27. Kuroiwa T, Sedia M, Tomida S, Hiratsuka H, Okeda R, Inaba Y. Discrepanceis among CT, histological, and blood-brain barrier findings in early cerebral ischemia. J Neurosurg 1986; 65:199–202.
28. Riggs JE. Tissue plasminogen activator should not be used in acute ischemic stroke. Arch Neurol 1996; 53:1306–1308.
29. von Kummer R, Holle R, Gryska U, et al. Interobserver agreement in assessing early CT signs of middle cerebral artery infarction. AJNR 1995; 17:1743–1748.
30. Inoue Y, Takemoto K, Miyamoto T, et al. Sequential computed tomography scans in acute cerebral infarct. Radiology 1980; 135:655–662.
31. Castillo M. Prethrombolysis brain imaging: trends and controversies. AJNR 1997; 18:1830–1834.
32. Libman RB, Wirkowski E, Alvir J, Rao TH. Conditions that mimic stroke in the emergency department. Arch Neurol 1995; 52:1119–1122.
33. Fisher M, Pessin MS, Furian AJ. ECASS: lessons for future thrombolytic stroke trials. European Cooperative Acute Stroke Study (editorial). JAMA 1995; 274:1058–1059.
34. Elster AD, Moody DM. Early cerebral infarction: gadopentetate dimeglumine enhancement. Radiology 1990; 177:627–632.
35. Fellner C, Geissler A, Held P, Strotzer M, Treibel W, Fellner F. Signal, contrast and resolution in optimized PD- and T2-weighted turbo SE images of the knee. J Comput Assist Tomogr 1995; 19:96–105.
36. Fellner F, Fellner C, Held, Schmitt R. Comparison of spin-echo pulse sequences for imaging of the brain. AJNR 1997; 18:1617–1625.
37. Atlas SW, Hackney DB, Yousem DM, Listerud J. Fast spin echo MR imaging: blinded comparison with conventional spin echo imaging for the detection of focal brain lesions (abstr). In: Book of abstracts: Society of Magnetic Resonance in Medicine 1991. Berkeley, Calif: Society of Magnetic Resonance in Medicine, 1991; 41.
38. Prorok RJ. Signa applications guide. Vol. 4. Milwaukee, Wis: GE Medical Systems, 1992; 30–35.
39. Wehrli FW, McGowan JC. The basis of MR contrast. In: Atlas SW, ed. Magnetic resonance imaging of the brain and spine. 2nd ed. Philadelphia, Pa: Lippincott-Raven, 1996; 29–48.
40. DeCoene B, Hajnal JV, Gatehouse P, et al. MR of the brain using fluid attenuated inversion-recovery (FLAIR) pulse sequence. AJNR 1992; 13:1555–1564.
41. Hajnal JV, Bryant DJ, Kasuboski L, et al. Use of fluid attenuated inversion recovery (FLAIR) pulse sequences in MRI of the brain. J Comput Assist Tomogr 1992; 16:841–844.
42. Alexander JA, Sheppard S, Davis PC, Salverda P. Adult cerebrovascular disease: role of modified rapid fluid-attenuated inversion-recovery sequences. AJNR 1996; 17:1507–1513.
43. Rydberg JN, Hammond CA, Grimm RC, et al. Initial clinical experience in MR imaging of the brain with a fast fluid-attenuated inversion-recovery pulse sequence. Radiology 1994; 193:173–180.
44. Post MJ. Fluid-attenuated inversion-recovery fast spin-echo MR: a clinically useful tool in the evaluation of neurologically symptomatic HIV-positive patients. AJNR 1997; 18:1611–1616.
45. Atlas SW, Mark AS, Grossman RI, Gomori JM. Intracranial hemorrhage: gradient-echo MR imaging at 1.5 T—comparison with spin-echo imaging and clinical applications. Radiology 1988; 168:803–807.
46. Hayman LA, McArdle CB, Taber KH. MR imaging of hyperacute intracranial hemorrhage in the cat. AJR 1989; 10:681–686.
47. Weingarten K, Filippi C, Zimmerman RD, Deck MDF. Detection of hemorrhage in acute cerebral infarction: evaluation with spin-echo and gradient echo MRI. Clin Imaging 1994; 18:43–55.
48. Noguchi K, Ogawa T, Ingami A. Acute subarachnoid hemorrhage: MR imaging with fluid-attenuated inversion-recovery pulse sequences. Radiology 1995; 196:733–737.
49. Noguchi K, Ogawa T, Seto H, et al. Subacute and chronic subarachnoid hemor-

rhage: diagnosis with fluid-attenuated inversion-recovery MR imaging. Radiology 1997; 203:257–262.
50. Astrup J, Siesjo B, Symon L. Thresholds in cerebral ischemia: the ischemic penumbra. Stroke 1981; 12:723–725.
51. Hossmann KA. Viability thresholds and the penumbra of focal ischemia. Ann Neurol 1994; 36:557–565.
52. Castillo J, Davalos A, Noya M. Progression of ischaemic stroke and excitotoxic aminoacids. Lancet 1997; 349:79–83.
52a. Koenig M, Klotz E, Luka B, Venderink DJ, Spittler JF, Heuser L. Perfusion CT of the brain: diagnostic approach for early detection of ischemic stroke. Radiology 1998; 209:85–93.
53. Frackowiak RSJ, Lenzi G, Jones T, Heather JD. Quantitative measurement of regional cerebral blood flow and oxygen metabolism in man using ^{15}O and positron emission tomography: the theory, procedure and normal values. J Comput Assist Tomogr 1980; 4:727–736.
54. Carr HY, Purcell EM. Effects of diffusion on free precession in nuclear magnetic resonance experiments. Physiol Rev 1954; 94:630–638.
55. Stejskal EO, Tanner JE. Spin diffusion measurements: spin echoes in the presence of a time-dependent field gradient. J Chem Phys 1965; 42:288–292.
56. Le Bihan D, Breton E, Lallemand D. MR imaging of intravoxel incoherent motions: application to diffusion and perfusion in neurologic disorders. Radiology 1986; 161:401–407.
57. Moseley ME, Cohen Y, Mintorovitch J, et al. Early detection of regional cerebral ischemia in cats: comparison of diffusion- and T2-weighted MRI and spectroscopy. Magn Reson Med 1990; 14:330–346.
58. Knight RA, Dereski MO, Helpern JA, Ordidge RJ, Chopp M. Magnetic resonance imaging assessment of evolving focal cerebral ischemia. Stroke 1994; 25:1252–1262.
59. Decanniere C, Eleff S, Davis D, van Zijl PC. Correlation of rapid changes in the average water diffusion constant and the concentrations of lactate and ATP breakdown products during global ischemia in cat brain. Magn Reson Med 1995; 34:343–352.
60. Kohno K, Hoehn-Berlage M, Mies G, Back T, Hossman KA. Relationship between diffusion-weighted MR images, cerebral blood flow, and energy state in experimental brain infarction. Magn Reson Imaging 1995; 13:73–80.
61. van der Toorn A, Sykova E, Skobisova I, et al. Dynamic changes in brain water ADC and extracellular space parameters induced by cardiac arrest in neonatal rats (abstr). In: Proceedings of the Second Meeting of the Society of Magnetic Resonance. Berkeley, Calif: Society of Magnetic Resonance, 1994; 141.
62. Davis D, Ulatowski J, Eleff S, et al. Rapid monitoring of changes in water diffusion coefficients during reversible ischemia in cat and rat brain. Magn Reson Med 1994; 31:454–460.
63. Benveniste H, Hedlund LW, Johnson GA. Mechanisms of detection of acute cerebral ischemia in rats by diffusion-weighted magnetic resonance microscopy. Stroke 1992; 23:746–754.
64. Norris DG, Niendorf TG, Leibfritz D. Healthy and infarcted brain tissue studies at short diffusion times: the origins of apparent restriction and the reduction in apparent diffusion constant. NMR Biomed 1994; 7:304–310.
65. Helpern JA, Ordidge RJ, Knight RA. The effect of cell membrane water permeability on the apparent diffusion coefficients of water (abstr). In: Book of abstracts: Society of Magnetic Resonance in Medicine 1992. Berkeley, Calif: Society of Magnetic Resonance in Medicine, 1992; 1201.
66. Duong TQ, Ackerman JJH, Ying HS, Neil JJ. Evaluation of extra and intracellular apparent diffusion in normal and intracellular apparent diffusion in normal and globally ischemic rat brains via 19F NMR. Magn Reson Med 1998; 40:1–13.
67. van der Toorn A, Sykova' EDRM, Vorisek I, et al. Dynamic changes in water ADC, energy metabolism, extracellular space volume, and tortuosity in neonatal rat brain during global ischemia. Magn Reson Med 1996; 36:52–60.
68. van Gelderen P, de Vleeschouwer MHM, DesPres D, Pekar J, van Zijl PCM, Moonen CTW. Water diffusion and acute stroke. Magn Reson Med 1994; 31:154–163.
69. Moonen CTW, Pekar J, de Vleeschouwer MHM, van Gelderen P, van Zijl PCM, DesPres D. Restricted and anisotropic diffusion of water in healthy cat brain and in stroke studied by NMR diffusion imaging. Magn Reson Med 1991; 19:327–332.
70. Moseley ME, Cohen Y, Kucharczyk J, et al. Diffusion-weighted imaging of anisotropic water diffusion in the cat central nervous system. Radiology 1990; 176:439–446.
71. Busza AL, Allen KL, King MD, van BN, Williams SR, Gadian DG. Diffusion-weighted imaging studies of cerebral ischemia in gerbils: potential relevance to energy failure. Stroke 1992; 23:1602–1612.
72. Branston NM, Symon L, Crockard HA, Pasztor E. Relationship between cortical evoked potential and local cortical blood flow following acute middle cerebral artery occlusion in the baboon. Exp Neurol 1974; 45:195–208.
73. Pierpaoli C, Righini A, Linfante J, Tao-Cheng H, Alger J, Di Chiro G. Histopathological correlates of abnormal water diffusion in cerebral ischemia: diffusion-weighted MR imaging and light and electron microscopic study. Radiology 1993; 189:439–448.
74. Gyngell ML, Back T, Hoehn-Berlage M, Kohno K, Hossmann KA. Transient cell depolarization after permanent middle cerebral artery occlusion: an observation by diffusion-weighted MRI and localized 1H-MRS. Magn Reson Med 1994; 31:337–341.
75. Miyabe M, Mori S, van Zijl PCM, et al. Correlation of the average water diffusion constant with cerebral blood flow and ischemic damage after transient middle cerebral artery occlusion in cats. J Cereb Blood Flow Metab 1996; 881–891.
76. Minematsu K, Li L, Fisher M, Sotak CH, Davis MA, Fiandaca MS. Diffusion-weighted magnetic resonance imaging: rapid and quantitative detection of focal brain ischemia. Neurology 1992; 42:235–240.
77. Hasegawa Y, Fisher M, Latour LL, Dardzinski BJ, Sotak CH. MRI diffusion mapping of reversible and irreversible ischemic injury in focal brain ischemia. Neurology 1994; 44:1484–1490.
78. Baird AE, Benfield A, Schlaug G, Siewert B, Lovblad KO, Edelman RR, et al. Enlargement of human cerebral ischemic lesion volumes measured by diffusion-weighted magnetic resonance imaging. Ann Neurol 1997; 41:581-589.
79. Beauchamp NJ, Ulug AM, Passe TJ, van Zijl PCM. MR diffusion imaging in stroke: review and controversies. RadioGraphics 1998; 18:1269–1283.
80. van Zijl PCM, Davis D, Moonen CTW. Diffusion spectroscopy in living systems. In: Gillies RJ, ed. NMR in physiology and biomedicine. San Diego, Calif: Academic Press, 1994; 185–198.
81. Warach S, Boska M, Welch KM. Pitfalls and potential of clinical diffusion-weighted MR imaging in acute stroke (editorial). Stroke 1997; 28:481–482.
82. Welch KMA, Windham J, Knight RA, et al. A model to predict the histopathology of human stroke using diffusion and T2-weighted magnetic resonance imaging. Stroke 1995; 26:1983–1989.
83. Knight RA, Ordidge RJ, Helpern JA, Chopp M, Rodolosi LC, Peck D. Temporal evolution of ischemic damage in rat brain measured by proton nuclear magnetic resonance imaging. Stroke 1991; 22:802–808.
84. Lutsep HL, Albers GW, DeCrespigny A, Kamat GN, Marks MP, Moseley ME. Clinical utility of diffusion-weighted MRI in the assessment of ischemic stroke. Ann Neurol 1997; 41:574–580.
85. Schlaug G, Siewert B, Benfield A, Edelman RR, Warach S. Time course of the apparent diffusion coefficient (ADC) abnormality in human stroke. Neurology 1997; 49:113–119.
86. Koroshetz WJ, Gonzalez G. Diffusion-weighted MRI: an ECG for "brain attack"? Ann Neurol 1997; 41:565–566.
87. Singer MB, Chong J, Lu D, Schonewille WJ, Turhim S, Atlas SW. Diffusion-weighted MRI in acute subcortical infarction. Stroke 1998; 29:133–136.
88. Lovblad KO, Baird AE, Schlaug G, et al. Ischemic lesion volumes in acute stroke by diffusion-weighted magnetic resonance imaging correlate with clinical outcome. Ann Neurol 1997; 42:164–170.
89. Warach S, Dashe JF, Edelman RR. Clinical outcome in ischemic stroke predicted by early diffusion-weighted and perfusion magnetic resonance imaging: a preliminary analysis. J Cereb Blood Flow Metab 1996; 16:53–59.
90. Warach S, Gaa J, Siewert B, Wielopolski P, Edelman RR. Acute human stroke studied by whole brain echo planar diffusion-weighted magnetic resonance imaging. Ann Neurol 1995; 37:231–241.
91. Sorenson AG, Buonanno FS, Gonzalez RG, et al. Hyperacute stroke: evaluation with combined multisection diffusion-weighted and hemodynamically weighted echo-planar MR imaging. Radiology 1996; 391–401.
92. Soher BJ, Gillard JH, Bryan RN, Oppenheimer SM, Barker PB. MR perfusion imaging in acute middle cerebral artery stroke: comparison of blood volume and bolus arrival time. J Stroke Cerebrovasc Dis 1998; 7:17–23.

93. Toole JF. Cerebral Embolism. In: Toole JF, ed. Cerebrovascular disorders. New York: Raven, 1990; 240–255.
94. Wang PY, Beauchamp NJ, Ulug AM, Barker PB, van Zijl PCM. Diffusion negative MR in acute stroke (abstr). In: Proceedings of the Annual Meeting of the American Society of Neuroradiology. Philadelphia, Pa: American Society of Neuroradiology, 1997.
95. Feinberg DA, Kiefer B, Johnson G. GRASE improves spatial resolution in single shot imaging. Magn Reson Med 1995; 33:529–533.
96. Haase A, Frahm J, Matthei D, Haenicke W, Merboldt KD. FLASH imaging: rapid NMR imaging using low flip-angle pulses. J Magn Reson 1986; 67:258–266.
97. Ordidge RJ, JA, Qing ZX, Knight RA, Nagesh V. Correction of motional artifacts in diffusion-weighted MR images using navigator echoes. Magn Reson Imag 1994; 12:455–460.
98. Wimberger DM, Roberts TP, Barkovich AJ, Prayer LM, Moseley ME, Kucharczyk J. Identification of "premyelination" by diffusion-weighted MRI. J Comput Assist Tomogr 1995; 19:28–33.
99. Pierpaoli C, Choi B, Schiffmann R, Di Chiro G. Diffusion tensor MRI in Pelizaeus-Merzbacher disease (abstr). In: Proceedings of the Fifth Meeting of the International Society for Magnetic Resonance in Medicine. Berkeley, Calif: International Society for Magnetic Resonance in Medicine, 1997; 664.
100. Ulug AM, Beauchamp N, Bryan RN, van Zijl PCM. Absolute quantitation of diffusion constants in human stroke. Stroke 1997; 28:483–490.
101. Ulug AM, van Zijl PCM. Orientation-independent isotropic and anisotropic diffusion tensor imaging without tensor diagonalization. Magn Reson Imaging 1999; 9:804–813.
102. Mori S, van Zijl PCM. Diffusion weighting by the trace of the diffusion tensor within a single scan. Magn Reson Med 1995; 33:41–52.
103. Chun T, Ulug AM, van Zijl PCM. Single-scan isotropic diffusion weighting on a clinical scanner (abstr). In: Proceedings of the Fifth Meeting of the International Society for Magnetic Resonance in Medicine. Berkeley, Calif: International Society for Magnetic Resonance in Medicine, 1997; 1735.
104. Beauchamp NJ Jr, Ulug AM, Wang P, Chun T, Barker PB, van Zijl PCM. Single-shot diffusion-weighted trace imaging of acute stroke (abstr). In: Proceedings of the Annual Meeting of the American Society of Neuroradiology. Philadelphia, Pa: American Society of Neuroradiology, 1998; 345.
105. Benfield A, Prasad PV, Edelman RR, Warach S. On the optimal β-value for measuring lesion volumes in ischemic stroke using diffusion-weighted MR imaging (abstr). In: Proceedings of the Fourth Meeting of the International Society for Magnetic Resonance in Medicine. Berkeley, Calif: International Society for Magnetic Resonance in Medicine, 1996; 1344.
106. Basser PJ, Mattiello J, LeBihan D. Estimation of the effective self-diffusion tensor from the NMR spin echo. J Magn Reson B 1994; 103:247–254.
107. Rosen BR, Belliveau JW, Vevea JM, Brady TJ. Perfusion imaging with NMR contrast agents. Magn Reson Med 1990; 14:249–265.
108. Villringer A, Rosen BR, Belliveau JW, et al. Dynamic imaging with lanthanide chelates in normal brain: contrast due to magnetic susceptibility effects. Magn Res Med 1988; 6:164–174.
109. Belliveau JW, Kennedy DN, McKinstry RC, et al. Functional mapping of the human visual cortex by magnetic resonance imaging. Science 1990; 254:716–721.
110. Conturo TE, Barker PB, Mathews VP, Monsein LH, Bryan RN. MR imaging of cerebral perfusion by phase-angle reconstruction of bolus paramagnetic-induced proton frequency shifts. Magn Reson Med 1992; 27:375–390.
111. Hacklander T, Reichenbach JR, Hofer M, Modder U. Measurement of cerebral blood volume via the relaxing effect of low-dose gadopentetate dimeglumine during bolus transit. AJNR 1996; 17:821–830.
112. Kuppusamy K, Lin W, Cizek GR, Haacke EM. In vivo regional cerebral blood volume: quantitative assessment with 3D T1-weighted pre- and post-contrast MR imaging. Radiology 1996; 201:106–112.
113. Bruening R, Kwong KK, Vevea MJ, et al. Echo-planar MR determination of relative cerebral blood volume in human brain tumors: TI versus T2 weighting. AJNR 1996; 17:831–840.
114. Zierler KL. Equations for measuring blood flow by external monitoring of radioisotopes. Circ Res 1965; 16:309–321.
115. Weisskoff RM, Chesler D, Boxerman JL, Rosen BR. Pitfalls in MR measurements of tissue blood flow with intravenous tracers: which mean transit time? Magn Reson Med 1993; 29:553–559.
116. Rempp KA, Brix G, Wenz F, Becker CR, Guckel F, Lorenz WJ. Quantification of regional cerebral blood flow and volume with dynamic susceptibility contrast-enhanced MR imaging. Radiology 1994; 193:637–641.
117. Aronen HJ, Glass J, Pardo FS, et al. Echo-planar MR cerebral blood volume mapping of gliomas: clinical utility. Acta Radiol 1995; 36:520–528.
118. Ostergaard L, Sorensen AG, Kwong KK, Weisskoff RM, Gyldensted C, Rosen BR. High resolution measurement of cerebral blood flow using intravascular tracer bolus passages. II. Experimental comparison and preliminary results. Magn Reson Med 1996; 36:726–736.
119. Thompson HK, Starmer CF, Whalen RE, McIntosh HD. Indicator transit time considered as a gamma variate. Circ Res 1964; 14:502–514.
120. Powers W. Cerebral hemodynamics in ischemic cerebrovascular disease. Ann Neurol 1991; 29:231–240.
121. Maeda M, Crosby DL, Magnotta VA, et al. Cerebral hemodynamics in patients with major cerebral artery occlusion or severe stenosis: evaluation with perfusion MR imaging (abstr). In: Proceedings of the Fourth Meeting of the International Society for Magnetic Resonance in Medicine. Berkeley, Calif: International Society for Magnetic Resonance in Medicine, 1996; 594.
122. Warach S, Li W, Ronthal M, Edelman RR. Acute cerebral ischemia: evaluation with dynamic contrast-enhanced MR imaging and MR angiography. Radiology 1992; 182:41–47.
123. Warach S, Dashe JF, Edelman RR. Clinical outcome in ischemic stroke predicted by early diffusion-weighted and perfusion magnetic resonance imaging: a preliminary analysis. J Cereb Blood Flow Metab 1996; 16:53–59.
124. Sorensen AG, Koroshetz WJ, Buonanno FS, et al. Diffusion/perfusion mismatch in MRI of acute human stroke (abstr). In: Proceedings of the Fourth Meeting of the International Society for Magnetic Resonance in Medicine. Berkeley, Calif: International Society for Magnetic Resonance in Medicine, 1996; 91.
125. Lavy S, Melamed E, Portnoy Z. The effect of cerebral infarction on the regional cerebral blood flow of the contralateral hemisphere. Stroke 1975; 6:160–163.
126. Feeney DM, Baron JC. Diaschisis. Stroke 1986; 17:817–830.
127. Baron JC, Frackowiak RSJ, Herholz K, et al. Use of PET methods for measurements of cerebral energy metabolism and hemodynamics in cerebrovascular disease. J Cereb Blood Flow Metab 1989; 9:723–742.
128. Edelman RR, Mattle HP, Atkinson DJ, et al. Cerebral blood flow: assessment with dynamic contrast-enhanced T2*-weighted MR imaging at 1.5 T. Radiology 1990; 176: 211–220.
129. Duyn JH, van Gelderen P, Liu G, Moonen CTW. Fast volume scanning with frequency-shifted BURST MRI. Magn Reson Med 1993; 32:429–432.
130. Edelman RR, Siewert B, Darby DG, et al. Qualitative mapping of cerebral blood flow and functional localization with echo-planar MR imaging and signal targeting with alternating radiofrequency. Radiology 1994; 192:513–520.
131. Duyn JH, van Gelderen P, Barker PB, Frank JA, Mattay VS, Moonen CTW. 3D bolus-tracking with frequency-shifted BURST MRI. J Comput Assist Tomogr 1994; 18:680–687.
132. Yang Y, Glover GH, van Gelderen P, et al. Fast 3D functional magnetic resonance imaging at 1.5 T with spiral acquisition. Magn Reson Med 1996; 36:620–626.
133. Duyn JH, Yang Y. Single-shot spiral magnetic resonance imaging with trapezoidal gradients. J Magn Reson 1997; 4:130-134.
134. Birken DL, Oldendorf WH. *N*-acetyl-L-aspartate: a literature review of a compound prominent in 1H-NM spectroscopic studies of the brain. Neurosci Biobehav Rev 1989; 13:23–31.
135. Simmons ML, Frondoza CG, Coyle JT. Immunocytochemical localization of *N*-acetyl-aspartate with monoclonal antibodies. Neuroscience 1991; 45:37–45.
136. Gadian DG, Frackowiak RS, Crockard HA, et al. Acute cerebral ischaemia: concurrent changes in cerebral blood flow, energy metabolites, pH and lactate measured with hydrogen clearance and 31P and 1H nuclear magnetic resonance spectroscopy. I. Methodology. J Cereb Blood Flow Metab 1987; 7:199–206.
137. Crockard HA, Gadian DG, Frackowiak RS, et al. Acute cerebral ischaemia: concurrent changes in cerebral blood flow, energy metabolites, pH, and lactate mea-

sured with hydrogen clearance and 31P and 1H nuclear magnetic resonance spectroscopy. II. Changes during ischaemia. J Cereb Blood Flow Metab 1987; 7:394–402.
138. Allen K, Busza AL, Crockard HA, et al. Acute cerebral ischaemia: concurrent changes in cerebral blood flow, energy metabolites, pH and lactate measured with hydrogen clearance and 31P and 1H nuclear magnetic resonance spectroscopy. III. Changes following ischaemia. J Cereb Blood Flow Metab 1988; 8:816–821.
139. Petroff OA, Prichard JW, Ogino T, Shulman RG. Proton magnetic resonance spectroscopic studies of agonal carbohydrate metabolism in rabbit brain. Neurology 1988; 38:1569–1574.
140. Rehncrona S, Rosen I, Siesjo BK. Brain lactic acidosis and ischemic cell damage. I. Biochemistry and neurophysiology. J Cereb Blood Flow Metab 1981; 1:297–311.
141. Monsein LH, Mathews VP, Barker PB, et al. Irreversible regional cerebral ischemia: serial MR imaging and proton MR spectroscopy in nonhuman primate model. AJNR 1993; 14:963–970.
142. Sager TN, Laursen H, Hansen AJ. Changes in *N*-acetyl-aspartate content during focal and global brain ischemia of the rat. J Cereb Blood Flow Metab 1995; 15:639–646.
143. Higuchi T, Fernandez EJ, Maudsley AA, Shimizu H, Weiner MW, Weinstein PR. Mapping of lactate and *N*-acetyl-L-aspartate predicts infarction during acute focal ischemia: in vivo 1H magnetic resonance spectroscopy in rats. Neurosurgery 1996; 38:121–129.
144. Bizzi A, Righini A, Turner R, Le Bihan D, Bockhorst KH, Alger JR. Imaging focal reperfusion injury following global ischemia with diffusion-weighted magnetic resonance imaging and 1H-magnetic resonance spectroscopy. Magn Reson Imaging 1996; 14:581–592.
145. van Zijl PCM, Moonen CTW. In situ changes in purine nucleotide and *N*-acetyl concentrations upon inducing global ischemia in cat brain. Magn Reson Med 1993; 29:381–385.
146. Guimaraes A, Schwartz P, Prakash MR, et al. Quantitative in vivo 1H magnetic resonance spectroscopic imaging of neuronal loss in rat brain. Neuroscience 1995; 69:1095–1101.
147. Strauss I, Williamson JM, Bertram EH, Lothman EW, Fernandez EJ. Histological and 1H magnetic resonance spectroscopic imaging analysis of quinolinic acid-induced damage to the rat striatum. Magn Reson Med 1997; 37:24–33.
148. Graham GD, Blamire AM, Rothman DL, et al. Early temporal variation of cerebral metabolites after human stroke: a proton magnetic resonance spectroscopy study. Stroke 1993; 24:1891–1896.
149. Lanfermann H, Kugel H, Heindel W, Herholz K, Heiss WD, Lackner K. Metabolic changes in acute and subacute cerebral infarctions: findings at proton MR spectroscopic imaging. Radiology 1995; 196:203–210.
150. Siesjo BK. Lactic acidosis in the brain: occurrence, triggering mechanisms and pathophysiological importance. In: Metabolic acidosis. London, England: Pitman, 1982; 77–100.
151. Petroff OAC, Graham GD, Blamire AM, et al. Spectroscopic imaging of stroke in humans: histopathological correlates of spectral changes. Neurology 1992; 42: 1349–1354.
152. Barker PB, Gillard JH, van Zijl PCM, et al. Acute stroke: evaluation with serial proton magnetic resonance spectroscopy. Radiology 1994; 192:723–732.
153. Gillard JH, Barker PB, van Zijl PCM, Bryan RN, Oppenheimer SM. Proton spectroscopic imaging in acute middle cerebral stroke. AJNR 1996; 17:873–886.
154. Hakim AM. The cerebral ischemic penumbra. Can J Neurol Sci 1987; 14:557–559.
155. Hakim AM, Hogan MJ, Carpenter S. Time course of cerebral blood flow and histological outcome after focal cerebral ischemia in rat. Stroke 1992; 23:1138-1143.
156. Berkelbach van der Sprenkel JW, Luyten PR, van Rijen PC, Tulleken CA, den Hollander JA. Cerebral lactate detected by regional proton magnetic resonance spectroscopy in a patient with cerebral infarction. Stroke 1988; 19:1556–1560.
157. Bruhn H, Frahm J, Gyngell ML, Merboldt KD, Hanicke W, Sauter R. Cerebral metabolism in man after acute stroke: new observations using localized proton NMR spectroscopy. Magn Reson Med 1989; 9:126–131.
158. Hugg JW, Duijn JH, Matson GB, et al. Elevated lactate and alkalosis in chronic human brain infarction observed by 1H and 31P MR spectroscopic imaging. J Cereb Blood Flow Metab 1992; 12:734–744.
159. Duijn JH, Matson GB, Maudsley AA, Hugg JW, Weimer MW. Human brain infarction: proton MR spectroscopy. Radiology 1992; 183:711–718.
160. Duyn JH, Gillen J, Sobering G, van Zijl PCM, Moonen CTW. Multisection proton MR spectroscopic image of the brain. Radiology 1993; 188:277–282.
161. Duyn JH, Moonen CTW. Fast proton spectroscopic imaging of the human brain using multiple spin-echoes. Magn Reson Med 1994; 30:409–414.
162. Posse S, Tedeschi G, Risinger R, Ogg R, Le Bihan D. High speed 1H spectroscopic imaging in human brain by echo planar spatial-spectral encoding. Magn Reson Med 1995; 33:34–40.
163. Posse S, Dager SR, Richards TL, et al. In vivo measurement of regional brain metabolic response to hyperventilation using magnetic resonance: proton echo planar spectroscopic imaging (PEPSI). Magn Reson Med 1997; 37:858–865.
164. Thulborn KR, Waterton JC, Matthews PM, Radda GK. Oxygenation dependence of the transverse relaxation time of water protons in whole blood at high field. Biochim Biophys Acta 1982; 714: 265–270.
165. Ogawa S, Lee TM, Kay AR, Tank DW. Brain magnetic resonance imaging with contrast dependent on blood oxygenation. Proc Natl Acad Sci USA 1990; 87:9868–9872.
166. Detre JA, Leigh JS, Williams DS, Koretsky AP. Perfusion imaging. Magn Reson Med 1992; 23:37–45.
167. Kwong KK, Belliveau JW, Chesler DA, et al. Dynamic magnetic resonance imaging of human brain activity during primary sensory stimulation. Proc Natl Acad Sci USA 1992; 89:5675–5679.
168. Ogawa S, Lee TM, Barrere B. The sensitivity of magnetic resonance image signals of a rat brain to changes in the cerebral venous blood oxygenation. Magn Reson Med 1993; 29:205–210.
169. Kim SG. Quantification of relative cerebral blood flow change by flow-sensitive alternating inversion recovery (FAIR) technique: application to functional mapping. Magn Reson Med 1995; 34: 293–301.
170. Schwarzbauer C, Morrissey SP, Haase A. Quantitative magnetic resonance imaging of perfusion using magnetic labeling of water proton spins within the detection slice. Magn Reson Med 1996; 35: 540–546.
171. Ye FQ, Pekar JJ, Jezzard P, Duyn J, Frank JA, McLaughlin AC. Perfusion imaging of the human brain at 1.5T using a single-shot EPI tagging approach. Magn Reson Med 1996; 36:217–224.
172. van Zijl PCM, Eleff SM, Ulatowski JA, et al. Quantitative assessment of blood flow, blood volume and blood oxygenation effects in functional magnetic resonance imaging. Nat Med 1998; 4:159–167.
173. Gröhn OHJ, Lukkarinen JA, Oja JME, et al. Noninvasive detection of cerebral hypoperfusion and reversible ischemia from reductions in the magnetic resonance imaging relaxation time T2. J Cereb Blood Flow Metab 1998; 18:911–920.
174. de Crespigny AJ, Wendland MF, Deruguin N, Koziewska E, Moseley ME. Real time observation of transient focal ischemia and hyperemia in cat brain. Magn Reson Med 1992; 27:391–397.
175. van der Toorn A, Verheul HB, van der Sprenkel JW, Tulleken CA, Nicolay K. Changes in metabolites and tissue water status after focal ischemia in cat brain assessed with localized proton MR spectroscopy. Magn Reson Med 1994; 32:685–691.
176. Roussel SA, van Bruggen N, King MD, Gadian DG. Identification of collaterally perfused areas following focal cerebral ischemia in the rat by comparison of gradient echo and diffusion-weighted MRI. J Cereb Blood Flow Metab 1995; 15:578–586.
177. Boada FE, Shen GX, Chang SY, Thulborn KR. Spectrally weighted twisted projection imaging: reducing T2 signal attenuation effects in fast three-dimensional sodium imaging. Magn Reson Med 1997; 38:1022–1028.

Jeffrey L. Sunshine, MD, PhD
Robert W. Tarr, MD
Charles F. Lanzieri, MD
Dennis M. D. Landis, MD
Warren R. Selman, MD
Jonathan S. Lewin, MD

Index terms:
Brain, infarction, 13.781, 13.782
Brain, MR, 13.121411, 13.121412, 13.121413, 13.121416, 13.12143, 13.12144
Magnetic resonance (MR), comparative studies, 13.121411, 13.121412, 13.121413, 13.121416, 13.12143, 13.12144
Magnetic resonance (MR), diffusion study, 13.12144
Magnetic resonance (MR), perfusion study, 13.12144

Radiology 1999; 212:325–332

Abbreviations:
FLAIR = fluid-attenuated inversion-recovery
GRASE = gradient- and spin-echo
TR = repetition time

[1] From the Departments of Radiology (J.L.S., R.W.T., C.F.L., J.S.L.), Neurology (D.M.D.L.), and Neurosurgery (W.R.S.), University Hospitals of Cleveland and Case Western Reserve University, Lakeside Basement, 11000 Euclid Ave, Cleveland, OH 44106. Received August 14, 1998; revision requested October 15; revision received November 12; accepted January 25, 1999. **Address reprint requests to** J.L.S.

Author contributions:
Guarantor of integrity of entire study, J.L.S.; study concepts, J.L.S.; study design, J.L.S., R.W.T., J.S.L.; definition of intellectual content, J.L.S., R.W.T.; literature research, J.L.S.; clinical studies, all authors; data acquisition, J.L.S., D.M.D.L.; data and statistical analyses, J.L.S.; manuscript preparation, J.L.S.; manuscript editing, J.L.S., R.W.T., J.S.L.; manuscript review, J.L.S., R.W.T., C.F.L., J.S.L.

Hyperacute Stroke: Ultrafast MR Imaging to Triage Patients prior to Therapy[1]

PURPOSE: To test diffusion- and perfusion-weighted MR imaging techniques within the extreme time constraints of stroke evaluation before therapy, and then, with MR imaging, stratify patients into those without ischemia, those with noncortical ischemia, and those with cortical ischemia.

MATERIALS AND METHODS: T2-weighted turbo gradient- and spin-echo images and echo-planar diffusion- and perfusion-weighted images were obtained. Trace diffusion-weighted images and time-to-peak perfusion maps were automatically postprocessed and immediately available for interpretation.

RESULTS: Forty-one patients with acute stroke symptoms underwent imaging within 6 hours of symptom onset; 35 were eligible for the therapy protocol. The mean time from entering the emergency department to beginning MR imaging was 45 minutes; the mean total MR imaging time was less than 15 minutes. Immediate image analysis directly affected individual clinical management. Four patients showed evidence of no infarct; seven, of lacunar infarct; and 24, of acute cortical infarct. Sixteen patients underwent angiography, thirteen had large-vessel occlusion, eleven were treated intraarterially, and in seven, recanalization was achieved.

CONCLUSION: Echo-planar diffusion- and perfusion-weighted MR imaging for acute stroke is feasible and applicable before therapy decisions. Ultrafast MR imaging permitted immediate triage of 35 patients with symptoms of hyperacute stroke and thus helped avoid the risks from angiography and thrombolytic agents in some or spurred the judicious use of more aggressive intervention in others.

Magnetic resonance (MR) imaging can be used objectively to identify patients who have cerebral ischemia among those who meet the initial clinical diagnostic criteria for stroke. This specifically requires the use of diffusion- and perfusion-weighted MR imaging, because conventional MR sequences, even with contrast material, are limited by their relative insensitivity during the initial hours following the onset of deficit (1). The application of diffusion-weighted MR imaging to acute stroke therapy in humans is the logical extension from the previous efforts of others. Diffusion-weighted images were initially used to demonstrate the earliest changes of cerebral infarct in animal models (2–5). When used in humans, the sensitivity of diffusion weighting relative to that of the previous reference standard, T2 weighting, was confirmed (6,7). Most recently, the usefulness of diffusion weighting in staging human subcortical infarcts has been shown (8).

The addition of perfusion data in the evaluation of stroke was suggested even as the efficacy of diffusion-weighted imaging of stroke in humans was becoming apparent (9–12). Several groups (7,13,14) then showed the ability of ultrafast echo-planar diffusion- and perfusion-weighted MR imaging to demonstrate cerebral infarct and ischemia during the early hours after onset of stroke symptoms. The potential to illuminate an ischemic penumbra, or region of ischemic tissue at risk of infarct, by using relative subtraction of diffusion disruptions from perfusion deficits has been hypothesized previously (13,15).

First, we sought to test the feasibility of using diffusion- and perfusion-weighted MR imaging techniques within the extreme time constraints of stroke evaluation prior to the initiation of therapeutic intervention. We strongly believed that because every moment of delay carried the potential for greater brain tissue death, the total time devoted to MR imaging—including the time for transporting the patient to and from imaging, transferring the patient on and off the imager, imager setup, and data acquisition—must never exceed 20 minutes and preferably should conclude in 15 minutes. We believed equally strongly that if the information was to have any use in acute management decisions, then all postprocessing algorithms had to be online and capable of delivering output to the console within that same allotted time.

Then, we sought to assess the potential added diagnostic value these tests offered to patients in the setting of emergent stroke once we had achieved the technical and logistic goals. We hoped to prospectively stratify patients into the following three groups: those without MR imaging–confirmed cerebral ischemia in whom no additional risks were justified, those with evidence of ischemia exclusive to the cortical gray matter in whom we believed that risks of intravenous recombinant tissue-type plasminogen activator only were reasonable, and those with cortical ischemia for whom the greatest potential benefit existed and thus catheter angiography and potential intraarterial thrombolytic therapy were justified.

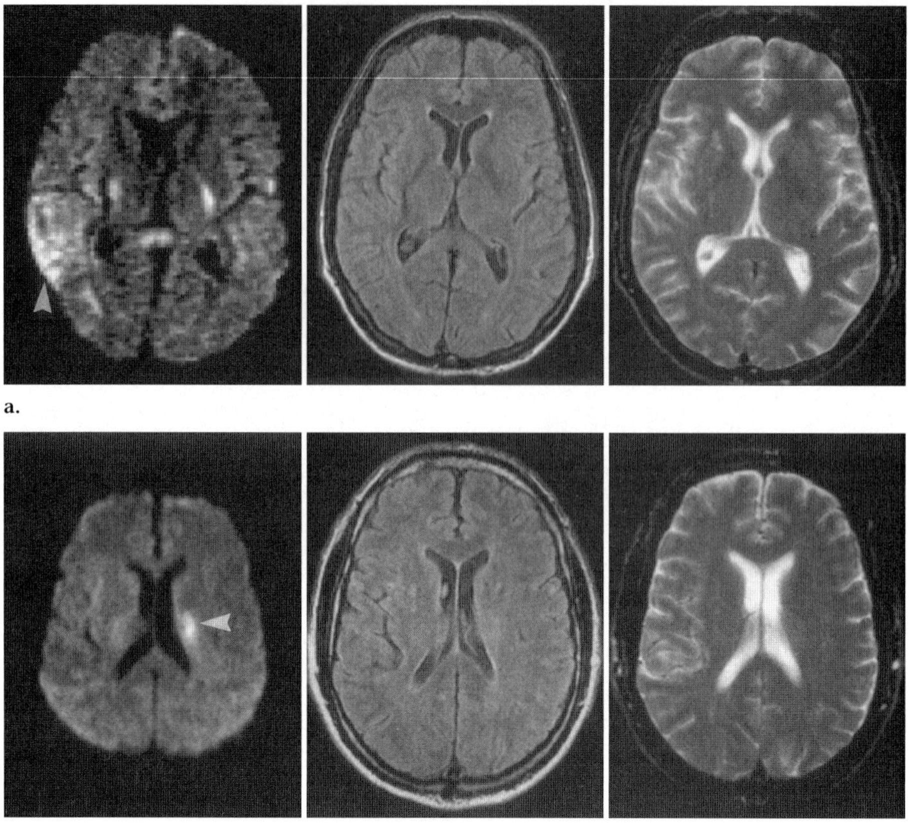

a. b.

Figure 1. **(a)** Temporal sensitivity. Axial diffusion-weighted image (b = 1,000 sec/mm^2) (left) obtained 45 minutes after the onset of symptoms shows a right temporal cortical infarct (arrowhead). **(b)** Spatial sensitivity. Axial diffusion-weighted image (b = 1,000 sec/mm^2) (left) obtained in a different patient 5 hours and 50 minutes after the onset of symptoms shows a left corona radiata lacunar infarct (arrowhead). Note the absence of detectable signal intensity changes on the FLAIR (9,000/110/2,500) (**a** and **b**, middle) and T2-weighted GRASE (4,480/108) (**a** and **b**, right) images obtained at the same position and within the same time period as the diffusion-weighted images (**a** and **b**, left).

MATERIALS AND METHODS

Patients with acute neurologic changes suspicious for stroke were entered into our stroke therapy protocol group; appropriate patient informed consent and institutional review board approval were obtained. Head CT scans were obtained if they were not available. Patients then either underwent MR imaging on an emergent basis before therapy or underwent MR imaging on an urgent basis following the onset of or attempt at therapy. A clinical 1.5-T whole-body imager with a 24-mT/m gradient strength, 300-msec rise time, and echo-planar–capable receiver (Magnetom Vision; Siemens Medical Systems, Erlangen, Germany) was used. The images obtained included sagittal Tl-weighted scout (repetition time [TR] msec/echo time msec, 15/6; matrix, 128 × 256; section thickness, 8 mm; field of view, 300 mm; one signal acquired), axial T2-weighted turbo gradient- and spin-echo (GRASE) (4,480/108, 132 × 256 matrix, 5-mm section thickness, 230-mm field of view, one signal acquired), and axial echo-planar diffusion- and perfusion-weighted images. Standard axial T1-weighted and turbo fluid-attenuated inversion-recovery (FLAIR) (9,000/110/2,500 [TR/echo time/inversion time], 198 × 256 matrix, 5-mm section thickness, one signal acquired) images were obtained when possible.

The diffusion-weighted images were obtained with a single-shot, gradient-echo, echo-planar pulse sequence with diffusion gradient b values of 0 and 1,000 sec/mm^2 along all three orthogonal axes over 18 axial sections (TR, 6,000 msec; 18 7-mm-thick sections with no intersection gap; matrix, 96 × 128; field of view, 240 mm with one acquisition). Perfusion-weighted images were obtained during the first pass of a 0.1 mmol/kg bolus of gadolinium-based contrast material (Omniscan; Nycomed, Oslo, Norway or Magnevist; Berlex Laboratories, Wayne, NJ) by using a gradient-echo, echo-planar sequence set for a selected 12 of the 18 section positions measured 30 times sequentially, for a total imaging time of 49 seconds to ensure imaging during the entire duration of the first passage of contrast material. The following imaging parameters were used: per-section image acquisition rate, approximately seven axial images per second; TR, 1,680 msec; 4-mm-thick sections with a 0.5 intersection gap; matrix, 64 × 128; field of view, 300 mm with one acquisition.

The total image acquisition and reconstruction processing time with the described sequences was approximately 6 minutes. This permitted a total imaging time, including patient transfer to and from the table, patient positioning, and coil tuning, of 15–20 minutes. Diffusion-weighted image data were automatically postprocessed to yield trace images at each section position from the primary data. The perfusion-weighted sequence generated a time-to-peak map for each section position. These maps were immediately available for interpretation at the console with all the other images. All

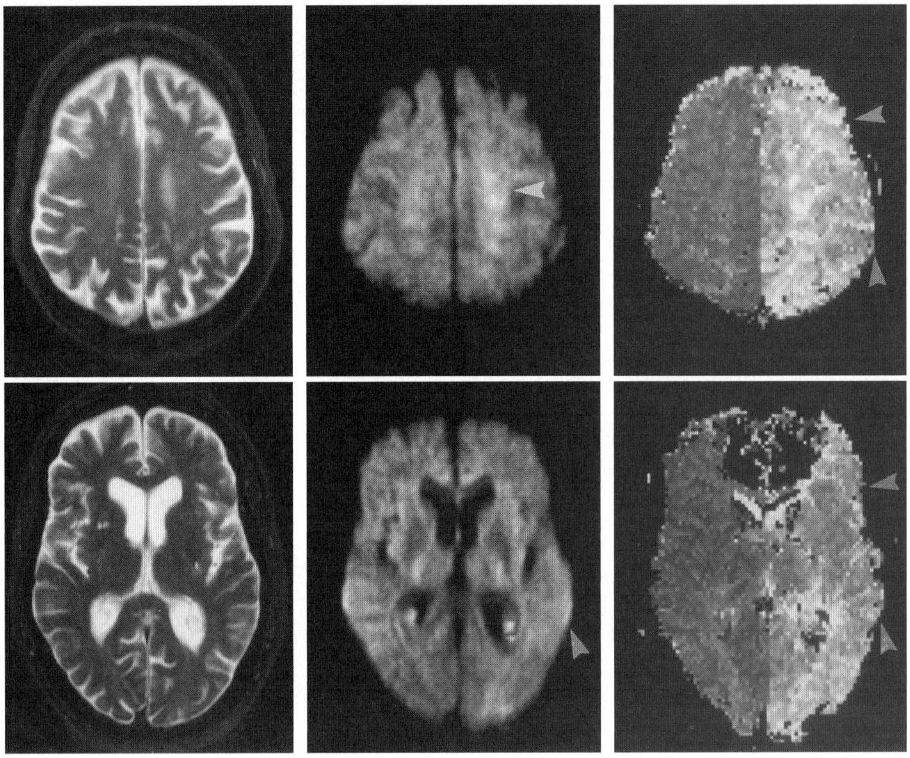

a. b. c.

Figure 2. Representative **(a)** T2-weighted turbo GRASE images (4,480/108), **(b)** diffusion-weighted images (b = 1,000 sec/mm^2), and **(c)** time-to-peak perfusion maps obtained in the same position 55 minutes after the onset of an extensive right hemiparesis, hemiplegia, aphasia, and unresponsiveness. Note the lack of apparent signal intensity abnormality on the GRASE images, the subtle early changes (arrowheads in **b**) on the diffusion-weighted images, and the unmistakable holohemispheric perfusion deficit (arrowheads in **c**) on the time-to-peak maps.

image interpretations were performed by a single attending-level board-certified radiologist (J.L.S., C.F.L., R.W.T., or J.S.L.) who has added qualifications in neuroradiology and training in reading diffusion- and perfusion-weighted MR images. The areas of hyperintensity were noted on the diffusion-weighted trace images, and areas of decreased (hyperintense) or increased (hypointense) perfusion were noted on the time-to-peak maps. The times of symptom onset, arrival in the emergency department, CT, MR, and angiography were tabulated for each patient.

The data collected included the site and distribution of ischemic changes on diffusion-weighted images, presence of concordant or discordant perfusion abnormality, and changes on T2-weighted images. These data were then used to decide for or against anticoagulation therapy, guide catheter placement toward the involved distribution, or decide whether to proceed with intraarterial thrombolysis. The images obtained in the patients in the stroke protocol group were immediately evaluated at the console and used to place these patients in one of the following three categories: no MR imaging evidence of infarct, evidence of infarct limited to the perforating arterial distributions only, or evidence of acute infarct involving cortical or brain stem tissue.

Thrombolytic therapy was administered to patients after MR imaging within the following guidelines. Intravenous recombinant tissue-type plasminogen activator was administered only within the first 3 hours following symptom onset. This therapy was used with a full dose of 0.9 mg/kg gadolinium-based contrast material in those patients with small-vessel (perforating arteries) disease. Patients with evidence of large-vessel (first- through fourth-order arteries) occlusion were given an initial dose of 0.6 mg/kg. These patients then underwent angiography for potential additional intraarterial lysis. Patients who presented with symptoms after 3 hours but before 6 hours were limited to intraarterial therapy. Urokinase, in aliquots of 125,000–250,000 U, was used in all intraarterial treatments, with an expected maximum of 1,000,000 U.

RESULTS

Forty-one patients with acute symptoms consistent with cerebral infarct underwent MR imaging, by means of some or all of the described sequences, within 6 hours of symptom onset. These patients can be subdivided further. Extremely early MR imaging was performed in four patients within 1 hour of symptom onset. Very early MR imaging was performed in nine patients in the 1–3-hour window following symptom onset. Early MR imaging, which was still within our therapeutic window, was performed in 28 additional patients during the 3–6-hour window after symptom onset. In sum and at the time this article was written, these methods had enabled the successful acquisition of high-speed MR images within the currently accepted therapeutic window in a total of 41 patients, 35 of whom were entered into our active stroke therapy protocol group.

Diffusion-weighted imaging was far more temporally and spatially sensitive for the earliest changes in cerebral ischemia in the acute setting relative to conventional T2-weighted or FLAIR imaging. Diffusion-weighted imaging alone demonstrated 26 cortical infarcts in 24 patients (Fig 1a). In 10 patients, the images showed ischemia in 13 deep gray matter structures. Abnormally increased signal intensity appeared in the deep white matter regions consistent with acute small-vessel ischemia in six patients (Fig 1b). Six patients had no visible abnormalities. Signal intensity changes in the same regions were apparent prospectively on T2-weighted images (or turbo FLAIR images when acquired) in two patients (Fig 1).

Perfusion maps were obtained following the administration of gadolinium-based contrast material in 32 patients. Twenty-two patients demonstrated an increased time-to-peak effect on postprocessed maps consistent with relative hypoperfusion (Fig 2). Eight patients showed no evident abnormality in perfusion, even in the regions of abnormal diffusion signal intensity. The remaining two patients had a decreased time-to-peak effect in the regions corresponding to the relative hyperperfusion; this was probably a direct or "luxury" response to the immediately preceding ischemic insult. In four of the patients who did not undergo perfusion imaging, this procedure was attempted, but other factors precluded accurate acquisition. The problems encountered included technical difficulties, such as injection tube leak and venous extravasation, and physiologic issues—for example, unsuspected slow cardiac output from cardiomyopathy, which caused a delayed and diluted contrast material bolus, and involuntary parkinsonian tremors.

Six of the 41 patients were not included in our therapy protocol for a variety of reasons. One patient clinically seemed to have a postoperative seizure with a Todd paralysis. Three patients had deficits that clinically resolved, which is consistent with transient ischemic attacks. These four patients were clinically excluded from therapy, and the results of their MR examinations confirmed the absence of ischemic changes. The two remaining patients were examined very early in our experience. One patient demonstrated a clinically suspected acute lacunar infarct, but this was prior to our protocol's inclusion of intravenous recombinant tissue-type plasminogen activator for treatment of that disease. The last patient actually underwent angiography but did so prior to the MR examination, and thus prospective information was not available and the therapeutic decision was made prior to MR imaging.

For the 35 patients entered into our stroke protocol group for potential therapy, imaging represented a potential delay in therapy, so we tracked our time efficiency. For patients transferred from the emergency department as candidates for potential intraarterial thrombolysis, we summed the time spent for taking the clinical history, performing the physical examination, taking vital signs, performing blood work, performing electrocardiography, and performing nonenhanced head CT prior to MR imaging. The average time expended, from entering the emergency department to beginning MR imaging, was 45 minutes (range, 15–75 minutes).

Furthermore, we logged the total time in the MR suite, from leaving the emergency department to returning from MR imaging. In all but three patients, the total MR imaging time was less than 15 minutes. These three patients had extreme morbidity and were delayed because of ventilation constraints prior to adequate training of all respiration therapists in the use of MR-compatible units. Thus, those patients who required angiography arrived in the interventional angiography suite 1 hour or sooner after arriving in the emergency department, with all evaluations, including CT and MR imaging, completed. In sum, we were able to perform imaging in 35 patients during their acute assessment period and prior to the final therapeutic decision, with only a limited time delay.

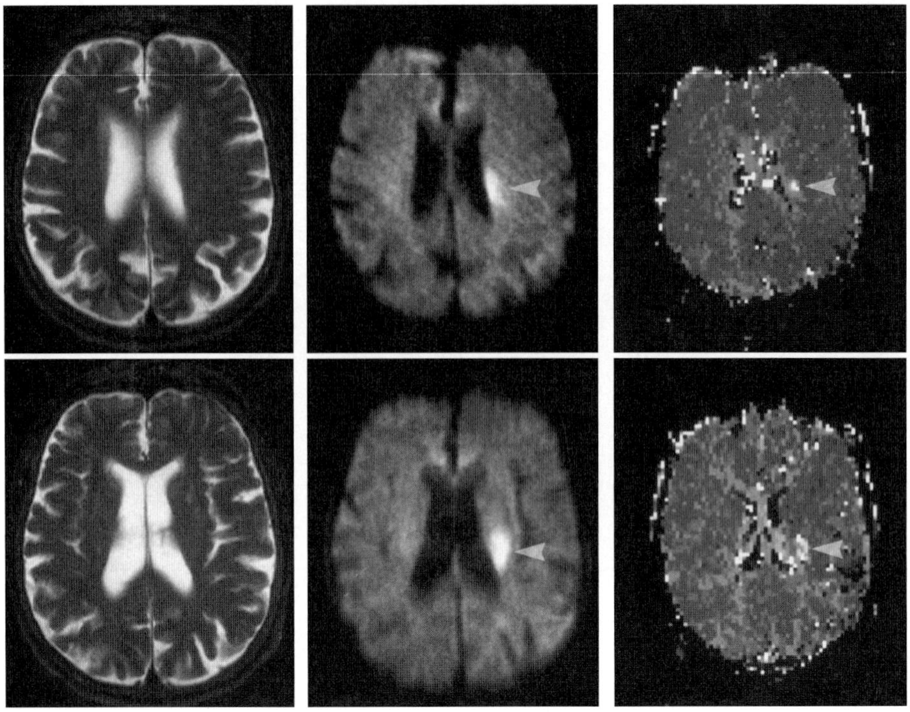

a. b. c.

Figure 3. **(a)** T2-weighted GRASE images (4,480/108), **(b)** diffusion-weighted images (b = 1,000 sec/mm^2), and **(c)** perfusion time-to-peak maps obtained at the same level 4 hours and 45 minutes after the onset of right hemiparesis. Given the patient's presentation, angiography would have been required to exclude large-vessel or branch occlusion. On **(a)** the T2-weighted GRASE images, no corona radiata lacunar infarct is seen, but on **(b)** the diffusion-weighted images (b = 1,000 sec/mm^2), a left corona radiata lacunar infarct (arrowheads) is apparent. **(c)** The perfusion time-to-peak maps show a matched volume of abnormal perfusion (arrowheads) that confirms the small infarct but suggests no further tissue at risk, or penumbra. Therefore, this patient did not undergo angiography, but rather was treated with a neuroprotective agent.

In the 35 stroke patients, we were able to compare perfusion deficits to regions with abnormal diffusion to produce an estimate of brain tissue at risk, or penumbra. Immediate imaging analysis directly affected individual clinical management; we were able to triage critical patients into groups directed toward and away from aggressive therapy with its inherent risks (Table). Four patients were triaged into group 1, in which no infarct was evident following image interpretation, and our therapy protocol was effectively terminated despite suggestive symptoms. As an example, one of these four patients subsequently demonstrated seizure activity, which confirmed the presence of a Todd paralysis that had mimicked an acute stroke, and further risk associated with therapy was avoided. Seven patients were triaged into group 2, in which imaging demonstrated the presence of acute lacunar infarcts in deep gray or white matter structures (Fig 3). For these individuals, treatment was limited to intravenous therapy for two patients, who presented with symptoms within the initial 3-hour window, or to conservative options for five patients, who presented at later time periods.

All of the remaining patients (n = 24) were triaged into group 3, because their images showed evidence of acute cortical infarct; these individuals were therefore considered candidates for our most aggressive therapy. However, eight of these patients were treated conservatively for the following reasons: Two had minimal clinical deficits (National Institutes of Health stroke scale <5), four had contraindications to treatment (end-stage cancer, iodine allergy, marked hemispheric edema at CT, late arrival with high morbidity), and two had hyperperfusion at MR imaging that was consistent with resolving ischemia. The final 16 patients underwent angiography after the MR imaging findings confirmed the clinical assessment of acute cortical ischemia or challenged it with findings in excess of the initial clinically suspicious symptoms (Fig 4). Thirteen (81%) of these patients had

Triage of Stroke Patients

Patient No.	Time from Symptom Onset to Arrival in ED	Time from Symptom Onset to MR Imaging (h)	Anatomic Region with Abnormality at MR	Perfusion	Treatment*	Comments
No infarcts (group 1)						
1	NA	1–3	Negative	Normal	None	None
2	4 h 15 min	3–6	Negative	Normal	None	None
3	NA	3–6	Negative	Normal	None	None
4	NA	3–6	Negative	NA	None	None
Lacunar infarcts (group 2)						
5	40 min	1–3	Right putamen, left posterior limb internal capsule	NA	Conservative	None
6	2 h 10 min	3–6	Right thalamus	NA	Conservative	None
7	1 h 10 min	3–6	Right corona radiata	Normal	Conservative	None
8	1 h 45 min	3–6	Right cerebellum	Normal	IV thrombolysis	None
9	3 h 30 min	3–6	Left corona radiata	Decreased	Conservative	None
10	5 h	3–6	Left corona radiata	Normal	Conservative	None
11	45 min	1–3	Left posterior limb internal capsule	Normal	IV thrombolysis	None
Cortical infarcts (group 3)†						
12	5 h	3–6	Right MCA	Decreased	Conservative	None
13	3 h 25 min	3–6	Right basal ganglia, MCA	Decreased	IA thrombolysis and lysis	None
14	2 h 40 min	3–6	Left MCA	Decreased	Conservative	None
15	20 min	0–1	Right MCA, posterior division	Decreased	IV and IA thrombolysis	None
16	3 h 5 min	3–6	Left thalamus	Decreased	Conservative	None
17	1 h 45 min	1–3	Right thalamus, cerebellum, PCA	Decreased	Conservative	None
18	15 min	3–6	Left MCA	NA	IA thrombolysis	None
19	3 h 45 min	3–6	Right MCA	NA	IA thrombolysis and lysis	None
20	1 h 30 min	1–3	Right thalamus, right PCA	Decreased	Conservative	None
21	3 h 30 min	3–6	Left MCA	NA	IA thrombolysis and lysis	None
22	0 h 0 min	1–3	Right MCA	NA	IA thrombolysis and lysis	None
23	3 h 25 min	3–6	Left MCA	Decreased	IA thrombolysis and lysis	None
24	2 h 25 min	3–6	Right cerebellum, brain stem	Decreased	IA thrombolysis and lysis	None
25	50 min	1–3	Right MCA	Decreased	IA thrombolysis	None
26	10 min	0–1	Left inferior cerebral artery	Decreased	IA thrombolysis	None
27	3 h 30 min	3–6	Left MCA	Decreased	IA thrombolysis and lysis	None
28	4 h 40 min	3–6	Left MCA	Increased	Conservative	Hyperperfusion
29	2 h 35 min	1–3	Left MCA	Increased	Conservative	Hyperperfusion
30	1 h	3–6	Left MCA	Decreased	Conservative	High morbidity
31	NA	3–6	Right MCA	Decreased	Conservative	Marked edema
32	4 h	3–6	Right MCA	Decreased	Conservative	Iodine allergy
33	10 min	1–3	Right MCA	Decreased	Conservative	End-stage cancer
34	6 h 30 min	3–6	Left thalamus, left PCA	Decreased	Conservative	Minimal deficit
35	3 h	3–6	Left basal ganglia, left MCA	Decreased	Conservative	Minimal deficit

Note.—ED = emergency department, IA = intraarterial, IV = intravenous, MCA = middle cerebral artery, NA = not available, PCA = posterior cerebral artery.

* Lysis refers to full or at least partial recanalization of the lumen with active flow.

† Patients 12 through 27 underwent angiography. Patients 28 through 35 did not undergo angiography and received conservative treatment.

objective evidence of large-vessel (internal carotid artery, middle cerebral artery [M1 or M2], posterior cerebral artery, or basilar artery) occlusion at angiography. We treated 11 (69%) of the 16 patients in whom angiograms were obtained with intraarterial thrombolytic therapy, which ultimately achieved recanalization in seven of these patients. The remaining five patients received conservative treatment.

DISCUSSION

We have demonstrated that echo-planar diffusion- and perfusion-weighted MR imaging in the setting of acute stroke is feasible and applicable to an active therapy protocol. At our institution, this imaging has been performed before making final triage decisions and most often before beginning definitive therapy. In the present study, MR imaging was performed, on average, within 45 minutes after the patient's arrival in the emergency department, with less than 15 minutes of total time diverted from the care path and a total image acquisition and processing time of less than 6 minutes. This imaging revealed cortical and deep gray matter ischemia, as well as hypoperfusion, in a time-efficient manner before more conventional sequences were performed; these findings confirmed the results in previous reports (13,14,16).

To our knowledge, for the first time, the early availability of this information permitted the immediate triage of 35 patients with hyperacute symptoms and thus influenced the decisions of whether to treat, whether to administer only intravenous thrombolytic agents, and whether to advance to angiography and attempt intraarterial thrombolysis. Therefore, diffusion- and perfusion-weighted MR imaging can be performed within the time constraints of an acute stroke protocol and provide valuable data to guide criti-

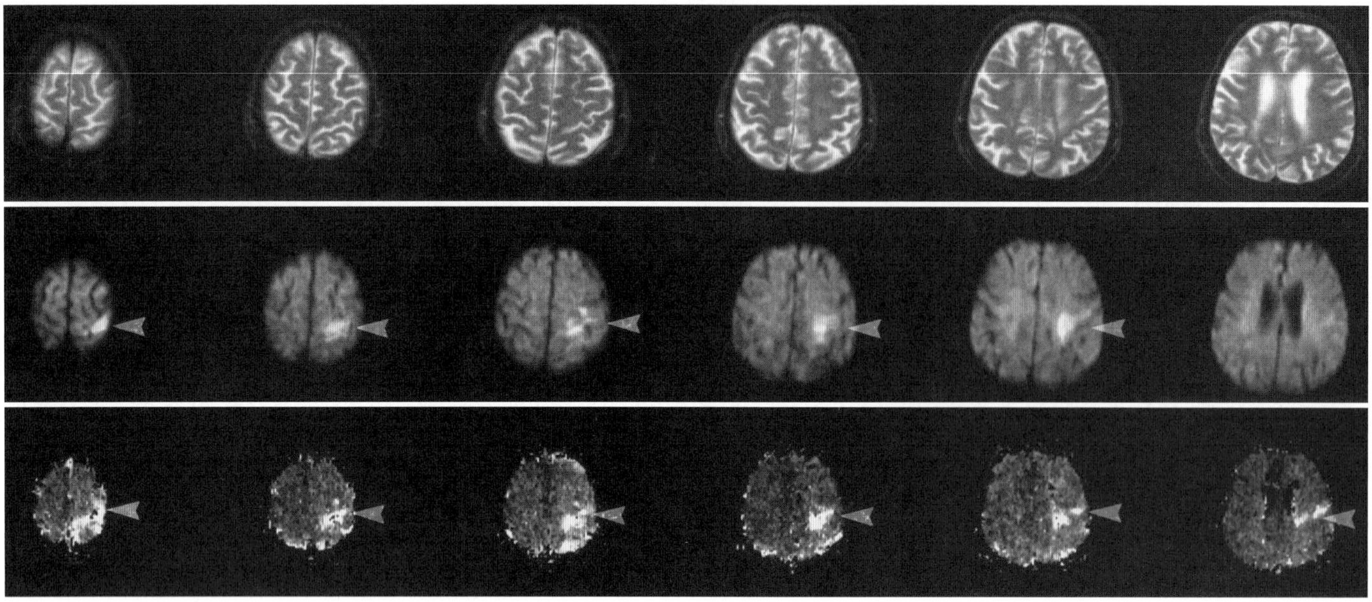

a.

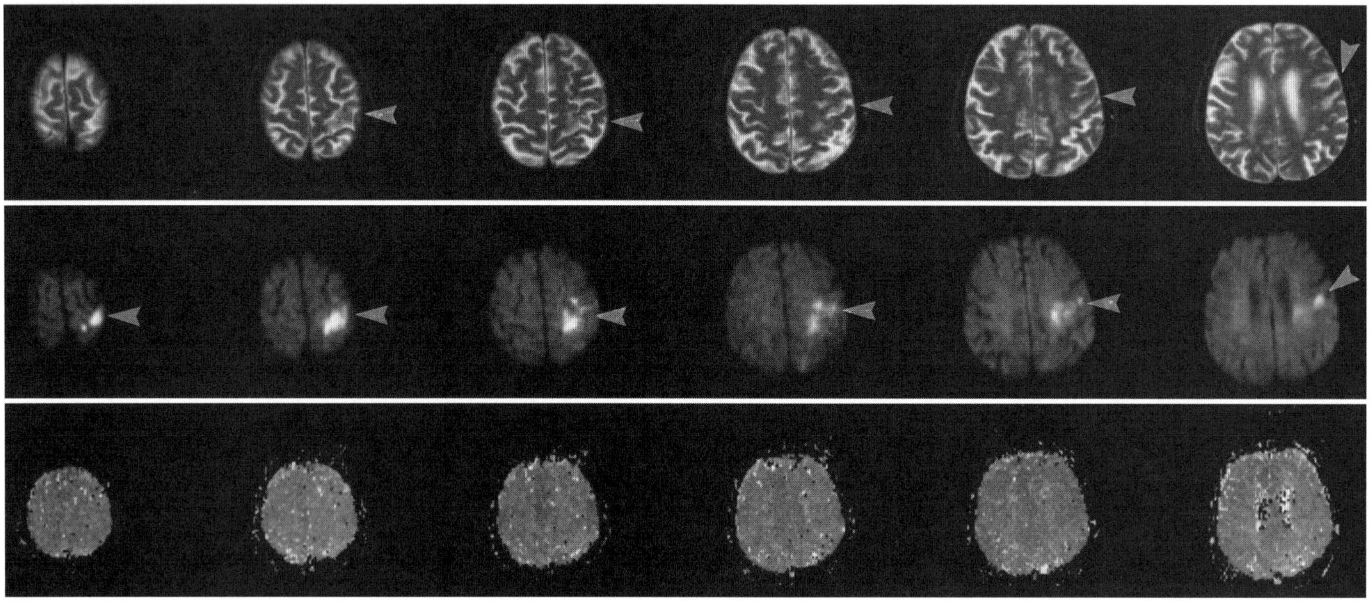

b.

Figure 4. **(a)** T2-weighted GRASE images (4,480/108) (top row), diffusion-weighted images (b = 1,000 sec/mm^2) (middle row), and time-to-peak perfusion maps (bottom row) obtained in a patient with dysphagia and right arm paresis that began 3 hours and 55 minutes before MR imaging. Results of clinical assessment concluded that these symptoms reflected an acute left hemispheric white matter lacunar infarct. These images demonstrate the unexpected finding of a cortical infarct (arrowheads, middle row) on the diffusion-weighted images, with an even greater volume of cortex with diminished perfusion (arrowheads, bottom row) seen on the time-to-peak maps. These findings suggested a penumbra that might be salvaged according to our working hypotheses. The patient underwent angiography, in which 500,000 U of urokinase was infused intraarterially into the occluded posterior parietal branches of the left middle cerebral artery, with the result of improved blood flow. **(b)** T2-weighted GRASE images (4,480/108) (top row), diffusion-weighted images (b = 1,000 sec/mm^2) (middle row), and time-to-peak perfusion maps (bottom row) obtained in the same patient 1 day after thrombolysis. The diffusion-weighted images (middle row) still show abnormal signal intensity (arrowheads), but there has been a clear resolution of the perfusion deficit, and there are only minimal areas of signal intensity change (arrowheads, top row) on the T2-weighted GRASE images.

cal patient triage and therapeutic decisions.

This study advances previous efforts along several lines. Foremost, we performed imaging in the majority of our patients prospectively, during the interval of the therapeutic decision rather than following it. This allowed the MR images to be of additional diagnostic value to the acutely ill patient, and in some cases, it enabled us to avoid risky interventions when they were not necessary. Furthermore, compared with previous work (14), multisection analysis of each patient's brain, in both the diffusion- and perfusion-weighted modes, was used in this study, which minimized sampling errors. It is worth noting that we administered intraarterial thrombolytic agents to 11 (69%) of the patients who underwent angiography in the population reported herein. In comparison, the findings in a previous series of acute stroke angiograms, which were obtained without MR imaging being performed beforehand, resulted in the administration of intraarterial thrombolytic agents to 51 (38%) of the 136 patients who underwent angiography. Our use of MR imaging to triage patients resulted in a much higher rate of true-positive angiograms and thus helped us to clearly exclude a number of patients in whom risky invasive treatment was not necessary.

Diffusion-weighted images can be obtained and viewed variably. We used a set of parameters designed to maximize lesion conspicuity and minimize both acquisition and processing times. For these reasons, we obtained images in only three orthogonal planes, and from these, trace images were generated. Although the use of apparent diffusion coefficient maps in the evaluation of acute stroke has been reported (13,16), these cannot yet be generated on our system in a manner that is applicable to our time constraints.

The reader should note that perfusion data obtained during the first passage of the contrast material bolus can be evaluated by examining multiple variables other than the time-to-peak effect, as was used here. Currently at our institution, a time-efficient processing algorithm for perfusion-weighted MR imaging is available for the time-to-peak option only. Measurements of mean transit time, as well as relative cerebral blood volumes or flow, are possible (12,13,17). However, in our experience, these have not proved to be as sensitive or conspicuous in the acute setting. For some, the transfer of data offline for processing, which is not practical for hyperacute triage, has been required to obtain these measurements. For others, these measurements have involved longer reconstruction times—for example, 10 minutes for one group (13), which alone exceeds our total acquisition and processing time. However, in at least one center (18), relative cerebral blood flow and mean transit time maps are generated from multiple sets of 11 sections in less than 4 minutes. Although this is not truly time prohibitive, it is approximately twice the time required to process our image data. We continue to obtain high-speed turbo GRASE images because of their sensitivity to blood susceptibility effects and because of the requirement to exclude the "shine through" of T2-weighted signal intensity that occurs on diffusion-weighted images (19).

We have encountered patients with no or minimal abnormal signal intensity on diffusion-weighted images who ultimately had very large infarcts that involved whole cerebral vessel distributions. These patients had marked perfusion abnormalities at these distributions. Thus, in our series, diffusion-weighted imaging alone was, on occasion, insufficiently sensitive to allow exclusion of substantial risk of infarct (Fig 2). This finding confirms those in other reports (13,20) yet demonstrates further the potential to miss large volumes of tissue that may ultimately become infarcted if only diffusion-weighted images are relied on.

Our study results confirm the finding in previous reports (16,20) that most unremarkable diffusion-weighted images help delineate patients who present with stroke symptoms but do not have cerebral ischemia and will recover without intervention, but only when these images are coupled with normal perfusion-weighted images. Furthermore, in several instances in our study, MR images alone demonstrated the presence of cortical tissue at risk of infarct when the clinical assessment suggested the presence of only small deep white matter at risk. Although these patients may be treated with intravenous thrombolytic therapy efficaciously within the first 3 hours after symptom onset (21), we currently will not use the invasive, aggressive, and ultimately successful measures described without MR imaging evidence of their necessity (Fig 4).

Although MR imaging offers clear advantages over the more widely available CT scanning (22,23), CT still can be used to characterize early stroke. The "dense middle cerebral artery sign" at CT continues to indicate a poor prognosis that possibly can be improved with aggressive therapy (24,25). CT, in combination with xenon gas inhalation, can be used for imaging and quantitative measurement of cerebral perfusion (26). Furthermore, in settings where MR images may not be obtainable, CT data may help predict outcome (27). Alternatively, because MR imaging can help identify hemorrhagic stroke on T2-weighted images (28), there may come a time when CT can be safely bypassed in the hyperacute evaluation of stroke.

Currently, MR perfusion and diffusion techniques demonstrate cerebral infarct and ischemia earliest and best. For example, FLAIR imaging techniques have shown improvement over conventional T1- and T2-weighted imaging in cerebral infarct evaluation (29), but the FLAIR sequence has not shown the early temporal sensitivity of diffusion- and perfusion-weighted sequences when performed in our patient populations. Furthermore, MR spectroscopy can help identify the abnormal accumulation of intracellular lactate and the associated drop in the pH level that occurs with ischemic damage to cellular sodium-potassium pumps (18). However, this technique's current lack of spatial resolution renders it much less useful in delineating the boundaries of parenchymal ischemia.

Our work could be strengthened in several ways in the future. First, a greater degree of follow-up imaging would better test the estimation of penumbra. In those patients who do not undergo successful therapeutic intervention, images obtained later would be expected to demonstrate an infarct size that approaches that of the perfusion deficit. Similarly, in those patients in whom arterial therapy produces successful recanalization, later images should show infarcts that are no larger than the region of diffusion abnormality. The addition of online, rapidly available apparent diffusion coefficient maps (13,30) potentially could allow better identification of ischemic cores because of the additional demarcation of threshold boundaries within the regions of abnormal diffusion. Absolute quantification may be possible (31).

Similarly, the quantification of perfusion and regions of deficit (32), and, thus, the acquisition of better images of the degrees of ischemic risk, may be possible in the future. In addition, if our treatment populations become larger, then a certain number of parenchymal hemorrhages will be encountered. Review of initial imaging findings from the subset of patients with parenchymal hemorrhage may allow the identification of imaging conditions that are suggestive of a higher risk of bleeding, and this could lead to improved pretreatment stratification of patients. The results of current animal studies (33) suggest that early gadolinium-based contrast material enhancement following reperfusion may represent an increased risk of hemorrhagic transformation. Similarly, because an underlying threat of increased tissue damage from reperfusion injury exists (34), we should encounter a group of patients whose condition worsens despite adequate therapy. Again, a review of their initial images may reveal predictive characteristics.

In conclusion, rapidly acquired and processed echo-planar diffusion- and perfusion-weighted MR imaging can be used successfully in patients with the most acute symptoms of stroke. The available image and image map data can then be incorporated into emergency triage protocols. This may exclude some patients from the risks of invasive testing and hemorrhage from thrombolytic agents or spur the judicious use of more aggressive interventions to improve the outcome of patients with the greatest burden of risk based on the natural history of their disease.

Acknowledgments: The authors thank the following dedicated magnetic resonance technologists: Ginger Haddad, Mark Clampitt, Roberta Koss, Vicki Tabor, Robin Fumich, Dera Ewing-Collins, Mark Brandt, Larry Lasky, Deann Caswell, Earl Brown, and Deana Tabor. They also thank secretaries Betty Little and Cynthia Bosse. The authors are also grateful to MR physicists Jeffrey Duerk, PhD, and Dee Wu, PhD for their dedication and tireless support.

References

1. Yuh WT, Crain MR, Loes DJ, Greene GM, Ryals TJ, Sato Y. MR imaging of cerebral ischemia: findings in the first 24 hours. AJNR 1991; 12:621–629.
2. Minematsu K, Li L, Fisher M, Sotak CH, Davis MA, Fiandaca MS. Diffusion-weighted magnetic resonance imaging: rapid and quantitative detection of focal brain ischemia. Neurology 1992; 42:235–240.
3. Mintorovitch J, Moseley ME, Chileuitt L, Shimizu H, Cohen Y, Weinstein PR. Comparison of diffusion- and T2-weighted MRI for the early detection of cerebral ischemia and reperfusion in rats. Magn Reson Med 1991; 18:39–50.
4. Moonen CT, Pekar J, de Vleeschouwer MH, van Gelderen P, van Zijl PC, DesPres D. Restricted and anisotropic displacement of water in healthy cat brain and in stroke studied by NMR diffusion imaging. Magn Reson Med 1991; 19:327–332.
5. Moseley ME, Kucharczyk J, Mintorovitch J, et al. Diffusion-weighted MR imaging of acute stroke: correlation with T2-weighted and magnetic susceptibility–enhanced MR imaging in cats. AJNR 1990; 11:423–429.
6. Chien D, Kwong KK, Gress DR, Buonanno FS, Buxton RB, Rosen BR. MR diffusion imaging of cerebral infarction in humans. AJNR 1992; 13:1097–1102.
7. Warach S, Chien D, Li W, Ronthal M, Edelman RR. Fast magnetic resonance diffusion-weighted imaging of acute human stroke. Neurology 1992; 42:1717–1723. [Erratum: Neurology 1992; 42:2192.]
8. Singer MB, Chong J, Lu D, Schonewille WJ, Tuhrim S, Atlas SW. Diffusion-weighted MRI in acute subcortical infarction. Stroke 1998; 29:133–136. [Erratum: Stroke 1998; 29:731.]
9. Edelman RR, Mattle HP, Atkinson DJ, et al. Cerebral blood flow: assessment with dynamic contrast-enhanced T2*-weighted MR imaging at 1.5 T. Radiology 1990; 176:211–220.
10. Fisher M, Sotak CH, Minematsu K, Li L. New magnetic resonance techniques for evaluating cerebrovascular disease. Ann Neurol 1992; 32:115–122.
11. Lee C, Dean BL, Kirsch JE, et al. Cerebral infarction: assessment of patterns using ultra-fast MR contrast imaging. AJNR 1992; 13:277–279.
12. Warach S, Li W, Ronthal M, Edelman RR. Acute cerebral ischemia: evaluation with dynamic contrast-enhanced MR imaging and MR angiography. Radiology 1992; 182:41–47.
13. Sorensen AG, Buonanno FS, Gonzalez RG, et al. Hyperacute stroke: evaluation with combined multisection diffusion-weighted and hemodynamically weighted echo-planar MR imaging. Radiology 1996; 199: 391–401.
14. Warach S, Dashe JF, Edelman RR. Clinical outcome in ischemic stroke predicted by early diffusion-weighted and perfusion magnetic resonance imaging: a preliminary analysis. J Cereb Blood Flow Metab 1996; 16:53–59.
15. Fisher M, Takano K. The penumbra: therapeutic time window and acute ischaemic stroke. Baillieres Clin Neurol 1995; 4:279–295.
16. Warach S, Gaa J, Siewert B, Wielopolski P, Edelman RR. Acute human stroke studied by whole-brain echo-planar diffusion-weighted magnetic resonance imaging. Ann Neurol 1995; 37:231–241.
17. Rother J, Guckel F, Neff W, Schwartz A, Hennerici M. Assessment of regional cerebral blood volume in acute human stroke by use of single-slice dynamic susceptibility contrast-enhanced magnetic resonance imaging. Stroke 1996; 27:1088–1093.
18. Maeda M, Maley JE, Crosby DL, et al. Application of contrast agents in the evaluation of stroke: conventional MR and echo-planar MR imaging. JMRI 1997; 7:23–28.
19. Warach S, Boska M, Welch KM. Pitfalls and potential of clinical diffusion-weighted MR imaging in acute stroke (editorial). Stroke 1997; 28:481–482.
20. Lovblad K, Laubach H, Baird A, et al. Clinical experience with diffusion-weighted MR in patients with acute stroke. AJNR 1998; 19:1061–1066.
21. The National Institute of Neurological Disorders and Stroke rt-PA Stroke Study Group. Tissue plasminogen activator for acute ischemic stroke. N Engl J Med 1995; 333:1581–1587.
22. Russell EJ. Diagnosis of hyperacute ischemic infarct with CT: key to improved clinical outcome after intravenous thrombolysis? (editorial). Radiology 1997; 205: 315–318.
23. von Kummer R, Allen KL, Holle R, et al. Acute stroke: usefulness of early CT findings before thrombolytic therapy. Radiology 1997; 205:327–333.
24. Tomsick T, Brott T, Barsan W, et al. Prognostic value of the hyperdense middle cerebral artery sign and stroke scale score before ultra-early thrombolytic therapy. AJNR 1996; 17:79–85.
25. Bendszus M, Urbach H, Ries F, Solymosi L. Outcome after local intra-arterial fibrinolysis compared with the natural course of patients with a dense middle cerebral artery on early CT. Neuroradiology 1998; 40:54–58.
26. Nambu K, Suzuki R, Hirakawa K. Cerebral blood flow: measurement with xenon-enhanced dynamic helical CT. Radiology 1995; 195:53–57.
27. Toni D, Fiorelli M, Bastianello S, et al. Acute ischemic strokes improving during the first 48 hours of onset: predictability, outcome, and possible mechanisms—a comparison with early deteriorating strokes. Stroke 1997; 28:10–14.
28. Ebisu T, Tanaka C, Umeda M, et al. Hemorrhagic and nonhemorrhagic stroke: diagnosis with diffusion-weighted and T2-weighted echo-planar MR imaging. Radiology 1997; 203:823–828.
29. Brant-Zawadzki M, Atkinson D, Detrick M, Bradley WG, Scidmore G. Fluid-attenuated inversion recovery (FLAIR) for assessment of cerebral infarction: initial clinical experience in 50 patients. Stroke 1996; 27:1187–1191.
30. Marks MP, de Crespigny A, Lentz D, Enzmann DR, Albers GW, Moseley ME. Acute and chronic stroke: navigated spin-echo diffusion-weighted MR imaging. Radiology 1996; 199:403-408. [Erratum: Radiology 1996; 200:289.]
31. Ulug AM, Beauchamp NJ, Bryan RN, van Zijl PC. Absolute quantitation of diffusion constants in human stroke. Stroke 1997; 28:483–490.
32. Rosen BR, Belliveau JW, Vevea JM, Brady TJ. Perfusion imaging with NMR contrast agents. Magn Reson Med 1990; 14:249–265.
33. Knight RA, Barker PB, Fagan SC, Li Y, Jacobs MA, Welch KM. Prediction of impending hemorrhagic transformation in ischemic stroke using magnetic resonance imaging in rats. Stroke 1998; 29: 144–151.
34. Aronowski J, Strong R, Grotta JC. Reperfusion injury: demonstration of brain damage produced by reperfusion after transient focal ischemia in rats. J Cereb Blood Flow Metab 1997; 17:1048–1056.

Jonathan H. Burdette, MD
Allen D. Elster, MD
Peter E. Ricci, MD

Index terms:
Brain, infarction, 10.78
Brain, MR, 10.12144
Magnetic resonance (MR), diffusion study, 10.12144

Radiology 1999; 212:333–339

Abbreviations:
ADC = apparent diffusion coefficient
DW = diffusion weighted
SI = signal intensity

[1] From the Department of Radiology, Wake Forest University School of Medicine, the Bowman Gray Campus, Medical Center Blvd, Winston-Salem, NC 27157. From the 1998 RSNA scientific assembly. Received August 26, 1998; revision requested November 2; revision received November 30; accepted March 1, 1999. Supported in part by a grant from GE Medical Systems. **Address reprint requests to** J.H.B. (e-mail: *jburdett@rad.wfubmc.edu*).

Author contributions:
Guarantor of integrity of entire study, J.H.B.; study concepts and design, A.D.E., J.H.B., P.E.R.; definition of intellectual content, J.H.B., A.D.E., P.E.R.; literature research, J.H.B., A.D.E., P.E.R.; clinical studies, J.H.B., P.E.R., A.D.E.; data acquisition, J.H.B.; data analysis, J.H.B., P.E.R., A.D.E.; statistical analysis, J.H.B., A.D.E.; manuscript preparation, J.H.B., A.D.E.; manuscript editing and review, J.H.B., A.D.E., P.E.R.

Acute Cerebral Infarction: Quantification of Spin-Density and T2 Shine-through Phenomena on Diffusion-weighted MR Images[1]

PURPOSE: To quantify the relative contributions of spin density and T2 effects ("shine through") on diffusion-weighted (DW) magnetic resonance (MR) images of acute and subacute cerebral infarction.

MATERIALS AND METHODS: In 30 patients, 1.5-T imaging was performed within the first 7 days after onset of cerebral infarction. Estimates of T2, spin density, and apparent diffusion coefficient (ADC) in the region of stroke and contralateral normal brain were computed by means of standard regression techniques after quadruple-echo conventional MR imaging and single-shot echo-planar DW imaging with a maximum *b* value of 1,000 sec/mm^2. Expected signal intensity (SI) enhancement ratios resulting from independent changes in T2, spin density, and ADC were then calculated for the DW sequence.

RESULTS: The overall SI of cerebral infarction on DW images was significantly higher than that of normal brain throughout the 1st week after stroke (mean relative SI enhancement ratio, 2.29; $P < .001$). During the first 2 days after stroke, decreased ADC within the stroke region made the dominant contribution to increased SI on DW images. By day 3, increased T2 values in the stroke region became equally important, and, from days 3–7, the contribution to SI from T2 effects became dominant. A slight increase of spin density in the stroke region made a relatively small and constant contribution to DW SI over the 1st week.

CONCLUSION: The increased SI of subacute cerebral infarction on DW images reflects not only a shortening of ADC but a prolongation of T2 and spin-density values.

The utility of diffusion-weighted (DW) magnetic resonance (MR) imaging for the diagnosis of acute cerebral infarction has now been thoroughly established (1–19). DW imaging is a relatively new technique that uses powerful imaging gradients coupled with rapid spin-echo or echo-planar data acquisition to accentuate phase differences between protons of varying mobility. In regions of recent cerebral infarction, the diffusion of tissue water becomes restricted, as manifested by a decrease in its apparent diffusion coefficient (ADC).

Alterations in brain diffusion by disease can be represented in an anatomically meaningful format by using either of two methods: (*a*) display of a DW image, in which the brightness of each pixel is proportional to the magnitude of the MR signal intensity (SI) recorded under maximum strength application of the diffusion-sensitizing gradient, or (*b*) display of an ADC map, in which the brightness of each pixel is proportional to its calculated ADC value.

The diagnostic information provided by DW images and ADC maps is not identical. For example, the time course of SI changes after an acute infarction differs markedly depending on the display method employed (8,11,13,14,16,17). Specifically, ADC maps typically

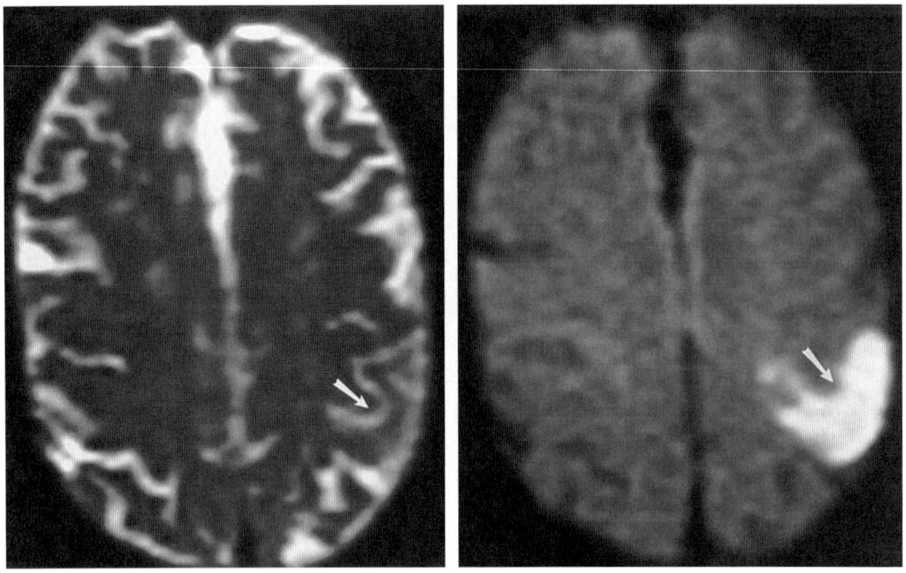

a. b.

Figure 1. Case 5. Echo-planar MR images in a 71-year-old man with a 36-hour-old cerebral infarction in the left anterior parietal region. **(a)** On the T2-weighted image (10,000/97 with *b* value of 1 sec/mm^2), the infarct (arrow) is extremely subtle. **(b)** However, on the DW image (10,000/97 with *b* value of 1,000 sec/mm^2), the infarct (arrow) is very conspicuous. When the infarct is compared with normal contralateral brain, there is only a 7% increase in the T2 value within the infarct, whereas there is a 55% decrease in ADC value. Thus, almost all of the abnormal increased SI in **b** arises from diffusion effects.

return to normal within 7–10 days after stroke, whereas DW images may remain abnormal for up to 14 days (14).

Just as a so-called T2-weighted image is not a simple map of T2 values, a DW image is not a simple map of diffusion constants. Rather, DW images contain mixed contributions from changes in T2, spin density, and ADC. We refer to these spillover effects of T2 and spin density on the DW image as MR "shine through." The purpose of this study was to quantify MR shine-through effects in the DW imaging of acute and subacute cerebral infarction.

MATERIALS AND METHODS

Our study population comprised 30 patients (16 male and 14 female patients; age range, 4–84 years; mean age, 64 years). All had been referred for MR imaging from March 1998 through June 1998 with definitive clinical evidence of a cerebral infarction less than 7 days old. A reliable time of clinical ictus could be established in all patients to within plus or minus 6 hours, as determined by means of review of the medical records, consultation with the referring physician, and/or direct patient interview. Ten patients underwent imaging during the first 48 hours after clinical stroke, 12 patients between 48 and 96 hours, and eight patients between 4.5 and 7 days.

MR imaging was performed in all subjects with a commercially available echo-planar instrument operating at 1.5 T (Signa EchoSpeed Horizon; GE Medical Systems, Milwaukee, Wis). Conventional axial spin-echo MR images were obtained with a multiecho technique, with a repetition time of 4,000 msec and echo times of 40, 80, 120, and 160 msec (4,000/40, 80, 120, 160). Other imaging parameters included one signal acquired, field of view of 24 cm, acquisition matrix of 256 × 128, and section thickness of 5 mm with a 2.5-mm intersection gap. A single-shot echo-planar DW imaging sequence was then performed with the following parameters: 10,000/97, one signal acquired, field of view of 30 cm, acquisition matrix of 128 × 128, and section thickness of 5 mm with a 2.5-mm intersection gap. Diffusion gradients were sequentially activated in each of the three principal anatomic axes to obtain DW images sensitive to diffusion in the x, y, and z planes. Gradient strengths corresponding to *b* values of 1 and 1,000 sec/mm^2 were used. This commercially available diffusion imaging software produced 20 axial images, covering the entire brain in 40 seconds.

For the two *b* value image sets and the quadruple echo time image sets, region-of-interest SIs were obtained in the core of the cerebral infarction and within normal contralateral brain by a neuroradiologist (J.H.B.). Within the infarct and normal brain for each patient, the size and location of the region of interest remained constant (ie, maintained the same size for the two *b* value image sets and the quadruple echo time image sets). The trace value of the estimated diffusion tensor

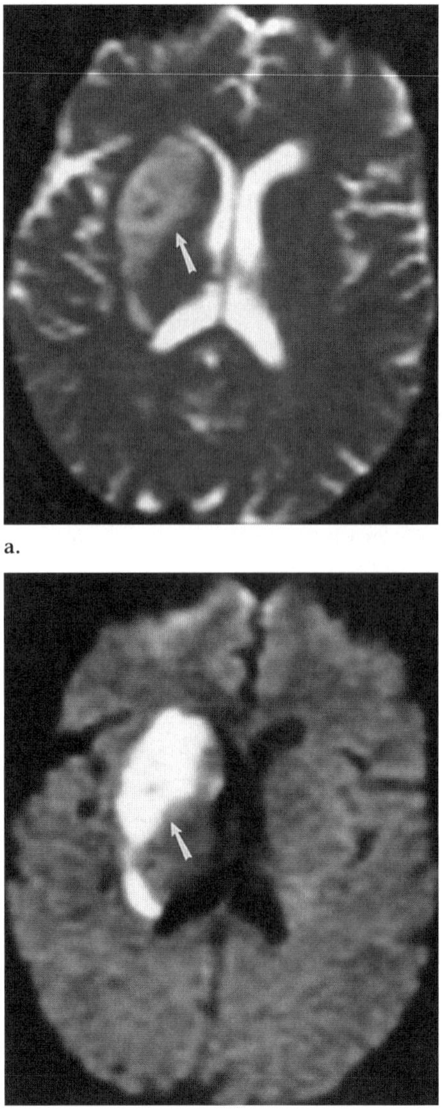

a.

b.

Figure 2. Case 18. Echo-planar MR images in an 80-year-old man with a 4-day-old cerebral infarction in the right basal ganglia (arrow). The infarct is apparent on both the **(a)** T2-weighted image (10,000/97 with *b* value of 1 sec/mm^2) and **(b)** DW image (10,000/97 with *b* value of 1,000 sec/mm^2). With a T2 increase of 36%, ADC decrease of 33%, and spin-density increase of 38% within the infarct, there is similar contribution to the increased SI within the infarct in **b** from each parameter.

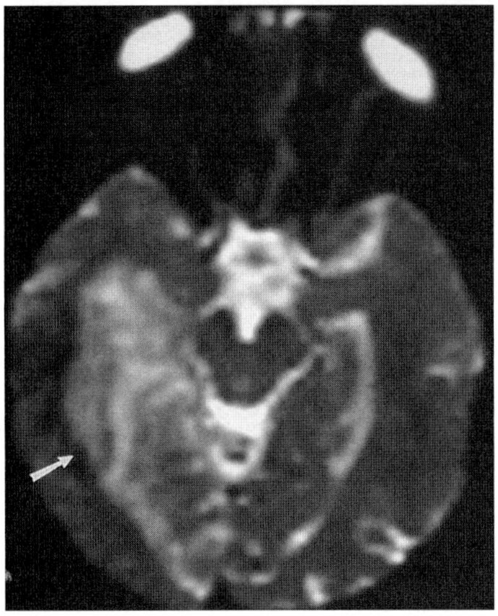

a.

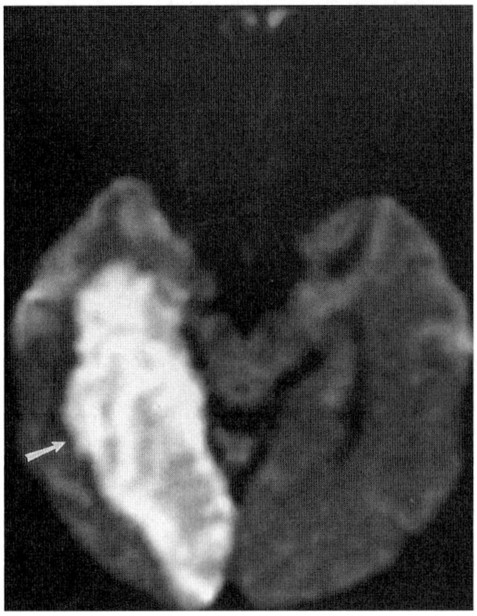

b.

Figure 3. **Case 29.** Echo-planar MR images in a 60-year-old man with a 7-day-old cerebral infarction (arrow) in the right occipital and medial temporal lobes. The infarct is apparent on both the **(a)** T2-weighted (10,000/97 with b value of 1 sec/mm^2) and **(b)** DW (10,000/97 with b value 1,000 sec/mm^2) images. These images show the decreasing contribution of ADC and increasing contribution of T2 effects to SI within infarcts on DW images with increasing time. In this case, there was an increase in T2 of 58%, ADC decrease of 26%, and spin density increase of 38% within the infarct, indicating dominance of the T2 effects in **b**.

was used for each ADC measurement, representing the average of region-of-interest values along the three principal diffusion axes.

The data were analyzed by means of standard linear and nonlinear regression models by using commercially available statistical software (Systat, Evanston, Ill). Calculations of ADC values were obtained for infarct and normal brain by applying the Stejskal-Tanner equation (20) with two b values of 1 and 1,000 sec/mm^2. This two-point estimation of ADC values has recently been shown to be highly accurate by two independent groups of investigators (21,22). Estimates of T2 and relative spin density were obtained by using measurements from the long repetition time, quadruple echo time sequence. These estimates were obtained by means of nonlinear parameter fitting to the well-recognized formula for spin-echo SI derived from the Bloch equations (23,24). For each patient, therefore, six estimated tissue parameters were calculated: three in the region of stroke (spin density [SD_S], $T2_S$, and ADC_S) and three in normal brain contralateral to the stroke (SD_N, $T2_N$, and ADC_N).

TABLE 1
Tissue Parameters Measured in Normal Brain and the Stroke Region

Parameter	Normal Brain	Stroke Region
Spin density (relative units)	0.88 ± 0.13	1.07 ± 0.20
T2 (msec)	85 ± 12	120 ± 17
ADC ($\times 10^{-4}$ mm^2/sec)	7.9 ± 1.1	5.1 ± 1.2

Note.—Numbers are the mean ± SD (n = 30). Differences in the means between normal brain and stroke region for each parameter are all statistically significant (paired t test, $P < .01$).

Descriptive statistics (means and SDs) for spin density, T2, and ADC were computed, and differences in these parameters between the stroke region and normal brain were analyzed by means of a paired Student t test. As outlined in the Appendix, percentage changes in each tissue parameter as a function of infarct age were computed. These percentage changes in tissue parameters were also displayed graphically with simple linear or quadratic least squares regression lines added to assist visualization of trends as a function of time after infarction.

To understand the individual contributions of these changes in spin density, T2, and ADC to overall SI on DW images, these measured values were substituted one at a time into the model (22,23) for MR SI of the DW imaging sequence as shown in the Appendix. With this model, expected ratios of SI in the stroke region to normal brain resulting from differences in spin density, T2, and ADC could then be independently calculated and represented as SI enhancement ratios due to each parameter (spin density, T2, and ADC).

RESULTS

Each infarction imaged during the 1st week was noted to be markedly hyperintense to normal brain on DW images (Figs 1–3), with an average stroke-to-brain SI enhancement ratio (SIR_{total}) of 2.29. This increased total SI from stroke, also documented in multiple previous reports (6,17,21–23), is consistent with measured differences in spin density, T2, and ADC between stroke region and normal brain. On the average, we found that spin density and T2 increased by approximately 22% and 41%, respectively, whereas ADC values decreased by about 35% (Table 1).

Examination of the time course of these changes is even more enlightening. As seen in Figure 4a, the stroke-to-brain SI ratio on DW images remained relatively constant over the 1st week, decreasing only 1.5% per day (on the basis of the equation for the regression line). However, the relative values of spin density, T2, and ADC differed markedly as a function of time during this period (Table 2, Fig 4b–4d). Spin-density values became elevated above baseline by about 20% on day 1, with only a minimal further increase noted throughout the remainder of the 1st week. T2 values were elevated less than 20% in the first 2 days, but they rose to 70%–80% by the end of the 1st week. ADC values had a time course opposite that of T2 values, initially falling by approximately 60% but returning nearly to normal by the end of the 1st week.

The individual effects on total SI of these time-dependent changes in spin density, T2, and ADC can be analyzed by looking at their SI enhancement ratios (Fig 5). With our diffusion sequence with echo time of 97 msec and b value of 1,000 sec/mm^2, overall SI is dominated by diffusion effects for the first 2–3 days. Thereafter, T2 effects account for most of the high SI seen on the DW images. By day 7, almost all of the increased SI on DW images within the infarction was due to T2 effects, with only a modest contribution from spin-density effects.

DISCUSSION

DW MR imaging has become an important component of the modern imaging

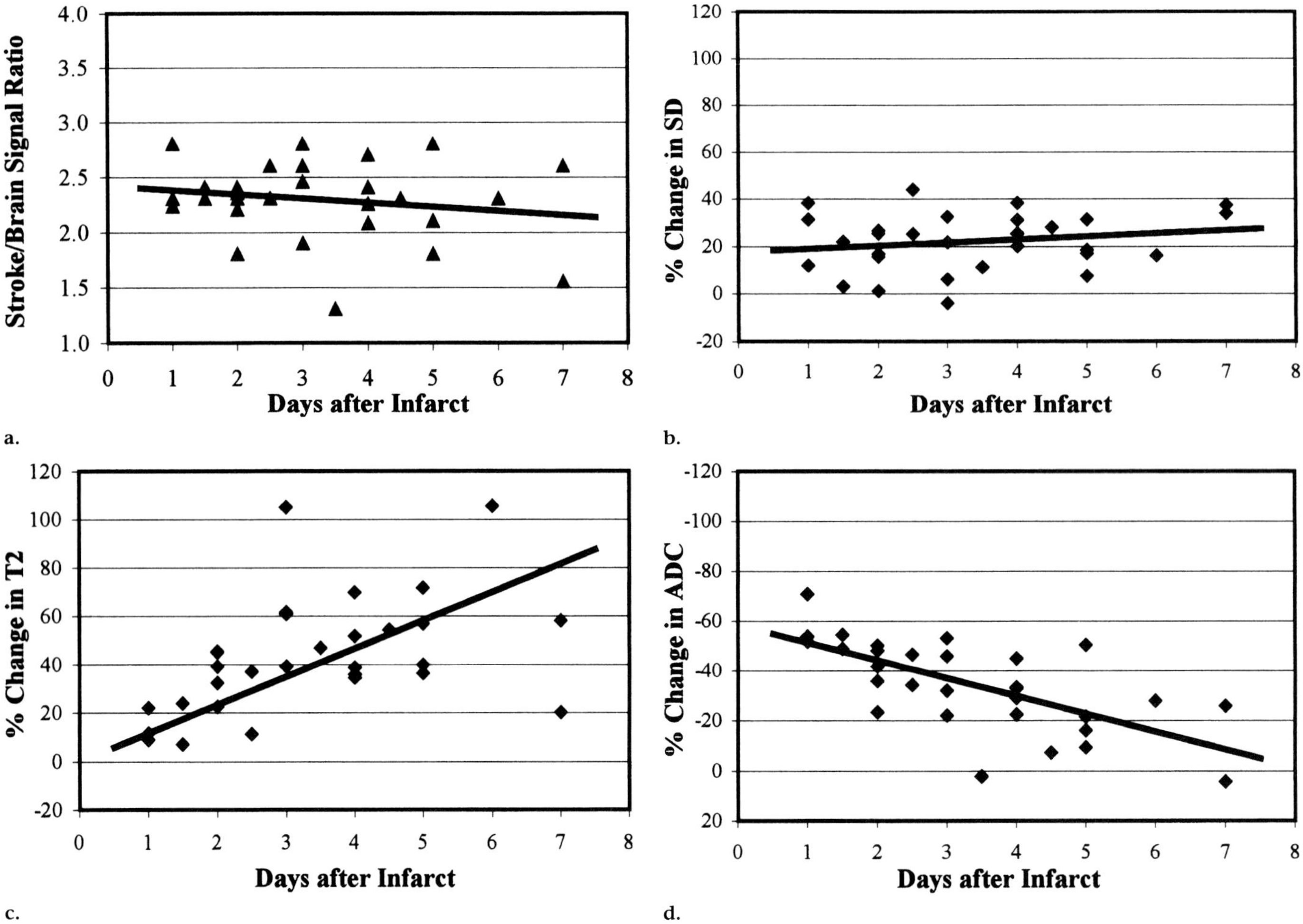

Figure 4. Changes in DW SI and tissue parameters as a function of time show the greatest initial change to be in ADC values and the greatest change by the end of the 1st week to be in T2 values. **(a)** Stroke-to-brain SI ratio is seen to remain relatively constant over the entire week. **(b)** Spin-density (*SD*) values remain elevated by approximately 20%–25% throughout the 1st week. **(c)** T2 values progressively increase over the 1st week. **(d)** ADC values are sharply reduced immediately after infarction, returning to nearly normal by the end of the week.

armamentarium for the diagnosis of acute cerebral infarction (1–18). In animal models, DW images can reliably reveal infarcted areas within minutes of experimental vascular occlusion (3,5,6). Although only a few clinical examples are available of human strokes imaged at such short time intervals, many positive DW images in patients with strokes only a few hours old have been published (8–14).

In addition to evaluating DW images, several investigators have used stepped gradient techniques to estimate changes in ADC after acute cerebral infarction. Reith et al (16) noted changes in ADC values within 5 minutes of onset of ischemia. Schlaug et al (17) found reduction, pseudonormalization, or even elevation of ADC values after the 7th day after infarction. Lutsep et al (11) found that ADC values remained low for the 1st week after infarction and normalized or became elevated at more chronic time points. Warach et al (8) and Marks et al (13) both found that after the initial decrease in the acute stroke period, ADC values gradually increased and became elevated after 10 days.

Although calculation of ADC values and production of ADC maps yields quantifiable results, it currently requires a level of data processing and complexity more extensive than is commonly available in most clinical MR centers. In current practice at most sites today, visual assessment of DW images (rather than ADC maps) is commonly employed for the diagnosis of stroke. The analogy is that even though it is possible to generate T1 and T2 maps from the MR raw data, this step is seldom performed. Radiologists prefer to use T1- or T2-weighted images for diagnosis, even though such images lack parameter "purity" and contain mixed contributions to overall SI (25).

As with T1- and T2-weighted images, DW images are not pure maps of ADC but contain mixed contributions from spin-density and T2 effects. We have referred to this phenomenon as MR shine through and have attempted to quantify its importance in clinical DW imaging. Other investigators have also recognized that shine-through effects exist in the DW imaging of stroke but have not thoroughly quantified them. Because of these shine-through effects, the DW images should be interpreted with reference to images obtained with other sequences, such as T2-weighted images, fluid-attenuated inversion-recovery, or FLAIR, images, and ADC maps (18).

Without actually calculating T2 values, Lutsep et al (11) noted a discrepancy in the temporal evolution of ADC and SI

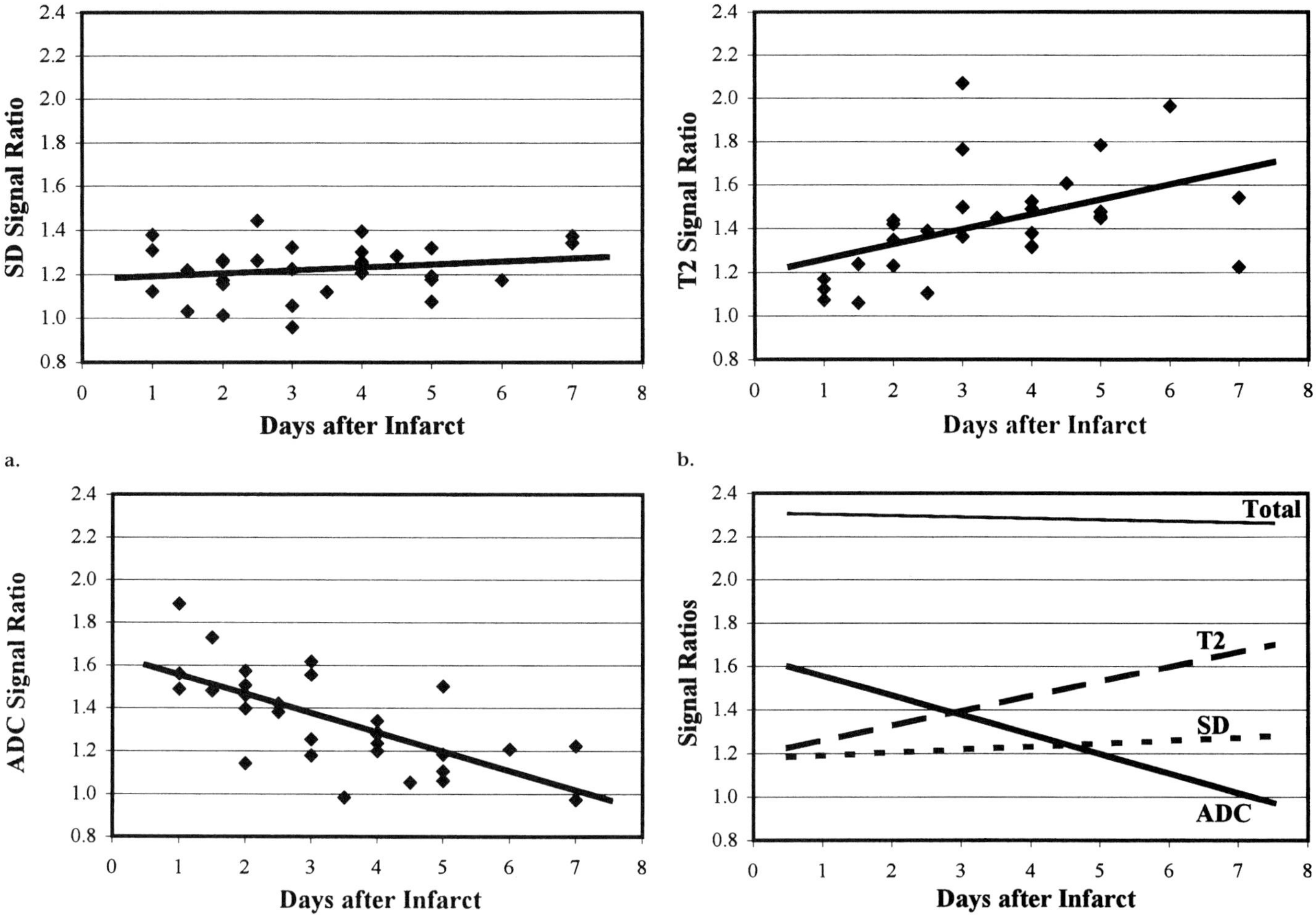

Figure 5. SI enhancement contributions to total DW SI by individual parameter and day. With our DW sequence, the overall SI is dominated by diffusion effects in the first 2–3 days; thereafter, T2 effects account for most of the high SI with only a modest contribution from spin-density (*SD*) effects. **(a)** Spin-density effects. **(b)** T2 effects. **(c)** ADC effects. **(d)** Individual contributions displayed together.

changes on T2-weighted images within 10 days after stroke (11). Burdette et al (14) noted the discrepancy in time course of SI changes of subacute cerebral infarction on T2-weighted and DW images; whereas ADC maps return to normal by 7–10 days, DW images may remain abnormal for up to 2 weeks. Knight et al (19) calculated ADC, T2, and T1 values in ischemic regions in rats after occlusion of the middle cerebral artery and found behavior of T1, T2, and spin density independent from that of ADC. They noted that the hyperintense appearance of infarcts on DW images cannot be attributed solely to ADC values and that care must be taken when SI abnormalities on DW images are interpreted.

By extending the work of these investigators, we quantified the independent contributions of ADC, T2, and spin density to the SI changes seen on DW images

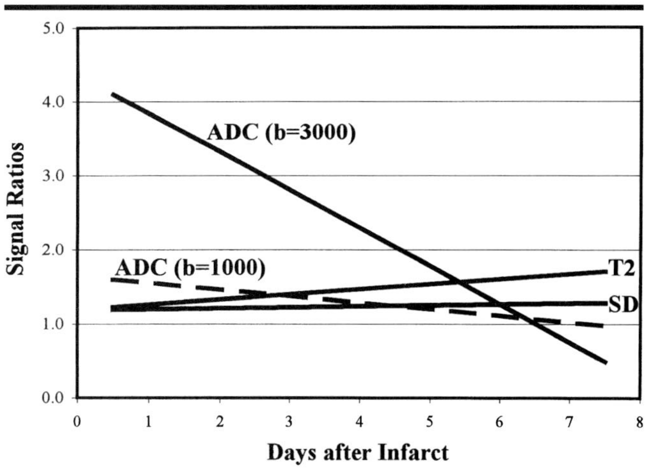

Figure 6. Theoretic individual contributions of ADC, T2, and spin density (*SD*) to DW image contrast for *b* values of 3,000 versus 1,000 sec/mm^2. The threefold increase in *b* value markedly increases the relative contribution of ADC to overall SI, but, by day 6, T2 and spin-density shine through still occur, eventually dominating the MR SI.

as a function of time during the 1st week after cerebral infarction. Our findings show that with use of current diffusion gradients with maximum b values of 1,000 sec/mm^2, all three components contribute to increased SI within the infarct on DW images. For the first 2–3 days, the increased SI on DW images results principally from restricted diffusion (ie, shortening of ADC). Thereafter, T2 effects, and to a lesser degree spin-density effects, provide the dominant mechanism of image contrast.

With advancing technology, stronger gradients will allow higher b values and consequently more ADC contrast to be present on DW images. The quantitative data in this report allow predictions of the degree of spin-density and T2 shine through that will be present on the next generation of diffusion-sensitive images. The SI enhancement ratio due to diffusion scales exponentially with b value (20). For example, each doubling of gradient b values squares the SI contribution of ADC to the DW image.

By using our model and data, it is possible to calculate the anticipated effect of increasing gradient strength on T2 shine through and the time course of total stroke SI on DW images. In Figure 6, we plotted the expected SI enhancement ratios of cerebral infarction for spin density, T2, and ADC in a high-performance gradient system with a b value of 3,000 sec/mm^2. As expected, this threefold increase in b value dramatically increased the relative contribution of ADC to the overall MR SI. By day 6, however, T2 and spin-density shine through still occurred, eventually dominating the MR SI.

In summary, with use of current gradient strengths with b values of 1,000 sec/mm^2, T2 (and to a lesser degree spin-density) shine-through effects account for a substantial component of the total MR SI observed on DW images of subacute cerebral infarction, especially beyond 3–4 days. The future use of gradients with higher strength will shift the timing of this effect but will not eliminate it.

TABLE 2
Changes in Spin Density, T2, and ADC due to Infarction

Case No.	Time after Infarct (day)	Percentage Change in Spin Density	Percentage Change in T2	Percentage Change in ADC
1	1.0	12	9	−71
2	1.0	38	11	−54
3	1.0	31	22	−52
4	1.5	22	24	−49
5	1.5	3	7	−55
6	2.0	26	32	−48
7	2.0	16	23	−50
8	2.0	1	46	−23
9	2.0	17	39	−42
10	2.0	27	45	−36
11	2.5	44	11	−34
12	2.5	25	37	−47
13	3.0	33	39	−46
14	3.0	6	61	−53
15	3.0	22	62	−22
16	3.0	−4	105	−32
17	3.5	11	47	+2
18	4.0	38	36	−33
19	4.0	25	52	−23
20	4.0	26	70	−45
21	4.0	20	35	−34
22	4.0	31	39	−29
23	4.5	28	54	−7
24	5.0	17	72	−16
25	5.0	8	40	−9
26	5.0	31	37	−22
27	5.0	19	57	−28
28	6.0	16	106	−28
29	7.0	38	58	−26
30	7.0	34	20	+4

APPENDIX

The percentage changes in each tissue parameter (P) as a function of infarct age were computed with the following formula:

$$\%\Delta P - \frac{P_{\text{Stroke}} - P_{\text{Normal}}}{P_{\text{Normal}}} \times 100$$

where P is spin density, T2, or ADC, respectively. These percentage changes in tissue parameters were also displayed graphically, with simple linear or quadratic least squares regression lines added to assist visualization of trends as a function of time after infarction.

To understand the individual contributions of these changes in spin density (SD), T2, and ADC to overall SI on DW images, these measured values were substituted one at a time into the following model (22,23) for MR SI of the DW imaging sequence:

$$\text{SI} = k \cdot \text{SD} \cdot e^{-\text{TE/T2}} \cdot e^{-b \cdot \text{ADC}}.$$

For our experiments, k is an arbitrary scaling constant, echo time (TE) is 97 msec, and the b value is 1,000 sec/mm^2. Note that because we used a single-shot, echo-planar diffusion technique, the repetition time is effectively infinite, and T1 effects make no significant contributions to the MR SI.

By using this model, expected ratios of SI in the stroke region to normal brain resulting from differences in spin density, T2, and ADC could then be independently calculated. For example, we defined the SI enhancement ratio (SIR) due to T2 effects alone (SIR_{T2}) in stroke region (S) relative to normal (N) brain as

$$\text{SIR}_{\text{T2}} = \frac{k \cdot \text{SD}_{\text{N}} \cdot e^{-\text{TE/T2}_{\text{S}}} \cdot e^{-b \cdot \text{ADC}_{\text{N}}}}{k \cdot \text{SD}_{\text{N}} \cdot e^{-\text{TE/T2}_{\text{N}}} \cdot e^{-b \cdot \text{ADC}_{\text{N}}}} = \frac{e^{-\text{TE/T2}_{\text{S}}}}{e^{-\text{TE/T2}_{\text{N}}}}.$$

Similarly, the SI enhancement ratios due to spin-density effects alone (SIR_{SD}) and ADC effects alone (SIR_{ADC}) were defined as

$$\text{SIR}_{\text{SD}} = \frac{\text{SD}_{\text{S}}}{\text{SD}_{\text{N}}} \quad \text{and} \quad \text{SIR}_{\text{ADC}} = \frac{e^{-b \cdot \text{ADC}_{\text{S}}}}{e^{-b \cdot \text{ADC}_{\text{N}}}}.$$

Note that the total SI enhancement ratio of stroke to normal brain with the DW pulse sequence ($\text{SIR}_{\text{total}}$) is merely the product of the individual enhancement ratios:

$$\text{SIR}_{\text{TOT}} = \frac{\text{SI}_{\text{S}}}{\text{SI}_{\text{N}}} = \text{SIR}_{\text{SD}} \cdot \text{SIR}_{\text{T2}} \cdot \text{SIR}_{\text{ADC}}.$$

This formulation provided a useful check on individual SI enhancement ratio calculations and on the overall consistency of our results.

Acknowledgments: The authors thank Hugh Howards, PhD, for help with the statistical analysis, Shona Simpson, PhD, for editorial comments, and the MR imaging technologists for their patience and support for clinical MR imaging research.

References

1. Kucharczyk J, Mintorovitch J, Asgari HS, Moseley M. Diffusion/perfusion MR imaging of acute cerebral ischemia. Magn Reson Med 1991; 19:311–315.
2. Jones SC, Perez-Trepichio AD, Xue M, Furlan AJ, Awad IA. Magnetic resonance diffusion-weighted imaging: sensitivity and apparent diffusion constant in stroke. Acta Neurochir Suppl (Wien) 1994; 60: 207–210.
3. Minematsu K, Li L, Sotak CH, Davis MA, Fisher M. Reversible focal ischemic injury demonstrated by diffusion-weighted magnetic resonance imaging in rats. Stroke 1992; 23:1304–1311.
4. Moseley ME, Kucharczyk J, Mintorovitch J, et al. Diffusion-weighted MR imaging of acute stroke: correlation with T2-weighted and magnetic susceptibility–enhanced MR imaging in cats. AJNR 1990; 11:423–429.
5. Moseley ME, Cohen Y, Mintorovitch J, et al. Early detection of regional cerebral ischemia in cats: comparison of diffusion- and T2-weighted MRI and spectroscopy. Magn Reson Med 1990; 14:330–346.
6. Mintorovitch J, Moseley ME, Chileuitt L, Shimizu H, Cohen Y, Weinstein PR. Comparison of diffusion- and T2-weighted MRI for the early detection of cerebral ischemia and reperfusion in rats. Magn Reson Med 1991; 18:39–50.
7. Moonen CT, Pekar J, de Vleeschouwer MH, van Gelderen P, van Zijl PC, DesPres D. Restricted and anisotropic displacement of water in healthy cat brain and in stroke studied by NMR diffusion imaging. Magn Reson Med 1991; 19:327–332.
8. Warach S, Gaa J, Siewert B, Wielopolski P, Edelman RR. Acute human stroke studied by whole brain echo planar diffusion-weighted magnetic resonance imaging. Ann Neurol 1995; 37:231–241.
9. Warach S, Dashe JF, Edelman RR. Clinical outcome in ischemic stroke predicted by early diffusion-weighted and perfusion magnetic resonance imaging: a preliminary analysis. J Cereb Blood Flow Metab 1996; 16:53–59.
10. Sorensen AG, Buonanno FS, Gonzalez RG, et al. Hyperacute stroke: evaluation with combined multisection diffusion-weighted and hemodynamically weighted echo-planar MR imaging. Radiology 1996; 199:391–401.
11. Lutsep HL, Albers GW, DeCrespigny A, Kamat GN, Marks MP, Moseley ME. Clinical utility of diffusion-weighted magnetic resonance imaging in the assessment of ischemic stroke. Ann Neurol 1997; 41: 574–580.
12. Warach S, Chien D, Li W, Ronthal M, Edelman RR. Fast magnetic resonance diffusion-weighted imaging of acute human stroke. Neurology 1992; 42:1717–1723.
13. Marks MP, de Crespigny A, Lentz D, Enzmann DR, Albers GW, Moseley ME. Acute and chronic stroke: navigated spin-echo diffusion-weighted MR imaging. Radiology 1996; 199:403–408.
14. Burdette JB, Ricci PE, Petitti N, Elster AD. Cerebral infarction: time course of signal changes on diffusion-weighted MR images. AJR 1998; 171:791–795.
15. Le Bihan D, Breton E, Lallemand D, Grenier P, Cabanis E, Laval-Jeantet M. MR imaging of intravoxel incoherent motions: application to diffusion and perfusion in neurologic disorders. Radiology 1986; 161:401–407.
16. Reith W, Hasegawa Y, Latour LL, Dardzinski BJ, Sotak CH, Fisher M. Multislice diffusion mapping for 3-D evolution of cerebral ischemia in a rat stroke model. Neurology 1995; 45:172–177.
17. Schlaug G, Siewert B, Benfield A, Edelman RR, Warach S. Time course of the apparent diffusion coefficient (ADC) abnormalities in human stroke. Neurology 1997; 49:113–119.
18. Beauchamp NJ, Bryan RN. Acute cerebral ischemic infarction: a pathophysiologic review and radiologic perspective. AJR 1998; 171:73–84.
19. Knight RA, Dereski MO, Helpern JA, Ordidge RJ, Chopp M. Magnetic resonance imaging assessment of evolving focal cerebral ischemia: comparison with histopathology in rats. Stroke 1994; 25:1252–1262.
20. Stejskal EO, Tanner JE. Spin diffusion measurements: spin echoes in the presence of a time-dependent field gradient. J Chem Phys 1965; 42:288–292.
21. Burdette JH, Elster AD, Ricci PE. Calculation of apparent diffusion coefficients (ADCs) in brain using two-point and six-point methods. J Comput Assist Tomogr 1998; 22:792–794.
22. Xing D, Papadakis NG, Huang CL, Lee VM, Carpenter TA, Hall LD. Optimized diffusion-weighting for measurement of apparent diffusion coefficient (ADC) in human brain. Magn Reson Imaging 1997; 15:771–784.
23. Kjos BO, Ehman RL, Brant-Zawadski M, Kelly WM, Norman D, Newton TH. Reproducibility of relaxation times and spin density calculated from routine MR imaging sequences: clinical study of the CNS. AJR 1985; 144:1165–1170.
24. Breger RK. Reproducibility of relaxation and spin-density parameters in phantoms and the human brain measured by MR imaging at 1.5 T. Magn Reson Med 1986; 3:649–662.
25. Elster AD. An index system for comparative parameter weighting in MR imaging. J Comput Assist Tomogr 1988; 12:130–134.

Moyamoya Disease: Evaluation with Diffusion-weighted and Perfusion Echo-planar MR Imaging[1]

Ichiro Yamada, MD
Yoshiro Himeno, MD
Tsukasa Nagaoka, MD
Hideaki Akimoto, MD
Yoshiharu Matsushima, MD
Toshihiko Kuroiwa, MD
Hitoshi Shibuya, MD

Index terms:
Carotid arteries, MR, 17.121416, 17.12144
Cerebral angiography, 17.1243, 17.1246, 17.1247
Cerebral blood vessels, MR, 17.121416, 17.12144
Cerebral blood vessels, stenosis or obstruction, 17.72134
Moyamoya disease, 17.72134, 17.781

Radiology 1999; 212:340–347

Abbreviations:
ADC = apparent diffusion coefficient
ICA = internal carotid artery
PCA = posterior cerebral artery
ΔR2* = change in the effective transverse relaxation rate

[1] From the Departments of Radiology (I.Y., Y.H., H.S.) and Neurosurgery (T.N., H.A., Y.M.), Faculty of Medicine, and the Department of Neuropathology (T.K.), Medical Research Institute, Tokyo Medical and Dental University, 1-5-45 Yushima, Bunkyo-ku, Tokyo 113-8519, Japan. Received June 2, 1998; revision requested August 5; final revision received November 10; accepted February 22, 1999. **Address reprint requests to** I.Y. (e-mail: *yamada.crad@med.tmd.ac.jp*).

PURPOSE: To determine the clinical efficacy of diffusion-weighted and perfusion echo-planar magnetic resonance (MR) imaging in the evaluation of moyamoya disease.

MATERIALS AND METHODS: Seventeen patients with moyamoya disease were examined prospectively with diffusion-weighted and perfusion echo-planar MR imaging and conventional angiography. The change in the effective transverse relaxation rate (ΔR2*) peak value, ΔR2* peak time, and ΔR2* integral were calculated to assess regional cerebral perfusion. The MR images were compared with angiographic images.

RESULTS: Of the 34 posterior cerebral arteries (PCAs) of the 17 patients, 14 PCAs (41%) in 11 patients showed stenosis or occlusion. The ΔR2* peak value ratio in the cerebral hemispheres decreased significantly, and the ΔR2* peak time ratio increased significantly, with PCA stenosis and occlusion. However, no correlation was apparent between perfusion and extent of the stenotic or occlusive lesions of the internal carotid artery bifurcation. The frequency of cerebral infarctions was significantly increased in patients with stenotic or occlusive PCA lesions. For three acute infarctions, a decrease in the apparent diffusion coefficient was significantly correlated with a decrease in the ΔR2* peak value, an increase in the ΔR2* peak time, and a decrease in the ΔR2* integral.

CONCLUSION: Regional cerebral perfusion in moyamoya disease is decreased and delayed with PCA stenosis, with greater decrease and delay with PCA occlusion. Diffusion-weighted and perfusion imaging are useful for evaluating cerebral ischemia in moyamoya disease.

Moyamoya disease is a rare cerebrovascular occlusive disease of unknown cause that occurs predominantly in the Japanese, although cases in other ethnic groups have also been described (1–4). The angiographic features of this disease include (*a*) bilateral stenosis or occlusion of the supraclinoid portion of the internal carotid artery (ICA) that extends to the proximal portions of the anterior cerebral artery and the middle cerebral artery and (*b*) the presence of parenchymal, leptomeningeal, or transdural collateral vessels that supply the ischemic brain (5,6).

Diffusion-weighted and perfusion echo-planar magnetic resonance (MR) imaging have recently been applied to evaluate occlusive cerebrovascular diseases (7–10). However, to our knowledge, few studies have described the application of such imaging in patients with moyamoya disease (11). We now present the results of a prospective study that was undertaken to determine the clinical efficacy of diffusion-weighted and perfusion echo-planar MR imaging, compared with that of conventional angiography, in the evaluation of moyamoya disease.

Author contributions:
Guarantor of integrity of entire study, I.Y.; study concepts, I.Y.; study design, I.Y., Y.H.; definition of intellectual content, I.Y.; literature research, I.Y., T.K.; clinical studies, I.Y., Y.M.; data acquisition, I.Y., T.N.; data analysis, I.Y., H.A.; statistical analysis, I.Y., T.K.; manuscript preparation, I.Y., Y.H.; manuscript editing, I.Y.; manuscript review, I.Y., H.S.

MATERIALS AND METHODS

Patients

Over the past 2 years (October 1997 to April 1998), 17 consecutive patients with idiopathic moyamoya disease at cerebral angiography were examined in our department of radiology. Eleven of these subjects were female, and six were male; their ages ranged from 3 to 48 years (mean, 22 years ± 18 [SD]). None of the 17 patients exhibited underlying disease, thereby confirming the diagnosis of idiopathic moyamoya disease. Fourteen patients had not previously undergone surgical treatment, whereas three had undergone duraencephalosynangiosis, an external carotid artery–to-ICA bypass operation. The study protocol was approved by the institutional review board, and informed consent was obtained from all patients.

Imaging Examinations

All MR images were obtained with a 1.5-T superconducting system with a 25 mT/m maximal gradient capability (Magnetom Vision; Siemens, Erlangen, Germany) and a circularly polarized head coil. Initially, all patients underwent conventional MR imaging. Axial T1-weighted images were obtained with a spin-echo sequence (600/14 [repetition time msec/ echo time msec]), a matrix of 192 × 256, and two signals acquired. Axial T2-weighted images were obtained with a turbo spin-echo sequence (4,000/96, echo train length of seven), a matrix of 210 × 512, and two signals acquired. All images were acquired with a field of view of 165 × 220 mm and a section thickness of 5 mm, with a 1-mm intersection gap.

Diffusion-weighted imaging.—Diffusion-weighted imaging was performed with a multisection, single-shot, spin-echo, echo-planar sequence, which included an echo time of 123 msec, a bandwidth of 1,250 Hz per pixel, a matrix of 128 × 200, a field of view of 230 × 230 mm, a section thickness of 5 mm with a 1-mm intersection gap, and one signal acquired. Fat suppression was performed by applying the frequency-selective radio-frequency pulse before imaging with the pulse sequence.

The diffusion gradient was applied along the section-select direction and had a duration of 26 msec, a separation time of 59.7 msec, and a gradient strength of 3.5 or 21.1 mT/m. The resultant values for the gradient factor b were 30 or 1,100 sec/mm^2. Apparent diffusion coefficient (ADC) maps were calculated by using the following equation: $ADC = \ln(S_0/S)/(b - b_0)$, where S_0 and S are the signal intensities of the two diffusion-weighted images, and the gradient factors b_0 and b are 30 and 1,100 sec/mm^2, respectively.

Perfusion imaging.—Perfusion imaging was performed with a multisection, single-shot, free induction decay, echo-planar sequence, which included an echo time of 54 msec, a bandwidth of 1,190 Hz per pixel, a matrix of 128 × 128, a field of view of 230 × 230 mm, a section thickness of 5 mm, and one signal acquired. We obtained 50 images every 1.2 seconds, with seven sections in each image. The seven sections were set to cover both cerebral hemispheres.

At the beginning of the image acquisition, a bolus of 0.1 mmol of gadodiamide (Omniscan; Daiichi Seiyaku, Tokyo, Japan) per kilogram of body weight was administered intravenously by means of manual injection over approximately 5 seconds, followed by a saline flush. Injection was performed with an 18-gauge intravenous catheter in an antecubital vein to minimize resistance to the injection.

Images based on the change in the effective transverse relaxation rate (ΔR2*) were constructed from each time series at each time point along the first pass of the contrast agent bolus. The ΔR2* was computed on a pixel-by-pixel basis according to the following formula: $\Delta R2^* = -\ln(S_t/S_0)/TE$, where S_t is signal intensity at time t, S_0 is the precontrast baseline signal intensity, and TE is the sequence echo time. ΔR2* is proportional to the concentration of the contrast agent and can be used to estimate perfusion parameters.

On ΔR2* images, regions of large signal change appear as areas of high signal intensity, whereas regions of small signal change appear as areas of low signal intensity. These images were processed to create maps of the ΔR2* peak value, ΔR2* peak time, and ΔR2* integral, with the use of a numerical integration technique similar to those described previously (12).

Conventional angiography.—All patients also underwent cerebral angiography that included bilateral internal and external carotid arteriography and unilateral or bilateral vertebral arteriography, with the use of the transfemoral catheterization technique for both carotid and vertebral arteriography. Conventional angiograms were obtained with a digital subtraction technique. Digital subtraction images were obtained with a 0.6-mm focal spot and a 10-inch (25.4-cm) cesium iodide image-intensifying tube (KXO-80C/D and DFP-2000A; Toshiba Medical Systems, Tokyo, Japan). Images were displayed and printed with a 1,024 × 1,024 matrix. A dose of 8–10 mL of ioxaglate (Hexabrix 320; Eiken Kagaku, Tokyo, Japan) was injected for each arteriographic examination. Conventional angiography was performed within 1 month before (n = 14) or after (n = 3) MR imaging. In these three patients, the diagnosis was made with conventional angiography after MR imaging.

Image Analysis

On the basis of the angiographic findings, we classified stenotic or occlusive lesions of the ICA bifurcation, according to the extent of narrowing in the supraclinoid portion of the ICA and the proximal portions of the anterior cerebral artery and middle cerebral artery, into five different stages: stage 1, mild to moderate stenosis of the ICA bifurcation (≤80% reduction in diameter); stage 2, severe stenosis of the ICA bifurcation (>80% reduction in diameter); stage 3, occlusion of either the anterior cerebral artery or middle cerebral artery; stage 4, occlusion of the ICA bifurcation, with partial retention of the anterior cerebral artery or middle cerebral artery main trunk; and stage 5, occlusion of the ICA bifurcation, with no detectable anterior cerebral arterial or middle cerebral arterial main trunk (6). Stenotic or occlusive lesions in the posterior cerebral artery (PCA) were also identified. Thus, the PCA was graded as normal, stenotic, or occluded.

We also classified the basal cerebral moyamoya vessels on the basis of their presence and appearance into four grades: none, slight, moderate, or marked. "Marked" indicated the moyamoya vessels formed a vascular network that showed high contrast and that extended above the basal ganglia, with visualization of the medullary arteries. "Moderate" meant the moyamoya vessels formed an intermediate vascular network localized in the basal ganglia, without visualization of the medullary arteries. "Slight" indicated the moyamoya vessels showed less contrast and a more orderly arrangement near only the internal carotid bifurcation, and they assumed the appearance of unusually dilated perforating arteries.

The ΔR2* images were reviewed by two radiologists (I.Y., Y.H.) for the distribution of areas that showed decreased regional cerebral perfusion. Circular regions of interest were thus set on ΔR2* images in the frontal, temporal, parietal, and occipital lobes and in the basal ganglia, and the mean value of three or four regions of interest was calculated in these five cerebral regions. Ratios of the ΔR2* peak value, ΔR2* peak time, and ΔR2* integral were calculated by dividing the value in these regions by the mean cerebral value obtained from both cerebral hemispheres to assess the regional cerebral perfusion parameters. Values were expressed as means ± 1 SD.

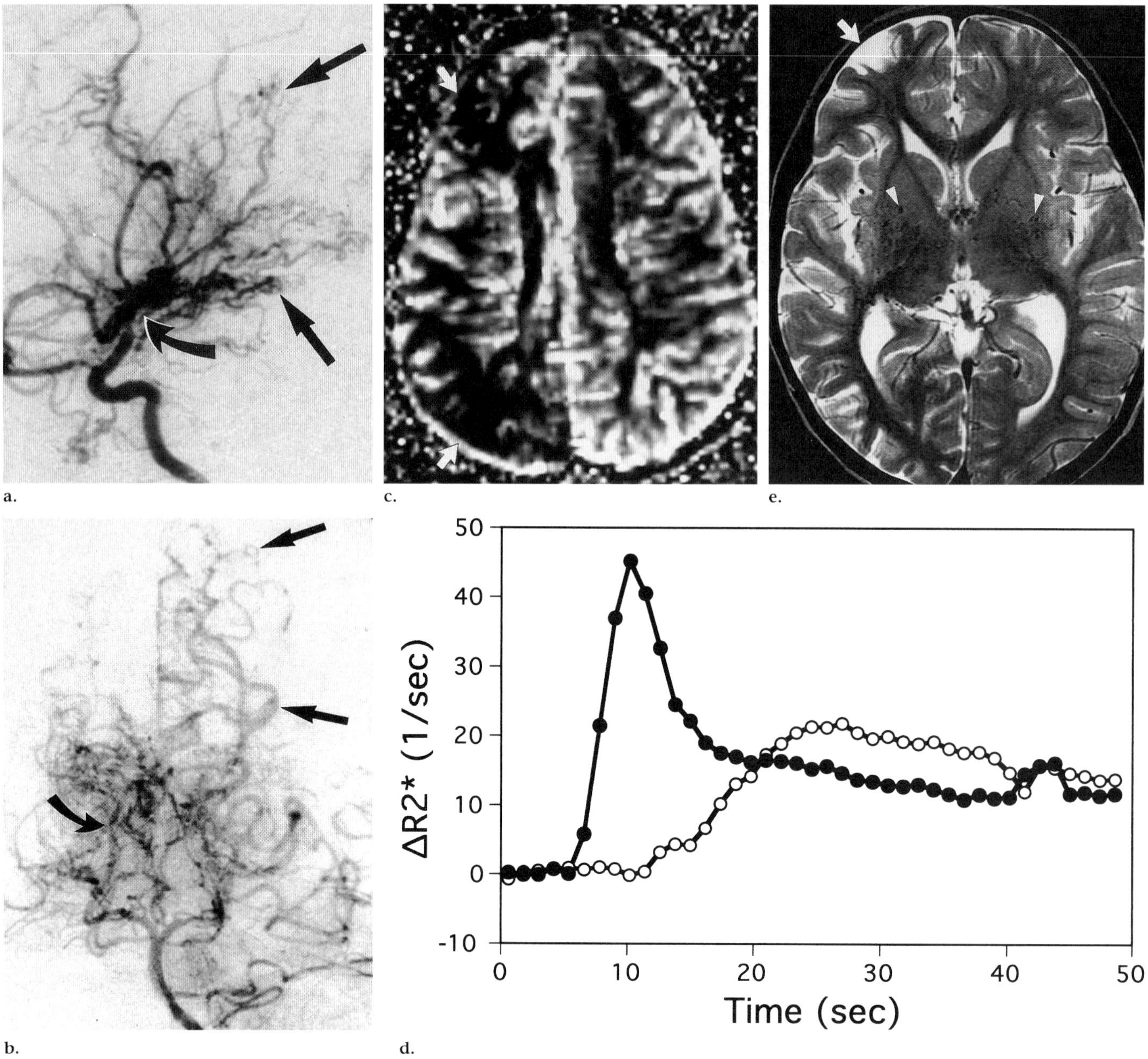

Figure 1. Moyamoya disease in a 4-year-old girl. **(a)** Right internal carotid arteriogram in lateral projection shows the right ICA (curved arrow) is occluded, and thus the anterior cerebral and middle cerebral arteries are occluded. Marked moyamoya vessels (straight arrows) are seen, and peripheral branches of the anterior cerebral and middle cerebral arteries are delineated by the collateral vessels. **(b)** Left vertebral arteriogram in frontal projection shows the right PCA (curved arrow) is occluded. There were no leptomeningeal collateral vessels to the anterior circulation of the right cerebral hemisphere. However, the enlarged branches of the left PCA have developed numerous leptomeningeal collateral vessels (straight arrows) to the anterior circulation of the left cerebral hemisphere. **(c)** Axial ΔR2* image (∞/54) shows areas of decreased perfusion (arrows) in the right cerebral hemisphere, which has PCA occlusion, as compared with the left cerebral hemisphere. **(d)** Time-ΔR2* curves show a decreased peak value and a delayed peak time for the right cerebral hemisphere (○), which had PCA occlusion, as compared with the left cerebral hemisphere (●). **(e)** Axial T2-weighted turbo spin-echo MR image (4,000/96) shows infarctions in the right frontal (arrow) and parietal lobes. There are numerous moyamoya vessels (arrowheads) in the bilateral basal ganglia.

Diffusion-weighted and conventional MR images were reviewed by two radiologists (I.Y., Y.H.) for cerebral infarctions. At conventional MR imaging, an infarction was diagnosed for lesions that showed an abnormal signal intensity on both T1- and T2-weighted images but not for lesions that showed an abnormal signal intensity in the deep white matter on only T2-weighted images. On diffusion-weighted MR images, an acute infarction was diagnosed for lesions that showed a high signal intensity on heavily diffusion-weighted images with a gradient factor b of 1,100 sec/mm^2.

The ADC values were estimated for these lesions, and the ADC ratios were calculated by dividing the ADC value in these regions by the normal ADC value in the anatomically matched site of the contralateral cerebral hemisphere. To examine the relationships between the perfu-

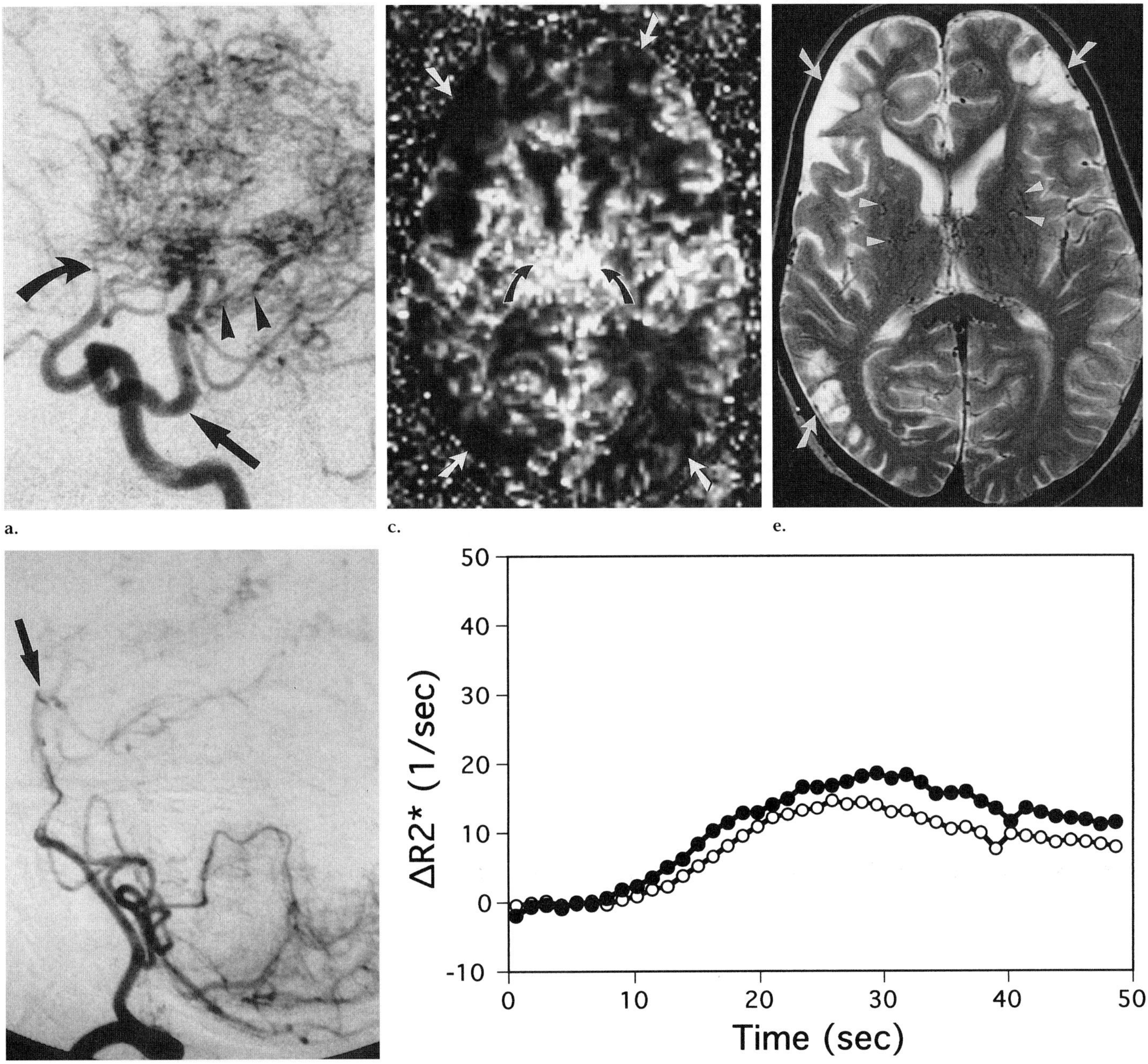

a. c. e. b. d.

Figure 2. Moyamoya disease in a 9-year-old boy. **(a)** Right internal carotid arteriogram in lateral projection shows the right ICA (curved arrow) is occluded, and thus the anterior cerebral and middle cerebral arteries are occluded. There are marked moyamoya vessels. Through the persistent primitive trigeminal artery (straight arrow), the basilar artery and its branches are opacified, but both PCAs are occluded in their proximal portions (arrowheads). **(b)** Left vertebral arteriogram in lateral projection shows both PCAs (arrow) are occluded. There were no leptomeningeal collateral vessels to the anterior circulation. **(c)** Axial ΔR2* image (∞/54) shows extensive areas of decreased perfusion (straight arrows) in both cerebral hemispheres, which have PCA occlusions, as compared with perfusion in the basal ganglia (curved arrows). **(d)** Time-ΔR2* curves show a decreased peak value and a delayed peak time for the right (○) and left (●) cerebral hemispheres, which had PCA occlusions. **(e)** Axial T2-weighted turbo spin-echo MR image (4,000/96) shows extensive infarctions (arrows) in bilateral frontal and right parietal lobes. There are numerous moyamoya vessels (arrowheads) in the bilateral basal ganglia.

sion parameters and ADC values, we selected several regions of interest for these acute infarctions.

Imaging studies were evaluated on the basis of blinded, separate interpretations by two independent radiologists (I.Y., Y.H.). Furthermore, MR images were interpreted independently, without knowledge of the angiographic findings. In instances in which the radiologists did not fully agree, diagnosis was achieved by consensus.

Finally, a statistical analysis of the comparisons between groups was performed with the Spearman rank correlation test, unpaired Student *t* test, χ^2 test, or Mann-Whitney *U* test. The statistical tests were corrected for multiple comparisons. Linear regression analysis was used to assess the relationships between the perfusion parameters and ADC values. A P value of less than .05 was considered to indicate a statistically significant difference.

RESULTS

Stenotic or Occlusive Lesions and ΔR2* Images

In all 17 patients, stenosis or occlusion of the supraclinoid portion of the ICA and of the proximal portions of the anterior cerebral artery and middle cerebral artery was detected bilaterally (Figs 1, 2). The stages of stenotic or occlusive lesions in the 34 ICA bifurcations were as follows: stage 1, three arteries; stage 2, seven arteries; stage 3, 16 arteries; stage 4, five arteries; and stage 5, three arteries. Furthermore, of the 34 PCAs, six arteries were found to be stenotic, and eight arteries were occluded (Figs 1, 2). Thus, a total of 14 PCAs (41%) in 11 patients had stenotic or occlusive lesions.

As shown in Table 1, the ΔR2* peak value ratios for the frontal, temporal, parietal, and occipital lobes decreased significantly with PCA stenosis, with a greater decrease with PCA occlusion (Spearman rank correlation test) (Figs 1, 2). In contrast, the ΔR2* peak value ratio for the basal ganglia increased with PCA stenosis or occlusion (Spearman rank correlation test). Furthermore, the ΔR2* peak time ratios for the frontal, temporal, parietal, and occipital lobes increased significantly with PCA stenosis, with a greater increase with PCA occlusion (Spearman rank correlation test).

However, the ΔR2* integral ratios did not significantly correlate with PCA stenosis and occlusion, with the exception of that for the occipital lobe, which increased with PCA stenosis or occlusion (Spearman rank correlation test). Thus, the presence of stenotic or occlusive PCA lesions was markedly related to both the ΔR2* peak value and ΔR2* peak time ratios in patients with moyamoya disease.

In contrast, on ΔR2* images, the stage of stenotic or occlusive lesions of the ICA bifurcation did not correlate significantly with the ΔR2* peak value, ΔR2* peak time, or ΔR2* integral ratios ($P > .05$ for all, Spearman rank correlation test). When stages 1, 2, and 3 were grouped as stenotic and stages 4 and 5 were grouped as occluded, there was no significant difference between the two groups of the ICA bifurcation lesions for the ΔR2* peak value, ΔR2* peak time, and ΔR2* integral ratios ($P > .05$ for all, unpaired Student t test).

TABLE 1
ΔR2* Ratios and Grade of PCA Lesion in Patients with Moyamoya Disease

Region	Grade of PCA Lesion: Normal (n = 20)	Stenotic (n = 6)	Occluded (n = 8)	P Value*
ΔR2* Peak Value Ratio				
Frontal	0.93 ± 0.14	0.81 ± 0.18	0.71 ± 0.10	<.001
Temporal	1.15 ± 0.19	1.04 ± 0.10	0.78 ± 0.35	<.01
Parietal	1.09 ± 0.18	1.01 ± 0.24	0.80 ± 0.27	<.05
Occipital	1.11 ± 0.21	0.85 ± 0.11	0.77 ± 0.19	<.001
Basal ganglia	1.04 ± 0.13	1.07 ± 0.25	1.33 ± 0.31	<.05
All	1.06 ± 0.11	0.96 ± 0.10	0.88 ± 0.12	<.001
ΔR2* Peak Time Ratio				
Frontal	1.04 ± 0.11	1.02 ± 0.15	1.22 ± 0.14	<.05
Temporal	0.89 ± 0.12	1.00 ± 0.14	1.21 ± 0.40	<.01
Parietal	0.99 ± 0.14	1.16 ± 0.17	1.53 ± 0.33	<.001
Occipital	0.87 ± 0.16	1.06 ± 0.05	1.18 ± 0.23	<.001
Basal ganglia	0.84 ± 0.15	0.80 ± 0.10	0.72 ± 0.16	>.05
All	0.93 ± 0.12	1.01 ± 0.04	1.17 ± 0.16	<.001
ΔR2* Integral Ratio				
Frontal	0.96 ± 0.14	0.83 ± 0.12	0.92 ± 0.17	>.05
Temporal	1.00 ± 0.28	1.21 ± 0.18	0.98 ± 0.53	>.05
Parietal	1.06 ± 0.45	1.15 ± 0.24	1.17 ± 0.62	>.05
Occipital	0.91 ± 0.23	1.03 ± 0.12	1.15 ± 0.34	<.05
Basal ganglia	0.96 ± 0.20	0.84 ± 0.21	1.02 ± 0.30	>.05
All	0.98 ± 0.80	1.01 ± 0.06	1.05 ± 0.11	>.05

Note.—Data are means ± SD.
* Based on the Spearman rank correlation test.

Collateral Vessels and ΔR2* Images

In all 17 patients, basal cerebral moyamoya vessels were detected bilaterally in the cerebral hemispheres (Figs 1, 2). The grades of the moyamoya vessels in the 34 cerebral hemispheres were as follows: slight, 20 hemispheres; moderate, eight hemispheres; and marked, six hemispheres. Furthermore, leptomeningeal collateral vessels from the PCA to the anterior circulation were detected in 18 cerebral hemispheres (53%) (Fig 1). However, in hemispheres that had occlusion of the PCA, no leptomeningeal collateral vessels from the PCA to the anterior circulation were apparent (Figs 1, 2).

As shown in Table 2, the ΔR2* peak value ratios for the frontal, temporal, parietal, and occipital lobes were significantly greater when leptomeningeal collateral vessels were present than when they were not (unpaired Student t test) (Figs 1, 2). The ΔR2* peak time ratios for the frontal, temporal, parietal, and occipital lobes were significantly smaller when leptomeningeal collateral vessels were present than when they were not (unpaired Student t test). However, the ΔR2* integral ratios did not significantly correlate with the presence of the leptomeningeal collateral vessels, with the exception of that for the occipital lobe, which was smaller in the presence of such vessels (unpaired Student t test). Thus, the presence of leptomeningeal collateral vessels was closely related to both the ΔR2* peak value and ΔR2* peak time ratios.

However, on ΔR2* images, the grade of the basal cerebral moyamoya vessels did not significantly correlate with the ΔR2* peak value, ΔR2* peak time, or ΔR2* integral ratios, with the exception of the ΔR2* peak time ratio for the basal ganglia, which decreased as the grade of moyamoya vessels increased ($P < .01$, unpaired Student t test).

Cerebral Infarctions on Diffusion-weighted and Conventional MR Images

Of the 34 cerebral hemispheres in the 17 patients, cerebral infarctions were detected in 14 hemispheres (41%) on conventional MR images (Figs 1, 2). As shown in Table 3, the frequency of cerebral infarction significantly increased with PCA stenosis, with a greater increase with PCA occlusion (Mann-Whitney U test) (Figs 1, 2). Thus, the presence of stenotic or occlusive PCA lesions was related to the occurrence of cerebral infarction in patients

TABLE 2
ΔR2* Ratios and Leptomeningeal Collateral Vessels in Patients with Moyamoya Disease

Region	Leptomeningeal Collateral Vessels: Absent (n = 16)	Leptomeningeal Collateral Vessels: Present (n = 18)	P Value*
	ΔR2* Peak Value Ratio		
Frontal	0.78 ± 0.15	0.93 ± 0.15	<.01
Temporal	0.95 ± 0.30	1.13 ± 0.20	<.05
Parietal	0.91 ± 0.26	1.10 ± 0.19	<.05
Occipital	0.84 ± 0.18	1.12 ± 0.22	<.001
Basal ganglia	1.19 ± 0.30	1.05 ± 0.13	>.05
All	0.93 ± 0.12	1.06 ± 0.11	<.01
	ΔR2* Peak Time Ratio		
Frontal	1.13 ± 0.16	1.03 ± 0.11	<.05
Temporal	1.08 ± 0.30	0.89 ± 0.13	<.05
Parietal	1.34 ± 0.31	0.98 ± 0.14	<.001
Occipital	1.12 ± 0.18	0.86 ± 0.16	<.001
Basal ganglia	0.77 ± 0.14	0.84 ± 0.16	>.05
All	1.09 ± 0.14	0.92 ± 0.12	<.001
	ΔR2* Integral Ratio		
Frontal	0.90 ± 0.15	0.95 ± 0.15	>.05
Temporal	1.10 ± 0.39	0.97 ± 0.29	>.05
Parietal	1.13 ± 0.46	1.08 ± 0.47	>.05
Occipital	1.08 ± 0.25	0.90 ± 0.24	<.05
Basal ganglia	0.96 ± 0.26	0.95 ± 0.20	>.05
All	1.03 ± 0.08	0.97 ± 0.08	<.05

Note.—Leptomeningeal collateral vessels extend from the PCA to the anterior circulation. Data are means ± SD.
* Based on the Student t test.

TABLE 3
Angiographic Findings and Cerebral Infarction on MR Images in Patients with Moyamoya Disease

Angiographic Findings	Cerebral Infarction: Absent (n = 20)	Cerebral Infarction: Present (n = 14)	P Value*
PCA lesion			
Normal (n = 20)	18	2	...
Stenotic (n = 6)	2	4	<.001
Occluded (n = 8)	0	8	...
Stage of ICA bifurcation			...
1 (n = 3)	3	0	...
2 (n = 7)	4	3	...
3 (n = 16)	11	5	>.05
4 (n = 5)	2	3	...
5 (n = 3)	0	3	...

* Based on the Mann-Whitney U test.

with moyamoya disease. However, the stage of stenotic or occlusive lesions of the ICA bifurcation did not significantly correlate with cerebral infarction.

Furthermore, acute-phase infarctions were identified in three hemispheres (9%) on diffusion-weighted MR images (Fig 3). All three acute-phase infarctions detected on diffusion-weighted MR images also occurred in cerebral hemispheres with stenotic or occlusive PCA lesions; two occurred with PCA occlusion, and one occurred with PCA stenosis. These acute infarctions were readily apparent as areas of high signal intensity on heavily diffusion-weighted MR images (Fig 3). The calculated ADC values for these infarctions ranged from 0.158×10^{-3} to 0.656×10^{-3} mm²/sec, and the ADC ratios ranged from 0.199 to 0.711.

With the use of linear regression analysis, we also examined the relationships between the perfusion parameters and ADC values for these acute infarctions (Fig 4). The ΔR2* peak value ratio was postively correlated with the ADC value (r = 0.872, P < .01), and the ΔR2* peak time ratio was negatively correlated with the ADC value (r = −0.680, P < .05). The ΔR2* integral ratio also was positively correlated with the ADC value (r = 0.831, P < .01). Thus, the decrease in the ΔR2* peak value ratio, the increase in the ΔR2* peak time ratio, and the decrease in the ΔR2* integral ratio correlated significantly with the decrease in the ADC value for acute infarctions in patients with moyamoya disease.

DISCUSSION

We have shown that, of the 34 PCAs in the 17 patients with moyamoya disease that were examined, 14 arteries (41%) in 11 patients exhibited stenotic or occlusive lesions. When the PCA had stenotic or occlusive lesions, the ΔR2* peak value ratio for the cerebral hemispheres decreased significantly and the corresponding ΔR2* peak time ratio increased significantly. Thus, the presence of stenotic or occlusive PCA lesions is significantly associated with a decrease in the ΔR2* peak value and an increase in the ΔR2* peak time in patients with moyamoya disease. However, no significant correlation was apparent between the stenotic or occlusive lesions of the ICA bifurcation and the ΔR2* peak value or ΔR2* peak time.

These data indicate cerebral ischemia in individuals with moyamoya disease increases with stenotic or occlusive lesions of the posterior circulation, rather than with stenotic or occlusive lesions of the anterior circulation. To our knowledge, the role of the posterior circulation in moyamoya disease has not previously been evaluated at perfusion echo-planar MR imaging.

Furthermore, the presence of leptomeningeal collateral vessels from the PCA to the anterior circulation was shown to be significantly correlated with the ΔR2* peak value and ΔR2* peak time for the cerebral hemispheres. In patients with moyamoya disease in whom both ICA bifurcations are occluded, the leptomeningeal collateral vessels become a major provider of a compensatory cerebral blood supply (13,14). Thus, any decrease in the number of leptomeningeal collateral vessels would critically influence the cerebral blood flow. The reduction in the

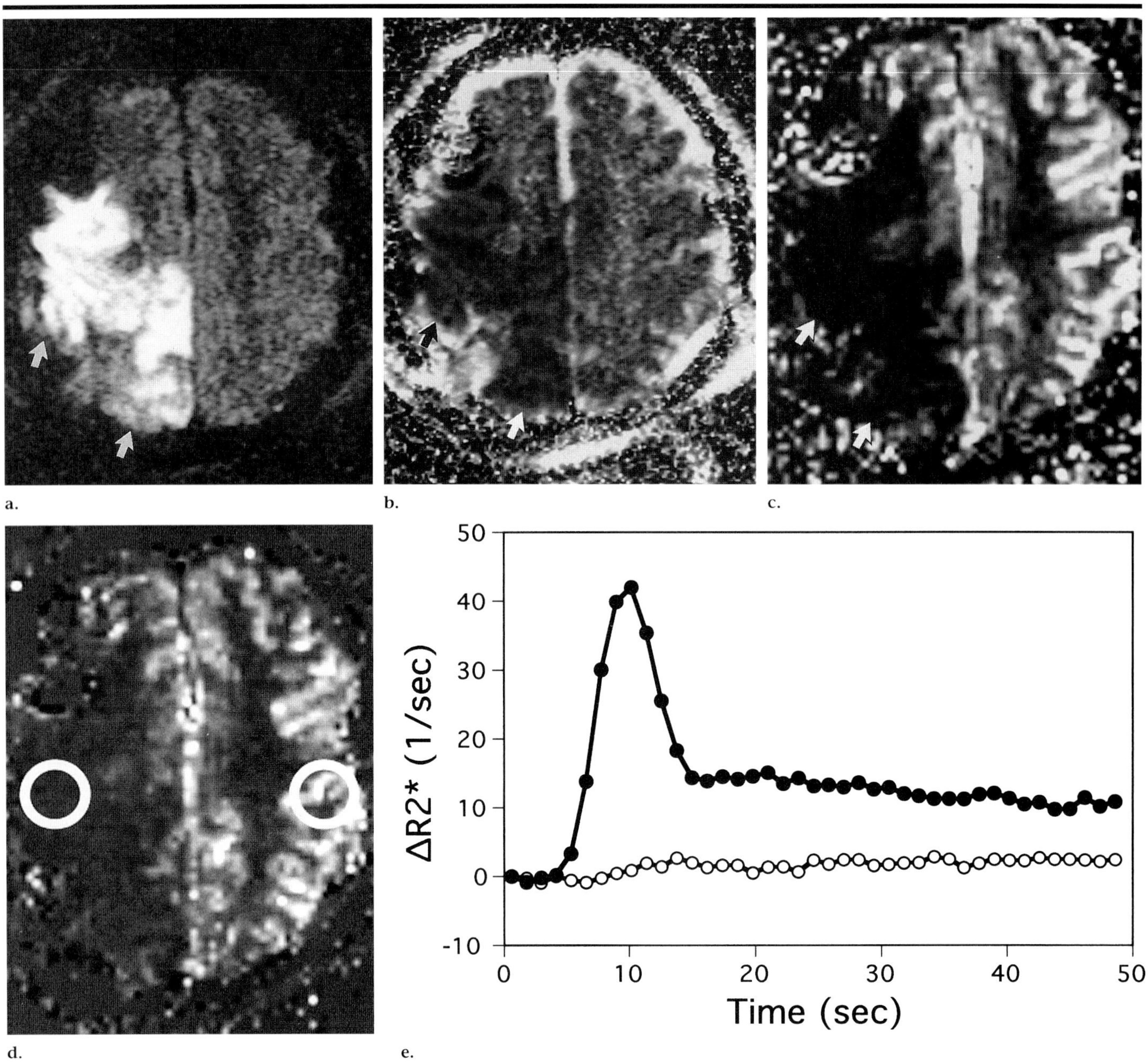

Figure 3. Moyamoya disease manifesting acute cerebral infarction in a 45-year-old woman. **(a)** Axial diffusion-weighted MR image (∞/123) with a gradient factor b of 1,100 sec/mm^2 shows irregularly shaped areas of high signal intensity (arrows) in the right parietal lobe. **(b)** Axial ADC map (∞/123) shows areas of decreased ADC (arrows) in the right parietal lobe. **(c)** Axial ΔR2* image (∞/54) shows areas of decreased perfusion (arrows) for the acute infarction, as compared with perfusion in the contralateral cerebral hemisphere. **(d)** Axial ΔR2* image (∞/54) demonstrates how the regions of interest (○) were drawn to assess the regional cerebral perfusion parameters. **(e)** Time-ΔR2* curves show a markedly decreased peak value and a delayed peak time for the acute infarction (○), as compared with those in the contralateral cerebral hemisphere (●).

number of leptomeningeal collateral vessels may be due to the progressive stenotic or occlusive lesions of the PCA. When the PCA finally becomes occluded, the leptomeningeal collateral vessels presumably disappear, thereby resulting in severe cerebral ischemia.

In contrast, the grade of the basal cerebral moyamoya vessels in patients with moyamoya disease did not correlate with the ΔR2* peak value or ΔR2* peak time. Thus, although the presence of basal cerebral moyamoya vessels is a characteristic of moyamoya disease (1,2), the contribution of the basal cerebral moyamoya vessels to the cerebral blood flow appears to be much less than that of the leptomeningeal collateral vessels.

On the basis of the conventional MR images, the frequency of cerebral infarction significantly increased with PCA stenosis, with a greater increase with PCA occlusion. Thus, the presence of stenotic or occlusive PCA lesions appears to be significantly related to the occurrence of cerebral infarction in patients with moyamoya disease. However, no significant correlation was apparent between the stage of stenotic or occlusive lesions of the ICA bifurcation and cerebral infarction.

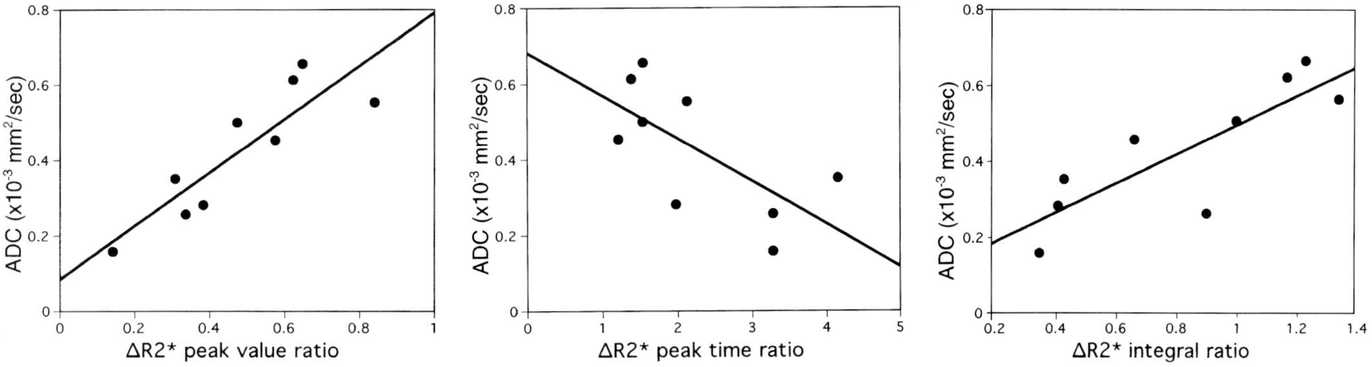

a. b. c.

Figure 4. Relationships between the perfusion parameters and ADC values in three acute cerebral infarctions in patients with moyamoya disease. Note that there are multiple points per patient, as explained in Materials and Methods. **(a)** Plot of the ΔR2* peak value ratio versus the ADC shows a significant positive correlation (r = 0.872, $P < .01$). **(b)** Plot of the ΔR2* peak time ratio versus the ADC shows a significant negative correlation (r = -0.680, $P < .05$). **(c)** Plot of the ΔR2* integral ratio versus the ADC shows a significant positive correlation (r = 0.831, $P < .01$).

Our data demonstrate that diffusion-weighted MR images were useful for the detection of acute cerebral infarctions in patients with moyamoya disease. The acute infarctions also occurred in cerebral hemispheres with stenotic or occlusive PCA lesions. Furthermore, the decrease in the ΔR2* peak value ratio, the increase in the ΔR2* peak time ratio, and the decrease in the ΔR2* integral ratio correlated significantly with the decrease in ADC value for these acute infarctions.

Results of recent studies (15–18) with animal models of ischemia have revealed an important relationship between the peak ΔR2* ratios and ADC values. The results of these studies and our data indicate reduced and delayed perfusion is directly related to the mechanism of ADC reduction in acute infarctions due to moyamoya disease.

Diffusion-weighted and perfusion echo-planar MR imaging may affect the treatment of patients with moyamoya disease. The noninvasive assessment of cerebral ischemia with diffusion-weighted and perfusion echo-planar MR imaging may have value in following up disease progression, planning surgical treatment, and evaluating patients postoperatively.

In conclusion, regional cerebral perfusion in patients with moyamoya disease is decreased and delayed with PCA stenosis, with a greater decrease and delay with PCA occlusion. If the PCA is occluded, the number of leptomeningeal collateral vessels to the anterior circulation presumably decreases, thereby causing severe cerebral ischemia that results in an infarction. In acute infarctions, the ADC reduction correlates with decreased and delayed perfusion. Thus, diffusion-weighted and perfusion echo-planar MR imaging are useful methods for evaluating cerebral ischemia in patients with moyamoya disease.

References

1. Nishimoto A, Takeuchi S. Abnormal cerebrovascular network related to the internal carotid arteries. J Neurosurg 1968; 29:255–260.
2. Suzuki J, Takaku A. Cerebrovascular "moyamoya" disease: disease showing abnormal net-like vessels in base of brain. Arch Neurol 1969; 20:288–299.
3. Taveras JM. Multiple progressive intracranial arterial occlusions: a syndrome of children and young adults. AJR 1969; 106:235–268.
4. Pecker J, Simon J, Guy G, Herry JF. Nishimoto's disease: significance of its angiographic appearances. Neuroradiology 1973; 5:223–230.
5. Takahashi M. Magnification angiography in moyamoya disease: new observations on collateral vessels. Radiology 1980; 136: 379–386.
6. Yamada I, Himeno Y, Suzuki S, Matsushima Y. Posterior circulation in moyamoya disease: angiographic study. Radiology 1995; 197:239–246.
7. Warach S, Dashe JF, Edelman RR. Clinical outcome in ischemic stroke predicted by early diffusion-weighted and perfusion magnetic resonance imaging: a preliminary analysis. J Cereb Blood Flow Metab 1996; 16:53–59.
8. Sorensen AG, Buonanno FS, Gonzalez RG, et al. Hyperacute stroke: evaluation with combined multisection diffusion-weighted and hemodynamically weighted echo-planar MR imaging. Radiology 1996; 199: 391–401.
9. Marks MP, de Crespigny A, Lentz D, Enzmann DR, Albers GW, Moseley ME. Acute and chronic stroke: navigated spin-echo diffusion-weighted MR imaging. Radiology 1996; 199:403–408.
10. Gückel FJ, Brix G, Schmiedek P, et al. Cerebrovascular reverse capacity in patients with occlusive cerebrovascular disease: assessment with dynamic susceptibility contrast-enhanced MR imaging and the acetazolamide stimulation test. Radiology 1996; 201:405–412.
11. Tsuchiya K, Inaoka S, Mizutani Y, Hachiya J. Echo-planar perfusion MR of moyamoya disease. AJNR 1998; 19:211–216.
12. Aronen HJ, Gazit IE, Louis DN, et al. Cerebral blood volume maps of gliomas: comparison with tumor grade and histologic findings. Radiology 1994; 191:41–51.
13. Yamada I, Matsushima Y, Suzuki S. Childhood moyamoya disease before and after encephalo-duro-arterio-synangiosis: an angiographic study. Neuroradiology 1992; 34:318–322.
14. Yamada I, Murata Y, Umehara I, Suzuki S, Matsushima Y. SPECT and MRI evaluations of the posterior circulation in moyamoya disease. J Nucl Med 1996; 37:1613–1617.
15. Kucharczyk J, Vexler ZS, Roberts TP, et al. Echo-planar perfusion-sensitive MR imaging of acute cerebral ischemia. Radiology 1993; 188:711–717.
16. Roberts TP, Vexler Z, Derugin N, Moseley ME, Kucharczyk J. High-speed MR imaging of ischemic brain injury following stenosis of the middle cerebral artery. J Cereb Blood Flow Metab 1993; 13:940–946.
17. Pierce AR, Lo EH, Mandeville JB, Gonzalez RG, Rosen BR, Wolf GL. MRI measurements of water diffusion and cerebral perfusion: their relationship in a rat model of focal cerebral ischemia. J Cereb Blood Flow Metab 1997; 17:183–190.
18. Kuroiwa T, Nagaoka T, Ueki M, Yamada I, Miyasaka N, Akimoto H. Different apparent diffusion coefficient: water-content correlations of gray and white matter during early ischemia. Stroke 1998; 29: 859–865.

Christophe Cognard, MD
Alain Weill, MD
Laurent Spelle, MD
Michel Piotin, MD
Lina Castaings, MD
Alain Rey, MD
Jacques Moret, MD

Long-term Angiographic Follow-up of 169 Intracranial Berry Aneurysms Occluded with Detachable Coils[1]

PURPOSE: To evaluate the stability of aneurysm occlusion at follow-up angiography after endovascular treatment (EVT) with detachable coils in intracranial berry aneurysms.

MATERIALS AND METHODS: A total of 203 berry aneurysms (<1.5 cm) were treated with EVT. Follow-up angiography at least 3 months later was performed in 169 cases.

RESULTS: Complete occlusion of the aneurysm sac and neck was achieved in 148 aneurysms, subtotal occlusion in 18, and incomplete occlusion in three. Recurrence occurred between 3 and 40 months in 20 (14%) of the 148 totally occluded aneurysms. A second treatment was performed in five cases, was scheduled in one, and failed in one. The small neck remnant increased in size but did not require any retreatment in three cases, and the size of the neck remnant remained stable in 10 cases. Remnant regrowth occurred in six of the 18 subtotally occluded aneurysms. A second treatment was performed in three. Of the 169 cases, last follow-up angiography showed total occlusion in 133 cases, subtotal in 30, and incomplete in six. No rebleeding occurred.

CONCLUSION: A very small recurrence may be observed at the level of the neck of the aneurysm at long-term follow-up angiography despite achieving total occlusion initially with detachable coils.

Index terms:
Aneurysm, intracranial, 1728.73
Angiography, 1722.1247
Arteries, therapeutic blockade 1723.1264, 1731.1264, 1733.1264, 174.1264, 175.1264
Brain, hemorrhage, 10.367

Radiology 1999; 212:348–356

Abbreviation:
EVT = endovascular treatment

[1] From the Department of Interventional Neuroradiology, Fondation Ophtalmologique Adolphe de Rothschild, 25 rue Manin, 75940 Paris 19, France (C.C., A.W., L.S., M.P., L.C., J.M.) and Department of Neurosurgery, Hopital Beaujon, Clichy, France (A.R.). Received November 12, 1997; revision requested February 16, 1998; revision received July 10; accepted February 12, 1999. **Address reprint requests to** J.M. (e-mail: *moretnri@fo-rothschild.fr*).

Author contributions:
Guarantors of integrity of entire study, A.R., J.M.; study concepts and design, C.C., J.M.; definition of intellectual content, C.C., J.M.; literature research, C.C., L.S.; clinical studies, C.C., A.W., L.S., M.P., L.C.; data acquisition, C.C., A.W.; data analysis, C.C.; statistical analysis, C.C.; manuscript preparation and review, C.C., J.M.; manuscript editing, C.C.

The therapeutic treatment plan for intracranial berry (<1.5-cm) aneurysms is, at the present time, extremely variable from one country to another, and even from one institution to another, and remains tremendously questionable. Selective endovascular treatment (EVT) with Gugliemi detachable coils (GDC; Target Therapeutics, Fremont, Calif) is now the treatment of choice for nonsurgical aneurysms (1–7). Treatment of surgical aneurysms is much more controversial. The comparison between surgical clipping and EVT poses two main questions. The first question revolves around providing protection against rebleeding for ruptured aneurysms, the feasibility of the treatment in the acute phase after the rupture, its morbidity and mortality, and technical complications of the treatment. Results of EVT compared with those of surgery were recently reported and, although much debated, may be accurately evaluated (8–15). The second question is stability of the occlusion with detachable coils and the efficacy in providing protection against growth or regrowth of the aneurysm and consequent bleeding, in ruptured or nonruptured aneurysms. To our knowledge, there are no answers to these questions at this time.

The aim of this study was to document the preliminary results of evaluating the long-term angiographic stability of the occlusion of intracranial aneurysms with detachable coils.

MATERIALS AND METHODS

All the patients were enrolled in a clinical study for the treatment of intracranial aneurysms with detachable coils (Gugliemi detachable coils [GDC]; Target Therapeutics) in France.

TABLE 1
Location of the 169 Aneurysms

Location	No. of Aneurysms
Internal carotid artery	59 (35)
Anterior communicating artery	41 (24)
Middle cerebral artery	34 (20)
Vertebrobasilar artery	27 (16)
Pericallosal artery	3 (2)
Posteroinferior cerebellar artery	3 (2)
Posterior cerebral artery	2 (1)
Total	169 (100)

Note.—Numbers in parentheses are percentages.

TABLE 2
Evolution of the 148 Aneurysms with Total Occlusion

Follow-up Angiography	Mean Delay* (mo)	No. of Recurrences†	Total‡
First	3	8 (5)	148
Second	18	9 (9)	99
Third	38	3 (8)	39

* Time interval between treatment and follow-up angiography.
† Numbers in parentheses are percentages.
‡ Total number of aneurysms followed up.

The French National Ethics Committee (Loi Hurier) allowed four different centers in the entire country to participate in this clinical study. All patients were apprised of the study protocol and signed an informed consent form.

From November 1992 to November 1996, 236 berry aneurysms (<1.5 cm) in 208 patients were intended to be treated with detachable coils. Treatment was achieved in 203 aneurysms in 182 patients (9). Sixteen patients died—nine of subarachnoid hemorrhage, four of complications of the treatment, one of rebleeding of an incompletely occluded aneurysm, one of aneurysm rupture during surgery of an associated aneurysm, and one of a nonrelated disease. Thus, 166 patients with 187 aneurysms were treated and could be followed up. Each patient was scheduled for follow-up angiography at 3 months, 18 months, and 3–4-year intervals after treatment. Angiography was planned for all patients with subtotal or incomplete occlusions. Eighteen patients, mostly those who lived outside France, were lost to follow up. Of the 187 aneurysms treated, 169 (90%) had at least one follow-up angiography at 3 months.

Clinical symptoms, location of the aneurysm, size of the first coil, and aneurysm sac size–to–neck diameter ratio were all taken into consideration. In this series, we evaluated the evolution of the occlusion on follow-up angiograms in these 169 treated aneurysms; all were reevaluated at 3 months. Of the 169 aneurysms, 107 aneurysms were ruptured and 62 were not ruptured. The locations of all the aneurysms are detailed in Table 1. The size of the first coil was taken in 161 aneurysms as an indirect measurement of the aneurysm sac size. Aneurysms were classified as small berry (2- or 3-mm-diameter coils; 52 cases [32%]), medium berry (4- or 5-mm-diameter coils; 57 cases [35%]), or large berry (6-, 7-, or 8-mm-diameter coils; 52 cases [32%]). The ratio between aneurysm sac size and neck diameter was classified as 1, between 1 and 2, and 2, for the small, medium, and large berry classifications, respectively. We were able to accurately estimate the size of the neck and obtain the ratio in 136 (84%) of the 161 aneurysms. The ratio was 1 in 37 cases (27%), between 1 and 2 in 66 cases (49%), and 2 in 33 cases (24%).

The percentage occlusion rate at the end of the procedure and at follow-up angiography was classified as follows: 100% or total occlusion when the sac and neck were densely packed (Fig 1), 95%–99% or subtotal occlusion when the sac was occluded but there was a suspicion of a neck remnant or an obvious tiny neck remnant (Fig 2), less than 95% or incomplete occlusion when there was loose packing and/or persistent opacification of the sac or neck remnant.

An aneurysm was considered recurrent if a previously totally occluded aneurysm was seen to have a change in the coil mesh and partial or even small recanalization of the neck at follow-up angiography (Fig 1). In addition, an aneurysm was considered remnant regrowth if a subtotally occluded aneurysm was found to have an increasing neck remnant at follow-up angiography (Fig 2).

The results were subjected to statistical analysis by using a standard χ^2 test. Recurrence rate was correlated to clinical presentation, ratio between aneurysm sac size and neck diameter, aneurysm location, and aneurysm size. The significant P value was less than .05.

RESULTS

Overall Findings

At the end of the initial procedure, occlusion of the 169 aneurysms was total in 95 cases (56%), subtotal in 66 cases (39%), and incomplete in eight cases (5%). Because of initial subtotal or incomplete occlusion, a second procedure was performed in 18 cases, with total occlusion in 14 (Fig 2), subtotal in three, and incomplete in one. Furthermore, the first follow-up angiogram confirmed total occlusion in 39 aneurysms, the occlusion of which was considered uncertain at the end of the first treatment. To clarify the analysis, these aneurysms were initially considered subtotally occluded because we were not able to accurately assess a total occlusion, but they were retrospectively included into the group of initially totally occluded cases. Overall then, total occlusion was obtained in 148 (88%) of the 169 aneurysms: 95 initially, 14 after a second treatment, and 39 with occlusion initially uncertain but confirmed to be total on the first follow-up angiogram. A subtotal occlusion was obtained in 18 cases ([11%] in three cases despite a second treatment), and an incomplete occlusion was obtained in three cases ([2%] in one case despite a second treatment).

Evolution of the 148 Aneurysms with Total Occlusion

At the first follow-up angiographic examination (mean, 3 months), a recurrence was observed in eight of the 148 aneurysms (5%) (Table 2). Ninety-nine aneurysms totally occluded at first follow-up angiography underwent second follow-up angiography (mean, 18 months), and a recurrence was observed in nine (9%). Thirty-nine aneurysms totally occluded at second follow-up angiography underwent third angiography (mean, 38 months), and a recurrence was observed in three (8%) (Fig 3).

Overall, a recurrence was observed in 20 of the 148 aneurysms (14%). A second treatment was required in five aneurysms: Total occlusion was attained in four of these five. In the remaining case, a second selective treatment was considered impossible to perform due to the morphology of the sac (laterobasilar wide-neck aneurysm), and occlusion of the basilar artery was performed. At the time of this writing, a second treatment was scheduled in one case; in another case, the second treatment failed. In 10 cases, the small remnant at the level of the aneurysm neck was followed for 12–46 months (mean, 25 months) and remained stable. The very tiny neck recurrence did not require (or allow) retreatment (Fig 4).

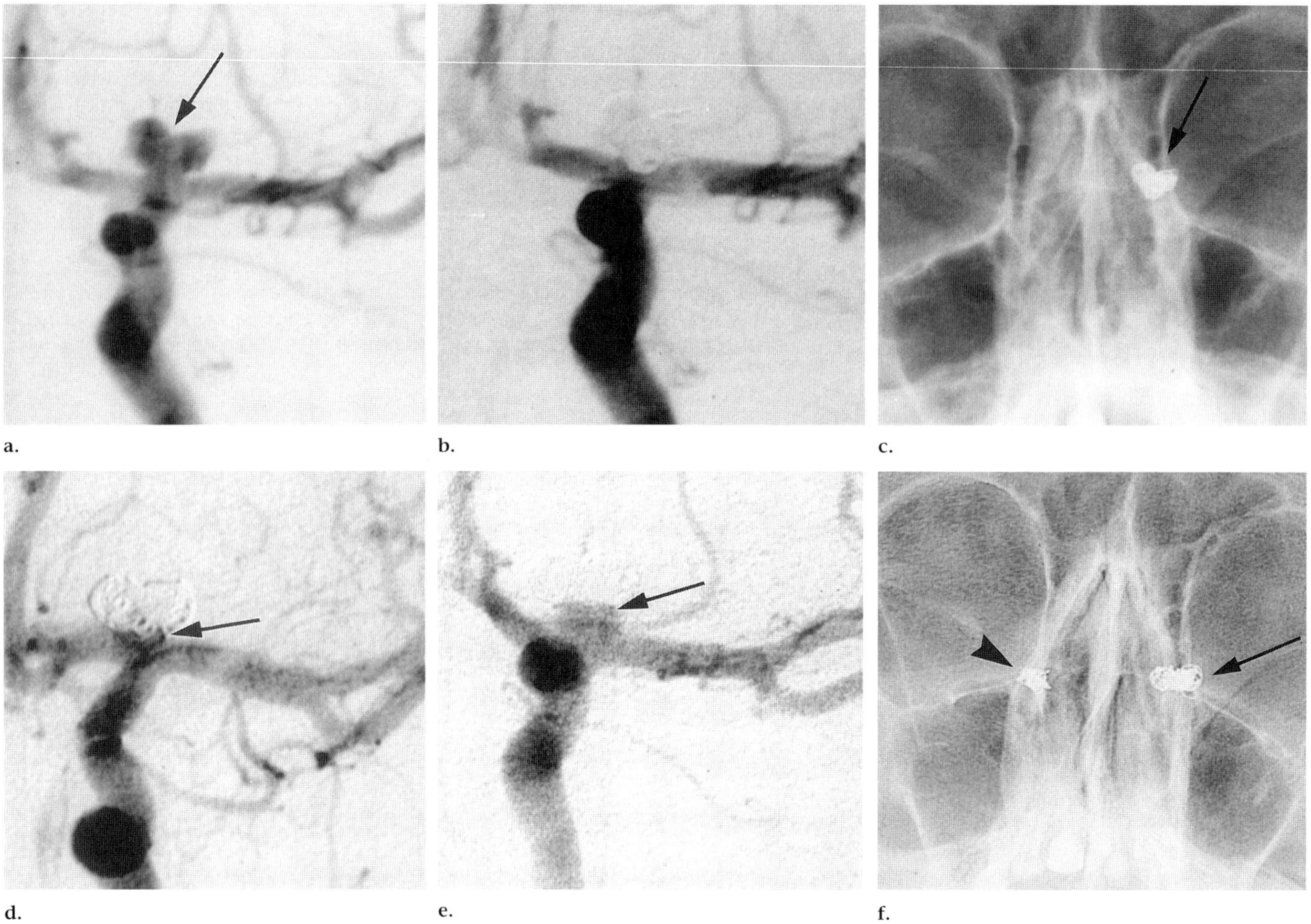

Figure 1. (a) Pretreatment angiogram shows a bilobular ruptured aneurysm (arrow) of the left internal carotid bifurcation. (b, c) Initial angiograms at the end of the treatment show total occlusion with dense packing (arrow in c). (d) Three-month follow-up angiogram demonstrates a small recurrence at the level of the neck (arrow). (e, f) Angiograms obtained 46 months after treatment show (e) an increased remnant size (arrow) and (f) substantial compaction of the coils (arrow). Note that a contralateral aneurysm was treated (arrowhead) at previous angiography. Follow-up angiography was scheduled for 1 year after e and f were obtained.

In the three remaining cases, the small remnant increased slightly in size on a later follow-up angiogram but was too small to be re-treated. At the time of this writing, further follow-up angiography was scheduled in all these cases for 1–2 years later.

The rate of recurrence in these 148 aneurysms was analyzed depending on the following factors:

Clinical presentation (ruptured or nonruptured aneurysms).—The frequency of recurrence was 17% in ruptured aneurysms and 7% in nonruptured aneurysms (Table 3). At first follow-up angiography (eight recurrences in 148 aneurysms), seven occurred in the 94 ruptured aneurysms (7%) and one in the 54 nonruptured aneurysms (2%). At second follow-up angiography (nine recurrences in 99 cases), there were eight recurrences in 66 ruptured aneurysms (12%) and one recurrence in the 33 nonruptured ones (3%). At the third follow-up angiography (three recurrences in 39 cases), there was only one recurrence in 26 ruptured aneurysms (4%), and there were two recurrences in 13 nonruptured ones (15%).

Location.—There was no difference in frequency of recurrence according to the location (Table 4).

Size of the sac.—Recurrence was observed in 8% of small berry (2- or 3-mm-diameter coils), in 9% of medium berry (4- or 5-mm-diameter coils), and in 22% of large berry (6-, 7-, or 8-mm-diameter coils) aneurysms (Table 5). There was no significant difference in the recurrence rates according to sac size ($P = .1$).

Ratio between aneurysm sac size and neck diameter.—Recurrences were observed in two (6%) of 31 cases with a ratio of 1, in eight (14%) of the 59 cases with a ratio between 1 and 2, and in seven (22%) of the 32 cases with a ratio of 2 (Table 6). There was no significant difference in the recurrence rates according to this ratio ($P = .2$).

TABLE 3
Rate of Recurrence Depending on the Initial Symptoms (Ruptured or Nonruptured Aneurysms)

	Ruptured	Nonruptured	Total
Recurrence*	16 (17)	4 (7)	20
Total occlusion	78	50	128
Total	94	54	148

* Number in parentheses is the percentage of total ruptured or nonruptured aneurysms.

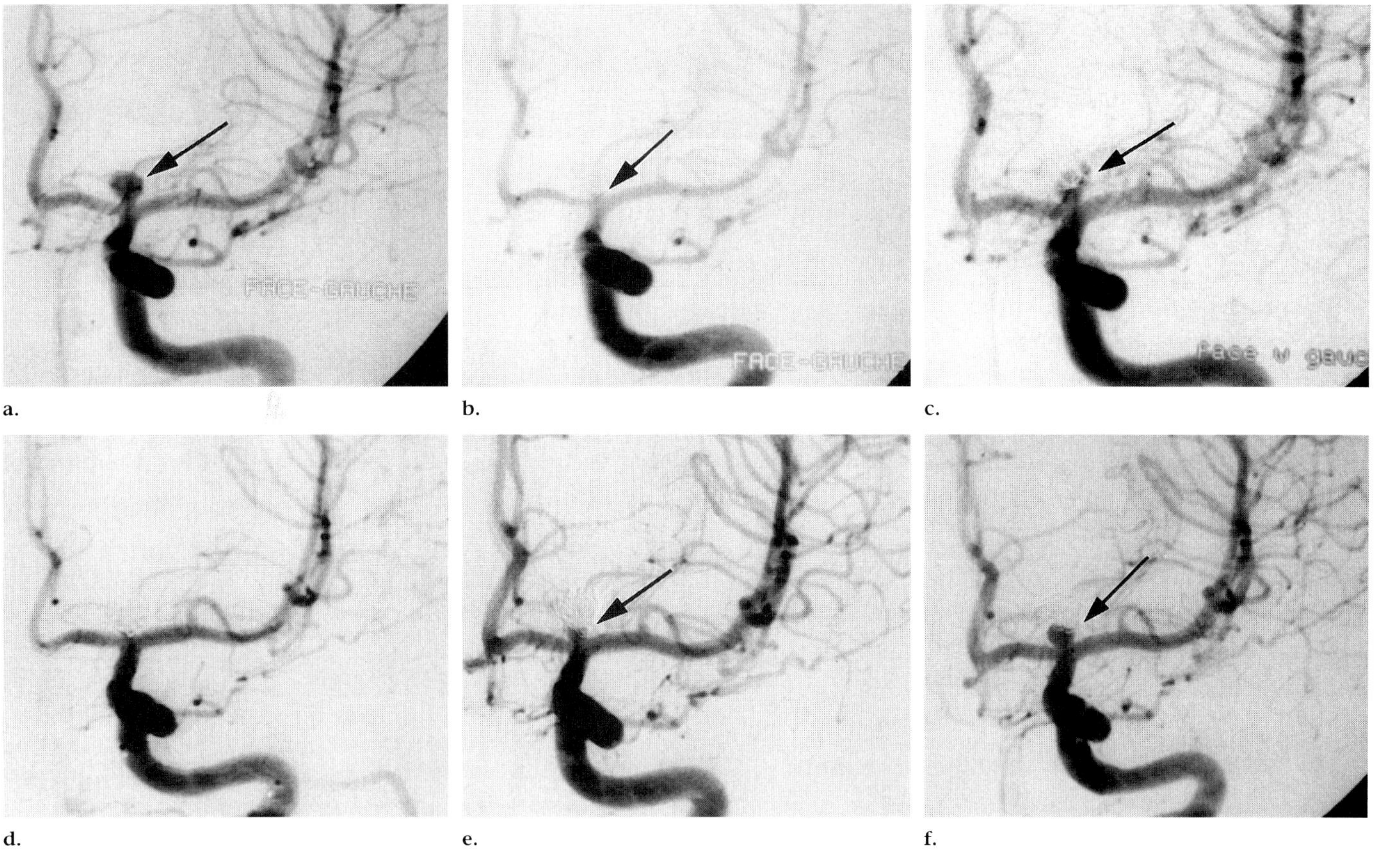

Figure 2. (a) Pretreatment angiogram shows a ruptured aneurysm (arrow) of the left internal carotid bifurcation. (b) Initial angiogram at the end of the treatment shows subtotal occlusion with a small neck remnant (arrow). (c) Follow-up angiogram obtained 3 months later shows wide regrowth of the remnant (arrow). (d) Retreatment was performed, and angiogram shows that total occlusion was attained. (e) Follow-up angiogram at 6 months shows recurrence (arrow). (f) The remnant increased in size (arrow) as seen on this 1-year follow-up angiogram. In this case, the coil mesh appearance did not change despite recurrence, and coil compaction did not occur. Retreatment was scheduled.

TABLE 4
Rate of Recurrence Depending on the Aneurysm Location

Location	Recurrence	No Recurrence	Total	Rate of Recurrence (%)
Internal carotid artery	6	47	53	11
Anterior communicating artery	3	32	35	9
Middle cerebral artery	5	26	31	16
Vertebrobasilar artery	5	19	24	20
Pericallosal artery	1	2	3	33
Posteroinferior cerebellar artery	0	2	2	0
Total	20	128	148	14

Evolution of the 18 Aneurysms with Subtotal Occlusion

In 12 cases, the very tiny remnant did not change at follow-up angiography (range, 12–29 months later; mean, 18 months). At the time of this writing, a late follow-up was scheduled for 2 years later. In six cases (30%), the remnant regrew, resulting in an incomplete occlusion (Fig 2). Regrowth occurred in three cases at the first angiography (3 months), in one case at the second, and in two cases at the third (38 and 42 months). In three cases, the remnant did not allow or require any retreatment. In three cases, a second treatment was performed, with a subtotal occlusion in two and an incomplete occlusion in one.

Evolution of the Three Aneurysms with Incomplete Occlusion

In one case, the occlusion was stable at 18 months. In the second case, despite a second treatment, the occlusion was still incomplete. In the third case, the aneurysm remnant decreased, resulting in a subtotal occlusion (stable 39 months later).

Final Results

Finally, the last follow-up angiogram showed a total occlusion in 133 cases (79%), subtotal in 30 cases (18%), and incomplete in six cases (4%). All the cases with subtotal occlusion will be reevaluated, depending on the size of the remnant, 1–3 years later. For the six incompletely occluded aneurysms, a surgical clipping was never proposed because of the location of the aneurysm or because the remnant size was too small.

Clinical Evolution

No rupture occurred in this series of 169 treated and reevaluated aneurysms during a follow-up from 3 to 50 months

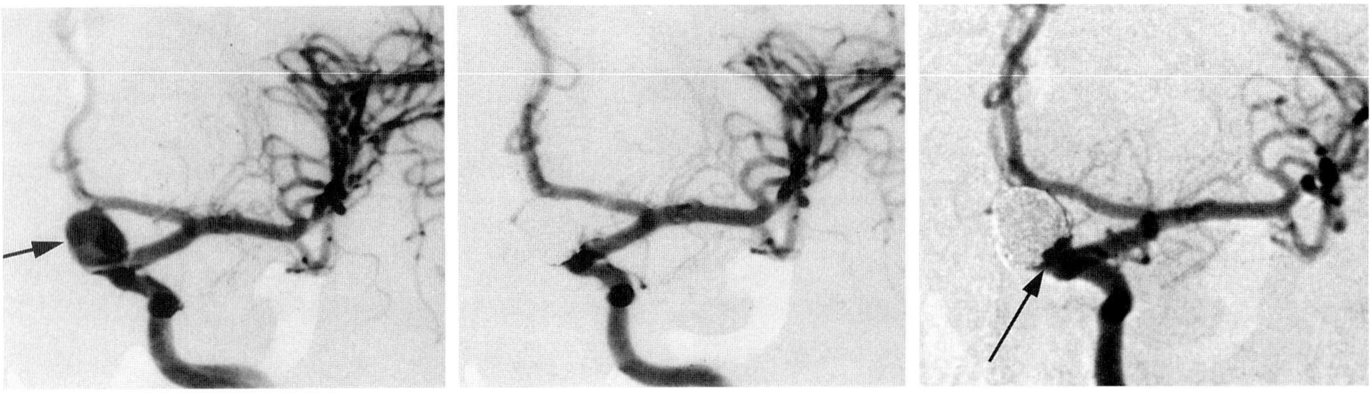

a. b. c.

Figure 3. (a) Pretreatment angiogram shows a large symptomatic berry aneurysm (arrow) of the left carotid ophthalmic artery. (b) The aneurysm was considered totally occluded on this angiogram obtained at the end of the procedure. (c) Last follow-up angiogram at 31 months shows recurrence (arrow). In this case, the aneurysm neck is very difficult to precisely delineate from the parent artery within the loop of the carotid siphon. Recurrence was probably already present at the first follow-up angiography but only became obvious at the last one. One-year follow-up angiography is scheduled.

later (mean, 20.2 months), for a cumulative follow-up of 3,419 months.

DISCUSSION

Since the introduction of detachable coils, EVT has become the reference standard in the management of aneurysms not amenable to surgical clipping (1–7,16,17). We recently published results of EVT as the primary treatment for berry intracranial aneurysms even though they were amenable to a surgical approach (9). In that series, EVT was performed in 86% of the cases (203 of 236 aneurysms), with a good level of total (123 [81%] of 152 aneurysms) or subtotal (26 [17%] of 152 aneurysms) occlusion and with few technical complications. The morbidity rate due to the technique was low and only due to thromboembolic (4% [seven of 189 surviving patients) or anticoagulation-related (0.5% [one of 189 patients) complications. EVT in the acute phase of ruptured aneurysms was performed without substantially increased technical difficulties and with a low mortality rate due to perioperative rupture (1% [two of 182 patients]). Regardless of the initial clinical grade of the patient, EVT may be performed very early after subarachnoid hemorrhage, to protect against early rebleeding (15). If the results with EVT are good in the short-term follow-up period, the question remains regarding long-term occlusion rates and protection against late rebleeding. It is well known that occlusion of intracranial aneurysms with a balloon or free coils only partially protects against further growth of the aneurysm and subsequent bleeding (18,19).

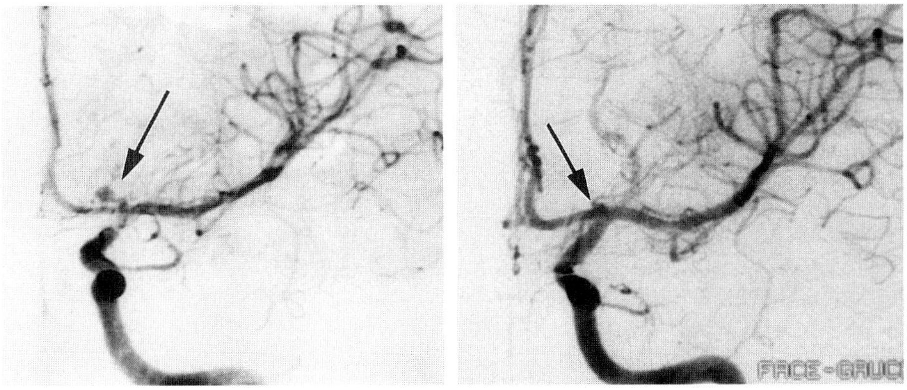

a. b.

Figure 4. (a) Pretreatment angiogram shows an aneurysm (arrow) of the left internal carotid artery bifurcation. (b) Fifteen-month follow-up angiogram shows the very tiny remnant at the level of the neck (arrow) without any modification over the months. This stable small remnant corresponds to what may be called a "residual deformation of the parent artery."

In a recent study (8), we reported the evolution of the occlusion rate in 55 aneurysms treated with mechanical detachable spirals. The results in the short-term period were disappointing, with a recurrence in 15% of the cases (two of 13) despite initial total occlusion and with 69% regrowth of the remnant in cases that were subtotally occluded. These spirals are no longer used in berry aneurysms.

To our knowledge, little is reported about long-term angiographic follow-up after treatment with detachable coils. Graves et al (15) reported that all of the completely occluded aneurysms in their series remained 100% occluded during follow-up (eight aneurysms with a mean follow-up of 7.7 months). In the series of Gurian et al (20), surgical clipping was required after partial occlusion or recanalization in 5.7% (eight of 141) of aneurysms treated with detachable coils. The frequency of recanalization was not addressed. In their recent study, Raymond et al (6) reported results of 31 aneurysms of the basilar bifurcation. Twenty-seven of the 29 surviving patients underwent 6-month follow-up angiography, and 12 patients underwent another follow-up angiographic examination 1 year later. Recurrence or regrowth of the remnant was shown in seven patients (24%).

Evaluation of the Occlusion

It is very difficult to assess the occlusion rate of the aneurysms after EVT.

TABLE 5
Rate of Recurrence Depending on the Size of the Aneurysm

	2–3 mm	4–5 mm	6–8 mm	Total
Recurrence*	4 (9)	5 (9)	9 (22)	18
Total occlusion	42	50	32	124
Total	46	55	41	142

Note.—Size of the aneurysm was estimated by the size of the first coils (noted in 142 cases).
* Number in parentheses is the percentage of total aneurysms in that size category.

TABLE 6
Rate of Recurrence Depending on the Ratio between Aneurysmal Sac Size and Neck Diameter

	Ratio $\leq$ 1	1 $<$ Ratio $<$ 2	Ratio $>$ 2	Total
Recurrence	2 (6)	8 (14)	7 (22)	17
Total occlusion	29	51	25	105
Total	31	59	32	122

Note.—The ratio could be measured in 122 of the 148 totally occluded aneurysms.

Evaluation is very subjective and must include both the density of the coil packing and amount of possible neck remnant. It is impossible to compare from one institution to another and then from one article to another what the authors define as complete occlusion with dense packing. In fact, when an aneurysm is already filled with a few large coils, the deposition of several small coils inside the coil mesh does not substantially change the appearance of the coil mesh on radiographs. At our institution, we try to pack the aneurysms as much as possible and stop the procedure only when the last coil cannot be introduced inside the sac. The last coil is always wasted for each procedure. The ability to introduce the last coil is completely dependant on the operator's skill level and experience. In addition, assessment of the neck remnant is made more difficult at the end of the procedure due to the mass of coils that frequently hides the aneurysm neck.

Evaluation of long-term angiographic follow-up is more reliable because aneurysm occlusion is evaluated by the same observers and with the same angiographic machine under exactly the same projections. However, the evaluation remains subjective, and it is sometimes difficult to assess slight modifications of the coil mesh and a very tiny neck remnant. In the current study, occlusion rates could not be determined in 39 aneurysms at the end of the first treatment because vasospasm due either to subarachnoid hemorrhage or to the catheterization made it impossible to assess the occlusion at the level of the neck. Total occlusion was confirmed at the first follow-up angiography when arteries had returned to their normal appearance.

Recurrences

Despite total occlusion obtained in 148 cases, recurrences were observed in 20 aneurysms (14%). It appears that even densely packed, totally occluded aneurysms may recanalize. It is difficult to understand the mechanism of the origin of the coil mesh changes and recanalization of the neck, but probably recurrences may be due to two causes: (*a*) coil compaction due to arterial blood flow and (*b*) true persistent growth of the aneurysm due to the initial disease of the arterial wall. These two phenomena are probably interrelated since as soon as a coil compaction occurs it may produce neck remnant growth by the arterial blood flow. However, a regrowth of the neck may produce a change in the coil mesh.

These recurrences are probably much less frequently encountered after surgical clipping and are at least partially related to the principle of the EVT. With intrasaccular occlusion of the aneurysm as in EVT, contact between the arterial walls does not occur as it does in surgical clipping. Nevertheless, true recurrences after complete surgical clipping have been described (21–24). Sasaki et al (23) reported seven cases of rebleeding of previously clipped aneurysms, 4–7 years after treatment. Five of them had initial complete clipping confirmed at angiography. Ebina et al (22) reported two cases of recurrence after complete clipping.

Histologic findings in animal aneurysm models treated with detachable coils are unclear (2,25–28). Mawad et al (25) demonstrated, in a canine lateral venous pouch model, regrowth of a new intimal layer over the neck of all aneurysms filled with coils. Both completely occluded and recanalized aneurysms were isolated from the circulation by this neointima composed of three well-identifiable layers. Reul et al (26) showed different results in a rabbit carotid bifurcation model. No intraluminal thrombi were found adhering to the coils, and in only the most densely packed cases were the coils covered by granulation tissue, with endothelial cells seen on the intraluminal surface of this tissue. Byrne et al (27) reported increased cellularity in the thrombus in a swine aneurysm model, but the importance of this finding is unclear because all the aneurysms in their model thrombosed, indicating that in pigs a vigorous cellular response is not necessary for aneurysms to thrombose and heal. The durability of an aneurysm healing with detachable coils probably cannot be inferred directly from these animal studies, given the very complex phenomena they involve. Coagulation in these animals is not identical to that in humans. Furthermore, in these animal aneurysm models the authors did not study the mechanism at the origin of aneurysm formation and its role in regrowth after treatment (29).

Molyneux et al (28) reported pathologic and histologic findings in two patients with giant partially thrombosed aneurysms. Histologic findings (2 and 6 months after treatment) showed coils embedded in a largely unorganized thrombus with no evidence of endothelialization at the neck. Nevertheless, EVT of large or giant aneurysms is known to be ineffective in the long term, and histologic findings would probably be completely different after treatment of berry aneurysms.

Delay between Treatment and Recurrence

In the current study, recurrence occurred at the third follow-up angiographic examination when postprocedural first and second follow-up angiography showed a total occlusion. In the surgical literature, the mean time between surgical clipping and clinical symptoms of recurrence is approximately 10 years (22,23,30).

Factors Influencing the Rate of Recurrence

Recurrences were more frequent after treatment of ruptured aneurysms (17%) than in nonruptured aneurysms (7%). The more important rate of recurrence in ruptured aneurysms may be due to alterations in anatomic conditions. It is probable that, in ruptured aneurysms, coils are frequently packed due to the spontaneous lysis of the clot at the rupture site and in a false, partially thrombosed aneurysm sac (8). Clinically important changes in the aneurysm sac appearance may be observed when angiography is performed at two separate times within a few days after the rupture (Fig 5). This is probably due to the spontaneous lysis of the clot at the rupture site and in the false aneurysm sac. When lysis of the clot occluding the rupture site occurs in the days after the rupture, this may induce the coils to compact to the back of the aneurysm and in the false aneurysm sac.

Location.—Some aneurysms are frequently described as "in-flow aneurysms." For example, aneurysms of the basilar or internal carotid artery bifurcations are known to be more prone to the arterial flow stresses than are middle cerebral or anterior communicating artery aneurysms. Most interventionalists have the common belief that this phenomenon induces more frequent recanalization. This was not true in this series; the rate of recurrence was not higher in these locations.

Size of the sac.—It is well known that EVT of large and giant aneurysms frequently fails to obtain a total and durable occlusion of the aneurysm sac (6,13,31). EVT for large berry aneurysms obtains less favorable initial results than for small or medium berry aneurysms (9). In our study, the rate of recurrence was higher in large berry aneurysms (22% vs 8% for small and 9% for medium aneurysms). A dense packing was less frequently obtained, and depositing the last small coils inside the basket of larger coils was very difficult.

Ratio between aneurysm sac size and neck diameter.—The size of the neck was not measured in this series. Previous studies assessed the role of the aneurysm neck size on the occlusion rate (5,6,13). The remodeling technique allowed the same results to be obtained whatever the size of the neck (32). The influence of this ratio on final results was disappointing. In aneurysms with a ratio of 2 (the best morphology for EVT), results were less favorable (rate of recurrence = 22%). This morphology was more frequently encountered in large berry aneurysms in which EVT did not perform optimally.

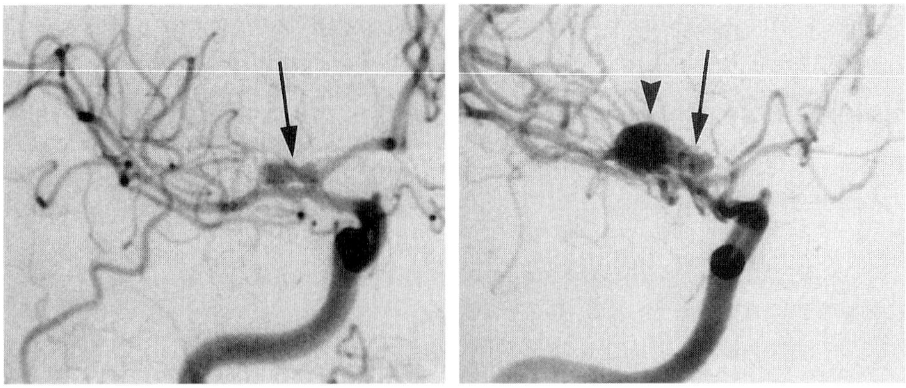

a. b.

Figure 5. Aneurysm of the right internal carotid artery bifurcation. (**a**, **b**) Angiograms obtained the day after the rupture (arrow) and 10 days later, respectively. The changes in the size and morphology of the sac are probably related to the spontaneous lysis of the clot at the rupture site. The large external pouch (arrowhead in **b**) probably corresponds to a false aneurysm sac. The size of the first coil and final appearance of the coil mesh would not have been the same if the treatment had been done the day after the bleeding and not 10 days later.

Evolution of the Recurrences

The indication for retreatment is primarily dependent on the aneurysm remnant size, shape, and angiographic evolution. At our institution, as soon as the remnant seems accessible to an endovascular retreatment, a second procedure is attempted. Nevertheless, a very small remnant (1 or 2 mm) carries a very low risk of rebleeding, and treatment may be very tricky to perform either surgically or with EVT. In cases with very small neck remnants in which retreatment seems impossible or very difficult, legitimate concern regarding rebleeding exists in the very long term period. These aneurysms are reevaluated 1 year later for any remnant growth indicating retreatment. Retreatment after recanalization may be very difficult to perform because the aneurysm remnant frequently has a square shape with a large neck and a small residual sac. The remodeling technique is frequently required to allow for dense coil packing (32). Clipping after incomplete embolization has been described (as has coil placement after incomplete clipping) (20,33–35). Surgical clipping was never required in our cases. In 10 cases, the small remnant at the level of the aneurysm neck was followed for 12–46 months (mean, 25 months) and remained stable. The very tiny neck recurrence did not require (or allow for) any retreatment. A very long term follow-up will be necessary to assess whether a residual deformation of the parent artery does not change over the years.

Evolution of Aneurysms with Subtotal or Incomplete Occlusion

Subtotal initial treatment may lead more frequently to remnant regrowth than total occlusion may lead to true recurrence. Nevertheless, to our knowledge the evolution of such remnants over the years remains unknown.

Comparison with the Surgical Literature

The frequency and long-term consequences of incomplete surgical clipping has been debated for a long time. In 1967, Drake and Vanderlinden (36) reported results of routine postoperative angiography after surgery in 70 cases. They confirmed that no episodes of recurrent hemorrhage occurred from the 45 aneurysms completely obliterated (64%). In 12 (17%) of the 70 aneurysms, a "small" remnant was shown at angiography. Aneurysms rebled in two of these patients; one of the patients died soon after discharge and the other 11 years later. In 13 of the 70 aneurysms (18%), a "large" remnant was revealed. In six cases, the aneurysms rebled and the patients died, three soon after discharge and three in the long-term period. In 1973, Drake and Allcock (37) reported on 329 patients with postoperative angiograms that demonstrated contrast material filling of a substantial part of the sac in 43 patients, and at least 12 aneurysms rebled. Katakura et al (38) reported 41 remnants in 578 cases (7%).

Our search of the recent microneurosurgery literature revealed only a few studies that deal with the rate of inadequate clipping (39–43). Surgical clipping has been the reference standard for intracranial aneurysms, and in the absence of alternative therapy, very little is known concerning routine postoperative angiography. Although it is commonly believed that postoperative angiography may only accurately document the results of clipping, standard practice is to perform angiography only in cases in which the surgery was difficult. Furthermore, up to 50% of the neurosurgeons believe that a second surgical approach should not be required, as shown by Feuerberg et al (41). In 1987, they reported on 715 patients who were operated on with microsurgical technique and in whom postoperative angiography was performed. Residual filling was observed in 28 patients (4%). MacDonald and co-workers (42) reported on a series of patients with 78 aneurysms in whom routine postoperative angiography was performed. They reported unclipped aneurysms in three cases (4%), incomplete clipping in eight (10%), and unexpected major vessel occlusion in nine (12%). In the series by Martin et al (40), inadequate clipping was disclosed during intraoperative angiography in five (9%) of 57 cases and during postoperative angiography in two other cases.

The evolution of these aneurysm rests, the frequency of remnant growth, and the risk of bleeding, as well as indications for reoperation, have been discussed (23,24,30,36,37,41,44–46). In the series of Feuerberg et al (41), 27 aneurysm remnants disclosed at angiography were followed over an 8-year period, with 62% unchanged, 24% resolved, 10% decreased, and only 5% (one case) enlarged and with rebleeding. They found that the incidence of rebleeding from an aneurysm remnant is 3.7% and that the risk of rupture is 0.8% per year. Lin et al (46) reported on 19 patients in which a neck remnant regrew to become symptomatic (14 aneurysms with rebleeding). They stated that even a 1- or 2-mm residual neck seen on postoperative angiograms, previously thought to be a small risk, may dilate over a long period to form another dangerous aneurysm. However, they did not address the number of treated and angiographically reevaluated aneurysms that showed remnants and consequently the rate of remnant regrowth. In 1995, Giannotta and Litofsky (30) discussed reoperative management in 20 recurrent or residual aneurysms. The lag time between initial treatment and clinical recurrence (bleeding or mass effect) was around 10 years. Here again, the rate of recurrence was not discussed. The results of these series suggest that reoperation should be performed on residual aneurysms to avoid further growth and rupture. However, these data must be related to the risk of reoperation given by Drake et al (45), with a 7% operative morbidity rate and a 5% mortality rate. Residual aneurysms were shown despite reoperation in 15 (13%) of the 115 cases (45).

Conclusion

A true recurrence was observed in 20 (14%) of the 148 totally occluded aneurysms. Recurrences may be observed in the very late follow-up, although previous follow-up angiography may have shown persistent total occlusion. Treatment of ruptured aneurysms and of large berry aneurysms is more likely to induce recurrences. In this series, the ratio between the size of the sac and size of the neck and the location of the aneurysm did not correlate with the frequency of recurrences. Recurrences are probably much more frequently encountered after EVT than after surgical clipping, probably due to coil compaction by arterial blood flow. Furthermore, the arterial walls are kept apart with coiling, while after clipping they are closely appositioned. Seven of the 20 recurrences required a second treatment, which was performed without any clinical complications and resulted in total occlusion in five aneurysms. Retreatment may be performed in the course of follow-up angiography. Remnant regrowth after subtotal occlusion was more frequent than true recurrences (30% vs 14%, respectively) and may indicate retreatment. Evolution of aneurysm remnants remains unclear in the very long term follow-up. In some cases, after tiny coil compaction, late follow-up did not show any changes and occlusion remained stable (residual deformation of the parent artery). In others, the small remnant increased in size over the years and required retreatment.

At our institution, patients with total occlusion at the second follow-up angiography (at least 15 months after the procedure) are scheduled for final angiography 3 years later. Patients with subtotal occlusion are followed up angiographically (depending on the remnant) for 1 or 2 years after the second follow-up angiography to assess whether the occlusion remains stable in the long term or if the remnant regrowth requires another procedure to complete the occlusion. It is too early to speculate when repeat angiography will no longer be needed. Magnetic resonance angiography will certainly replace conventional angiography in the future (47). Our results indicate that if thorough angiographic follow-up is performed to look for any recurrence or remnant growth, long-term clinical follow-up remains excellent with no late rebleeding.

References

1. Halbach VV, Higashida RT, Dowd CF, et al. The efficacy of endosaccular aneurysm occlusion in alleviating neurological deficits produced by mass effect. J Neurosurg 1994; 80:659–666.
2. Guglielmi G, Vinuela F, Dion J, Duckwiler G. Electrothrombosis of saccular aneurysms via endovascular approach. II. Preliminary clinical experience. J Neurosurg 1991; 75:8–14.
3. Guglielmi G, Vinuela F, Duckwiler G, et al. Endovascular treatment of posterior circulation aneurysms by electrothrombosis using electrically detachable coils. J Neurosurg 1992; 77:515–524.
4. Massoud T, Guglielmi G, Vinuela F, Duckwiler G. Endovascular treatment of multiple aneurysms involving the posterior intracranial circulation. AJNR 1996; 17: 549–554.
5. Zubilaga A, Gugliemi G, Vinuela F, Duckwiler G. Endovascular occlusion of intracranial aneurysms with electrically detachable coils: correlation of aneurysm neck size and treatment results. AJNR 1994; 15:815–820.
6. Raymond J, Roy D, Bojanowski M, Moumdjian R, L'Esperance G. Endovascular treatment of acutely ruptured and unruptured aneurysms of the basilar bifurcation. J Neurosurg 1997; 86:211–219.
7. Pierot L, Boulin A, Castaing L, Rey A, Moret J. Selective occlusion of the basilar artery aneurysms using controlled detachable coils: report of 35 cases. Neurosurgery 1996; 38:948–954.
8. Cognard C, Pierot L, Boulin A, et al. Intracranial aneurysms: endovascular treatment with mechanical detachable spirals in 60 aneurysms. Radiology 1997; 202:783–792.
9. Cognard C, Weill A, Castaings L, Rey A, Moret J. Intracranial berry aneurysms: angiographic and clinical results after endovascular treatment. Radiology 1998; 206: 499–510.
10. Pierot L, Boulin A, Castaing L, Rey A, Moret J. Endovascular treatment of pericallosal artery aneurysms. Neurol Res 1996; 18:49–53.
11. Moret L, Pierot L, Boulin A, Castaings L, Rey A. Endovascular treatment of anterior communicating artery aneurysms using Guglielmi detachable coils. Neuroradiology 1996; 38:800–805.
12. Roy D, Raymond J, Bouthillier A, Bojanowski MW, Moumdjian R, L'Esperance G. Endovascular treatment of ophthalmic segment aneurysms with Guglielmi detachable coils. AJNR 1997; 18:1207–1215.
13. Vinuela F, Duckwiler G, Mawad M. Guglielmi detachable coil embolization

of acute intracranial aneurysm: perioperative anatomical and clinical outcome in 403 patients. J Neurosurg 1997; 86:475–482.
14. Richling B, Bazinzski G, Gross C, Gruber A, Killer G. Early clinical outcome of patients with ruptured cerebral aneurysms treated by endovascular (GDC) or microsurgical techniques: a single center experience. Intervent Neuroradiol 1995; 1:19–27.
15. Graves VB, Strother CM, Duff TA, Perl J. Early treatment of ruptured aneurysms with Guglielmi detachable coils: effects on subsequent bleeding. Neurosurgery 1995; 37:640–648.
16. Ahuja A, Graves VB, Barnwell SL, et al. Endovascular treatment of basilar tip aneurysms with Guglielmi detachable coils. AJNR (in press).
17. McDougall C, Halbach V, Dowd C, Higashida R, Larsen D, Hieshima G. Endovascular treatment of basilar tip aneurysms using electrolytically detachable coils. J Neurosurg 1996; 84:393–399.
18. Hodes JE, Fox AJ, Pelz DM, Peerless SJ. Rupture of aneurysms following balloon embolization. J Neurosurg 1990; 72:567–571.
19. Casasco AE, Aymard A, Gobin YP, et al. Selective endovascular treatment of 71 intracranial aneurysms with platinum coils. J Neurosurg 1993; 79:3–10.
20. Gurian JH, Martin NA, King W, Duckwiler G, Guglielmi G, Vinuela F. Neurosurgical management of cerebral aneurysms following unsuccessful or incomplete embolization. J Neurosurg 1995; 83:843–853.
21. Adamson T, Batjer H. Aneurysm recurrence associated with induced hypertension and hypervolemia. Surg Neurol 1988; 29:57–61.
22. Ebina K, Suzuki M, Andoh A. Recurrence of cerebral aneurysm after initial neck clipping. Neurosurgery 1982; 11:764–768.
23. Sasaki T, Takeshima T, Tominaga M, Hashimoto H, Kawagichi S. Recurrence of ICA-PCoA aneurysms after neck clipping. J Neurosurg 1994; 80:58–63.
24. Weir B, Drake CG. Rapid growth of residual aneurysmal neck during pregnancy. J Neurosurg 1991; 75:780–782.
25. Mawad ME, Mawad JK, Cartwright J, Gokaslan Z. Long-term histologic changes in canine aneurysms embolized with Guglielmi detachable coils. AJNR 1995; 16:7–13.
26. Reul J, Weis J, Spetzger U, Konert T, Fricke C, Thron A. Long term angiographic and histopathologic findings in experimental aneurysms of the carotid bifurcation embolized with platinium and tungsten coils. AJNR 1997; 18:35–42.
27. Byrne JV, Hubbard N, Morris JH. The nature of thrombosis induced by platinium and tungsten coils in saccular aneurysms. AJNR 1997; 18:29–33.
28. Molyneux AJ, Ellison DW, Morris J, Byrne JV. Histological findings in giant aneurysms treated with Guglielmi detachable coils. J Neurosurg 1995; 83:129–132.
29. Stehbens WE. Etiology of intracranial berry aneurysms. J Neurosurg 1989; 70:823–831.
30. Giannotta SL, Litofsky S. Reoperative management of intracranial aneurysms. J Neurosurg 1995; 83:387–393.
31. Gobin Y, Vinuela F, Gurian J, et al. Treatment of large and giant fusiform intracranial aneurysms with Guglielmi detachable coils. J Neurosurg 1996; 84:55–62.
32. Moret J, Cognard C, Weill A, Castaings L, Rey A. The "remodelling technique" in the treatment of wide neck intracranial aneurysms. Intervent Neuroradiol 1997; 3:21–35.
33. Forsting M, Albert FK, Jansen O, et al. Coil placement after clipping: endovascular treatment of incompletely clipped cerebral aneurysms. J Neurosurg 1996; 85:966–969.
34. Civit T, Auque J, Marchal JC. Aneurysm clipping after endovascular treatment with coils: a report of eight patients. Neurosurgery 1996; 38:955–961.
35. Chavis TD, Hopkins LN. Comments on Graves VB, Strother CM, Duff TA, et al. Early treatment of ruptured aneurysms with Guglielmi Detachable coils: effects on subsequent bleeding. Neurosurgery 1995; 37:647–648.
36. Drake CG, Vanderlinden RG. The late consequences of incomplete surgical treatment of cerebral aneurysms. J Neurosurg 1967; 27:226–238.
37. Drake CG, Allcock JM. Postoperative angiography and the "slipped" clip. J Neurosurg 1973; 39:683–689.
38. Katakura K, Kwak R, Hatanaka M, Suzuki J. Angiographical consideration of residual aneurysms following direct operations on intracranial aneurysms. Neurol Surg (Tokyo) 1979; 7:139–148.
39. Alexander TD, MacDonald RL, Weir B, Kowalczuk BA. Intraoperative angiography in cerebral aneurysm surgery: a prospective study of 100 craniotomies. Neurosurgery 1996; 39:10–18.
40. Martin NA, Bentson J, Vinuela F, et al. Intraoperative digital substraction angiography and the surgical treatment of intracranial aneurysms and vascular malformations. J Neurosurg 1990; 73:526–533.
41. Feuerberg I, Linquist C, Linquist M. Natural history of postoperative aneurysmal rests. J Neurosurg 1987; 66:30–34.
42. MacDonald RL, Wallace MC, Kestle JR. Role of angiography following aneurysm surgery. J Neurosurg 1993; 79:826–832.
43. Barrow DL, Boyer KL, Joseph GJ. Intraoperative angiography in the management of neurovascular disorders. Neurosurgery 1992; 30:153–159.
44. MacKissoc W. Recurrence of an intracranial aneurysm after excision. J Neurosurg 1964; 23:547–548.
45. Drake CG, Friedman AH, Peerless SJ. Failed aneurysms surgery: reoperation in 115 cases. J Neurosurg 1984; 61:848–856.
46. Lin T, Fox AJ, Drake CG. Regrowth of aneurysm sacs from residual neck following aneurysm clipping. J Neurosurg 1989; 70:556–560.
47. Derdeyn CP, Graves VB, Turski PA, Masaryk AM, Strother CM. MR Angiography of saccular aneurysms after treatment with GDC coils: preliminary experience. AJNR 1997; 18:279–286.

Diagnosis Please

Noriko Salamon-Murayama, MD ▮ Eric J. Russell, MD ▮ Barry M. Rabin, MD

Case 17[1]

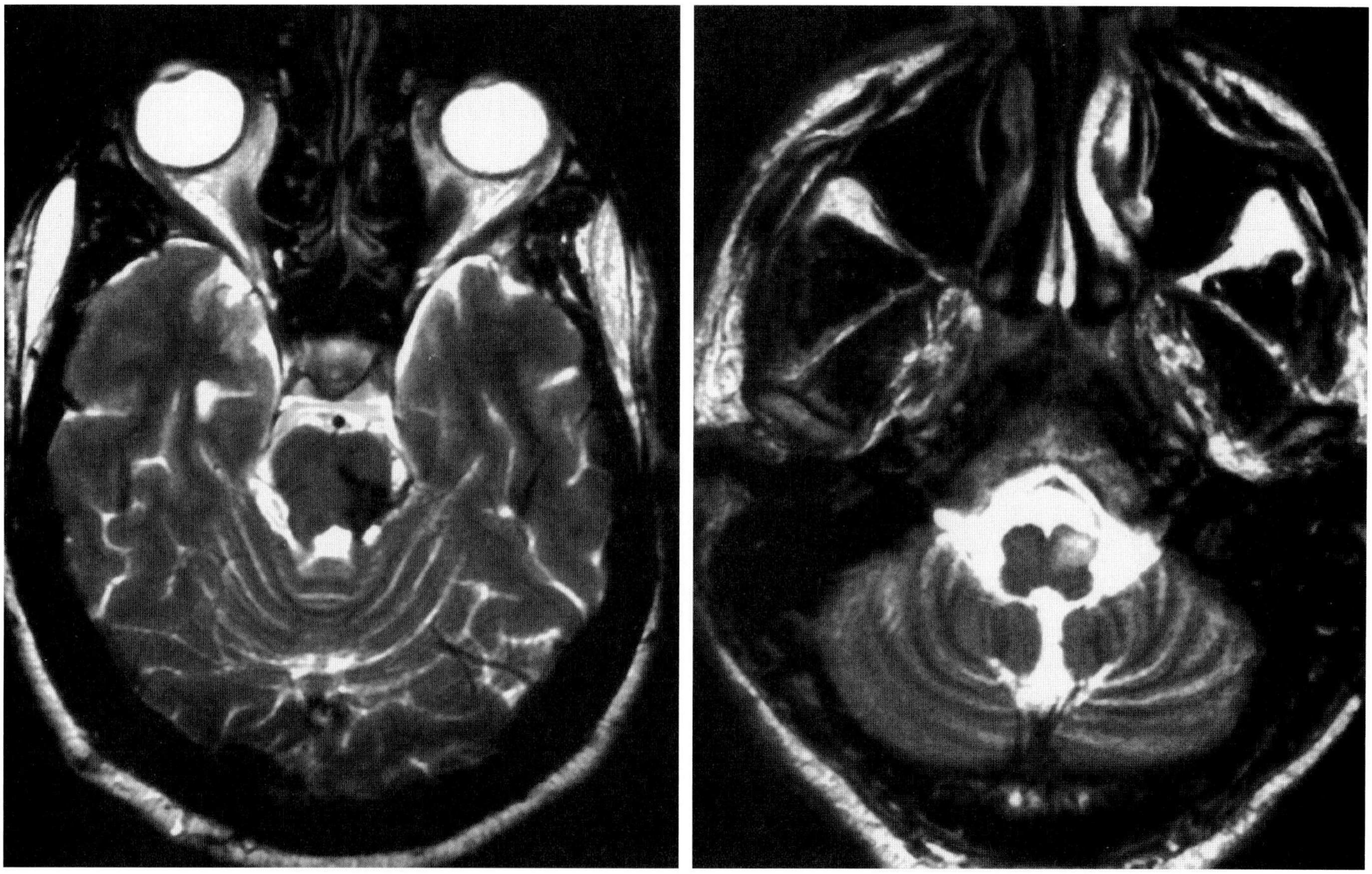

a. b.

Figure 1. Axial transverse T2-weighted (repetition time, 6,500 msec; echo time, 119 msec; number of signals acquired, two) fast spin-echo MR images of the brain obtained through **(a)** the pontomesencephalic junction and **(b)** the lower medulla.

Index term:
Diagnosis please

Radiology 1999; 212:357

[1] From the Department of Radiology, Section of Neuroradiology, Northwestern University Medical School and Northwestern Memorial Hospital, Olson Pavilion 3426, 710 N Fairbanks Ct, Chicago, IL 60611. Received August 4, 1998; revision requested September 11; revision received October 23; accepted March 16, 1999. **Address reprint requests to** N.S.M. (e-mail: *n-salamon@nwu.edu*).

HISTORY

The patient, a 36-year-old man with a history of hypertension and a prior stroke, developed right upper extremity rhythmic tremor (dentatorubral tremor).

E-mail the most likely diagnosis to *dxplease@rsna.org* (use ***only*** for submission of diagnosis). Include case number, your name (as you would want it to appear in the journal), address, phone and fax numbers. Only one case, one name, and one diagnosis per e-mail submission. Multiple diagnoses, multiple submissions, submissions without a case number will not be considered. ***Deadline:*** October 15, 1999. Answer will appear in the December issue. Authors wishing to submit cases for Diagnosis Please should first write to the Editor to obtain approval for the case and further information.

Swaggering Aorta

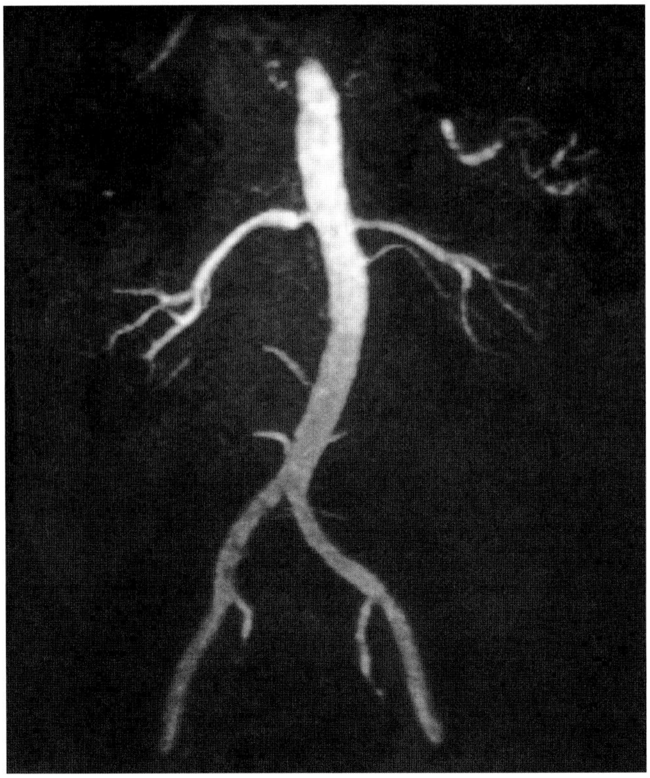

Courtesy of Stephen J. Riederer, MD, Rochester, Minn

Klaus D. Hagspiel, MD
J. Fritz Angle, MD
David J. Spinosa, MD
Alan H. Matsumoto, MD

Case 13: Polyarteritis Nodosa—Systemic Necrotizing Vasculitis with Involvement of Hepatic and Superior Mesenteric Arteries[1]

HISTORY

A 56-year-old woman fell and fractured her right ankle. After 2 days of bed rest, she presented to an outside institution with acute onset of shortness of breath, epigastric and right upper quadrant pain radiating to the back, and severe nausea and vomiting. She was afebrile, and her other vital signs were normal. She had a long medical history of "fibromyalgia," for which she received disability benefits. She also had a history of erythema nodosum that had been clinically quiescent. One year prior to this hospitalization, a temporal artery biopsy was performed because of chronic severe headaches. The biopsy results were negative. Four-vessel cerebral angiography and brain magnetic resonance imaging were performed at that time, and the results were unremarkable. The patient has a remote history of hypertension, although her blood pressure has been normal recently without antihypertensive medications. She also has been taking tricyclic antidepressants for chronic depression. She has no history of drug abuse or clinically important abdominal trauma.

The patient was hospitalized, and a myocardial infarction was ruled out. A perfusion lung scan showed no perfusion defects, and findings of a lower extremity ultrasonographic examination were negative for deep venous thrombosis. A contrast material–enhanced computed tomographic (CT) scan of the abdomen (Fig 1) was obtained, and the patient was then transferred to our institution (University of Virginia Health Sciences Center) for further evaluation. Throughout her hospitalization, she was afebrile and normotensive.

Results of laboratory tests performed at the time of admission revealed an erythrocyte sedimentation rate of 84 mm/h (normal range, 0–20 mm/h), a C-reactive protein level of 5.2 mg/dL (normal level, below 0.8 mg/dL), a serum albumin level of 3.0 g/dL (normal level, 3.5–5.0 g/dL), and a hemoglobin level of 10.0 g/dL (normal level, 12.0–16.0 g/dL), with a normal white cell and differential blood cell count. The total eosinophil count was normal. The results of liver function tests at the initial visit to the outside institution were grossly abnormal, with alanine aminotransferase and aspartate aminotransferase levels both above 400 U/L. At the patient's admission to our institution, the alanine aminotransferase level was 234 U/L (normal level, 11–66 U/L), and the aspartate aminotransferase level was normal. The alanine aminotransferase level subsequently normalized during her hospitalization. The results of an extensive serologic panel for a collagen vascular disease or an autoimmune disorder were negative. All hepatitis serologic and urine test results were normal.

Index terms:
Arteries, hepatic, 952.621
Arteries, superior mesenteric, 955.621
Arteritis, 761.621
Diagnosis please
Hepatic arteries, 952.122, 952.621
Hepatic arteries, CT, 761.12112, 761.12115
Liver, diseases, 761.621
Liver, infarction
Vasculitis, 761.621

Radiology 1999; 212:359–364

[1] From the Department of Radiology, Division of Angiography and Interventional Radiology, University of Virginia Health Sciences Center, Box 170, Charlottesville, VA 22908. Received June 24, 1998; revision requested July 10; revision received July 27; accepted October 26. **Address reprint requests to** K.D.H. (e-mail: *kdh2n@virginia.edu*).

IMAGING FINDINGS

Four noncontiguous 10-mm images from a contrast-enhanced helical CT scan of the liver are shown. Figure 1a demonstrates a focal, wedged-shaped area of low attenuation in the periphery of the liver. There is a round 1.5-cm lesion with the same attenuation as that of the aorta immediately adjacent to the described wedge-shaped defect. In addition, there is slight prominence of the intrahepatic bile ducts seen on all images. The patient had undergone cholecystectomy; no other biliary abnormality was present clinically or radiologically. Figure 1b shows the same abnormalities as Figure 1a. Figure 1c shows fusiform dilatation of a right hepatic arterial branch. Obtained immediately caudad to Figure 1c, Figure 1d demonstrates a

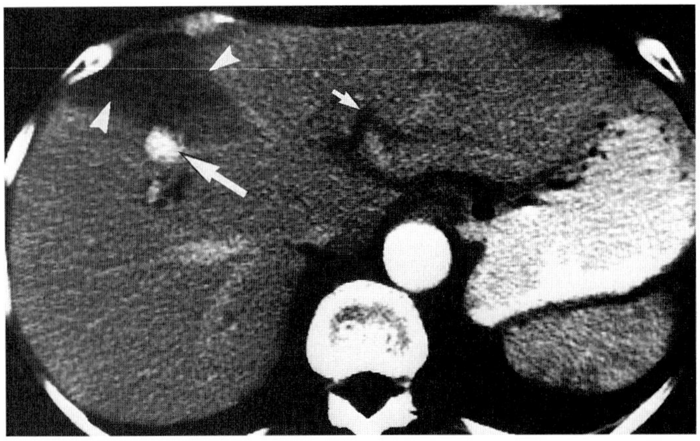

a.

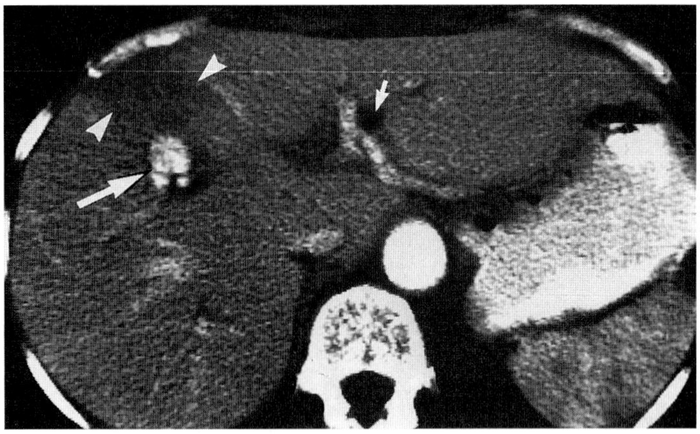

b.

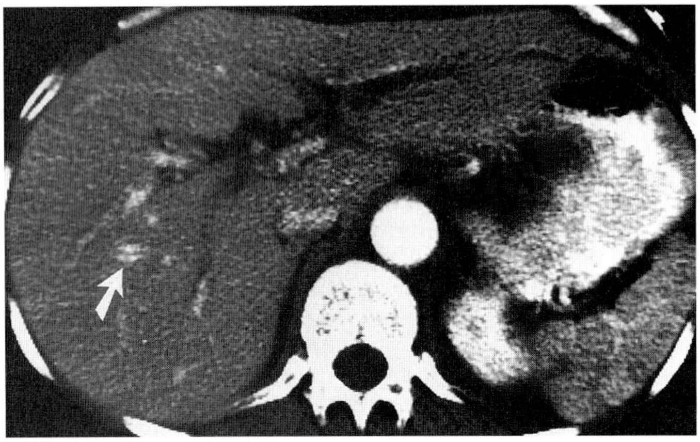

c.

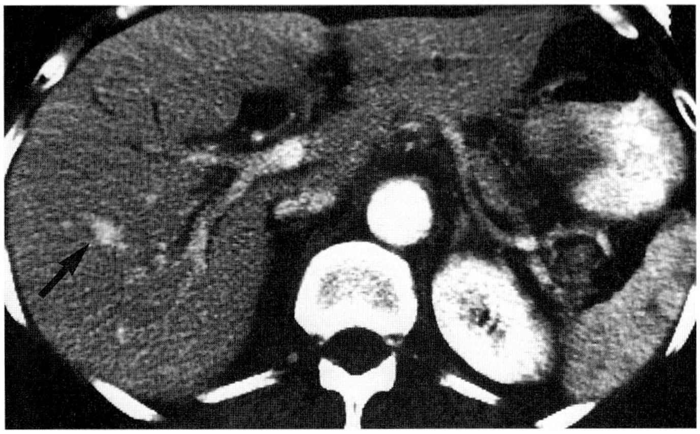

d.

Figure 1. **(a–d)** Four noncontiguous 10-mm images from a contrast-enhanced helical CT scan of the liver. **(a, b)** Images show a wedge-shaped area of low attenuation that represents an infarct (arrowheads) in the periphery of the liver. A round focal 1.5-cm lesion (large arrow) with the same attenuation as that of the aorta is seen immediately adjacent to the infarct. There is also slight prominence of the intrahepatic bile ducts (small arrow) on both images. **(c)** Image shows fusiform dilatation of the right hepatic arterial branch (arrow). **(d)** Image obtained immediately caudad to **c** shows a large contrast-filled structure (arrow) contiguous with a right hepatic arterial branch; this structure represents an aneurysm.

large contrast material–filled structure that is contiguous with a right hepatic arterial branch.

Figures 2–5 are arteriograms. Figure 2 is a celiac arteriogram that shows multiple saccular and fusiform aneurysms of the hepatic arteries; the largest aneurysm corresponds to that seen in Figure 1a and 1b. Other abnormal findings include smooth tapering and dilatation and occlusions of the intrahepatic arteries. Figure 3 shows subtle luminal irregularities and caliber changes in superior mesenteric arterial branches, and Figure 4 shows pleating of the main renal artery typical for fibromuscular dysplasia. Figure 5 is an arteriogram obtained 11 months after the study in Figure 2 and shows almost complete resolution of the aneurysms owing to immunosuppressive treatment.

The most likely diagnosis is systemic necrotizing vasculitis with multiple intrahepatic arterial aneurysms and an associated segmental liver infarct.

DISCUSSION

Multiple intrahepatic arterial aneurysms can be seen with trauma, mycotic infection, intravenous drug abuse (heroin, amphetamines), autoimmune disorders, fibromuscular dysplasia, or a primary necrotizing vasculitis or after viral infection (1–6). The patient in this case had no history of clinically important abdominal trauma or drug use. The patient's serum cryoglobulin levels and the results of a hepatitis serologic test and an extensive autoimmune serologic panel (antinuclear antibodies, antineutrophil cytoplasmic antibody, rheumatoid arthritis factor, etc) were all normal. Infections (mycotic aneurysms) were an unlikely cause because of the absence of febrile illness or a history of endocarditis. Therefore, the primary differential diagnostic considerations were a vasculitis or fibromuscular dysplasia.

Fibromuscular dysplasia can involve the mesenteric arteries, but typically the proximal celiac trunk and superior mesenteric artery are affected. However, tubular stenoses and aneurysms appear to be more common in the mesenteric arteries, in contrast to the classic "string-of-beads" appearance characteristic of medial fibroplasia in the renal arteries (6).

A variant of fibromuscular dysplasia is an entity termed "segmental mediolytic arteriopathy." Segmental mediolytic arteriopathy can mimic systemic necrotizing vasculitides angiographically (7). Segmental mediolytic arteriopathy is a rare, noninflammatory disease of small and medium arteries and is characterized by focal segmental disruption of the medial

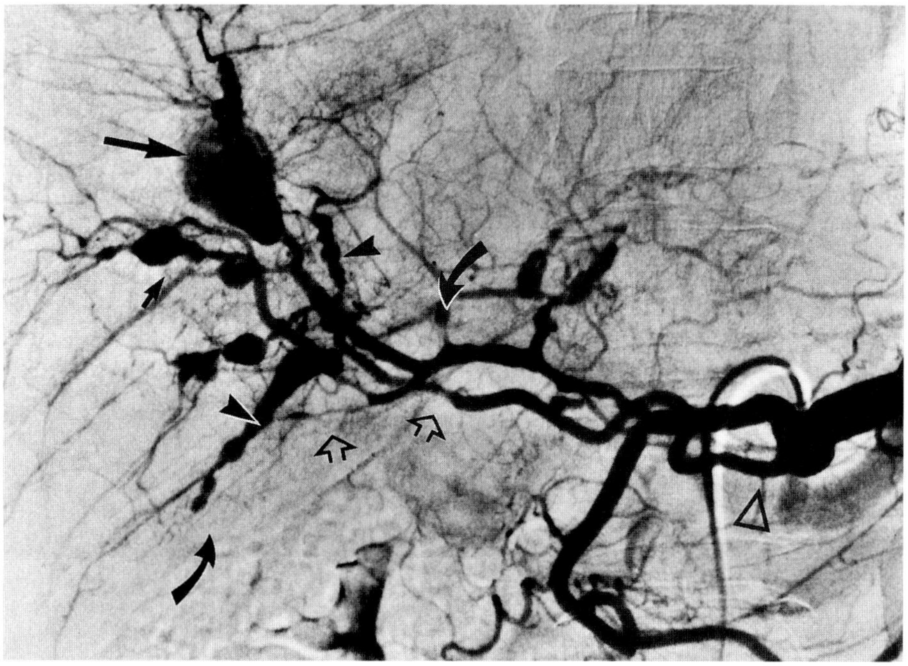

Figure 2. Manually subtracted image from a celiac arteriogram shows multiple saccular (small solid arrow) and fusiform (solid arrowheads) aneurysms of the medium and small hepatic arteries. The largest aneurysm (large solid arrow) is approximately 2 cm and corresponds to the aneurysm seen in Figure 1a and 1b. Many of the aneurysms have a predilection for hepatic arterial branching points. Other abnormal findings include smooth tapering and dilatation (open arrows) and occlusions (curved arrows) of the intrahepatic arteries. Of note, there is a normal variant with a separate origin of an accessory right hepatic artery from the celiac trunk (open arrowhead).

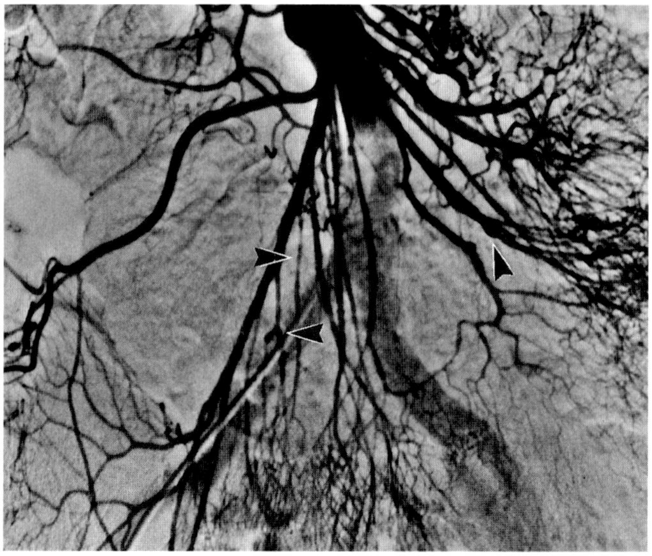

Figure 3. Manually subtracted image from a superior mesenteric arteriogram reveals subtle luminal irregularities and caliber changes in medium and small arterial branches (arrowheads). Mesenteric involvement in polyarteritis nodosa has been found angiographically in up to 54% of patients (1).

smooth muscle cells with mediolysis, which leads to dissection, intramural hemorrhage, and aneurysm formation (7–9). Although the string-of-beads is the classic angiographic appearance, irregular stenoses and aneurysms can occur (10). However, the typical clinical and laboratory findings seen with a systemic necrotizing vasculitis are not associated with this entity. This differentiation is important because immunosuppressive treatment is ineffective in segmental mediolytic arteriopathy. The clinical (diffuse muscle aches and headaches) and laboratory (elevated erythrocyte sedimentation rate and C-reactive protein levels, anemia, and hypoalbuminemia) findings in this patient militate against the diagnosis of segmental mediolytic arteriopathy (10).

The finding of multiple intrahepatic aneurysms and a hepatic infarct are hallmark findings of a systemic necrotizing vasculitis (2,11). The clinical presentation (abdominal pain, the diagnosis of fibromyalgia, and the history of erythema nodosum) and laboratory findings (elevated erythrocyte sedimentation rate and C-reactive protein levels, moderate anemia, and low serum albumin levels) all support this diagnosis.

Systemic necrotizing vasculitides are characterized by inflammation and necrosis of the blood vessels (12,13). Vasculitides are classified according to the clinical features and pathologic findings, but a universally accepted classification is lacking and there is substantial overlap between the individual entities (14,15). Polyarteritis nodosa, hypersensitivity vasculitis, Churg-Strauss syndrome, Wegener granulomatosis, Takayasu arteritis, and giant cell arteritis are the vasculitides that most commonly involve the hepatic arteries. The absence of a history of respiratory disease, eosinophilia, and palpable cutaneous purpura and negative temporal artery biopsy results make the diagnoses of Wegener granulomatosis, Churg-Strauss syndrome, giant cell arteritis, and hypersensitivity angiitis, respectively, extremely unlikely.

The diagnosis of a necrotizing vasculitis typically is made from the results of a biopsy. However, biopsy results may provide information only about the small arteries, thereby

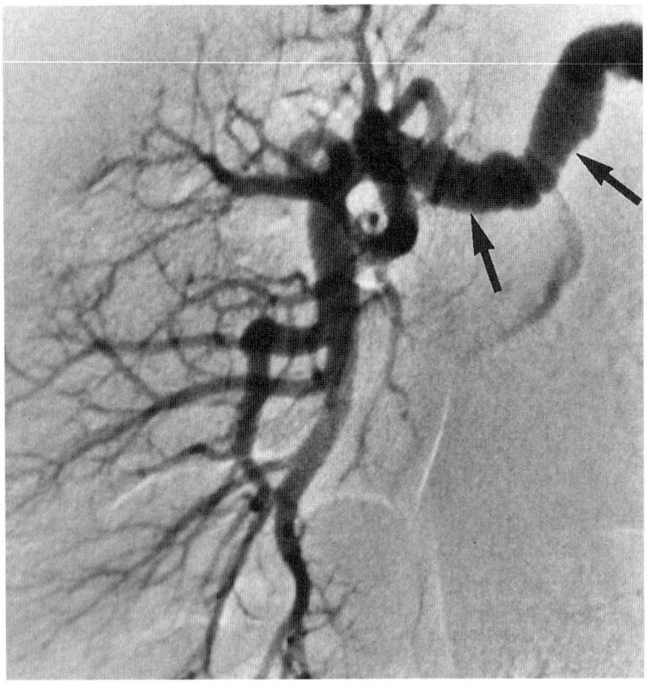

Figure 4. Selective right renal digital subtraction arteriogram shows pleating (arrows) of the main renal artery (string-of-beads sign) typical for fibromuscular dysplasia. The kidney is otherwise normal in size, and there are no aneurysms within the intrarenal arterial vasculature. The arteriogram of the left kidney (not shown) also showed a mild change of fibromuscular dysplasia of the main renal artery but no other abnormal findings.

missing the pathologically involved medium-sized vessels. In addition, performance of a biopsy in the affected organs occasionally is considered too high risk. Therefore, the diagnosis is based on the clinical and angiographic findings and response to treatment (11). The physical findings and symptoms in patients with a vasculitis are nonspecific and quite variable. Fever of unknown origin, weight loss, anorexia, fatigue, unexplained abdominal pain, arthralgias, or cerebrovascular or coronary events in young patients without other risk factors, polymyalgia, nondestructive oligoarthritides, and psychiatric disorders all have been reported as manifestations of a vasculitis (12,13,16,17).

Common abnormal laboratory test results include an elevated erythrocyte sedimentation rate, anemia, leukocytosis, thrombocytosis, reduced serum albumin concentration, and abnormal urinalysis results. There are no laboratory parameters that are specific for the diagnosis of a vasculitis (11,18).

Because the clinical and laboratory findings are so nonspecific, angiography plays an important role in the diagnosis of these disease entities. Polyarteritis nodosa is the prototypical systemic necrotizing vasculitis. It affects small and medium arteries. Transmural inflammation can result in arterial occlusions, which can lead to ischemia and widespread organ dysfunction (12,17,19,20). The exact pathogenesis of the disease is unknown, but some, if not all vasculitides, are thought to be the result of immune processes affecting blood vessels (21). The diagnosis can be based on tissue biopsy results, but not infrequently angiography is used to make the diagnosis. The diagnostic procedure in this case was angiography of the abdominal aorta, the celiac artery, the superior mesenteric artery, and both renal arteries (Figs 2–4).

The prognosis of patients with polyarteritis nodosa that involves multiple organ systems is poor, with a reported 5-year

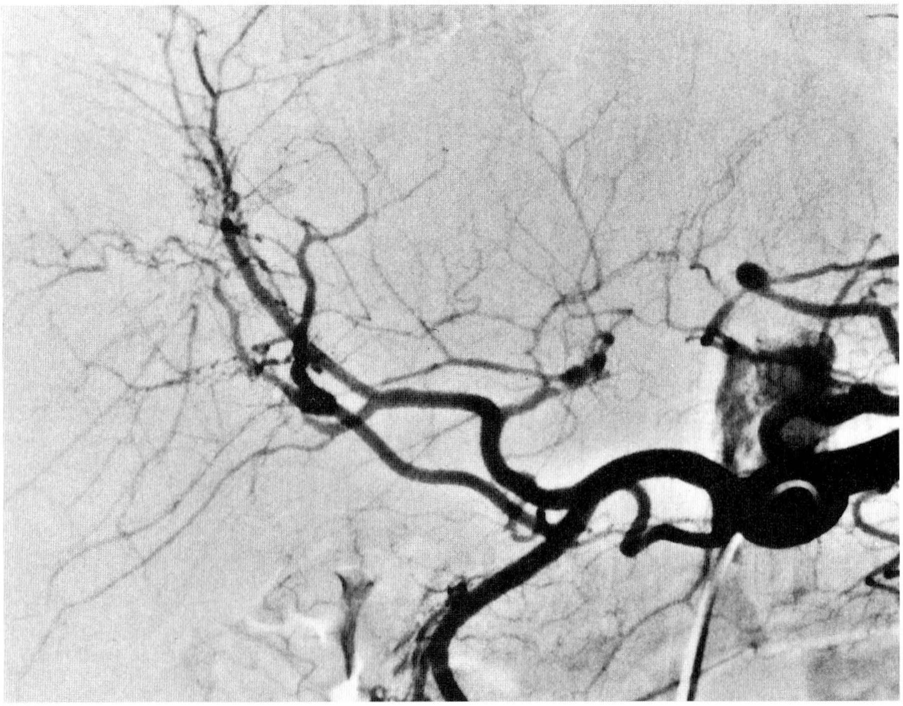

Figure 5. Manually subtracted image from a celiac arteriogram obtained 11 months after the study in Figure 2. The patient underwent immunosuppressive treatment in the interim, and there is almost complete resolution of the multiple aneurysms of the medium and small hepatic arteries.

survival rate of only 13%. Immunosuppressive treatment is effective and has been reported to increase 5-year survival rates to 48% (13). Resolution of aneurysms on follow-up angiograms in response to immunosuppressive treatment has been considered a favorable sign (11,13) (Fig 5).

The angiographic findings in polyarteritis nodosa are well described (1,2,4,5,11). However, they are not pathognomonic and can be found in any necrotizing vasculitis. Multiple saccular aneurysms that result from pannecrosis of the internal elastic lamina of the medium and small arteries are the most common findings. The aneurysms are typically 1–5 mm in diameter, but larger ones, as in this case, have been described (1,5,18). Fusiform aneurysms also have been reported (11). The aneurysms tend to occur at branching points of the affected arteries. The affected arteries can be as large as primary branches of the aorta or as small as arteriolar vessels (16). The main target organs are the kidneys and liver, but polyarteritis nodosa also has been found in the heart, brain, gallbladder, mesenteric circulation, muscles, spleen, and skin (18). Aneurysms have been found during angiography in 12.5%–94% of patients with an established diagnosis of polyarteritis nodosa (2,4). The majority of patients with aneurysms have multiple aneurysms, typically 10 or more (5). These aneurysms commonly involve multiple organs but may be present in only one system (22).

Other less specific angiographic findings in polyarteritis nodosa include stenoses, intraarterial thrombosis, areas with intermittent smooth tapering and dilatation, and occlusions. Luminal irregularities have been described in up to 90% of patients with polyarteritis nodosa (11) (Fig 3). The arterial occlusions can result in organ infarcts, which can be detected readily at CT (20). The small aneurysms typically encountered in polyarteritis nodosa usually cannot be visualized with CT. Alterations of vascular flow during angiography also have been described (11). In the kidneys, changes in the vascular flow pattern are seen in up to 86% of patients and manifest as irregular nephrograms, radiolucent cortical areas, and prolonged contrast material washout (11). In the liver, prolonged washout due to an increase in peripheral hepatic arterial resistance and hepatic infarcts has been described (11).

The sensitivity and specificity of angiography in polyarteritis nodosa have been reported to be 89% and 90%, respectively, with a positive predictive value of 55% and a negative predictive value of 98% (2). It is estimated that angiography establishes the presence of polyarteritis nodosa in 80% of all patients with the disease (13). However, it is important to remember that a negative angiogram does not exclude the presence of polyarteritis nodosa (13).

In summary, this patient presents with clinical, laboratory, and CT findings consistent with a systemic necrotizing vasculitis such as polyarteritis nodosa. The angiographic findings confirm this diagnosis. There were also incidental findings of fibromuscular dysplasia of the renal arteries, but to the best of our knowledge there is no known association between polyarteritis nodosa and fibromuscular dysplasia. Immunosuppressive treatment was started, and the patient improved both clinically and angiographically.

References

1. Travers RL, Allison DJ, Brettle RP, Hughes GRV. Polyarteritis nodosa: a clinical and angiographic analysis of 17 cases. Semin Arthritis Rheum 1979; 8:184–199.
2. Hekali P, Kajander H, Pajari R, Stenman S, Somer T. Diagnostic significance of angiographically observed visceral aneurysms with regard to polyarteritis nodosa. Acta Radiol 1991; 32:143–148.
3. Scully RE, Mark EJ, McNeely BU. Case records of the Massachusetts General Hospital. N Engl J Med 1985; 313:622–631.
4. Nove-Josserand R, Durand DV, Ninet J, Pasquier J, Levrat R. Clinical study and diagnostic criteria of periarteritis nodosa: apropos of 27 cases. Rev Med Interne 1991; 12:111–115.
5. Capasso P, Dondelinger RF. Vascular disorders of the liver. In: Gazelle GS, Saini S, Mueller PR, eds. Hepatobiliary and pancreatic radiology: imaging and intervention. New York, NY: Thieme, 1998; 294–334.
6. Luscher TF, Lie JT, Stanson AW, Houser OW, Hollier LH, Sheps SG. Arterial fibromuscular dyplasia. Mayo Clin Proc 1987; 62:931–952.
7. Chan RJ, Goodman TA, Aretz TH, Lie JT. Segmental mediolytic arteriopathy of the splenic and hepatic arteries mimicking systemic necrotizing vasculitis. Arthritis Rheum 1998; 41:935–938.
8. Lie JT. Systemic, cerebral, and pulmonary segmental mediolytic arteriopathy: villainous masqueraders of vasculitis. Cardiovasc Pathol 1996; 5:305–314.
9. Heritz DM, Butany J, Johnston KW, Sniderman KW. Intraabdominal hemorrhage as a result of segmental mediolytic arteritis of an omental artery: case report. J Vasc Surg 1990; 12:561–565.
10. Lee SI, Chew FS. Splanchnic segmental arterial mediolysis. AJR 1998; 170:122.
11. Vazquez JJ, San Martin P, Barbado FJ, et al. Angiographic findings in systemic necrotizing vasculitis. Angiology 1981; 32:773–779.
12. Conn DL. Update on systemic necrotizing vasculitis. Mayo Clin Proc 1989; 64:535–543.
13. Cupps TR, Fauci AS. Systemic necrotizing vasculitis of the polyarteritis nodosa group. In: Cupps TR, Fauci AS, eds. The vasculitides. Philadelphia, Pa: Saunders, 1981; 26–49. Smith LH Jr, ed. Major problems in internal medicine; Vol 21.
14. Leavitt RY, Fauci AS. Polyangiitis overlap syndrome: classification and prospective clinical experience. Am J Med 1986; 81:79–85.
15. Karanjia ND, Cawthorn SJ, Giddings AE. The diagnosis and management of arteritis. J R Soc Med 1993; 86:267–270.
16. Rosen S, Falk RJ, Jennette CJ. Polyarteritis nodosa, including microscopic form and vasculitis. In: Churg A, Churg J, eds. Systemic vasculitides. New York, NY: Igaku-Shoin, 1991; 57–77.
17. Fauci AS, Haynes BF, Katz P. The spectrum of vasculitis: clinical, pathologic, immunologic and therapeutic considerations. Ann Intern Med 1978; 89:660–676.
18. Kandarpa K, Chopra PS, Chakrabarti J, Mandell V. The vasculitides: current imaging and clinicopathologic correlation. J Vasc Med Biol 1991; 3:419–431.
19. Ewald EA, Griffin D, McCune WJ. Correlation of angiographic abnormalities with disease manifestations and disease severity in polyarteritis nodosa. J Rheumatol 1987; 14:952–956.
20. Jaques PF, Parker LA, Mauro MA. Fulminant systemic necrotizing arteritis: CT findings. J Comput Assist Tomogr 1988; 12:104–108.
21. Churg A, Churg J. Introduction. In: Churg A, Churg J, eds. Systemic vasculitides. New York, NY: Igaku-Shoin, 1991; 1–5.
22. Stanson AW. Roentgenographic findings in major vasculitic syndromes. Rheum Dis Clin North Am 1990; 16:293–308.

Our congratulations to the 38 individuals who submitted the most likely diagnosis (polyarteritis nodosa—systemic necrotizing vasculitis with involvement of hepatic and superior mesenteric arteries) for Diagnosis Please, Case 13. The names and locations of the individuals, as submitted, are as follows:

Gholamali Afshang, MD, *Tinley Park, Ill*
David R. Anderson, MD, *Richmond, Va*
Roger L. Antonelli, MD, *Dayton, Ohio*
Lionel Arrivé, MD, *Paris, France*
Edward L. Baker, MD, *San Francisco, Calif*
Maria Elena Castrillon, *Cordoba, Argentina*
Seyed A. Emamian, MD, PhD, *Washington, DC*
Keith D. Epperson, MD, *Milwaukee, Wis*
Andrew J. Fisher, *Denver, Colo*
Thomas Grant, DO, *Chicago, Ill*

Helen T. Ho, MD, *Chicago, Ill*
Lowrey H. Holthaus, MD, *Richmond, Va*
Douglas S. Katz, MD, *Mineola, NY*
Louis S. Magagna, MD, *Ann Arbor, Mich*
Andrew J. McDonnell, MD, *Corning, NY*
Peter Miltner, MD, *Heidelberg, Germany*
Manabu Minami, MD, *Tokyo, Japan*
Sergio Moguillansky, MD, *Rio Negro, Argentina*
James A. Newcomb, MD, *Allentown, Pa*
Sanford M. Ornstein, MD, *Phoenix, Ariz*
David M. Panicek, MD, *New York, NY*
Narendrakumar Patel, MD, *Newburgh, NY*
Victor Pérez-Candela, MD, *Las Palmas, Spain*
Dr. Roberto E. Perez Gautrin, *Sonora, Mexico*
John M. Plotke, *Naperville, Ill*
Shawn P. Quillin, MD, *Charlotte, NC*
M. R. Ramakrishnan, MD, *Big Stone Gap, Va*
Enrique Remartinez Escobar, MD, *Melilla, Spain*
Pierre Schmit, *l'Hay les Roses, France*
Steven M. Schultz, MD, *Fort Worth, Tex*
Matt Shapiro, MD, *Boxborough, Mass*
James E. Silberzweig, *New York, NY*
J. Takasugi, *Mercer Island, Wash*
J. Keith Thompson, MD, *Richmond, Va*
John To, MD, *Iron Mountain, Mich*
Carlos E. Triana Rodriguez, *Santafe de Bogota, Colombia*
H. Wouter van Es, MD, *Nieuwegein, The Netherlands*
Joe Yut, MD, *Olathe, Kan*

Kai E. Wilhelm, MD
Ulrich Hofer, MD
Hans J. Textor, MD
Thorsten Böker, MD
Holger M. Strunk, MD
Hans H. Schild, MD

Dacryoliths: Nonsurgical Fluoroscopically Guided Treatment during Dacryocystoplasty[1]

Index terms:
Catheters and catheterization, 223.1263
Fluoroscopy, 223.11
Lacrimal gland and duct, 223.1492, 223.818
Lacrimal gland and duct, interventional procedures, 223.1262, 223.1263, 223.1267, 223.1295
Lacrimal gland and duct, radiography, 223.11, 223.1295

Radiology 1999; 212:365–370

[1] From the Departments of Radiology (K.E.W., U.H., H.J.T., H.M.S., H.H.S.) and Ophthalmology (T.B.), University Hospital Bonn, Sigmund-Freud-Strasse 25, D-53127 Bonn, Germany. From the 1997 RSNA scientific assembly. Received July 20, 1998; revision requested September 4; final revision received February 4, 1999; accepted March 1. **Address reprint requests to** K.E.W. (e-mail: *wilhelm@uni-bonn.de*).

See also the editorial by Weissman (pp 305–306) in this issue.

Author contributions:
Guarantors of integrity of entire study, all authors; study concepts and design, K.E.W., U.H., T.B.; definition of intellectual content, all authors; literature research, K.E.W.; clinical studies, K.E.W., U.H., T.B., H.J.T.; data acquisition, K.E.W., T.B.; data analysis, K.E.W., U.H., T.B.; manuscript preparation, K.E.W.; manuscript editing and review, all authors

PURPOSE: To evaluate dacryocystoplasty with fluoroscopically guided nonsurgical removal of dacryoliths in the treatment of dacryolithiasis.

MATERIALS AND METHODS: Ten patients with severe epiphora due to partial (n = 8) or complete (n = 2) obstruction of the nasolacrimal duct system associated with dacryolithiasis underwent fluoroscopically guided removal of dacryoliths during dacryocystoplasty. Balloon dilation was performed initially to widen the nasolacrimal duct obstructions and to fragment dacryoliths. This was followed by forced irrigation with saline solution through the canaliculi. In patients with incomplete dacryolith washout, a 6.3-F sheath was advanced in a retrograde fashion into the nasolacrimal sac, and forced irrigation was repeated with aspiration of the fragments through the sheath. In two patients with therapy-resistant dacryoliths, additional fragmentation of the concrements was performed with a gooseneck snare.

RESULTS: Removal of dacryoliths was technically successful in all patients (complete removal, n = 6; partial removal, n = 4). During a follow-up period of up to 18 months, complete resolution of epiphora was achieved in five patients, and five patients showed partial resolution of their symptoms.

CONCLUSION: Fluoroscopically guided removal of dacryoliths during dacryocystoplasty is a feasible nonsurgical therapy with good clinical results and may be used as an alternative to dacryocystorhinostomy.

Epiphora is a common ophthalmologic problem composing 3% of clinical visits (1,2). Tearing may have several causes. There may be excessive lacrimation, neoplastic processes, or congenital malformation (1,2). Alternatively, and much more commonly, tearing is caused by obstructive epiphora, which results from complete or incomplete obstruction of the lacrimal system (1). Dacryolithiasis is a sequela of chronic infection in up to 30% of patients (3). Stasis secondary to an anatomic obstruction is likely to be the precipitating factor (4). In most cases, flushing out of the dacryoliths as a sole procedure is not a sufficient therapy because the stenosis of the nasolacrimal duct system persists or because of the size of the dacryoliths. Therefore, surgical removal of the dacryoliths along with dacryocystorhinostomy is still the standard therapy (5).

Recently, fluoroscopically guided nonsurgical dacryocystoplasty has shown encouraging results in the treatment of nasolacrimal duct obstruction (6–10). However, filling defects indicating dacryoliths on dacryocystograms are regarded as a relative contraindication for dacryocystoplasty because dacryoliths are a common cause of reobstruction (11).

Although there have been clinical reports of dacryoliths passing spontaneously through the stenosed nasolacrimal duct into the nasal cavity (12,13) or being removed by forced irrigation, to our knowledge, removal of dacryoliths has never been performed as an interventional radiologic procedure. The purpose of this study was to evaluate fluoroscopically guided nonsurgical removal of dacryoliths during dacryocystoplasty for symptomatic nasolacrimal duct obstruction associated with dacryolithiasis.

MATERIALS AND METHODS

Patient Population

Between July 1995 and March 1998, 60 consecutive patients (41 women, 19 men; age range, 21–85 years; mean age, 56 years) who presented with severe epiphora to the department of ophthalmology were referred for dacryocystoplasty. In 10 of these patients (eight women, two men; age range, 28–71 years; mean age, 58 years), dacryolithiasis was diagnosed at dacryocystography. For diagnostic purposes, 1–2 mL iopamidol (Solutrast 300; Bracco-Byk Gulden, Konstanz, Germany) was injected manually during the acquisition of the digital subtraction dacryocystographic series at a frame rate of 2 per second (14). In these patients, preinterventional dacryocystography demonstrated nasolacrimal duct obstruction associated with prestenotic dacryolithiasis (partial obstruction, $n = 8$, complete obstruction, $n = 2$). The obstruction was located at the junction between the lacrimal sac and the nasolacrimal duct in eight patients and at the outlet of the nasolacrimal duct near the valve of Hasner in two patients. The valve of Hasner is a mucosal constriction at the distal end of the nasolacrimal duct, just before the duct empties into the inferior meatus of the nose, beneath the inferior turbinate (Fig 1).

The obstructions were due to idiopathic inflammation and scarring in all patients. At the time of dacryocystoplasty, however, no active inflammation was present. Lacrimal fistula or diverticula, neoplastic processes, or other abnormalities of the lid were not observed. In our study, epiphora was evaluated subjectively according to a scale similar to that of Munk et al (15); in our scale, the grade 4 defined by Munk et al was divided into grades 4 and 5. All patients complained of severe epiphora. Three required dabbing more than 10 times a day (grade 4), and seven had constant tearing (grade 5). The history of epiphora varied 1–4 years (mean, 2.5 years). The patients gave their written informed consent to dacryocystoplasty, which is an established procedure in our hospital, after they had been informed about the interventional procedure, risks, and alternatives.

Technique

Dacryocystoplasty was performed on an outpatient basis after the administration of topical anesthesia. For this, two to four drops of benoxinate hydrochloride 0.4% (Novesine 0.4; CIBA Vision Ophthalmics, Germering, Germany) were applied to the conjunctival sac followed by an irrigation of the nasolacrimal duct system with 1 mL benoxinate hydrochloride 0.4% through the canaliculi. For local anesthesia of the nasal mucosa, a nasal pack was placed in the inferior nasal meatus. This pack consisted of two cotton pledgets moistened with oxybuprocaine hydrochloride 1% (Novesine Wander 1%; Wander Pharma, Nürnberg, Germany) and was left in place for 5–10 minutes. Infratrochlear nerve block was performed with the subcutaneous injection of 1–2 mL of mepivacaine hydrochloride 2% (Scandicain 2%; Astra, Wedel, Germany). Additional sedation with 5 mg of midazolam hydrochloride (Dormicum 5/1 mL; Hoffmann-La Roche, Grenzach-Wyhlen, Germany) was administered intravenously in two patients during fragmentation of the dacryoliths.

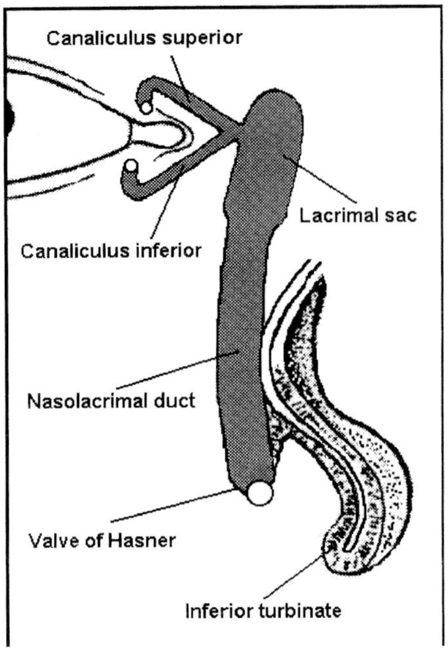

Figure 1. Drawing of the anatomy of the normal nasolacrimal drainage system of the right eye viewed frontally.

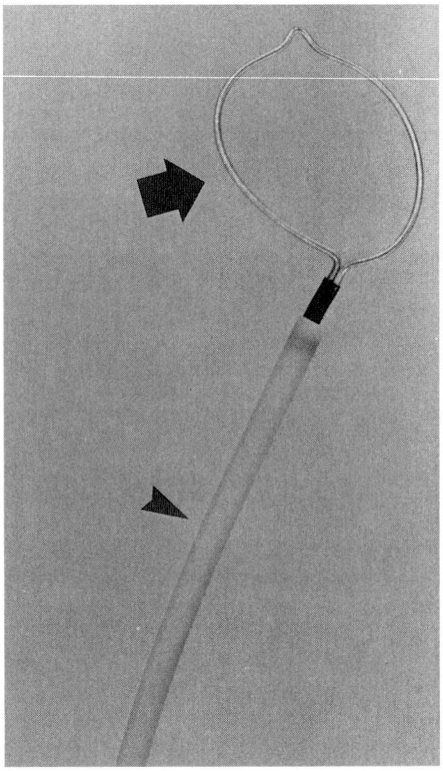

Figure 2. Photograph of a 6.0-F gooseneck snare with a radiopaque loop (arrow), 15-mm loop diameter, and a multipurpose catheter (arrowhead).

For diagnostic purposes and to plan the intervention, dacryocystography was performed in anteroposterior (Fig 1) and lateral views after intubation of the inferior canaliculus with a 27-gauge polyvinyl chloride tubing catheter with a stainless steel cannula (dacryocystography catheter; Cook Europe, Bjaerverskov, Denmark).

In patients with incomplete obstructions ($n = 8$), a 5-F salivary gland catheter with a 23-gauge tapered tip (Rüschelit; Rüsch, Kernen, Germany) was introduced into the superior canaliculus. Recanalization of the stenoses was performed with lateral fluoroscopic guidance by using a 0.014-inch flexible wire (Skipper steerable guide wire; Invatec, Concesio, Italy), which was advanced through the catheter. The guide wire was advanced through the stenoses into the inferior meatus of the nasal cavity. Subsequently, the guide wire was grasped with a 6.0-F gooseneck snare (Amplatz Goose Neck snare; Microvena, White Bear Lake, Minn) with fluoroscopic control and pulled out of the external nares.

In patients with complete obstruction ($n = 2$), a 0.018-inch rigid, double-ended, ball-tipped guide wire (Cook) was used for recanalization. With lateral tension on the lid to prevent kinking of the canaliculus, the guide wire was advanced through the canaliculus to the nasal wall of the lacrimal sac. The guide wire was slightly withdrawn and rotated 90° to point the ball-tipped end caudad. With lateral fluoroscopic guidance, the guide wire was advanced gently across the obstruction into the inferior meatus. The ball-tipped guide wire was then grasped, with lateral fluoroscopic guidance, with a retrieval hook (Cook) and pulled out. The distal ball tip was then cut with a wire-cutting scissors (Storz, St Louis, Mo).

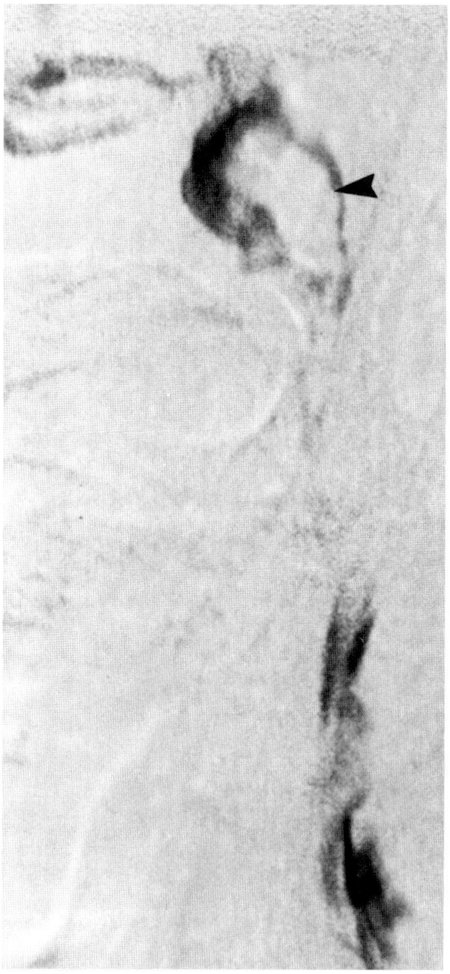

a.

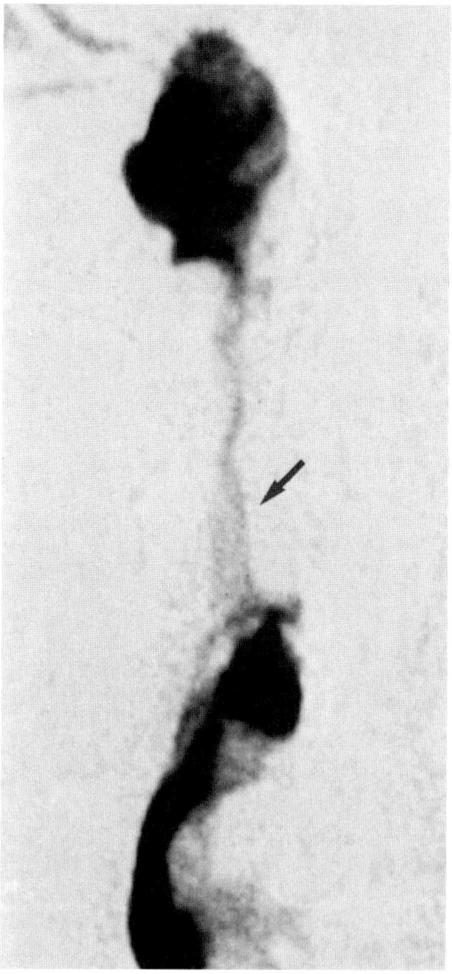

b.

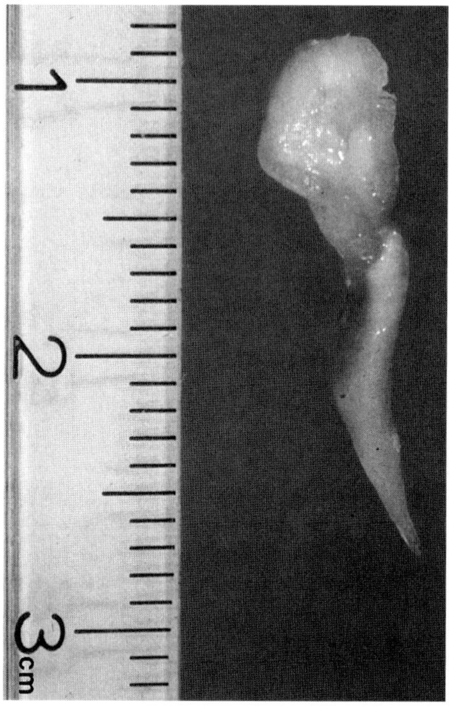

c.

Figure 3. **(a)** Dacryocystogram (frontal view) of the right nasolacrimal duct system shows a large filling defect (arrowhead) in an abnormally dilated lacrimal sac. **(b)** Dacryocystogram (frontal view) after balloon dilation of the stenosed nasolacrimal duct demonstrates improvement of the passage of contrast medium (arrow) through the nasolacrimal duct system. **(c)** Photograph of the dacryolith spontaneously washed out by forced irrigation with saline solution.

With lateral fluoroscopic guidance, a 3-mm-diameter angioplasty balloon catheter (Cook) was passed retrograde over the wire into the nasolacrimal duct and nasolacrimal sac. Dilation of the stenoses was performed by repeated inflation of the balloon for approximately 15 seconds in all 10 patients. After removal of the balloon catheter, washout of the dacryoliths was performed by means of forced antegrade irrigation with saline solution.

In patients with failed dacryolith washout (n = 8) due to dacryolith size, additional balloon dilation was performed to crush the dacryoliths. After the procedure, a 6.3-F sheath (Cook) was passed retrograde over the wire across the stenosed nasolacrimal duct until the tip of the dilator was lying in the nasolacrimal sac below the dacryolith. After withdrawal of the guide wire, the dilator was removed from the sheath, and stone removal was followed by repeated forced irrigation with saline solution with active aspiration of the fragments at the distal end of the sheath with a 50-cm^3 syringe (Plastipak; Becton Dickinson, Drogheda, Ireland).

In two patients with nonfragmented dacryoliths in the nasolacrimal sac after balloon dilation, additional fragmentation of the dacryoliths was performed with a gooseneck snare (Amplatz Snare) (Fig 2). The gooseneck catheter was passed transnasally through the 6.3-F sheath into the nasolacrimal sac, and stone fragmentation was performed by twirling the snare with lateral fluoroscopic control. Afterward, forced irrigation with saline solution was repeated with active aspiration of the fragments at the distal end of the sheath.

In patients with preinterventional complete obstruction of the nasolacrimal duct system, stent (nasolacrimal duct stent; SNDS-600 Song; Cook Australia, Brisbane, Queensland, Australia) implantation was performed according to the technique described by Song et al (7) to restore drainage function and patency. Control dacryocystography was performed in all patients immediately after the procedure.

Prophylactic local antibiotic therapy was performed postinterventionally with gentamicin sulfate antibiotic eyedrops (Refobacin; Merck, Darmstadt, Germany) four times a day. In addition, patients were treated with xylometazoline hydrochloride decongestant eyedrops (Otriven; Zyma, Munich, Germany) for at least 1 week (two drops, four to five times a day) to avoid mucosal swelling. Follow-up dacryocystography and clinical examination were performed 2 weeks and at intervals of 3 months after dacryocystoplasty to assess the function and patency of the nasolacrimal duct system. In addition, clinical success was evaluated by interviewing the patients at the end of the follow-up period (June 5, 1998).

RESULTS

Fluoroscopically guided dacryocystoplasty was technically successful in all patients. During dacryocystoplasty, complete removal of dacryoliths was achieved in six patients, and partial removal was achieved in four patients. The average fluoroscopy

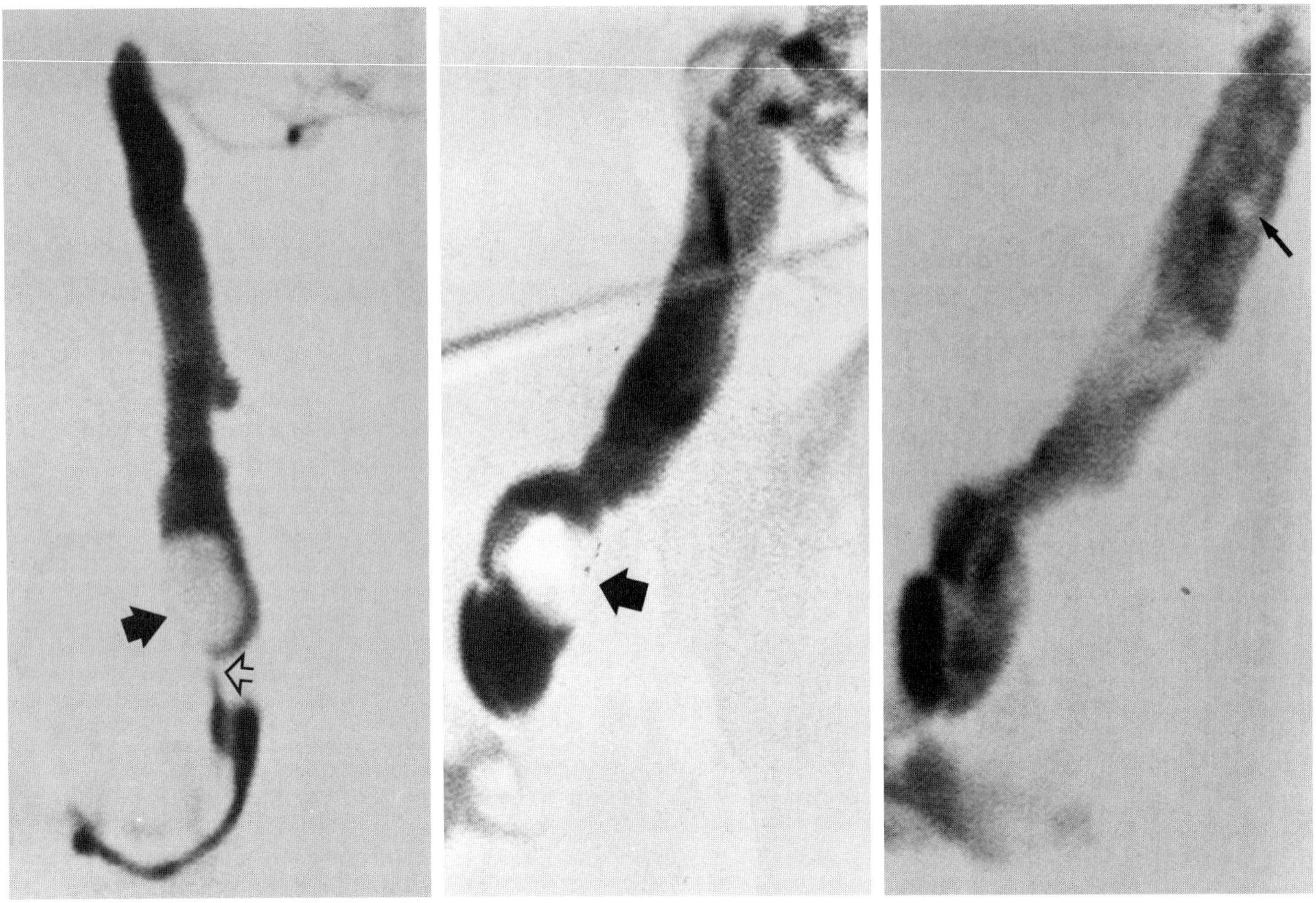

a. b. c.

Figure 4. **(a)** Dacryocystogram (frontal view) of the left nasolacrimal duct system shows a discrete rounded prestenotic filling defect (solid arrow) at the outlet of the nasolacrimal duct near the valve of Hasner (open arrow). **(b)** Dacryocystogram (lateral view) demonstrates the dacryolith (arrow) in a dependent (posterior) position in the nasolacrimal duct, not floating in the lacrimal sac. **(c)** Control dacryocystogram (lateral view) shows a patent nasolacrimal duct system after balloon dilation and removal of the dacryolith. The small filling defect near the upper end of the duct represents an air bubble (arrow) inadvertently injected during dacryocystography.

time of the procedure was 5.7 minutes (range, 3.1–11.5 minutes). There were no major complications. All patients described mild pain during fragmentation of the dacryoliths with the balloon catheter or gooseneck snare. Three patients had slightly blood-stained nasal discharge during and after dacryocystoplasty, which stopped spontaneously within 1–2 hours after the procedure.

The dacryoliths were flushed out completely in two patients, without having to deal with the dacryoliths directly (Figs 3, 4). However, both patients needed dilation of the obstructed nasolacrimal duct segment prior to flushing so that the dacryoliths could be passed.

In patients with failed dacryolith washout (n = 8) due to dacryolith size, additional balloon dilation was performed to crush the dacryoliths. Fragmentation of the dacryoliths was achieved in six patients. Complete removal of the crushed dacryoliths was achieved by aspirating the fragments in three patients. Partial removal of the crushed dacryoliths was achieved in three patients.

In the two patients with unsuccessful balloon fragmentation, additional fragmentation of the dacryoliths with a gooseneck snare was performed (Fig 5). Fragmentation of the dacryoliths was achieved by using the snare in both patients. Complete removal of the crushed dacryoliths was achieved by aspirating the fragments in one patient.

Postinterventional dacryocystography showed adequate widening of all incomplete obstructions after balloon dilation (n = 8). Nasolacrimal duct stents were deployed successfully in the two patients with preexistent complete nasolacrimal duct obstruction after complete extraction of the dacryoliths (n = 2).

The clinical results of the procedure were evident after dacryocystoplasty in all cases. Within a follow-up period up to 18 months (average follow-up, 6 months; range, 3–18 months), five patients showed complete resolution of epiphora, and the remaining five patients showed partial resolution. In three of these patients, the procedure resulted in epiphora requiring dabbing less than twice a day (grade 1, according to Munk et al [15]), and two patients demonstrated occasional epiphora that required dabbing two to four times a day (grade 2, according to Munk et al [15]). In these two patients, clinical examination results demonstrated chronic infective canaliculitis and scarring of the canaliculi.

DISCUSSION

Dacryolithiasis has been considered a clinically important cause of lacrimal duct occlusion (16,17). Cranial movement of

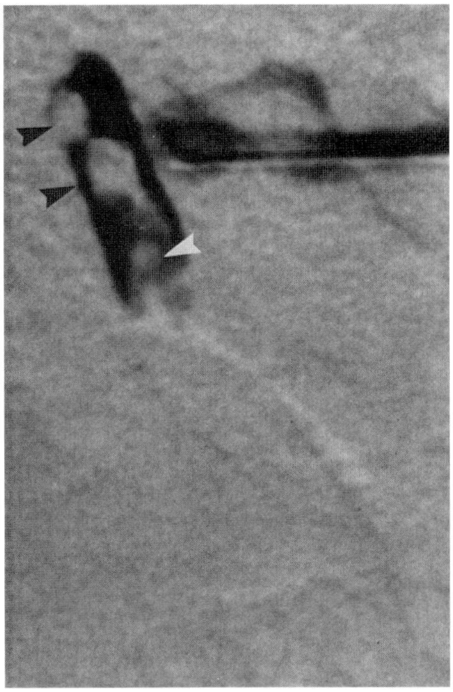

a.

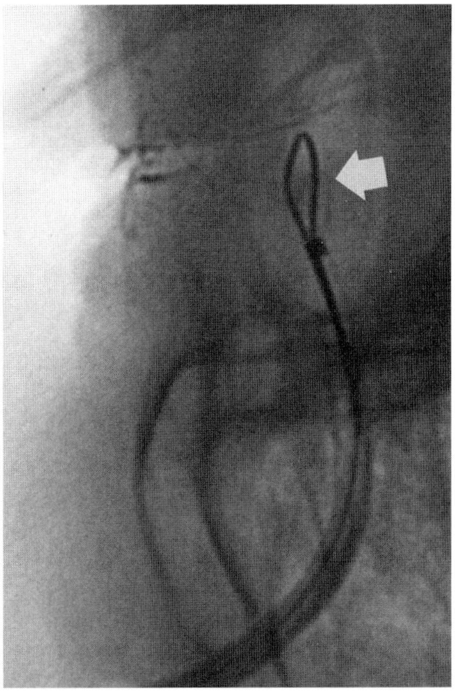

b.

Figure 5. (a) Dacryocystogram (frontal view) shows complete obstruction of the left nasolacrimal duct system at the junction between the lacrimal sac and the nasolacrimal duct, with prestenotic filling defects (arrowheads) representing dacryoliths. (b) Dacryocystogram (lateral view) shows a gooseneck snare (arrow) has been passed transnasally through the 6.3-F sheath in the nasolacrimal sac, and fragmentation of the dacryoliths is performed by twirling the snare. (c) Dacryocystogram (lateral view) obtained during forced irrigation and aspiration at the distal end of the sheath shows fragmented dacryoliths (arrows) flowing through the sheath. (d) Dacryocystogram (frontal view) obtained after stent implantation shows good passage of the contrast medium (arrows) through the stent into the nasal cavity. (e) Photograph shows multiple small fragments aspirated into the syringe.

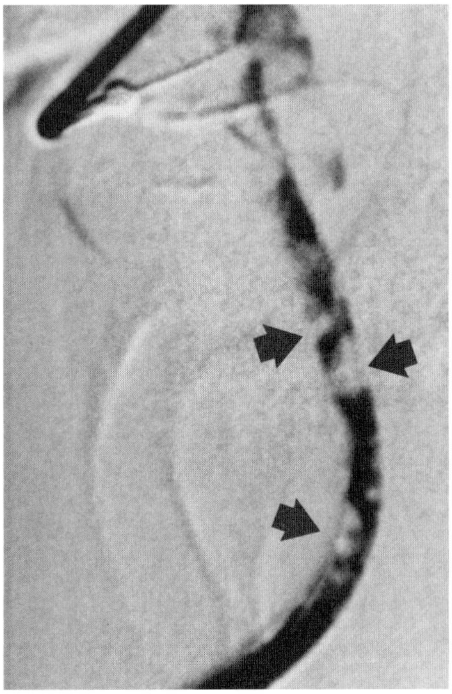

c.

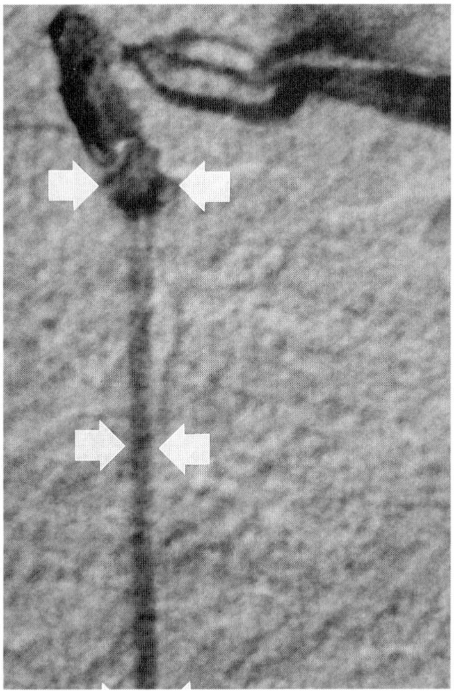

d.

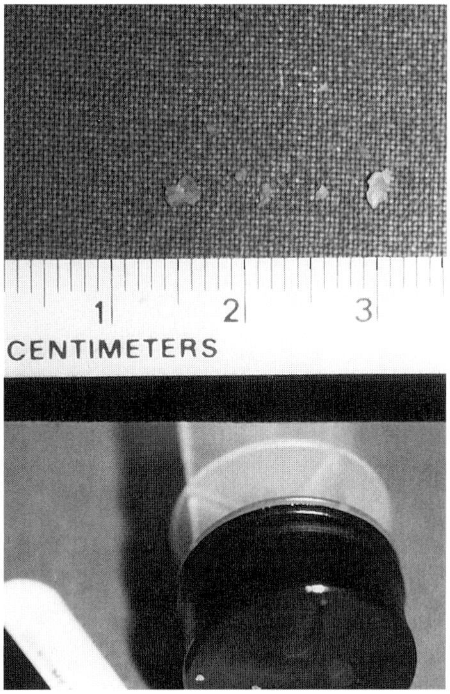

e.

free dacryoliths will allow free flow of tears, while caudal movement of the dacryoliths creates a ball-valve effect that results in complete nasolacrimal obstruction (17,18). Patients complain of chronic intermittent epiphora frequently associated with mucopurulent discharge (17,19,20). Stasis secondary to an anatomic irregularity is a frequent predisposing factor (21,22). Additional chronic infective canaliculitis is frequently associated with dacryolithiasis because organisms, such as an *Actinomyces* species or, less frequently, *Staphylococcus aureus,* form filamentous aggregates (sulfur granules) (17,23).

Dacryocystography frequently shows dilatation and irregularity of the affected nasolacrimal duct system with an appearance of sacculation, beading, or diverticula (17). Prestenotic filling defects representing dacryoliths typically are located in the lacrimal sac (Figs 3a, 5a) (11,14). However, air bubbles injected into the nasolacrimal system during dacryocystography represent an artifact that can simulate dacryoliths. In these cases, a cross-table lateral view will demonstrate the air bubble floating in the lacrimal sac, while dacryoliths tend to settle in the more dependent (posterior) position (Fig 4b) (17).

In 1995, Song et al (5) reported nonsurgical management of dacryolithiasis in a 51-year-old woman with epiphora caused by a complete obstruction of the nasolacrimal duct system. Preinterventional dacryocystography showed an obstruction at the level of the neck of the lacrimal sac at its junction with the nasolacrimal duct, with filling defects in the prestenotic dilated nasolacrimal sac. During stent implantation, the authors discovered that the concrements were broken into fragments. While the lacrimal system was irrigated with saline solution, the fragments passed into the pharynx. The authors were unable to save the dacryoliths because the patient swallowed them during the irrigation.

Removal of dacryoliths as a sole procedure is not a sufficient therapy because the stenosis of the duct system persists and results in continued epiphora. Therefore, surgical removal of dacryoliths along with dacryocystorhinostomy has still been necessary (5). Dacryocystorhinostomy, however, usually requires general anesthesia combined with hospitalization of the patient and may leave a permanent facial scar. Moreover, failure still occurs in 6%–13% (13 of 103) of patients (21,24). The previous studies (15,21) of nasolacrimal duct stent implantation or balloon dilation showed encouraging results in the treatment of the obstructed nasolacrimal duct system. However, the extraction of associated dacryoliths was not mentioned as an interventional radiologic procedure in these reports.

In cases of dacryolithiasis associated with an incomplete obstruction of the nasolacrimal duct system, patients may be treated by means of balloon dilation followed by forced irrigation with saline solution. In these cases, balloon dilation primarily is used to widen the stenosed lacrimal duct segment so that dacryoliths can pass into the nasal cavity. If stone passage is not achieved because of the size of the dacryoliths, or because of a persistent stenosis of the nasolacrimal duct system, balloon dilation also may be used to crush the concrements. In cases of incomplete washout of concrements by means of forced irrigation with saline solution, a 6.3-F sheath is advanced retrograde over the wire, across the stenosed nasolacrimal duct, until the tip of the dilator is lying below the dacryolith. After the guide wire is withdrawn, repeated forced irrigation with saline solution is performed with active aspiration of the fragments through the sheath.

During these procedures, fluoroscopy is necessary to avoid damage of the nasolacrimal duct system, to observe the position of the balloon catheter and sheath, and to control the aspiration of the fragmented dacryoliths. When bending of the sheath occurs or fragments are too large to pass through the sheath, attempts of stone removal may be ineffective. However, according to our observations, aspiration of the fragments during forced irrigation with saline solution is sufficient in most cases.

In a few cases, control dacryocystography will show persistent concrements in the lacrimal sac. In these cases, additional fragmentation with a gooseneck snare is possible. A snare is passed transnasally through a 6.3-F sheath into the lacrimal sac, and stone fragmentation is performed by twirling the snare (Fig 5b). During this intervention, fluoroscopy is necessary to identify the exact level of the dacryolith so that the twirling of the gooseneck snare is effective and to avoid damage of the nasolacrimal duct system. The procedure is very effective but causes more discomfort for the patients than balloon dacryocystoplasty alone. Therefore, in addition to the routinely administered topical anesthesia, the patient should be sedated. After the fragmented dacryoliths have been completely washed out, control dacryocystography must be performed to verify nasolacrimal duct patency. In cases of preinterventional complete obstruction of the nasolacrimal duct system, stent implantation is necessary to restore the drainage function.

In conclusion, the results of our study demonstrate that dacryocystoplasty is a feasible form of therapy with good clinical outcome even in nasolacrimal duct obstructions associated with dacryolithiasis. This procedure offers the following advantages over the invasive surgical procedure: General anesthesia is not needed, there is no alteration of the anatomy, the therapy is feasible on an outpatient basis, and no facial scar is produced. The interventional radiologic procedure we describe should be considered as an alternative to dacryocystorhinostomy in the treatment of dacryolithiasis, and dacryocystorhinostomy can be used in case of failure.

Acknowledgment: We thank William P. Gray, MD, FRCSI, FRCS(SN), Senior Lecturer, University Department of Clinical Neurosciences, Southampton General Hospital, Southampton, England, for correcting the manuscript.

References

1. Linberg JV, McCormick SA. Primary acquired nasolacrimal duct obstruction: a clinicopathologic report and biopsy technique. Ophthalmology 1986; 93:1055–1063.
2. Traquair HM. Chronic dacryocystitis: its causation and treatment. Arch Ophthalmol 1941; 26:165–180.
3. Hawes MJ. The dacryolithiasis syndrome. Ophthalmol Plast Reconstr Surg 1988; 4:87–90.
4. Herzig S, Hurwitz JJ. Lacrimal sac calculi. Can J Ophthalmol 1979; 14:17-20.
5. Song HY, Jin YH, Lee HK, Sung KB. Nonoperative management of dacryolithiasis. JVIR 1995; 6:647–650.
6. Janssen AG, Mansour K, Bos JJ. Obstructed nasolacrimal duct system in epiphora: long-term results of dacryocystoplasty by means of balloon dilatation. Radiology 1997; 205:791–796.
7. Song HY, Jin YH, Kim JH, et al. Placement of a nasolacrimal polyurethane stent. Radiology 1995; 194:233–237.
8. Wilhelm KE, Textor J, Hofer U, Schild HH. Nasolacrimal duct obstructions: treatment with balloon dilatation and stent implantation (abstr). Radiology 1997; 205(P):430.
9. Wilhelm K, Textor J, Hofer U, Böker T, Strunk H, Schild H. Nasolacrimal duct obstructions: treatment with balloon dilatation and stent implantation. Fortschr Röntgenstr 1997; 167: 486–490. [German]
10. Song HY, Jin YH, Kim JH, et al. Nonsurgical placement of a nasolacrimal polyurethane stent: long-term effectiveness. Radiology 1996; 200:759–763.
11. Berkefeld J, Kirchner J, Müller HM, Fries U, Kollath J. Balloon dacryocystoplasty: indications and contraindications. Radiology 1997; 205:785–790.
12. Jones LT. Tear-sac foreign bodies. Am J Ophthalmol 1965; 60:111–113.
13. Wilkis RB, Pressly JP. Diagnosis and incidence of lacrimal calculi. Ophthalmic Surg 1980; 11:787–789.
14. Wilhelm K, Krämer S, Textor J, Ewen K, Schüller H, Schild H. Radiation dose to the ocular lens, parotid and thyroid glands during dacryocystography and fluoroscopy-guided dacryocystoplasty. Fortschr Röntgenstr 1998; 168:270–274. [German]
15. Munk PL, Lin DTC, Morris DC. Epiphora: treatment by means of dacryocystoplasty with balloon dilation of the nasolacrimal drainage apparatus. Radiology 1990; 177:687–690.
16. Baratz KH, Bartley GB, Campbell RJ, Garrity JA. An eyelash nidus for dacryoliths of the lacrimal excretory and secretory systems. Am J Ophthalmol 1991; 111:624–627.
17. Kassel EE, Schatz CJ. Lacrimal apparatus. In: Som PM, Curtin HD, eds. Head and neck imaging. 3rd ed. St Louis, Mo: Mosby-Year Book, 1995; 1129–1183.
18. Berlin AJ, Rath R, Rich L. Lacrimal system dacryoliths. Surgery 1980; 11:435–436.
19. Francois J, Elewault-Ryssellaere M, De Vos E. Mycose et pseudomycoses des voies lacrymales. Ann d'Oculistique 1966; 199:1129–1142.
20. Sathananthan N, Sullivan TJ, Rose GE, Moseley IF. Intubation dacryocystography in patients with a clinical diagnosis of chronic canaliculitis ("streptothrix"). Br J Radiol 1993; 66:389–393.
21. Becker BB, Berry FD. Balloon catheter dilatation in lacrimal surgery. Ophthalmic Surg 1989; 20:193–198.
22. Maltzmann BA, Favetta JR. Dacryolithiasis. Ann Ophthalmol 1979; 11:473–475.
23. Kaye-Wilson LG. Spontaneous passage of a dacryolith (case report). Br J Ophthalmol 1991; 75:564.
24. Walther EK, Herberhold C, Lippel R. Digitale subtraktions-dacryozystographie (DS-DCG) und ergebnisbilanz endonasaler tränenwegschirurgie. Laryngorhinootologie 1994; 73: 609–613.

Johann Link, MD
Johann C. Steffens, MD
Joachim Brossmann, MD
Joachim Graessner, PhD
Stephanie Hackethal, MD
Martin Heller, MD

Index terms:
Arteries, grafts and prostheses, 922.1268, 984.1268, 986.1268
Arteries, stenosis or obstruction, 922.721, 984.721, 986.721
Magnetic resonance (MR), comparative studies
Magnetic resonance (MR), vascular studies, 922.12942, 922.12943, 984.12942, 984.12943, 986.12942, 986.12943
Stents and prostheses, 922.1268, 984.1268, 986.1268

Radiology 1999; 212:371–377

Abbreviation:
DSA = digital subtraction angiography

[1] From the Department of Radiology, Christian-Albrechts-University of Kiel, Germany (J.L., J.C.S., J.B., S.H., M.H.); and Siemens Medical Systems, Hamburg, Germany (J.G.). Received December 1, 1997; revision requested February 23, 1998; final revision received November 16; accepted February 22, 1999. **Address reprint requests to** J.L., Institut für Röntgendiagnostik, Universitätsklinikum Regensburg, Regensburg 93042, Germany (e-mail: *johann.link@klinik.uni-regensburg.de*).

Author contributions:
Guarantor of integrity of entire study, J.L.; study concepts, J.L.; study design, J.L., J.C.S.; definition of intellectual content, J.L., M.H.; literature research, S.H.; clinical studies, J.L., J.C.S., J.B.; data acquisition, J.C.S., J.B.; data analysis, J.L., J.C.S.; statistical analysis, S.H.; manuscript preparation, J.L., J.G.; manuscript editing, J.B.; manuscript review, M.H.

Iliofemoral Arterial Occlusive Disease: Contrast-enhanced MR Angiography for Preinterventional Evaluation and Follow-up after Stent Placement[1]

PURPOSE: To evaluate the efficacy of contrast material–enhanced magnetic resonance (MR) angiography for the diagnosis of peripheral arterial occlusion and follow-up after stent placement.

MATERIALS AND METHODS: Sixty-seven patients (21 women, 46 men; mean age, 64.6 years) were examined. Digital subtraction angiography and contrast-enhanced MR angiography were performed in 28 patients for preinterventional evaluation of iliofemoral arterial occlusion and in 39 patients for follow-up after stent placement in the iliac or femoral arteries, which had been performed several months before.

RESULTS: All 24 occlusions were correctly diagnosed with contrast-enhanced MR angiography. Of the 59 stenoses, 36 were greater than 50% and 23 were 50% or less. Sensitivity and specificity for the detection of stenoses greater than 50% were 100% and 83%, respectively. Patency of the different stents was determined correctly with contrast-enhanced MR angiography. Some stents caused signal intensity dropout, which made MR evaluation of stents difficult. Generally, these signal intensity artifacts were most severe in stainless steel stents and mild in some nitinol stents.

CONCLUSION: Contrast-enhanced MR angiography is comparable to digital subtraction angiography for the detection of stenosis greater than 50% and occlusion in the iliofemoral arteries. Stent patency can be determined, but contrast-enhanced MR angiography is not suitable for stent evaluation owing to signal intensity dropout; however, it provides information about the vascular anatomic areas proximal and distal to the stent.

Magnetic resonance (MR) angiography is an alternative to intraarterial digital subtraction angiography (DSA) for the diagnosis of peripheral arterial occlusive disease. The limitations of MR angiography have been long imaging times and artifacts caused by elongated vessels, superimposed venous structures, and slow and pulsatile flow (1–3).

With the advent of contrast material–enhanced MR angiography, a technique is available that makes use of the shortened T1 relaxation times of blood after the administration of gadopentetate dimeglumine and thus achieves high signal intensity from blood with the use of three-dimensional gradient-echo sequences and short relaxation times (4–13).

The goals of this prospective study were to determine the role of contrast-enhanced MR angiography in the evaluation of iliofemoral arterial occlusive disease and to evaluate its accuracy in assessing the patency of iliofemoral arterial stents by using DSA as the reference standard.

MATERIALS AND METHODS

Sixty-seven patients (21 women, 46 men; age range, 29–87 years; mean age ± SD, 64.6 years ± 11) who were referred to our hospital for angiography and underwent contrast-enhanced MR angiography of the iliac and femoral arteries in addition to intraarterial DSA were included in this study. MR angiography was performed in all patients the day before intraarterial DSA. Informed consent was obtained from all patients, and institutional approval to perform contrast-enhanced MR angiographic studies for comparison with DSA was obtained. The contrast-enhanced MR angiographic studies were performed by using a three-dimensional gradient-echo sequence (repetition time msec/echo time msec, 7.8/2.1; flip angle, 30°; effective section thickness, 1.82 mm; slab thickness, 116 mm; field of view, 438 × 500 mm; matrix, 224 × 512) with a 1.5-T MR imaging unit (Magnetom Vision; Siemens Medical Systems, Erlangen, Germany). The circular polarized body coil served as a transmit-receive coil. The data acquisition time was 1 minute 54 seconds. Owing to the field of view limitation of 500 mm, contrast-enhanced MR angiography enabled the assessment of only the iliofemoral region; popliteal and infrapopliteal arteries were not evaluated with this imaging modality.

Seven targeted views were reconstructed with the maximum intensity projection technique in intervals of 0° and 180° (left lateral–to–right lateral view) and in steps of 30°. In all patients, the maximum intensity projection images and raw data were analyzed together. Thirty milliliters of gadodiamide (Omniscan; Nycomed, Oslo, Norway) was injected with an MR-compatible injector (Spectris; Medrad, Volkach, Germany) at a flow rate of 0.6 mL/sec and an injection delay of 10 seconds.

Indications for DSA were preinterventional evaluation of iliofemoral arterial occlusive disease in 28 (42%) symptomatic patients and follow-up after stent placement in 39 (58%) patients in whom 41 stents had been implanted several months before. In each patient who underwent DSA, for either preinterventional evaluation of iliofemoral occlusive disease or follow-up after stent placement, additional contrast-enhanced MR angiography was performed. Intraarterial DSA was performed in five steps, from the iliac region to the lower limb, in an anteroposterior view. Occasionally, in cases of uncertainty, multiple views were obtained. A 4-F pigtail catheter was inserted above the aortic bifurcation. In each step, 30 mL of iomeprol (300 mg/mL) (Imeron 300; Byk Gulden, Konstanz, Germany) was injected at a flow rate of 14 mL/sec.

With DSA only anteroposterior views were available; however, contrast-enhanced MR angiography provided anteroposterior views and additional views of 30°, 60°, and 90° projections on each side. In both contrast-enhanced MR angiography and DSA, narrowing of the vessels was measured with calipers on the film hard-copy images. The most severe narrowing was related to the normal diameter of the artery above and below the lesion.

Twenty-four occlusions and 59 stenoses were observed in all 67 patients. The grade of stenoses was 50% or less in 23 (39%) of 59 cases and greater than 50% in 36 (61%) of 59 cases. Five occlusions, 14 stenoses greater than 50%, and 16 stenoses of 50% or less were observed in the iliac region. The other 19 occlusions, 22 stenoses greater than 50%, and seven stenoses of 50% or less were located in the superficial femoral arteries.

In the 39 patients with 41 stents, follow-up angiography was performed. The 24 stents implanted in the iliac arteries

Stent Sizes and Lengths

Stent	Size (mm)	Length (cm)
Wallstent	8.9 ± 0.7 (8.0–10.0)	3.8 ± 0.8 (3.0–4.5)
Memotherm	9.8 ± 1.5 (8.0–12.0)	5.4 ± 1.9 (4.0–8.0)
Palmaz	6.0 ± 0.6 (4.0–6.0)	3.4 ± 0.4 (3.0–3.9)
Cragg	10.0 ± 1.1 (8.0–12.0)	4.5 ± 1.6 (3.0–6.0)
Cragg Endopro	5.5 ± 0.5 (5.0–6.0)	9.0 ± 2.3 (3.0–10.0)

Note.—Data are the mean ± SD. Numbers in parentheses are the range.

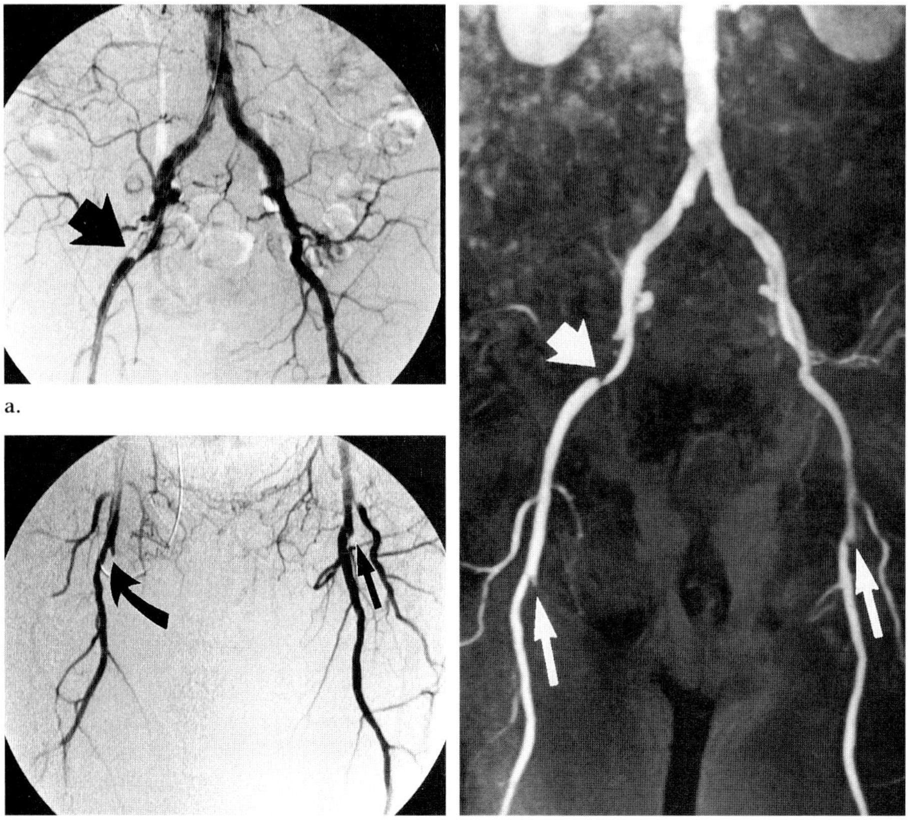

a. b. c.

Figure 1. (**a**, **b**) Anteroposterior digital subtraction angiograms obtained in a 72-year-old man show high-grade stenosis of the right external iliac artery (arrow in **a**) and occlusion of the right (curved arrow in **b**) and left (straight arrow in **b**) superficial femoral arteries. (**c**) Anteroposterior contrast-enhanced MR angiogram (7.8/2.1, 30° flip angle) obtained in the same patient shows high-grade stenosis of the right external iliac artery (short arrow) to the same extent as that in **a**. The occlusions of both superficial femoral arteries (long arrows), which were seen in **b**, are depicted equally well at contrast-enhanced MR angiography.

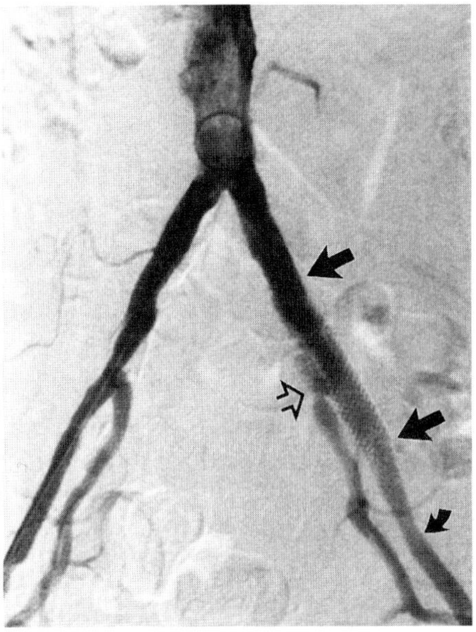

a.

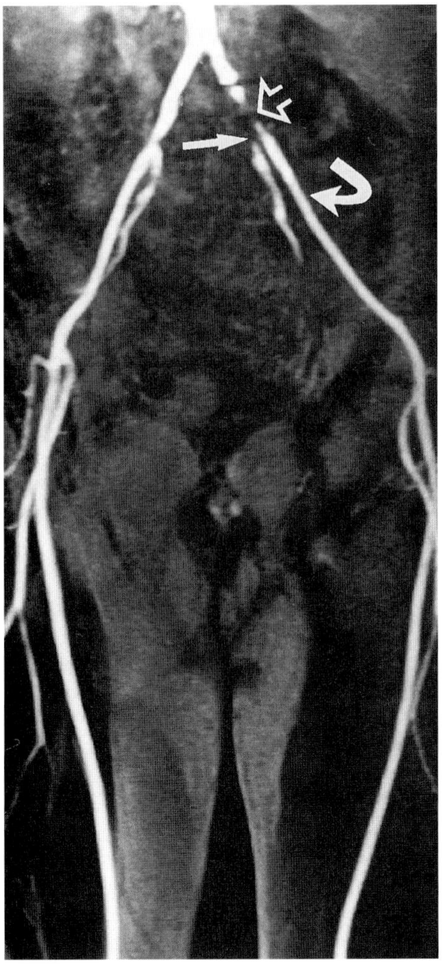

b.

Figure 2. (a) Follow-up anteroposterior digital subtraction angiogram obtained in a 61-year-old man 6 months after placement of a Wallstent (solid straight arrows) that extends from the distal common iliac artery to the external iliac artery. Although the Wallstent is crossing the origin of the left internal iliac artery (open arrow), DSA shows patency of the left internal and external (curved arrow) iliac arteries. (b) Follow-up anteroposterior contrast-enhanced MR angiogram (7.8/2.1, 30° flip angle) obtained in the same patient shows signal intensity voids at the proximal and distal ends of the left common iliac arterial segment treated with a Wallstent. There is complete signal intensity dropout in the center of the Wallstent (open arrow). The origin of the left internal iliac artery (solid straight arrow) is not visible owing to the signal intensity loss caused by the stent placement. Patency of the Wallstent is defined by the high signal intensity of the external iliac artery (curved arrow) without the presence of collateral vessels.

were as follows: eight Cragg and two Cragg Endopro stents (Boston Scientific, Watertown, Mass), seven Memotherm stents (Bard-Angiomed, Karlsruhe, Germany), and seven Wallstents (Schneider, Buelach, Switzerland). The 17 stents placed in the femoral arteries were Cragg Endopro (n = 12) and Palmaz (Johnson & Johnson Interventional Systems, Warren, NJ) (n = 5) stents. The sizes of these stents are shown in the Table.

The evaluation criteria for the comparative study were the quality of contrast-enhanced MR versus intraarterial digital subtraction angiograms with regard to venous superimposition, and the accuracy of contrast-enhanced MR angiography versus that of DSA in depicting occlusions and stenoses of 50% or less and greater than 50% in the iliac and femoral region and in assessing patency and stenosis after stent placement at 6-month follow-up.

All digital subtraction angiograms and MR angiograms were evaluated separately by two experienced cardiovascular radiologists (J.L., J.C.S.) in a blinded manner. The entire vascular tree, from the distal aorta to the femoral arteries, was assessed. Discrepancies were resolved by consensus. Statistical analyses were performed by calculating sensitivity and specificity values. Overestimations of stenosis were considered to be false-positive findings, and underestimations were considered to be false-negative findings. To determine interobserver variability, the Spearman-rank correlation test was used.

RESULTS

All of the arteries could be evaluated. All of the nondiseased arteries were assessed correctly, and no stenosis was overestimated as an occlusion. Veins were enhanced in eight examinations; however, there was no superimposition on the arteries.

The mean length of the stenoses and occlusions (± SD) were 2.7 cm (± 1.7) and 3.5 (± 2.3), respectively. The results of analyses of all the lesions, including the 59 stenoses and 24 occlusions, with contrast-enhanced MR angiography and intraarterial DSA agreed in 79 (95%) of the 83 cases. In the evaluation of the 36 high-grade (greater than 50%) stenoses and 24 occlusions, there was 100% agreement between contrast-enhanced MR angiography and intraarterial DSA; both the sensitivity and specificity of MR angiography were 100%.

Stenoses of 50% of less were overestimated with MR angiography—that is, interpreted as stenoses greater than 50%—in four (17%) of 23 cases. Thus, the sensitivity of MR angiography for the detection of stenoses greater than 50% was 100%, and the specificity was 83% (19 of 23 cases).

The overall agreement between contrast-enhanced MR angiography and intraarterial DSA was 93% in the iliac region (Fig 1); the sensitivity and specificity of MR angiography for the detection of stenosis greater than 50% in this region were 100% and 88%, respectively. There was 93% agreement between contrast-enhanced MR angiography and intraarterial DSA in depicting stenosis greater than 50% in the femoral region, with a sensitivity of 100% and specificity of 71%. The interobserver variability for identifying and grading all lesions was 0.93 ($P < .001$).

Four femoral stents were incompletely visualized with contrast-enhanced MR angiography because of their location at the distal end of the field of view. The depiction of the remaining different stents on contrast-enhanced MR angiograms was heterogeneous. The Wallstent caused a reduction in signal intensity in four of seven cases (Fig 2) and a complete loss of signal intensity in three of seven cases (Fig 3). The Palmaz stent caused a total loss of signal intensity in the area in which it was placed in all five cases (Fig 3). The Memotherm stent caused a loss of signal intensity in four cases (Fig 4) and reduced signal intensity in three cases. The Cragg and Cragg Endopro stents caused discrete reductions in signal intensity along the stents and circumscribed signal intensity voids at the ends of these prostheses (Fig 3).

Four occlusions that were visible after the placement of Cragg Endopro stents in the femoral arteries were detected with both contrast-enhanced MR angiography and DSA. Furthermore, eight restenoses of greater than 70% were observed at intraarterial DSA. These occurred at the ends of the Cragg Endopro stent in four cases and inside the Cragg stent in two cases, Palmaz stent in one case, and Wallstent in one case. Only one of the four restenoses that occurred at the ends of the Cragg Endopro stent was detected with contrast-enhanced MR angiography (Fig 5).

DISCUSSION

Contrast-enhanced MR angiography is a promising technique that may have the potential to replace angiography in the assessment of peripheral arterial occlusive disease (13). Usually, only stenoses greater than 50% require surgical or interventional treatment; however, some 50% stenoses may be hemodynamically relevant, as proved by pressure measurements obtained before and after the administration of vasodilators. In the present study, the maximum intensity projection reconstruction of targeted parts of the vessels allowed an unobstructed view of the arteries in all cases. Veins were visible on eight contrast-enhanced MR angiographic studies, but the diagnostic value of these images was not reduced. No false-positive overestimations of normal arteries as stenosed or of high-grade stenoses as occluded occurred in this study. However, four stenoses of 50% or less were given false-positive evaluations as stenoses greater than 50%. These four overestimated stenoses were interpreted as 40%–45% stenoses on the DSA studies.

Compared with contrast-enhanced MR angiography, the time-of-flight MR angiographic technique that we used previously often had disadvantages in imaging of the iliac arteries; the transversal orientation of vessel branches was hardly visualized owing to inplane saturation effects on the original axial sections. This effect causes normal arteries to be misinterpreted as stenosed or occluded (3). Another cause of problems with time-of-flight MR angiography is turbulent blood flow in the poststenotic region, which causes an overestimation of stenosis. Good agreement between conventional angiography and time-of-flight MR angiography in the detection of 50%–90% stenoses has been reported in the literature (3,14–16).

In previous studies (2,3), use of thin transaxial sections in combination with segmented and triggered acquisition in two-dimensional time-of-flight MR angiography caused a reduction of saturation effects. This technique, however, requires a long acquisition time for the examination of iliac and femoral vessels (2,3). Nevertheless, there are reports that two-dimensional time-of-flight MR angiography may depict stenoses and occlusions in elongated iliac vessels when there is slow blood flow (1,3).

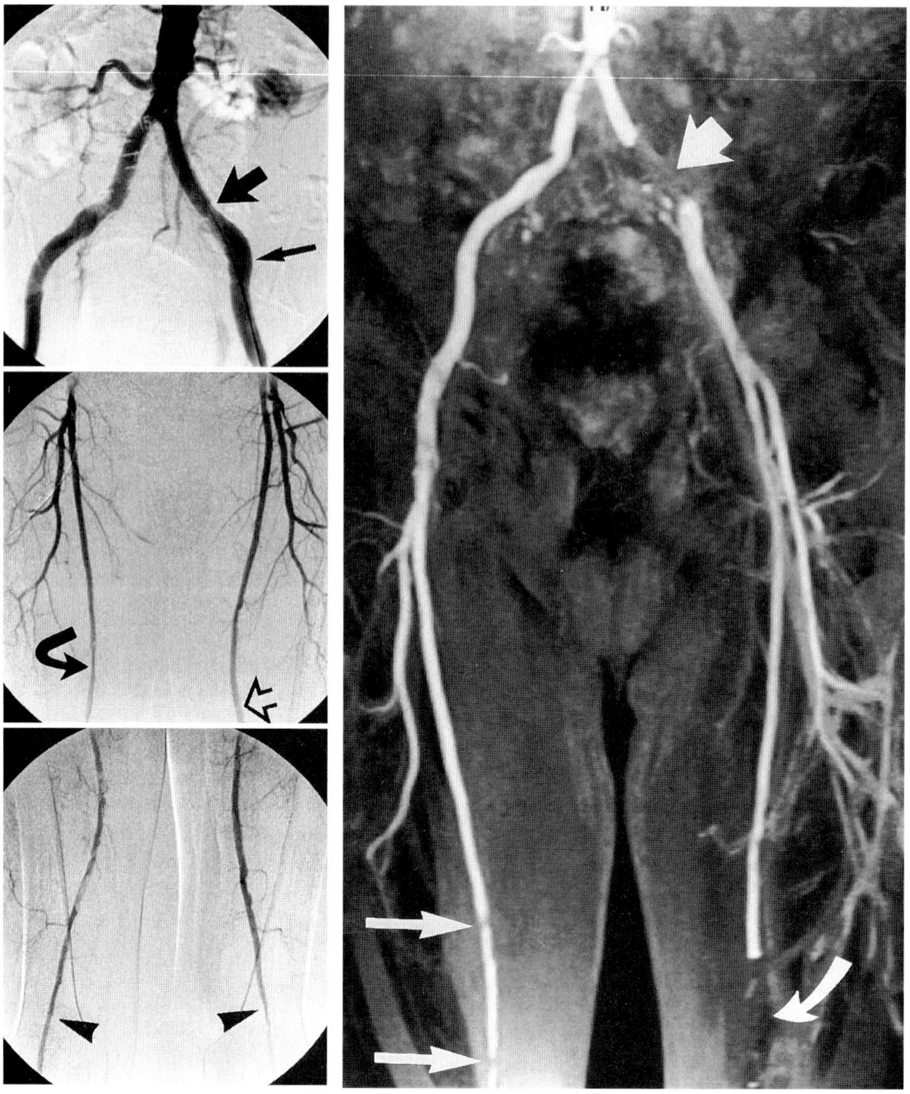

a. b.

Figure 3. (a) Follow-up anteroposterior digital subtraction angiograms obtained in a 64-year-old man after placement of a Wallstent (thick arrow) in the left common iliac artery, Palmaz stent (open arrow) in the left superficial femoral artery, and Cragg Endopro stent (curved arrow) in the right superficial femoral artery. The angiograms show patency of the stents in the left iliac artery (thin arrow) and in both superficial femoral arteries (arrowheads). (b) On the follow-up anteroposterior contrast-enhanced MR angiogram (7.8/2.1, 30° flip angle) obtained in the same patient, complete signal intensity loss is seen in the left common iliac artery segment treated with a Wallstent (thick arrow) and in the left superficial femoral artery treated with a Palmaz stent (curved arrow). There are circumscribed signal intensity voids (thin arrows) at the ends of the Cragg Endopro stent in the right superficial femoral artery.

The contrast mechanism of contrast-enhanced MR angiography circumvents all of the obstacles mentioned above. With the use of very short repetition and echo times at moderate (25°–40°) flip angles, the shortening of the T1 relaxation time of blood, from normally about 1,200 msec at 1.5 T to less than 50 msec, results in high signal intensity in the entire vessel lumen (4–13). Because of its independence from inflow effects, contrast-enhanced MR angiography enables the acquisition of data in the coronal plane. This allows a long vessel segment to be depicted with one short sequence

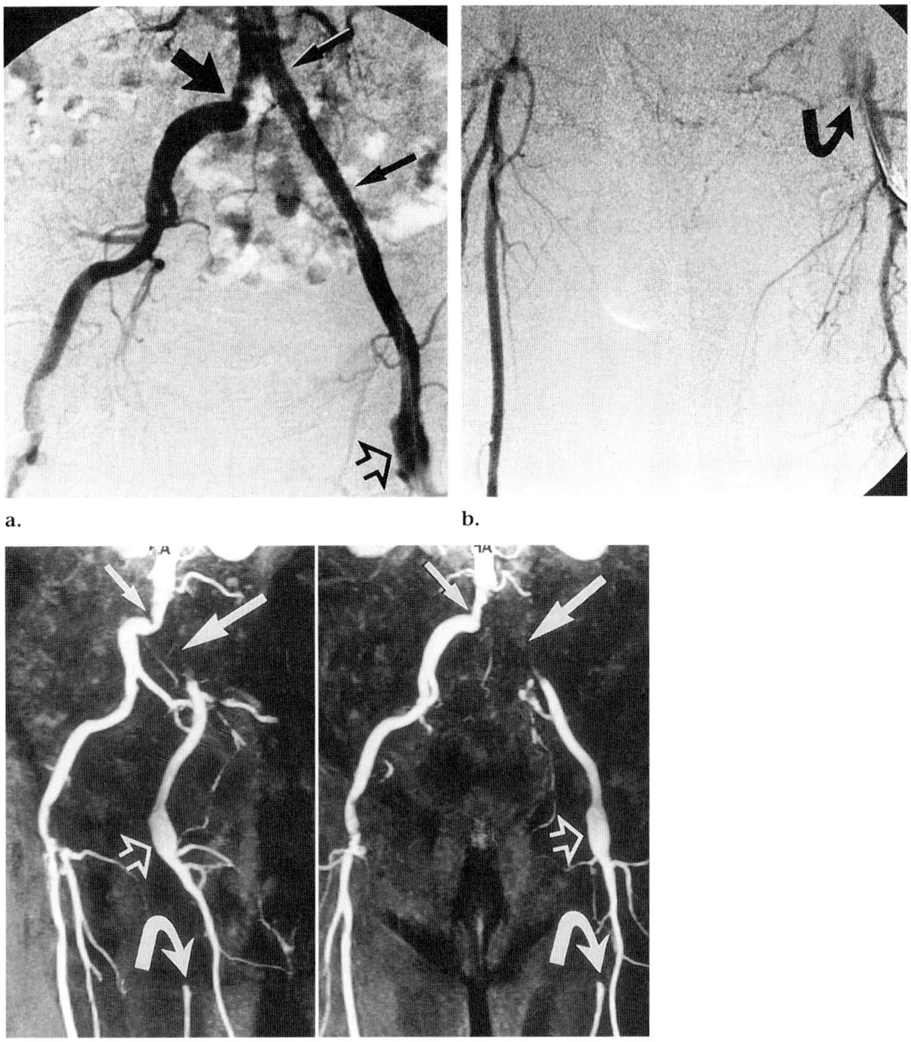

a. b. c.

Figure 4. (**a**, **b**) Follow-up anteroposterior digital subtraction angiograms obtained in a 69-year-old man 6 months after placement of a Memotherm stent (thin arrows in **a**) show patency of the left common iliac artery and an elongated right common iliac artery with stenosis greater than 50% (thick arrow in **a**). There is an aneurysm (open arrow in **a**) in the distal common femoral artery. The left superficial femoral artery (curved arrow in **b**) is occluded. (**c**) Follow-up left anterior oblique (60°)(left) and anteroposterior (right) contrast-enhanced MR angiograms (7.8/2.1, 30° flip angle) obtained in the same patient show complete signal intensity loss in the left common iliac artery (large arrow) due to the placement of the Memotherm stent. The high-signal-intensity vessel distal to the stent makes stent patency evident. There is an aneurysm (open arrow) at the origin of the occluded left superficial femoral artery. High signal intensity can be seen distally in the superficial femoral artery (curved arrow). Elongation of the right common iliac artery with stenosis greater than 50% (small arrow) also is seen.

(17). The measurement time was less than 2 minutes in our study. Two-dimensional segmented and triggered time-of-flight MR angiography, as well as thick-slab triggered two-dimensional phase-contrast MR angiography, requires 10–30 minutes to cover the same range of anatomy (2,3). The three-dimensional phase-contrast MR angiographic technique is generally no longer used because it involves extremely long acquisition times in imaging the peripheral arteries. Two-dimensional phase-contrast MR angiography has yielded good results in the depiction of peripheral arterial occlusive disease in the coronal plane, but it also has caused overestimations of stenoses in the region of the vessel branches owing to turbulence (2).

The advantage of contrast-enhanced MR angiography compared with two-dimensional triggered phase-contrast MR angiography is its capability to enable one to view multiple reconstructed maximum intensity projection images from the three-dimensional data without venous superimposition in most cases. Two-dimensional phase-contrast MR angiography tends to cause underestimations of stenoses owing to superimposed venous structures (2,18). Another advantage of the described contrast-enhanced MR angiographic technique is the use of a 512 matrix, which provides better resolution and improved suppression of stent artifacts because of the smaller voxels and results in decreased dephasing effects.

Four reocclusions of femoral arteries treated with Cragg Endopro stents were diagnosed owing to a lack of enhancement within the stent and distinct collateralization around the narrowed region. On the other hand, the patency of Palmaz stents was evaluated despite the complete loss of signal intensity in the stent. When there is signal intensity loss in the area of stent placement, the patency of the prosthesis can be determined when there is a high-signal-intensity vessel distal to the stent with no collateral vessels present.

The composition and orientation of the stent influence the imaging artifacts caused by stents at contrast-enhanced MR angiography. Contrast-enhanced MR angiography revealed signal intensity loss in all cases in which stainless steel Palmaz stents were placed. However, in all cases of nitinol Cragg and Cragg Endopro stent placement, there was slightly diminished signal intensity along the stent at contrast-enhanced MR angiography but circumscribed signal intensity voids at the ends owing to the platinum markers. Olree et al (19) observed a variety of susceptibility artifacts with different stent designs. These artifacts were most severe with stainless steel stents and mild with nitinol stents. Similar to Schuermann et al (20), we observed different signal intensity behaviors in the nitinol stents from different manufacturers. This was probably due to the different compositions of the nickel-titanium alloy in these devices.

The signal intensity characteristics of the nitinol Memotherm stent and of the metallic cobalt-chromium-nickel alloy in the Wallstent were nonuniform at contrast-enhanced MR angiography. The different signal intensity behaviors of stents made of the same alloy are due to the orientation of the stents to the main magnetic field. Artifacts increase when a stent is angulated more perpendicularly to the main magnetic field (19). There is higher potential for artifacts when high field strengths and gradient-echo sequences are used (21,22).

A limitation of the current contrast-

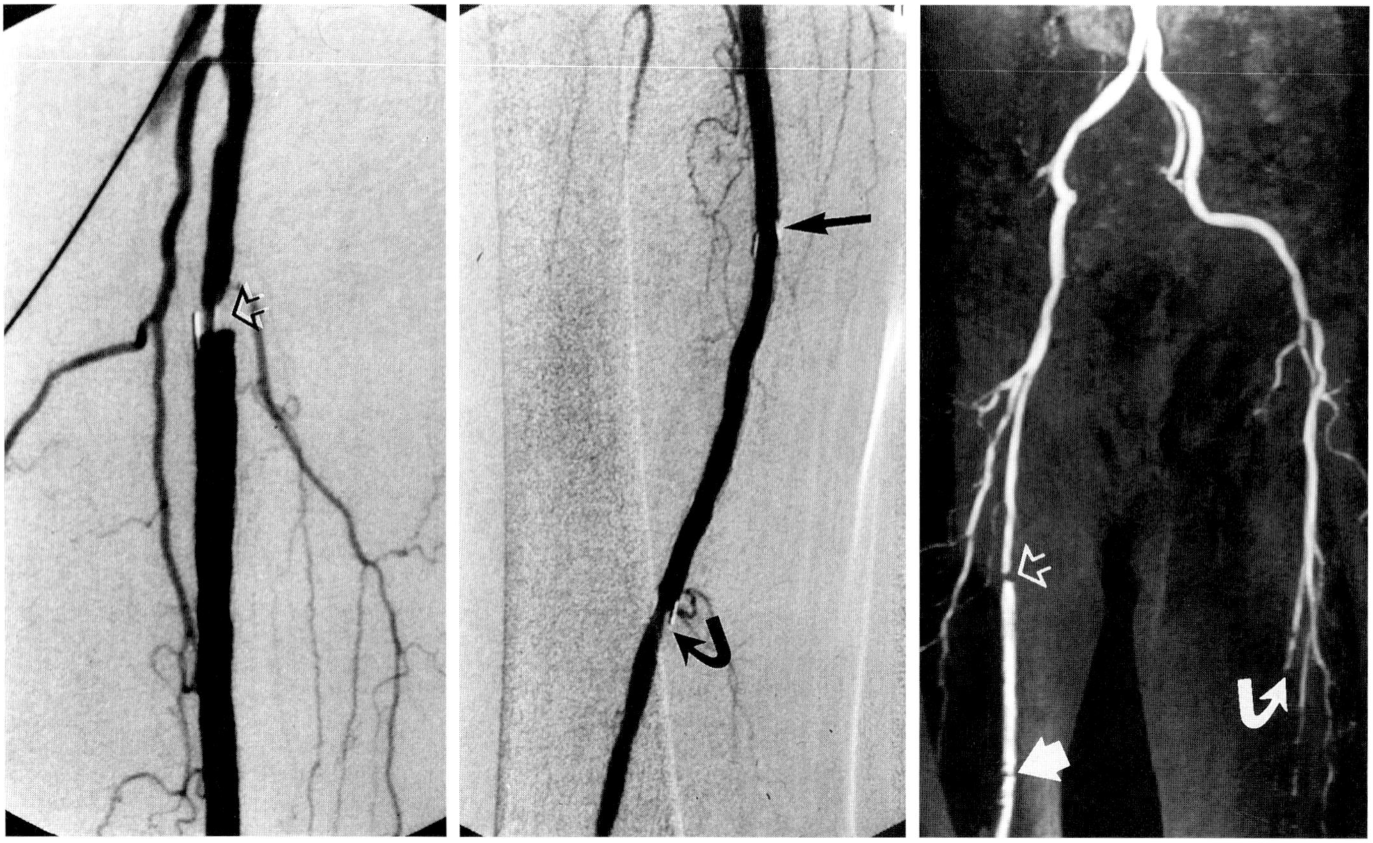

a. b. c.

Figure 5. (a, b) Anteroposterior digital subtraction angiograms obtained in a 58-year-old man after placement of two Cragg Endopro stents in the right superficial femoral artery show high-grade stenosis (open arrow in a) at the upper end of the proximal Cragg Endopro stent. The platinum markers at the overlap of the two stents (straight arrow in b) are indicated. There is restenosis (curved arrow) at the lower end of the distal Cragg Endopro stent. (c) Right anterior oblique (30°) contrast-enhanced MR angiogram (7.8/2.1, 30° flip angle) obtained in the same patient shows circumscribed signal intensity loss (open arrow) at the upper end of the proximal Cragg Endopro stent; high-grade restenosis in this area was presumed. The decreased signal intensity at the overlap of the two stents (solid arrow) was caused by the platinum markers. An occlusion (curved arrow) of the left superficial femoral artery also is seen. The lower end of the distal Cragg Endopro stent was not depicted at contrast-enhanced MR angiography.

enhanced MR angiographic technique is the 500-mm field of view for the examination of the lower limb arteries. At present, this technique allows demonstration of only the iliac and femoral region. In four patients, the stent in the femoropopliteal region was not completely depicted because of the height of the patient. The missing demonstration of the runoff vessels is a further disadvantage of contrast-enhanced MR angiography in treatment planning. Information about the runoff vessels is less important for lesions in the iliac arteries, but it is essential for long segmented femoropopliteal lesions. The distal runoff is an indication of the success of a bypass or interventional procedure. When information about the runoff vessels is missing, only conservative treatment or amputation is considered. In the future, this shortcoming can be overcome by carrying out a second contrast-enhanced MR angiographic study in which the popliteal and lower limb arteries are imaged, with a slight overlap in the femoropopliteal area. The advantages of contrast-enhanced MR angiography compared with the older nonenhanced MR angiographic techniques are dramatically reduced susceptibility artifacts and extremely short acquisition times.

In conclusion, contrast-enhanced MR angiography can enable highly accurate diagnosis of occlusion and stenosis greater than 50% in the iliac and femoral arteries; the patency of stents can be determined, but restenoses within stents may not be detected.

References

1. Carpenter JP, Baum RA, Holland GA, Barker CF. Peripheral vascular surgery with magnetic resonance angiography as the sole preoperative imaging modality. J Vasc Surg 1994; 20:861–871.
2. Steffens JC, Link J, Mueller-Huelsbeck S, Brinkmann G, Heller M. Cardiac gated two-dimensional phase-contrast MR angiography of lower extremity occlusive disease. AJR 1997; 169:749–754.
3. Vosshenrich R, Fischer U, Funke M, Grabbe E. 2-D-time-of-flight-MR-angiographie der peripheren gefaesse: experimentelle und klinische studien zur wertigkeit der methode bei AVK. ROFO 1996; 164:25–30.
4. Bosmans H, Marchal G. Contrast-enhanced MR angiography. Radiologe 1996; 36:115–123.
5. Earls JP, Rofsky NM, DeCorato DR, Krinsky GA, Weinreb JC. Breath-hold single-dose gadolinium-enhanced three-dimensional MR aortography: usefulness of a timing examination and MR power injector. Radiology 1996; 201:705–710.
6. Holland GA, Dougherty L, Carpenter JP, et al. Breath-hold ultrafast three-dimensional gadolinium-enhanced MR angiography of the aorta and the renal and other visceral abdominal arteries. AJR 1996; 166: 971–981.
7. Krinsky GA, Rofsly NM, DeCorato DR, et al. Thoracic aorta: comparison of gadolin-

ium-enhanced three-dimensional MR angiography with conventional MR imaging. Radiology 1997; 202:183–193.
8. Link J, Steffens JC, Brossmann J, Loose R, Heller M. Contrast-enhanced MR angiography in Leriche's syndrome. ROFO 1998; 169:22–26.
9. Prince MR, Yucel EK, Kaufman JA, Harrison DC, Geller SC. Dynamic gadolinium-enhanced three-dimensional abdominal MR arteriography. JMRI 1993; 3:877–881.
10. Prince MR. Gadolinium-enhanced MR aortography. Radiology 1994; 191:155–164.
11. Prince MR, Narasimham DL, Stanley JC, et al. Breath-hold gadolinium-enhanced MR angiography of the abdominal aorta and its major branches. Radiology 1995; 197:785–792.
12. Shetty AN, Shirkhoda A, Kostaki GB, Alcantara A. Contrast-enhanced three-dimensional MR angiography in a single breath hold: a novel technique. AJR 1995; 165:990–992.
13. Snidow JJ, Johnson MS, Harris VJ, et al. Three-dimensional gadolinium-enhanced MR angiography for aortoiliac inflow assessment plus renal artery screening in a single breath hold. Radiology 1996; 198: 725–732.
14. Quinn SF, Demlow TA, Hallin RW, Eidemiller LR, Szumowski J. Femoral MR angiography versus conventional angiography: preliminary results. Radiology 1993; 189:181–184.
15. Schnall MD, Holland GA, Baum RA, Cope C, Schiebler ML, Carpenter JP. MR angiography of the peripheral vasculature. RadioGraphics 1993; 13:920–930.
16. Yucel EK, Kaufmann JA, Geller SC, Waltmann AC. Atherosclerotic occlusive disease of the lower extremity: prospective evaluation with two-dimensional time-of-flight MR angiography. Radiology 1993; 187:637–641.
17. Steffens JC, Link J, Graessner J, et al. Contrast-enhanced k-space centered breath hold MR angiography of the renal arteries and the abdominal aorta. JMRI 1997; 7:617–622.
18. Dumoulin CL, Yucel EK, Vock P. Two- and three-dimensional phase contrast MR angiography of the abdomen. J Comput Assist Tomogr 1990; 14:779–784.
19. Olree M, Bakker CJG, van Leeuwen MS, Mali WTPM. MCI of endovascular stents: in vitro analysis of imaging artifacts (abstr). Cardiovasc Intervent Radiol 1997; 20(suppl):60.
20. Schuermann K, Vorwerk D, Buecker A, Uppenkamp R, Grosskortenhaus R, Guenther RW. Monitoring the patency of iliac artery endoluminal prostheses: comparison of angiography and MR-angiography in an experimental study (abstr). Cardiovasc Intervent Radiol 1997; 20(suppl):59.
21. Lewin JS, Duerk JL, Jain VR, Petersilge CA, Chao CP, Haaga JR. Needle localization in MR-guided biopsy and aspiration: effects of field strength, sequence design, and magnetic field orientation. AJR 1996; 166: 1337–1345.
22. Frahm C, Gehl HB, Melchert UH, Weiss HD. Visualization of magnetic resonance-compatible needles at 1.5 and 0.2 Tesla. Cardiovasc Intervent Radiol 1996; 19:335–340.

Outcome and Cost Comparison of Percutaneous Transluminal Renal Angioplasty, Renal Arterial Stent Placement, and Renal Arterial Bypass Grafting[1]

Feyiu Xue, MD, PhD
Michael A. Bettmann, MD
David R. Langdon, MD
Wayne A. Wivell, MD

Index terms:
Arteries, transluminal angioplasty, 961.1282
Cost-effectiveness
Grafts, 961.452
Hypertension, renovascular, 81.72
Renal arteries, stenosis or obstruction, 961.721, 961.722
Stents and prostheses, 961.1268, 961.1269

Radiology 1999; 212:378–384

Abbreviations:
PTRA = percutaneous transluminal renal angioplasty
PTSP = percutaneous transluminal stent placement
RABG = renal arterial bypass grafting

[1] From the Department of Radiology, Dartmouth-Hitchcock Medical Center, One Medical Center Dr, Lebanon, NH 03756. From the 1998 RSNA scientific assembly. Received June 8, 1998; revision requested July 27; revision received December 11; accepted March 4, 1999. Supported in part by the Hitchcock Foundation. **Address reprint requests to** M.A.B. (e-mail: *MAB@Hitchcock.org*).

PURPOSE: To compare the outcomes and costs of percutaneous transluminal renal angioplasty (PTRA), percutaneous transluminal stent placement (PTSP) of renal arteries, and renal arterial bypass grafting (RABG) in treatment of renovascular hypertension.

MATERIALS AND METHODS: Medical records and angiograms of 130 patients who underwent PTRA, PTSP, or RABG were retrospectively studied to determine success and complication rates, angiographic stenoses, blood pressures, antihypertensive medications, and serum creatinine levels. Actual costs were analyzed in detail.

RESULTS: Technical success rates for PTRA, PTSP, and RABG were 91%, 98%, and 92%, respectively. Complication rates were 13%, 16%, and 38%, respectively. The mean arterial pressure was initially lowered by 29.2 mm Hg, 30.3 mm Hg, and 27.3 mm Hg, respectively, and maintained at 21.0 mm Hg, 19.8 mm Hg, and 20.2 mm Hg below baseline at 12 months. The number of antihypertensive medications was initially reduced on average by 0.63, 0.72, and 0.58, respectively, but returned to baseline in all patients by 12 months. The serum creatinine level did not change substantially with any treatment. Initial treatment costs were $1,402, $2,573, and $15,393, respectively.

CONCLUSION: PTRA, PTSP, and RABG were equally efficacious for control of renovascular hypertension. The initial treatment cost for bypass grafting was substantially higher than that for PTRA and PTSP of renal arteries.

Renal arterial stenosis is the most common cause of secondary hypertension; it is responsible for hypertension in 1%–5% of the 60 million people with this condition in the United States (1). Hypertension caused by renal arterial stenosis is usually poorly controlled by medications (2). Severe renal arterial stenosis may lead to chronically insufficient blood flow to the kidneys and result in renal failure (3).

Percutaneous transluminal renal angioplasty (PTRA) and percutaneous transluminal stent placement (PTSP) of renal arteries have become the frontline treatments for renovascular hypertension and largely replaced renal arterial bypass grafting (RABG), the more invasive surgical revascularization option. Although PTRA and PTSP have been shown to be safe and effective for treatment of most renal arterial stenoses (4–12), the clinical outcomes and costs of these two interventional radiologic procedures compared with those of their surgical alternative have been compared in few studies. In this study, we analyzed and compared the technical results; immediate, 6-month, and 12-month clinical outcomes; and initial treatment costs of PTRA, PTSP of renal arteries, and RABG at a university hospital.

Author contributions:
Guarantors of integrity of entire study, F.X., M.A.B.; study concepts and design, M.A.B., F.X.; definition of intellectual content, M.A.B., F.X.; literature research, F.X., M.A.B.; clinical studies, all authors; data acquisition, F.X., D.R.L., W.A.W.; data analysis, F.X., M.A.B.; statistical analysis, F.X.; manuscript preparation, editing, and review, F.X., M.A.B.

TABLE 1
Treatment Group Patient Characteristics

Characteristic	PTRA	PTSP	RABG	*P* Value
No. of patients	70	39	21	
No. of male/female patients	26/44	21/18	4/17	.027
Age (y)*†	64.2 ± 16.6 (6–92)	68.6 ± 9.8 (42–84)	67.4 ± 8.6 (51–80)	.305
Patients with azotemia (%)‡	27 (19/70)	36 (14/39)	33 (7/21)	.613
No. of coexistent morbidities*	2.37 ± 0.95	2.65 ± 0.92	2.76 ± 0.85	.165
Baseline blood pressure (mm Hg)*				
Systolic	188.0 ± 34.0	182.1 ± 30.5	176.7 ± 17.7	.327
Diastolic	98.0 ± 16.9	95.4 ± 16.8	91.5 ± 12.9	.390
Baseline no. of blood pressure medications*	2.12 ± 1.05	2.31 ± 0.66	2.48 ± 0.81	.311
Baseline creatinine level (mg/dL)*§	1.74 ± 1.95	1.71 ± 1.47	1.85 ± 0.76	.744

* Data are the mean ± SD.
† The numbers in parentheses are the age range.
‡ The numbers in parentheses are the number of patients.
§ For SI conversion (μmol/L), multiply by 76.25.

MATERIALS AND METHODS

Patients

This was a retrospective study of the medical records and angiograms of 130 patients who underwent PTRA, PTSP, or RABG between June 1992 and February 1998 in a single tertiary medical center. The number of male versus female patients and the mean age and age range of patients are shown in Table 1.

PTRA was performed in 90 renal arteries in 70 patients. The indications for PTRA were severe hypertension refractory to medications, with or without renal insufficiency, and angiographic evidence of renal arterial stenosis. Renal arterial stenosis was defined as a greater than 50% reduction in the luminal diameter of the renal artery. All 70 patients were included in the subsequent analysis, even if angioplasty was unsuccessful, for example, because of failure to cross the stenosis or resolve the narrowing.

PTSP was performed in 45 renal arteries in 39 patients. The indications for this procedure were failure to satisfactorily eliminate the stenosis after repeat balloon dilation (24 arteries), intimal dissection with luminal compromise (two arteries), recurrent stenosis after previous PTRA (three arteries), and stenosis involving the renal arterial ostium (16 arteries).

RABG was performed in 26 renal arteries in 21 patients for treatment of renovascular hypertension. The indications for primary RABG were diffuse stenosis or stenosis involving branches of the renal artery that were not treatable with PTRA or PTSP (four arteries). This group also included patients who had recurrent renal arterial stenosis after PTRA (nine arteries in eight patients) or PTSP (one artery in one patient), severe atherosclerosis involving other abdominal aortic branches in addition to renal arterial stenosis (four arteries in two patients), or a concurrent abdominal aortic aneurysm that needed surgical repair (eight arteries in six patients).

Techniques

To assess the degree of stenosis, renal angiography was performed in all cases prior to the intervention. Angiography was also performed after PTRA and PTSP. Angiography was not routinely performed after RABG; rather, duplex ultrasonography (US) was usually performed to confirm graft patency.

All patients who underwent interventional radiologic treatments received intraarterial boluses of heparin (1,000–5,000 U) and nitroglycerin (0.1–0.4 mg) during the procedure. Some patients also received 10 mg of nifedipine sublingually. Aspirin (325 mg daily) was the only postprocedural medication used routinely.

PTRA.—Standard balloon angioplasty techniques were used in all PTRA procedures. Typically, a lesion was dilated with a 5-F angioplasty balloon catheter that was passed through a valved 6–8-F introducer sheath by using the femoral approach. The immediate technical result after angioplasty was evaluated with repeat angiography and measurement of the postdilation transstenotic gradient. Balloon dilation was repeated when the residual stenosis was greater than 30% or the gradient was 10 mm Hg or more.

PTSP.—All procedures were performed by using the femoral approach with metallic stents (Palmaz stents [Johnson & Johnson Interventional Systems, Warren, NJ] or Wallstents [Medi-tech/Boston Scientific, Natick, Mass]). All Palmaz stents were 1.5 cm in length; the Wallstents, which were used in two cases, were 2 cm in length. The stents were then positioned through a vascular 7- or 8-F sheath or 8- or 9-F guiding catheter over a Rosen guide wire (Cook, Bloomington, Ind). For ostial lesions, a 1-mm protrusion of the stent into the aortic lumen was attempted to cover the lesion. For more distal lesions, the stent was deployed entirely within the renal arterial lumen. After predilation and standard deployment, the stents were dilated to what was thought to be the normal renal arterial size (5–8 mm).

RABG.—The standard surgical technique was used. Typically, vein grafts or polytetrafluoroethylene grafts were placed to one or both major renal arteries. Some patients also underwent bypass grafting of the celiac axis or superior mesenteric artery or repair of abdominal aortic aneurysms.

Evaluation of Technical Results

The technical results of PTRA and PTSP were determined by evaluating angiograms obtained before and after the procedures. The angiograms were evaluated by one observer (F.X.). If there was disagreement between his findings and those in the dictated report, a consensus was reached between this observer and another reviewer (M.A.B.). Technical success for PTRA and PTSP was defined as residual stenosis of 30% or less; technical failure was defined as residual stenosis of greater than 30% or failure to cross the stenosis. Technical success for RABG was defined as graft patency at duplex US. Angiographic stenosis was characterized by type (atherosclerosis or fibromuscular dysplasia), distribution (focal or diffuse), location, and severity. Lesions within 5 mm of the aortic lumen were classified as ostial. Nonostial lesions were further classified as proximal or distal with respect to the renal arterial ostium and bifurcation. Stenosis severity was measured on hardcopy images and expressed quantitatively as a percentage of the main renal artery. Complications directly related to the procedure were noted.

Evaluation of Clinical Outcomes

The blood pressure, number of antihypertensive medications, and serum creatinine level were evaluated as functional outcomes. The immediate response was determined by comparing the values obtained before and after the procedures. Most preprocedural values were obtained on the day of the procedure; postprocedural values were obtained within 48 hours after the procedure. Six- and 12-month values were obtained from medical records. The clinical benefit was evaluated according to the criteria of the Standards of Practice Committee of the Society of Cardiovascular and Interventional Radiology (13).

Cure of hypertension was defined as diastolic pressure less than 90 mm Hg without administration of antihypertensive medication. Improvement of hypertension was defined as (*a*) diastolic pressure less than 90 mm Hg with administration of antihypertensive medication or (*b*) diastolic pressure of 90–109 mm Hg with a decrease of at least 15 mm Hg with the patient receiving the same or fewer medications at the same or a lower dose. The effect of intervention on renal function was assessed by measuring serum creatinine values. A serum creatinine level of 1.5 mg/dL (114 µmol/L) or higher (normal = 0.7–1.4 mg/dL [53–107 µmol/L]) was defined as the presence of azotemia.

TABLE 2
Treatment Group Technical Results

Result	PTRA	PTSP	RABG	*P* Value
Successes (%)*	91 (82/90)	98 (44/45)	92 (24/26)	.345
Complications (%)*	13 (12/90)	16 (7/45)	38 (10/26)†	.012
Type of Lesion‡				
Atherosclerosis	82 (91)	45 (100)	22 (85)	.044
Fibromuscular dysplasia	8 (9)	0 (0)	4 (15)	
Distribution‡				
Diffuse	5 (6)	0 (0)	3 (12)	.091
Focal	85 (94)	45 (100)	26 (88)	
Location‡				
Ostial	15 (17)	16 (36)	5 (19)	.042
Proximal	71 (79)	26 (58)	19 (73)	
Distal	4 (4)	3 (7)	2 (8)	
Stenosis (%)§				
Preintervention	72 (45–99)	78 (50–95)	81 (60–99)	.102
Postintervention	11 (0–43)‖	2 (0–25)‖	Patency#	

Note.—PTRA data are based on a total of 90 arteries, PTSP data are based on a total of 45 arteries, and RABG data are based on a total of 26 arteries.

* Numbers in parentheses are the number of arteries.

† The complication rate with RABG was significantly higher than that with PTRA (*P* = .004) or with PTSP (*P* = .029).

‡ Data are the number of arteries. Numbers in parentheses are the percentage.

§ Data are the mean percentage of stenosis. Numbers in parentheses are the range of percentages.

‖ *P* = .007 for the difference in mean percentage of postsurgical stenosis between the arteries treated with PTRA and those treated with PTSP.

\# Postsurgical angiography was not routinely performed in the RABG group; rather duplex US was performed to confirm graft patency.

Cost Analysis

To analyze the actual initial treatment cost, we broke down the total cost for each procedure into procedural costs and postprocedural hospitalization costs. The procedural costs for PTRA and PTSP were calculated by using the calculated hourly rate multiplied by the duration of the procedure, plus the cost of consumable supplies. The hourly rate was the all-inclusive rate for running the cardiovascular and interventional radiology suite at our hospital, which had been calculated to be $519 per hour (Langdon and Bettmann, manuscript in preparation). This hourly rate was derived from the direct costs for labor (physicians, technicians, nurses, receptionists, and secretaries), equipment, and supplies and from the indirect cost for administrative support, facility maintenance, and other overhead. It also included the cost for postprocedural monitoring and observation of patients who were not hospitalized after PTRA or PTSP. The physician and related administrative support portion of the hourly rate was $215 per hour. The durations of PTRA and PTSP were determined by averaging the time to perform these procedures in 10 uncomplicated unilateral cases.

The actual cost for RABG was obtained in a similar manner (Wivell and Bettmann, manuscript in preparation). The procedural cost was calculated as an hourly vascular surgery rate multiplied by the duration of the surgery, plus the costs of material and anesthesia. The hourly vascular surgery rate, excluding physician and related vascular surgery administrative costs, was $377. We estimated the physician and related vascular surgery administrative costs for vascular surgery to be at least equal to those for interventional radiology. The all-inclusive hourly rate for vascular surgery was therefore estimated to be $602 per hour. The average anesthesia cost for RABG, including physician costs, was $2,506. The average duration of RABG was determined from four cases of uncomplicated unilateral RABG without other surgical interventions.

Exact postprocedural hospital costs were difficult to calculate; they were determined mainly on the basis of the duration of hospital stay. To get an accurate estimate of these costs, we calculated the intensive care unit and regular hospital costs separately. The average daily cost in the intensive care unit for patients undergoing vascular surgery at our hospital was estimated to be $1,650. The average daily cost of regular hospitalization at our hospital was approximately $800. Thus, by knowing the average duration of stay in the intensive care unit and in the regular hospital after each procedure, we were able to determine the cost of postprocedural hospitalization.

Statistical Analyses

Quantitative values are given as the mean ± SD. Statistical analyses were performed by using analysis of variance or the Student *t* test for continuous variables and the χ^2 test for categorical variables. *P* values of less than .05 were considered to be statistically significant.

RESULTS

Patient Characteristics

The characteristics of the patients are shown in Table 1. There was no statistically significant difference in age, percentage of patients with azotemia, or number of coexistent morbidity factors among

TABLE 3
Treatment Group Clinical Outcomes

Outcome	PTRA	PTSP	RABG	*P* Value
Mean arterial blood pressure (mm Hg)				
Baseline	127.7 ± 20.8	123.9 ± 17.6	118.1 ± 12.9	.135
Immediate	98.5 ± 18.4*	93.6 ± 13.5*	90.8 ± 9.2*	.122
6 months	103.6 ± 19.2*	97.6 ± 17.2*	96.1 ± 10.2*	.294
12 months	106.7 ± 13.9*	104.1 ± 11.9*	97.9 ± 13.0*	.091
No. of blood pressure medications				
Baseline	2.12 ± 1.05	2.31 ± 0.66	2.48 ± 0.81	.311
Immediate	1.49 ± 0.79*	1.59 ± 0.70*	1.90 ± 0.62*	.147
6 months	1.76 ± 0.72*	1.63 ± 0.81*	2.35 ± 0.86†	.028
12 months	2.21 ± 0.80†	2.44 ± 0.51†	2.26 ± 0.87†	.738
Creatinine level (mg/dL)‡				
Baseline	1.74 ± 1.95	1.71 ± 1.47	1.85 ± 0.76	.744
Immediate	2.20 ± 2.42†	1.59 ± 1.41†	1.93 ± 2.09†	.299
6 months	1.85 ± 1.59†	1.44 ± 1.03†	2.36 ± 2.75†	.150
12 months	1.57 ± 1.65†	1.53 ± 1.11†	1.80 ± 1.27†	.320

Note.—Data are the mean ± SD.
* $P < .05$ for the difference between these values and the baseline values.
† The difference between these values and the baseline values was not significant.
‡ For SI conversion (μmol/L), multiply by 76.25.

the treatment groups. There also was no significant difference among the treatment groups with respect to baseline systolic or diastolic blood pressures, number of antihypertensive medications, or serum creatinine levels. The male-to-female ratio was significantly different among the treatment groups: Relative to the PTSP group, the percentage of women was higher in the RABG group ($P = .009$).

Technical Results

Technical results are summarized in Table 2. The overall success rate of PTRA was 91%; PTSP, 98%; and RABG, 92%. There was no statistically significant difference in the success rate among groups ($P = .345$). Elastic recoil was responsible for the majority of the technical failures of PTRA (six cases), and failure to cross the stenosis and intimal dissection were responsible for the remaining failures (two cases). The only failure of PTSP resulted from failure to cross the stenosis. None of the patients in whom PTRA or PTSP failed underwent emergent surgical bypass grafting. Occlusion from thrombus formation within the graft was the cause of the two RABG failures.

The overall complication rates were 13% for PTRA, 16% for PTSP, and 38% for RABG. The differences in complication rates were statistically significant ($P = .012$). The most common complications from PTRA and PTSP were nausea and vomiting, local hematoma at the site of arterial puncture, and transient spasm of a renal artery with no clinical consequences. The more serious complications of PTRA and PTSP included intimal dissection (two cases in PTRA and one case in PTSP), thrombus formation (one case in PTRA), perforation (two cases in PTSP), excessive blood loss requiring transfusion (one case in PTSP), periprocedural non–Q-wave myocardial infarction (one case in PTSP), and cerebral vascular accident (one case in PTSP). The rate of complications with RABG was significantly higher than that with PTRA ($P = .004$) or with PTSP ($P = .029$). The complications with RABG also tended to be more serious than those with PTRA or PTSP; they included excessive blood loss requiring transfusion (two cases), wound infection (one case), urinary tract infection (one case), pseudomembranous colitis (one case), occlusive thrombosis (two cases), transmural myocardial infarction (one case), cardiovascular collapse due to unknown causes (one case), and prolonged stay in the intensive care unit (two cases). These 11 complications occurred in 10 patients. No deaths within 30 days occurred as a direct consequence of any of the three procedures.

All of the lesions treated with PTSP and the majority of those treated with PTRA (91%) and RABG (85%) were atherosclerotic. Nine percent of the lesions treated with PTRA and 15% of those treated with RABG were fibromuscular dysplasia. A higher percentage of lesions treated with PTSP involved the ostium, which reflected a bias toward the use of stents for ostial stenoses.

Angiographic stenosis improved on average from 72% to 11% with PTRA, from 78% to 2% with PTSP, and from 81% to patency with RABG. Compared with PTRA, PTSP yielded significantly superior angiographic results ($P = .007$).

Clinical Outcomes

Cure of hypertension was achieved with PTRA in six (9%) patients, with PTSP in four (10%) patients, and with RABG in four (19%) patients. The differences among the groups were not statistically significant ($P = .395$). Improvement of hypertension was noted in 53 (76%) patients who underwent PTRA, 28 (72%) who underwent PTSP, and 16 (76%) who underwent RABG. No change was observed in 11 (16%) patients who underwent PTRA, seven (18%) who underwent PTSP, and one (5%) who underwent RABG. Overall, 59 (84%) of the patients treated with PTRA, 32 (82%) of those treated with PTSP, and 20 (95%) of those treated with RABG were either cured or improved. The differences in rates of cure and improvement among the groups were not statistically significant ($P = .359$).

The immediate, 6-month, and 12-month clinical outcomes in all patients are summarized in Table 3. The mean blood pressures immediately, 6 months, and 12 months after treatment were significantly lower than were the mean baseline blood pressures in all groups. Immediately after PTRA, PTSP, and RABG, the mean arterial pressures were lowered by 29.2 mm Hg (22.9%), 30.3 mm Hg (24.5%), and 27.3 mm Hg (23.1%), respectively. There was no statistically significant difference in the initial mean arterial pressure response among the groups. Mean arterial pressures showed persistent diminutions of 24.1 mm Hg (18.9%), 26.3 mm Hg (21.2%), and 22.0 mm Hg (18.6%) at 6 months after PTRA, PTSP, and RABG, respectively, compared with the baseline values, and they remained at 21.0 mm Hg (16.4%), 19.8 mm Hg (16.0%), and 20.2 mm Hg (17.1%) below the baseline values, respectively, at 12 months. The differences among the groups in maintaining a lower mean arterial blood pressure at 6 and 12 months were not statistically significant.

The number of antihypertensive medications taken by patients immediately after all three treatments was significantly fewer than the baseline number. The number of antihypertensive agents taken was reduced on average by 0.63, 0.72, and 0.58 following PTRA, PTSP, and RABG, respectively. There was no statistically significant difference among the groups. At 6 months after PTRA and PTSP, the mean number of antihypertensive medications taken by patients in each group was, respectively, 0.36 and 0.68 fewer than that before the procedures, but for the surgical group, the number of medications had essentially returned to baseline. By 12 months, the number of antihypertensive medications taken by patients had returned to the baseline level for all three groups.

After the procedures, 10 (14%) of the 70 patients who underwent PTRA, four (10%) of the 39 who underwent PTSP, and two (10%) of the 21 patients in the surgical group had improvement in renal function. Fifty-six (80%) patients in the PTRA group, 32 (82%) in the PTSP group, and 15 (71%) in the surgical group had no change in renal function. Four (6%) patients in the PTRA group, three (8%) in the PTSP group, and four (19) in the RABG group had worsening of renal function. Overall, the mean serum creatinine levels did not change significantly and were stable for the 12 months following all three treatments. In two patients, who had acute renal failure in addition to hypertension, the renal function returned to baseline after PTRA (one case) and PTSP (one case).

Among the patients with azotemia, two (10%) in the PTRA group, two (14%) in the PTSP group, and none in the RABG group had normalization of renal function (creatinine level <1.5 mg/dL [<114 μmol/L]) over the next 12 months. In the PTRA group, five (26%) additional patients with azotemia had temporary or permanent improvement, nine (47%) had no change, and three (16%) had worsening of renal function. In the PTSP group, three (21%) additional patients with azotemia had improvement, seven (50%) had no change, and two (14%) had worsening of renal function. In the RABG group, two (29%) patients had improvement, three (38%) had no change, and three (43%) had worsening of renal function. Overall, the creatinine levels did not change significantly in patients with azotemia following any of the treatments, except a subgroup of patients who underwent PTSP and had moderately elevated creatinine levels (1.5–3.5 mg/dL [114–267 μmol/L]). The mean creatinine level in these patients decreased from 2.03 mg/dL (155 μmol/L) to 1.49 mg/dL (114 μmol/L) after treatment (P = .018), but went up to 1.61 mg/dL (123 μmol/L) by 6 months (P = .072 compared with baseline) and to 1.94 mg/dL (148 μmol/L) by 12 months (P = .824 compared with baseline). No patients who were on hemodialysis improved sufficiently to allow cessation of dialysis.

TABLE 4
Procedural and Immediate Postprocedural Costs

Costs	PTRA	PTSP	RABG
Procedural			
Hourly rate ($)	519	519	602
Mean duration (h) ± SD	2.0 ± 0.4	2.3 ± 0.6	5.75 ± 1.0
Material cost ($)	364	1,379	1,700
Anesthesia cost ($)	NA	NA	2,506
Average cost ($)	1,402	2,573	7,668
Immediate postprocedural in all cases			
Patients hospitalized (%)*	17 (12/70)	15 (6/39)	100 (21/21)
Mean duration (d) ± SD	0.6 ± 1.6	2.0 ± 6.6	15.2 ± 8.7
Duration range (d)	0–7	0–35	6–37
Average cost ($)	540	1,779	16,325
Postprocedural in cases of uncomplicated unilateral treatment			
Patients hospitalized (%)*	0 (0/10)	0 (0/10)	100 (4/4)
Mean duration (d) ± SD	NA	NA	7.0 ± 1.8
Duration range (d)	NA	NA	5–9
Average cost ($)	0	0	7,725

Note.—NA = not applicable.
* Numbers in parentheses are the number of patients.

Cost Analysis and Comparison

The actual procedural costs and immediate postprocedural hospital costs are summarized in Table 4. The average procedural cost for PTRA was $1,402, and for PTSP, $2,573; the difference in these costs was mainly secondary to material (ie, the cost of the stents). The calculated average procedural cost for RABG was $7,668. Postprocedural hospitalization was required for 12 (17%) patients who underwent PTRA, six (15%) patients who underwent PTSP, and all (100%) who underwent RABG. The average hospital stay was 0.6 day (0–7 days) for patients in the PTRA group, 2.0 days (0–35 days) for patients in the PTSP group, and 15.2 days (6–37 days) for patients in the RABG group. Of these hospitalizations, time in the intensive care unit accounted for 0.07 day (one patient, 5 days) for the PTRA group, 0.21 day (one patient, 7 days) for the PTSP group, and 4.9 days (all 21 patients, 2–14 days) for the RABG group.

The estimated average costs for immediate postprocedural care were $540, $1,779, and $16,325 following PTRA, PTSP, and RABG, respectively. The difference in postoperative hospitalization cost between PTRA and PTSP ($540 vs $1,779) was related to the prolonged hospitalization of a single patient (35 days) in the latter group.

When only uncomplicated unilateral procedures were considered, no hospitalization was needed for PTRA or PTSP, whereas an average of 7.0 days of hospitalization were required for RABG. The postprocedural care for uncomplicated PTRA and PTSP was minimal; 2–5 hours of monitoring and observation with basic nursing were required. The postprocedural costs for space, equipment, and personnel were factored into the procedural costs. The immediate postprocedural care of patients who underwent uncomplicated unilateral RABG involved, on average, 2.5 days in the intensive care unit and 4.5 additional days of regular hospitalization. The average postoperative hospitalization cost for uncomplicated unilateral RABG was calculated to be $7,725. The total initial treatment cost for this surgical procedure, including postoperative hospital costs, was $15,393, which was almost 11 times the cost of uncomplicated unilateral PTRA and six times that of PTSP (Table 4).

DISCUSSION

In this retrospective study, we analyzed and compared the technical results; the initial, 6-month, and 12-month functional outcomes; and the costs of PTRA, PTSP, and RABG at one tertiary care center. The results of our study support the conclusion of numerous previously published studies (4–12): PTRA and PTSP are safe and effective treatments for hypertension caused by renal arterial stenosis. The technical success rate of PTRA in our study was higher than that in several earlier reports, probably because of the added experience and improvements in equipment and techniques since the previous studies were published. For ex-

TABLE 5
Treatment Group Real Costs, Hospital Charges, and Medicare Reimbursements

Variable	PTRA	PTSP
Real cost ($)	1,402	2,573
Hospital charge ($)	5,785	3,461
Medicare reimbursement ($)	2,319	1,943

ample, a large number of technical failures in PTRA in the past involved atherosclerotic lesions of the renal arterial ostium (4,6). There is some evidence that PTSP is a more effective treatment for ostial lesions than is PTRA (10,11). Consequently, at our institution, as reflected in the numbers, ostial lesions have been routinely treated with stent placement rather than with simple angioplasty since 1995.

We also found no statistically significant difference in the initial functional outcomes among PTRA, PTSP, and RABG. All three treatments resulted in a decreased mean arterial blood pressure and reduced requirements for antihypertensive medications; none of the procedures resulted in significant changes in the mean serum creatinine concentration. These findings are essentially in agreement with the results of the 1993 prospective randomized study by Weibull et al (12); their results showed no difference between PTRA and surgical reconstruction of renal arteries with respect to primary blood pressure response or influence on renal function.

The results of our study also demonstrated no statistically significant difference in outcome with regard to blood pressure and renal function at 6 months and 12 months between the two interventional procedures and surgery. Although all three treatments were successful in maintaining lower blood pressure at 12 months, the number of antihypertensive medications required for this returned to baseline in 6 months following RABG and in 12 months following PTRA and PTSP. Renal function, as measured by using the serum creatinine level, improved in several patients, but it did not change significantly following any of the procedures among the patients who were treated primarily for hypertension rather than for renal failure.

It may not be surprising that, statistically, PTRA and PTSP had fewer complications than did RABG, because percutaneous, catheter-based procedures are generally much less invasive than are open surgeries. The complications with PTRA and PTSP also tended to be less severe than those with RABG. For example, although the most common complications with PTRA and PTSP were local hematoma at the site of arterial puncture, blood loss of up to 500 mL was not even considered as a complication with RABG. It is important to note, however, that six of the 21 patients who underwent RABG had concurrent abdominal aortic aneurysm repairs, and two others underwent bypass procedures of other vessels at the time of RABG. In addition, nine of these 21 patients had previously undergone PTRA or PTSP.

Although there was no significant difference among the groups with regard to mean age, baseline blood pressure, number of antihypertensive medications, creatinine level, and number of coexistent morbidities (Table 1), it is possible that the patients in the RABG group had more severe visceral vascular disease than did those in the other two groups. All of these factors may have contributed to the increased prevalence and severity of complications with RABG, although they are not likely to provide a complete explanation.

To our knowledge, this study is the first attempt to directly compare the outcomes and costs between two interventional radiologic procedures and surgery for treatment of renovascular hypertension. Although PTRA and PTSP are as safe and efficacious as RABG in the initial treatment of renal arterial stenosis, they cost a fraction of what surgical interventions do.

Because many patients in the RABG group also underwent other concurrent surgical procedures, such as abdominal aortic aneurysm repair or revascularization of other vessels, we included only cases of uncomplicated unilateral RABG in our calculation of the procedural cost. The procedural cost for PTRA was less than one-fifth that for RABG, and that for PTSP was one-third that for RABG (ie, $6,266 less and $5,095 less, respectively). When the cost for postprocedural hospitalization was taken into account, PTRA and PTSP offered even more substantial savings over RABG. When the cases of uncomplicated unilateral treatment in all three groups were compared, the procedural and immediate postprocedural hospital costs for PTRA and PTSP were, respectively, $13,991 and $12,820 less than those for RABG.

Savings in the costs of using interventional radiologic procedures compared with surgical revascularization were due to the (*a*) shortened procedure duration, (*b*) elimination of the need for general anesthesia, and (*c*) minimal postoperative care, with the limitation or elimination of hospitalization. The average duration for performing PTRA and PTSP was more than 3 hours shorter than that for performing uncomplicated RABG.

The single most important factor in the reduction of costs for PTRA and PTSP compared with those for RABG, however, was the difference in postprocedural hospitalization costs. In most cases, minimal postoperative care was needed after interventional radiologic procedures; in contrast, both intensive care unit stay and regular hospitalization were necessary following all of the surgical procedures, including the uncomplicated cases. Savings in postprocedural hospital costs with PTRA and PTSP were over $7,700 when these procedures were compared with the surgical option.

Because of their less invasive nature, endovascular techniques often offer reduced risks, shorter hospital stays, and substantially lower costs to patients compared with open surgery. The argument against the use of these techniques has centered around their reduced long-term success compared with that of surgery, which, some argue, may not offer real savings in the long run. Interestingly, in our study, there was no indication of potentially increased costs attributable to PTRA or PTSP as a result of their shorter duration of effectiveness at 12 months compared with that of RABG. In fact, a more rapid return to the baseline number of medications following RABG may further increase the costs in this group of patients. The question of added cost because of the need to cross over from PTRA or PTSP to surgery is an important one. The data from our study raise the possibility, as supported by Weibull et al (12), that failure of PTRA or PTSP should be treated by using repeat percutaneous intervention.

To our knowledge, few studies in the literature have addressed the issues of true costs in comparing treatments for renovascular hypertension. In one study (14), the cost of PTRA was compared with that of renal revascularization surgery by using hospital charges as the measure of cost in a cost-effective analysis. Another similar study (15) did not provide details on how the cost information was obtained. It is not uncommon in the literature to find hospital charges or insurance reimbursements used as surrogates for the true costs of medical procedures (16,17). Both of these measures, however, may misrepresent the true costs substantially. Table 5 shows an example of such discrepancies in hospital charges, Medicare reimbursements, and true costs between PTRA and PTSP in our hospital. It is important to attempt to study the true costs of medical procedures, because only when these are known can valid cost-effective analyses be undertaken.

This study has limitations in that it was a retrospective outcome study and had a relatively small sample size. Furthermore, there may have been biases in the assigning of patients to treatment groups. This is supported by the differences in the type and location of lesions among the treatment groups. For example, the PTSP group had disproportionately more patients with atherosclerotic ostial lesions, because such lesions have been selectively treated with stent placement in our hospital since 1995. Second, patients with an abdominal aortic aneurysm or disease of multiple branches of the abdominal aorta were often preferentially treated with RABG; therefore, they might have had more severe vascular disease than did the patients in the other two groups.

Another confounding factor in this study is that some patients in the PTSP group had undergone prior PTRA (three patients, one within 12 months), and some in the RABG group had previously undergone either PTRA (eight patients, one within 6 months and another within 12 months) or PTSP (one patient). Consequently, these patients in the PTSP and RABG groups might have had more advanced disease. It is conceivable that these biases and confounding factors could have negatively influenced the outcomes of RABG and PTSP. As a group, however, the patients in the stent placement and surgical groups did not differ substantially from those in the PTRA group with regard to baseline blood pressure, number of antihypertensive medications, serum creatinine level, percentage with azotemia, or number of coexistent morbidities.

The higher complication rate of RABG might have been partially secondary to the fact that six of the 21 patients who underwent this procedure had concurrent abdominal aortic aneurysm repairs, which are inherently larger and longer procedures than is simple RABG. Conversely, all patients who underwent RABG required both intensive care unit stay and regular hospitalization. Another potentially confounding variable is that the male-to-female ratio among the treatment groups was significantly different, with more women (n = 17) than men (n = 4) in the RABG group. This sex discrepancy in the surgical group is not easily explained, and its influence on outcome is difficult to predict.

The cost analysis in this study was strictly limited to that of initial treatment costs, which included the calculated actual procedural costs and an estimation of the postprocedural hospitalization costs. The costs for preprocedural workup and long-term postprocedural follow-up were not studied here. It is reasonable to assume, however, that the costs of the preprocedural workup for renal arterial hypertension were similar no matter what treatment was used, because the diagnosis was made on the same clinical and technical grounds. On the other hand, the long-term follow-up cost could have differed substantially among the groups. In several studies (12,18,19) conducted by surgical groups, PTRA and PTSP were found to have a higher restenosis rate than that of RABG. Our results, however, did not confirm this difference. Repeat PTRA or the need for stent placement or surgery increases the total cost of PTRA. Because the actual cost of PTRA itself is about one-eleventh of that for RABG, the total cost of repeat PTRA is still substantially less than that for the primary RABG. Our results suggest that there is no increase in follow-up costs for PTRA or PTSP at up to 12 months, and there is evidence in the literature (12) that the long-term efficacy of repeat PTRA is as good as that of primary surgical revascularization. Nevertheless, the total long-term costs of PTRA, PTSP, and RABG deserve further study.

In conclusion, in our study population, PTRA, PTSP of renal arteries, and RABG had similar success rates and were equally efficacious for treatment of renovascular hypertension; however, the two percutaneous treatments cost substantially less than RABG. Although it is perhaps indicated in certain clinical settings (eg, concurrent abdominal aortic aneurysm), overall, RABG did not result in more favorable clinical outcomes at 12 months compared with PTRA and PTSP. The initial treatment costs for PTRA or PTSP are substantially lower than those for uncomplicated RABG. A large portion of the cost for RABG is related to expected complications and unavoidable postoperative hospitalization.

References

1. Mitty HA, Shapiro RS, Parsons RB, Silberzweig JE. Renovascular hypertension. Radiol Clin North Am 1996; 34:1017–1036.
2. Derkx FH, Schalekamp MA. Renal artery stenosis and hypertension. Lancet 1994; 344:237–239.
3. Hansen KJ. Prevalence of ischemic nephropathy in the atherosclerotic population. Am J Kidney Dis 1994; 24:615–621.
4. Sos TA, Pickering TG, Phil MB, et al. Percutaneous transluminal renal artery angioplasty in renovascular hypertension due to atheroma or fibromuscular dysplasia. N Engl J Med 1983; 309:274–279.
5. Losinno F, Zuccala A, Busato F, Zucchelli P. Renal artery angioplasty for renovascular hypertension and preservation of renal function: long-term angiographic and clinical follow-up. AJR 1994; 162:853–857.
6. Bonell FS, McKusick MA, Textor SC, et al. Renal artery angioplasty: technical results and clinical outcome in 320 patients. Mayo Clin Proc 1995; 70:1041–1052.
7. von Knorring J, Edgren J, Lepantalo M. Long-term results of percutaneous transluminal angioplasty in renovascular hypertension. Acta Radiol 1996; 37:36–40.
8. Hennequin LM, Joffre FG, Rousseau HP, et al. Renal artery stent placement: long-term results with the Wallstent endoprosthesis. Radiology 1994; 191:713–719.
9. Boisclair C, Therasse E, Oliva VL, et al. Treatment of renal angioplasty failure by percutaneous renal artery stenting with Palmaz stents: midterm technical and clinical results. AJR 1997; 168:245–251.
10. van de Ven PJ, Beutler JJ, Kaatee R, et al. Transluminal vascular stent for ostial atherosclerotic renal artery stenosis. Lancet 1995; 346:672–673.
11. Blum U, Krumme B, Flugel P, et al. Treatment of ostial renal-artery stenoses with vascular endoprostheses after unsuccessful balloon angioplasty. N Engl J Med 1997; 336:459–465.
12. Weibull H, Bergqvist D, Bergentz SE, Jonsson K, Hulthen L, Manhem P. Percutaneous transluminal renal artery angioplasty versus surgical reconstruction of atherosclerotic renal artery stenosis: a prospective randomized study. J Vasc Surg 1993; 18:841–852.
13. Standards of Practice Committee of the Society of Cardiovascular and Interventional Radiology. Guidelines for percutaneous transluminal angioplasty. Radiology 1990; 177:619–626.
14. England WL, Roberts SD, Grim CE. Surgery or angioplasty for cost-effective renal revascularization? Med Decis Making 1987; 7:84–91.
15. Weibull H, Bergquist D, Jendteg S, et al. Clinical outcome and health care costs in renal revascularization: percutaneous transluminal renal angioplasty versus reconstructive surgery. Br J Surg 1991; 78: 620–624.
16. Dacey LJ, Dow RW, McDaniel MD, Walsh DB, Zwolak RM, Cornenwett JL. Cost-effectiveness of intra-arterial thrombolytic therapy. Arch Surg 1988; 123:1218–1223.
17. Hunink MG, Cullen KA, Donaldson MC. Hospital costs of revascularization procedures for femoropopliteal arterial disease. J Vasc Surg 1994; 19:632–641.
18. Erdoes LS, Berman SS, Hunter GC, Mills JL. Comparative analysis of percutaneous transluminal angioplasty and operation for renal revascularization. Am J Kidney Dis 1996; 27:496–503.
19. Tullis MJ, Zierler RE, Glickerman DJ, et al. Results of percutaneous transluminal angioplasty for atherosclerotic renal artery stenosis: a follow-up study with duplex ultrasonography. J Vasc Surg 1997; 25:46–54.

Secondary Postpartum Hemorrhage: Treatment with Selective Arterial Embolization[1]

Jean-Pierre Pelage, MD
Philippe Soyer, MD, PhD
Danielle Repiquet, MD
Denis Herbreteau, MD, PhD
Olivier Le Dref, MD
Emmanuel Houdart, MD
Denis Jacob, MD
Mourad Kardache, MD
Patrick Schurando, MD
Jean-Bernard Truc, MD
Roland Rymer, MD

Index terms:
Arteries, therapeutic blockade, 98.1264, 98.41
Arteries, uterine, 98.1264, 98.41
Pregnancy, complications, 854.41, 854.82, 854.8255
Uterus, hemorrhage, 854.41, 854.8255, 854.8269

Radiology 1999; 212:385–389

[1] From the Departments of Vascular Imaging (J.P.P., P. Soyer, D.H., O.L.D., E.H., M.K., R.R.), Obstetrics and Gynecology (D.R., D.J., J.B.T.), and Critical Care (P. Schurando), Hôpital Lariboisière, AP-HP, 2 rue Ambroise Paré, 75475 Paris 10, France. Received June 11, 1998; revision requested July 30; revision received September 10; accepted February 12, 1999. **Address reprint requests to** J.P.P. (e-mail: *jean-pierre.pelage@lrb.ap-hop.paris.fr*).

Author contributions:
Guarantors of integrity of entire study, J.P.P., R.R.; study concepts, J.P.P., D.R.; study design, J.P.P., P. Soyer, R.R.; definition of intellectual content, J.P.P., O.L.D., J.B.T., R.R.; literature research, J.P.P., D.H., D.R., D.J.; clinical studies, J.P.P., O.L.D., D.H., E.H., P. Soyer, M.K., D.J., D.R., P. Schurando; data acquisition, J.P.P., O.L.D., D.R., D.J., P. Schurando; data analysis, J.P.P., O.L.D., D.H.; manuscript preparation, J.P.P., D.R.; manuscript editing and review, J.P.P., P. Soyer.

PURPOSE: To evaluate the efficacy and safety of selective arterial embolization of the uterine arteries in the management of intractable delayed postpartum hemorrhage.

MATERIALS AND METHODS: Fourteen consecutive women with secondary postpartum hemorrhage were treated with selective embolization of the uterine arteries. In all cases, hemostatic embolization was performed because of intractable hemorrhage that could not be controlled with the administration of uterotonic drugs or with uterine curettage.

RESULTS: The causes of bleeding included genital tract tears in four women and endometritis in eight women; the endometritis was associated with proved, retained portions of placenta in four women. In two women, no evident cause of bleeding was found before angiography. Angiography revealed extravasation in three women. A false aneurysm of the uterine artery was found in two women. In one patient, an arteriovenous fistula was observed. Immediate resolution of external bleeding was observed in all women. No complication related to embolization was found. Normal menstruation resumed in all women.

CONCLUSION: Selective arterial embolization of the uterine arteries is a safe and effective means of controlling secondary postpartum hemorrhage.

Postpartum hemorrhage remains one of the major worldwide causes of maternal mortality (1). The postpartum period is typically defined as the 6 weeks after delivery of the infant (2,3). Postpartum hemorrhage may occur immediately or several hours or days after delivery. In most published studies about puerperal bleeding, primary and secondary postpartum hemorrhage were treated in the aggregate when clinical presentations, causes, and maternal mortality rates were different.

Postpartum hemorrhage that occurs during the first 24 hours following delivery is termed primary, or early, postpartum bleeding (4,5). Secondary, or delayed, postpartum hemorrhage is usually defined as excessive bleeding from the genital tract, with a blood loss of 500 mL or more, that occurs after the first 24 hours following delivery until the 6th week of the puerperium (4,5).

This uncommon complication, which affects 1%–3% (4) of all deliveries, is underestimated because of difficulties in evaluating blood loss by only visual observation (6,7). In most cases, postpartum hemorrhage can be managed with conservative treatment by using uterotonic drugs. Curettage is both a diagnostic and a therapeutic tool in the management of delayed postpartum hemorrhage. However, in the case of persistent bleeding, vascular ligation or hysterectomy may be needed (3). For these reasons, transcatheter embolization of the uterine arteries may be an interesting alternate treatment for intractable bleeding.

The goal of our study was to evaluate the efficacy and safety of selective arterial embolization of the uterine arteries in the management of intractable delayed postpartum hemorrhage.

MATERIALS AND METHODS

Fourteen consecutive women with uncontrollable secondary postpartum hemorrhage who were referred for pelvic angiography and possible treatment with selective arterial

Patient Data, Treatment, and Findings

Patient No.	Age (y)	Mode of Delivery	Onset of Bleeding*	Suspected Cause†	Preembolization Treatment	Angiographic Findings	Arteries Embolized	Material
1	32	Vaginal	8	Retention endometritis	Resuscitation, uterotonic drugs, curettage, antibiotics	Normal	Both uterine arteries	Absorbable gelatin sponge
2	32	Vaginal	10	Genital tract laceration	Resuscitation, uterotonic drugs	Extravasation, left uterine artery, left vaginal artery	Both uterine arteries, left vaginal artery	Absorbable gelatin sponge
3	26	Cesarean	22	Genital tract laceration	Resuscitation, uterotonic drugs, antibiotics	Extravasation, right uterine artery	Both uterine arteries	Absorbable gelatin sponge
4	32	Vaginal	13	Retention endometritis	Resuscitation, uterotonic drugs, curettage, antibiotics	Normal	Both uterine arteries	Absorbable gelatin sponge
5	28	Vaginal	45	Genital tract laceration	Uterotonic drugs, curettage	False aneurysm	Both uterine arteries	Absorbable gelatin sponge
6	24	Vaginal	9	Retention endometritis	Uterotonic drugs, curettage, antibiotics	Normal	Both uterine arteries	Absorbable gelatin sponge
7	29	Cesarean	14	Endometritis	Uterotonic drugs, curettage, antibiotics	Normal	Both uterine arteries	Absorbable gelatin sponge
8	28	Cesarean	28	None	Uterotonic drugs, curettage, antibiotics	False aneurysm	Left uterine artery	*n*-butyl-2-cyanoacrylate
9	25	Cesarean	21	None	Uterotonic drugs, antibiotics	Arteriovenous fistula	Left uterine artery	Absorbable gelatin sponge
10	35	Cesarean	5	Retention endometritis	Resuscitation, uterotonic drugs, antibiotics	Normal	Both uterine arteries	Absorbable gelatin sponge
11	36	Cesarean	5	Endometritis	Resuscitation, uterotonic drugs, curettage, antibiotics	Normal	Both uterine arteries	Absorbable gelatin sponge
12	26	Vaginal	8	Retention endometritis	Uterotonic drugs, curettage, antibiotics	Normal	Both uterine arteries	Absorbable gelatin sponge
13	28	Vaginal	30	Genital tract laceration	Resuscitation, uterotonic drugs, curettage	Extravasation, left uterine artery	Both uterine arteries	Absorbable gelatin sponge
14	36	Vaginal	10	Retention endometritis	Resuscitation, uterotonic drugs, antibiotics	Normal	Both uterine arteries	Absorbable gelatin sponge

* Day of puerperium.
† Before embolization.

embolization were included in the study. The mean age of the women was 29.8 years ± 4.1 (SD; age range, 24–36 years). The women were referred to our department of radiology between July 1994 and December 1997.

Initial evaluation and resuscitation, when needed, were performed in the intensive care unit of our institution before the patient was transferred to the department of radiology. The evaluation of the seriousness of the hemorrhage was based on the clinical and hemodynamic status of the women. The decision to perform embolization was made on the basis of active continuing hemorrhage in spite of appropriate medical and obstetric treatment. No patient underwent vascular ligation before the procedure. The potential risks and benefits of the procedure were explained, and informed consent was obtained in all cases.

Digital subtraction angiography (iohexol [Omnipaque 300]; Nycomed, Paris, France) was performed by a vascular radiologist (J.P.P., P. Soyer, D.H., O.L.D., E.H., M.K.), who used a right-sided unifemoral approach in all cases. Contralateral internal iliac angiography and selective study of the anterior division of the internal iliac artery were then performed with a 5-F cobra-shaped catheter (Cobra; Terumo, Tokyo, Japan) and a 0.032-inch-diameter hydrophilic polymer–coated guide wire (Radifocus; Terumo) for the analysis of the uterine arteries. Superselective angiography of the left uterine artery was achieved in all cases.

Other anastomotic vessels, such as the vaginal branches, were studied when necessary. The ipsilateral internal iliac artery and the right uterine artery were also systematically catheterized. Pledgets of absorbable gelatin sponge (Gelfoam; Pharmacia and Upjohn, Bridgewater, NJ) of increasing sizes were introduced under fluoroscopic control in a free-flowing manner (Table). In one patient with a false aneurysm, *n*-butyl-2-cyanoacrylate (Embucrilate Histoacryl; Braun, Melsungen, Germany) was chosen as the embolic material because the lesion would not have been treated satisfactorily by using pledgets of absorbable gelatin sponge, in view of the difficulty to completely fill a false aneurysm with a resorbable agent. A postembolization angiographic study was performed to ensure the complete occlusion of the vessels.

RESULTS

The time of onset of the bleeding was 16.3 days ± 11.6 after delivery. The major clinical indication for transcatheter embo-

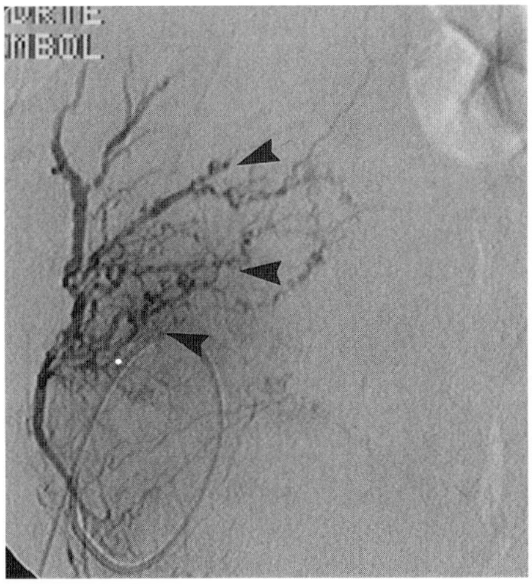

a.

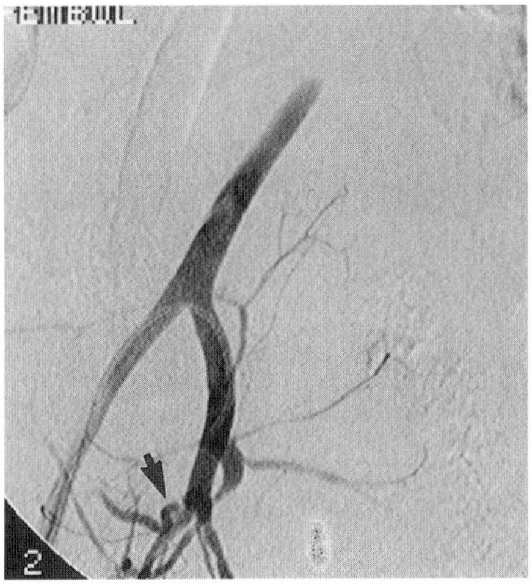

b.

Figure 1. Patient 1. (**a**) Right uterine angiogram in a 25° left anterior oblique projection shows uterine hypervascularity (arrowheads) but no extravasation. (**b**) Postembolization angiogram shows complete occlusion (arrow) of the right uterine artery.

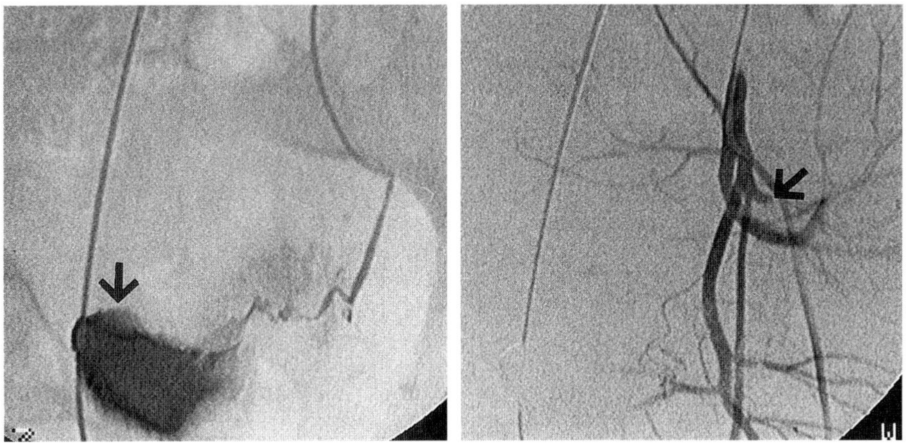

a. b.

Figure 2. Patient 13. (**a**) Left uterine angiogram in a right anterior oblique projection shows massive extravasation (arrow) of iodinated contrast material. (**b**) Postembolization angiogram shows the left uterine artery is occluded (arrow) and the extravasation has disappeared.

lization was endometritis, which was encountered in eight women (57%) and which was associated with histopathologically proved retained portions of placenta in four women (Table). Genital tract lacerations were encountered in four women. In two women, no cause of bleeding was found before angiography. In six women (43%), babies were born by means of cesarean delivery, and in eight women (57%), babies were born by means of spontaneous vaginal delivery. All children were liveborn and were in good health at the time this article was written.

At the time of admission to our institution, seven women presented with symptoms of severe hypovolemic shock; disseminated intravascular coagulopathy was biologically present in five of these seven women.

Medical management consisted of intravenous administration of uterotonic drugs, oxytocin or prostaglandin-E_2 analogues (sulprostone), in all women. Obstetric procedures consisted of manual exploration of the uterus in all women and curettage of the uterine cavity in nine women. Antibiotics were administered to 11 women.

Angiography showed no extravasation in eight (57%) women (Fig 1). Active bleeding was shown in three women; the bleeding arose from the uterine artery (n = 3) (Fig 2) and/or from the vaginal artery (n = 1). A false aneurysm of the uterine artery was found in two women (Fig 3), and an arteriovenous fistula was found in one woman.

Selective embolization of both uterine arteries was performed in 12 women (86%). In two women (14%), unilateral embolization of a false aneurysm (n = 1) or the arteriovenous fistula (n = 1) was performed. Absorbable gelatin sponge that was cut into particles of increasing sizes was used as the embolic material in 13 women. n-butyl-2-cyanoacrylate was used in one woman with a false aneurysm.

The embolization procedure lasted 50–80 minutes. In all women, external bleeding disappeared immediately. In all cases of severe initial bleeding, hemodynamic stability and immediate correction of the coagulopathy was obtained. No general or local complications were noticed.

DISCUSSION

In our study, we found that selective arterial embolization of the uterine arteries is an effective and safe treatment for the control of secondary postpartum hemorrhage. Uterine atony, which accounts for 75% of reported cases, is the main cause of primary postpartum hemorrhage, which is often associated with life-threatening situations (8,9). In contrast, secondary postpartum bleeding is most commonly caused by retained placental fragments (4,5). Delayed postpartum bleeding may also be caused by endometritis and vaginal or uterine tears. Hypofibrinogenemia (10) and endometrial carcinoma (11) may also be responsible for late postpartum bleeding.

In our article, we report two uncommon causes of delayed hemorrhage. False aneurysm and arteriovenous fistula are sometimes associated with menorrhagia and postpartum bleeding (12,13). These lesions, which developed following cesarean delivery, are probably of posttraumatic origin related to hysterotomy (12).

Until now, secondary postpartum hemorrhage had received little attention, probably because of its low incidence and because it tended to be more frequently associated with maternal morbidity rather than mortality (4). However, secondary postpartum bleeding may sometimes become nearly fatal, as we noticed in six of the women. Bleeding occurs most frequently between the 8th and the 14th day of the puerperium, so the patient often will have been discharged from the hospital and will require readmission (4).

In the case of hypovolemic shock and coagulopathy, initial resuscitation with volume replacement and blood transfusion is required. Uterotonic drugs, such as oxytocin and prostaglandin-E_2 analogues, are commonly used (2). If endometritis is suspected, a combination of ampicillin and metronidazole is administered (4,5). The lower genital tract should be carefully inspected to rule out laceration or to find placental fragments (4). In such a case, suction evacuation and curettage is often successful in stopping the hemorrhage, but it may also increase placental bleeding (2).

For women whose condition is still deteriorating, ligation of the internal iliac artery or its branches (14) or even hysterectomy is often considered the ultimate therapeutic option (15). However, vascular ligation often fails to stop the bleeding because ligation is proximal, so collateral vessels, such as the middle sacral, the last lumbar, and the inferior epigastric arteries, can provide an alternate blood supply to the uterus (16).

Many reports have emphasized the usefulness of transcatheter embolization in the control of intractable bleeding that is associated with pelvic trauma (17), tumors (18,19), or vascular malformation (20,21). Arterial embolization has also been successfully used for the management of postoperative (22), postabortion (23), and postpartum (19,24–26) intractable bleeding. To our knowledge, the first case of uterine embolization in the management of severe postpartum hemorrhage was reported by Brown et al (27) in the obstetrics and gynecology literature.

Angiographic study helps to localize the bleeding site in the case of extravasation of iodinated contrast material. If the bleeding is intermittent or is in a patient with endometritis, angiography may often fail to demonstrate active bleeding (28). Embolization should be selective, either in the pathologic vessel or in the uterine artery, even when no active bleeding is detected. Embolization of the vaginal artery should be performed in the case of identified extravasation.

In other situations, bleeding related to a genital tract tear is usually controlled after embolization of both uterine arteries because the cervicovaginal branches often originate from the arches of the uterine arteries. In our study, embolization of both uterine arteries in the cases of endometritis immediately stopped the external bleeding.

Several agents for embolization are currently available. They include gelatin sponge pledgets, polyvinyl alcohol particles, steel coils, and *n*-butyl-2-cyanoacrylate. Most authors use gelatin sponge as the embolic material because of semipermanent occlusion of the vessels with a potential for recanalization 3 weeks later (25,26). Particles of increasing sizes are particularly suitable for leaving the capillary bed intact. Inert particles of polyvinyl alcohol are also short-term occlusive agents at the level of the small arteries, but they have a limited potential for restoring vascular continuity (20). Steel coils were used in several studies (20,24,28). *n*-butyl-2-cyanoacrylate may be suitable when more definitive devascularization is required, especially in the case of a false aneurysm (21).

The use of arterial embolization to control hemorrhage has a reported success rate of 90%–95%, which is even higher in our series. In the literature, failures are likely to occur in cases of unilateral treatment (22) and in women who have undergone bilateral hypogastric arterial ligation before embolization (19). In this last situation, it is likely that prior surgical ligation obliterates the direct access route for the embolization catheter. However, successful embolization via the pelvic collateral vessels has already been reported (19,27,29,30).

Although no complication was noted in our study, arterial embolization is not side-effect free. The size of the particles used and the location of the injection during embolization influence the safety of the procedure. Arterial catheterization is easy in young and healthy women. In addition, high blood flow in the uterine arteries tends to protect against the unexpected reflux of embolic material. However, the interventional radiologist should be aware of possible variations in pelvic vascular anatomy and anastomotic channels (31).

Ischemic complications were reported in two women with postpartum bleeding who underwent arterial embolization after unsuccessful internal iliac artery ligation was performed (19). Other complications following pelvic embolization have been reported in the literature. They include muscle pain (22), neurologic damage (32), bladder necrosis (33), and vesicovaginal fistula (34). All of these complications were found in elderly women with pelvic neoplasm or who had previously received radiation therapy of the pelvis.

Numerous cases of pregnancy after ligation of the internal iliac arteries have been reported in the literature (35). Pregnancies are also possible after pelvic embolization (19,36).

In conclusion, our results show that selective arterial embolization of the uterine arteries should be the preferred treatment for intractable secondary postpartum hemorrhage when conservative treatment fails. Even though retention of gestational products and endometritis are the most frequent causes of secondary postpartum bleeding, angiographic exploration often demonstrates a bleeding artery that is related to previously unsuspected genital tract lesions. We have reported three cases in which acquired false aneurysm or arteriovenous fistula caused postpartum bleeding.

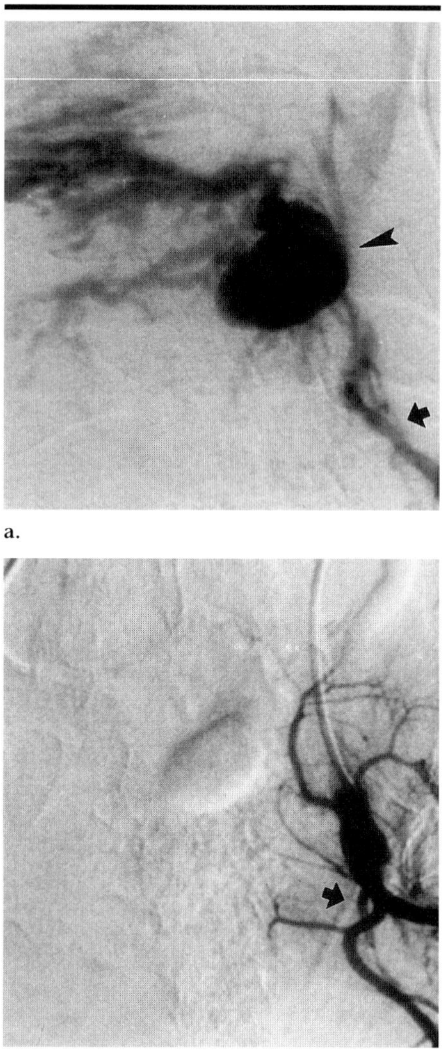

a.

b.

Figure 3. Patient 8. **(a)** Left uterine arteriogram with a right anterior oblique projection demonstrates a false aneurysm (arrowhead) of the uterine artery (arrow). **(b)** Postembolization angiogram confirms complete occlusion (arrow) of the left uterine artery.

References

1. Gilbert L, Porter W, Brown VA. Postpartum haemorrhage: a continuing problem. Br J Obstet Gynaecol 1987; 94:67–71.
2. Gilstrap LC III, Ramin SM. Postpartum hemorrhage. Clin Obstet Gynecol 1994; 37:824–830.
3. Herbert WP, Cefalo RC. Management of postpartum hemorrhage. Clin Obstet Gynecol 1984; 27:139–147.

4. King PA, Duthie SJ, Dong ZG, Ma HK. Secondary postpartum haemorrhage. Aust N Z J Obstet Gynecol 1989; 29:394–398.
5. Rome RM. Secondary postpartum hemorrhage. Br J Obstet Gynaecol 1975; 82:289–292.
6. Ghares EE, Albert SN, Dodek SM. Intrapartum blood loss measured with Cr 51-tagged erythrocytes. Obstet Gynecol 1962; 19:455–462.
7. Newton M, Mosey LM, Egli GE, Gifford WB, Hull CT. Blood loss during and immediately after delivery. Obstet Gynecol 1961; 17:9–18.
8. Combs CA, Murphy EL, Laros RK Jr. Factors associated with postpartum hemorrhage with vaginal birth. Obstet Gynecol 1991; 77:69–76.
9. Combs CA, Murphy EL, Laros RK Jr. Factors associated with hemorrhage in cesarean deliveries. Obstet Gynecol 1991; 77: 77–82.
10. Strickland DM, Galey WT, Hauth JC. Hypofibrinogenemia as a cause of delayed postpartum hemorrhage. Am J Obstet Gynecol 1982; 143:230–231.
11. Ojomo EO, Ezimokhai M, Reale FR, Nwabineli NJ. Recurrent postpartum hemorrhage caused by endometrial carcinoma co-existing with endometrioid carcinoma of the ovary in a full term pregnancy. Br J Obstet Gynaecol 1993; 100:489–491.
12. Sergent F, Clavier E, Rachet B, Marpeau L. Late post-partum hemorrhage after cesarean section due to rupture of a false aneurysm of the uterine pedicle. J Gynecol Obstet Biol Reprod 1997; 26:641–644. [French]
13. Ramin KD, Ramin SM, Webb LS, Radford LR, Sewall LE. Antepartum diagnosis of pelvic arteriovenous malformation. Obstet Gynecol 1996; 88:647–650.
14. Evans S, McShane P. The efficacy of internal iliac artery ligation in obstetric hemorrhage. Surg Gynecol Obstet 1985; 160: 250–253.
15. Clark SL, Yeh SY, Phelan JP, Bruce S, Paul RH. Emergency hysterectomy for obstetric hemorrhage. Obstet Gynecol 1984; 64:376–380.
16. Burchell RC. Physiology of internal iliac artery ligation. J Obstet Gynaecol Br Commonwealth 1968; 75:642–651.
17. Ring EJ, Athanasoulis C, Waltman AC, Margolies MN, Baum S. Arteriographic management of hemorrhage following pelvic fractures. Radiology 1973; 109:65–70.
18. Goldstein HM, Medellin H, Ben-Menachem Y, Wallace S. Transcatheter arterial embolization in the management of bleeding in the cancer patient. Radiology 1975; 115:603–608.
19. Greenwood LH, Glickman MG, Schwartz PE, Morse SS, Denny DF. Obstetric and nonmalignant gynecologic bleeding: treatment with angiographic embolization. Radiology 1987; 164:155–159.
20. Lang EK. Transcatheter embolization of pelvic vessels for control of intractable hemorrhage. Radiology 1981; 140:331–339.
21. Markoff G, Quagliarello J, Rosen RJ, Beckman EM. Uterine arteriovenous malformation successfully embolized with a liquid polymer, isobutyl 2-cyanoacrylate. Am J Obstet Gynecol 1986; 155:659–660.
22. Rosenthal DM, Colapinto, R. Angiographic arterial embolisation in the management of postoperative vaginal hemorrhage. Am J Obstet Gynecol 1985; 151: 227–231.
23. Haseltine FP, Glickman MG, Marchesi S, Spitz R, Dlugi A, DeCheney AA. Uterine embolization in a patient with postabortal hemorrhage. Obstet Gynecol 1984; 63(3 suppl):78–80.
24. Chin HG, Scott DR, Resnik R, et al. Angiographic embolization of intractable puerperal hematomas. Am J Obstet Gynecol 1989; 160:434–438.
25. Mitty HA, Sterling KM, Alvarez M, Gendler R. Obstetric hemorrhage: prophylactic and emergency arterial catheterization and embolotherapy. Radiology 1993; 188: 183–187.
26. Yamashita Y, Takahashi M, Ito M, Okumura H. Transcatheter arterial embolization in the management of postpartum hemorrhage due to genital tract injury. Obstet Gynecol 1991; 77:160–163.
27. Brown BJ, Heaston DK, Poulson AM, Gabert HA, Mineau DE, Miller FJ Jr. Uncontrollable postpartum bleeding: a new approach to hemostasis through angiographic arterial embolization. Obstet Gynecol 1979; 54:361–365.
28. Yamashita Y, Harada M, Yamamoto H, et al. Transcatheter arterial embolization of obstetric and gynaecological bleeding: efficacy and clinical outcome. Br J Radiol 1994; 67:530–534.
29. Collins CD, Jackson JE. Pelvic arterial embolization following hysterectomy and bilateral internal iliac artery ligation for intractable primary post partum haemorrhage. Clin Radiol 1995; 50:710–714.
30. Sproule MW, Bendomir AM, Grant KA, Reid AW. Embolisation of massive bleeding following hysterectomy, despite internal iliac artery ligation. Br J Obstet Gynaecol 1994; 101:908–909.
31. Chait A, Moltz A, Nelson JH Jr. The collateral arterial circulation in the pelvis: an angiographic study. AJR 1968; 102:392–400.
32. Hare WSC, Holland CJ. Paresis following internal iliac artery embolization. Radiology 1983; 146:47–51.
33. Sieber PR. Bladder necrosis secondary to pelvic artery embolization: case report and literature review. J Urol 1994; 151: 422.
34. Behnam K, Jarmolowski CR. Vesicovaginal fistula following hypogastric embolization for control of intractable pelvic hemorrhage. J Reprod Med 1982; 27:304–306.
35. Mengert WF, Burchell RC, Blumstein RW, Daskal JL. Pregnancy after bilateral ligation of the internal iliac and ovarian arteries. Obstet Gynecol 1969; 34:664–666.
36. Stancato-Pasik A, Mitty HA, Richard HM III, Eshkar N. Obstetric embolotherapy: effect on menses and pregnancy. Radiology 1997; 204:791–793.

Jae-Kyu Kim, MD
Yong-Yeon Jeong, MD
Yun-Hyeon Kim, MD
Young-Chul Kim, MD
Heoung-Keun Kang, MD
Ho-Sun Choi, MD

Index terms:
Cyst, percutaneous drainage, 992.1263
Lymphatic system, interventional procedure, 992.123, 992.1263
Lymphocele, 992.842

Radiology 1999; 212:390–394

[1] From the Departments of Diagnostic Radiology (J.K.K., Y.Y.J., Y.H.K., Y.C.K., H.K.K.) and Obstetrics and Gynecology (H.S.C.), Chonnam University Medical School, 8 Hakdong, Dongku, Kwangju, 501-757 South Korea. Received May 18, 1998; revision requested July 14; revision received September 9; accepted February 12, 1999. **Address reprint requests to** J.K.K. (e-mail: *kjkrad@chonnam.chonnam.ac.kr*).

Author contributions:
Guarantor of integrity of entire study, J.K.K.; study concepts, J.K.K., Y.Y.J.; study design, J.K.K., H S.C.; definition of intellectual content, J.K.K., Y.H.K.; literature research, J.K.K., Y.C.K.; clinical studies, J.K.K.; data acquisition, J.K.K., Y.H.K.; data analysis, J.K.K., H.K.K.; statistical analysis, Y.C.K.; manuscript preparation and editing, J.K.K., H.K.K.; manuscript review, J.K.K.

Postoperative Pelvic Lymphocele: Treatment with Simple Percutaneous Catheter Drainage[1]

PURPOSE: To evaluate the effectiveness of simple percutaneous catheter drainage in the treatment of postoperative lymphocele.

MATERIALS AND METHODS: Percutaneous catheter drainage of 23 symptomatic lymphoceles was performed with ultrasonographic (US) guidance in 20 patients who had undergone radical pelvic lymphadenectomy because of uterine malignancy. All lymphoceles were diagnosed on the basis of biochemical and cytologic findings in aspirated fluid. The drainage catheter was removed when the amount of daily drainage was less than 10 mL per day and when the lymphocele was seen at imaging to have resolved. Follow-up US was performed at 1, 3, and 6 months after catheter removal. The results were classified as success, partial success, or failure.

RESULTS: Lymphoceles ranged in size from 5 × 4 × 3 to 25 × 10 × 10 cm. Mean total drainage volume was 2,012 mL (range, 300–17,240 mL). Fluid from 10 lymphoceles (43%) was positive at Gram staining and bacteriologic culture; fluid from 13 (57%) was sterile. Duration of catheter drainage was 3–49 days (mean, 22 days). Twenty (87%) lymphoceles resolved completely; three (13%) recurred. Two recurrent lymphoceles were again treated with percutaneous catheter drainage; the third resolved spontaneously 5 months after catheter removal. Successful treatment was ultimately achieved in all patients. Postprocedural complications occurred in four patients. One had a secondary infection of lymphocele; one, catheter dislodgment; and two, skin infection at the site of catheter insertion.

CONCLUSION: Percutaneous catheter drainage is safe and effective for treatment of symptomatic postoperative lymphoceles.

Pelvic or retroperitoneal lymphoceles are bothersome postoperative complications and have been reported in up to 30% of cases of lymphadenectomy performed because of prostatic or gynecologic malignancy and in 2%–18% of cases of renal transplantation (1–3). Small or sterile lymphoceles often are asymptomatic and spontaneously resorbed (4). Large or infected lymphoceles, however, may cause serious complications that necessitate treatment (4–7). Several methods of treatment for postoperative lymphocele, such as conservative observation, surgical treatment, and percutaneous catheter drainage with or without sclerotherapy, have been introduced, with various results (4–12).

The purpose of this study was to analyze the results and evaluate the effectiveness of simple percutaneous catheter drainage of pelvic or retroperitoneal lymphoceles in patients who had undergone radical pelvic lymph node dissection because of uterine malignancy.

MATERIALS AND METHODS

Between January 1995 and December 1996, 23 lymphoceles developed in 20 women after radical hysterectomy with pelvic lymphadenectomy. Sixteen patients had undergone surgery for treatment of uterine cervical carcinoma, and four had undergone surgery for treatment of uterine endometrial carcinoma. The patients were aged 24–62 years (mean, 48

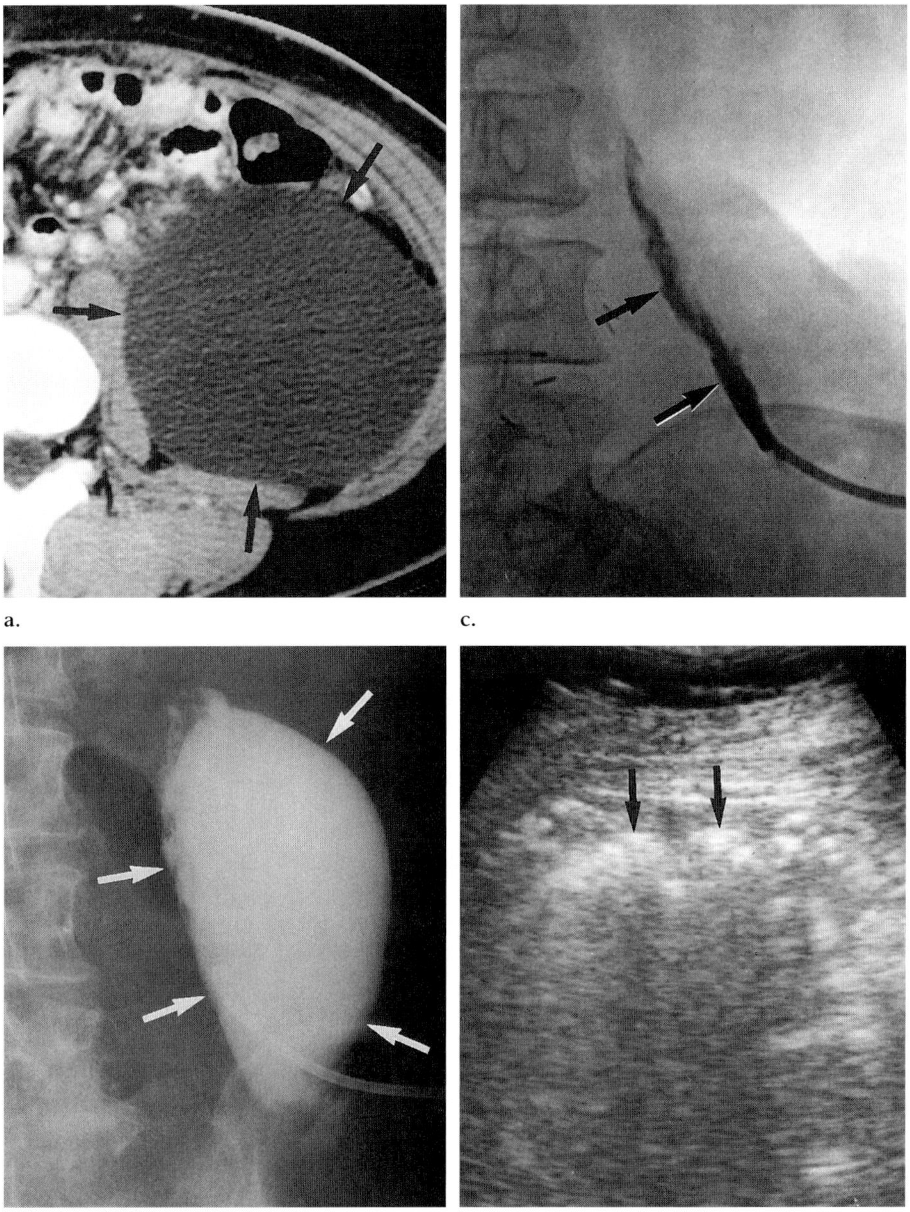

Figure 1. Sterile lymphocele. (a) Axial contrast medium–enhanced CT image shows a large, well-defined, homogeneous, low-attenuating mass (arrows) in the left side of the infrarenal retroperitoneum. (b) Initial lymphograph obtained after catheter insertion shows a lymphocele (arrows) in left side of the abdomen. (c) Follow-up lymphograph obtained 15 days later shows nearly complete collapse of the lymphocele (arrows). (d) Follow-up oblique sagittal transabdominal US image obtained 6 months after catheter removal shows a focal fibrotic remnant (arrows) of the lymphocele.

years). Written informed consent was obtained from all patients prior to percutaneous catheter drainage.

Fifteen lymphoceles were detected at ultrasonography (US); three, at computed tomography (CT); and five, at both US and CT. Lymphoceles were located in the pelvic cavity (n = 8), retroperitoneal cavity (n = 6), or both cavities (n = 9). The time between surgery and catheter drainage was 7–219 days (mean, 68 days). No patient had previously undergone surgery for treatment of a lymphocele. Indications for drainage were abdominal pain in all patients, fever and chills in 13 patients, edema of lower extremities and external genitalia in 10 patients, palpable pelvic mass in eight patients, and ipsilateral hydronephrosis in two patients.

Before the procedure, a complete blood count and biochemical analysis was performed to evaluate for the likelihood of bleeding. Prophylactic antibiotics (piperacillin sodium and amikacin sulfate) were administered 24 hours before the procedure. The patients received nothing by mouth for 6 hours before the procedure.

In all patients, US was performed to determine the relationship between the lymphocele(s) and adjacent abdominal organs and to choose the safest and shortest approach. Routes of approach were transperitoneal in 16 cases amd retroperitoneal in seven.

By using sterile procedures and US guidance, the lesion was punctured with a 21-gauge Chiba needle (Jung Sung, Seoul, South Korea). Approximately 15 mL of fluid was aspirated for the purposes of biochemical, cytologic, and bacteriologic examinations. A lymphocele was diagnosed when the creatinine, urea nitrogen, protein, and electrolyte components of aspirated fluid were similar to those of serum at the biochemical examination and when the aspirated fluid had few leukocytes, predominant lymphocytes, and no cancer cells at the cytologic examination (4–8).

For initial lymphography, the lymphocele was opacified with diluted contrast medium (Urografin 60%; Schering, Berlin, Germany) injected through the Chiba needle. Insertion of a 0.018-inch guide wire was followed by removal of the puncture needle. A 6.3-F sheath (MEDIKIT; Jung Sung) was then inserted over the wire. As much fluid as possible was aspirated through this sheath to prevent contamination from adjacent organs.

The second lymphographic procedure was performed through the 6.3-F sheath to evaluate the size of the lesion and internal septation. A 0.038-inch guide wire (Boston Scientific/Medi-tech, Natick, Mass) was inserted. If internal septation was seen, the septum was broken by using the guide wire with fluoroscopic guidance. Next, an 8.0–10.2-F pigtail drainage catheter (Boston Scientific/Microvasive, Natick, Mass) was inserted into the cavity after removal of sheath. The tip of the catheter was left at the most dependent position of the cavity to facilitate spontaneous drainage by means of gravity. The drainage catheter was irrigated three to five times per day with 5–10 mL of physiologic saline solution, and the amount of drainage was recorded. Follow up US (n = 15) or lymphography (n = 8) was performed 1 week later to help evaluate the size of the lymphocele.

The catheter was removed when the following criteria were met: Drainage had stopped or was less than 10 mL per day for more than 3 days and when the cavity was seen to be collapsed at US or lymphography. The patient was discharged when lymphocele-related symptoms were relieved. All patients were followed up with US in the outpatient department at 1, 3, and 6 months after catheter removal.

Results were defined as follows: Complete success was achieved when abnormal fluid collections seen at US had collapsed, lymphocele-related symptoms were relieved, there was no recurrence at follow-up, and there was no need for surgical management. Partial success was achieved when a lymphocele recurred but resolved without surgical management. The result was classified as a failure when clinical symptoms were aggravated, and the lymphocele was managed with surgical intervention.

The correlations of duration of drainage with size of lymphocele and presence of secondary infection were analyzed by using the Spearman correlation method.

RESULTS

Lymphoceles were demonstrated as well-marginated, cystic lesions at US and as well-delineated, low-attenuating lesions with a nonenhancing, thin wall at CT (Fig 1). Septation was seen in nine infected lymphoceles and in two noninfected lymphoceles.

Aspirated or drained fluids were clear and yellow in noninfected lesions and turbid and gray in infected lymphoceles. The results of biochemical and cytologic analyses showed the protein, urea nitrogen, creatinine, and electrolyte levels of aspirated fluid to be same as or less than those of serum; in some lesions, lipids and triglycerides were found. A few leukocytes and predominant lymphocytes were found in all lymphoceles. Aspirates from 10 lesions (43%) with clear, yellowish fluid were gram-positive and produced positive bacteriologic cultures. Aspirates in 13 lesions (57%) with turbid, gray fluid were bacteriologic culture–negative and gram-negative. Cytologic examination results showed that all lymphoceles were negative for malignant cells.

Lymphocele size varied between 5 × 4 × 3 cm and 25 × 10 × 10 cm. The total volume of drained fluid was 300–17,240 mL (mean, 2,012 mL). Lymphocele-related symptoms were relieved within 3 days after the procedure in all patients. The duration of catheter drainage was 3–49 days (mean, 22 days). There were no significant differences between lesion size and drainage duration (P = .072) and between mean drainage duration in noninfected lymphoceles (18.8 days) and that in infected lymphoceles (24.9 days) (P = .9688).

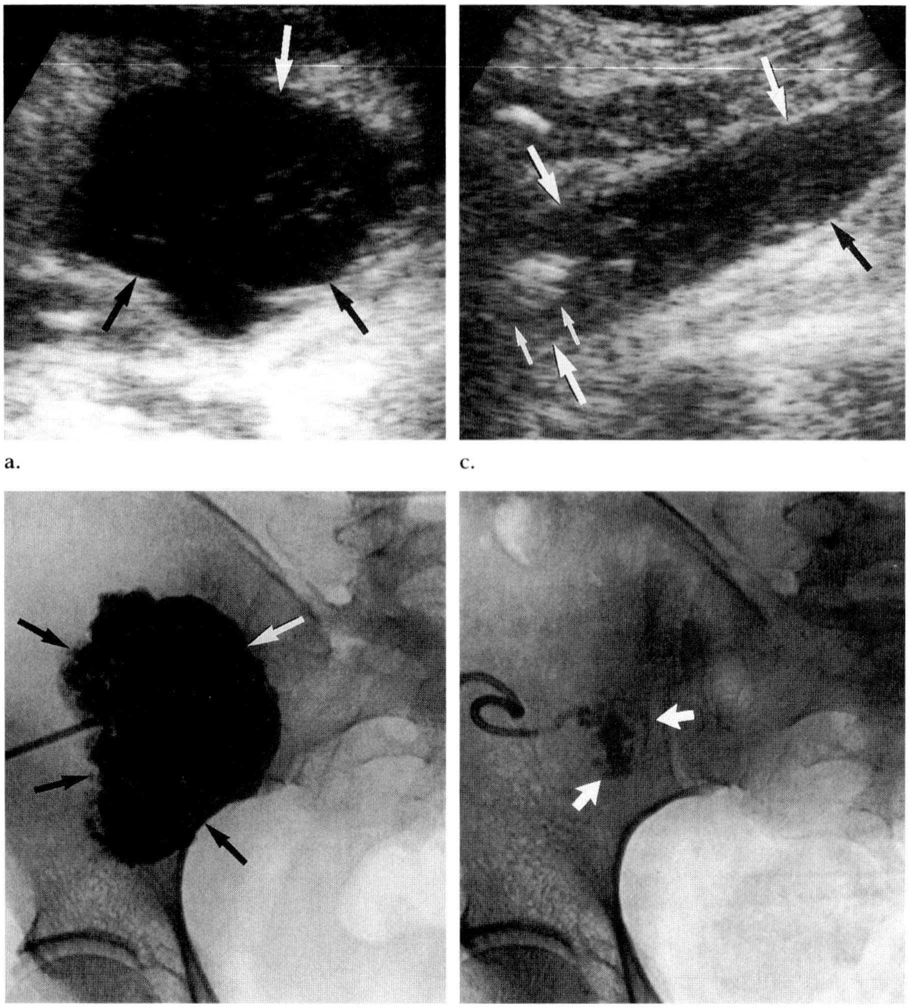

a. c. b. d.

Figure 2. Infected lymphocele. **(a)** Axial pelvic US image shows a septated lymphocele (arrows) with hyperechoic debris in the right side of the pelvic cavity. **(b)** Initial lymphograph shows an irregularly marginated lymphocele (arrows) with septation in the right side of the pelvic cavity. **(c)** Follow-up oblique axial pelvic US image obtained 1 week after catheter drainage shows the shrunken lymphocele (large arrows). Small arrows = catheter. **(d)** Follow-up lymphograph obtained 23 days after catheter drainage shows nearly complete collapse of the lymphocele (arrows).

Twenty lymphoceles (87%) were completely obliterated after initial catheter drainage. Recurrence was noted in three lymphoceles (13%). In two of these, obliteration occurred after a second catheter drainage procedure; the third lymphocele, which was small and produced no symptoms, completely resolved after 5 months without any further treatment (Fig 2). As a result, successful percutaneous catheter drainage was attained in all cases.

Complications occurred in four patients: a secondary skin infection at the catheter entry site in two patients with an infected lymphocele, a secondary infection of a previously noninfected lymphocele in one patient, and dislodgment of the catheter in an infected lymphocele in one patient. This last patient was treated with reinsertion of the drainage catheter and antibiotic therapy for 1 week (Fig 3). There was no significant difference between the number of complications in infected lymphoceles versus that in noninfected lymphoceles.

DISCUSSION

Pelvic or retroperitoneal lymphoceles occur as a complication after renal trans-

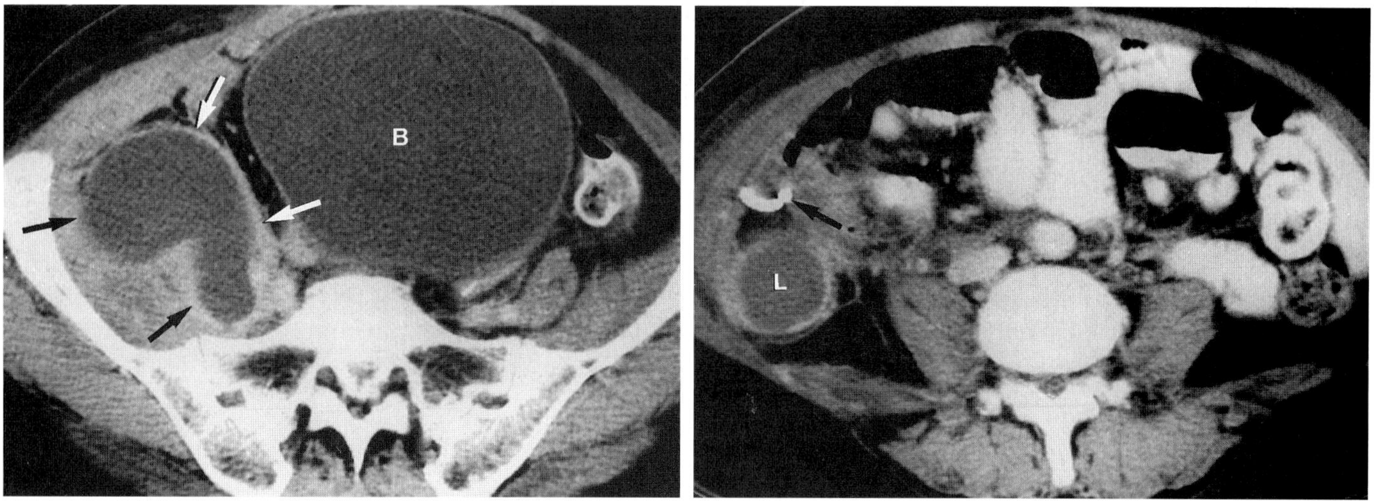

a. b.

Figure 3. Catheter dislodgment. **(a)** Axial contrast-enhanced CT image shows a well-defined lymphocele (arrows) with an enhancing wall along the right side of the pelvic cavity. *B* = urinary bladder. **(b)** Follow-up contrast-enhanced axial CT image obtained 15 days after catheter drainage reveals dislodgment of the catheter (arrow) from the lymphocele (*L*).

plantation or extensive surgery with radical lymphadenectomy performed because of prostatic or gynecologic malignancy (1–3). Pelvic lymphocele after radical pelvic lymphadenectomy is believed to result from surgical transection or inadequate ligation of lymphatic vessels during lymph node dissection. If the injury to the lymphatic vessels is mild, lymph flow will continue through collateral pathways, with eventual reestablishment or regeneration of the lymphatic network (13). If the disruption is severe, however, this process may not occur, and lymphatic fluid from transected afferent vessels may accumulate in various anatomic compartments, such as the pelvic or retroperitoneal space, and result in lymphocele formation (6).

In histologic terms, the wall of a lymphocele consists of dense fibrotic tissue with no lining of epithelial cells. The wall of a lymphocele does not infiltrate adjacent structures (3). A lymphocele must be differentiated from a postoperative urinoma, hematoma, seroma, or abscess, but this is difficult on the basis of radiologic results alone. At biochemical analysis, a lymphocele has the same levels of protein, urea nitrogen, creatinine, electrolytes, and, occasionally, lipids as serum has, so differentiation from urinoma, hematoma, seroma, or abscess is possible (4–9). In our study, the urea nitrogen, creatinine, and electrolytes levels in lymphoceles were similar to those in serum in all cases, and three retroperitoneal lymphoceles had levels of lipids and triglycerides that were higher than those of serum.

The natural course of a lymphocele usually is dependent on the size of the lesion and the presence of infection. When a lymphocele is small and sterile, it usually heals by means of spontaneous resorption. When it is large, however, the lymphocele may compress adjacent structures such as the iliac vessels, bladder, ureter, or rectosigmoid (3–8). This compression causes manifestations that include abdominal distention, abdominal and pelvic pain, hydronephrosis, bladder dysfunction, constipation, tenesmus, edema of the ipsilateral leg and of the genitalia, and thromboembolism of iliac vessels.

When complications such as abdominal pain, fever, chills, and sepsis develop (3–8), surgical treatment or catheter drainage is necessary. Indications for treatment usually are determined on the basis of the severity of clinical symptoms and the presence of functional compromise of adjacent vital structures (10–15). In our study, all 23 lymphoceles produced clinical symptoms. Ten lymphoceles (43%) produced symptoms associated with infection of the lymphocele.

There are several methods for treatment of a lymphocele, including surgical drainage, peritoneal marsupialization, simple aspiration, percutaneous catheter drainage, and percutaneous catheter drainage with sclerotherapy (4–12). When surgery was the only available therapeutic option, surgical drainage resulted in a success rate of 50%–70%, and peritoneal marsupialization resulted in a success rate of greater than 90% (16). However, these methods have some disadvantages, such as surgical morbidity and mortality, economic burden, and the need for long hospitalization (3,4).

Simple aspiration is safer and more effective than surgical therapy, but repeated procedures are necessary in 80%–90% of patients, and an infection rate of 25%–50% has been reported (5,7,9). Conte et al (9) reported a mean drainage duration of 14.5 days and a success rate of 100% with simple percutaneous catheter drainage. White et al (6) and vanSonnenberg et al (5) reported catheter drainage durations, either with or without sclerotherapy, of 4–120 days and 5–32 days, respectively, and success rates of 82% and 79%, respectively.

Sclerotherapy with the use of tetracycline, ampicillin, povidone-iodine, or alcohol usually results in a high success rate of 79%-93% (3,4,7,8). Akhan et al (7), Zuckerman and Yeager (8), and Sawhney et al (4) reported that percutaneous catheter drainage combined with alcohol sclerotherapy results in average drainage durations of 9, 19, and 36 days, respectively, and success rates of 88%, 94%, and 100%, respectively. In our study, the mean duration of lymphocele drainage was 22 days. Inflammatory changes in an infected lymphocele render the lymphocele adhesive, which results in a short drainage duration. We achieved successful treatment of postoperative lymphoceles by means of simple catheter drainage in all cases, with no important complications and no need for secondary surgical treatment.

Percutaneous catheter drainage has some advantages; namely, no need to perform sclerotherapy and an only infrequent need for a repeated procedure. These advantages result in a lower economic burden for the patient. Sclerotherapy with absolute alcohol causes an intense inflammatory reaction during the obliteration of injured lymphatic channels that maintain persistent fluid output. Absolute alcohol dehydrates cells and degrades proteins in the layers of tissue. The effects of alcohol are followed by inflammatory changes and scarring (4,8). Other sclerosing agents, including tetracycline and povidone-iodine, cause similar inflammatory effects (4).

In our study, there was no statistical correlation between the size of the lymphocele and the duration of drainage. Drainage duration was longer for infected lymphoceles (mean, 24.9 days) than for sterile lymphoceles (mean, 18.8 days), but this difference was not significant.

No serious catheter-related complications necessitating further therapy have been reported (8). Likewise, no major complications were encountered in this study; minor complications included skin infection, secondary infection of the lymphocele, and dislodgment of the catheter.

In conclusion, percutaneous catheter drainage without sclerotherapy is a simple and effective therapeutic method that results in a high success rate in the treatment of a symptomatic lymphocele after radical pelvic lymphadenectomy performed because of uterine malignancy.

References

1. Dodd GD, Rutledge F, Wallace S. Postoperative pelvic lymphocysts. AJR 1970; 108:312–323.
2. Sweizer R, Cho S, Kountz SL, Belzer FO. Lymphoceles following renal transplantation. Arch Surg 1972; 104:42–45.
3. Petru E, Tamussino K, Lahousen M, et al. Pelvic and paraaortic lymphocysts after radical surgery because of cervical and ovarian cancer. Am J Obstet Gynecol 1989; 161:937–941.
4. Sawhney R, D'Agostino HB, Zinck S, et al. Treatment of postoperative lymphoceles with percutaneous drainage and alcohol sclerotherapy. JVIR 1996; 7:241–245.
5. vanSonnenberg E, Wittich GR, Casola G, et al. Lymphocele: imaging characteristics and percutaneous management. Radiology 1986; 161:593–596.
6. White M, Mueller PR, Ferrucci JT, et al. Percutaneous drainage of postoperative abdominal and pelvic lymphoceles. AJR 1985; 145:1065–1069.
7. Akhan O, Cekirge S, Ozmen M, Besim A. Percutaneous transcatheter sclerotherapy of postoperative pelvic lymphoceles. Cardiovasc Intervent Radiol 1992; 15:224–227.
8. Zuckerman DA, Yeager TD. Percutaneous ethanol sclerotherapy of postoperative lymphoceles. AJR 1997; 169:433–437.
9. Conte M, Panici PB, Guariglia L, et al. Pelvic lymphocele following radical paraaortic and pelvic lymphadenectomy for cervical carcinoma: incidence rate and percutaneous management. Obstet Gynecol 1990; 76:268–271.
10. Kay R, Fechs E, Barry JM, et al. Management of postoperative pelvic lymphoceles. Urology 1980; 15:345–347.
11. Gilliland JD, Spies JB, Brown SB, et al. Lymphoceles: percutaneous treatment with povidone-iodine sclerosis. Radiology 1989; 171:227–229.
12. Lin JJ, Sorbi D, Uy JP, et al. Doxycycline sclerotherapy of lymphocele after renal transplantation and its inhibition of gelatinase activity. Transplant Proc 1993; 25:3320–3324.
13. Braun WE, Banowsky LH, Straffon RA, et al. Lymphoceles associated with renal transplantation: report of 15 cases and review of the literature. Am J Med 1974; 57:714–719.
14. Ojeda L, Sharifi R, Lee M, et al. Lymphocele formation after extraperitoneal pelvic lymphadenectomy: possible predisposing factors. J Urol 1986; 136:616–618.
15. vanSonnenberg E, Mueller PR, Ferrucci JT Jr. Percutaneous drainage of 250 abdominal abscesses and fluid collections: results, failures, and complications. Radiology 1984; 151:337–341.
16. Meyers AM, Levine E, Myburgh JA, et al. Diagnosis and management of lymphoceles after renal transplantation. Urology 1977; 10:497–502.

Role of MR Imaging in the Selection of Patients with Early Cervical Carcinoma for Fertility-preserving Surgery: Initial Experience[1]

P. Delia Peppercorn, MB, ChB
Arjun R. Jeyarajah, MB, BS
Robert Woolas, MB, BS
John H. Shepherd, MB, BS
David H. Oram, MB, ChB
Ian J. Jacobs, MD
Peter Armstrong, MB, BS
David Lowe, MD
Rodney H. Reznek, MB, ChB

Index terms:
Pelvic organs, MR, 854.121411, 854.121415, 854.12143
Sterility, 854.32
Uterine neoplasms, MR, 854.121411, 854.121415, 854.12143
Uterine neoplasms, staging, 854.32
Uterus, interventional procedures, 854.1267

Radiology 1999; 212:395–399

Abbreviation:
FIGO = International Federation of Gynecology and Obstetrics

[1] From the Departments of Radiology (P.D.P., P.A., R.H.R.), Gynaecological Oncology (A.R.J., R.W., J.H.S., D.H.O., I.J.J.), and Pathology (D.L.), St. Bartholomew's Hospital, West Smithfield, London EC1 7BE, UK. From the 1997 RSNA scientific assembly. Received June 17, 1998; revision requested July 30; final revision received November 10; accepted February 22, 1999. **Address reprint requests to** R.H.R. (e-mail: *jkjessop@mds.qmw.ac.uk*).

Author contributions:
Guarantor of integrity of entire study, R.H.R.; study concepts, R.W., R.H.R.; study design, P.D.P., A.R.J.; definition of intellectual content, R.H.R., P.A., J.H.S.; literature research, P.D.P., R.H.R.; clinical studies, P.D.P., R.H.R., D.L., J.H.S., D.H.O., I.J.J.; data acquisition, P.D.P.; data analysis, P.D.P., A.R.J., I.J.J.; statistical analysis, P.D.P., A.R.J., I.J.J.; manuscript preparation, P.D.P., A.R.J.; manuscript editing, I.J.J., P.A., R.H.R.; manuscript review, R.W., J.H.S., D.H.O., I.J.J., P.A., D.L., R.H.R.

PURPOSE: To assess whether magnetic resonance (MR) imaging can be used for reliable prediction of proximal extension of cervical carcinoma into the myometrium.

MATERIALS AND METHODS: Thirty patients with early cervical carcinoma underwent MR imaging with use of a 1.5-T magnet prior to surgery. The MR images were analyzed by two radiologists, unaware of the histopathologic findings, for the relationship of the tumor to the internal os and extension of the tumor into the myometrium. Findings at MR imaging were compared with those at histopathologic examination.

RESULTS: At MR imaging, 24 patients were considered not to have tumor extension proximal to the internal os and into the myometrium. All tumors were confirmed histopathologically. In six patients thought to have myometrial tumor invasion at MR imaging, five tumors were confirmed histopathologically; in one, tumor extended up to the internal os but did not involve the myometrium.

CONCLUSION: This is a small study, but MR imaging appears accurate in the prediction of myometrial tumor involvement and in showing the relationship of cervical carcinoma to the internal os and, hence, the patient's suitability for trachelectomy.

The standard treatment for stage IA2 and stage IB cervical carcinoma in most centers in Europe and the United States is radical hysterectomy and pelvic lymphadenectomy. Most patients with cervical carcinoma are either postmenopausal or have completed their families, and for these patients the consequent loss of fertility is not a major issue. The primary purpose of cervical screening is to detect preinvasive disease; however, it has also led to earlier diagnosis of cervical carcinoma, often at a superficial stage. This has been reflected in the new International Federation of Gynecology and Obstetrics (FIGO) staging system (Table) (1). Approximately 30% of women with cervical carcinoma are less than 35 years of age, and for many of these women preservation of fertility is a major issue (2). Consequently, surgical approaches that combine radical excision of the tumor with conservation of the uterus have been explored. Our group and others (3,4) recently have reported on the performance of radical trachelectomy in this situation.

Trachelectomy involves a vaginal surgical approach to radical removal of the cervix along with parametrial tissue and a cuff of the vagina. Either a laparoscopic or retroperitoneal pelvic lymphadenectomy is performed at the same time (5,6). The uterine body is left intact, and a nonabsorbable suture, a cervical cerclage, is placed around the uterine isthmus. This suture is used to maintain the competency of the uterus in subsequent pregnancies. Although the number of these operations is small to date, it seems to be possible to achieve satisfactory surgical clearance, and pregnancies and term deliveries have been achieved (3,7).

The performance of radical trachelectomy introduces a new surgical resection margin and consequently a new consideration into preoperative assessment and staging. Prior to radical hysterectomy, the staging process is directed toward assessment of the parametrium and pelvic lymph node status, and little attention is directed toward documenting extension of the primary cervical tumor to the uterus.

The relationship of the proximal extent of the tumor to the internal os and lower portion of the uterine body is, however, a critical consideration in preoperative assessment of patients who may wish to undergo radical trachelectomy. Extension of tumor beyond the internal os and therefore into the body of the uterus indicates that the patient is not suitable for trachelectomy. The exact location of the internal os may not be critical for the surgeon, who is guided by the uterine arteries, especially as the length and shape of the cervix vary from patient to patient owing to previous obstetric events or surgery. In this study, we evaluate the predictive value of magnetic resonance (MR) imaging in the assessment of proximal tumor extension beyond the internal os into the body of the uterus, and hence patient suitability for radical trachelectomy.

MATERIALS AND METHODS

All patients presenting to our hospital with primary carcinoma of the cervix, regardless of stage, between January 1996 and October 1997 were entered into this prospective study, and 39 patients were recruited. The diagnosis was confirmed by means of biopsy performed 10–28 days before evaluation with MR imaging. Nine patients with inoperable, advanced disease at MR imaging or examination under anesthesia were excluded. Thirty patients (age range, 25–66 years; mean, 41 years) were included. Five patients subsequently were found to have no residual disease at the time of definitive surgery, all tumor having been removed at the time of biopsy; however, these patients were included as this was not known when the patients entered the study.

MR imaging was performed with use of a 1.5-T imager (Signa; GE Medical Systems, Milwaukee, Wis). Pulse sequences performed were axial and sagittal T2-weighted fast spin-echo sequences, 5,000–6,000/119 (repetition time msec/echo time msec), 7-mm section thickness, 2-mm gap; axial and sagittal T1-weighted spin-echo sequences with fat saturation before and after the intravenous administration of gadopentetate dimeglumine, 500/11; and oblique T2-weighted fast spin-echo sequences, 6,000/114, 5-mm section thickness, and 1-mm gap. The oblique plane was selected by the radiologist and was perpendicular to the cervical canal.

A 24 × 24-cm field of view was used for the axial and oblique sequences, and a 32 × 32-cm field of view was used for the sagittal sequences. A matrix of 256 × 256 or 516 × 256 was used, with three or four signals acquired. All sequences were performed by using a phased-array pelvic coil. The axial and sagittal sequences covered the whole of the abdomen and pelvis, and the oblique sequences were confined to the pelvis. Intravenous administration of 10 mL of gadopentetate dimeglumine (Magnevist; Schering Health Care, West Sussex, UK) was performed by hand injection over 15 seconds. All the injections were performed by the same radiologist (P.D.P.). The sagittal contrast medium–enhanced T1-weighted sequence was performed immediately after the injection of contrast medium. Each sequence took between 3 minutes 30 seconds and 5 minutes to perform.

The MR images were interpreted by the consensus of two radiologists (P.D.P., R.H.R.). They were aware of the diagnosis of cervical carcinoma but not of the histopathologic type or clinical staging. All the MR images from the various sequences were viewed together. The images obtained before and after contrast enhancement were assessed for depiction of the tumor, the relationship of the tumor to the internal os, and extension of tumor into the myometrium. Abnormal areas of intermediate to high signal intensity on T2-weighted images, with or without mass effect, were considered to represent tumor and were measured in the maximum dimension.

On the sagittal images, the internal os was defined as the waist of the uterine contour and entrance of the uterine vessels, where the low signal intensity of the cervical stroma changed to the uterine appearance with myometrium of intermediate signal intensity. On the oblique images, the internal os was defined as the point of transition from the low signal intensity of the cervix to the intermediate signal intensity of the myometrium. Tumor extension into the uterine body was defined as tumor extending across the internal os, expanding the endometrial cavity, or disrupting the endometrial-myometrial zones and their normal signal intensities.

The size of any demonstrable pelvic lymph node was recorded. All nodes were measured in the short axis on the axial images, and their exact locations were recorded.

FIGO Staging of Early Cervical Cancer

Stage	Description
I	Carcinoma confined strictly to the cervix; extension into the uterine corpus should be disregarded
IA1	Invasion of the stroma no greater than 3 mm in depth and no wider than 7 mm in diameter
IA2	Invasion of the stroma greater than 3 mm, no greater than 5 mm in depth, and no wider than 7 mm in diameter
IB1	Clinical lesions no greater than 4 cm
IB2	Clinical lesions greater than 4 cm
II	Carcinoma extends beyond the cervix but not to the pelvic side wall or the lower third of the vagina
IIA	No parametrial involvement or extension into the lower third of the vagina
IIB	Obvious parametrial involvement but not to the pelvic side wall

All patients underwent definitive surgery within 14 days of the MR study. In patients who underwent hysterectomy, the surgically excised uterus was sectioned sagittally, corresponding to the MR images, to assess the extent of tumor beyond the internal os. The cervix was then amputated and sectioned radially. The depth of tumor invasion was determined with the use of the Vwenier scale of the microscope. In patients who underwent trachelectomy, the cervix was handled in exactly the same manner. The locations of all lymph nodes removed at surgery were recorded. Each node was examined histopathologically for metastatic involvement and was measured by using a dissecting microscope.

The sensitivity, specificity, and positive predictive value of MR imaging in the assessment of the proximal extension of cervical tumor into the body of the uterus and the sensitivity and specificity of MR imaging in the detection of nodal involvement with tumor were calculated.

RESULTS

Histopathologic confirmation was obtained in 27 patients who underwent Wertheim hysterectomy with pelvic lymphadenectomy and in three patients who had radical trachelectomy and laparoscopic or extraperitoneal lymphadenectomy. Disease in all patients was classified as FIGO stage IIB or less. The histopathologically diagnosed tumor types were

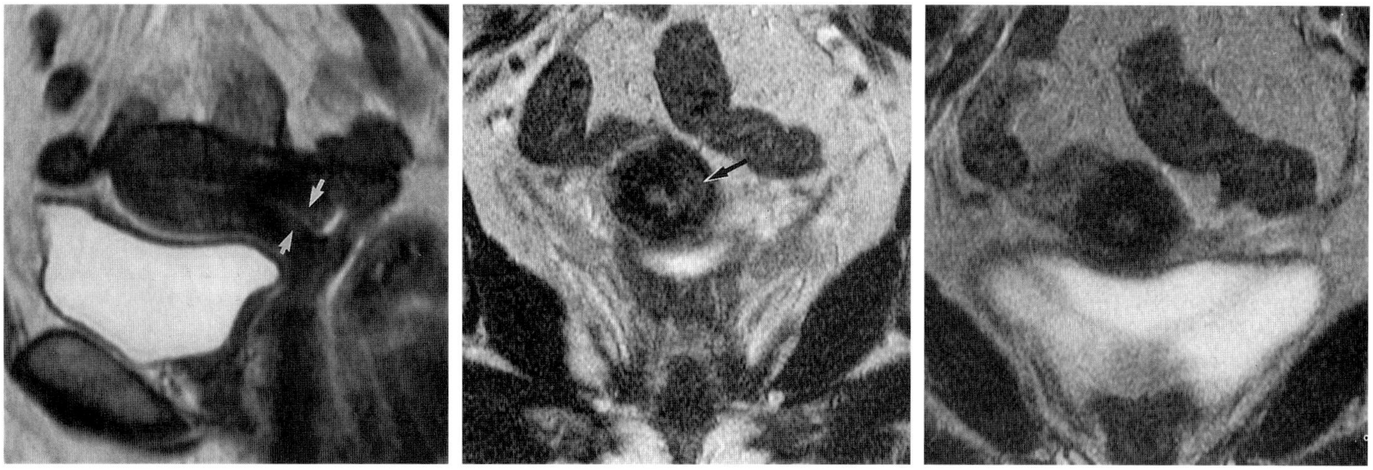

a. b. c.

Figure 1. Images obtained in 42-year-old woman. **(a)** Sagittal T2-weighted MR image (4,000/85) shows a small area of intermediate signal intensity (arrows) in the cervix, which is consistent with tumor. **(b)** Oblique T2-weighted MR image (6,000/84) shows the small area of intermediate-signal-intensity tumor (arrow) that is adjacent to normal low-signal-intensity cervix. **(c)** Oblique T2-weighted MR image (6,000/84) obtained just above **b** at the level of the internal os shows no evidence of disease.

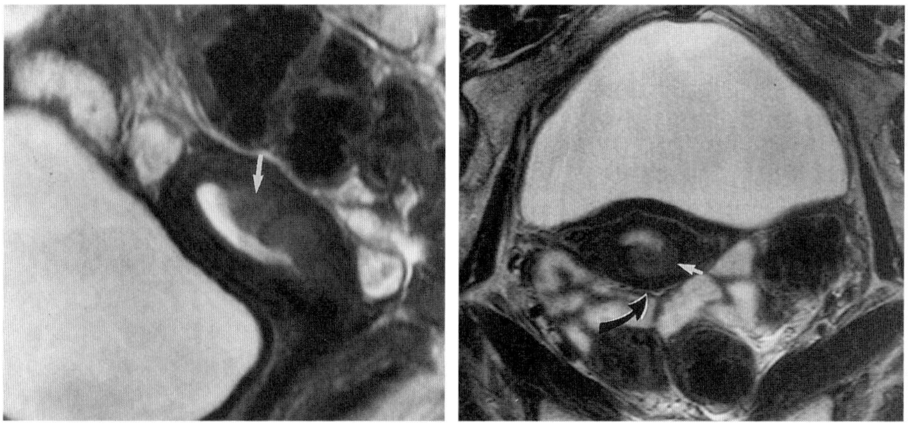

a. b.

Figure 2. Images obtained in 37-year-old woman. **(a)** Sagittal T2-weighted MR image (4,000/128) shows a tumor (arrow) that is of intermediate signal intensity in the cervix and that extends superiorly into the uterine cavity. **(b)** Oblique T2-weighted MR image (4,000/128) shows that the tumor (straight arrow) does not extend into the normal parametrium (curved arrow).

squamous cell carcinoma ($n = 26$), adenocarcinoma ($n = 3$), and adenosquamous carcinoma ($n = 1$).

The primary tumor could not be identified on MR images in nine of 30 patients. In five of these nine patients, no tumor was apparent at histopathologic examination because all of the tumor had been removed at the time biopsy was performed, and in the other four patients the tumor was less than 3 mm in maximum diameter.

In a further five patients, it was not possible to differentiate on MR images between small-volume tumor and inflammatory changes in the cervix as a consequence of performance of biopsy, although the proximal extent of abnormal signal intensity could still be assessed. In three of these five patients, inflammation with focal ulceration and no residual tumor was seen at histopathologic examination, and in the other two the tumor was less than 6 mm in maximum diameter.

Overall, at MR imaging 24 of 30 patients were considered not to have tumor invasion beyond the internal os into the myometrium (Fig 1). This interpretation was confirmed histopathologically. Of the six tumors considered to have invaded the myometrium at MR imaging, five were confirmed histopathologically (Fig 2). In the sixth patient, tumor extended up to the internal os but did not involve the uterine isthmus at histopathologic examination (Fig 3). This last patient was not considered suitable for trachelectomy as there would have been an inadequate resection margin.

The sensitivity of MR imaging for the detection of tumor beyond the internal os was 100% (five of five), and the specificity was 96% (24 of 25). The positive predictive value was 83% (five of six). One of the five patients with tumor extension into the uterine body also had parametrial tumor extension at MR imaging that was confirmed at histopathologic examination.

With the axial T1-weighted sequence, the tumor could be identified in only one of the 30 patients. With the axial T2-weighted sequence, the tumor was depicted in three patients, but the relationship to the internal os could not be determined. With the sagittal T2-weighted sequence, the tumor could be identified in all patients, but in one patient the relationship to the internal os was incorrectly assessed (Fig 3). With the oblique T2-weighted sequence, the tumor and its relationship to the internal os were correctly identified in all patients. Use of intravenously administered gadopentetate dimeglumine increased observer confidence in three patients and in one patient helped to differentiate between tumor and the site of recent biopsy.

Eight patients had lymph nodes demonstrable at MR imaging. Of these patients, one had a 1.2-cm right external iliac node at MR imaging, with histopathologic confirmation of the size of the node, but no tumor infiltration was demonstrated. Seven patients had 5–9-mm lymph nodes at MR imaging; three were right internal iliac nodes, two were left internal iliac nodes, and two were left external iliac nodes. Four of these seven nodes showed metastatic involvement at histopathologic examination. Three other patients had nodal involvement at histopathologic examination, but the nodes did not exceed 5 mm and were not demonstrated at MR imaging. These nodes were in the right obturator region (one patient) and in both external iliac regions (two patients). By using the criterion of 1 cm in the short axis, we found that the sensitivity for detection of nodal involvement at MR imaging was 0% (zero of seven), and the specificity was 96% (22 of 23). Using the lymph node size of 5 mm or greater in the short axis, we found that the sensitivity of MR imaging for the detection of nodal involvement was 57% (four of seven), and the specificity was 83% (19 of 23).

Two of the patients who underwent trachelectomy had nodal involvement at histopathologic examination. In one patient, no enlarged nodes could be identified at MR imaging, but bilateral external iliac involvement was found at histopathologic examination. In the other patient, an 8-mm left external iliac node was demonstrated at MR imaging; at histopathologic examination, subcapsular tumor infiltration was shown. Neither of these patients had histopathologically demonstrable tumor in the cervix at the time of surgery. In the patient with subcapsular involvement of a single node, it was decided to pursue a "watch and wait" policy, and no further treatment was undertaken; and the other patient, with bilateral nodal involvement, subsequently was treated with a combination of chemotherapy and radiation therapy.

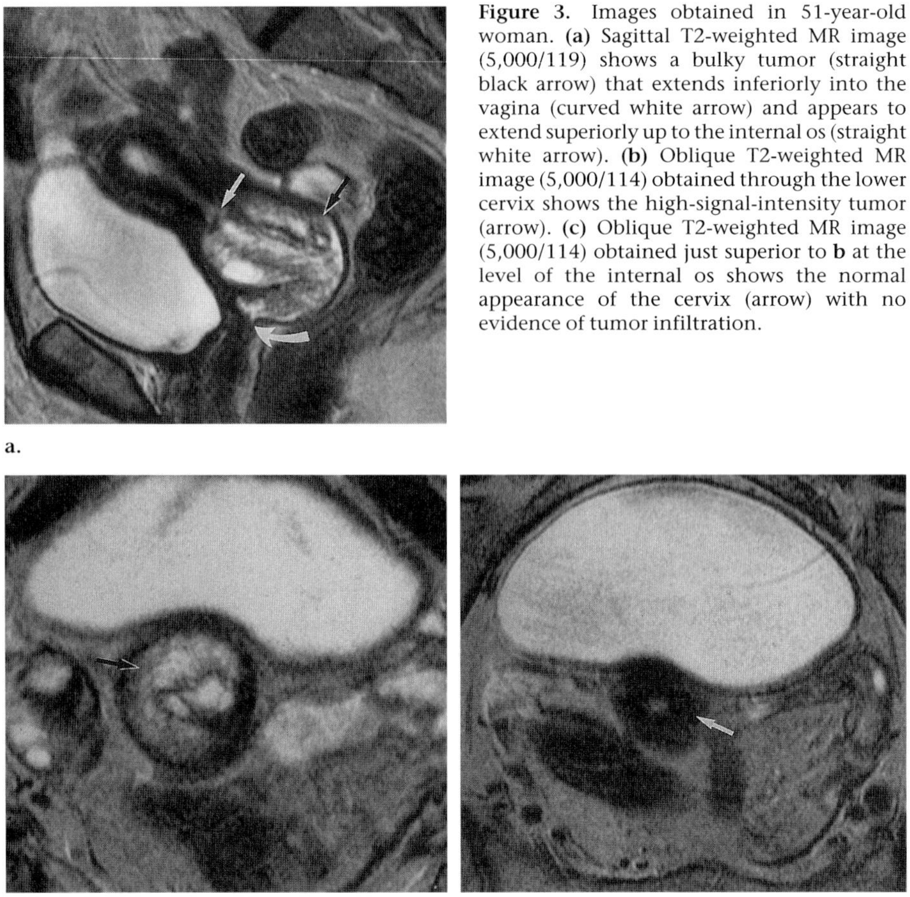

a. b. c.

Figure 3. Images obtained in 51-year-old woman. **(a)** Sagittal T2-weighted MR image (5,000/119) shows a bulky tumor (straight black arrow) that extends inferiorly into the vagina (curved white arrow) and appears to extend superiorly up to the internal os (straight white arrow). **(b)** Oblique T2-weighted MR image (5,000/114) obtained through the lower cervix shows the high-signal-intensity tumor (arrow). **(c)** Oblique T2-weighted MR image (5,000/114) obtained just superior to **b** at the level of the internal os shows the normal appearance of the cervix (arrow) with no evidence of tumor infiltration.

DISCUSSION

In previous MR imaging studies (8) of cervical carcinoma, much attention has been paid to the accuracy of staging with respect to parametrial tumor extension and tumor volume; indeed the FIGO staging system concentrates on the factors that affect resectability with conventional surgical techniques. The proximal extension of the tumor into the body of the uterus is not relevant to patients undergoing hysterectomy, and the detection of proximal tumor extension at MR imaging has not been studied widely.

However, there is a small group of young patients with early-stage disease who wish to preserve their fertility. This now can be achieved with a radical trachelectomy rather than a hysterectomy, and in these patients extension of the tumor proximal to the internal os becomes crucial. Assessment of tumor extent by means of clinical examination is known to be poor (8), and tumor extension into the uterine body cannot be accurately assessed clinically. There is therefore the need for an imaging modality that can demonstrate proximal extension of tumor to ensure a clear surgical resection margin.

The results of our study, which included only patients with both early disease and histopathologic correlation, show that MR imaging can be used to assess the relation of the tumor to the internal os accurately, with a sensitivity of 100% (five of five) and a specificity of 96% (24 of 25).

These results compare well with those of a previous study (9) in which a sensitivity of 86% (12 of 14) and a specificity of 100% were reported for invasion of the lower uterine segment. This previous study, however, included several patients with advanced disease (greater than stage IIB), the majority of whom also had parametrial disease. In our study, only 20% (one of five) of the patients with uterine involvement also had parametrial invasion. We confirmed that the sagittal plane was most helpful in assessing proximal tumor extension, even though we also used the oblique rather than the coronal plane.

Both computed tomography and MR imaging have difficulty depicting nodal metastases, as both techniques rely on size criteria, and our data for sensitivity and specificity reflect this problem. Our data for sensitivity and specificity with use of the criterion of 1 cm have little meaning, as there was only one node larger than this depicted at MR imaging. Using the size criterion of 5 mm or greater, we found that our data are more meaningful but continue to reflect the longstanding problem found in many other studies (10–12) in which size alone was used to detect nodal involvement.

Despite the very low probability of nodal involvement in small-volume disease (less than 16% for stage IB disease or less [8]), two patients who underwent trachelectomy in our study, and who had no residual cervical disease at the time of surgery, had nodal involvement, and one required further treatment that destroyed her fertility. Nevertheless, we have demonstrated that MR imaging can be used to accurately predict cervical tumor confined to the cervix, which enables patients with early disease who wish to attempt to preserve their fertility to be offered trachelectomy and laparoscopic lymphadenectomy with the understanding that further treatment occasionally may be required.

References

1. Shepherd JH. Cervical and vulva cancer: changes in FIGO definitions of staging. Br J Obstet Gynaecol 1996; 103:405–406.
2. Office of National Statistics. Cancer statistics: registrations of cancer diagnoses 1991, England and Wales. Series MB1, no. 24. London, England: Her Majesty's Stationery Office, 1997.
3. Shepherd JH, Crawford RF, Oram DH. Radical trachelectomy: a way to conserve fertility in the treatment of early stage cervical cancer. Br J Obstet Gynaecol 1998; 105:912–916.
4. Dargent D. Laparoscopic surgery in gynaecologic cancer. Curr Opin Obstet Gynecol 1993; 5:294–300.
5. Dargent D. A new future for Schauta's operation through a pre-surgical retroperitoneal pelviscopy. Eur J Gynaecol Oncol 1987; 8:292–296.
6. Querleu D, LeBlanc E, Castelain B. Laparoscopic pelvic lymphadenectomy in the staging of early carcinoma of the cervix. Am J Obstet Gynecol 1991; 164:579–581.
7. Dargent D, Brun JL, Roy M, Remy I. Pregnancies following radical trachelectomy for invasive cancer (abstr). Gynecol Oncol 1994; 52:105.
8. Hricak H, Yu KK. Radiology in invasive cervical cancer. AJR 1996; 167:1101–1108.
9. Hricak H, Lacey CG, Sandles LG, Chang YCF, Winkler ML, Stern JL. Invasive cervical carcinoma: comparison of MR imaging and surgical findings. Radiology 1988; 166:623–631.
10. Kim SH, Choi B, Han JK, et al. Preoperative staging of uterine cervical carcinoma: comparison of CT and MR imaging in 99 patients. J Comput Assist Tomogr 1993; 17:633–640.
11. Kim SH, Choi BI, Lee PH, et al. Uterine cervical carcinoma: comparison of CT and MR findings. Radiology 1990; 175:45–51.
12. Subak LL, Hricak H, Powell CB, Aziz L, Stern JL. Cervical carcinoma: computed tomography and magnetic resonance imaging for preoperative staging. Obstet Gynecol 1995; 86:43–50.

Intestinal Worm

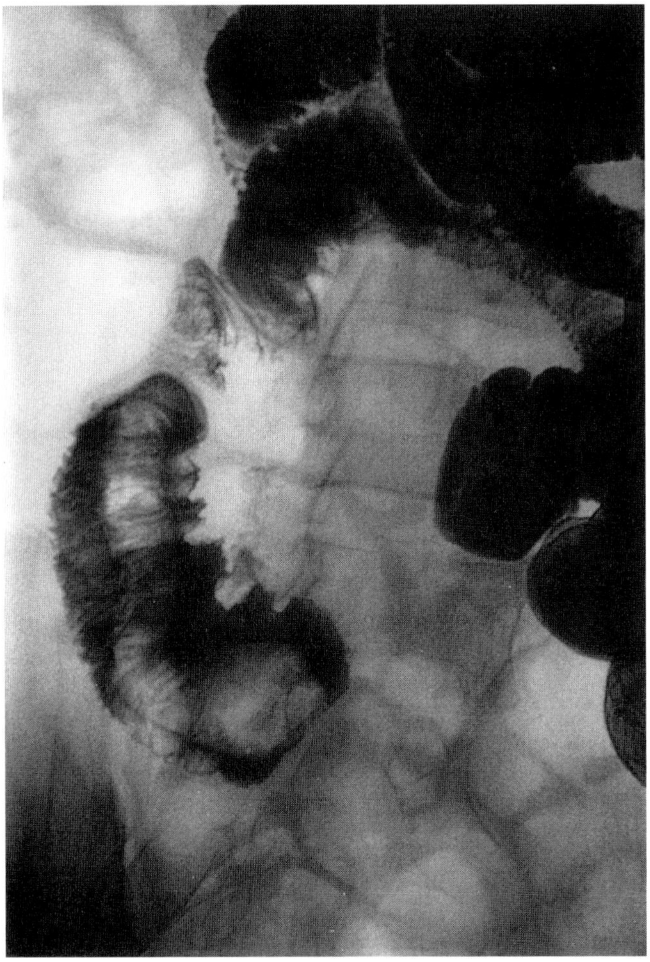

Courtesy of Gerd Bodner, MD, Innsbruck, Austria

Ovarian Cancer: Comparison of Observer Performance for Four Methods of Interpreting CT Scans[1]

Patrick J. Fultz, MD
Christina V. Jacobs, MD[2]
W. Jackson Hall, PhD
Ronald Gottlieb, MD
Deborah Rubens, MD
Saara M. S. Totterman, MD, PhD
Steven Meyers, MD, PhD
Cynthia Angel, MD
Giuseppe Del Priore, MD, MPH[3]
David P. Warshal, MD[4]
Kelly H. Zou, PhD[5]
David E. Shapiro, PhD[6]

Index terms:
Diagnostic radiology, observer performance, 852.12112
Images, interpretation, 852.12112
Ovary, CT, 852.12112
Ovary, neoplasms, 852.32

Radiology 1999; 212:401–410

[1] From the Depts of Radiology (P.J.F., C.V.J., R.G., D.R., S.M.S.T., S.M.), Obstetrics and Gynecology (C.A., G.D.P., D.P.W.), and Biostatistics (W.J.H., K.H.Z., D.E.S.), University of Rochester Medical Center, 601 Elmwood Ave, Rochester, NY 14642. Received May 7, 1997; revision requested May 27; final revision received Sep 2, 1998; accepted Feb 12, 1999. Supported in part by a grant from Innovations in Patient Care Program, Univ of Rochester Medical Center. **Address reprint requests to** P.J.F.

Current addresses:
[2] Elmendorf Hospital, Alaska
[3] Dept of Obstetrics and Gynecology, New York University Medical School, NY.
[4] Dept of Obstetrics and Gynecology, Cooper Health System, Camden, NJ
[5] Dept of Health Care Policy, Harvard Medical School and Dept of Radiology, Brigham and Women's Hospital, Boston, Mass
[6] Center for Biostatistics in AIDS Research, Harvard School of Public Health, Boston, Mass

Author contributions:
Guarantor of integrity of entire study, P.J.F.; study concepts, P.J.F., C.V.J.; study design, P.J.F., D.E.S., W.J.H.; definition of intellectual content, P.J.F., W.J.H.; literature research, P.J.F., W.J.H., K.H.Z.; clinical studies, P.J.F., C.V.J., R.G., D.R., S.M.S.T., S.M., C.A., G.D.P., D.P.W.; data acquisition, P.J.F., C.V.J., R.G., D.R., S.M.S.T., S.M., C.A., G.D.P., D.P.W.; data analysis, P.J.F., W.J.H., K.H.Z., C.V.J.; statistical analysis, W.J.H., K.H.Z.; manuscript preparation, P.J.F., W.J.H., K.H.Z., D.E.S.; manuscript editing, P.J.F., C.V.J., W.J.H., R.G., S.M.S.T., G.D.P., D.P.W., K.H.Z., D.E.S.; manuscript review, all authors

PURPOSE: To assess the effects of four interpretative methods on observers' mean sensitivity and specificity by using computed tomography (CT) of ovarian carcinoma as a model.

MATERIALS AND METHODS: CT scans in 98 patients with ovarian carcinoma and 49 women who were disease free were retrospectively reviewed by four experienced blinded radiologists to compare single-observer reading, single-observer reading with an anatomic checklist, paired-observer reading (simultaneous double reading), and replicated reading (combination of two independent readings). Confidence level scoring was used to identify three possible disease forms in each patient: extranodal tumor, lymphadenopathy, and ascites. Patient conditions were then categorized as abnormal or normal.

RESULTS: There were no significant improvements in sensitivity or specificity for classification of patient conditions as abnormal or normal when comparing single-observer interpretation with single-observer interpretation with a checklist or paired-observer interpretation. Although there was no significant improvement in the mean sensitivity (93% vs 94%) by using the replicated reading method, there was a statistically significant improvement in mean specificity (85% vs 79%) for the replicated readings compared with single-observer interpretations ($P < .05$).

CONCLUSION: Diagnostic aids such as checklists and paired simultaneous readings did not lead to an improved mean observer performance for experienced readers. However, an increase in the mean specificity occurred with replicated readings.

More than 50 years have passed since Birkelo et al (1) illuminated inconsistencies among radiologists in interpretations of radiographs of the chest for the assessment of tuberculosis. In that study, 1,256 radiographs were obtained for screening for tuberculosis, and five readers independently interpreted the radiographs. The number of positive diagnoses for the five readers ranged from 56 to 100. Since the initial work by Birkelo et al (1), a number of studies (2–6) have raised concerns regarding the variability and/or accuracy of radiologic interpretations for examinations such as chest radiography, mammography, computed tomography (CT), and magnetic resonance (MR) imaging.

Ovarian carcinoma is estimated to be the fifth leading cancer cause of death in women in the United States (7). While CT has some inherent limitations in the detection of ovarian carcinoma and its metastases, it is often used preoperatively and/or in postoperative follow-up in these patients (8,9). Findings of a previous study (5) of CT in patients with ovarian carcinoma showed that in paired comparisons of three independent reviews of the images in 100 cases, there were up to 26 cases with discrepancy between two reviewers for the presence of a mass. We therefore chose to use CT in the setting of ovarian carcinoma as a model to investigate the effects of four methods of image interpretation on observer performance.

This project was designed to assess the effects of a variety of methods of image interpretation on interobserver agreement, mean sensitivity, and mean specificity. Methods to potentially improve the efficacy of standard single-observer image interpretation included an observer checklist, paired simultaneous reading by two observers, and combining two independent readings in the form of a replicated reading. Comparison of these various methods was performed by using a group of experienced radiologists (R.G., D.R., S.M.S.T., S.M.) in an effort to identify the most efficacious approach to CT interpretations in patients with ovarian carcinoma.

MATERIALS AND METHODS

Patient Population

Our focus was on the effects of four interpretative methods on mean observer performance with use of CT of ovarian cancer as a model and not on the accuracy of CT as a modality in this setting. Therefore, we included only patients with disease judged as recognizable at CT in the study group and only patients whose CT scans showed no recognizable disease in the control group.

CT studies from January 1990 to February 1995 in 98 patients with a history of active ovarian cancer and in 19 patients with disease in remission were selected from our gynecologic oncology clinic and surgery records. All patients who presented to the clinic and those who underwent surgery performed by our gynecologic oncologists (including C.A., G.D.P., D.P.W.) were identified from a computer printout of patients examined in this time frame. Thirty women without a history of gynecologic malignancy who had undergone body CT examinations during this same period were selected from the general adult patient population. Therefore, the study comprised 147 patients (98 with abnormal and 49 with normal conditions) who had undergone abdominal and/or pelvic CT.

The 98 patients with abnormal CT findings were the 17 patients with ovarian cancer at initial presentation and the 81 patients with disease recurrence recognizable at CT examination. Normal CT examinations were those in the 19 patients with ovarian cancer in remission and the 30 women with no history of gynecologic malignancy who underwent abdominal or pelvic CT examinations at our hospital for various indications.

The mean age of patients with ovarian cancer was 60 years (SD, 12 years; age range, 30–82 years); the mean age of patients free of disease was 62 years (SD, 14 years; age range, 30–86 years).

The patients with ovarian cancer and those free of ovarian cancer after treatment were identified from consecutive CT examinations that fulfilled specific diagnostic criteria for confirmation of active disease or remission at the time of the CT examination. The inclusion criteria in 58 patients included timely (within less than 1 month) surgical and/or percutaneous biopsy confirmation of CT findings. The inclusion criteria for the remaining 59 patients included findings of serial clinical examinations and serum tumor marker analysis and/or follow-up CT examinations over intervals of at least 6 months that corroborated the findings of the specific CT examinations included in this study.

A total of 261 patients with a history of ovarian cancer were excluded because of lack of complete CT examinations (some patients underwent no CT or only limited CT for percutaneous biopsy guidance), the presence of concomitant disease (eg, other malignancy, abscess, or lymphocele) at CT, insufficient follow-up to document the true status of the disease, and/or surgically documented disease with no recognizable disease at CT.

By using the aforementioned diagnostic information, the confirmation of CT findings for each of the 147 patients was established by means of a consensus review of all data by investigators (P.J.F., C.V.J.) who were not involved in the subsequent blinded comparative CT examination interpretations. By using all available clinical and radiologic data, the CT scans in each of the 147 patients were then reviewed to create the standard interpretations to which the blinded interpretations were compared.

Three forms of possible disease were defined: extranodal tumor mass, nodal disease, and ascites. When an abnormality was present, it was localized to the upper or lower part of the abdomen or to the upper or lower part of the pelvis so that four sites of abnormality were possible for each form of disease. The total numbers of normal and abnormal areas for each of the three forms of disease are presented in Table 1.

The majority of patients with a history of ovarian carcinoma had typical epithelial cell cancer; the remaining patients had tumors of low malignant potential or nonepithelial malignancies.

All 147 CT examinations (CT HiSpeed Advantage, HiLight Advantage, model 9800, and model 8800 scanners; GE Medical Systems, Milwaukee, Wis) were performed at our hospital between January 1990 and February 1995. More than half

TABLE 1
Patients with Abnormalities for Each of Three Forms of Disease

No. of Abnormal Areas*	Extranodal Tumor Mass (n = 147)	Nodal Disease (n = 147)	Ascites (n = 147)
0	53	93	93
1	10	19	6
2	20	10	12
3	12	16	11
4	52	9	25

* Each patient's disease was localized to the upper part of the abdomen, lower part of the abdomen, upper part of the pelvis, and/or lower part of the pelvis for a total of four possible abnormal areas.

Reader	Reading Session 1			Reading Session 2			Reading Session 3			Reading Session 4
1	**G2**	G3✓	G1	G3	**G1**	G2✓	G1✓	G2	**G3**	Single observer review of 30 exams (10 each from G1, G2, G3)
2	**G2**	G3	G1✓	G3✓	**G1**	G2	G1	G2✓	**G3**	Single observer review of 30 exams (10 each from G1, G2, G3)
3	G3	**G1**	G2✓	G1✓	G2	**G3**	**G2**	G3✓	G1	Single observer review of 30 exams (10 each from G1, G2, G3)
4	G3✓	**G1**	G2	G1	G2✓	**G3**	**G2**	G3	G1✓	Single observer review of 30 exams (10 each from G1, G2, G3)

G1 G2 = paired reading, G1✓ = reading with a checklist

Figure 1. Diagram shows the format for the review of images from CT examinations and the reader (observer) assignments. For reading sessions 1–3, the 147 examinations were divided into three groups of examinations: group 1 (*G1*), 49 examinations; group 2 (*G2*), 49 examinations; and group 3 (*G3*), 49 examinations.

Observer #: Date:

Patient #:

	Findings:		Normal	Abnormal (Explain, then transfer information to attached data sheet)
ABDOMEN	• Liver	Parenchyma		
		Biliary system		
	• Spleen	Parenchyma		
	• Pancreas	Parenchyma		
	• Adrenals	Right		
		Left		
	• Kidneys	Right		
		Left		
		Collecting System		
	• Retroperitoneum	Nodes		
		Retroperitoneal Fat		
		Aorta		
		IVC		
	• Abdominal GI Tract (including mesentery)			
	• Abdominal Peritoneal Cavity			
PELVIS	• Adnexa	Right		
		Left		
	• Uterus			
	• Bladder			
	• Other Extraperitoneal Structures	Nodes		
		Vessels		
		Extraperitoneal Fat		
	• Pelvic GI Tract (including mesentery)			
	• Pelvic Peritoneal Cavity			

Figure 2. Abdominal-pelvic CT checklist. Modified from Kinard et al (10). *GI* = gastrointestinal, *IVC* = inferior vena cava.

the patients (n = 78) received contrast material intravenously, orally, and rectally, with most of the remaining patients receiving contrast material intravenously and orally (n = 46). The remaining examinations (n = 23) were performed with at least one of these three routes of contrast material administration. Most (n = 117) examinations were performed with 10-mm contiguous images, with the remaining examinations performed with a variety of section thicknesses (5 or 7 mm) and scanning intervals (7 or 10 mm).

CT Scan Review and Replicated Reading Method

Images from the 147 CT examinations were intermixed randomly, and the examinations were subdivided into three groups as follows: group 1, 49 examinations; group 2, 49 examinations; and group 3, 49 examinations. Images from these 147 examinations were then reviewed without clinical information in a blinded retrospective manner by four attending cross-sectional imaging radiologists (including R.G., D.R., S.M.S.T., S.M.) in three sessions at three different times. Subsequently, in a fourth reading session, each of four observers reviewed images from 30 of the CT examinations (10 from each of the three original groups of examinations) to allow evaluation of calculations of intraobserver agreement. Each reading session was separated by at least 2 months. This CT scan review method is summarized in Figure 1.

With this format, a different interpretative method was used by each reader for each of the three groups of CT examinations within each session. The randomized order within each reading session and the 2-month interval between the different review methods applied to a given group of examinations diminished the potential for learning biases (reading-order effects) that could be introduced by using only one specific order of application of the various methods.

Three direct methods of interpretation were employed in the first three reading sessions, and the four radiologists actively participated in each of these three image reviews by using confidence level scoring. The three direct methods were (*a*) the standard single-observer approach, (*b*) the single-observer interpretation with a predesigned CT checklist (Fig 2), and (*c*) simultaneous consensus interpretation by two observers (paired reading). By using this review format, images from each of the 147 examinations were reviewed three times by each observer (alone, with a checklist, and as pairs of readers) in the first three reading sessions, with each session separated by at least 2 months.

As noted earlier, the fourth reading session was an independent review of images from 30 of the original 147 CT examinations. This final interpretative method was a form of replicated reading (11). The replicated reading used in this study was a mathematic retrospective pairing of earlier single-observer interpretations in all possible combinations. For the purposes of this analysis, the original confidence level scores were dichotomized into a "yes or no" response (discussed further in Statistical Methods, Sensitivity and Specificity). Because these artificial reader pairings will at times result in disagreement, a pseudoarbitration method (12) was used when the pair disagreed about a classification as normal or abnormal. Therefore, each replicated reading pair was evaluated by alternatively combining readings of this pair with one of the two remaining readers, who then served as an arbitrator only when a disagreement occurred between the original pair of readers. The arbitrator's patient assessment thus served as a tiebreaker when needed. This design yielded a total of 12 possible reader combinations when dispute arbitrators were included in the replicated reading calculations. A mean sensitivity and specificity were then calculated from these 12 reader combinations.

The four individual readers were randomly designated as reader 1, 2, 3, or 4. The pairs of observers for the double-reading sessions were randomly assigned and were constant throughout the study. The four readers varied in duration of specialized body imaging experience from

2 to 10 years when this study was initiated. The random reader assignments coincidentally resulted in pairing the two radiologists least experienced in body imaging (2 and 5 years experience) and the two radiologists most experienced (9 and 10 years).

Prior to the reading sessions, the observers received an overview of the use of a data collection form and confidence level scoring method: 0 indicated definitely absent, 1 indicated probably absent, 2 indicated possibly present, 3 indicated probably present, and 4 indicated definitely present. The observers assessed each patient CT study for the presence of three categories of possible disease by using confidence level scoring for each disease category, regardless of the number of sites involved. These three categories of disease included extranodal tumor mass, nodal disease, and ascites (5). At subsequent questioning, there was also agreement among all the readers that in a "forced choice" situation (normal vs abnormal) a confidence level score of 0 or 1 generally corresponded to a diagnosis of normal and scores of 2–4 corresponded to a diagnosis of abnormal. The division between abdomen and pelvis was defined as the iliac crest, and the division between the upper and lower parts of the abdomen or pelvis was the midway point in each area. If a mass crossed a boundary, it was scored in each area. Actual observer time per examination interpretation was also recorded.

Only those observers who used the CT checklist (Fig 2) in a given session received instruction regarding its use. Observers could use the checklist as a simple reminder to review all listed anatomic areas, or they could formally complete the form and then transfer information to the data collection form. Other detailed information given to all observers included instructions to omit chest cavity findings from their analysis, a review of CT nodal size criteria for this study, and instructions that cysts contiguous with the liver margin and all mesenteric nodules should be considered extranodal tumor masses and that centrally located simple liver cysts, along with hepatic hemangiomas and renal or adrenal lesions, should be considered incidental findings. In addition, a review of a pseudoarbitration method (12) was provided to resolve potential disputes during the paired-observer simultaneous reading sessions.

Statistical Methods

Modeling the confidence level scores.—To assess the magnitude and statistical significance of the effects of various factors on the ordinal scores assigned by the readers for each of the three forms of disease, we fit a linear model to the scores (SAS Institute, "SAS/STAT Software: Changes and Enhancements through Release 6.11," SAS Institute, Cary, NC, 1996)(Appendix 1). We thus treated the scores as if continuous just for this purpose; regrettably, software modeling of ordinal scores in a complex design (with pairing) is not to our knowledge currently available. Results from ordinal regression modeling of subsets of the data agreed well with results from continuous modeling.

The results of these analyses helped in guiding the agreement and observer performance analyses. Moreover, other results of tests of significance about various measures of observer performance were in agreement with results of tests associated with this modeling.

Intraobserver and interobserver agreement.—Intraobserver agreement information for the single-observer review method for each of the three forms of disease was obtained by comparing earlier single-reader observations (from reading sessions 1–3) with individual reinterpretations of examinations of 30 patients in reading session 4, the final session. By using the various combinations of paired comparisons, the mean interobserver agreement was calculated for each of the three direct interpretative methods (single observer, single observer with anatomic checklist, and paired observers). Intraobserver agreement and interobserver agreement were initially calibrated by using the weighted κ statistic (13), in which we assigned weight w to a disagreement for which the two readings were w confidence levels apart. Also, a simple κ analysis for the three direct interpretative methods was performed for dichotomized patient condition categorizations of normal versus abnormal.

Sensitivity and specificity.—Analysis of sensitivity and specificity was carried out to estimate observer performance in the context of the more commonly used measures of a method's utility. In this analysis, sensitivity and specificity were defined with respect to the true status of the patient's condition (diseased vs normal).

To achieve a dichotomy of yes or no responses (ie, disease present or absent) for this analysis, the observers' confidence level scores for a patient's three possible forms of disease were redefined as absent (score of 0 or 1) or present (score of 2–4). Our readers were in agreement that this was the most appropriate format for dichotomizing their confidence level responses.

The localization data for each of the three forms of disease in each of the four body areas were then tabulated by categorizing the observer responses for detection of disease as true-positive, true-negative, false-positive, or false-negative findings in a comparison with our previously defined standards of reference (see Materials and Methods, Patient Population). Subsequent data analysis for the 98 patients with abnormal and the 49 patients with normal CT findings (in contrast with normal and abnormal areas on CT scans) was accomplished by using a 0 or 1 confidence level score for all of the three forms of disease as a diagnosis of normal and scores of 2–4 for any of the three forms of disease as a diagnosis of abnormal.

The mean sensitivities and specificities for a given reading method were obtained by averaging the various observer's respective results within that reading method.

When comparing two or more proportions (eg, sensitivities across observers or across interpretative methods), McNemar χ^2 tests were used. When comparing mean proportions—that is, proportions averaged across observers—mean proportions and differences in mean proportions were evaluated relative to an estimated standard error (Appendix 2). All tests accounted for inherent dependence because several methods were evaluated in the same patients. Effects were considered statistically significant if P values (two-sided) were less than .05 (with no adjustments for multiple comparisons).

Receiver operating characteristic analysis.—In addition, Receiver operating characteristic (ROC) analyses were performed on the data from the three direct interpretative methods to analyze the confidence level scores without dichotomizing the observer responses. Separate analyses were carried out for each observer and each method, but only pooled (across observers) data curves are presented, as conclusions from the others were similar to those from the traditional sensitivity and specificity analyses. A ROC analysis could not be performed for the replicated reading methods, as the data for this interpretative form were obtained by dichotomizing the original confidence level scores.

ROC curves were constructed by using ROCFIT (Metz CE, Shen JH, Wang PL, Kronman HB, Fortran program ROCFIT, Department of Radiology, University of Chicago, Ill, 1994) and CORROC2 (Metz CE, Shen JH, Kronman HB, Wang PL, Fortran program CORROC2, Department of Radiology, University of Chicago, Ill, 1994) software (14,15) for fitting binormal models

TABLE 2
κ Analysis of Intraobserver and Interobserver Agreement for the Three Forms of Disease and for Categorization of Normal and Abnormal CT Studies

Disease	Intraobserver Agreement	Interobserver Agreement: Single Observers	Checklist	Paired Observers (1 and 2 vs 3 and 4)
Extranodal tumor mass				
Range	0.75–0.84	0.61–0.70	0.58–0.70	. . .
Mean	0.79	0.66	0.62	0.66
Nodal disease				
Range	0.22–0.75	0.32–0.46	0.37–0.50	. . .
Mean	0.49	0.43	0.43	0.52
Ascites				
Range	0.76–0.98	0.80–0.88	0.76–0.80	. . .
Mean	0.88	0.83	0.78	0.78
Normal vs abnormal CT studies				
Range	0.44–0.85	0.57–0.74	0.59–0.72	. . .
Mean	0.69	0.67	0.64	0.75

Note.—For the three forms of disease, weighted κ analyses were used for the confidence level scoring. For the dichotomized results (normal vs abnormal condition), κ analysis was used.

to rating data. ROC curves were constructed for each reader or reader pair and for each of the first three direct interpretative methods. When comparing two interpretative methods, CORROC2 software was used, with recognition that data from the same 147 patients were being studied. To construct a summary curve, by summarizing over readers, we used the ad hoc method of simply pooling all readings together as if they were single readings in different patients rather than multiple readings in the same patients. No significance testing was done with these summary curves.

ROC analyses were performed by using the overall classification of patient conditions as abnormal or normal (rather than abnormalities in separate forms of disease). The overall confidence level score (rating) of a patient condition along the confidence level spectrum from abnormal to normal was defined as the highest of the scores for the three forms of disease.

To compare curves, three summary characteristics were considered: area under the curve, true-positive rate at a false-positive rate of 0.1, and false-positive rate at a true-positive rate of 0.9. When comparing characteristics of two curves, significance testing was done by comparing the difference between characteristics with an estimated standard error. When comparing characteristics of three (or four) curves simultaneously, we treated the sum of squared deviations from the mean characteristic divided by a pooled variance estimate as a χ^2 with 2 (or 3) degrees of freedom. Similar significance testing methods were used for comparing true-positive rates and false-positive rates across readers or across methods. Effects were considered statistically significant if P values were less than .05.

Analysis of the time to read images.—Each observer's mean time to read images from an examination for each of the four methods of interpretation was compared to those of the other observers. The mean times to read images from examinations for all observers combined within each of the various reading methods were also compared. The replicated reading session times are the sum of the mean times to read for each single observer that were artificially paired to create the various replicated readings. Some of the time data are not available because the data collection form was simplified during the first reading session; therefore, 60% (294 of 490) of the image interpretation times from reading session 1 were disregarded. Furthermore, the time to read was not recorded by the observers on some occasions.

RESULTS

Modeling the Confidence Level Scores

The modeling of the confidence level scores (Appendix 1) led to the following general conclusions, which are consistent among the three forms of disease (details omitted). There was a slight increase in confidence level scores from reading session 1 to reading session 2 and a further increase at reading session 3 (ie, there was a trend of observers perceiving more abnormal findings in the later reading sessions), but these effects were not statistically significant. Consequently, no attempts at adjustments for reading sessions were made in further analyses. There were scoring differences among readers; some tended to give higher scores than others, but generally in a consistent way across methods; this is addressed further below.

When comparing confidence level scores among the three direct interpretive methods for each reader, no statistically significant differences were found. Other comparisons of the methods are considered below.

Intraobserver and Interobserver Agreement

Table 2 summarizes the two κ analyses of intraobserver and interobserver agreement for recognition of each of the three forms of disease and for categorization of patient conditions as normal or abnormal for the three direct interpretative methods. There was very good intraobserver agreement for categorization of patient conditions with respect to extranodal tumor masses (mean weighted κ statistic of 0.79) and ascites (mean weighted κ statistic of 0.88). There was less intraobserver agreement among observers for recognition of nodal disease; the mean weighted κ statistic of 0.49 reflects a moderate or fair level of mean intraobserver agreement. Generally, the intraobserver agreement was greater than interobserver agreement for the three possible forms of disease.

The κ analysis for intraobserver and interobserver agreement for the dichotomized confidence level scores (disease present or absent) yielded a mean intraobserver κ of 0.69. This was similar to the mean interobserver agreements for each of the three direct interpretative methods, which ranged from 0.64 to 0.75.

Sensitivity and Specificity

The means and ranges across observers for sensitivity and specificity for the various interpretative methods are shown in Table 3. There were statistically significant differences among observers for sensitivity (range, 87%–97%, $P < .01$) and specificity (range, 65%–92%, $P < .01$), both for single reading and reading with the checklist, but there were no statistically significant differences among the first three methods for any particular observer. The largest differences in sensitivity and specificity between single readers for classification of patient conditions as abnormal or normal were for observers 1 and 3: Sensitivities for these observers were 97% and 87%, respectively, and specificities were 67% and 92%, respectively.

When averaging sensitivity or specificity over observers, there was no statistically significant improvement for the increment over single-observer interpretations for single observers reading with a checklist or for paired observers. There was a statistically significant improvement in mean specificity (84.7% vs 79.1%) for the replicated reading method when compared with the single-observer reading. However, there was no statistically significant improvement in the mean sensitivity (93.9% vs 93.1%).

We estimate (by using information in Table 3 [details omitted]) that the power to detect a 5% improvement in sensitivity in any of the alternative reading methods compared with the single observer method was 90% or more; the power to detect a 3% improvement was around 50%. We estimate that the power to detect a 17% improvement in specificity in any of the alternative reading methods compared with the single-observer method was 90% or more; the power to detect a 10% improvement was around 50%.

ROC Analysis

Figure 3 presents the ROC analyses of abnormal versus normal patient condition assessment for each observer by using each of the three direct interpretative methods; ROC curves of reading method 1 (single observer) were compared with those of reading method 2 (checklist) and with reading method 3 (paired reading). There were no statistically significant differences between these curves or in the areas under the curves for any reader when comparing method 1 with method 2 or method 1 with method 3.

Table 4 presents the true-positive rate at a false-positive rate of 0.1, and Table 5 presents the false-positive rate at a true-positive rate of 0.9 for each observer by using each reading method. These were determined from fitted binormal ROC curves. By using these measures, the checklist was generally unhelpful or detrimental. Pairing observers 1 and 2 had almost no effect, but pairing observers 3 and 4 resulted in false-positive rates and true-positive rates that were, approximately, means of the rates for each observer. This improved the performance of observer 3 at the expense of that of observer 4.

Figure 4 is the overall ROC analysis of

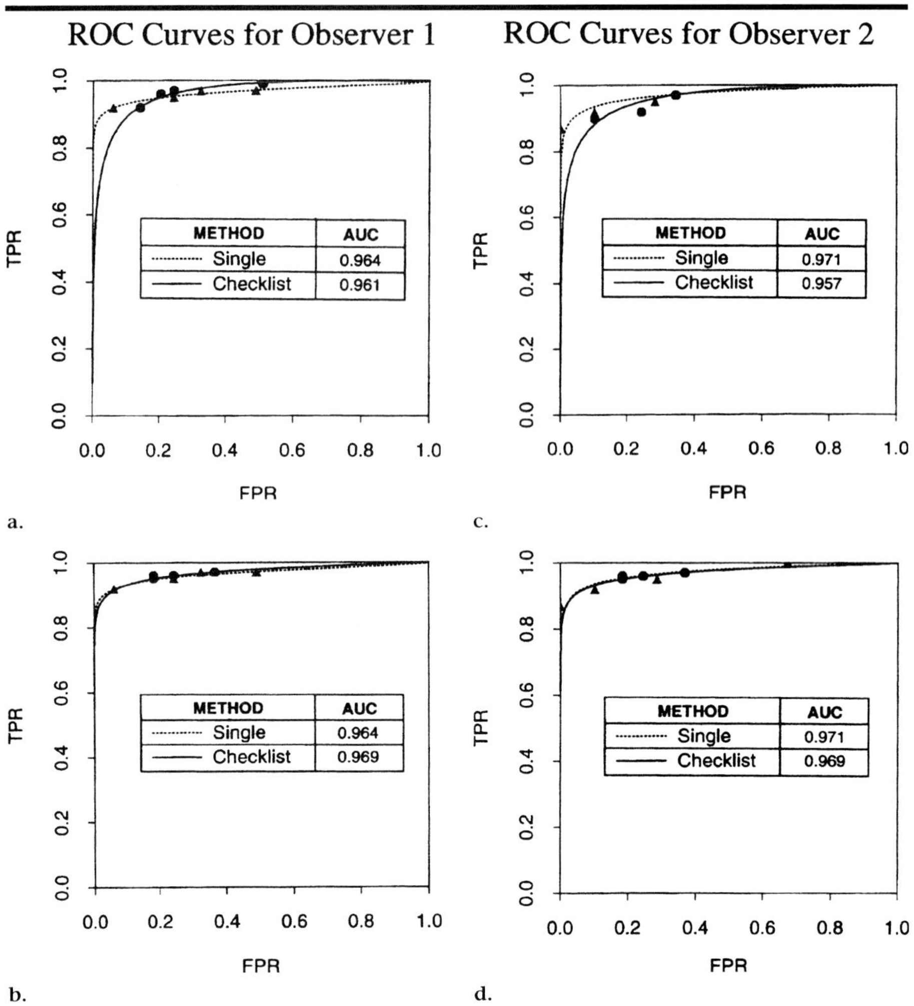

Figure 3. ROC curves and areas under the curves (*AUC*) for overall patient CT study evaluation (abnormal vs normal) for each observer in comparisons of single observer with single observer plus checklist and of single observer with paired observers. **(a, b)** Observer 1. **(c, d)** Observer 2 (*Fig 3 continues*).

TABLE 3
Sensitivity and Specificity for Each Interpretative Technique

Parameter	Single Observer	Single Observer with Checklist	Paired Observers	Replicated Readings
Sensitivity				
Mean (%)	93.1	93.4	93.9	93.9
Range (%)	87–97	87–97	92–95	93–95
Increment over single observer	. . .	0.3 ± 2.1	0.8 ± 2.8	0.8 ± 1.7
Specificity				
Mean (%)	79.1	79.6	81.6	84.7
Range (%)	67–92	65–92	76–88	82–90
Increment over single observer	. . .	0.5 ± 7.4	2.6 ± 8.4	5.6 ± 4.1

Note.—Data are the means and ranges for the four observers, the two paired observers, or the 12 replicated reader combinations. Each increment over the single observer is the mean for the reading method minus the mean for the single observer; the number that follows each plus or minus sign is 1.96 times the estimated standard error of the difference, thereby enabling 95% confidence limits for the difference (eg, for replicated readings vs single-observer sensitivity, the true difference is between −0.9 and +2.5 percentage points, with 95% confidence).

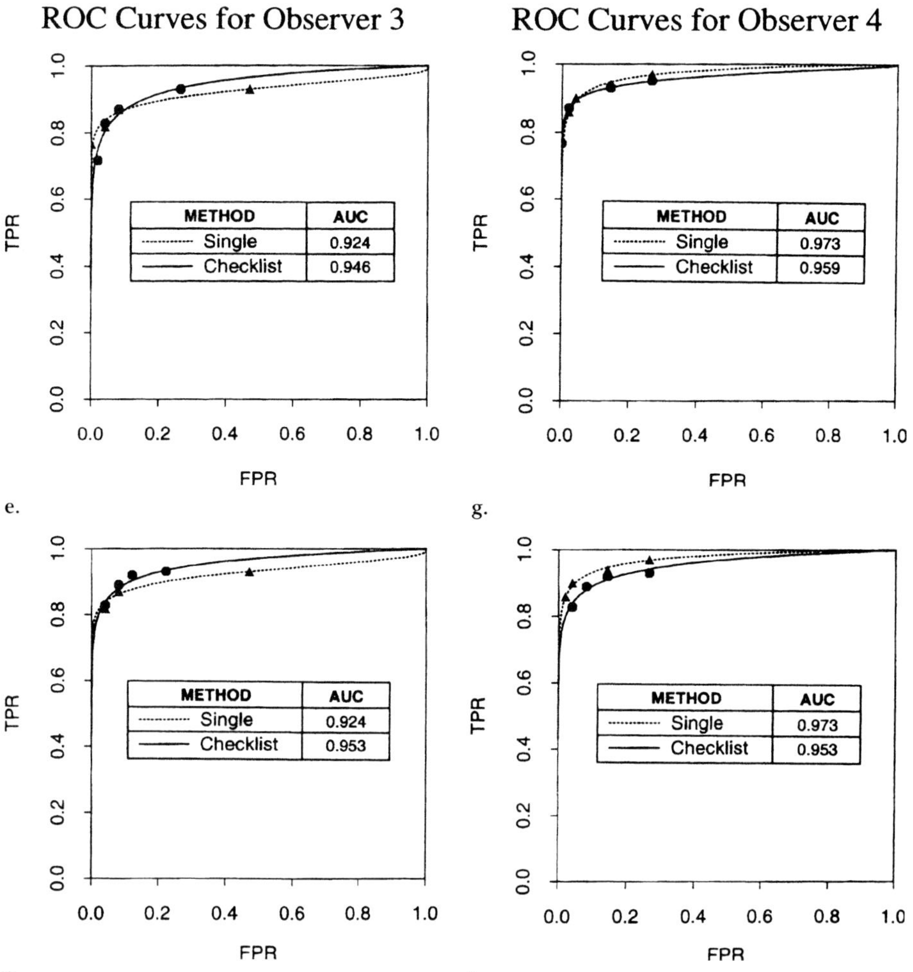

Figure 3 (*continued*). **(e, f)** Observer 3. **(g, h)** Observer 4. *FPR* = false-positive rate, *TPR* = true-positive rate.

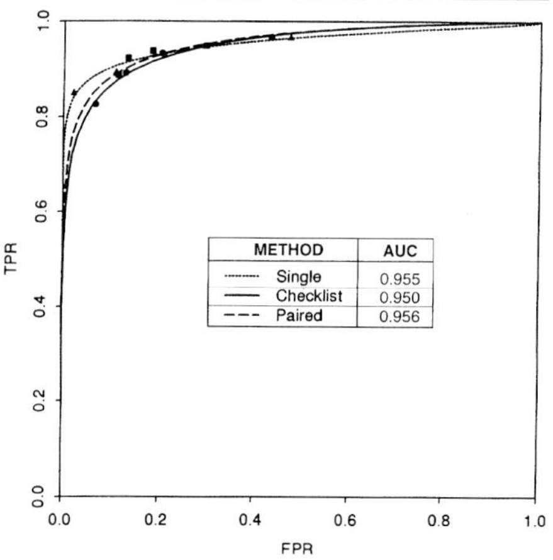

Figure 4. ROC curves and areas under the curve (*AUC*) for categorizing abnormal and normal patient CT studies for the three interpretative methods. These curves were constructed by pooling all readings for each method. *FPR* = false-positive rate, *TPR* = true-positive rate.

abnormal versus normal patient condition assessments for the three direct interpretative methods constructed by pooling all readings by using each interpretative method. The curves are very similar; if anything, the single-observer curve appears best. No significance testing was feasible here, due to the pooling across readers. However, no statistically significant differences were found when analyzed reader by reader (Fig 3).

Analysis of the Time to Read Images

The mean time to read images from an examination for each of the interpretative methods was as follows: single observer, 3.44 minutes (range, 2.35–4.89 minutes); checklist, 3.99 minutes (range, 3.54–4.61 minutes); paired observers, 5.07 minutes (range, 3.12–6.99 minutes); and replicated readings, 6.53 minutes (range, 5.04–8.02 minutes). This last time estimate does not include the additional time commitment of the third independent reader when the pseudoarbitration method was applied. There were statistically significant differences in these times between all observers within and among reading methods. As expected, on average it was more time-consuming to read with a checklist or as pairs of readers and, because of the design, for replicated readings.

DISCUSSION

Other investigators have also addressed various aspects of radiologic diagnostic efficacy as they relate to interobserver agreement, sensitivity, and specificity, and some (5,16) have evaluated methods to improve on these measures of observer performance. In a previous study (5), investigators assessed interobserver reliability for the interpretation of CT scans of advanced ovarian cancer. These authors did not assess the effect of improving CT techniques or other approaches for resolving discrepancies. We found somewhat lower, but nevertheless striking levels of disagreement between various pairs of independent observers (up to 17% [25 of 147]) for the presence of a mass. It is of interest that interobserver agreement has also been investigated in a wide variety of clinical situations (17,18), with similar striking variability among individual observers.

Other investigators (1,3,4) have shown a wide spectrum of observer sensitivities and specificities for other radiologic examinations. To our knowledge, much of the previous literature on this topic has been in the area of mammography. In one review (3) of 10 radiologists' independent mammographic interpretations in 150 patients (for a mixture of screening and diagnostic studies), there was a median sensitivity for a diagnosis of "suggestive of cancer" of 70% with a range of 37%–85% and a median specificity of 93% with a range of 85%–99%. Furthermore, in 33% of patients recommended for additional work-up in this study (3), at least one of the 10 radiologists differed with regard to the side of the possible abnormality. In a different project (4) in which the variability in breast cancer detection was assessed for a group of 108 radiologists reviewing images from 79 screening mammographic examinations, a range of sensitivity of 47%–100% and a range of specificity of 36%–99% were found. In our study, the results were less variable than the aforementioned mammographic assessments; the individual reader sensitivities ranged from 87% to 97% and the individual reader specificities ranged from 67% to 92% for classification of patient conditions as abnormal or normal.

Reproducibility of interpretation results is an important feature of diagnostic efficacy. We used the weighted κ statistic for analysis of intraobserver and interobserver agreements or reliabilities for our confidence level scoring system. The critical issue in the comparison of these weighted κ values relates to determining which methods of interpretation will yield the highest level of interobserver agreement. However, neither using the checklist when interpreting studies nor the paired readings yielded an increase in mean interobserver agreement over that for the standard independent interpretations for our experienced readers. Given the lack of improvement in mean sensitivity and specificity for the three direct interpretative methods in our study, a more detailed discussion of the differences in interobserver agreement among those methods becomes moot. We did not assess interobserver agreement for the replicated reading method because by design this method forces interpretations to be in greater agreement.

Several previous investigators (10–12,19–31) have addressed methods ranging from simple to more complex to improve individual observer performances. These methods have included use of various checklists; simultaneous pairing of observers; sequential pairing of observers, with the second independent observer either aware or unaware of the first interpretation; replicated readings; group consensus; group consultation followed by independent diagnoses; the Delphi technique; computerized noninteractive consultation; mathematic combinations of different interpretations; computerized sequential decision making; and computer-assisted interpretations (10–12,19–31). We chose to emphasize three of these methods to potentially improve the single-observer performance of CT interpretation in light of the improved observer performance previously reported with these methods (6,10,12,21,22).

A checklist worksheet has been suggested as a method to improve diagnostic accuracy for body CT examinations (10). It is of interest that, on the basis of our ROC analysis, three of our four readers had poorer results when using a checklist than they did with their independent readings.

Furthermore, on the basis of the ROC analysis, there were variable effects recognized when pairing our observers. There was no benefit to pairing observers 1 and 2. Pairing observers 3 and 4 yielded mean false-positive rates and true-positive rates, with the performance of observer 3 improving at the expense of that of observer 4. The net result was no significant improvement in overall mean sensitivity or specificity. Representative examples of false-negative and false-positive diagnoses in our study are illustrated in Figures 5 and 6.

TABLE 4
ROC Analysis: True-Positive Rates for Each Observer and Reading Method at a False-Positive Rate of 0.1

Observer	Single Observer	Single Observer with Checklist	Paired Observers (1 and 2 or 3 and 4)
1	0.93	0.89	0.93
2	0.93	0.88	. . .
3	0.87	0.87	0.89
4	0.93	0.92	. . .

TABLE 5
ROC Analysis: False-Positive Rates for Each Observer and Reading Method at a True-Positive Rate of 0.9

Observer	Single Observer	Single Observer with Checklist	Paired Observers (1 and 2 or 3 and 4)
1	0.03	0.11	0.04
2	0.04	0.13	. . .
3	0.24	0.16	0.12
4	0.05	0.06	. . .

The only interpretative method in our study that yielded an improvement in mean observer performance (via an improved mean specificity) was the replicated reading method. In a prior study (12) of 100 randomly selected chest radiographs independently interpreted by eight radiologists, various pairings of the independent reviews were reviewed to produce independent replicated "double readings." The pseudoarbitration method was used as a third independent opinion to settle disputes that arose with the reader pairings; this yielded a 37% improvement in accuracy (12).

An earlier investigation compared single readings of chest photofluorograms obtained for tuberculosis screening with a combination of two separate interpretations (replicated readings) to improve accuracy (20). In those cases where the combined single readings differed, a third opinion was used, with an additional 10% improvement in sensitivity when compared with the sensitivity of individual interpretations and without a change in specificity (20).

Sequential double reading, where the second observer often had knowledge of the original interpretation (21), and independent sequential double readings (22) of screening mammograms have yielded increases in cancer detection sensitivity of 10%–15%, with variable effects on specificity. However, using data from their previous mammographic study (4), Beam et al (23) examined the effects of a form of independent double reading and concluded that radiologists may form complementary or noncomplementary pairs. The average radiologist in their study (23) had an increase in the true-positive rate of 0.11 accompanied by an increase in the false-positive rate of 0.07. As in our study, some observer pairings in their study resulted in no change or in small changes in sensitivities and specificities.

The accuracy of radiologic examinations for recognizing abnormalities requires the identification and proper interpretation of various examination findings. Some studies of observer performance have purposely focused on interpretation by identifying the radiologic abnormality for the observers (24,28). In addition, the cognitive methods used to influence observer performance have had varied levels of complexity. We focused on three of the simpler interpretative methods (checklists, paired observers, and replicated readings) supplementary to the standard single-observer approach and used experienced observers who were required to both identify and interpret abnormal findings. Contrary to what might be inferred from most of the published literature, these approaches

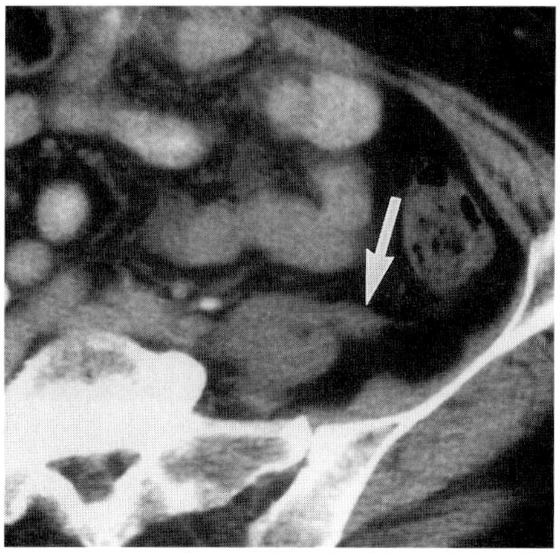

Figure 5. False-negative diagnosis. CT image shows a tumor implant (arrow) at the psoas margin that was unrecognized at six of 10 reviews.

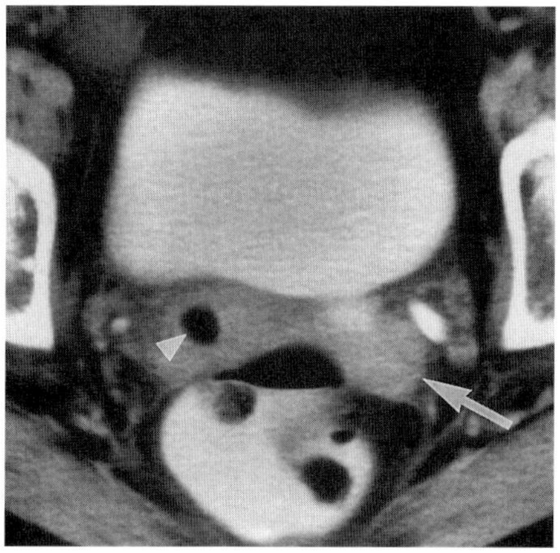

Figure 6. False-positive diagnosis. Pelvic CT image shows a mildly asymmetric vaginal cuff (arrow), which was mistaken for a tumor implant at three of 10 reviews. A vaginal tampon (arrowhead) is present on the right.

are not always successful in improving the performance of experienced observers.

There is also a potential cost in time that may occur with any supplemental interpretative methods. It should be noted that in the context of a study such as this, observers' times to read do not incorporate the time involved in developing a protocol or monitoring CT examinations, patient preparation, review of clinical data or prior studies, report dictation, and review or consultation with clinicians. In our investigation, the greatest cost in terms of physician time occurred with paired and replicated readings. In the absence of documented improvements in sensitivity and/or specificity, the cost of paired readings is not justified in this patient population for our readers. Replicated readings, or some modification thereof, may be more justifiable.

The limitations of studies such as ours are well outlined in the project of Elmore et al (3), who assessed variability of mammographic interpretations. These limitations include the effects of a study situation, where radiologists may be more (or less) diligent in their examination reviews than they are in daily practice and where the images from previous examinations are unavailable for comparison (3).

Another limitation of our study was that each disease site (upper vs lower abdomen or pelvis) was not documented with surgery in every case. As our focus was on observers categorizing patients with any evidence of ovarian cancer on CT scans versus patients with no disease on CT scans, the effect of lack of surgical confirmation at all anatomic sites was minimized. We believe our combined verification criteria listed in Materials and Methods were sufficiently accurate standards of reference for the CT findings to enable us to address the objectives of this study.

It is also important to note that these results may apply only to our four readers for this particular indication for CT examination. In addition, the results might have differed if only the more difficult cases had been addressed. Furthermore, a variety of CT scanning protocols were used in our patient population, which may have influenced our results. Continued refinements and standardization of CT protocols should serve to minimize observer variability and improve observer performance.

Most research in radiology focuses on applications of technologic improvements in complex imaging modalities including CT, MR imaging, and ultrasonography. Less effort has been devoted to improving the methods of image interpretation on the part of the radiologist, the human element in the process. Methods to improve interobserver reliability and observer performance for complex examinations, such as CT, may improve on delays in diagnosis, which contribute to delays in hospital discharge and lead to additional costly diagnostic testing. Independent replicated readings slightly increased the mean specificity of the CT interpretations, but this was the most time-consuming interpretative method.

Diagnostic aids such as anatomic checklists and paired simultaneous readings did not lead to improved mean interobserver agreement, sensitivity, or specificity for experienced readers in our study. Potential benefits of various forms of paired reading and other diagnostic aids must be weighed carefully against the increased physician time commitment. While some methods may assist less experienced readers or even experienced individuals for certain possible diseases or radiologic examinations, their universal application may not be efficacious. Certain interpretative methods, such as the integration of independent readings to form a noninteractive replicated reading, may be helpful for improving observer performance for experienced readers.

APPENDIX 1

For each of the three forms of disease (with each form analyzed separately), there were 1,470 confidence level scores (10 observer-group combinations in each of three reading sessions, with 49 patients per group [Fig 1]). Each score was represented as a base mean score for single-observer readings of normal CT studies in the first reading session, plus linear and quadratic effects for the true number of areas with abnormalities in patients with abnormalities, plus an effect of deviation from the single-observer method for checklist or for paired-reading methods, plus linear and quadratic effects for second and third reading sessions, plus a random patient effect for each of the 147 patients, plus a random observer effect for each of the 10 observer-method combinations, plus a random error.

Differing error variances for differing methods and normal-versus-diseased conditions were allowed, as were correlations between random effects involving the same observers. The 27 parameters (seven fixed effects, 11 variances of random effects, three correlation coefficients, and six error variances) were fitted by using mixed-effect linear-model methods, and then submodels were fitted after the finding of many nonsignificant parameters.

The true number of areas with abnormalities and the random patient effects removed a major part of the variability of the scores, which enabled inference about the effects of interest—in particular, about the reading methods.

APPENDIX 2

There were four reading methods evaluated (Table 3), with four versions (readers) for the single-observer method, four versions for the checklist method, two versions for the paired-observer method, and 12 versions for the replicated reading method (six different pairings, each with two possible tiebreakers). We refer to these

22 versions as "systems." Of special interest are the mean sensitivity and mean specificity of each of the four methods (with averaging over the versions) and the differences between two such mean sensitivities or mean specificities. Other comparisons may be treated similarly.

To assess precision, a standard error is needed. Since all systems were evaluated in the same 98 patients with disease or the same 49 healthy persons, dependencies need to be accounted for. We illustrate with consideration of the difference between mean paired-observer sensitivity and mean single-observer sensitivity in six of the 22 systems.

We labeled the two versions of paired observers as systems 1 and 2 and the four versions of single observers as systems 3–6. We let p_i represent the proportion of the 98 patients with disease classified correctly with system i, and, for later use, we let p_{ij} represent the proportion classified correctly with both system i and system j. (Note that $p_i = p_{ii}$.) Then, interest centered on the difference d in mean sensitivities: $d = [(p_1 + p_2)/2] - [(p_3 + p_4 + p_5 + p_6)/4]$. Writing this as the inner product of two vectors, we had $d = c'p$, with c having elements ½, ½, −¼, −¼, −¼, and −¼ and with p having elements p_1 to p_6.

We let V represent the 6 × 6 matrix of variances and covariances, with (i,j)-element $v_{ij} = \mathrm{cov}(p_i,p_j)$. Then, the variance of the difference d was $c'Vc$ (the double summation of $c_i c_j v_{ij}$). Moreover, the variance v_{ii} of p_i was estimated by using the familiar $p_i(1 - p_i)/n$, while the covariance v_{ij} was $(p_{ij} - p_i p_j)/n$; here n is 98. This enabled estimation of the variance of d, and the desired standard error was the square root thereof. Finally, d was evaluated relative to its standard error by reference to a standard normal distribution. (Notice that this method uses two 22 × 22 matrices of proportions p_{ij}, one for sensitivities and one for specificities.)

To evaluate differences among several means simultaneously, an appropriate quadratic form is constructed and evaluated against a χ^2 distribution.

Acknowledgments: We thank Margaret Kowaluk, BS, for secretarial assistance in the preparation of this manuscript and Roberta Montanaro for clerical assistance.

References

1. Birkelo CC, Chamberlain WE, Phelps PS, Schools PE, Zacks D, Yerushalmy J. Tuberculosis case findings: a comparison of the effectiveness of various roentgenographic and photofluorographic methods. JAMA 1947; 133:359–366.
2. Muhm JR, Miller WE, Fontana RS, et al. Lung cancer detected during a screening program using four-month chest radiographs. Radiology 1983; 148:609–615.
3. Elmore JG, Wells CK, Lee CH, Howard DH, Feinstein AR. Variability in radiologists' interpretations of mammograms. N Engl J Med 1994; 331:1493–1499.
4. Beam CA, Layde PM, Sullivan DC. Variability in the interpretation of screening mammograms by U.S. radiologists. Arch Intern Med 1996; 156:209–213.
5. Warde P, Rideout DF, Herman S, et al. Computed tomography in advanced ovarian cancer: inter- and intraobserver reliability. Invest Radiol 1986; 21:31–33.
6. Wakeley CJ, Jones AM, Kabala JE, Prince D, Goddard PR. Audit of the value of double reading magnetic resonance imaging films. Br J Radiol 1995; 68:358–360.
7. Landis SH, Murray T, Bolden S, Wingo PA. Cancer statistics, 1998. Cancer 1998; 47:6–29.
8. Forstner R, Hricak H, White S. CT and MRI of ovarian cancer. Abdom Imaging 1995; 20:2–8.
9. Nelson RC, Frederick MG. Peritoneal carcinomatosis. Abdom Imaging 1995; 20:56–57.
10. Kinard RE, Orrison WW, Brogdon BG. The value of a worksheet in reporting body-CT examinations. AJR 1986; 147:848–849.
11. Metz CE, Shen JH. Gains in accuracy from replicated readings of diagnostic images: prediction and assessment in terms of ROC analysis. Med Decis Making 1992; 12:60–75.
12. Hessel SJ, Herman PG, Swensson RG. Improving performance by multiple interpretations of chest radiographs: effectiveness and cost. Radiology 1978; 127:589–594.
13. Fleiss JL. Statistical methods for rates and proportions. 2nd ed. New York, NY: Wiley, 1981.
14. Dorfman DD, Alf E. Maximum-likelihood estimation of parameters of method data. J Math Psych 1969; 6:487–496.
15. Metz CE, Wang PL, Kronman HB. A new approach for testing the significance of differences between ROC curves measured from correlated data. In: Proceedings of the Eighth Information Processing in Medical Imaging Conference. The Hague, the Netherlands: Nijhoff, 1984; 432–454.
16. Webb RW, Sarin M, Zerhouni EA, Heelan RT, Glazer GM, Gatsonis C. Interobserver variability in CT and MR staging of lung cancer. J Comput Assist Tomogr 1993; 17:841–846.
17. Koran LM. The reliability of clinical methods, data and judgments. I. N Engl J Med 1975; 293:642–648.
18. Koran LM. The reliability of clinical methods, data and judgments. II. N Engl J Med 1975; 293:695–701.
19. Markus JB, Somers S, O'Mally BP, Stevenson GW. Double-contrast barium enema studies: effect of multiple reading on perception error. Radiology 1990; 175:155–156.
20. Yerushalmy J, Harkness JT, Cope JH, Kennedy BR. The role of dual reading in mass radiography. Am Rev Tuberc 1950; 61:443–463.
21. Anderson ED, Muir BB, Walsh JS, Kirkpatrick AE. The efficacy of double reading mammograms in breast screening. Clin Radiol 1994; 49:248–251.
22. Thurfjell EL, Lernevall KA, Taube AA. Benefit of independent double reading in a population-based mammography screening program. Radiology 1994; 191:241–244.
23. Beam CA, Sullivan DC, Layde PM. Effect of human variability on independent double reading in screening mammography. Acad Radiol 1996; 3:891–897.
24. Hillman BJ, Swensson RG, Hessel SJ, Gerson DE, Herman PG. The value of consultation among radiologists. AJR 1976; 127:807–809.
25. Hillman BJ, Hessel SJ, Swensson RG, Herman PG. Improving diagnostic accuracy: a comparison of interactive and Delphi consultations. Invest Radiol 1977; 12:112–115.
26. Curtis PB, Ferrell WR, Hillman BJ. Improved imaging diagnosis by sequentially combined confidence judgments. Invest Radiol 1988; 23:342–347.
27. Ferrell WR, Hillman BJ, Brewer ML, Amendola MA, Thornbury JR. Interactive, mathematical, and sequential consultative methods in diagnosing renal masses on excretory urograms. Invest Radiol 1989; 24:456–462.
28. Getty DJ, Pickett RM, D'Orsi CJ, Swets JA. Enhanced interpretation of diagnostic images. Invest Radiol 1988; 23:240–252.
29. Swets JA, Getty DJ, Pickett RM, D'Orsi CJ, Seltzer SE, McNeil BJ. Enhancing and evaluating diagnostic accuracy. Med Decis Making 1991; 11:9–18.
30. Baker JA, Kornguth PJ, Lo JY, Floyd CE Jr. Artificial neural network: improving the quality of breast biopsy recommendations. Radiology 1996; 198:131–135.
31. Seltzer SE, Getty DJ, Tempany CM, et al. Staging prostate cancer with MR imaging: a combined radiologist-computer system. Radiology 1997; 202:219–226.

Angelo Luca, MD
Gennaro D'Amico, MD
Roberto La Galla, MD
Massimo Midiri, MD
Alberto Morabito, MS
Luigi Pagliaro, MD

Index terms:
Liver, cirrhosis, 761.794
Liver, hemorrhage, 761.458. 761.75
Liver, interventional procedures, 761.1299
Radiology and radiologists, outcomes studies
Shunts, portosystemic, 95.1268
Varices, 71.75

Radiology 1999; 212:411–421

Abbreviation:
TIPS = transjugular intrahepatic portosystemic shunt

[1] From the Departments of Radiology (A.L., R.L.G., M.M.) and Internal Medicine (G.D.) and the Institute of Internal Medicine and Pneumology (A.L., L.P.), University of Palermo, Ospedale V Cervello, Via Trabucco 180, 90146 Palermo, Italy, and the Institute of Medical Statistics and Biometry, University of Milan, Italy (A.M.). Received May 1, 1998; revision requested July 6; revision received August 26; accepted January 25, 1999. **Address reprint requests to** A.L.

Author contributions:
Guarantors of integrity of entire study, A.L., G.D.; study concepts, A.L., G.D., L.P.; study design, G.D.; definition of intellectual content, A.L., G.D., L.P.; literature research, R.L.G., M.M.; data acquisition, R.L.G., M.M.; data analysis, A.L., G.D.; statistical analysis, A.M., G.D.; manuscript preparation and editing, G.D., A.L.; manuscript review, G.D.

TIPS for Prevention of Recurrent Bleeding in Patients with Cirrhosis: Meta-analysis of Randomized Clinical Trials[1]

PURPOSE: To compare the effects of transjugular intrahepatic portosystemic shunt (TIPS) creation with those of endoscopic treatment with or without propranolol administration (ie, conventional treatment) on recurrent bleeding, encephalopathy, and mortality by using meta-analysis of 11 published randomized clinical trials.

MATERIALS AND METHODS: Data from 11 relevant studies were retrieved by means of computerized and manual search. The combinability of the studies was assessed in terms of clinical and statistical criteria. Data were extracted on the basis of the intention-to-treat principle, and treatment effects were measured as risk differences between TIPS creation and conventional treatment. Pooled estimates were computed according to a random-effects model.

RESULTS: A total of 750 patients were included in 11 trials. No significant heterogeneity was found for any of the outcomes. Pooled risk differences were recurrent bleeding, −31% (95% CI, −39%, −23%); encephalopathy, +16% (95% CI, +10%, +22%); death due to all causes, +2% (95% CI, −4%, +9%); and death due to bleeding, −5% (95% CI, −11%, +6%). Clinically important complications occurred in 22% of patients and were associated with both treatments. TIPS dysfunction occurred in 55% of patients.

CONCLUSION: TIPS creation markedly reduces risk of rebleeding but increases risk of encephalopathy without affecting survival. Therefore, TIPS creation may not be the best first-choice therapy for prevention of recurrent variceal bleeding. Criteria for selection of candidates for TIPS creation should be assessed in future prospective studies.

In 1990, Richter et al (1) reported preliminary clinical results of percutaneous transjugular intrahepatic portosystemic shunt (TIPS) creation with use of a balloon-expandable metallic stent. TIPS creation is an interventional radiologic procedure that results in decompression of the splanchnic venous system in patients with portal hypertension by creating a low-resistance channel between an intrahepatic branch of the portal vein and a main hepatic vein. This technique has gained wide popularity for management of portal hypertension because it is relatively noninvasive, has a low frequency of procedure-related complications, and does not preclude future liver transplantation. However, the initial enthusiasm for this procedure has been dampened because of results from several uncontrolled studies in which a remarkable frequency of stent dysfunction (2–5) and increased risk of encephalopathy (5–8) after TIPS creation were reported.

In an early randomized study (9), published in abstract form in 1994, TIPS creation was compared with endoscopic sclerotherapy for the prevention of recurrent variceal bleeding. The results of this study showed an increased mortality rate in patients treated with TIPS. In 1994, a consensus conference sponsored by the National Digestive Advisory Board (10) recommended guidelines for TIPS creation. It was recommended that until the role of TIPS has been identified in randomized clinical trials, the procedure should be clinically used only in patients with acute variceal bleeding that cannot be controlled with endoscopic and pharmacologic therapy and in patients with recurrent bleeding despite adequate

TABLE 1
Patient Characteristics and Control Treatments in Randomized Clinical Trials in the Meta-analysis

Trial	Year	No. of Patients*	Mean Age (y)*	Male Patients (%)*	Alcoholic Cirrhosis (%)*	Child-Pugh Class (%)†	Ascites (%)*	Bleeding-Assignment Interval (d)	Type of Control Treatment
Cabrera et al (17)‡	1996	32/31	56/56	72/65	54/65	44/46/10	34/32	≤ 3	Sclerotherapy
Rössle et al (18)‡	1997	65/61	57/54	68/66	65/69	31/51/18	NR	≤ 14	Sclerotherapy, banding ligation, β-blockers
Sauer et al (19)‡	1997	41/42	60/53	52/64	63/60	33/43/24	NR	≤ 3	Sclerotherapy, β-blockers
Sanyal et al (20)‡	1997	39/41	52/48	69/63	44/39	16/35/49	31/34	3–21	Sclerotherapy
Cello et al (21)‡	1997	25/24	46/49	68/79	68/67	NR	44/54	≤ 1	Sclerotherapy
Jalan et al (22)‡	1997	27/31	60/55	59/67	77/83	12/40/48	78/90	≤ 2	Banding ligation
Merli et al (23)‡	1998	43/38	50/60	72/71	40/24	35/56/12	63/71	1–180	Sclerotherapy
Groupe d'Etude des Anastomoses Intra-Hépatic (24)§	1995	33/32	51‖	NR	NR	0/0/100	NR	≤ 4	Sclerotherapy, β-blockers
García-Villareal et al (25)§	1996	19/18	NR	NR	NR	16/52/32	NR	≤ 14	Sclerotherapy
Sauer et al (26)§	1997	17/16	NR	NR	NR	NR	NR	NR	Banding ligation
Pomier-Layargues et al (27)§	1997	37/38	NR	NR	NR	NR	NR	≤ 3	Banding ligation

Note.—NR = not reported.
* Data are for patients receiving conventional treatment/patients treated with TIPS creation.
† Data are for Child-Pugh class A/class B/class C.
‡ Results published in a full report.
§ Results published in an abstract.
‖ Only the mean age for all patients (in both groups) was reported.

treatment with β-adrenergic blocking agents (hereafter, β-blockers) and endoscopic therapy. Thus far, however, randomized clinical trials usually have included small sample sizes and have shown conflicting results, which hinder the drawing of conclusions for clinical practice.

The aim of this meta-analysis was to assess the effectiveness of TIPS as compared with sclerotherapy or banding ligation of esophageal varices, with or without administration of propranolol hydrochloride, for the prevention of recurrent bleeding. Because these endoscopic treatments and the use of propranolol are well established and widely used for the prevention of recurrent bleeding in patients with cirrhosis (11), they are referred to as conventional treatment throughout this article.

TABLE 2
Technical Results of Treatment in Full Reports of Randomized Clinical Trials

Trial	Successful Stent Placement (%)	Portocaval Pressure Gradient (mm Hg)*	TIPS Dysfunction (%)	Variceal Eradication after Conventional Treatment (%)	Variceal Recurrence after Conventional Treatment (%)†
Cabrera et al (17)	97	20.8 ± 5.6/10.5 ± 2.8	55	63	55
Rössle et al (18)	100	22 ± 5/8 ± 4	30	80	NR
Sauer et al (19)	100	23.6 ± 7.2/12.8 ± 1.8	76	74	32
Sanyal et al (20)	95	23 ± 3/11 ± 2	59	78	28
Cello et al (21)	100	23.9 ± 1.9/7.7 ± 0.5	18	56	NR
Jalan et al (22)	90	19.4 ± 1.1/8.8 ± 1.1	31	61	NR
Merli et al (23)	92	24 ± 0.9/10 ± 0.7	66	51	NR

* Data are pressure gradients (±SD) before TIPS/after TIPS.
† NR = not reported.

MATERIALS AND METHODS

This meta-analysis was performed according to a protocol determined before the study, and we followed widely accepted methodological recommendations (12–15). Measurement of treatment effectiveness was determined on the basis of four clinically relevant outcomes: recurrence of gastrointestinal bleeding due to any cause, portosystemic encephalopathy, mortality due to any cause, and mortality due to recurrent bleeding. Although recurrent bleeding from esophageal varices may be a more clinically important measure of treatment effectiveness, we used recurrent bleeding from any source because, in some of the available studies, the information on the source of recurrent bleeding is incomplete and because TIPS is expected to reduce recurrent bleeding due to any portal hypertensive cause.

Selection of the Trials

Studies that fulfilled the following criteria were included in the present meta-analysis: (*a*) TIPS was compared with endoscopic treatment (sclerotherapy or banding ligation) alone or with propranolol; (*b*) patients were randomly assigned to the treatment regimen, and prospective follow-up was included; (*c*) patients with cirrhosis and previous variceal bleeding were included; (*d*) two or more of the following outcomes were assessed: (i) recurrent bleeding, (ii) encephalopathy, and (iii) death; and (*e*) results were published in English as abstracts or full reports.

Study Identification

Pertinent studies were retrieved from the MEDLINE database (January 1991–February 1998) by using the search terms "TIPS," "sclerotherapy," "variceal band ligation," and "beta-blockers" and by limiting the search to reports of clinical trials and studies with human patients. In addition, a manual search was performed by checking the reference lists from articles

TABLE 3
Outcome Rates in Randomized Clinical Trials and Pooled Risk Differences

Trial and Statistic	Recurrent Bleeding: No. of Patients*	Recurrent Bleeding: Rate Difference†	Encephalopathy: No. of Patients*	Encephalopathy: Rate Difference†	Deaths due to All Causes: No. of Patients*	Deaths due to All Causes: Rate Difference†	Deaths due to Recurrent Bleeding: No. of Patients*	Deaths due to Recurrent Bleeding: Rate Difference†
Trial								
Cabrera et al (17)‡	21 (66)/7 (23)§	−43 (−65, −21)	4 (13)/10 (32)	20 (−1, 40)	6 (19)/5 (16)	4 (−15, 23)	3 (9)/0 (0)	−9 (−19, 1)
Rössle et al (18)‡	33 (51)/15 (25)‖	−26 (−42, −10)	12 (18)/22 (36)	18 (2, 33)	8 (12)/8 (13)	1 (−11, 12)	2 (3)/2 (3)	0 (−6, 6)
Sauer et al (19)‡	24 (59)/6 (14)§	−44 (−63, −26)	3 (7)/14 (33)	26 (10, 42)	11 (27)/12 (29)	2 (−18, 21)	5 (12)/0 (0)	−12 (−22, −2)
Sanyal et al (20)‡	10 (26)/10 (24)‖	−1 (−20, 18)	5 (13)/12 (29)	16 (−1, 34)	7 (18)/12 (29)	11 (−7, 30)	3 (8)/5 (12)	5 (−9, 18)
Cello et al (21)‡	12 (48)/3 (13)§	−36 (−59, −12)	11 (44)/14 (58)	14 (−13, 42)	4 (16)/5 (21)	5 (−17, 27)	Not reported	Not reported
Jalan et al (22)‡	14 (52)/3 (10)§	−42 (−64, −21)	3 (11)/5 (16)	5 (−12, 23)	10 (37)/13 (42)	5 (−20, 30)	2 (7)/0 (0)	−7 (−17, 2)
Merli et al (23)‡	22 (51)/9 (24)‖	−27 (−48, −7)	10 (26)/21 (55)	32 (12, 52)	8 (19)/9 (24)	5 (−13, 23)	4 (9)/4 (11)	1 (−12, 14)
Groupe d'Etude des Anastomoses Intra-Hépatic (24)#	20 (61)/13 (41)**	−20 (−44, 4)	Not reported	Not reported	14 (42)/16 (50)	8 (−17, 32)	7 (21)/8 (25)	4 (−17, 24)
García-Villareal et al (25)#	9 (47)/2 (11)**	−36 (−63, −10)	5 (26)/4 (22)	−4 (−32, 23)	8 (42)/1 (6)	−37 (−61, −12)	5 (26)/0 (0)	−26 (−46, −7)
Sauer et al (26)#	9 (53)/3 (19)**	−34 (−65, −4)	2 (12)/4 (25)	13 (−13, 39)	2 (12)/2 (13)	1 (−22, 23)	Not reported	Not reported
Pomier-Layargues et al (27)#	22 (59)/10 (26)**	−33 (−54, −12)	10 (27)/13 (34)	7 (−14, 28)	20 (54)/26 (68)	14 (−8, 36)	Not reported	Not reported
Statistic								
Pooled risk difference (%)	. . .	−31 (−39, −23)	. . .	16 (10, 22)	. . .	2 (−4, 9)	. . .	−5 (−11, 6)
χ^2 value for heterogeneity	. . .	11.79	. . .	6.87	. . .	9.53	. . .	13.74
P value for heterogeneity	. . .	>.25	. . .	>.5	. . .	>.25	. . .	>.05
τ^2 value	. . .	0.0061	. . .	0.0001	. . .	0.0021	. . .	0.0029

* Data are for patients treated conventionally/patients treated with TIPS. Numbers in parentheses are percentages.
† Value is the rate in patients treated with TIPS minus the rate in patients treated conventionally. Numbers in parentheses are the lower and upper limits of the 95% CI.
‡ Results published in a full report.
§ Bleeding was from esophageal varices.
‖ Bleeding was from any source.
Results published in an abstract.
** Source of bleeding not reported.

or reviews to identify studies not yet included in the MEDLINE database (16). Finally, the abstracts from international congresses on liver diseases underwent peer review to identify trials still in progress. When the results of a single study were reported in more than one publication, only the most recent and complete data were included in the meta-analysis. Eleven randomized clinical trials that fulfilled the criteria were identified, seven published in full form (17–23) and four published in abstract form (24–27).

Data Extraction

Data from each randomized clinical trial were extracted by two independent reviewers (A.L., G.D.). For each study and each type of treatment, the following data were extracted: number of patients, mean age, sex, prevalence of alcoholic cirrhosis, Child-Pugh score, presence of ascites, time between index bleeding and random assignment to treatment, type and modality of control treatment, rate of technical success of the procedures, portacaval pressure gradient before and after TIPS creation, mean length of follow-up, incidence of TIPS dysfunction, and definition and number of each outcome (Tables 1–4). Numeric discrepancies between the two independent data extractions were resolved after discussion.

Qualitative Assessment

The quality of randomized clinical trials published in full reports was assessed by two independent observers (A.L., G.D.) who used a previously reported (28) quality-assessment system that was partially modified according to the treatments under study (see Appendix). The system was based on the following principal criteria: clearly defined inclusion and exclusion criteria, blinded treatment assignment, baseline comparability of treatment groups, clearly defined outcome variables, treatment for acute bleeding equal in the two groups, and assessment of treatment side effects and complications. To assess baseline comparability of patient groups in each trial, we made an arbitrary and a priori decision to consider the trial groups to be similar at baseline if none of the baseline variables showed either a statistically significant difference or a difference of 40% or greater (28).

Any discrepancy in the qualitative assessment between the two observers was discussed, and a consensus was achieved.

TABLE 4
Methodologic Characteristics of Randomized Clinical Trials Published as Full Reports

Trial	No. of Centers	Follow-up (mo)*	Modality and Schedule for TIPS Surveillance	Definition of TIPS Dysfunction†	Definition of Recurrent Bleeding	Treatment for Active Recurrent Bleeding
Cabrera et al (17)	1	15/15	Angiography every 6 mo	PPG >25% of value obtained after TIPS if PPG >12 mm Hg	Endoscopically confirmed variceal rebleeding; bleeding from ulcer after endoscopy was not considered to be rebleeding	Not reported
Rössle et al (18)	1	14/13	Doppler ultrasonography (US) at 1, 3, 6, 9, and 12 mo, thereafter every 6 mo; angiography if no shunt flow or if portal flow velocity <50% of pretreatment value	Angiographic shunt occlusion or stenosis and PPG >12 mm Hg	Rebleeding 24 h after random assignment and after 24 h of hemodynamic stabilization	Not reported
Sauer et al (19)	1	17/19	Angiography every 3 mo	PPG >15 mm Hg	Endoscopically confirmed variceal rebleeding, independent of severity, within 24 h of index bleeding	Sclerotherapy and/or balloon tamponade and/or octreotide administration
Sanyal et al (20)	1	33/32	Doppler US at 1 d, 1 wk, 1 and 3 mo, and every 3 mo thereafter; angiography every 6 mo	Angiographic shunt occlusion or stenosis and/or PPG >12 mm Hg or PPG increased more than 25% if posttreatment PPG >12 mm Hg	Hematemesis or melena after random assignment	Sclerotherapy in all patients; balloon dilation and/or further stent placement in some cases in TIPS group
Cello et al (21)	1	19/19	Doppler US	Decreased portal flow velocity	Hematemesis or melena with decrease in hematocrit value sufficient to warrant transfusion	Not reported
Jalan et al (22)	1	17/16	Angiography at 1 mo and every 6 mo thereafter	PPG >12 mm Hg or PPG >20% of posttreatment value	Hematemesis or melena after random assignment	Banding or sclerotherapy in all patients; balloon dilation and/or further stent placement in some cases in TIPS group
Merli et al (23)	4	18/18	Doppler US every 6 mo, angiography at 6 mo or when stent malfunction was suspected	Angiographic shunt occlusion or stenosis and/or PPG >15 mm Hg	Hematemesis or melena after 24 h of hemodynamic stabilization	Not reported

* Data for conventional treatment/TIPS creation.
† PPG = portocaval pressure gradient.
‡ Conn Ho. Trailmaking and number-connection tests in assessment of mental state in portal systemic encephalopathy. Am J Dig Dis 1977; 22:541–550.
§ Parsons-Smith GB, Summerskill WHJ, Dawson AM, Sherlock S. The electroencephalograph in liver disease. Lancet 1952; 2:867.

The total score of each trial also was expressed as a percentage of the maximum achievable score.

Statistical Methods

We assumed that variceal endoscopic sclerotherapy and banding ligation with or without the use of β-blockers were equivalent control interventions. Although the results of previous meta-analyses (29,30) do not support this assumption, there were no significant differences between the control groups of the trials included in the present analysis in terms of the incidence of outcomes of interest during the study period (Table 3). Thus, in an attempt to improve the power of the meta-analysis, we considered the control treatments to be equivalent.

All comparisons were performed according to the randomly assigned treatment (intended-treatment analysis). Because of differing clinical characteristics among study groups, varying sample sizes, and different control treatments, we assumed that heterogeneity was present even when not statistically significant, and we decided to combine data by using a random-effects model (31) whenever the τ^2 value (a measure of the between-study variability of the treatment effect) was greater than 0 (32,33), to achieve more conservative pooled estimates.

For all outcomes, the pooled risk difference was computed with the method of DerSimonian and Laird (31). Summary point estimates and 95% CIs, χ^2 statistics for heterogeneity, and τ^2 values are reported. For statistically significant risk differences (that is, if the 95% CI of the summary risk difference did not include 0), the number needed to treat was calculated (34). The number needed to treat is the number of patients who must be treated to avoid one unfavorable event; it is calculated by using the reciprocal of the weighted difference in rates between treat-

Cause of Crossover Treatment	Definition of Encephalopathy	Definition of Death due to Rebleeding
Conventional: uncontrolled rebleeding, three or more variceal bleeding episodes in 4 mo, rebleeding from gastric varices; TIPS: no crossover	Spontaneous episode of clinical changes in mental state after exclusion of all other precipitate factors; chronic encephalopathy if three or more such episodes per y	Not reported
Conventional: uncontrolled acute rebleeding of three or more important rebleedings in 1 y; TIPS: no crossover	Grade 1, minor limitation of concentration, fatigue; grade 2, somnolence, asterixis; grade 3, deep somnolence or stupor; grade 4, coma	Not reported
Conventional: uncontrolled acute variceal rebleeding or more than two rebleedings in 6 mo; TIPS: no crossover	Impairment of mental status and trailmaking scores‡, classified as induced or spontaneous; chronic encephalopathy if worsening of mental state refractory to medical treatment	Any death during rebleeding, independent of possible liver failure
Conventional: any rebleeding; TIPS: failure to place stent	New onset or acutely worsening encephalopathy	Not reported
Conventional: recurrent variceal hemorrhage with no response to sclerotherapy; TIPS: stent placement technically impossible	Asterixis, gross disorientation, agitation; frank somnolence or coma in absence of identifiable cause	Not reported
Conventional: uncontrolled rebleeding; TIPS: failure to place stent	New onset or deterioration of encephalopathy according to Parsons-Smith criteria§	Not reported
Uncontrolled acute rebleeding in both groups; conventional: recurrent variceal bleeding with no response to repeated sclerotherapy or gastric variceal rebleeding; TIPS: failure to place stent, rebleeding not treatable with stent dilation or replacement, or rebleeding after previous intervention	Defined and graded according to Parsons-Smith criteria§ as grade I–II (moderate) and grade III–IV (severe)	Any death within 6 wk of rebleeding episode

ment and control groups. The 95% CIs for number needed to treat also are reported.

To determine the consistency of results, two sensitivity analyses were performed according to type of publication (abstract or full article) and control treatment. The data were processed by using the META-ANALYST program (version 0.989; Lau J, Boston, Mass).

RESULTS

Reports of 11 pertinent randomized clinical trials were retrieved; these trials included a total of 750 patients: 372 treated with TIPS and 378 treated conventionally. Clinical and methodological characteristics of the 11 trials are summarized in Tables 1 and 4. In one trial (24), only patients assigned to Child-Pugh class C were enrolled. The time from cessation of bleeding to random assignment to treatment was less than 4 days in six trials (17,19,21,22,24,27), less than 3 weeks in three trials (18,20,25), and 1 day to 6 months in one trial (23) (Table 1).

TIPS creation was compared with sclerotherapy in five trials (17,20,21,23,24), with sclerotherapy and propranolol administration in three trials (18,19,24), and with band ligation in three trials (22,26,27). In one trial (18), eventual embolization of the varices was performed in half the patients in the TIPS group. The mean follow-up was 15.9 months in the TIPS groups and 16.3 months in the conventional treatment groups.

Treatment for episodes of recurrent bleeding was reported to be the same in the two treatment groups in one trial (19). In two trials (20,22), emergency sclerotherapy was performed in both groups, and balloon dilatation and/or further stent placement were also performed in the TIPS group. In the other trials, no information about treatment

TABLE 5
Treatment Complications in Seven Randomized Clinical Trials Published as Full Reports

Complication	Conventional Treatment (n = 272)	TIPS Creation (n = 268)
Bleeding	13*	9†
Infection	20‡	23§
Hemolysis	0	6
Heart failure	0	2
Cardiac arrest	0	1
Pulmonary embolism	0	1
Stent dislocation	0	7
Portal thrombosis	0	2
Dysphagia	14	0
Esophageal stenosis	9	0
Embolic stroke	1	0
Abdominal pain	0	6

Note.—Data are number of complications.
* Includes five cases that occurred after endoscopy and eight due to esophageal ulcer.
† Bleeding was intraperitoneal in three cases, due to hemobilia in four, and intrahepatic in two.
‡ Includes six cases of sepsis, 11 of pneumonia, and three of spontaneous bacterial peritonitis.
§ Includes 14 cases of sepsis, seven of pneumonia, and two of spontaneous bacterial peritonitis.

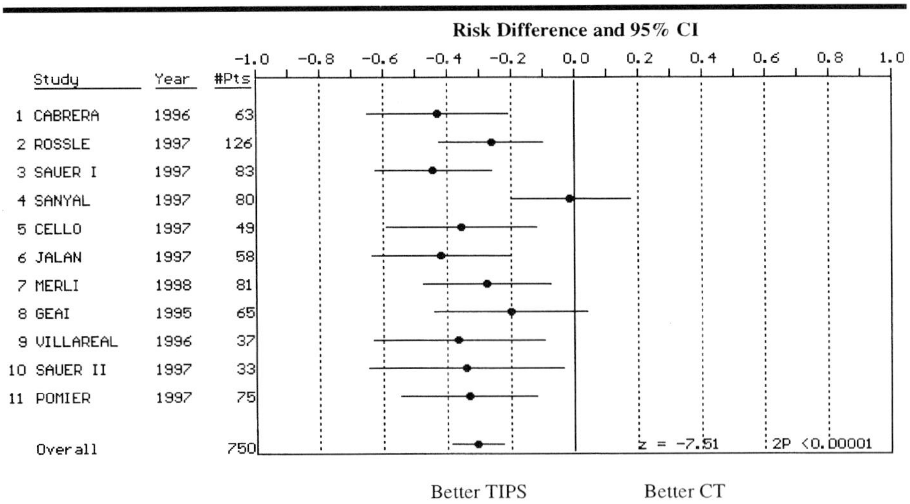

Figure 1. Point estimates (●) and 95% CIs (horizontal bars) of the risk difference between TIPS creation and conventional treatment show that TIPS creation significantly reduces the risk of recurrent bleeding. Risk differences represented to the left of the 0-difference line (the equivalence line) denote an advantage for TIPS creation; those to the right denote an advantage for conventional therapy (*CT*). CI bars that do not cross the 0-difference line denote a statistically significant advantage. "Overall" denotes the pooled risk difference. Trials reported in full articles are listed before those reported in abstracts, and all are listed in ascending order of year of publication. Each trial is identified by the name of the first author. z = z value, $2P$ = two-sided P value, *#Pts* = number of patients included in each trial.

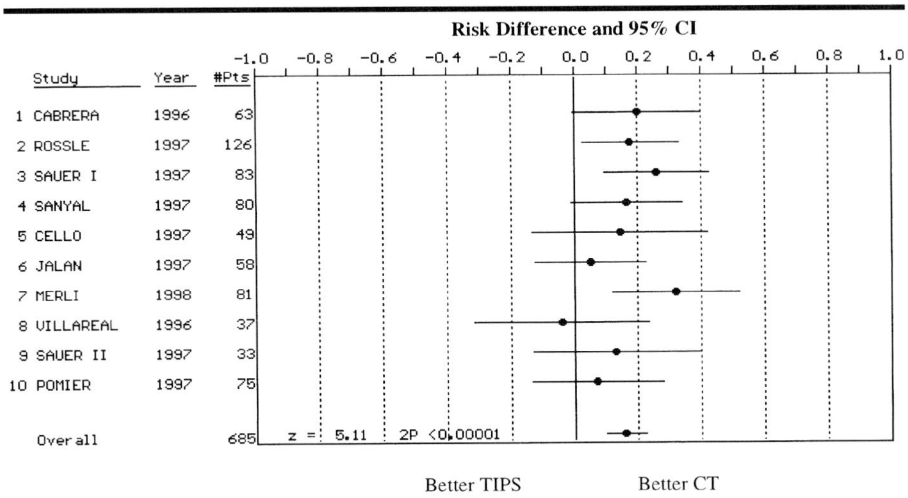

Figure 2. Point estimates (●) and 95% CIs (horizontal bars) of the risk difference between TIPS creation and conventional treatment show that TIPS creation significantly increases the risk of portosystemic encephalopathy. Risk differences represented to the left of the 0-difference line (the equivalence line) denote an advantage for TIPS creation; those to the right denote an advantage for conventional therapy (*CT*). CI bars that do not cross the 0-difference line denote a statistically significant advantage. "Overall" denotes the pooled risk difference. Trials reported in full articles are listed before those reported in abstracts, and all are listed in ascending order of year of publication. Each trial is identified by the name of the first author. z = z value, $2P$ = two-sided P value, *#Pts* = number of patients included in each trial.

for recurrent bleeding was reported. The definition of death due to recurrent bleeding was reported in only two trials (19,23), although the number of patients who died of recurrent bleeding was reported in six of the seven studies published as full articles. The definitions of the other three outcomes in this meta-analysis were fairly comparable across the trials described in full reports (Table 4).

The quality score for the seven trials published as full reports and assessed for methodological quality ranged from 51% to 88%, which was indicative of fair to good quality. Details on the single components of the quality score for each trial are reported in the Appendix.

No significant heterogeneity of treatment effect was found for any of the assessed outcomes (even when the analyses were repeated by using odds ratios [data not shown]), and the τ^2 value was greater than 0 in all analyses.

Technical Results and Complications of Treatment

TIPS creation was successful in 90%–100% (median, 98.5%) of patients. The reduction of the portosystemic pressure gradient ranged from 10.3 to 16.2 mm Hg (median, 13.0 mm Hg). At stent surveillance (Table 4), narrowing or occlusion of the stent lumen, defined as stent dysfunction (Table 4) and necessitating shunt revision, was found in 18%–76% (median, 55%) of patients (Table 2).

Endoscopic sclerotherapy or banding ligation of varices resulted in variceal obliteration in 51%–80% (median, 66%) of patients. Recurrence of varices in endoscopically treated patients was reported in three studies and was 28% (20), 32% (19), and 55% (17).

Complications of treatment published

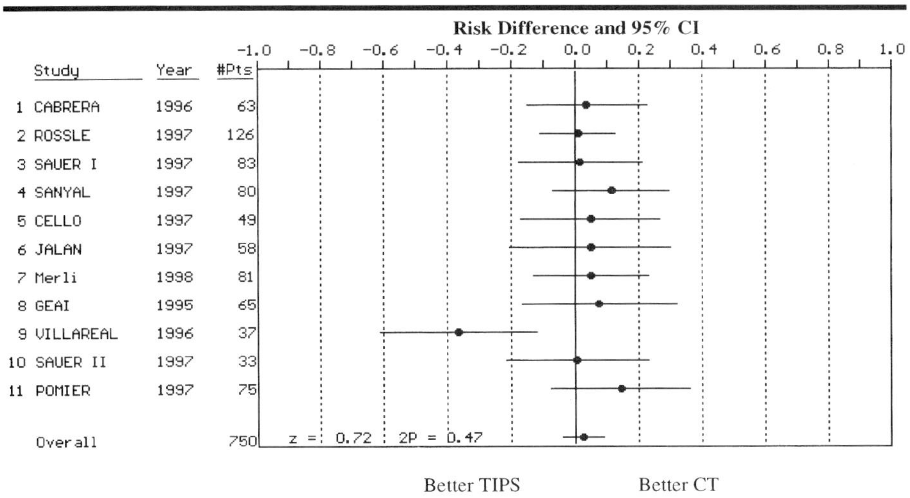

Figure 3. Point estimates (●) and 95% CIs (horizontal bars) of the risk difference between TIPS creation and conventional treatment show that TIPS creation does not affect the risk of death due to all causes. Risk differences represented to the left of the 0-difference line (the equivalence line) denote an advantage for TIPS creation; those to the right denote an advantage for conventional therapy (*CT*). CI bars that do not cross the 0-difference line denote a statistically significant advantage. "Overall" denotes the pooled risk difference. Trials reported in full articles are listed before those reported in abstracts, and all are listed in ascending order of year of publication. Each trial is identified by the name of the first author. *z* = *z* value, *2P* = two-sided *P* value, *#Pts* = number of patients included in each trial.

TABLE 6
Cause of Death in Full Reports of Randomized Clinical Trials

Cause of Death	Conventional Treatment (*n* = 247)	TIPS Creation (*n* = 244)
Liver failure	15	20
Variceal rebleeding	21	9
Ulcerative bleeding	0	2
Hemoperitoneum	0	3
Hemothorax	1	0
Sepsis	5	10
Spontaneous bacterial peritonitis	0	1
Aspiration pneumonia	3	1
Hepatocellular carcinoma	3	4
Intestinal occlusion	0	1
Pulmonary edema	0	1
Cerebrovascular accident	0	2
Cardiomyopathy	0	1
Myocardial infarction	1	0
Other	1	5

Note.—Data are from six of the seven trials published as full reports. Cause of death was not reported in the study by Cello and colleagues (21).

in the seven full reports are summarized in Table 5. After TIPS creation, 60 of 268 (22%) patients experienced complications, the most serious of which were hemorrhage in nine patients (intraperitoneal in three, intrahepatic in two, and hemobilia in four) and infections in 23 patients. Complications of endoscopic therapy occurred in 61 of 272 (22%) patients, including bleeding in 13 patients (due to esophageal ulcer in eight and immediately after a sclerotherapy session in five); infection in 20; and dysphagia in 14, nine of whom had esophageal stenosis necessitating dilation.

Recurrent Bleeding

Data on recurrent bleeding were available for all 11 trials (17–27) (Table 3). In five (17–19,21,22) of the full reports, the rate of recurrent bleeding from esophageal varices was reported; in one of these (18), the total number of patients who experienced recurrent bleeding from any source also was reported. In the remaining two studies (20,23), the rate of recurrent bleeding from any source was reported: In one of these (23), the mean number of episodes of recurrent bleeding from esophageal varices (but not the number of patients with recurrent bleeding from esophageal varices) also was reported. No detailed information on the source of recurrent bleeding was reported in the studies published in abstract form.

TIPS creation resulted in a significant reduction in the rate of recurrent bleeding in nine trials (17–19,21–23,25–27) and a nearly significant reduction in another (24) (Fig 1), whereas there was no effect in one trial (20). The overall weighted recurrent bleeding rate was 21% for TIPS creation and 52% for endoscopic treatment. The pooled risk difference was −31% (95% CI, −39%, −23%) (Fig 1). The χ^2 value for heterogeneity was 11.79 ($df = 10$, $P > .25$). The "number needed to treat" (ie, number of patients who need to be treated with TIPS to prevent one episode of recurrent bleeding) was 3.3 (95% CI, 2.6, 4.4), which indicates that, compared to conventional therapy, two to five patients needed to be treated with TIPS to prevent one recurrent bleeding episode.

Encephalopathy

The encephalopathy rate was reported in 10 studies (17–23,25–27) involving 685 patients, 340 treated with TIPS creation and 345 treated with conventional therapy (Table 3). TIPS creation increased the frequency of encephalopathy in all but one trial (25); we found a statistically significant increase in three trials (18,19,23) (Fig 2) and a nearly significant increase in two (17,20). The overall weighted encephalopathy rate was 35% after TIPS creation and 19% after conventional treatment. The pooled risk difference was 16% (95% CI, 10%, 22%). The χ^2 value for heterogeneity was 6.87 ($df = 9$, $P > .5$). The number needed to treat was 6.0 (95% CI, 4.5, 10.0), which indicates that for every four to 10 patients treated with TIPS, one more episode of encephalopathy occurs more than if they had been treated conventionally.

Mortality

Mortality data were reported for all 11 trials (17–27) (Table 3). TIPS creation resulted in a significant reduction in the mortality rate in one study (25) and had no significant effect in the others (Fig 3). The overall weighted mortality rate was 28% for TIPS creation and 26% for endoscopic treatment. The pooled risk difference was +2% (95% CI, −4%, +9%) (Figure 3). The χ^2 value for heterogeneity was 9.53 ($df = 10$, $P > .25$). Causes of death are reported in Table 6.

Death due to Recurrent Bleeding

Data from eight trials (17–20,22–25) involving 594 patients, 294 treated with TIPS creation and 299 treated conventionally, were available for this end point (Table 3). TIPS creation resulted in a significant reduction in the mortality rate due to recurrent bleeding in two studies

(19,25), a nearly significant reduction in one (17), and no effect in the other five (18,20,22–24) (Fig 4). The overall weighted recurrent bleeding–related mortality rate was 5% for TIPS creation and 10% for endoscopic treatment. The pooled risk difference showed a trend (−5% [95% CI, −11%, +6%]) toward a reduction in mortality rate due to bleeding after TIPS creation, but this result was not statistically significant (Fig 4). The χ^2 value for heterogeneity was 13.74 ($df = 7$, $P > .05$).

Treatment Crossover

In nine trials (17–23,26,27) involving 648 patients, the number of patients who underwent conventional treatment after TIPS creation or who underwent TIPS creation because of failure of conventional treatment (ie, treatment crossover) was reported. Of 321 patients randomly assigned to undergo TIPS creation, eight (2%) also underwent conventional treatment mainly because of failure to place the stent. Of 327 patients randomly assigned to undergo conventional treatment, 58 (18%) also underwent TIPS creation mainly because of uncontrolled or recurrent bleeding. Indications for crossover treatment in the trials published as full reports are summarized in Table 4.

Sensitivity Analyses

Sensitivity analyses showed consistency of results for type of publication (full report or abstract) and type of conventional treatment (sclerotherapy, sclerotherapy with propranolol administration, or endoscopic band ligation). However, the increased risk of encephalopathy after TIPS creation was not statistically significant in abstract reports and in trials in which banding ligation was the conventional therapy. Results of the sensitivity analyses are shown in Table 7.

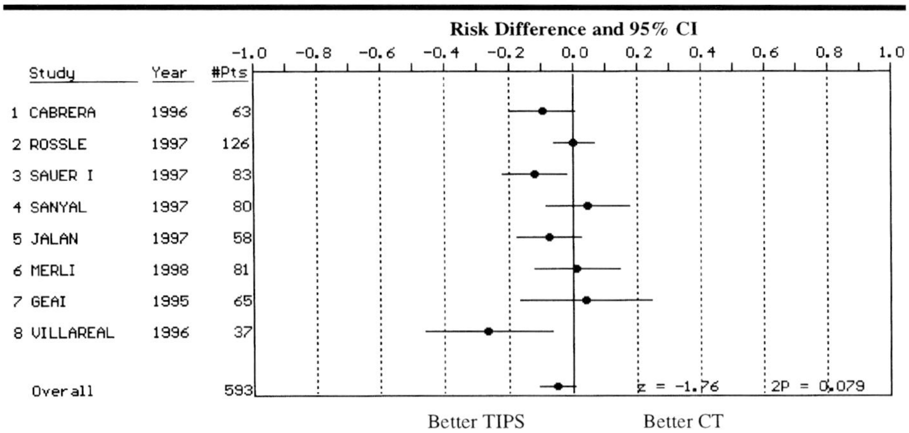

Figure 4. Point estimates (●) and 95% CIs (horizontal bars) of the risk difference between TIPS creation and conventional treatment show that TIPS creation does not significantly reduce the risk of death due to recurrent bleeding. Risk differences represented to the left of the 0-difference line (the equivalence line) denote an advantage for TIPS creation; those to the right denote an advantage for conventional therapy (*CT*). CI bars that do not cross the 0-difference line denote a statistically significant advantage. "Overall" denotes the pooled risk difference. Trials reported in full articles are listed before those reported in abstracts, and all are listed in ascending order of year of publication. Each trial is identified by the name of the first author. *z* = *z* value, *2P* = two-sided *P* value, *#Pts* = number of patients included in each trial.

TABLE 7
Results of Sensitivity Analyses

Variable	No. of Trials*	Pooled Risk Difference (%)†	*P* Value‡
	Recurrent Bleeding		
Type of report			
Full article	7 (17–23)	−31 (−43, −19)	<.001
Abstract	4 (24–27)	−30 (−43, −18)	<.001
Type of therapy			
Sclerotherapy	5 (17,20,21,23,25)	−27 (−43, −12)	<.001
Sclerotherapy plus propranolol	3 (18,19,24)	−31 (−45, −17)	<.001
Banding ligation	3 (22,26,27)	−37 (−50, −24)	<.001
	Encephalopathy		
Type of report			
Full article	7 (17–23)	+19 (+12, +26)	<.001
Abstract	3 (25–27)	+6 (−8, +20)	NS
Type of therapy			
Sclerotherapy	5 (17,20,21,23,25)	+18 (+8, +28)	<.001
Sclerotherapy plus propranolol	2 (18,19)	+21 (+10, +33)	<.001
Banding ligation	3 (22,26,27)	+7 (−4, +19)	NS
	Survival		
Type of report			
Full article	7 (17–23)	+4 (−3, +11)	NS
Abstract	4 (24–27)	−3 (−25, +19)	NS
Type of therapy			
Sclerotherapy	5 (17,20,21,23,25)	−1 (−15, +14)	NS
Sclerotherapy plus propranolol	3 (18,19,24)	+2 (−7, +11)	NS
Banding ligation	3 (22,26,27)	+7 (−6, +20)	NS

* Numbers in parentheses are reference numbers.
† Value is pooled risk difference (risk associated with TIPS minus risk associated with conventional treatment). Numbers in parentheses are the lower and upper limits of the 95% CI.
‡ NS = not significant.

DISCUSSION

In the present meta-analysis, we reviewed 11 randomized clinical trials in which TIPS creation was compared with endoscopic therapy (sclerotherapy in five trials, sclerotherapy plus administration of β-blockers in three, and banding ligation in three) for the prevention of recurrent variceal bleeding in patients with cirrhosis. Overall results showed that TIPS creation significantly reduced the risk of recurrent bleeding, with no effect on survival. TIPS creation significantly increased the risk of encephalopathy, however. Sensitivity analysis results suggested that this interpretation holds true even if we considered only those trials published as full reports and when TIPS creation was compared with sclerotherapy, with sclerotherapy plus β-blockers, or with banding ligation of esophageal varices. In fact, the lack of a statistically significant increase in the risk of encephalopathy after TIPS compared with that after banding ligation probably reflects a type II error due to insufficient sample size.

Although no significant heterogeneity was found for any of the assessed outcomes, differences in the ways in which the trials were conducted and in the methods used suggest that some caution is warranted as regards interpretation of the results of the pooled estimates. Although inclusion of data from trials published in abstract form (24–27) did not significantly affect the overall estimates of the effect of TIPS creation, the combinability of the included trials should be reassessed after full reports of all have been published.

The beneficial effect of TIPS creation on recurrent bleeding was observed in all but one of the trials. The average rate of recurrent bleeding was 20% in patients treated with TIPS creation, which suggests that this interventional radiologic procedure is highly effective for the prevention of recurrent bleeding. A comparably low frequency of recurrent bleeding was reported (35) only in trials where portosystemic shunts were surgically created. However, the comparability of the effect on recurrent bleeding rates associated with TIPS creation and that associated with surgical creation of other types of portosystemic shunt should be reassessed after longer follow-up in patients treated with TIPS creation.

Despite the low frequency of recurrent bleeding in patients treated with TIPS creation, the median rate of stent dysfunction reported in the seven full articles (17–23) was 55%. This finding suggests that other factors may contribute to the precipitation of recurrent bleeding. Of interest in this regard, Sanyal et al (4) recently reported that active alcoholism and high systemic venous pressure together with stent dysfunction are independent risk factors for recurrent bleeding in patients treated with TIPS creation. The wide variability in dysfunction rates across the studies is accounted for by the different definitions and surveillance modalities used, with higher rates found when dysfunction is defined on the basis of invasive hemodynamic measurements. A 2-year incidence of TIPS dysfunction of up to 90% has been reported (4) when invasive hemodynamic measurement was used. The best approach to monitoring of TIPS function in clinical practice is still unsettled, however, and further studies specifically designed for this aim are needed.

The most important side effect of TIPS creation is encephalopathy. Experience with the surgical creation of portosystemic shunts was predictive of this outcome (35). In fact, in hemodynamic terms, a TIPS behaves like a side-to-side portosystemic shunt: The greater the diversion of blood into the systemic circulation, the greater the reduction in portal venous pressure and, hence, the greater the protection against bleeding and the greater the risk of encephalopathy. For this reason, portosystemic shunt surgery, either total or selective, was almost completely abandoned in the past 2 decades. Other than ease of performance, TIPS creation has the advantage over shunt surgery of the ability to calibrate the shunt, which can be tailored in each patient to achieve the minimum portosystemic blood diversion with the optimal portal venous pressure reduction.

The 11 randomized clinical trials included in the present meta-analysis showed a significant increase in the frequency of encephalopathy in patients treated with TIPS creation. However, a conclusion on this crucial point is not possible for two important reasons. First, the optimal reduction in portal venous pressure still is undefined: A reduction below the threshold value of 12 mm Hg should represent maximal protection against the risk of bleeding (36). It has also been suggested (37) and prospectively validated (38) that a 20% reduction from baseline may be enough of a decrease; however, it is not known whether reductions of either more or less than 20% will provide better protection. In none of the 11 trials included in this meta-analysis was there an attempt to determine the optimal reduction in portal venous pressure, and the available data do not allow such an analysis.

The second reason we cannot draw conclusions about TIPS creation and encephalopathy is that encephalopathy was not blindly assessed in any of the studies included in this meta-analysis. Diagnostic bias, therefore, cannot be ruled out.

Thus, the frequency of encephalopathy after TIPS creation should probably be reassessed in further randomized clinical trials that have been more specifically designed to tailor portal venous pressure reduction to achieve the best decrease in the risk of bleeding with the lowest frequency of encephalopathy.

Until such studies are performed, it may be prudent to not perform TIPS creation or to use smaller-diameter stents in patients with known risk factors for encephalopathy, such as age older than 60 years, female sex, previous episodes of encephalopathy, nonalcoholic cause of cirrhosis, low albumin levels, and Child-Pugh class (6–8,17–19). Moreover, a portacaval pressure gradient of less than 10 mm Hg after TIPS creation is associated with a substantially higher risk of encephalopathy (8) and should be avoided. Finally, it is important to remark that in patients with severe and progressive encephalopathy, it is possible to reduce flow through the prosthesis by placing reducing stents or detachable balloons (39).

The overall incidence of complications that occurred during the reviewed trials was high and similar for the two types of treatment. Major complications were bleeding and sepsis for both, although bleeding was more frequent after endoscopic treatment, and sepsis was more frequent after TIPS creation. The available information does not allow assessment of whether the excess rate of encephalopathy after TIPS creation occurred in patients free of other complications. Thus, it is not possible to compare the numbers of patients without complications for each type of treatment.

The results of this meta-analysis showed that TIPS creation did not significantly affect survival, although the significant reduction in the rate of recurrent bleeding after TIPS creation was expected to result in a parallel reduction in deaths due to bleeding. In one study (25), a significant reduction in the risk of death was observed in patients treated with TIPS creation, but no data on cause of death are available because the study was reported in abstract form. In another study (20), a significant increase in the risk of death was reported; in this study, cumulative death proportions were compared by using the log rank test; however, the mortality rate related to recurrent bleeding after TIPS creation was unusually high (42% of all deaths). Overall, in patients who underwent TIPS creation, there was no significant trend toward a reduction in deaths due to bleeding, and there was an opposite trend toward an increase in deaths due to other causes. This combination of results seems to have balanced the overall mortality rate between the two treatment groups. The lack of a significant reduction in deaths caused by bleeding probably is due to type II error; also, the large number of patients who did not respond to conventional treatment and therefore crossed over to TIPS creation could have contributed to lessen this difference. However, whether TIPS creation has a substantial effect on cause of death should be reassessed when all the studies included in this meta-analysis have been published as full reports.

TABLE A1
Quality Scoring Components for Fully Reported Randomized Clinical Trials

	Quality Score Component*												Score	
Trial	1	2	3	4	5	6	7	8	9	10	11	12	Overall	Percentage†
Cabrera et al (17)	4	6	0	0	3	6	6	6	0	6	0	9	46	64
Rössle et al (18)	0	6	6	6	3	6	6	6	0	6	0	9	54	75
Sauer et al (19)	4	6	6	0	3	6	6	6	6	6	0	9	58	81
Sanyal et al (20)	4	6	6	3	3	6	3	3	6	6	0	9	55	76
Cello et al (21)	4	0	6	0	3	6	6	3	0	0	0	9	37	51
Jalan et al (22)	4	6	6	6	3	6	6	6	6	6	0	9	64	88
Merli et al (23)	4	6	6	6	3	6	6	6	0	3	0	9	54	75

* Definitions of quality score components are provided in the text of the Appendix.
† Score expressed as a percentage of the maximum possible score of 72.

In conclusion, the results of this meta-analysis show that in patients with cirrhosis and previous variceal bleeding, TIPS creation is more effective than endoscopic therapy with or without propranolol administration for the prevention of recurrent bleeding but significantly increases the risk of encephalopathy and does not affect survival.

Because of the significant excess risk of encephalopathy, TIPS creation is far from the ideal therapy for prevention of recurrent bleeding and, in our opinion, cannot be considered a first-choice treatment. However, several considerations suggest that the efficiency of TIPS creation can probably be much improved. First, the optimal reduction in portal venous pressure to achieve the highest protection against bleeding and the lowest risk of encephalopathy still is unsettled. Second, there may be improvements in the selection criteria for patients at lower risk for encephalopathy who may benefit more from TIPS creation. Third, technical advances are expected to reduce the frequency of TIPS dysfunction. In some respects, further meta-analysis of the available trials, in which individual patient data are used, will be most helpful, and the authors who conduct such trials should be encouraged to combine their data.

APPENDIX

The following is the quality scoring system used in this meta-analysis. The number in parentheses for each item is the score assigned for that item. The score for each trial was reported as a percentage of the maximum possible score of 72 (Table A1).

1. Randomization
   - A (6). By telephone contact with a central or independent source
   - B (4). By sealed opaque envelopes
   - C (0). Other or not reported
2. Efficacy of randomization
   - A (6). Treated and control groups comparable for the following prognostic variables: age, sex, Child-Pugh class (or score), etiology of cirrhosis
   - B (3). Relative difference for Child-Pugh class (or score) >0.40, but not statistically significant
   - C (0). Child-Pugh class (or score) statistically different between TIPS or conventional treatment, or information not reported
3. Time between randomization and treatment
   - A (6). Same in the two groups
   - B (0). Different interval of time in the two groups or no information reported
4. Withdrawals
   - A (6). Intention-to-treat analysis; number of patients withdrawn from treatment and reasons of withdrawal reported; less than 15% of randomized patients lost to follow-up
   - B (3). One of the above conditions not fulfilled or information not reported
   - C (0). Two or all of the above conditions not fulfilled or information not reported
5. Sample size
   - A (3). A priori estimate of sample size reported
   - B (0). A priori assessment of sample size not reported or not done
6. Definition of treatment failure (as indication to other therapy)
   - A (6). Clear and reproducible
   - B (3). Incomplete information
   - C (0). No information reported
7. Definition of hepatic encephalopathy
   - A (6). Clear and reproducible
   - B (3). Incomplete information
   - C (0). No information reported
8. Definition of the necessity to modify the treatment
   - A (6). Clear and reproducible
   - B (3). Incomplete information
   - C (0). No information reported
9. Treatment of the rebleeding
   - A (6). Same in the two groups
   - B (3). Information lacking for less than 20% of bleeding episodes
   - C (0). Information lacking for 20% or more than 20% of bleeding episodes. Different treatment in the two groups or no information reported
10. Side effects and complications
    - A (6). Number, type, and outcome of side effects
    - B (3). Incomplete information
    - C (0). No information reported
11. Prophylactic treatment of hepatic encephalopathy
    - A (6). Reported in the two groups
    - B (0). Reported only in one group or no information reported
12. External validity
    - A (9). Inclusion and exclusion criteria clearly stated; adequate description of patient characteristics; source of population reported
    - B (6). Only two of the above conditions fulfilled
    - C (3). Only one of the above conditions fulfilled
    - D (0). No information reported

Acknowledgment: The present meta-analysis was carried out by using the META-ANALYST program (version 0.989, July 2, 1996) written by Joseph Lau, MD (Division of Clinical Care Research, New England Medical Center Hospitals, Boston, Mass). The authors thank Dr Lau for having made his program available.

References

1. Richter GM, Noeldge G, Palmaz JC, et al. Transjugular intrahepatic portocaval stent shunt: preliminary clinical results. Radiology 1990; 174:1027–1030.

2. Lind CD, Malisch TW, Chong WK, et al. Incidence of shunt occlusion or stenosis following transjugular intrahepatic portosystemic shunt placement. Gastroenterology 1994; 106:1277–1283.
3. LaBerge JM, Somberg KA, Lake JR, et al. Two-year outcome following transjugular intrahepatic portosystemic shunt for variceal bleeding: results in 90 patients. Gastroenterology 1995; 108:1143–1151.
4. Sanyal AJ, Freedman AM, Luketic VA, et al. The natural history of portal hypertension after transjugular intrahepatic portosystemic shunts. Gastroenterology 1997; 112:889–898.
5. Barton RE, Rösch J, Saxon RR, Lakin PC, Petersen BD, Keller FS. TIPS: short and long-term results—a survey of 1750 patients. Semin Intervent Radiol 1995; 12:364–367.
6. Somberg KA, Riegler JL, Doherty M, et al. Hepatic encephalopathy after transjugular intrahepatic portosystemic shunts: incidence and risk factors. Am J Gastroenterol 1995; 4:549–555.
7. Sanyal AJ, Freedman AM, Shiffman ML, Purdum PP III, Luketic VA, Cheatham AK. Portosystemic encephalopathy after transjugular intrahepatic portosystemic shunt: results of a prospective controlled study. Hepatology 1994; 20:46–55.
8. Riggio O, Merli M, Pedretti G, et al. Hepatic encephalopathy after transjugular intrahepatic portosystemic shunt: incidence and risk factors. Dig Dis Sci 1996; 41:578–584.
9. Sanyal AJ, Freedman AM, Purdum PP, et al. Transjugular intrahepatic portosystemic shunt (TIPS) vs sclerotherapy for prevention of recurrent variceal hemorrhage: a prospective trial (abstr). Gastroenterology 1994; 106:A975.
10. Shiffman ML, Jeffers L, Hoofnagle JM, Tralka TS. The role of transjugular intrahepatic portosystemic shunt (TIPS) for treatment of portal hypertension and its complications: a conference sponsored by the National Digestive Advisory Board. Hepatology 1995; 22:1591–1597.
11. Pagliaro L, D'Amico G, Pasta L, et al. Efficacy and efficiency of treatments in portal hypertension. In: De Franchis R, ed. Portal hypertension II: proceedings of the Second Baveno International Consensus Workshop on Definitions, Methodology and Therapeutic Strategies. Oxford, England: Blackwell Science, 1996; 159–179.
12. Sacks HS, Berrier J, Reitman D, Ancona-Berk VA, Chalmers TC. Meta-analyses of randomized controlled trials. N Engl J Med 1987; 316:450–455.
13. Egger M, Smith GD, Phillips AN. Meta-analysis: principles and procedures. BMJ 1997; 315:1533–1537.
14. Egger M, Smith GD. Meta-analysis: beyond the grand mean. BMJ 1997; 315: 1610–1614.
15. Pogue J, Yusuf S. Meta-analysis duet: overcoming the limitations of current meta-analysis of randomised controlled trials. Lancet 1998; 351:47–52.
16. Poynard T, Conn HO. The retrieval of randomized clinical trials in liver disease from the medical literature: a comparison of Medlars and manual methods. Control Clin Trials 1985; 6:271–279.
17. Cabrera J, Maynar M, Granados R, et al. Transjugular intrahepatic portosystemic shunt versus sclerotherapy in the elective treatment of variceal hemorrhage. Gastroenterology 1996; 110:832–839.
18. Rössle M, Deibert P, Haag K, et al. Randomised trial of transjugular-intrahepatic-portosystemic shunt versus endoscopy plus propranolol for prevention of variceal rebleeding. Lancet 1997; 249:1043–1049.
19. Sauer P, Theilmann L, Stremmel W, Benz C, Richter GM, Stiehl A. Transjugular intrahepatic portosystemic stent shunt versus sclerotherapy plus propranolol for rebleeding. Gastroenterology 1997; 113:1623–1631.
20. Sanyal AJ, Freedman AM, Velimir A, et al. Transjugular intrahepatic portosystemic shunt compared with endoscopic sclerotherapy for the prevention of recurrent variceal hemorrhage: a randomized, controlled trial. Ann Int Med 1997; 126:849–857.
21. Cello JP, Ring EJ, Olcott EW, et al. Endoscopic sclerotherapy compared with percutaneous transjugular intrahepatic portosystemic shunt after initial sclerotherapy in patients with acute variceal hemorrhage: a randomized, controlled trial. Ann Int Med 1997; 126:858–865.
22. Jalan R, Forrest EH, Stanley AJ, et al. A randomized trial comparing transjugular intrahepatic portosystemic stent-shunt with variceal band ligation in the prevention of rebleeding from esophageal varices. Hepatology 1997; 26:1115–1122.
23. Merli M, Salerno F, Riggio O, et al. Transjugular intrahepatic portosystemic shunt versus endoscopic sclerotherapy for the prevention of variceal bleeding in cirrhosis: a randomized multicenter trial. Hepatology 1998; 27:40–45.
24. Groupe d'Etude des Anastomoses Intra-Hépatic. TIPS vs sclerotherapy + propranolol in the prevention of variceal rebleeding: preliminary results of a multicenter randomized trial (abstr). Hepatology 1995; 22:A297.
25. García-Villareal L, Martínez-Lagares F, Sierra A, et al. TIPS vs sclerotherapy for the prevention of variceal rebleeding: preliminary results of a randomized study (abstr). Hepatology 1996; 24:208A.
26. Sauer P, Theilmann L, Benz C, Richter G, Stremmel W, Stiehl A. Transjugular intrahepatic portosystemic stent shunt versus endoscopic banding in the prevention of variceal rebleeding: interim analysis of a randomized study (abstr). Gastroenterology 1997; 111:A1374.
27. Pomier-Layrargues G, Dufresne MP, Bui B, et al. TIPS vs endoscopic variceal ligation in the prevention of variceal rebleeding in cirrhotic patients: a comparative randomized clinical trial (interim analysis) (abstr). Hepatology 1997; 26:A137.
28. Pagliaro L, D'Amico G, Sörensen TIA, et al. Prevention of first bleeding in cirrhosis: a meta-analysis of randomized trials of nonsurgical treatment. Ann Int Med 1992; 117:59–70.
29. Laine L, Cook D. Endoscopic ligation compared with sclerotherapy for treatment of esophageal variceal bleeding: a meta-analysis. Ann Intern Med 1995; 123: 280–287.
30. Bernard B, Lebrec D, Mathurin P, Opolon P, Poynard T. Propranolol and sclerotherapy in the prevention of gastrointestinal rebleeding in patients with cirrhosis: a meta-analysis. J Hepatol 1997; 26:312–324.
31. DerSimonian R, Laird N. Meta-analysis of randomized clinical trials. Control Clin Trial 1986; 7:177–188.
32. Whithead A, Whithead J. A general pragmatic approach to the meta-analysis of randomized clinical trials. Stat Med 1991; 10:1665–1677.
33. Lau J, Ioannidis JPA, Schmid HC. Summing up evidence: one answer is not always enough. Lancet 1998; 351:123–127.
34. Laupacis A, Sackett DL, Roberts AS. An assessment of clinically useful measures of the consequences of treatment. N Engl J Med 1988; 318:1728–1733.
35. D'Amico G, Pagliaro L, Bosch J. The treatment of portal hypertension: a meta-analytic review. Hepatology 1995; 22:332–354.
36. Groszmann RJ, Bosch J, Grace ND, et al. Hemodynamic events in a prospective randomized trial of propranolol versus placebo in the prevention of a first variceal hemorrhage. Gastroenterology 1990; 99:1401–1407.
37. Feu F, García-Pagán JC, Bosch J, et al. Relation between portal pressure response to pharmacotherapy and risk of recurrent variceal haemorrhage. Lancet 1995; 346: 1056–1059.
38. Villanueva C, Balanzó J, Novella MT, et al. Nadolol plus isosorbide mononitrate compared with sclerotherapy for the prevention of variceal rebleeding. N Engl J Med 1996; 334:1624–1629.
39. Hauensten KH, Haag K, Ochs A, Lange M, Rössle M. The reducing stent: treatment for transjugular intrahepatic portosystemic shunt–induced refractory hepatic encephalopathy and liver failure. Radiology 1995; 194:175–179.

Book Review

Intraoperative, Laparoscopic, and Endoluminal Ultrasound

Edited by Robert A. Kane, MD

Philadelphia, Pa: Churchill Livingstone, 1999. ISBN 0-443-07998-6.
Hardcover, $130.00; pp 236; 274 figures; tables.

Air, bone, fat, and distance are barriers to sound transmission that reduce the image quality of transcutaneous ultrasonography (US). These obstacles can be overcome by placing the probe inside the body so that it is in close proximity to the organ of interest. This has become feasible with the development of miniaturized, high-frequency transducers.

Dramatic improvements in probe design and computer power in recent years have resulted in probes that can produce high-quality images despite their small size and have color and power Doppler US capabilities. Miniature probes have been incorporated into endoscopes and used to image the gastrointestinal tract from the inside. Even smaller catheter-based probes have been placed into blood vessels and the genitourinary and respiratory tracts. US is becoming an important tool in the operating room, where specially designed probes are used in conventional and laparoscopic surgery.

Intraoperative, laparoscopic, and endoluminal US studies usually require a collaborative effort between the radiologist and surgeon or gastroenterologist. Small transducers and the constraint of working within a limited space mean that the operator needs to acquire scanning skills that are different from those for conventional US. This book is meant to be a comprehensive, state-of-the-art review of intracorporeal US. The authors are radiologists and the book is aimed at radiologists, but surgeons, ultrasonographers, and operating room nurses will also find it useful.

More than half of the book is devoted to intraoperative US. The first chapter deals with technical aspects of US in the operating room. Intraoperative probes are compared, and different methods of probe sterilization are discussed. Intraoperative studies can potentially disrupt the work of a radiology department because they are often requested on short notice and require the presence of a radiologist and/or ultrasonographer in the operating room. There is a useful section in this chapter on how to organize and schedule intraoperative studies. The technique of cryoablation is covered in detail.

Subsequent chapters deal with intraoperative US of the liver, pancreas, biliary tree, kidneys, vessels, breast, and central nervous system. There is one chapter on the newly emerging field of laparoscopic US. Endoscopic US of the gastrointestinal tract is covered in two chapters and prostatic US is covered in one. One chapter deals with catheter-based probes, but there is little discussion of intravascular US. Transesophageal US of the aorta is covered in a single paragraph.

Each chapter is succinct and well laid out. The book is a delight to read and practically oriented, and it contains valuable tips on scanning technique. The illustrations, obtained from up-to-date equipment, are of excellent quality. A lot of information has been packed into a slim volume, providing good value for the price.

Few radiologists have much experience with intraoperative, laparoscopic, or endoscopic US, and there is a learning curve even for veteran ultrasonographers. This book will be particularly useful for practicing radiologists with little experience who are called upon to provide service in these areas.

Reviewed by Wui K. Chong, MB, FRCR

Kathirkamanathan Shanmuganathan, MD
Stuart E. Mirvis, MD
Caroline D. Sherbourne, MD
William C. Chiu, MD
Aurelio Rodriguez, MD

Index terms:
Abdomen, CT, 70.12112, 70.12115, 80.12112, 80.12115
Abdomen, hemorrhage, 791.41
Abdomen, injuries, 70.41, 80.41
Abdomen, US, 70.1298, 80.1298
Trauma, 70.41, 80.41

Radiology 1999; 212:423–430

Abbreviation:
FAST = focused abdominal sonography for trauma

[1] From the Department of Diagnostic Radiology (K.S., S.E.M.) and the Shock Trauma Center (W.C.C., A.R.), University of Maryland Medical Center, 22 S Greene St, Baltimore, MD 21201 and the Department of Radiology, University of Texas Southwestern, Parkland Memorial Hospital, Dallas (C.D.S.). Received June 22, 1998; revision requested August 13; final revision received December 10; accepted January 19, 1999. **Address reprint requests to** K.S. (e-mail: *kshan@radiology.ab.umd.edu*).

Author contributions:
Guarantors of integrity of entire study, K.S., S.E.M.; study concepts and design, all authors; definition of intellectual content, all authors; literature research, K.S.; data acquisition, K.S., S.E.M.; manuscript preparation, editing, and review, K.S., S.E.M., C.D.S.

Hemoperitoneum as the Sole Indicator of Abdominal Visceral Injuries: A Potential Limitation of Screening Abdominal US for Trauma[1]

PURPOSE: To determine, at screening ultrasonography, the prevalence, severity, and clinical outcome of clinically important abdominal visceral injuries, without associated hemoperitoneum, that result from blunt abdominal trauma.

MATERIALS AND METHODS: Computed tomography (CT) was performed at admission in 466 patients with visceral injury. A retrospective review was performed of findings from surgery and contrast material–enhanced spiral and conventional CT performed to verify abdominal visceral injuries in 467 (4%) of 11,188 patients with blunt trauma. These patients were admitted to a level I trauma center over 33 months to determine the presence of hemoperitoneum and to identify the grade of injury. Medical records of patients with abdominal visceral injury without hemoperitoneum were reviewed for the management required and for results of focused abdominal sonography for trauma (FAST).

RESULTS: A total of 575 abdominal visceral injuries were identified at CT and/or surgery. Findings of CT at admission (n = 156) and of surgery (n = 1) revealed no evidence of hemoperitoneum in 157 (34%) patients with abdominal visceral injury; 26 (17%) of whom also had negative FAST studies. Abdominal visceral injuries diagnosed in patients without hemoperitoneum included 57 (27%) of 210 splenic injuries, 71 (34%) of 206 hepatic injuries, 30 (48%) of 63 renal injuries, four (11%) of 35 mesenteric injuries, and two (29%) of seven pancreatic injuries. Surgical and/or angiographic intervention was required in 26 (17%) patients without hemoperitoneum.

CONCLUSION: Reliance on the presence of hemoperitoneum as the sole indicator of abdominal visceral injury limits the value of FAST as a screening diagnostic modality for patients who sustain blunt abdominal trauma.

Clinical findings are often unreliable and have low sensitivity for diagnosis of intraperitoneal injuries following blunt abdominal trauma (1,2). It is challenging, even for an experienced trauma surgeon, to determine the extent of abdominal injury and the need for surgical intervention on the basis of clinical presentation alone. Historically, most trauma centers in the United States have used diagnostic peritoneal lavage and/or computed tomography (CT) to diagnose abdominal injuries in patients with acute blunt trauma. Ultrasonography (US) has been recognized as a valuable primary imaging modality in Europe and in Asia for more than 20 years, but it was not until the 1990s that it gained popularity in the United States for the evaluation of trauma injuries (2–12). In the United States, surgeons and emergency physicians have developed an interest in US and are attempting to incorporate it as an initial diagnostic study in the examination of patients with blunt trauma or as an ancillary study to either CT or diagnostic peritoneal lavage.

The use of bedside US to evaluate patients with blunt trauma is based on the assumption that clinically important abdominal injuries are associated with free intraperitoneal fluid or hemoperitoneum. Most studies of the use of US to evaluate injuries from blunt trauma to the torso have used hemoperitoneum as the sole criterion of abdominal organ injury. The reported sensitivity and negative predictive value for US in depicting hemoperitoneum vary from 78% to 99% and from 93% to 99%, respectively (8–10,12–16).

However, previous smaller studies have shown abdominal injuries can occur without hemoperitoneum in up to 7% of patients with blunt trauma (15–17), but none or only a few of these patients need laparotomy to treat their abdominal visceral injuries. At our level I trauma center, Shock Trauma Center, University of Maryland Medical Center, Baltimore, CT is primarily used to screen patients for organ injury following blunt trauma, and our experience with CT suggests a high number of clinically important abdominal organ injuries do occur without associated hemoperitoneum.

We undertook a large retrospective study of patients with blunt trauma who were admitted to our level I trauma center to determine the frequency, severity, and clinical outcome of important organ injuries that occur without free fluid or hemoperitoneum identified at the initial diagnostic evaluation.

MATERIALS AND METHODS

During 33 months, 11,188 patients with blunt trauma were admitted to our level I trauma center. The trauma registry database was reviewed (by K.S., S.E.M., and C.D.S.) to find all intraabdominal injuries involving the spleen, liver, kidney, diaphragm, mesentery, bowel, pancreas, urinary bladder, aorta, and inferior vena cava (18). During the study period, traumatic intraabdominal injuries were identified in 467 patients (4%).

CT was performed at admission in 466 patients with abdominal injuries. CT and surgery reports on the 467 patients with abdominal injuries were retrospectively reviewed (by C.D.S., S.E.M., and K.S.) to determine the presence of hemoperitoneum. Three radiologists (C.D.S., S.E.M., K.S.) retrospectively reviewed the CT scans at the same time, by consensus, and were blinded to the results of focused abdominal sonography for trauma (FAST) in all patients whose initial CT interpretation included no hemoperitoneum. The abdominal and pelvic CT scans were reviewed, and the presence of hemoperitoneum, its location, and the grades of organ injuries were determined by consensus.

TABLE 1
American Association for the Surgery of Trauma Splenic Injury Scale (1994 Revision)

Grade*	Type of Injury	Description of Injury
I	Hematoma	Subcapsular, <10% surface area
	Laceration	Capsular tear, <1-cm parenchymal depth
II	Hematoma	Subcapsular, 10%–50% surface area; intraparenchymal, <5 cm in diameter
	Laceration	1–3-cm parenchymal depth that does not involve a trabecular vessel
III	Hematoma	Subcapsular, >50% surface area or expanding; ruptured subcapsular or parenchymal hematoma
	Laceration	>3-cm parenchymal depth or involving trabecular vessels
IV	Laceration	Laceration involving segmental or hilar vessels producing major devascularization (>25% of spleen)
V	Laceration	Completely shattered spleen
	Vascular	Hilar vascular injury that devascularizes spleen

* Advance one grade for multiple injuries, up to grade III.

TABLE 2
American Association for the Surgery of Trauma Hepatic Injury Scale (1994 Revision)

Grade*	Type of Injury	Description of Injury
I	Hematoma	Subcapsular, <10% surface area
	Laceration	Capsular tear, <1-cm parenchymal depth
II	Hematoma	Subcapsular, 10%–50% surface area; intraparenchymal, <10 cm in diameter
	Laceration	1–3-cm parenchymal depth, <10 cm in length
III	Hematoma	Subcapsular, >50% surface area or expanding; ruptured subcapsular or parenchymal hematoma; intraparenchymal hematoma >10 cm or expanding
	Laceration	>3-cm parenchymal depth
IV	Laceration	Parenchymal disruption involving 25%–75% of hepatic lobe or 1–3 Couinaud segments within a single lobe
V	Laceration	Parenchymal disruption involving >75% of hepatic lobe or >3 Couinaud segments within a single lobe
	Vascular	Juxtahepatic venous injuries (ie, retrohepatic vena cava and/or central major hepatic veins)
VI	Vascular	Hepatic avulsion

* Advance one grade for multiple injuries, up to grade III.

The scale devised by the Organ Injury Scaling Committee of the American Association for the Surgery of Trauma was used to grade injuries of the spleen and liver (Tables 1, 2) (19). The method described by Mirvis and Gelman (20) was used to grade injuries to the kidney. Abdominal and pelvic extraperitoneal hematomas were diagnosed by consensus as small, moderate, or large. Large hematomas were those that distended the extraperitoneal compartment and exerted a mass effect on adjacent organs. Medical records were reviewed (by C.D.S., S.E.M., and K.S.) to determine the surgical findings, FAST results, management, and clinical outcome for all patients who had organ injury without hemoperitoneum diagnosed at CT, surgery, or US.

CT was performed with a Hi-Q or Somatom Plus 4 scanner (Siemens Medical

TABLE 3
Abdominal Injuries

Organ or System	No. of Injuries in All Patients	No. of Injuries in Patients without Hemoperitoneum*
Spleen	210	57 (27)
Liver	206	71 (34)
Kidney	63	30 (48)
Mesentery	35	4 (11)
Pancreas	7	2 (29)
Gastrointestinal	6	1 (17)
Bladder	21	0 (0)
Vascular and/or retroperitoneal hematoma	20	14 (70)
Gallbladder	7	0 (0)
Total	575	179 (31)

* Numbers in parentheses are percentages.

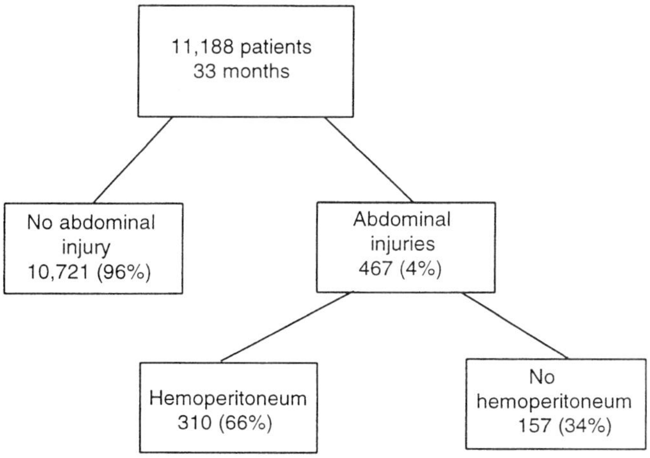

Figure 1. Flow diagram of patients admitted for blunt trauma.

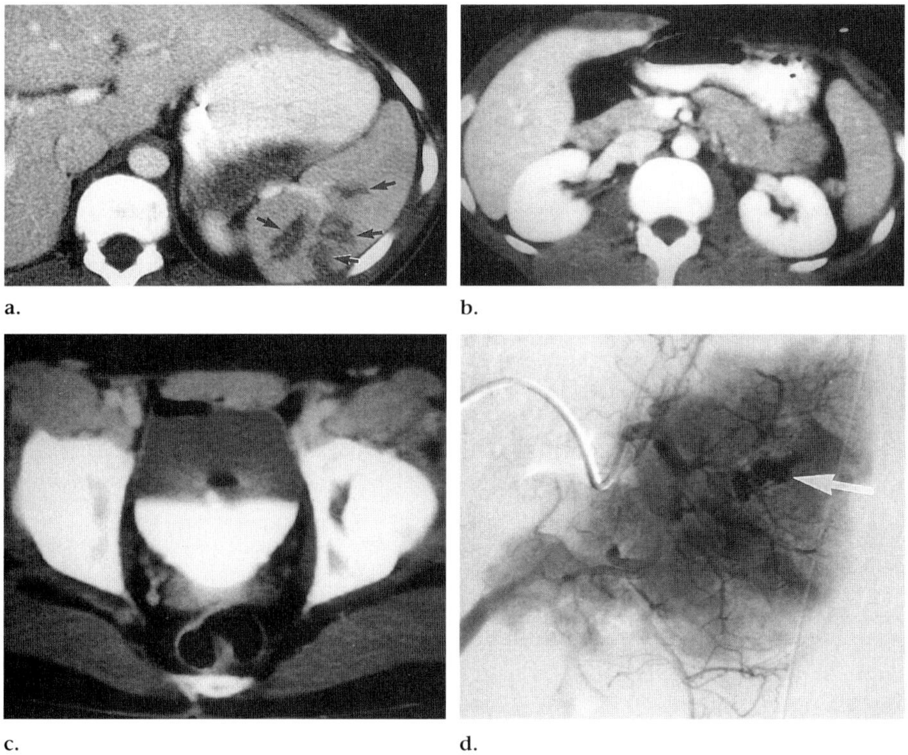

Figure 2. Grade IV splenic laceration without hemoperitoneum. **(a)** Axial CT image obtained at admission shows a grade IV splenic laceration (arrows). **(b, c)** Axial CT images show no hemoperitoneum in the **(b)** region of the hepatorenal fossa or **(c)** pelvis. **(d)** Angiogram shows a pseudoaneurysm (arrow) of the splenic artery with intraparenchymal extravasation of contrast material. The pseudoaneurysm was successfully embolized.

Systems, Iselin, NJ). The abdomen was scanned from the lower part of the chest to the iliac crest, and the pelvis was scanned from the iliac crest to the symphysis pubis. Spiral CT was performed with 10-mm collimation and a table speed of 10 mm/sec (pitch of 1). To visualize the excretion of contrast material in the pelvic ureters and bladder, a 100–120-second delay was instituted between abdominal and pelvic scanning.

Conventional CT was performed with a scanning time of 2.0 seconds or less, with contiguous axial scans obtained with 10-mm collimation from the lower part of the chest to the iliac crest and with 10-mm collimation at 20-mm table increments from the iliac crest to the symphysis pubis.

Contrast material (Hypaque 60% [diatrizoate meglumine] or Omnipaque 240 [iohexol]; Nycomed Amersham, Princeton, NJ) was intravenously power injected (Mark IV; Medrad, Indianola, Pa) as a 150-mL bolus at a rate of 3 mL/sec for spiral CT and as an initial bolus of 100 mL at a rate of 1.5–2.0 mL/sec followed by an injection of an additional 50-mL bolus at a rate of 1 mL/sec for conventional CT. All patients orally received contrast material consisting of 5 g of Hypaque powder (diatrizoate meglumine; Nycomed Amersham) in 300 mL of water 30–45 minutes prior to imaging, and, if time permitted, a second dose was given in the scanning suite, either orally or through a nasogastric tube.

FAST was performed and the images were interpreted by the attending trauma surgeon or trauma fellow in the admitting area during the initial evaluation of the patient. US was performed with a Sonoline model SI-400 system (Siemens Medical Systems) by using a 3.5-MHz convex sector transducer. Hard copies of the studies were not reviewed by either the radiology resident or the staff radiologist.

A nonrandomized, nonconsecutive subset of patients underwent FAST at the discretion of the attending trauma surgeon. FAST was aimed at the depiction of hemoperitoneum in three regions, including the hepatorenal fossa (Morison pouch) and right subdiaphragmatic space; the left upper quadrant, with attention to the splenorenal recess and left subdiaphragmatic space; and the pelvis, with attention to the rectouterine pouch (pouch of Douglas).

FAST results were interpreted as positive if hemoperitoneum was depicted in any of the three regions scanned and were interpreted as negative if no hemoperitoneum was found in these regions. All patients underwent further abdominal evaluation at CT or exploratory laparotomy, as indicated by the overall clinical presentation.

RESULTS

Of the 11,188 consecutive patients who were admitted with blunt abdominal trauma, 467 (4%) had visceral injuries that were ultimately diagnosed at contrast material–enhanced CT and/or surgery. A total of 575 injuries were identified (Table 3) among the 467 patients. Of these patients, 157 (34%) had visceral injuries without hemoperitoneum diagnosed at CT on admission (n = 156) or at laparotomy (n = 1) (Fig 1). FAST was also performed in 26 (17%) of the 157 patients without hemoperitoneum and revealed negative results in 25 patients and false-positive results in one patient with pelvic fractures and retroperitoneal and pelvic hematomas.

Among all the abdominal visceral injuries identified at CT or at surgery in the entire population of patients admitted with blunt trauma, hemoperitoneum was not seen in 27% of the splenic injuries (Fig 2), 34% of the hepatic injuries (Fig 3), 48% of the renal injuries, 11% of the mesenteric injuries, and 29% of the pancreatic injuries (Table 3).

Retrospective CT grades, determined by using the surgical scale of splenic and liver injuries diagnosed in patients without hemoperitoneum, are displayed in Table 4. Forty-one (58%) of the 71 hepatic and 23 (40%) of the 57 splenic injuries in patients without hemoperitoneum were classified as high-grade (grade III or higher) injuries on the American Association for the Surgery of Trauma scale.

Fourteen patients without hemoperitoneum also had large extraperitoneal hematomas that were diagnosed at CT on admission. Active hemorrhaging was seen in six of these patients (21,22). Eight of the extraperitoneal pelvic hematomas occurred as isolated injuries.

Among the 30 renal injuries that occurred in patients without hemoperitoneum were 19 (63%) minor and 11 (37%) major lesions. The major renal injuries included either large perinephric or subcapsular hematomas (n = 5), renal lacerations involving the collecting system or a transected kidney (n = 4), and renal vascular pedicle injuries (n = 2). The minor renal injuries included small perinephric or subcapsular hematomas (n = 8), segmental renal infarctions (n = 3), and renal lacerations without involvement of the collecting system with small or no perinephric hematoma (n = 8). Four major and six minor renal lesions occurred as isolated injuries, and the other renal lesions were associated with additional intraperitoneal traumatic lesions.

Three of the four mesenteric injuries in patients without hemoperitoneum were diagnosed at CT at admission and were managed conservatively with clinical examinations and follow-up CT. One of the patients had a mesenteric injury that was diagnosed at surgery to repair a ruptured left hemidiaphragm that was depicted at CT of the chest at admission. The mesenteric injury was directly repaired without resection of the bowel.

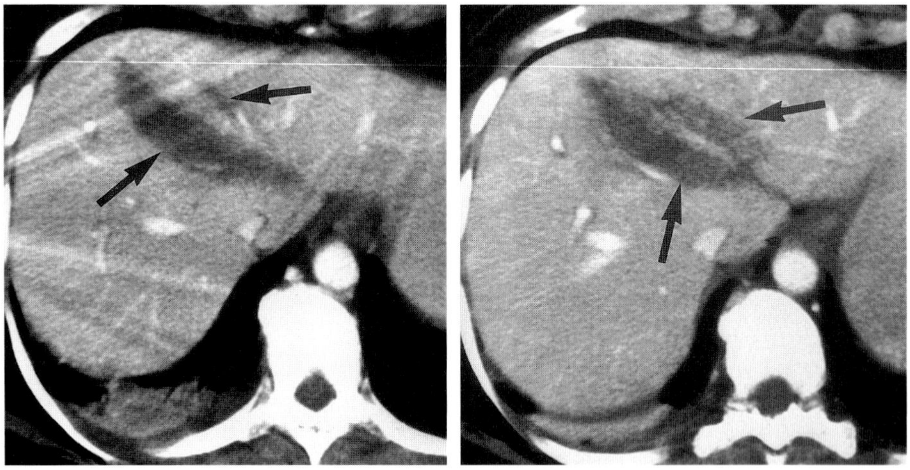

a. b.

Figure 3. Grade IV hepatic laceration in a patient without hemoperitoneum. **(a, b)** Axial CT images obtained at different levels in the hepatic region show multiple lacerations (arrows) involving the right and left lobes. No hemoperitoneum is seen.

Twenty-six (17%) of the 157 patients with abdominal injuries without hemoperitoneum required surgery (n = 19) or angiographic embolization (n = 8) to manage their injuries (Table 5). (One patient underwent both splenectomy and diaphragmatic repair.) Splenic injury (n = 14) was the most common reason (Table 5) for celiotomy (n = 9) or angiographic embolization (n = 5) (Figs 2, 4). Five patients without hemoperitoneum needed surgery, including nephrectomy in four patients and thrombectomy and reanastomosis of a renal arterial injury in one patient, for major renal injuries.

Three patients with pelvic fractures but no hemoperitoneum had sites of active bleeding within the extraperitoneal pelvic hematomas that required angiographic embolization. One patient underwent celiotomy to repair bilateral diaphragmatic injuries. In another patient, a transverse colostomy was performed for cecal and anal tears.

Nontherapeutic celiotomies, associated with pancreatic injury, were performed in two patients without hemoperitoneum. At surgery, one patient had a pancreatic contusion, a nonobstructive contusion of the duodenum, and a hemostatic grade III splenic injury, whereas the other patient had a pancreatic contusion and a hematoma of the proximal jejunal wall. None of the abdominal lesions in these patients required surgical repair. One of the patients without hemoperitoneum with a large retroperitoneal hematoma died of massive, uncontrolled hemorrhage into the retroperitoneum.

Twenty-nine (18%) patients without hemoperitoneum had combined abdominal injuries (Table 6). Thirteen patients had combined visceral injuries and 19 patients had intraperitoneal and retroperitoneal injuries. The most common combined visceral injuries involved the liver and kidney (n = 10). Five of the patients

TABLE 4
Injuries in Patients without Hemoperitoneum

Grade*	Splenic	Hepatic
I	4	10
II	30	20
III	18	25
IV	5	15
V	0	1

* American Association for the Surgery of Trauma classification.

TABLE 5
Surgery or Embolization Required in Patients without Hemoperitoneum

Procedure	No. of Patients (n = 26)
Splenorrhaphy	5
Splenectomy	4
Splenic embolization	5
Nephrectomy and/or renal arterial repair	5
Pelvic embolization	3
Diaphragmatic repair	3
Nontherapeutic laparotomy	2

Note.—One patient underwent both splenectomy and diaphragmatic repair.

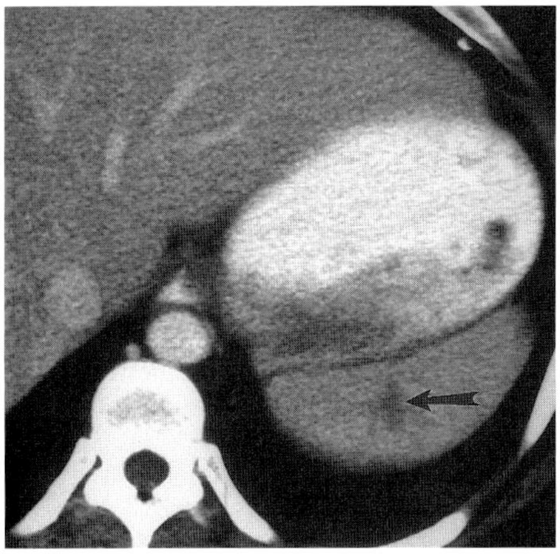
a.

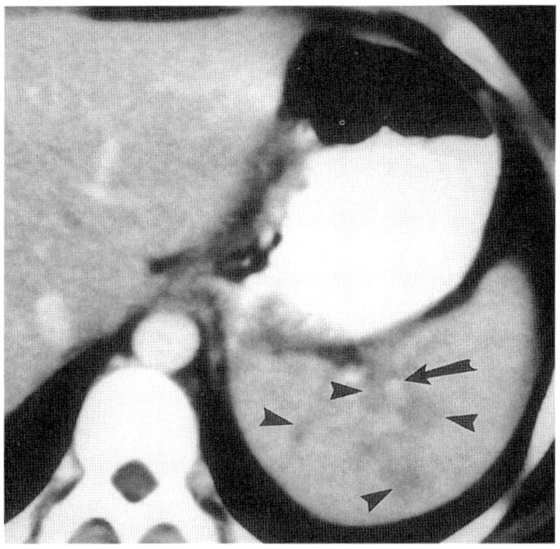
b.

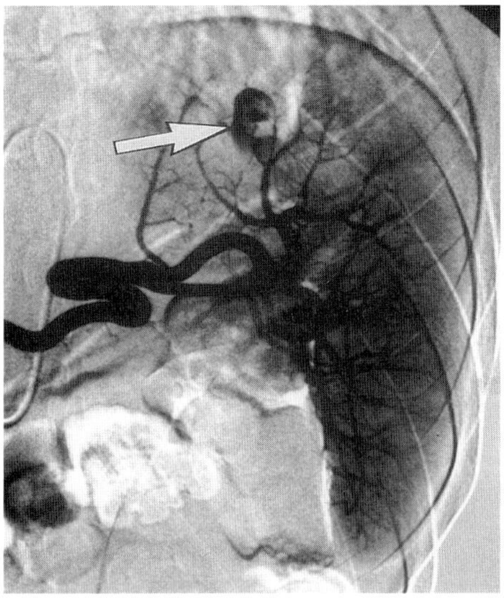
c.

Figure 4. Progression of low-grade splenic injury to a higher grade injury needing angiography. **(a)** Axial CT image obtained at admission shows a grade II intraparenchymal splenic laceration (arrow). **(b)** Follow-up axial CT image obtained 5 days after admission shows multiple splenic lacerations (arrowheads) with a splenic pseudoaneurysm (arrow), which indicates progression to higher-grade (grade IV) splenic injury. **(c)** Angiogram shows a pseudoaneurysm (arrow) of the upper pole branch of splenic artery. The splenic pseudoaneurysm was embolized.

without hemoperitoneum had three or more abdominal visceral injuries (Fig 5). Twelve (41%) of the 29 patients with combined abdominal injuries without hemoperitoneum needed laparotomy (n = 11) or angiographic embolization (n = 1) to manage their injuries.

DISCUSSION

The advantage of using US for the evaluation of patients with potential abdominal trauma is that it is a rapid, noninvasive modality that can be used at the bedside to depict hemoperitoneum. Serial US examinations can also be performed, if clinically warranted, at regular intervals.

Unlike previous studies, the current study demonstrated that 34% of patients with abdominal visceral injuries following blunt abdominal trauma did not have hemoperitoneum at CT on admission or at surgery. In 17% of patients without hemoperitoneum in whom visceral injuries were ultimately diagnosed, both admission FAST and CT findings confirmed the absence of associated hemoperitoneum. The high frequency of visceral injuries occurring without hemoperitoneum in this study could be attributed to the lack of a reference standard test (CT and/or surgery) in most previous studies (2,3,8–10,12,14–17) to verify US findings obtained at admission.

Also, the time from injury to diagnosis for most patients with trauma admitted to our trauma center is less than 1 hour. This brief time may not always be sufficient for intraperitoneal hemorrhaging to manifest from some intraperitoneal injuries. Since FAST relies on the presence of hemoperitoneum as the sole indicator of abdominal organ injury, 34% of the patients with blunt trauma and abdominal injuries (157 of 467 patients) would not have had their injuries diagnosed at US at admission if it were used as the sole screening modality.

Fifty-eight percent of the hepatic and 40% of the splenic injuries in patients without hemoperitoneum were a surgical grade of III or higher. Fourteen patients with large extraperitoneal hematomas and 11 (37%) of 30 patients with renal trauma had major injuries but no hemoperitoneum.

Our study findings demonstrate that substantial numbers of high-grade intraperitoneal or extraperitoneal injuries can occur without associated hemoperitoneum. Surgical or angiographic intervention was required to manage abdominal visceral injuries in 17% of patients who had no hemoperitoneum at CT on admission. The consequence of missing the injuries in the other 131 patients is difficult to extrapolate from our study findings, since all 131 patients were successfully managed with close observation of their hemodynamic status and with restricted activity.

Most trauma centers that use US as a primary screening modality rely on the assumption that any missed injuries are low-grade lesions without serious clinical consequence (13,23). Although this may be true for most hepatic injuries, splenic injuries have a more unpredictable course (24). It has been shown that the use of a CT-based grading system to select patients for nonsurgical management of splenic injuries is unreliable (24–28). In up to 15%–20% of patients with low-grade splenic injuries, conservative treatment has been shown to fail (24,29). It is well established that such injuries may clinically manifest later as delayed splenic ruptures (24,29,30).

In a recent study (29), conventional and spiral CT results demonstrated that nonsurgical management failed in 15% of patients with splenic injury, and 82% of these patients had low-grade splenic injuries with vascular abnormalities, including pseudoaneurysm or hemorrhage within the splenic parenchyma at CT either at admission or at follow-up. Early surgical or angiographic intervention in such patients could have reduced the failure rate of conservative management of splenic injury to 4% (29).

We have also observed the progression of initially low-grade splenic injuries to higher-grade injuries at follow-up CT (Fig 3). In this study, among the patients without hemoperitoneum with visceral injuries that were diagnosed at CT on admission, splenic injuries were the most common cause of hemorrhage that required surgery or angiographic embolization. Among patients with these injuries, six (43%) of 14 had grade I or grade II splenic injuries.

Our study findings validate the importance of diagnosing low-grade splenic injuries that occur without hemoperitoneum in hemodynamically stable patients. It is important to treat these patients with careful observation and with restricted activity and to document healing or progression of the splenic injury at follow-up CT.

Like diagnostic peritoneal lavage, US has known limitations in evaluating the retroperitoneum (2,8). Optimal evaluation of injuries to the kidney, pancreas, or duodenum and detection of retroperitoneal hematoma could be time-consuming and limited secondary to overlying bowel gas from the paralytic ileus that results from retroperitoneal injury, soft-tissue emphysema, difficulty in differentiating intra- and extraperitoneal soft-tissue planes, or inability to alter the patient's position.

A small amount of hemoperitoneum is not uncommon in patients with large retro- or extraperitoneal pelvic hematomas from red blood cells or plasma that enters the peritoneal cavity through a small tear or even through the intact serosal layer of the retroperitoneal lining (31). This could further add to the difficulty in determining the exact site of injury or hemorrhage (intra- vs retroperitoneal space). A large amount of hemorrhaging into the retroperitoneal structures is an important but not uncommon cause for the hemodynamic instability or occult blood loss in patients with blunt trauma.

In this study, 11 patients had major renal injuries and 14 patients had large retro- or extraperitoneal pelvic hematomas without hemoperitoneum. Five of the retroperitoneal and three of the extraperitoneal pelvic hematomas occurred as isolated injuries. Surgery, including nephrectomy and repair of a renal vascular pedicle injury, was required in five (45%) of 11 patients with major renal injuries. Three of the patients with large extraperitoneal pelvic hematomas had sites of active bleeding that required angiographic embolization.

At our trauma center, the FAST technique is not used routinely to evaluate the retroperitoneum. A substantial number of major retroperitoneal injuries that needed surgical or angiographic intervention occurred in this study. Although these injuries and sites of hemorrhage would have been missed at FAST, they were diagnosed correctly because, at our center, CT is used as the principal screening modality to evaluate these patients with blunt trauma.

Hemodynamically stable patients with blunt trauma could have concurrent injuries in multiple abdominal and pelvic regions. Prior knowledge of the precise extent and grades of the coexistent injuries is helpful in identifying the predominant injury, which guides the surgeon through the decision tree of clinical management. Although it produces highly sensitive findings in well-trained hands, FAST, unlike CT, is not specific to the site of origin and extent of injury.

TABLE 6
Combinations of Injuries in Patients without Hemoperitoneum

Patient No.	Hepatic*	Splenic*	Renal†	Retroperitoneal Hematoma	Other
1	II	III	Absent	Absent	Absent
2	III	Absent	Major	Absent	Absent
3‡	II	Absent	Major	Absent	Absent
4‡	III	II	Absent	Absent	Absent
5	Absent	II	Minor	Absent	Diaphragmatic
6‡	Absent	IV	Absent	Absent	Diaphragmatic
7	Absent	IV	Minor	Absent	Absent
8‡	Absent	Absent	Absent	Absent	Diaphragmatic and mesenteric
9‡	Absent	Absent	Absent	Present	Intestinal and mesenteric
10‡	III	II	Absent	Absent	Absent
11	II	Absent	Minor	Absent	Mesenteric
12	II	Absent	Minor	Absent	Mesenteric
13	II	II	Absent	Absent	Absent
14‡	Absent	III	Major	Absent	Absent
15‡	Absent	Absent	Major	Absent	Diaphragmatic
16	III	II	Absent	Absent	Absent
17	III	Absent	Minor	Absent	Absent
18	II	II	Absent	Absent	Absent
19‡	Absent	Absent	Minor	Absent	Diaphragmatic
20	IV	Absent	Major and minor	Absent	Absent
21	III	III	Minor	Absent	Absent
22	IV	Absent	Minor	Absent	Absent
23	Absent	III	Minor	Absent	Absent
24‡	III	Absent	Major	Absent	Absent
25§	Absent	IV	Minor	Absent	Absent
26	IV	Absent	Minor	Absent	Absent
27	Absent	III	Minor	Absent	Absent
28‡	Absent	Absent	Absent	Present	Diaphragmatic
29	Absent	Absent	Major	Absent	Mesenteric

* American Association for the Surgery of Trauma grade.
† Mirvis and Gelman (20) grade.
‡ Required surgery.
§ Required angiography.

Twenty-nine (18%) of 157 patients without hemoperitoneum had combined injuries, including concurrent intraperitoneal ($n = 19$) or intra- and retroperitoneal ($n = 7$) injuries (Table 6). CT was helpful in determining the predominant injury in 43% of the patients in the combined injury group and helped to prioritize patients for angiographic embolization or laparotomy.

The goal of this retrospective study was to ascertain the prevalence of abdominal visceral injuries that occur without hemoperitoneum and to determine if a substantial number of these injuries may need surgical or angiographic intervention. This study was not undertaken to measure the sensitivity, specificity, or accuracy of FAST at our level I trauma center.

Only 17% of 157 patients with blunt trauma who had abdominal visceral injury without hemoperitoneum underwent both FAST and CT and/or surgery at admission; FAST revealed false-negative results in 25 patients. A prospective study, in which FAST was performed at admission in all patients with blunt trauma who were evaluated consecutively with CT or surgical correlation, would have been optimal to determine the sensitivity, specificity, and accuracy of FAST at our trauma center.

CT and surgery are considered the standard or reference modalities for detecting hemoperitoneum in patients with trauma; CT and surgery were performed in all 157 patients with abdominal visceral injury without hemoperitoneum in this study (13,15,16,31–34). Prior study findings have indicated that a minimum of a liter of fluid should be present in the hepatorenal fossa for prompt, reliable detection of intraperitoneal fluid in 97% of patients at US in the trauma setting (11,35).

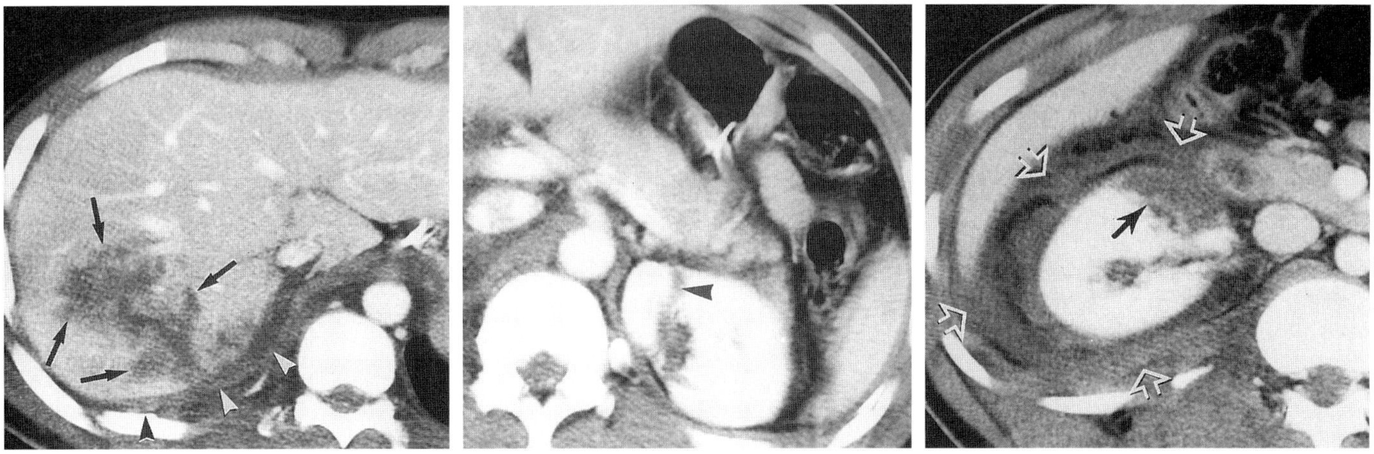

a. b. c.

Figure 5. Combined injuries of both kidneys. (**a**) Axial CT image shows a grade IV liver laceration (arrows) involving the right lobe. Posterior pararenal hematoma is adjacent to the bare area (arrowheads) of the liver. (**b**, **c**) Axial CT images show a minor left (arrowhead in **b**) and a major right (solid arrow in **c**) renal injury with a large right paranephric hematoma (open arrows in **c**). No hemoperitoneum is seen.

Most investigators in studies in which US is used as a screening tool for blunt abdominal injuries recommend clinical observation and monitoring of the patients with negative or indeterminate initial abdominal US results (23,36). None of these studies, however, define the indications for repeated US examinations, the intervals at which they should be repeated, and the number of negative results that are needed prior to discharging the patient.

At our trauma center, if no injury is identified at initial CT, patients may be discharged as soon as 3–4 hours following admission. Findings from a multicenter prospective study (37) also indicate that abdominal CT has a negative predictive value of 99.63% for the need for celiotomy following blunt trauma and that CT enables reliable identification of patients who do not require admission to the hospital. Abdominal CT can prevent the unnecessary and potentially costly admission of patients without documented injury for observation only and helps to more precisely select patients with multiple trauma injuries for surgical, angiographic, or expectant management.

Thirty-four percent of patients with abdominal visceral injury following blunt abdominal trauma had no hemoperitoneum at admission, but CT reliably depicted injuries that did not have associated hemoperitoneum. In this study, 17% of patients with abdominal and/or retroperitoneal injuries but without hemoperitoneum required surgical and/or angiographic intervention. Since FAST relies on the presence of hemoperitoneum as the sole indicator of abdominal visceral injury, it will fail to depict many intraperitoneal, as well as retroperitoneal, injuries.

References

1. Branney SW, Wolfe RE, Moore EE, et al. Quantitative sensitivity of ultrasound in detecting free intraperitoneal fluid. J Trauma 1995; 39:375–380.
2. Lentz KA, McKenney MG, Nunez DB Jr, Martin L. Evaluating blunt abdominal trauma: role for ultrasonography. J Ultrasound Med 1996; 15:447–451.
3. Kretschmer KH, Bohndorf K, Pohlenz O. The role of sonography in abdominal trauma: the European experience. Emerg Radiol 1997; 4:62–67.
4. Bode PJ, van Vugt AB. Ultrasound in the diagnosis of injury. Injury 1996; 27:379–383.
5. Bode PJ, Niezen RA, van Vugt AB, Schipper J. Abdominal ultrasound as a reliable indicator for conclusive laparotomy in blunt abdominal trauma. J Trauma 1993; 34:27–31.
6. Chambers JA, Pilbrow WJ. Ultrasound in abdominal trauma: an alternative to peritoneal lavage. Arch Emerg Med 1988; 5:26–32.
7. Rozycki GS. Abdominal ultrasonography in trauma. Surg Clin North Am 1995; 75:175–191.
8. Glaser K, Tschemelitsch J, Klingler P, Wetscher G, Borden E. Ultrasonography in the management of blunt abdominal and thoracic trauma. Arch Surg 1994; 129:743–747.
9. Goletti G, Ghiselli G, Lippolis PV, et al. The role of ultrasonography in blunt abdominal trauma: results in 250 consecutive cases. J Trauma 1994; 36:178–181.
10. Liu M, Lee CH, P'eng FK. Prospective comparison of diagnostic peritoneal lavage, computed tomographic scanning, and ultrasonography for the diagnosis of blunt abdominal trauma. J Trauma 1993; 35:267–270.
11. Huang MS, Liu M, Wu JK, Shih HC, Ko TJ, Lee CH. Ultrasonography for the evaluation of hemoperitoneum during resuscitation: a simple scoring system. J Trauma 1994; 36:173–177.
12. Rothlin MA, Naf R, Amgwered M, Candinas D, Frick T, Trerrtz O. Ultrasound in blunt abdominal and thoracic trauma. J Trauma 1993; 34:488–495.
13. Boulanger BR, McLellan BA, Brenneman FD, et al. Emergent abdominal sonography as a screening test in a new diagnostic algorithm for blunt trauma. J Trauma 1996; 40:867–874.
14. Gruessner R, Mentges B, Duber CH, Ruckert K, Rothmund M. Sonography versus peritoneal lavage in blunt abdominal trauma. J Trauma 1989; 29:242–244.
15. McKenney M, Lentz K, Nunez D, et al. Can ultrasound replace diagnostic peritoneal lavage in the assessment of blunt trauma? J Trauma 1994; 37:439–441.
16. Rozycki GS, Ochsner MG, Jaffin JH, Champion HR. Prospective evaluation of surgeons' use of ultrasound in the evaluation of trauma patients. J Trauma 1993; 34:516–527.
17. Lucciarini P, Ofner D, Weber F, Lugenschmid D. Ultrasonography in the initial evaluation and follow-up of blunt abdominal injury. Surgery 1993; 114:506–512.
18. Dunham CM, Cowley RA, Gens DR, et al. Methodologic approach for a large functional trauma registry. Md Med J 1989; 38:227–230.
19. Moore EE, Cogbill TH, Jurkovich GJ, Shackford SR, Malangoni MA, Champion HR. Organ injury scaling: spleen and liver (1994 revision). J Trauma 1995; 38:323–324.
20. Mirvis SE, Gelman R. Imaging of acute renal trauma. IX. Contemp Diagn Radiol 1992; 15:1–6.
21. Shanmuganathan K, Mirvis SE, Sover ER. Value of contrast-enhanced CT in detecting active hemorrhage in patients with blunt abdominal or pelvic trauma. AJR 1993; 161:65–69.
22. Cerva DS Jr, Mirvis SE, Shanmuganathan K, Kelley IM, Pais SO. Detection of bleeding in patients with major pelvic fractures: value of contrast-enhanced CT. AJR 1996; 166:131–135.
23. Boulanger BR, Brenneman FD, McLellan

BA, Rizoli SB, Culhane J, Hamilton P. Prospective study of emergent abdominal sonography after blunt trauma. J Trauma 1995; 39:325–330.
24. Mirvis SE, Whitley NO, Gens DR. Blunt splenic trauma in adults: CT-based classification and correlation with prognosis and treatment. Radiology 1989; 171:33–39.
25. Pappas D, Mirvis SE, Crepps JT. Splenic trauma: false-negative CT diagnosis in cases of delayed rupture. AJR 1987; 149: 727–728.
26. Buntain WL, Gould HR, Maull KI. Predictability of splenic salvage by computed tomography. J Trauma 1988; 28:24–34.
27. Becker CD, Sprin P, Glattli A, Schweizer W. Blunt splenic trauma in adults: can CT findings be used to determine the need for surgery? AJR 1994; 162:343–347.
28. Kohn JS, Clark DE, Isler RJ, Pope CT. Is computed tomographic grading of splenic injury useful in the nonsurgical management of blunt trauma? J Trauma 1994; 36:385–390.
29. Gavant ML, Schurr M, Flick PA, Croce MA, Fabian TC, Gold RE. Predicting clinical outcome of nonsurgical management of blunt splenic injury: using CT to reveal abnormalities of splenic vasculature. AJR 1997; 168:207–212.
30. Federle MP, Courcoulas AP, Powell M, Ferris JV, Peitzman AB. Blunt splenic injury in adults: clinical and CT criteria for management, with emphasis on active extravasation. Radiology 1998; 206:137–142.
31. Mirvis SE, Dunham CM. Abdominal/pelvic trauma. In: Mirvis SE, Young JWR, eds. Imaging in trauma and critical care. Baltimore, Md: Williams & Wilkins, 1992; 145–242.
32. Buzzas RG, Kern SJ, Smith RS, Harrison PB, Helmer SD, Reed JA. A comparison of sonographic examinations for trauma performed by surgeons and radiologists. J Trauma 1998; 44:604–608.
33. Ma OJ, Mateer JR, Ogata M, Kefer MP, Wittmann D, Aprahamian C. Prospective analysis of a rapid trauma ultrasound examination performed by emergency physicians. J Trauma 1995; 38:879–895.
34. Akgur FM, Aktug T, Olguner M, Kovanlikaya A, Hakguder G. Prospective study investigating routine usage of ultrasonography as the initial diagnostic modality for the evaluation of children sustaining blunt abdominal trauma. J Trauma 1997; 42:626–628.
35. Branney SW, Wolfe RE, Moore EE, et al. Quantitative sensitivity of ultrasound in detecting free intraperitoneal fluid. J Trauma 1995; 39:375–380.
36. McKenney KL, Nunez DB Jr, McKenney MG, Asher J, Zelnick K, Shipshak D. Sonography as the primary screening technique for blunt abdominal trauma: experience with 899 patients. AJR 1998; 170: 979–985.
37. Livingston DH, Lavery RF, Passannante MR, et al. Admission or observation is not necessary after a negative abdominal computed tomographic scan in patients with suspected blunt abdominal trauma: results of a prospective, multi-institutional trial. J Trauma 1998; 44:273–282.

Extravasation Detection Accessory: Clinical Evaluation in 500 Patients[1]

Bernard A. Birnbaum, MD
Rendon C. Nelson, MD
Judith L. Chezmar, MD
Seth N. Glick, MD

Index terms:
Angiography, complications, **.44[2]
Computed tomography (CT), contrast media
Contrast media, complications

Radiology 1999; 212:431–438

Abbreviation:
EDA = extravasation detection accessory

[1] From the Departments of Radiology, Hospital of the University of Pennsylvania, 3400 Spruce St, Philadelphia, PA 19104 (B.A.B.); Duke University Medical Center, Durham, NC (R.C.N.); Emory University Hospital, Atlanta, Ga (J.L.C.); and Hahnemann University Medical Center, Philadelphia, Pa (S.N.G.). Received July 30, 1998; revision requested September 4; revision received October 29; accepted February 15, 1999. **Address reprint requests to** B.A.B. (e-mail: *birnbaum@oasis.rad.upenn.edu*).

[2] **. Multiple body systems

PURPOSE: To assess the ability of an extravasation detection accessory (EDA) to detect clinically important (≥10 mL) extravascular injection of iodinated contrast material delivered with an automated power injector.

MATERIALS AND METHODS: Five hundred patients referred for contrast material–enhanced body computed tomography (CT) participated in a prospective, multi-institutional, observational study in which the EDA was used to identify and interrupt any injection associated with clinically important extravasation. The presence or absence of extravasation was definitively established with helical CT at the injection site (injection rate, from 1.0 to 5.0 mL/sec; mean, 2.9 mL/sec; median, 3.0 mL/sec).

RESULTS: There were four true-positive (extravasation volumes, 13–18 mL), 484 true-negative, 12 false-positive, and no false-negative cases. The prevalence of overall and clinically important (≥10 mL) extravasation was 3.6% (18 of 500 cases) and 0.8% (four of 500 cases), respectively. The EDA had a sensitivity of 100% (four of four cases; 95% CI: 51%, 100%) and a specificity of 98% (484 of 496 cases; 95% CI: 96%, 99%) in the detection of clinically important extravasation.

CONCLUSION: The EDA is easy to use, safe, and accurate in the monitoring of intravenous injections for extravasation, which could prove especially useful in high-flow-rate CT applications.

Automated power injectors have become standard equipment in radiology departments practicing state-of-the-art body computed tomography (CT) (1). These devices enable contrast material to be delivered as a uniform, high-flow-rate, nonfragmented bolus, which is essential for many contrast material–enhanced CT applications (2,3). This is particularly true for helical CT protocols such as CT angiography, hepatic biphasic CT, and pancreatic biphasic CT, in which contrast material infusion rates of 3.0–5.0 mL/sec have been recommended (4–7). The major risk associated with use of automated power injectors is the well-known complication of contrast material extravasation at the injection site. Previous articles (2,3,8–11) have shown that extravascular injection of contrast material occurs with a prevalence of 0.04%–1.3%. The vast majority of these extravasations involve small volumes of contrast material that result in mild soft-tissue injury and require only supportive care (8–14). Severe skin ulceration and necrosis are extremely rare but can result from extravasation volumes as small as 10 mL (15). Although conventional ionic contrast media are more toxic to the skin than are nonionic agents, extravasation of either type of contrast material may cause direct soft-tissue injury or neurovascular compromise secondary to compartment syndrome (13,16–24). These catastrophic injuries often necessitate plastic surgery or emergent fasciotomy and may place the radiologist at risk for litigation.

Traditionally, efforts to avoid morbidity from extravasation injuries have focused on prevention by identifying patients at risk and following recommended guidelines (13). We recently described an extravasation detection accessory (EDA) that is capable of detecting and interrupting automated injections complicated by extravasation (25). The purpose of this study was to assess the ability of this device to detect clinically important episodes of extravasation.

Author contributions:
Guarantors of integrity of entire study, all authors; study concepts, B.A.B.; study design, B.A.B.; definition of intellectual content, B.A.B., R.C.N., J.L.C.; literature research, B.A.B.; clinical studies, all authors; data acquisition, all authors; data analysis, B.A.B.; statistical analysis, B.A.B.; manuscript preparation, B.A.B.; manuscript editing, B.A.B., R.C.N., J.L.C.; manuscript review, B.A.B., R.C.N., J.L.C.

MATERIALS AND METHODS

We conducted a prospective, nonblinded, observational study in which the EDA was used to monitor automated injection of contrast material in 500 patients at four institutions. The research protocol was approved by an institutional review board at each of the participating centers.

Patients

The study population consisted of 500 adult patients who were referred for routine contrast-enhanced CT at the Hospital of the University of Pennsylvania (*n* = 125), Duke University Medical Center (*n* = 157), Emory University Hospital (*n* = 168), and Hahnemann University Medical Center (*n* = 50) between April 24, 1997, and November 6, 1997. There were 257 men and 243 women with a mean age of 58 years (range, 19–90 years), mean weight of 77 kg (range, 38–155 kg), and mean height of 170 cm (range, 137–206 cm). Patients were considered eligible for study participation if they were older than 18 years, willing and able to provide informed consent, scheduled to undergo routine contrast-enhanced CT (either as an inpatient or outpatient), and if they had at least one healthy, functioning arm without evidence of arterial, venous, or lymphatic insufficiency. Patients were excluded from participation if they were younger than 18 years, unable or unwilling to provide informed consent, unable or unwilling to comply with the protocol requirements, or if they had previously undergone mastectomy on the ipsilateral side of the injection site. The patients included in this study had not participated in any prior research involving the EDA and have not been previously reported on.

Scanning Protocol

All CT examinations (CT HiSpeed Advantage, GE Medical Systems, Milwaukee, Wis; CTI, GE Medical Systems; Somatom Plus 4; Siemens Medical Systems, Erlangen, Germany) were performed according to the standard of care as practiced in each institution. Intravenous access was established by a trained physician, nurse, or technologist. A new plastic venous cannula was placed in the peripheral arm vein in 479 (96%) of the 500 patients, whereas a preexistent intravenous catheter was secured for injection in 21 (4%). Existing catheters were used if they flushed easily with saline solution, demonstrated acceptable blood return, and showed no evidence of phlebitis. Injection sites for the 500 patients were located in the antecubital fossa in 391 (78%), the forearm in 49 (10%), the back of the hand in 37 (7%), and the wrist in 23 (5%). The left arm was used in 261 (52%) patients, and the right arm was used in 239 (48%). All intravenous cannulas were 20 or 22 gauge. Twenty-gauge cannulas, 1.0 inch (2.54 cm) in length, were used in 430 (86%) of the 500 patients, and 22-gauge cannulas, 1.25 inches (3.18 cm) in length, were used in 70 (14%). Metallic butterfly needles were not used in this study.

The appropriate type, concentration, and volume of intravenous contrast material was loaded into the power injector syringe (PercuPump II; E-Z-Em, Westbury, NY). Contrast material selection was based on patient history, the type of CT study to be performed, and individual institutional preference for contrast media class usage. Nonionic, low-osmolality contrast material (Omnipaque 300, Nycomed, Princeton, NJ; Isovue 300, Bristol-Myers Squibb, New Brunswick, NJ) was used in 349 (70%) of the 500 patients, whereas ionic, high-osmolality contrast material (Conray 60, Mallinckrodt Medical, St Louis, Mo; Hypaque 60, Nycomed, New York, NY) was used in 151 (30%). The mean intended volume of injection was 132 mL (range, 50–184 mL; median, 140 mL). The injection flow rate was determined by the supervising physician or nurse on the basis of the size of the venous cannula and the particular CT application. The injection rates used in this study were 1.0 mL/sec (*n* = 6), 1.2 mL/sec (*n* = 1), 1.5 mL/sec (*n* = 21), 1.8 mL/sec (*n* = 2), 2.0 mL/sec (*n* = 58), 2.2 mL/sec (*n* = 3), 2.3 mL/sec (*n* = 4), 2.5 mL/sec (*n* = 16), 3.0 mL/sec (*n* = 319), 3.5 mL/sec (*n* = 4), 4.0 mL/sec (*n* = 64), and 5.0 mL/sec (*n* = 2). The mean flow rate was 2.9 mL/sec (range, 1.0–5.0 mL/sec; median, 3.0 mL/sec). The distribution of flow rates appeared Gaussian (Fig 1). The maximal flow rate was 5.0 mL/sec for 20-gauge cannulas and 3.5 mL/sec for 22-gauge cannulas. A physician or nurse was available to manually palpate and visually monitor the injection site for extravasation during injection initiation (before scanning) in all patients (*n* = 500). At one institution (*n* = 157), a nurse remained with the patient to monitor the entire course of the intravenous injection. Radiation exposure to monitoring personnel was minimized in these cases with use of lead aprons.

The EDA was used to monitor electrical impedance at the percutaneous injection site in all patients. A detailed description of the appearance of this device and how it functions has been previously reported (25). In brief, the EDA consisted of a pliable, adhesive-backed electrode patch that was placed on the patient's arm directly above the tip of the cannula. The sensor patch was positioned so that the array of the electrode was in direct line with the tip of the cannula, with the axis of the cannula parallel to the axis of the array. The patch was then coupled, via connecting cable, to a dedicated power injector, where the EDA electronic processing module was located. Device setup

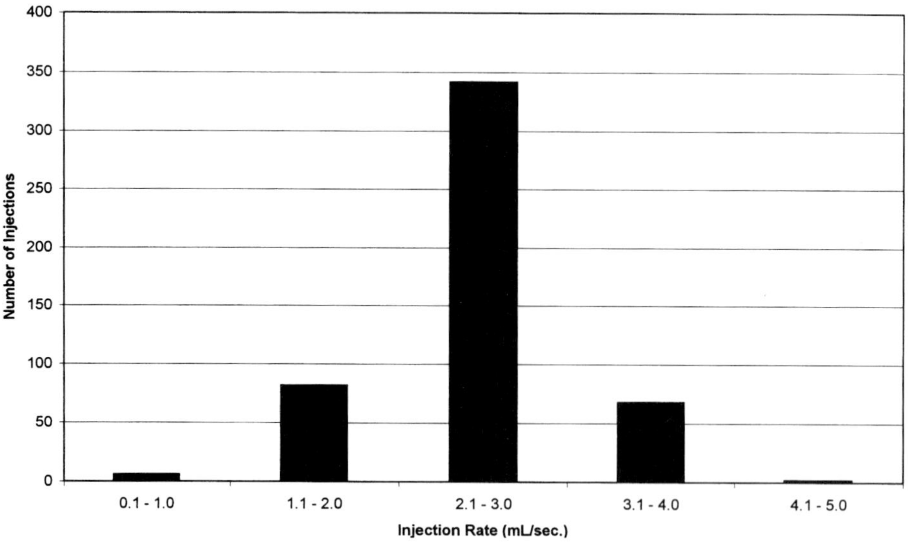

Figure 1. Frequency distribution of flow rates. A Gaussian distribution is identified, centered near the median injection rate of 3.0 mL/sec.

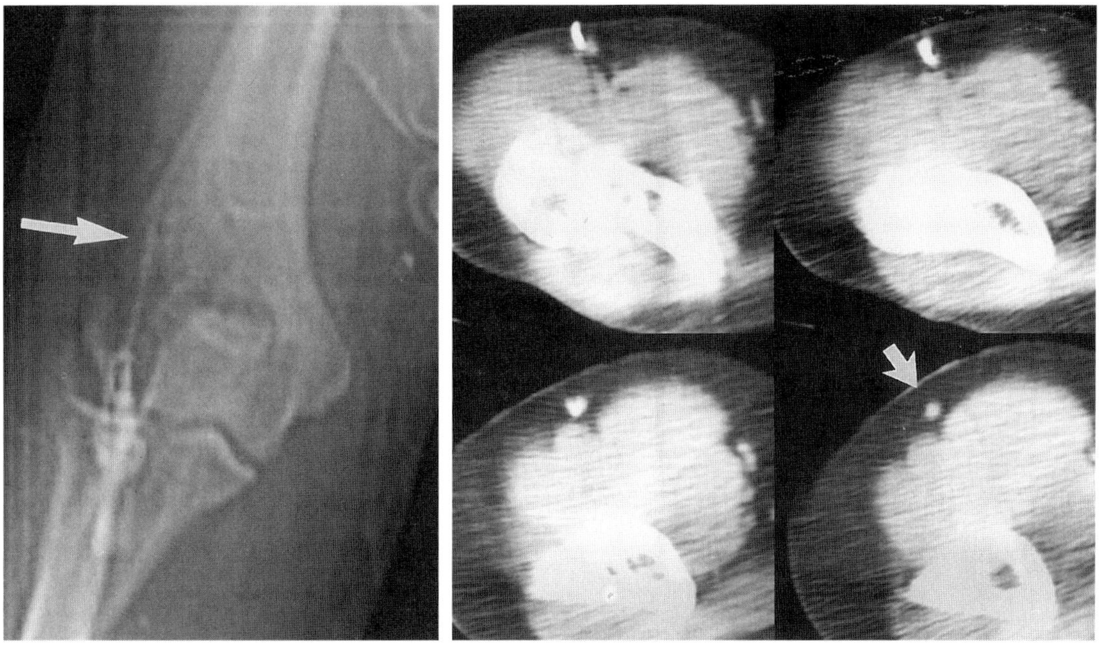

a. b.

Figure 2. True-negative case of nonextravasated injection. **(a)** CT scout view of the injection site shows no evidence of extravasated contrast material near the tip (arrow) of the radiopaque cannula. **(b)** Multiimage display of axial CT scans obtained at the injection site demonstrates that the injected vein (arrow) has a normal appearance, with no perivenous extravasation.

time for nursing personnel was less than 20 seconds. The EDA determined the baseline impedance of the skin and underlying subcutaneous tissues and then monitored the injection site for a change in this value during delivery of the contrast material. The rate of change or the slope of impedance over time was used to trigger an extravasation event, which automatically discontinued the injection and set the power injector into a pause mode (25). The EDA was calibrated to detect extravasation at a clinically important 10-mL threshold level.

If the injection was interrupted, as occurred in 16 patients, the injection site was evaluated by monitoring personnel to determine whether it was necessary to reposition the venous cannula to a new injection site and attempt another injection ($n = 2$), abort the injection entirely and continue CT with whatever amount of contrast material may have been successfully administered ($n = 6$), or reposition the arm and attempt another injection ($n = 8$). The power injection could not be reinstated unless it was deemed appropriate by the physician or nurse supervising the study. Impedance monitoring was halted and the sensor electrode removed at the conclusion of the injection. The power injectors used in this study were coupled to computer equipment, which collected the impedance data on floppy disks. This enabled ex post facto data analysis of concurrent clinical observations and device recordings and provided the device manufacturer with impedance data that could be used to analyze and improve the software algorithm of the EDA.

Proof of Diagnosis

After each patient underwent conventional contrast-enhanced CT, he or she underwent limited, low-dose (multiple scan average dose to arm, 0.42 cGy), 3-second helical CT of the injection site to definitively determine the presence or absence of extravascular contrast material. This CT examination was prescribed after a scout radiograph of the arm was acquired to precisely locate the cannula tip and was performed with 120 kVp, 120 mAs, 10-mm section collimation, 2:1 helical pitch, and contiguous section reconstruction. If extravasation was identified radiologically, its volume was quantitatively estimated by an investigator (B.A.B., R.C.N., J.L.C., S.N.G.) at each clinical site. This was accomplished by using the trace function software of the CT scanner to manually draw a line around the periphery of the extravasated contrast material on each axial image in which extravasation was identified. The trace function software automatically calculated the area of the region of interest. Data for the regions of interest containing extravasated contrast material were then summed together to provide an estimate of total extravasation volume.

Definitions

Extravasation was defined as the presence of any amount of extravascular contrast material at CT. Extravasation was considered clinically important if the volume of extravasation was at least 10 mL. Study definitions of outcome classification were based on the fact that the EDA was calibrated to detect extravasation at a threshold of 10 mL. True-positive cases were defined as those in which the EDA interrupted the injection and CT demonstrated clinically important extravasation. False-positive cases were defined as those in which the EDA interrupted the injection and CT demonstrated either no extravasation or extravasation of less than 10 mL. True-negative cases were defined as those in which the injection proceeded without interruption and CT demonstrated either no extravasation or extravasation of less than 10 mL. False-negative cases were defined as those in which the injection proceeded without interruption

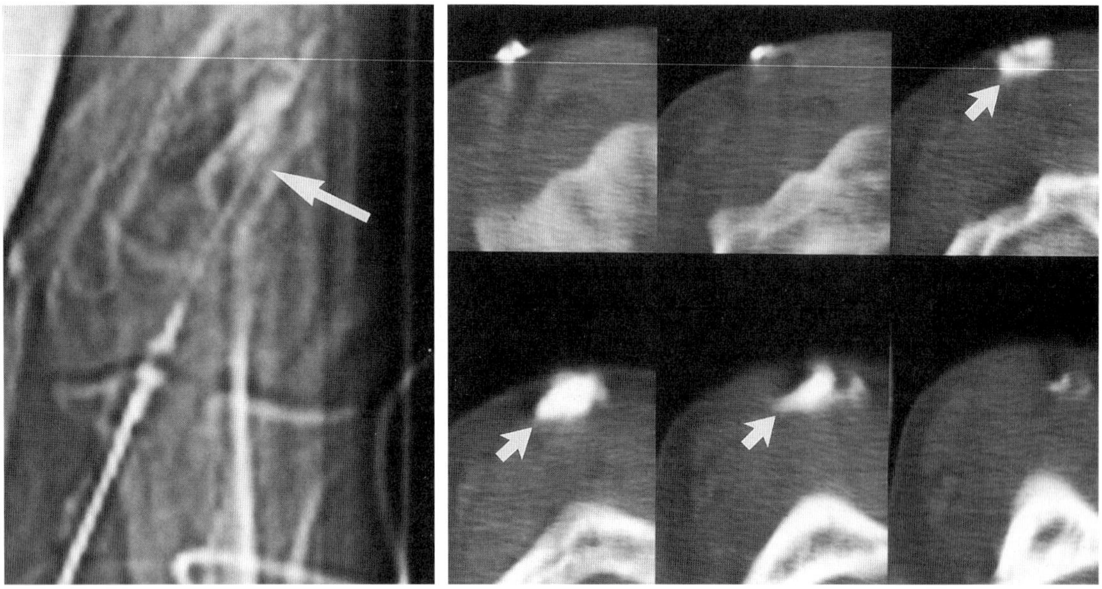

a. b.

Figure 3. True-negative case with trace extravasation. **(a)** CT scout view of the injection site shows a very small amount of extravasated contrast material (arrow) adjacent to the tip of the cannula. **(b)** Multiimage display of axial CT scans obtained at the injection site demonstrates perivenous extravasation (arrow), which was estimated to have a volume of 1.7 mL.

and CT demonstrated clinically important extravasation.

Statistical Analysis

The primary outcomes analyzed for the study population were the prevalence of overall extravasation and the prevalence of clinically important extravasation. In addition, the sensitivity, specificity, positive predictive value, and negative predictive value of the EDA for detecting clinically important extravasation were determined by using the foregoing definitions for outcome classification; 95% CIs were calculated.

RESULTS

Four hundred eighty-four (96.8%) of the 500 injections were determined to be true-negative cases. These included 470 cases in which the injection proceeded without interruption, the patient was asymptomatic, and CT demonstrated no radiologic evidence of contrast material extravasation (Fig 2). Also included in this category were 13 cases in which the injection proceeded without interruption and the patient remained asymptomatic; however, CT demonstrated trace extravasation of contrast material at the tip of the venous cannula (Fig 3). The volumes of these "subclinical" extravasations ranged from 0.5 to 3.0 mL. The last true-negative case involved a patient who received an antecubital fossa injection of nonionic contrast material delivered at 3 mL/sec through a newly established, 20-gauge intravenous catheter. This injection was interrupted by the nurse monitoring the injection site, who noted visual evidence of extravasation after 17 mL of contrast material had been administered. CT helped confirm the presence of extravasation, which was estimated to be 8–9 mL. Presumably, 8–9 mL remained within the intravascular space in this patient. Analysis of the impedance data from this injection revealed that the extravasation threshold of the EDA algorithm had not been reached and that the nurse detected the extravasation before the EDA was configured to trigger.

Four (0.8%) of the 500 injections were true-positive cases in which the EDA interrupted the injection and CT documented clinically important extravasation (Fig 4) (Table). These extravasations occurred at initiation of injection in one patient and during the course of the injection in three patients. This determination was made by comparing the volumes of extravasation (range, 13–18 mL) with the volumes of contrast material actually delivered with the power injector (range, 18–77 mL). Visual signs of extravasation (swelling or discoloration at the percutaneous injection site) were noted in all four cases, although this was very subtle in one asymptomatic patient and was identified only in retrospect after the EDA paused the injection. Most extravasations occurred in patients with newly established intravenous catheters (n = 3), 20-gauge cannulas injected at 3.0 mL/sec (n = 3), and nonionic contrast material (n = 3). Extravasation sites included the wrist (n = 2), antecubital fossa (n = 1), and forearm (n = 1).

There were no false-negative cases. All injections complicated by extravascular injection of at least 10 mL of contrast material were correctly detected and interrupted by the EDA .

Twelve (2.4%) of the 500 injections were determined to be false-positive cases because the EDA interrupted the injection and CT failed to document extravasation. All false-positive injections occurred at the antecubital fossa in patients with newly established intravenous catheters. These injections were primarily performed by using 20-gauge cannulas (n = 11) and nonionic contrast material (n = 11), with flow rates varying from 3.0 to 5.0 mL/sec (mean, 3.5 mL/sec; median, 3.0 mL/sec). The volume of contrast material delivered at suspension of injection varied from 8.0 to 124 mL (mean, 53 mL). In four (33%) of these 12 cases, the EDA paused the injection after only 8–9 mL of contrast material had been delivered. Nursing personnel monitoring the injec-

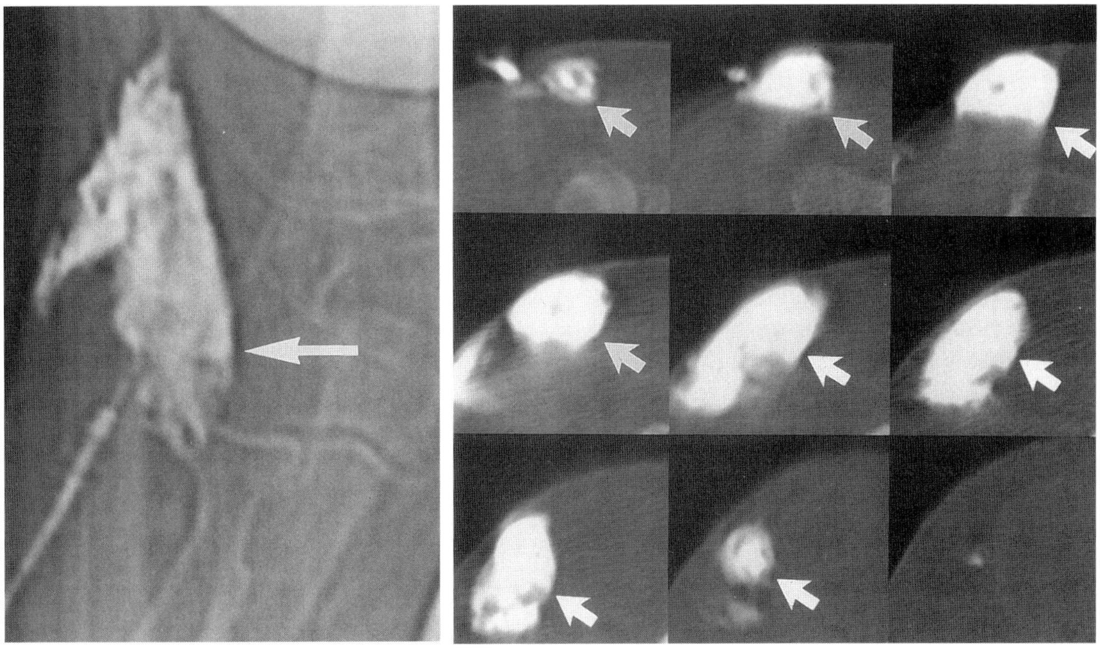

a. b.

Figure 4. Patient 1. True-positive case of clinically important extravasation. **(a)** CT scout view of the injection site shows extravasated contrast material (arrow) within the subcutaneous tissue surrounding the cannula. **(b)** Multiimage display of axial CT scans obtained at the injection site demonstrates perivenous extravasation (arrow), which was estimated to have a volume of 18 mL.

tion site were believed to have palpated the EDA sensor patch in these four cases as well as in five others during impedance monitoring as contrast material was being infused. One false-positive case was believed to have resulted from vigorous patient tremors during the injection. The cause of the EDA miscue in the remaining two cases is unknown.

The prevalence of overall extravasation and clinically important (≥10 mL) extravasation was 3.6% (18 of 500 cases) and 0.8% (four of 500 cases), respectively. The EDA demonstrated a sensitivity of 100% (four of four cases; 95% CI: 51%, 100%) and a specificity of 98% (484 of 496 cases; 95% CI: 96%, 99%) in the detection of clinically important extravasation. The positive predictive value of an EDA response was 25% (four of 16 cases; 95% CI: 10%, 50%), whereas the negative predictive value was 100% (484 of 484 cases; 95% CI: 99%, 100%).

DISCUSSION

Traditionally, efforts to avoid extravasation have focused on prevention by exercising special care in high-risk groups. These groups include patients who are uncommunicative or unlikely to complain of pain (infants and children, elderly, or unconscious) and severely debilitated or chronically ill patients who are at increased risk for extravasation and severe sequelae (12,13). Extravasation is more common when tourniquets are not released (24), contrast material is administered with metallic cannulas (26), multiple attempts are made to secure intravenous access (27), and injections are performed by using indwelling intravenous catheters that have been in place for more than 20 hours (28). In addition, substantial morbidity may result when extravasation occurs in the dorsum of the hand, foot, and wrist (24,29) or in an injected limb compromised by arterial, venous, or lymphatic insufficiency (13). As a result, it is advised that automated injection of contrast material be performed by using newly established intravenous catheters located at acceptable percutaneous injection sites and that trained personnel directly monitor the injection site for signs of extravasation (9,13).

Extravascular injection of contrast material is a well-known complication of contrast-enhanced CT (8–14). In most practices, the reported frequency of extravasation is less than 1% (3,8–11). Although the number of reported extravasations has increased since automated injection of contrast material replaced drip-infusion and hand-bolus injection techniques, the relationship between extravasation frequency and injection rate remains controversial. Sistrom et al (9) detected extravasation in six (0.1%) of 5,598 patients examined with an injection rate of 0.5 mL/sec and noted that the extravasation rate more than doubled (13 [0.25%] of 5,294) when the rate of infusion increased to 1.0–1.5 mL/sec. Recent studies performed with higher injection rates suitable for helical CT, however, have failed to demonstrate such a relationship (10,11). Federle et al (10) retrospectively identified extravasation in 48 (0.9%) of 5,106 patients examined with injection rates of 1.0–5.0 mL/sec and were unable to identify a linear trend between extravasation frequency and injection rate. Similarly, Jacobs et al (11) prospectively detected extravasation in 41 (0.6%) of 6,660 patients examined with injection rates of 0.5–4.0 mL/sec and showed no correlation between flow rate and frequency of extravasation. Neither study demonstrated correlation between volume of extravasation and injection rate.

Although most radiologists exercise diligence and follow recommended guidelines, extravasation of radiologic contrast material continues to be an event that occurs on the order of three to four times per month during contrast-enhanced CT. Moreover, automated power injection of

True-Positive Cases: Clinically Important Extravasation

Patient No./Age (y)/Sex	Injection Site	Injection Rate (mL/sec)	Cannula Gauge	New versus Existing Catheter	Type of Contrast Material	Volume (mL) Attempted	Volume (mL) Delivered	Volume (mL) of Extravasation	Time (sec) of Extravasation*
1/77/F	Antecubital fossa	1.5	22	New	Nonionic	147	18	18	0
2/60/M	Wrist	3.0	20	New	Nonionic	136	23	13	3
3/75/F	Wrist	3.0	20	New	Ionic	140	61	15	15
4/73/M	Forearm	3.0	20	Existing	Nonionic	92	77	15	21

* Onset of extravasation was determined as follows: time of extravasation (in seconds) = (volume delivered [in milliliters] − extravasation volume [in milliliters])/injection rate [in milliliters per second].

contrast material may result in large-volume (50–150 mL) extravasation because the mechanical injector will continue to infuse the contrast material at a fixed pressure regardless of whether the injection is intra-or extravascular (8,13). Modern injectors, such as the device used in this investigation, have the ability to automatically suspend an injection when a maximum pressure limit is exceeded; however, this technique has never been shown to be an effective means of detecting or preventing clinically important extravasation. Large-volume extravasation may result in severe damage to extravascular tissue. This complication is most likely to occur when the injection site is not monitored throughout injection of the entire bolus and when uncommunicative or asymptomatic patients experience a "silent" extravasation. In the first instance, monitoring personnel may leave the CT room to avoid radiation exposure and are unavailable to detect a delayed extravasation event that occurs after initiation of injection of the bolus of contrast material. In the second instance, monitoring personnel may fail to detect nonsuperficial extravasation if the patient appears to be in no distress. In our experience, this most commonly occurs in patients who experience painless extravasation of nonionic contrast material in the antecubital fossa (14).

Results of recent studies have shown that the overwhelming majority of patients who develop an extravasation tolerate it well and experience only brief and self-limited symptoms (10,14). Severe extravasation injuries are rare, but they can cause substantial morbidity. Severe injuries usually manifest as tissue necrosis and may require extensive débridement with split- or full-thickness skin graft procedures (9,13,14). Subfascial extravasation of large volumes of contrast material may result in compartment syndrome, which may necessitate emergency fasciotomy to relieve neurovascular compromise (10,13). Other reported sequelae of extravasation include hypoesthesia, marked extremity deformity, weakness, persistent pain, decreased range of motion, and difficulty performing activities of daily living (13,14). Many radiologists prefer to inject low-osmolality, nonionic contrast material to reduce the risk of severe extravasation injury. This practice is based, in part, on results in animal studies that have demonstrated nonionic agents are less toxic to the skin and subcutaneous tissues than are conventional ionic contrast media (16–19). Unfortunately, extravasation of moderate to large volumes of nonionic contrast material may still result in clinically important soft-tissue injury (14,21–23). Because the risk of injury often correlates with extravasation volume, every effort should be made to limit the extent of extravasation regardless of the type of contrast material used.

The EDA evaluated in this study is a U.S. Food and Drug Administration–approved, commercially available product designed to detect and interrupt intravenous injections complicated by low-volume extravasation (25). The EDA electrode patch serves to monitor tissue impedance at the percutaneous injection site and is configured to detect the change in impedance that characteristically occurs with extravascular injection of contrast material. The device is calibrated to detect extravasation at a threshold of 10 mL and to suspend the injection before 20 mL of contrast material is extravasated.

We found the EDA to be easy to use, safe, and accurate for monitoring intravenous injections for extravasation. The prevalence of clinically important extravasation in this study was 0.8% (four of 500 cases), which is comparable to extravasation rates recently reported in the literature (10,11). The device demonstrated a sensitivity of 100% (95% CI: 51%, 100%) and a specificity of 98% (95% CI: 96%, 99%) in the detection of clinically important extravasation. All true-positive injections were detected and suspended by the EDA, which limited the volume of extravasation to 13–18 mL. No false-negative cases occurred; therefore, the negative predictive value of an uninterrupted injection was 100% (95% CI: 99%, 100%).

The prevalence of overall extravasation in this study was 3.6% (18 of 500 cases), a finding that exceeds all previously reported extravasation rates (2,3,8–11). This reflects the fact that we used CT as the standard of reference, which enabled detection of 13 (2.6%) cases of trace extravasation (0.5–3.0 mL) of contrast material at the cannula tip in totally asymptomatic patients. These extravasations would have gone undetected if we had used clinical criteria for diagnosis. These cases were classified as true-negative because the extravasation volume did not reach the EDA threshold. The device functioned properly in these patients because the EDA algorithm was specifically designed to prevent clinically unimportant trace extravasation from interrupting the injection of contrast material (25). There was one additional true-negative case in which CT demonstrated radiologic evidence of low-volume extravasation (8.0–9.0 mL). This injection was suspended by a monitoring nurse who identified a very small, superficial extravasation before the EDA was activated. Ex post facto analysis of this patient's impedance data revealed that the EDA algorithm was functioning properly and that the nurse interrupted the injection before the EDA reached the required threshold for triggering interruption of the bolus injection. This case emphasizes the fact that diligent monitoring personnel will occasionally detect a superficial extravasation before the EDA. This will result in a slight reduction in extravasation volume, which may theoretically benefit the patient.

The posttest probability or predictive value of a positive test in this study was only 25%, which reflects the presence of the four true-positive and 12 false-positive cases. The low positive predictive value was not unexpected given the fact that we applied a very sensitive (100%) and specific (98%) test to a population with a very low (0.8%) pretest probability of disease (extravasation). It is not unusual for most positive test results to be false-positive when an excellent screening test is applied to a population with a low pretest probability of disease (30). Nevertheless, it is important to understand why these false-positive cases occurred because unnecessary interruption of uncomplicated injections can adversely affect scan quality and patient throughput.

Nine (75%) of the 12 false-positive cases were believed to have resulted from inadvertent manipulation of the EDA electrode patch during infusion of contrast material. This occurred when nursing personnel vigorously palpated the sensor patch within seconds of bolus initiation in four patients and while monitoring the course of the injection in five. Motion at the percutaneous injection site may have contributed to a 10th false-positive case in which a patient experienced multiple tremors during the injection. Ex post facto analysis of the impedance data in these 10 cases revealed that the false-positive findings caused by motion at the injection site may be averted by modifying the EDA software algorithm. As a result, the device manufacturer has since implemented this improvement to the EDA system. The cause of the last two false-positive readings is unknown. Further research is necessary to determine whether additional physiologic factors contribute to the impedance characteristics of intravenous injections. If this is the case, it may be possible to filter out additional signals that cause false-positive readings.

Several limitations of our study must be addressed. First, although the 0.8% prevalence of clinically important extravasation in this study is comparable to recently reported extravasation rates (10,11), we identified only four true-positive cases. It would have been optimal if a greater number of true-positive injections occurred, since this would have helped verify the ability of the EDA to detect all cases of clinically important extravasation. The small number of true-positive cases also precluded us from attempting to correlate injection variables with extravasation. Second, we determined the volume of extravasation by drawing area tracings around extravascular contrast material on axial CT scans and then summing data from these regions of interest together. This is not an exact measurement technique and may have resulted in slight under- or overestimation of extravasation volume. We believe that this technique allowed us to reasonably approximate extravasation volume to within 1.0–1.5 mL in those cases in which extravasation exceeded 10 mL, and it may have been more accurate for smaller extravasations in which it was easier to identify and trace the entire periphery of the extravasation. Finally, our study population was biased toward patients who received new intravenous catheters. Only 4% of our study subjects received injections via preexisting catheters. It is possible that our results may not be directly applicable to an inpatient population preferentially presenting with preexisting intravenous access. Nevertheless, it is encouraging that the EDA functioned properly and suspended an intravenous injection complicated by delayed extravasation in a patient studied with an existing intravenous catheter.

In summary, the EDA evaluated in this study demonstrated a sensitivity of 100% (95% CI: 51%, 100%) and a specificity of 98% (95% CI: 96%, 99%) in the detection of clinically important extravasation. Extravasation volume was limited to a maximum of 18 mL, and use of CT as the standard of reference helped confirm that the bolus of contrast material was not interrupted in patients who experienced inconsequential extravasation at the cannula tip. We believe that this device represents a technologic breakthrough in dynamic contrast-enhanced CT and has the potential to eliminate nearly all clinically important contrast material extravasation events, whether with ionic or nonionic contrast media. The device should prove especially useful for high-flow-rate CT applications because the EDA algorithm is configured to suspend extravasated injections at a threshold of 10 mL, regardless of injection rate. Its use may be particularly efficacious in patients who are at increased risk for extravasation and severe sequelae, including patients with preexisting intravenous catheters.

Further study is needed to assess whether successful implementation of the device will obviate support personnel to monitor the injection site. If so, the device has the potential to reduce radiation exposure to support personnel and simultaneously reduce costs and improve efficiency by permitting these individuals to be reassigned to other tasks (25). Although the EDA detected all cases of clinically important extravasation in this study, the number of extravasations was small. Additional investigation in a patient population with a higher prevalence of extravasation is necessary to confirm the high sensitivity that we report. A large-scale multicenter clinical trial is currently under way to determine the sensitivity and specificity of the modified EDA algorithm. This software enhancement should reduce the false-positive rate of the EDA while maintaining the high sensitivity and specificity shown in this study. If this is achieved, radiologists will be able to power inject contrast material with a higher level of safety and confidence.

References

1. Silverman PM, Kohan L, Ducic I, et al. Imaging of the liver with helical CT: a survey of scanning techniques. AJR 1998; 170:149–152.
2. Shuman WP, Adam JJ, Shoenecker SA, Tazioli PR, Moss AA. Use of a power injector during dynamic computed tomography. J Comput Assist Tomogr 1986; 10: 1000–1002.
3. Miles SG, Rasmussen JF, Litwiller T. Safe use of an intravenous power injector for CT: experience and protocol. Radiology 1990; 176:69–70.
4. Rubin GD, Dake MD, Napel S, et al. Spiral CT of renal artery stenosis: comparison of three-dimensional rendering techniques. Radiology 1994; 190:181–189.
5. Hollett MD, Jeffrey RB Jr, Nino-Murcia M, et al. Dual-phase helical CT of the liver: value of arterial phase scans in the detection of small (≤1.5 cm) malignant hepatic neoplasms. AJR 1995; 164:879–884.
6. Oliver JH III, Baron RL. Helical biphasic contrast-enhanced CT of the liver: technique, indications, interpretation and pitfalls. Radiology 1996; 201:1–14.
7. Lu DSK, Vedantham S, Krasny RM, Kadell B, Berger WL, Reber HA. Two-phase helical CT for pancreatic versus hepatic phase enhancement of tumor, pancreas and vascular structures. Radiology 1996; 199:697–701.
8. Cohan RH, Dunnick NR, Leder RA, Baker ME. Extravasation of nonionic radiologic contrast media: efficacy of conservative treatment. Radiology 1990; 176:65–67.
9. Sistrom CL, Gay SB, Peffley L. Extravasation of iopamidol and iohexol during contrast-enhanced CT: report of 28 cases. Radiology 1991; 180:707–710.
10. Federle MP, Chang PJ, Confer S, Ozgun B. Frequency and effects of extravasation of ionic and nonionic contrast media during rapid bolus injection. Radiology 1998; 206:637–640.
11. Jacobs JE, Birnbaum BA, Langlotz CP. Contrast media reactions and extravasation: relationship to intravenous injection rates. Radiology 1998; 209:411–416.
12. Burd DAR, Santis G, Milward TM. Severe extravasation injury: an avoidable iatrogenic disaster. BMJ 1985; 290:1579–1580.
13. Cohan RH, Ellis JH, Garner WL. Extravasation of radiologic contrast material: recognition, prevention, and treatment. Radiology 1996; 200:593–604.
14. Cohan RH, Bullard MA, Ellis JH, et al. Local reactions after injection of iodinated contrast material: detection, management and outcome. Acad Radiol 1997; 4:711–718.

15. Ayre-Smith G. Tissue necrosis following extravasation of contrast media (letter). J Can Assoc Radiol 1982; 33:104.
16. Kim SH, Park JH, Kim YI, Kim CW, Han MC. Experimental tissue damage after subcutaneous injection of water-soluble contrast media. Invest Radiol 1990; 25: 678–685.
17. McAlister WH, Kissane JM. Comparison of soft-tissue effects of conventional ionic, low osmolar ionic and nonionic iodine containing contrast material in experimental animals. Pediatr Radiol 1990; 20: 170–174.
18. Cohan RJ, Leder RA, Bolick D, et al. Extravascular extravasation of radiographic contrast media: effects of conventional and low-osmolar agents in the rat thigh. Invest Radiol 1990; 25:504–510.
19. Elam EA, Dorr RT, Lagel KE, Pond GE. Cutaneous ulceration due to contrast extravasations: experimental assessment of injury and potential antidotes. Invest Radiol 1991; 26:13–16.
20. Leung PC, Cheng CY. Extensive local necrosis following the intravenous use of x-ray contrast medium in the upper extremity. Br J Radiol 1980; 53:361–364.
21. Pond GD, Dorr TR, McAleese KA. Skin ulceration from extravasation of low-osmolality contrast medium: a complication of automation. AJR 1992; 158:915–916.
22. Memolo M, Dyer R, Zagoria RJ. Extravasation injury with nonionic contrast material (letter). AJR 1993; 160:203–204.
23. Young RA. Injury due to extravasation of nonionic contrast material (letter). AJR 1994; 162:1499.
24. Upton J, Mulliken JB, Murray JE. Major intravenous extravasation injuries. Am J Surg 1979; 137:497–506.
25. Nelson RC, Anderson FA Jr, Birnbaum BA, Chezmar JC, Glick SN. Contrast media extravasation during dynamic CT: detection with an extravasation detection accessory. Radiology 1998; 209:837–843.
26. Gothlin J. The comparative frequency of extravasal injection at phlebography with steel and plastic cannulas. Clin Radiol 1972; 23:183–184.
27. Stanley MD, Meister E, Fuschuber K. Infiltration during intravenous therapy in neonates: comparison of Teflon and Vialon catheters. South Med J 1992; 85:883–886.
28. Lewis GBH, Heckler JF. Radiological examination of failure of intravenous infusions. Br J Surg 1991; 78:500–501.
29. Gault DT. Extravasation injuries. Br J Plast Surg 1993; 46:91–96.
30. Riegelman RK, Hirsch RP. Studying a study and testing a test: how to read the health science literature. 3rd ed. New York, NY: Little, Brown, 1996; 183–191.

Corinne B. Winston, MD
June W. Chen, MD
Yuman Fong, MD
Lawrence H. Schwartz, MD
David M. Panicek, MD

Index terms:
Abdominal wall, 762.331
Cholecystectomy, 762.1267
Gallbladder, CT, 762.12112, 762.12115
Gallbladder, MR, 762.121411
Gallbladder, neoplasms, 762.32
Laparoscopic surgery, 762.1267
Surgery, complications, 762.458

Radiology 1999; 212:439–444

[1] From the Department of Radiology, Memorial Sloan-Kettering Cancer Center, 1275 York Ave, New York, NY 10021. Received July 31, 1998; revision requested September 10; revision received October 28; accepted January 11, 1999. **Address reprint requests to** C.B.W. (e-mail: *winstonc@mskcc.org*).

Author contributions:
Guarantors of integrity of entire study, C.B.W., J.W.C., D.M.P.; study concepts, C.B.W., J.W.C., Y.F., D.M.P.; study design, C.B.W., J.W.C., D.M.P.; definition of intellectual content, all authors; literature research, C.B.W.; data acquisition, C.B.W., J.W.C., D.M.P.; data analysis, C.B.W.; manuscript preparation, C.B.W., D.M.P.; manuscript editing and review, all authors.

Recurrent Gallbladder Carcinoma along Laparoscopic Cholecystectomy Port Tracks: CT Demonstration[1]

PURPOSE: To describe the computed tomographic (CT) appearance of recurrent gallbladder carcinoma along port tracks after laparoscopic cholecystectomy and to assess the effect of recurrence on patient care.

MATERIALS AND METHODS: Seventeen abdominal CT scans in 16 of 19 consecutive patients who underwent hepatic resection for gallbladder carcinoma diagnosed at laparoscopic cholecystectomy were reviewed retrospectively. Medical records were reviewed to determine the clinical effect of tumor recurrence along a port track.

RESULTS: CT revealed 12 tumor recurrences along laparoscopic port tracks in six (32%) patients (mean, two recurrences per patient; range, one to four per patient). Eight (67%) CT-depicted recurrences appeared homogeneous, and nine (75%) directly involved subjacent omental fat. The mass was the only site of recurrence at CT in two (33%) patients. The presence of an abdominal wall tumor recurrence affected patient care in four (67%) of six patients. Histopathologic examination results confirmed recurrent tumor in all five (100%) patients who underwent biopsy.

CONCLUSION: Tumor recurrence along port tracks is a potential complication of laparoscopic cholecystectomy when gallbladder carcinoma is present, even after subsequent hepatic resection is performed for attempted cure. Recurrences appear as a new or enlarging abdominal wall mass, often involving subjacent omental fat, and may be the only site of recurrent disease at CT. Demonstration of abdominal wall tumor recurrence affects patient care.

Laparoscopic cholecystectomy has become increasingly accepted in the treatment of uncomplicated symptomatic cholelithiasis (1). Complications of laparoscopic cholecystectomy previously described include bile duct injury, retained stones, spilled gallstones throughout the abdomen, bowel perforation from trocar insertion, and abdominal wall hematoma (2). An additional serious complication of laparoscopic cholecystectomy with delayed manifestations is the inadvertent dissemination of unsuspected gallbladder carcinoma (3–16).

Approximately 15%–30% of gallbladder carcinomas are detected incidentally at microscopic review of cholecystectomy specimens (16). Hepatic resection, common bile duct excision, and portal lymphadenectomy have been suggested as treatment for gallbladder carcinoma that is incidentally detected at cholecystectomy (17). Patients are often followed up with computed tomography (CT) after hepatic resection to assess for tumor recurrence. The purpose of our study was to describe the CT appearance of laparoscopic port track tumor recurrences in patients who underwent definitive hepatic resection for gallbladder carcinoma diagnosed at laparoscopic cholecystectomy and to assess the effect of the abdominal wall tumor recurrence on patient care.

MATERIALS AND METHODS

Patient Population

In a search of the hepatobiliary tumor database at our institution, we identified 42 patients referred from January 1991 to November 1996 for definitive hepatic resection of

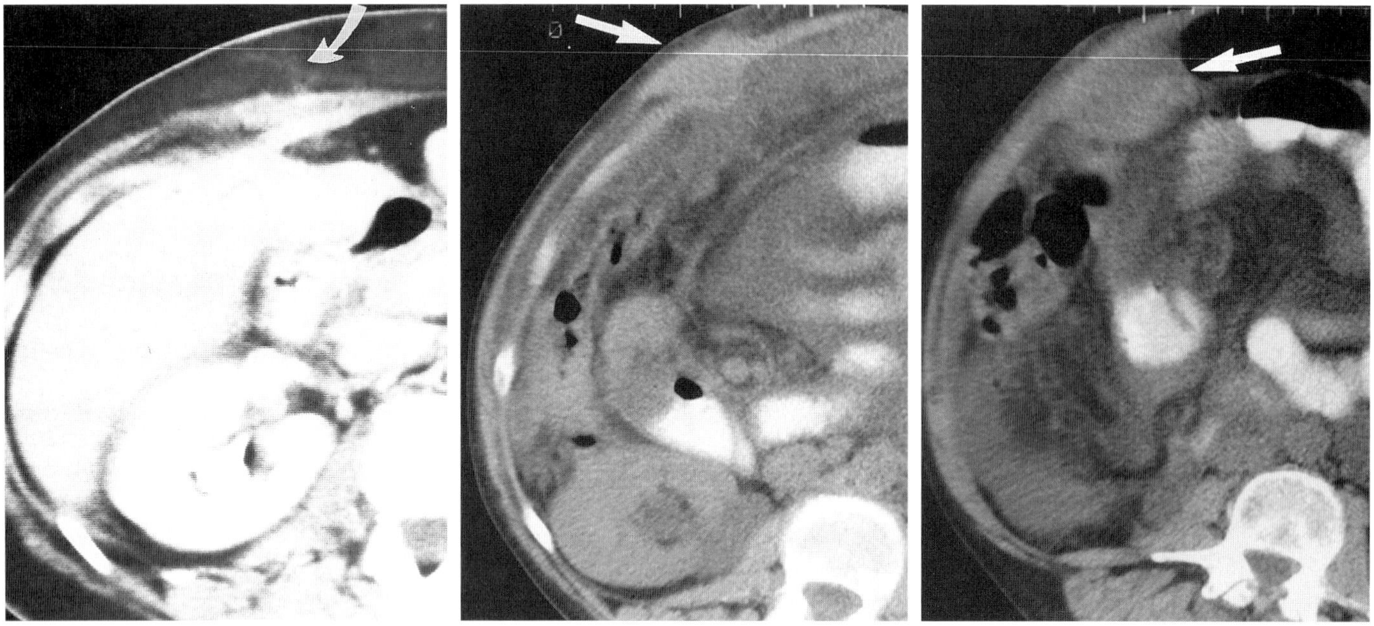

a. b. c.

Figure 1. Tumor recurrence along the port track near the lateral border of the right rectus abdominis muscle. **(a)** Axial CT image obtained following laparoscopic cholecystectomy reveals postsurgical change in the anterior abdominal wall along the laparoscopic port site (arrow). **(b, c)** Follow-up axial CT images obtained 6 months after **a** reveal a new mass along the initial laparoscopic port track (arrow, **b**); the mass extends into the omental fat (arrow, **c**). Histopathologic examination results confirmed the presence of recurrent gallbladder carcinoma.

gallbladder carcinoma that was diagnosed at laparoscopic cholecystectomy. Carcinoma was suspected prior to the laparoscopic cholecystectomy in three (7%) patients. Laparoscopic cholecystectomy was converted to open cholecystectomy in five patients owing to extensive inflammation within the gallbladder fossa ($n = 2$), discovery of unsuspected gallbladder carcinoma intraoperatively ($n = 2$), and detection of unsuspected hepatic metastases ($n = 1$).

One (2%) patient had a T1 gallbladder carcinoma (ie, tumor confined to the mucosal or muscular layer) (18) for which no additional surgery was considered necessary. Twenty-two patients had lesions that were deemed unresectable at imaging after laparoscopic cholecystectomy or at exploratory laparotomy. Nineteen patients (14 women, five men; mean age, 60 years; age range, 34–78 years) underwent a definitive surgical procedure for potential cure. The mean interval between laparoscopic cholecystectomy and definitive hepatic surgery was 40 days (range, 18–94 days).

Thirteen patients underwent an extended right hepatectomy, common bile duct excision, portal lymphadenectomy, and hepaticojejunostomy. Five patients underwent resection of hepatic segments 4 and 5, excision of the common bile duct, lymphadenectomy, and hepaticojejunostomy. One patient underwent a limited en bloc resection of the liver surrounding the gallbladder fossa, common bile duct excision, lymphadenectomy, and hepaticojejunostomy. The final histopathologic diagnoses were adenocarcinoma ($n = 17$) and adenosquamous carcinoma ($n = 2$).

Of the 19 patients who underwent definitive surgical resection, one patient had a T1 tumor with a positive lymph node, eight had T2 tumors (tumor invading the perimuscular connective tissue without extension into the liver), and eight had T3 tumors (tumor invading the serosa and one adjacent organ, or invading into liver less than 2 cm). Two patients had a T4 tumor (more than 2-cm invasion into liver). Seventeen port tracks were resected in eight patients at definitive surgery: Three patients underwent resection of one track, two patients underwent resection of two tracks, two underwent resection of three tracks, and one underwent resection of four tracks. Gallbladder carcinoma was identified at histopathologic examination in three (18%) of the tracks resected.

CT Findings

Retrospective review of abdominal CT scans obtained following definitive hepatic resection was performed by two experienced oncologic radiologists (C.B.W., D.M.P.) in consensus to assess for the presence of anterior abdominal wall tumor recurrence. If multiple postoperative CT scans had been obtained in a single patient, the most recent scan (ie, the examination performed the longest time after hepatic resection) was reviewed. All CT scans were evaluated in conjunction with a prior CT ($n = 15$) or magnetic resonance (MR) ($n = 2$) image for comparison. If the comparison examination revealed evidence of an additional anterior abdominal wall mass, data also were obtained from that study ($n = 1$).

Seventeen CT examinations in 16 (84%) patients (11 women, five men; age range, 34–78 years) were included in this study. No postoperative CT scans were available in three (16%) patients. The mean interval between the definitive hepatic resection and follow-up CT was 18 months (range, 1–62 months). Fifteen CT examinations were performed with use of intravenous contrast material; 17 scans were obtained with use of oral contrast material. Ten of 17 examinations were performed by using a helical technique.

A new or enlarging anterior abdominal wall mass was considered diagnostic of tumor recurrence. Linear infiltration within the anterior abdominal wall was considered to represent postoperative change. The radiologists (C.B.W., D.M.P.) determined the location of the mass and assessed for associated involvement of subjacent omental fat. The relative size of the mass was calculated as the product of

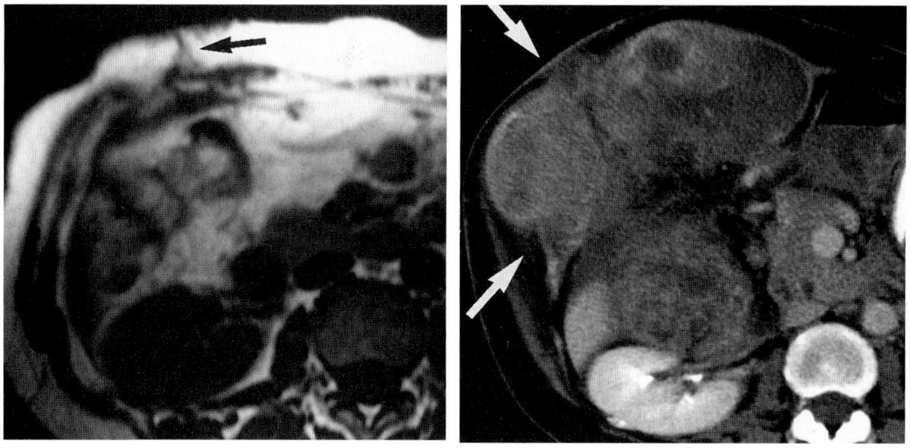

a. b.

Figure 2. Tumor recurrence along the large laparoscopic port track. **(a)** Axial spin-echo T1-weighted (repetition time, 650 msec; echo time, 9 msec) MR image obtained following laparoscopic cholecystectomy reveals linear postsurgical change within the subcutaneous fat along the laparoscopic track (arrow). **(b)** Axial CT image obtained 1 year after definitive hepatic surgery reveals a large mass (arrows) in the location of the laparoscopic track seen in **a**; the mass involves subcutaneous fat, abdominal wall muscles, and omental fat.

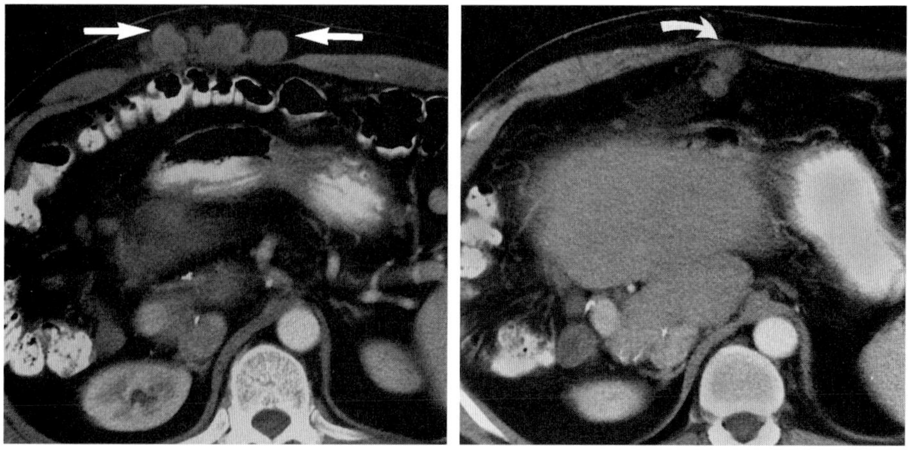

a. b.

Figure 3. Tumor recurrence along the subxiphoid port track. **(a)** Axial CT image reveals soft-tissue nodules within the subcutaneous fat of the anterior abdominal wall along the subxiphoid laparoscopic port track (arrows). **(b)** Axial CT image obtained 2 cm caudad to **a** reveals soft-tissue nodules (arrow) within the omental fat. Histopathologic examination results confirmed the presence of recurrent gallbladder carcinoma.

the greatest perpendicular diameters obtained from an axial image. Masses were categorized as homogeneous or heterogeneous. The presence of a mesh prosthesis, lymphadenopathy, hepatic metastases, and peritoneal carcinomatosis was recorded.

Clinical Follow-up

Medical records were reviewed to assess for clinical evidence of abdominal wall tumor recurrence and the effect of an abdominal wall tumor recurrence on patient care. Review of histopathology reports and surgical notes was performed to confirm the presence of recurrent tumor in those patients who underwent biopsy and to determine whether any of the laparoscopic port tracks were resected at the time of definitive surgery.

RESULTS

CT revealed 12 abdominal wall tumor recurrences along the laparoscopic port tracks in six (32%) patients. Five (83%) of the six patients had more than one recurrence (four patients had two recurrences and one patient had three). The mean interval between definitive hepatic resection and abdominal wall tumor recurrence seen at CT was 17 months (range, 6–41 months). Four recurrences were along the port track near the lateral aspect of the right rectus abdominis muscle, four were located just anterior to or within the right rectus abdominis muscle port track, and two were located within the left rectus abdominis muscle port track. One recurrence was located along the periumbilical port track, and one was along the subxiphoid port track. Two patients had a prior abdominal wall tumor recurrence surgically resected with placement of a mesh prosthesis; CT revealed recurrent tumor along the prosthesis in both patients.

The mean bidimensional product of the abdominal wall mass was 29.7 cm^2 (range, 1.2–217.0 cm^2). Nine (75%) recurrent masses directly involved the subjacent omental fat (Figs 1–3). All nine of these recurrences had peritoneal carcinomatosis elsewhere in the abdomen at CT. None of the anterior abdominal wall tumor recurrences without extension into the omental fat had peritoneal carcinomatosis at CT. Eight (67%) masses were of homogeneous soft-tissue attenuation. Ten patients had no evidence of recurrent tumor within the anterior abdominal wall muscles at CT.

Histopathologic examination results confirmed the presence of recurrent gallbladder carcinoma in all five (100%) of the patients with CT evidence of anterior abdominal wall tumor who underwent biopsy, three by means of fine-needle aspiration and two by means of wide excisional biopsy. Because one patient refused treatment, no biopsy was performed; however, an abdominal wall tumor recurrence was suspected clinically. Five (42%) of the 12 abdominal wall tumor recurrences appeared in port tracks that were surgically resected at definitive surgery; only three (60%) of these sites had revealed foci of tumor at initial resection.

The abdominal wall tumor recurrence was the only site of recurrent abdominal disease seen at CT in two (33%) of the six patients. One of these patients developed additional anterior abdominal wall masses and peritoneal carcinomatosis at a subsequent CT examination. Information from that subsequent CT examination was included in the data. Four patients (67%) had disease elsewhere seen at CT (two patients had carcinomatosis; two had both lymphadenopathy and carcinomatosis). None of the six had hepatic metastases.

Clinical follow-up results obtained a minimum of 1 month following definitive hepatic resection were available in 17 (89%) patients: in six (100%) patients with CT evidence of port track tumor recurrences and in 10 (100%) patients without CT evidence of abdominal wall tumor recurrence. One patient had clinical follow-up but no postoperative CT scan. The two patients without clinical follow-up did not have a postoperative CT scan available for evaluation. None of the 10 patients without CT evidence of recurrent tumor in the anterior abdominal wall had clinical evidence of an abdominal wall mass (mean clinical follow-up, 22 months; range, 1–63 months after definitive hepatic resection). One of these patients died of sepsis 1 month following surgery.

The presence of an abdominal wall tumor recurrence affected patient care in four (67%) of six patients. One patient underwent chemotherapy, one underwent surgical resection of the abdominal wall mass, one underwent surgical resection and chemotherapy, and one underwent radiation therapy. An abdominal wall tumor recurrence potentially affected management in all patients; one patient died of sepsis prior to the initiation of therapy, and one patient refused treatment.

DISCUSSION

Laparoscopic cholecystectomy has become increasingly accepted as an alternative treatment for symptomatic uncomplicated cholelithiasis owing to the decreased postoperative pain, shorter hospitalization, and lower cost as compared with open cholecystectomy (1,19,20). It has been estimated that approximately 80% of cholecystectomies nationwide are performed laparoscopically (21). However, if gallbladder carcinoma is suspected preoperatively, on the basis of either clinical or radiologic findings, laparoscopic cholecystectomy should not be performed and open cholecystectomy, hepatic resection, and lymph node dissection may be indicated (3,4,10,12,13,16,22–25).

Typically, 3–4 L of carbon dioxide is introduced into the peritoneal cavity via a periumbilical port site. A laparoscopic camera usually is placed through this port site. After insufflation of the peritoneal cavity, three additional trocars are introduced into the anterior abdominal wall with direct laparoscopic visualization, which provides portals for the laparoscopic instruments. One portal usually is located in the subxiphoid region, one in the right upper quadrant (along the right midclavicular line), and the third further caudad, lateral to the right rectus abdominis muscle (19). If additional traction is required, a trocar may be inserted in the left upper quadrant (26). This procedure enables the surgeon to remove the gallbladder without a large abdominal wall incision. An estimated 70,000 laparoscopic cholecystectomies were performed in 1990 (16).

A potentially serious complication of laparoscopic cholecystectomy is the inadvertent dissemination of unsuspected gallbladder carcinoma. Clinical symptoms of gallbladder carcinoma are similar to chronic cholecystitis; include weight loss, pain, and jaundice; and often mask the preoperative diagnosis of gallbladder carcinoma. In a study of 50 patients by Kumar and Aggarwal (27), a preoperative clinical diagnosis of gallbladder carcinoma was made in less than half of the patients with histopathologic proof of gallbladder carcinoma. Shirai et al (18) examined 241 consecutive patients with gallbladder carcinoma treated with surgical resection; only 102 (42%) of these patients had disease diagnosed correctly preoperatively. Even with thorough preoperative evaluation, 15%–30% of gallbladder carcinomas are detected incidentally at microscopic review of the surgical specimens (16). The subgroup of patients with only microscopic evidence of disease has a better prognosis (16).

Because all 19 patients in our study underwent laparoscopic cholecystectomy at outside institutions, we did not have access to the preoperative imaging studies and could not assess whether findings suggestive of gallbladder carcinoma were present. However, even if gallbladder carcinoma is not evident on preoperative imaging studies, the surgeon needs to scrutinize the surgical specimen carefully at the time of the laparoscopic cholecystectomy and obtain a frozen section if a suspicious lesion is detected (10,16,24,28). If gallbladder carcinoma is detected intraoperatively, a more complete staging procedure and hepatic resection, as well as resection of the port sites, may be indicated.

In our study, three (18%) of the 17 port tracks resected at subsequent definitive surgery revealed foci of adenocarcinoma, which likely resulted from seeding at laparoscopy. Han-Joo and Tapan (29) reported a case of microscopic tumor foci detected in a port track that was resected at the time of definitive hepatic surgery performed 18 days after laparoscopic cholecystectomy.

Six (32%) of the 19 patients in our study who underwent definitive hepatic surgery for potential cure had tumor recurrence along a laparoscopic track seen at CT a mean of 17 months after the initial laparoscopic procedure. Because most outside surgical reports were not available, it was not possible to determine the specific port site through which the gallbladder was laparoscopically removed. However, given the presence of multiple abdominal wall tumor recurrences in a single patient (five [83%] patients had more than one anterior abdominal wall tumor recurrence), we conclude that tumor also recurred along other laparoscopic port tracks. Nine (75%) of the 12 anterior abdominal wall masses extended directly into the subjacent omental fat, presumably along the track of the laparoscopic instruments.

There are surgical case reports (3–8,10–16,30) of abdominal wall tumor recurrence following laparoscopic cholecystectomy and occurring both at the site through which the gallbladder was removed as well as along trocar sites through which the laparoscopic instruments were inserted. Several hypotheses have been proposed to explain these findings. Direct tumor spread to the anterior abdominal wall may occur at removal of the gallbladder. The laparoscopic instruments used to mobilize the gallbladder during surgery may be inoculated with tumor cells and may seed the anterior abdominal wall at their removal (3,23,28). In addition, tumor cells may undergo aerosolization at insufflation of the peritoneum and may seed the port sites at the time of deflation (31).

The gallbladder may be torn when extensive retraction is required to obtain adequate exposure of the porta hepatis or at extraction through the anterior abdominal wall incision site (32). The rate of gallbladder rupture at removal from the abdomen during laparoscopic cholecystectomy has been reported to be as high as 24%–33% (32). It has been suggested that the wound site has increased capillary formation and thus provides an ideal milieu for tumor implantation (7,28,30).

Wibbenmeyer et al (24) have reported that gallbladder carcinoma recurs more rapidly after laparoscopic cholecystectomy than after open cholecystectomy. The pattern of tumor recurrence also differs between these procedures. Whereas local peritoneal tumor recurrence by direct tumor extension is more common after open cholecystectomy, port site tumor recurrence and diffuse peritoneal disease is more common after laparoscopic cholecystectomy (24).

Owing to increased awareness of laparoscopic port site tumor recurrence, it has now become the standard surgical practice at our institution to excise the laparoscopic port sites at the time of definitive hepatic resection. Five (42%) of the 12 abdominal wall tumor recurrences in our study occurred at port tracks that had been resected at the time of definitive surgery. No tumor was detected at histopathologic examination in two of the sites resected in which gallbladder carcinoma subsequently recurred.

A possible explanation for this is that the spatial relation of the skin, anterior abdominal wall muscles, and the intervening fascia changes at the time of the laparoscopic surgery; when the abdomen is insufflated with carbon dioxide, the abdominal wall muscles are in a different position in relation to the skin incision site than when the abdomen is deflated (as it is at definitive hepatic resection). Thus, when the surgeon excises the port track on the basis of the skin incision, the actual oblique track through the abdominal wall may not be completely excised. In addition, tumor may seed the fascial planes at the time of the laparoscopic cholecystectomy and spread between the muscle layers.

The goals of definitive resection of gallbladder carcinoma following routine cholecystectomy include removal of any potential residual tumor within the gallbladder bed, resection of portal and paraaortic lymph nodes, and reestablishment of biliary drainage (17). Patients with T2 or greater gallbladder carcinoma that is detected incidentally at cholecystectomy have improved survival if a radical second operation is performed (17,18). For patients with T1 tumor with clear surgical margins obtained at cholecystectomy, close-interval follow-up without a second resection is recommended (28).

The actual prevalence of abdominal wall tumor recurrence in the patient group in our study is likely higher than our data suggest. Patients who underwent treatment on the basis of physical examination without CT documentation were not included in our study group. One patient who had three port track tumor recurrences at CT had a fourth recurrence that was detected at physical examination and that was resected immediately prior to CT, which then revealed only a postoperative fluid collection in that region. In addition, it is possible that if we obtained CT follow-up in those patients considered to have inoperable gallbladder carcinoma after laparoscopic cholecystectomy, the number of abdominal wall tumor recurrences would have been even higher. However, we chose to evaluate that subgroup of patients who were treated with definitive hepatic surgery—theoretically, the group with the best prognosis.

Several other limitations of our study should be noted. We did not have access to the surgical reports from the laparoscopic cholecystectomies performed at other institutions and cannot determine if the gallbladder was torn at surgery or if gallstones were spilled into the abdomen. As this is a retrospective study, the interval we report between definitive hepatic surgery and CT evidence of recurrent tumor is an overestimation of the true interval before the abdominal wall tumor recurrence might have been visible at CT. Some patients may have undergone CT examinations elsewhere that were not available to us or may have had clinical evidence of a mass prior to the CT examination. In at least one patient, CT provided the initial depiction of an abdominal wall tumor recurrence. A prospective study with CT scans obtained at frequent, regular intervals would be required to determine the rate of tumor recurrence. Our study was not intended to determine the sensitivity or specificity of CT in the detection of abdominal wall recurrence of gallbladder carcinoma but rather to assess the CT appearance of tumor seeding along laparoscopic tracks.

Finally, it is possible that recurrences in some patients may have occurred along surgical drain tracks rather than along laparoscopic port tracks. However, when surgical drains are inserted at laparoscopic cholecystectomy, they usually are placed through a laparoscopic port incision. Regardless, the principles involved in both types of recurrence are essentially the same.

In conclusion, gallbladder carcinoma can recur in laparoscopic port tracks even if surgical resection of the port sites is performed at subsequent hepatic resection for attempted cure. Recurrent tumor may appear as a new or enlarging mass along the anterior abdominal wall with extension into the subjacent omental fat. Owing to the increasing performance of laparoscopic cholecystectomy, port site tumor recurrence of unsuspected gallbladder carcinoma may become a more common event. Our findings underscore the desirability for preoperative identification of gallbladder carcinoma, as this will substantially affect initial surgical planning. In addition, the anterior abdominal wall should be closely scrutinized at postoperative CT, as the discovery of tumor recurrence affects patient care.

References

1. Grace PA, Quereshi A, Coleman J, et al. Reduced postoperative hospitalization after laparoscopic cholecystectomy. Br J Surg 1991; 78:160–162.
2. McGahan JP, Stein M. Complications of laparoscopic cholecystectomy: imaging and intervention. AJR 1995; 165:1089–1097.
3. Coltar AM, Mueller MC, Pettit JW, Schmidt ER, Villar HV. Trocar site seeding of inapparent gallbladder carcinoma during laparoscopic cholecystectomy. J Laparoendosc Surg 1996; 6:35–45.
4. Lomis KD, Vitola JV, Delbeke D, et al. Recurrent gallbladder carcinoma at laparoscopy port sites diagnosed by positron emission tomography: implications for primary and radical second operations. Am Surg 1997; 63:341–345.
5. O'Rourke N, Price PM, Kelly S, Sikora K. Tumour inoculation during laparoscopy (letter). Lancet 1993; 342:368.
6. Pezet D, Fondrinier E, Rotman N. Parietal seeding of carcinoma of the gallbladder after laparoscopic cholecystectomy (case report). Br J Surg 1992; 79:230.
7. Jacobi CA, Keller H, Monig S, Said MS. Implantation metastasis of unsuspected gallbladder carcinoma after laparoscopy (case report). Surg Endosc 1995: 9:351–352.
8. Karayiannakis AJ, Knight MJ. Umbilical port metastasis from gallbladder carcinoma after laparoscopic cholecystectomy (case report). Eur J Surg Oncol 1997; 23: 186–187.
9. Fligelstone LJ, Johnson RC, Stiff GJ, Wheeler MH. Laparoscopy and gastrointestinal cancer (letter). Am J Surg 1993; 166:571.
10. Copher JC, Rogers JJ, Dalton ML. Trocar-site metastasis following laparoscopic cholecystectomy for unsuspected carcinoma of the gallbladder. Surg Endosc 1995; 9:348–350.
11. Drourad F, Delamarre J, Capron J. Cutaneous seeding of gallbladder cancer after laparoscopic cholecystectomy (letter). N Engl J Med 1991; 325:1316.
12. Landen SM. Laparoscopic surgery and tumor seeding (letter). Surgery 1993; 114: 131–132.
13. Shibata N, Kagotani K, Noguchi S, Tamai M. Portsite and intraabdominal metastases of unsuspected gallbladder carcinoma after laparoscopic cholecystectomy: report of a case. Surg Today 1996; 26:1014–1016.
14. Nally C, Pershaw R. Tumour implantation at umbilicus after laparoscopic cholecystectomy for unsuspected gallbladder carcinoma (case report). Can J Surg 1994; 37:243–244.
15. Baer HU, Metzger A, Glattli A, Klaiber C, Ruchti C, Czerniak A. Subcutaneous periumbilical metastasis of a gallbladder carcinoma after laparoscopic cholecystectomy. Surg Laparosc Endosc 1995; 5:59–63.
16. Clair DG, Lautz DB, Brooks DC. Rapid development of umbilical metastases after laparoscopic cholecystectomy for unsuspected gallbladder carcinoma. Surgery 1993; 113:355–358.
17. Fong Y, Heffernan N, Blumgart LH. Gall-

bladder cancer discovered during laparoscopic cholecystectomy: aggressive resection is beneficial. Cancer 1998; 83:423–427.
18. Shirai Y, Yoshida K, Tsukada K, Muto T. Inapparent carcinoma of the gallbladder: an appraisal of a radical second operation after simple cholecystectomy. Ann Surg 1992; 215:326–331.
19. Zucker KA, Bailey RW, Gadacz TR, Imbembo AL. Laparoscopic guided cholecystectomy. Am J Surg 1991; 161:36–44.
20. The Southern Surgeons Club. A prospective analysis of 1,518 laparoscopic cholecystectomies. N Engl J Med 1991; 324:1073–1078.
21. NIH Consensus Conference. Gallstones and laparoscopic cholecystectomy. JAMA 1993; 269:1018–1024.
22. Nishizaki T, Matsumata T, Hashizume M, Maeda T, Otsuka K, Sugimachi K. Hepatic metastasis after laparoscopic cholecystectomy for polypoid gallbladder cancer followed by radical surgery. Surg Endosc 1994; 8:1436–1438.
23. Principe A, Lugaresi RC, Golfieri R, et al. Unsuspected carcinoma of the gallbladder: case report of trocar-site metastasis following laparoscopic cholecystectomy. Hepatogastroenterology 1997; 44:990–993.
24. Wibbenmeyer LA, Wade TP, Chen RC, Meyer RC, Turgeon RP, Andrus CH. Laparoscopic cholecystectomy can disseminate in situ carcinoma of the gallbladder. J Am Coll Surg 1995; 181:504–510.
25. Fong Y, Brennan MF, Turnbull A, Colt D, Blumgart LH. Gallbladder cancer discovered during laparoscopic surgery: potential for iatrogenic tumor dissemination. Arch Surg 1993; 128:1054–1056.
26. Berci G, Sackier JM. Laparoscopic cholecystectomy and laparoscopic choledocholithotomy. In: Blumgart LH, ed. Surgery of the liver and biliary tract. 2nd ed. London, Great Britain: Churchill-Livingstone, 1994; 633–661.
27. Kumar A, Aggarwal S. Carcinoma of the gallbladder: CT findings in 50 cases. Abdom Imaging 1994; 19:304–308.
28. Yamaguchi K, Chijiiwa K, Ichimiya H, et al. Gallbladder carcinoma in the era of laparoscopic cholecystectomy. Arch Surg 1996; 131:981–984.
29. Han-Joo K, Tapan R. Unsuspected gallbladder cancer with cutaneous seeding after laparoscopic cholecystectomy. South Med J 1994; 87:817–820.
30. Fligelstone L, Rhodes M, Flook D, Puntis M, Crosby D. Tumour inoculation during laparoscopy (letter). Lancet 1993; 342:368–369.
31. Nduka CC, Monson JR, Menzies-Gow N, Darzi A. Abdominal wall metastases following laparoscopy. Br J Surg 1993; 81:648–652.
32. Fitzgibbons RJ, Annibali R, Litke BS. Gallbladder and gallstone removal, open versus closed laparoscopy, and pneumoperitoneum. Am J Surg 1993; 165:497–504.

Local Extension of Pancreatic Carcinoma: Assessment with Thin-Section Helical CT versus with Breath-hold Fast MR Imaging—ROC Analysis[1]

Taiji Nishiharu, MD
Yasuyuki Yamashita, MD
Yasuko Abe, MD
Katsuhiko Mitsuzaki, MD
Tadatoshi Tsuchigame, MD
Yoshiharu Nakayama, MD
Mutsumasa Takahashi, MD

Index terms:
Computed tomography (CT), comparative studies, 77.12111, 77.12112, 77.12115, 77.12118
Magnetic resonance (MR), comparative studies, 77.121411, 77.121415, 77.121416, 77.12143
Pancreas, CT, 77.12111, 77.12112, 77.12115, 77.12118
Pancreas, MR, 77.121411, 77.121415, 77.121416, 77.12143
Pancreas, neoplasms, 77.291, 77.321, 77.33
Receiver operating characteristic curve (ROC)

Radiology 1999; 212:445–452

Abbreviations:
FLASH = fast low-angle shot
ROC = receiver operating characteristic

[1] From the Department of Radiology, Kumamoto University Hospital, 1-1-1 Honjo, Kumamoto City 860-0811, Japan. Received December 24, 1997; revision requested March 24, 1998; final revision received November 24; accepted March 2, 1999. **Address reprint requests to** Y.Y. (e-mail: *yama@kaiju.medic.kumamoto-u.ac.jp*).

PURPOSE: To compare contrast material–enhanced thin-section helical CT with breath-hold contrast-enhanced MR imaging for sensitivity in the detection of pancreatic adenocarcinoma and for accuracy in local tumor staging.

MATERIALS AND METHODS: Fifty-seven patients (37 men, 20 women aged 42–28 years) suspected of having pancreatic adenocarcinoma were examined. The final diagnosis was confirmed at surgery to be pancreatic cancer in 31 patients; the other 26 patients were deemed not to have pancreatic cancer. All patients underwent both CT and MR imaging (turbo spin-echo and fast low-angle shot) studies. Image quality and pancreatic enhancement were subjectively evaluated. All CT scans and MR images were assessed by two independent observers by using a five-point scale for the detection of tumor and of invasion into the peripancreatic tissue, portal vein, and/or peripancreatic artery. Receiver operating characteristic curves for CT and MR imaging were analyzed.

RESULTS: At visual analysis, pancreatic enhancement at CT and at MR imaging was comparable, but depiction of vessels was superior at helical CT. Detectability of tumor was comparable. Helical CT was significantly superior to MR imaging in diagnostic imaging of invasion into the peripancreatic tissue, portal vein, and/or peripancreatic artery ($P < .01$).

CONCLUSION: Thin-section dynamic CT is more sensitive than MR imaging for detection of peripancreatic and vascular invasion in patients with pancreatic cancer.

Computed tomography (CT) or magnetic resonance (MR) imaging of the pancreas provides a means of determining whether a neoplasm is localized within the pancreas, has metastasized to the liver or local lymph nodes, or has invaded the surrounding vessels. This determination allows preoperative assessment of whether a patient is a candidate for attempted resection or a palliative procedure. Dynamic contrast material–enhanced CT is the technique most frequently performed to confirm the clinical diagnosis and assess for resectability. CT should be performed with protocols directed at optimal imaging of the pancreas (1–6). Thin-section CT of the pancreas can be achieved by using thin sections and a small field of view (7–9).

Among the several potential advantages of MR imaging are high tissue contrast, which might increase the conspicuity of the pancreatic lesions, and the option to manipulate pulse sequence parameters to improve depiction of structures such as blood vessels and the pancreas (10–16).

Although the findings of studies (10–12,14–17) suggest the superiority of MR imaging, especially dynamic imaging, over CT in the assessment of pancreatic neoplasms, to our knowledge, this superiority has not been recognized in clinical situations: With the exception of a report by Ichikawa et al (11), in which helical CT was used, all prospective studies were conducted before helical CT became widely available (14–16). Thus, the goal of this study was to compare, by means of receiver operating characteristic (ROC) analysis,

Author contributions:
Guarantor of integrity of entire study, Y.Y.; study concepts and design, Y.Y.; definition of intellectual content, T.T., M.T.; literature research, T.N.; clinical studies, T.N.; data acquisition, K.M.; data analysis, Y.N., Y.A.; statistical analysis, Y.A.; manuscript preparation, Y.Y.; manuscript editing, T.N.; manuscript review, M.T.

technically optimized thin-section helical CT with technically optimized MR imaging for sensitivity in the detection of pancreatic adenocarcinoma and for accuracy in assessing vascular invasion or invasion into peripancreatic tissue.

MATERIALS AND METHODS

Patient Population

All of the patients at our institution between April 1995 and September 1997 who were suspected of having pancreatic cancer were included. On the basis of the results of screening for symptoms, which included measuring for elevated tumor marker levels (CA–19-9 [colorectal cancer antigen], carcinoembryonic antigen) and/or ultrasonography (US), these patients underwent both helical CT and MR imaging according to the recommendations of their surgeons. Patients with adenocarcinoma of the Vater ampulla, duodenum, or distal bile duct who had imaging findings that did not seem to indicate pancreatic cancer at endoscopy, endoscopic pancreatography, or US were excluded from the beginning, as were patients with islet cell tumors, cystic tumors, and other rare tumors of the pancreas. There were 37 men (age range, 42–78 years; mean age, 66 years) and 20 women (age range, 56–75 years; mean age, 62 years), for a total of 57 patients in the study. We obtained informed consent from all patients. The CT studies were performed within 1 week after the MR studies. We did not exclude cases because of image quality. We did not perform preoperative biopsy in any of the patients.

The preoperative criteria for definitely nonresectable cancer included the presence of distant metastasis, multiple liver metastases, peritoneal dissemination with massive ascites, and involvement of the neighboring major vascular system (ie, encasement of the celiac axis and superior mesenteric artery). Involvement of the superior mesenteric vein or main portal vein was not a contraindication to resectability, because resection of tumor and reconstruction of the portal venous system could be performed, if necessary. If the tumor was nonresectable, surgical biopsy followed by bypass surgery (ie, gastrojejunostomy combined with biliary-jejunostomy) was performed.

Histopathologic evaluation included the notation of the size, location, appearance, and histologic features of the mass and associated complications (eg, pancreatitis). When a pancreatic tumor was completely resected, the pathologic results were used as the standard of reference for diagnosis. When the lesion was nonresectable, the operative findings were used as the standard of reference. When the mass was not resected, the pathologist indicated the histologic nature of the tissue sampled at biopsy. Surgeons indicated whether a mass was present at palpation and at intraoperative US. We could not spatially localize the pathologic conditions of the actual vessels and of the actual peripancreatic fat to compare them with the imaging findings. Intraoperative US was performed to confirm vascular encasement by the tumor. Manual palpation of a pancreatic mass fixed to retropancreatic vessels or structures, with intraoperative US–based confirmation of vascular encasement, was considered adequate surgical confirmation of extrapancreatic invasion and therefore of nonresectability. No attempt was made at surgery to visualize every liver lesion depicted on the images. Infiltration of the pancreatic capsule was assessed, as was invasion into the surgical resection margins.

Imaging Techniques

CT protocol.—All CT examinations were carried out by using a helical CT scanner (CT HiSpeed Advantage; GE Medical Systems, Milwaukee, Wis). Each patient was asked to drink 300 mL of water to fill the duodenum. We did not use any other oral contrast material. For the intravenous contrast material, 300 mg of iodine per milliliter of iopamidol (Iopamiron 300; Schering, Osaka, Japan) was injected at a rate of 3 mL/sec for 30 seconds (total dose, 2 mL/kg). A 20-gauge needle was positioned in a medial antecubital vein, and the rate of flow was controlled with a power injector. After nonenhanced CT scanning, cephalocaudal scanning through the pancreatic region was begun 35 seconds (early phase), 70 seconds (portal venous phase), and 240 seconds after the start of the contrast material injection.

For thin-section helical CT imaging of the pancreas, the examination began at the level of the splenic hilum just cephalad to the pancreatic tail. The position of the pancreas was determined by obtaining axial images of the entire pancreas before the administration of contrast material (ie, precontrast images). Patients were prepared for the breath hold with three coached, deep respiratory excursions before scanning. In one breath hold, an area of 7 or 8 cm was scanned; this coverage included the pancreas in all patients.

Helical CT scanning during the early phase and portal venous phase was performed with a breath-hold technique in a 1 second per gantry rotation with a table feed of 4.5 mm/sec, section thickness of 3 mm, pitch of 1.5, 120 kVp, and either 240 or 220 mA. The scans were reconstructed in 2-mm section increments with a retrospectively targeted small (25-cm) field of view and a pixel size of 0.49×0.49 mm by using a standard reconstruction algorithm. Because we focused on imaging of the pancreas, the entire liver was not evaluated in the early and portal venous phases. For precontrast and delayed phase imaging of both the liver and pancreas, a craniocaudal scanning direction with a beam collimation of 7 mm was used in the nonhelical mode.

MR imaging protocol.—All imaging was performed with a 1.5-T superconducting magnet (Magnetom Vision; Siemens Medical Systems, Erlangen, Germany) by using a standard phased-array coil (Siemens Medical Systems) with four elements. After axial, fat-saturated T1-weighted fast low-angle shot (FLASH) (repetition time msec/echo time msec, 150/4.1) and respiratory-triggered turbo spin-echo (3,000–5,000/90) sequences were performed, dynamic MR images with gadopentetate dimeglumine (Magnevist; Schering) enhancement were obtained. Before and after rapid (2 mL/sec) manual injection of gadopentetate dimeglumine (0.1 mmol/kg), axial T1-weighted FLASH (150/6, 75° flip angle) MR images were obtained at 30, 60, 90, and 240 seconds in a breath hold. Arterial phase images were usually obtained at 30 seconds; portal venous phase images, at 90 seconds; and delayed phase images, at 240 seconds.

In some patients, the timing at 30 seconds was too early to obtain arterial phase images. In these cases, we used images obtained at 60 seconds as arterial phase images. A rectangular field of view of 213 (phase) $\times$ 340 (frequency) mm and a matrix of either 160×256 (matrix size, 2.04×1.03 mm) for fat-saturated FLASH and turbo spin-echo imaging or of 160×512 (size, 1.33×0.66 mm) for dynamic MR imaging were used. For the dynamic study, the frequency resolution was increased while limiting the phase-encoding steps to result in nonsquare pixels. A section thickness of 8 mm, intersection gap of 20%, and identical section locations were used in all acquisitions (subject to any inconsistencies in breath hold).

The imaging time was 18 seconds for the fat-saturated FLASH sequences and 19 seconds for the dynamic FLASH sequence. In the respiratory-triggered turbo spin-echo sequence, the acquisition time varied, depending on the repetition time; it ranged from 149 to 319 seconds (mean, 251 seconds) for 14 sections. The total examination time was approximately 30 minutes.

Image Analyses

CT and MR reading sessions were carried out separately and independently by two abdominal radiologists who have similar experience (more than 7 years) in both CT and MR imaging and had not seen these cases previously; the interval between the two readings was 3 weeks. For the CT and MR image readings, both arterial and portal venous phase images were simultaneously read, but combined readings of the two types of images were not performed for the ROC analysis. The readers did not know the surgical or histopathologic examination findings or the intraoperative US results, but the transabdominal US findings were made available at the time of the CT scan and MR image readings.

Initially, the two independent readers evaluated the image quality for the dynamic studies during the CT and MR examinations. Film hard-copy images in each examination were reviewed. The readers assessed the images for enhancement of the normal pancreas, vascular opacification, and presence of artifacts (chemical shift, susceptibility, and vascular ghosting artifacts on MR images and respiratory blurring on CT scans and MR images) by using a scoring system of 0 to 2, where 0 indicated a poorly enhanced pancreas, poorly depicted vessels, or severe artifacts; 1, a moderately enhanced pancreas, moderately depicted vessels, or slight artifacts; and 2, a well-enhanced pancreas, clearly depicted vessels, or the absence of artifacts. Discrepancies in scores were solved by using consensus. Nonparametric rank tests were used to compare scores in both imaging groups for every parameter, and a P value of .05 or less was considered to be statistically significant.

Second, local tumor extension was evaluated. Peripancreatic invasion was diagnosed when irregular signal intensity or soft-tissue streaks and strands in the peripancreatic fat layer were seen (1,11). Because a histopathologic examination could not be performed when the lesions were nonresectable, we could not tell whether the peripancreatic invasion was due to the tumor itself or to associated fibrosis. A vessel was considered to be nonresectable if it showed a focal reduction in caliber, circumferential encasement by the tumor, or frank thrombosis. We assumed that a vessel was involved with the tumor when more than half the circumference of the vessel was seen (7). No analysis of lymph nodes was performed.

To estimate the likelihood that a certain finding was present, the readers used a five-point confidence scale in which 5 indicated definitely present; 4, probably present; 3, indeterminate; 2, probably absent; and 1, finding not present. Each of the determinants of resectability—that is, tumor detection and invasion into the peripancreatic tissue, peripancreatic artery (celiac, hepatic, splenic, or superior mesenteric artery), and/or portal vein (main portal, splenic, or superior mesenteric vein)—was assessed.

To compare CT and MR imaging performance, we compared the ROC curves constructed for the two techniques. For each imaging method, a binominal ROC curve was fitted to each observer's confidence rating data by using a maximum likelihood estimation. The diagnostic accuracy of each imaging technique was determined by calculating the area under each reader-specific binominal ROC curve (A_z). The differences between ROC curves for the individual readers were tested for significance by using the CORROC (statistical comparison of ROC curves estimated from correlated data sets) algorithm. The differences between the imaging techniques in terms of mean A_z scores were analyzed statistically by using the Student two-tailed t test for paired data (18,19). The number of lesions correctly judged to be probably present ($n = 4$) or definitely present ($n = 5$) with ROC analysis by each reviewer was regarded as the number of correctly diagnosed lesions. The sensitivity, specificity, and accuracy of each sequence were evaluated.

For analysis of interobserver variability in the detection of lesions and evaluation of invasion with each imaging modality, κ statistics were used to measure the degree of agreement between the two observers. κ values greater than 0 were considered to be indicative of a positive correlation. Values of up to 0.40 were considered to be indicative of a positive but poor correlation; 0.41–0.75, a good correlation; and greater than 0.75, an excellent correlation.

RESULTS

Surgical and Pathologic Results

Among the 57 patients in the study, surgery was performed in 36. Thirty-one of these 36 patients proved to have adenocarcinoma, and five proved to have chronic pancreatitis, as confirmed at surgical and histopathologic examinations. The carcinomas were resectable in 20 patients and nonresectable in 11 patients, in whom only bypass surgery was performed. Eighteen patients had lymph node involvement confirmed at surgery or pathologic examination. However, because most of the lymph nodes were microscopic and lymph nodes were not explored or sampled in 10 patients, lymph node metastasis was not analyzed. In the 21 patients who did not undergo surgery, the tumors were deemed to be noncancerous because there was no definite abnormality at follow-up more than 1 year later. In all of these patients, the imaging findings, including those of both CT and MR imaging, did not change during that period.

Image Quality

The image quality results are shown in Table 1. The pancreatic enhancement on helical CT scans was subjectively given a mean grade of 1.2, and that on dynamic MR images was subjectively given a mean grade of 1.3; this difference was not statistically significant. Peripancreatic vessels were significantly more clearly depicted on helical CT scans (mean grade, 1.8) than on dynamic MR images (mean grade, 1.2). Image blurring was seen in two patients at helical CT; it was more frequently seen at dynamic MR imaging (in 10 patients). The susceptibility, chemical shift, and vascular ghosting artifacts seen on MR images occasionally caused difficulty in interpreting the images (in 15 patients).

Lesion Detection

At precontrast MR imaging, the pancreatic carcinomas were hypointense (20 patients) or isointense (11 patients) relative to the surrounding pancreas on T1-weighted images with or without fat saturation; the lesions were hyperintense (17 patients) or isointense (14 patients) on T2-weighted images. The lesions were most conspicuous during the early dynamic phase of both CT and MR imaging. At dynamic MR imaging, ringlike enhancement of the tumor was seen in lesions confined to the pancreas. These findings were not evident at helical CT.

The results of analysis of lesion detection with CT and MR imaging are shown in Tables 2 and 3. Helical CT was slightly more accurate than was dynamic MR imaging in the detection of lesions (Table 2), and the area under the ROC curve was greater with helical CT (Table 3), but neither difference was significant. In lesions confined to the pancreas (in 11 patients), the tumor was somewhat more conspicuous on the MR images, but its detectability with MR imaging was simi-

TABLE 1
Enhancement of the Pancreas, Vessels, and Artifacts

Structure or Finding	Helical CT	Dynamic MR Imaging
Pancreas	1.2 ± 0.7	1.3 ± 0.7
Peripancreatic vessels*	1.8 ± 0.4	1.2 ± 0.6
Respiratory blurring*	1.0 ± 0.2	1.8 ± 0.5
Artifacts (chemical shift, vascular ghosting, or susceptibility)	. . .	1.7 ± 0.4

Note.—Data are mean enhancement scores (± SD) based on a scoring system of 0–2, in which 0 = poorly enhanced pancreas, poorly depicted vessels, or severe artifacts; 1 = moderately enhanced pancreas, moderately depicted vessels, or slight artifacts; and 2 = well-enhanced pancreas, clearly depicted vessels, or absence of artifacts.

* $P < .05$ for the difference between helical CT and dynamic MR imaging.

TABLE 2
Comparison of CT and MR Imaging in the Detection of Pancreatic Adenocarcinoma: Sensitivity, Specificity, and Accuracy Values

	Reviewer 1			Reviewer 2		
Diagnosis	Sensitivity	Specificity	Accuracy (%)	Sensitivity	Specificity	Accuracy (%)
Cancer (n = 31)						
Helical CT	25 (96)	25 (81)	88	24 (83)	25 (89)	86
Dynamic MR imaging	20 (80)	25 (78)	79	21 (95)	25 (71)	81
Tumor invasion into peripancreatic tissue						
Helical CT	25 (89)	26 (90)	89	25 (86)	25 (89)	88
Dynamic MR imaging	15 (75)	23 (64)	67	15 (68)	22 (63)	65
Tumor invasion into portal vein						
Helical CT	22 (76)	24 (94)	86	25 (77)	25 (89)	84
Dynamic MR imaging	14 (40)	18 (64)	58	15 (42)	20 (66)	58
Tumor invasion into peripancreatic artery						
Helical CT	18 (74)	27 (87)	81	17 (80)	30 (88)	84
Dynamic MR imaging	12 (71)	25 (75)	74	14 (75)	29 (71)	72

Note.—Sensitivity and specificity data are the number of patients. The numbers in parentheses are the percentage.

lar to that with CT (Fig 1); eight tumors each were detected with CT and MR imaging. Neither CT nor MR imaging depicted three tumors less than 1.5 cm in diameter that were confined to the pancreas; however, these lesions were detected at endoscopic US or intraoperative palpation. A false-positive diagnosis of cancer was made in four (reviewer 1) and five (reviewer 2) patients at CT and in nine (reviewer 1) and eight (reviewer 2) patients at MR imaging. When the lesion extended beyond the pancreas (20 patients), detectability of the pancreatic tumor itself was greater on the CT scans (Fig 2). Nineteen such tumors were detected at CT compared with 14 detected at MR imaging by reviewer 1. Reviewer 2 detected 18 tumors that extended beyond the pancreas at CT compared with 14 detected at MR imaging.

Invasion into Peripancreatic Tissue

In patients with nonresectable tumor due to peripancreatic tissue invasion, including serosal or retroperitoneal extension at surgical palpation, the peripancreatic invasion was depicted as a signal intensity irregularity or as soft-tissue streaks and strands of the peripancreatic fat layer on both CT scans and MR images. The depiction of peripancreatic invasion on helical CT scans was significantly more certain than that on the MR images, as assessed by both reviewers (Table 3). Image blurring or chemical shift artifacts on the MR images occasionally obscured the peripancreatic tissue invasion.

TABLE 3
Comparison of CT and MR Imaging in the Detection of Pancreatic Adenocarcinoma: A_z and P Values

	Reviewer 1		Reviewer 2	
Diagnosis	A_z Value	P Value	A_z Value	P Value
Cancer		.24		.46
Helical CT	0.94		0.92	
Dynamic MR imaging	0.88		0.88	
Tumor invasion into peripancreatic tissue		<.01		<.01
Helical CT	0.92		0.89	
Dynamic MR imaging	0.65		0.62	
Tumor invasion into portal vein		<.01		<.01
Helical CT	0.99		0.94	
Dynamic MR imaging	0.65		0.74	
Tumor invasion into peripancreatic artery		<.01		<.01
Helical CT	0.88		0.88	
Dynamic MR imaging	0.60		0.61	

Resectability of Major Peripancreatic Vessels and Portal Veins

At surgery, 20 peripancreatic major arteries (nine common hepatic arteries, five superior mesenteric arteries, three celiac arteries, and three splenic arteries) in 18 patients were nonresectable, and 21 portal or superior mesenteric veins in 21 patients were nonresectable; these findings were confirmed by means of surgical palpation with US assistance. Among the nonresectable arteries, 15 were detected with CT and nine were detected with MR imaging by reviewer 1; 16 nonresectable arteries were detected with CT and seven were detected with MR imaging by reviewer 2. Among the nonresectable portal venous systems, 19 veins were detected with CT and six were detected with MR imaging by reviewer 1; 17 nonresectable veins were detected with CT and eight were detected with MR imaging by reviewer 2. The results of ROC analysis revealed that CT was significantly more accurate than MR imaging (Fig 3) ($P < .01$) in the detection of both arterial invasion and portal venous invasion.

Interobserver Agreement on Tumor Detection and Determination of Tumor Extension

The interobserver agreement on tumor detection with CT was excellent (κ = 0.92). The κ values for the detection of peripancreatic extension (0.74) and invasion into the portal vein (0.72) or peripancreatic artery (0.65) indicated good agree-

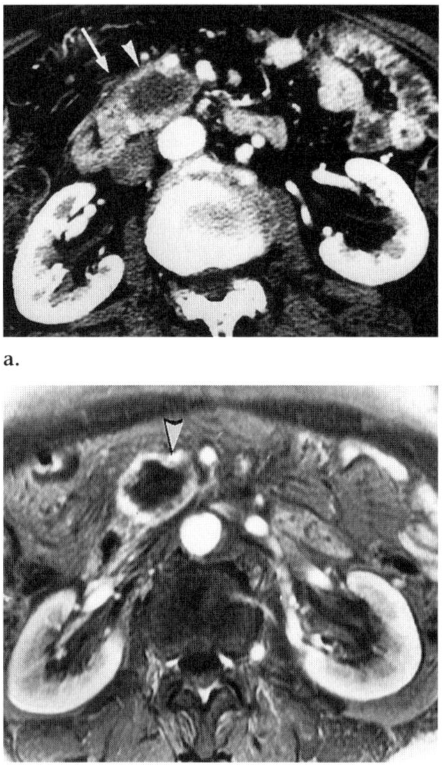

a. b.

Figure 1. (a) Axial helical CT scan and (b) axial contrast-enhanced dynamic T1-weighted FLASH MR image (150/4.1), both of which were obtained during the early phase in a 68-year-old woman with pancreatic cancer. In both **a** and **b**, a mass (arrowhead) in the inferior pancreatic head and uncinate process is clearly seen, and the superior mesenteric vein is almost encased. Peripancreatic invasion is suggested by the irregularity of the peripancreatic fatty tissue (arrow) in **a**; however, in **b**, the mass is delineated clearly, but invasion into the peripancreatic fat is not evident. Operative findings confirmed invasion into the superior mesenteric vein and peripancreatic tissue.

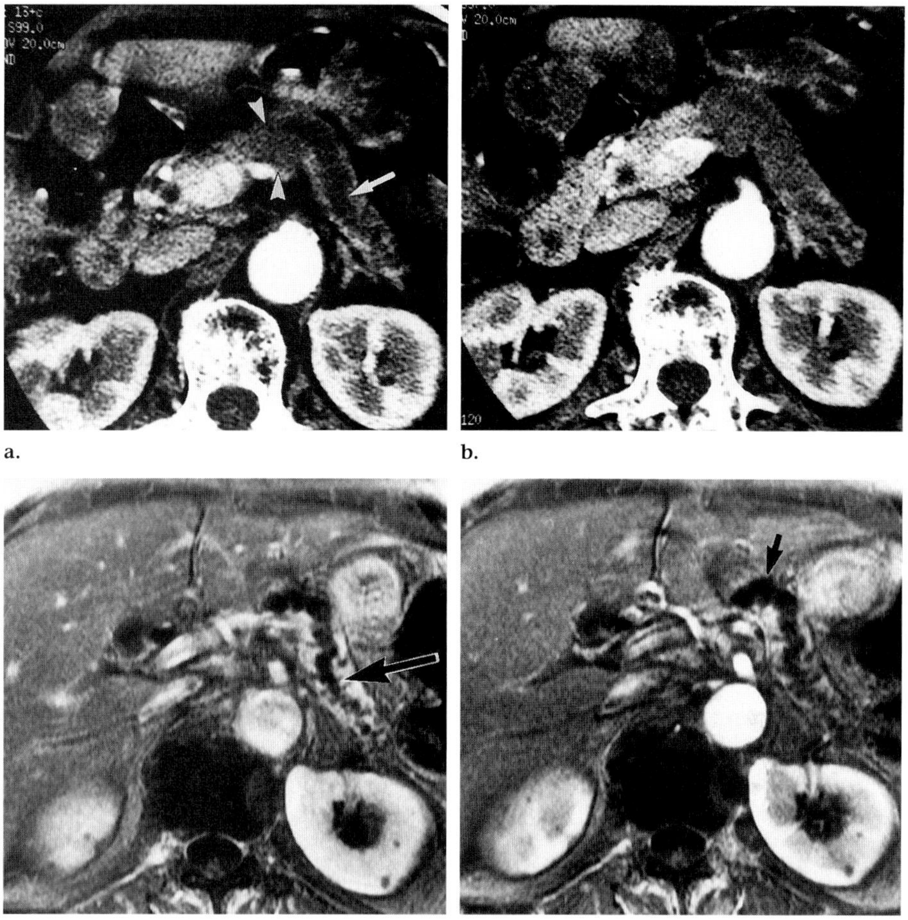

a. b. c. d.

Figure 2. (**a, b**) Axial helical CT scans and (**c, d**) axial contrast-enhanced dynamic T1-weighted FLASH images (150/4.1), both of which were obtained during the early phase in an 80-year-old woman with pancreatic cancer. Dilatation of the main pancreatic duct (arrow in **a**, **c**, and **d**) is seen on both the helical CT scans and MR images. In **a**, at the distal portion of the dilated pancreatic duct, a hypoattenuating mass (arrowheads) is seen in the pancreatic body. The mass is difficult to detect in **c** and **d**, probably because of the susceptibility and motion blurring artifacts and limited spatial resolution. Operative findings confirmed the presence of the tumor in the body of the pancreas. They also revealed duodenal invasion, which was not detected at either CT or MR imaging.

ment. These values with MR imaging indicated excellent agreement for tumor detection (0.92) and good agreement for the detection of peripancreatic invasion (0.71), portal venous invasion (0.60), and peripancreatic arterial involvement (0.51).

DISCUSSION

Surgical resection remains the treatment of choice for pancreatic cancer and is currently the only potentially curative therapy. Although the criteria for tumor resectability differ among institutions, important determinants of tumor resectability include peripancreatic tumor extension and vascular involvement. CT, particularly dynamic CT, is a useful tool that can help detect and stage pancreatic cancers (1–3,5,6), but small tumors occasionally are not detected owing to limited contrast resolution (11,15,20). Because of its superb contrast resolution, MR imaging, especially gadolinium–enhanced dynamic studies, has been confirmed to be useful for the evaluation of pancreatic diseases (10–12,16,17).

Helical CT has been used successfully in imaging of the pancreas because it provides excellent depiction of the details of pancreatic tissue and small vessels and a high level of parenchymal enhancement without respiratory misregistration (3,7,20–24). Because data are acquired from a volume of tissue in helical CT rather than section by section, this modality is suitable for the evaluation of small cancers, which theoretically could be overlooked on nonhelical CT scans, even with 5-mm section widths, because of respiratory misregistration. A high degree of vascular and tumor opacification was achieved by using helical CT compared with the previously routinely used dynamic CT examination (3,21). In this study, we obtained thin-section images of the pancreas by means of retrospective targeting with a narrow (3-mm) collimation protocol. In our phantom study (9), increased resolution with acceptable reduction in the signal-to-noise ratio was achieved by using this technique. The thin-section technique also enables better evaluation of vascular involvement by the tumor (25).

In the past, MR imaging had a limited role in the detection and staging of pancreatic cancers because of phase-shift artifacts and limited spatial resolution. The fat suppression technique reduces phase-shift artifacts, increases the dynamic ranges of the signal intensities of abdominal organs, and depicts the pancreas with higher signal intensity relative to that of the surrounding tissue (10,12,26). With recent advances in MR pulse sequences, small pixel size, gradient-echo T1-weighted MR images can be obtained in a breath hold. Anatomic details are now more clearly depicted, and lesions become conspicuous with reduced chemical shift and ringing artifacts. In addition, with the use of a phased-array coil, the signal-to-noise ratio remains within an acceptable range (11).

Because the pancreas is a vascular organ with an abundant arterial supply and rich network of capillaries, the characteristic parenchymal "blush" that appears during dynamic contrast-enhanced studies has enabled the depiction of tumors at CT or MR imaging. Investigating the differences in vascularity and background tissue between cancers by using nonspecific extracellular contrast material in CT or MR studies permits optimal tumor detection. With either CT or MR imaging, dynamic imaging after the administration of contrast material has proved to be useful in detecting and staging pancreatic cancer. In the early phase of the dynamic study, the pancreas shows markedly uniform enhancement; in the later phase, its signal intensity (at MR imaging) or attenuation (at CT) gradually diminishes. On the other hand, pancreatic cancers are usually desmoplastic and hypovascular and thus appear at MR imaging as low-signal-intensity areas or at CT as low-attenuating areas during the early phase.

There have been few studies, however, in which dynamic helical CT was compared with dynamic MR imaging (10,12). Ichikawa et al (11) performed their dynamic MR study by using a 256 × 512 matrix and thin sections. Their MR imaging technique showed better performance than did helical CT in the identification of tumor, peripancreatic extension, and vascular involvement. However, in the present study, we found significantly better performance in the detection of peripancreatic tissue invasion and peripancreatic vascular invasion with helical CT, but the tumors were somewhat more conspicuous on the dynamic MR images. The difference between the results of the study by Ichikawa et al and those of this study may be due to the difference in CT technique. Ichikawa et al used 5-mm collimation with a standard field of view, whereas we used 3-mm collimation with a small field of view. The difference in spatial resolution between these two collimation techniques is substantial.

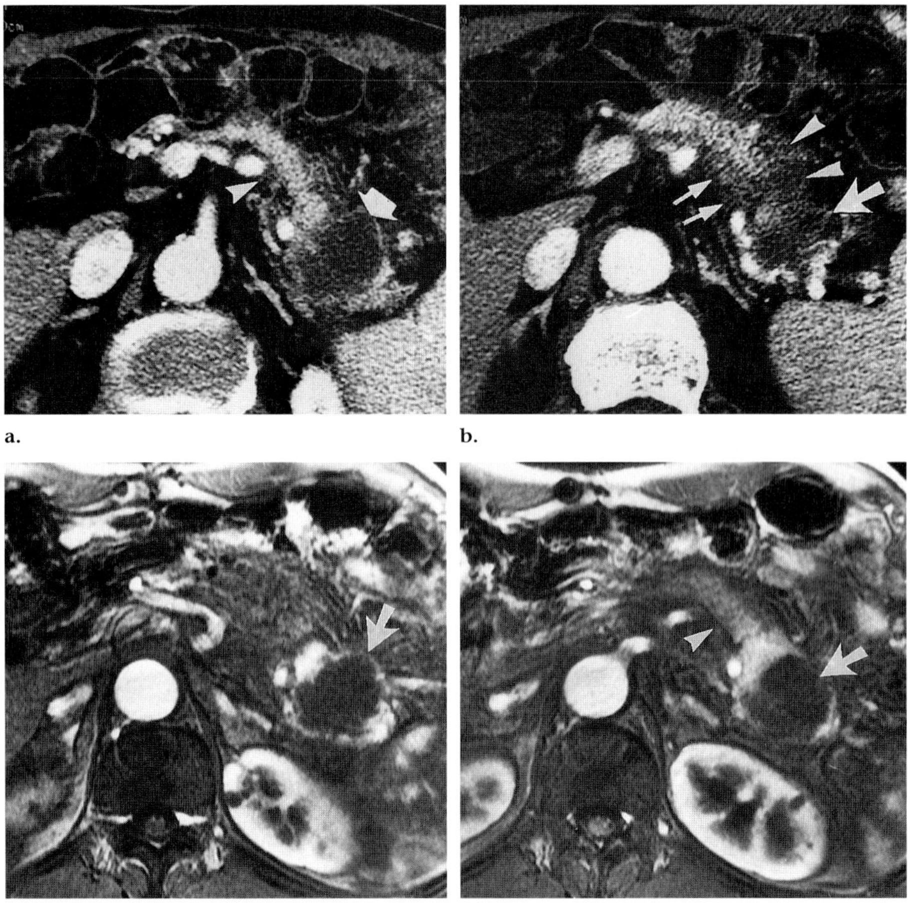

a. b. c. d.

Figure 3. **(a, b)** Axial helical CT scans and **(c, d)** axial contrast-enhanced dynamic T1-weighted FLASH MR images (150/4.1), both of which were obtained during the early phase in a 61-year-old woman with pancreatic cancer. **(a–d)** A mass lesion (large arrow) is seen in the tail of the pancreas on both the helical CT scans and dynamic MR images. Splenic vein encasement (arrowheads in **a**, **b**, and **d**) is seen on the CT scan obtained during the early phase and on the MR image obtained during the late phase. **(b)** Encasement of the splenic artery (small arrows) is seen. However, it is difficult to estimate the degree of peripancreatic arterial invasion in **c** and **d**, because these images have intersection gap and chemical shift artifacts, which are always seen between the pancreas and peripancreatic fat at MR imaging. Tumor invasion into the body of the pancreas and into the peripancreatic tissue also is seen, but it is not evident on the dynamic MR images. The operative findings confirmed invasion into the splenic vein, splenic artery, and peripancreatic tissues.

Theoretically, dynamic MR imaging has several potential advantages over dynamic CT. MR imaging has better contrast enhancement sensitivity and temporal resolution for whole-organ coverage and allows the administration of a more compact bolus for the contrast material injection. Breath-hold MR imaging provides better image quality than does the non–breath-hold technique. However, because imaging must be completed within a breath-hold period, the spatial resolution at MR imaging is substantially lower than that at CT owing to limited phase-encoding steps. The spatial resolution at CT can be increased by using the targeted thin-section technique. Furthermore, a breath hold of at least 16 seconds is required in multisection dynamic MR imaging, and this occasionally causes image blurring. In our study, there were several patients who could not hold their breath for 16 seconds and thus started to breathe. With helical CT, even if the patient cannot tolerate breath holding at the end of scanning, the quality of the majority of the sections will not be degraded by the resultant artifact. In our study, chemical shift, susceptibility, and vascular ghosting artifacts were unavoidable with MR imaging and caused difficulty in interpreting the fine details of peripancreatic and vascular invasion.

We found the three-dimensional data acquisition in helical CT to be useful in assessing vascular invasion. Although definite criteria for vascular invasion have not been established, thin-section helical CT after the intravenous administration of a bolus of contrast material reportedly increases the ability to assess vascular involvement by pancreatic cancer (25,27). In our study, at MR imaging, including dynamic studies, data were acquired with the two-dimensional multisection technique. Evaluation of vascular invasion was extremely difficult owing to the large section thickness and intersection gaps. Three-dimensional gradient-echo sequences have been used for vascular imaging. However, these sequences are mainly designed for imaging the vessels. We used this technique several times, but the signal-to-noise ratio and soft-tissue contrast were poor because of the extremely short repetition time. In the future, a fast three-dimensional data acquisition technique optimized for nonvascular imaging may help resolve the potential drawbacks of two-dimensional MR imaging.

Although diagnostic capability has substantially improved with recent developments in CT and MR imaging techniques, it is often difficult to detect very small tumors confined to the pancreas. Neither CT nor MR imaging demonstrated three tumors smaller than 1.5 cm in diameter that were confined to the pancreas. These tumors were detected only by using endoscopic US or at intraoperative palpation. The false-positive diagnosis of cancer of the pancreas in patients with chronic pancreatitis remains a diagnostic dilemma (14). Unless ancillary features of chronic pancreatitis are evident, differentiating these two entities may be impossible with the current techniques.

By taking advantage of the fine spatial resolution and consistency provided by the current CT technology, one can successfully use CT in tumor detection and staging. The sensitivity and accuracy of MR imaging seem to be inferior to those of CT owing to the limited spatial resolution and various artifacts, including chemical shift, motion, pulsation, and susceptibility artifacts, associated with MR imaging. The circumstances in which MR imaging may be useful include those in which (*a*) the clinical and CT findings are discordant, (*b*) the CT findings are indeterminate (16), or (*c*) the patient is allergic to iodinated contrast material.

A major disadvantage of the CT imaging protocol in this study is that the liver could not be fully evaluated by using our scanning parameters. We performed liver imaging before contrast material administration and during the delayed phase. Ideally, a CT protocol in which staging of pancreatic carcinoma is attempted should involve scanning of the liver to assess for the presence of hepatic metastases. However, the importance of the portal venous phase in imaging pancreatic carcinoma has been reported (8,28). Therefore, we chose to reduce the collimation in the early and portal venous phases to 3 mm and used a narrow field of view to increase the spatial resolution. Multisection helical scanners will make it possible to perform both portal venous phase hepatic imaging and thin-section pancreatic imaging.

The second limitation of our study is that histopathologic confirmation of all the imaging findings could not be obtained because 11 of the 31 tumors were nonresectable; however, a diagnosis of the tissue was made in all patients. Manual palpation of a pancreatic mass fixed to retropancreatic vessels indicates tumor resectability. In this study, although vascular involvement was confirmed at surgical palpation, the results of histologic examination confirmed the absence of invasion. Abundant fibrosis and many inflammatory changes surrounded the vessels. Further histopathologic comparison with helical CT or dynamic MR imaging findings would be necessary to establish the criteria for tumor invasion. Third, we did not evaluate lymph node swelling. This is because most of the metastatic tumors were small, and sometimes they were microscopic. This may have created a bias toward better results with both CT and MR imaging.

In conclusion, our study results demonstrated that, compared with MR imaging, thin-section helical CT may have more useful applications in the diagnostic imaging of pancreatic tumor. Thin-section helical CT of the pancreas enables detection of the tumor and evaluation of invasion into the peripancreatic tissue, peripancreatic artery, and/or portal vein.

References

1. Freeny PC, Marks WM, Ryan JA, Traverso LW. Pancreatic ductal adenocarcinoma: diagnosis and staging with dynamic CT. Radiology 1988; 166:125–133.
2. Bonaldi VM, Bret PM, Atri M, Garcia P, Reinhold C. A comparison of two injection protocols using helical and dynamic acquisitions in CT examinations of the pancreas. AJR 1996; 167:49–55.
3. Dupuy DE, Costello P, Ecker CP. Spiral CT of the pancreas. Radiology 1992; 183:815–818.
4. Vernacchia FS, Jeffrey RB Jr, Federle MP, et al. Pancreatic abscess: predictive value of early abdominal CT. Radiology 1987; 162: 435–438.
5. Zeman RK, Davros WJ, Berman P, et al. Three-dimensional models of the abdominal vasculature based on helical CT: usefulness in patients with pancreatic neoplasms. AJR 1994; 162:1425–1429.
6. Hollett MD, Jorgensen MJ, Jeffrey JB Jr. Quantitative evaluation of pancreatic enhancement during dual-phase helical CT. Radiology 1995; 195:359–361.
7. Lu DS, Reber HA, Krasny RM, Kadell BM, Sayre J. Local staging of pancreatic cancer: criteria for unresectability of major vessels as revealed by pancreatic-phase, thin-section helical CT. AJR 1997; 168:1439–1443.
8. Graf O, Boland GW, Warshaw AL, Fernandez-del-Castillo C, Hahn PF, Mueller PR. Arterial versus portal venous helical CT for revealing pancreatic adenocarcinoma: conspicuity of tumor and critical vascular anatomy. AJR 1997; 169:119–123.
9. Nishiharu T, Yamashita Y, Ogata I, Sumi S, Mitsuzaki K, Takahashi M. Spiral CT of the pancreas: the value of small field-of-view targeted reconstruction. Acta Radiol 1998; 39:60–63.
10. Gabata T, Matsui O, Kadoya M, et al. Small pancreatic adenocarcinomas: efficacy of MR imaging with fat suppression and gadolinium enhancement. Radiology 1994; 193:683–688.
11. Ichikawa T, Haradome H, Hachiya J, et al. Pancreatic ductal adenocarcinoma: preoperative assessment with helical CT versus dynamic MR imaging. Radiology 1997; 202:655–662.
12. Semelka RC, Kroeker MA, Shoenut JP, Kroeker R, Yaffe CS, Micflikier AB. Pancreatic disease: prospective comparison of CT, ERCP, and 1.5-T MR imaging with dynamic gadolinium enhancement and fat suppression. Radiology 1991; 181:785–791.
13. Semelka RC, Simm FC, Retch M, Delmming M, Lenz G, Laug GA. MR imaging of the pancreas at high field strength: a comparison of six sequences. J Comput Assist Tomogr 1991; 15:966–971.
14. Megibow AJ, Zhou XH, Rotterdam H, et al. Pancreatic adenocarcinoma: CT versus MR imaging in the evaluation of resectability—report of the Radiology Diagnostic Oncology Group. Radiology 1995; 195: 327–332.
15. Vellet AD, Romano W, Bach DB, Passi RB, Taves DH, Munk PL. Adenocarcinoma of the pancreatic ducts: comparative evaluation with CT and MR imaging at 1.5 T. Radiology 1992; 183:87–95.
16. Semelka RC, Kelekis NL, Molina PL, Sharp TJ, Calvo B. Pancreatic masses with inconclusive findings on spiral CT: is there a role for MRI? JMRI 1996; 6:585–588.
17. Irie H, Honda H, Kaneko K, Kuroiwa T, Yoshimitsu K, Masuda K. Comparison of helical CT and MR imaging in detecting and staging small pancreatic adenocarcinoma. Abdom Imaging 1997; 22:429–433.
18. Metz CE. ROC methodology in radiologic imaging. Invest Radiol 1986; 21:720–733.
19. Hanley JA, McNeil BJ. The meaning and use of the area under a receiver operating characteristic (ROC) curve. Radiology 1982; 143:29–36.
20. Bluemke DA, Cameron JL, Hruban RH, et al. Potentially resectable pancreatic adeno-

carcinoma: spiral CT assessment with surgical and pathologic correlation. Radiology 1995; 197:381–385.

21. Raptopoulos V, Steer ML, Sheiman RG, Vrachliotis TG, Gougoutas CA, Movson JS. The use of helical CT and CT angiography to predict vascular involvement from pancreatic cancer: correlation with findings at surgery. AJR 1997; 168:971–977.
22. Choi BI, Chung MJ, Han JK, Han MC, Yoon YB. Detection of pancreatic adenocarcinoma: relative value of arterial and late phases of spiral CT. Abdom Imaging 1997; 22:199–203.
23. Coley SC, Strickland NH, Walker JD, Williamson RC. Spiral CT and the preoperative assessment of pancreatic adenocarcinoma. Clin Radiol 1997; 52:24–30.
24. Zeman RK, Cooper C, Zeiberg AS, et al. TNM staging of pancreatic carcinoma using helical CT. AJR 1997; 169:459–464.
25. Loyer EM, David CL, Dubrow RA, Evans DB, Charnsangavej C. Vascular involvement in pancreatic adenocarcinoma: reassessment by thin-section CT. Abdom Imaging 1996; 21:202–206.
26. Mitchell DG, Vinitski S, Saponaro S, et al. Liver and pancreas: improved spin-echo Tl contrast by shorter TE and fat suppression at 1.5 T. Radiology 1991; 178:68–71.
27. Kaneko K, Honda H, Hayashi T, et al. Helical CT evaluation of arterial invasion in pancreatic tumors: comparison with angiography. Abdom Imaging 1997; 22: 204–207.
28. Keogan MT, McDermott VG, Paulson EK, et al. Pancreatic malignancy: effect of dual-phase helical CT in tumor detection and vascular opacification. Radiology 1997; 205:513–518.

Elena Rociu, MD
Jaap Stoker, MD
Marinus J. C. Eijkemans, MSc
W. Ruud Schouten, MD
Johan S. Laméris, MD

Index terms:
Anus, abnormalities, 757.411
Anus, MR, 757.121411, 757.121412
Anus, US, 757.12981, 757.12989
Magnetic resonance (MR), comparative studies

Radiology 1999; 212:453–458

[1] From the Departments of Radiology (E.R.) and General Surgery (W.R.S.), University Hospital Rotterdam, the Netherlands; the Department of Radiology, Academic Medical Center, University of Amsterdam, G 1-211, Meibergdreef 9, 1105 AZ Amsterdam, the Netherlands (J.S., J.S.L.); and the Department of Public Health, Erasmus University, Rotterdam, the Netherlands (M.J.C.E.). Received June 18, 1998; revision requested August 5; final revision received November 23; accepted March 1, 1999. **Address reprint requests to** J.S. (e-mail: *j.stoker@amc.uva.nl*).

Author contributions:
Guarantor of integrity of entire study, E.R.; study concepts and design, E.R., J.S., J.S.L.; definition of intellectual content, E.R., J.S., J.S.L.; literature research, E.R.; clinical studies, E.R., J.S., J.S.L., W.R.S.; data acquisition and analysis, E.R., J.S., M.J.C.E.; statistical analysis, M.J.C.E.; manuscript preparation, E.R., J.S.; manuscript editing, E.R.; manuscript review, E.R., J.S., J.S.L., M.J.C.E.

Fecal Incontinence: Endoanal US versus Endoanal MR Imaging[1]

PURPOSE: To assess endoanal ultrasonography (US) and endoanal magnetic resonance (MR) imaging for mapping of anal sphincter defects that have been validated at surgery in patients with fecal incontinence.

MATERIALS AND METHODS: US, MR imaging, and surgical findings in 22 women with fecal incontinence who underwent sphincter repair were retrospectively reviewed. US and MR imaging had been performed before surgery. The findings were evaluated separately and validated with surgical results.

RESULTS: Endoanal MR imaging findings showed better agreement with surgical results than did endoanal US findings for diagnosis of lesions of the external sphincter (κ value, 0.85 vs 0.53) and of the internal sphincter (κ value, 0.64 vs 0.49). Endoanal US could not accurately demonstrate thinning of the external sphincter. MR imaging results correlated moderately with US results (κ = 0.39). If endoanal MR images alone had been considered, the correct surgical decision would have been made in 21 (95%) patients; if endoanal US images alone had been considered, the correct decision would have been made in 17 (77%) patients.

CONCLUSION: MR imaging is more accurate than US for demonstration of sphincter lesions. MR imaging provides higher spatial resolution and better inherent image contrast for lesion characterization. Endoanal MR imaging allows more precise description of the extent and structure of complex lesions and is superior for help in decisions about optimal therapy.

Fecal incontinence, the inability to voluntarily control the anal sphincter, may severely affect a person's quality of life and eventually lead to social isolation (1). The prevalence reported in a number of studies (2,3) has ranged from three to 10 cases per thousand but may actually be much higher. The most common causes include traumatic sphincter defects (obstetric, surgical), neurogenic dysfunction of the pelvic floor musculature, and rectal prolapse (4,5).

The main cause of fecal incontinence in women is childbirth, which can lead to mechanical or neurologic injury to the anal sphincter (6), especially the external anal sphincter. After vaginal delivery, only 0.7% of women have clinically overt sphincter damage (7). Sultan et al (8) reported that 35% of primiparous women have occult sphincter damage after vaginal delivery, and one-third of these women also have direct disturbances of anal continence. An occult sphincter defect may precipitate overt symptoms later, in middle age, as the effects of menopause (9), neuropathy, and muscle loss accumulate (10).

In treating fecal incontinence, the physician can choose from several modalities (11). Patients with sphincter damage may benefit from surgical repair (12). The choice of an optimal therapy is determined on the basis of accurate images of the anal sphincter complex. Currently, endoanal ultrasonography (US) is the preferred diagnostic technique and has replaced the invasive method of electromyography (13,14). Recently, endoanal magnetic resonance (MR) imaging was introduced and was shown to be accurate in demonstrating the anatomy of the sphincter complex (15–19).

The aim of this study was to determine which imaging technique was preferable by assessing the amount of agreement between endoanal US and endoanal MR imaging findings for mapping of external sphincter defects that had been validated with surgical results.

MATERIALS AND METHODS

Patients

Twenty-two consecutive, nonselected women (median age, 49 years; range, 22–74 years) with fecal incontinence who underwent surgical repair of the sphincter were included in this retrospective study. Informed consent was obtained from all patients, and the medical ethics committee approved the research. All of the patients were parous (median, three deliveries; range, one to eight deliveries). The degree of fecal incontinence was determined by using the grading system of Parks (20): Three patients had grade II incontinence (incontinent for flatus alone), eight had grade III incontinence (incontinent for loose stool at any time), and 11 had grade IV incontinence (incontinent for solid stool). Incontinence occurred in the women after childbirth (19 patients), anorectal surgery (two patients), or rape (one patient). All patients underwent endoanal US and endoanal MR imaging on the same day, per the standard procedure at the University Hospital Rotterdam (the Netherlands). Before US, the patients underwent limited rectal cleansing. The mean and median interval between imaging and surgery were both 189 days. The same surgeon (W.R.S.) treated all patients.

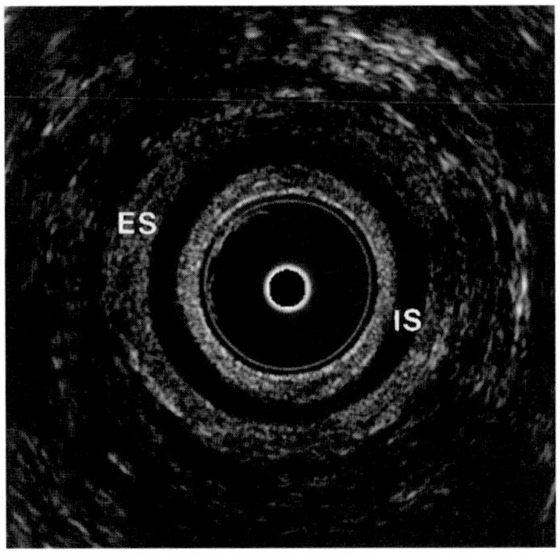

Figure 1. Axial endoanal US image shows a normal sphincter complex. *ES* = external sphincter, *IS* = internal sphincter.

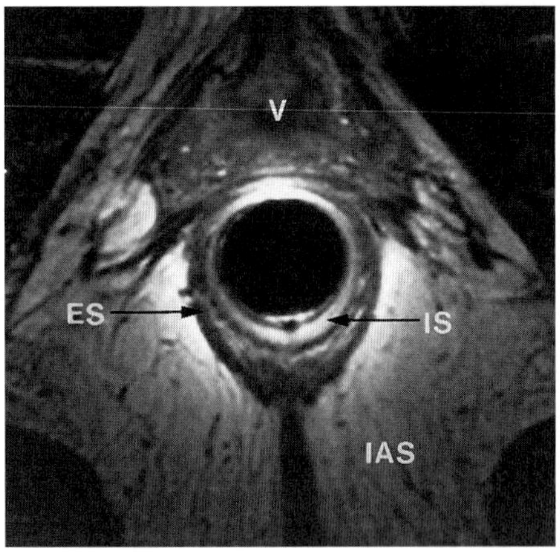

Figure 2. Axial endoanal gradient-echo MR image (30/13) shows a normal sphincter complex. *ES* = external sphincter, *IAS* = ischioanal space, *IS* = internal sphincter, *V* = vagina.

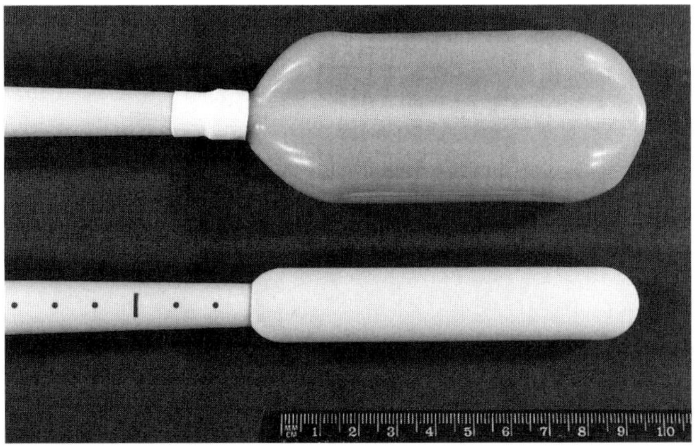

Figure 3. The endorectal coil is shown at top with a balloon. The rigid endoanal coil is shown at bottom.

Endoanal US

Endoanal US was performed with a scanner (Brüel & Kjaer, Naerum, Denmark) equipped with a rotating probe that provides a 360° image. A 7-MHz transducer with a minimum beam width of 1.1 mm and a focal length of 3 cm was used. The transducer was covered with a hard, plastic cone 18 mm in diameter. This cone was filled with degassed water for acoustic coupling and was covered with a condom after lubricant was applied to the surfaces of the condom and the cone.

The probe was inserted into the rectum while the patient was in the left lateral position and was rotated so that the 12 o'clock position was anterior. The probe was then withdrawn until the highly reflective puborectal muscle was seen; this structure was used as the main landmark. Hard copies of axial images of the puborectal muscle and the internal and external anal sphincters were recorded at four levels in the anal canal. Figure 1 is an endoanal US image of a normal sphincter complex.

The internal sphincter appears as a symmetric ring of low reflectiveness. Any break in the continuity of this ring is abnormal and indicative of direct trauma (21,22). The external anal sphincter classically shows a fibrillar pattern of fine parallel lines that becomes more homogeneous at lower levels. Tears are defined by an interruption of the fibrillar echotexture. Scarring is characterized by loss of the normal architecture, with an area of amorphous texture that usually has low reflectiveness. The sphincter muscles may also show local thickening or thinning. Generalized external sphincter atrophy is difficult to appreciate because of the vague contours of the muscle ring.

Endoanal MR Imaging

Endoanal MR imaging was performed at 1.5 T (Gyroscan ACS-NT; Philips Medical Systems, Best, the Netherlands) without bowel preparation. Figure 2 is an endoanal MR image of a normal sphincter complex. Before imaging, 1 mL of butylscopolamine bromide (Buscopan, 20 mg/mL; Boehringer Ingelheim, Germany) was injected intramuscularly to reduce bowel motion. The endoanal coil (Philips Medical Systems) (Fig 3), which was 19 mm in diameter, was covered with a condom, and lubricant was applied to the surface of the condom.

Axial three-dimensional gradient-echo MR imaging (30/13 [repetition time msec/echo time msec]; acquisition time, 6.5 minutes; flip angle, 60°; field of view , 140 × 112 mm; imaging matrix, 205 × 256; section thickness, 2 mm with contiguous sections; two signals acquired) was performed perpendicular to the long axis of the endoanal coil. For sagittal and coronal images, T2-weighted turbo spin-echo MR imaging was performed (2,800/120 [repetition time msec/effective echo time msec]; acquisition time, 5.0 minutes; echo train length, 10; echo spacing, 21.8 msec; field of view, 120 × 90 mm; imaging

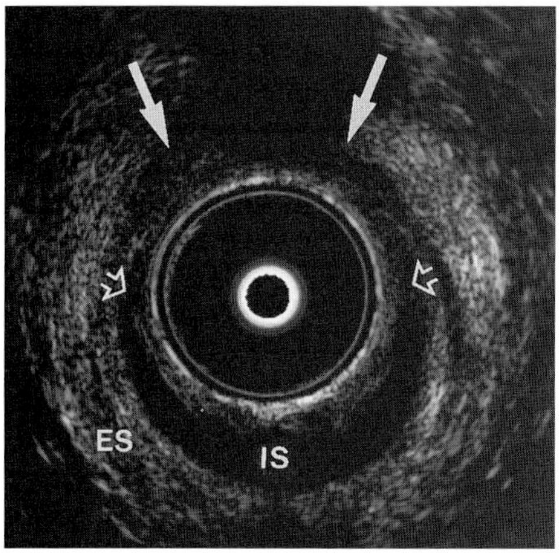

a.

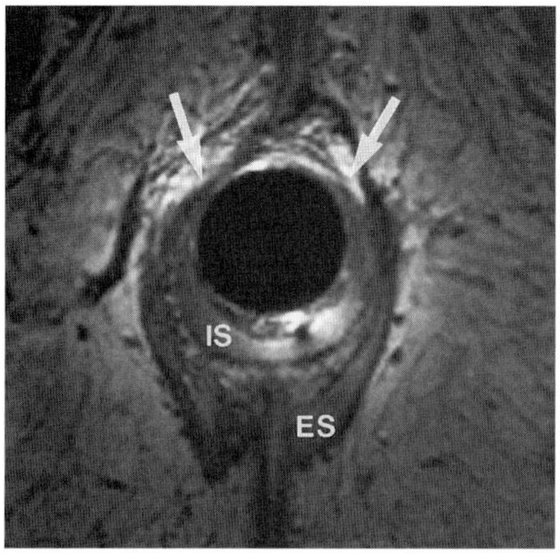

b.

Figure 4. **(a)** Axial endoanal US image in a 53-year-old woman with fecal incontinence shows a defect (solid arrows) of the external sphincter (*ES*) and a defect (open arrows) of the internal sphincter (*IS*). **(b)** Axial endoanal gradient-echo MR image (30/13) in the same patient also shows defects (arrows) of the external sphincter (*ES*) and the internal sphincter (*IS*).

TABLE 1
Endoanal US, Endoanal MR Imaging, and Surgical Diagnoses of External Sphincter Conditions

External Sphincter Condition	US Diagnosis		MR Imaging Diagnosis		Surgical Diagnosis
	Reported	Correct	Reported	Correct	
Defect	13	11	13	12	13
Scarring	5	4	5	4	4
Thinning	0	0	2	2	2
Normal	4	1	2	2	3
Total	22	16	22	20	22

TABLE 2
Endoanal US, Endoanal MR Imaging, and Surgical Diagnoses of Internal Sphincter Conditions

Internal Sphincter Condition	US Diagnosis		MR Imaging Diagnosis		Surgical Diagnosis
	Reported	Correct	Reported	Correct	
Defect	12	10	11	10	12
Scarring	1	1	1	1	1
Thinning	1	1	8	5	5
Normal	8	3	2	1	4
Total	22	15	22	17	22

matrix, 186 × 256; section thickness, 4.0 mm with an intersection gap of 0.4 mm; eight signals acquired). The coronal and sagittal sections were parallel to the long axis of the endoanal coil.

A sphincter defect was defined as a discontinuity of the muscle ring. Scarring was defined as a hypointense deformation of the normal pattern of the muscle layer due to replacement of muscle cells by fibrous tissue. Local thinning and generalized atrophy were scored on MR images.

Image Analysis

Before surgery, two radiologists evaluated the images separately: One radiologist (J.S.L.) evaluated the US images, and the other (J.S.) evaluated the MR images. Each radiologist was blinded to the results of the other technique. The decision to perform surgery was made by the surgeon on the basis of medical history, physical examination findings, and the existence of any kind of lesion of the external sphincter on MR or US images.

Because atrophy of the sphincter is not visible on endoanal US images, this condition was not considered in the correlation with MR imaging results. The quality of the images (good, moderate, or poor) and the presence, location, and type of lesions were thoroughly evaluated and recorded. The results of the imaging methods were compared with the detailed description of the surgical findings.

Statistical Analyses

Differences between US and MR imaging in the quality of images were tested with the χ^2 statistic. The categoric agreement between US, MR imaging, and surgical findings was assessed by calculating unweighted κ values. A κ value of 0.20 or less indicated poor agreement; a κ value of 0.21–0.40, moderate agreement; a κ value of 0.61–0.80, good agreement; and a κ value of 0.81–1.00, very good agreement.

In this retrospective study, all patients underwent surgery because a lesion was detected at imaging. There may have been patients with a lesion that was not detected at imaging who consequently did not undergo surgery. Therefore, the positive predictive value of the imaging techniques was considered to be a more appropriate measure than the sensitivity. The operation revealed only those parts of the sphincter that needed to be repaired. To avoid the possibility of iatrogenic incontinence, undamaged parts of the sphincter were not dissected. This rendered the negative predictive value more appropriate than the specificity. Therefore the positive and negative predictive values for detecting damage on both US and MR images were calculated.

RESULTS

Image Quality

The quality of the US images was good in 17 (77%) of 22 patients, moderate in two (9%), and poor in three (14%). The quality of the MR images was good in eighteen (82%) patients, moderate in three (14%), and poor in one (4%). The differences in image quality between US and MR imaging were not statistically significant (χ^2 test for comparison, $P = .5$; χ^2 test for trend, $P = .6$). No disturbing artifacts were present on the images.

External Sphincter

At surgery, an external sphincter defect was detected in 13 patients; isolated scarring, in four patients; and local thinning

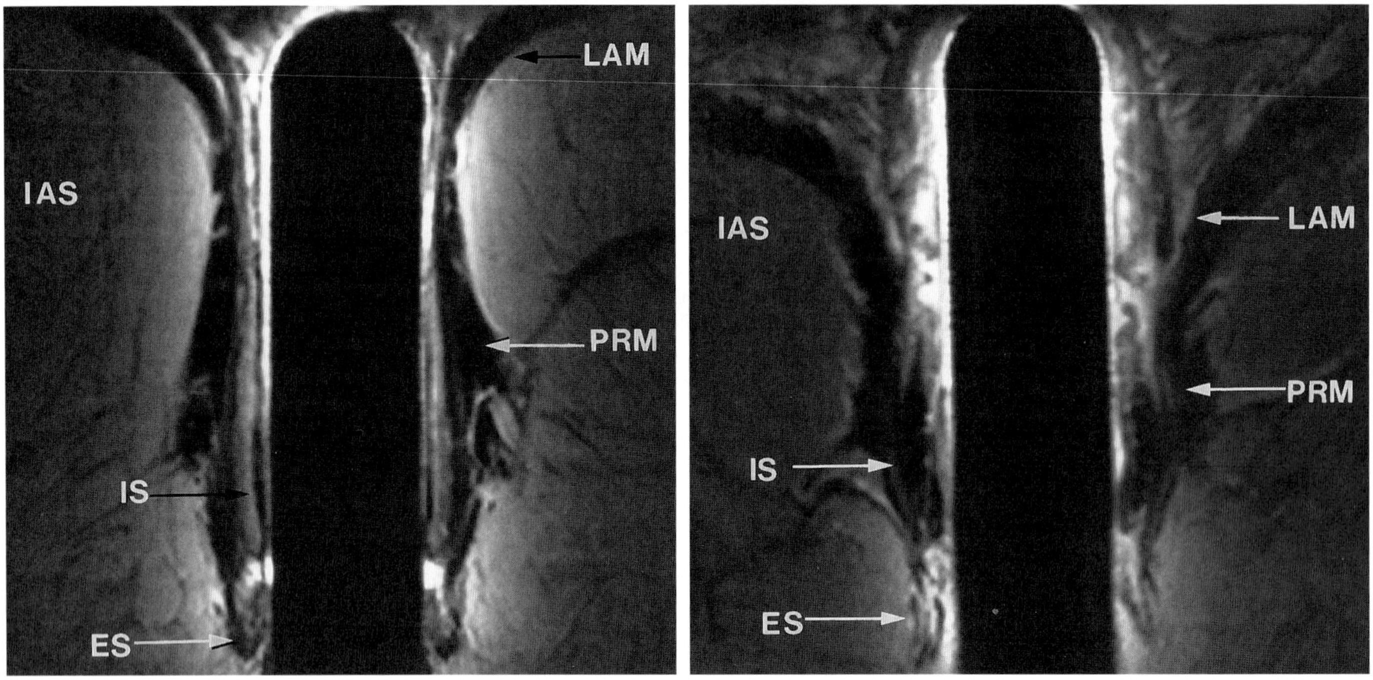

a. b.

Figure 5. **(a)** Coronal T2-weighted turbo spin-echo endoanal MR image (2,800/120 [effective]) in a 46-year-old woman with a normal anal sphincter. The external sphincter (*ES*), internal sphincter (*IS*), puborectal muscle (*PRM*), and levator ani muscle (*LAM*) are shown. *IAS* = ischioanal space. **(b)** Coronal T2-weighted turbo spin-echo endoanal MR image (2,800/120 [effective]) in a 61-year-old woman with atrophy of the external sphincter (*ES*). *IAS* = ischioanal space, *IS* = internal sphincter, *LAM* = levator ani muscle, *PRM* = puborectal muscle. Scarring causes low signal intensity in the internal sphincter.

of the sphincter, in two patients. Three patients had a normal sphincter. An external sphincter defect was correctly assessed at endoanal US in 16 (73%) of 22 patients, which was indicative of moderate agreement with surgical results (κ = 0.53) (Fig 4a). An external sphincter defect was correctly assessed at endoanal MR imaging in 20 (91%) patients, which was indicative of very good agreement with surgical results (κ = 0.85) (Fig 4b). At surgery, the position of one defect was different from that seen at MR imaging, and the imaging-determined position was considered to be incorrectly reported. External sphincter atrophy was detectable only with MR imaging and was seen in nine patients, in whom atrophy was confirmed at surgery (Fig 5). The surgeon did not find external sphincter atrophy in any patient in whom atrophy was not detected on MR images. The distribution of reported and correct diagnoses for the imaging techniques is shown in Table 1.

In this retrospective study, the decision to perform surgery was based on the presence of any kind of lesion of the external sphincter (defect, scar, or thinning) as seen on MR or US images. In this regard, there were no false-negative MR images and one false-positive MR image (Fig 6). US images were false-negative in three patients and false-positive in two. If MR imaging findings alone had been considered, the correct decision would have been made in 21 (95%) of 22 patients; if US findings alone had been considered, the correct decision would have been made in 17 (77%) patients.

Internal Sphincter

At surgery, an internal sphincter defect was found in 12 patients; local thinning, in five; isolated scarring, in one; and a normal sphincter, in four. On the basis of endoanal US findings, thinning was correctly reported in one patient and incorrectly reported as a normal internal sphincter in three patients and as a defect in one patient. All cases of thinning found at surgery were seen on MR images. In three additional patients, thinning was seen on MR images but was not validated at surgery. Endoanal US results were indicative of a correct diagnosis in 15 (68%) of 22 patients (Fig 4a); the agreement with surgical results was moderate (κ = 0.49). Endoanal MR imaging results were indicative of a correct diagnosis in 17 (77%) patients; the agreement with surgical results was good (κ = 0.64) (Fig 4b). The distribution of reported and correct diagnoses for the imaging techniques is shown in Table 2.

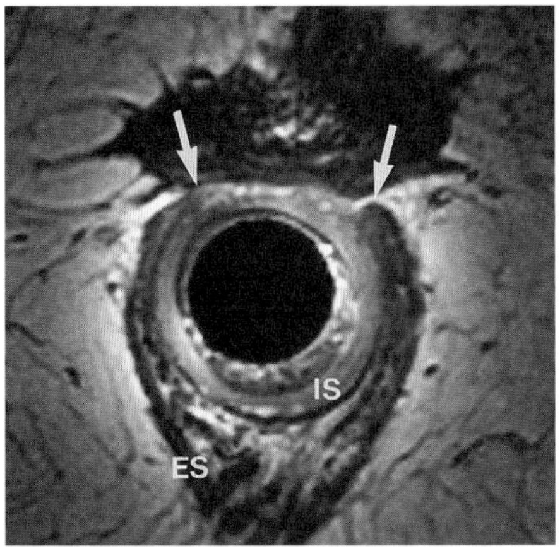

Figure 6. Axial endoanal gradient-echo MR image (30/13) in a 40-year-old woman with fecal incontinence shows a subtle decrease in signal intensity and altered texture (arrows) of the external sphincter (*ES*). These findings were suggestive of a diagnosis of scarring. Surgical results did not validate this diagnosis. *IS* = internal sphincter.

Agreement between US and MR Imaging Results

For the diagnosis of the external sphincter conditions (defects, scarring, thinning, or normal), endoanal US findings

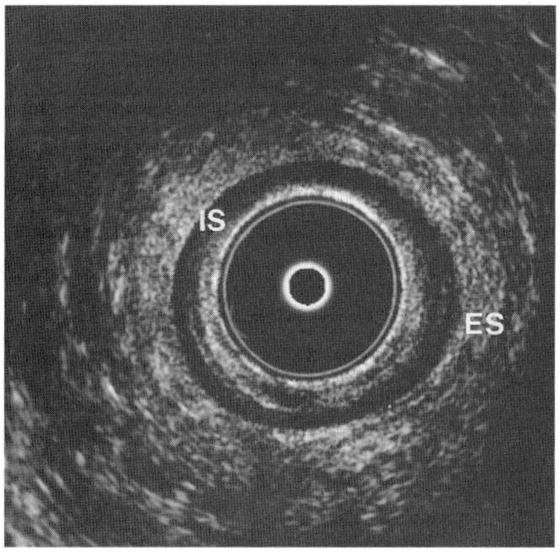

a.

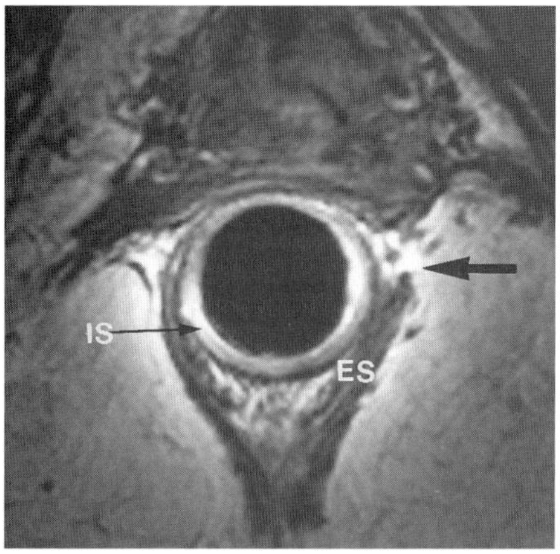

b.

Figure 7. (a) Axial endoanal US image in a 41-year-old woman with fecal incontinence shows no evidence of a lesion of the external sphincter (*ES*) or the internal sphincter (*IS*). At surgery, an external sphincter defect was found. **(b)** Axial endoanal gradient-echo MR image (30/13) in the same patient shows the defect (thick arrow) of the external sphincter (*ES*), which was validated with surgical results. The internal sphincter (*IS*) is normal on the MR image, and this finding was confirmed at surgery.

corresponded with endoanal MR imaging findings in 14 (64%) of 22 patients, which was indicative of fair to moderate agreement (κ = 0.38) (Fig 7). For mapping of internal sphincter damage, results from the two imaging techniques corresponded in 13 (59%) of 22 patients, again indicative of fair to moderate agreement (κ = 0.39).

Atrophy or thinning of the sphincter could not be correctly detected with endoanal US. The positive and negative predictive values for each diagnostic method for the demonstration of damage (excluding atrophy or thinning) of the external and internal sphincters are given in Table 3.

TABLE 3
Predictive Values of US and MR Imaging for Demonstration of Damage to the External and Internal Sphincters

Sphincter and Value	US	MR Imaging
External		
Positive predictive value	15 of 18 (83)	18 of 20 (90)
Negative predictive value	1 of 4 (25)	2 of 2 (100)
Internal		
Positive predictive value	12 of 14 (86)	16 of 20 (80)
Negative predictive value	3 of 8 (38)	1 of 2 (50)

Note.—Number in parentheses is the percentage.

For conditions of the external sphincter, MR imaging findings yielded good positive and negative predictive values, both higher than those of US findings. For conditions of the internal sphincter, the imaging techniques yielded comparable predictive values.

The positive predictive values for demonstration of any damage to the anal sphincter complex (external or internal sphincter) were 89% (32 of 36) for US and 95% (38 of 40) for MR imaging. Likewise, the negative predictive values were 25% (two of eight) for US and 100% (four of four) for MR imaging. Endoanal MR imaging results showed good agreement with surgical results (κ = 0.75), whereas US results showed moderate agreement (κ = 0.52).

DISCUSSION

Patients with fecal incontinence who may benefit from surgical therapy are selected on the basis of the detection and type of sphincter damage. To perform optimal surgery, an accurate description of the position, extent, and type of lesion is necessary. In previous studies (22), endoanal US findings validated with surgical results have been shown to be more accurate than findings from electromyography and manometry for the diagnosis of fecal incontinence. Other authors (23) have reported that endoanal US was also superior to MR imaging with a body coil for evaluation of the anatomy of the sphincter.

The limitation of endoanal US, however, is poor inherent contrast on images, which makes characterization of the external anal sphincter difficult. Surgery often damages this anal muscle, which is of major importance for continence. The recently developed technique of endoanal MR imaging produces images with high inherent contrast and high spatial resolution and enables detailed demonstration of normal sphincter anatomy and pathologic conditions (muscle tears, abscesses, fistulous tracks, scars, atrophy, and hypertrophy) (24). In a study (25) with seven patients who had obstetric sphincter trauma, endoanal MR imaging findings validated with surgical results provided a 100% accurate description of the site and extent of the sphincter tears.

Our aim, therefore, was to select the best imaging technique for the work-up in patients with a sphincter defect. To our knowledge, this is the first study in which endoanal MR imaging and endoanal US have been directly compared in relation to surgical findings in patients with fecal incontinence. In our study, the sphincter lesion in all but three patients was the result of childbirth. The position of the majority of lesions, therefore, was anterior. In the three patients with a lesion not caused by childbirth, the position of the lesion also was anterior. The surgical technique (anterior anal repair) allowed a good description of the lesion, which was used as the reference standard for the comparison between the two imaging methods.

Lesion Detection

For the detection of lesions, MR imaging findings showed very good agreement with surgical results as regards the external sphincter and good agreement as regards the internal sphincter. US findings showed moderate agreement with surgical results for detection of lesions of both the external sphincter and the internal sphincter. The correlation between MR imaging and US findings was moderate.

The negative predictive value of both techniques was relatively low. This can be explained by the fact that our study included a small number of patients with lesions that could not be detected on either on MR or US images. If, for instance, the lesion in one additional patient could have been detected on MR images, the negative predictive value of MR imaging would have doubled. Further study with a larger number of patients will result in a more accurate determination of the negative predictive value. Nevertheless, MR imaging yielded a combination of high positive and negative predictive values for lesions of the external sphincter, which suggests that MR imaging is a good preoperative diagnostic method in patients who require anterior sphincter repair.

Lesion Characterization

US and MR imaging were comparable with regard to characterization of damage to the internal sphincter. With regard to characterization of damage to the external sphincter, however, endoanal MR imaging allowed good distinction among different types of tissue (muscle, scar, fat). This facilitated accurate detection of local thinning, which was not possible with US, and more precise description of the extent and structure of complex lesions. In a recent study (26), it was shown that thinning and atrophy of the external sphincter seen on endoanal MR images is predictive of the outcome of anterior sphincteroplasty.

Surgical Decision Making

The two imaging techniques were complementary with regard to surgical decision making. The advantage of US is that it is a cheaper, more widely available, and quicker technique than MR imaging. Nevertheless, if only one technique is to be used, then MR imaging findings will result in the optimal decision more often than will US findings. This could prevent unnecessary surgery and may make MR imaging cost-effective.

A prospective study is currently underway to assess all the aspects presented in this report. In the current study, the use of endoanal MR imaging findings was superior to the use of endoanal US findings with regard to decisions about the optimal therapy.

References

1. Haugen V, Moore A. "I will manage": promoting continence through community education. J Wound Ostomy Continence Nurs 1995; 22:291–295.
2. Gordon PH, Nivatvongs S. Principles and practice of surgery for the colon, rectum, and anus. St Louis, Mo: Quality Medical, 1992.
3. Johanson JF, Lafferty J. Epidemiology of fecal incontinence: the silent affliction. Am J Gastroenterol 1996; 91:33–36.
4. Jorge JM, Wexner SD. Etiology and management of fecal incontinence. Dis Colon Rectum 1993; 36:77–97.
5. Vernava AM III, Longo WE, Daniel GL. Pudendal neuropathy and the importance of EMG evaluation of fecal incontinence. Dis Colon Rectum 1993; 36:23–27.
6. Wells M. Continence following childbirth. Br J Nurs 1996; 5:353–354.
7. Sultan AH, Kamm MA, Hudson CN, Bartram CI. Third-degree obstetric anal sphincter tears: risk factors and outcome of primary repair. BMJ 1994; 308:887–891.
8. Sultan AH, Kamm MA, Hudson CN, Thomas JM, Bartram CI. Anal-sphincter disruption during vaginal delivery. N Engl J Med 1993; 329:1905–1911.
9. Laurberg S, Swash M. Effects of aging on the anorectal sphincters and their innervation. Dis Colon Rectum 1989; 32:737–742.
10. Snooks SJ, Swash M, Mathers SE, Henry MM. Effect of vaginal delivery on the pelvic floor: a 5-year follow-up. Br J Surg 1990; 77:1358–1360.
11. Norton C. Faecal incontinence in adults. II. Treatment and management. Br J Nurs 1997; 6:23–26.
12. Briel JW, de Boer LM, Hop WC, Schouten WR. Clinical outcome of anterior overlapping external anal sphincter repair with internal anal sphincter imbrication. Dis Colon Rectum 1998; 41:209–214.
13. Enck P, von Giesen HJ, Schafer A, et al. Comparison of anal sonography with conventional needle electromyography in the evaluation of anal sphincter defects. Am J Gastroenterol 1996; 91:2539–2543.
14. Tjandra JJ, Milsom JW, Schroeder T, Fazio VW. Endoluminal ultrasound is preferable to electromyography in mapping anal sphincteric defects. Dis Colon Rectum 1993; 36:689–692.
15. Hussain SM, Stoker J, Laméris JS. Anal sphincter complex: endoanal MR imaging of normal anatomy. Radiology 1995; 197:671–677.
16. Hussain SM, Stoker J, Zwamborn AW, et al. Endoanal MRI of the anal sphincter complex: correlation with cross-sectional anatomy and histology. J Anat 1996; 189: 677–682.
17. deSouza NM, Puni R, Gilderdale DJ, Bydder GM. Magnetic resonance imaging of the anal sphincter using an internal coil. Magn Reson Q 1995; 11:45–56.
18. deSouza NM, Puni R, Zbar A, Gilderdale DJ, Coutts GA, Krausz T. MR imaging of the anal sphincter in multiparous women using an endoanal coil: correlation with in vitro anatomy and appearances in fecal incontinence. AJR 1996; 167:1465–1471.
19. Stoker J, Laméris JS. Endoanal magnetic resonance imaging. Acta Gastroenterol Belg 1997; 60:274–277.
20. Parks AG. Royal Society of Medicine, section of proctology; meeting 27 November 1974: president's address—anorectal incontinence. Proc R Soc Med 1975; 68:681–690.
21. Sultan AH, Kamm MA, Nicholls RJ, Bartram CI. Prospective study of the extent of internal anal sphincter division during lateral sphincterotomy. Dis Colon Rectum 1994; 37:1031–1033.
22. Sultan AH, Kamm MA, Talbot IC, Nicholls RJ, Bartram CI. Anal endosonography for identifying external sphincter defects confirmed histologically. Br J Surg 1994; 81: 463–465.
23. Schafer A, Enck P, Furst G, Kahn T, Frieling T, Lubke HJ. Anatomy of the anal sphincters: comparison of anal endosonography to magnetic resonance imaging. Dis Colon Rectum 1994; 37:777–781.
24. deSouza NM, Kmiot WA, Puni R, et al. High resolution magnetic resonance imaging of the anal sphincter using an internal coil. Gut 1995; 37:284–287.
25. deSouza NM, Hall AS, Puni R, Gilderdale DJ, Young IR, Kmiot WA. High-resolution magnetic resonance imaging of the anal sphincter using a dedicated endoanal coil: comparison of magnetic resonance imaging with surgical findings. Dis Colon Rectum 1996; 39:926–934.
26. Rociu E, Stoker J, Briel JW, Hop WC, Schouten WR, Laméris JS. Endoanal MR imaging evaluation of sphincter atrophy (abstr). Radiology 1997; 205(P):453.

Effects of Superparamagnetic Iron Oxide on Radiofrequency–induced Temperature Distribution: In Vitro Measurements in Polyacrylamide Phantoms and in Vivo Results in a Rabbit Liver Model[1]

Elmar M. Merkle, MD
S. Nahum Goldberg, MD
Daniel T. Boll, MD
Ajit Shankaranarayanan, BS
Travis Boaz, MD
Gretta H. Jacobs, MD
Michael Wendt, PhD
Jonathan S. Lewin, MD

Index terms:
Iron
Liver, interventional procedures, 761.1269
Liver neoplasms, therapy, 761.1269
Magnetic resonance (MR), utilization, 761.1269, 761.121412
Radiofrequency (RF), ablation, 761.1269, 761.33

Radiology 1999; 212:459–466

Abbreviations:
RF = radio frequency
SE = spin echo
SPIO = superparamagnetic iron oxide
STIR = short inversion time inversion recovery

[1] From the Depts of Radiology and MR Imaging (E.M.M., D.T.B., A.S., T.B., M.W., J.S.L.), Biomedical Engineering (A.S., M.W.), Pathology (G.H.J.), and Oncology (J.S.L.), University Hospitals of Cleveland/Case Western Reserve University, 11100 Euclid Ave, Cleveland, OH 44106; Dept of Diagnostic Radiology, University of Ulm, Germany (E.M.M.); and Dept of Radiology, Beth Israel Deaconess Medical Center, Harvard Medical School, Boston, Mass (S.N.G.). Received July 29, 1998; revision requested Aug 28; final revision received Dec 9; accepted Jan 21, 1999. Supported in part by grants from the Whitaker Foundation, Siemens Medical Systems, Radionics, American Cancer Society, Mary Ann S. Swetland Fund, M.E. and F.J. Callahan Foundation, and Deutsche Forschungsgemeinschaft grant Me 1593/1-1. **Address reprint requests to** J.S.L. (e-mail: *lewin@uhrad.com*).

Author contributions:
Guarantors of integrity of entire study, J.S.L., E.M.M.; study concepts and design, J.S.L., E.M.M., M.W., S.N.G., D.T.B.; definition of intellectual content, J.S.L., E.M.M., M.W., S.N.G., D.T.B.; literature research, J.S.L., E.M.M., D.T.B.; experimental studies, E.M.M., G.H.J., T.B., D.T.B., A.S.; data acquisition, J.S.L., E.M.M., G.H.J.; data analysis, J.S.L., E.M.M., G.H.J., S.N.G.; statistical analysis, J.S.L., E.M.M., S.N.G.; manuscript preparation, editing and review, J.S.L., E.M.M., M.W., G.H.J., S.N.G.

PURPOSE: To determine whether contrast medium containing superparamagnetic iron oxide (SPIO) alters radio-frequency (RF)–related temperature distribution in acrylamide phantoms and in an in vivo model.

MATERIALS AND METHODS: In nine acrylamide phantoms with increasing SPIO content, RF was applied with simultaneous measurement of temperature profile along the probe track. Additionally, magnetic resonance imaging–guided RF ablation was performed in the liver of six rabbits after the intravenous administration of SPIO (0.05 mL per kilogram of body weight) 40 minutes prior to ablation (SPIO group) and in another six rabbits without prior SPIO administration (control group). Coagulation diameter was evaluated on the basis of postprocedural imaging and subsequent gross pathologic findings. Statistical analysis was performed with the Student *t* test.

RESULTS: In the phantoms, progressive increases in iron content resulted in higher temperatures along the RF electrode track ($P < .05$). In the in vivo model, however, SPIO at physiologic concentrations did not significantly increase the diameter of coagulation on the basis of either postprocedural imaging or subsequent gross pathologic findings. Additionally, no significant differences were seen in other RF-related parameters including impedance, voltage, current, and grounding pad temperature.

CONCLUSION: Administration of SPIO in conjunction with RF ablation of focal liver lesions is feasible and safe, but no significant difference in the extent of induced coagulation can be expected.

Minimally invasive treatment of malignant liver lesions has become an area of considerable interest during the past few years. In addition to percutaneous ethanol injection and transcatheter chemoembolization, localized thermal energy can be delivered by using many different energy sources such as laser, cryotherapy, radio frequency (RF), microwaves, or focused ultrasound to induce coagulation necrosis (1–5). The common limitation of these interstitial thermotherapies is the extent of induced coagulation necrosis. With use of conventional probes, lesion diameter is usually limited to approximately 15 mm in the liver (6). Subsequently, technical modifications such as perfused laser or RF systems have

TABLE 1
Content of SPIO in Different Acrylamide Samples

Sample No.	Amount (mL) of Ferumoxides (80-g sample)	Percentage of Physiologic Concentration
1	0.00	0
2	0.05	25
3	0.10	50
4	0.15	75
5	0.20	100
6	0.39	200
7	0.98	500
8	1.96	1,000
9	9.80	5,000

Note.—SPIO content in physiologic human liver was calculated considering the following parameters: recommended dose of ferumoxides, 0.05 mL/kg; body weight, 70 kg; hepatic SPIO uptake, 80%; human liver weight, 1.15 kg.

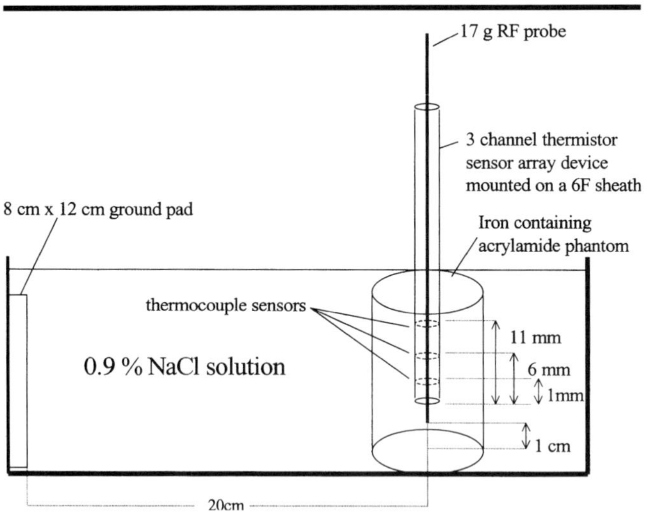

Figure 1. Standardized experimental setup for in vitro measurements performed in 0.9% saline solution. The distance between the RF probe tip and the bottom of the acrylamide phantom is 1 cm; the grounding pad is 20 cm away.

been developed to increase energy deposited into the tissue with a resultant increase in the diameter of coagulation to 4.5 and 2.4 cm in ex vivo and in vivo liver, respectively (7,8).

Other strategies to increase efficacy of interstitial RF thermotherapy have focused on changing the characteristics of the tissue to be ablated in an attempt to increase electric or thermal conductivity (eg, by means of intraparenchymal injection of saline solution during RF application) (9). Findings in prior studies have demonstrated altered heat transmission during RF application in the presence of iron compounds, which in part are also used as contrast media in diagnostic magnetic resonance (MR) imaging (10–13). We therefore sought to determine (*a*) whether contrast medium containing superparamagnetic iron oxide (SPIO) alters the temperature distribution in an in vitro model, (*b*) whether RF ablation is safe after intravenous administration of SPIO in an in vivo rabbit liver model, and (*c*) whether these iron compounds alter the volume of resultant coagulation.

MATERIALS AND METHODS

In Vitro Phantom Studies

Polyacrylamide phantoms.—Nine cylindric acrylamide phantoms were constructed (E.M.M.). Each phantom was 4.5 cm in diameter and 5.0 cm high, for a total volume of approximately 80 mL. Each of these phantoms contained 24 mL of 40% acrylamide-bis solution (37.5:1.0, 2.6% carbon) (Bio-Rad Laboratories, Hercules, Calif) mixed with 0.12 mL TEMED *N,N,N′N′*-tetra-methylethylenediamine (Bio-Rad Laboratories) with different concentrations of ferumoxides (Feridex IV; Berlex Laboratories, Wayne, NJ) added (Table 1). A 0.9% saline solution was then added up to a volume of 70 mL. Finally, 0.12 mg ammonium persulfate (Bio-Rad Laboratories) diluted in 10 mL distillated water was used as a polymerization initiator.

RF application.—The standardized experimental setup for in vitro measurements, performed in 0.9% saline solution, is shown in Figure 1. RF was applied for 6 minutes with use of a 50-W RF generator operating at 500 kHz and a custom MR-compatible 17-gauge monopolar electrode with 3-cm-long exposed tip (Radionics, Burlington, Mass). Tip temperature was maintained at 90°C ± 2 throughout the procedure. Parameters of RF application were documented, including impedance, voltage, current, and power. Each phantom was tested in a minimum of three trials, and phantom samples 1 (no SPIO added), 5 (physiologic SPIO concentration), and 9 (superphysiologic SPIO) were each tested eight times. Thus, a total of 42 RF applications were studied in this phase of experimentation. Temperature measurements along the probe track were determined by using a modified MR-compatible three-channel thermocouple sensor array device, which was mounted on a 6-F sheath (14) (Fig 1). This thermistor array provided temperature measurements during RF deposition at 1, 6, and 11 mm from the exposed electrode tip along the probe track. All other values were provided as output parameters on a display built in the RF generator. Statistical analysis was performed with the Student *t* test. A *P* value less than .05 was considered statistically significant.

In Vivo Studies

MR imaging system.—MR imaging guidance and monitoring for the RF probe insertion and ablation were performed with a low-field-strength, clinical C-arm, 0.2-T imaging system (Magnetom Open; Siemens Medical Systems, Erlangen, Germany) with three modifications to enable RF ablation.

First, an in-room 1,024 × 1,280-pixel RF-shielded liquid crystal monitor was installed to allow image viewing at the side of the magnet, in a manner analogous to the setup of an x-ray fluoroscopy suite. Second, control of the imager from within the imaging suite was enabled by means of an MR-compatible mouse and foot pedal. Third, rapid gradient-echo sequences were applied (fast imaging with steady-state precession, or FISP, with repetition time msec/echo time msec of 18/7, one signal acquired, flip angle of 90°, section thickness of 5 mm, field of view of 200 × 200, matrix of 128 × 256) to produce images with clinically adequate signal-to-noise ratio and spatial resolution. These images were acquired in 1.5–3.0 seconds per section in a single-section mode, or 4–9 seconds in a three-section mode.

A belt-shaped 12-cm-diameter multiturn solenoid receive-only coil was used for signal reception. The whole-body reso-

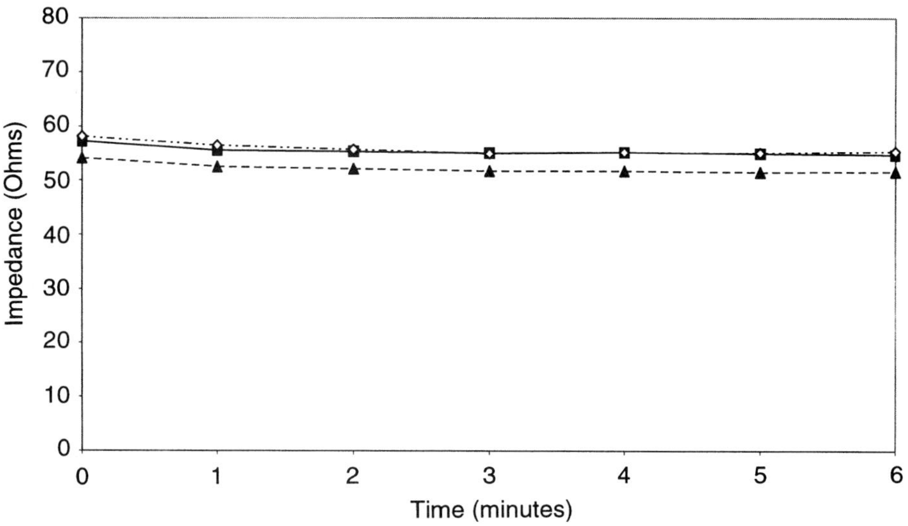

Figure 2. In vitro relationship between RF impedance and SPIO content. Phantom 1 (■) contains no SPIO; phantom 5 (▲), a standard concentration; and phantom 9 (◇), a superphysiologic dose (50 × standard dose). Mean values, on the basis of eight measurements in each phantom, are displayed at each time point (SEM values are in the range of 20% and are not displayed for clarity). Differences are not statistically significant.

nators incorporated in the imager were used for RF transmission.

Animal model.—On the basis of a protocol approved by the animal research committee at Case Western Reserve University, 12 male white New Zealand rabbits (weight range, 2.0–3.2 kg) were anesthetized by using a combination of xylazine (5 mg per kilogram of body weight) and ketamine (50 mg/kg) (both manufactured by Phoenix Scientific, St Joseph, Mo) in an intramuscular injection. A 22-gauge, 1-inch-long intravenous catheter (Terumo Medical, Elkton, Md) was inserted in a dorsal ear vein of the rabbits. In six rabbits, ferumoxides diluted with 5% dextrose solution (Baxter Health Care, Deerfield, Ill) was administered intravenously 40 minutes prior to the RF ablation procedure at a dose of 0.05 mL/kg (SPIO group). The other six rabbits received no SPIO and served as a control group.

The thighs and abdomen of each animal were shaved. The rabbits were positioned right side down within the gantry of the MR imager. An 8 × 12-cm wire mesh grounding pad coated with conductive gel was placed on each thigh bilaterally. A custom MR-compatible 17-gauge monopolar thermistor was inserted between the skin of the rabbit and the right grounding pad to measure the temperature in this area.

RF ablation.—After prospective determination of a desired ablation site (with a lot of parenchyma surrounding the electrode) on axial T2-weighted turbo spin-echo (SE) images (2,000/96, one signal acquired, echo train length of seven, total acquisition time of 3 minutes 49 seconds, section thickness of 5 mm, field of view of 200 × 200, matrix of 196 × 256), the target was localized by using a fluid-filled syringe on the skin surface. A custom MR-compatible 17-gauge monopolar electrode with 2-cm-long exposed tip (Radionics) was advanced with a continuous imaging mode that consisted of the sequential acquisition, reconstruction, and display of multiple sets of three parallel 5-mm-thick sections. This set of sections was centered on the predicted probe position to allow rapid detection of probe bending or deflection. After the probe was placed at the target site, the position was confirmed by means of T1-weighted SE imaging (480/26, three signals acquired, total acquisition time of 4 minutes 39 seconds, section thickness of 5 mm, field of view of 200 × 200, matrix of 192 × 256). In all rabbits, RF was applied for 8 minutes with the tip temperature maintained at 90°C ± 2. During RF application, impedance, voltage, current, power, and grounding pad temperatures were documented every 60 seconds.

Postprocedural imaging included turbo SE T2-weighted imaging (2,000/96, one signal acquired, echo train length of seven, total acquisition time of 3 minutes 49 seconds, section thickness of 5 mm, field of view of 200 × 200, matrix of 196 × 256), turbo short inversion time inversion-recovery (STIR) imaging (3,190/48/110 [inversion time msec], two signals acquired, echo train length of seven, total acquisition time of 5 minutes 19 seconds, section thickness of 5 mm, field of view of 200 × 200, matrix of 210 × 256), and SE T1-weighted imaging (480/26 with three signals acquired, total acquisition time of 4 minutes 39 seconds, section thickness of 5 mm, field of view of 200 × 200, matrix of 192 × 256) before and after intravenous administration of gadopentetate dimeglumine (Magnevist [0.1 mmol/kg]; Berlex Laboratories, Wayne, NJ). These sequences were chosen on the basis of prior findings that demonstrate the usefulness of T2-weighted turbo STIR and contrast material–enhanced T1-weighted images for visualization of thermally induced lesions (15,16). Gadopentetate dimeglumine was injected after ablation to help depict the area of hyperemia that surrounds the newly formed thermal lesion. Coagulation diameter perpendicular to the RF probe track was evaluated by means of postprocedural imaging and subsequent gross pathologic findings.

The background signal intensity (noise) and the signal intensities of the RF thermal lesion and liver were measured for all the previously mentioned sequences after RF application. Regions of interest were placed on homogeneous structures in artifact-free regions. Regions of interest representative of the tissue were chosen. Measurements were made at the same anatomic level for each image sequence for each rabbit. Regions of interest for signal intensity of RF thermal lesions included at least 20 pixels. Regions of interest for noise included at least 500 pixels. For the measurement of liver signal intensity (SI), three separate regions of interest from different areas of the same section were used, and the results were averaged. Mean background noise was measured for each image ventral to the liver outside the rabbit along the phase-encoding axis and included ghost artifacts that might have been propagated over the image (17). For all images, the RF-induced lesion-to-liver contrast-to-noise ratio was calculated for each sequence as $(SI_{liver} - SI_{lesion})/SI_{noise}$.

Statistical analysis was performed with the Student *t* test. A *P* value less than .05 was considered statistically significant.

RESULTS

In Vitro Phantom Studies

RF parameters including current and impedance reached steady state within 4 minutes of energy application (Figs 2, 3). Phantoms with a higher concentration of iron demonstrated higher temperatures

TABLE 2
RF-induced Lesion-to-Liver Contrast-to-Noise Ratios for Each Sequence

Sequence	SPIO Group	Control Group
Turbo STIR	1.07 ± 0.51	1.02 ± 0.64
T2 weighted	0.62 ± 0.59	0.63 ± 0.29
T1 weighted	1.21 ± 1.08	1.57 ± 1.78
Gadolinium-enhanced T1 weighted	2.58 ± 2.36	1.61 ± 0.94

Note.—Differences in contrast-to-noise ratios between groups were not statistically significant.

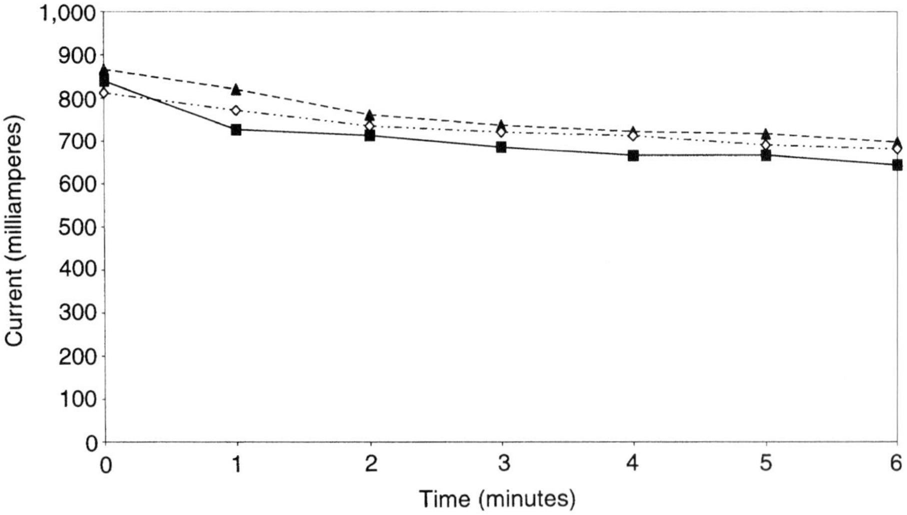

Figure 3. In vitro relationship between RF current and SPIO content. Phantom 1 (■) contains no SPIO; phantom 5 (▲), a standard concentration; and phantom 9 (◇), a superphysiologic dose. Mean values, on the basis of eight measurements in each phantom, are displayed at each time point (SEM values are in the range of 20% and are not displayed for clarity). Differences are not statistically significant.

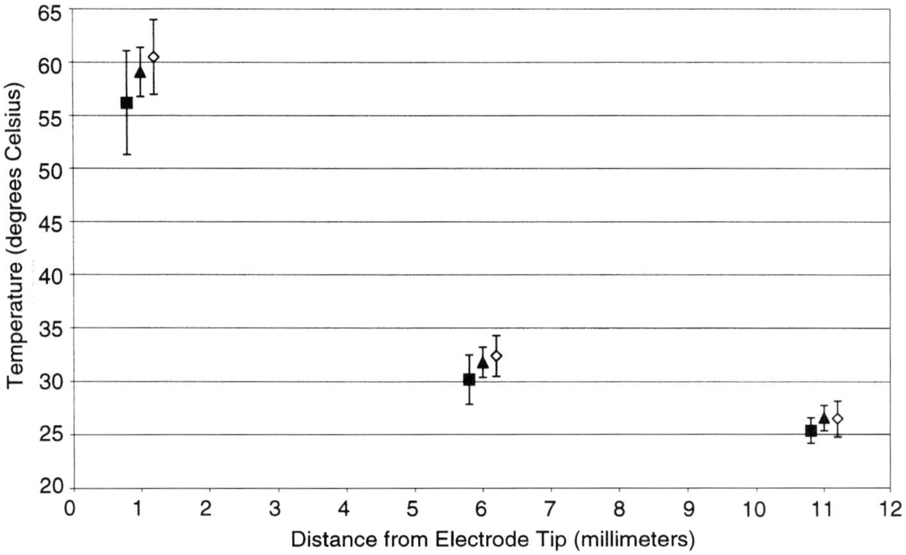

Figure 4. In vitro relationship between temperature profile along the RF probe track and SPIO content. Phantom 1 (■) contains no SPIO; phantom 5 (▲), a standard concentration; and phantom 9 (◇), a superphysiologic dose. Mean values plus or minus SEM, on the basis of eight measurements in each phantom, are displayed. Temperatures were measured at 1, 6, and 11 mm from the electrode tip (data points are expanded along the x axis for clarity). Differences are statistically significant between phantom 1 and phantom 5, and between phantom 1 and phantom 9. No statistically significant differences are found between phantom 5 and phantom 9.

along the RF electrode track (Fig 4). At a physiologic concentration of SPIO (phantom with 0.196 mL SPIO and total volume of 80 mL), temperatures increased by 2.9°C, 1.6°C, and 1.2°C over baseline at 1, 6, and 11 mm from the electrode tip, respectively. These differences were statistically significant (1 mm, $P = .04$; 6 mm, $P = .02$; 11 mm, $P = .01$). Superphysiologic concentrations of SPIO (phantom with 9.8 mL SPIO and total volume of 80 mL) increased heat deposition by 4.3°C, 2.3°C, and 1.1°C over baseline at 1, 6, and 11 mm from the electrode tip, respectively. These differences were also statistically significant (1 mm, $P < .01$; 6 mm, $P < .01$; 11 mm, $P = .04$).

However, no significant differences were observed between samples 5 (physiologic concentration) and 9 (superphysiologic concentration) (1 mm, $P = .18$; 6 mm, $P = .30$; 11 mm, $P = .90$). Baseline impedance (defined as the impedance before RF application) did not demonstrate any dependence on the concentration of SPIO. In all phantoms, the reduction in impedance after RF application for 6 minutes varied from 3 to 6 Ω (Fig 2). No significant differences were observed for the other RF-related parameters such as voltage, current, or power (Fig 3).

In Vivo Animal Studies

With MR guidance in all rabbits, the desired site for ablation in the liver was accessed without difficulty or complications.

On contrast-enhanced coronal SE T1-weighted images, coagulation, characterized as a central hypointense nonenhancing zone, ranged in diameter from 0.7 to 1.1 cm (0.87 cm ± 0.15 [mean ± SD]) and from 0.7 to 1.2 cm (0.97 cm ± 0.21) in the SPIO and control groups, respectively (Figs 5, 6). These differences in diameter were not statistically significant ($P = .36$). The foci of coagulation were also visible on nonenhanced SE T1-weighted images, but were poorly detected on turbo SE T2-weighted and turbo STIR images, as they were demarcated only by the surrounding edema. Contrast-to-noise ratios were highest for contrast-enhanced SE T1-weighted images in both groups (SPIO group, 2.58 ± 2.36; control group, 1.61 ± 0.94), but no statistically significant inter- or intragroup differences were seen (Table 2).

At pathologic analysis, coagulation diameter varied from 1.0 to 1.3 cm (1.15 cm ± 0.14) in the SPIO group and from 0.9 to 1.4 cm (1.22 cm ± 0.21) in the control group. These differences were also not statistically significant ($P = .54$). At

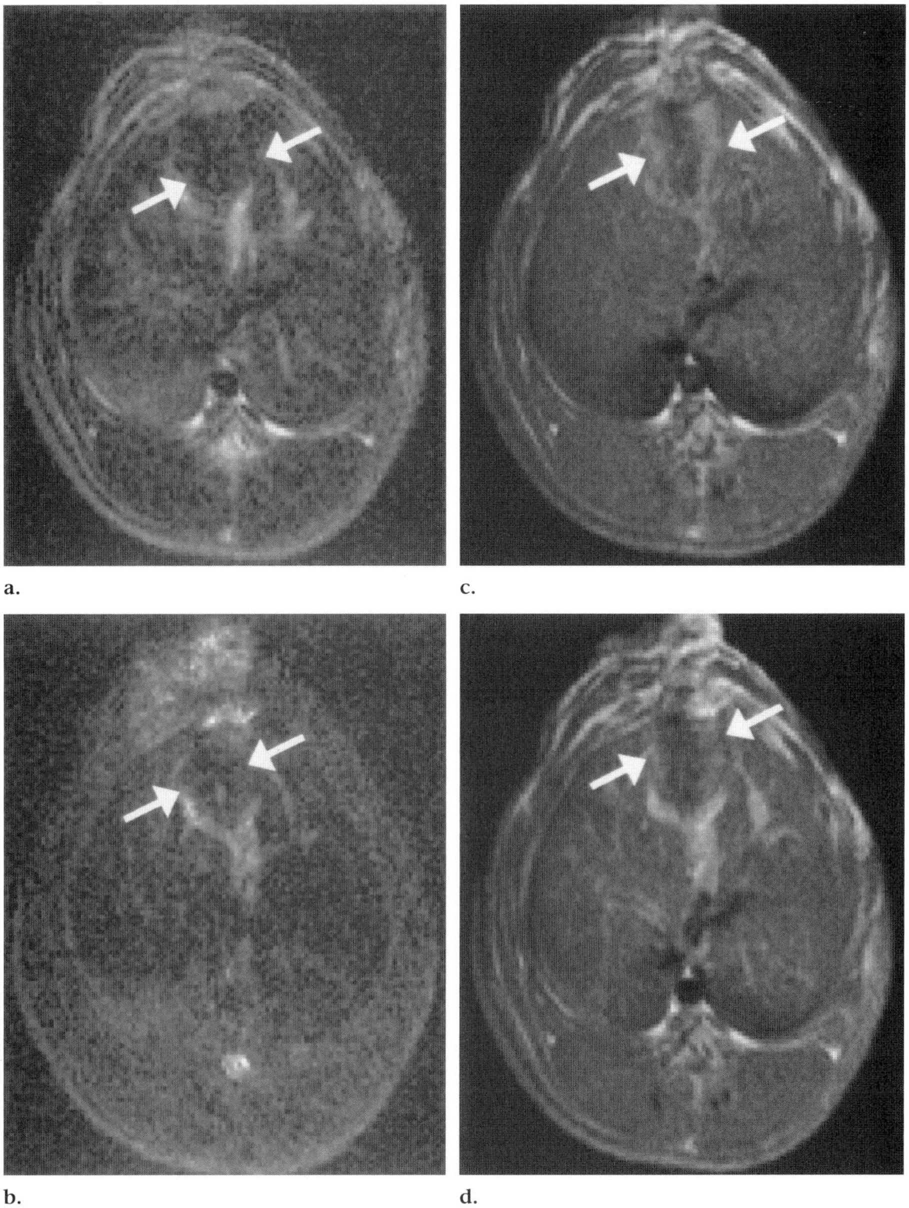

Figure 5. In vivo rabbit liver after intravenous administration of SPIO followed by RF application for 8 minutes. **(a)** Axial turbo SE T2-weighted image (2,000/96 with one signal acquired and echo train length of seven) and **(b)** axial turbo STIR image (3,190/48/110 with one signal acquired and echo train length of seven) depict coagulated tissue (arrows), which is poorly delineated by the surrounding edema. **(c)** Nonenhanced T1-weighted SE image (480/26 with three signals acquired) allows better visualization of the hypointense RF-induced lesion (arrows). **(d)** Gadolinium-enhanced T1-weighted SE image (480/26 with three signals acquired) clearly depicts the thermal lesion, which appears as a hypointense nonenhancing area with rim enhancement (arrows). The region of coagulation appears bigger in **a**.

gross examination in both groups, specimens demonstrated a central area of white tissue with a peripheral rim (1–2 mm thick) of pinkish tissue surrounded by normal liver parenchyma. The lesion border was assessed as well demarcated in two rabbits from each group, as irregular in three rabbits each, and as fuzzy in one rabbit each (Fig 7). At histologic examination, the central white zone corresponded to tissue coagulation, and the pink zone represented hyperemia.

Contrast-enhanced coronal SE T1-weighted images slightly underestimated the pathologic diameter of the thermal lesion, with a correlation coefficient of 0.67 for the SPIO group and 0.65 for the control group.

Differences in RF parameters were not statistically significant between the SPIO and control groups. The baseline impedance ranged from 90 to 103 Ω (96.33 Ω ± 5.81) in the SPIO group and from 87 to 103 Ω (97.00 Ω ± 5.59) in the control group; this difference was not statistically significant (P = .84). The drop in impedance after RF application for 8 minutes varied from 4 to 12 Ω (8.33 Ω ± 3.27) and from 4 to 11 Ω (7.00 Ω ± 2.61) in the SPIO and control groups, respectively (P = .45). Furthermore, significant differences were not observed for the other RF-related parameters such as voltage, current, and power. Grounding pad temperatures ranged from 37°C to 40°C, with no differences observed between the two groups.

DISCUSSION

RF ablation is a safe, minimally invasive modality that has been used in stereotactic neurosurgical procedures for more than 30 years (18). During the past decade, RF-induced tumor ablation has also been used in early clinical trials for the treatment of hepatocellular carcinoma (19), hepatic (9,20,21) and cerebral (15) metastases, and benign bone lesions such as osteoid osteomas (22). Typically, with cross-sectional imaging guidance, a thin (usually 14–21-gauge) electrode is placed percutaneously directly in the tumor. Coagulation necrosis results from resistive heating in the tissue adjacent to the noninsulated part of the electrode.

A key aim of tumor ablation therapy is eradication of the entire tumor with a minimum number of treatments. Yet, conventional monopolar RF electrodes can ablate tissue only 1.5 cm in diameter. As a result, multiple electrode insertions are required to treat all but the smallest tumors. Therefore, several approaches have been developed to increase the diameter of coagulation necrosis achieved when RF techniques are used, including multiprobe (23), hooked (24), and bipolar (25) arrays. Internally cooled RF electrodes have also been developed, and they are used without and with pulsed RF deposition (7,26,27). These techniques are all based on the premise of increasing energy deposition into the tumor from a single electrode or multiple electrodes.

Another strategy to increase the extent of coagulation is the injection of normal saline solution into the tumor through tiny holes at the distal end of the electrode during RF application in an attempt to alter tissue electric and thermal conductivity. With use of this technique with continuous infusion of saline solution at 1 mL/min in experimental animal models, Livraghi et al (9) reported coagulation as large as 4.1 cm in diameter. This strategy seems to confirm the supposition that high local ion concentration from saline solution injection could potentially increase the extent of coagulation necrosis by effectively increasing the area of the active surface electrode. Clinical results with this technique, however, have been somewhat disappointing. In the clinical study by Livraghi et al (9) of 14 patients with tumors up to 4.5 cm in diameter, coagulation volume was unpredictable and irregularly shaped. The authors offered two possible explanations: (*a*) uneven diffusion of saline solution results in nonuniform impedance and/or (*b*) diffusion of heated saline solution differentially through tissue leads to necrosis along the diffusion path.

Findings in prior studies have also demonstrated altered heat transmission during RF application in the presence of iron compounds (10–13). Ikenaga et al (13) report localized treatment in a rabbit bone tumor model with use of an alternating magnetic field. Hyperthermia of the tumor was accomplished after insertion of a ferromagnetic ceramic pin as an iron compound. These results were confirmed by Akagi et al (12), who report statistically significant antitumor effects of localized hyperthermia on an experimental bone tumor with use of an intramedullary nail and an RF generator system working with a maximum power of 5 kW at 100 kHz. The same effects were demonstrated when commercial powders of magnetite were investigated (10,11).

In the most common theory, high local ion concentration from iron oxide uptake is postulated to increase the extent of coagulation necrosis by effectively increasing the area of the active surface electrode. Another possible causative factor is the inductive heating of ferromagnetic particles and magnetic fluids after they are exposed to alternating magnetic fields. This effect is described in detail by Jordan and co-workers (10).

The biologic effects of magnetic microparticles exposed to an alternating magnetic field have been previously investigated in animal tumor systems with use of ferric hydroxide (28). The magnetically heated particles were shown to have tumoricidal effects.

In vitro, progressive increase of SPIO content within the acrylamide phantoms resulted in higher temperatures along the RF electrode track in our study (Fig 4). At a physiologic concentration of SPIO (on the basis of a liver uptake of 80%), temperatures increased over baseline at all measured points in a statistically significant manner ($P < .05$). Further increase in the iron content showed increased heat deposition over baseline, but no significant differences when compared to that with a physiologic concentration of SPIO.

Neither baseline impedance nor impedance decrease demonstrated any degree of dependence on the concentration of SPIO (Fig 2). Therefore, the explanation that high local ion concentration from iron oxide uptake could increase the extent of coagulation necrosis by effectively increasing the area of the active surface electrode seems unlikely, and other effects such as inductive heating of magnetic fluids after alternating magnetic field exposure might be responsible for increased heat distribution in acrylamide phantoms containing SPIO. This hypothesis is supported by the data provided by Jordan et al (10) and Hilger et al (11). These groups used an external alternating magnetic field, and they demonstrated tissue heating around the magnetite samples.

In our study, no statistically significant differences in the diameter, shape, or border of the induced coagulation were observed between the SPIO and control groups at image evaluation or at pathologic analysis (Figs 5–7). Additionally, neither baseline impedance nor impedance decrease demonstrated any variation due to administration of SPIO. Similarly, other RF-related parameters such as voltage, power, and current did not demonstrate any differences between the SPIO and control groups.

The most likely reason for the discrepancy between significant differences in heat deposition seen in vitro and the nonsignificant difference in coagulation diameter observed in vivo can be attributed to perfusion-mediated tissue cooling (vascular flow within the liver), which reduces the extent of coagulation necrosis produced by RF energy (7,24). Furthermore, although heat deposition was greater in the presence of iron, the overall difference was limited, with an average increase in temperature of only 1.6°C (equivalent to a 5% change) 6 mm from the electrode and a maximum change of 18% (defined as the minimum value of sample 1 [at 6 mm] and the maximum value of sample 5 [at 6 mm]). If these observed changes are applied to the in vivo measurements, the interpolated differences would be in the range of 1 mm, which lies within the range of measurement accuracy, especially when the lesion border is irregularly shaped rather than well delineated. Although a significant increase in the volume of coagulation necrosis was not observed with this SPIO agent, it is possible that administration of other iron-containing compounds could result in an increase in the effective-

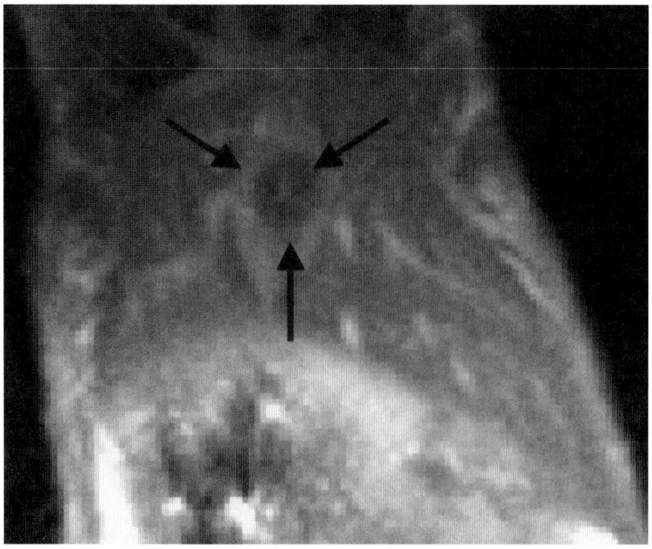

Figure 6. In vivo rabbit liver after intravenous administration of SPIO followed by RF application for 8 minutes. Coronal gadolinium-enhanced T1-weighted SE image (480/26 with three signals acquired) clearly depicts the coagulated tissue, which appears as a hypointense nonenhancing area (arrows) with rim enhancement. The bright spot within the thermal lesion represents blood within the RF probe track.

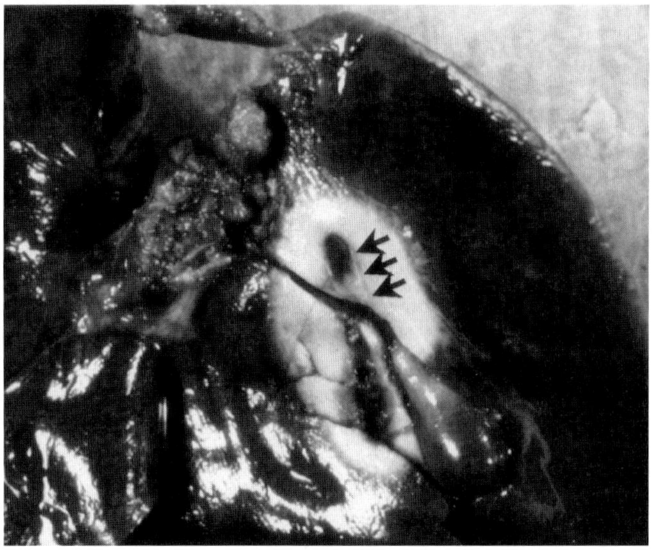

Figure 7. Rabbit liver gross specimen after RF application for 8 minutes, sliced in an axial direction. The central area of whitish-appearing tissue represents the thermal lesion, which is 11 mm perpendicular to the probe track (arrows).

ness of RF ablation, and further investigation may be warranted.

The RF-induced coagulation could be delineated on turbo STIR, T2-weighted, and nonenhanced SE T1-weighted images, but it was visible most clearly on contrast-enhanced T1-weighted images in both groups (Figs 5, 6; Table 2). The ability of MR imaging, including T2-weighted imaging, to depict RF-induced thermal lesions in livers with a high iron content is an important observation of this investigation, as MR imaging is currently the only imaging modality that allows visualization of the developing thermal lesion during RF ablation (4). Furthermore, MR images obtained immediately after thermal ablation can help predict the diameter of thermal coagulation necrosis. Boaz et al (16) reported a correlation coefficient of 0.87 when gross pathologic measurement of lesion diameter was compared to image findings (T2-weighted images). With contrast-enhanced coronal T1-weighted images in our study, correlation coefficients were 0.67 and 0.65 for SPIO and control groups, respectively. This lower correlation allows prediction of lesion diameter, but it needs to be explained. One reason for this discrepancy is that different sequences were used for evaluation (T2 weighted vs contrast-enhanced T1 weighted [cf Fig 5]). A second and potentially more important cause is that on T1-weighted contrast-enhanced images, only the nonenhancing hypointense zone was considered as thermal lesion. It is well known that there is also irreversible cell damage at the border zone of the lesion, but this area, which enhances on contrast-enhanced T1-weighted images, was not included in the diameter measurements. This might further explain why MR images underestimated the diameter of the coagulated foci at pathologic examination.

Regarding safety, there is, to our knowledge, only one report in the literature concerning thermal stability of SPIO (29). In that study, a dextran-coated Fe_3O_4 complex was exposed to temperatures ranging from 80°C to 121°C, to reduced pH, and to high-intensity light in an effort to approximate conditions in a tumor during RF or laser ablation. MR assessment after diameter and cation chromatography and tumor cell cytotoxicity assays indicated high photothermal stability of SPIO. SPIO particles are therefore not considered dangerous for use in conjunction with thermal ablation therapies.

Another safety issue during RF application is the possibility of raised temperature between skin and ground pad, which might cause thermal injury. The temperatures in our study ranged from 37°C to 40°C in the SPIO and control groups, and differences were not significant.

Practical application: Our in vitro data suggest that local temperatures can be increased in tissues surrounding an RF electrode when ablation is performed in the presence of SPIO particles. However, these agents did not increase the diameter of RF-ablation–induced coagulation at physiologic concentrations in our in vivo rabbit model. The most likely causes for this discrepancy are the limited increase (1.6°C) in temperature observed at the border of the lesion (at 6 mm from the electrode tip) and the cooling effects of tissue perfusion, which may overcome this modest increase in heat deposition.

Regarding safety, neither our in vitro nor in vivo data demonstrate any reasons that would contraindicate the use of RF ablation techniques in SPIO-enhanced human livers.

References

1. Vogl TJ, Muller PK, Hammerstingl R, et al. Malignant liver tumors treated with MR imaging-guided laser-induced thermotherapy: technique and prospective results. Radiology 1995; 196:257–265.
2. Murakami R, Yoshimatsu S, Yamashita Y, Matsukawa T, Takahashi M, Sagara K. Treatment of hepatocellular carcinoma: value of percutaneous microwave coagulation. AJR 1995; 164:1159–1164.
3. Tacke J, Adam G, Speetzen R, et al. MR-guided interstitial cryotherapy of the liver with a novel, nitrogen-cooled cryoprobe. Magn Reson Med 1998; 39:354–360.
4. Lewin JS, Connell CF, Duerk JL, et al. Interactive MRI-guided radiofrequency interstitial thermal ablation of abdominal tumors: clinical trial for evaluation of safety and feasibility. JMRI 1998; 8:40–47.
5. McDannold NJ, Hynynen K, Wolf D, Wolf G, Jolesz F. MRI evaluation of thermal ablation of tumors with focused ultrasound. JMRI 1998; 8:91–100.
6. Goldberg SN, Gazelle GS, Dawson SL, Rittman WJ, Mueller PR, Rosenthal DI. Tissue ablation with radiofrequency: effect of probe size, gauge, duration, and temperature on lesion volume. Acad Radiol 1995; 2:399–404.
7. Goldberg SN, Gazelle GS, Solbiati L, Rittman WJ, Mueller PR. Radiofrequency tissue ablation: increased lesion diameter with a perfusion electrode. Acad Radiol 1996; 3:636–644.
8. Vogl TJ, Mack MG, Straub R, Roggan A, Knappe V, Felix R. Internally cooled laser applicator system for MR-guided laser-induced thermotherapy (abstr). Radiology 1997; 205(P):177–178.
9. Livraghi T, Goldberg SN, Monti F, et al. Saline-enhanced radio-frequency tissue ablation in the treatment of liver metastases. Radiology 1997; 202:205–210.
10. Jordan A, Wust P, Fahling H, John W, Hinz A, Felix R. Inductive heating of ferromagnetic particles and magnetic fluids: physical evaluation of their potential for hyperthermia. Int J Hyperthermia 1993; 9:51–68.
11. Hilger I, Andre W, Hergt R, Kaiser WA. Suitability of iron oxides as contrast media in interventional radiology (abstr). Radiology 1997, 205(P):258–259.
12. Akagi M, Tsuboyama T, Ikenaga M, Matsusue Y, Hiraoka M, Nakamura T. Antitumour effects of localized hyperthermia on an experimental bone tumour using an intramedullary nail. Int J Hyperthermia 1997; 13:387–400.
13. Ikenaga M, Ohura K, Yamamuro T, Kotoura Y, Oka M, Kokubo T. Localized hyperthermic treatment of experimental

bone tumors with ferromagnetic ceramics. J Orthop Res 1993; 11:849–855.
14. Shankaranarayanan A, Duerk JL, Lewin JS. Developing a multichannel temperature probe for interventional MRI. JMRI 1998; 8:197–202.
15. Anzai Y, Lufkin R, DeSalles A, Hamilton DR, Farahani K, Black KL. Preliminary experience with MR-guided thermal ablation of brain tumors. AJNR 1995; 16:39–52.
16. Boaz TL, Lewin JS, Chung YC, Duerk JL, Clampitt ME, Haaga JR. MR monitoring of MR-guided radiofrequency thermal ablation of normal liver in an animal model. JMRI 1998; 8:64–69.
17. Ros PR, Freeny PC, Harms SE, et al. Hepatic MR imaging with ferumoxides: a multicenter clinical trial of the safety and efficacy in the detection of focal hepatic lesions. Radiology 1995; 196:481–488.
18. Brodkey JS, Miyazaki Y, Ervin FR, Mark VH. Reversible heat lesions with radio frequency current: a method of stereotactic localization. J Neurosurg 1964; 21:49–53.
19. Rossi S, Buscarini E, Garbagnati F, et al. Percutaneous treatment of small hepatic tumors by an expandable RF needle electrode. AJR 1998; 170:1015–1022.
20. Solbiati L, Ierace T, Goldberg SN, et al. Percutaneous US-guided radio-frequency tissue ablation of liver metastases: treatment and follow-up in 16 patients. Radiology 1997; 202:195–203.
21. Solbiati L, Goldberg SN, Ierace T, et al. Hepatic metastases: percutaneous radiofrequency ablation with cooled-tip electrodes. Radiology 1997; 205:367–373.
22. Rosenthal DI, Springfield DS, Gebhardt MC, Rosenberg AE, Mankin HJ. Osteoid osteoma: percutaneous radio-frequency ablation. Radiology 1995; 197:451–454.
23. Goldberg SN, Gazelle GS, Dawson SL, Rittman WJ, Mueller PR, Rosenthal DI. Tissue ablation with radiofrequency using multiprobe arrays. Acad Radiol 1995; 2:670–674.
24. Siperstein AE, Rogers SJ, Hansen PD, Gitomirsky A. Laparoscopic thermal ablation of hepatic neuroendocrine tumor metastases. Surgery 1997; 122:1147–1155.
25. McGahan JP, Gu WZ, Brock JM, Tesluk H, Jones CD. Hepatic ablation using bipolar radiofrequency electrocautery. Acad Radiol 1996; 3:418–422.
26. Lorentzen T. A cooled needle electrode for radiofrequency tissue ablation: thermodynamic aspects of improved performance compared with conventional needle design. Acad Radiol 1996; 3:556–563.
27. Goldberg SN, Solbiati L, Mueller PR, Conrad JE, Hahn PF, Gazelle GS. Radiofrequency ablation: larger volume tissue necrosis using a pulsed, high current technique (abstr). Radiology 1997; 205(P):258.
28. Lerch IA, Pizzarello DJ. The physics and biology of tumor-specific particle-induction hyperthermia (abstr). Med Phys 1986; 13:786.
29. Saxton RE, Huang A, Anzai Y, Castro DJ, Lufkin RB. Laser photothermal effects on stability and toxicity of magnetic resonance contrast agents. J Clin Laser Med Surg 1995; 13:363–366.

Infarcted Myocardium in Pigs: MR Imaging Enhanced with Slow-Interstitial-Diffusion Gadolinium Compound P760[1]

Lucia J. M. Kroft, MD
Joost Doornbos, PhD
Rob J. van der Geest, MSc
Soraya Benderbous, PhD
Albert de Roos, MD

Index terms:
Contrast media, comparative studies, 511.12143
Contrast media, experimental studies, 511.121411, 511.121412, 511.12143
Gadolinium, 511.12143
Heart, experimental studies, 511.121411, 511.121412, 511.12143
Myocardium, infarction, 511.771
Myocardium, MR, 511.121411, 511.121412, 511.12143

Radiology 1999; 212:467–473

Abbreviation:
ROI = region of interest

[1] From the Department of Radiology (L.J.M.K., J.D., A.d.R.) and the Department of Radiology, Division of Image Processing (R.J.v.d.G.), Leiden University Medical Center, C2-S, Albinusdreef 2, 2333 ZA Leiden, the Netherlands; and Laboratoire Guerbet, Aulnay-sous-Bois, France (S.B.). Received May 27, 1998; revision requested July 16; final revision received November 13; accepted January 27, 1999. Supported in part by a grant from Laboratoire Guerbet. **Address reprint requests to** A.d.R.

Author contributions:
Guarantor of integrity of entire study, L.J.M.K.; study concepts, L.J.M.K., A.d.R.; study design, L.J.M.K.; definition of intellectual content, A.d.R., L.J.M.K., J.D., R.J.v.d.G., S.B.; literature research, L.J.M.K., J.D.; experimental studies, L.J.M.K., J.D., S.B.; data acquisition, L.J.M.K., J.D.; data analysis, L.J.M.K., J.D., R.J.v.d.G., S.B.; statistical analysis, L.J.M.K.; manuscript preparation and editing, L.J.M.K.; manuscript review, J.D., A.d.R., S.B.

PURPOSE: To assess the value of P760, a gadolinium chelate with slow interstitial diffusion and high relaxivity, for magnetic resonance (MR) imaging of acute myocardial infarction in pigs.

MATERIALS AND METHODS: First-pass gradient-echo MR imaging and spin-echo MR imaging were performed with P760 and then with gadoterate meglumine in eight pigs with occlusive acute myocardial infarction. P760 signal intensity enhancement and clearance were compared with those of gadoterate meglumine.

RESULTS: The first-pass enhancement ratio of P760 in normal myocardium was higher than that in infarcted myocardium (1.37 ± 0.06 [SEM] vs 1.05 ± 0.03, P = .03). The myocardial first pass showed a blood pool–like curve for P760. The blood pool enhancement ratio 40 seconds after injection was higher for P760 than for gadoterate meglumine (left ventricular cavity, 1.75 ± 0.06 vs 1.45 ± 0.06, P = .009). Spin-echo MR imaging showed improved contrast between normal and infarcted myocardium after P760 administration: The ratio before contrast material administration was 0.21 ± 0.03, that at 15 minutes was 0.48 ± 0.05 (P = .002), and that at 25 minutes was 0.47 ± 0.07 (P = .003).

CONCLUSION: P760 is an MR imaging contrast agent characterized by low diffusion, a blood pool effect soon after low-dose administration, and fast elimination. This agent is useful for improved myocardial perfusion MR imaging of acute myocardial infarction.

To improve the distinction between normal and infarcted myocardium, extracellular gadolinium-based contrast agents have successfully been used in magnetic resonance (MR) imaging (1,2). After diffusion of the contrast agent into the interstitial space, infarctions are visible as regions of high signal intensity at T1-weighted spin-echo MR imaging. In combination with a first-pass perfusion technique, information can be obtained about regional blood flow and volume during the passage of a contrast agent bolus through the myocardium (3–5).

P760 (Laboratoire Guerbet, Aulnay-sous-Bois, France [6]) is a newly designed extracellular contrast agent with two major improvements over conventional extracellular contrast agents. First, its relaxivity in plasma is seven to eight times higher than that of other currently available extracellular contrast agents (7). This means that a substantially lower dose is required to obtain similar signal intensity–enhancing effects. Second, P760 has a lower diffusion rate, which produces a transient blood pool effect, although it is not a true blood pool contrast agent. These characteristics may be clinically relevant for the functional assessment of ischemic myocardium by using MR perfusion imaging.

We performed this experimental study to examine the value of low-dose P760 for first-pass gradient-echo and delayed spin-echo MR imaging in a model of acute myocardial infarction in pigs.

MATERIALS AND METHODS

Contrast Medium

P760 is a macrocyclic gadolinium chelate with a molecular mass of 5,293 Da. The size restricts fast diffusion through capillary membranes, although it is small enough to pass through the glomerular membrane, which allows rapid renal excretion. The compound, containing one gadolinium atom per molecule, is based on a tetraazacyclododecanetetraacetic acid structure that is substituted by hydrophilic bulky groups branched on the amino-acetic residues. The substituents are synthesized from a halogenated aromatic derivative. The hydrophilicity of the substituent is provided by the addition of polyhydroxylated amines on the aromatic derivative. The relaxivities of P760 are high: r1 is 24.9 $L \cdot mmol^{-1} \cdot sec^{-1}$ and r2 is 29.4 $L \cdot mmol^{-1} \cdot sec^{-1}$ in water at 37°C and 0.47 T. To compare, the relaxivities of gadoterate meglumine (Dotarem; Laboratoire Guerbet) are as follows: r1 is 3.8 $L \cdot mmol^{-1} \cdot sec^{-1}$, and r2 is 4.0 $L \cdot mmol^{-1} \cdot sec^{-1}$. Also, gadoterate meglumine has a molecular mass of 561 Da. In plasma, a dose of only 0.0065 mmol of P760 per kilogram of body weight is isoefficient with 0.05 mmol/kg gadoterate meglumine.

Surgical Procedure

All animal experiments were performed within the guidelines established by the Committee on Animal Experiments of Leiden University Medical Center, the Netherlands (8). Eight domestic female pigs with a mean weight of 31.6 kg (27.3–33.6 kg) were anesthetized with an intramuscular injection of azaperone (Stresnil; Janssen Pharmaceutica, Tilburg, the Netherlands; 2.0 mg/kg) and atropine sulfate (Atropinesulfaat, AUV Coöperatie, Cuyk, the Netherlands; 0.05 mg/kg) and an intraperitoneal injection of metomidate (Hypnodil; Janssen Pharmaceutica; 20.0 mg/kg). The animals received ventilation with a gas mixture containing 1:1 (vol:vol) oxygen and nitrous oxide and with 3%–4% isoflurane (Forene; Abbott, Amstelveen, the Netherlands) for muscle relaxation. Then they were intubated and received ventilation artificially with the same gas mixture but with 1% isoflurane. A 4-mg bolus of pancuronium bromide (Pavulon; Organon Teknika, Boxtel, the Netherlands) was intravenously injected for muscle relaxation.

A venous catheter (Truwave PX-600F; Baxter, Utrecht, the Netherlands) was introduced into the right jugular vein and advanced into the superior vena cava just above the right atrium. An arterial pressure catheter (Truwave PX-600F; Baxter) was introduced into the right carotid artery and advanced into the ascending aorta.

Midsternal thoracotomy was performed, and the thorax was opened. To prevent arrhythmia, lidocaine hydrochloride (AUV Coöperatie) was administered as a 50-mg bolus injection followed by a continuous 2 mg/min intravenous infusion. The pericardium was opened, and one or two diagonal branches of the left anterior descending coronary artery were ligated with a suture. The presence of occlusion was confirmed with development of myocardial cyanosis and electrocardiographic changes. After 30 minutes, the thorax was closed.

Immediately after extubation and on the 1st postoperative day, 3–10 mL of Prisantol (Intervet Nederland, Boxmeer, the Netherlands; 120 mg of phenylbutazone and 240 mg of isopropyl aminopyrine per milliliter [analgesic]) was administered subcutaneously. Antibiotics were administered daily: penicillin G procaine (Procpen [AUV Coöperatie], 300,000 IU administered intramuscularly) and gentamicin sulfate (Gentamicin 5% [AUV Coöperatie], 3 mL of a 5% solution, 50 mg of gentamicin administered intravenously). The animals recovered for 5 days.

During MR imaging, 5 days after coronary artery occlusion, the animals were anesthetized with the same medication as was administered for surgery. Midazolam hydrochloride (Dormicum; Roche Nederland, Mijdrecht, the Netherlands) was administered when necessary.

After the imaging procedure, the animals were sacrificed with a bolus injection of 20 mL of 7.5% potassium chloride (Kaliumchloride 7.5%; Fresenius 'sHertogenbosch, the Netherlands; 1.429 g of potassium chloride) and 4 mg of pancuronium bromide. The hearts were excised, rinsed with saline solution, filled with 1% agar, and cooled to 4°C for 10 hours. The agar-rigid hearts were cut into 1-cm slices perpendicular to the interventricular groove and were stained with nitroblue tetrazolium chloride (Sigma Chemie, Zwijndrecht, the Netherlands) to demarcate the infarcted region. Nitroblue tetrazolium chloride stains normal myocardium dark blue or purple, while severely ischemic or infarcted tissue remains unstained (9).

MR Imaging

First-pass fast gradient-echo MR imaging and delayed spin-echo MR imaging of the myocardium were performed at 1.5 T (Gyroscan NT 15; Philips Medical Systems International, Best, the Netherlands). The animals were placed on their left side and examined with a 17-cm-diameter circular surface coil. For cardiac triggering of the MR imaging acquisition, the up slope of the aortic pressure was used, the signal for which was obtained from the catheter placed in the ascending aorta. Breath holds were achieved by turning off the respirator at end expiration. The systolic and diastolic blood pressures and pulse rate were monitored continuously during the study via the intraarterial catheter.

Baseline gradient-echo images were obtained in the coronal, sagittal, and transverse planes. The images were used to obtain oblique horizontal and vertical myocardial images in the long-axis plane. These images were used to obtain a double-oblique orientation to define the short-axis plane through the left ventricle.

Short-axis cine MR imaging was used to localize the section level with the largest area of infarction for first-pass perfusion imaging, with visual determination of the region with abnormal wall motion and wall thickening, markers of infarction (10). The following imaging parameters were used: 330-mm field of view; 128 × 128 matrix; 550/4.8 (repetition

TABLE 1
Comparison of First-Pass Gradient-Echo MR Imaging Maximum Ventricular Blood Pool Enhancement Ratios for P760 and Gadoterate Meglumine

Ventricle	P760	Gadoterate Meglumine	*P* Value
Right	2.83 ± 0.22	1.86 ± 0.12	.032
Left	2.13 ± 0.22	1.73 ± 0.19	.059
P value	.018	.496	. . .

Note.—Data were obtained in five pigs and are the mean ± SEM.

TABLE 2
Comparison of Ventricular Blood Pool Enhancement Ratios at Gradient-Echo MR Imaging for P760 and Gadoterate Meglumine at 40 Seconds after Injection

Ventricle	P760	Gadoterate Meglumine	*P* Value
Right	1.97 ± 0.13	1.50 ± 0.05	.029
Left	1.75 ± 0.06	1.45 ± 0.06	.009
P value	.251	.193	. . .

Note.—Data were obtained in five pigs and are the mean ± SEM. The nonsignificant differences between the right ventricle and the left ventricle indicate homogeneous distribution in the circulation for both contrast agents.

time msec [R-R aortic pressure up-slope interval]/echo time msec); 22–33-msec temporal resolution; echo-planar imaging factor of three k-y lines per echo-planar imaging, or EPI, segment; 30° flip angle; 7-mm section thickness; 11–14 phases per section; five to 10 section levels; and one breath hold per section level.

First-pass fast gradient-echo perfusion imaging was performed during P760 administration. The imaging parameters were as follows: 300–350-mm field of view, 113 × 128 to 128 × 128 matrix, 6.0–6.3/2.1, 15° flip angle, and 8-mm section thickness. During the breath hold, 100 images were obtained at one image per heartbeat, with a temporal resolution of approximately 550 msec. The contrast agent injection was initiated after acquisition of the fifth image to allow imaging of a steady-state baseline situation. A presaturation pulse was used to suppress the myocardial and ventricular cavity signals. The trigger delay was adjusted per animal to null the signal from the myocardium, and it was chosen to image in diastole.

First-pass imaging requires fast central venous bolus injection of the contrast agent to obtain adequate first-distribution imaging (11). The animals received P760 as a 3-mL compact bolus (0.0065 mmol/kg) followed by a 3-mL physiologic saline flush by manual injection within 2 seconds into the right atrium via the central venous catheter. In five pigs, the first-pass sequence was repeated 1 hour after P760 injection by using a 3-mL bolus of 0.05 mmol of the extracellular contrast agent gadoterate meglumine per kilogram, followed by a 3-mL physiologic saline flush.

T1-weighted spin-echo images were obtained before and after P760 administration by using the following imaging parameters: 330-mm field of view, 256 × 256 matrix, 550/30 (repetition time = aortic pressure up-slope interval), 7-mm section thickness, 0.7-mm intersection gap, five to eight sections acquired. The acquisition order of the k-y lines depended on the amount of respiratory motion to minimize artifacts due to respiration.

Image Analysis

The MR images were transferred to an UltraSPARC-1 workstation (Sun Microsystems, Mountain View, Calif). Image data were analyzed by using the MR Analytical Software System (MASS 3.0; R. J. Van der Geest, Leiden University Medical Center, Leiden, the Netherlands) (12). Photographed ventricular slices of excised nitroblue tetrazolium chloride–stained hearts, containing the maximal area of infarction, were digitized and transferred to the workstation.

A region of interest (ROI), as determined on the corresponding nitroblue tetrazolium chloride–stained slice, was drawn by one of the authors (L.J.M.K.) in the infarcted myocardium on gradient-echo and spin-echo images. The ROI for normal myocardium was drawn at a distance from the infarcted myocardium.

First-pass images.—The image analysis included the construction of the curves of signal intensity versus time for both ventricular cavities and the myocardium. Ventricular and myocardial contours were drawn on the initial image and were subsequently copied to all other images. To avoid artifactual measurements, the ROI within the infarcted myocardium was taken into account only when the ROI contained at least 15 pixels (in four pigs). First-pass maximum enhancement ratios of contours and ROIs were calculated as (maximum SI_{FP})/SI_{pre}, where maximum SI_{FP} is the maximum signal intensity during the first pass and SI_{pre} is the precontrast signal intensity.

The enhancement ratio after the second pass at 40 seconds was measured in the right ventricle, the left ventricle, and the normal myocardium as SI_{40}/SI_{pre}, where SI_{40} is the signal intensity at 40 seconds after contrast agent injection and SI_{pre} is the precontrast signal intensity.

Spin-echo images.—The difference between the signal intensities in the ROIs in the infarcted myocardium and those in the normal myocardium was calculated as the contrast ratio according to the following: $(SI_{infarct} - SI_{normal})/SI_{normal}$, where $SI_{infarct}$ is the signal intensity of the infarcted myocardium and SI_{normal} is the signal intensity of the normal myocardium. The enhancement percentage of the contrast ratio was measured as follows: [(contrast ratio after injection − contrast ratio before injection)/(contrast ratio before injection)] × 100.

The infarcted region revealed a "doughnut" pattern of enhancement in two animals. This doughnut pattern is characterized by an enhancing rim with a dark nonenhancing core. In these two animals, measurements were performed in the enhancing ring. In general, ROI measurements of infarcted myocardium contained at least 31 pixels.

Blood Samples

In two pigs, arterial blood samples were obtained before and at multiple intervals up to 1 hour after P760 and gadoterate meglumine injection to obtain plasma clearance curves. The gadolinium concentrations of P760 and gadoterate meglumine were quantified by means of atomic emission spectrometry by using direct-current plasma. Pharmacokinetic parameters were calculated according to a bicompartmental model, with adjustment to experimental points with the weighted least-squares method.

Statistical Analysis

The MR imaging values are expressed as the mean ± SEM. The paired two-tailed Student *t* test was used to determine the differences between enhancement of the right ventricle and that of the left ventricle and enhancement of the normal myocardium and that of the infarcted myocardium and the differences between P760 and gadoterate meglumine. *P* values less than .05 were considered to indicate a significant difference.

RESULTS

MR imaging was successfully completed in seven animals; one animal was excluded from analysis due to inadequate and incomplete data acquisition. P760 bolus injections were hemodynamically well tolerated, as confirmed with electrocardiographic and blood pressure readings.

Fast Gradient-Echo Imaging

First-pass blood pool enhancement of the right ventricular cavity was significantly higher with P760 than with gadoterate meglumine (Table 1). Although a similar difference was observed for the left ventricular cavity during the first pass, it did not reach statistical significance. At 40 seconds after injection, blood pool enhancement for both ventricles was significantly higher with P760 than with gadoterate meglumine (Table 2).

The evolution of normal myocardial enhancement for both contrast agents is shown in Figure 1. Note the more pronounced enhancement in the myocardium for gadoterate meglumine than for P760 (Fig 1, *I* vs Fig 1, *D*), which is due to the diffusion of gadoterate meglumine into the interstitium. The remaining blood pool enhancement at 40 seconds is higher for P760, with less background enhancement, due to its slow interstitial diffusion (Fig 1, *E* vs Fig 1, *J*).

The contrast agent enhancement dur-

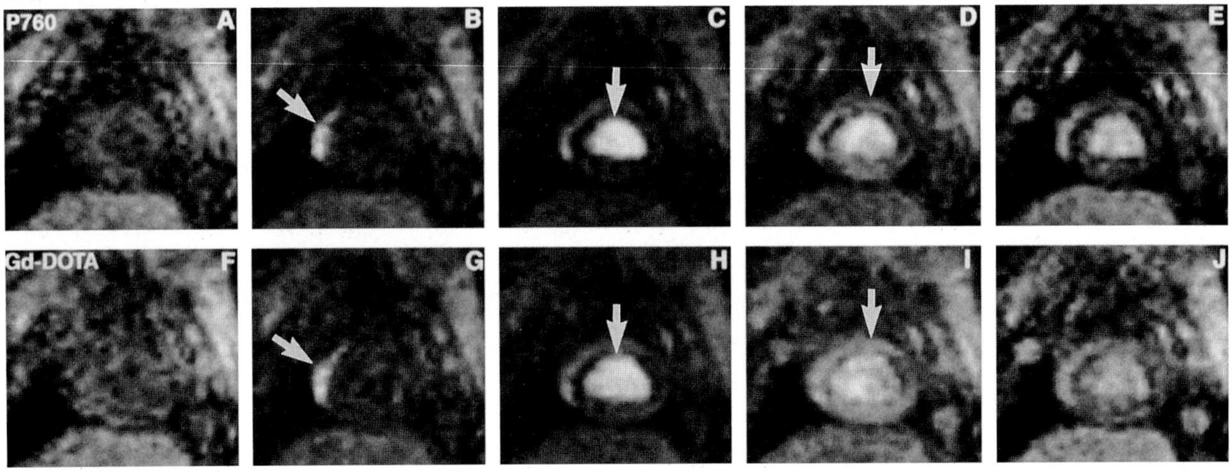

Figure 1. Selected fast gradient-echo MR images (6.3/2.1, 15° flip angle) obtained in the myocardial short-axis view during the first pass of *A–E,* 0.0065 mmol/kg P760 and *F–J,* 0.05 mmol/kg gadoterate meglumine. *A* and *F,* Images obtained prior to injection. *B* and *G,* Images obtained at peak enhancement of the right ventricular blood pool (arrows). *C* and *H,* Images obtained at peak enhancement of the left ventricular blood pool (arrows). *D* and *I,* Images obtained at peak enhancement of the myocardium (arrows). *E* and *J,* Images obtained 40 seconds after contrast agent injection. Note that the evolution of enhancement for both contrast agents is similar, with more pronounced enhancement of the myocardium with gadoterate meglumine, which is related to a more pronounced extravascular diffusion. The blood pool signal intensity is higher in *E* than in *J.*

ing the first pass in normal myocardium is illustrated by marked differences in curve shapes for P760 and gadoterate meglumine (Fig 2). Note that the curve shape for gadoterate meglumine is that for a true extracellular contrast agent, with pronounced enhancement followed by a slow decrease in myocardial signal intensity, whereas the curve shape for P760 is more like that for a blood pool agent, with a lower maximum enhancement of the myocardium and a decrease in signal intensity before recirculation. These results are supported by statistical analysis of P760 and gadoterate meglumine curve shapes (Table 3) and indicate lower diffusion into the extracellular space for P760 than for gadoterate meglumine.

P760 was useful for identifying first-pass enhancement differences between normal myocardium and infarcted myocardium. The first-pass maximum enhancement ratio was significantly higher for normal myocardium than for infarcted myocardium (1.37 ± 0.06 vs 1.05 ± 0.03, $P = .03$, $n = 4$). Figure 3c shows P760 first-pass signal intensity–time curves for normal myocardium and for infarcted myocardium. Note the distinct increase in myocardial signal intensity during the P760 first pass in the normal myocardium, whereas the infarcted myocardium shows no enhancement (Fig 3c).

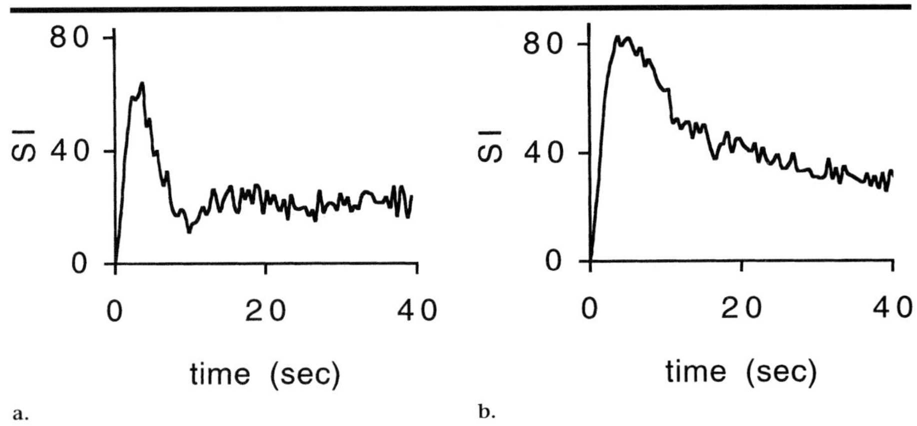

Figure 2. First-pass perfusion curves in myocardial tissue (raw data) after injection of isoefficient doses of **(a)** P760 (0.0065 mmol/kg) and **(b)** gadoterate meglumine (0.05 mmol/kg). The signal intensity (*SI*) is in arbitrary units. The maximum first-pass signal intensity is higher in **b** than in **a.** In **a,** note the recirculation minimum at 10 seconds, after which the second pass occurs and the curve continues horizontally. In **b,** no recirculation minimum is seen, and the signal intensity decreases continuously. The curves are in accordance with the fast extravasation of gadoterate meglumine, whereas P760 remains in the blood pool during the imaging time window.

Spin-Echo Imaging

Spin-echo images were obtained before, within 5 minutes, and approximately 15 and 25 minutes after P760 injection. Figure 4 summarizes the myocardial contrast ratios before and after injection ($n = 7$). There was a significant increase from the precontrast ratio (0.21 ± 0.03) to the postcontrast ratios at 15 and 25 minutes. At 2–5 minutes after P760 injection, the contrast ratio was 0.67 ± 0.30 ($P = .163$, not significant); at 15 minutes after injection, it was 0.48 ± 0.05 ($P = .002$); and at 25 minutes after injection, it was 0.47 ± 0.07 ($P = .003$). Figure 5 shows P760-enhanced infarcted myocardium on a delayed spin-echo image.

Blood Samples

Figure 6 shows the P760 and gadoterate meglumine elimination curves, and Table 4 shows the extrapolated perfusion parameters in the anesthetized pigs. Note that the pharmacokinetic parameters of P760 and gadoterate meglumine are similar.

DISCUSSION

Findings of the present study show the usefulness of the gadolinium compound

TABLE 3
Comparison of First-Pass Enhancement Curve Data in Normal Myocardium for P760 and Gadoterate Meglumine at Gradient-Echo MR Imaging

Parameter	P760	Gadoterate Meglumine	*P* Value
(Maximum SI_{FP})/SI_{pre}			
Gamma variate–raw data	1.33 ± 0.04	1.48 ± 0.05	.025
Gamma variate–fitted data	1.32 ± 0.03	1.49 ± 0.05	.010
Recirculation minimum	1.07 ± 0.02	. . .	. . .
SI_{40}/SI_{pre}	1.14 ± 0.03	1.21 ± 0.02	.050

Note.—Data were obtained in four pigs and are the mean ± SEM. SI_{FP} = signal intensity during the first pass. The P760 recirculation minimum in the time–signal intensity curve between the first pass and the second pass was not present after gadoterate meglumine injection because of the fast extravasation of gadoterate meglumine into the extracellular space. For P760, the recirculation minimum was significant, as compared with the enhancement at 40 seconds (P = .012). The results support the hypothesis of slower diffusion of P760 in the early phase as compared with diffusion of gadoterate meglumine.

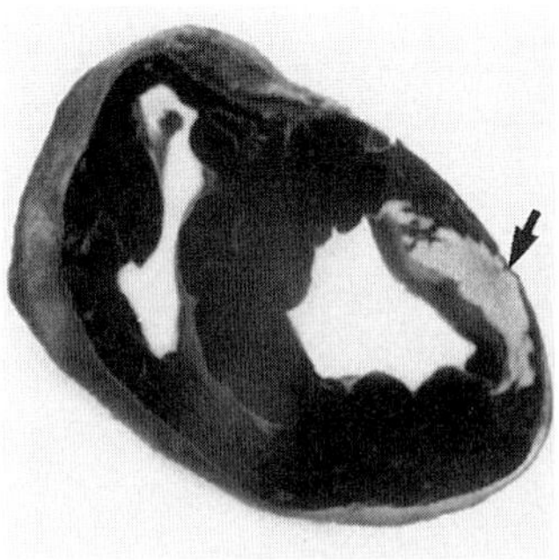

a.

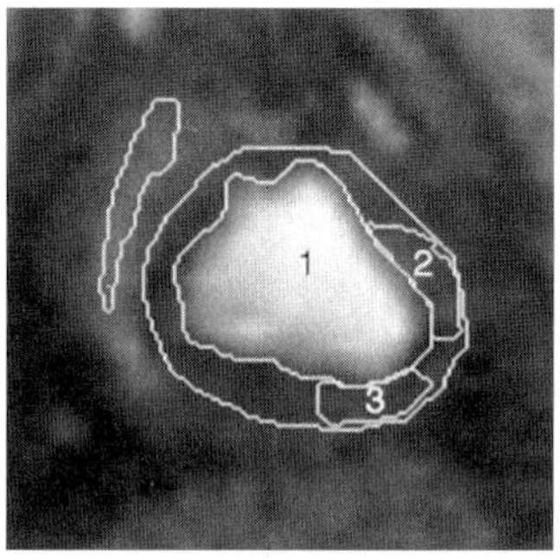

b.

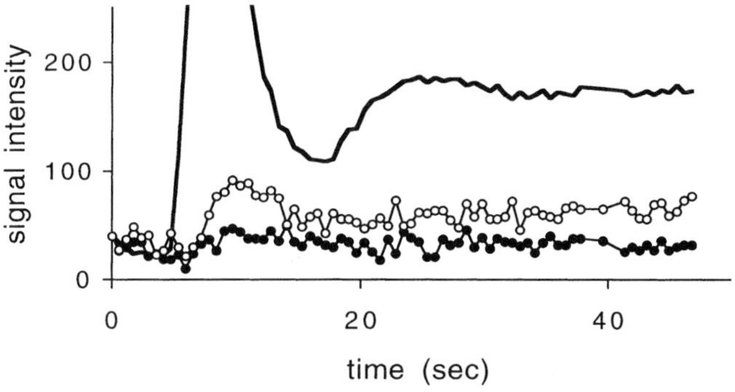

c.

Figure 3. **(a)** Short-axis pathologic nitroblue tetrazolium chloride–stained slice with myocardial infarction (arrow) in the left ventricular free wall. **(b)** Contours and ROIs drawn on a first-pass dynamic fast gradient-echo MR image (6.3/2.1, 15° flip angle) obtained in the myocardial short-axis view. The ROIs correspond to the left ventricular blood pool (ROI *1*), infarction (ROI *2*), and normal myocardium (ROI *3*) on the nitroblue tetrazolium chloride–stained slice. **(c)** Corresponding P760 first-pass raw data curve of signal intensity (in arbitrary units) versus time shows the signal intensity in the left ventricular blood pool (solid line, corresponds to ROI 1), the infarcted myocardium (●, corresponds to ROI 2), and the normal myocardium (○, corresponds to ROI 3). Note the clear increase in signal intensity during the first pass of P760 in the normal myocardium at 10–15 seconds, which is not seen in the infarcted myocardium.

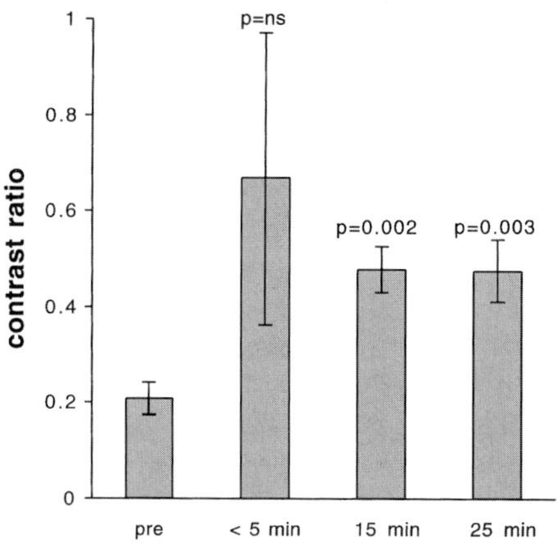

Figure 4. Bar graph (bars ± SEM) demonstrates the mean contrast ratio between infarcted myocardium and normal myocardium on spin-echo images (550/30) before (*pre*) and after injection of 0.0065 mmol/kg P760 (in seven pigs). Within 5 minutes after P760 injection, the contrast ratio was improved, but this improvement was not statistically significant (*ns*) due to the variation within the group. The contrast ratio was significantly improved according to enhancement percentages of 129% at approximately 15 minutes (P = .002) and 124% at approximately 25 minutes (P = .003).

P760 for first-pass and equilibrium MR imaging of infarcted myocardium. The major findings are as follows:

1. The high r1 of P760 causes pronounced blood pool enhancement with one-seventh of the normal dose of extracellular gadolinium compounds.
2. P760 has marked blood pool retention during the first pass, causing excellent blood pool enhancement and a blood pool–like curve for the myocardial first pass.
3. P760 is useful for identifying regional perfusion differences between normal myocardium and infarcted myocardium at first-pass gradient-echo imaging.
4. The late extracellular distribution improves the contrast between normal myocardium and infarcted myocardium at delayed spin-echo imaging.
5. P760 is eliminated quickly, which is comparable with an extracellular gadolinium compound.

P760 is classified as a slow-interstitial-diffusion or low-diffusion contrast agent. Its larger molecular size as compared with the sizes of conventional extracellular contrast agents prevents fast diffusion through the capillary membranes. Its enhancement during the first pass and during early circulation is therefore more like that of a blood pool agent. The distribution volume of the contrast agent is similar to the distribution volumes of conventional extracellular contrast agents and allows rapid renal clearance.

Fast Gradient-Echo First–Pass Imaging

There was a significantly higher first-pass maximum enhancement in the right

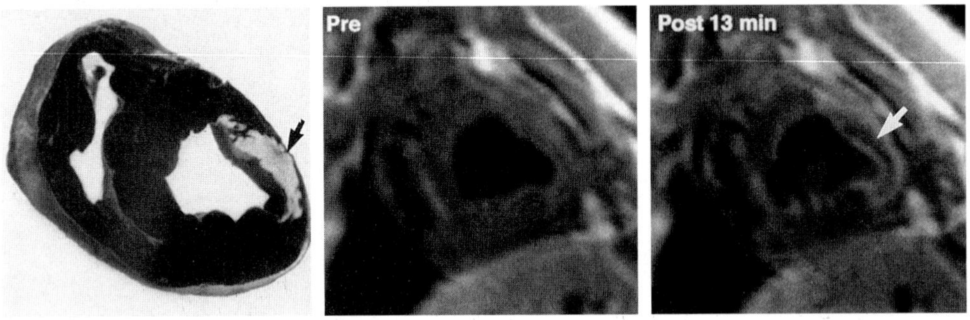

a. b. c.

Figure 5. (**a**) Short-axis pathologic nitroblue tetrazolium chloride–stained slice of infarcted myocardium (arrow). (**b, c**) T1-weighted spin-echo images (550/30) in the short-axis view show the corresponding level of myocardium (**b**) before and (**c**) 13 minutes after injection of P760. In **b**, the large infarction is not recognized. In **c**, the necrotic area is recognized as a dark core (arrow) surrounded by an enhancing rim.

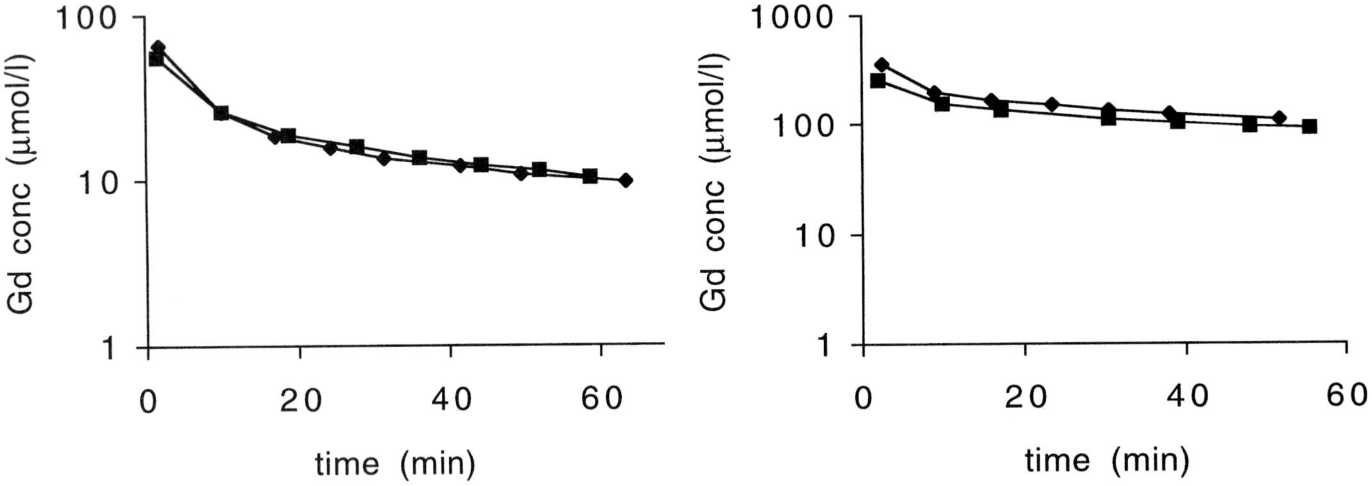

a. b.

Figure 6. Semilogarithmic plots of plasma concentration versus time for (**a**) P760 and (**b**) gadoterate meglumine in two anesthetized pigs (◆ = pig 1, ■ = pig 2). Note that the curve shapes in **a** and **b** are similar, in spite of the few data points soon after injection. The distribution into the extracellular compartment is mainly represented in the first phase after injection (fast decrease in gadolinium concentration [*Gd conc*] in micromoles per liter), whereas the excretion is mainly represented in the later (linear) phase (slower decrease in gadolinium concentration).

ventricle than in the left ventricle for P760 that was not seen with gadoterate meglumine. The results suggest that there is less T2*-based signal intensity loss in the blood pool for P760 than for gadoterate meglumine, as the T2* effect is due to the local gadolinium concentration, which is lower for P760 than for gadoterate meglumine at an isoefficient dose.

TABLE 4
Plasma Pharmacokinetics of P760 and Gadoterate Meglumine in Two Anesthetized Pigs

	P760		Gadoterate Meglumine	
Parameter	Pig 1	Pig 2	Pig 1	Pig 2
Distribution half-life (min)	3	4	2	3
Elimination half-life (min)	58	51	58	70
Distribution volume (mL/kg)	234	226	223	299
Clearance (mL/min/kg)	3.3	3.4	2.8	3.1

In a comparison of the myocardial first-pass curves for P760 with those for gadoterate meglumine, there was a substantially higher normal myocardial enhancement for gadoterate meglumine than for P760. However, the higher enhancement for gadoterate meglumine can be explained by the fast extravasation (diffusion) into the interstitial space. Diffusion of any contrast agent from the blood pool into the myocardial interstitial space plays an important role in myocardial signal intensity measurements and hampers adequate quantification of myocardial perfusion (13). Intravascular contrast agents may simplify perfusion analysis (14). The blood pool–like enhancement of P760 during the first pass could be advantageous for quantitative evaluation of first-pass perfusion imaging. The peak intensity of passage of a contrast agent bolus is an efficient parameter for evaluating relative inhomogeneity of regional myocardial perfusion (3). In the present study, regional perfusion differences were identified between normal myocardium and infarcted myocardium at first-pass gradient-echo imaging by using P760.

The elimination half-life of currently experimental blood pool contrast agents is long (15,16). This limits repetitive injections during the same session. Repeat injections are needed to determine myocardial perfusion reserve in perfusion imaging under rest and stress conditions (17). The blood pool enhancement, in combination with the low dose and fast elimination rate that allow repeated injections, makes P760 a promising contrast agent for quantitative perfusion measurements.

Spin-Echo Imaging

Before P760 injection, there was little difference between the signal intensity of normal and that of infarcted myocardium. After P760 injection and diffusion of the contrast agent into the interstitial space, a clear enhancement of the infarcted area, confirmed pathologically, was shown at 15 and 25 minutes. Small infarctions were homogeneously enhanced, whereas large infarctions appeared as a dark core surrounded by an enhancing ring. These enhancement patterns are in agreement with those of extracellular contrast agents such as gadopentetate dimeglumine (2).

In conclusion, P760 is a newly designed extracellular contrast agent with improvements over conventional extracellular contrast agents for MR myocardial perfusion imaging. The strength of the product is based on the combination of high relaxivity and slow diffusion, which allow low-dose administration and cause a blood pool effect with improved enhancement. We believe that the slow-interstitial-diffusion contrast agent P760 warrants further investigation as a potential contrast agent for various MR applications.

Practical application: P760 is a promising contrast agent for perfusion studies. Its blood pool retention with less background enhancement during a myocardial first pass is expected to be advantageous for quantitative perfusion measurements. The low dose and fast elimination allow repetitive injections as needed during stress testing. In addition, the combination of initial slow extravasation, high relaxivity, and low-dose administration is potentially valuable for MR imaging.

References

1. Nishimura T, Kobayashi H, Ohara Y, et al. Serial assessment of myocardial infarction by using gated MR imaging and Gd-DTPA. AJR 1989; 153:715–720.
2. de Roos A, Van Rossum AC, Van der Wall EE, et al. Reperfused and nonreperfused myocardial infarction: diagnostic potential of Gd-DTPA–enhanced MR imaging. Radiology 1989; 172:717–720.
3. Lombardi M, Jones RA, Westby J, et al. MRI for the evaluation of regional myocardial perfusion in an experimental animal model. JMRI 1997; 7:987–995.
4. Judd RM, Lugo-Olivieri CH, Arai M, et al. Physiological basis of myocardial contrast enhancement in fast magnetic resonance images of 2-day-old reperfused canine infarcts. Circulation 1995; 92:1902–1910.
5. Wilke N, Jerosch-Herold M, Wang Y, et al. Myocardial perfusion reserve: assessment with multisection, quantitative, first-pass MR imaging. Radiology 1997; 204:373–384.
6. Meyer D, Rousseaux O, Schaefer M, Simonot C; Laboratoire Guerbet France, assignee. P760. International patent WO.97/01359. January 16, 1997.
7. Port M, Meyer D, Bonnemain B, Corot C. MRI contrast agents characterized by new pharmacokinetic properties. MAGMA (in press).
8. deGreeve PCM, deLeeuw WA. Wettelijeke aspecten van dierproeven. In: Van Zuthphen LFM, Baumans V, Beynen AC, eds. Proefdieren en dierproeven. 2nd ed. Utrecht, the Netherlands: Wetenschappelijke Uitgeverij Bunge, 1995; 10–19.
9. Feldman S, Glagov S, Wissler RW, Hughes RH. Postmortem delineation of infarcted myocardium. Arch Pathol Lab Med 1976; 100:55–58.
10. Holman EH, Vliegen HW, van der Geest RJ, et al. Quantitative analysis of regional left ventricular function after myocardial infarction in the pig assessed with cine magnetic resonance imaging. Magn Reson Med 1995; 34:161–169.
11. Keijer JT, Van Rossum AC, Van Eenige MJ, et al. Semiquantitation of regional myocardial blood flow in normal human subjects by first-pass magnetic resonance imaging. Am Heart J 1995; 130:893–901.
12. van der Geest RJ, Buller VGM, Jansen E, et al. Comparison between manual and semiautomated analysis of left ventricular volume parameters from short axis MR images. J Comput Assist Tomogr 1997; 21:756–765.
13. Burstein D, Taratuta E, Manning WJ. Factors in myocardial "perfusion" imaging with ultrafast MRI and Gd-DTPA administration. Magn Reson Med 1991; 20:299–305.
14. Wilke N, Kroll K, Merkle H, et al. Regional myocardial blood volume and flow: first-pass MR imaging with polylysine-Gd-DTPA. JMRI 1995; 5:227–237.
15. McLachlan SJ, Morris MR, Lucas MA, et al. Phase I clinical evaluation of a new iron oxide MR contrast agent. JMRI 1994; 4:301–307.
16. Parmelee DJ, Walovitch RC, Ouellet HS, Randall B, Lauffer B. Preclinical evaluations of the pharmacokinetics, biodistribution, and elimination of MS-325, a blood pool agent for magnetic resonance imaging. Invest Radiol 1997; 32:741–747.
17. Eichenberger AC, Shuiki E, Kochli VD, Amann FW, McKinnon GC, von Schulthess GK. Ischemic heart disease: assessment with gadolinium-enhanced ultrafast MR imaging and dipyridamole stress. JMRI 1994; 4:425–431.

Marc W. Münter, MD
Christian P. Karger, PhD
Wolfgang Reith, MD
H. Michael Schneider, MD
Peter Peschke, PhD
Jürgen Debus, MD, PhD

Index terms:
Brain, effects of irradiation on, 10.47, 17.47
Brain, necrosis, 10.47
Radiobiology, 10.47, 17.458, 17.47
Therapeutic radiology, experimental studies, 10.47, 17.47

Radiology 1999; 212:475–482

[1] From the Departments of Radiation Oncology (M.W.M., P.P., J.D.) and Medical Physics (C.P.K.), German Cancer Research Center, Im Neuenheimer Feld 280, 69120 Heidelberg, Germany; the Department of Neuroradiology, University of Heidelberg, Germany (W.R.); and the Department of Pathology, St Vincentius Hospital, Karlsruhe, Germany (H.M.S.). Received June 19, 1998; revision requested September 3; revision received October 30; accepted January 15, 1999. C.P.K. is supported by Deutsche Forschungsgemeinschaft grant DFG HA 1426/3-2. **Address reprint requests to** J.D. (e-mail: *j.debus@dkfz-heidelberg.de*).

Author contributions:
Guarantors of integrity of entire study, P.P., J.D.; study concepts, C.P.K., J.D., P.P.; study design, M.W.M., W.R., H.M.S.; definition of intellectual content, C.P.K., P.P., J.D.; literature research, M.W.M., C.P.K.; experimental studies, M.W.M., W.R., H.M.S.; statistical analysis, C.P.K.; manuscript preparation, M.W.M.; manuscript editing, M.W.M., P.P., C.P.K.; manuscript review, C.P.K., W.R., H.M.S., P.P.

Delayed Vascular Injury after Single High-Dose Irradiation in the Rat Brain: Histologic, Immunohistochemical, and Angiographic Studies[1]

PURPOSE: To investigate structural and functional changes in rats after focal brain irradiation by using histologic, immunohistochemical, and angiographic methods.

MATERIALS AND METHODS: Sixty rats were irradiated stereotactically with photons from a 15-MeV linear accelerator. Two collimators and single doses ranging from 20 to 100 Gy were used to treat stereotactically defined areas of 3.7- and 4.7-mm cross section (80% isodose) in the right frontal lobe. The dose-response relationship for the end-point necrosis at 19 months revealed a mean tolerance dose (D_{50}) of 34.2 Gy (standard errors: +4.1, −3.7 Gy). Histologic, immunohistochemical, and angiographic examinations were performed to evaluate delayed radiation effects.

RESULTS: All animals irradiated with 100 Gy developed radiation necrosis after 9 months. Microangiography and immunohistochemical fluorescence staining of the endothelial cells revealed dose-dependent vascular dilatation and rarefaction. Animals irradiated with 20–50 Gy showed no morphologic changes after 9 months. With irradiation of 30–50 Gy, histologic vascular changes that increased with dose were found after 19 months. At that time, no changes were detected after irradiation with 20 Gy with both field sizes and after irradiation with 30 Gy and the 2-mm collimator. Radiation-induced functional disturbances of the brain vasculature could be demonstrated by extravasation of contrast medium by using a microangiographic technique.

CONCLUSION: The observed effect had a definite dependence on dose, volume, and time after treatment.

Delayed radiation injury is of major concern in radiation therapy, since it is known to lead to permanent lesions in normal tissue. Evaluation of delayed radiation effects in patients is difficult, so various experimental studies have been carried out to study radiation injury in large and in small animals. Monkeys are comparable to humans with respect to the volume and morphologic structure of the brain (1). Difficulty in procuring and in working with the animals, however, often limits the number of animals available for study and hence the statistical significance of the results. With the technical possibility of attaining very small treatment volumes with stereotactic radiosurgery (2), interest in determining radiation-induced alterations in the brain, even in smaller species (3,4), increases.

Numerous investigators have described the pathophysiologic changes in the central nervous system following irradiation (4–8). Radiation injury has been classified by Van der Kogel (9) as acute, early-delayed, and late-delayed reactions. Until now, to our knowledge, there has been no general agreement about the underlying mechanisms leading to delayed effects, such as demyelination and white matter necrosis. It is generally accepted, however, that radiation injury is the result of a proceeding cell degeneration and metabolic disturbance.

The vascular system, together with the blood-brain barrier, is believed to be the main target structure for the development of delayed radiation effects (4,10). Other observations have resulted in the postulation that certain cell populations, especially oligodendrocytes, are specific targets for ionizing radiation (11).

In the literature, some excellent early work about the tolerance of human brain after irradiation is available. Hindo et al (12) tested large, single fractions for palliative treatment. Other authors evaluated acute or late radiation effects and complications after irradiation (13,14) and found distinguishing sensitivities to radiation in different areas of the human brain (15). Eifel et al (16) compared the outcomes of radiation treatment for tumors of the brainstem and for tumors of the midbrain in children.

In early animal studies (17,18), the sensitivity of the brain following irradiation and the relationship between fractionation and total dose in causing brain damage was evaluated. Studies in humans, as well as in animals, concerning late radiation effects after heavy-particle therapy have also been performed (7,19–21).

Stereotactic radiosurgery with a linear accelerator is a new technique for delivering focal high-dose radiation to the brain. The goal of this study was to investigate structural and functional changes after focal brain irradiation by using histologic, angiographic, and immunohistochemical methods. A stereotactic device was designed for experimental radiosurgery of the rat brain (2,22) and was applied to enable focal irradiation of the rat frontal lobe. Of central interest were radiation-induced perturbations of the vascular system, which we studied by using a series of clinically relevant doses; we focused on the influence of dose and posttreatment time of up to 19 months.

MATERIALS AND METHODS

Animals

The study was performed with a total of 66 male Copenhagen rats that were, at the time of irradiation, 67 days old ± 7 (mean ± SD) and 216 g ± 14 in weight. For stereotactic positioning and irradiation, the rats were first lightly anesthetized with ketamine hydrochloride (Ketanest; Parke-Davis, Berlin, Germany; 80 mg/kg) and then maintained under general anesthesia by using a gaseous mixture of halothane (Halothan; Hoeschst, Frankfurt, Germany; 0.6% volume), oxygen (1,500 mL/min), and nitrous oxide (800 mL/min). The study was approved by an appropriate external animal protection committee, Regierungspraesidium, Karlsruhe, Germany. Rats were kept two per cage under temperature- and light-controlled conditions with free access to food and water according to the guidelines established for laboratory animals by the German government.

Fixation and Localization Device

The procedure of fixation, target localization, and irradiation is described in detail elsewhere (2,22) and thus will be outlined only briefly: The rat was immobilized in prone position with two ear pins and a bar with a hole for the front teeth. The target was localized in each rat by using two perpendicular x-ray radiographs. Stereotactic positioning in the isocenter was accomplished by attaching the fixation device to a modified Riechert and Mundinger head frame (23,24).

The spatial uncertainty of the position of the treatment volume was 1.0 mm ± 0.2. The target area, which was chosen to be in the right hemisphere of the frontal lobe of the rat, was located laterally on the x axis at 3.0 mm, anteroposteriorly on the y axis at 6.0 mm, and craniocaudally on the z axis at 10.7 mm. Coordinates were taken from the stereotactic atlas of the rat brain (25): This target region contains white (frontal cortex, area 1) and gray (caudate putamen) matter.

Irradiation

A convergent photon-beam technique consisting of six converging arcs was applied by using a 15-MeV linear accelerator (Mevatron 77; Siemens, Erlangen, Germany). We applied arcs at the following table positions: at 0°, two arcs, 20° to 160° and −20° to −160°; at +36°, one arc, −20° to −160°; at −36°, one arc, 20° to 160°; at +72°, one arc, −20° to −160°; and at −72°, one arc, 20° to 160°. The radiation fields were defined by using cylindric collimators with apertures of 2 or 3 mm (corresponding to a 3.9- or 5.9-mm aperture projected to the isocenter). The diameters of the resultant spherical 80% isodoses within the rat brain were 3.7 or 4.7 mm. Dosimetry was performed with acquisition of a therapy-verification film image in a water-equivalent depth of 10 mm. During the treatment period, the dose remained constant within 2%.

Sixty animals were randomized into 10 groups of six animals each and were treated with doses of 20, 30, 40, 50, and 100 Gy by using two different volumes (2- or 3-mm collimation). An extra group of six age-matched rats served as control animals.

Histologic Examination

Histologic examination was performed in 57 animals selected with random sampling. Treated rats were sacrificed 9 or 19 months after irradiation and were processed for histologic examination. Before sacrificing, intravascular perfusion was performed in anesthetized animals with a mixture of 2% paraformaldehyde and 2% glutaraldehyde in phosphate buffer (pH 7.6) by using a polyethylene catheter (PE 50) inserted by performing an arteriectomy of the common carotid artery. After opening the skull carefully, the brain was removed, cut into two coronal sections 4 mm rostral of the interaural line, fixed for 48 hours in buffered formalin, dehydrated with alcohol and xylene, and finally embedded in paraffin. Sections of 4–6-μm thickness were cut by using a microtome (Autocut; Reichert and Jung, division of Leica Mikrosysteme Vertrieb, Bensheim, Germany) and stained with hematoxylin-eosin or cresyl violet acetate for Nissl staining.

The histologic sections were used to study the morphology of the brain following different doses of radiation, with observation for gliosis, telangiectasia, proliferation, inflammation, necrosis, and any other alterations associated with central nervous system radiation injury.

For cryofixation, the brains were rapidly removed from the rat skull and frozen in isopentane, at liquid-nitrogen temperature. Coronal sections of 20 μm were produced with a cryomicrotome (2800 Frigocut; Reichert and Jung, division of Leica Mikrosysteme Vertrieb) and were mounted on glass slides coated with 2% silane. Frozen sections were fixed in acetone for 60 seconds and were then air dried.

Immunohistochemical Examination

A polyclonal anti–human fibronectin antibody (1:40 dilution, 30 minutes exposure) developed in sheep (Biotrend Chemikalien, Cologne, Germany) and conjugated to fluorescein isothiocyanate was used as the primary antibody in a direct immunofluorescent technique. In addition, the labeled-avidin binding method was used according to the following brief description: 10–20-μm-thick tissue sections placed on silane-coated slides were saturated with normal serum to block binding sites (30 minutes) and were incubated with anti–human fibronectin antibody (1:100, 1 hour). Both methods were used for 11 animals (one animal from each dose and collimator group). We used a biotinylated rabbit anti–sheep immunoglobulin G antibody (Vector Laboratories, Burlingame, Calif) (1:100, 1 hour) followed by fluorescein isothiocyanate–conjugated streptavidin (Dianova, Hamburg, Germany) (1:50, 30 minutes) as a reporter system.

All staining procedures were performed at room temperature. The sections were embedded in Vectashield (mounting medium with DAPI counterstain; Vector Laboratories), and coverslips were applied. Histologic evaluation was performed with a fluorescence microscope (Axiophot; Carl Zeiss, Jenna, Germany). For photographic documentation, Ektachrome 400 ASA film (Eastman Kodak, Rochester, NY) was used.

The immunohistologic evaluation was conducted to investigate alterations of the vascular system following irradiation, such as dilatation of the vessels and destruction of the vessels.

Angiographic Examination

Angiographic examination was performed in 11 animals (one from each dose and collimator group) selected with random sampling. Anesthetized rats were immobilized in dorsal position in a specially designed jig. A thoracotomy was performed, and a cannula was transcardially pushed into the ascending aorta and was fixed. The contrast medium (Mikropaque; Guerbet, Suzlbach, Germany) consisted of an aqueous suspension of barium sulfate, which was mixed in a ratio of 8:2 with 25 g of gelatin and dissolved in 100 mL of physiologic saline solution at 40°C. Ten milliliters of the solution was administered continuously through the cannula over 1 minute. To avoid overloading the circulatory system with fluid, the right ventricle of the heart was opened. Immediately after perfusion, the brains were removed and fixed in 4% formaldehyde for at least 5 days.

To assess the quality of vascular filling with contrast medium and to define a sectional plane for microangiography, macroangiograms of the whole brains were obtained by using a Faxitron (radiographic inspection unit; Faxitron X-ray, Wheeling, Ill). For this soft-tissue technique, the brains were put directly on a piece of mammographic film (Ready Pack; Eastman Kodak) and were exposed to 40-kV x rays.

For microangiography, the brains were cut with a specially designed cutting device into 3–6-mm-thick frontal sections. Contact radiographs were obtained from formaldehyde-fixed sections exposed to 20-kV x rays in a microstructure x-ray system (PW 1170; Philips, Eindhoven, the Netherlands). High-resolution (2,000 lines per millimeter) x-ray emulsion-coated glass plates (type 1A; Eastman Kodak) were used in direct contact with the histologic sections.

The radiographs were evaluated with a computer-assisted analysis system (MCID; Imaging Research, St Catharines, Ontario, Canada) with a magnification power of up to ×10. For higher magnifications, a photomicroscope (Axiophot; Carl Zeiss) was used. The aim was to observe the structure of the vascular system and the integrity of vessels by detecting leakage of contrast medium.

Statistical Analysis of the Dose-Response Relationship

The histologic findings at 9 and 19 months were classified according to slightly modified scoring criteria, which were originally established by Rubin et al (10). The dose-response relationship was calculated for the irradiation with the 3-mm collimator by using two different end points: (*a*) any necrosis (including mild, moderate, or severe necrosis) at 19 months and (*b*) severe necrosis at 19 months. A logistic dose-response model was defined by the following equation:

$$P(D) = \frac{1}{1 + \left(\frac{D_{50}}{D}\right)^k} \quad (1)$$

where P is the probability of complication, D_{50} is the dose level with a 50% complication probability, D is the dose, and k reflects the slope of the dose-response curve. The equation was adjusted by using a maximum likelihood procedure. The uncertainties provided for the parameters D_{50} and k are the single standard errors. The asymptotic 95% CIs are also provided. This standard procedure of adjusting dose-response curves was not applicable to the data of the 2-mm collimator, since it requires at least two data points that are different from 0% and 100%.

RESULTS

Anesthesia and radiosurgery were well tolerated by all animals, as described earlier (22). Development of neurologic dysfunctions was restricted to animals treated with 100 Gy, independent of collimator size, and occurred 7 months after stereotactic irradiation.

Histologic Findings

Histologic processing within the 100-Gy group was possible in six of 12 animals. Within the observation period of 19 months, one rat died during a magnetic resonance (MR) imaging procedure, and two animals died of unknown causes.

Brain tissue of the nonirradiated control animals showed a normal morphologic appearance. Similarly, the nonirradiated hemisphere of all stereotactically treated rats did not exhibit any pathologic alterations. Macroscopically, an increase in volume was observed in the irradiated hemisphere in all animals treated with 100 Gy.

Table 1 summarizes the extent of necrosis after single high-dose irradiation that was classified according to the slightly modified criteria of Rubin et al (10). A clear cystic necrosis seen in all animals treated with 100 Gy was restricted to the irradiated region of the brain (Fig 1a). The effect was more pronounced after using the 3-mm collimator, which resulted in even larger necrotic areas.

The deteriorated regions were surrounded by gliosis, were predominantly located in the white matter of the medullary layer, and were rarely located in the basal ganglia. Hemorrhages were visible either within the necrotic areas or were restricted to areas surrounding the cystic necrosis. No hemorrhages were found in the contralateral nonirradiated hemisphere.

Perivascular lymphocytic infiltrations were observed, and the necrotic areas showed only minor signs of glial inflammatory cell reaction. Nissl staining showed complete necrosis of the neuronal structures. The blood vessels around the necrotic area were abnormally dilatated and exhibited degeneration of the endothelial cells, swelling of the vessel walls, and varying degrees of adjoining edema. Occasionally, endothelial-cell nuclei were enlarged. Close to the blood vessels, hypertrophic and proliferating astrocytes were detectable.

No sign of necrosis was visible 9 months after irradiation in animals exposed to 50 Gy, yet marginal morphologic alterations, such as slight telangiectasia, tissue swelling, and mild abnormalities of glial and neuronal architecture, were observed

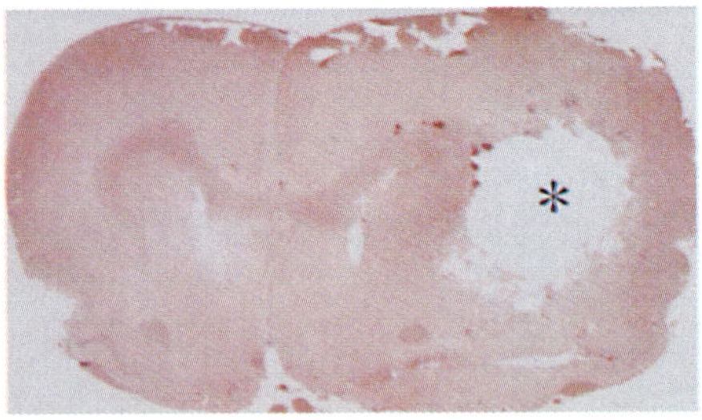

a.

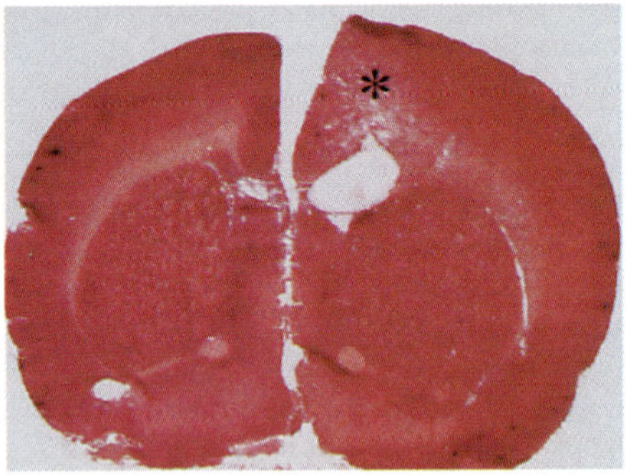

b.

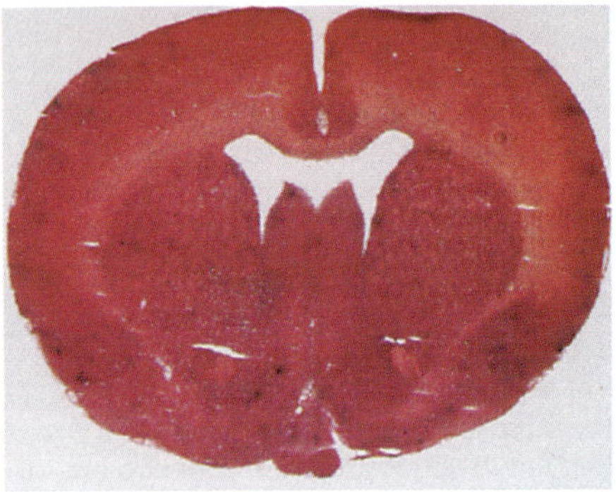

c.

Figure 1. Radiation-induced morphologic changes in the normal rat. Brain sections from different animals depict **(a)** a large area of radiation necrosis (*) of the right frontal lobe 9 months after irradiation with 100 Gy and 2-mm collimation and **(b)** radiation necrosis (*) near the lateral ventricle after 19 months in an animal irradiated with 50 Gy and 3-mm collimation. **(c)** Brain section obtained 19 months after irradiation with 20 Gy shows no radiologic alterations. (Hematoxylin-eosin stain; cross section, 10 µm; original magnification, ×5.)

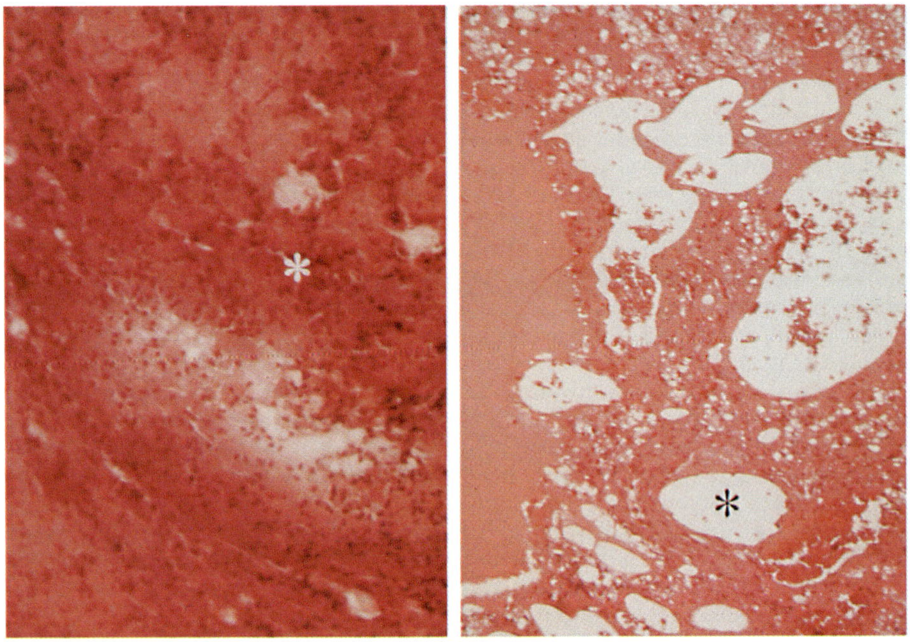

a. b.

Figure 2. Morphologic alterations in a stereotactically irradiated brain. Photomicrographs from different animals depict **(a)** necrosis with local inflammatory glial cell reaction (*) 19 months after treatment with 50 Gy and 2-mm collimation (hematoxylin-eosin stain; original magnification, ×320) and **(b)** telangiectatic vessels (*) close to a necrotic area in the focus of irradiation after 19 months in an animal irradiated with 30 Gy and 3-mm collimation (hematoxylin-eosin stain; original magnification, ×160).

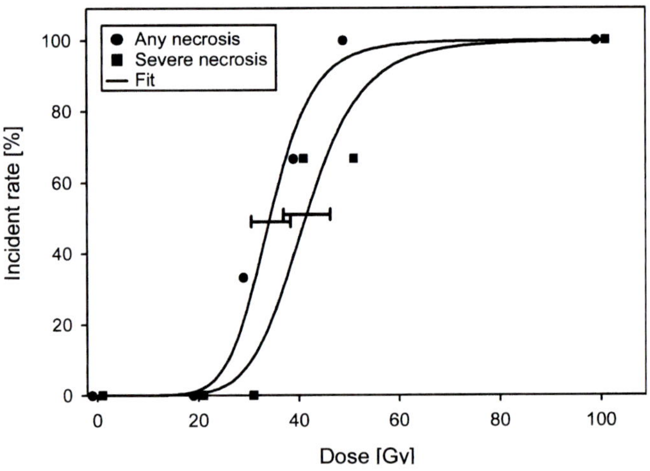

Figure 3. Dose-response curve at 19 months after irradiation for two slightly different histologic end points that were derived for the animals treated with 3-mm collimation. Solid lines are the result of a maximum-likelihood fit of the logistic model to the data. Error bars are single standard errors. Note: Animals irradiated with 100 Gy were included in the calculation, since they had severe necrosis already at 7 months after irradiation. For better visibility, data points and error bars are slightly shifted horizontally and vertically, respectively.

within the treatment volume. Animals exposed to less than 50 Gy did not exhibit any morphologic perturbation at all at this observation point.

In contrast, radiation necrosis was detected in animals that were sacrificed 19 months after irradiation (50 Gy and less) and was dependent on the size of the collimator and on the dose (Fig 1b, Table 1). The extent of the necrosis found after 19 months was clearly smaller than the cystic necrosis seen after 9 months in the animals irradiated with 100 Gy (Fig 2a). Moreover, the incidence and the extent of necrosis were variable. Although some animals within one group showed large areas of focal acellular necrosis (severe necrosis), others exhibited only small diffuse spongiform areas (mild necrosis) or telangiectasia and rarefaction of tissue structure (Fig 2b).

No morphologic changes were ob-

TABLE 1
Classification of Necrosis after Single High-Dose Irradiation

Dose (Gy)	No. of Rats	Grade of Necrosis* after 9 Months	Grade of Necrosis* after 19 Months
	2-mm Collimation Group		
100	4	Severe† (4)	Not done
50	6	None (3)	Severe (1) Moderate (1) Mild (1)
40	6	None (3)	Mild (1) None (2)
30	6	None (3)	None (3)
20	5	None (3)	None (2)
	3-mm Collimation Group		
100	2	Severe† (2)	Not done
50	6	None (3)	Severe (2) Mild (1)
40	6	None (3)	Severe (2) None (1)
30	6	None (3)	Mild (1) None (2)
20	6	None (3)	None (3)
	Control Group		
0	4	None (2)	None (2)

* Number of rats appear in parentheses. To classify necrotic areas in the rat brain after single high-dose irradiation in different dose and volume groups, a modified classification system (10) was used. Mild = small, diffuse spongiform areas; moderate = areas of mixed focal and/or diffuse spongiform necrosis; severe = large areas of focal acellular necrosis.
† Rats were sacrificed after 7 months because of neurologic deficits.

TABLE 2
Estimates of the Model Parameters and the 95% CIs

Parameter	Estimate	Standard Error	95% CI
Any necrosis at 19 mo			
D_{50}	34.2*	+4.1 −3.7	26.9, 42.2
k	7.9	±4.4	0, 16.5
Severe necrosis at 19 mo			
D_{50}	41.3*	+4.9 −4.4	32.7, 50.9
k	7.3	±4.4	0, 15.9

* In gray units.

served in animals irradiated with 20 Gy, independent of field size, and in animals irradiated with 30 Gy by using the 2-mm collimator (Fig 1c). Figure 3 shows the dose-response curves for 3-mm collimation, which were calculated for the end points "any necrosis at 19 months" and "severe necrosis at 19 months." The values of the parameters used to fit the data, resulting from the maximum likelihood procedure, are displayed in Table 2.

Immunohistochemical Findings

Vascular structure after irradiation was assessed with the immunohistochemical detection of fibronectin. Both techniques, direct as well as indirect immunofluorescence, were highly sensitive. Specific vascular staining was restricted to cryofixed brains, and capillary structures could be detected, with high contrast to the surrounding tissue. Even vessels cut in longitudinal orientation could be examined over some length (micrometers).

No morphologic alterations of the capillary and arterial patterns were found in the control animals (Fig 4a). Similarly, animals exposed to 30 Gy or less exhibited undisturbed vascular architecture. Necrotic areas within the irradiated hemisphere showed a marked destruction of the vascular structure. Endothelial remnants were found in these regions (Fig 4b) and were accompanied by a gross vasodilatation of capillaries and arterioles, with varying diameters, as well as by thickened endothelial walls.

Beyond the necrosis, telangiectasia was less pronounced, whereas in cortical areas of the temporal lobe, the capillary structure appeared normal. In animals irradiated with 40 or 50 Gy, without necrosis, vasodilatation was visible in the center of the treatment field.

Angiographic Findings

Structural-functional relationships of the vasculature were evaluated with brain macroangiograms. Shape and distribution of the vascular system appeared normal in the nonirradiated hemisphere. Figure 5 shows branches of the central brain artery, the lenticular artery, and parts of capillaries in a rat brain after exposure to 100 Gy. In the irradiated region (Fig 5, magnified section of angiogram), destroyed vessels and extravasation of contrast medium were observed. Microangiographic specimens cut in frontal orientation offered a more detailed depiction of the vascular architecture and allowed for the assessment of morphologic alterations after irradiation (Fig 6).

Vascular structure was totally lost in animals irradiated with 50 or 100 Gy and developed a visible cystic necrosis. In regions surrounding the necrosis, dilated vessels and extravasation of contrast medium occurred. Microangiographic findings thus confirmed our immunohistochemical results.

DISCUSSION

Animal Model

To study delayed radiation effects on normal tissue in the rat brain, a method of stereotactic radiosurgery was developed and applied (2,22). The present article summarizes our results of radiation-induced vascular alterations as well as the time course of delayed radiation effects in the sense of Van der Kogel's definition (9) of effects that appear after a nonlethal dose of radiation within about 1 year.

From a biologic point of view, the rat central nervous system is regarded as an acceptable model in which to study the radiation effects in normal tissue (26,27). Unfortunately, to our knowledge, most of the published articles deal with irradiation of the whole brain or at least a hemisphere of the brain (5,7,28), which does not allow for the evaluation of volume effects.

Because, to our knowledge, studies of stereotactically guided irradiation of small volumes are scarce (29–31), we initiated an experimental study using collimators with 2- and 3-mm apertures that lead to spherical dose distributions with 80% isodose contours of 3.7 and 4.7 mm, respectively. In combination with isocentric multiple arc treatment, a high dose can be concentrated in a small target volume, with reasonable sparing of the surrounding tissue, as exemplified recently with a 1-mm collimator (2).

As expected, the histologic examination revealed a higher incidence of late structural changes in the brain in the 3-mm collimation group compared with the 2-mm collimation group. Volume effects are described in the literature by Lo et al (7), who irradiated a complete brain hemisphere in rabbits nonstereotactically with 60 Gy and who found necrotic alterations after 10 weeks. Similarly, necrosis occurred after 9 months in the white matter following bilateral irradiation (22.5 Gy) of the rat brain (3). Kondziolka and co-workers (31) observed no histologic changes after 90 days in the frontal lobe in rats irradiated stereotactically (4-mm-diameter treatment field at the isocenter) with 60 Gy. This discrepancy might be attributed to volume effects.

Radiation dose appears to be another important parameter for delayed radiation effects. Increasing the dose to 100 Gy or more, Kondziolka et al (31) found clear radiation-induced alterations after 90 days, under the experimental conditions described previously. Our study findings showed vascular changes increasing with dose. Furthermore, a uniform appearance of radiation-induced necrosis was found at the histologic level in the 100-Gy groups after 7 months, compared with a nonuniform appearance after 19 months. Delayed radiation injury in the 100-Gy group after 9 months and in animals irradiated with 50-Gy or less also revealed a strong time dependence.

Within the observational period, we excluded aging effects of the brain, which were not visible in the irradiated hemisphere, in the nonirradiated hemisphere, or in the age-matched control animals. Nevertheless, some animals showed visible telangiectasia without further vascular or cellular damage in the irradiated hemisphere. These can be interpreted (9) as beginning delayed radiation effects, in the lower-dose groups, that have not completely manifested yet. In species with higher life expectancies, however, angiectatic changes progress with time (eg, in humans, over 5–10 years) (32).

Evaluation of Treatment Effects

In the present study, we focused our histologic and immunohistochemical investigations on vascular alterations. It is well accepted that radiation-induced vascular damage can result in the breakdown of the blood-brain barrier, an important factor that leads to the development of a late radiation response in the central nervous system, although an alternative hypothesis focuses on oligodendrocytes as the main radiation target (11).

The normal or pathologic physiology of the blood-brain barrier depends mainly on the tight junctions between endothelial cells. Alterations of glial cells have only a minor effect on the blood-brain barrier (6). Our present structural and functional results are in accordance with study findings that show a strong correlation between functional radiation effects and vascular alterations, which suggests vascular injury is a major factor that contributes to the pathogenesis of delayed radiation injury in normal tissues (33,34).

The fibronectin staining of the vascular endothelium turned out to be sensitive and specific by both direct and indirect detection techniques, as described by former investigators (35,36). All animals with radiation necrosis verified by using hematoxylin-eosin and Nissl staining also showed substantial vascular abnormalities at immunodetection. The vessel structure of the irradiated hemisphere was totally destroyed. Including the 40-Gy groups, all animals exhibited severe dila-

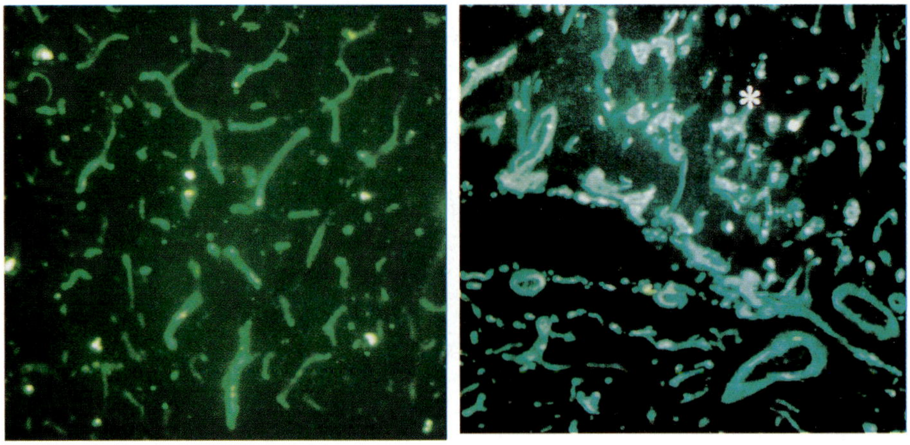

a. b.

Figure 4. Immunodetection of fibronectin in brain capillaries. Photomicrographs depict **(a)** normal capillary morphology in a control animal (original magnification, ×25) and **(b)** severe alterations of the capillary structure (*) 19 months after exposure to 50 Gy and 3-mm collimation in another animal (original magnification, ×50).

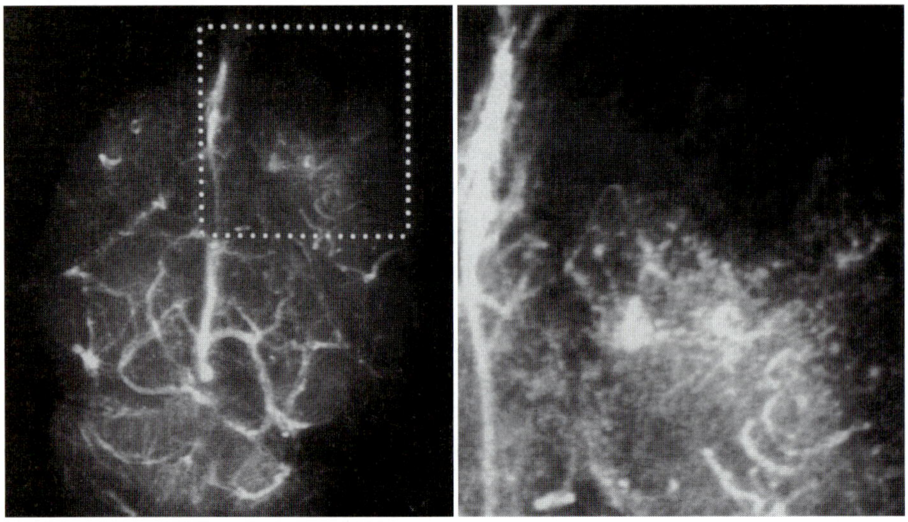

Figure 5. Anteroposterior macroangiogram of a rat brain irradiated with 100 Gy and 3-mm collimation depicts extravasation of contrast medium in the right frontal lobe after 9 months. A region of the right frontal lobe from the survey radiograph (left) was magnified (right) to distinguish details.

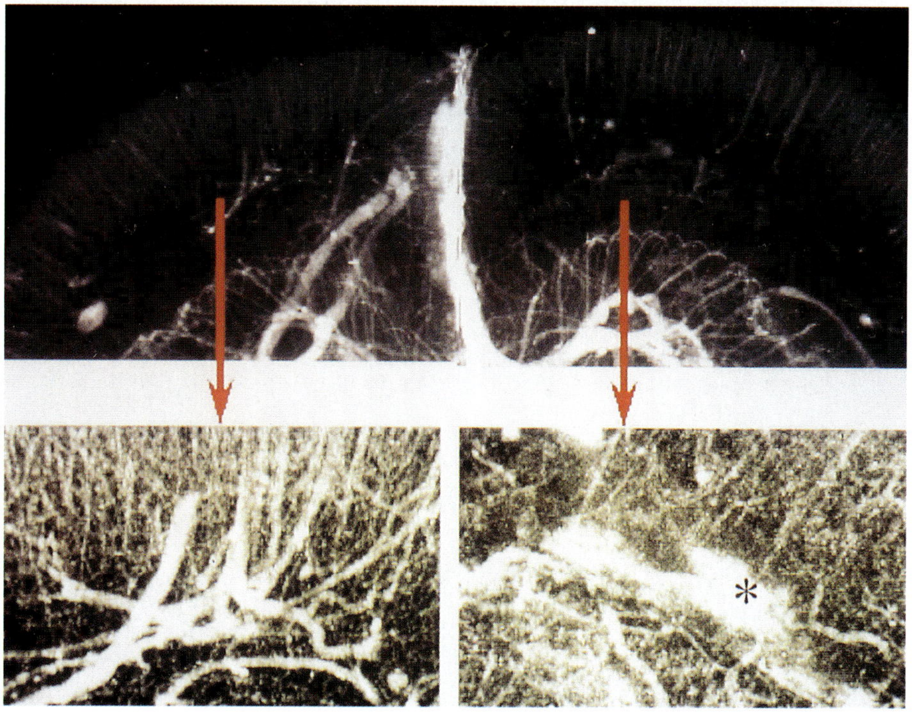

Figure 6. Microangiogram of the focus of irradiation after 7 months in an animal irradiated with 100 Gy and 3-mm collimation shows the nonirradiated hemisphere with a normal vascular morphology (left) and extravasation (*) of the contrast medium and a deterioration of the capillary structure (right).

tation of the vessels in the irradiated target volume. These alterations were definitely time dependent. Telangiectatic vessels were seen after 9 months in only the 50-Gy, 3-mm-collimation group and in the 100-Gy groups.

The largest extension of vascular damage preceded the development of a radiation necrosis (7). The pathogenesis of telangiectasia can be explained by microvascular occlusion (3,5,37) or decreased venous draining (38). These changes increase the intraluminal pressure, which, in turn, leads to the dilatation of the capillaries and arterioles.

The vascular changes after high-dose irradiation were also detected by using macro- and microangiographic techniques. These methods were used mainly to describe the vascularization after the transplantation of brain tumors or after experimental brain trauma (39,40). Compared with conventional histologic examination, microangiography could easily depict functional alterations of telangiectasia as well as vascular obliteration and vasoconstriction.

The present experiment was not designed to describe the acute effects of irradiation. All animals irradiated with 100 Gy showed cystic necrosis in the treated hemisphere after 9 months. Necrotic areas appeared exclusively in the white matter of the brain, which is known to be preferentially sensitive to radiation (41,42). Radiation necrosis was surrounded by areas of enlargement of the endothelial cells, blood vessel dilatation, thickening of the blood vessel wall, and hypertrophy of adjacent astrocytes. These four morphologic criteria have been defined as the "tissue injury unit" by Calvo (5) and are correlated with the development of radiation necrosis.

Findings from brain tissue irradiated with 50 Gy and 3-mm collimation confirmed the correlation between the tissue injury unit after 9 months and the radiation necrosis after 19 months. In contrast, it was difficult to assign the morphologic changes that occurred in the 100-Gy group to Calvo's criteria because all animals had already developed complete radiation necrosis within 9 months.

The dose-response curves that were calculated for the end points of "any necrosis at 19 months" and "severe necrosis at 19 months" show different tolerance doses, although the difference of 7 Gy was not significant with respect to the 95% CI. An experiment with a larger number of animals and smaller dose intervals would allow the discrimination between these two curves. In addition, it would be of interest to compare these curves with dose-response curves obtained at serial MR imaging, since MR imaging enables the detection of small vascular lesions and can be applied easily to patients.

Practical application: Our experimental study on delayed radiation effects in normal brain tissue used a series of clinically relevant doses combined with an extended follow-up of up to 19 months. The steep dose-response relationship suggests dose-escalation studies in radiosurgery have to be performed with caution, that is, by allowing only moderate escalation steps. Normal tissue tolerance of the brain is strongly volume dependent. Hence, quantification of radiation tolerance has to be specified relative to treatment volume. Moreover, it became evident that morphologic disturbances have a longer latency period after a low dose of radiation, whereas the development of radiation necrosis is accelerated by higher doses and larger volumes. Vascular changes seem to be major factors that contribute to radiation-induced late effects.

Acknowledgments: The authors are indebted to Annemarie Schroedersecker and Alexandra Tietz for technical assistance and to Gerd Wolber, PhD, for the critical reading of the manuscript.

References

1. Lunsford LD, Altschuler EM, Flickinger JC, Wu A, Martinez AJ. In vivo biological effects of stereotactic radiosurgery: a primate model. Neurosurgery 1990; 27:373–382.
2. Karger CP, Hartmann GH, Hoffmann U, Lorenz WJ. A system for stereotactic irradiation and MR evaluations in the rat brain. Int J Radiat Oncol Biol Phys 1995; 33:485–492.
3. Calvo W, Hopewell JW, Reinhold HS, Yeung TK. Time- and dose-related changes in the white matter of the rat brain after single dose of x rays. Br J Radiol 1988; 61:1043–1052.
4. Yoshii Y, Phillips TL. Late vascular effects of whole brain X-irradiation in the mouse. Acta Neurochir 1982; 64:87–102.
5. Calvo W. Experimental radiation damage of central nervous system. In: Hinkelmann W, Bruggmoser G, Frommhold H, Wannenmacher M, eds. Acute and long-term side-effects of radiotherapy: biological basis and clinical relevance. Recent Result Cancer Res, vol 130. Berlin, Germany: Springer-Verlag 1993; 175–188.
6. Hopewell JW. Late radiation damage to the central nervous system: a radiobiological interpretation. Neuropathol Appl Neurobiol 1979; 5:329–343.
7. Lo EH, Frankel KA, Steinberg GK, DeLaPaz RL, Fabrikant JI. High-dose single-fraction brain irradiation: MRI, cerebral blood flow, electrophysiological, and histological studies. Int J Radiat Oncol Biol Phys 1991; 22:47–55.

8. Blatt DR, Friedmann WA, Bova FJ, Theele DP, Mickle JP. Temporal characteristics of radiosurgical lesions in an animal model. J Neurosurg 1994; 80:1046–1055.
9. Van der Kogel AJ. Central nervous system injury in small animal models. In: Gutin PH, Leibel SA, Sheline GE, eds. Radiation injury to the nervous system. New York, NY: Raven, 1991; 91–112.
10. Rubin P, Gash DM, Hansen JT, Nelson DF, Williams JP. Disruption of the blood-brain barrier as the primary effect of CNS irradiation. Radiother Oncol 1994; 31:51–60.
11. Schultheiss TE, Stephens LC. Permanent radiation myelopathy. Br J Radiol 1992; 65:737–753.
12. Hindo WA, DeTrana FA III, Lee MS, Hendrickson FR. Large dose increment irradiation in treatment of cerebral metastases. Cancer 1970; 26:138–141.
13. Cohen L, Hendrickson F, Mansell JA, et al. Late reactions and complications in patients treated with high energy neutrons p (66 MeV)be(40 MeV). Int J Radiat Oncol Biol Phys 1981; 7:179–184.
14. Sheline GE, Wara WM, Smith V. Therapeutic irradiation and brain injury. Int J Radiat Oncol Biol Phys 1980; 6:1215–1228.
15. Aristizabal S, Caldwell WL, Avila J. The relationship of time-dose fractionation factors to complications in the treatment of pituitary tumors by irradiation. Int J Radiat Oncol Biol Phys 1977; 2:667–673.
16. Eifel PJ, Cassady JR, Belli JA. Radiation therapy of tumors of the brainstem and midbrain in children: experience of the Joint Center for Irradiation Therapy and Children's Hospital Medical Center (1971–1981). Int J Radiat Oncol Biol Phys 1987; 13:847–852.
17. Kagan AR, Steckel RJ, Cancilla P, Juillard G, Patin T. The pathogenesis of brain necrosis: time and dose parameters. Int J Radiat Oncol Biol Phys 1976; 1:729–732.
18. Hornsey S, Morris CC, Myers R. The relationship between fractionation and total dose for x ray induced brain damage. Int J Radiat Oncol Biol Phys 1981; 7:393–396.
19. Lo EH, DeLaPaz RL, Frankel KA, et al. MRI and PET of delayed heavy-ion radiation injury in the rabbit brain. Int J Radiat Oncol Biol Phys 1991; 20:689–696.
20. Steinberg GK, Fabrikant JI, Marks MP, et al. Stereotactic helium ion Bragg peak radiosurgery for intracranial arteriovenous malformations: detailed clinical and neurologic outcomes. Stereotact Funct Neurosurg 1991; 57:36–49.
21. Cox AB, Keng PC, Glass NL, Lett JT. Effects of heavy ions on rabbit tissues: alopecia. Int J Radiat Biol Relat Stud Phys Chem Med 1981; 40:645–657.
22. Karger CP, Hartmann GH, Peschke P, et al. Dose-response relationship for late functional changes in the rat brain after radiosurgery evaluated by magnetic resonance imaging. Int J Radiat Oncol Biol Phys 1997; 39:1163–1172.
23. Sturm V, Pastyr O, Schlegel W, et al. Stereotactic computer tomography with modified Riechert-Mundinger device as the basis for integrated stereotactic neuroradiological investigations. Acta Neurochir 1983; 68:11–17.
24. Pastyr O, Hartmann GH, Schlegel W, et al. Stereotactically guided convergent beam irradiation with a linear accelerator: localization-technique. Acta Neurochir 1989; 99:61–64.
25. Paxinos G, Watson C. The rat brain in stereotaxic coordinates. 2nd ed. San Diego, Calif: Academic Press, 1986.
26. Fowler JF. Review: total doses in fractionated radiotherapy—implications of new radiobiological data. Int J Radiat Biol Relat Stud Phys Chem Med 1984; 46:103–120.
27. Van der Kogel AJ. Mechanisms of late radiation injury in the spinal cord. In: Meyn RE, Withers HR, eds. Radiation biology in cancer research. New York, NY: Raven, 1980; 461–470.
28. Remler MP, Marcussen WH, Tiller-Borsich, J. The late effects of radiation on the blood brain barrier. Int J Radiat Oncol Biol Phys 1986; 12:1965–1969.
29. Kamiryo T, Kassell NF, Thai QA, Lopes MB, Lee KS, Steiner L. Histological changes in the rat brain after gamma irradiation. Acta Neurochir 1996; 138:451–459.
30. Kamiryo T, Lopes MB, Berr SS, Lee KS, Kassell NF, Steiner L. Occlusion of the anterior cerebral artery after gamma knife irradiation in a rat. Acta Neurochir 1996; 138:983–991.
31. Kondziolka D, Lunsford LD, Claassen D, Maitz AH, Flickinger JC. Radiobiology of radiosurgery. I. The normal rat brain model. Neurosurgery 1992; 31:271–279.
32. Turesson I, Notter G. Dose-response and dose-latency relationships for human skin after various fractionation schedules. Br J Cancer 1986; 53(suppl 7):67–72.
33. Phillips TL. Early late effects of radiation on normal tissue. In: Gutin PH, Leibel SA, Sheline GE, eds. Radiation injury to the nervous system. New York, NY: Raven, 1991; 37–55.
34. Schneider BF, Eberhard DA, Steiner LE. Histopathology of arteriovenous malformations after gamma knife radiosurgery. J Neurosurg 1997, 87:352–357.
35. Göbel U, Theilen H, Kuschinsky W. Congruence of total and perfused capillary network in rat brains. Circ Res 1990; 66:271–281.
36. Theilen H, Kuschinsky W. Fluorescence labeling of the capillary network in rat brains. J Cereb Blood Flow Metab 1992; 12:347–350.
37. Law MP. Radiation-induced vascular injury and its relation to late effects in normal tissues. Adv Radiat Biol 1981; 9:37–73.
38. Baker DG, Krochak RJ. The response of the microvascular system to radiation: a review. Cancer Invest 1989; 7:287–294.
39. Brecht G, Schwinger E, Gebhardt M. Early changes in the microangiogram of the rabbit brain after experimental skull and cerebral trauma. I. Methods. ROFO 1980; 132:124–132. [German]
40. Schumacher M, Mennel HD, Weisser G, Voigt K. Neuroradiology of the normal and pathological anatomy of the rat brain. II. Microangiographic investigations of the vascularization of transplanted malignant brain tumors. ROFO 1980; 133:514–520. [German]
41. Clemente CD, Holst EA. Pathological changes in neurons, neuroglia and blood-brain-barrier induced by x-irradiation of heads of monkeys. Arch Neurol Psychiatry 1954; 71:66–79.
42. Vogel FS, Pickering JE. Demyelinization induced in the brains of monkeys by means of fast neutrons: pathogenesis of the lesion and comparison with the lesion of multiple sclerosis and Schilder's disease. J Exp Med 1956; 104:435–442.

Hannu I. Manninen, MD, PhD
Heikki T. Räsänen, MD
Ritva L. Vanninen, MD, PhD
Pauli Vainio, PhL
Mikko Hippeläinen, MD, PhD
Veli-Matti Kosma, MD, PhD

Index terms:
Carotid arteries, MR, 172.121411, 904.129411
Carotid arteries, stenosis or obstruction, 172.721, 904.721
Carotid arteries, transluminal angioplasty, 172.126, 904.1282, 904.1286
Carotid arteries, US, 172.1298, 904.1298
Stents and prostheses, 172.126, 904.1268

Radiology 1999; 212:483–492

Abbreviation:
PTA = percutaneous transluminal angioplasty

[1] From the Departments of Clinical Radiology (H.I.M., H.T.R., R.L.V., P.V.), Surgery (M.H.), and Pathology (V.M.K.), Kuopio University Hospital, Puijonlaaksontie 2, SF-70210 Kuopio, Finland, and the Department of Pathology and Forensic Medicine, University of Kuopio, Finland (V.M.K.). Received June 5, 1998; revision requested July 31; final revision received November 2; accepted February 9, 1999. **Address reprint requests to** H.I.M. (e-mail: *hannu.manninen@kuh.fi*).

Author contributions:
Guarantor of integrity of entire study, H.I.M.; study concepts, H.I.M., H.T.R.; study design, H.I.M., H.T.R., M.H.; definition of intellectual content, H.I.M.; literature research, H.I.M.; experimental studies, H.I.M., H.T.R., R.L.V., P.V., M.H.; data acquisition, H.I.M., H.T.R., R.L.V., P.V.; data analysis, H.I.M., P.V., V.M.K.; statistical analysis, H.I.M.; manuscript preparation, H.I.M., H.T.R., V.M.K.; manuscript editing, R.L.V., P.V.; manuscript review, M.H.

Stent Placement versus Percutaneous Transluminal Angioplasty of Human Carotid Arteries in Cadavers in Situ: Distal Embolization and Findings at Intravascular US, MR Imaging, and Histopathologic Analysis[1]

PURPOSE: To compare endovascular stent placement with percutaneous transluminal angioplasty (PTA) of carotid arteries with respect to distal embolization and findings at intravascular ultrasonography (US), magnetic resonance (MR) imaging, and histopathologic analysis.

MATERIALS AND METHODS: PTA was performed in situ in one carotid artery, and stent placement was performed in the other, in ten cadavers (age range, 57–82 years; mean age, 68 years) with severe atherosclerosis by using fluoroscopic and intravascular US guidance. The carotid artery was connected to a pressurized tubing system in which a pulsatile pump circulated water. The effluent water was collected during the interventions, and after filtration and staining, the embolic material was analyzed histologically. After the interventions, the arteries were excised and 1.5-T spin-echo MR imaging was performed.

RESULTS: No difference in severity of distal embolization during stent placement versus during PTA was found. The embolic particles were composed mainly of intimal strips and cellular constituents of the atherosclerotic plaques. MR imaging accurately depicted postinterventional changes, and the findings correlated closely with those of intravascular US and histopathologic analysis.

CONCLUSION: Although stent placement and PTA were associated with equal distal embolization, the smooth surface and fully patent arterial lumen depicted at intravascular US and MR imaging postinterventionally may indicate that stent placement is preferable to PTA.

Percutaneous endovascular interventions are rapidly evolving as alternatives to surgical endarterectomy of atherosclerotic stenoses of carotid arteries. The results of several studies (1–4) indicate that balloon angioplasty (ie, percutaneous transluminal angioplasty [PTA]) effectively resolves stenoses of the carotid arterial bifurcation. Stents provide an effective means of improving the primary success and long-term patency of peripheral and coronary arteries compared with PTA, and reports (5,6) show very promising results in atherosclerotic lesions of the carotid arterial bifurcation. Although distal embolism is seldom encountered in peripheral and coronary arteries, it is a feared complication during endovascular procedures in carotid arteries because of its potentially serious consequences. In trials with selected patients, clinically important embolism seems to occur in 3.0%–6.5% of patients during PTA and/or stent placement in internal carotid arteries (2,4–6), but asymptomatic embolization detected at transcranial Doppler ultrasonography (US) is much more common (7). To our knowledge, there have been no analyses of the frequency of distal embolization during PTA compared with that during endovascular stent placement.

Intravascular US is widely used in peripheral and coronary arteries (8,9) for guiding complex endovascular interventions; the technique is considered to be the standard of reference for imaging arterial wall and atherosclerotic plaque (10). Intravascular US seems to be feasible and safe for imaging carotid arteries that are "protected" with a stent (11,12) and "unprotected" carotid arteries that have mild atherosclerotic changes (13). However, intravascular US is an invasive technique that currently cannot be used to image severely diseased carotid arteries or performed during PTA of carotid arteries. Thus, there is a definite need for a noninvasive and safe imaging technique for monitoring carotid arteries after PTA or stent placement. Although magnetic resonance (MR) imaging has shown promise in quantitating and characterizing carotid atherosclerosis in vivo (14), to our knowledge, its use in evaluating carotid arteries after PTA and stent placement has not been reported on.

The present study was undertaken to (*a*) compare the severity of distal embolization during carotid arterial stent placement with that during PTA by means of experimental interventions in cadavers in situ, (*b*) correlate the distal embolization with the intravascular US appearance and histopathologic findings of the atherosclerotic arterial wall, and (*c*) compare T1-, T2-, and intermediate-weighted spin-echo MR imaging with intravascular US for the postinterventional evaluation of the carotid arteries.

MATERIALS AND METHODS

Ten cadavers (nine men, one woman; age range at time of death, 57–82 years; mean age, 68 years) with histories of severe cardiovascular disease and/or calcified plaques identified at external US performed after death were selected for the study. The cause of death was acute myocardial infarct in five cases, stroke in two cases, rupture of an abdominal aortic aneurysm in two cases, and gastrointestinal bleeding in one case. The study protocol was approved by the ethics committee of our hospital.

Carotid Arterial PTA and Stent Placement

The experimental endovascular interventions were performed in conjunction with the autopsies within 48 hours after death. The aortic arch was cannulated by using visual guidance after the removal of the manubrium sterni and costal cartilages, and an 8-F introducer sheath was advanced into the proximal common carotid artery with contrast medium–enhanced digital fluoroscopic guidance (at the lateral projection). To eliminate backflow, the proximal part of the common carotid artery was tightly ligated around the sheath. Postmortem thrombi were removed by vigorously flushing the artery with water through the side port of the sheath by means of manual injections. After all friable material had been removed, the intracranial internal carotid artery was tightly cannulated at the base of the skull. The artery was connected to a circulating tubing system in which a pulsatile pump circulated water. Carotid arterial angiography was performed by manually injecting contrast medium into the side port of the introducer sheath.

At the beginning of the intervention, the extracranial internal carotid artery was traversed with a 0.018-inch guide wire with the aid of digital road map control. A 3.5-F, 30-MHz intravascular US catheter (Sonicath; Medi-tech/Boston Scientific, Watertown, Mass) was introduced into the distal internal carotid artery, and intravascular US (Sonos; Hewlett Packard, Andover, Mass) was performed while the catheter was slowly pulled back. The US scans were registered on super-VHS tape, as described in greater detail elsewhere (13). The mean intravascular pressure during imaging was maintained at 70–100 mm Hg to provide full expansion of the carotid artery. To register the exact longitudinal location of the US probe within the artery, several single x-ray exposures were obtained during imaging, and the corresponding time points were marked with annotations on the intravascular US videotape.

The right and left carotid arteries in each cadaver were randomized for PTA or stent placement. The sizes of the PTA balloon and the stent were determined on the basis of the measurement at intravascular US. The PTA balloon diameter was selected to match the luminal diameter of the normal internal carotid arterial segment adjacent to the diseased segment. The nominal diameter of the self-expanding stent (Wallstent; Schneider, Bulach, Switzerland) was 1–2 mm bigger than the luminal diameter of the artery. If angiographically detected residual stenosis persisted after stent placement, then complementary balloon dilation was performed. Conventional 5-F PTA balloon catheters and dilation pressures of 8–10 atmospheres were used. The results were monitored with contrast-enhanced angiography, and intravascular US was repeated at the end of the procedure.

Collection of Embolic Material

The effluent water was collected during the intervention, from the point when the lesion was traversed with the guide wire to the time of final angiography, excluding intravascular US. If the stent placement procedure ended with balloon dilation, another fraction of effluent water was collected during this stage. At the end of the intervention, 20–40 mL of water was forcefully injected by hand into the side port of the sheath to flush the remaining friable material into the tubing system. Then, a volume of 99% ethanol equivalent to the volume of water collected was added to the solution. Immediately after the intervention, the extracranial carotid arteries were excised, and the specimens were immersed in 10% buffered formalin.

MR Imaging

MR imaging of the excised arterial samples was performed at room temperature by using 1.5-T equipment (Magnetom Vision; Siemens Medical Systems, Erlangen, Germany). A 40-mm solenoid radio-frequency coil was used as a receiver. After sagittal T1-weighted localizer images (repetition time msec/echo time msec, 15/6; flip angle, 70°) were obtained, T1-weighted spin-echo (400/14) and fast intermediate- and T2-weighted images (2,500/17–102) were obtained in the axial plane by using the following parameters: field of view, 31 × 50 mm; section thickness, 2 mm; and matrix, 160 × 256. A total length of 5–6 cm, which covered the treated area, was imaged.

Analysis of Intravascular US Findings

All of the intravascular US videotapes were analyzed at a consensus reading by two vascular radiologists (H.I.M., H.T.R.) with prior experience in intravascular US of the coronary, carotid, and peripheral arteries. The inter- and intraobserver variabilities of these two readers in interpreting carotid arterial intravascular US findings are presented elsewhere (13). The percentage diameter of stenosis before and after the intervention was measured at intravascular US by using the analysis program provided with the equipment software. The morphology of the atherosclerotic plaques was classified at intravascular US on the basis of established criteria as soft, fibrotic, or mixed (13,15,16). The intravascular US appearance of the surface of the plaques was classified as smooth, irregular, or ulcerated. Hyperechoic intralesional areas with acoustic shadowing were interpreted as calcifications. The total number of macroscopic calcifications at the treated segments were calculated. The degree of lesion calcification was visually assessed on a four-point scale as not calcified, minimally calcified, moderately calcified, or heavily calcified.

The postinterventional intravascular US scans were analyzed for the presence of dissections, which were defined as separations of the components of the arterial wall. The site of the dissection in relation to the atherosclerotic plaque and the extension of the dissection were graded as minor or major. We also searched for fractures in the inner parts of the plaque. Partly loosened intimal flaps and other components of the atherosclerotic arterial wall floating inside the arterial lumen were registered.

In the arterial segments treated with stents, we evaluated the contact between the stent and arterial wall and searched for protrusion of the plaque material through the stent. The extension of the stent over the whole diseased segment was assessed.

Analysis of MR Imaging Findings

The axial MR images were analyzed by one radiologist (H.I.M.) 2 months before the intravascular US analysis by using a classification similar to that used in the analysis of the postinterventional intravascular US videotapes. Furthermore, T1-, T2-, and intermediate-weighted MR images were compared side by side and given a grade of 1–3 relative to each other for the depiction of the following anatomic and diagnostic details: calcifications, dissections, demarcation of the arterial wall from the periadventitial tissues, demarcation of the atherosclerotic plaque from the arterial wall, and absence of artifacts due to the stent.

Histologic Analysis of the Embolic Material

The histologic analyses were performed by an experienced pathologist (V.M.K.). The effluent fluid collected during each intervention was micropore filtered, and the sediment was stained with Papanicolaou stain. To characterize the distal embolism, the material captured by the filters was analyzed under a light microscope. The composition of the filtered particles was classified into the following three categories: clusters of unspecified cells, lipid-filled foam cells or other material of the fragmented atherosclerotic plaque, and intimal strips. The number of these elements in each sample was calculated, and the dimensions of the largest particles were measured with an image analyzer (Quantimet 570; Leica, Cambridge, England) operated in an interactive mode. In addition, the relative amounts of lipid-filled foam cells or other fragmented atherosclerotic plaque material were classified as scanty (less than 10), numerous, or abundant (unmeasurable). On the basis of the abundance of the components described above, the overall severity of embolism was assessed on a three-point scale as mild, moderate, or severe. Finally, in each cadaver, the severity of embolism between the right and left carotid arteries, with consideration of the amount of embolic material and the particle size, was compared pairwise by using a rating system in which a score of −2 indicated the embolism was much more severe on the stent-treated side; −1, the embolism was slightly more severe on the stent-treated side; 0, the embolism was equal on both sides; 1, the embolism was slightly more severe on the PTA-treated side; and 2, the embolism was much more severe on the PTA-treated side.

Histopathologic Analysis of Arterial Specimens

To locate the anatomic landmarks, fine-resolution native film hard-copy images of the air-filled carotid arterial specimens were obtained at 30 kVp in the lateral projection. On the basis of findings on these images, the MR images, and the intravascular US scans, two or three anatomic locations were selected in the area of the treated (with stent placement or balloon dilation) segment. The stents were carefully removed from the excised, formalin-buffered arteries. Five-micrometer-thick slices were cut in the marked locations. The slices were stained with either hematoxylin-eosin or Masson trichrome stain and analyzed under a light microscope. Other constituents of the plaques that were registered included the presence of a necrotic core, hemorrhage or remarkable neovascularity, and intraplaque calcifications (hematoxylin-eosin stain). The calcifications were classified as microscopic (punctate) or large (either deep or superficial).

Plaques with a fibrotic superficial part and middle and basal cell layers that contained foam cells, cellular debris, and cholesterol crystals were classified as fibrous cap lesions (13). The fibrous cap was further classified as complete, thin, or incomplete. Dissections, which were defined and classified analogously to those on the imaging studies, were registered. Plaque disruption was defined as intraplaque material protruding outside the plaque.

Statistical Analyses

The Spearman correlation coefficient for the continuous and ordinal scale variables between the two treatment groups was calculated. The differences between the two groups were tested by using the Wilcoxon rank sum *W* test for the continuous and ordinal scale variables and the Fisher exact test for the dichotomized variables. The Wilcoxon matched pairs signed rank test was used to perform paired comparisons between the right and left carotid arteries in each cadaver. The Friedman two-way analysis of variance was used to test differences between the three MR imaging sequences. Differences with a *P* value of less than .05 were considered to be statistically significant.

RESULTS

Comparability of Study Groups

The preinterventional intravascular US and histopathologic characteristics of the treated lesions in the two treatment groups are shown in Tables 1 and 2. The stenotic lesions in the PTA and stent placement groups were comparable with respect to all the analyzed parameters; however, the lesions in the stent placement group tended to be slightly more atherosclerotic. In five arteries, the surface of the plaque was irregular at intravascular US, but no ulcerated lesions were detected in either treatment group.

Experimental PTA and Stent Placement

The endovascular interventions were successfully completed in 19 of the 20 arteries. In one cadaver, the right carotid artery that was randomized for stent placement proved to be chronically occluded and thus could not be traversed with the guide wire. Thus, 10 arteries were included in the PTA group, and nine arteries were included in the stent placement group for the comparative analyses. The main part of the lesion that was treated was at the bifurcation or bulbar segment of the internal carotid artery in all arteries. The diameter of the balloon was 6 mm in five, 7 mm in three, and 8 mm in two arteries. The diameter of the stent was 7 mm in five and 8 mm in four arteries. The nominal lengths of the fully open stents were 29–37 mm. No predilation of the lesion was performed before stent placement; however, in four cases, balloon dilation was performed inside the stent because of residual stenosis (Fig 1).

TABLE 1
Preinterventional Intravascular US Characteristics of the Treated Lesions

Parameter	Stent Placement Group	PTA Group	*P* Value
Mean diameter of stenosis (%)*	52 (34–85)	44 (32–80)	.16
Intravascular US morphology of the lesion†			.41
Fibrotic	3 (33)	5 (50)	
Soft	1 (11)	3 (30)	
Mixed	5 (56)	2 (20)	
Calcified lesions at intravascular US†			.58
Total	7 (78)	8 (80)	
Minimally calcified	NA	1	
Moderately calcified	6	5	
Heavily calcified	1	2	
Mean number of calcifications*	3.7 (0–10)	3.8 (0–11)	.97

Note.—Data are based on nine arteries treated with stent placement and 10 arteries treated with PTA. NA = not available.
* Numbers in parentheses are the range.
† Data are the number of arteries. Numbers in parentheses are the percentage.

TABLE 2
Histopathologic Characteristics and Postinterventional Changes in the Atherosclerotic Plaques

Parameter	Stent Placement Group	PTA Group	*P* Value
Fibrous cap lesions	7 (78)	7 (70)	.99
Complete	5	6	
Incomplete	2	1	
Lesions with a necrotic core	5 (56)	2 (20)	.17
Intraplaque hemorrhages	6 (67)	2 (20)	.07
Calcified lesions			.90
Total	8 (89)	8 (80)	
Only punctate	2	1	
Larger	6	7	
Postinterventional dissections	5 (56)	8 (80)	.19
Minor	2	2	
Major	3	6	
Postinterventional plaque disruption	3 (33)	4 (40)	.87

Note.—Data are based on nine lesions treated with stent placement and 10 lesions treated with PTA. Numbers in parentheses are the percentage.

Distal Embolization during PTA and Stent Placement

Table 3 shows the results of the analyses of the embolic material in the two treatment groups. As can be seen from the results, there were no statistically significant differences between the groups with regard to the severity or composition of the embolic material. Furthermore, the paired comparison between the right and left arteries in the nine cadavers in whom the two interventions were performed did not reveal any clear differences. In each of the four cases in which balloon dilation was performed inside the stent, the results of analysis of the embolic contents in the two collected fluid fractions (during stent placement and during additional dilation) revealed further embolization during the balloon dilation. However, the overall severity and type of distal embolization in these four cases did not differ from those in the other five arteries in the stent placement group.

The largest and potentially most dangerous embolic constituents were the intimal strips (Fig 2) that were found in all nine arteries in the stent placement group and in seven of the 10 arteries in the PTA group. Some of these strips contained cellular material, probably from the superficial part of the atherosclerotic arterial wall. The three arteries with the greatest number of embolic intimal strips were in the PTA group. The length of the intimal strips was up to 5 mm. There was a positive correlation between the number of intimal strips in the arteries treated with stents and that in the arteries treated with PTA for each subject (nine subjects treated with both treatments, $r = 0.62$ and $P = .06$).

Determinants of Distal Embolization

Because the frequency and severity of distal embolization in the two treatment groups was equal, all 19 arteries were considered in a single group for the analysis of the predictors of distal embolization. The greater abundance of lipid-filled foam cells in the filtrate was associated with the presence of intraplaque hemorrhage histopathologically ($P = .04$). Furthermore, the abundance of unspecified cells in the embolic filtrate correlated positively with the number of calcifications at intravascular US ($r = 0.42$, $P = .07$). Severe distal embolization caused by intimal strips was encountered in one artery (seven intimal strips) in the stent placement group and in two arteries (eight and 11 intimal strips, respectively) in the PTA group; at postprocedural intravascular US, these vessels had partly loosened intimal flaps floating inside the arterial lumen (Fig 3).

Postprocedural Intravascular US and MR Imaging

Residual stenosis.— The mean diameter of stenosis of the 10 PTA-treated lesions measured by using intravascular US decreased from 44% before the procedure to 34% after the treatment (range, 24%–51%) ($P < .01$). The residual diameter of stenosis after PTA measured by using MR imaging correlated significantly with that measured by using intravascular US ($r = 0.71$, $P < .05$). The lumen was fully patent at both intravascular US and MR imaging after stent placement in each case. Sagittal MR images depicted well the longitudinal extension of the plaques and stents (Figs 1, 4). There was agreement between intravascular US and MR imaging in the detection of five arteries in which the

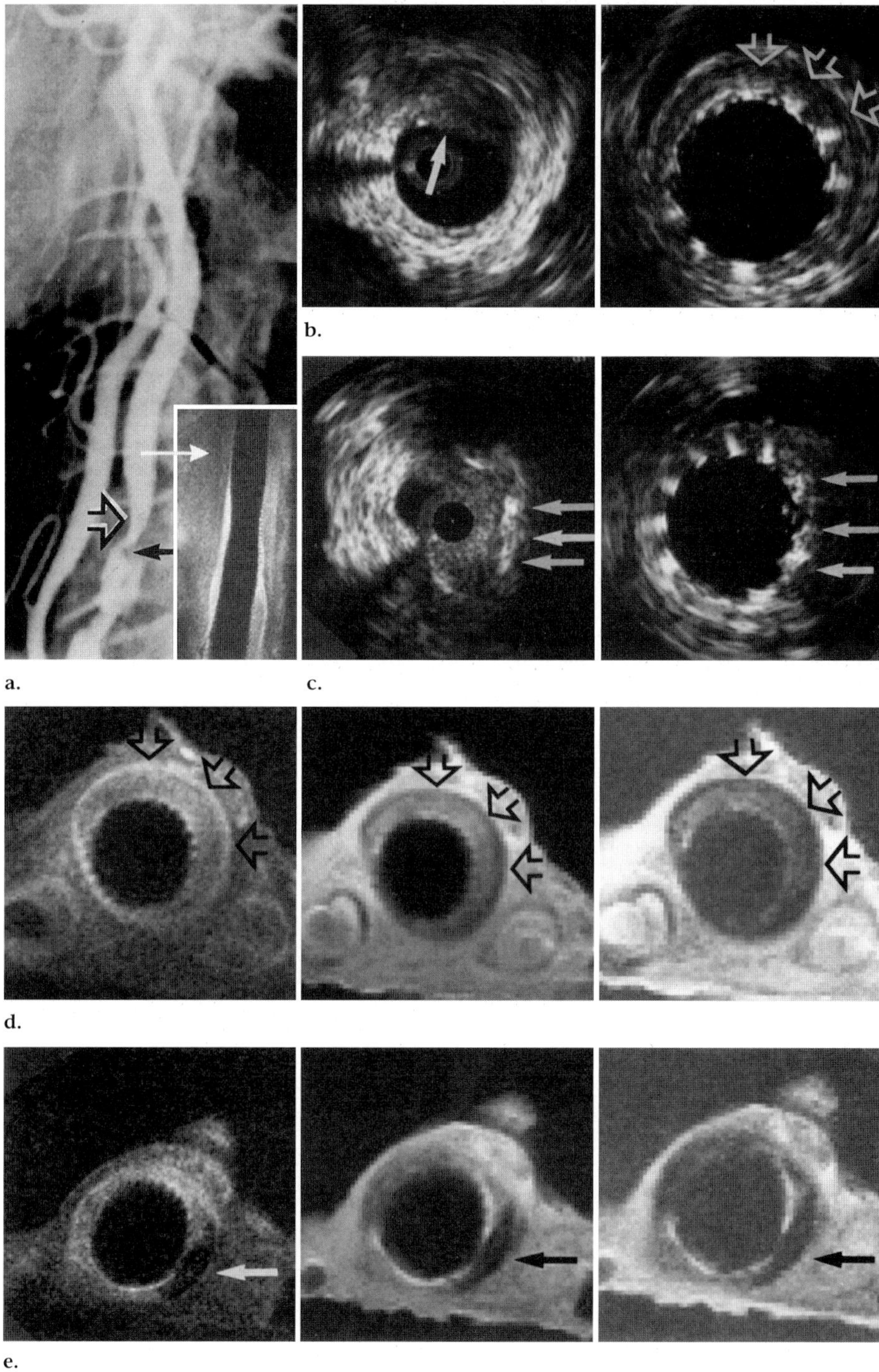

Figure 1. **(a)** X-ray angiogram at lateral projection shows a complex stenotic lesion at the bulbar segment of the internal carotid artery. Corresponding sagittal T1-weighted MR image (400/14) (boxed insert) demonstrates a fully patent, smooth arterial lumen after stent placement and complementary balloon dilation, but the stent does not entirely cover the proximal edge of the plaque. The white arrow denotes the end of the stent. The open arrow and black arrow denote the levels at which the corresponding **(b, c)** axial intravascular US scans and **(d, e)** axial MR images were obtained. **(b)** Axial intravascular US scan obtained at the level of the open arrow in **a** before treatment (left) shows an eccentric, hypoechoic lesion (solid arrow) consistent with a "soft" plaque. The intravascular US scan obtained after stent placement (right) shows an excellent result. The extension of the plaque (open arrows) is satisfactorily seen through the stent mesh. **(c)** Intravascular US scan obtained at the level denoted by the black arrow in **a** before treatment (left) reveals a tight stenosis with a deep calcification (arrows). The intravascular US scan obtained after stent placement (right) reveals good contact between the stent and the arterial wall, but the calcification (arrows) hinders visualization of the deeper part of the plaque. **(d)** Axial T1- (400/14)(left), intermediate- (2,500/17) (middle), and T2-weighted (TR/TE 2,500/102) (right) MR images obtained at the level of the open arrow in **a** show the full extension of the plaque (arrows) in the stent-treated artery. **(e)** T1- (400/14) (left), intermediate- (2,500/17) (middle), and T2-weighted (2,500/102) (right) MR images obtained at the level denoted by the black arrow in **a** show the calcification (arrow) and plaque behind the stent.

stent did not cover the whole length of the diseased arterial segment (Fig 1). Intravascular US revealed one artery in which the contact of the stent with the vessel wall was not adequate despite additional balloon dilation (Fig 5), apparently because of heavy calcifications. This was not detected at MR imaging.

Findings of arterial damage.— In six of 10 lesions, the surface of the plaque was irregular after PTA at intravascular US and MR imaging. Moreover, in two cases, intravascular US depicted plaque fracture, one of which was also detected at MR imaging. After stent placement, the surface of the treated segment was smooth at intravascular US and MR imaging in each case. Intravascular US revealed dissection in eight of 10 arteries in the PTA group. Three dissections were restricted to the shoulder area of the atherosclerotic lesions, which is characteristic of calcified lesions, and five of the dissections were major. The findings at MR imaging were much more subtle, but in five (62%) of the eight cases, the crescent-shaped dissection was also detected at axial MR imaging (Fig 6). Neither intravascular US nor MR imaging depicted any of the five dissections within the segments treated with stent placement that were evident in the histopathologic specimens (Table 2), but intravascular US revealed a small dissection adjacent to the segment treated with stent placement in two of four arteries in which balloon dilation was performed inside the stent. These dissections were not depicted at MR imaging.

Other findings.— Intravascular US depicted 15 calcified lesions, 13 (87%) of which were also visible at postinterventional MR imaging (Figs 1, 4, 6). Although heavy superficial calcifications severely hampered assessment of the inner structures of the atherosclerotic plaque at intravascular US in two cases, MR imaging consistently depicted the whole extension of the plaque. Similarly, depiction of the atherosclerotic arterial wall and plaque morphology through the stent at intravas-

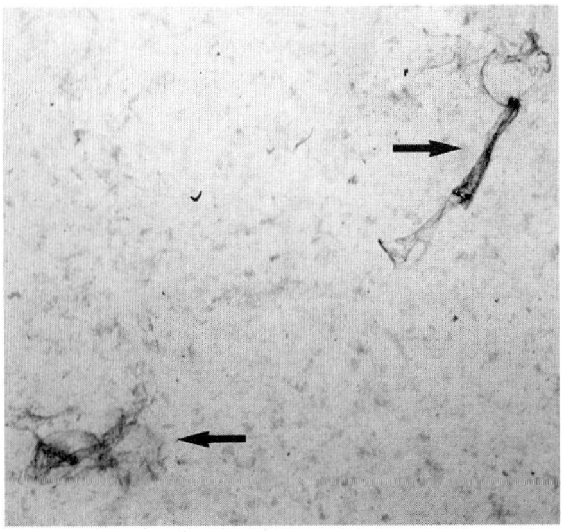

Figure 2. Photomicrograph of two embolic intimal strips (arrows) filtered from the effluent obtained during stent placement in the lesion in Figure 1. (Papanicolaou stain; original magnification, ×2.)

TABLE 3
Distal Embolization during Endovascular Stent Placement and PTA

Embolic Constituents	Stent Placement Group	PTA Group	*P* Value
Intimal strips*	4.8 (1–8)	4.2 (0–11)	.55
Lipid-filled foam cells†			.68
None	6 (67)	5 (50)	
Scanty	1 (11)	4 (40)	
Numerous	2 (22)	1 (10)	
Clusters of unspecified cells†			.39
Scanty	3 (33)	3 (30)	
Numerous	5 (56)	3 (30)	
Abundant	1 (11)	4 (40)	
Overall severity of distal embolization†			.17
Mild	1 (11)	2 (20)	
Moderate	5 (56)	6 (60)	
Severe	3 (33)	2 (20)	

Note.—Data are based on nine lesions treated with stent placement and 10 lesions treated with PTA.
* Data are the mean number of strips. Numbers in parentheses are the range.
† Data are the number of lesions. Numbers in parentheses are the percentage.

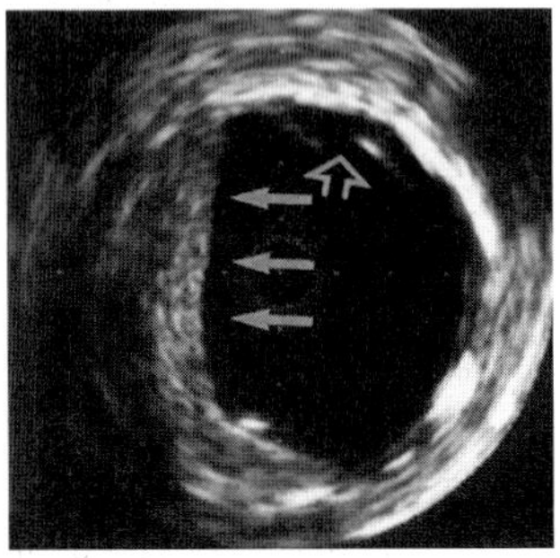

Figure 3. Axial intravascular US scan at the bulbar segment of the internal carotid artery shows a partly loosened intimal flap (open arrow) floating in the lumen beside the eccentric plaque (closed arrows) after PTA.

TABLE 4
Relative Mean Grades of the Three MR Imaging Sequences for Depiction of Anatomic Structures of the Atherosclerotic Carotid Artery after Endovascular Intervention

Analyzed Parameter	MR Imaging Sequence Grade: T1-weighted	T2-weighted	Intermediate-weighted
Depiction of calcifications	1.0	2.4*	1.6†
Demarcation of the plaque	1.0	1.2	1.0
Depiction of dissection	1.0	2.0	1.5
Demarcation of the arterial wall	1.0	1.3	1.2
Absence of stent artifacts	1.7	1.1	1.0

Note.—The three MR imaging sequences were given a grade of 1.0–3.0, with 1.0 indicating the best depiction of a given structure and 3.0 indicating the poorest depiction.
* $P < .01$ for the difference between T1- and T2-weighted sequences.
† $P < .05$ for the difference between T2- and intermediate-weighted sequences.

cular US was often severely restricted, but the anatomic details were delineated at MR imaging (Fig 1).

Comparison of MR Imaging Sequences

Table 4 shows the main results of comparisons between T1-, T2-, and intermediate-weighted MR imaging sequences for the depiction of the postinterventional status of the carotid arteries. The differences in usefulness between the sequences were small. Overall, the T1-weighted images depicted best the calcifications of the plaques (Figs 1, 4), but in one artery, the depiction of a deep calcification was poorest on the T1-weighted image (Fig 6c). The stent mesh caused minimal artifacts with all three sequences, and T2- and intermediate-weighted images in particular were almost free of artifacts (Fig 4).

DISCUSSION

Although the results of several large randomized multicenter trials (17,18) have demonstrated the beneficial effects of surgical carotid endarterectomy in the prevention of ischemic brain infarction, the indications for endovascular treatment of carotid stenoses have not yet been established. Endovascular treatment seems to be associated with a complication rate comparable to that associated with carotid endarterectomy, but the clinical criteria for the selection of endovascular treatment rather than carotid endarterectomy remain uncertain. In addition, it remains uncertain whether PTA or stent placement is the most effective endovascular technique (4,6). Although stent placement provides superior angiographic primary results, PTA is technically easier, and the primary angiographic result is often improved by the remodeling process within 1 year after PTA (19).

Distal Embolization during Carotid Arterial Interventions

The frequency of complications, especially ischemic stroke caused by distal embolization, is of fundamental importance when selecting the therapeutic intervention. Transcranial Doppler US of the middle cerebral artery has been reported (20) to register more microembolic signals during PTA than during surgical carotid endarterectomy. However, transcranial Doppler US cannot enable differentiation between microembolic signals caused by particulate and those caused by contrast media injections or inflation and deflation of the angioplastic balloon, and it does not offer any information about the pathologic type of the emboli.

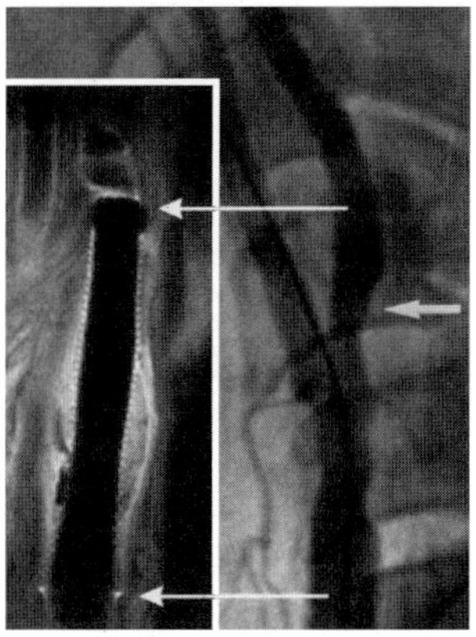

a.

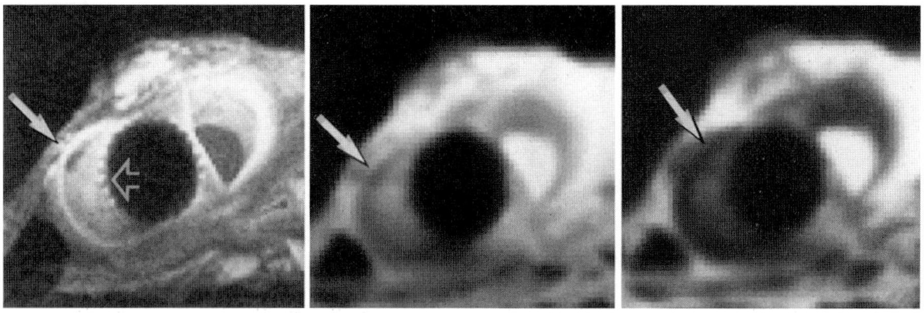

b.

Figure 4. **(a)** X-ray angiogram of the extracranial carotid artery obtained at the lateral projection before intervention and corresponding sagittal T1-weighted (400/14) MR image (boxed insert) obtained after stent placement. The long arrows indicate the ends of the stent that covers the whole length of the lesion. The short arrow denotes the level at which the corresponding axial MR images in **b** were obtained. **(b)** On the axial T1-weighted image (400/14) (left), the deep calcification (solid arrow) of the internal carotid bulb (at the level of the short arrow in **a**) is clearly depicted. However, the calcification is hardly recognized on the intermediate- (2,500/17) (middle) and T2-weighted (2,500/102) (right) images. A slight artifact due to the stent (open arrow) is seen on the T1-weighted image, but the stent has no signal intensity on the intermediate- and T2-weighted images.

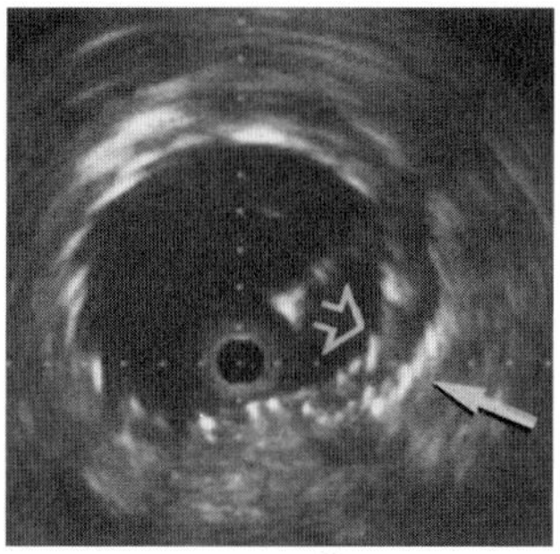

Figure 5. Axial intravascular US scan shows poor contact between the stent (open arrow) and the calcified arterial wall (solid arrow) despite balloon dilation inside the stent.

An in vitro model with specimens of carotid plaque encased in a vascular graft wrap was used to quantitate embolic material during experimental stent placement (21). Unfortunately, in such models, when the intervention is not performed in situ, the atherosclerotic lesions are exposed to mechanical handling during surgical excision, and the normal elasticity of human carotid adventitia and periadventitial tissues is missing. Our experimental setup, in which the endovascular therapies were performed in situ in fresh cadavers, simulates better a clinical intervention and thus facilitates the accurate collection and histologic analysis of embolic constituents. The interventions were performed under pressurized conditions that provided an opportunity to assess the imaging findings after carotid arterial PTA with intravascular US. Intravascular US cannot be used to guide carotid angioplasty in living humans because of the risk of embolization.

The most common stent currently used in carotid arteries is the self-expandable Wallstent. One might expect the distal embolization during self-expanding stent placement to occur less frequently than that during balloon dilation. First, the Wallstent has the ability to expand during placement, beginning from the distal end and encompassing the atherosclerotic plaque and possibly the embolic fragments against the vessel wall. Second, the results of intravascular US and autopsy studies (22,23) on peripheral and coronary arteries have shown that the inner surface of vessels treated with stents is smooth, whereas extensive irregularity due to plaque ruptures and dissections are frequently encountered after PTA. Although intravascular US and MR imaging confirmed this in the present study, the severity of distal embolization was similar in the stent and PTA groups. Because the atherosclerotic lesions and other characteristics of the arterial wall (ie, vulnerability to catheter and/or guide-wire manipulation) of the two carotid arteries in each cadaver were interrelated, a paired analysis of the stent-treated arteries compared with the PTA–treated arteries in each cadaver also was performed. Not even the pairwise comparison revealed definite differences.

We did not perform predilation of any arteries in the stent group, but we performed balloon dilation inside the stent after stent placement in four arteries because of residual stenosis. It seems to be commonly assumed that embolization occurs most often during balloon dilation. However, although we found some embolic material during the complementary balloon dilation in each case, the overall severity of distal embolization in these arteries did not clearly differ from those in which dilation inside the stent was not performed. It should be noted that dilation inside the stent is a part of the placement of balloon-expanding stents and commonly is mandatory after the clinical deployment of self-expanding stents in carotid atherosclerotic lesions (6).

The most potentially dangerous embolic constituents encountered in the present study were intimal strips, the largest of which were several millimeters long. Similar particles have been found in experimental atheroablations of lower limb arteries with the Kensey atherectomy catheter (24). On the other hand, the embolic particles found by Ohki et al (21) during experimental carotid arterial stent placement did not include intimal strips. In the present study, the three cases with the greatest numbers of embolic intimal strips were encountered in the PTA group, but the mean numbers of intimal strips in the two study groups were almost equal (Table 3).

In three cases with large numbers of embolic strips, postinterventional intravascular US revealed partly loosened intimal flaps floating in the vessel lumen. One of these flaps was on the normal side of the arterial wall (Fig 3), and another was adjacent to the segment treated with a stent, which implied that the balloon dilation or stent deployment was not necessarily the reason for the strips, but rather guide-wire and/or catheter manipulation may have been the causative factor. The behavior of cadaveric arteries may not be identical to that of in vivo arteries, and postmortem autolysis probably contributed to the vulnerability of the arterial intima and increased friability of the plaque. Our experimental setup may have therefore overestimated the abundance of embolic intimal strips and other embolic constituents that manifest during clinical endovascular carotid interventions.

Recognition of the imaging features that correspond to the histopathologic constituents of carotid plaques associated with increased risk of distal embolization during endovascular intervention would be very useful before deciding on the therapy in individual cases. We correlated the histopathologic and intravascular US characteristics of such plaques with the distal embolism. The presence of histopathologic intraplaque hemorrhage and/or remarkable neovascularity was associated with a greater abundance of lipid-filled foam cells in the embolic filtrate. Intraplaque hemorrhage indicates an unstable lesion, which is prone to spontaneous rupture (25). One could postulate that the compression of such plaques makes the inner constituents more prone to disperse as embolic particles.

Ohki et al (21) found an increased risk of distal embolization in lesions that were hypoechoic at external US and "soft" at histopathologic analysis. We did not find such correlation; however, it should be noted that only about one-fifth (four of 19) of the lesions in the present study were "soft" at intravascular US (Table 1), whereas almost three-fourths (14 of 19) of the lesions had a fibrous cap at histopathologic analysis (Table 2). On the other hand, in the present study the abundance of unspecified cells in the embolic filtrate correlated positively with the number of calcifications at intravascular US. Ohki et al (21) found that plaques with a more than 90% diameter of stenosis produced a higher number of embolic particles during experimental stent placement. The embolic material in our study did not include such tight lesions: The diameter of stenosis at intravascular US in the arteries treated with interventions ranged from 32% to 85%.

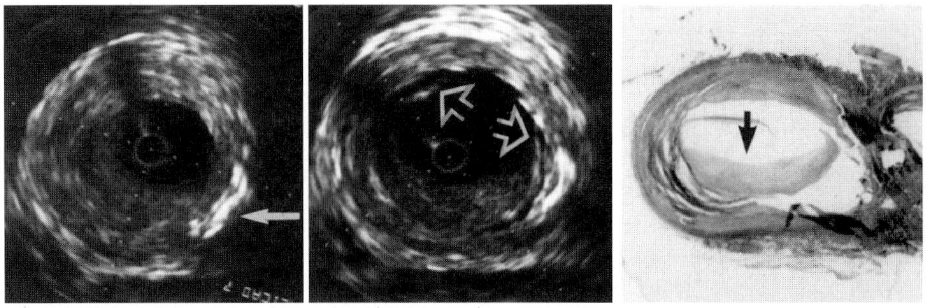

a. b.

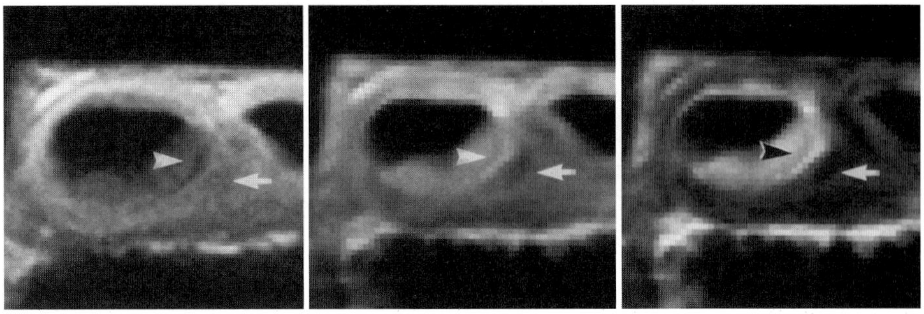

c.

Figure 6. **(a)** Axial intravascular US scan of the internal carotid artery bulb obtained before balloon PTA (left) demonstrates an eccentric lesion with a deep calcification (solid arrow). The intravascular US scan obtained after angioplasty (right) reveals major dissections (open arrows) originating from the shoulder regions of the plaque and extending deep behind the plaque. **(b)** Histopathologic specimen confirms separation of the fibrotic plaque (arrow) from the medial layer. (Masson trichrome stain; original magnification, ×2.) **(c)** On the axial T1- (400/14) (left), intermediate- (2,500/17) (middle), and T2-weighted (2,500/102) (right) MR images, the crescent outline of the dissection (arrowhead) can be discerned, but the deep calcification (arrow), delineated as a definite hypointense lesion on the T2- and intermediate-weighted images, is hardly discernable on the T1-weighted image.

Postinterventional Changes at Intravascular US and MR Imaging

The intravascular US appearance of the arterial wall after coronary and peripheral arterial PTA and stent placement in vivo has been established by several authors (9,22,26). Our findings during ex vivo, in situ interventions in human carotid arteries were very similar: There was substantial residual stenosis in every case, and the surface of the arterial plaque was mainly irregular or the plaque was fractured after PTA, with dissections in the majority of the arteries. The lumen was fully patent and the surface of the treated segment was smooth in all arteries after stent placement. It should be noted that the long-term patency of carotid arteries treated with stents compared with that of arteries treated with PTA is still unknown.

Neither intravascular US nor MR imaging depicted any dissections or plaque fractures at the area of segments treated with stents, even though the histopathologic specimens revealed dissection in five cases and plaque disruption in three. Although it is possible that these damages were partly due to excision of the vessels and removal of the stent from the formalin-buffered artery, it is evident that they were mainly caused by the active radial expansion force of the self-expanding Wallstent and/or the additional balloon dilation. It remains uncertain whether these damages, which were isolated by the stent mesh, were the cause of the distal embolization.

Reports on the use of MR imaging for postinterventional evaluation of PTA are sparse. Although time-of-flight MR angiography accurately depicts the degree of stenosis with reference to x-ray angiography, its poor soft-tissue contrast reduces its potential to enable assessment of postinterventional morphologic changes in the treated lesion (27). Toussaint et al (28) used spin-echo sequences at 9.4-T to image samples of atherosclerotic arteries treated with balloon compression and found fibrous cap lesions to be resistant to compression; however, substantial reduction and redistribution occurred in the lipid cores of the fatty plaques. We did not find any association between the histopathologic type of the lesion and the post-PTA status at MR imaging or intravascular US. This might be owing to the small total number of lesions in our study and to the fact that the majority of the plaques had a fibrous cap (Table 2). Toussaint et al (28) reported that the compression often dissected the calcified plaques at shoulder level; we also encountered this finding (Fig 6).

Metallic stents are a concern during MR imaging, especially during the immediate postinterventional period, because they can theoretically move, induce electrical currents, or heat tissues (29,30). The key determinant in the safeness of a metallic stent in MR imaging is its ferromagnetic properties. According to the manufacturer, the self-expanding Wallstent used in our study is made of an alloy of cobalt and tantalum and hence is nonferromagnetic and safe for MR imaging. However, to our knowledge, the safeness of MR imaging immediately after the deployment of a Wallstent in a human carotid artery in vivo has not been assessed. Minimal artifacts were seen at spin-echo MR imaging in the present study (Figs 1, 4), but they did not interfere with the diagnostic quality of the images. On the contrary, the diagnostic value of external US for assessment after stent placement was considerably deteriorated by the acoustic shadowing caused by the stent mesh. However, our experimental setup with MR imaging of excised carotid arteries was highly contrived; greater degradation of image quality would be expected at clinical spin-echo MR imaging owing to flow and motion artifacts.

T2-weighted MR imaging has shown promise in differentiating lipid-rich, necrotic, hemorrhagic, and fibrotic constituents of atherosclerotic plaque in vivo (14). Because our study focused on the evaluation of post-PTA and post–stent placement changes, we did not correlate in detail the MR imaging findings and histopathologic constituents of the lesions. Overall, MR imaging depicted accurately most of the postinterventional changes after stent placement and PTA and correlated well with intravascular US imaging: The residual stenosis, extent of the plaques and stents, and surface of the treated segments were precisely assessed. However, it appears that intravascular US is superior to MR imaging for depicting dissection; intravascular US depicted eight dissections in the PTA group, whereas MR imaging depicted five. In addition, the findings were often more subtle at MR imaging than at intravascular US. It should be noted that the arteries were not pressurized during imaging, and this may have contributed to the findings being more subtle at MR imaging.

The T1-weighted images were slightly superior to the T2- and intermediate-weighted images, especially in the depiction of calcifications; the deep, hypointense calcifications in particular were demarcated better, because the adventitia has high signal intensity on T1-weighted images but low signal intensity on intermediate- and T2-weighted images (Fig 4) (31). In one case (Fig 6c), however, the calcification was almost isointense on the T1-weighted image, whereas a distinct signal intensity void was seen on the T2- and intermediate-weighted images. In this particular focus, this phenomenon, which is familiar in intervertebral disks, probably indicates a relatively low concentration of calcium, which occurs when the simultaneously shortened T1 and T2 relaxation times due to the calcium are in equilibrium (32).

Practical application: Distal embolization was common during both PTA and stent placement in situ in the carotid arteries of cadavers, and there was no substantial difference in the severity of distal embolization between the treatments. Intravascular US and MR imaging revealed substantial residual stenosis, dissections, plaque fractures, and irregularity on the surface of the treated segments after PTA, but showed fully patent lumens and smooth surfaces after stent placement; these findings might lead us to favor stent placement over PTA. MR imaging with spin-echo sequences, because of its noninvasiveness, clarity of image presentation, and ability to depict the whole extension of the atherosclerotic plaque despite calcifications or stent mesh, has potential for postinterventional imaging.

Acknowledgments: We thank Schneider for providing the stents used in this study and Asta Rikkonen and Irma Väänänen for their technical assistance in the staining of the histologic specimens.

References

1. Tsai FY, Matovich V, Hieschima G, et al. Percutaneous transluminal angioplasty of the carotid artery. AJNR 1986; 7:349–358.
2. Kachel R, Basche ST, Heerklotz I, Grossman K, Endler S. Percutaneous transluminal angioplasty (PTA) of supra-aortic arteries especially the internal carotid artery. Neuroradiology 1991; 33:191–194.
3. Mathias KD, Jaeger HJ, Man C, Goetz F. Problems and complications of internal carotid artery percutaneous transluminal angioplasty and stent placement (abstr). Radiology 1995; 197(P):650.
4. Gil-Perelta A, Mayol A, Gonzalez M Jr, et al. Percutaneous transluminal angioplasty of the symptomatic atherosclerotic arteries. Stroke 1996; 27:2271–2273.
5. Theron JG, Payelle GG, Coscun O, Huet HF, Guirmaraens L. Carotid artery stenosis: treatment with protected balloon angioplasty and stent placement. Radiology 1996; 201:627–636.
6. Yadav JS, Roubin GS, Iyer S, et al. Elective stenting of the extracranial carotid arteries. Circulation 1997; 95:376–381.
7. Markus HS, Clifton A, Buckenham T, Brown MM. Carotid angioplasty: detection of embolic signals during and after the procedure. Stroke 1994; 25:2403–2406.
8. Vorwerk D, Neuerburg J, Klein M, et al. Intravascular ultrasound in interventional procedures. Semin Intervent Radiol 1995; 12:47–52.
9. Hall P, Nakamura S, Maiello L, et al. Clinical and angiographic outcome after Palmaz-Schatz stent implantation guided by intravascular ultrasound. J Invasive Cardiol 1995; 7:12–22.
10. Waller BF, Pinkerton CA, Slack JD. Intravascular ultrasound: a histological study of vessels during life—the new "gold standard" for vascular imaging. Circulation 1992; 85:2305–2310.
11. Reid DB, Dietrich EB, Marx P, Wrasper R. Intravascular ultrasound assessment in carotid interventions. J Endovasc Surg 1996; 3:203–210.
12. Manninen HI, Koivisto T, Saari T, et al. Dissecting aneurysms of all four cervicocranial arteries in fibromuscular dysplasia: treatment with self-expanding endovascular stents, coil embolization, and surgical ligation. AJNR 1997; 18:1216–1220.
13. Manninen HI, Räsänen H, Vanninen RL, et al. Human carotid arteries: correlation of intravascular US with angiographic and histopathologic findings. Radiology 1998; 206:65–74.
14. Toussaint JF, la Muraglia GM, Southem JF. Magnetic resonance images lipid, fibrous, calcified, hemorrhagic, and thrombotic components of human atherosclerosis in vivo. Circulation 1996; 94:932–938.
15. Gussenhoven EJ, Essed CE, Lancee CT, et al. Arterial wall characteristics determined by intravascular ultrasound imaging: an in vitro study. J Am Coll Cardiol 1989; 14:947–952.
16. Nishimura RA, Edwards WD, Warnes CA, et al. Intravascular ultrasound imaging: in vitro validation and pathological correlation. J Am Coll Cardiol 1990; 16:145–154.
17. European Carotid Surgery Trialists' Collaborative Group. MRC European carotid surgery trial: interim results for symptomatic patients with severe (70-99%) or with mild (0-29%) carotid stenosis. Lancet 1991; 337:1235–1243.
18. North American Symptomatic Carotid Endarterectomy Trial Collaborators. Beneficial effect of carotid endarterectomy in symptomatic patients with high-grade carotid stenosis. N Engl J Med 1991; 325: 445–453.
19. Crawley F, Clifton A, Markus H, Brown MM. Delayed improvement in carotid artery diameter after carotid angioplasty. Stroke 1997; 28:574–579.
20. Crawley F, Clifton A, Buckenham T, Loosemore T, Taylor RS, Brown MM. Comparison of hemodynamic cerebral ischemic and microembolic signals detected during carotid endarterectomy and carotid angioplasty. Stroke 1997; 28:2460–2464.
21. Ohki T, Marin NL, Lyon RT, et al. Ex vivo human carotid artery bifurcation stenting: correlation of lesion characteristics with embolic potential. J Vasc Surg 1998; 27:463–471.
22. Goldberg SL, Colombo A, Nakamura S, et al. Benefit of intracoronary ultrasound in the deployment of Palmaz-Schatz stents. J Am Coll Cardiol 1994; 24:996–1003.
23. Peters RJ, Kok VEM, van der Wal AG, et al. In vitro validation of intravascular ultrasound imaging after balloon angioplasty of coronary artery stenoses. Ultrasound Med Biol 1996; 22:999–1005.
24. Coleman CC, Posalaky IP, Robinson JD, Payne WD, Vlodaver ZA, Amplatz K. Ath-

eroablation with the Kensey catheter: a pathologic study. Radiology 1989; 170: 391–394.
25. Fisher M, Blumenfeld M, Smit TW. The importance of carotid artery plaque disruption and hemorrhage. Arch Neurol 1987; 44:1086–1089.
26. Korogi Y, Hirai T, Takahashi M. Intravascular ultrasound imaging of peripheral arteries as an adjunct to balloon angioplasty and atherectomy. Cardiovasc Intervent Radiol 1995; 19:1–9.
27. Laissy JP, Liniot 0, Henry-Feugeas MC, et al. Iliac artery patency before and immediately after percutaneous transluminal angioplasty: assessment with time-of-flight MR angiography. Radiology 1995; 197: 455–459.
28. Toussaint JF, Southem JF, Kantor IHL, Jang IK, Fuster V. Behavior of atherosclerotic plaque components after in vitro angioplasty and atherectomy studied by high field MR imaging. Magn Reson Imaging 1998; 16:175–183.
29. Davis PL, Crooks L, Arakawa M, McRee R, Kaufinan L, Maqulis AR. Potential hazards in NMR imaging: heating effects of changing magnetic fields and RF fields on small metallic implants. AJR 1981; 137: 857–860.
30. Sheflock FG, Curtis JS. MR imaging and biomechanical implants, materials, and an updated review. Radiology 1991; 180: 541–550.
31. Martin AJ, Ryan LK, Gotlieb AI, Henkelman RM, Foster FS. Arterial imaging: comparison of high-resolution US and MR imaging with histologic correlation. RadioGraphics 1997; 17:189–202.
32. Bangert BA, Modic MT, Ross JS. Hyperintense disks on T1-weighted MR images: correlation with calcification. Radiology 1995; 195:437–443.

Vivian S. Lee, MD, PhD
Barbara S. Hertzberg, MD
Mark A. Kliewer, MD
Barbara A. Carroll, MD

Assessment of Stenosis: Implications of Variability of Doppler Measurements in Normal-appearing Carotid Arteries[1]

Index terms:
Carotid arteries, flow dynamics, 172.12984
Carotid arteries, stenosis or obstruction, 172.721
Carotid arteries, US, 172.12983, 172.12984

Radiology 1999; 212:493–498

Abbreviations:
CCA = common carotid artery
EDV = end diastolic velocity
ICA = internal carotid artery
PSV = peak systolic velocity

[1] From the Department of Radiology, Duke University Medical Center, PO Box 3808, Durham, NC. Received August 13, 1998; revision requested September 25; revision received October 21; accepted January 11, 1999. **Address reprint requests to** V.S.L., Department of Radiology-MRI, New York University Medical Center, 530 First Ave, HCC Basement, New York, NY 10016.

Author contributions:
Guarantor of integrity of entire study, V.S.L.; study concepts and design, all authors; definition of intellectual content, all authors; literature research, V.S.L., B.A.C.; clinical studies, all authors; data acquisition, all authors; data and statistical analyses, V.S.L.; manuscript preparation, V.S.L.; manuscript editing and review, all authors.

PURPOSE: To examine the variability of Doppler measurements along the extracranial courses of the nondiseased common carotid artery (CCA) and internal carotid artery (ICA) and determine the effect of this variability on assessment of carotid arterial stenosis.

MATERIALS AND METHODS: During the study period, 580 patients were referred for carotid arterial ultrasonography (US), including Doppler measurements of flow velocities in the proximal, middle, and distal portions of the CCA, in the bulb, and in the proximal and distal portions of the ICA. Eighty-five patients (average age, 59 years) with normal ICAs and CCAs formed the cohort for this study.

RESULTS: The range of peak systolic velocity (PSV) measurements (maximum minus minimum) averaged 20 cm/sec ± 13 in the CCA and 15 cm/sec ± 13 in the ICA. ICA/CCA velocity ratios varied, depending on the CCA measurement location. In five arteries, PSV ratios exceeded a threshold of 1.8 (suggesting ≥60% stenosis); in 23 arteries, end diastolic velocity ratios exceeded a threshold of 2.4 (also suggesting ≥60% stenosis). Right-to-left CCA PSV ratios were abnormal in up to 26 patients (suggesting >50% ICA stenosis), depending on where CCA measurements were obtained. When the CCA ratios were obtained at the same level, 16 were in the abnormal range.

CONCLUSION: Variability of Doppler measurements in the CCA and ICA in patients without visible disease is substantial and could lead to inaccuracies in carotid arterial stenosis assessment.

Duplex ultrasonography (US) has become a widely used means of detecting and characterizing carotid arterial atherosclerotic disease. For quantitative assessment of the degree of stenosis, the most frequently used Doppler parameters include peak systolic velocity (PSV) and end diastolic velocity (EDV) in the internal carotid artery (ICA), as well as ICA-to-common carotid artery (CCA) PSV and EDV ratios. Despite the common use of these quantitative parameters, there has been no consensus between laboratories on the interpretation of clinical measurements: No universal table of measurement standards that reliably estimates the degree of stenosis found with contrast material–enhanced angiography has been established (1–10). The differences in measurement standards between laboratories may reflect methodologic differences in protocol or imaging technique (11,12), physiologic differences between patient populations (eg, prevalence of cardiac dysfunction or hypertension), or the random variation in measurement. Velocity ratios may provide more robust estimates than do absolute velocity measurements by reducing the effects of differences in technique or equipment and compensating, at least in part, for physiologic differences (2).

We suspected that variability in velocity measurements along the courses of the ICA and CCA might influence the interpretation of ratio parameters. Therefore, we performed a prospective study to measure the variability of velocity measurements in patients without visible evidence of disease and determine the likelihood that this variability would produce spuriously elevated velocity ratios in this setting.

MATERIALS AND METHODS

Between September 1996 and March 1997, 580 patients were referred for carotid arterial US. All patients who had prior carotid endarterectomy, cardiac arrhythmia, or any visible disease of either the CCA or ICA at gray-scale or color Doppler US imaging were excluded. Eighty-five patients (47 women, 38 men; average age ± SD, 59 years ± 12) formed the cohort for this study. Indications for study in these patients were as follows: stroke or transient ischemic attack (n = 49), dizziness or syncope (n = 12), asymptomatic carotid bruit (n = 9), mental status changes (n = 1), headache (n = 1), retinal arterial occlusion (n = 1), and preoperative evaluation for heart surgery (n = 1). Indications were either unknown or not recorded in 11 patients.

TABLE 1
Mean PSV and EDV Values on the Right and Left Sides in Patients without US Evidence of Carotid Disease

	Right		Left	
Artery	PSV	EDV	PSV	EDV
Distal ICA	65.1 ± 19.1 (23–107)	23.4 ± 9.0 (8–54)	65.2 ± 17.1 (26–100)	23.9 ± 8.3 (8–48)
Proximal ICA	59.9 ± 19.9 (22–105)	18.7 ± 7.9 (5–43)	59.5 ± 17.3 (28–100)	19.6 ± 7.3 (6–38)
Bulb	63.9 ± 21.4 (30–154)	17.6 ± 7.8 (0–43)	64.6 ± 23.6 (21–137)	18.1 ± 8.6 (4–49)
Distal CCA	75.2 ± 22.1 (37–182)	19.9 ± 8.5 (4–62)	77.0 ± 22.8 (29–147)	21.1 ± 8.0 (5–46)
Middle CCA	82.7 ± 24.3 (39–191)	19.4 ± 7.8 (6–43)	87.6 ± 23.6 (43–207)	21.5 ± 8.3 (6–54)
Proximal CCA	83.6 ± 23.8 (35–182)	17.1 ± 7.3 (4–45)	90.3 ± 25.1 (36–197)	19.5 ± 8.6 (3–50)

Note.—The values (cm/sec) given, expressed as the mean ± SD, were obtained in 85 patients. The numbers in parentheses are the range.

TABLE 2
Range of Velocities (Maximum minus Minimum Values) along the Course of Each Individual CCA and ICA

Artery	PSV	EDV
ICA	15.4 ± 13.2 (0–83)	6.7 ± 6.0 (0–38)
CCA	19.8 ± 12.9 (1–76)	6.2 ± 4.5 (0–21)

Note.—All values (cm/sec) are expressed as the mean ± SD. Numbers in parentheses are the range.

US Examination

Prior to the US examination, the heart rate and blood pressure were recorded with the patient in the supine position. Bilateral carotid arterial US was performed with HDI 3000 (Advanced Technology Laboratories, Bothell, Wash) and model 128 (Acuson, Mountain View, Calif) units by using a variety of broadband linear-array transducers with frequencies ranging from 4 to 7 MHz. Each examination was performed by an experienced sonographer with a radiologist in attendance. The ICA and CCA were examined initially by using gray-scale and color Doppler US imaging. Spectral Doppler waveform measurements were obtained at multiple locations: three locations in the CCA (as close to the aortic arch as possible, in the middle portion, and before the widening of the bulb), one location in the bulb, and two locations in the ICA (just beyond the bulb widening and in the most distal part visible). A single measurement was recorded at each location. In all cases, the measured angle of insonation was kept below 60°.

The PSV and EDV were determined from velocity waveforms at all locations by using electronic calipers during the examination. The following velocity ratios were calculated for each possible combination of locations: ICA/CCA PSV ratio, ICA/CCA EDV ratio, and right-to-left CCA ratio. The following published thresholds were used to predict 60% or greater ICA stenosis: ICA PSV greater than 130 cm/sec, ICA EDV greater than 40 cm/sec, ICA/CCA PSV ratio greater than 1.8, and ICA/CCA EDV greater than 2.4 (3). The right-to-left CCA PSV ratios also were computed, and a threshold of less than 0.7 or greater than 1.3 was used to predict stenosis greater than 50% (13).

For each side of each patient, the maximum ICA/minimum CCA and minimum ICA/maximum CCA ratios were computed for the PSV and EDV to determine the effects of sampling location on ICA/CCA ratios. We then determined the number of patients whose values (maximum ICA/minimum CCA) would have exceeded the published thresholds.

For example, consider a patient whose PSV measurements on the right side were as follows: proximal CCA, 95 cm/sec; middle CCA, 63 cm/sec; distal CCA, 64 cm/sec; bulb, 43 cm/sec; proximal ICA, 56 cm/sec; and distal ICA, 33 cm/sec. The two limits for ICA/CCA PSV ratios on the right can be computed as follows: maximum ICA/minimum CCA = 56 cm/sec ÷ 63 cm/sec = 0.89 and minimum ICA/maximum CCA = 33 cm/sec ÷ 95 cm/sec = 0.35. For this particular patient, both values would fall within the range of normal (<1.8) on the basis of published criteria (3). The difference in velocity ratio values in this patient is calculated to be 0.54 (0.89 − 0.35). This analysis was performed for all carotid arteries studied (n = 170). A similar analysis was performed to determine right-to-left CCA PSV ratios.

Statistical Analyses

The statistical significance of differences in velocity measurements along the course of the ICA was assessed by using the two-tailed Student t test, and that of differences along the course of the CCA was assessed by using analysis of variance. The correlation between left and right measurements was evaluated by using Pearson correlation coefficients. To assess the effects of patient age, blood pressure, and heart rate on Doppler parameters, patients were stratified into the following pairs of groups: age 60 years or older or age older than 60 years, hypertensive (systolic blood pressure ≥160 mm Hg or diastolic blood pressure ≥95 mm Hg)

TABLE 3
Heart Rates and PSVs in the CCA and ICA

Artery	Heart Rate <75 bpm	Heart Rate ≥75 bpm	P Value*
CCA			
Proximal	80.6 ± 21.2	93.9 ± 26.1	<.001
Middle	77.5 ± 19.2	93.0 ± 26.2	<.001
Distal	69.1 ± 17.8	83.4 ± 24.5	<.001
Range	18.9 ± 12.1	20.7 ± 14.0	.37
ICA			
Proximal	56.2 ± 17.9	63.2 ± 19.2	.02
Distal	62.6 ± 17.6	67.6 ± 18.0	.07
Range	14.7 ± 12.8	15.8 ± 13.5	.59

Note.—Data are the mean PSV (cm/sec) ± SD.
* *P* values were calculated by using the Student *t* test.

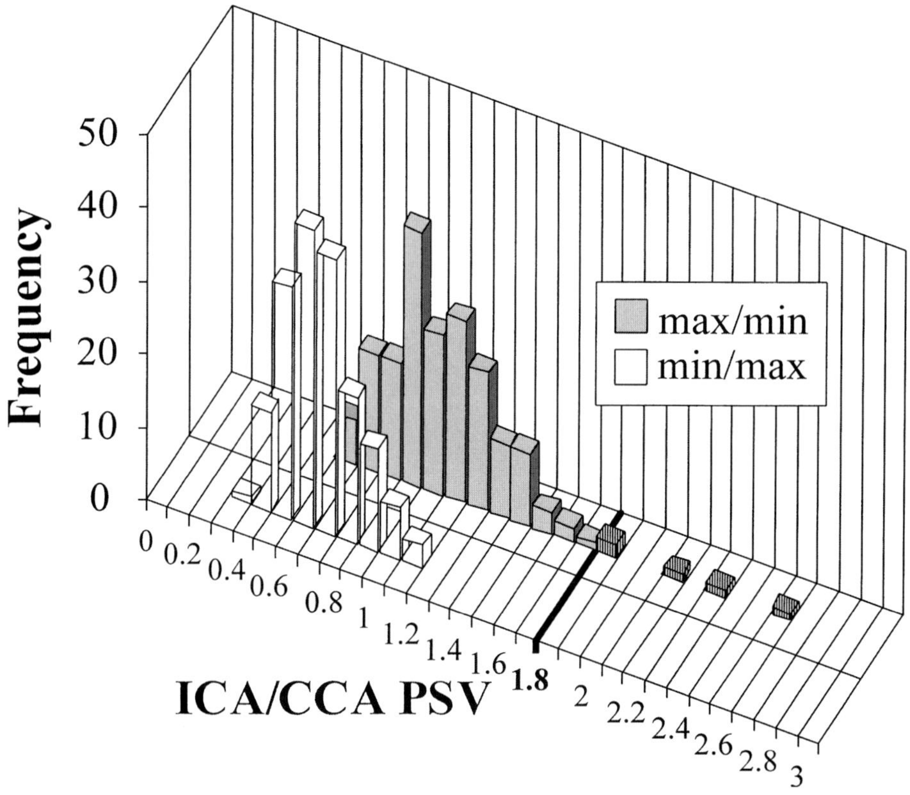

Figure 1. Histogram of the highest (maximum/minimum) and lowest (minimum/maximum) ICA/CCA PSV ratios based on measurements of velocities in different locations along each ipsilateral vessel. The published ICA/CCA PSV threshold of greater than 1.8 was used to indicate 60% or greater stenosis (3). *max/min* = maximum ICA velocity divided by minimum ipsilateral CCA velocity, *min/max* = minimum ICA velocity divided by maximum ipsilateral CCA velocity, striped bars = all values exceeding the threshold (>1.8).

or normotensive, and heart rate 75 beats per minute or higher or less than 75 beats per minute. The two-tailed Student *t* test was used to compare velocity measurements in each pair of groups. For all statistical tests, which were performed with Excel software (Microsoft, Redmond, Wash), a *P* value of less than .05 was used to assign statistical significance.

RESULTS

Eighty-five of the patients who were referred for evaluation for possible carotid arterial disease were found to have no visible evidence of extracranial carotid disease at gray-scale and color Doppler US imaging. In this ostensibly disease-free population, the systolic and diastolic velocities demonstrated wide variability along the course of each individual CCA and ICA, as summarized in Tables 1 and 2.

A trend in PSV was observed along the course of the CCA: The more distal the measurement, the lower the velocity (Table 1). The average PSV (± SD) in the distal CCA (75.2 cm/sec ± 23.7) was significantly lower than that in the proximal CCA (86.9 cm/sec ± 25.6) ($P < .001$). The range of PSVs along each individual CCA (maximum value minus minimum value) averaged 19.8 cm/sec ± 12.9 (Table 2). In eight (5%) of the 170 arteries, the velocities within a single CCA differed by 50 cm/sec or more. In 74 (44%) arteries, the velocity values in the CCA differed by more than 20 cm/sec. There was no correlation between the ranges of PSV in the CCA on the left and right sides ($r = 0.09$). In contrast, EDV values increased along the course of the CCA. The average proximal CCA EDV was 18.2 cm/sec ± 8.0 compared with the average distal CCA EDV of 19.9 cm/sec ± 8.6 ($P = .04$).

A variability of measurements in the ICA also was observed (Table 2). The mean range of PSV measurements (greater minus lesser PSV value) in each individual ICA was 15.4 cm/sec ± 13.2 (range, 0–83 cm/sec). Unlike in the CCA, in the ICA, the more distal PSV measurements (65.1 cm/sec ± 18.0) exceeded the proximal measurements (59.0 cm/sec ± 19.6) ($P = .003$). In five (3%) vessels, the difference in PSV between the proximal and distal portions of the ICA differed by 50 cm/sec or more; in 48 (28%) vessels, the difference was 20 cm/sec or more. No correlation was observed between the range of PSV measurements obtained in the right ICA compared with those obtained in the left ICA ($r = 0.15$).

The EDVs in the ICA also varied substantially. The average distal value (23.4 cm/sec ± 8.6) was significantly higher than the average proximal value (18.9 cm/sec ± 7.8; $P < .001$).

The effects of age, blood pressure, and heart rate on differences in velocity measurements also were considered. The range of PSV measurements along the ICA and CCA did not differ significantly in patients older than 60 years ($n = 35$, 41%) compared with those 60 years or younger ($n = 50$, 59%) ($P > .05$). Eighteen (21%) patients were considered to be hypertensive (systolic blood pressure ≥160 mm Hg or diastolic blood pressure ≥95 mm Hg), and no statistically significant difference in variability of velocities was observed when patients were stratified by blood pressure. The absolute PSV values were also not significantly different among patients stratified by age or blood pressure. However, although we did observe that patients with heart rates of 75 beats per minute or greater (n = 43, 51%) had higher velocity measurements in the carotid arteries than did patients with lower rates (n = 42, 49%), there was no significant difference in the range or variability of velocities in the ICA or CCA (Table 3).

Subsequently, we examined the effects of variability in velocities on the parameters used to estimate the degree of carotid arterial stenosis. In none of the patients did the PSV in the ICA exceed a threshold of 130 cm/sec. In 12 (7%) arteries, the EDV in the ICA exceeded 40 cm/sec, which is a published threshold for moderate to severe (≥60%) stenosis (3).

To evaluate whether variability in velocity measurements along a vessel can affect stenosis estimates based on ICA/CCA ratios, we determined the number of patients whose calculated ratios would have exceeded published thresholds. Figures 1 and 2 demonstrate the effects of sampling location on ICA/CCA ratios. By using an ICA/CCA PSV ratio threshold of greater than 1.8 to indicate 60% or greater ICA stenosis, five (3%) vessels in a total of three (4%) patients had maximum ICA/minimum CCA values that were abnormal without other visible US evidence of disease (Fig 1). By using an ICA/CCA EDV ratio threshold of greater than 2.4, 23 (14%) vessels in 19 (22%) patients had ICA/CCA EDV values that exceeded the threshold, which suggested 60% or greater ICA stenosis (Fig 2). The mean difference in velocity ratio (ICA/CCA) values, depending on the location of the CCA measurements, was 0.2 ± 0.1 for the PSV ratio and 0.4 ± 0.4 for the EDV ratio.

We further assessed whether the use of CCA velocities obtained at one of the three locations tended to result in fewer misleading ratio values. When distal CCA values were used, three (2%) vessels (in two [2%] patients) had elevated ICA/CCA PSV ratios, and seven (4%) arteries (in six [7%] patients) had elevated EDV ratios. When middle CCA values were measured, the ICA/CCA PSV was elevated in one (1%) vessel, and the ICA/CCA EDV was elevated in five (3%) vessels (in five [6%] patients). When proximal CCA values were measured, one (1%) vessel demonstrated an abnormally elevated ICA/CCA PSV ratio, whereas 13 (8%) vessels (in 11 patients [13%]) had ICA/CCA EDV ratio values that exceeded the normal range. The statistical significance of these differences was not assessed because of the small sample sizes.

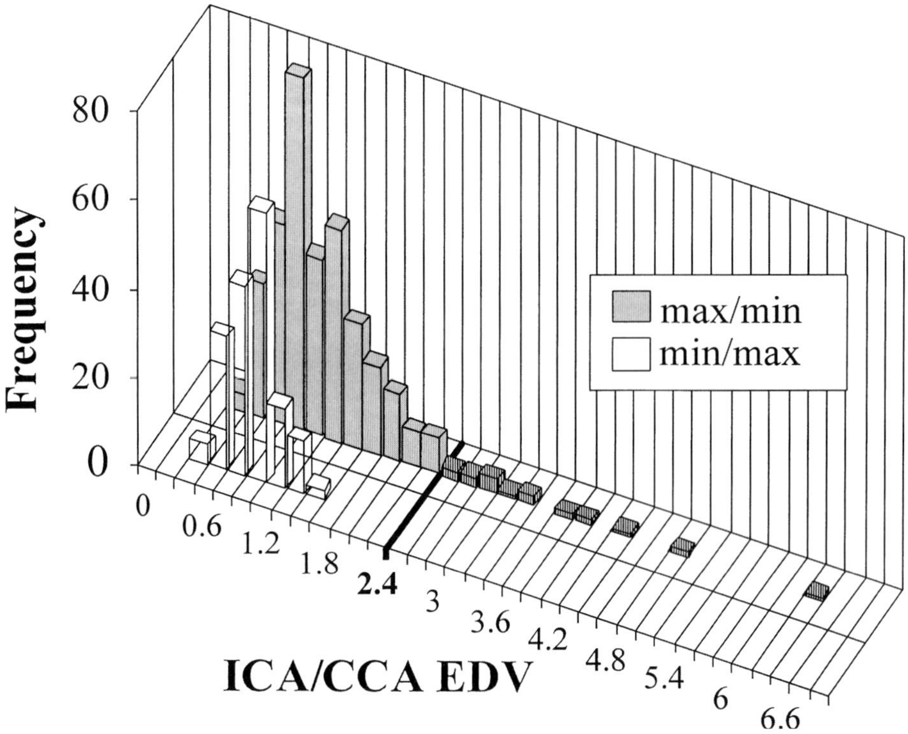

Figure 2. Histogram of the highest (maximum/minimum) and lowest (minimum/maximum) ICA/CCA EDV ratios based on measurements of velocities in different locations along each ipsilateral vessel. Values of greater than 2.4, the threshold, were considered to indicate 60% or greater stenosis (3). *max/min* = maximum ICA velocity divided by minimum ipsilateral CCA velocity, *min/max* = minimum ICA velocity divided by maximum ipsilateral CCA velocity, striped bars = all values exceeding the threshold (>2.4).

Right-to-left CCA PSV ratios demonstrated wide variability that was based on the location in the CCA that the measurements were obtained (Fig 3). By using maximum CCA (right) PSV/minimum CCA (left) PSV ratios, 26 (31%) patients had abnormal values (<0.7 or >1.3), which suggested stenosis of greater than 50% (13). When velocity ratio measurements were taken from matching locations, from side to side (ie, proximal CCA/proximal CCA, middle CCA/middle CCA, and distal CCA/distal CCA), the ratios fell in the abnormal range in 16 (19%) patients.

DISCUSSION

In carotid US, velocity measurements and ratios can provide quantitative estimates of the percentage of luminal narrowing. We set out to determine the variability of velocities along the courses of the CCA and ICA, with the intent of assessing the effect of such variation on various parameters used to estimate carotid arterial stenosis. We specifically selected a subset of our patients who demonstrated no gray-scale or color Doppler US evidence of carotid plaque so that we could better assess the intrinsic variability of velocity measurements without the confounding effects of plaque-related flow disturbance or variation in luminal cross-sections. Clearly, the diagnosis of carotid arterial stenosis does not rely entirely on parameter measurements; Doppler values are intended to complement assessments based on gray-scale and color Doppler US findings. Therefore, despite having Doppler measurements that exceeded published thresholds for hemodynamically significant carotid arterial disease, all patients in this study had a diagnosis of "disease-free" on the basis of the absence of carotid arterial disease at gray-scale and color Doppler US imaging.

The results of our study demonstrated a progressive decline in PSV from the proximal to distal CCA. This result is in agreement with that reported by Meyer et al (14), who examined 20 healthy volunteers and found an average decrease in PSV of 9 cm/sec for each centimeter increment in distance from the proximal CCA to the distal CCA (approaching the bifurcation). Because the age of their volun-

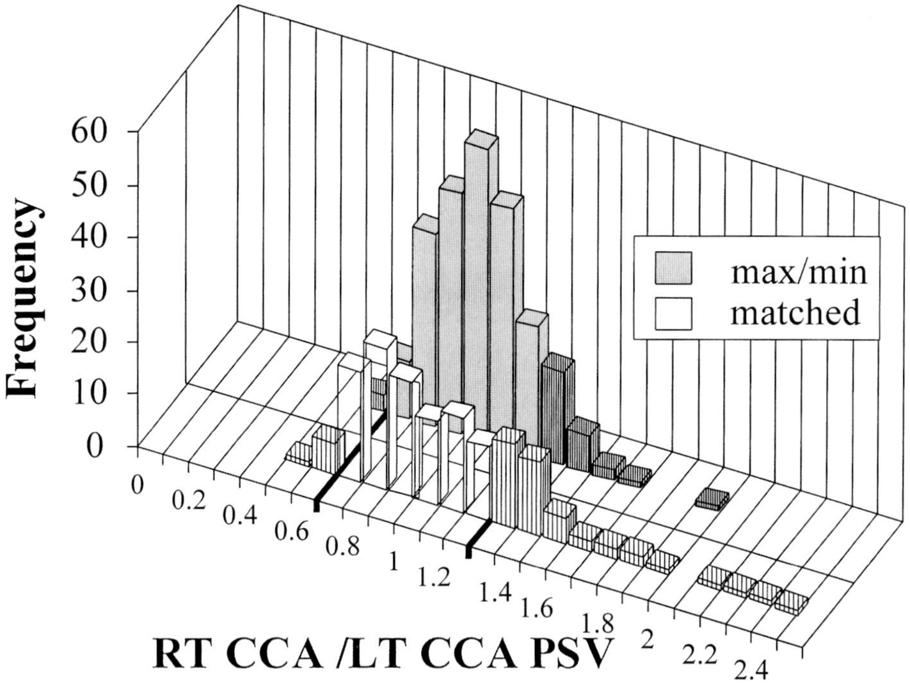

Figure 3. Histogram of the maximum and minimum and matched values for right CCA/left CCA PSV ratios. Values less than 0.7 or greater than 1.3, the thresholds, were considered to indicate ICA stenosis of greater than 50% (13). *max/min* = maximum right CCA PSV divided by minimum left CCA PSV or maximum left CCA PSV divided by minimum right CCA PSV, *matched* = all values in which the velocity ratios were matched at the same level (right proximal CCA/left proximal CCA, right middle CCA/left middle CCA, and right distal CCA/left distal CCA), striped bars = all values less than the 0.7 threshold or greater than the 1.3 threshold.

teers ranged from 25 to 43 years, the authors provided the caveat that the applicability of their results to an older or symptomatic population is uncertain. Our study results substantiate the presence of a similar velocity change in patient populations that are more representative of those who are referred for carotid arterial US.

The results of our study further demonstrate that the effect of this variability on velocity measurements such as ICA/CCA PSV and EDV ratios and right-to-left CCA ratios is substantial and could lead to diagnostic error. Interestingly, none of the 85 patients had ICA PSV measurements that exceeded 130 cm/sec, a commonly used threshold for the indication of 60% or greater stenosis (3); this supports claims that the PSV may be the most reliable Doppler measurement for estimating stenosis (15–17). Nevertheless, the absolute PSV is potentially influenced by differences in equipment and technique (11,12) and by physiologic factors such as cardiac output and contralateral restriction of blood flow (10,18). Velocity ratios have been promoted as a means of providing an internal standard that can account for some of these systematic (nonrandom) effects. As such, these ratios provide valuable complementary information, assuming that the variability of CCA velocities is considered in the interpretation.

When we evaluated whether ICA/CCA ratios would be less likely to be misleading if we obtained CCA measurements from each of the three locations, we found no substantial difference in ratios. Although some authors (3,8,17) have advocated the routine practice of obtaining CCA measurements just below the bifurcation (which corresponds to the distal CCA in our study) for ICA/CCA velocity ratios, our results do not clearly substantiate this preference. However, our results may be limited because of the small sample size.

The variability of velocities along the course of the CCA may be a result of several factors. Laminar (nonturbulent) flow within a rigid tube is governed by the law of conservation of momentum: $A1 \times V1 = A2 \times V2$, where A1 and A2 are cross-sectional areas at two points in the tube, and V1 and V2, the corresponding mean velocities in the two areas. Thus, velocity changes along the course of a vessel may, in part, correspond to changes in cross-sectional area. In the CCA and ICA, however, blood flow is not laminar where the vessel is tortuous, or where it bifurcates (18). Furthermore, the normal compliance of the vessel wall may serve to dampen velocities and thereby contribute to the progressive decline in velocity along the course of the CCA (14).

Our study results did not reveal statistically significant effects based on age or hypertension. Although Hansen et al (19) observed decreased vessel compliance with age, we did not observe an age-related pattern in ICA or CCA velocities. Similarly, we did not observe a substantial difference in velocity measurements when patients were stratified by blood pressure; our findings in the CCA are essentially in agreement with those reported by Ferrara et al (20), although in our study, we did not reproduce their finding of slightly increased mean velocities in the ICA in hypertensive patients. It is possible that differences exist but could not be detected with our sample size. Nonetheless, the magnitude of the effect is likely to be small and possibly not of clinical importance. We did find that patients with higher heart rates had higher velocities at all locations. However, there was no difference in the variability of velocities in the CCA or in the ICA/CCA PSV ratios between the two groups.

The criteria for hemodynamically significant carotid arterial stenosis vary among laboratories (8,10,11,16,17). These different criteria may stem from differences in equipment and measurement techniques, as well as differences in the test characteristics (sensitivity vs specificity) of particular patient populations and practice patterns. Although the use of slightly different thresholds could have shifted the percentage of cases that were regarded as abnormal in our study, it is unlikely that the use of different criteria would alter the basic conclusions of this study.

One limitation of this study is the assumption that patients who did not have visible disease on gray-scale and color Doppler US images were truly disease-free. Although it is possible that a minority of patients had imperceptible carotid plaque, this is unlikely to have been a common occurrence, given the high correlation between color Doppler US and angiographic findings in patients without visible carotid arterial disease (9,21). Still, vessel compliance can be focally or segmentally altered in the early stages of atherosclerosis.

It is also possible that some patients may have had disease beyond the areas visualized. In the Joint Study of Extracranial Arterial Occlusion (22), more than 4,000 patients were evaluated with conventional angiography, and stenosis was observed in the brachiocephalic artery in 4.2%, in the proximal left CCA in 4.8%, and in the intracranial portion of the ICA, on the left and right sides, in 6.6% and 6.7%, respectively. However, these data would likely be an overestimation of the prevalence of stenosis in our population, given the complete absence of discernible disease over the examined length of the extracranial carotid system in our study patients.

In conclusion, we have demonstrated a statistically significant variability in PSV and EDV along the course of the CCA in patients without visible US evidence of disease. This result is important because it was found in a patient population representative of those who are referred for carotid arterial US and because the observed variability of velocity measurements along the CCA was shown to affect Doppler velocity ratios and result in misleadingly abnormal values. If such variation is present in an ostensibly healthy group of patients, one is left to wonder how much more variation might exist in patients with demonstrable disease. Our findings may explain, in part, the inconsistent results reported between different laboratories when fixed thresholds for Doppler parameters are used. For improved consistency and comparability, a consensus in the community may need to be reached with regard to the optimal location of CCA measurements; further evaluation of Doppler criteria based on carefully defined and reproducible CCA measurements may then be justified.

References

1. Garth KE, Carroll BA, Sommer FG, Oppenheimer DA. Duplex ultrasound scanning of the carotid arteries with velocity spectrum analysis. Radiology 1983; 147:823–827.
2. Zweibel WJ. Spectrum analysis in carotid sonography. Ultrasound Med Biol 1987; 13:625–636.
3. Bluth EI, Stavros AT, Marich KW, Wetzner SM, Aufrichtig D, Baker JD. Carotid duplex sonography: a multicenter recommendation for standardized imaging and Doppler criteria. RadioGraphics 1988; 8:487–506.
4. Robinson ML, Sacks D, Perlmutter GS, Marinelli DL. Diagnostic criteria for carotid duplex sonography. AJR 1988; 151: 1045–1049.
5. Friedman SG, Hainline B, Feinberg AW, Lesser ML, Napolitano BA. Use of diastolic velocity ratios to predict significant carotid artery stenosis. Stroke 1988; 19:910–912.
6. Withers CE, Gosink BB, Keightley AM, et al. Duplex carotid sonography: peak systolic velocity in quantifying internal carotid artery stenosis. J Ultrasound Med 1990; 9:345–349.
7. Hunink MGM, Polak JF, Barlan MM, O'Leary DH. Detection and quantification of carotid artery stenosis: efficacy of various Doppler velocity parameters. AJR 1993; 160:619–625.
8. Carpenter JP, Lexa FJ, Davis JT. Determination of sixty percent or greater carotid artery stenosis by duplex Doppler ultrasonography. J Vasc Surg 1995; 22:697–705.
9. Srinivasan J, Mayberg MR, Weiss DG, Eskridge J. Duplex accuracy compared with angiography in the Veterans Affairs Cooperative Studies Trial for Symptomatic Carotid Stenosis. Neurosurgery 1995; 36:648–655.
10. Zwiebel WJ. New Doppler parameters for carotid stenosis. Semin Ultrasound CT MR 1997; 18:66–71.
11. Howard G, Baker WH, Chambless LE, Howard VJ, Jones AM, Toole JF. An approach for the use of Doppler ultrasound as a screening tool for hemodynamically significant stenosis (despite heterogeneity of Doppler performance): a multicenter experience. Stroke 1996; 27:1951–1957.
12. Wolstenhulme S, Evans JA, Weston MJ. The agreement between colour Doppler systems in measuring internal carotid artery peak systolic velocities. Br J Radiol 1997; 70:1043–1052.
13. Vaisman U, Wojciechowski M. Carotid artery disease: new criteria for evaluation by sonographic duplex scanning. Radiology 1986; 158:253–255.
14. Meyer JI, Khalil RM, Obuchowski NA, Baus LK. Common carotid artery: variability of Doppler US velocity measurements. Radiology 1997; 204:339–341.
15. Schwartz SW, Chambless LE, Baker WH, Broderick JP, Howard G. Consistency of Doppler parameters in predicting arteriographically confirmed carotid stenosis. Stroke 1997; 28:343–347.
16. Faught WE, Mattos MA, van Bemmelen PS, et al. Color-flow duplex scanning of carotid arteries: new velocity criteria based on receiver operator characteristic analysis for threshold stenoses used in the symptomatic and asymptomatic carotid trials. J Vasc Surg 1994; 19:818–828.
17. Moneta GL, Edwards JM, Papanicolaou G, et al. Screening for asymptomatic internal carotid artery stenosis: Duplex criteria for discriminating 60% to 99% stenosis. J Vasc Surg 1995; 21:989–994.
18. Steinke W, Kloetzsch C, Hennerici M. Variability of flow patterns in the normal carotid bifurcation. Atherosclerosis 1990; 84:121–127.
19. Hansen F, Mangell P, Sonesson B, Länne T. Diameter and compliance in the human common carotid artery: variations with age and sex. Ultrasound Med Biol 1995; 21:1–9.
20. Ferrara LA, Mancini M, Iannuzzi R, et al. Carotid diameter and blood flow velocities in cerebral circulation in hypertensive patients. Stroke 1995; 26:418–421.
21. Zierler RE, Kohler TR, Strandness DE Jr. Duplex scanning of normal or minimally diseased carotid arteries: correlation with arteriography and clinical outcome. J Vasc Surg 1990; 12:447–455.
22. Hass WK, Fields WS, North RR, Kricheff II, Chase NE, Bauer RB. Joint study of extracranial arterial occlusion. II. Arteriography, techniques, sites, and complications. JAMA 1968; 203:961–968.

Count-based PET Method for Predicting Ischemic Stroke in Patients with Symptomatic Carotid Arterial Occlusion[1]

Colin P. Derdeyn, MD
Tom O. Videen, PhD
Nicholas R. Simmons, BA
Kent D. Yundt, MD
Susanne M. Fritsch, RN
Robert L. Grubb, Jr, MD
William J. Powers, MD

Index terms:
Brain, emission CT (ECT), 10.12163
Brain, ischemia, 10.781
Carotid arteries, stenosis or obstruction, 172.721, 175.721
Emission CT (ECT), experimental studies, 10.12163

Radiology 1999; 212:499–506

Abbreviations:
OEF = oxygen extraction fraction
ROC = receiver operating characteristic
STLCOS = St Louis Carotid Occlusion Study

[1] From the Section of Neuroradiology (C.P.D.) and Div of Radiological Sciences (C.P.D., T.O.V., N.R.S., R.L.G., W.J.P.), Mallinckrodt Institute; Dept of Neurology and Neurological Surgery (T.O.V., K.D.Y., S.M.F., R.L.G., W.J.P.); and Lillian Strauss Institute of the Jewish Hospital of St Louis (W.J.P.), Washington University School of Medicine, 510 S Kingshighway Blvd, St Louis, MO 63110. From the 1998 RSNA scientific assembly. Received Sep 16, 1998; revision requested Nov 17; revision received Dec 7; accepted Mar 2, 1999. Supported by National Institutes of Health grants NS02029 (C.P.D.), NS28947 (T.O.V., S.M.F., R.L.G., W.J.P.), and NS34050 (W.J.P.) and Charles A. Dana Foundation (C.P.D., K.D.Y., W.J.P.) and by RSNA Research and Education Foundation as a 1994 Siemens Medical Systems/RSNA Fellow (C.P.D.). Address reprint requests to C.P.D. (e-mail: *derdeyn@mirlink.wustl.edu*).

Author contributions:
Guarantor of integrity of entire study, C.P.D.; study concepts and design, W.J.P., C.P.D.; definition of intellectual content, W.J.P., C.P.D.; literature research, C.P.D., W.J.P.; clinical studies, W.J.P., R.L.G., C.P.D., S.M.F., K.D.Y.; experimental studies, C.P.D., W.J.P., T.O.V.; data acquisition, C.P.D., S.M.F., K.D.Y., W.J.P., R.L.G., T.O.V.; data analysis, C.P.D., W.J.P., T.O.V., N.R.S.; statistical analysis, C.P.D., W.J.P.; manuscript preparation, C.P.D.; manuscript editing, W.J.P.; manuscript review, W.J.P., R.L.G., T.O.V.

PURPOSE: To test the ability of a count-based positron emission tomographic (PET) method, without arterial sampling, for the measurement of regional cerebral oxygen extraction fraction (OEF) to predict ischemic stroke in patients with symptomatic carotid arterial occlusion.

MATERIALS AND METHODS: The outcome analysis of a blinded prospective study designed to determine if increased OEF was an independent predictor of stroke in patients with symptoms and with carotid occlusion was repeated by substituting a count-based method of OEF measurement for the original quantitative technique. The performance of the quantitative and count-based methods was assessed by using Kaplan-Meier cumulative survival functions (log-rank, [$P < .05$]). Receiver operating characteristic (ROC) curves for both methods were generated.

RESULTS: Thirteen ipsilateral strokes occurred during a mean follow-up of 3.1 years for 81 patients. All ipsilateral strokes occurred in 50 patients with increased count-based OEF ($P = .002$, sensitivity 100%, specificity 46%). Sixty-eight patients underwent complete quantitative studies, which allowed comparison of OEF methods. Both the count-based and the quantitative methods were predictive of stroke in this subgroup ($P = .005$ and .025, respectively). ROC analysis demonstrated a greater area under the curve for the count-based OEF method.

CONCLUSION: Count-based PET measurement of OEF without arterial sampling accurately predicts stroke in patients with carotid occlusion.

The hemodynamic effect of ipsilateral carotid arterial occlusion has been categorized into three stages (1). The rationale for this scheme is based on the known compensatory responses made by the cerebrovasculature to progressive reductions in cerebral perfusion pressure. When cerebral perfusion pressure is normal (stage 0), cerebral blood flow is closely matched to the resting metabolic rate of the tissue. As a consequence of this resting balance between flow and metabolism, the oxygen extraction fraction (OEF) shows little regional variation. Moderate reductions in cerebral perfusion pressure have little effect on cerebral blood flow. Dilatation of arterioles reduces cerebrovascular resistance, thus maintaining a constant blood flow (stage 1). This phenomenon is known as cerebrovascular autoregulation.

With more severe reductions in cerebral perfusion pressure, the capacity for compensatory vasodilation is exceeded, and cerebral blood flow begins to decline (Fig 1). A progressive increase in OEF then maintains cerebral oxygen metabolism and brain function (stage 2, Fig 1). This most severe form of cerebral hemodynamic failure also has been termed "misery perfusion" (2). At present, OEF can be measured only with PET and oxygen 15–labeled radiotracers.

Severe atherosclerotic disease of the carotid and vertebral arteries or their intracranial branches can lead to reduced perfusion pressure in the distal cerebral circulation, which depends primarily on the adequacy of collateral sources of blood flow (3). While the relative role of hemodynamic factors in the pathogenesis of ischemic stroke has become a moot question for patients with carotid stenosis, it remains an important issue for many patients with cerebrovascular disease, particularly those with occlusion of the carotid artery

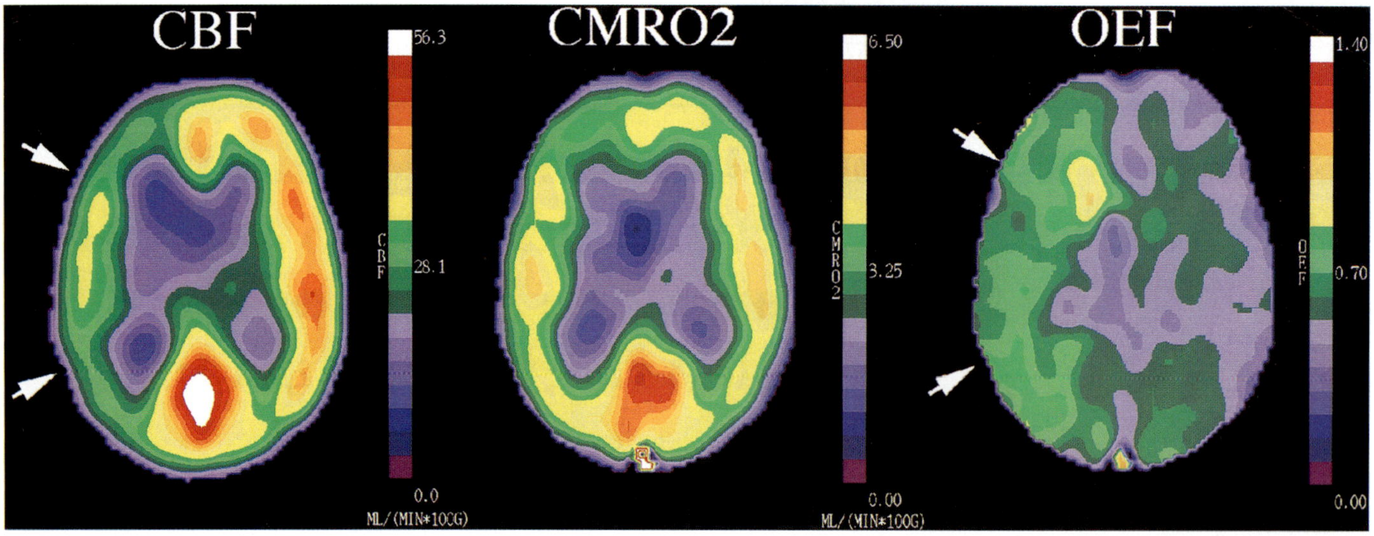

Figure 1. Positron emission tomographic (PET) scans show increased OEF, or "misery perfusion." This patient was 65 years old when he enrolled in the STLCOS after several transient ischemic attacks involving his right leg. His first symptoms occurred approximately 4 months prior to enrollment and PET examination. A CT scan at the time of the PET study demonstrated a small lacunar infarction of the right internal capsule. Neurologic examination results were normal. Cerebral angiography revealed an occlusion of the left internal carotid artery. The quantitative map of cerebral blood flow (*CBF*) on the far left demonstrates diffuse decrease in flow throughout the left cerebral hemisphere (arrows; note that left and right are reversed on these PET images relative to CT and MR conventions). The image depicting cerebral metabolic rate of oxygen consumption (*CMRO2*) in the middle shows normal and symmetric metabolism of oxygen. The quantitative OEF image on the far right shows increased OEF in the left hemisphere (arrows). The ability of the brain to increase the fraction of oxygen extracted from the blood allows normal oxygen metabolism and neurologic function, once the capacity for autoregulatory vasodilation has been exceeded and blood flow begins to decrease. This patient was treated with aspirin and had a fatal ipsilateral ischemic stroke 525 days after enrollment.

(4). Up to 15% of patients presenting with symptoms of acute cerebral or ocular ischemia have occlusion of the ipsilateral carotid artery (5–7). Their annual risk for subsequent stroke is 5%–7% (8). The presence of hemodynamic compromise long has been suspected as a factor in the pathogenesis of recurrent ischemic stroke in these patients, but without conclusive proof (3,4,9–11).

Findings of the St Louis Carotid Occlusion Study (STLCOS) recently demonstrated that increased OEF was an independent predictor of subsequent stroke in patients with symptomatic carotid occlusion in a blinded longitudinal study (12). In PET studies in patients with carotid occlusion before and after extracranial-to-intracranial arterial bypass, the OEF elevation has been shown to be reversible (2,13–15). Consequently, a clinical trial of surgical revascularization for patients with increased OEF has been proposed (12).

The quantitative measurement of an in vivo physiologic process, such as cerebral OEF, with PET is complicated (16). Three basic components are necessary: (*a*) a radiotracer, (*b*) a radiation detection system, and (*c*) a mathematic model relating the physiologic process to the detected radiation. For the quantitative measurement of OEF, a subject first inhales trace amounts of ^{15}O-labeled oxygen mixed with air. The ^{15}O-labeled oxygen is then bound to hemoglobin and transported throughout the body where some of it is used for oxidative metabolism. Some ^{15}O-labeled oxygen is metabolized to water, which returns to the bloodstream and recirculates.

As these processes are occurring, the ^{15}O radionuclides are decaying by emission of a positron. These positively charged particles can travel a few millimeters within a tissue before encountering an electron. This interaction leads to annihilation of both the positron and the electron and generates two photons of equal energy heading in opposite directions. The PET scanner uses data from detector pairs to create an image of regional activity, or PET counts, and this PET image of regional counts must be processed to translate regional activity to a physiologic measurement.

The quantitative measurement of OEF requires time-activity data acquired from arterial sampling during scanning and quantitative values of blood flow and blood volume provided from separate PET examinations (17). This information is used to correct for the PET counts measured in the head owing to unextracted ^{15}O-labeled oxygen, which remains bound to hemoglobin, and the PET counts from recirculating ^{15}O-labeled water owing to metabolism of ^{15}O-labeled oxygen.

Metabolic processing of PET images is complicated and time-consuming. Percutaneous arterial cannulation may not be possible in some patients. Arterial sampling requires additional equipment and adds time to the PET procedure. In the STLCOS, complete arterial time-activity data were not available owing to technical factors in 13 of 81 subjects. These 13 subjects were therefore assigned to categories on the basis of the count-based method of OEF measurement presented in this report, while the remaining 68 subjects were assigned to categories by using the quantitative OEF processing. A count-based technique that does not require arterial time-activity data would be useful, particularly in the setting of a multiinstitutional trial in which standardization of complicated quantitative PET techniques might be difficult.

In this article, we present a further evaluation of the count-based PET technique to measure relative OEF (Fig 2). The count-based OEF image is generated by dividing the PET counts in an ^{15}O-labeled oxygen scan by the PET counts in an ^{15}O-labeled water scan on a pixel-by-pixel basis. The ratio of the counts in the ^{15}O-labeled oxygen image and the ^{15}O-labeled water image are linearly propor-

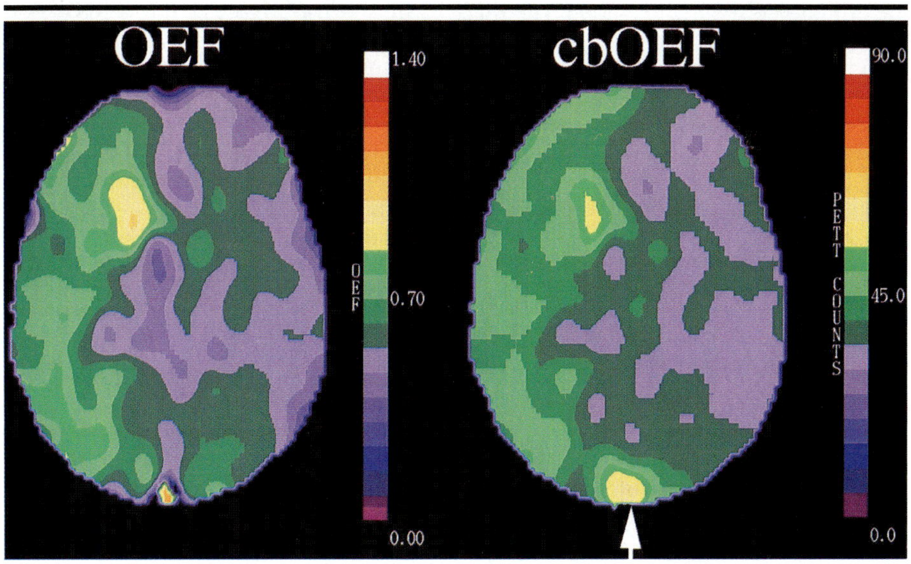

Figure 2. PET scans show the similarity of quantitative (on the left) and count-based (on the right) OEF images in the same patient as in Figure 1. The image on the right is the count-based oxygen extraction (*cbOEF*) image, which was generated by dividing the ^{15}O-labeled oxygen image by the ^{15}O-labeled water image. With the exception of the sagittal sinus (arrow on the *cbOEF* image), the regional map of oxygen extraction is very similar to that of the quantitative OEF image on the left. As the count-based OEF image is not corrected for intravascular ^{15}O-labeled oxygen, the sagittal sinus has more activity than on the quantitatively processed OEF image. High values of OEF can be seen in the center of the sagittal sinus on the quantitative OEF image, which may be owing to misregistration of the cerebral blood volume scan during processing.

tional to quantitative regional OEF except for the small contributions from intravascular oxygen and recirculating labeled water. The errors are small when regional oxygen metabolism is normal (17–19).

In the present study, we compared the results of repeating the outcome analysis of the STLCOS by using both the count-based method and the quantitative method of OEF measurement. The purpose of this study was to evaluate the accuracy of the count-based OEF method to predict ischemic stroke in patients with symptomatic carotid arterial occlusion.

MATERIALS AND METHODS

Patients and Control Subjects

Eighty-one patients with symptomatic unilateral atherosclerotic carotid arterial occlusion were enrolled in the STLCOS, a blinded prospective study of cerebral hemodynamics and ischemic stroke. The study was designed to test the hypothesis that increased OEF measured in the cerebral hemisphere distal to the occluded carotid artery was an independent predictor of stroke in these patients. Enrollment began in 1992 and ended in 1996. Analysis of both the baseline risk factors and of the long-term follow-up of these patients has been published (12,20). Details of the study design, patient population, and inclusion and exclusion criteria can be found in these two reports.

Patients were followed-up by the study coordinator (S.M.F.) for the duration of the study by telephone contact every 6 months with the patient or next of kin. The occurrence of any symptoms suggesting a stroke was thoroughly evaluated by one designated investigator (R.L.G.), who remained blinded to the PET data. All living patients were followed-up for the duration of the study. The primary end point of the original prospective study was subsequent ischemic stroke defined clinically as a neurologic deficit of presumed ischemic cerebrovascular cause lasting more than 24 hours in any cerebrovascular territory. Secondary end points were ipsilateral ischemic stroke and death.

Eighteen healthy control subjects (eight women, 10 men; age range, 19–77 years; mean age ± SD, 45 years ± 18) were recruited by means of public advertisement. All underwent neurologic evaluation, magnetic resonance (MR) imaging of the head, and duplex ultrasonographic (US) imaging of the extracranial carotid arteries. None had (*a*) signs or symptoms of neurologic disease other than mild distal sensory loss in the legs consistent with age, (*b*) pathologic lesions on MR images (mild atrophy and punctate asymptomatic white matter abnormalities were not considered pathologic), or (*c*) more than 50% stenosis of the extracranial carotid arteries.

A computed tomographic (CT) scan of the brain was obtained without contrast enhancement if CT or MR imaging had not been performed as part of the usual clinical care sufficiently long after an ischemic event to permit accurate definition of infarction location. This CT scan was used to determine the site of tissue infarction to exclude these regions from subsequent PET analysis.

This research was approved by the human studies committee and written informed consent was obtained from all subjects.

PET Examination

Hemodynamic PET studies in patients with carotid occlusion were performed at study entry. Blood pressure was measured in the clinic prior to walking to the scanner suite. After positioning the patient in the scanner gantry, an individually molded thermoplastic face mask was applied to ensure that the patient's head remained in a constant position during the scanning period. The exact position of the patient's head relative to the scanning plane was recorded on a lateral skull radiograph obtained after head immobilization. Venous and, when possible, arterial catheters were placed for the intravenous administration of the radiotracer and for arterial blood gas analyses and arterial time-activity curve determination, respectively (21). All PET studies were performed with use of one of two scanners (ECAT 953B or ECAT EACT HR; Siemens/CTI, Knoxville, Tenn). A transmission scan was obtained by using the two-dimensional mode (intersection septa extended) before radiotracer administration by using germanium 68/gallium 68 rotating rod sources.

Each PET study consisted of three separate physiologic studies. During each, arterial blood samples were drawn by hand or automatically to convert quantitative regional radioactivity data to quantitative physiologic measurements. Additional arterial samples were drawn at intervals during the examination for determination of Pa_{CO_2} stability, mean arterial oxygen content calculations, and carboxyhemoglobin content.

A 5-minute scan was obtained 1 minute and 45 seconds after inhalation of one to two breaths of air containing trace amounts of ^{15}O-labeled carbon monoxide. After allowing this activity to decay for approximately 15 minutes, a 40-second scan was obtained after inhalation of one to two breaths of air containing trace amounts of ^{15}O-labeled oxygen. After another 15 minutes, the last scan was acquired after the injection of a bolus of ^{15}O-labeled water.

Both the ^{15}O-labeled oxygen scans and ^{15}O-labeled water scans acquired counts for 40 seconds, beginning when the radiotracer reached the brain. The circulation time for intravenously administered or inhaled radiotracer to reach the brain varies greatly from person to person, so accurate online monitoring of brain radioactivity is necessary to start data acquisition at the proper time. Both scanners used in this study provide such online monitoring of coincidence events within the field of view, but the temporal resolution is poor unless data acquisition is underway.

Another potential problem is that there is a delay after scan initiation before data are acquired. This delay does not occur during advancement from one dynamic frame of data acquisition to another, however. Thus, it was necessary to modify the scan acquisition protocols to include two dynamic frames: Frame 1 had no preset duration and was begun 5–10 seconds prior to radiotracer administration. Frame 2 was preset to be 40 seconds in duration and was begun by the scanner operator when the coincidence events in the field of view sharply increased and indicated the arrival of the radiotracer bolus in the brain. Only the data from frame 2 was reconstructed and used in subsequent analysis.

The entire PET examination could be performed within 1 hour because of the short half-life (122.2 seconds) of ^{15}O. All radionuclides were produced in the Washington University cyclotron facility (22,23).

Image Processing and Analysis

All images were reconstructed by using filtered backprojection and scatter correction with a ramp filter at the Nyquist frequency. They were then filtered with a three-dimensional Gaussian filter to a uniform resolution of 16 mm full width at half maximum. These images subsequently were transformed to stereotactic atlas space (24) by using the lateral skull radiograph and the transmission scan. This was done to allow reproducible placement of regions of interest.

When combined with the arterial time-activity curve data and the hematocrit values, the ^{15}O-labeled carbon monoxide image provided the quantitative regional measurement of cerebral blood volume on a pixel-by-pixel basis (25). A regional map of quantitative cerebral blood flow was generated from the ^{15}O-labeled water image by using arterial time-activity data (21,26,27). The ^{15}O-labeled oxygen image provided the quantitative regional measurement of OEF, once combined with data from processed cerebral blood flow and cerebral blood volume images and the arterial time-activity curve information (17). Images depicting cerebral metabolic rate for oxygen were generated as the product of OEF, cerebral blood flow, and Pa_{O_2} content (17).

The count-based OEF image was generated as the ratio image of the counts in the filtered and atlas-transformed ^{15}O-labeled oxygen and ^{15}O-labeled water images, normalized to a whole-brain mean of 0.40—this value was the mean whole-brain quantitative OEF measured in the 68 patients with arterial time-activity curve data. This was performed in the following manner.

First, the normalization factor was calculated: (*a*) A template was created by using brain edges defined by isointensity contours at approximately 30% of the whole-brain maximum counts of the ^{15}O-labeled water image to eliminate extracranial noise—the water image was used rather than the oxygen image because of the greater number of counts (ie, less noise); (*b*) this template was saved and used to mask the extracranial noise in the ^{15}O-labeled oxygen image; (*c*) whole-section mean counts for 21 PET sections that included the middle cerebral arterial territories were calculated from both the ^{15}O-labeled water and ^{15}O-labeled oxygen scans by using the saved templates to mask the extracranial noise; (*d*) the ratio of the ^{15}O-labeled oxygen counts to the ^{15}O-labeled water counts was calculated; and (*e*) 0.40 was divided by this ratio to yield the normalization factor (0.40 = normalization factor × [whole-brain ^{15}O-labeled oxygen counts/whole-brain ^{15}O-labeled water counts]).

Next, a second mask was created in a similar manner to eliminate extracranial noise from the ^{15}O-labeled oxygen images and ^{15}O-labeled water images prior to the pixel-by-pixel division of the counts in the images: (*a*) A mask image was created from the ^{15}O-labeled water image by using the same threshold percentage used for the template in the calculation of the normalization factor and in an identical manner (brain edges identified by means of isointensity contours at a specified threshold percentage of maximum whole-brain counts), and (*b*) this mask was applied to the ^{15}O-labeled oxygen image.

Finally, the counts in the masked ^{15}O-labeled oxygen image were multiplied by the normalization factor and divided by the counts in the masked ^{15}O-labeled water image on a pixel-by-pixel basis. This resulted in the count-based OEF image used in the subsequent regional analyses (Fig 2).

For each patient and healthy volunteer, seven separate spherical regions of interest 19 mm in diameter were placed in the territory of the middle cerebral artery in each hemisphere. Each region included gray and white matter and was placed by using stereotactic coordinates (1,28). Areas of prior infarction were identified by two investigators (C.P.D., W.J.P.) by review of images depicting cerebral metabolic rate for oxygen (or ^{15}O-labeled images for the 13 patients without arterial data) and CT or MR images. Neither the regions within these areas nor the corresponding contralateral regions were used for analysis. Left-to-right ratios of mean hemispheric values of both quantitative OEF images and count-based OEF images were calculated for patients and control subjects. For each patient, the ratio was considered abnormal if it decreased beyond the range observed in the normal sample.

Data Analysis

Several analyses were performed. First, the ability of the count-based OEF ratio to predict subsequent stroke was examined. The 81 patients were divided into two groups on the basis of comparison with the range of normal values: those with abnormal count-based OEF ratios and those with normal count-based OEF ratios. The primary analysis compared the two groups with respect to the length of time before reaching the end point of ipsilateral stroke by means of Kaplan-Meier survival curves and the log-rank statistic.

Second, the count-based technique was compared directly with the quantitative method in predicting ipsilateral stroke. In these analyses, the image data of the 68 patients with arterial time-activity curves was processed by using both count-based and quantitative methods. Quantitative and count-based OEF ratios were compared for each patient by means of a paired Student *t* test.

Finally, receiver operating characteristic (ROC) curves for the prediction of subsequent ischemic stroke were generated by varying the threshold ratio used for a positive test for both quantitative and count-based techniques. This was done by progressively increasing the threshold for an abnormal test result from a left-to-right OEF ratio of 1.00 ± 0.01 (0.99 to 1.01) to 1.00 ± 0.28 (0.72 to 1.28) by increments of 0.01. A value of $P < .05$ was used as the criterion of statistical significance. Statistical analyses were performed with SPSS 7.0 (SPSS, Chicago, Ill) for Windows.

RESULTS

Clinical

Eighty-one patients were followed up for a mean of 3.1 years. All patients had unilateral carotid occlusion. Fifteen strokes were recorded during the follow-up period, and all of them were ischemic. Thirteen of these strokes were ipsilateral to the occluded carotid artery.

Normal Range

The range for left-to-right hemispheric ratios for the quantitative OEF observed in the 18 healthy subjects was 0.914–1.084. The normal range of left-to-right hemispheric ratios for count-based OEF was 0.935–1.062 in these subjects.

Results of Count-based OEF for All 81 Patients

Fifty of the 81 patients with symptomatic carotid occlusion had abnormal results, with left-to-right hemispheric count-based ratios that fell outside of the range observed in the healthy subjects. In all 50, the hemisphere with the increased count-based OEF was ipsilateral to the occluded carotid artery. All 13 ipsilateral ischemic strokes occurred in the 50 patients with an increased count-based OEF ($P = .002$). The sensitivity of the count-based method for the prediction of subsequent ipsilateral stroke was 100% (95% CI = −23%) (29) with use of the range observed in the healthy subjects to define the normal range. However, 37 of the 68 patients who did not have an ipsilateral stroke had increased OEF (specificity of 46% [95% CI: 40.5%, 51.5%]). The Kaplan-Meier cumulative failure curve is shown in Figure 3. The ROC curve generated by progressively increasing the threshold at which the count-based OEF ratio was defined as abnormal is shown in Figure 4.

Comparison of Count-based and Quantitative Methods

Complete quantitative metabolic processing of PET images could not be performed for 13 of the 81 patients. Difficulty with arterial access or with the measurement of arterial blood counts during the PET examination accounted for 11 of these 13 studies. Arterial access could not be established in six: Four patients were taking warfarin sodium (Coumadin; Du Pont Pharma, Wilmington, Del) and failed Allen tests bilaterally, and in two patients several attempts at both radial and brachial arterial catheterization failed. Technical problems related to the quantitative processing of PET data accounted for the remaining seven patients. These problems involved malfunctioning of the device used to measure the arterial blood counts automatically in five patients.

Nine ipsilateral strokes occurred in the 68 patients with complete quantitative data. By using the normal range of values observed in the healthy volunteers to define the threshold, 31 of the 68 patients had abnormal results with use of quantitative OEF ratios. Seven ipsilateral ischemic strokes occurred in this group of 31 patients, compared with two strokes in the 37 patients with quantitative OEF ratios within the normal range ($P = .025$; sensitivity of 78% [95% CI: 64.5%, 91.5%]; specificity of 59% [95% CI: 52.2%, 65.8%]). The count-based OEF ratio was less specific (specificity of 48% [95% CI: 41.2%, 54.8%]) and more sensitive (sensitivity of 100% [95% CI = −33%]) than the quantitative method. Forty-one patients had abnormal results, and all strokes occurred in this group ($P = .005$). Kaplan-Meier cumulative failure curves of the quantitative and count-based analyses for these 68 patients are shown in Figure 5a and 5b, respectively.

Comparison of the count-based OEF ratio with the quantitative OEF ratio for each of the 68 patients demonstrated no significant difference at paired Student t test analysis ($P = .299$). The mean absolute difference between count-based OEF and quantitative OEF ratios was 0.034 (95% CI: 0.025, 0.043). ROC curves were generated for both methods (Fig 6). The area under the curve for the count-based OEF method (0.815) was greater than that for the quantitative OEF method (0.737).

DISCUSSION

In this retrospective analysis of STLCOS data, we have demonstrated that the count-based measurement of OEF can be used to identify patients at increased risk of ischemic stroke with accuracy similar to that of the quantitative method. By using the count-based OEF ratio instead of the quantitative OEF ratio for all 81 patients, we found that all 13 subsequent ipsilateral strokes occurred in the 50 patients with abnormal ratios. When the Kaplan-Meier survival functions of the two OEF processing methods were compared directly in the 68 patients with complete quantitative data, both achieved statistical significance. Direct comparison of count-based and quantitative OEF ratios showed no statistical difference (mean absolute difference = 0.034; 95% CI: 0.025, 0.043).

Why does the count-based method presented in this article perform as well as, if not better than, the quantitative OEF technique in the prediction of subsequent stroke? The data from the count-based OEF image are linearly proportional to the quantitative OEF image except for the small contributions from intravascular oxygen and recirculating labeled water.

The equation for quantitative OEF developed by Mintun et al (17) is as follows:

$$\mathrm{OEF} = [\mathrm{PET}_{\mathrm{obs}} - \mathrm{CBF} \times \int_{t1}^{t2} C_{\mathrm{art}}^{\mathrm{H_2O}}(t) * e^{-kt}\,\mathrm{d}t - R \times \mathrm{CBV} \times \int_{t1}^{t2} C_{\mathrm{art}}^{\mathrm{O_2}}(t)\,\mathrm{d}t] \div [\mathrm{CBF} \times \int_{t1}^{t2} C_{\mathrm{art}}^{\mathrm{O_2}}(t) * e^{-kt}\,\mathrm{d}t - (0.835) \times R \times \mathrm{CBV} \int_{t1}^{t2} C_{\mathrm{art}}^{\mathrm{O_2}}(t)\,\mathrm{d}t].$$

$\mathrm{PET}_{\mathrm{obs}}$ is the regional, decay-corrected PET counts measured in the brain after inhalation of a bolus of ^{15}O-labeled oxygen summed over a 40-second scan; obs is "observed." $\mathrm{CBF} \times \int_{t1}^{t2} C_{\mathrm{art}}^{\mathrm{H20}}(t) * e^{-kt}\mathrm{d}t$ is the activity due to the recirculating labeled water owing to ^{15}O-labeled oxygen metabolism, where CBF is cerebral blood flow, $t1$ and $t2$ are the scanning time, and $C_{\mathrm{art}}^{\mathrm{H20}}$ is the time-dependent concentration of ^{15}O-labeled water in the arterial blood. The term $R \times \mathrm{CBV} \times \int_{t1}^{t2} C_{\mathrm{art}}^{\mathrm{O2}}(t)\mathrm{d}t$ defines the post midcapillary activity of the intravascular ^{15}O-labeled oxygen where R is the ratio of small-vessel to large-vessel hematocrit values used in the calculation of CBV, CBV is the cerebral blood volume, and $C_{\mathrm{art}}^{\mathrm{O2}}$ is the time-dependent concentration of ^{15}O-labeled oxygen in the arterial blood.

The two terms in the denominator of the equation are the blood flow delivering the oxygen ($\mathrm{CBF} \times \int_{t1}^{t2} C_{\mathrm{art}}^{\mathrm{O2}}[t] * e^{-kt}\mathrm{d}t$) minus the intravascular ^{15}O-labeled oxygen ($0.835 \times R \times \mathrm{CBV} \int_{t1}^{t2} C_{\mathrm{art}}^{\mathrm{O2}}[t]\mathrm{d}t$). This method requires separate measurements

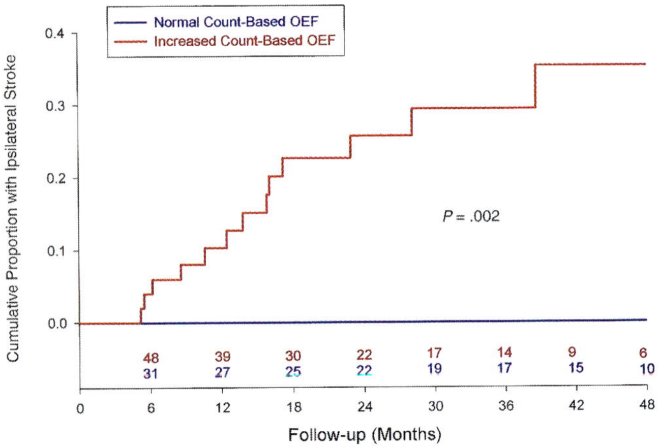

Figure 3. Graph shows Kaplan-Meier cumulative failure curves for the end point of ipsilateral stroke for all 81 patients with symptomatic carotid occlusion who were examined by using the count-based OEF method. None of the patients with normal count-based OEF ratios had an ipsilateral stroke (blue line). All 13 ipsilateral strokes occurred in the 50 patients with increased OEF (red line). The number of patients remaining event free and available for follow-up evaluation at each 6-month interval is shown at the bottom of the graph. The numbers in blue correspond to patients with normal OEF and the numbers in red to those with increased OEF. The vertical axis shows the cumulative proportion of patients with ipsilateral stroke. The difference in outcome was highly statistically significant.

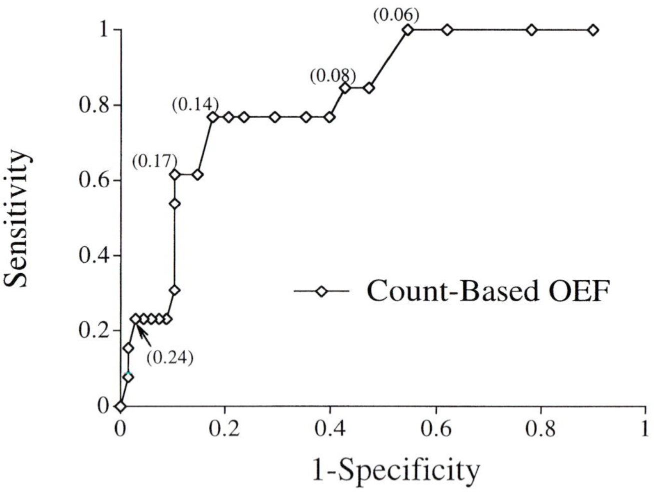

Figure 4. Graph shows ROC curve for the count-based OEF method for all 81 patients. Sensitivities and specificities of the count-based OEF ratio for the prediction of ipsilateral stroke were calculated at progressively larger thresholds from 1.00 ± 0.01 (0.99–1.01) to 1.00 ± 0.28 (0.72–1.28) by increments of 0.01. Several of these thresholds are indicated in parentheses next to their corresponding points on the curve. At threshold ratios up to 1.06 (in parentheses as 0.06, fourth point from the right), all subsequent ipsilateral strokes occur in the patients who have abnormal OEF ratios. However, the specificity of the count-based method at these thresholds is very low, as nearly all patients are considered to have abnormal OEF ratios. As specificity improves (moving to the left on the curve), sensitivity begins to decrease.

of cerebral blood flow and cerebral blood volume to yield an accurate quantitative measurement of OEF. It has been validated in nonhuman primates by using intracarotid injections of ^{15}O-labeled oxygen (17). In addition, it has been rigorously validated in nonhuman primates against direct measurements of arteriovenous oxygen difference in pathologic conditions (30).

The contribution of the recirculating labeled water of metabolism and the intravascular labeled oxygen to the counts measured in the brain is small in areas of normal cerebral oxygen metabolism (discussed later). Without these terms, the equation for OEF becomes the observed PET counts from the ^{15}O-labeled oxygen image divided by the cerebral blood flow delivering the oxygen.

In the tissue autoradiographic technique of blood flow measurement used in our laboratory, the relationship between the tissue concentration of ^{15}O-labeled water to the local blood flow is almost linear (21,26). In the count-based OEF method, therefore, we use the regional PET counts observed during the ^{15}O-labeled oxygen scanning for the numerator and the regional PET counts observed during the ^{15}O-labeled water scanning for the denominator: count-based OEF = PET_{obs} (^{15}O-labeled oxygen)/PET_{obs} (^{15}O-labeled water). Because we are comparing the ratio of the counts from the ^{15}O-labeled oxygen images and the counts from the ^{15}O-labeled water images from one hemisphere to the other, rather than using the absolute values for comparison between patients, the left-to-right ratio for the count-based estimate of OEF should be very similar to the left-to-right ratio of quantitative OEF.

In the first PET methods for OEF measurement, the ratio of counts from a steady-state or equilibrium ^{15}O-labeled oxygen image to a steady-state ^{15}O-labeled water image was used. This method was proposed by Jones and co-workers (31) before implementation and validation by Frackowiak et al (32). In this technique, blood flow is measured by using a continuous inhalation of ^{15}O-labeled carbon dioxide. The labeled carbon dioxide is converted to labeled water by carbonic anhydrase in the lung and enters the blood. A steady-state situation in which the delivery of labeled water to the brain becomes equal to the washout and decay of tracer is reached after several half-lives.

The measured activity in the brain at this point is directly proportional to the blood flow. Quantitative values are provided by converting PET counts to milliliters per gram per minute by means of an arterial sample for the measurement of activity in the blood. A similar steady-state scan is obtained during the continuous inhalation of ^{15}O-labeled oxygen. The ratio of the counts obtained during the oxygen scan to the counts measured during the water scan is linearly proportional to the OEF, except for the contribution of intravascular activity.

Baron and co-workers (18) compared the results of the steady-state ^{15}O PET technique, uncorrected for intravascular ^{15}O, with direct measurements of arteriovenous oxygen differences while changing Pa_{CO_2} in baboons. They found a linear relationship between the measured PET OEF and the arteriovenous oxygen difference. A consistent 13.3% overestimation of OEF by PET was found: OEF (arteriovenous oxygen difference) = 1.009 OEF (PET) + 13.3 ($P < .001$). To our knowledge, the first published description of misery perfusion used this uncorrected count-based technique of OEF measurement (2). In subsequent steady-state PET studies (19,33) that incorporated a correction for the intravascular ^{15}O-labeled oxygen, the mean percentage of overestimation of actual quantitative OEF in uninfarcted tissue by using the uncorrected count-based method was 11%–14% in gray matter and 8%–9% in white matter.

The ROC analysis demonstrates similar

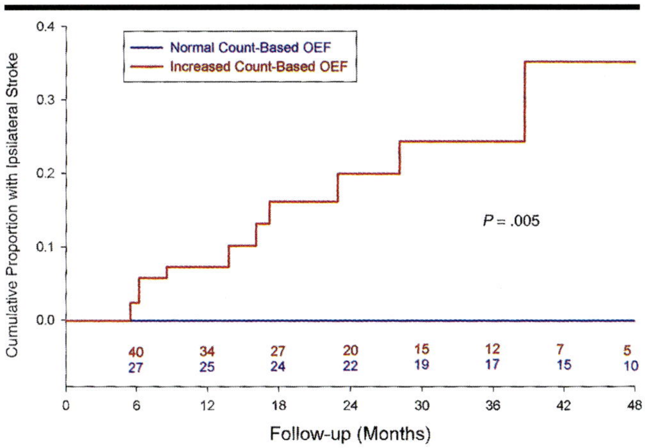

a.

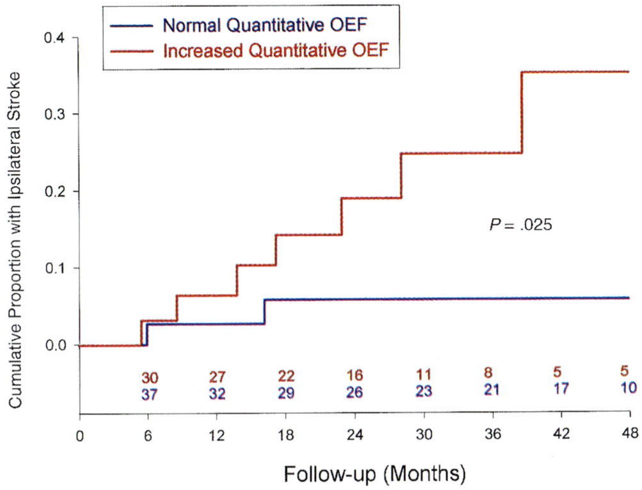

b.

Figure 5. Graphs show Kaplan-Meier cumulative failure curves for the 68 patients with complete quantitative data allowing comparison of count-based OEF and quantitative OEF methods. **(a)** Graph demonstrates the results for count-based OEF. **(b)** Graph shows the results for quantitative OEF. The vertical axis shows the cumulative proportion of patients with ipsilateral stroke. The numbers above the time intervals indicate the total number of patients remaining for follow-up at each 6-month period. The numbers in blue correspond to patients with normal OEF and the numbers in red to those with increased OEF. While the difference in outcome remains statistically significant for both techniques in this smaller group of patients, by using the threshold range of normal OEF established in the healthy volunteers the count-based method is 100% sensitive (all nine ipsilateral strokes occurred in the 41 patients with abnormal OEF), while the quantitative OEF method is not (two strokes occurred in the 37 patients with OEF inside the normal range). Fewer patients have abnormal OEF with the quantitative technique, however (31 compared with 41).

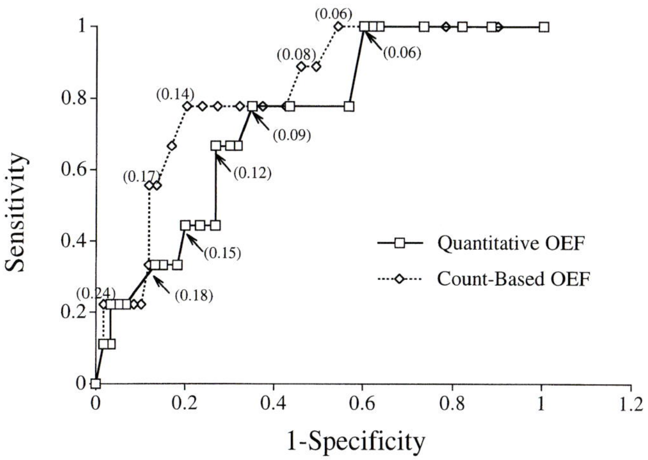

Figure 6. Graph shows ROC curves for the count-based (dotted line) compared with the quantitative (solid line) methods of OEF processing for the 68 patients with complete quantitative data. Sensitivities and specificities of both methods for the prediction of ipsilateral stroke were calculated at progressively greater thresholds from left-to-right ratios of 1.00 ± 0.01 (0.99–1.01) to 1.00 ± 0.28 (0.72–1.28) by increments of 0.01. Several of these thresholds are indicated in parentheses next to their corresponding points on the curve. Higher values of both sensitivity and specificity are seen with the count-based method compared with those of the quantitative technique at nearly all points along the curve. However, owing to the small number of strokes, it is not possible to determine if this apparent improvement in accuracy is real.

sensitivity and specificity of the quantitative and count-based methods. In fact, the area under the curve is greater with the count-based technique. Thus, the count-based method performs as well as, if not better than, the quantitative technique in the prediction of subsequent ipsilateral stroke. With the relatively small number of patients examined with both methods with subsequent strokes at follow-up (nine patients), however, we cannot conclude with any confidence that the count-based OEF technique is better than the quantitative OEF method (34).

One aspect of the count-based OEF method that may provide greater accuracy is the use of the normalizing factor. Quantitative OEF values can vary widely between subjects with normal cerebral hemodynamics but are relatively uniform within individual patients. For example, one subject may have a quantitative OEF of 0.40 in both hemispheres, and another may have a value of 0.30. These absolute values of OEF are within the range of normal. Because of this normal variation in absolute values, we use the hemispheric ratio of OEF to identify abnormally increased OEF. An individual with a mean OEF of 0.30 in the left middle cerebral arterial territory and 0.40 in the right would have a very abnormal OEF ratio: left-to-right ratio of 0.30/0.40 = 0.75, well outside of the normal range.

However, in patients with low absolute values of quantitative OEF, the left-to-right ratio is more likely to fall beyond the normal range than in patients with higher OEF values. For example, a mean OEF of 0.40 on the left and 0.42 on the right would be categorized as normal (ratio = 0.95) while a mean OEF of 0.20 on the left and 0.22 on the right (ratio = 0.909) would be categorized as abnormal. In other words, although the absolute difference in quantitative OEF between the hemispheres is the same in both patients, the relative difference is greater in the patient with lower absolute values. By normalizing the count-based OEF image to a whole-brain mean of 0.40 before calculating the hemispheric ratio, this potential bias in categorization of patients with low absolute values is avoided.

If a multicenter trial is organized to test the effect of surgical revascularization in selected patients with high OEF, the count-based method presented here would hold several advantages over the quantitative technique. First, it may be possible to successfully enroll more patients. It may not be possible or safe to place an arterial catheter in many patients with carotid occlusion. This occurred in six of the 13 patients in whom quantitative processing could not be completed. Also, technical problems may render the arterial time-activity curve data useless, as occurred in five of the remaining seven patients.

Second, processing the count-based images is less complicated. The processing of the PET images, arterial activity curves, and other necessary laboratory data (hematocrit values, etc) required to yield quantitative metabolic data is both time and labor intensive (17,27). Third, the count-based technique does not require the synthesis and administration of ^{15}O-labeled carbon monoxide for a cerebral blood volume scan. Finally, issues of standardization of PET methodology between institutions would be greatly simplified by using this count-based technique, as the software programs used for quantitative metabolic processing would need to be installed on different computer systems.

In summary, we have demonstrated that a count-based method of OEF measurement can be used to predict stroke in patients with symptomatic carotid occlusion. The sensitivity and specificity of this technique for the identification of patients at risk for stroke are comparable to those of the more complicated quantitative method. If a multicenter trial of surgical revascularization for patients with symptomatic carotid occlusion is organized, the count-based method of OEF measurement presented in this article should be used to select patients for surgery. The optimal threshold of the count-based OEF ratio used to select patients for surgery in such a trial will need to be determined through cost-effectiveness analysis.

References

1. Powers WJ, Press GA, Grubb RL Jr, Gado M, Raichle ME. The effect of hemodynamically significant carotid artery disease on the hemodynamic status of the cerebral circulation. Ann Intern Med 1987; 106: 27–35.
2. Baron JC, Bousser MG, Rey A, Guillard A, Comar D, Castaigne P. Reversal of focal "misery perfusion syndrome" by extra-intracranial artery bypass in hemodynamic cerebral ischemia: a case study with O-15 positron emission tomography. Stroke 1981; 12:454–459.
3. Powers WJ. Cerebral hemodynamics in ischemic cerebrovascular disease. Ann Neurol 1991; 29:231–240.
4. Barnett HJ. Hemodynamic cerebral ischemia: an appeal for systematic data gathering prior to a new EC/IC trial. Stroke 1997; 28:1857–1860.
5. Balow J, Alter M, Resch JA. Cerebral thromboembolism: a clinical appraisal of 100 cases. Neurology 1966; 16:559–564.
6. Pessin MS, Duncan GW, Mohr JP, Poskanzer DC. Clinical and angiographic features of carotid transient ischemic attacks. N Engl J Med 1977; 296:358–362.
7. Thiele BL, Young JV, Chikos PM, Hirsch JH, Strandness DE Jr. Correlation of arteriographic findings and symptoms in cerebrovascular disease. Neurology 1980; 30: 1041–1046.
8. Hankey GJ. Prognosis of symptomatic carotid artery occlusion. Cerebrovasc Dis 1991; 1:245–256.
9. Yonas H, Smith HA, Durham SR, Pentheny SL, Johnson DW. Increased stroke risk predicted by compromised cerebral blood flow reactivity. J Neurosurg 1993; 79:483–489.
10. Widder B, Kleiser B, Krapf H. Course of cerebrovascular reactivity in patients with carotid artery occlusions. Stroke 1994; 25:1963–1967.
11. Klijn CJ, Kappelle LJ, Tulleken CA, van Gijn J. Symptomatic carotid artery occlusion: a reappraisal of hemodynamic factors. Stroke 1997; 28:2084–2093.
12. Grubb RL Jr, Derdeyn CP, Fritsch SM, et al. Importance of hemodynamic factors in the prognosis of symptomatic carotid occlusion. JAMA 1998; 280:1055–1060.
13. Powers WJ, Martin WR, Herscovitch P, Raichle ME, Grubb RL Jr. Extracranial-intracranial bypass surgery: hemodynamic and metabolic effects. Neurology 1984; 34:1168–1174.
14. Samson Y, Baron JC, Bousser MG, et al. Effects of extra-intracranial arterial bypass on cerebral blood flow and oxygen metabolism in humans. Stroke 1985; 16:609–615.
15. Gibbs JM, Wise RJ, Thomas DJ, Mansfield AO, Russell RW. Cerebral haemodynamic changes after extracranial-intracranial bypass surgery. J Neurol Neurosurg Psychiatry 1987; 50:140–150.
16. Derdeyn CP, Powers WJ. Positron emission tomography: experimental and clinical applications. In: Batjer HH, ed. Cerebrovascular disease. Philadelphia, Pa: Lippincott-Raven, 1997; 239–253.
17. Mintun MA, Raichle ME, Martin WR, Herscovitch P. Brain oxygen utilization measured with O-15 radiotracers and positron emission tomography. J Nucl Med 1984; 25:177–187.
18. Baron JC, Steinling M, Tanaka T, Cavalheiro E, Sousaline F, Collard P. Quantitative measurement of CBF, oxygen extraction fraction (OEF) and CMRO2 with the O-15 continuous inhalation technique and positron emission tomography (PET): experimental evidence and normal values in man. J Cereb Blood Flow Metab 1981; 1(suppl 1):5–6.
19. Pantano P, Baron JC, Crouzel C, Collard P, Sirou P, Samson Y. The O-15 continuous-inhalation method: correction for intravascular signal using O-15 CO. Eur J Nucl Med 1985; 10:387–391.
20. Derdeyn CP, Yundt KD, Videen TO, Carpenter DA, Grubb RL Jr, Powers WJ. Increased oxygen extraction fraction is associated with prior ischemic events in patients with carotid occlusion. Stroke 1998; 29:754–758.
21. Raichle ME, Martin WR, Herscovitch P, Mintun MA, Markham J. Brain blood flow measured with intravenous H2(15)O. II. Implementation and validation. J Nucl Med 1985; 24:790–798.
22. Welch MJ, Ter-Pogossian MM. Preparation of short half-lived radioactive gases for medical studies. Radiat Res 1968; 36: 580–587.
23. Welch MJ, Lifton JF, Ter-Pogossian MM. The preparation of millicurie quantities of oxygen-15 labeled water. J Lab Clin Med 1969; 5:168–172.
24. Talairach J, Tournoux P. Co-planar stereotactic atlas of the human brain. New York, NY: Thieme Medical, 1988.
25. Grubb RL Jr, Raichle ME, Higgins CS, Eichling JO. Measurement of regional cerebral blood volume by emission tomography. Ann Neurol 1978; 4:322–328.
26. Herscovitch P, Markham J, Raichle ME. Brain blood flow measured with intravenous H2(15)O. I. Theory and error analysis. J Nucl Med 1983; 24:782–789.
27. Videen TO, Perlmutter JS, Herscovitch P, Raichle ME. Brain blood volume, blood flow, and oxygen utilization measured with O-15 radiotracers and positron emission tomography: revised metabolic computations. J Cereb Blood Flow Metab 1987; 7:513–516.
28. Fox PT, Perlmutter JS, Raichle ME. A stereotactic method of anatomical localization for positron emission tomography. J Comput Assist Tomogr 1985; 9:141–153.
29. Hanley JA, Lippman-Hand A. If nothing goes wrong, is everything all right? Interpreting zero numerators. JAMA 1983; 249: 1743–1745.
30. Altman DI, Lich LL, Powers WJ. Brief inhalation method to measure cerebral oxygen extraction fraction with PET: accuracy determination under pathologic conditions. J Nucl Med 1991; 32:1738–1741.
31. Jones T, Chesler DA, Ter-Pogossian MM. The continuous inhalation of oxygen-15 for assessing regional oxygen extraction in the brain of man. Br J Radiol 1976; 49:339–343.
32. Frackowiak RS, Lenzi GL, Jones T, Heather JD. Quantitative measurement of regional cerebral blood flow and oxygen metabolism in man using 15O and positron emission tomography: theory, procedure, and normal values. J Comput Assist Tomogr 1980; 4:727–736.
33. Lammertsma AA, Wise RJ, Heather JD, et al. Correction for the presence of intravascular oxygen-15 in the steady-state technique for measuring regional oxygen extraction ratio in the brain. II. Results in normal subjects and brain tumour and stroke patients. J Cereb Blood Flow Metab 1983; 3:425–431.
34. Hanley JA, McNeil BJ. The meaning and use of the area under a receiver operating characteristic (ROC) curve. Radiology 1982; 143:29–36.

Martin Charron, MD, FRCPC
Fernando J. del Rosario, MD
Samuel A. Kocoshis, MD

Index terms:
Children, gastrointestinal tract, 75.261
Colitis, ulcerative, 75.261
Colon, radionuclide studies, 75.1265
Gastrointestinal tract, radionuclide studies, 75.1265
Inflammation, radionuclide studies, 74.1265, 75.1265
Intestines, radionuclide studies, 74.1265, 75.1265
Leukocytes
Radionuclide imaging, in infants and children, 74.1265, 75.1265

Radiology 1999; 212:507–513

Abbreviations:
CD = Crohn disease
HMPAO = hexamethylpropyleneamine oxime
IBD = inflammatory bowel disease
UC = ulcerative colitis
WBC = white blood cells

[1] From the Departments of Radiology (M.C.) and Gastroenterology (F.J.d.R., S.A.K.), Children's Hospital of Pittsburgh and University of Pittsburgh School of Medicine, Pittsburgh, Pa. Received July 15, 1998; revision requested September 24; final revision received January 13, 1999; accepted February 16. **Address reprint requests to** M.C., 335 S Linden Ave, Pittsburgh, PA 15208 (e-mail: *charron@pop.pitt.edu*).

Author contributions:
Guarantor of integrity of entire study, M.C.; study concepts and design, M.C., F.J.d.R., S.A.K.; definition of intellectual content, M.C., F.J.d.R., S.A.K.; literature research, M.C.; clinical studies, S.A.K., F.J.d.R.; data acquisition, M.C.; data analysis, M.C., F.J.d.R.; statistical analysis, M.C.; manuscript preparation, editing, and review, M.C., F.J.d.R., S.A.K.

Pediatric Inflammatory Bowel Disease: Assessment with Scintigraphy with ^{99m}Tc White Blood Cells[1]

PURPOSE: To evaluate the sensitivity and specificity of scintigraphy with technetium 99m white blood cells (WBC) for detection of colonic inflammation in children with and children without inflammatory bowel disease (IBD).

MATERIALS AND METHODS: In 215 patients, uptake of ^{99m}Tc WBC in 3,440 bowel segments was graded. In 137 of the 215 patients, the ^{99m}Tc WBC scans were interpreted blindly and findings compared with results at colonoscopy and endoscopic biopsy. Planar, single photon emission computed tomographic, and maximum-activity-projection images were reviewed together. In 78 children without recent endoscopic biopsy results, ^{99m}Tc WBC scan findings were compared with laboratory values, the gastroenterologist's initial clinical assessment, and findings at long-term clinical follow-up.

RESULTS: In 128 of 137 children with recent biopsies, findings at histologic examination and on ^{99m}Tc WBC scans were correlated. There were seven false-negative and two false-positive studies. Sensitivity was 90%, specificity 97%, positive predictive value 97%, negative predictive value 93%, prevalence of disease 53%, and overall accuracy 93%. In 75 of 78 (96%) children without recent biopsies, ^{99m}Tc WBC scan findings were consistent with the laboratory values, gastroenterologist's clinical assessment, and long-term clinical follow-up findings.

CONCLUSION: Scintigraphy with ^{99m}Tc WBC is a useful noninvasive diagnostic test to determine the extent and distribution of inflammation in children with IBD.

The treatment of patients with inflammatory bowel disease (IBD) depends on knowledge of the location, extent, and activity of the inflammation. The diagnosis of IBD in children is often complex and difficult. For many years, barium enema examination was the cornerstone of diagnostic testing; recently, colonoscopy is used more liberally.

Promising results have been published about the clinical use of technetium 99m white blood cells (WBC) in the assessment of IBD in adults (1,2) and in a small series of children (3,4). The purpose of this retrospective study was to evaluate the accuracy of ^{99m}Tc WBC scintigraphy for detection of acute inflammation in a large population of children with and children without IBD. In a smaller group of children without recent biopsy results, we compared the scintigraphic result with the laboratory values, the gastroenterologist's clinical assessment, and the long-term clinical follow-up findings.

MATERIALS AND METHODS

Patients

We retrospectively reviewed the charts of 215 consecutive children (100 boys and 115 girls; average age, 12 years; median age, 13 years) who underwent ^{99m}Tc WBC scintigraphy between September 16, 1992, and December 12, 1996.

Diagnoses in 132 of the 215 patients were based on standard colonoscopic, histologic, or radiologic criteria (5,6) and included Crohn disease (CD) in 80 patients, ulcerative colitis

(UC) in 34, and miscellaneous colitis in 18 (indeterminate colitis in 11, infectious colitis in three, autoimmune colitis in three, and toxic colitis in one).

In the 132 patients with IBD, a ^{99m}Tc WBC study was performed to assess the intensity of inflammation in 113, and/or the extent of disease in 98, and/or the presence of small-bowel disease in 72.

Fifty-two of the 215 children had a very low probability of IBD (low-probability group) on the basis of nonspecific gastrointestinal symptoms and no demonstrable findings of IBD with conventional diagnostic methods (ie, radiography, colonoscopy, clinical follow-up). Final diagnoses in this group included lactose intolerance, anal fissure, postviral gastroparesis, gastritis, mesenteric adenitis, duodenogastric reflux, hepatitis, protein-losing enteropathy, duodenitis, chronic constipation, appendicitis, ulcer, irritable bowel syndrome, rectal polyp, and gluten enteropathy. Colonoscopy was performed in 29 of these children and surgery in one. Colonoscopic results were normal in this group, and we arbitrarily chose not to reclassify them into the control group.

Thirty-one control subjects (20 boys and 11 girls; average age, 10 years; median age, 11 years) underwent ^{99m}Tc WBC scanning for nonabdominal problems (the final diagnoses included osteomyelitis, cellulitis, trauma, myocarditis, fever of unknown origin, painful hip, and peritonitis).

The medication regimen of each patient in the week before ^{99m}Tc WBC scintigraphy was recorded, but not that of each control subject. Laboratory values (eg, sedimentation rate and levels of WBC, hemoglobin, hematocrit, platelets, serum albumin, protein, amylase, alanine aminotransferase, aspartate aminotransferase, and γ-glutamyl transpeptidase) were recorded when available. The time between initial diagnosis of IBD and performance of the imaging examination was as long as 62 months (mean, 277 days).

TABLE 1
Number of Children Who Underwent Various Examinations

Examination	CD	UC	Miscellaneous Colitis	Control Subjects	Low Probability	Total
Endoscopic biopsy	36	23	12	31	29	131
Surgery	7*	2*	2*	0	1	12†
Clinical follow-up	39	11	6	0	22	78
Total	80	34	18	31	52	215

* Two children also underwent colonoscopy.
† Six children underwent only surgery (ie, no colonoscopy).

Colonoscopy and Surgery

Colonoscopy and endoscopic biopsy were performed within 30 days (average, 10 days; mode, 7 days) of ^{99m}Tc WBC scintigraphy in 137 of the 215 patients. Diagnoses in 106 of the 137 patients included CD in 41, UC in 23, miscellaneous colitis in 12, and low probability of IBD in 30. Table 1 shows the number of children who underwent surgery, endoscopic biopsy, or both.

Total colonoscopy (models CF100TL or PCF20; Olympus Optical, Tokyo, Japan) was performed by an experienced endoscopist to assess the extent and activity of the mucosal inflammatory changes in eight intestinal segments (rectum, sigmoid, descending, transverse, ascending, cecum, terminal ileum, and small bowel). The endoscopic findings of inflammatory activity were classified as absent (noninflamed mucosa), mild (granularity, edema, invisible vascular pattern), moderate (hyperemia, friability, and all features of mild inflammatory activity), or severe (ulcerations, in addition to features of moderate inflammatory activity) (7).

Surgery was performed in 12 of the 137 patients, within an average of 15 days before ^{99m}Tc WBC scintigraphy. Six of the patients who underwent surgery also underwent colonoscopy. Macroscopic findings at surgery and microscopic details at biopsy of resected segments were compared with the grade for the ^{99m}Tc WBC scan.

Patients without Colonoscopic Data: Clinical Follow-up

The remaining 78 children (22 with low probability, 56 with IBD [CD in 39, UC in 11, and miscellaneous colitis in six]) underwent colonoscopy longer than 1 month before ^{99m}Tc scintigraphy. Findings on the ^{99m}Tc WBC scans were compared with laboratory values, the gastroenterologist's initial assessment, and findings at clinical follow-up in the 56 children with IBD (average follow-up, 398 days) and in the 22 low-probability patients (average follow-up, 336 days).

Scanning Examinations

Venous blood (20–45 mL) was withdrawn into a 60-mL syringe containing 7 mL of acid citrate dextrose solution. Six percent hetastarch (5 mL) was added and mixed. The syringe was inverted and allowed to settle for 40–60 minutes. The leukocyte-rich plasma was collected and centrifuged at 300 *g* for 5 minutes. A vial with 0.5 mg of hexamethyl-propylene-amine oxime (HMPAO) (Cerentec; Nycomed Amersham, Princeton, NJ) was reconstituted with 1,110 MBq ^{99m}Tc (3 mL), and radiochemical purity was tested. The ^{99m}Tc HMPAO (2.5 mL [925 MBq]) was added to the leukocyte button, mixed gently, and incubated for 15 minutes. Platelet-rich plasma (5 mL) was added, and the entire preparation was centrifuged for 5 minutes. The ^{99m}Tc leukocyte button was reconstituted in 5 mL platelet-rich plasma and assayed in a dose calibrator. The adult dose of 740 MBq per kilogram of body weight was adjusted for children to 20 MBq/kg. The average efficiency of labeling was 62%. The blood was then reinjected intravenously.

In all patients, imaging was performed at ½ to 1 hour after injection, with a gamma camera (Large Field of View; Siemens Orbiter, Des Plaines, Ill) fitted with a low-energy, high-resolution collimator. Anterior and posterior 8-minute images of the abdomen and pelvis were recorded in analog and digital form. Pelvic outlet, or caudal, views were also obtained to distinguish bladder from rectal inflammation activities. Anterior views of the abdomen were obtained with the patient standing, to separate the liver from the transverse colon. At 2–4 hours after injection in all patients, an 8-minute anterior view of the abdomen was acquired.

Also at 2–4 hours after injection in 97 patients, single photon emission computed tomography (SPECT) was performed with a newly purchased double-headed camera (model dst-xl; SMV, Twinsburgh, Ohio). SPECT was performed with the following acquisition parameters: 30 seconds per stop; 60 stops; 120 projections; 1.6 magnification; Hanning-Nyquist prefilter, 1.515; cut-off, 1.315; Nyquist ramp filter, 1.515; cut-off, 1.31. SPECT was not performed in the 31 control subjects. Volume-rendered images were derived from the SPECT data by means of the maximum-activity-projection technique. When scan findings were

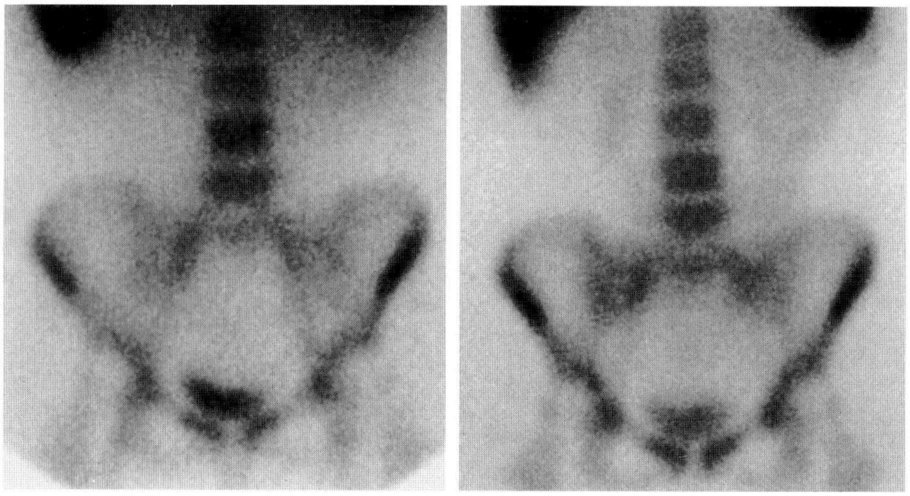

a. b.

Figure 1. Normal ^{99m}Tc WBC studies at **(a)** 30 minutes and **(b)** 3 hours.

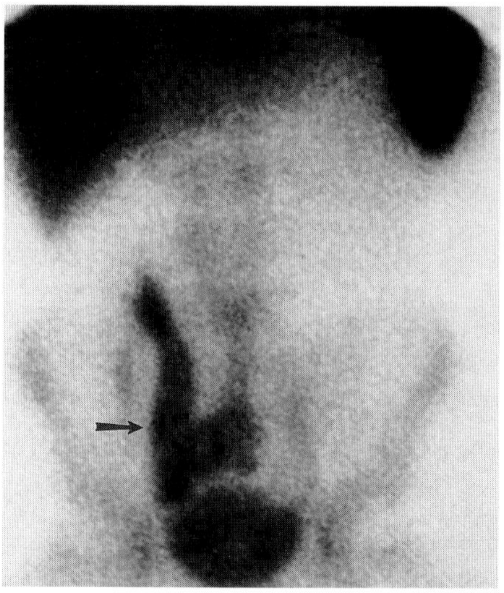

Figure 2. Abnormal uptake of ^{99m}Tc WBC in the terminal ileum (arrow) in a child with CD. The uptake is intense, bowel-shaped, and appears early (at 30 minutes). On the late scan (not shown), the uptake did not move or change shape, which suggests active inflammation (proved at endoscopic biopsy).

equivocal, delayed imaging was performed at 6–8 hours and, rarely, at 24 hours, to differentiate active CD from late accumulation of ^{99m}Tc WBC in the right lower quadrant. Cinematic representations of some of the maximum-activity-projection ^{99m}Tc WBC images are available for review at our Internet site: *http://128.147.46.201.*

Analysis of Scans

To assess the sensitivity and specificity of ^{99m}Tc WBC scintigraphy with each set of scans (½ to 1 hour and 2–4 hours) in the 215 patients, the bowel was divided into eight segments (rectum, sigmoid, descending, transverse, ascending, cecum, terminal ileum, and small bowel). This resulted in 3,440 bowel segments to be scored (ie, eight segments × two images × 215 patients = 3,440 segments). The inflammatory activity in each segment on the planar images was graded semiquantitatively by one reviewer (M.C.) by comparing the uptake in the bowel with that in the liver and the bone marrow in the iliac crest (8–11). The following grading scale was used: grade 0, no inflammatory activity; grade 1, inflammatory activity less than that in the iliac crest; grade 2, activity similar to that in the iliac crest; grade 3, activity greater than that in the iliac crest; grade 4, activity equal to that in the liver; grade 5, activity greater than that in the liver; grade 6, activity equal to that in the spleen.

The grade of uptake on the planar images was compared with the endoscopic biopsy result. Planar, orthogonal SPECT, and maximum-activity-projection images were reviewed together on a workstation with ad lib manipulation of intensity scale, contrast, color scale, and cine display. Maximum-activity-projection images were used to help interpret the SPECT images (12–14).

A ^{99m}Tc WBC scintigram was considered false-negative if there was a difference in the degree of inflammation depicted and the result at endoscopic biopsy (ie, mild inflammation [grade 1 or 2] depicted but severe inflammation seen at colonoscopy). A ^{99m}Tc WBC scintigram was considered false-positive if it depicted increased uptake of ^{99m}Tc WBC in an area that was seen to be normal at endoscopic biopsy. Thus, ^{99m}Tc WBC scans in one patient with active gastrointestinal bleeding were considered to be false-positive despite movement of inflammatory activity over time at colonoscopy. Inflammatory activity seen at a colostomy or ileostomy site was excluded from analysis.

RESULTS

Findings at ^{99m}Tc WBC Scintigraphy and Biopsy

In the 137 children with endoscopic biopsy results, the sensitivity of ^{99m}Tc WBC scintigraphy was 90%, the specificity 97%, the positive predictive value 97%, and the negative predictive value 93% (Table 2). The prevalence of disease was 53%, and the accuracy of ^{99m}Tc WBC scintigraphy was 93%. When children with miscellaneous colitis were excluded from analysis, the sensitivity of ^{99m}Tc WBC scintigraphy was 93% (57 of 61 patients). The number of normal (Fig 1) and positive and negative scans is also given in Table 2.

In 128 of the 137 patients with a biopsy specimen, the intensity and location of inflammation were consistent with those on the ^{99m}Tc WBC scan (Figs 2, 3). In this group, there were two false-positive studies and seven false-negative studies (two in patients with CD, two with UC, and three with miscellaneous colitis). Note that four of the children with a false-negative ^{99m}Tc WBC study had normal laboratory values and a visually normal colonic mucosa during colonoscopy, with mild chronic inflammation seen at biopsy. These findings suggest that minute microscopic inflammation may not be scintigraphically evident. The remaining three false-negative ^{99m}Tc WBC studies were seen in children with miscellaneous colitis (three with autoimmune colitis), who had moderately to severely abnormal laboratory values and moderate to severe inflammation at colonoscopy.

In five patients (two with CD, one with low probability, one with miscellaneous colitis), the ^{99m}Tc WBC studies underestimated the amount of inflammation in one segment; other segments were positive in these patients. Labeling efficiency in the false-negative ^{99m}Tc WBC study was greater than 50% and thus did not account for the lack of uptake. False-positive ^{99m}Tc WBC studies were seen in a child who was actively bleeding from the

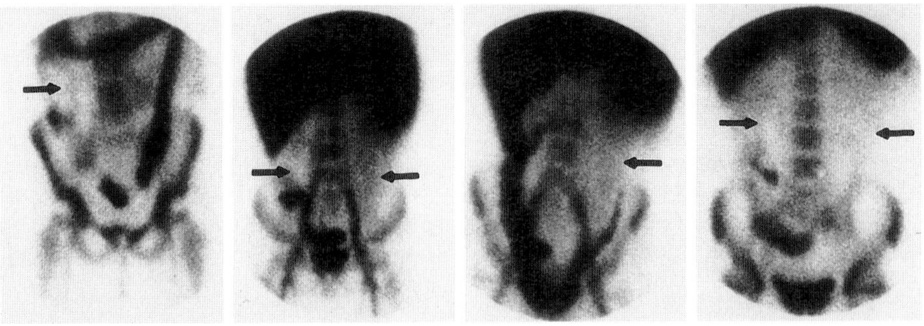

Figure 3. Skip areas of inflammation (arrows) are depicted on the ^{99m}Tc WBC scans obtained in four children with CD (proved at endoscopic biopsy).

TABLE 2
Results with ^{99m}Tc WBC Scintigraphy

Result	CD	UC	Miscellaneous Colitis	Control Subjects	Low Probability	Total
Number of biopsies	41	23	12	31	30	137
^{99m}Tc WBC findings						
Positive	38	21	8	0	0	67
Negative	3	2	4	31	30	70
Biopsy findings						
Negative	2	1	1	31	30	65
Positive	39	22	11	0	0	72
Findings						
False-positive (FP)	1	1	0	0	0	2
False-negative (FN)	2	2	3	0	0	7
True-positive (TP)	37	20	8	0	0	65
True-negative (TN)	1	0	1	31	30	63
Sensitivity	95	91	73	NA	NA	90*
Specificity	50†	0	100	100	100	97
Positive predictive value	97	95	100	NA	NA	97
Negative predictive value	50†	0	25†	100	100	93

Note.—Data are the number of patients. Accuracy = 93% (TP + TN) × 100)/(TP + FN + FP + TN). NA = not applicable. Negative predictive value (%) = (TN × 100)/(TN + FN). Positive predictive value (%) = (TP × 100)/(TP + FP). Prevalence = 53% = (TP + FN) × 100)/(TP + FN + FP + TN). Sensitivity (%) = (TP × 100)/(TP + FN). Specificity (%) = (TN × 100)/(TN + FP).
* 93% when analysis excludes miscellaneous colitis.
† Calculated with results in four or fewer patients.

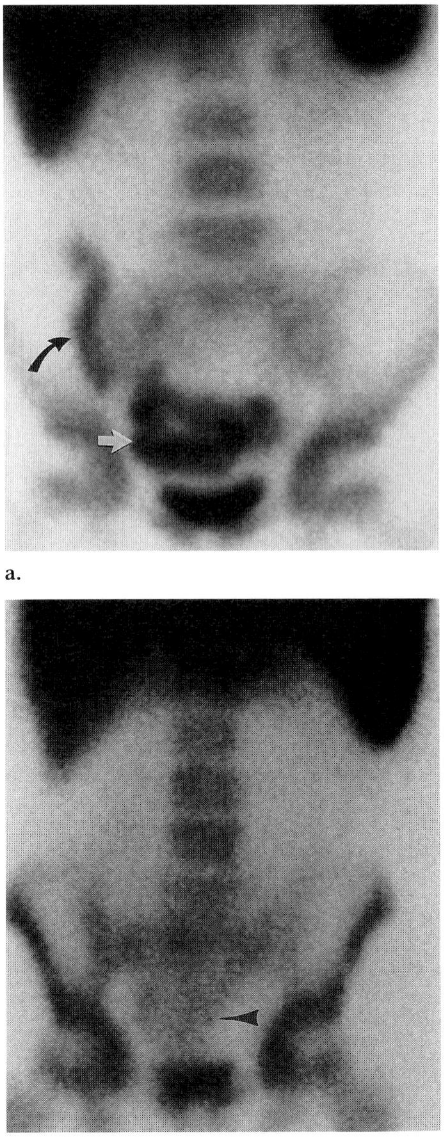

a.

b.

Figure 4. CD depicted on ^{99m}Tc WBC scans. **(a)** At 3 hours after injection, inflammation is depicted in the terminal ileum (curved arrow) and small bowel (straight arrow). This pattern of uptake contrasts singularly with **(b)** the late physiologic excretion (mild ill-defined uptake) (arrowhead) seen in a different patient at 3 hours.

gastrointestinal tract and in a child with a new surgical anastomosis. In the patient with gastrointestinal bleeding, delayed images revealed movement of inflammatory activity in the distal bowel, a finding not suggestive of active inflammation.

No false-positive ^{99m}Tc WBC studies were seen in the 31 control subjects or in the 30 children in the low-probability group (SPECT images were normal) who had undergone biopsy. One child in the low-probability group had a rectal polyp with associated acute and chronic inflammation seen at biopsy, yet the ^{99m}Tc WBC scan was normal.

Surgery

The ^{99m}Tc WBC scan showed the same intensity and distribution of inflammation as was seen in the surgical specimens in all but one patient, in whom the scan underestimated the inflammation in the cecum while accurately showing inflammation in the rest of the colon.

One child's resected ileum and ascending colon showed an area of focal ulceration and increased lymphoid inflammatory cells within the lamina propria and inflammatory cells in the muscularis externa at the margin of resection. In this patient, the ^{99m}Tc WBC scan acquired after surgery correctly depicted increased accumulation of ^{99m}Tc WBC at the anastomotic site.

Another child underwent exploratory laparoscopy that revealed a macroscopically normal ileum, and 3 days later, a ^{99m}Tc WBC scan showed abnormal localization in the terminal ileum. Three days after the ^{99m}Tc WBC scan was acquired, colonoscopy revealed inflammation in the terminal ileum.

One of the children in the low-probability group underwent appendectomy, and both the pathologic specimen and the ^{99m}Tc WBC scan were normal.

Patients without Colonoscopic Data

In 75 (96%) of 78 children (39 with CD, 11 with UC, six with miscellaneous colitis, 22 with low probability [Table 1]) without recent endoscopic biopsy results, the laboratory values, gastroenterologist's initial assessment, and findings at clinical follow-up (average, 398 days) were consistent with the results at ^{99m}Tc WBC scintigraphy.

In the 39 children with CD and without recent endoscopic biopsy results, 38 studies were abnormal. In 37 of these children, the scan results were congruent with the laboratory values, gastroenterologist's initial assessment, and findings at clinical follow-up (average, 464 days). In the two children with positive ^{99m}Tc WBC studies that were not consistent with the findings at clinical follow-up, laboratory values were normal at presentation, and the prednisone dose was lowered. At clinical follow-up, however, these children did not experience any exacerbation of their symptoms. In three patients with CD, small-bowel uptake of ^{99m}Tc WBC was seen due to gastrointestinal bleeding. Uptake was also noted in an abdominal scar in a child who underwent surgery 9 days prior to scanning. In four different children, uptake of ^{99m}Tc WBC was seen at a stricture site, as documented at upper gastrointestinal and small-bowel follow-through examinations. Recent endoscopic biopsy results were not available to document the histologic nature of the strictured areas. Similarly, uptake was seen in a perirectal abscess and fistula in two children with CD. In four other children, uptake of ^{99m}Tc WBC was seen at an anastomotic site, and we could not differentiate active CD from normal inflammatory repair.

In all six children with miscellaneous colitis and 10 of the 11 children with UC, results at ^{99m}Tc WBC scintigraphy were congruent with laboratory values, the gastroenterologist's initial assessment, and clinical follow-up findings. In one child with UC, uptake of ^{99m}Tc WBC was seen in the right lower quadrant, and we could not exclude subclinical appendicitis or CD. In a 14-year-old girl with UC and known pancreatitis, the ^{99m}Tc WBC study did not show any uptake in the pancreas.

Twenty-one children in the low-probability group had a normal ^{99m}Tc WBC study, and there was no evidence of IBD on the basis of laboratory values or findings at clinical follow-up (average, 336 days). In one child in the low-probability group, ^{99m}Tc WBC uptake was seen in a loop of small bowel, but there was no clinical suggestion of IBD on the basis of findings at prolonged follow-up (558 days). In one child in this group, inflammatory activity was seen in a dilated ureter that could have been ascribed to small-bowel uptake.

Miscellaneous Colitis

The initial disease classification prior to ^{99m}Tc WBC scintigraphy was incorrect in two patients. The correct classifications were suggested by findings on the ^{99m}Tc WBC scan, and they were subsequently proved at surgery. One of these two patients was referred to our center with a diagnosis of UC, but the ^{99m}Tc WBC scan depicted small-intestine disease indicative of Crohn disease (Fig 4). Disease in the other patient was initially diagnosed as indeterminate colitis, but grade 3 rectosigmoid involvement and the lack of skip areas or small-intestine involvement helped correct prediction of the surgical diagnosis of UC.

In eight children, a segment with increased uptake of ^{99m}Tc WBC depicted on the SPECT and maximum-activity-projection images was depicted as normal on the planar images. In all these children, planar images depicted abnormal uptake of ^{99m}Tc WBC in other segments of the bowel (sum of scores for each segment, 24, 6, 9, 27, 18, 3, 12, 14, respectively). Three of these children underwent colonoscopy, which revealed very mild inflammation in the segment missed on the planar images.

In 11 other patients, SPECT and maximum-activity-projection images revealed uptake of ^{99m}Tc WBC at colostomy or ileostomy sites. We were able to identify all patients with active gastrointestinal bleeding on the basis of movement of inflammatory activity depicted over time, without interfering with the interpretation of inflammation in patients with IBD.

No side effect of ^{99m}Tc WBC was reported in any children. Among 120 of the 184 patients, 105 (88%) had abnormal ^{99m}Tc WBC studies at 30 minutes and 15 (12%) had abnormal studies only later.

DISCUSSION

IBD is an important category of chronic gastrointestinal disease. The approach to treatment of a child with suspected IBD is intricate. The accuracy of colonoscopic diagnosis of IBD ranges from 80% to 90% (15–17). One weakness with colonoscopy and biopsy as the reference method is that the biopsy specimen may not be representative of an entire colorectal segment, particularly in patients with CD, in whom the inflammatory changes are often patchy. There appears to be no justification for repeated routine endoscopic assessment of colonic inflammation, since there is poor correlation between clinical symptoms and endoscopic and histologic findings (15,16). Endoscopic and radiologic methods of disease localization are more invasive than is ^{99m}Tc WBC scintigraphy, and they tend to produce more discomfort related to instrumentation and preparation for the procedure (eg, bowel cleansing). Moreover, several studies are needed to analyze the entire bowel, since colonoscopy cannot be used to analyze the entire small bowel.

A noninvasive technique is needed that can be used in the follow-up of pediatric patients. Scintigraphy with ^{99m}Tc WBC seems ideally suited to obtain a precise temporal snapshot of the distribution and intensity of inflammation, whereas radiographic modalities tend to depict more chronic changes. An additional advantage is high patient acceptability, especially in children. Patients prefer ^{99m}Tc WBC scintigraphy to barium follow-through study or enteroclysis. The effective dose equivalent for a ^{99m}Tc WBC study is approximately 3 mSv, whereas it is on the order of 6 mSv for a barium small-bowel follow-through study or 8.5 mSv for a barium enema examination (18). A positive ^{99m}Tc WBC study occurs by 30 minutes in most children (88%). The examination can be terminated if there is a clinical need.

Scintigraphy with ^{99m}Tc WBC has been reported to be sensitive for the detection of inflammation in adults (1,2,8–10,19–23) and small series of children (4,22,24,25). The correlation between scintigraphic and endoscopic findings is sufficiently close that scintigraphy can supplement left-side colonoscopy if total colonoscopy is technically impossible (2,8,10,26–30). Scintigraphy with ^{99m}Tc WBC may replace colonoscopy as a monitoring tool for inflammatory activity. Scintigraphy can also be used to document proximal extension of ulcerative proctosigmoiditis (31) (Fig 5) or postoperative recurrence of CD (32). Scintigraphy with ^{99m}Tc WBC is useful to assess the inflammatory component of a stricture seen on a small-bowel follow-through study.

However, ^{99m}Tc WBC scintigraphy has limitations. It is not useful to define anatomic details such as strictures, prestenotic dilations, or fistulas, which are best evaluated with barium radiographic studies. In a patient with CD, distinction of the large from the small bowel can be difficult if the uptake is focal, since landmarks disappear. The presence of gastrointestinal bleeding during the ^{99m}Tc WBC study can complicate the interpretation of findings. Clearance of uptake from the initial site on the delayed images indicates the presence of gastrointestinal bleeding.

Our experience suggests that inflammation on a ^{99m}Tc WBC scan is bowel shaped, does not move on the late scan, and increases in intensity over time. Three-dimensional display of SPECT data by means of the maximum-activity-projection technique increases continuity of structures and facilitates understanding of spatial relationships (14). This technique, used routinely at our institution, has advantages and limitations that have been enumerated (12,13). Maximum-activity-projection images are not a substitute for SPECT images, and both sets of images should be reviewed together (12). In eight children, a segment of bowel with increased uptake of ^{99m}Tc WBC was depicted on only the SPECT and maximum-activity-projection images. On the planar images for these children, however, uptake of ^{99m}Tc WBC was abnormal in other bowel segments. Therefore, the routine use of SPECT is probably not indicated. The detection of one additional segment with minimal inflammation is unlikely to change patient treatment.

In this study, we found high accuracy for ^{99m}Tc WBC scintigraphy in the evaluation of inflammation in children with IBD. We compared the findings at ^{99m}Tc WBC scintigraphy to those at biopsy in three groups of children: patients with known IBD, control subjects, and patients with a low probability of IBD. This variation in pretest probability of disease allowed us to accurately calculate the positive and negative predictive values of ^{99m}Tc WBC scintigraphy in children with and children without IBD. Compared with the accuracy of colonoscopy (17), the accuracy of ^{99m}Tc WBC scintigraphy is more than 90%. Compared with the accuracy of laboratory values, the gastroenterologist's initial assessment, and clinical follow-up findings (15), the accuracy of ^{99m}Tc WBC scintigraphy is even higher, although in a small number of children there was no standard of reference that could corroborate the ^{99m}Tc WBC scan findings of uptake at fistulas and anastomoses. We had no false-positive ^{99m}Tc WBC scintigraphic findings in 79 control subjects, which helps confirm a high positive predictive value for ^{99m}Tc WBC scintigraphy. False-negative ^{99m}Tc WBC studies or scans that underestimated the amount of inflammation were seen in a few cases of early CD with a few small aphthoid ulcers and in cases of autoimmune colitis. In most of the children without recent endoscopic biopsy findings, laboratory values, the gastroenterologist's initial assessment, and clinical follow-up findings agreed with the ^{99m}Tc WBC scan findings.

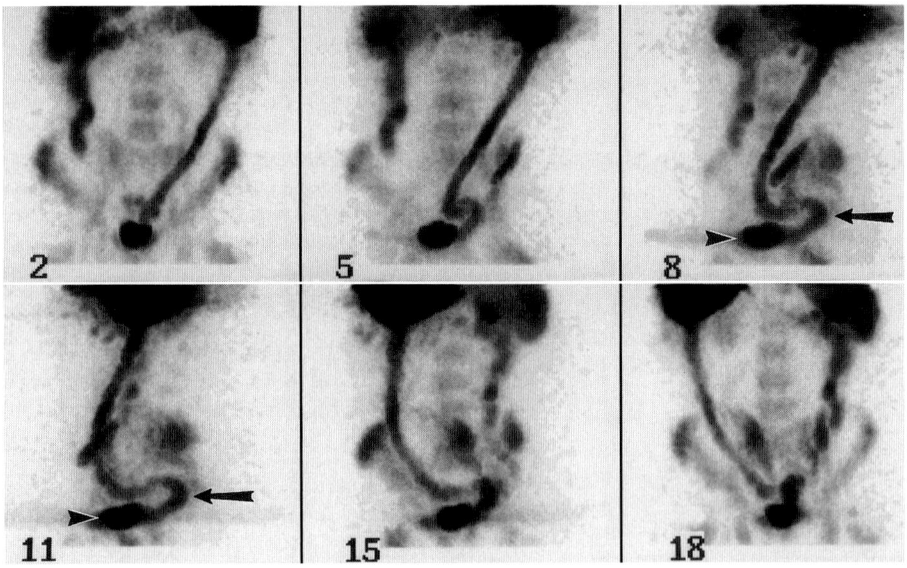

Figure 5. Multiple continuous ^{99m}Tc WBC projections from a three-dimensional cine display on our Internet site (see Materials and Methods) show separation of inflammatory activity in the rectum (arrow) from that in the bladder (arrowhead).

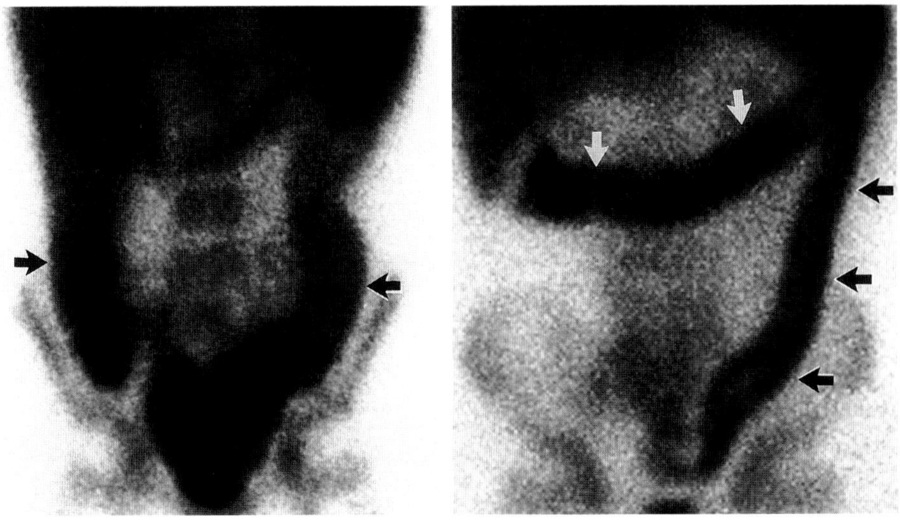

a. b.

Figure 6. **(a,b)** Continuous uptake (arrows) is depicted on ^{99m}Tc WBC scans obtained in two different children with UC.

In a few children, uptake of ^{99m}Tc WBC was depicted at anastomotic sites. Because of the lack of biopsy data at these sites, we could not document the nature of these findings. In a recent prospective study in 17 patients, Biancone et al (32) evaluated ^{99m}Tc WBC scintigraphy for the early detection of postoperative, asymptomatic recurrence of CD. They found the ^{99m}Tc WBC studies to be accurate. We observed focal uptake of ^{99m}Tc WBC in fistulas and in one polyp, as reported by others (33). Because of the punctiform nature of the findings, this is easily distinguishable from uptake in IBD. An exception is the presence of focal inflammatory activity near the cecum; the differential diagnosis then also includes appendicitis. Appendiceal involvement was recently reported (34–37) to occur in UC, and this could have been the case in one of our patients.

This study has three potential limitations. Colonoscopy is not a perfect standard of reference, and thus some discrepancies between ^{99m}Tc WBC scintigraphy and colonoscopy can be expected. Also, only one nuclear physician interpreted each scan blindly, albeit the scans are easy to interpret (Fig 6). Finally, SPECT data in this series were not obtained in control subjects. Since SPECT findings may decrease the specificity of ^{99m}Tc WBC scintigraphy, it is conceivable that we might have seen some false-positive results if SPECT had been performed in the control subjects. SPECT images were obtained in the low-probability group, however, and no false-positive results were seen.

In conclusion, ^{99m}Tc WBC scintigraphy is an accurate technique to assess inflammation in children with IBD. Scintigraphy should play an important role in the follow-up of IBD patients, especially in cases of suspected recurrence and in the monitoring of treatment, which would reduce the need for repeated colonoscopy. Scintigraphy with ^{99m}Tc WBC is a rapid, relatively painless test that requires no bowel preparation. The minimal invasiveness of ^{99m}Tc WBC scintigraphy makes it a practical modality for the evaluation of children with IBD. It is economical, and its diagnostic sensitivity is excellent.

Acknowledgments: We thank Ricki Smith and Melanie Fitzgerald for their help with the manuscript. We also thank A. Delbert Bowen, MD, Thomas Foley, MD, Patty Murtha, PhD, David Townsend, PhD, and Nick Bohnen, MD, PhD, for their helpful comments about the manuscript.

References

1. Reynolds JH, Graham D, Smith FW. Imaging inflammation with ^{99m}Tc HMPAO labelled leucocytes. Clin Radiol 1990; 42: 195–198.
2. Kennan N, Hayward M. Tc HMPAO-labelled white cell scintigraphy in Crohn's disease of the small bowel. Clin Radiol 1992; 45:331–334.
3. Bhargava SA, Orenstein SR, Charron M. Technetium-99m hexamethylpropylene-amine-oxime–labeled leukocyte scintigraphy in inflammatory bowel disease in children. J Pediatr 1994; 125:213–217.
4. Charron M, Ironstone SR, Bhargava S. Detection of inflammatory bowel disease in pediatric patients with technetium-99m-HMPAO-labeled leukocytes. J Nucl Med 1994; 35:451–455.
5. Lennard-Jones JE. Classification of inflammatory bowel disease. Scand J Gastroenterol Suppl 1989; 170:2–6.
6. Lennard-Jones JE. Classification of inflammatory bowel disease. Scand J Gastroenterol Suppl 1989; 170:16–19.
7. Sninsky CA, Cort DH, Shanahan F, et al. Oral mesalamine (Asacol) for mildly to moderately active ulcerative colitis: a multicenter study. Ann Intern Med 1991; 115:350–355.
8. Giaffer MH, Tindale WB, Holdsworth D. Value of technetium-99m HMPAO-labelled leucocyte scintigraphy as an initial screening test in patients suspected of having inflammatory bowel disease. Eur J Gastroenterol Hepatol 1996; 8:1195–2000.
9. Middleton SJ, Li D, Wharton S, Reynolds PD, Wraight EP, Hunter JO. Validation of ^{99m}Tc-HMPAO leucocyte scintigraphy in ulcerative colitis by comparison with histology. Br J Radiol 1995; 68:1061–1066.
10. Sciarretta G, Furno A, Mazzoni M, Basile C, Malaguti P. Technetium-99m hexamethyl propylene amine oxime granulocyte scintigraphy in Crohn's disease: diagnostic and clinical relevance. Gut 1993; 34:1364–1369.
11. Kolkman JJ, Falke TH, Roos JC, et al. Computed tomography and granulocyte scintigraphy in active inflammatory bowel disease: comparison with endoscopy and operative findings. Dig Dis Sci 1996; 41: 641–650.
12. Keyes JW Jr. Three-dimensional display of SPECT images: advantages and problems (editorial). J Nucl Med 1990; 31:1428–1430.
13. Wallis JW, Miller TR. Three-dimensional display in nuclear medicine and radiology. J Nucl Med 1991; 32:534–546.
14. Wallis JW, Miller TR. Volume rendering in three-dimensional display of SPECT images. J Nucl Med 1990; 31:1421–1428.
15. Gomes P, du Boulay C, Smith CL, Holdstock G. Relationship between disease activity indices and colonoscopic findings in patients with colonic inflammatory bowel disease. Gut 1986; 27:92–95.
16. Landi B, Anh TN, Cortot A, et al. Endoscopic monitoring of Crohn's disease treatment: a prospective, randomized clinical trial—the Groupe d'Etudes Therapeutiques des Affections Inflammatoires Digestives. Gastroenterology 1992; 102: 1647–1653.
17. Pera A, Bellando P, Caldera D, et al. Colonoscopy in inflammatory bowel disease: diagnostic accuracy and proposal of an endoscopic score. Gastroenterology 1987; 92:181–185.
18. Shields RA, Lawson RS. Effective dose equivalent. Nucl Med Commun 1987; 8:851–855.
19. Arndt JW, Grootscholten MI, van Hogezand RA, Griffioen G, Lamers CB, Pauwels EK. Inflammatory bowel disease activity assessment using technetium-99m-HMPAO leukocytes. Dig Dis Sci 1997; 42:387–393.
20. Gibson P, Lichtenstein M, Salehi N, Hebbard G, Andrews J. Value of positive technetium-99m leucocyte scans in predicting intestinal inflammation. Gut 1991; 32:1502–1507.
21. Charron M, Fernando del Rosario J, Kocoshis S. Distribution of acute bowel inflammation determined by technetium-labeled white blood cells in children with inflammatory bowel disease. Inflamm Bowel Dis 1998; 4:84–88.
22. Jobling JC, Lindley KJ, Yousef Y, Gordon I, Milla PJ. Investigating inflammatory bowel disease: white cell scanning, radiology, and colonoscopy. Arch Dis Child 1996; 74:22–26.
23. Papos M, Nagy F, Lang J, Csernay L. Technetium-99m hexamethylpropylene-amine oxime labelled leucocyte scintigraphy in ulcerative colitis and Crohn's disease. Eur J Nucl Med 1993; 20:766–769.
24. Jewell FM, Davies A, Sandhu B, Duncan A, Grier D. Technetium-99m-HMPAO labelled leucocytes in the detection and monitoring of inflammatory bowel disease in children. Br J Radiol 1996; 69:508–514.
25. Papos M, Varkonyi A, Lang J, et al. HMPAO-labeled leukocyte scintigraphy in pediatric patients with inflammatory bowel disease. J Pediatr Gastroenterol Nutr 1996; 23:547–552.
26. Allan RA, Sladen GE, Bassingham S, Lazarus C, Clarke SE, Fogelman I. Comparison of simultaneous ^{99m}Tc-HMPAO and ^{111}In-oxine labelled white cell scans in the assessment of inflammatory bowel disease. Eur J Nucl Med 1993; 20:195–200.
27. Becker W, Schomann E, Fischbach W, Borner W, Gruner KR. Comparison of ^{99m}Tc-HMPAO and ^{111}In-oxine labelled granulocytes in man: first clinical results. Nucl Med Commun 1988; 9:435–447.
28. Roddie ME, Peters AM, Danpure HJ, et al. Inflammation: imaging with Tc-99m HMPAO-labeled leukocytes. Radiology 1988; 166:767–772.
29. Spinelli F, Milella M, Sara R, et al. The ^{99m}Tc-HMPAO leukocyte scan: an alternative to radiology and endoscopy in evaluating the extent and the activity of inflammatory bowel disease. J Nucl Biol Med 1991; 35:82–87.
30. Giaffer MH. Labelled leucocyte scintigraphy in inflammatory bowel disease: clinical applications. Gut 1996; 38:1–5.
31. Almers S, Granerus G, Franzen L, Strom M. Technetium-99m scintigraphy: more accurate assessment of ulcerative colitis with exametazime-labelled leucocytes than with antigranulocyte antibodies. Eur J Nucl Med 1996; 23:247–255.
32. Biancone L, Scopinaro F, Ierardi M, et al. ^{99m}Tc-HMPAO granulocyte scintigraphy in the early detection of postoperative asymptomatic recurrence in Crohn's disease. Dig Dis Sci 1997; 42:1549–1556.
33. Figa M, Acero D, Gonzalez-Huix F, Berna L. Tc-99m HMPAO labeled leukocyte uptake by an inflammatory fibroid polyp of the ileum. Clin Nucl Med 1994; 19:356.
34. Kroft SH, Stryker SJ, Rao MS. Appendiceal involvement as a skip lesion in ulcerative colitis. Mod Pathol 1994; 7:912–914.
35. Davison AM, Dixon MF. The appendix as a 'skip lesion' in ulcerative colitis. Histopathology 1990; 16:93–95.
36. Cohen T, Pfeffer RB, Valensi Q. Ulcerative appendicitis occurring as a skip lesion in chronic ulcerative colitis: report of a case. Am J Gastroenterol 1974; 62:151–155.
37. Groisman GM, George J, Harpaz N. Ulcerative appendicitis in universal and nonuniversal ulcerative colitis. Mod Pathol 1994; 7:322–355.

Patient with a Frog in His Throat

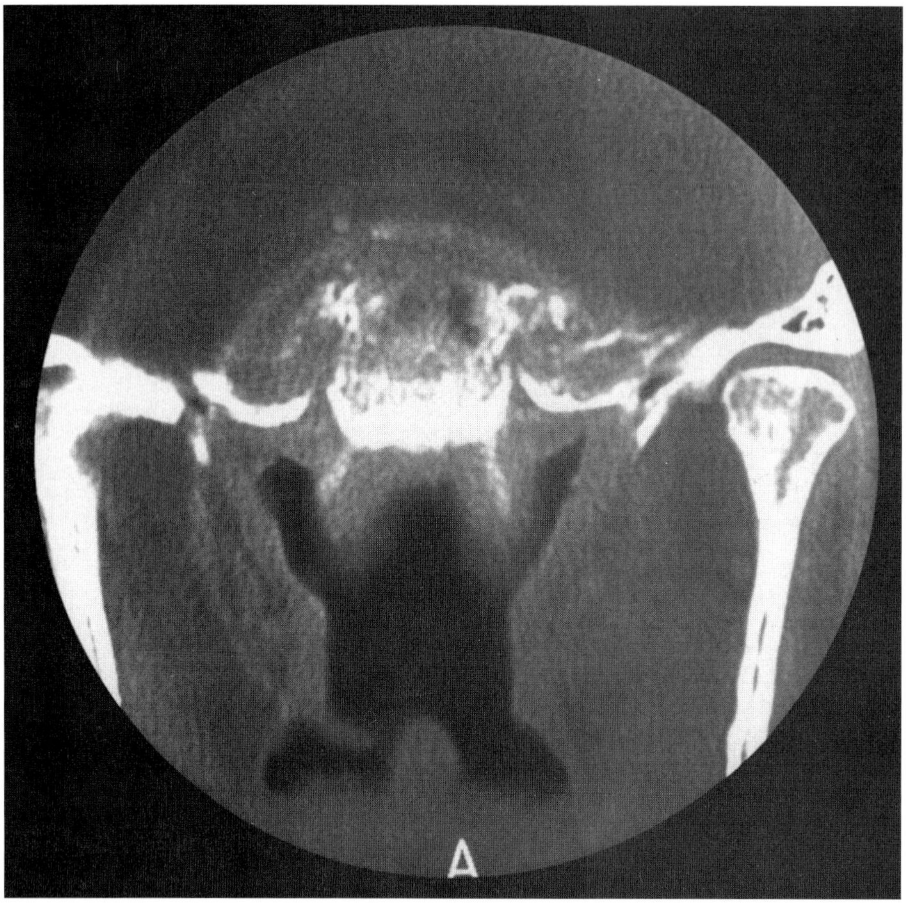

Courtesy of Bruce N. Troup, MD, PhD, Napa, Calif

Splenic Injury Diagnosed with CT: US Follow-up and Healing Rate in Children and Adolescents[1]

Kathleen H. Emery, MD
Diane S. Babcock, MD
Andrea S. Borgman, MD
Victor F. Garcia, MD

Index terms
Spleen, CT, 775.12112
Spleen, injuries, 775.411, 775.43
Spleen, neoplasms, 775.3121
Spleen, US, 775.1298

Radiology 1999; 212:515–518

[1] From the Departments of Radiology (K.H.E., D.S.B., A.S.B.) and Pediatric Surgery (V.F.G.), Children's Hospital Medical Center, 3333 Burnet Ave, Cincinnati, OH 45229-3039. From the 1997 RSNA scientific assembly. Received August 12, 1998; revision requested September 25; revision received December 22; accepted February 12, 1999. **Address reprint requests to** K.H.E.

PURPOSE: To determine if pediatric splenic injury healing observed during ultrasonography (US) is related to the computed tomographic (CT) grade of injury severity, to review any delayed complications, and to formulate a grade-specific timetable for follow-up imaging.

MATERIALS AND METHODS: Sixty-eight children and adolescents with CT-documented blunt splenic injury underwent US at approximate 6-week intervals to document injury healing (normal parenchyma or linear echogenic "scar"). Medical records of those not followed up to complete healing were reviewed.

RESULTS: Forty-eight patients were followed up to complete injury healing: 14 of injury grade 1 (mean, 7 weeks; range, 4–12 weeks), 24 of injury grade 2 (mean, 9.5 weeks; range, 6–17 weeks), and 10 of injury grade 3 (mean, 16 weeks; range, 6–29 weeks). The difference in mean time to healing among all grades was significant ($P <$ .02). Only two cysts were found; one decreased in size over time. No complications occurred in the 68 study patients.

CONCLUSION: The time course to US-documented healing of blunt pediatric splenic injury is related to injury severity. This information can be used to tailor follow-up imaging and provide cost savings.

In the child with hemodynamically stable blunt injury to the spleen, nonsurgical management has become the standard of care (1–3). However, there is no consensus regarding the length of time to restrict physical activity in these patients. Documentation of injury healing with noninvasive imaging is often the benchmark cited. Several researchers in the literature have examined the use of computed tomography (CT) for this purpose (4–6). Questions have even been raised about the necessity of routine follow-up imaging in pediatric (6) and adult (4) patients in clinically stable condition, as CT results do not appear to contribute to clinical management.

The late complications of blunt splenic injury, while rare, are real. These include delayed rupture (7), pseudoaneurysm formation (8,9), and enlarging posttraumatic cyst formation (10,11). Surgeons caring for these patients must balance the risk of missing late sequelae with the economic pressure to decrease utilization of resources. Ultrasonography (US) may be useful in fulfilling this need, since it is less costly than CT and uses no radiation or contrast material. The purpose of our study was to determine if US-documented healing of the pediatric spleen is related to the CT grade of injury, to review any posttraumatic complications, and to formulate an optimum grade-specific timetable for US follow-up of these injuries, with the goal of minimizing the number of scans obtained per patient.

MATERIALS AND METHODS

At our level I trauma center between January 1991 and March 1997, 157 children and adolescents were evaluated for blunt traumatic splenic injury. Eight of these children and adolescents required surgical management; the remaining 149 were treated nonsurgically. Criteria for conservative management were hemodynamic stability, absence of peritoneal

Author contributions:
Guarantor of integrity of entire study, K.H.E.; study concepts, K.H.E., D.S.B.; study design, K.H.E., D.S.B., V.F.G.; definition of intellectual content, K.H.E., D.S.B., V.F.G.; literature research, K.H.E., A.S.B.; clinical studies, K.H.E., D.S.B., A.S.B.; data acquisition, K.H.E., D.S.B., A.S.B.; data analysis, K.H.E.; statistical analysis, K.H.E.; manuscript preparation, K.H.E.; manuscript editing, K.H.E., D.S.B., V.F.G.

irritation, and absence of other abdominal injuries requiring surgery. Eighty patients did not return for US follow-up. Of the 69 patients who returned for follow-up US of their splenic injury, one had CT results that could not be obtained for review. The remaining 68 patients formed the study population (43 male, 25 female; age range, 1–16 years; mean age, 9 years). The distribution of injury grades was similar in this study group and the group that did not return for US follow-up.

At the time of injury, 54 of the 68 patients underwent CT at our institution with either a model 9800 Quick or CT HiSpeed Advantage system (GE Medical Systems, Milwaukee, Wis). The remaining 14 patients underwent CT at neighboring institutions on third- or fourth-generation units. All scans were obtained during or immediately after intravenous bolus administration of contrast material with 7–10-mm section collimation. In 66 of the 68 patients, scanning included the entire abdomen and pelvis. In two patients with outside studies, scanning included only the abdomen.

All CT scans were retrospectively reviewed, and splenic injuries were graded with the consensus of two radiologists (K.H.E., D.S.B.). A variation of the grading classification proposed by Brick et al (12) (Table 1) with estimation of the percentage of parenchymal involvement was used. Where only a laceration was visible, the classification by Mirvis et al (13) (Table 1) was used to grade the injury. The presence of peritoneal fluid was noted.

Per clinical routine, follow-up abdominal US was performed 6 weeks after discharge from the hospital and then every 4–6 weeks. All studies were performed with a model 128 unit (Acuson, Mountain View, Calif) or an HDI scanner (Advanced Technology Laboratories, Bothell, Wash). Color Doppler US was not performed.

The images were retrospectively reviewed by the same two radiologists with knowledge of the CT findings. Degree of healing was determined by the presence of either normal homogeneous splenic parenchymal echogenicity or a thin linear echogenic band presumably representing scar (14) (Fig 1). The presence of heterogeneous echogenicity, a hypoechoic collection (Fig 2), or an anechoic structure (presumably a cyst) was labeled as not healed.

Activity restrictions were maintained until the US results documented healing. The medical records of 20 study patients who underwent initial US but were not followed up until healing was complete were reviewed to determine if there were any delayed sequelae.

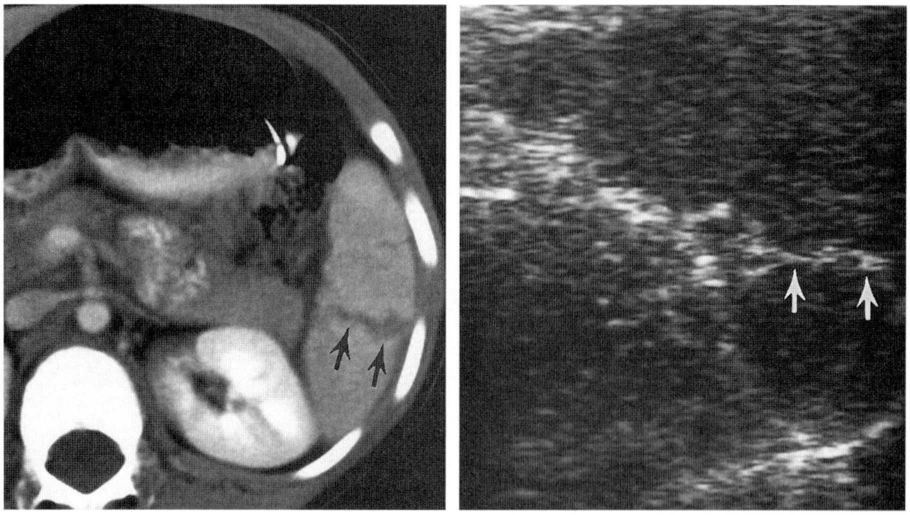

a. b.

Figure 1. Healing with scar. **(a)** CT scan of grade 2 splenic laceration (arrows). **(b)** Transverse follow-up US image shows thin, linear echogenic scar (arrows) at 9 weeks after injury.

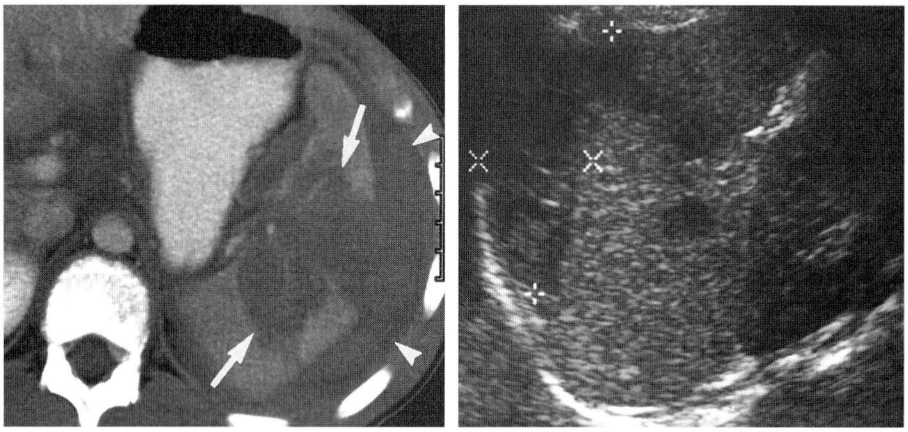

a. b.

Figure 2. Incomplete splenic healing. **(a)** CT scan shows grade 3 splenic injury (arrows) with moderate hemoperitoneum (arrowheads). **(b)** Follow-up US image at 7 weeks after injury shows that an irregular hypoechoic region remains (cursors).

RESULTS

In the 68 children and adolescents who returned for follow-up US, the distribution of splenic injury grade according to CT findings was as follows: 15 with grade 1, 33 with grade 2, 20 with grade 3, and 0 with grade 4 injuries. Forty-eight of these were followed up to complete US-documented healing: 14 of 15 with grade 1 (range, 4–12 weeks; mean, 7.0 weeks ± 0.6 [SD]), 24 of 33 with grade 2 (range, 6–17 weeks; mean, 9.5 weeks ± 0.7), and 10 of 20 with grade 3 (range, 6–29 weeks; mean, 16.6 weeks ± 2.6) injuries. When the Wilcoxon rank sum test was applied, the difference between the times to mean healing among the grades of injury was significant ($P < .02$).

Thirty-six of the 48 patients (75%) com-

TABLE 1
Method of Splenic Injury Grading

Grade	Parenchymal Involvement (%)*	Laceration† (cm)
1	<25	<1
2	25–50	1–3
3	>50	>3
4	Rupture	. . .

* Brick et al (12).
† Mirvis et al (13).

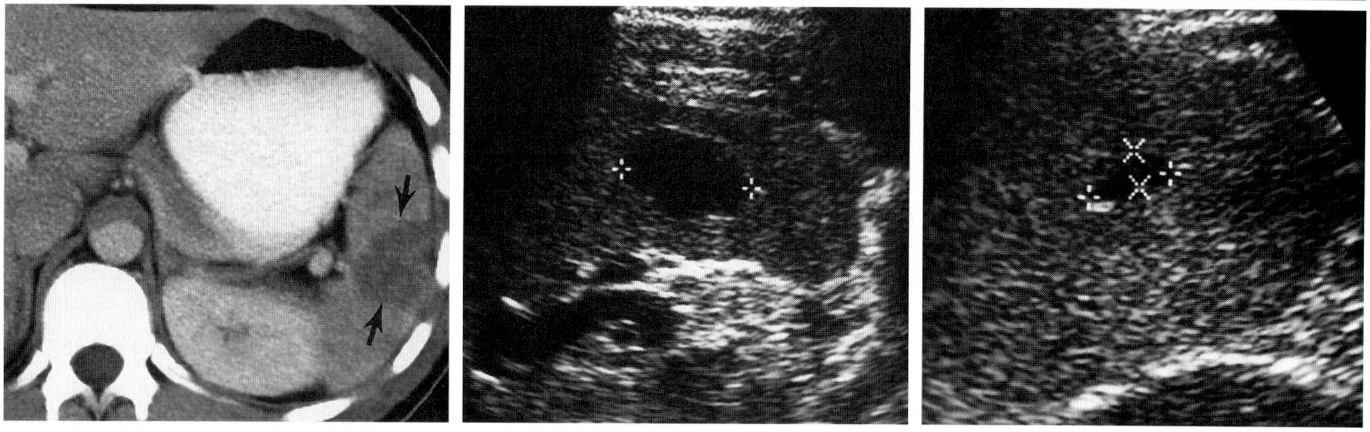

a. b. c.

Figure 3. Involuting posttraumatic fluid collection. **(a)** CT scan of grade 2 splenic injury (arrows). **(b)** Initial US image at 6 weeks after injury shows that the injury has developed a small anechoic fluid collection (cursors). **(c)** Delayed US image at 23 weeks after injury shows only a tiny residual cystic structure (cursors).

TABLE 2
Healing Pattern

Grade	Normal	Scar	Total
1	12	2	14
2	19	5	24
3	5	5	10
Total	36 (75)	12 (25)	48

Note.—Data are the number of patients. The numbers in parentheses are percentages.

pleting follow-up had normal homogeneous parenchymal echogenicity at healing (Table 2). The remaining 12 (25%) demonstrated a visible echogenic scar: two of 14 patients with grade 1 injuries, five of 24 with grade 2 injuries, and five of 10 with grade 3 injuries. While there was an increased incidence of scar formation with higher-grade injuries, the increase was not statistically significant ($P > .05$).

Only two patients developed anechoic structures meeting the criteria for a cyst; both had grade 2 injuries. Neither of these patients was followed up to complete resolution. One patient had a 2.6-cm cyst at initial US at 6 weeks, which decreased to 1.2 cm by his third US examination 23 weeks after injury (Fig 3). The other patient had only a 0.4-mm cyst at an 8-week postinjury US examination. Neither patient has returned to our institution with clinical sequelae of an enlarging posttraumatic cyst. The remaining 18 patients not meeting the criteria for healing had residual hypoechoic or heterogeneously echogenic areas within the spleen. Review of medical records in this group also failed to reveal any delayed sequelae.

Eight of the 68 patients (12%) had no visible peritoneal fluid at CT at the time of injury. Four of these had grade 1 splenic injury and four had grade 2 injury. Neither of the two patients lacking pelvic CT scans from outside institutions was included in this group, as both had visible peritoneal fluid in the upper abdomen or paracolic gutter. No free fluid was seen on any of the follow-up US scans.

With our current protocol of follow-up imaging at 6 weeks, 10 of the 48 patients with documented healing (21%) required more than one US examination (grade 1, one of 14 patients [7%]; grade 2, three of 24 patients [13%]; and grade 3, six of 10 patients [60%]).

DISCUSSION

The issue of follow-up imaging of blunt splenic injury in the era of nonsurgical management has been a source of controversy throughout the literature (4–6,15). While pseudocyst formation, delayed splenic rupture as the result of subcapsular hematoma, and pseudoaneurysm formation remain rare (7–11), the potential consequences of missing even one case remain formidable. It is this concern that drives most surgeons caring for these patients to seek objective documentation of injury healing before removing physical activity restrictions. Given the high degree of physical activity in the pediatric population as compared with that in adults (often including contact sports), this concern is valid.

If imaging documentation of healing of blunt splenic injury is required, one ideally minimizes costs and relative risk (radiation, intravenous contrast material, etc) while maximizing yield (ie, documenting healing with one examination). In studies in the literature, CT has been the predominant imaging modality (4–6). An informal survey (Emery KH, unpublished data, 1997) of the membership of the Society for Pediatric Radiology, or SPR, for which 95 radiology departments in North America responded, revealed that in nearly 80% routine follow-up imaging is performed to document splenic injury healing. The majority, approximately 65%, stated that they use CT.

However, US may be better suited to document injury healing at lower cost and risk. As these study findings have shown, there are significantly different healing times dependent on graded severity of injury. This relationship has been documented in children and adolescents with both CT (5) and US, as noted in a recent article in the surgery literature (15).

To our knowledge, there have been no direct comparative studies of CT and US to determine the relative accuracy of these two modalities for confirming splenic injury healing. One limitation of our study, as well as that of Lynch et al (15), is the assumption that use of the term "US-documented healing" implies that the organ has completely healed. To our knowledge, there have been no correlative US and histologic studies performed to confirm the assumption that normal parenchymal echogenicity equates to normal, functioning splenic tissue.

Researchers in a prior study (14) examining the use of US to observe healing in the traumatized spleen discovered that intrasplenic hematomas and contusions were resorbed over several months, and in two of 26 patients, linear echogenic bands were observed, which they attributed to fibrous scarring (14). While to our knowledge there is no histopathologic proof, the spleen is known to heal with fibrosis and scarring in areas of hemorrhage and infarction in patients with sickle cell disease (16). Realizing that hemorrhage and infarction occur in the traumatized spleen, it is reasonable to assume that scarring may also occur in this setting. Of interest, in the 58 patients examined by Lynch and colleagues (15) (including four with grade 4 injuries equivalent to complete splenic rupture), no echogenic parenchymal scars were reported. The reasons for this are not clear but may be related to equipment differences and scanning techniques, neither of which is specified in their article.

By combining the numbers of patients in the study by Lynch et al (15) with ours, we found that of the 106 patients followed up to complete US-documented healing, no complications were encountered. This emphasizes the rarity of these complications.

The two cysts in the patients in our study were likely resolving hematomas. Of interest, the patient with the decreasing posttraumatic cyst on serial US scans (Fig 3) had incurred a splenic injury 6 years earlier. We had no imaging documentation of complete healing of this prior injury. The possibility that this earlier injury was a precipitating factor for subsequent cyst development is interesting. None of the 20 patients who did not complete US follow-up subsequently presented to our institution with delayed injuries during the follow-up of 1–6 years.

In light of our results, we propose a more tailored approach to US follow-up of splenic injuries on the basis of injury grade to minimize the number of scans necessary to document healing (Table 3). Ten of our 48 patients with documented healing (21%) required more than one US examination following the current protocol of follow-up imaging at 6 weeks. While it is impossible to predict accurately the number of examinations that would not have been performed by using this revised protocol (given the relative variability of timing of the repeat studies), at least five of the six patients with grade 3 injuries who underwent two or more examinations would have required only one.

At our institution, the cost of an abdominal US examination is $81, as compared to $176 for an abdominal CT examination. A detailed cost analysis is beyond the scope of this article. However, the 68 patients in our study underwent a total of 86 US examinations. Had these all been CT examinations, the total cost would have been $15,136 instead of the $6,966 for US examinations, an increased cost of $8,170.

TABLE 3
Injury Grade and Recommended US Follow-up

Injury Grade	95% Likelihood of Healing: Range (wk)	95% Likelihood of Healing: Mean (wk)	Initial US (wk)	Follow-up (wk)
1	5.8–8.2	7.0	6	9
2	8.1–10.9	9.5	9	12
3	11.4–23.8	16.6	16	24

More important, since no complications were encountered in the 149 pediatric patients with blunt splenic trauma treated nonsurgically at our institution over approximately 6 years, the next logical question would be whether follow-up imaging of these injuries is even necessary in asymptomatic patients. Given healing rates documented here and in other studies in which CT or US has been performed (4–6,15) without complication noted, logical times for activity restriction could be devised on the basis of injury severity with a high degree of confidence for patient safety. Some of our colleagues in trauma surgery (17) are beginning to critically examine this issue, noting that results of routine serial abdominal CT examinations do not influence management or outcome.

In summary, we have shown that there is a clear relationship between the severity of blunt splenic injury in children and adolescents and the time course to US-documented healing; this information may be used to tailor the timing of follow-up imaging. While some question remains as to the need for follow-up imaging of these injuries, US provides the necessary information in a more cost-effective way than CT. While we encountered no clinically important complications, gathering further data in a larger patient population is necessary to confirm the efficacy of this approach.

Acknowledgments: We thank Sallie Kroeger for her assistance in manuscript preparation and Jane C. Khoury, MS, for assistance with the statistical analysis.

References

1. Ein SH, Shandling B, Simpson JS, Stephens CA. Nonoperative management of traumatized spleen in children: how and why. J Pediatr Surg 1978; 13:117–119.
2. Keller MS, Vane DW. Management of pediatric blunt splenic injury: comparison of pediatric and adult trauma surgeons. J Pediatr Surg 1995; 30:221–225.
3. Powell M, Courcoulas A, Gardner M, et al. Management of blunt splenic trauma: significant differences between adults and children. Surgery 1997; 122:654–660.
4. Lawson DE, Jacobson JA, Spizarny DL, Pranikoff T. Splenic trauma: value of follow-up CT. Radiology 1995; 194:97–100.
5. Benya EC, Bulas DI, Eichelberger MR, Sivit CJ. Splenic injury from blunt abdominal trauma in children: follow-up evaluation with CT. Radiology 1995; 195:685–688.
6. Pranikoff T, Hirschl RB, Schlesinger AE, Polley TZ, Coran AG. Resolution of splenic injury after nonoperative management. J Pediatr Surg 1994; 29:1366–1369.
7. Kluger Y, Paul DB, Raves JJ, et al. Delayed rupture of the spleen: myths, facts, and their importance—case reports and literature review. J Trauma 1994; 36:568–571.
8. Hiraide A, Yamamoto H, Yahata K, Yoshicka T, Sugimoto T. Delayed rupture of the spleen caused by an intrasplenic pseudoaneurysm following blunt trauma: case report. J Trauma 1994; 36:743–744.
9. Sugg SL, Gerndt SJ, Hamilton BJ, Francis IR, Taheri PA, Rodriguez JL. Pseudoaneurysms of the intraparenchymal splenic artery after blunt abdominal trauma: a complication of nonoperative therapy and its management. J Trauma 1995; 39:593–595.
10. Edmond RE, Rochon BR, McPhail JF. Case report: a traumatic splenic pseudocyst—historical review, diagnoses, and current mode of treatment. J Trauma 1990; 30:349–352.
11. Pachter JL, Hofstetter SR, Elkowitz A, Harris L, Liang HG. Traumatic cysts of the spleen: the role of cystectomy and splenic preservation—experience with seven consecutive patients. J Trauma 1993; 35:430–436.
12. Brick SH, Taylor GA, Potter BM, Eichelberger MR. Hepatic and splenic injury in children: role of CT in the decision for laparotomy. Radiology 1987; 165:643–646.
13. Mirvis SE, Whitley NO, Gens DR. Blunt splenic trauma in adults: CT-based classification and correlation with prognosis and treatment. Radiology 1989; 171:33–39.
14. Lupien C, Sauerbrei EE. Healing in the traumatized spleen: sonographic investigation. Radiology 1984; 151:181–185.
15. Lynch JM, Meza MP, Newan B, Gardner MJ, Albanese CT. Computed tomographic grade of splenic injury is predictive of the time required for radiographic healing. J Pediatr Surg 1997; 32:1093–1096.
16. Miale JB. Hematopoietic system: reticuloendothelium, spleen, lymph nodes, blood, and bone marrow. In: Anderson WA, ed. Pathology. 6th ed. St Louis, Mo: Mosby, 1971; 1316.
17. Alonso M, Braithwaite C, Garcia VF, et al. Patient management guidelines for the nonoperative management of blunt injury to the liver and spleen. [Eastern Association for the Surgery of Trauma Web site.] Available at: http://www.east.org/tpg/chap6body.html. Accessed October 26, 1998.

Legg-Calvé-Perthes Disease: MR Imaging Evaluation during Manual Positioning of the Hip—Comparison with Conventional Arthrography[1]

Diego Jaramillo, MD
Tamara A. Galen, MS
Carl S. Winalski, MD
James DiCanzio, MS
David Zurakowski, PhD
Robert V. Mulkern, PhD
Patricia A. McDougall, MD
Olga L. Villegas-Medina, MD, MPH
Ferenc A. Jolesz, MD
James R. Kasser, MD

Index terms:
Bones, necrosis, 442.443
Hip, arthrography, 442.122
Hip, MR, 442.121411, 442.121412
Hip, necrosis, 442.443
Magnetic resonance (MR), comparative studies, 442.121411, 442.121412
Magnetic resonance (MR), in infants and children, 442.121411, 442.121412, 442.443

Radiology 1999; 212:519–525

[1] From the Departments of Radiology (D.J., T.A.G., D.Z., R.V.M., O.L.V.M.), Orthopaedic Surgery (P.A.M., J.R.K.), and Research Computing and Biostatistics (J.D.), Children's Hospital, 300 Longwood Ave, Boston, MA 02115; and the Department of Radiology, Brigham and Women's Hospital and Harvard Medical School, Boston, Mass (C.S.W., R.V.M., F.A.J.). Received May 14, 1998; revision requested July 13; final revision received December 2; accepted February 9, 1999. Supported in part by National Institutes of Health grant AR42396-04 (D.J., T.A.G., O.L.V.M.) and GE Medical Systems (all authors). **Address reprint requests to** D.J. (e-mail: *jaramillo@a1.tch.harvard.edu*).

Author contributions:
Guarantor of integrity of entire study, D.J.; study concepts, D.J., T.A.G., C.S.W., R.V.M., F.A.J., J.R.K.; study design, D.J., T.A.G., C.S.W., J.D., D.Z., R.V.M., O.L.V.M., J.R.K.; definition of intellectual content, D.J., T.A.G., C.S.W., J.R.K.; literature research, D.J., T.A.G.; clinical studies, D.J., C.S.W., P.A.M., O.L.V.M., J.R.K.; experimental studies, D.J., C.S.W., R.V.M., O.L.V.M., F.A.J.; data acquisition, D.J., T.A.G., C.S.W., R.V.M., P.A.M., O.L.V.M., J.R.K.; data analysis, D.J., T.A.G., C.S.W., J.R.K.; statistical analysis, J.D., D.Z.; manuscript preparation, D.J., T.A.G.; manuscript editing, all authors; manuscript review, D.J., T.A.G.

PURPOSE: To evaluate the use of magnetic resonance (MR) imaging during manual positioning of the hip, or multipositional MR imaging, in an open-magnet configuration to study femoral head containment, articular congruency, and femoral head deformity in Legg-Calvé-Perthes disease.

MATERIALS AND METHODS: In 12 children with advanced Legg-Calvé-Perthes disease, multipositional MR imaging and conventional arthrography were compared in the assessment of containment, femoroacetabular congruency, and femoral head deformity. Images of the hips in several positions were compared subjectively and objectively.

RESULTS: MR imaging correlated well with arthrography for overall subjective assessment of severity of disease ($r = 0.71$, $P = .01$), with good interobserver agreement ($\kappa = 0.65$, $P < .001$). MR images demonstrated all cases of hinge abduction shown arthrographically. However, MR imaging failed to depict one case of femoral head flattening. MR imaging correlated well with arthrography in the objective evaluation of joint fluid and lateral subluxation ($r = 0.80$, $P < .01$). MR imaging correlated poorly with arthrography in the measurement of sphericity of the femoral head.

CONCLUSION: Multipositional MR imaging with an open-magnet configuration was comparable to arthrography for demonstration of femoral head containment and congruency of the articular surfaces of the hip. In the evaluation of deformity, it performed less well.

Legg-Calvé-Perthes disease is an idiopathic avascular necrosis of the growing femoral epiphysis, which results in progressive deformity and outward displacement of the femoral head (1,2). One of the main goals of therapy is to maximize containment so that the femoral head can heal adequately within the acetabulum (3). It is also important to position the articular surfaces so that they remain congruent to decrease the risk of osteoarthritis. Patients ultimately may require osteotomies of the femur or the ilium to optimize femoroacetabular relationships.

Arthrography is often performed in severe Legg-Calvé-Perthes disease to decide whether the hips require bracing or surgery and to assess the best position for immobilization (4–7). Arthrography helps to show containment of the femoral head by the acetabulum, congruency of the femoral head and the acetabulum, and deformity of the cartilaginous femoral head. Arthrography of the hip in children usually requires general anesthesia, placing a needle into the joint, injecting contrast material in the joint space, and exposing the pelvis to radiation (8,9). Although magnetic resonance (MR) imaging has been used increasingly to evaluate Legg-Calvé-Perthes disease, it has not yet been used to show the positional variation of femoral head containment and congruency within the acetabulum.

We have performed multipositional MR imaging in a magnet system with an open configuration and compared the findings with those from arthrography. Our goal was to evaluate MR imaging as a possible substitute for arthrography in children with advanced Legg-Calvé-Perthes disease.

MATERIALS AND METHODS

Experimental Design

The study was a prospective comparison of multipositional MR imaging and conventional arthrography in children with Legg-Calvé-Perthes disease. Containment of the femoral head by the acetabulum, congruency between the femoral head and acetabulum, and deformity of the femoral head were each evaluated objectively and subjectively in many positions.

Subjects

From April 1996 to October 1997, we performed multipositional MR studies in 17 children with advanced Legg-Calvé-Perthes disease. Five subjects were not included in the analysis. The first three children were examined solely with fast gradient-recalled-echo sequences that did not allow adequate differentiation between joint fluid and epiphyseal cartilage. We subsequently used fast spin-echo T2-weighted sequences that provided excellent contrast between fluid and cartilage and therefore became the standard. One 12-year-old girl refused to undergo arthrography after the MR imaging study. One 3-year-old boy did not complete the study because it was impossible to perform imaging adequately without sedation.

The remaining 12 children (11 boys, one girl; age range, 4.3–11.5 years; median, 6.8 years) were the subjects of the study. All but one of the children underwent intraoperative arthrography within 1 week of MR imaging. This child, by parental decision, delayed the arthrography for 3 months after the MR imaging study. Because the radiographs had not changed substantially in the interval, we included this child in the results. The study was approved by the hospitals' institutional review boards, and informed consent was obtained from the parents for all patients.

Imaging

All MR imaging was performed with a 0.5-T open configuration MR system (Signa SP; GE Medical Systems, Milwaukee, Wis) (10). The imaging field of the system is within a 56-cm wide vertically oriented space; this allows ample space for manipulation of the hips by the examiner and close contact with one or both parents (Fig 1). A circular 25-cm rigid transmit-receive coil was placed around the affected hip from the groin to the anterior superior iliac spine.

An initial coronal fast gradient-recalled-echo sequence of the involved hip (16.9/7.9 [repetition time msec/echo time msec]; flip angle, 40°) was used as a localizer. Fast spin-echo T2-weighted images (2,500/108 [effective]; echo train length, eight; bandwidth, 16 kHz) were then obtained in the coronal plane with the hip in several positions and in the sagittal plane in the neutral position. Imaging parameters for the multipositional sequence were as follows: field of view, 24 × 24 cm; section thickness, 5 mm; intersection gap, 1 mm; matrix, 256 × 192; two signals acquired. Imaging time in each position was 1 minute 58 seconds. Fat saturation, although available, was not used in the open-magnet configuration owing to the low field strength and unavoidable magnetic field inhomogeneities over the field of view.

The patients were examined in the lateral decubitus position with the hip and knee supported with foam pads (Fig 1). Six hip positions in the multipositional series were studied: neutral, 5° of adduction, 20° of abduction, 40° of abduction, 30° of abduction with 45° of flexion, and 45° of abduction with 90° of flexion and maximal external rotation. Different foam pads were used for each position to maintain reproducible degrees of abduction. We standardized the plane of the coronal section by placing a marker on the patient, which was kept in alignment with the laser light during the imaging. A coronal T1-weighted (500/17) image of both hips was then obtained to show any contralateral avascular necrosis.

The spot radiographs from the hip arthrogram were obtained in positions closely matching those of the multipositional MR study. The arthrograms were obtained with use of general anesthesia in the operating room. With fluoroscopic guidance, a 22-gauge needle was placed into the joint at the level of the lower aspect of the femoral neck. Injection of 10–15 mL of iopamidol (Isovue 300; Bracco Diagnostics, Princeton, NJ) was performed with fluoroscopic control until full distention of the joint was achieved. Images were obtained by using a digital C-arm unit (BV29; Phillips Medical Systems, Shelton, Conn).

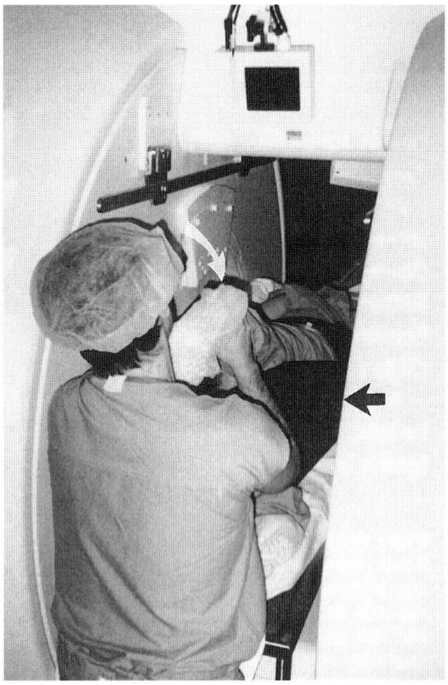

Figure 1. Photograph obtained during abduction and flexion. The child is in the lateral decubitus position. The knee is supported by a foam pad (straight arrow). The curved arrow points to the patient's foot.

Image Analysis

Three main parameters were analyzed subjectively and objectively: containment of the femoral head by the acetabulum, congruency of the articular surfaces of the femoral head and acetabulum, and deformity of the femoral head.

Subjective Evaluation

The subjective evaluation was performed by two observers, one pediatric radiologist (D.J.) and one pediatric orthopedic surgeon (J.R.K.), who analyzed the images independently and then by consensus. The observers were blinded to the identity of the patients. The scoring followed two practice sessions during which the observers agreed on the grading systems by using the images of the five patients who were not included in the final comparison. Evaluation of the overall severity of the disease is outlined in the Table. In addition, several parameters were graded separately.

Containment was analyzed by assessing whether with abduction the medial joint space was increased (graded 0 or 1) and whether abduction resulted in improved containment or hinging. Congruency of the articular surfaces was determined by assessing the degree of medial pooling of joint fluid or contrast material between the femoral head and acetabulum and grading it from 0 (absent) to 3

Grading of Severity of Legg-Calvé-Perthes Disease by Means of Arthrography and Multipositional MR Imaging

Grade	Femoral Head Flattening	Incongruity of Articular Surfaces	Medial Pooling of Joint Fluid	Containment in Abduction	Medial Joint Space
0	Absent	Congruent	Absent	Increased	Normal
1	Mild	Mild	Mild	Increased	Mildly increased
2	Moderate	Moderate	Moderate	Unchanged	Moderately increased
3	Severe	Severe	Severe	Decreased (hinge abduction)	Severely increased

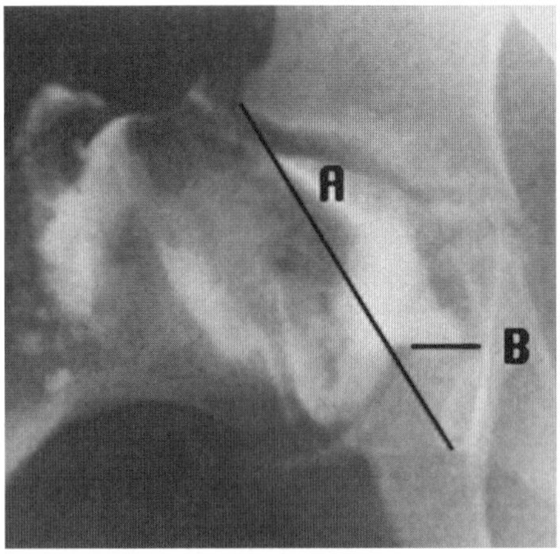

a.

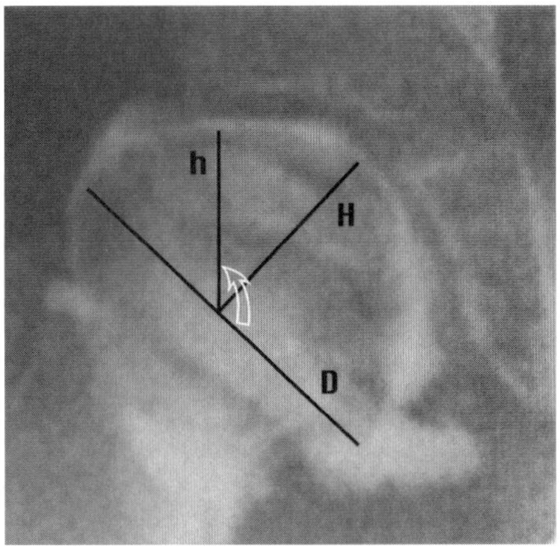

c.

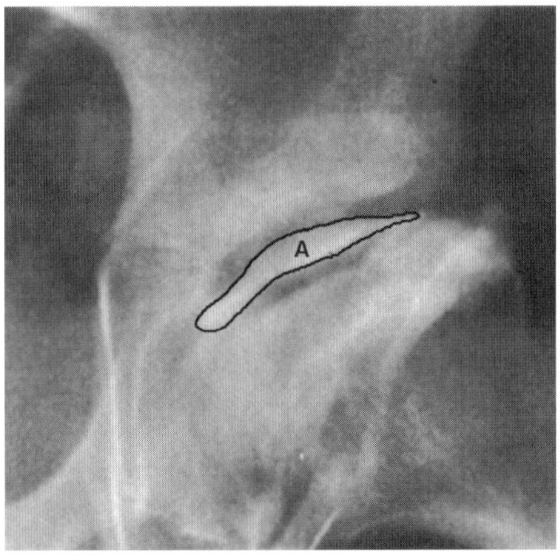

b.

Figure 2. (a) Anteroposterior arthrogram obtained with the hip in 40° of abduction shows a technique for measuring containment of the femoral head by the acetabulum. Subluxation is determined by dividing the femoroacetabular gap, *B*, by the bony acetabular diameter, *A*. (b) Anteroposterior arthrogram obtained with the hip in 40° of abduction shows a technique for measuring congruency of the femoral head and the acetabulum. The area, *A*, of fluid between the femoral head and the acetabulum is measured and divided by the square of the acetabular diameter (see **a** and the text). (c) Anteroposterior arthrogram obtained with the hip in the neutral position shows a technique for measuring femoral head sphericity. Sphericity is determined by dividing the height, *H*, by half of the maximal transverse diameter, *D*. The sphericity of the weight-bearing aspect of the head is measured by dividing the height, *h*, by the maximal transverse diameter, *D*. The height is measured at 135° from the maximal diameter; the 135° arc is identified by the arrow.

(severe). Femoral head deformity was evaluated by grading the degree of flattening of the femoral head from 0 to 3, depending on whether flattening was absent, mild, moderate, or severe. In addition, we determined whether flattening remained the same (grade 0) or became more apparent with abduction (grade 1).

Objective Evaluation

The objective evaluation also was based on containment, congruency, and femoral head deformity. Two observers (D.J., T.A.G.) independently performed measurements on the MR images and the arthrograms. MR imaging measurements were obtained with use of a workstation with version 2.0 software (Advantage Windows; GE Medical Systems). The arthrograms were digitized and analyzed on a computer (Power Macintosh 8500; Apple Computer, Cupertino, Calif) with NIH Image version 1.60 software (National Institutes of Health, Bethesda, Md). Each of the three parameters was measured by using the arthrograms and MR images from each subject for all available positions.

For evaluation of containment, we calculated a subluxation ratio (6) (Fig 2a), defined as the quotient of the gap between the acetabulum and femoral head, which was defined as the distance between the most medial surface of the femoral head and the lateral border of the acetabular teardrop, and the greatest acetabular diameter. Acetabular diameter was measured from the tip of the teardrop, on arthrograms, or from the corresponding inferior tip of the bony acetabulum, on MR images, to the most lateral portion of the bony acetabular rim. The subluxation ratio is independent of image magnification.

The evaluation of congruency was based on the measurement of the area of joint fluid or contrast material that was detectable between the femoral head and acetabulum (Fig 2b). This area was divided by the square of the greatest acetabular diameter defined earlier, again to make the measurement independent of image magnification.

Assessment of deformity of the femoral head was based on the determination of the sphericity ratio. Sphericity of the femoral head was calculated as the ratio of the height to half of the greatest transverse diameter as defined by Jonsäter (11) (Fig 2c). To evaluate whether the MR imaging–arthrography correlation varied with location of the height measurement of the femoral head, one observer (T.A.G.) also obtained measurements of femoral head height at an angle of 135° with respect to the greatest transverse femoral diameter (Fig 2c).

Statistical Analysis

For the subjective ratings, the κ statistic was used to measure chance-corrected agreement between readers for both MR imaging and arthrography and intermethod agreement for each reader: poor agreement, κ less than 0.40; fair agreement, κ = 0.40–0.59; good agreement, κ = 0.60–0.74; excellent agreement, κ = 0.75–1.00 (12). Spearman rank correlation coefficients (r_s) were calculated to determine the strength of association between MR imaging and arthrography for grade of disease, medial space widening, hinging with abduction, medial pooling of joint fluid, flattening in the neutral position, and flattening with abduction.

For the objective measurements, linear association between methods and readers for the three parameters (containment, congruency, and deformity) was analyzed by least squares regression analysis and the Pearson correlation coefficient (r). A comparison between arthrography and MR imaging was performed for the neutral position, positions of simple abduction (including 20° and 40°), and positions of flexion-abduction; this comparison between imaging modalities also was performed for all positions combined. For each parameter, agreement between MR imaging and arthrography was investigated by using the approach of Bland and Altman (13). Arthrography was considered to be the standard, and differences between the methods were calculated and plotted. A slope test was used to assess whether these differences varied systematically over the range of measurements (14). An α level of .05 was used to indicate statistical significance. SAS version 6.11 (SAS Institute, Cary, NC) and SPSS version 7.0 (SPSS, Chicago, Ill) software packages were used. All statistical tests were two tailed.

RESULTS

MR Imaging Appearance

T2-weighted fast spin-echo images allowed clear differentiation between the low-signal-intensity epiphyseal and articular cartilage and the high-signal-intensity articular fluid (Fig 3). The physis was seen as a low-signal-intensity area between the high signal intensities of the epiphyseal and metaphyseal marrow. Osteonecrotic marrow was generally of low signal intensity and often difficult to differentiate from the adjacent epiphyseal cartilage (Figs 4, 5). This was particularly noticeable in the younger children. In all cases, the contour of the femoral head changed with changes in position (Figs 3, 4). The ligamentum teres femoris, the transverse acetabular ligament, the fibrocartilaginous labrum, and the joint capsule were readily identified (Fig 3).

Eight patients showed interruption of the physis on coronal MR images (Fig 4a), three showed physeal irregularity, and one had an apparently normal physis. Sagittal images revealed that the deformity of epiphyseal contour was predominantly anterior in 11 patients and central in one. The marrow of the contralateral epiphysis was normal in all patients.

Subjective Analysis

MR imaging correlated well with arthrography for the determination of the overall grade of disease as evidenced by the scoring of the consensus evaluation ($r_s = 0.71$, $P = .01$) and of that of each independent reader ($r_s = 0.75$ and $r_s = 0.86$, $P < .01$). There was fair interobserver agreement for the two observers for the scoring of the overall grade of disease as determined by means of arthrography ($\kappa = 0.44$, $P < .01$), and interobserver agreement was good with MR imaging ($\kappa = 0.65$, $P < .001$).

The evaluation of containment showed a high correlation for hinging with abduction ($r_s = 0.78$, $P < .01$) (Fig 6) but no correlation between modalities for medial space widening ($r_s = 0.00$, $P = .99$). The evaluation of congruency showed a high correlation between modalities for medial pooling of joint fluid ($r_s = 0.80$, $P < .01$ for the consensus data). There was better agreement between observers for the evaluation of pooling with arthrography ($\kappa = 0.87$, $P < .001$) than with MR imaging ($\kappa = 0.31$, $P = .12$). The evaluation of deformity showed marginally significant correlation for flattening in the neutral position ($rs = 0.59$, $P = .04$) and no significant correlation for improved detection of flattening with abduction ($r_s = 0.43$, $P = .17$) (Fig 5).

Objective Analysis

The evaluation of containment by means of the subluxation ratio showed good correlation between modalities ($r = 0.64$, $P < .001$ for observer 1; $r = 0.50$, $P < .001$ for observer 2). The evaluation of congruency revealed good correlation for measurements of joint fluid area ($r = 0.45$, $P < .001$; $r = 0.37$, $P = .004$). Correlation of joint fluid area was the best for positions of simple abduction ($r = 0.60$, $P < .001$) and the worst for the neutral position ($r = -0.17$, $P = .32$). For the evaluation of deformity, MR imaging and arthrography correlated poorly. The sphericity index correlations were $r = 0.07$ ($P = 0.62$) and $r = 0.28$ ($P = .03$) for the two observers. The correlation improved when measurement was calculated by using the height of the femoral head along a line at 135° from the femoral head diameter ($r = 0.39$, $P = .003$).

The correlation between the two observers was statistically significant for all parameters and for both modalities. The interobserver correlation coefficients for arthrograms and MR images were 0.56 and 0.74 for subluxation ratio, 0.82 and 0.63 for joint fluid area, and 0.55 and 0.41 for sphericity ratio.

For all parameters, the difference between the measurements of the two modalities depended on the magnitude of the measurements. By using arthrography as the standard, a slope test indicated overestimation with MR imaging at small measurements and underestimation at large measurements (all $P < .001$).

DISCUSSION

The study shows that multipositional MR imaging can provide useful information about containment and congruency of the femoral head in children with Legg-Calvé-Perthes disease. It can reveal whether abduction causes the femoral head to come into the acetabulum or hinge out of it. MR images depict the contour of the femoral head in the coronal and sagittal planes, but our data suggest that there is poor correlation between the MR imaging and the arthrographic depiction of deformity.

The role of MR imaging in the evaluation of Legg-Calvé-Perthes disease varies according to the severity and duration of the disease (15,16). In early Legg-Calvé-Perthes disease, when radiographs are normal, the role of MR imaging is to detect the presence of ischemic marrow (17). In more advanced Legg-Calvé-Perthes disease, MR imaging can demonstrate the extent of marrow involvement (18), the degree of cartilaginous or synovial hypertrophy (19,20), and the extent of physeal and metaphyseal cartilaginous abnormalities (21). The main limitation of static MR imaging is its inability to demonstrate how the deformed femur relates to the acetabulum in various positions. For this reason, arthrography is still widely used prior to bracing or surgery (15).

The main imaging questions in advanced Legg-Calvé-Perthes disease are (*a*) what is the containment of the femoral head and what are the causes of decreased containment (22), (*b*) how congruent are the femoral head and the acetabulum, and (*c*) how severe is the femoral head deformity. Under most circumstances, containment of the femoral head improves with abduction (Fig 4). Abduction bracing and redirecting osteotomies of the ilium or proximal femur result in a greater portion of the femoral head lying within the acetabulum, which in turn facilitates the remodeling of the femoral head (22). A notable exception is hinge abduction. In this situation, the deformed femoral head hinges against the lateral margin of the acetabulum (Fig 6). With greater abduction, the femoral head tends to come out of the acetabulum (23). Therefore, hinge abduction is a contraindication to conventional bracing or surgical therapy.

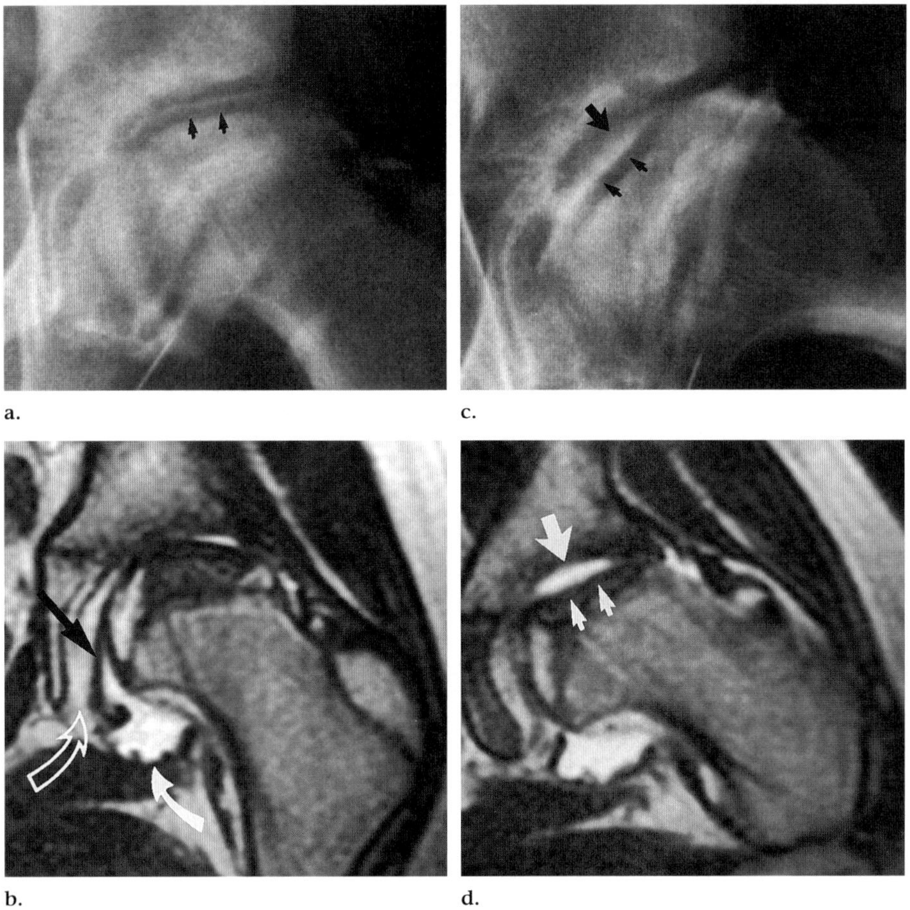

Figure 3. Images obtained in an 11-year-old boy with severe limitation of abduction and rotation of the left hip. The series of images shows that femoral head flattening may be demonstrated only in abduction with MR imaging. **(a)** Anteroposterior arthrogram obtained with the hip in the neutral position shows flattening of the femoral head (arrows). The femoral head is displaced laterally. **(b)** Coronal fast spin-echo T2-weighted MR image (2,500/108; echo train length, eight) obtained in the same position as **a** shows that the medial joint space contains tissue of high signal intensity, presumably representing thick synovium (open white arrow). The image shows joint fluid (solid white arrow) with the ligamentum teres femoris (black arrow) lying between the fluid and the acetabular tissues. The femoral epiphysis has abnormal signal intensity but is not far from round, and there is good congruency between the femoral head and the acetabulum. **(c)** Anteroposterior arthrogram obtained with the hip in 40° of abduction shows medial pooling (large arrow) of the contrast material. The femoral head (small arrows) is flattened. **(d)** Coronal fast spin-echo T2-weighted MR image (2,500/108; echo train length, eight) obtained in the same position as **c** helps confirm that the femoral head (small arrows) is flat. The large arrow shows joint fluid pooled between the femoral head and the acetabulum.

In advanced Legg-Calvé-Perthes disease, there is little correspondence between the contour of the ossified epiphysis and that of the cartilaginous femoral head, especially when the ossified femoral head undergoes fragmentation and resorption. Assessment of femoroacetabular relationships requires imaging that can define the contour of the cartilaginous femoral head, such as arthrography or MR imaging.

MR imaging offers some important advantages over arthrography. It is not invasive and allows simultaneous imaging of the joint space, the epiphyseal and physeal cartilage, and the marrow of both the affected side and the contralateral epiphysis. Furthermore, it allows a more physiologic evaluation of the range of motion without anesthetic relaxation and without added fluid. With multipositional MR imaging, however, femoral head contour is sometimes difficult to evaluate (Fig 5), and extreme positions are less well tolerated. Motion degradation of the MR images may require repetition of some imaging sequences. It is possible that with improvements in imaging sequences (such as the use of more rapid fast spin-echo acquisitions) and improvements in coil design, the imaging can be improved to the point where multipositional MR imaging is superior to arthrography in all aspects.

MR imaging was successfully performed without sedation and with, at most, mild discomfort. Most children complained about the duration of the study but otherwise tolerated the examination well. By comparison, arthrography is much more invasive and requires general anesthesia. The use of anesthesia allows for the evaluation of more extreme positions of the hip. We believe that multipositional MR imaging should be used instead of arthrography in patients who are at risk with anesthesia, arthrocentesis, or administration of contrast material.

The data suggest that the only substantial discrepancy between the modalities was in the evaluation of femoral head deformity. This was particularly evident in one of the patients (Fig 5) for whom the MR imaging evaluation suggested only mild deformity whereas the arthrography showed clear flattening. When there is little joint fluid, the contrast material injected during arthrography allows better differentiation between joint fluid and cartilage than that provided by MR imaging. In addition, when the deformity involves predominantly the anterior femoral head, the deformity is more apparent in projectional images, such as those obtained with arthrography, than in sectional images, such as coronal MR images.

The actual information about deformity provided by the MR images is better than what is suggested by our comparative study, as the anterior flattening could be seen best on sagittal images. However, we could not evaluate these images in the comparative analysis because it is difficult to obtain good arthrograms in a similar plane. We performed the objective comparison by using the sphericity ratio, widely used in the literature (16), which can be used to assess flattening only perpendicular to the greatest diameter of the femoral head. This measurement also varies owing to subjective differences in assessment of the greatest diameter of the femoral head. The statistically significant interobserver correlation, however, suggests that this is a reproducible way of assessing deformity.

There were differences in the assessment of medial joint fluid pooling. This is not surprising because the amount of joint fluid is much greater during the arthrographic study. Arthrography optimizes the demonstration of fluid distribution because of the injection of addi-

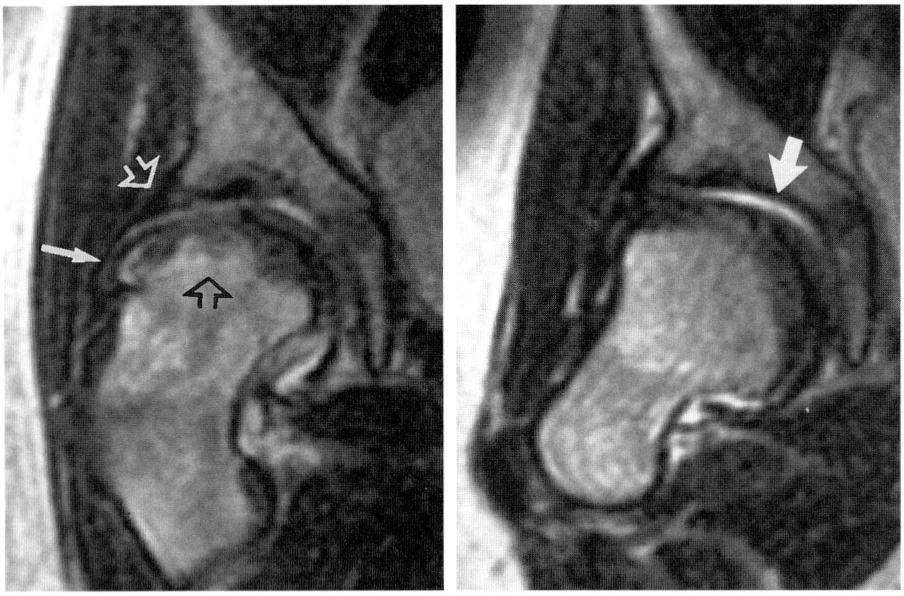

a. b.

Figure 4. Images obtained in a 6-year-old boy show poor containment of the femoral head and improvement with abduction. **(a)** Coronal fast spin-echo T2-weighted MR image (2,500/108; echo train length, eight) obtained with the hip in the neutral position shows that the most lateral part of the flattened femoral head (solid arrow) is lateral to the hypointense acetabular labrum (open white arrow) and helps confirm the poor containment. Most of the physis (open black arrow) is prematurely fused. **(b)** Coronal fast spin-echo T2-weighted MR image (2,500/108; echo train length, eight) obtained with the hip in 40° of abduction shows improved containment and also demonstrates the mild accumulation of fluid (arrow) in the joint space.

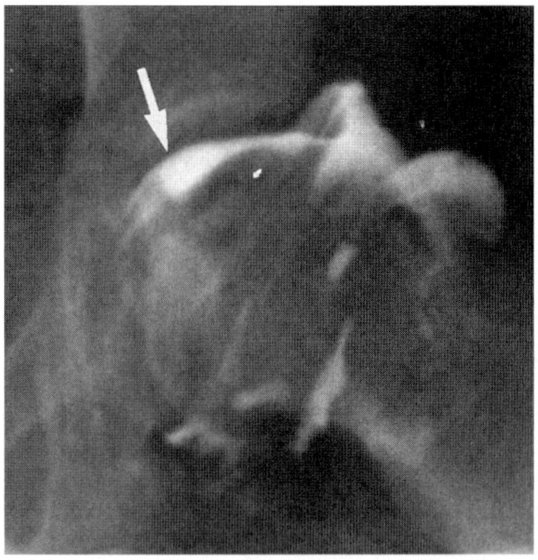

a.

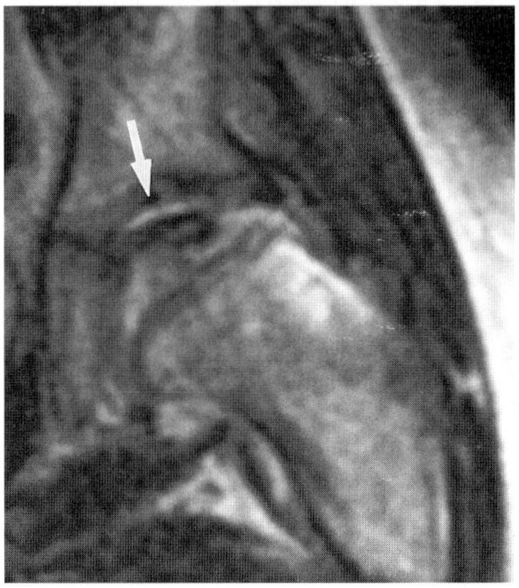

b.

Figure 5. Images obtained in a 9-year-old boy prior to Petrie abduction casting shows the failure of multipositional MR imaging to demonstrate severe femoral head deformity. **(a)** Anteroposterior arthrogram obtained with the hip in 20° of abduction shows that there is substantial pooling of fluid (arrow) between the femoral head and the acetabulum. This indicates lack of congruency. **(b)** Corresponding coronal fast spin-echo T2-weighted MR image (2,500/108; echo train length, eight) shows only minimal accumulation of fluid (arrow) between what appear to be relatively congruent surfaces. Although **a** and **b** were obtained with comparable abduction maneuvers, greater abduction was achieved during arthrography, which may explain the differences between the images.

tional fluid; MR imaging, however, shows the kinematics of the joint with its usual amount of fluid. Although arthrography was taken as the standard, both observers agreed that the MR images allowed better depiction of what occupied that space by showing the edematous synovial membrane, the ligamentum teres femoris, and acetabular fat as causes of lateral femoral head displacement. MR imaging and arthrography were comparable for the objective evaluation of lateral displacement of the femoral head. The differences in the assessment of the fluid pooled between the femur and acetabulum can be explained in the same fashion as the subjective differences already discussed.

The main limitation of this study was the small number of patients examined. The cases were collected from a very busy practice (Children's Hospital, Boston, Mass) with a large number of patients with Legg-Calvé-Perthes disease, yet it took 2 years to obtain 12 volunteers who would undergo both procedures sequentially. Further evaluation may require a multicenter trial. Great efforts were made to obtain the images in comparable positions by keeping the abduction foam pads constant and marking the plane of the coronal section on the patients. Nonetheless, the images obtained differed between modalities (Fig 5) and between patients.

Our data suggest that the more complex positions that involved flexion and abduction were more difficult to reproduce, although the images were clinically informative. The study was performed in a 0.5-T magnet with a vertically oriented open configuration that allows ample access to the patients; it is likely that similar results can be obtained in other open magnets with different configurations.

Our data show that MR imaging with use of manual positioning of the hip in an open-configuration magnet system in children with Legg-Calvé-Perthes disease is comparable to conventional arthrography for overall assessment of femoroacetabular relationships (containment and congruency) and detection of hinge abduction. Fast spin-echo T2-weighted MR imaging was necessary to show adequate contrast between fluid and cartilage. We hope further improvements such as faster imaging and better resolution will allow widespread use of MR imaging and may resolve some of the challenges in the evaluation of femoral head deformity. Future studies should evaluate a larger population and address cost and benefit. Improved multipositional MR imaging, a noninvasive, possibly less expensive modality that allows concurrent assessment of marrow, physis, and contralateral femoral head, clearly would be the modality of choice over conventional arthrography.

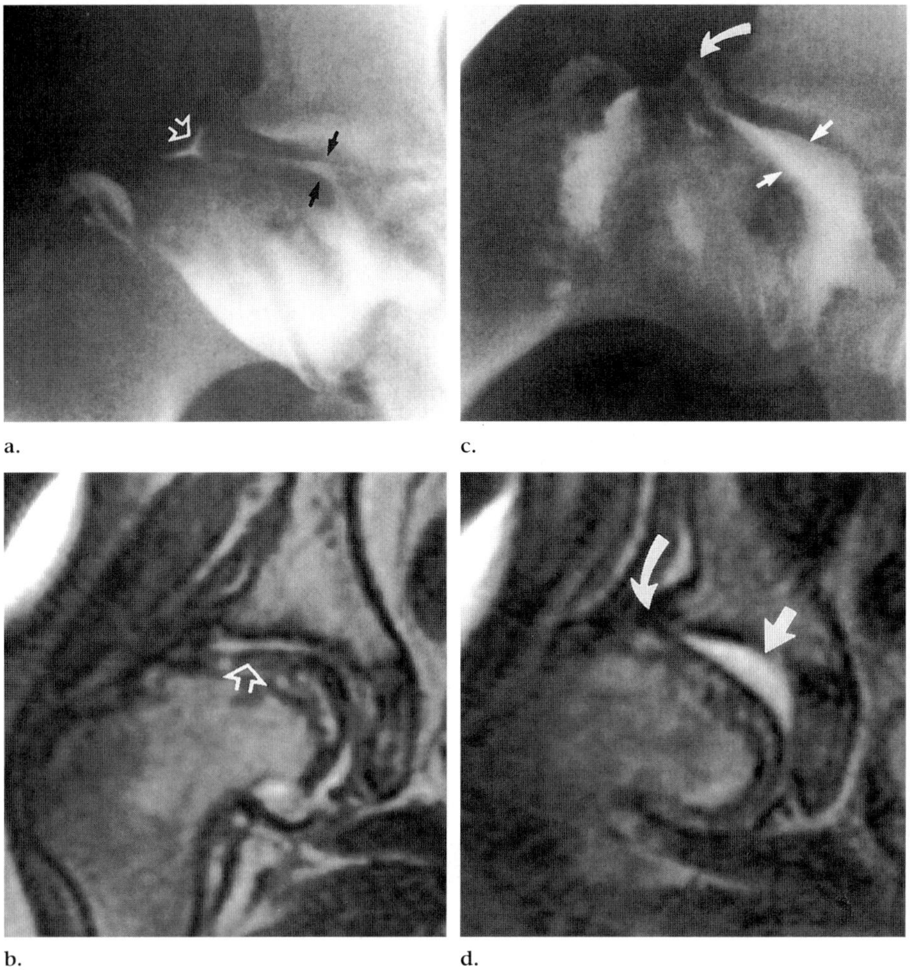

Figure 6. Images obtained in a 9-year-old boy show hinge abduction with marked deformity of the right hip. **(a)** Anteroposterior arthrogram obtained with the hip in a neutral position shows flattening of the femoral head. The contours of the femoral head and the acetabulum (black arrows) are nearly parallel. The white arrow shows the end of the acetabular labrum defined by the "rose thorn" (capsuloacetabular recess). **(b)** Coronal fast spin-echo T2-weighted MR image (2,500/108; echo train length, eight) obtained in the same position as **a** helps confirm the severe flattening of the femoral head (arrow). The articular surfaces appear congruent. The epiphyseal marrow is nearly normal, which indicates that healing has occurred. **(c)** Anteroposterior arthrogram obtained with the hip in 40° of abduction shows that the joint opens by hinging on the acetabular margin (curved arrow). There is medial joint pooling between the articular surfaces (straight arrows). **(d)** Coronal fast spin-echo T2-weighted MR image (2,500/108; echo train length, eight) obtained in the same position as **c** helps confirm severe medial pooling of fluid (straight arrow) and hinging of the femoral head on the acetabular margin (curved arrow).

References

1. Catterall A. The natural history of Perthes' disease. J Bone Joint Surg [Br] 1971; 53:37–53.
2. Herring JA, Williams JJ, Neustadt JN, Early JS. Evolution of femoral head deformity during the healing phase of Legg-Calvé-Perthes disease. J Pediatr Orthop 1993; 13:41–45.
3. Herring JA. The treatment of Legg-Calvé-Perthes disease: a critical review of the literature. J Bone Joint Surg [Am] 1994; 76:448–458.
4. Gallagher JM, Weiner DS, Cook AJ. When is arthrography indicated in Legg-Calvé-Perthes Disease? J Bone Joint Surg [Am] 1983; 65:900–905.
5. Hochbergs P, Eckerwall G, Egund N, Jonsson K, Wingstrand H. Femoral head shape in Legg-Calvé-Perthes disease: correlation between conventional radiography, arthrography and MR imaging. Acta Radiol 1994; 35:545–548.
6. Kamegaya M, Moriya H, Tsuchiya K, Akita T, Ogata S, Someya M. Arthrography of early Perthes' disease: swelling of the ligamentum teres as a cause of subluxation. J Bone Joint Surg [Br] 1989; 71:413–417.
7. Kaniklides C, Lonnerholm T, Moberg A, Sahlstedt B. Legg-Calvé-Perthes disease: comparison of conventional radiography, MR imaging, bone scintigraphy and arthrography. Acta Radiol 1995; 36:434–439.
8. Wilkinson R. Hip arthrography in children. In: Dalinka M, ed. Arthrography. New York, NY: Springer-Verlag, 1980; 119–126.
9. Lonnerholm T. Arthrography of the hip in children: technique, normal anatomy and findings in unstable hip joints. Acta Radiol 1980; 21:279–292.
10. Schenck JF, Jolesz FA, Roemer PB, et al. Superconducting open-configuration MR imaging system for image-guided therapy. Radiology 1995; 195:805–814.
11. Jonsäter S. Coxa plana: a histo-pathologic and arthrographic study. Acta Orthop Scand 1953; (suppl 12):58–88.
12. Landis JR, Koch GG. The measurement of observer agreement for categorical data. Biometrics 1977; 33:159–174.
13. Bland JM, Altman DG. Statistical methods for assessing agreement between two methods of clinical measurement. Lancet 1986; 1:307–310.
14. Zar JH. Biostatistical analysis. 3rd ed. Upper Saddle River, NJ: Prentice-Hall, 1996.
15. Hubbard AM, Dormans JP. Evaluation of developmental dysplasia, Perthes disease, and neuromuscular dysplasia of the hip in children before and after surgery: an imaging update. AJR 1995; 164:1067–1073.
16. Kaniklides C. Diagnostic radiology in Legg-Calvé-Perthes disease. Acta Radiol 1996; 406:1–28.
17. Sebag G, Ducou le Pointe H, Klein I, et al. Dynamic gadolinium-enhanced subtraction MR imaging: a simple technique for the early diagnosis of Legg-Calvé-Perthes disease—preliminary results. Pediatr Radiol 1997; 27:216–220.
18. Bos CF, Bloem JL, Bloem RM. Sequential magnetic resonance imaging in Perthes' disease. J Bone Joint Surg [Br] 1991; 73:219–224.
19. Rush BH, Bramson RT, Ogden JA. Legg-Calvé-Perthes disease: detection of cartilaginous and synovial changes with MR imaging. Radiology 1988; 167:473–476.
20. Ducou le Pointe H, Haddad S, Silberman B, Filipe G, Monroc M, Montagne JP. Legg-Perthes-Calvé disease: staging by MRI using gadolinium. Pediatr Radiol 1994; 24:88–91.
21. Jaramillo D, Kasser JR, Villegas-Medina OL, Gaary E, Zurakowski D. Cartilaginous abnormalities and growth disturbances in Legg-Calvé-Perthes disease: evaluation with MR imaging. Radiology 1995; 197:767–773.
22. Weinstein SL. Legg-Calvé-Perthes syndrome. In: Morrissy RT, Weinstein SL, eds. Pediatric orthopedics. Vol 2. Philadelphia, Pa: Lippincott-Raven, 1996; 951–991.
23. Reinker KA. Early diagnosis and treatment of hinge abduction in Legg-Perthes disease. J Pediatr Orthop 1996; 163:3–9.

Bruno C. Vande Berg, MD, PhD
Jacques J. Malghem, MD
Frederic E. Lecouvet, MD
Jacques Jamart, MD
Baudouin E. Maldague, MD

Index terms:
Alcohol, 443.869
Bone marrow, edema, 443.499
Hip, MR, 443.121411, 443.12143
Hip, necrosis, 443.44
Myeloma, 443.34
Osteoporosis, 443.56
Osteomalacia, 443.57
Steroids, complications, 443.542

Radiology 1999; 212:527–535

Abbreviation:
ROC = receiver operating characteristic

[1] From the Department of Radiology and Medical Imaging, Cliniques Universitaires St Luc, Universite catholique de Louvain, 10 Avenue Hippocrate, 1200 Brussels, Belgium (B.C.V.B., J.J.M., F.E.L., B.E.M.) and the Center for Biostatistics and Medical Documentation, Universite catholique de Louvain, Cliniques Universitaires de Mont Godinne, Yvoir, Belgium (J.J.). Received June 29, 1998; revision requested August 5; final revision received November 11; accepted February 22, 1999. **Address reprint requests to** B.C.V.B. (e-mail: *vandeberg@rdgn.ucl.ac.be*).

Author contributions:
Guarantor of integrity of entire study, B.C.V.B.; study concepts, B.E.M., J.J.M.; study design, B.C.V.B.; definition of intellectual content, B.C.V.B., J.J.M.; literature research, B.C.V.B.; clinical studies, B.C.V.B., J.J.M., F.E.L.; data acquisition, B.C.V.B., J.J.M., F.E.L.; data analysis, B.C.V.B., F.E.L.; statistical analysis, J.J.; manuscript preparation, B.C.V.B.; manuscript editing, B.C.V.B., J.J.M., B.E.M., F.E.L.; manuscript review, all authors.

Idiopathic Bone Marrow Edema Lesions of the Femoral Head: Predictive Value of MR Imaging Findings[1]

PURPOSE: To determine the frequency of several subchondral magnetic resonance (MR) imaging features observed in bone marrow edema lesions of the femoral head and to determine their value for differentiation of irreversible from transient lesions.

MATERIALS AND METHODS: The authors reviewed MR images of 72 femoral head lesions in 42 men and 25 women (median age, 48 years) with equivocal radiographic findings and bone marrow edema seen at MR imaging (T1- and T2-weighted images in all patients and contrast material–enhanced T1-weighted images in 39 patients). Follow-up MR images showed 57 lesions to be transient and 15 to be irreversible. The presence and size of subtle subchondral features observed on initial MR images were compared for both types of lesion.

RESULTS: Lack of any additional subchondral change on T2-weighted or contrast-enhanced T1-weighted images had 100% positive predictive value for transient lesions. For irreversible lesions, presence of a subchondral area of low signal intensity at least 4 mm thick or 12.5 mm long had positive predictive values of 85% and 73%, respectively, on T2-weighted images and 87% and 86%, respectively, on contrast-enhanced T1-weighted images.

CONCLUSION: Careful assessment of subchondral changes enables confident differentiation between early irreversible lesions and transient bone marrow edema lesions.

Magnetic resonance (MR) imaging greatly contributes to the assessment of symptomatic hip joints when inconclusive radiographs have been obtained (1). One of most outstanding advantages of MR imaging is the ability to depict radiographically occult femoral head osteonecrosis (2–5).

Typically, femoral head osteonecrosis is characterized by a subchondral lesion of variable signal intensity that is demarcated from the surrounding tissue by a rim of low signal intensity on T1-weighted MR images and of low and high signal intensity on T2-weighted MR images (2,3,6–10). This lesion pattern differs from the bone marrow edema pattern that is characterized by an ill-defined epiphyseal marrow area of low signal intensity on T1-weighted MR images and of intermediate to high signal intensity on T2-weighted images (11–14). The bone marrow edema pattern is nonspecific and can be observed in association with several conditions, including transient osteoporosis (12,15–17), transient bone marrow edema syndrome (12,13,16), and epiphyseal stress fracture (18,19). These conditions are self-limiting disorders that necessitate no specific therapy other than palliative measures.

Femoral head osteonecrosis occasionally manifests with the bone marrow edema pattern at MR imaging, with, however, no visible reactive interface between necrotic and viable tissue (3,12,20–22). Therefore, when the bone marrow edema pattern is present in a femoral head, early differentiation between irreversible epiphyseal osteonecrosis and a spontaneously transient lesion is important to prevent overtreatment of spontaneously resolving lesions and reserve more aggressive therapy for lesions that are associated with a poor prognosis (1,13,14,23–26).

On T2-weighted and contrast material–enhanced T1-weighted MR images of bone marrow edema lesions of the femoral head, several discrete features can occasionally be observed in the subchondral area of the femoral head (12,17,19,26). In hypothetical terms, assessment of the presence of these subchondral changes and precise determination of their spatial characteristics on MR images could help differentiate irreversible from transient epiphyseal lesions. We previously demonstrated the prognostic value of MR imaging in the setting of lesions of the femoral condyle (27), and we now address lesions of the femoral head that show the bone marrow edema pattern.

In January 1989, we started a prospective study that included all patients in whom MR imaging demonstrated the bone marrow edema pattern in the femoral head and in whom radiographs were inconclusive; these patients were treated conservatively and were followed up to determine the outcome of the lesions. Our aims were to compare irreversible and transient lesions for the frequency and extent of subchondral changes observed at MR imaging and to determine the features that most reliably enable differentiation between these lesions.

MATERIALS AND METHODS

Patients

The study population consisted of 67 patients (42 men and 25 women; median age, 48 years; age range, 29–84 years) with a total of 72 lesions. Five patients had bilateral epiphyseal abnormalities that occurred simultaneously (n = 4) or successively (n = 1). Inclusion criteria were (*a*) spontaneous hip pain with no history of trauma or no clinical suspicion of inflammatory disorder, (*b*) normal or inconclusive radiographs, (*c*) an ill-defined area of low signal intensity involving the femoral head on T1-weighted MR images and intermediate to high signal intensity on T2-weighted MR images, (*d*) no surgical treatment, and (*e*) available imaging proof of the outcome of the lesion. Patients with femoral head lesions with joint-space narrowing on conventional radiographs or cartilage lesions on MR images were excluded. Patients with lesions with a reactive interface on MR images also were excluded.

All patients underwent an initial MR study performed at our institution between January 1989 and January 1997. None of the patients had been referred for consultation. In addition, 10 other lesions (in 10 patients) that fulfilled the inclusion criteria at the onset of the disease were excluded from the current study because of the lack of definite imaging proof of lesion outcome. Of the 10 patients with no available imaging follow-up, seven, who were contacted by phone, reported no residual pain, and three were lost to follow-up.

Nine lesions occurred during or immediately after pregnancy. Other associated findings were frank, diffuse osteoporosis seen on conventional radiographs (n = 5); osteomalacia (n = 5); history of alcohol abuse (n = 5), steroid therapy (n = 4), or fluoride therapy (n = 1); renal transplantation (n = 5); chronic renal failure (n = 1); radiation therapy (n = 1); and untreated multiple myeloma (n = 2). Because all patients were not primarily evaluated for the presence of these conditions, we cannot verify the importance of the conditions in the pathogenesis of the lesions. In the other 34 patients (34 lesions), the medical history was unremarkable.

Conventional radiographs, including anteroposterior views of the pelvis and anteroposterior and lateral views of the symptomatic hips, showed either no abnormality (n = 22) or nonspecific findings, which were described as discrete subchondral sclerosis (n = 10), subchondral bone rarefaction (n = 25), or both (n = 15). Forty-seven patients had undergone technetium 99m bone scanning that consistently demonstrated increased isotope uptake in the femoral heads, which corresponded to the bone marrow edema pattern seen at MR imaging.

Initial MR Imaging

MR imaging was performed at a mean (±SD) of 9.7 weeks ± 6.4 (median interval, 8 weeks; range, 2–32 weeks) after the onset of symptoms by using a 1.5-T (56 lesions) or a 0.5-T (16 lesions) superconducting magnet (Gyroscan; Philips Medical Systems, Best, the Netherlands).

After acquisition of sets of transverse T1-weighted scout MR images and comparative coronal T1-weighted MR images of both hips, coronal T1-weighted images of the symptomatic hips were systematically obtained by using a 40 × 20-cm supple receiver-only surface coil (Philips Medical Systems) wrapped around the symptomatic hip joint. In 57 lesions, sagittal T1-weighted images were obtained in a plane with approximately 10° of internal rotation with respect to the plane perpendicular to the femoral neck.

T1-weighted spin-echo MR images were obtained with the following parameters: 350–550/20–25 (repetition time msec/echo time msec), 14–20-cm field of view, 3.5–5.0-mm section thickness, 0.5-mm intersection gap, two to four signals acquired, and a 230 × 256 matrix.

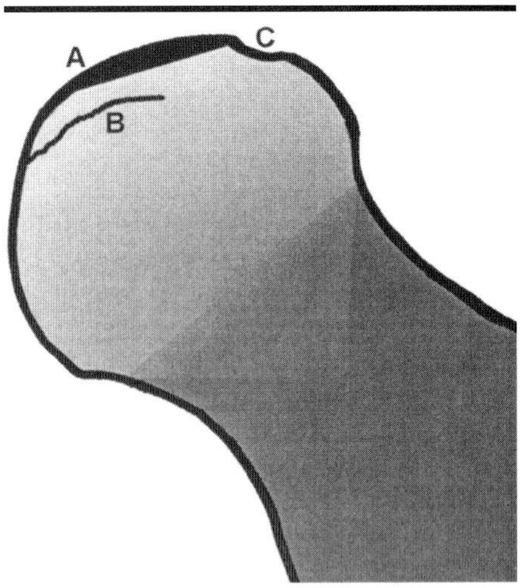

Figure 1. Schematic view of a coronal T2-weighted MR image of the proximal end of the femur depicts a subchondral area of low signal intensity (*A*), a thin line of low signal intensity (*B*), and a focal deformity of the epiphyseal contour (*C*), all within an ill-defined area of intermediate to high signal intensity suggestive of edema.

T2-weighted spin-echo MR images also were obtained by using the surface coil. Coronal or sagittal images were obtained as necessary, depending on the topography of the marrow changes on the T1-weighted images. The sagittal plane was favored when femoral head changes predominated anteriorly or posteriorly, and the coronal plane was selected when the predominant area of involvement was the upper aspect of the femoral head. Both sagittal and coronal images were obtained in 21 lesions.

Fifty-four sets of sagittal and 39 sets of coronal T2-weighted spin-echo images were obtained with the following parameters: 2,000–2,500/100–120, 16–20-cm field of view, 4–5-mm section thickness, 0.5-mm intersection gap, one to two signals acquired, and a 180 × 256 matrix.

T1-weighted spin-echo MR images were obtained after administration of 0.1 mmol/kg gadoterate dimeglumine (Dotarem; Guerbet, Roissy, France) in 39 consecutive lesions observed between 1989 and 1993. In these patients, the technique and spatial parameters were identical to those used for nonenhanced T1-weighted sagittal (n = 29) or coronal (n = 32) MR imaging. At the time of the study, fat-saturated T1-weighted MR images were

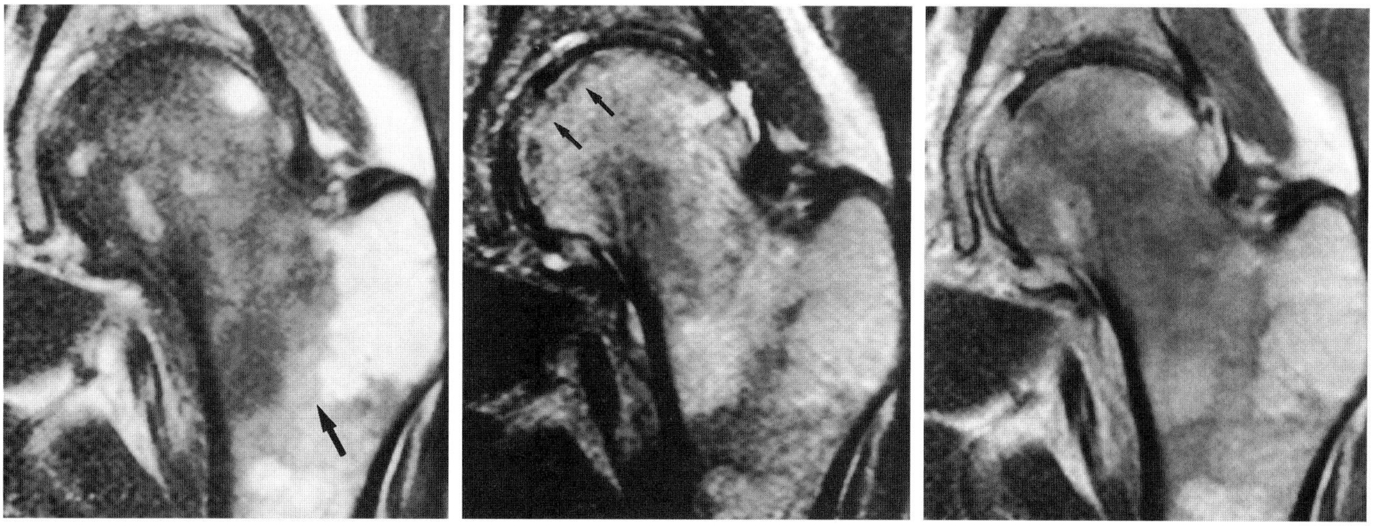

a. b. c.

Figure 2. MR images in a 43-year-old woman with left hip pain of 7 weeks duration. **(a)** Coronal T1-weighted (415/20) image of the left hip shows an ill-defined area of reduced signal intensity in the femoral head and neck (arrow). **(b)** Corresponding coronal T2-weighted image (2,200/120) shows increased signal intensity in the same area and a low signal intensity line (arrows). **(c)** Corresponding coronal contrast-enhanced T1-weighted (415/20) image shows a homogeneous increase in signal intensity. A follow-up MR study obtained 11 months later (not shown), when the patient was asymptomatic, demonstrated normal epiphyseal marrow.

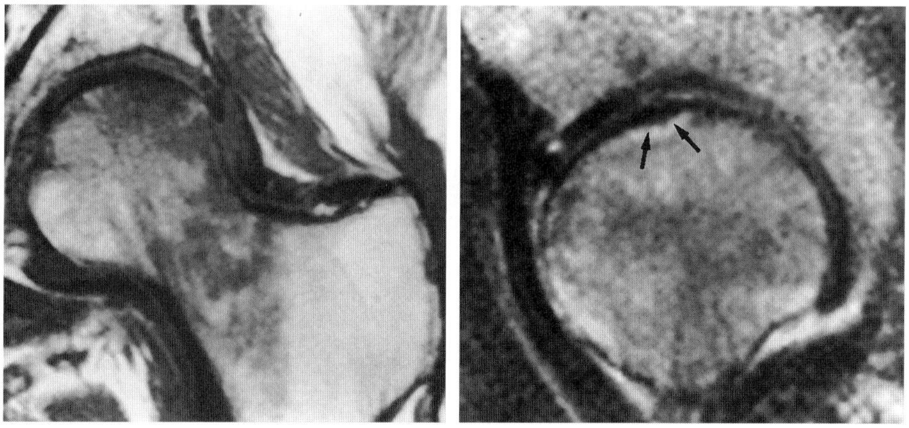

a. b.

Figure 3. MR images in a 70-year-old woman with left hip pain of 12 weeks duration. **(a)** Coronal T1-weighted (510/22) image of the left hip shows an ill-defined area of low signal intensity in the femoral head and neck. **(b)** Sagittal T2-weighted image (2,200/120) shows intermediate to high signal intensity in the femoral head. A low-signal-intensity subchondral area (arrows) is depicted in the upper pole of the femoral head. This 2.5-mm-thick, 10-mm-long area is compatible with a transient lesion. Follow-up MR study obtained 6 months later (not shown) demonstrated complete resolution of femoral head marrow changes.

not available at our MR unit. The duration of the MR examination was 25–45 minutes.

Other sequences included T2*-weighted gradient-echo, T2-weighted fast spin-echo, fat-saturated fast spin-echo, intermediate-weighted, and T2-weighted imaging sequences. These sequences were performed in some patients during the study period, but the images were not included in the review process.

Patient Follow-up and Determination of Lesion Outcome

All patients were advised to reduce weight bearing by using two crutches and then one crutch during 3–5 weeks. Nonsteroid analgesics were prescribed. Patients were not confined to bed rest. All patients were informed of the prospective study and consented to undergo future MR or radiographic studies to determine lesion outcome. At the time of this study, our ethical committee did not mandate its approval for noninvasive diagnostic procedures of potential clinical importance, provided that informed consent had been obtained from the patients.

Follow-up imaging was performed regardless of whether symptoms persisted and continued for at least 24 months, unless either conventional radiographs showed typical osteonecrosis with epiphyseal collapse or MR images showed complete resolution of marrow abnormalities. A total of 111 follow-up MR studies were obtained, including 64 studies obtained within 6 months after the initial study, 24 obtained 6–12 months after the initial study, and 23 obtained more than 12 months after the initial study. Seven patients did not come to the scheduled follow-up MR examination but decided to undergo follow-up MR imaging during 1997, 15–72 months (mean, 46 months) after the initial study. Follow-up MR studies included sagittal and coronal T1-weighted images obtained with the same technical parameters as for the initial studies. Follow-up T2-weighted images were obtained when persistent abnormalities were present on T1-weighted images.

A lesion was considered to be transient if normal signal intensity was observed in the femoral head on follow-up T1-weighted MR images, with resolution of the abnormalities that had been seen on initial MR studies. A lesion was considered to be irreversible if typical osteonecrosis occurred or if residual changes were demonstrated at MR imaging after at least 2 years of follow-up.

Analysis of Initial MR Images

The 283 sets of initial MR images (129 sets of T1-weighted images, 93 sets of T2-weighted images, and 61 sets of contrast-enhanced T1-weighted images) were reviewed independently by two musculoskeletal radiologists (B.C.V.B., F.E.L.) who were unaware of patient name, age, and sex and of lesion outcome. Initial radiographs, bone scans, initial large-field-of-view comparative T1-weighted coronal MR images, and all follow-up imaging studies were not available. All sets of images from each case were reviewed separately from each other. To assess intraobserver reproducibility, one radiologist (B.C.V.B.) reviewed the 283 sets of images 6 months after initial analysis.

Bone marrow edema was a common MR imaging feature of all lesions, and no lesion manifested with the demarcation rim or reactive interface typical of avascular necrosis. Because of previously reported (12,17,19,26) additional subchondral findings, we studied three parameters to determine their prognostic significance: low-signal-intensity subchondral areas, epiphyseal lines, and contour deformities (Fig 1).

On all MR images, the following characteristics observed in the subchondral area of the involved femoral heads were determined: (*a*) the presence, length, and thickness of subchondral areas of low signal intensity immediately adjacent to subchondral bone; (*b*) the presence, length, and distance from subchondral bone of low-signal-intensity lines that coursed in the vicinity of and approximately parallel to the articular surface; and (*c*) subtle focal contour deformities of the subchondral bone plate. These deformities were graded with a four-point scale: grade of 0, absent; grade of 1, possible flattening; grade of 2, possible depression; or grade of 3, frank depression.

Measurements were performed on the images, which were printed on separate films with a 1.2–1.4 zoom factor, by using a 0.5-mm–graduated ruler. In addition, the extent of the ill-defined area of low signal intensity was determined on coronal T1-weighted MR images and was considered to involve either the epiphysis alone or both the epiphysis and the femoral neck. These subchondral changes are illustrated in Figures 2–5.

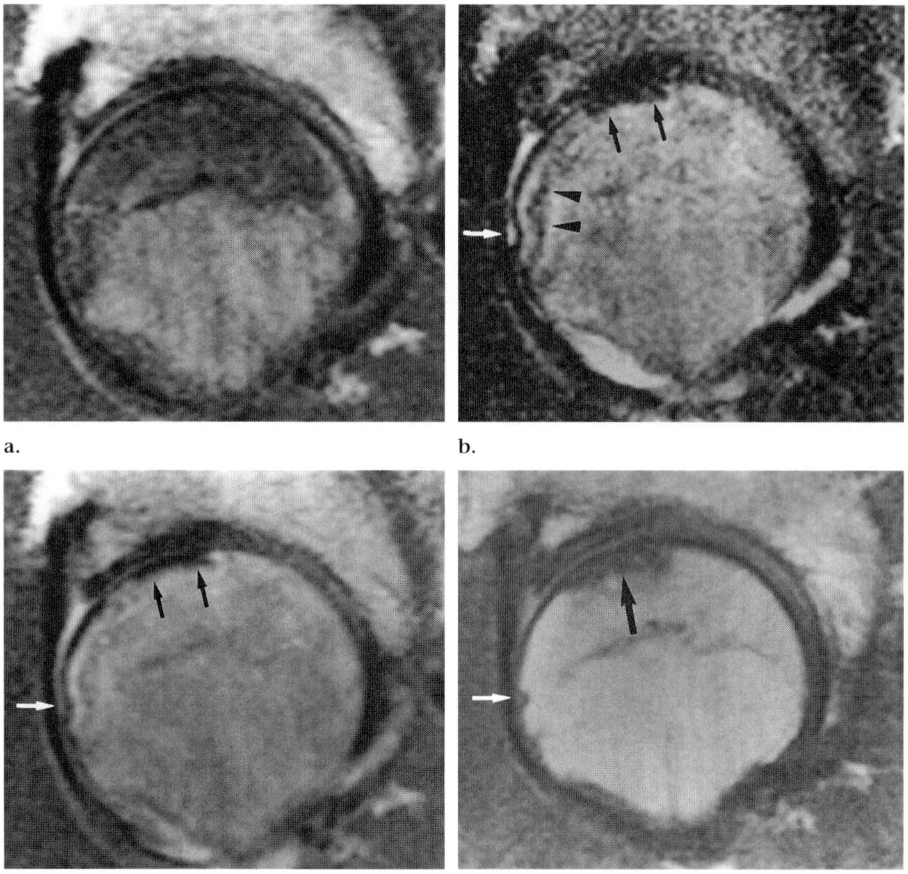

a. b. c. d.

Figure 4. MR images in a 34-year-old man with right hip pain of 14 weeks duration. **(a)** Sagittal T1-weighted (450/20) image of the right hip shows an ill-defined area of low signal intensity in the femoral head. **(b)** Corresponding sagittal T2-weighted (2,100/120) image shows a 3-mm-thick, 12-mm-long area of low signal intensity (black arrows) adjacent to the subchondral bone plate. A grade 2 deformity of the subchondral bone plate (white arrow) is well depicted at the anterior aspect of the femoral head, with a 25-mm-long line of low signal intensity (arrowheads). **(c)** Corresponding sagittal contrast-enhanced T1-weighted (450/20) image better depicts the low-signal-intensity subchondral area (black arrows) and the epiphyseal deformity (white arrow). **(d)** Sagittal T1-weighted (415/20) image obtained 2 years later, when the patient was asymptomatic, demonstrates irreversibility of the lesion. A small subchondral area of low signal intensity (black arrow) is present at the upper pole of the femoral head, and minor residual changes can be seen at the anterior aspect of the epiphysis (white arrow).

Statistical Analyses

Statistical comparisons were performed by using the χ^2 test for independent categoric variables, the Student *t* test for numeric variables, and the Wilcoxon rank sum test for ordinal variables. All tests were two tailed. A *P* value of less than .05 was considered to indicate a significant difference.

The ability of the statistically significant parameters to aid in differentiation of irreversible from transient lesions was assessed by calculating the sensitivity, specificity, and positive and negative predictive values for qualitative parameters and receiver operating characteristic (ROC) curves for quantitative measurements. ROC curves obtained for the length and the thickness of the subchondral low-signal-intensity component on T2-weighted and contrast-enhanced T1-weighted images were constructed for both observers by using maximum likelihood estimation calculated with the Labroc 1 program (C. Metz, Chicago, Ill). Values measured by the first observer were used to calculate sensitivities, specificities, and predictive values.

Reproducibility of findings between observers was assessed with the κ coefficient for categoric parameters and with correlation coefficients for numeric variables. In general, a κ value of less than 0.4 represented a poor level of agreement; a κ value of 0.41–0.60, fair agreement; a κ value of 0.61–0.80, good agreement; and a κ value of 0.81–1.00, excellent agreement (28). To study intra- and interobserver reproducibility, parameters derived from all sagittal and coronal images were

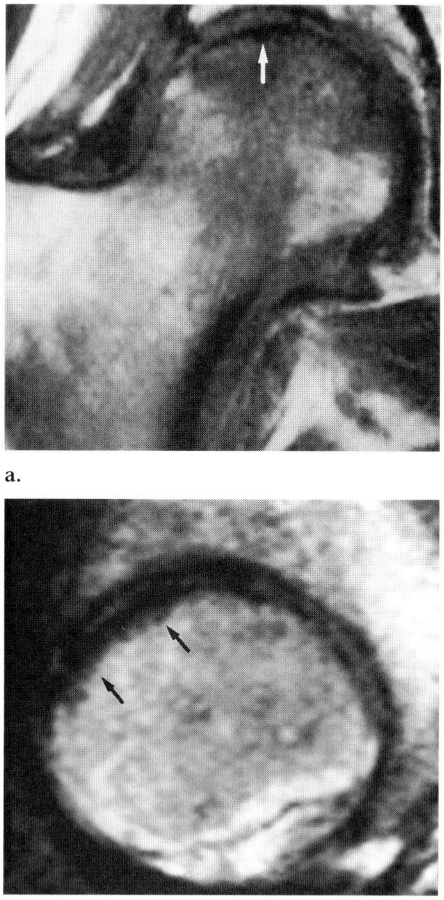

a.

b.

Figure 5. MR images in a 62-year-old woman with right hip pain of 10 weeks duration. **(a)** Coronal T1-weighted (415/20) image of the right hip shows an ill-defined area of low signal intensity in the femoral head and neck and a subchondral area with a more pronounced decrease in signal intensity (arrow). **(b)** Sagittal T2-weighted (2,140/120) image shows increased signal intensity in the femoral head, with a 4-mm-thick, 20-mm-long area of low signal intensity (arrows) at the anterosuperior pole of the femoral head. Follow-up radiographs (not shown) demonstrated femoral head osteonecrosis with a subchondral bone fracture. Total hip replacement was performed 7 months later.

used. To study the prognostic significance of MR parameters, the more elevated values from either the sagittal or the coronal images were used for statistical analysis.

RESULTS

Outcome of Femoral Head Lesions

In 57 lesions, normal epiphyseal signal intensity was seen on follow-up MR images. Of 50 lesions that were prospectively followed, 48 were healed within 12 months and two were healed within 24 months after acquisition of the initial study. The seven patients who did not come to the scheduled follow-up MR examination but who agreed to undergo follow-up MR imaging 15–72 months (mean, 46 months) after the initial study had normal findings at follow-up.

Fifteen lesions were irreversible. Nine lesions (in eight patients) showed epiphyseal collapse with a subchondral bone fracture on conventional radiographs after 2–18-month follow-up (mean, 6.3 months). Seven patients, each with one lesion, were treated with total hip replacement. Two lesions in the same patient were well tolerated 47 months after disease onset. Six other lesions (in six patients) showed small, residual subchondral changes at MR imaging but no definite signs of osteonecrosis on radiographs. These six lesions were well tolerated clinically, and none of these patients had undergone surgery at the time of this writing. These six lesions were followed with MR imaging (20 studies) for a mean of 41 months (range, 24–76 months) after the initial MR study.

TABLE 1
Clinical Findings in Patients with Transient Lesions and Patients with Irreversible Lesions

Finding	Transient Lesions (n = 57)	Irreversible Lesions (n = 15)
Sex (M/F)	35/22	10/5
Side of lesion		
Right	30	5
Left	27	10
Age (y)*	49 ± 12	54 ± 17
Time between symptom onset and initial MR imaging (wk)*	9 ± 6	11 ± 7
Radiographic appearance		
Osteopenia	20	5
Osteopenia and sclerosis	11	4
Sclerosis	7	3
Normal	19	3

Note.—There were no significant differences between types of lesion.
* Data are the mean plus or minus the SD.

Clinical and Radiographic Findings

There were no significant differences between the group of patients with irreversible lesions (n = 15) and the group with transient lesions (n = 57) in terms of sex, age, side of the lesion, and interval between the onset of symptoms and the time of initial MR imaging (Table 1). Sixteen (46%) of 35 transient lesions observed in men and 13 (59%) of 22 transient lesions observed in women involved the left femoral head. The frequencies of the different patterns of changes determined on radiographs (osteopenia, subchondral sclerosis, mixed osteopenia and sclerosis, and normal appearance) were not significantly different between the groups.

Frequency of Additional Subchondral Changes on MR Images

On T1-weighted images, lack of additional subchondral changes and presence of low-signal-intensity subchondral areas, epiphyseal lines, and epiphyseal deformity, respectively, were observed in 21 (29%), 14 (19%), 32 (44%), and 32 (44%) of 72 lesions. On T2-weighted images, lack of subchondral changes and presence of low-signal-intensity subchondral areas, epiphyseal lines, and epiphyseal deformity, respectively, were observed in 24 (33%), 32 (44%), 21 (29%), and 37 (51%) of 72 lesions. On contrast-enhanced T1-weighted images, these features were observed in seven (18%), 17 (44%), 21 (54%), and 21 (54%) of 39 lesions, respectively (Figs 2–5).

Frequency of Subchondral Changes in Irreversible and Transient Lesions

On T1-weighted images, there was no difference in the frequency of subchondral changes between irreversible and transient lesions, and the usefulness of T1-weighted images for help in predicting the outcome was not further studied. Lack of additional subchondral changes was significantly more frequent in transient lesions than in irreversible lesions on T2-weighted images (24 [42%] of 57 transient and none [0%] of 15 irreversible lesions; $P < .001$) and contrast-enhanced T1-weighted images (seven [23%] of 30 transient and none [0%] of nine irreversible lesions; $P < .001$).

Low-signal-intensity subchondral areas (Figs 3–5) were significantly more frequent in irreversible than in transient lesions on T2-weighted images (15 [100%] of 15 irreversible and 17 [30%] of 57 transient lesions; $P < .001$) and on contrast-enhanced T1-weighted images (nine [100%] of nine irreversible and nine [29%] of 30 transient lesions; $P < .001$).

Epiphyseal deformities (Fig 4) were significantly more frequent in irreversible than in transient lesions on T2-weighted images (10 [66%] of 15 irreversible and 11 [19%] of 57 transient lesions; $P = .002$) and on contrast-enhanced T1-weighted images (nine [100%] of nine irreversible and eight [25%] of 30 transient lesions; $P < .001$).

Frequency of epiphyseal lines (Figs 2, 4) was not significantly different between irreversible and transient lesions on either T2-weighted (10 [66%] of 15 irreversible and 28 [49%] of 57 transient lesions) or contrast-enhanced T1-weighted (six [66%] of nine irreversible and 15 [50%] of 30 transient lesions) images.

Prognostic Value of the Subchondral Changes on MR Images

Lack of subchondral changes.—Lack of additional subchondral changes on both T2-weighted and contrast-enhanced T1-weighted images had excellent positive predictive value for the recognition of transient lesions (Table 2).

Subchondral low-signal-intensity areas.—Presence of subchondral low-signal-intensity areas on T2-weighted and contrast-enhanced T1-weighted images had excellent negative predictive value and poor positive predictive value for the recognition of irreversible lesions (Table 3). To discriminate irreversible from transient lesions, acceptable cutoff values for measurement of the subchondral low-signal-intensity component were a thickness of 4 mm or more (positive predictive value, 85% on T2-weighted and 87% on contrast-enhanced T1-weighted images) and a length of 12.5 mm or more (positive predictive value, 73% on T2-weighted and 86% on contrast-enhanced T1-weighted images) (Table 4). Areas under ROC curves were greater than 0.942 for measurements of the length and thickness on T2-weighted and contrast-enhanced T1-weighted images (Table 5). Intra- and interobserver reproducibility for detection and measurement of the thickness of the subchondral low-signal-intensity area were greater than 0.842 (Table 6).

Epiphyseal contour deformity.—Presence of epiphyseal deformity as an indicator of an irreversible lesion on either T2-weighted or contrast-enhanced T1-weighted images had poor positive predictive value and satisfactory to excellent negative predictive value (Table 3). The importance of epiphyseal deformity was significantly different between irreversible and transient lesions, with discrete and frank deformities more frequent in irreversible than in transient lesions ($P < .01$). Areas under ROC curves for the degree of deformity were 0.788 on T2-weighted images and 0.925 on contrast-enhanced T1-weighted images (Table 5). The κ coefficients for intra- and interobserver reproducibility of the degree of epiphyseal deformity were moderate (Table 6).

Epiphyseal lines.—Presence of epiphyseal lines had poor positive predictive value as an indicator of an irreversible lesion (Table 3). Length and distance of epiphyseal lines from the epiphyseal contour were not significantly different between transient and irreversible lesions.

DISCUSSION

Since the advent of MR imaging for evaluation of the symptomatic hip, the meaning of the diffuse pattern of abnormal marrow signal intensity has proved to be controversial (1,14). This abnormality is

TABLE 2
Sensitivity, Specificity, and Predictive Values for the Lack of Subchondral Changes as an Indicator of Transient Lesions

Type of MR Image	Sensitivity (%)	Specificity (%)	Positive Predictive Value (%)	Negative Predictive Value (%)
T1-weighted	31	80	86	23
T2-weighted	42	100	100	31
Contrast-enhanced T1-weighted	23	100	100	28

TABLE 3
Sensitivity, Specificity, and Predictive Values for T2-weighted and Contrast-enhanced T1-weighted MR Imaging Findings Indicative of Irreversible Lesions

Finding	Sensitivity (%)		Specificity (%)		Positive Predictive Value (%)		Negative Predictive Value (%)	
	T2-weighted	T1-weighted	T2-weighted	T1-weighted	T2-weighted	T1-weighted	T2-weighted	T1-weighted
Low-signal-intensity subchondral area	100	100	68	71	45	53	100	100
Epiphyseal deformity	60	100	79	57	43	43	88	100
Epiphyseal line	60	44	60	39	28	19	85	68

TABLE 4
Sensitivity, Specificity, and Predictive Values for Selected Cutoff Values for T2-weighted and Contrast-enhanced T1-weighted MR Imaging Findings Indicative of Irreversible Lesions

Cutoff Value of Low-Signal-Intensity Subchondral Area	Sensitivity (%)		Specificity (%)		Positive Predictive Value (%)		Negative Predictive Value (%)	
	T2-weighted	T1-weighted	T2-weighted	T1-weighted	T2-weighted	T1-weighted	T2-weighted	T1-weighted
Thickness ≥ 2.5 mm	100	89	86	89	65	73	100	89
Thickness ≥ 4.0 mm	73	78	96	96	85	87	93	93
Length ≥ 9.5 mm	87	89	86	89	62	73	96	96
Length ≥ 12.5 mm	73	67	93	96	73	86	93	90

characterized by an ill-defined area of decreased signal intensity in the femoral head and neck on T1-weighted MR images and increased signal intensity on T2-weighted images. In this popularly known bone marrow edema pattern, there is no evidence of a reactive interface, which is considered to be specific for osteonecrosis (3,13). The bone marrow edema pattern has been described (3,12,13,15–22) in association with a number of conditions, including transient osteoporosis of the hip, transient bone marrow edema syndrome, epiphyseal stress fracture, and epiphyseal osteonecrosis. The distinction between these conditions is crucial because of considerable differences in treatment and prognosis (1). Actually, the first three conditions are self limiting and resolve with conservative treatment. In contrast, epiphyseal osteonecrosis usually is not spontaneously reversible and can lead to epiphyseal collapse (29–31).

In the current prospective study, the spontaneous outcome in 72 femoral head lesions that were not treated surgically and that showed the bone marrow edema pattern was determined by using serial imaging. The features observed at initial MR imaging in 57 transient lesions and 15 irreversible lesions were reviewed to determine whether initial MR studies enabled early differentiation of irreversible lesions from transient lesions.

The results of our study allowed us to draw the following conclusions. First, absence of additional subchondral changes other than the bone marrow edema pattern on T2-weighted or contrast-enhanced T1-weighted images had excellent specificity and positive predictive value for transient lesions. Actually, all 24 (33%) lesions that showed no subchondral marrow changes other than the bone marrow edema pattern on T2-weighted images were found to be transient on follow-up MR studies. The transformation of a lesion that initially showed only the bone marrow edema pattern into an irreversible lesion was not observed in the current study.

Second, in about two-thirds of 72 bone marrow edema lesions, additional focal changes were depicted in the area adjacent to the subchondral bone plate on T2-weighted and contrast-enhanced T1-weighted MR images obtained with a small field of view. Actually, subchondral areas of low signal intensity, subtle deformity of the epiphyseal contours, and epiphyseal lines of low signal intensity were seen on T2-weighted images in 44%, 29%, and 52% of lesions, respectively. These three additional changes in signal intensity were observed in both transient and irreversible lesions. Subchondral low-signal-intensity areas and contour deformity, but not epiphyseal lines, were significantly more frequent in irreversible lesions than in transient lesions.

Finally, determination of the length and thickness of low-signal-intensity subchondral areas and of the importance of contour deformity on either T2-weighted or contrast-enhanced T1-weighted images helped differentiate irreversible from transient lesions. The presence and extent of epiphyseal lines of low signal intensity, however, had poor prognostic value.

Subchondral areas of low signal intensity had the greatest prognostic importance. In our study, a low-signal-intensity subchondral area with a thickness of at least 4 mm on T2-weighted or contrast-enhanced T1-weighted images had a positive predictive value of greater than 85% for prediction of lesion irreversibility. Similarly, a low-signal-intensity subchondral area with a length of at least 12.5 mm had a positive predictive value of greater than 73%. The κ values were indicative of excellent reproducibility of the size measurements obtained with both types of images but were greater with contrast-enhanced T1-weighted images than with T2-weighted images, probably because of better signal intensity contrast between epiphyseal marrow, subchondral changes, and articular cartilage on the contrast-enhanced T1-weighted images.

The magnitude of epiphyseal contour deformity also helped with recognition of irreversible lesions, with frank deformity more frequently associated with irreversible lesions than with transient lesions. However, because reproducibility of the determination of the degree of deformity was fair, the value of this criterion warrants further assessment. Computed tomography is superior to MR imaging for demonstrating changes in the sphericity of the femoral head (32,33) and could be used to assess epiphyseal contours when findings of bone marrow edema lesions are equivocal.

TABLE 5
Area under the ROC Curve for Measurements of Low-Signal-Intensity Areas and Importance of Epiphyseal Deformity as Indicators of Irreversible Lesions

Finding	T1-weighted Images	T2-weighted Images	Contrast-enhanced T1-weighted Images
Low-signal-intensity area measurement			
Thickness	0.652 ± 0.073	0.964 ± 0.021	0.963 ± 0.038
Length	0.630 ± 0.089	0.942 ± 0.026	0.952 ± 0.041
Epiphyseal deformity	0.712 ± 0.108	0.788 ± 0.083	0.925 ± 0.043

Note.—Data are area under the ROC curve plus or minus the standard error.

TABLE 6
Intra- and Interobserver Reproducibility for Detection and Measurement of Subchondral Changes on MR Images

Imaging Finding and Result	T1-weighted Images		T2-weighted Images		Contrast-enhanced T1-weighted Images	
	Intraobserver	Interobserver	Intraobserver	Interobserver	Intraobserver	Interobserver
Low-signal-intensity area						
Presence (κ)	0.756	0.468	0.757	0.843	1.000	0.827
Thickness (*r*)	0.638	0.546	0.863	0.898	0.976	0.892
Length (*r*)	0.660	0.466	0.692	0.672	0.905	0.880
Epiphyseal deformity						
Presence (κ)	0.665	0.616	0.687	0.570	0.734	0.726
Degree (κ)	0.560	0.504	0.579	0.502	0.555	0.466

MR imaging techniques, patient selection criteria, and outcome definitions used in the current study must be emphasized to avoid misinterpretation of our results. First, all images were obtained by using a surface coil and a small field of view. The higher spatial resolution achieved on these images than on large-field-of-view images could account for the high detection rate and good reproducibility of measurement of subchondral changes. It is possible that previously described (20) irreversible bone marrow edema lesions also had additional subchondral changes that were underestimated on the relatively low-resolution images obtained in the early era of MR imaging.

Second, we deliberately focused our investigation on ambiguous clinical and imaging conditions. Femoral head osteonecrosis lesions with obvious epiphyseal collapse seen on radiographs or with well-delimited marrow changes seen on MR images were not included in this study. Bone marrow edema lesions observed in association with joint-space narrowing on conventional radiographs or with cartilage lesions on MR images also were excluded. However, we did include 20 bone marrow edema lesions with radiographic features characteristic of transient osteoporosis of the hip. These lesions were included because focal osteopenia was rarely recognized by referring physicians and radiologists.

Finally, irreversible lesions did not systematically correspond to typical osteonecrosis, which was observed in nine of 15 irreversible lesions. The other six such lesions showed small residual subchondral signal intensity heterogeneities at MR imaging after a follow-up of 24–72 months. These small subchondral bone lesions were well tolerated clinically. A further study with a larger series of patients is needed to determine whether initial MR studies enable differentiation of lesions that will progress to typical osteonecrosis from relatively more benign lesions that will show only small residual changes at follow-up.

The fact that contrast-enhanced T1-weighted images helped differentiate irreversible from transient lesions does not imply that contrast material is necessary: Prognostic features depicted on T2-weighted images were similar to those observed on contrast-enhanced T1-weighted images. Our initial experience with contrast-enhanced T1-weighted images definitely helped by increasing confidence for detection of low-signal-intensity areas and focal deformities on T2-weighted images, because changes were often more conspicuous on contrast-enhanced T1-weighted images. In our current routine clinical practice, we reserve the performance of contrast-enhanced MR imaging for rare cases of equivocal findings on T2-weighted images. Furthermore, in our more recent experience, subchondral changes observed on standard T2-weighted spin-echo MR images also were well depicted on fast spin-echo T2-weighted and fat-saturated fast intermediate-weighted and T2-weighted images. These observations must be addressed in future studies.

The current study has several limitations inherent to the study design. First, implicit in the determination of a spontaneous lesion course is that no surgical intervention was performed. No correlation with histologic results can thus be provided. Results from previous studies (6,34,35) have demonstrated that subchondral areas of low signal intensity on either T2-weighted or contrast-enhanced T1-weighted images correspond to bone and marrow necrosis. Our observation that the size of these subchondral low-signal-intensity areas was directly related to outcome supports those previous results. The bone marrow edema pattern in itself is nonspecific, and histologic findings (36,37) from biopsy specimens of bone marrow edema lesions have demonstrated a range of features, including immature fibrovascular tissue, interstitial edema, bone and marrow necrosis, and variable changes in the trabecular network. The prognostic importance of the finding of bone and marrow necrosis at microscopic examination remains to be assessed, because bone and marrow cell death is a sign observed not only in epiphyseal osteonecrosis (38) but also in fractures (39), degenerative disease (40,41), and transient osteoporosis (20, 37,42).

Second, the effect on lesion outcome of a decrease in physical activity, which was recommended to all patients, remains unknown. Early recognition of a lesion and a subsequent decrease in physical activity could have influenced lesion outcome.

Finally, we addressed intra- and interobserver reproducibility of the identification of features that were helpful for determination of the prognosis. As in any single-center study, reproducibility is biased due to the experience that is progressively acquired by the reviewers. A multicenter study is mandatory to validate our observations.

Results from the current study of idiopathic femoral head lesions that show the bone marrow edema pattern at MR imaging demonstrate that precise analysis of the subchondral marrow changes depicted on T2-weighted or contrast-enhanced T1-weighted images helps differentiate irreversible lesions from transient lesions. Absence of subchondral low-signal-intensity areas on T2-weighted or contrast-enhanced T1-weighted images is invariably indicative of a spontaneous favorable outcome with resolution of the lesions. Thickness and length of the subchondral areas of low signal intensity on T2-weighted or contrast-enhanced T1-weighted images are the most important reproducible features for differentiation of irreversible lesions from transient lesions.

Acknowledgments: We are greatly indebted to the clinicians at our institution who collaborated in this study, including the orthopedic surgeons A. Vincent, MD, J. J. Rombouts, MD, P. De Nayer, MD, and colleagues, and the rheumatologists J. P. Devogelaer, MD, D. Manicourt, MD, and colleagues. We also thank Patrick Schmitz, Benoit Dehon, Eric Ligot, Françoise Martin, and Martine Milecan for technical and secretarial support.

References

1. Conway WF, Totty WG, McEnery KW. CT and MR imaging of the hip. Radiology 1996; 198:297–307.
2. Totty WG, Murphy WA, Ganz WI, Kumar B, Daum WJ, Siegel BA. Magnetic resonance imaging of the normal and ischemic femoral head. AJR 1984; 143:1273–1280.
3. Mitchell DG, Rao VM, Dalinka MK, et al. Femoral head avascular necrosis: correlation of MR imaging, radiographic staging, radionuclide imaging, and clinical findings. Radiology 1987; 162:709–715.
4. Mitchell DG, Kressel HY, Arger PH, Dalinka M, Spritzer CE, Steinberg ME. Avascular necrosis of the femoral head: morphologic assessment by MR imaging, with CT correlation. Radiology 1986; 161:739–742.
5. Mitchell MD, Kundel HL, Steinberg ME, Kressel HY, Alavi A, Axel L. Avascular necrosis of the hip: comparison of MR, CT, and scintigraphy. AJR 1986; 147: 67–71.
6. Lang P, Jergesen HE, Moseley ME, Block JE, Chafetz NI, Genant HK. Avascular necrosis of the femoral head: high-field-strength MR imaging with histologic correlation. Radiology 1988; 169:517–524.
7. Beltran J, Herman LJ, Burk JM, et al. Femoral head avascular necrosis: MR imaging with clinical-pathologic and radionuclide correlation. Radiology 1988; 166: 215–220.
8. Markisz JA, Knowles RJ, Altchek DW, Schneider R, Whalen JP, Cahill PT. Segmental patterns of avascular necrosis of the femoral heads: early detection with MR imaging. Radiology 1987; 162:717–720.
9. Coleman BG, Kressel HY, Dalinka MK, Scheibler ML, Burk DL, Cohen EK. Radio-

graphically negative avascular necrosis: detection with MR imaging. Radiology 1988; 168:525–528.
10. Tervonen O, Mueller DM, Matteson EL, Velosa JA, Ginsburg WW, Ehman RL. Clinically occult avascular necrosis of the hip: prevalence in an asymptomatic population at risk. Radiology 1992; 182:845–847.
11. Vogler JB III, Murphy WA. Bone marrow imaging. Radiology 1988; 168:679–693.
12. Vande Berg BC, Malghem JJ, Labaisse MA, Noel HM, Maldague BE. MR imaging of avascular necrosis and transient marrow edema of the femoral head. RadioGraphics 1993; 13:501–520.
13. Hayes CW, Conway WF, Daniel WW. MR imaging of bone marrow edema pattern: transient osteoporosis, transient bone marrow edema syndrome, or osteonecrosis. RadioGraphics 1993; 13:1001–1011.
14. Mitchell DG. Using MR imaging to probe the pathophysiology of osteonecrosis (editorial). Radiology 1989; 171:25–26.
15. Bloem JL. Transient osteoporosis of the hip: MR imaging. Radiology 1988; 167: 753–755.
16. Wilson AJ, Murphy WA, Hardy DC, Totty WG. Transient osteoporosis: transient bone marrow edema? Radiology 1988; 167:757–760.
17. Higer HP, Grimm J, Pedrosa P, Apel R, Bandilla K. Transitorische osteoporose oder femurkopfnekrose? frühdiagnose mit der MRT. ROFO 1989; 150:407–412.
18. Vande Berg BC, Malghem J, Goffin EJ, Duprez TP, Maldague BE. Transient epiphyseal lesions in renal transplant recipients: presumed insufficiency stress fractures. Radiology 1994; 191:403–407.
19. Rafii M, Mitnick H, Klug J, Firooznia H. Insufficiency fracture of the femoral head: MR imaging in three patients. AJR 1997; 168:159–163.
20. Turner DA, Templeton AC, Selzer PM, Rosenberg AG, Petasnick JP. Femoral capital osteonecrosis: MR finding of diffuse marrow abnormalities without focal lesions. Radiology 1989; 171:135–140.
21. Mitchell DG, Kressel HY. MR imaging of early avascular necrosis (letter). Radiology 1988; 169:281–282.
22. Thickman D, Axel L, Kressel HY, et al. Magnetic resonance imaging of avascular necrosis of the femoral head. Skeletal Radiol 1986; 15:133–140.
23. Froberg PK, Braunstein EM, Buckwalter KA. Osteonecrosis, transient osteoporosis, and transient bone marrow edema: current concepts. Radiol Clin North Am 1996; 34:273–291.
24. Stutley JE, Conway WF. Magnetic resonance imaging of the pelvis and hips. Orthopedics 1994; 17:1053–1062.
25. MacDougall L, Conway WF. Controversies in magnetic resonance imaging of the hip. Top Magn Reson Imaging 1996; 8:44–50.
26. Maldague BE, Vande Berg BC, Duprez TP, et al. Avascular necrosis, transient osteoporosis, and presumed stress fractures of the femoral head: imaging approach and differential diagnosis. In: Baert AL, Grenier P, Willi UV, Bloem JL, eds. Musculoskeletal imaging: an update. Berlin, Germany: Springer-Verlag, 1995; 45–56.
27. Lecouvet FE, Vande Berg BC, Maldague BE, et al. Early irreversible osteonecrosis versus transient lesions of the femoral condyles: prognostic value of subchondral bone and marrow changes on MR imaging. AJR 1998; 170:71–77.
28. Landis JR, Koch GG. The measurement of observer agreement for categorical data. Biometrics 1977; 33:159–174.
29. Shimizu K, Moriya H, Akita T, Sakamoto M, Suguro T. Prediction of collapse with magnetic resonance imaging of avascular necrosis of the femoral head. J Bone Joint Surg [Am] 1994; 76:215–223.
30. Lafforgue P, Dahan E, Chagnaud C, Schiano A, Kasbarian M, Acquaviva PC. Early-stage avascular necrosis of the femoral head: MR imaging for prognosis in 31 cases with at least 2 years of follow-up. Radiology 1993; 187:199–204.
31. Takatori Y, Kokubo T, Ninomiya S, Nakamura S, Morimoto S, Kusaba I. Avascular necrosis of the femoral head: natural history and magnetic resonance imaging. J Bone Joint Surg [Br] 1993; 75:217–221.
32. Magid D, Fishman EK, Scott WW Jr, et al. Femoral head avascular necrosis: CT assessment with multiplanar reconstruction. Radiology 1985; 157:751–756.
33. Lang P, Genant HK, Jergesen HE, Murray WR. Imaging of the hip joint: computed tomography versus magnetic resonance imaging. Clin Orthop 1992; 274:135–153.
34. Jergesen HE, Lang P, Moseley M, Genant HK. Histologic correlation in magnetic resonance imaging of femoral head osteonecrosis. Clin Orthop 1990; 253:150–163.
35. Vande Berg BC, Malghem J, Labaisse MA, Noel H, Maldague B. Avascular necrosis of the hip: comparison of contrast-enhanced and nonenhanced MR imaging with histologic correlation—work in progress. Radiology 1992; 182:445–450.
36. Plenk H, Hofmann S, Eschberger J, et al. Histomorphology and bone morphometry of the bone marrow edema syndrome of the hip. Clin Orthop 1997; 334:73–84.
37. Hofmann S, Engel A, Neuhold A, Leder K, Kramer J, Plenk H Jr. Bone marrow oedema syndrome and transient osteoporosis of the hip: an MRI-controlled study of treatment by core decompression. J Bone Joint Surg [Br] 1993; 75:210–216.
38. Ficat RP. Idiopathic bone necrosis of the femoral head: early diagnosis and treatment. J Bone Joint Surg [Br] 1985; 67:3–9.
39. Lichtenstein L. Fractures and their sequelae. In: Diseases of bone and joints. St Louis, Mo: Mosby 1970; 1–9.
40. Ahuja SC, Bullough PG. Osteonecrosis of the knee: a clinicopathological study in twenty-eight patients. J Bone Joint Surg [Am] 1978; 60:191–197.
41. Kiaer T, Pedersen NW, Kristensen KD, Starklint H. Intra-osseous pressure and oxygen tension in avascular necrosis and osteoarthritis of the hip. J Bone Joint Surg [Br] 1990; 72:1023–1030.
42. Dunstan CR, Evans RA, Somers NM. Bone death in transient regional osteoporosis. Bone 1992; 13:161–165.

Khaled I. El-Noueam, MD
Mark E. Schweitzer, MD
Roberto Blasbalg, MD
Aly A. Farahat, MD
Randall W. Culp, MD
Lee A. Osterman, MD
Amaar Malik, BA

Is a Subset of Wrist Ganglia the Sequela of Internal Derangements of the Wrist Joint? MR Imaging Findings[1]

Index terms:
Ganglion, 434.361
Wrist, abnormalities, 434.361, 434.483
Wrist, injuries, 434.419, 434.483
Wrist, MR, 434.121411, 434.121412, 434.121415, 434.12143

Radiology 1999; 212:537–540

[1] From the Department of Diagnostic Radiology, Faculty of Medicine, Alexandria University, Egypt (K.I.E.N., A.A.F.); and the Departments of Radiology (K.I.E.N., M.E.S., R.B., A.M.) and Orthopedic Surgery (R.W.C., L.A.O.), Thomas Jefferson University Hospital, Jefferson Medical College, 132 S 10th St, 1096 Main Bldg, Philadelphia, PA 19107. Received March 6, 1998; revision requested April 14; final revision received October 13; accepted March 16, 1999. **Address reprint requests to** M.E.S. (e-mail: *mark.schweitzer@mail.tju.edu*).

Author contributions:
Guarantor of integrity of entire study, K.I.E.N.; study concepts and design, M.E.S.; definition of intellectual content, M.E.S.; literature research, A.A.F., A.M.; clinical studies, R.W.C., L.A.O.; data acquisition, K.I.E.N., R.B.; data analysis, K.I.E.N., A.M.; statistical analysis, K.I.E.N.; manuscript preparation, K.I.E.N.; manuscript editing and review, M.E.S.

PURPOSE: To determine if there is an association between wrist ganglia and internal derangements of the wrist joint by reviewing magnetic resonance (MR) images.

MATERIALS AND METHODS: Two observers retrospectively reviewed MR images of the wrist obtained in 625 patients at 1.5 T for the presence of ganglia and associated triangular fibrocartilage complex, scapholunate ligamentous, or lunotriquetral ligamentous tears that were within 3 mm of the ganglion. When available, surgery and/or pathology records were reviewed.

RESULTS: There were 122 ganglia and 37 internal derangements. Of the 22 ulnar-sided ganglia, 10 (45%) demonstrated associated triangular fibrocartilage complex tears. Of the 97 radial-sided ganglia, 27 (28%) demonstrated ligamentous tears related to the site of the ganglion. The radial-sided tears involved the radial aspect of the triangular fibrocartilage complex in 12 ganglia; the scapholunate ligament, in isolation, in eight ganglia; and both the triangular fibrocartilage complex and the scapholunate ligament in six ganglia. Only one of the ganglia demonstrated an associated lunotriquetral ligamentous tear. Surgical findings confirmed the ligamentous tears in 25 patients.

CONCLUSION: Wrist ganglia are associated, not infrequently, with internal derangements of the wrist.

A ganglion is a cystic swelling that usually occurs in proximity to joints or tendon sheaths. Ganglia are frequent in the wrist and are often asymptomatic (1,2). The pathogenesis of ganglia remains obscure; many different causes (in particular, trauma) have been proposed (3,4).

In the knee joint, a portion of the paraarticular cysts initially thought to be ganglia is presently believed to be meniscal cyst (5). Similarly, it has recently been noted that a subset of paraarticular cysts in the shoulder represents the sequela of labral tears (6). Since ganglia are most common in the wrist, we hypothesized that a subset of cystic lesions related to the wrist may be secondary to internal derangements. Consequently, the aim of this study was to determine if a fraction of the cystic lesions about the wrist are associated with internal derangements of the wrist.

MATERIALS AND METHODS

We (M.E.S., K.I.E.N.) retrospectively reviewed magnetic resonance (MR) images of the wrist, obtained from 1993 to 1997, in 625 patients. Images were obtained by using a 1.5-T superconducting magnet (Signa; GE Medical Systems, Milwaukee, Wis) with a dedicated wrist coil (ICG Medical Advances, Milwaukee, Wis).

Wrists were imaged in the coronal and axial planes, with a combination of a T1-weighted spin-echo (400–900/10–30 [repetition time msec/echo time msec]) sequence, an intermediate-weighted spin-echo (4,000/40) sequence, a T2-weighted spin-echo (1,800/70) or fast spin-echo (5,300/140) sequence, and a three-dimensional coronal gradient-echo sequence

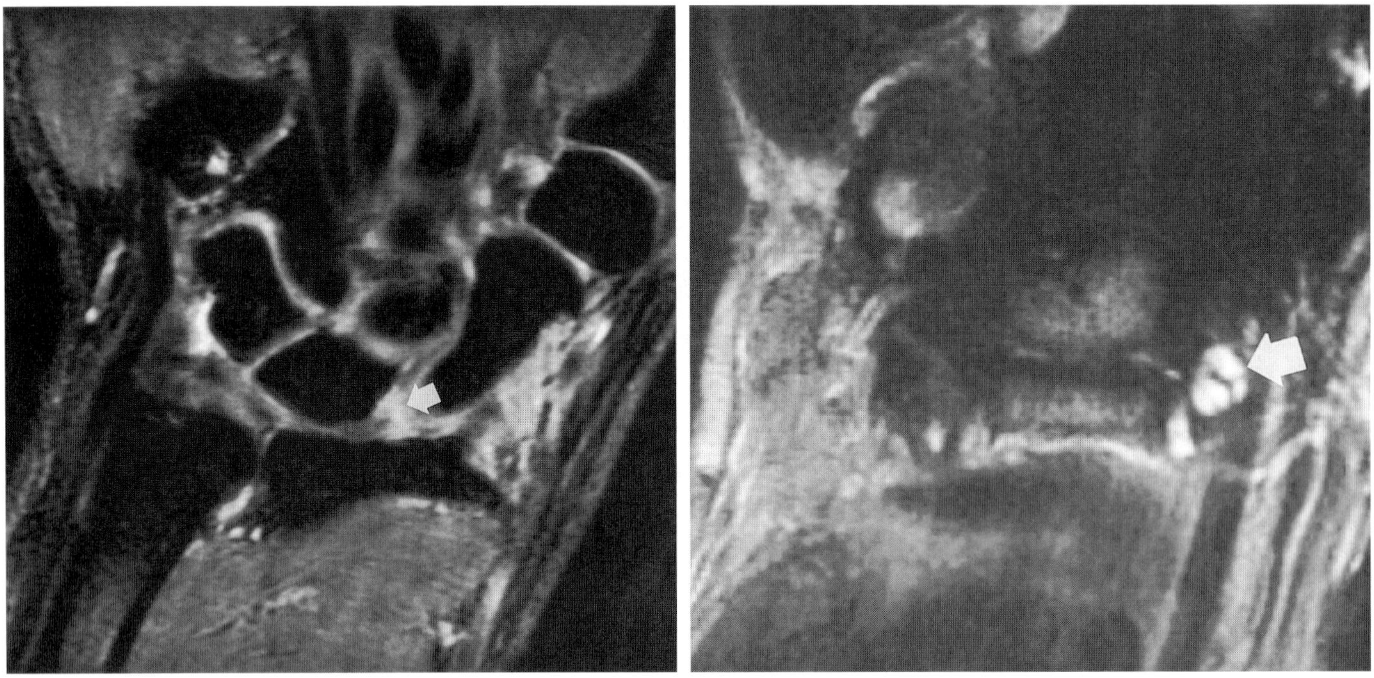

a.

b.

Figure 1. Coronal MR images of the left wrist in a 33-year-old man with pain in the left wrist. **(a)** Three-dimensional T1-weighted gradient-echo image (45/15) obtained after intravenous injection of a gadolinium-based contrast material demonstrates a tear of the scapholunate ligament (arrow). **(b)** Fast spin-echo T2-weighted image (3,116/115) shows a ganglion (arrow) protruding from the scapholunate interval.

(45/15 or 30/12, 20° flip angle). Other parameters included a 256 × 128–256 acquisition matrix and a 3–5-mm section thickness with a 1-mm intersection gap. For the gradient-echo sequence, the section thickness was 1.2 mm with no intersection gap. The field of view was 10–12 cm.

The clinical indication for MR imaging was wrist pain in 614 patients. However, 11 of the patients had a clinical presentation of a palpable wrist mass. In nine of these patients, additional T1-weighted images obtained after the intravenous administration of 20 mL of contrast material (Magnevist [gadopentetate dimeglumine]; Berlex Laboratories, Wayne, NJ) were available.

Two patients underwent fluoroscopically guided direct MR arthrography; two additional patients underwent indirect (intravenous) MR arthrography (Fig 1a). The MR images were evaluated by two observers (M.E.S, K.I.E.N.) working in consensus to determine the presence of paraarticular ganglia and associated triangular fibrocartilage complex, scapholunate ligamentous, or lunotriquetral ligamentous tears in proximity to the ganglion. A ganglion was considered to be related to the ligamentous tear if it was seen within 3 mm of the ligament. Demonstration of a direct communication was not considered a prerequisite for the diagnosis of synovial herniation through the ligamentous tear.

Medical records were reviewed (R.W.C., L.A.O.) to determine the presenting symptoms. Surgery reports and histopathologic results were also reviewed, when available, for the confirmation of ligamentous tears in proximity to the ganglion.

RESULTS

In 120 patients (19.2%), 122 wrist ganglia were demonstrated. Only 11 of these ganglia (9.0%) were clinically palpable. The ganglia were encountered in the following locations: 97 ganglia (79.5%) were on the radial side, 22 ganglia (18.0%) were ulnar-sided, and three ganglia (2.5%) were in the region of the lunotriquetral articulation. Of the 122 ganglia, 75 ganglia (61.5%) were on the volar aspect of the wrist, whereas 47 ganglia (38.5%) were on the dorsal aspect of the wrist. Two patients each had two ganglia; in each patient's wrist, one ganglion was radial-sided, and the other was ulnar-sided.

Of the 22 ganglia on the ulnar side of the wrist, 10 (45%) demonstrated triangular fibrocartilage complex tears that were contiguous with the site of the ganglion. Of the 97 ganglia on the radial side of the wrist, 26 (27%) demonstrated ligamentous tears related to the ganglion; the tears involved the radial aspect of the triangular fibrocartilage complex in 12 ganglia (46%), combined triangular fibrocartilage complex and scapholunate ligamentous tears in six ganglia (23%), and isolated scapholunate ligamentous tear in eight ganglia (31%) (Figs 1, 2). Only one of the three patients with ganglia related to the lunotriquetral ligament demonstrated perforation of this ligament.

Surgery reports were available for 30 patients and confirmed the ligamentous tear in 25 patients. In the other five patients, no ligamentous tears were demonstrated surgically; these were primarily interpreted as triangular fibrocartilage complex tears. Histopathologic analysis in four patients revealed an appearance similar to that of meniscal cysts in the knee, with a fibrous wall not lined with synovial membrane.

DISCUSSION

A ganglion is a lesion of unknown origin that arises in the paraarticular tissues. Ganglia about the wrist are common; they may be asymptomatic or may cause

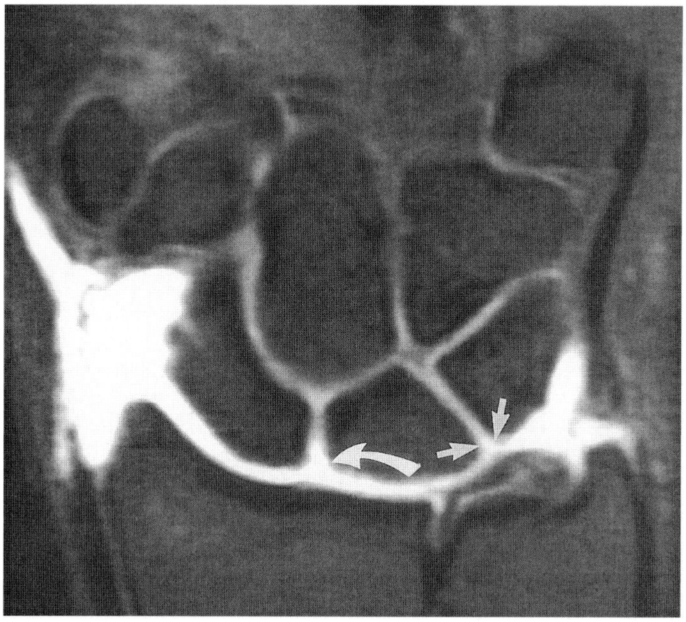

a.

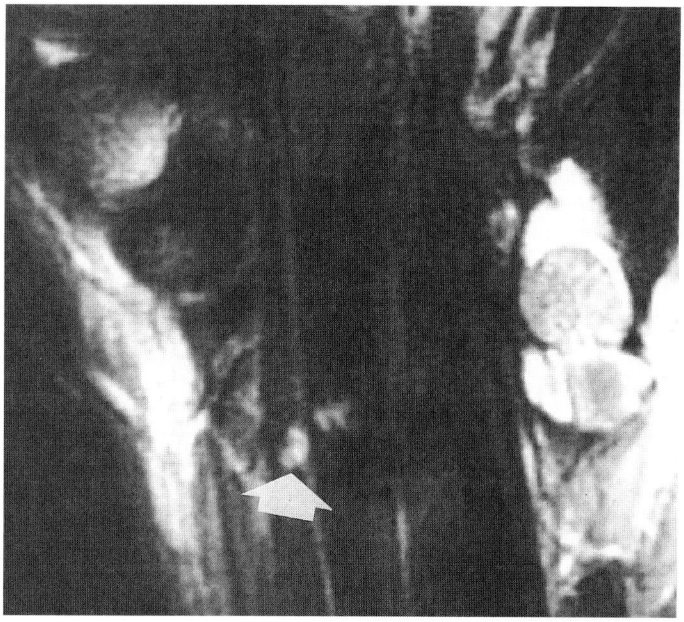

b.

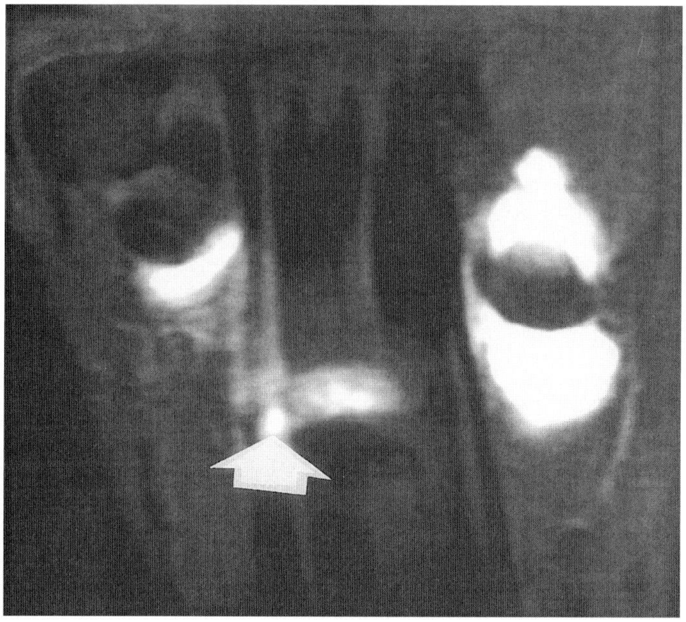

c.

Figure 2. Coronal MR images of the wrist in a 27-year-old woman with wrist pain. **(a)** T1-weighted fat-suppressed spin-echo image (500/16) obtained following a radiocarpal arthrographic injection demonstrates tears of the scapholunate ligament (curved arrow) and of the lunotriquetral ligament (straight arrows). **(b)** Fat-suppressed image (5,400/70 [effective]) shows fluid in a ganglion (arrow) just anterior to the scapholunate interval. **(c)** Postarthrographic T1-weighted fat-suppressed spin-echo image (500/16) anterior to **a** demonstrates that the injected contrast material goes through the scapholunate interval into the ganglion (arrow).

tenderness or pain due to pressure and inflammation of adjacent structures, such as tendons and tendon sheaths (1,3).

Ultrasonography (US) and MR imaging are both effective in depicting ganglia. The lower cost of US makes it useful as the first imaging modality. US will readily depict even small ganglia, which are identified as well-defined, homogeneously anechoic masses (7,8). MR imaging clearly aids in the localization of the ganglia and in the identification of their relationship to adjacent structures, which include vessels, tendons, and nerves (9).

Ganglia have been recognized since antiquity and were described by Hippocrates as a knot of tissue containing mucoid flesh (1). Repeated trauma that results in the degeneration and liquefaction of the periarticular connective tissue has been hypothesized as a possible cause (3). Volkmann, in 1882, considered the ganglion to be a prolapse of synovial tissue, basing his view on the fact that the ganglion occurs in the proximity of joints and tendon sheaths. He hypothesized that the bulging synovial membrane maintains its function of producing synovial fluid, with impaired outflow that results in gradual widening of the synovial pouch (3,10).

There are two groups of paraarticular cystic lesions: ganglia and synovial cysts. Ganglia are thin-walled cysts that contain viscous mucoid fluid and are found usually in the hand and wrist. Synovial cysts are herniations of the synovial lining of a disrupted joint space (3).

A portion of paraarticular cysts, which were initially thought to be ganglia, is currently considered to be synovial cyst associated with internal derangements. This was first noted in the knee, where meniscal cysts, initially believed to be ganglia, are presently believed to represent encapsulated paraarticular fluid collections associated with horizontal meniscal tears. It is believed that the synovial fluid is forced out between the leaves of a complete horizontal meniscal tear and collects at the meniscocapsular border. Medial cysts may be more likely to be symptomatic because of the greater pressure they produce beneath the medial collateral ligament (5,11).

Similarly, paralabral cysts in the shoulder are synovial fluid–filled cysts that are related to the glenoid labrum. There is a strong correlation between paralabral cysts, which have a posterior location, and posterosuperior labral tears. These cysts may communicate with the joint via the posterosuperior glenoid labrum, and they may extend medially into the spinoglenoid notch. The posterosuperior paralabral cyst is thus a common location for a cyst that is seen in association with a posterior capsulolabral injury, including superior labral tears extending anterior to posterior, or SLAP lesions (6,12).

We hypothesized that a subset of the cysts that occur around the wrist, although they are commonly called ganglia, represents the sequela of internal derangements of the wrist joint. We believe these wrist ganglia are more accurately termed synovial cysts and are similar to meniscal cysts in the knee and paralabral cysts in the shoulder.

In our study, 30% (37 of 122) of the paraarticular cysts reviewed were related to ligamentous tears. Surgical findings confirmed this association in 25 of 30 patients. Histopathologic findings, which were available for only four patients, indicated an appearance similar to that of meniscal cysts.

We acknowledge a number of limitations with this study. First, the surgical correlation of the imaging findings was available in only 30 patients, and the histopathologic findings were available in only four patients. Perhaps the most important limitation is that, since this is a retrospective study, only cases with ganglia were evaluated for ligamentous tears. Therefore, we did not determine the true incidence of ganglia in patients with internal derangements of the wrist.

Historically, synovial herniation as a cause of ganglia has been conjectured (10). In addition, it is well known that ganglia in the wrist have a characteristic location close to the scapholunate ligament, which is frequently torn. Arthrography occasionally reveals a one-way communication between the opacified joint fluid and the paraarticular ganglia (13). Constrast-enhanced tenography also may reveal communication between an opacified tendon sheath and the ganglion (14).

On the basis of the results of this study, we conclude that a subset of paraarticular cysts around the wrist may be the sequela of internal derangements. Although many of these perforations may be asymptomatic, a local ganglion may be a secondary sign of an internal derangement of the wrist. We believe this hypothesis is closely related to the pathophysiology of meniscal cysts in the knee and of labral cysts in the shoulder.

References

1. Feldman F, Singson RD, Staron RB. Magnetic resonance imaging of para-articular and ectopic ganglia. Skeletal Radiol 1989; 18:353–358.
2. Kransdorf MJ, Murphey MD. MR imaging of musculoskeletal tumors of the hand and wrist. Magn Reson Imaging Clin N Am 1995; 3:327–344.
3. Enzinger FM, Weis SW. Soft tissue tumors. 2nd ed. St Louis, Mo: Mosby, 1988.
4. Butt WP, McIntyre JL. Double-contrast arthrography of the knee. Radiology 1969; 92:487–499.
5. Rubin DA. MR imaging of the knee menisci. Radiol Clin North Am 1997; 35:21–44.
6. Stoller DS. MR arthrography of the glenohumeral joint. Radiol Clin North Am 1997; 35:97–116.
7. Cardinal E, Buckwalter KA, Braunstein EM, Mih AD. Occult dorsal wrist ganglion: comparison of US and MR imaging. Radiology 1994; 193:259–262.
8. Hashimoto BE, Hayes AS, Ager JD. Sonographic diagnosis and treatment of ganglion cysts causing suprascapular nerve entrapment. J Ultrasound Med 1994; 13: 671–674.
9. Weiss KL, Beltran J, Lubbers LM. High-field MR surface-coil imaging of the hand and wrist. II. Pathologic correlations and clinical relevance. Radiology 1986; 160: 147–152.
10. Volkmann R. Ganglion. In: v. Pitha-Billroth's hand buch der allgemeinen und speziellen chirurgie. Vol 2. 1882; 838.
11. Burk DL Jr, Dalinka MK, Kanal E, et al. Meniscal and ganglion cysts of the knee: MR evaluation. AJR 1988; 150:331–336.
12. Tirman PF, Feller JF, Janzen DL, Peterfy CG, Bergman AG. Association of glenoid labral cysts with labral tears and glenohumeral instability: radiologic findings and clinical significance. Radiology 1994; 190:653–658.
13. Andren L, Eiken O. Arthrographic studies of wrist ganglions. J Bone Joint Surg [Am] 1971; 53:299–302.
14. Resnick D, Kang HS. Wrist. In: Resnick D. Internal derangements of joints: emphasis on MR imaging. Philadelphia, Pa: Saunders, 1997; 387–472.

John V. Zurlo, MD

The Double-Line Sign[1]

APPEARANCE

The double-line sign is seen on T2-weighted magnetic resonance (MR) images of medullary bone as a high-signal-intensity line within a parallel rim of decreased signal intensity, often with serpentine borders (Fig 1). Corresponding T1-weighted images demonstrate both (high- and low-signal-intensity) zones together as a single low-signal-intensity band (Fig 2).

EXPLANATION

The double-line sign is seen with AVN (osteonecrosis) on MR images. The high-signal-intensity inner zone represents hyperemic granulation tissue. The low-signal-intensity outer zone represents adjacent sclerotic bone (1,2). Chemical shift misregistration may accentuate the low signal intensity of the outer rim in some cases (3).

DISCUSSION

AVN has many causes; trauma is the most common. Other causes include hemoglobinopathies, Cushing syndrome, and exogenous steroid use; alcoholism; pancreatitis; human immunodeficiency virus; Gaucher disease; and Caisson disease (4,5). AVN may also be idiopathic. The epiphysis and metaphysis of long tubular bones are susceptible because of their limited arterial supply and limited venous drainage. The hip is the most common site, but the knee, shoulder, and carpal and tarsal bones can be affected. The location of AVN may be influenced by the underlying disease (eg, the shoulder in sickle cell disease).

AVN may be initiated by a traumatic disruption of a vessel or by other factors that cause ischemia, such as thromboembolism or venous stasis. After an initial traumatic insult, hematopoietic cells die within 6–12 hours; fat marrow cells die in 2–5 days. Ischemic bone eventually undergoes repair from its periphery to its infarcted center. Healing begins with hyperemia at the ischemic periphery; the hyperemia is subsequently replaced by reactive tissue and sclerosis. Microfractures and bony collapse may occur as trabeculae are reabsorbed. Articular cartilage is spared from injury because its nutrient supply is from synovial fluid; however, with loss of subchondral bone, cartilage may be damaged owing to frank collapse or altered mechanics. It is the reparative process that is best depicted on MR images and on conventional radiographs (6).

The depiction of findings on conventional radiographs lags several months behind the time of injury. These findings include areas of radiolucency, sclerosis, bone collapse, joint space narrowing, and, in the femoral head, a characteristic subchondral radiolucent crescent. Some of these findings indicate a late, irreversible stage of disease. A modification of the system proposed by Ficat can be used to classify the radiographic appearance of AVN of the hip (4). In stage 0, the patient is suspected of having AVN without clinical or radiographic findings. In stage 1, the patient has clinical symptoms of AVN but no radiographic findings. In stage 2, the patient has osteopenia, cystic areas, and sclerosis. In stage 3, the patient has flattening of the femoral head; a subchondral crescentic area of radiolucency also may be seen. In stage 4, secondary osteoarthritis of the hip with associated joint space narrowing develops.

MR imaging is reported (7) to have a sensitivity of 97% and specificity of 98% in the diagnosis of AVN of the hip when a variety of findings are used to aid in the diagnosis. This is more sensitive than computed tomography, scintigraphy, or conventional radiography (8). MR imaging may help detect the bone marrow edema associated with early AVN, which is seen as decreased signal intensity with poorly defined margins on T1-weighted images. The characteristic appearance of AVN, the double-line sign, occurs later in the disease process, after the start of osseous repair. It is seen in up to 80% of cases (2). MR imaging may also help detect the associated joint effusions and risk factors, such as early fatty conversion of red bone marrow and prominent physeal scars (6).

The MR imaging findings of AVN of the hip may be classified

Index terms:
Bones, MR, 48.12141
Bones, necrosis, 48.44, 48.542, 48.65, 48.671, 77.291

Radiology 1999; 212:541–542

Abbreviation:
AVN = avascular necrosis

[1] From the UMDNJ-New Jersey Medical School, Newark, NJ. Received May 22, 1998; revision requested July 14; revision received July 28; accepted August 26. **Address reprint requests to** the author, Department of Radiology, University of Pittsburgh Medical Center, 200 Lothrop St, Pittsburgh, PA 15213.

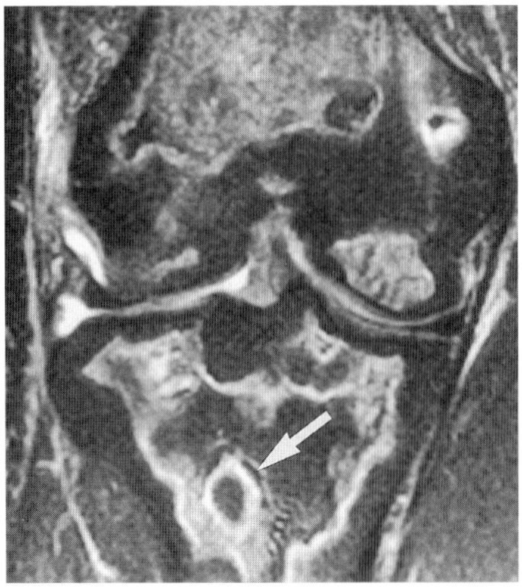

Figure 1. The double-line sign in a patient with multifocal avascular necrosis (AVN) secondary to steroid therapy. Coronal T2-weighted fast spin-echo MR image (3,000/75 [repetition time msec/effective echo time msec]) of the knee shows high signal intensity in the inner zone and a low-signal-intensity line (arrow) in the parallel outer zone.

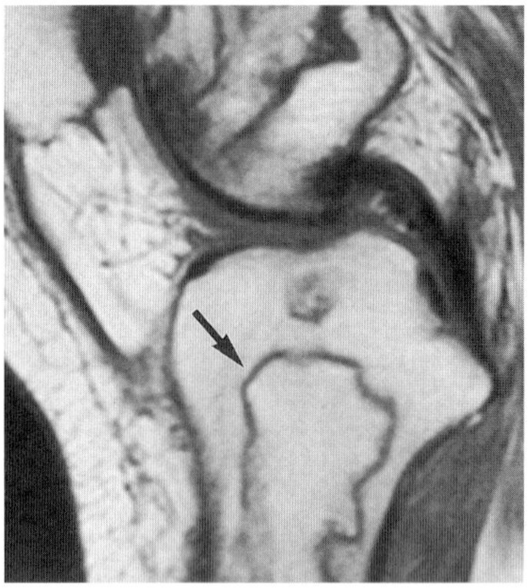

Figure 2. Sagittal T1-weighted spin-echo MR image (600/20) of the knee in Figure 1 shows an abnormal low-signal-intensity band (arrow) in the proximal tibia.

according to a system proposed by Mitchell et al (2). Class A lesions have signal intensity characteristics analogous to those of fat—that is, high signal intensity on T1-weighted images and intermediate signal intensity on T2-weighted images. Class B lesions demonstrate signal intensity characteristics that are similar to those of blood, which has high signal intensity on both T1- and T2-weighted images. Class C AVN lesions in the hips have signal intensity properties that are similar to those of fluid—that is, low signal intensity on T1-weighted images and high signal intensity on T2-weighted images. The signal intensity characteristics of class D lesions are similar to those of fibrous tissue, which has low signal intensity on both T1- and T2-weighted images (2). Class A signal intensity tends to reflect early disease, and class D signal intensity tends to reflect late disease.

MR imaging is helpful in planning treatment for AVN; imaging performed in multiple planes allows determination of the volume of tissue involved. In the hip, treatment is geared toward saving the joint, especially in young patients. Early detection enables early intervention and may help avoid prosthetic hip replacement. Treatment options include core decompression, which is most commonly used in early disease, bone grafts, osteotomy, and electrical stimulation (6). MR imaging may also be used to evaluate the hip after treatment.

With or without treatment, AVN may progress to cystic degeneration, intraarticular osseous bodies, and collapse of articular surfaces with subsequent secondary osteoarthritis. Patients may ultimately require joint replacement (6).

References

1. Mitchell DG, Kressel HY, Rao VM, et al. The unique MRI appearance of the reactive interface in avascular necrosis: the double-line sign. Magn Reson Imaging 1987; 5(suppl 1):41.
2. Mitchell DG, Rao VM, Dalinka MK, et al. Femoral head avascular necrosis: correlation of MR imaging, radiographic staging, radionuclide imaging, and clinical findings. Radiology 1987; 162:709–715.
3. Sugimoto H, Okubu RS, Ohsawa T. Chemical shift and the double-line sign in MRI of early femoral avascular necrosis. J Comput Assist Tomogr 1992; 16:727–730.
4. Deely DM, Schweitzer ME. MR imaging of bone marrow disorders. Radiol Clin North Am 1997; 35:202–208.
5. Blacksin MF, Kloser P, Simon J. Avascular necrosis of bone in human immunodeficiency virus (HIV)-infected patients (abstr). Presented at the First International Symposium of Musculoskeletal MRI, San Francisco, Calif, January 22–25, 1996.
6. Resnick D, Sweet DE, Madewell JE. Osteonecrosis and osteochondrosis. In: Resnick D, ed. Bone and joint imaging. 2nd ed. Philadelphia, Pa: Saunders, 1996; 941–959.
7. Glickstein MF, Burk DL, Schiebler ML, et al. Avascular necrosis versus other diseases of the hip: sensitivity of MR imaging. Radiology 1988; 169:213–215.
8. Coleman BG, Kressel HY, Dalinka MK, et al. Radiographically negative avascular necrosis: detection with MR imaging. Radiology 1988; 168:525–528.

Susan G. Orel, MD
Susan P. Weinstein, MD
Mitchell D. Schnall, MD
Carol A. Reynolds, MD
Lynn M. Schuchter, MD
Douglas L. Fraker, MD
Lawrence J. Solin, MD

Breast MR Imaging in Patients with Axillary Node Metastases and Unknown Primary Malignancy[1]

Index terms:
Breast neoplasms, diagnosis, 00.121412, 00.121415, 00.12143, 00.30
Breast neoplasms, localization, 00.121412, 00.121415, 00.12143, 00.30
Breast neoplasms, metastases, 997.33
Breast neoplasms, MR, 00.121412, 00.121415, 00.12143, 00.30
Breast neoplasms, staging, 00.30

Radiology 1999; 212:543–549

[1] From the Departments of Radiology (S.G.O., S.P.W., M.D.S.), Surgery (D.L.F.), and Radiation Oncology (L.J.S.) and the Hematology-Oncology Division (L.M.S.), University of Pennsylvania Medical Center, 3400 Spruce St, Philadelphia, PA 19104; and the Department of Anatomic Pathology, Mayo Clinic, Rochester, Minn (C.A.R.). Received July 8, 1998; revision requested August 18; final revision received October 22; accepted February 10, 1999. **Address reprint requests to** S.G.O. (e-mail: *orel@oasis.rad.upenn.edu*).

PURPOSE: To assess the usefulness of magnetic resonance (MR) imaging of the breast in patients with malignant axillary adenopathy and unknown primary malignancy.

MATERIALS AND METHODS: Between October 1993 and December 1997, 38 women with malignant axillary adenopathy and negative mammographic and physical examination findings underwent contrast material–enhanced MR imaging. Sixteen patients were excluded due to axillary tail cancer ($n = 7$), lack of follow-up ($n = 4$), second primary malignancy ($n = 3$), or chemotherapy before MR imaging ($n = 2$). The study population comprised the remaining 22 patients. Histopathologic findings were available in 20 patients; follow-up MR imaging findings were available in two patients.

RESULTS: MR imaging depicted a primary breast cancer in 19 patients (86%; identified at excisional biopsy or mastectomy in 17, resolved on follow-up MR images during treatment in two). MR imaging depicted 4–30-mm cancers (mean, 17 mm), which correlated closely with histopathologic size. Two patients (9%) had false-negative findings: (*a*) One had a 2-mm invasive ductal carcinoma, and (*b*) one had 17- and 20-mm invasive ductal carcinomas. Of the 19 patients, 11 underwent mastectomy, seven underwent breast-conservation therapy, and one did not undergo a surgical procedure.

CONCLUSION: MR imaging is very sensitive for the detection of mammographically and clinically occult breast cancer in patients with malignant axillary adenopathy. In these patients, MR imaging offers potential not only for cancer detection but also for staging the cancer within the breast, which may be useful for treatment planning.

Breast cancer can manifest as isolated axillary metastases, with no radiographic or clinical evidence of a primary tumor within the breast. The incidence of an axillary lymph node manifestation from an occult primary breast cancer is low, ranging from 0.3% to 0.8% of all patients with carcinoma of the breast at presentation (1).

The most commonly used treatment in patients with axillary node metastases and an unknown primary site has been mastectomy and axillary node dissection (1–3). However, there can be a reluctance to perform "blind" mastectomy, since in approximately one-third of cases, no tumor is found at microscopic evaluation of the mastectomy specimen (4,5). Articles reporting the results of breast-conservation therapy in these patients have shown no survival difference between those who undergo mastectomy and those who do not, which supports the use of breast-conservation therapy with breast irradiation as an alternative to mastectomy (1,3,6–8). Yet, there is concern that in those patients with a relatively large occult tumor burden, whole-breast irradiation is unlikely to control the disease (3).

The ability of mammography to depict a primary breast cancer and define its extent in patients with axillary node metastases at presentation has been disappointing (4,6,8,9). The reported incidence of finding an occult breast cancer at mammography has ranged from 0% to 56% (3). In two series (6,9), when a primary tumor was found in the breast at microscopic examination, the mammogram was positive in only 29% and 35% of the cases.

Author contributions:
Guarantor of integrity of entire study, S.G.O.; study concepts and design, S.G.O.; definition of intellectual content, S.G.O.; literature research, S.P.W., S.G.O.; clinical studies, M.D.S., C.A.R., S.G.O.; data acquisition and analysis, S.P.W., S.G.O.; manuscript preparation, L.M.S., D.L.F., L.J.S., S.G.O.; manuscript editing and review, L.M.S., D.L.F., L.J.S., S.P.W., S.G.O.

Findings of several studies now demonstrate the potential of magnetic resonance (MR) imaging to have greater sensitivity in the depiction of breast cancer than is possible with mammography, with multiple reported cases of MR imaging–detected mammographically and clinically occult carcinoma (10–15). The purpose of this study was to assess the usefulness of MR imaging of the breast in patients with axillary node metastases and negative clinical and mammographic findings at presentation.

MATERIALS AND METHODS

Between October 1993 and December 1997, 38 women with axillary node metastases and unknown primary malignancy underwent contrast material–enhanced MR imaging at 1.5 T. All of the women had palpable axillary adenopathy at initial presentation; biopsy was performed, and metastatic adenocarcinoma was found in each case. All patients had a negative mammogram and negative physical examination findings at presentation.

Of the 38 patients, 16 were excluded from the study due to axillary tail cancer (n = 7), lack of follow-up (n = 4), a second primary nonipsilateral breast cancer (n = 3), or chemotherapy prior to MR imaging (n = 2). In the seven patients with axillary tail cancer, the tumor was removed prior to the MR imaging examination in four patients, was identified at MR imaging in two patients, and was not identified at MR imaging in one patient. MR imaging findings were negative in all four patients in whom surgical and/or clinical follow-up was not available. Among the three patients with a second nonipsilateral breast tumor, one patient had a contralateral breast tumor with identical histologic findings; among the other two patients, the tumors were metastatic melanoma and metastatic salivary gland tumor. In two of these three patients, the MR imaging findings were negative. In one patient, an enhancing lesion was identified and localized with MR imaging guidance but was proved to be fat necrosis. In the two patients who received chemotherapy prior to MR imaging, no abnormality was identified at MR imaging.

The remaining 22 patients made up the study population. The women ranged in age from 37 to 66 years (mean age, 49 years). Diagnostic mammography was performed at an outside institution in 21 of the 22 patients and at the University of Pennsylvania Medical Center in one

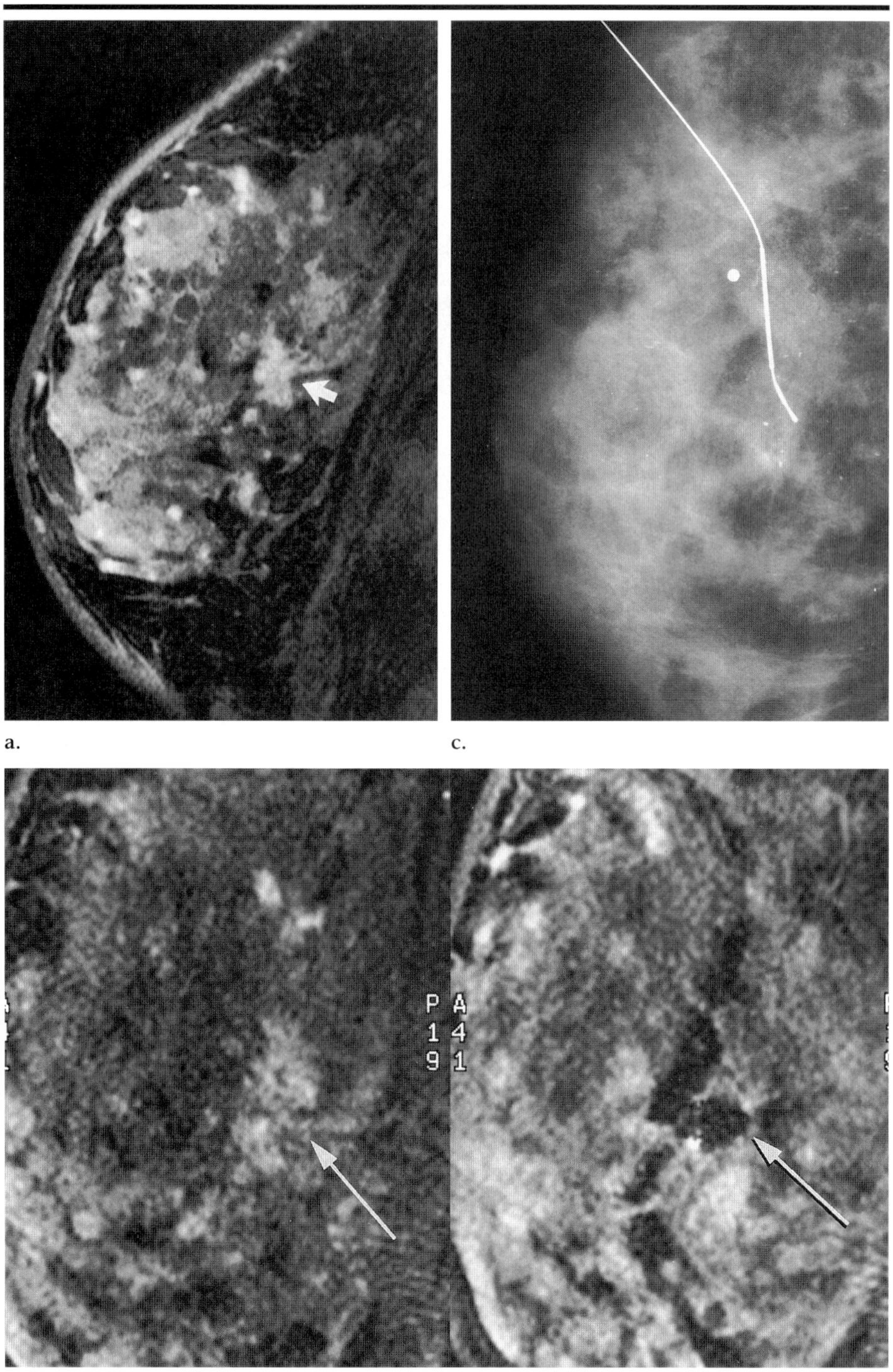

Figure 1. **(a)** Sagittal fat-suppressed contrast-enhanced three-dimensional fast spoiled gradient-recalled-echo MR image (15/2.2) demonstrates an enhancing 1-cm mass (arrow) with spiculated margins. **(b)** Sagittal fat-suppressed contrast-enhanced three-dimensional fast spoiled gradient-recalled-echo MR images (9.2/2.2) obtained during MR imaging–guided localization. The arrow in the image on the left marks the lesion. The arrow in the image on the right marks the artifact from the needle. **(c)** Postlocalization mediolateral mammogram reveals the hook wire in the central part of the breast and a skin marker (metallic bead). Scattered calcifications adjacent to and distant from the wire were present in both breasts and were stable. Excisional biopsy revealed a 6-mm infiltrating ductal carcinoma with associated ductal carcinoma in situ and extensive lymphatic invasion. On the basis of the histopathologic features, mastectomy was recommended. At mastectomy, minimal residual invasive ductal carcinoma and ductal carcinoma in situ were identified near the biopsy site. No other tumor was found in the breast.

patient. Reports were available for all of the outside mammograms. Eighteen of the 21 outside mammograms and the one inside mammogram were available for review. All available mammograms were retrospectively reviewed by one radiologist (S.G.O.) experienced in breast imaging who had knowledge of the clinical history. The mammograms were reviewed to ensure that no suspicious findings (mass, microcalcifications, or architectural distortion) could be identified in either the breast ipsilateral to the malignant axillary nodes or the contralateral breast. The time from mammography to MR imaging examination was 0–84 days, with a mean of 40 days.

MR imaging was performed with a 1.5-T Signa system (GE Medical Systems, Milwaukee, Wis) equipped with a prototype high-performance gradient system. All patients were imaged in the prone position by using a specially designed compression multicoil array (16). Sagittal T1-weighed spin-echo (500–600/17 [repetition time msec/echo time msec]) and sagittal fat-suppressed T2-weighted fast spin-echo (4,000/120 [effective echo time]) imaging was performed with a 12–16-cm field of view, 3-mm section thickness, 1-mm gap, and a 256 × 256 matrix. The entire breast was then imaged before and following the bolus administration of 20 mL of gadopentetate dimeglumine (Magnevist; Schering, Berlin, Germany) with a sagittal three-dimensional-volume fat-suppressed fast spoiled gradient-recalled-echo sequence (minimum repetition time/minimum echo time, 18-cm field of view, 2-mm section thickness, no gap, and a 256 × 512 matrix). Regardless of weight, each patient received 20 mL of gadopentetate dimeglumine as a bolus injection followed by 20 mL of physiologic saline. Imaging was initiated during the saline injection.

The three-dimensional-volume fast spoiled gradient-recalled-echo sequence evolved, and the imaging time for each three-dimensional volume decreased from 3 minutes 30 seconds to 90 seconds. For the 90-second sequence, the entire breast volume was imaged four times (total of 6 minutes).

The MR images were read prospectively by two radiologists (S.G.O., M.D.S.) experienced in MR imaging of the breast. The studies were read collectively, and a consensus was reached in each case. The images were read with knowledge of the clinical history of axillary node metastases and the negative mammographic and physical examination findings. The mammograms were not available at the time the MR images were reviewed.

A lesion was considered suspicious if it was enhanced on the first (90-second) postcontrast image and was visualized as (*a*) a mass with at least partially ill-defined or irregular borders, (*b*) an area of linear or branching enhancement suggestive of ductal enhancement, or (*c*) an area of regional enhancement where the borders of the enhancing area were ill-defined or irregular or there was associated architectural distortion. Scattered punctate (1–3-mm) foci of enhancement, patchy enhancement of fibroglandular tissue with no architectural distortion, enhancing masses with circumscribed smooth or lobulated borders with or without internal septations, and masses that demonstrated no contrast material enhancement were classified as benign findings. These architectural features and an MR interpretation model incorporating multiple architectural features identified on breast MR images have been previously reported (17,18).

Seven patients underwent MR imaging–guided wire localization. The details of this procedure have been previously described (19).

Twenty of the 22 patients underwent surgery following the MR imaging examination and prior to treatment with chemotherapy: excisional biopsy in nine patients, mastectomy in 10 patients, and excisional biopsy followed by mastectomy in one patient. In each of the patients who underwent surgery, the MR imaging findings were correlated with the histopathologic findings. In two of the 22 patients, surgery was not performed prior to treatment with chemotherapy. Both patients were followed up with sequential MR imaging examinations. One of the two patients subsequently underwent mastectomy following chemotherapy.

For excisional biopsy, including MR-guided wire localization, the specimen and the radiograph of the specimen were delivered to the pathology laboratory. In MR-guided wire localization cases, a radiologic-histopathologic correlation sheet accompanied the specimen to further clarify the relationship between the wire and the region of interest. The specimen was oriented by the surgeon, and the area of interest designated by the radiologist was inked with one color. The specimen was then measured, inked with several colors to correspond to the margins, and sectioned every 2–3 mm. Any lesion or lesions of interest were measured and photographed, and the entire specimen was submitted for histopathologic examination.

In cases in which mastectomy was performed, standard gross examination, including measurements, application of ink, sectioning, and lymph node dissection, was performed. Mastectomy specimens were sectioned every 0.5–1.0 cm, and each section was closely examined and palpated. Sections of tumor and all suspicious areas, with notation of the quadrant, were submitted for examination. In cases where the breast parenchyma was grossly unremarkable, a minimum of 12–15 sections were submitted for histopathologic examination. For all cases, two to three sections from the four quadrants, one section from the deep margin of resection, two sections of nipple, and all lymph nodes were microscopically examined.

RESULTS

Mammograms were available for retrospective review in 19 women. In 15 of the women, the breast parenchymal pattern was heterogeneously dense; in four women, the breast parenchymal pattern was scattered fibroglandular densities. In all patients, the mammogram demonstrated no suspicious findings. In the three patients for whom only the mammography report was available, the parenchymal pattern was described as dense.

In 19 (86%) of the 22 patients, a primary breast cancer was detected on MR images; the cancer was confirmed at excisional biopsy or mastectomy in 17 patients and had resolved on follow-up MR images obtained during chemotherapy in two patients. Of the 19 patients with MR imaging–detected cancers, 17 had cancers that appeared as a focal enhancing mass with spiculated (n = 5) or irregular (n = 12) borders (Figs 1–3). The enhancement pattern was homogeneous in nine patients and peripheral in eight patients. In the 17 patients with focal enhancing lesions, the lesions ranged in size from 5 to 30 mm, with a mean size of 17 mm. In two of the 19 patients, the enhancement was multifocal throughout the breast in one patient and in one quadrant in the second patient (Figs 4, 5). Due to the multifocality of the enhancement, an accurate measurement of tumor size was not possible.

Among the 17 women with histopathologically proved carcinoma, the diagnosis was established at excisional biopsy in eight women and at mastectomy in nine women. In four of the eight women who underwent excisional biopsy, the MR imaging–detected lesion was localized with MR imaging guidance (Figs 1, 2). In the remaining four women, the MR imaging–detected lesion was subsequently identified and localized at mammography in one woman, at US in one woman, and at physical examination in two women. Histopathologic diagnosis revealed invasive ductal carcinoma in 15 women and invasive lobular carcinoma in two women. The invasive ductal carcinomas ranged in size from 4 to 30 mm (mean, 15 mm) and in all women appeared on MR images as a focal enhancing lesion. In the two women with invasive lobular carcinoma, the carcinoma appeared histologically as multifocal disease. In the first woman, the overall tumor size was estimated to be 5 cm. In the second woman, due to the multifocality of the tumor, an accurate tumor size could not be measured. In both women, MR imaging demonstrated multifocal enhancing lesions. In all 17 women, the size and location of the enhancing lesion or lesions identified on MR images correlated closely with those found at histopathologic review.

In two of the 19 women in whom a suspicious lesion was identified on MR images, the lesion had resolved on MR images obtained during chemotherapy. In the first woman, an enhancing, irregular, 1.5-cm mass was identified on MR images. The mass appeared unchanged on follow-up MR images at 3 and 4 months but was no longer identified on follow-up MR images at 7 months (Fig 6). In the second woman, an enhancing, spiculated, 1.5-cm mass was identified at MR imaging. The lesion was not identified on follow-up MR images obtained at 3 months. Mastectomy was performed 7 months following the initial MR imaging, after the completion of chemotherapy, and no tumor was found in the breast.

False-positive enhancing lesions were identified in six women. In four of the six women, a true-positive lesion elsewhere in the breast was also identified (Fig 2). In three of the four women, MR imaging–guided wire localization and excisional biopsy were performed for both the true-positive and the false-positive lesions. At histopathologic review, atypical ductal hyperplasia, apocrine metaplasia, or a fibroadenoma was found. In the fourth woman, three enhancing lesions were identified on MR images. At mastectomy, invasive ductal carcinoma was identified, which appeared to correspond in size and location to one of the enhancing lesions identified on MR images. No additional lesions were found in the mastectomy specimen to correlate with the two additional enhancing lesions identified on MR images.

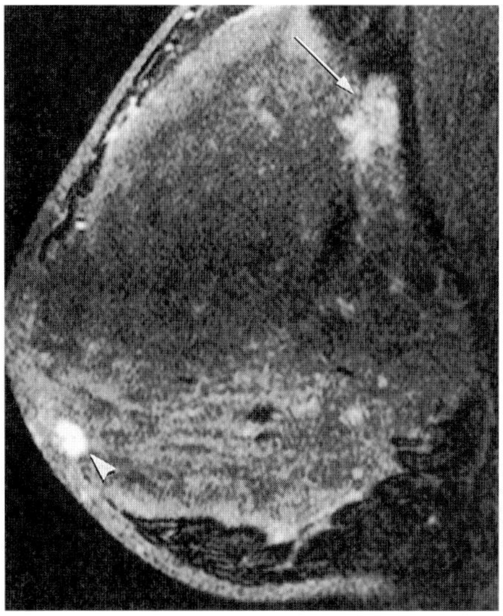

Figure 2. Sagittal fat-suppressed contrast-enhanced three-dimensional fast spoiled gradient-recalled-echo MR image (9.2/2.2) demonstrates a 2-cm enhancing mass (arrow) with irregular margins deep in the breast. A 5-mm enhancing mass (arrowhead) with irregular borders is also identified in the subareolar breast. MR imaging–guided localization of both lesions was performed. At excisional biopsy, the lesion deep in the breast was identified as a 1.8-cm infiltrating ductal carcinoma. In the subareolar excisional specimen, apocrine metaplasia was identified. The patient subsequently underwent breast-conservation therapy.

In two women, the only enhancing lesion or lesions proved to be false-positive. In the first woman, MR imaging–guided wire localization and excisional biopsy of an irregular 5-mm enhancing lesion revealed fibrocystic changes at histopathologic review. At mastectomy following chemotherapy, no tumor was found within the breast. In the second woman, MR imaging–guided wire localization and excisional biopsy of two irregular enhancing lesions (5 and 7 mm) revealed atypical ductal hyperplasia. Subsequent mastectomy revealed a 2-mm infiltrating ductal carcinoma. The location of the infiltrating carcinoma did not clearly correspond to the location of the MR imaging–detected lesions.

Two women had false-negative findings. In the first woman, two invasive ductal carcinomas were found at mastectomy and measured 17 mm in the lateral part of the breast and 20 mm in the axillary tail. At retrospective review of the MR images, the lateral lesion was not visible, and the axillary tail was not included in the field of view of the examination. The lesion in the second woman

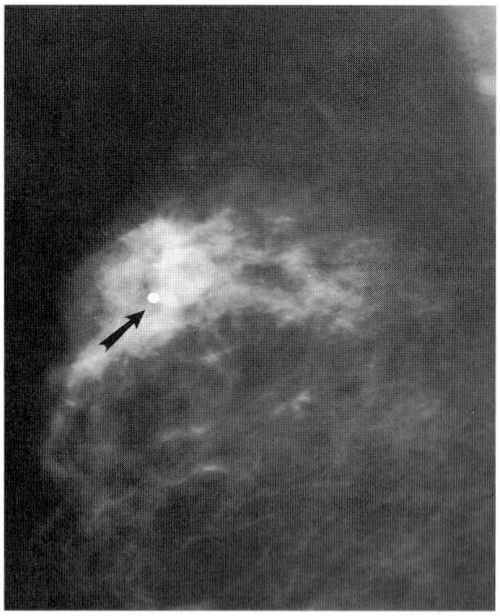

a.

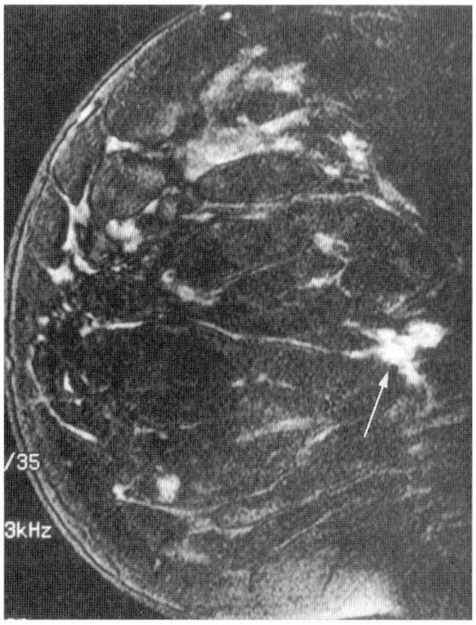

b.

Figure 3. Images in a patient with known axillary metastases and a palpable mass in the upper outer quadrant of the breast. (a) Mediolateral oblique mammogram reveals a mass (arrow) in the superior part of the breast near the skin marker. No other suspicious finding was identified. Ultrasonographic (US) examination of the palpable mass demonstrated a hypoechoic mass, which at core biopsy proved to be a metastatic intramammary node. (b) Sagittal fat-suppressed contrast-enhanced three-dimensional fast spoiled gradient-recalled-echo MR image (9.3/2.2) reveals an enhancing 1.5-cm mass (arrow) with irregular borders in the central part of the breast. At mastectomy, a 1.5-cm infiltrating ductal carcinoma was identified in a location corresponding to the MR imaging–detected lesion.

was described with the false-positive findings earlier; MR imaging–guided localization and excisional biopsy revealed atypical ductal hyperplasia, and a 2-mm infiltrating ductal carcinoma was found at mastectomy.

Of the 17 patients with a primary breast cancer identified on MR images and confirmed at surgery, 10 underwent mastectomy and seven underwent breast-conservation therapy. Of the two patients with a highly suspicious enhancing lesion that was identified on MR images and that resolved during treatment, one patient subsequently underwent mastectomy, and no tumor was found. The other patient did not undergo a surgical procedure.

DISCUSSION

MR imaging is an inherently expensive technology. For MR imaging to be used for breast imaging, it must be demonstrated that it can provide clinically valuable information that cannot be obtained with conventional imaging. While mammography is the primary imaging modality used for the detection of early, clinically occult breast cancer, the sensitivity of mammography is limited, largely due to the obscuration of cancer by dense breast parenchyma. There are now several studies with findings that demonstrate the potential of MR imaging for greater sensitivity than mammography in the detection and staging of breast cancer in patients with suspected or known breast cancer (10–14). The majority of patients in these series had either a suspicious mammographic or palpable abnormality or already had an established diagnosis of breast cancer at the time of the MR imaging examination.

As axillary node presentation of a clinically occult breast cancer is relatively uncommon, there have been very few reports of MR imaging–detected cancers in their clinical setting that we know of (11,15,20–22). In to our knowledge the largest published series to date, Morris et al (15) reported the MR imaging findings in 12 women with biopsy-proved metastatic adenocarcinoma to the axillary lymph nodes. In their series, a primary breast cancer was identified on MR images in nine (75%) of the 12 patients. In eight of the nine patients, cancers were visualized as a focal mass ranging from 9 to 20 mm (mean, 13 mm), and one cancer was visualized as an area of regional enhancement. The histopathologic findings in this series were invasive ductal carcinoma in seven patients, invasive lobular carcinoma in one patient, and ductal carcinoma in situ in one patient.

In our series, a primary breast cancer was detected on MR images in 19 (86%) of 22 patients. The MR imaging findings were similar to those reported by Morris et al. The most common MR imaging finding was that of a focal mass with irregular or spiculated borders, which was identified in 17 of the 19 patients in their study. The size of these lesions was also similar to that found by Morris et al, with a mean of 17 mm. In all 17 patients, the focally enhancing lesions proved to be invasive ductal carcinoma. In the remaining two patients, MR imaging demonstrated multiple enhancing lesions; in both patients, multifocal invasive lobular carcinoma was found at surgery.

The results of our series along with those of Morris et al (15), despite relatively small numbers of patients, suggest that MR imaging can be used to identify a primary breast cancer with high sensitivity in patients with isolated axillary metastases at presentation. However, the detection of a primary breast cancer is valuable clinically only if it will in some way affect patient care. The treatment of patients with isolated axillary metastases at presentation remains controversial. These patients are presumed to harbor an occult carcinoma in the ipsilateral breast (1,3). Review of the literature shows that 55%–100% of patients have an occult breast cancer (6). The traditional treatment of choice for this group of patients is mastectomy and axillary node dissection, which continues to be the most frequent treatment option (1–3). Most studies have shown long-term survival with mastectomy to be at least comparable with that for stage II breast cancer (1,3,5,6,9).

There are now reports demonstrating equivalent survival for patients with axillary node metastases and unknown primary malignancy who undergo breast-conservation therapy with breast irradiation and for those who undergo mastectomy (6–8). However, the recurrence rate in the breast in this population is higher than in the population undergoing breast-conservation therapy with radiation following excisional biopsy of the primary breast cancer (3,7,8). In two series (7,8), the recurrence rates in the breast were 23% and 12%. The failure rate in the breast is consistent with the expected failure rate that is based on the inability to control gross tumor in the breast with standard doses of radiation (3). With the exception of these two series (7,8), there is minimal information about the outcome of treatment with definitive radiation as an alternative to mastectomy (3).

Treatment recommendations for patients with newly diagnosed breast cancer are based on many factors, perhaps the most important being the extent of cancer within the breast. For patients with isolated axillary metastases at presentation, the extent of cancer within the breast is not known. As MR imaging appears to be very sensitive for the detection of an ipsilateral breast cancer in this population, MR imaging in these patients may provide information to help guide treatment planning. While overall survival appears to be similar for patients undergoing breast irradiation and for patients undergoing mastectomy, the detection and staging of an ipsilateral breast cancer provides clinical information that can allow the surgeon, radiation oncologist, and medical oncologist to determine whether breast-conservation therapy is a reasonable treatment option or whether the size and/or histopathologic features suggest a high rate of local recurrence following radiation, which makes mastectomy a better treatment choice.

In our series, the mean histopathologic lesion size was 17 mm, and in six women, the lesion measured less than 10 mm. In only two women was extensive cancer identified on MR images, and both women were proved to have multifocal invasive lobular carcinoma at mastectomy. Of the 17 patients with a primary breast cancer detected on MR images and surgically confirmed, seven (41%) underwent breast-conservation therapy. In these seven women, the information gained from the MR imaging study, namely the detection of a localized cancer on MR images, resulted in a change in clinical management; breast-conservation therapy was offered as an alternative to the traditional recommendation of mastectomy.

When breast cancer is suspected on an imaging study, the ability to offer lumpectomy with the potential for breast-conservation therapy is dependent on the localization of the suspicious lesion. In the setting of MR imaging–detected lesions, the lesion must either be localized with MR imaging guidance or be identified at mammography, US, or physical examination.

In our study, four of the eight excisional biopsies among the 17 patients with histopathologic proof were guided with MR imaging, while the remaining four were guided with mammography, US, or palpation. In our breast center, MR imaging–guided wire localization is readily available (19). Thus, for the lesions that were ultimately localized with MR imaging guidance, an attempt was

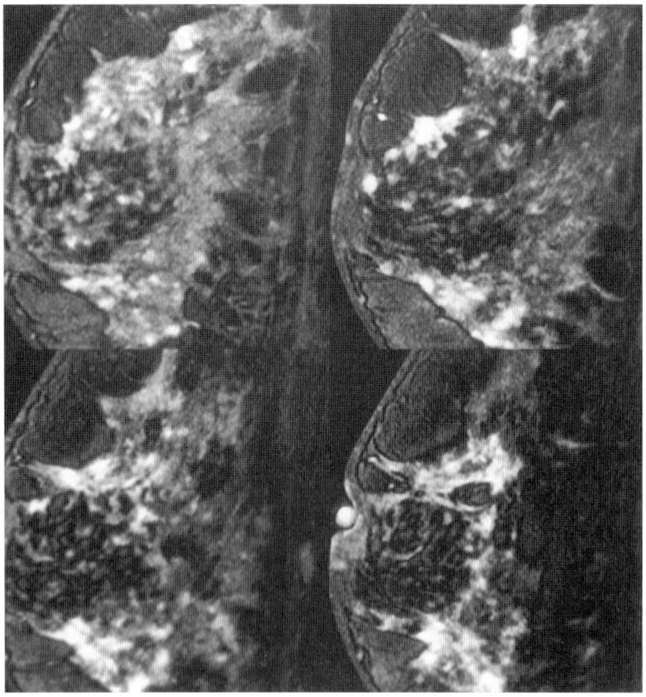

Figure 4. Sagittal fat-suppressed contrast-enhanced three-dimensional fast spoiled gradient-recalled-echo MR images (9.3/2.2) reveal multiple enhancing areas scattered throughout the breast. Mammography revealed dense tissue without a suspicious finding. At mastectomy, multifocal invasive lobular carcinoma was found in all quadrants of the breast.

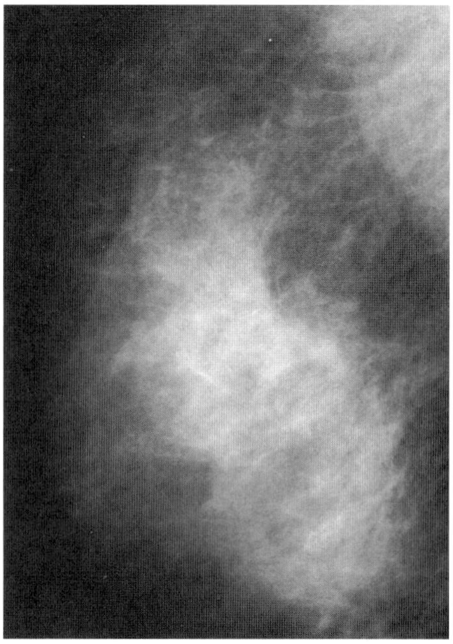

a.

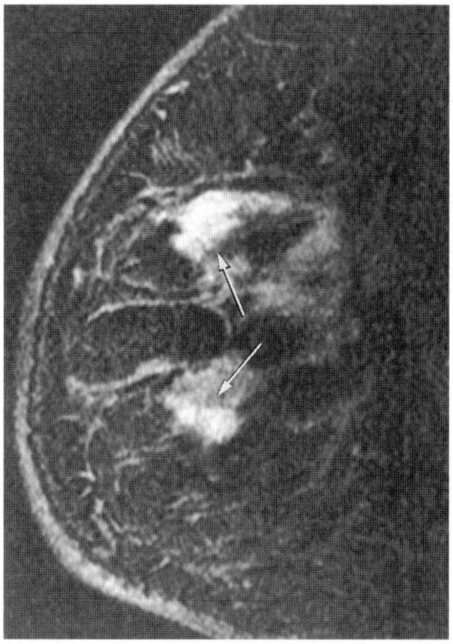

b.

Figure 5. **(a)** Mediolateral oblique mammogram reveals heterogeneously dense breast tissue. **(b)** Sagittal fat-suppressed contrast-enhanced three-dimensional fast spoiled gradient-recalled-echo MR image (9.3/2.2) demonstrates two areas (arrows) of ill-defined enhancement. At mastectomy, approximately 5-cm multifocal infiltrating lobular carcinoma was identified.

not made to localize the MR imaging–detected lesion with US. In the series reported on by Morris et al (15), an MR imaging–guided localization system was not available, and the authors were successful at identifying and localizing the MR imaging–detected lesion at US in six of nine patients. Ideally, an MR imaging–guided localization system should be available, as MR imaging–detected lesions may not be visible with US. However, as there is presently no commercially available MR imaging guiding system, directed US examination to the expected location of the MR imaging–detected lesion may allow for lesion identification and biopsy.

Two of the limitations of MR imaging previously reported (11,22), specifically, false-positive enhancement and the inability to document lesion removal following MR imaging–guided wire localization, were also present in this study. In six patients, a false-positive enhancing lesion was identified; in four patients, it occurred along with a true-positive enhancing lesion elsewhere in the breast. In two of these women, atypia was identified. There is, at the present time, no way to determine if a suspicious lesion localized with MR imaging is successfully removed at excisional biopsy unless cancer is found at histopathologic review. An MR imaging–compatible core biopsy system could both obviate a surgical procedure for a false-positive benign enhancing lesion and solve the problem of documenting lesion removal. Such systems are in development.

The clinical importance of a negative MR image in the setting of isolated axillary metastases is not clear. In this series, there were two patients with false-negative findings: one patient with two cancers measuring 17 and 20 mm and one patient with a cancer measuring 2 mm. The patient with the two cancers not identified on MR images was examined early in our study. In this patient, one of the cancers proved to be in the axillary tail, but the axillary tail was not included in the field of view of the MR imaging examination. With the present design of our breast coil, the axillary tail cannot always be compressed between the medial and lateral plates and is thereby excluded from the examination. Further coil development is needed so that the axillary tail can be fully evaluated.

The missed 2-mm cancer is our only recent false-negative case. Whether the axillary metastases in this case were secondary to this tiny cancer is not clear. Our inability to visualize the 2-mm cancer may reflect the ultimate imperfect

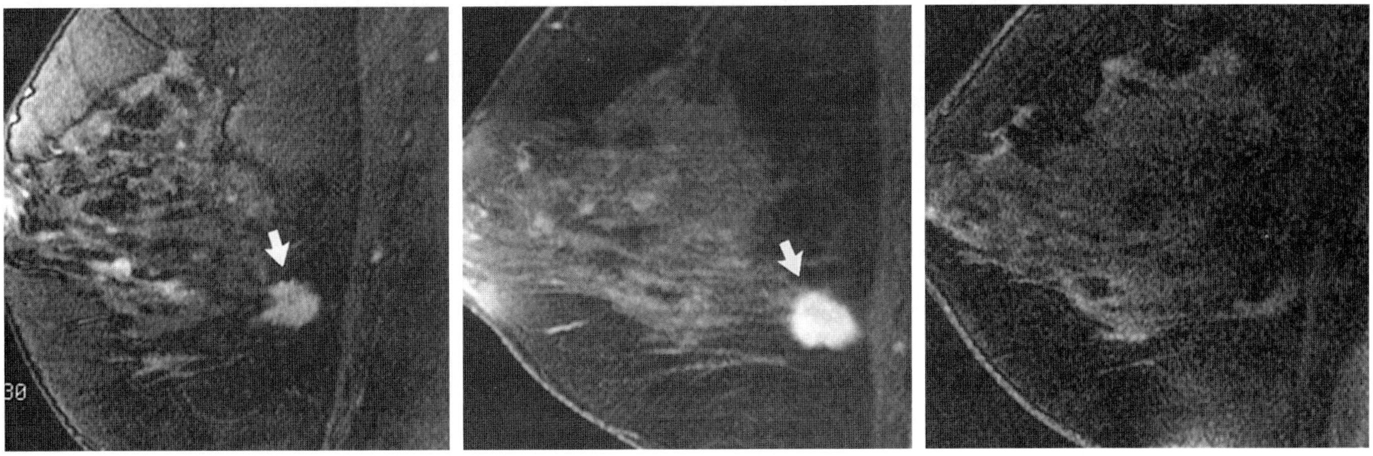

a. b. c.

Figure 6. Images in a patient with axillary node metastases and an MR imaging–detected suspicious mass that resolved during chemotherapy. Mammography revealed dense breast tissue without a suspicious finding. **(a)** Sagittal fat-suppressed contrast-enhanced three-dimensional fast spoiled gradient-recalled-echo MR image (11/2.2) shows a 1.5-cm, spiculated mass (arrow) deep in the breast. **(b)** Four-month follow-up sagittal fat-suppressed contrast-enhanced three-dimensional fast spoiled gradient-recalled-echo MR image (27.8/4) obtained during chemotherapy shows no substantial change in the size of the mass (arrow). **(c)** Seven-month follow-up sagittal fat-suppressed contrast-enhanced three-dimensional fast spoiled gradient-recalled-echo MR image (9.2/2.2) shows resolution of the mass. No surgical procedure was performed.

sensitivity of MR imaging. In our experience, multiple, scattered 2–3-mm enhancing foci are often identified on diagnostic breast MR images both in patients with known breast cancer and in those with no known breast cancer. In patients who undergo subsequent MR imaging examinations, these tiny foci commonly resolve and new foci appear. In the presence of these enhancing foci, it may not always be possible to identify a 2- or 3-mm breast cancer. The negative predictive value of MR imaging remains unknown. Whether a negative MR image can be used to support breast-conservation therapy with breast irradiation as an alternative to mastectomy needs to be determined with additional investigation.

Our results, along with those previously reported, support the use of MR imaging for the evaluation of patients who have axillary node metastases at presentation and negative mammographic and clinical examination findings. In this patient population, MR imaging offers potential not only for the detection of a primary ipsilateral breast cancer but also for staging, which may be used to guide treatment planning. The identification of localized disease may offer some women the option of breast-conservation therapy as an alternative to mastectomy.

References

1. Fourquet A, De La Rochefordiere A, Campana F. Occult primary cancer with axillary metastases. In: Harris JR, Lippman ME, Morrow M, Hellman S, eds. Diseases of the breast. Philadelphia, Pa: Lippincott-Raven, 1996; 892–896.
2. Halsted W. The results of radical operations for the cure of carcinoma of the breast. Ann Surg 1907; 46:1–19.
3. Solin LJ. Special considerations. In: Fowble B, Goodman RL, Glick JH, Rosato EF, eds. Breast cancer treatment: a comprehensive guide to management. St Louis, Mo: Mosby–Year Book, 1991; 523–528.
4. Jackson B, Scott-Conner C, Moulder J. Axillary metastasis from occult breast carcinoma: diagnosis and management. Am Surg 1995; 61:431–434.
5. Fortunato L, Sorrento JJ, Golub RA, Cantu R. Occult breast cancer. NY State J Med 1992; 92:555–557.
6. Baron PL, Moore MP, Kinne DW, Candela FC, Osborne MP, Petrek JA. Occult breast cancer presenting with axillary metastases. Arch Surg 1990; 125:210–214.
7. Campana F, Fourquet A, Ashby MA, et al. Presentation of axillary lymphadenopathy without detectable breast primary (T0 N1b breast cancer): experience at Institut Curie. Radiother Oncol 1989; 15:321–325.
8. Ellerbroek N, Holmes F, Singletary E, Evans H, Oswald SM, McNeese M. Treatment of patients with isolated axillary nodal metastases from an occult primary carcinoma consistent with breast origin. Cancer 1990; 66:1461–1467.
9. Knapper WH. Management of occult breast cancer presenting as an axillary metastasis. Semin Surg Oncol 1991; 7:311–313.
10. Harms SE, Flamig DP, Hesley K, et al. MR imaging of the breast with rotating delivery of excitation off resonance: clinical experience with pathologic correlation. Radiology 1993; 187:493–501.
11. Orel SG, Schnall MD, Powell CM, et al. Staging of suspected breast cancer: effect of MR imaging and MR-guided biopsy. Radiology 1995; 196:115–122.
12. Orel SG, Reynolds C, Schnall MD, Solin LJ, Fraker DL, Sullivan DC. Breast carcinoma: MR imaging before reexcisional biopsy. Radiology 1997; 205:429–436.
13. Mumtaz H, Hall-Craggs MA, Davidson T, et al. Staging of symptomatic primary breast cancer with MR imaging. AJR 1997; 169:417–424.
14. Rodenko GN, Harms SE, Pruneda JM, et al. MR imaging in the management before surgery of lobular carcinoma of the breast: correlation with pathology. AJR 1996; 167:1415–1419.
15. Morris EA, Schwartz LH, Dershaw DD, Van Zee KJ, Abramson AF, Liberman L. MR imaging of the breast in patients with occult primary breast carcinoma. Radiology 1997; 205:437–440.
16. Insko EK, Schnall MD, Connick TJ, Orel SG. Multi-coil array for high resolution imaging of the breast. Magn Reson Med 1997; 37:778–786.
17. Nunes LW, Schnall MD, Siegelman ES, et al. Diagnostic performance characteristics of architectural features revealed by high spatial-resolution MR imaging of the breast. AJR 1997; 169:409–415.
18. Nunes LW, Schnall MD, Orel SG, et al. Breast MR imaging: interpretation model. Radiology 1997; 202:833–841.
19. Orel SG, Schnall MD, Newman RW, Powell CM, Torosian MH, Rosato EF. MR imaging-guided localization and biopsy of breast lesions: initial experience. Radiology 1994; 193:97–102.
20. Harms SE, Flamig DP. Staging of breast cancer with MR imaging. Magn Reson Imaging Clin N Am 1994; 2:573–584.
21. Davis PL, Julian TB, Staiger M, et al. Magnetic resonance imaging detection and wire localization of an "occult" breast cancer. Breast Cancer Res Treat 1994; 32:327–330.
22. Orel SG, Hochman MG, Schnall MD, Reynolds C, Sullivan DC. High-resolution MR imaging of the breast: clinical context. RadioGraphics 1996; 16:1385–1401.

Book Review

Radiation Protection Dosimetry: A Radical Reappraisal

Jack A. Simmons and David E. Watt

Madison, Wis: Medical Physics Publishing, 1999. ISBN 0-944838-87-1.
Softcover, $35.95; pp 158; 17 figures; tables.

Simmons and Watt are radiation physicists who propose a new injury model based on fluence, where fluence describes the number of charged particles that traverse a specific biologic target such as a DNA molecule.

Since mostly x rays, gamma rays, and electrons (low linear energy transfer [LET] radiation) are used in radiation medicine, the fluence here describes the secondary electrons of primary ionizations. The biologic target size (where the injury occurs) can be described as a cross section. The probability of injury is then determined by multiplying the fluence by the biologic cross section. This model is simple in its construction, but it is not simple in its implementation. Cross sections vary with the biologic end point considered. They depend on the density of ionization caused by the charged particle fluence. Both low LET radiation and high LET radiation are addressed.

The authors believe their model unifies experimental and epidemiologic observations for both types of radiation. They address the well-known dependence of injury on dose rate or fluence rate (flux) with a time-sensitive "repair factor." This is especially important for low LET radiation.

The authors argue that absorbed dose (in rads or grays) does not provide a sound basis for studying the effects of radiation injury. Introducing "quality factors" and "distribution factors" to modify dose (in rems or sieverts) does not fix the problem. They conclude that this effectively invalidates the linear, no-threshold model of injury. Could a concept as widely accepted as the linear, no-threshold concept be wrong? The authors note that science sometimes requires "a fundamental reconsideration of . . . acceptable concepts." There is evidence that it is time for reappraisal of scientific beliefs regarding radiation injury.

Simmons and Watt conclude that for mammalian cells, injury is most critical when ionization events occur at spacings no greater than 2 nm. This roughly corresponds to the distance between strands of the double-helix DNA molecule and is likely the spacing at which double-strand breaks begin to occur. The 2-nm spacing can occur with a single high LET particle transversing a target, but, for low LET radiation, there is substantial occurrence of this spacing only when more than one primary charged particle interacts with the same biologic target. Low doses and/or low dose rates of low LET radiation may not cause injury because there is not enough charged particle fluence to cause unrepaired double-strand breaks.

This is an important and timely book. It contains descriptions of the models used today to describe radiation injury. There are chapters on the history and evolution of radiation protection policy by the International Commission for Radiological Protection and the International Commission on Radiation Units and Measurements. Policy positions that are not linked to science are identified.

The book can be read in a night, but it will take longer to understand. Concepts are evolving and difficult. Are the authors correct in their beliefs? I don't know. But like bold scientists of yesteryear, they have nailed their propositions on the "doors of the institution of science." We will decide to either excommunicate them as scientific heretics or embrace their proposals as having scientific merit. You will enjoy this book. Most will not understand all of it (I certainly did not), but you will feel enriched if you spend some time considering the authors' beliefs and proposals.

Reviewed by David S. Gooden, PhD, JD

James S. Michaelson, PhD
Elkan Halpern, PhD
Daniel B. Kopans, MD

Index terms:
Breast neoplasms, 00.32
Breast neoplasms, metastases, **.33[2]
Breast radiography, utilization
Cancer screening, 00.11
Computers, simulation

Radiology 1999; 212:551–560

[1] From the Departments of Pathology (J.S.M.) and Radiology (E.H., D.B.K.), Harvard Medical School, Boston, Mass, and the Massachusetts General Hospital Cancer Center, 149 13th St, Charlestown, MA 02129 (J.S.M.). From the 1998 RSNA scientific assembly. Received August 7, 1998; revision requested September 8; final revision received December 30; accepted February 9, 1999. **Address reprint requests to** J.S.M. (e-mail: *michaelj@helix.mgh.harvard.edu*).

[2] **. Multiple body systems

Author contributions:
Guarantor of integrity of entire study, J.S.M.; study concepts, J.S.M., E.H., D.B.K.; study design, J.S.M.; definition of intellectual content, J.S.M., E.H., D.B.K.; literature research, J.S.M., E.H., D.B.K.; statistical analysis, J.S.M., E.H.; manuscript preparation, editing, and review, J.S.M., E.H., D.B.K.

Breast Cancer: Computer Simulation Method for Estimating Optimal Intervals for Screening[1]

PURPOSE: To develop and evaluate a mathematic method that can be used to determine the optimal screening interval for detection of breast cancer prior to distant metastatic spread.

MATERIALS AND METHODS: A computer simulation was developed with the use of biologically based data from the literature on the rates of tumor growth and spread, which can be used to calculate the course of breast cancer growth and metastasis.

RESULTS: On the basis of the data available at this time, the results of the simulations suggested that a screening interval of 2 years would result in a 22% reduction in the rate of distant metastatic disease, an interval of 1 year would result in a 51% reduction, and an interval of 6 months would result in an 80% reduction.

CONCLUSION: These findings suggest that more frequent screening could dramatically reduce the death rate from breast cancer.

Invasive breast cancer is diagnosed in more than 180,000 women each year, and over 40,000 die of this disease annually. If these tumors can be identified while confined to the breast, then breast cancer usually can be cured by means of local treatment. It is distant metastatic disease, and the destruction of other organ systems, that causes death in women with breast cancer (1–14). Indeed, the results of randomized controlled trials of screening (9,10,13,14) have demonstrated that if breast cancer can be detected and treated before becoming metastatic, death due to breast cancer can be avoided.

Although the results of these trials have demonstrated that mammography can save lives, many aspects of screening remain undefined, including the optimal interval between screening sessions (15,16). The American College of Radiology and the American Cancer Society recommend that women aged 40 years and older undergo screening every year, whereas the National Cancer Institute recommends screening every 1–2 years (11,12). A 1-year interval has been chosen by several organizations, particularly for younger women, because the available data suggest that cancers grow faster in these women, and if the tumor is to be stopped prior to metastatic spread, a shorter time between screenings is needed (11,12).

Moskowitz (17) was one of the first to point out the importance of the screening interval. Subsequently, Tabar et al (18) demonstrated the same phenomenon by using interval cancer rates in which women aged 40–49 years underwent screening every 2 years, and women aged 50 years and older underwent screening every 3 years. More recently, Sickles (19) showed that the sensitivity of mammography was the same for women aged 40–49 years who underwent screening every year as it was for women aged 50 years and older who underwent screening every 2 years. Unfortunately, however, we are aware of no studies in which the issues of different screening intervals and how these intervals may influence mortality have directly and prospectively been addressed.

Although there has been a general appreciation that the rates of tumor growth and spread are fundamental to both the biology and the control of breast cancer, to our knowledge there has not been a mathematic model that could be used to determine such estimates in a quantitative fashion. In this article, we describe just such a computer simulation method, which is reliant on biologically based data on the rates of breast cancer growth and spread. The purpose of this study was to develop and evaluate a mathematic method that can be used to determine the optimal screening interval for detection of breast cancer prior to distant metastatic spread. This simulation method has allowed us to examine a variety of aspects of breast cancer screening, including the effect of various screening intervals on the reduction in the breast cancer death rate. The results of our simulations are generally in agreement with the results of randomized controlled trials of breast cancer screening and confirm the widely held belief in the benefit of yearly mammographic screening. In addition, our results raise the surprising possibility that considerable reductions in the breast cancer death rate might be achieved if breast cancer screening was performed more frequently.

MATERIALS AND METHODS

Data for Estimates of Breast Cancer Growth Rate

By using data from a variety of sources, it is possible to estimate the growth rate of breast cancer. Some of the most telling data are from studies (20–27) of serial mammograms; these studies are reliant on the fact that, in a small number of patients, the signs of the tumor can be found at a review of an earlier mammogram. von Fournier et al (20) studied mammograms in 147 such patients whose tumors could be seen on two or more serial mammograms and found these tumors to have a doubling time of 88–383 days. Heuser et al (26) used the same approach and observed 16 patients whose tumors had a doubling time of 109–270 days, eight patients whose tumors had a doubling time of more than 1 year (393–944 days), and nine patients whose tumors had an essentially infinite doubling time (ie, the tumors showed no growth). Lundgren (27) examined the growth rates of 15 tumors and found a doubling time of 42–406 days. In one of the largest such studies, Spratt et al (24) estimated tumor growth rates in 448 patients and found a mean doubling time of approximately 250 days and a range of 10–7,051 days.

The difficulty with estimates of cancer growth that are based on sequential mammographic data is that slow-growing tumors are more likely to be seen on two consecutive mammograms than are fast-growing tumors. This means that estimates derived from sequential mammographic data are likely to yield artificially low breast cancer growth rates. In part to generate estimates less susceptible to this bias, Peer et al (23) used data on breast cancers arising during a screening program. The growth of tumors that did not appear on two consecutive mammograms could be estimated by assuming that at the time of the previous mammogram, the tumor was just below the limit of detectability. Of course, these tumors could have been far smaller than this minimum size, so this approach is not entirely free of the tendency to underestimate growth rate, but bias with this method is of a smaller magnitude than bias with estimates determined on the basis of serial mammograms alone. Indeed, the estimates by Peer et al did result in a downward revision of the estimated growth rates of breast cancer. Peer et al also sorted the data by age and found that in patients younger than 50 years of age, tumors have a median doubling time of 80 days (with 95% of doubling times between 44 and 147 days), whereas the tumors in patients aged 50–70 years have a median doubling time of 157 days (with 95% of doubling times between 121 and 204 days), and tumors in patients older than 70 years have a median doubling time of 188 days (with 95% of doubling times between 120 and 295 days).

Of course, not all tumors grow at the same rate. However, there are excellent data on the distribution of growth rates. For example, the distribution of these doubling times has been characterized by Spratt et al (24), who found that roughly 50% of tumors have a doubling time close to the mean, whereas 25% of tumors have a doubling time of about twice the mean rate, and most of the remaining 25% have a doubling time of about half the mean rate.

There also are abundant data (28–38) that suggest that when breast cancers are much smaller than the size at which they become clinically evident, their growth is much more rapid than that during their clinical appearance. There also are data that indicate that breast cancers, if left untreated, will undergo a further decline in growth rate. Fortunately, however, as we shall report in this article, we have found that this so-called density-dependent change in growth rate, sometimes also called gompertzian growth (29), will not affect the general conclusions of our estimates on the outcome of breast cancer screening.

Tumor Size and Incidence of Metastasis

The probability that a breast cancer cell will leave the primary tumor and form a distant metastasis can be calculated from data on the relationship between tumor size and the incidence of distant metastatic disease. Many factors, including age and genotype, may play a role in the rate of metastasis. We can begin to gain some insight into this process from data collected by Tabar et al (9–11) and Tubiana and colleagues (6–8) on the relationship between the size of the primary breast cancer at the time of surgical removal and the subsequent incidence of distant metastatic disease (Table 1). By distant metastatic disease, we mean the spread and establishment of potentially lethal cancer to the periphery, beyond the breast and the regional lymph nodes. We emphasize that with this definition there are no assumptions about whether such spread occurs directly from the primary tumor or is mediated by an intervening step in the local lymph nodes.

A few simple mathematic tools are needed to extract an initial estimate of the probability of metastasis from the data collected by Tabar et al (9–11) and Tubiana et al (6–8). The number of cells n in a tumor can be roughly estimated from the tumor diameter by using the expression $n \approx B[4/3\pi(d/2)^3]$, where d is the tumor diameter, and B is the number of cells per cubic centimeter. Because most tumors cells are roughly 20 µm in diameter (39–41), a B value of approximately 10^8 cells per cubic centimeter is a reasonable approximation, although, as will become apparent later, our model does not require a precise estimate of B. The probability that a cell will leave the primary tumor and form a distant metastasis is defined as $1/P$, which is expressed in units of $\text{cell}^{-1} \cdot \text{day}^{-1}$. Thus, P may be thought of as the number cells for the number of days it takes until there will be, on average, one metastasis per tumor. P, therefore, is expressed with the unit "cell days." By definition, C is the number of cell days that a tumor with n cells has accumulated. If P should prove to be a constant, then it follows that the average number of metastases per tumor is equal to $C \times 1/P$.

To calculate the relationship between tumor size n and the number of cell days C that a tumor has accumulated requires consideration of the rate of tumor growth, as was discussed earlier. Such growth information can be incorporated into a simple computer simulation, and the relationship between n and C can be estimated. (The source code for these and other simulations described in this article is available at *http://webm9120.ntx.net/BreastCancerMath.html*. Accessed June 10, 1999.)

TABLE 1
Estimated Probability of Formation of Distant Metastasis from a Primary Breast Cancer Cell

Tumor Size (mm)	Fraction of Patients with Metastases	Constant Doubling Time 20 Days ($\times 10^{-12}$)	Constant Doubling Time 80 Days ($\times 10^{-12}$)	Constant Doubling Time 400 Days ($\times 10^{-12}$)	Density-dependent Growth with Terminal Doubling Time 20 Days ($\times 10^{-12}$)	Density-dependent Growth with Terminal Doubling Time 80 Days ($\times 10^{-12}$)	Density-dependent Growth with Terminal Doubling Time 400 Days ($\times 10^{-12}$)	Stochastic Process ($\times 10^{-12}$)*
12 (10–14)†	0.13	51.0	6.50	2.67	116.0	31.90	26.50	1,150
17 (15–19)†	0.20	29.0	7.50	1.50	57.6	15.40	3.12	865
17 (10–25)‡	0.27	41.0	10.60	2.10	80.0	22.00	4.40	1,225
25 (20–29)†	0.45	24.0	6.30	1.30	37.9	10.20	2.08	719
30 (26–35)‡	0.42	12.0	3.30	0.67	16.5	3.30	0.88	378
39 (30–49)†	0.55	8.4	2.20	0.44	9.5	2.40	0.48	251
40 (36–45)‡	0.56	8.3	2.10	0.43	9.1	2.10	0.50	245
50 (46–55)‡	0.66	5.6	1.40	0.29	5.9	1.40	0.31	167
60 (56–65)‡	0.78	3.9	0.99	0.20	4.0	0.99	0.21	114
70 (66–75)‡	0.83	3.4	0.87	0.18	3.4	0.87	0.18	99
80 (76–85)‡	0.81	2.1	0.53	0.11	2.1	0.53	0.11	62
90 (86–95)‡	0.92	2.2	0.57	0.12	2.2	0.57	0.12	64

Note.—Data are estimates of probability ($1/P$) expressed as number of metastases per cell day times 10^{-12}.
* Estimate determined on the basis of a stochastic process occurring once during each mitotic cycle.
† Data are from references 9–11. Numbers in parentheses are the range.
‡ Data are from references 6–8. Numbers in parentheses are the range.

TABLE 2
Estimated Reduction in Incidence of Distant Metastasis as a Function of Screening Frequency

Screening Frequency	Detection Method for Tumors with More than 10^8 Cells (%)*	Detection Method for Tumors with More than 10^7 Cells (%)†	Detection Method for Tumors with More than 10^6 Cells (%)‡
Every 3rd year	7	14	16
Every 2nd year	14	22	27
Every year	33	51	56
Every 6 months	62	78	84
Every 4 months	77	90	93
Every 3 months	86	96	98
Every 2 months	87	97	98

Note.—Reduction is relative to that in women who do not undergo screening.
* Corresponds to tumor diameter of approximately 12 mm.
† Corresponds to tumor diameter of approximately 3 mm.
‡ Corresponds to tumor diameter of approximately 1.2 mm.

For example, given a constant doubling time of 80 days, the simulation reveals that the various tumor sizes listed in the articles by Tabar et al (9–11) and Tubiana et al (6–8)—that is, 1.2, 1.7, 2, 2.5, 3, 3.9, 4, 5, 6, 7, 8, and 9 cm—correspond to C values of 0.1, 0.35, 0.48, 0.58, 1.6, 3.2, 3.8, 7.5, 13, 20, 31, and 44 $\times 10^{11}$ cell days, respectively. We also performed a similar calculation, taking into account the possibility that breast cancer may grow more rapidly when the tumor is small than when it is large (sometimes called gompertzian growth) (29,30); these estimates are shown in Table 2.

Now consider a group of patients whose tumors have grown to a size such that they have accumulated exactly P cell days ($C = P$). It would be expected in such a group of patients that, on average, there would be one metastasis per patient, since $C \times 1/P = P \times 1/P = 1$. Of course, this is an average. Although some of these patients would have one metastasis, others would have two metastases or four metastases, and some patients would have no metastases and would be free of metastatic disease. By using the Poisson distribution, it is possible to calculate that when the average number of metastases per patient is one, the fraction of patients with no metastases, that is, the fraction of metastatic disease–free patients is $1/e$, or about 37% of patients. On the other hand, for a different group of patients whose tumors are of sufficient size to have accumulated, for example, $C = 3P$ cell days—that is, in whom the average number of metastases per patient is three—it then follows that the fraction of metastatic disease–free patients is $1/e^3$. Thus, in general, if C equals the number of cell days a tumor has accumulated and P equals the number of cell days needed to cause one metastasis per patient, the fraction of metastatic disease–free patients fr is equal to $1/e^{C/P}$ or $\ln(fr) = -C/P$.

It follows from this latter equation that if $1/P$ is a constant, then a graph of the natural logarithm of fr versus C will form a straight, downward-pointing line that forms an intersection with the origin. In fact, the data of Tabar et al (9–11) and Tubiana et al (6–8) conform quite closely to the straight line predicted by $\ln(fr) = -C/P$, with an r^2 value of 0.8976, which thus provides direct empiric evidence that the value of $1/P$ is fairly constant (Fig 1).

From a biologic standpoint, this relative constancy of $1/P$ is what would be expected for mechanisms of metastasis formation that are dependent on processes such as mutation or simple mechanical events such as detachment from the primary tumor, dissemination, survival, and reengraftment (42–45). What is especially powerful about the results of Tabar et al (9–11) and Tubiana et al (6–8), however, is that their data provide a way to measure the value of this probability. Thus, the graph shown in Figure 1 can be used to develop a rough estimate of the value of $1/P$, which the equation $\ln(fr) = -C/P$ indicates will correspond to the point on the x axis where fr is equal to $1/e$, or about 37%, which yields an approximate value for $1/P$ from 10^{-11} to 10^{-13} metastases per cell day. Alterna-

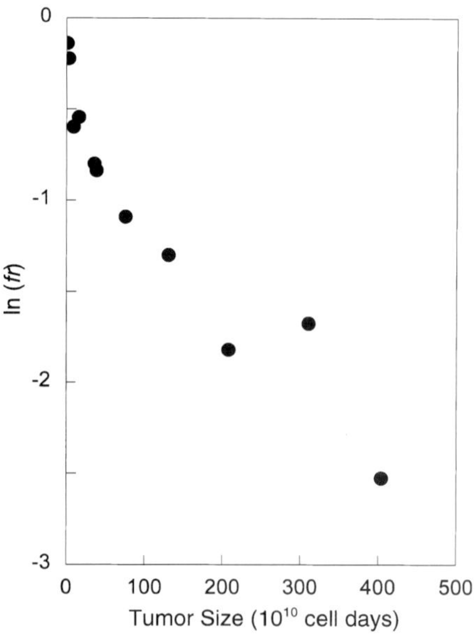

Figure 1. Graph shows the relationship between tumor size (in cell days) and the log of the incidence of metastatic disease (*fr*). The data are from studies by Tabar et al (9–11) and Tubiana et al (6–8). The number of cell days was calculated by using computer simulation in which a constant doubling time of 80 days was assumed. Tumor size (in number of cells *n*) was calculated on the basis of tumor diameter *d* by using the expression $n = B[4/3\pi(d/2)^3]$, with a *B* value of 10^8 cells per cubic centimeter. The r^2 value is 0.8976.

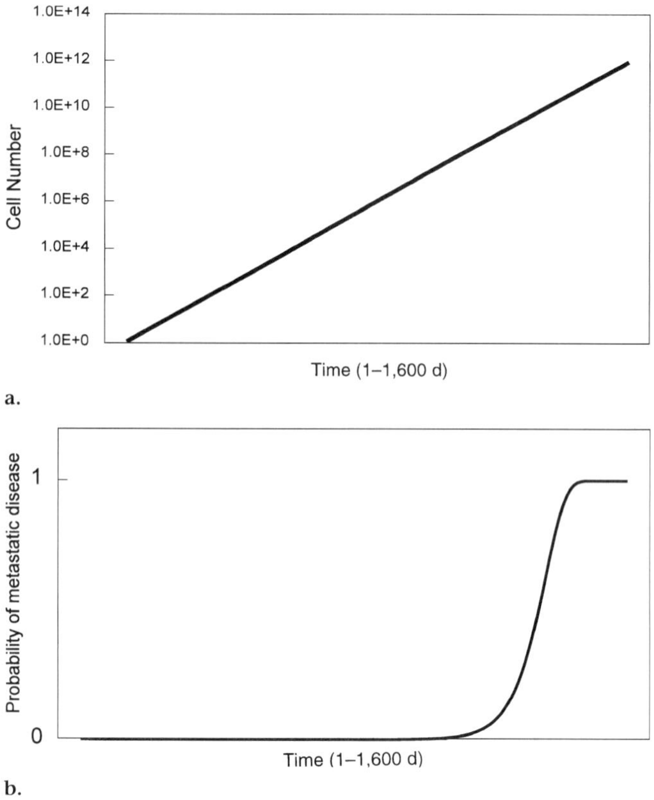

Figure 2. **(a)** Graph shows results of a computer simulation of breast cancer growth for a tumor with a doubling time of 80 days. This graph represents an idealized mean growth curve. The actual growth of tumors should be expected to display variation around this mean. **(b)** Graph shows computer simulation results for the development of distant metastatic disease. In this simulation, the probability that a cell will leave the primary tumor and form a distant metastasis ($1/P$) is 10^{-12} cell^{-1} · day^{-1}.

tively, the value of $1/P$ can be estimated directly with $\ln(fr) = -C/P$ for each tumor size and data point on the basis of metastatic disease incidence provided by Tabar et al (9–11) and Tubiana et al (6–8) (Table 1).

Estimates in Probability of Distant Metastasis

It is possible to estimate the degree of variability in the value of $1/P$. As already noted, if $1/P$ were perfectly constant, then it would follow from the expression $\ln(fr) = -C/P$ that a graph of the natural logarithm of *fr* versus *C* would form a straight, downward-pointing line that begins at the origin. Although close to this line, the data of Tabar et al (9–11) and Tubiana et al (6–8) display a slight curvature (Fig 1). There are a number of possible explanations for this rather subtle feature. For example, as tumors become larger, they may contain necrotic material, and this could cause overestimation of the number of cells in larger tumors and underestimation of the number of cells in smaller tumors, thus resulting in the curvature. Alternatively, cancer cells at the periphery of a tumor may have a slightly better chance of detaching from the primary tumor and forming a metastatic colony than might cells located in the interior of the tumor. This would mean that the value of $1/P$ would decrease slightly as the tumor became larger. It also is possible that small tumors have a slower growth rate than large tumors; examination of Table 1 reveals that because the growth rate is necessary for the calculation of $1/P$, this effect may account for the variability in $1/P$. Finally, there may be a small amount of tumor-to-tumor variation in the value of $1/P$. Indeed, the slight curvature seen in Figure 1 fits well with the type of curve we would expect if about 25% of tumors have a $1/P$ value of approximately 10^{-11}, another 50% of tumors have a value of approximately 10^{-12}, and the remaining 25% of tumors have a value of approximately 10^{-13}, as we have found by using a simulation that reconstructs a curve on the basis of a population of women with just this distribution of values (data not shown).

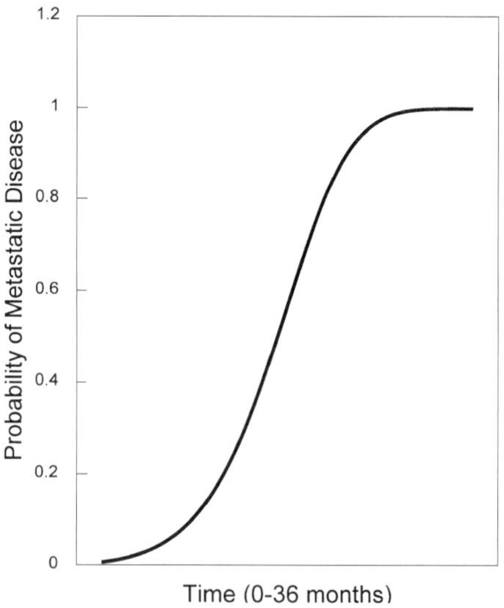

Figure 3. Graph shows computer simulation results for the probability of distant metastatic disease from the time when the primary tumor (doubling time, 80 days) is first detectable at mammography (tumor size, 10^7 cells). The $1/P$ value is approximately 10^{-12} cell^{-1} · day^{-1}.

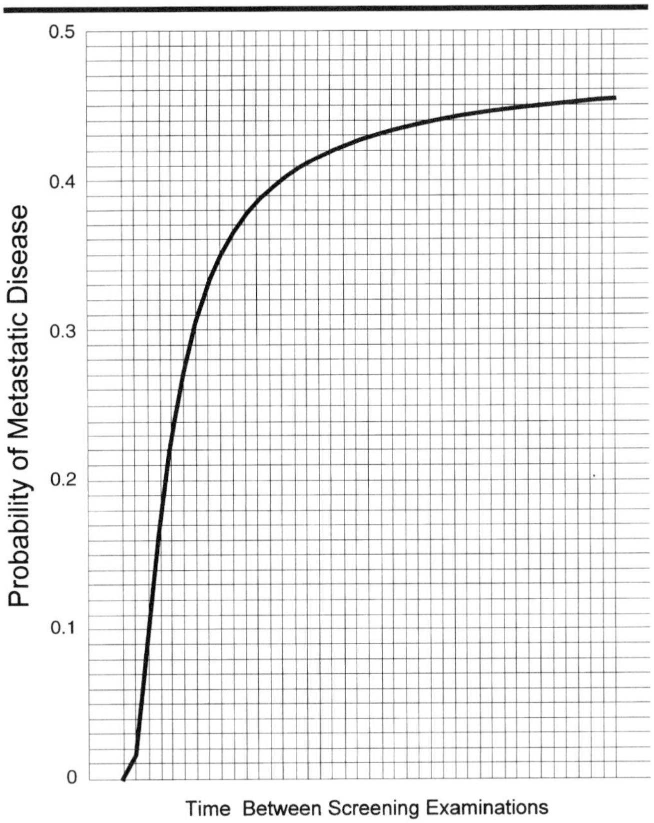

Figure 4. Graph shows the results of a computer simulation for the estimate of the effect of the interval, from 0 to 10 years in 3-month intervals, between screening examinations on the incidence of distant metastatic disease. For details about the simulation, see the text.

In the simulations that follow, we have adopted this as the most likely and accurate estimate of $1/P$ that we can achieve at this time.

We might wonder what the limits are to such variation in the value of $1/P$. That is, might there be subpopulations of tumors with very high or very low values of $1/P$? For example, by performing a simulation of the type shown in Figures 2 and 3, we found that tumors for which $1/P$ is 10^{-16} or less would essentially never metastasize, even if the primary tumor were to grow to a kilogram in mass (approximately 125 mm in diameter). However, the data from Tubiana et al (6–8) show that 92% of patients with tumors 86–95 mm in diameter develop distant metastases, so we can expect that there are very few tumors with such favorable $1/P$ values.

At the other extreme, we might wonder whether there are certain tumors that have such a high $1/P$ value that they would already have metastasized at the time of detection. No degree of surveillance can help identify such tumors before metastasis has occurred, and such tumors would thus be immune to the beneficial effects of screening. Simulation also revealed that tumors with a $1/P$ value of approximately 10^{-9} would have a 3% chance of metastasizing before they had reached a minimally detectable size of about 3 mm (approximately 10^7 cells), whereas tumors with larger $1/P$ values would have greater chances of metastasizing before detection. Fortunately, the data from Tabar et al (9–11) suggest that such tumors must be relatively rare. For example, in patients with tumors that are 1–9 mm in diameter, Tabar et al (9–11) found the frequency of distant metastatic disease to be about 7%. By using $\ln(fr) = -C/P$ and our simulation to calculate the number of cell days that are accumulated by a 9-mm tumor, it follows that the remaining 93% of these patients must have had tumors with $1/P$ values that were larger than 10^{-10} metastases per cell day. The screening simulations described earlier demonstrated that frequent screening can substantially reduce the incidence of distant metastatic disease even in patients with tumors with this value of $1/P$. This does not mean that no tumors will have such low $1/P$ values that there is no benefit to screening, but it does suggest that such tumors are likely to represent a small fraction of all breast cancers, which should not dampen the encouraging results that the simulations provide of the power of screening to reduce the death rate due to distant metastases.

Thus, these considerations suggest that for the majority of breast cancers, indeed for more than 93% of these tumors, $1/P$—the probability that each cancer cell will leave the primary tumor and form a distant metastasis—must have a value greater than 10^{-10} metastasis per cell day. As we shall show subsequently, this means that the overwhelming majority of patients with breast cancer will benefit from mammographic screening.

Estimates of Time Course of Cancer Growth

With the estimate of the probability of metastasis formation ($1/P \approx 10^{-12}$ metastases per cell day), it is possible to determine an initial rough estimate of the occurrence of metastases over time (Fig 2), because the average number of metastases formed each day is simply the probability that a single cell will form a metastasis (ie, $1/P$) times the number of cells in the tumor. By using such an approach, it is fairly straightforward to estimate the probability of distant metastatic disease from the time of occurrence of the first breast cancer cell (Fig 2b), as well as from the time when the tumor can first be detected (Fig 3).

The remarkable result of these simulations and the likely explanation as to why screening can reduce the death rate is that metastasis occurs late in the time course of breast cancer growth, generally after the minimal sizes usually detectable on mammograms (approximately 1–10 mm) have been reached (12). This suggests that breast cancer screening has the potential to help identify a large fraction of breast cancers before they metastasize, an impression that is borne out in the more detailed simulation described subsequently.

Practical Estimates of Relationship between Screening Interval and Incidence of Metastases

It is necessary to add several additional features to the simulation illustrated in Figures 2 and 3 before we can determine practical estimates of the influence of breast cancer screening on the reduction in distant metastatic disease.

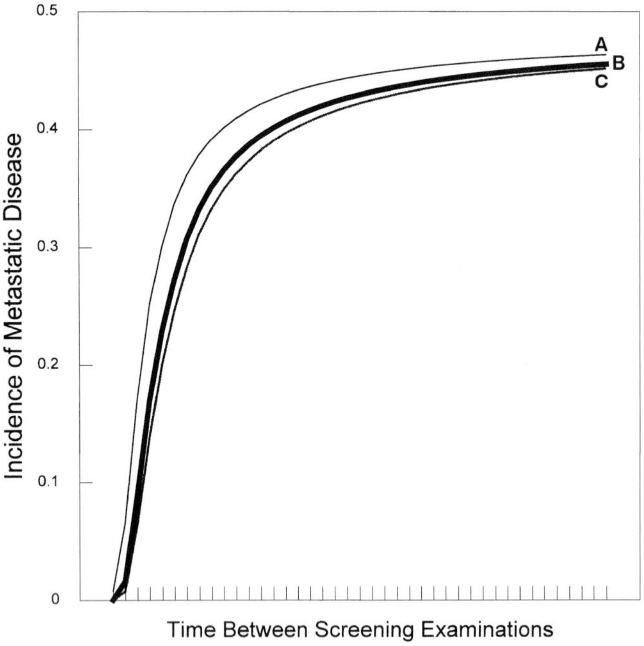

Figure 5. Graph shows the effect of physical sensitivity of the screening method on the incidence of distant metastatic disease. Details of this simulation were the same as those in Figure 4, except the three curves shown were calculated for detection sizes of 10^8 (*A*), 10^7 (*B*), and 10^6 (*C*) cells. The graph covers 0–10 years, and each hash mark represents 3 months.

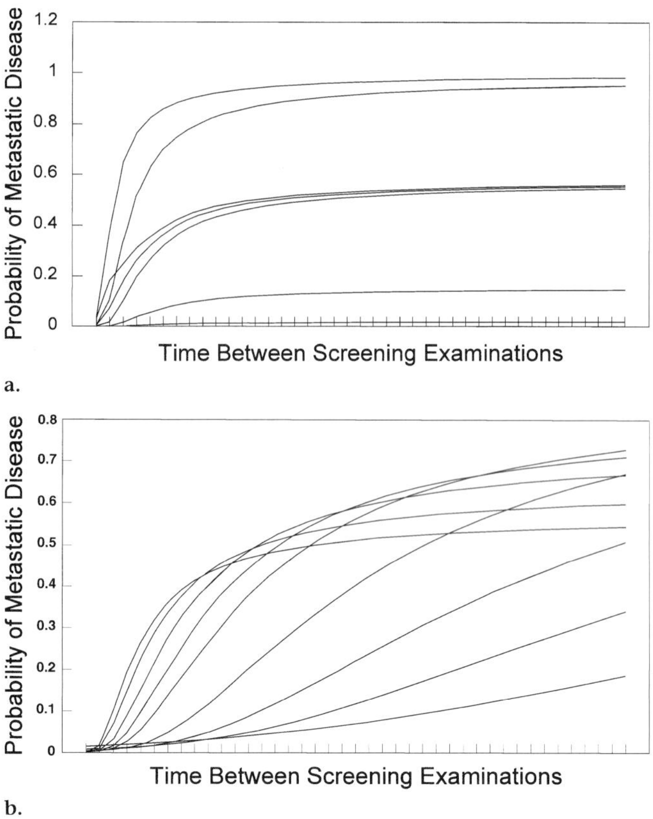

Figure 6. **(a)** Graph shows the effect of the value of the probability of metastasis formation ($1/P$) on the effectiveness of screening. Details of these simulations were the same as those in Figure 4, except mean values of $1/P$ were calculated for means of (from top to bottom) 10^{-9}, 10^{-10}, 10^{-11}, 10^{-12}, 10^{-13}, 10^{-14}, and 10^{-15}. The graph covers 0–10 years in 3-month intervals. **(b)** Graph shows the effect of tumor growth rate on the effectiveness of screening. Details of these simulations were the same as those in Figure 4, except that mean tumor doubling times were calculated for values (from steepest to shallowest curve) of 20, 30, 40, 60, 80, 200, 400, 800, and 2,000 days. The graph covers 0–10 years in 3-month intervals.

First, breast cancers that appear between screenings will be detected if they become palpable. This is the minimal size detectable with palpation, *Sp*. Bear in mind that *Sp* will likely represent a mean size and a distribution of sizes around that mean. Because the median size of breast cancers reported in studies by Tubiana and colleagues (9–11), which were conducted in the era before mammography, was approximately 10^{10} cells, the simulation assumes that tumors that had escaped detection at screening would be identified and removed when they reached this size ($Sp \approx 10^{10}$ cells).

Second, the simulation must take into account that breast cancers will eventually become detectable at mammography. The minimal size detectable at mammography, *Sd,* will also likely represent a mean size with a distribution of sizes around that mean, because not all tumors of the same size will be detectable.

Third, because, as already noted, tumors arise with a variety of growth rates and a variety of probabilities of metastasis, the simulation must incorporate a consideration of this feature of breast cancer biology.

Fourth, in a screening program, tumors detected with the aid of screening come to the attention of the physician at the time of the examination and not at the time when they reach minimum detectable size. Thus, the simulation was adapted to examine the case where a breast cancer might reach minimum detectable size on any day between mammographic examinations.

Figure 4 shows the results of our simulation for what we believe are the most likely features of breast cancer biology. Peer et al (23) selected 3 mm (approximately 10^7 cells) as a reasonable estimate of *Sd,* and the results of our simulation with this value of *Sd* are shown in Figure 4. Figure 5 displays the results of simulations in which *Sd* is 10^6 cells (approximately 1 mm) and 10^8 cells (approximately 12 mm). The simulation shown in Figure 4 illustrates the case where 25% of new breast cancers have a $1/P$ value of approximately 10^{-11}, 50% of tumors have a $1/P$ value of approximately 10^{-12}, and the remaining 25% of tumors have a $1/P$ value of approximately 10^{13}. The justification for the distribution of $1/P$ values was discussed earlier. Figure 6 shows the results of simulations with other mean values of $1/P$. The simulation in Figure 4 shows the case in which the mean tumor doubling time at the time of clinical detectability was 40 days, where 50% of tumors have a doubling time of this mean, 25% have a doubling time of twice the mean, and 25% have a doubling time of half the mean. These tumor doubling times and distributions were derived from the data of Peer et al (23) and Spratt et al (24), as already discussed. Figure 6 shows the results of simulations for other growth rates. The combination of these three metastasis probability groups and three tumor growth groups yields a total of nine groups, and the weighted contributions of each of these nine groups were summed.

Finally, a large number of observations (29–38) suggest that when breast cancers are small, they are likely to grow more rapidly than when they first become detectable at mammography. In the simulation shown in Figure 4, we incorporated such "density-dependent" growth, although equivalent simulations in which constant exponential growth was examined yielded essentially identical results (data not shown). (The precise schedule of such a density-dependent feature of breast cancer growth and the source code for these and other simulations described in this article are available at *http://webm9120.ntx.net/BreastCancerMath.html.* Accessed June 10, 1999.)

RESULTS

The results of the simulation designed to estimate the relationship between the screening interval and the incidence of distant metastases from breast cancer are shown in Figure 4 and Table 2. Results of this simulation suggest that in the absence of screening, the incidence of distant metastatic disease would be approximately 45%, which is in good agreement with the incidence actually seen in women with a diagnosis of breast cancer (1–8). Furthermore, the results of this simulation also predicted that for a screening method that can help detect tumors larger than 3 mm in diameter (approximately 10^7 cells), screening performed every 3 years would result in a 14% reduction in the incidence of distant metastatic disease (in comparison with that in women who do not undergo screening), screening performed every 2 years would be expected to result in a 22% reduction, and screening performed every year would be expected to result in a 51% reduction. This is also in general agreement with actual experience: In randomized mammographic screening trials (9–14), a reduction of approximately 30% in the breast cancer death rate has been achieved with screening intervals of 1–3 years.

Frequency of Screening

The results of the simulation shown in Figure 4 and Table 2 are of most interest where they show the consequences of screening at intervals not presently employed. Indeed, the simulation shown in Figure 4 suggests that more frequent screening could result in the identification of a much larger number of breast cancers before the onset of distant metastatic disease and thus a great reduction in the breast cancer death rate. Thus, the curve shown in Figure 4 and the summary in Table 2 suggest that, for a screening method that could help detect tumors larger than 3 mm in diameter (approximately 10^7 cells), there would be a 66% reduction in the frequency of distant metastatic disease in women who undergo screening every 9 months, as compared with that in women who do not undergo screening. Moreover, there would be a 78% reduction in the frequency of metastases in women who undergo screening every 6 months and a 96% reduction in frequency in women who undergo screening every 3 months. These are potentially enormous improvements in the effectiveness of screening, which thus deserve careful consideration.

Large Range of Values for Tumor Growth and Metastasis

One concern of any computer simulation study is that the results may not reflect the general features of the system but rather the specific values employed in the simulation. We could rule out this possibility by using a large range of values in the simulation shown in Figure 4. Thus, we found that the benefit of more frequent screening seen in Figure 4 was almost independent of the value of the probability of metastasis formation, with reductions in the incidence of distant metastatic disease to about 5% in simulations that incorporated $1/P$ values that ranged from 10^{-9} to 10^{-16} (Fig 6). As outlined earlier, the actual values of $1/P$ from most tumors probably range from 10^{-11} to 10^{-13}, so it appears likely that the general results of the simulations are relevant for the majority of breast cancers. Likewise, the ability to reduce the breast cancer mortality rate to less than 5% with more frequent screening was found for simulations in which tumor doubling times of 20–2,000 days were examined (Fig 6). We also did not find a substantial difference in the general results of the simulations, whether they were formulated to estimate a constant tumor growth rate (Fig 2) or a growth rate that declines with increasing tumor size (Fig 4) (24, 25,29–37).

Another detail of the model concerns the definition of $1/P$ in terms of $cell^{-1} \cdot days^{-1}$. One might wonder whether $1/P$ should be calculated in terms of mitotic cycles rather than cell days, because mutation is more likely to occur when cells divide. However, an estimate of the value of $1/P$ in terms of mitotic cycles revealed $1/P$ to be just as constant when calculated in terms of mitotic cycles as in terms of cell days (Table 1). Furthermore, a reformulation of the simulations in terms of mitotic cycles did not materially change the general results.

Finally, the outcome of the simulations also was found to be independent of the value of the density of cells per cubic centimeter (B). Identical curves resulted whether B was equal to 10^7, 10^8, or 10^9 cells per cubic centimeter.

Estimates of Physical Sensitivity of Screening

Both the detection method and the nature of the patient are likely to affect the minimal tumor size detectable at mammography. Some tumors may be detectable when very small, whereas others may not be detectable until they are much larger (12). The radiographic density of noncancerous breast tissues and possibly of the tumors themselves are likely to differ from woman to woman and to change with age (12). Presumably, *Sd,* the mean minimally detectable size, and the actual distribution of sizes around this mean must be reflections of the physics of depiction, the location and character of the tumor, and the nature of the surrounding tissue.

Our simulation allowed us to examine the effect of these limits of physical detectability on the capacity of mammography to help identify breast cancers before they spread distally. Figure 5 shows the results of simulations with cases where detection would occur for tumors larger than 10^6 cells (approximately 1.2 mm), 10^7 cells (approximately 3 mm), or 10^8 cells (approximately 12 mm); that is, *Sd* values of 10^6, 10^7, or 10^8 cells, respectively. Surprisingly, these three curves proved to be similar. This has two practical implications. First, the simulation results shown in Figure 5 revealed that although the capacity to identify smaller tumors results in greater ability to reduce the breast cancer death rate, such a reduction is more easily achieved by increasing the frequency of screening than by increasing the physical sensitivity of the screening method. Thus, the simple expedient of carrying out screening at more frequent intervals may be a more effective way to improve the outcome of screening than would be the development of improved screening technology. Consider the case where screening is performed every 2 years with a technology that can be used to detect tumors no smaller than 10^8 cells ($Sd = 10^8$ cells, or approximately 12 mm). Figure 5 shows that a screening program that used this method but with which examinations were performed every 3 months would achieve a reduction of approximately 80% in the breast cancer death rate in comparison with that in which examinations were performed every 2 years. On the other hand, even a hundredfold increase in detection sensitivity ($Sd = 10^6$ cells, or approximately 1 mm) would yield only a 20% reduction in mortality rate if the program maintained the 2-year screening interval. Second, not all breast cancer tumors of the same size will be detectable. Figure 5 reveals that a more realistic assessment of screening, in which the detection limit represents a distribution of values centered around a mean of about 10^7 cells, would yield roughly the same outcome as that shown in Figure 4 for the simple case of a single discrete detection limit of 10^7 cells.

Cost-Benefit Consequences of Different Screening Intervals

Because our simulations yielded data on the relationship between the frequency of mammographic screening and the reduction in the rate of distant metastatic disease and thus in the breast cancer death rate, it is fairly straightforward to use this information to calculate the cost per year of life saved for the various screening intervals. The results of these simulations, determined on the basis of an estimated cost per examination of $100 and the expected incidence of breast cancer in a 50-year-old woman, are shown in Table 3. These initial estimates indicate that, within limits, more frequent screening would appear to yield considerable reductions in the breast cancer death rate with only modest increases in cost per year of life saved. Thus, for example, a program in which 50-year-old women underwent screening every 3 years would reduce the incidence of distant metastatic disease by a modest 19% and would cost approximately $10,661 for every year of life saved, whereas screening twice a year would reduce the incidence of breast cancer by 81% and lead to only a small increase ($14,172) in cost per year of life saved. On the other hand, these estimates allow us to define screening intervals that are clearly too frequent for the marginal benefit derived. Indeed, the results shown in Table 3 indicate that screening more frequently than every 3 months is likely to be a waste of time and money.

TABLE 3
Cost-Benefit Estimates as a Function of Screening Frequency

Screening Frequency	Reduction in Incidence of Metastases*	Cost per Patient per Year ($)	Mean Cost per Year of Life Saved ($)	Marginal Cost per Year of Life Saved ($)
Every 3rd year	19.0	33	10,661	5,029
Every 2nd year	27.0	50	10,601	5,030
Every year	52.0	100	10,986	6,756
Every 6 months	81.0	200	14,172	16,973
Every 4 months	92.4	300	18,740	40,242
Every 3 months	97.0	400	23,927	118,312
Every 2 months	98.9	600	35,074	634,802
Every month	99.7	1,200	96,291	1,019,037

Note.—Estimates are based on data in Table 2. The estimated cost per mammogram is $100. The estimates are for the incidence of breast cancer and expected years of life in a 50-year-old woman. (Source code for these estimations is available at *http://webm9120.ntx.net/BreastCancerMath.html.* Accessed June 10, 1999.)

* Estimated reduction is for screening that can help detect a tumor larger than 10^7 cells (approximately 3 mm).

DISCUSSION

We developed a computer simulation model of breast cancer growth and spread, and the results of our model suggest that an increase in the frequency of breast cancer screening could lead to substantial reductions in the incidence of metastatic disease and, thus, in the breast cancer death rate. Of course, estimates for the optimal screening intervals that are shown in Figure 4 and Table 2 must be considered only as first approximations. Further work will be needed to improve the precision of the underlying data used in construction of these simulations and to test the results of these simulations against available clinical data. At a minimum, however, these results are in general agreement with the suggestions by many groups about the value of annual screening (12); the results also raise the question about whether more frequent screening might be of value.

The computer simulation approach described here can provide a method for quantitative evaluation of a number of aspects of screening both for breast cancer and for other tumors. One of the major areas of controversy and ambiguity in breast cancer screening concerns the question of when women should begin screening (9–14). Whereas some have argued that screening should begin at the age of 40 years, others have suggested that the age of 50 years is more appropriate (9–14,46). The simulation method we have outlined here should be helpful in assessing the effectiveness of screening in women with different genotypes and ages. For example, breast cancers in young women have been found to have faster growth rates than breast cancers in older women (23). Our simulations have revealed that this variation should not have an important influence on the effectiveness of screening (Fig 6), and this will certainly be an area for further analysis.

Although our simulations were developed with mammographic screening in mind, the general lessons should be applicable to other screening tests that can be used to identify breast cancers before they become clinically apparent (47). Of course, the potential beneficial effects of mammography must be considered together with the radiation required by this test, which is potentially carcinogenic (48,49). There are several ways to estimate this effect, one of the best of which uses epidemiologic data derived from studies with Japanese survivors of atomic bomb blasts (48,49). Although no effect of radiation on breast cancer incidence has been seen in individuals exposed to less than 250 mGy of radiation, survivors exposed to higher levels of radiation displayed a modest increase in breast cancer incidence. The current radiation dose per two-view mammogram is approximately 2.8 mGy (48,49). From these data, Mettler et al (48) estimated that yearly mammographic examinations in women from the age of 35 years to the age of 75 years would result in an increased incidence of breast cancer at the age of 75 years of 0.62%. By extrapolating from these data, we estimate that if these women underwent mammography four times a year, there would be a 2.5% increase in the incidence of cancer. By using this value and the data in Figure 4 and Table 2, it may be estimated that for every additional lethal breast cancer induced by the radiation associated with mammography four times a year, 32,333 lives would be saved because of screening.

Our initial cost-benefit estimates (Table 3), calculated for 50-year-old women, suggest that cost may not be a barrier to the possible benefit of more frequent screening (50). Of course, it remains to be seen what the cost-benefit estimates will be for women of other ages after taking into account other additional costs—both in terms of savings achieved from the prevention of distant metastatic disease and the additional costs raised by the discovery of these tumors (50).

More accurate assessments will also require us to take into account age-associated changes in breast cancer incidence, lead-time bias, age-associated change in life expectancy, and age-associated changes in the biologic properties of breast cancer, particularly changes in tumor growth rate. It also will be necessary to take into account the effect on the system as a whole, such as increases in the number of facilities, mammographic equipment, and radiology specialists, to determine whether the implications of our model can be accommodated in practice. This clearly will be a major task for investigators of the simulation approach in future studies.

In conclusion, we developed a computer simulation that calculated the time course of breast cancer growth and metastasis. These simulations were possible because the data from Tabar et al (9–11) and Tubiana et al (6–8) show that the probability of each cell in a breast cancer tumor leaving the primary tumor and forming a distant metastasis is relatively constant and measurable. With this information, as well as information on tumor growth rate (20–38), it was possible to estimate the effect screening can have on the incidence of distant metastatic disease and concomitantly on the breast cancer death rate. The results of these simulations suggest that screening may have a much greater potential for reduction in the breast cancer death rate than is presently achieved. Indeed, the findings described in this article suggest that screening, if used frequently enough, has the potential to convert breast cancer from a disease that is frequently fatal to a disease that can usually be cured.

Acknowledgment: Our appreciation is extended to the Marine Biological Laboratory, Woods Hole, Mass.

References

1. Hellman S. Natural history of small breast cancers. J Clin Oncol 1994; 12:2229–2234.
2. Russo J, Frederick J, Ownby HE, et al. Predictors of recurrence and survival of patients with breast cancer. Am J Clin Pathol 1987; 88:123–131.
3. Quiet CA, Ferguson DJ, Weichselbaum RR, Hellman S. Natural history of node-positive breast cancer: the curability of small cancers with a limited number of positive nodes. J Clin Oncol 1996; 14:3105–3111.
4. Quiet CA, Ferguson DJ, Weichselbaum RR, Hellmam S. Natural history of node-negative breast cancer: a study of 826 patients with long-term follow-up. J Clin Oncol 1995; 13:1144–1151.
5. Rosen PP, Groshen S, Saigo PE, Kine DW, Hellman S. A long-term follow-up study in stage I and stage II breast carcinoma. J Clin Oncol 1989; 7:355–366.
6. Koscielny S, Tubiana M, Le MG, et al. Breast cancer: relationship between the size of the primary tumor and the probability of metastatic dissemination. Br J Cancer 1984; 49:709–715.
7. Tubiana M, Koscielny S. Natural history of human breast cancer: recent data and clinical implications. Breast Cancer Res Treat 1991; 18:125–140.
8. Tubiana M, Koscielny S. The natural history of human breast cancer: implications for a screening strategy. Int J Radiat Oncol Biol Phys 1990; 19:1117–1120.
9. Tabar L, Fagerberg G, Duffy SW, Day NE, Gad A, Grontoft O. Update in the Swedish two-county program of mammographic screening for breast cancer. Radiol Clin North Am 1992; 30:187–210.
10. Tabar L, Fagerberg G, Chen HS, et al. Efficacy of breast cancer screening by age: new results from the Swedish two-county trial. Cancer 1995; 75:2507–2517.
11. Tabar L. Breast cancer screening with mammography in women aged 40–49 years. Int J Cancer 1996; 68:693–699.
12. Kopans DB. Breast imaging. 2nd ed. Philadelphia, Pa: Lippincott, 1997.
13. Smart CR, Byrnes C, Smith RA, et al. Twenty-year follow-up of the breast cancers diagnosed during the breast cancer detection demonstration project. CA Cancer J Clin 1997; 47:135–149.
14. Kopans DB. Updated results of the trials of screening mammography. Surg Oncol Clin North Am 1997; 6:233–263.
15. Milbrath JR, Moskowitz M, Bauermeister D. Breast cancer screening. Crit Rev Diagn Imaging 1981; 16:181–218.
16. Moskowitz M. Guidelines for screening for breast cancer: is a revision in order? Radiol Clin North Am 1992; 30:221–233.
17. Moskowitz M. Breast cancer: age-specific growth rates and screening strategies. Radiology 1986; 161:37–41.
18. Tabar L, Faberberg G, Day NE, Holmberg L. What is the optimum interval between screening examinations? an analysis based on the latest results of the Swedish two-county breast cancer screening trial. Br J Cancer 1987; 55:547–551.
19. Sickles EA. Breast cancer screening outcomes in women ages 40–49: clinical experience with service screening using modern mammography. Monogr Natl Cancer Inst 1997; 22:99–104.
20. von Fournier D, Weber E, Hoeffken W, Bauer M, Kubli F, Barth V. Growth rate of 147 mammary carcinomas. Cancer 1980; 45:2198–2207.
21. Gershoh-Cohen J, Berger SM, Klicksten HS. Roentgenography of breast cancer moderating the concept of "biologic determinism." Cancer 1963; 16:962–964.
22. Kuroishi T, Tominaga S, Morimoto T, et al. Tumor growth rate and prognosis of breast cancer mainly detected by mass screening. Jpn J Cancer Res 1990; 81:454–462.
23. Peer PG, van Dijck JA, Hendricks JH, Holland R, Verbeek AL. Age-dependent growth of primary breast cancer. Cancer 1993; 71:3547–3551.
24. Spratt JA, von Fournier D, Spratt JS, Weber EE. Mammographic assessment of human breast cancer growth and duration. Cancer 1993; 71:2020–2026.
25. Spratt JS, Spratt T. Rates of growth of pulmonary metastases and survival. Ann Surg 1964; 159:161–171.
26. Heuser L, Spratt JS, Polk HC. Growth rate of primary breast cancer. Cancer 1979; 43:1888–1894.
27. Lundgren B. Observations on the growth rate of breast carcinomas and its possible implications for lead time. Cancer 1977; 40:1722–1725.
28. Spang-Thomsen M, Nielsen A, Visfeldt J. Growth curves of three human malignant tumors transplanted to nude mice. Exp Cell Res 1980; 48:138–154.
29. Norton L. A gompertzian model of human breast cancer growth. Cancer Res 1988; 48:7067–7071.
30. Surbone A, Norton L. Kinetic concepts in the treatment of breast cancer. Ann NY Acad Sci 1993; 698:48–62.
31. Rae-Venter B, Reid LM. Growth of human breast carcinomas in nude mice and subsequent establishment in tissue culture. Cancer Res 1980; 40:95–100.
32. Kyriazias PA, Kyriazias AP. Preferential sites of growth of human tumors in nude mice following subcutaneous transplantation. Cancer Res 1980; 40:4509–4511.
33. Kristensen CA, Kristjansen PE, Brunner N, Clarke R, Spang-Thomsen M, Quistorff B. Effects of estrogen withdrawal on energy-rich phosphates and prediction of estrogen dependence monitored by in vivo 31P magnetic resonance spectroscopy of four human breast cancer xenografts. Cancer Res 1995; 55:1664–1669.
34. McManus MJ, Waelsch C. DNA synthesis of benign human breast tumors in untreated "nude" mouse: an in vivo model to study hormonal influences on growth of human breast tissues. Cancer 1980; 25:2160–2165.
35. Durbin PW, Jeung N, Williams MH, Arnold JS. Construction of the growth curves for mammary tumors of the rat. Cancer Res 1967; 27:1341–1347.
36. Huggins C, Yang NC. Induction and extinction of mammary cancer. Science 1962; 137:257–261.
37. Rockwell S. Effect of host age on the transplantation, growth, and radiation response of EMT6 tumors. Cancer Res 1981; 41:527–531.
38. Pearlman AW. Breast cancer: influence of growth rate on prognosis and treatment evaluation. Cancer 1976; 38:1826–1833.
39. Van der Linden HC, Baak JP, Smeulders AW, Lindeman J, Meyer CJ. Morphometry of breast cancer. I. Comparison of the primary tumours and the axillary lymph node metastases. Pathol Res Pract 1986; 181:236–242.
40. Boon ME, Trott PA, van Kaam H, Kurver PJ, Leach A, Baak JP. Morphometry and

cytodiagnosis of breast lesions. Virchows Arch [Pathol Anat] 1982; 396:9–18.
41. Pesce C, Colacino R. Morphometry of the breast fibroadenoma. Pathol Res Pract 1986; 181:718–720.
42. Folkman J. Angiogenesis in cancer, vascular, rheumatoid and other disease. Nat Med 1995; 1:27–31.
43. Folkman J, D'Amore PA. Blood vessel formation: what is its molecular basis? Cell 1996; 87:1153–1155.
44. Pluda JM. Tumor-associated angiogenesis: mechanisms, clinical implications, and therapeutic strategies. Semin Oncol 1997; 24:203–218.
45. Hanahan D, Folkman J. Patterns and emerging mechanisms of the angiogenic switch during tumorigenesis. Cell 1996; 86:353–364.
45. Hendrick RE, Smith RA, Rutledge JH III, Smart CR. Benefit of screening mammography in women aged 40–49: a new meta-analysis of randomized controlled trials. J Natl Cancer Inst Monogr 1997; 22:87–92.
47. D'Orsi CJ, Bartrum RJ, Moskowitz MM. Light-scanning of the breast. In: Bassett LW, Gold RH, eds. Breast cancer detection: mammography and other methods in breast imaging. 2nd ed. Orlando, Fla: Grune-Stratton, 1987; 169–177.
48. Mettler FA, Upton AC, Kelsey CA, Ashby RN, Rosenberg RD, Linver MN. Benefits versus risks from mammography: a critical reassessment. Cancer 1996; 77:903–909.
49. Feig SA, Ehrlich SM. Estimation of radiation risk from screening mammography: recent trends and comparison with expected benefits. Radiology 1990; 174:638–647.
50. Rosenquist CJ, Lindfors KK. Screening mammography beginning at age 40 years: a reappraisal of cost-effectiveness. Cancer 1998; 82:2235–2240.

David F. Yankelevitz, MD
Rajiv Gupta, PhD
Binsheng Zhao, DSc
Claudia I. Henschke, PhD, MD

Index terms:
Lung neoplasms, CT, 60.12118
Lung neoplasms, diagnosis, 60.31, 60.32

Radiology 1999; 212:561–566

[1] From the Department of Radiology, the New York Hospital–Cornell University Medical Center, 525 E 68th St, New York, NY 10021. Received March 19, 1998; revision requested May 19; final revision received October 25; accepted March 16, 1999. Supported in part by National Institutes of Health grant R01-CA-63393 and General Electric Corporate Research and Development. **Address reprint requests to** D.F.Y. (e-mail: *dyankele@mail.med.cornell.edu*).

Author contributions:
Guarantors of integrity of entire study, all authors; study concepts and design, all authors; definition of intellectual content, all authors; literature research, all authors; clinical studies, D.F.Y., C.I.H.; data acquisition and analysis, all authors; statistical analysis, C.I.H.; manuscript preparation, editing, and review, all authors.

Small Pulmonary Nodules: Evaluation with Repeat CT—Preliminary Experience[1]

PURPOSE: To assess the use of early repeat computed tomography (CT) of solitary pulmonary nodules to determine nodule growth.

MATERIALS AND METHODS: The authors performed repeat CT of nodule phantoms to assess the accuracy of their measurement technique. They then used this technique to assess nodule growth (nine malignant, six benign) in 15 patients (nine men, six women; age range, 60–79 years; average age, 66 years) who underwent repeat CT as part of their routine clinical protocol. The final diagnosis was established with surgical resection or follow-up for more than 2 years after an indeterminate biopsy.

RESULTS: Results of phantom experiments revealed that the method used to determine area change is sensitive enough to help detect nodule growth if one pixel is added around the entire circumference of a nodule. With use of standard exponential growth curves and known tumor growth rates, malignant growth could be detected in vivo within 30 days. All 15 in vivo nodules were correctly classified with early repeat CT.

CONCLUSION: Preliminary experience with early repeat CT suggests that a single repeat CT scan obtained 30 days after the first scan can depict growth in most malignant tumors as small as 5 mm.

The solitary pulmonary nodule is a common and challenging problem. In the United States, more than 150,000 new solitary pulmonary nodules are detected each year; one to two nodules are found on every 1,000 chest radiographs (1–3). With the introduction and continual improvement of computed tomography (CT) since the 1970s, the rate of detection of these nodules has increased. Once discovered, such nodules almost always lead to further diagnostic studies because a high percentage are malignant (2,3). Although the rate of benignity among resected nodules has decreased, it remains high—between 20% and 40% (4).

Small pulmonary nodules (those less than 1 cm in diameter) present an even greater diagnostic challenge because the accuracy of available diagnostic procedures is considerably decreased owing to their size. Given the virulence of lung cancer, the natural tendency is to err on the side of overdiagnosis, even for these small nodules. This explains, in part, the continued high rate of resection of benign nodules.

A key issue in patient treatment is balancing the trade-off between early versus unnecessary resection. Currently, only two radiologic criteria are widely accepted as proof of benignity: (*a*) nodule calcification in a benign pattern and (*b*) lack of growth (2). Curiously, although these two criteria were initially described at approximately the same time in the 1950s (5–8), most research to date, including a multicenter study involving CT densitometry and anthropomorphic phantoms (9), has dealt almost exclusively with obtaining additional information regarding calcification. To our knowledge, virtually no work has been done on refining measurement of growth. This is particularly puzzling because growth is a salient feature of malignancy.

In this study, we focused on rapid assessment of nodule growth, particularly of small pulmonary nodules, with repeat CT. We call this method early repeat CT. The feasibility of early repeat CT depends on (*a*) the expected nodule growth within a clinically acceptable delay between the initial and repeat scans and (*b*) the accuracy of the measurement technique. The growth observed with early repeat CT, or the lack of it, can be correlated with malignancy status.

The present study was conducted to assess the use of early repeat CT in determining pulmonary nodule growth. This study consisted of two parts. In the first part, we sought to demonstrate that there is a reliable way of measuring changes in small pulmonary nodules during a short follow-up period. This was achieved by using both theoretical considerations and in vitro experiments on nodule phantoms of known sizes. The second part consisted of actual clinical cases in which repeat CT data were available.

TABLE 1
Expected Nodule Diameter at Early Repeat CT based on Interval between Initial and Repeat CT, Initial Nodule Diameter, and Tumor Doubling Time

Interval between Initial and Early Repeat CT (d)	Initial Nodule Diameter (mm)	Expected Final Nodule Diameter (mm) according to Doubling Time				
		30 d	90 d	120 d	150 d	180 d
7	5	5.28	5.09	5.07	5.05	5.05
14	5	5.57	5.18	5.14	5.11	5.09
21	5	5.88	5.28	5.21	5.16	5.14
28	5	6.20	5.37	5.28	5.22	5.18
7	10	10.55	10.18	10.14	10.11	10.09
14	10	11.14	10.37	10.27	10.22	10.18
21	10	11.76	10.55	10.41	10.33	10.27
28	10	12.41	10.75	10.55	10.44	10.37
7	15	15.83	15.27	15.20	15.16	15.14
14	15	16.71	15.55	15.41	15.33	15.27
21	15	17.63	15.83	15.62	15.49	15.41
28	15	18.61	16.12	15.83	15.66	15.55
7	20	21.11	20.36	20.27	20.22	20.18
14	20	22.28	20.37	20.55	20.44	20.36
21	20	23.51	21.11	20.83	20.66	20.55
28	20	24.81	21.49	21.11	20.88	20.73

MATERIALS AND METHODS

Theoretical Growth Projections

To estimate tumor growth, we calculated the expected growth of nodules with different diameters by using an exponential growth model. Assuming the nodules were spherical and initially of diameters of 5, 10, 15, and 20 mm, we calculated the new diameters within 1–4 weeks by using doubling times of 30, 90, 120, 150, and 180 days (Table 1). These doubling times roughly correspond to those of a very aggressive small cell carcinoma (30-day doubling time), a squamous cell carcinoma (90-day doubling time), a large cell carcinoma (120-day doubling time), and an aggressive and average adenocarcinoma (150- and 180-day doubling time, respectively) (10).

As shown in Table 1, a nodule with a diameter of 5 mm and a doubling time of 30 days would reach a diameter of 5.57 mm after 14 days, 5.88 mm after 21 days, and 6.20 mm after 28 days. All of these diameter changes are greater than the CT resolution of 0.3 mm in the x and y planes. A larger nodule with a diameter of 10 mm and the same doubling time would reach a diameter of 10.55 mm after 7 days so that early repeat CT performed after 7 days could depict this change. Conversely, the same 10-mm-diameter nodule would have a barely discernible diameter change after 28 days if it had a doubling time of 180 days.

The data in Table 1 demonstrate that even the slowest growing 10-, 15-, and 20-mm-diameter nodules would register a measurable increase within 28 days for all listed growth rates. Thus, theoretically, repeat CT performed after 28 days would depict growth in these nodules. Nodules with a diameter of 5 mm would also demonstrate measurable growth within 28 days, except at the slowest growth rates of 150 and 180 days, at which the growth would be below the detection threshold. If a repeat scan were obtained after another 28 days, however, even such slowly growing nodules could be recognized.

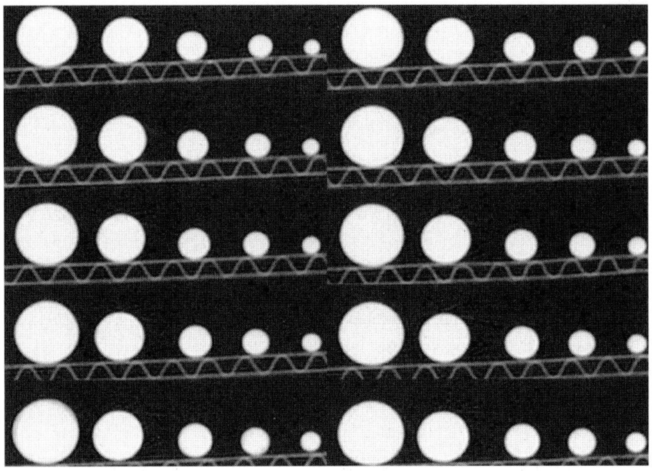

Figure 1. Ten cross-sectional CT scans of five polycarbonate rods with diameters of 3.17, 4.78, 6.24, 9.79, and 12.80 mm. The diameter of each group of rods increases from left to right and top to bottom in increments of 0.1 mm. The overall diameter change is about 1 mm between the smallest set of rods (top left) and the largest set of rods (bottom right).

Minimum Detectable Change

Nodule growth can be assessed on individual CT sections or on the whole volumetric stack. Our primary concern in this study was to determine the minimum detectable area change on individual CT sections because these are readily available for in vivo nodules and clinicians are used to analyzing nodules on a section-by-section basis.

To assess the area growth metric, we constructed CT phantoms by using polycarbonate rods with base diameters of 3.17, 4.78, 6.24, 9.79, and 12.80 mm. The rod diameters were incrementally increased by winding different numbers of turns of transparent adhesive tape around them, with each turn increasing the diameter by 0.1 mm. A total of 10 turns were applied to each rod. The rods were scanned with a CT HiSpeed Advantage (GE Medical Systems, Milwaukee, Wis) scanner by using a standard imaging protocol (1-mm collimation, spiral mode with a pitch of 1:1, and 9.6-cm field of view) (Fig 1).

TABLE 2
Comparison of Actual and Measured Areas of Rod Phantoms

Diameter (mm)	Actual Area (mm²)	Change in Actual Area (mm²)	Measured Area (no. of pixels)	Change in Measured Area (no. of pixels)
		Base Nodule Size of 3.17 mm		
3.17	7.889	0.000	203	0
3.27	8.394	0.506	213	10
3.36	8.862	0.974	221	18
3.47	9.452	1.564	248	45
3.58	10.061	2.172	255	52
3.68	10.631	2.742	275	72
3.81	11.395	3.507	293	90
3.91	12.001	4.113	305	102
4.07	13.003	5.115	327	124
4.11	13.260	5.372	341	138
		Base Nodule Size of 4.78 mm		
4.78	17.94	0.000	469	0
4.91	18.925	0.989	493	24
5.04	19.940	2.004	519	50
5.11	20.498	2.562	539	70
5.21	21.308	3.372	564	95
5.28	21.885	3.949	584	115
5.38	22.721	4.785	591	122
5.52	23.919	5.983	630	161
5.66	25.148	7.212	669	200
5.75	25.954	8.018	674	205
		Base Nodule Size of 6.24 mm		
6.24	30.566	0.000	806	0
6.37	31.853	1.287	822	16
6.54	33.576	3.010	850	44
6.62	34.402	3.836	877	71
6.60	34.195	3.629	889	83
6.64	34.610	4.044	902	96
6.80	36.298	5.732	947	141
7.01	38.575	8.009	992	186
7.16	40.243	9.677	1,038	232
7.36	45.523	11.957	1,071	265
		Base Nodule Size of 9.79 mm		
9.79	75.238	0.000	1,999	0
9.93	77.405	2.167	2,030	31
10.09	79.919	4.682	2,052	53
10.25	82.474	7.236	2,103	104
10.28	82.958	7.720	2,140	141
10.33	83.766	8.529	2,185	186
10.41	85.069	9.831	2,228	229
10.51	86.711	11.474	2,250	251
10.66	89.204	13.966	2,300	301
10.74	90.548	15.310	2,356	357
		Base Nodule Size of 12.80 mm		
12.80	128.614	0.000	3,372	0
12.90	130.632	2.017	3,416	44
13.00	132.665	4.051	3,464	92
13.13	135.332	6.717	3,534	162
13.20	136.778	8.164	3,603	231
13.32	139.277	10.662	3,658	286
13.51	143.278	14.664	3,775	403
13.66	146.478	17.863	3,840	468
13.71	147.552	18.937	3,942	570
13.76	148.630	20.016	3,903	531

Note.—Measured areas were determined with CT data.

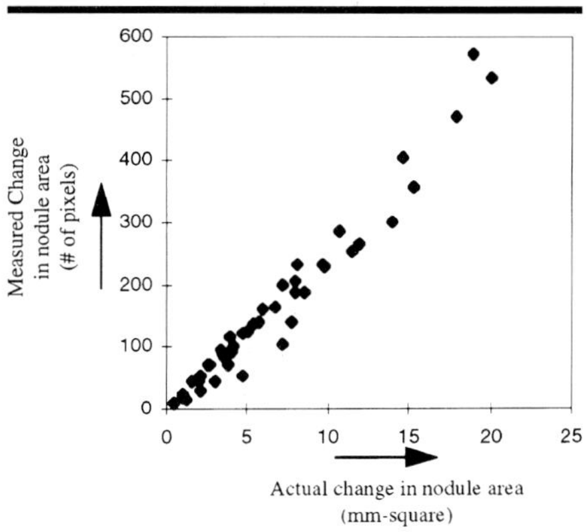

Figure 2. Graph shows actual versus measured change in the cross-sectional area of polycarbonate rod phantoms.

Each rod was then precisely measured with a micrometer (accuracy greater than 10 μm) to determine the actual area considered to have the true measurement. To determine the accuracy of the CT scanner, we measured the area of the rod phantom on the acquired image. The area was determined by segmenting its boundary with the k-means segmentation algorithm (11,12). The area was calculated by multiplying the number of pixels within the nodule boundary by the pixel size. The scans were analyzed with software that we developed on an Indy workstation (Silicon Graphics, Mountain View, Calif).

We used the k-means algorithm, which minimizes the sum of the Euclidean distances from all pixels in a cluster to the cluster center, because it is effective when there are marked differences between the structures being segmented—in this case between the rods and the surrounding air.

In Vivo Experiments

For the in vivo assessment of early repeat CT, we evaluated the nodule growth in 15 patients (nine men, six women; age range, 60–79 years; average age, 66 years) who underwent repeat CT during the course of their routine clinical work-up. According to routine clinical practice at our institution, biopsy was recommended for all nodules that demonstrated growth within the malignant range (Table 1); follow-up was recommended for all other nodules. Thus, except for those cases in which the second scan was obtained at biopsy, our recommendations were made before knowing the true status of the nodule. The actual malignancy status of the nodule was determined with resection or biopsy or after sufficient follow-up (minimum, 2 years) to ensure nodule stability, which is indicative of benignity.

Thin-section CT scans of the nodules were obtained, and the images from repeat CT were reconstructed at 0.5-mm intervals on the z axis to maximize the comparability of

TABLE 3
Results of in Vivo Studies of Malignant Nodules with Early Repeat CT

Case No.	Interval between Initial and Early Repeat CT (d)	Area (mm^2)		Final Diagnosis	Computed Diameter (mm)		Doubling Time (d)	Measurements Projected at 30 d		
		at T_0	at T_1		at T_0	at T_1		Diameter (mm)	Area (mm^2)	Change (%)
1	9	60.7	63.7	Adenocarcinoma	8.8	9.0	86	9.5	71.2	27
2	18	20.9	24.2	Adenocarcinoma	5.1	5.6	53	5.8	26.7	44
3	28	40.1	44.5	Adenocarcinoma	7.1	7.5	124	7.6	44.8	18
4	35	27.1	33.2	Adenocarcinoma	5.9	6.5	80	6.4	32.2	30
5	102	76.3	142.2	Adenocarcinoma	9.8	13.5	75	10.8	91.5	32
6	44	10.3	14.8	Adenocarcinoma	3.6	4.3	56	4.1	13.2	45
7	55	27.4	38.5	Adenocarcinoma	5.9	7.0	75	6.5	33.0	32
8	14	38.5	42.6	Adenocarcinoma	7.0	7.4	64	7.8	47.8	38
9	169	14.0	54.4	Adenocarcinoma	4.2	8.3	58	4.8	17.8	44

Note.—Nodule doubling time is based on the number of days between initial and repeat CT and the area and diameter at each time. The final diagnosis also is given. The projected diameter, area, and percentage of area change also are given, with the assumption that early repeat CT would have been performed 30 days after the initial finding. T_0 = initial CT, T_1 = early repeat CT.

the repeat and initial images. The image from the initial scan with the maximal area was compared with the image from the repeat scan with the maximal area. This comparison was done by displaying the two image sets side by side.

Once the nodule was segmented, the area could be readily calculated. Because there are marked differences between the attenuation (in Hounsfield units) of the nodule and that of the surrounding lung tissue, which is predominantly air, we again used the k-means algorithm for the segmentation of the nodule. Because this segmentation algorithm requires a predefined number of clusters, we compared the results obtained by using different numbers of clusters and found that 18 clusters were optimal for the segmentation of these nodules. Two experienced chest radiologists (D.F.Y., C.I.H.) also carefully compared each segmented nodule with the original CT scans to ensure that the nodule had been correctly and consistently identified with the segmentation procedure.

We used the calculated nodule area to determine nodule diameter. The exponential growth model was used to calculate the doubling time for each nodule and the projected area and corresponding diameter if the repeat scan had been obtained after 30 days. We also compared our calculated diameter with that obtained from the pathologic specimen for all resected nodules.

RESULTS

Minimum Detectable Change

Figure 1 shows that even a change of about 100 μm all around the simulated nodules, although only faintly perceptible to the human eye, can be measured on CT scans. Larger changes, those on the order of one pixel dimension (about 300 μm), are both visually discernible and quantitatively measurable. In addition, a measurement of this amount of change, that is, one pixel dimension all around the nodule, is robust in the sense that it is unlikely to be confused with other effects such as partial volume effects, detector quantum noise, and misregistration.

Table 2 shows the actual and measured areas and the corresponding changes from the base values for the various nodule phantoms shown in Figure 1. As mentioned earlier, the actual area was computed from the diameter of the rod phantom. The change in area (in square millimeters) from the base value is shown in column 3. The nodule area was also estimated from the acquired image. The image was segmented, and the number of pixels within the nodule were counted. The change in measured area (in number of pixels) from the base value also is shown. As can be seen in Table 2, even for the smallest change in area, the corresponding change in the image area is measurable.

Figure 2 shows the plot of the actual area change for the phantoms on the x axis and the corresponding measured change on the y axis. This graph demonstrates the linear relationship between the actual and measured change. In addition, even the smallest increment in the diameter is discernible on the image. Thus, the results shown in Table 2 demonstrate that we are able to discern change as small as a third of a pixel, provided it occurs around the entire circumference of the nodule. In other words, for a nodule with diameter D, a change of πD times the pixel size is detectable. Thus, an area change of 9 mm or 12% (assuming a pixel size of 0.3 mm) can be detected in a nodule with a diameter of 10 mm.

Validation of Early Repeat CT with in Vivo Nodules

Table 3 gives the intervals between acquisitions of the two CT scans, the nodule areas obtained at each time, and the final diagnosis for malignant nodules (nine malignant, six benign). All nine malignant nodules had growth well above the minimal detectable change. In addition, their growth rates correlated with the generally accepted growth rates for this type of malignancy. With use of the projected growth in 30 days, all of these nodules could have been detected with repeat CT after 30 days. Although the repeat CT scan obtained in case 9 does not qualify as "early," it does demonstrate rapid growth and, as can be seen from the projected 30-day growth, the change at that time was well within the limits of growth detection. Because all of these cases were treated according to current clinical practice, we did not control the scheduling of repeat scans.

Table 4 gives the same information for benign nodules. Cases 10–12, 14, and 15 are nodules that have now been followed-up for more than 2 years and have shown no growth. In case 10, biopsy of the nodule was performed; no malignant cells were found. In case 11, biopsy of the nodule was performed twice within a 3-year period, and the lesion did not demonstrate malignant cells. At all of these biopsies, the needle tip was confirmed to be in the lesion. In cases 10 and 11, repeat CT added substantial confi-

TABLE 4
Stability of Early Repeat CT in Benign Nodules

Case No.	Interval between Initial and Early Repeat CT (d)	Area (mm^2)		Final Diagnosis	Computed Diameter (mm)		Doubling Time (d)	Measurements Projected at 30 d		
		at T_0	at T_1		at T_0	at T_1		Diameter (mm)	Area (mm^2)	Change (%)
10	23	50.7	51.0	No growth in 2 y	8.0	8.0	1,801	8.0	51.1	1.0
11	377	54.7	53.8	No growth in 3 y	8.3	8.3	−10,500	8.3	54.6	−0.1
12	757	15.9	16.5	No growth in 3 y	4.5	4.6	9,443	4.5	15.9	0.2
13	102	30.4	29.3	Scar	6.2	6.1	−1,278	6.2	30.1	−1.0
14	216	29.0	30.4	No growth in 2 y	6.1	6.2	2,117	6.1	29.2	1.0
15	301	46.2	42.9	No growth in 2 y	7.7	7.4	−1,877	7.6	45.9	−1.0

Note.—Nodule doubling time is based on the number of days between initial and repeat CT and the area and diameter at each time. The final diagnosis also is given. The projected diameter, area, and percentage of area change also are given, with the assumption that early repeat CT would have been performed 30 days after the initial finding. T_0 = initial CT, T_1 = early repeat CT.

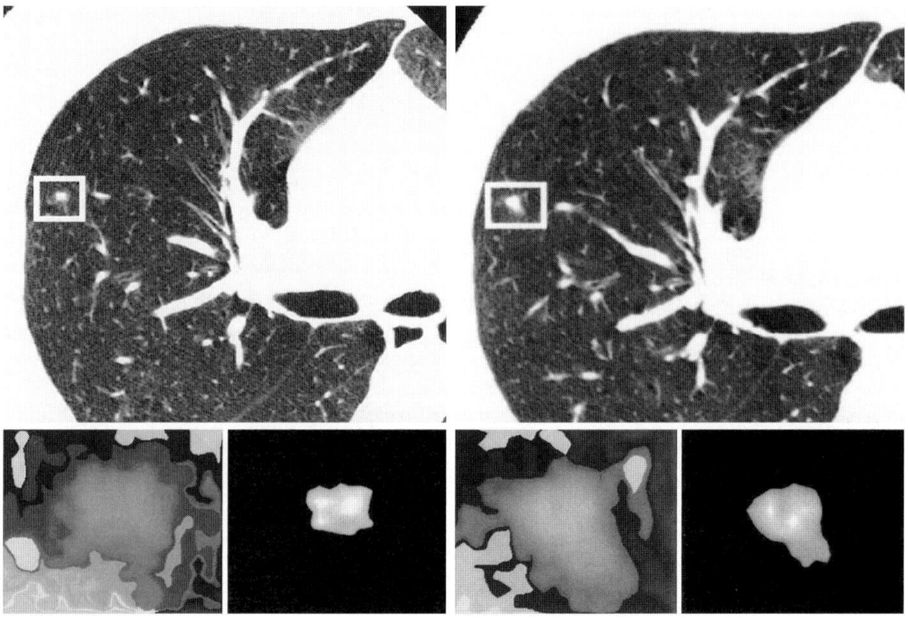

a. b.

Figure 3. Case 6. **(a)** Initial axial CT scan of the right upper lobe of the lung (nodule diameter, 3.6 mm) and **(b)** early repeat axial CT scan of the right upper lobe obtained 44 days later (nodule diameter, 4.3 mm) showing the selected region of interest (top), and the corresponding k-means classification of the region of interest (bottom left) and resultant segmented nodule (bottom right). The nodule was confirmed at pathologic evaluation to be an adenocarcinoma in the right upper lobe.

dence, so that surgical resection was avoided for these benign nodules. Cases 11 and 15 demonstrated a decrease in size, as represented by negative growth rates. Thus, a negative growth rate is also within the limits of variation in our current technique.

Early repeat CT depicted nodule growth within 6 weeks in the six patients who underwent repeat CT within that time. Early repeat CT depicted growth even for the smallest nodule (case 6 in Table 3 and Fig 3). Conversely, the increase in the area of the six benign nodules, even over long periods, was minimal and well below the CT detection limit.

DISCUSSION

The results of our experiments with phantoms and in vivo nodules show that early repeat CT can depict change within 30 days for malignancies that double within 30–180 days and are larger than 5 mm at initial presentation. To our knowledge, no study has documented a deleterious effect to the final outcome of the patient by observing a nodule for less than one doubling time before surgery. Although the policy of "watchful waiting" has come under scrutiny in the past, leading authorities in the field now advocate that "under certain circumstances, a decision to observe the nodule for a period of time with serial chest films may be appropriate, but this must be a considered approach and not a 'default' position" (2,13). Herein, we present one such approach, in which we established the usefulness of early repeat CT by demonstrating that growth in a nodule can be reliably detected with repeat CT performed within a clinically acceptable interval.

Early repeat CT also supplements information from the biopsy procedure by enabling direct confirmation of the presence or absence of growth. This is important because the accuracy of CT-guided needle biopsy in these small nodules is questionable (14). Needless to say, early repeat CT can be performed as part of the percutaneous CT-guided biopsy procedure. Our preliminary experience has shown that early repeat CT is highly desirable for determining the appropriate management actions when the biopsy result is indeterminate—allowing for confident continued observation when scans demonstrate lack of growth or suggesting further action when the malignant growth rate is determined. Thus, early repeat CT may be combined with a decision theoretical approach that enables determination of the probability of malignancy based on the initial CT findings. Results of early repeat CT can then be used to modify the baseline probability.

Gurney and colleagues (15,16) recommended using the Bayes theorem, which allows for the incorporation of likelihood ratios of various test results or clinical findings in determining the probability of malignancy of a given nodule. On the basis of a large literature survey, Gurney (15) found that the most important radiologic characteristics of malignant nodules were cavity wall thickness, spiculated edge, and nodule diameter greater than 3 cm; important characteristics for benignity were benign growth rate and benign pattern of calcification. As Swensen (17) noted, however, it is difficult to fully incorporate the combined information of many variables by using the Bayes theorem, and other techniques may be even more appropriate.

Additional advantages of early repeat CT include its potential for widespread availability and the fact that it does not require the specialized skills needed for accurate and safe percutaneous needle biopsy procedures or other more invasive diagnostic studies. In addition, early repeat CT entails a much lower cost.

In all of our in vivo studies, we relied on images that were obtained as part of routine clinical management. Repeat scans were typically obtained before biopsy. The routine clinical use of early repeat CT, however, would require a well-defined protocol for follow-up scanning. Ideally, this protocol would take into account the probability of malignancy based on both the patient's clinical characteristics and the nodule's initial morphologic features, as well as the parameters that describe the capabilities of the CT scanner. This task is complicated, because a complex interaction between these parameters determines when growth will become discernible. These parameters include (*a*) the initial size of the small pulmonary nodule, (*b*) the resolution of the imaging technique, (*c*) the measurement parameter used to assess growth, and (*d*) the doubling time of the tumor.

Any prespecified interval between initial and repeat CT (eg, 30 days) would enable only tumors growing faster than a certain rate to be reliably diagnosed. Thus, a single repeat scan might not depict the slower-growing tumors, and additional CT scans might be required. The scheduling function to determine when to obtain these additional repeat scans is a topic of current research.

Because volume changes as a function of the cube of the diameter, the proportional change in the nodule volume is much greater than the proportional change in the nodule diameter. Because the precision of these volume measurements is on the same order as that of diameter measurements, an increase in the nodule volume can be detected even earlier. For example, a 10-mm-diameter nodule with a doubling time of 30 days would show an increase of 1 mm in 12.4 days (a 10% increase), whereas the corresponding volume increase (33%) would be much larger. The larger the initial diameter, the greater the corresponding change in volume. Thus, determination of nodule volume directly from three-dimensional images is preferable.

Our current software implementation allows us to measure area change at the maximum cross section to assess growth as well as volumetric change in the overall nodule size. To analyze the capabilities of volumetric early repeat CT, we are currently gathering such volumetric data from appropriate clinical cases.

References

1. Lillington GA, Caskey CC. Evaluation and management of solitary and multiple pulmonary nodules. Clin Chest Med 1993; 14:111–119.
2. Lillington GA. Management of solitary pulmonary nodules. Postgrad Med 1997; 101:145–150.
3. Viggiano RW, Swensen SJ, Rosenow EC. Evaluation and management of solitary and multiple pulmonary nodules. Clin Chest Med 1992; 13:83–95.
4. Midthun DE, Swensen SJ, Jett JR. Clinical strategies for solitary pulmonary nodule. Annu Rev Med 1992; 43:195–208.
5. Hood RT Jr, Good CA, Clagett OT, McDonald JR. Solitary circumscribed lesions of the lung. JAMA 1953; 152:1185–1191.
6. Good CA, Hood RT Jr, McDonald JR. Significance of a solitary mass in the lung. AJR 1953; 70:543–554.
7. Good CA. Management of patient with solitary mass in lung. Chicago Med Soc Bull 1953; 55:893–896.
8. Good CA, Wilson TW. The solitary circumscribed pulmonary nodule. JAMA 1958; 166:210–215.
9. Zerhouni EA, Stitik FP, Siegelman SS, et al. CT of the pulmonary nodule: a cooperative study. Radiology 1986; 160:319–327.
10. Geddes DM. The natural history of lung cancer: a review based on rates of tumor growth. Br J Dis Chest 1979;73:1–17.
11. Russ JC. The image processing handbook. 2nd ed. Boca Raton, Fla: CRC, 1995.
12. Haralick RM, Shapiro LB. Survey-image segmentation techniques. Comp Vis Graphics Imaging Processing 1985; 29: 100–132.
13. Cumming SR, Lillington GA, Richard RJ. Managing solitary pulmonary nodules: the choice of strategy is a "close call." Am Rev Respir Dis 1986; 134:453–460.
14. Yankelevitz DF, Henschke CI, Koizumi J, Altorki N, Libby D. CT-guided transthoracic needle biopsy of small solitary pulmonary nodules. Clin Imaging 1997; 21: 107–110.
15. Gurney JW. Determining the likelihood of malignancy in solitary pulmonary nodules with Bayesian analysis. I. Theory. Radiology 1993; 186:405–413.
16. Gurney JW, Lyddon DM, McKay JA. Determining the likelihood of malignancy in solitary pulmonary nodules with Bayesian analysis. II. Application. Radiology 1993; 186:415–422.
17. Swensen SJ. The probability of malignancy in solitary pulmonary nodules: application to small radiologically indeterminate nodules. Arch Intern Med 1997; 157:849–855.

Lymphocytic Interstitial Pneumonia: Thin-Section CT Findings in 22 Patients[1]

Takeshi Johkoh, MD
Nestor L. Müller, MD, PhD
Heather A. Pickford, MD
Thomas E. Hartman, MD
Kazuya Ichikado, MD
Masanori Akira, MD
Osamu Honda, MD
Hironobu Nakamura, MD

Index terms:
Acquired immunodeficiency syndrome (AIDS), 60.206, 60.2068, 60.2518
Castleman disease, 60.314, 60.391
Eye, diseases, 22.696
Lung, CT, 60.12112, 60.12118
Pneumonitis, lymphocytic interstitial, 60.795
Sjögren syndrome, 22.696, 60.795

Radiology 1999; 212:567–572

Abbreviation:
AIDS = acquired immunodeficiency syndrome

[1] From the Department of Radiology, Vancouver Hospital and Health Sciences Center and University of British Columbia, 855 W 12th Ave, Vancouver, British Columbia, Canada V5Z 1M9 (T.J., N.L.M.); the Department of Radiology, Osaka University Medical School, Japan (T.J., O.H., H.N.); the Department of Radiology, Mayo Clinic, Rochester, Minn (H.A.P., T.E.H.); the First Department of Internal Medicine, Kumamoto University School of Medicine, Japan (K.I.); and the Department of Radiology, National Kinki Chuo Hospital for Chest Disease, Osaka, Japan (M.A.). Received March 25, 1998; revision requested June 18; final revision received October 23; accepted February 12, 1999. **Address reprint requests to** N.L.M.

Author contributions:
Guarantor of integrity of entire study, T.J.; study concepts and design, T.J., N.L.M.; definition of intellectual content, N.L.M., T.E.H.; literature research, T.J., K.I.; clinical studies, T.J., N.L.M., O.H., H.A.P., T.E.H., K.I., M.A.; data acquisition, T.J., N.L.M., K.I.; data analysis, T.J., N.L.M.; manuscript preparation, T.J., N.L.M.; manuscript editing, N.L.M., H.N.; manuscript review, N.L.M., T.E.H.

PURPOSE: To assess the thin-section computed tomographic (CT) findings of lymphocytic interstitial pneumonia.

MATERIALS AND METHODS: The study included 22 patients (five men, 17 women; age range, 24–83 years; mean age, 50 years) with biopsy-proved lymphocytic interstitial pneumonia. The CT scans were obtained by using 1–3-mm collimation and reconstructed by using a high-spatial-frequency algorithm.

RESULTS: The predominant abnormalities consisted of areas of ground-glass attenuation and poorly defined centrilobular nodules present in all 22 patients and subpleural small nodules seen in 19 patients. Other common findings included thickening of bronchovascular bundles ($n = 19$), interlobular septal thickening ($n = 18$), cystic airspaces ($n = 15$), and lymph node enlargement ($n = 15$). Less common findings included large nodules, emphysema, airspace consolidation, bronchiectasis, architectural distortion, honeycombing, and pleural thickening.

CONCLUSION: Lymphocytic interstitial pneumonia is characterized by the presence of ground-glass attenuation, poorly defined centrilobular nodules, and thickening of the interstitium along the lymphatic vessels. Lymph node enlargement is more common than previously recognized; it was seen in 68% of patients.

Lymphocytic interstitial pneumonia is a benign lymphoproliferative disorder characterized by a diffuse and exquisitely interstitial proliferation of small lymphocytes and plasma cells (1). Lymphocytic interstitial pneumonia occurs most commonly in patients who have Sjögren syndrome, autoimmune thyroid disease, acquired immunodeficiency syndrome (AIDS), or Castleman disease (2–8).

The natural history of lymphocytic interstitial pneumonia is highly variable (1,2,9). Some patients recover or have slowly improving or stable respiratory disease following treatment with corticosteroids. Over one-third of reported patients have progressive disease. Lymphoma has supervened in some patients, although it is likely that this group of patients had malignant lymphoma from the outset (10).

The appearance of lymphocytic interstitial pneumonia on chest radiographs has been reported to range from interstitial reticular opacities to nodular opacities (11,12). The computed tomographic (CT) findings of lymphocytic interstitial pneumonia have been described in a small number of isolated cases (6,7,13–15). The aim of this study was to assess the thin-section CT findings in 22 patients who had biopsy-proved lymphocytic interstitial pneumonia.

MATERIALS AND METHODS

We retrospectively identified 22 patients who had biopsy-proved lymphocytic interstitial pneumonia and had undergone CT examination at one of our five institutions between December 1989 and December 1997. The study group consisted of five men and 17 women, with a mean age of 50 years (age range, 24–83 years).

The diagnosis of lymphocytic interstitial pneumonia was obtained by performing open lung biopsy in 13 patients and transbronchial lung biopsy in nine patients. Transbronchial biopsy was performed in six patients with Sjögren syndrome and three patients with Castleman disease. In all patients, tissue diagnosis was obtained within 2 weeks of the CT

Chief CT Findings in Patients with Lymphocytic Interstitial Pneumonia

Patient No./ Age (y)/Sex	Underlying Disease	Centrilobular Nodules (n = 22)	Subpleural Nodules (n = 19)	Bronchovascular Thickening (n = 19)	Septal Thickening (n = 18)	Ground-Glass Attenuation (n = 22)	Cyst (n = 15)	Lymph Node Enlargement (n = 15)
1/28/F	Sjögren syndrome	Yes	Yes	Yes	Yes	Yes	No	No
2/76/M	Sjögren syndrome	Yes	Yes	Yes	Yes	Yes	Yes	No
3/56/F	Sjögren syndrome	Yes	Yes	Yes	Yes	Yes	No	Yes
4/43/F	Sjögren syndrome	Yes	Yes	Yes	Yes	Yes	Yes	Yes
5/59/F	Sjögren syndrome	Yes	No	No	No	Yes	Yes	No
6/61/F	Sjögren syndrome	Yes	Yes	Yes	Yes	Yes	No	Yes
7/28/F	Sjögren syndrome	Yes	Yes	Yes	No	Yes	Yes	Yes
8/50/F	Sjögren syndrome	Yes	Yes	Yes	Yes	Yes	Yes	No
9/49/F	Sjögren syndrome	Yes	Yes	No	Yes	Yes	No	No
10/64/F	Sjögren syndrome	Yes	Yes	Yes	Yes	Yes	Yes	Yes
11/44/F	Multicentric Castleman disease	Yes	Yes	Yes	Yes	Yes	Yes	Yes
12/50/F	Multicentric Castleman disease	Yes	No	Yes	Yes	Yes	Yes	Yes
13/49/F	Multicentric Castleman disease	Yes	Yes	Yes	Yes	Yes	Yes	Yes
14/32/F	Multicentric Castleman disease	Yes	Yes	Yes	Yes	Yes	No	Yes
15/53/F	Multicentric Castleman disease	Yes	Yes	Yes	Yes	Yes	Yes	Yes
16/24/F	Multicentric Castleman disease	Yes	Yes	Yes	Yes	Yes	Yes	Yes
17/55/F	Multicentric Castleman disease	Yes	Yes	Yes	Yes	Yes	Yes	Yes
18/50/M	AIDS	Yes	No	Yes	No	Yes	Yes	No
19/83/M	AIDS	Yes	Yes	No	No	Yes	No	No
20/28/F	None	Yes	Yes	Yes	Yes	Yes	No	Yes
21/81/M	None	Yes	Yes	Yes	Yes	Yes	Yes	Yes
22/36/F	None	Yes	Yes	Yes	Yes	Yes	Yes	Yes

scans. Ten patients had Sjögren syndrome, seven had Castleman disease, two had AIDS, and three had no underlying disease. All patients with Castleman disease had multicentric disease and hypergammaglobulinemia.

All patients underwent thin-section CT of the chest. The CT scans consisted of 1–3-mm-collimation sections reconstructed by using a high-spatial-frequency algorithm. The protocols consisted of thin sections obtained at 1-cm (18 patients) or 2-cm (three patients) intervals and five thin sections obtained in addition to contiguous 7–10-mm-collimation (conventional) scans obtained through the chest (one patient). In 14 patients, selected images were targeted to a single lung by using a small field of view (13–20 cm).

The CT scans were obtained with a variety of scanners. These included a model 8800, 9800, or CT HiSpeed Advantage scanner (GE Medical Systems, Milwaukee, Wis); X-Vigor scanner (Toshiba, Tokyo, Japan); Quantex scanner (Yokogawa, Hino, Japan); C 100 scanner (Imatron, San Francisco, Calif); and model 1200SX scanner (Picker International, Highland Heights, Ohio). Nine patients received intravenous injections of contrast medium.

The CT images were reviewed by two observers (T.J., N.L.M), and final decisions on the findings were reached by consensus. The observers assessed the presence, extent, and distribution of areas of ground-glass attenuation, airspace consolidation, parenchymal nodules, interlobular septal thickening, thickening of bronchovascular bundles, and cystic airspaces. The presence, extent, and distribution of associated findings such as emphysema, bronchiectasis, honeycombing, architectural distortion, lymph node enlargement, pleural thickening, and pleural effusion were also assessed. Ground-glass attenuation was defined as an area of hazy increased attenuation without obscuration of underlying vascular markings. Airspace consolidation was considered present when the opacities obscured the underlying vessels. Lymphadenopathy was considered present when the short-axis diameter of the nodes was greater than 1 cm. Because only nine patients received intravenous contrast material, the assessment of lymphadenopathy was limited to the mediastinal lymph nodes.

RESULTS

CT findings of lymphocytic interstitial pneumonia are summarized in the Table. Areas of ground-glass attenuation were present in all 22 patients (Fig 1). The areas of ground-glass attenuation were bilateral in 21 patients (95%) and unilateral in one patient (5%). The areas of ground-glass attenuation had a diffuse distribution in 14 patients (64%), a patchy random distribution in five patients (23%), and a peripheral distribution in three patients (14%).

Poorly defined centrilobular nodules were identified in all 22 patients (Figs 1–3). The centrilobular nodules were bilateral in 20 patients (91%) and unilateral in two patients (9%). The poorly defined centrilobular nodules were diffuse in 19 patients (86%) and had a patchy random distribution in three patients (14%).

Histologic assessment of pathologic specimens obtained from areas that contained centrilobular nodules demonstrated peribronchiolar infiltration with lymphocytes and plasma cells (Fig 1). Subpleural small nodules were found in 19 patients (86%). Thickening of bronchovascular bundles was present in 19 patients (86%) (Figs 2,4). The thickening was bilateral in 15 patients (68%) and unilateral in four patients (18%). In all patients with thickening of bronchovascular bundles, the thickening showed a patchy random distribution.

Interlobular septal thickening was

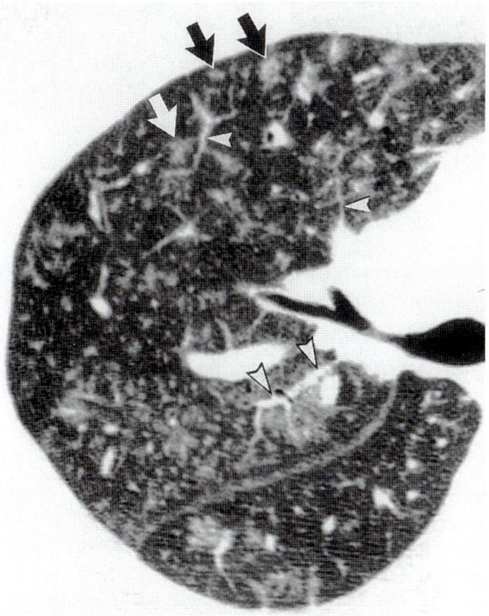

a.

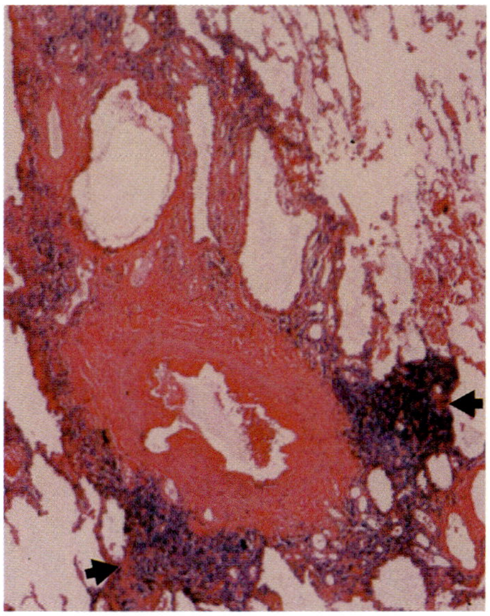

c.

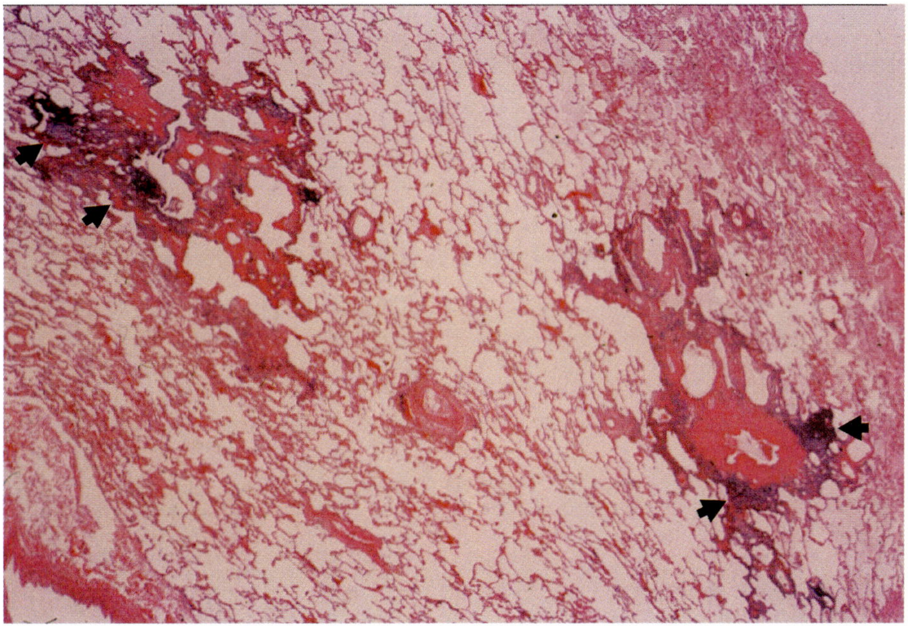

b.

Figure 1. Lymphocytic interstitial pneumonia in a 24-year-old woman with multicentric Castleman disease. **(a)** Thin-section (1-mm-collimation) CT scan obtained at the level of the carina demonstrates diffuse distribution of poorly defined centrilobular nodules (arrows) and areas of ground-glass attenuation and thickening of interlobular septa (arrowheads). **(b)** Histologic section. (Hematoxylin-eosin stain; original magnification, ×40.) **(c)** Same section as in **b** but at a higher power magnification. (Hematoxylin-eosin stain; original magnification ×100.) **b** and **c** show peribronchiolar infiltration with lymphocytes and plasma cells (arrows). This peribronchiolar infiltration accounts for the centrilobular nodules seen in **a**.

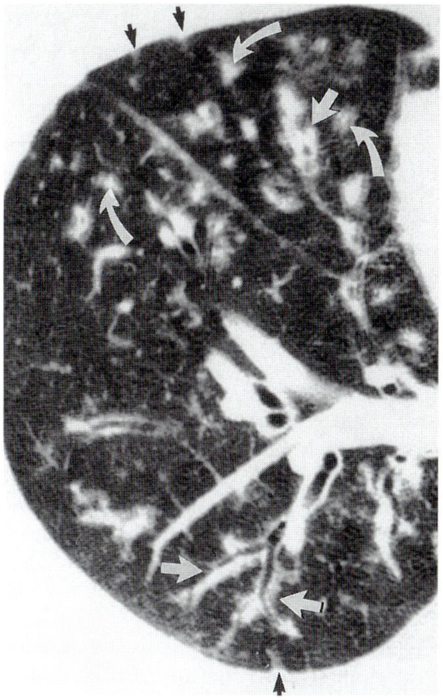

Figure 2. Lymphocytic interstitial pneumonia in a 32-year-old woman with multicentric Castleman disease. Thin-section (1-mm-collimation) CT scan obtained at the level of the right inferior pulmonary vein demonstrates diffuse distribution of thickened bronchovascular bundles (straight white arrows). Small, poorly defined centrilobular nodules (curved arrows) and subpleural nodules (black arrows) are also found.

found in 18 patients (82%) (Fig 5). It was bilateral in 14 patients and unilateral in four patients. The interlobular septal thickening had diffuse distribution in one patient and a patchy random distribution in the remaining 17 patients. Histologic assessment of pathologic specimens obtained from areas that had interlobular septal thickening showed infiltration of the interlobular septa and adjacent alveolar septa by lymphocytes and plasma cells (Fig 5).

Cystic airspaces ranging from 1 to 30 mm were seen in 15 patients (68%) (Fig 4). The average size of the cystic airspaces was 6.4 mm ± 2.9. The cystic airspaces were bilateral in 10 patients and unilateral in five patients. In all patients, the cystic airspaces had a random distribution and involved less than 10% of the lung parenchyma.

Lymph node enlargement was found in 15 patients (68%), including both mediastinal and hilar lymphadenopathy in 12 patients, mediastinal lymphadenopathy in two patients, and hilar lymphadenopathy in one patient. In all but one patient, lymph node enlargement was present in multiple nodal stations.

Less common findings included nodules 1–2 cm in diameter (n = 9 [41%]), airspace consolidation (n = 9 [41%]), architectural distortion (n = 8 [36%]), emphysema (n = 5 [23%]), bronchiectasis (n = 4 [18%]), pleural thickening (n = 4 [18%]), and honeycombing (n = 1 [5%]).

DISCUSSION

Previous reports on lymphocytic interstitial pneumonia have focused primarily on the histologic appearance, with reference to the clinical course and the findings on the chest radiograph (1–6). At histologic examination, lymphocytic interstitial pneumonia is characterized by a diffuse interstitial cellular infiltrate composed of a mixture of mature small lymphocytes and plasma cells that widen the alveolar septa (1–3,10,16). Although the process is diffuse, lymphocytic interstitial pneumonia has a propensity to be most severe in the perilymphatic interstitium, that is, along bronchovascular bundles, interlobular septa, and pleura (17). The appearance of lymphocytic interstitial pneumonia on radiographs is nonspecific and includes interstitial reticular opacities and nodular opacities (11,12). The CT findings reported in a small number of cases included areas of ground-glass attenuation, thin-walled cystic airspaces, focal airspace consolidation, centrilobular or peribronchiolar small nodules, and bronchiectasis (6,7,13–15).

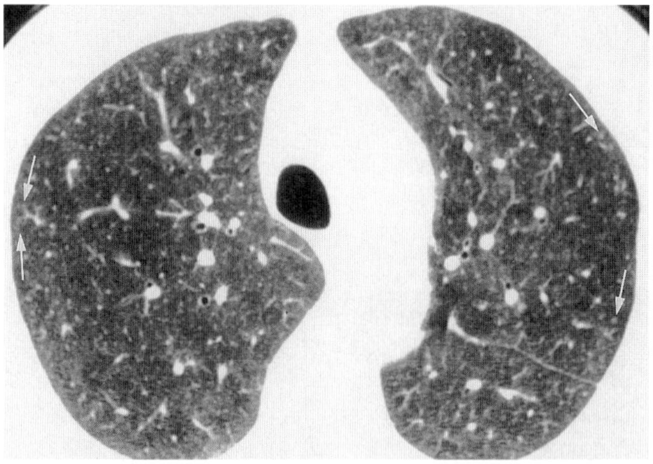

Figure 3. Lymphocytic interstitial pneumonia in an 83-year-old man with AIDS. Thin-section (1-mm-collimation) CT scan obtained at the level of the aortic arch shows extensive bilateral areas of ground-glass attenuation and small, poorly defined centrilobular nodules (arrows).

In our study, both ground-glass attenuation and poorly defined centrilobular nodules were present in all 22 patients. The areas of ground-glass attenuation and poorly defined centrilobular nodules were usually bilateral and involved all lung zones. These findings are not surprising, given the distribution of lymphocytic interstitial pneumonia along the alveolar septa and adjacent to small airways and vessels (10,16). The pulmonary lymphatic vessels extend along the centrilobular bronchioles (18). The peribronchiolar distribution accounts for the centrilobular nodules seen at thin-section CT. Thickening of bronchovascular bundles, interlobular septa, and subpleural small nodules was seen in the majority of patients. These findings also correspond to the distribution of lymphatic vessels (18,19).

Cystic airspaces were found in 15 patients in our study. Ichikawa et al (14) correlated thin-section CT findings of two cases of lymphocytic interstitial pneumonia with histologic findings obtained through open lung biopsy. Histologic specimens showed nodular infiltrates of lymphoid cells that were peribronchovascular in distribution. It was postulated that the mechanism of cystic airspace formation is partial airway obstruction caused by the peribronchiolar cellular infiltration. Desai et al (15) described three cases of lymphocytic interstitial pneumonia associated with multiple nodules and thin-walled cystic airspaces.

Lymph node enlargement was present in the majority of patients in the current study. This observation differs from the results of radiography of the chest in previous studies that indicated that lymphadenopathy is uncommon in lymphocytic interstitial pneumonia (20,21). The difference is presumably due to the greater sensitivity of CT in demonstrating mediastinal lymph node enlargement. It should be noted, however, that our study is weighted toward patients who had lymphocytic interstitial pneumonia in association with Sjögren syndrome or Castleman disease. Enlarged nodes were present in all seven patients with Castleman disease but in only five of the 10 patients with Sjögren syndrome and three of the five patients with AIDS or no underlying disease.

Hypersensitivity pneumonitis characteristically contains mixed mononuclear cell infiltrates with numerous small lymphocytes, which may resemble lymphocytic interstitial pneumonia (10,16). The characteristic thin-section CT findings of hypersensitivity pneumonitis consist of areas of ground-glass attenuation and small centrilobular nodules (22,23). Both findings are also typically seen in lymphocytic interstitial pneumonia. However, cystic airspaces, interlobular septal thickening, thickening of bronchovascular bundles, and lymph node enlargement are rarely seen in hypersensitivity pneumonitis (22,23).

Multiple cystic airspaces are typically seen at thin-section CT in patients with pulmonary Langerhans histiocytosis and lymphangioleiomyomatosis (24–26). The characteristic CT findings of Langerhans histiocytosis consist of cystic airspaces and multiple nodules (24,25). The nodules sometimes show a centrilobular distribution. Distinguishing features of lymphocytic interstitial pneumonia from Langerhans histiocytosis include the presence of interlobular septal thickening and lymphadenopathy. The absence of centrilobular nodules in lymphangioleiomyomatosis allows ready distinction of this

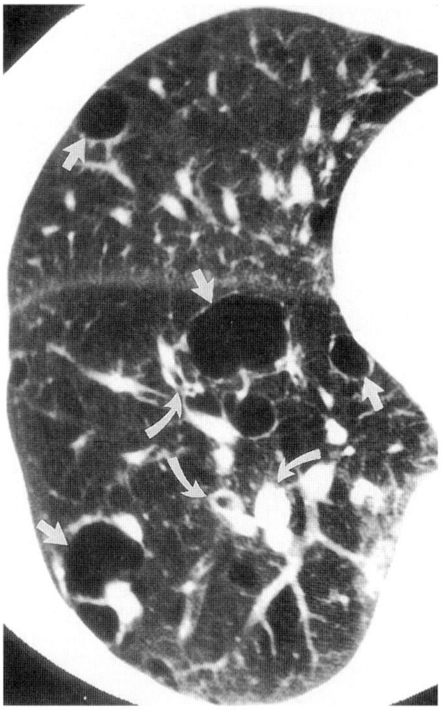

Figure 4. Lymphocytic interstitial pneumonia in a 76-year-old woman with Sjögren syndrome. Thin-section (1.5-mm-collimation) CT scan demonstrates several thin-walled cystic airspaces (straight arrows) in the right middle and lower lobes. Thickened bronchovascular bundles (curved arrows) are also found.

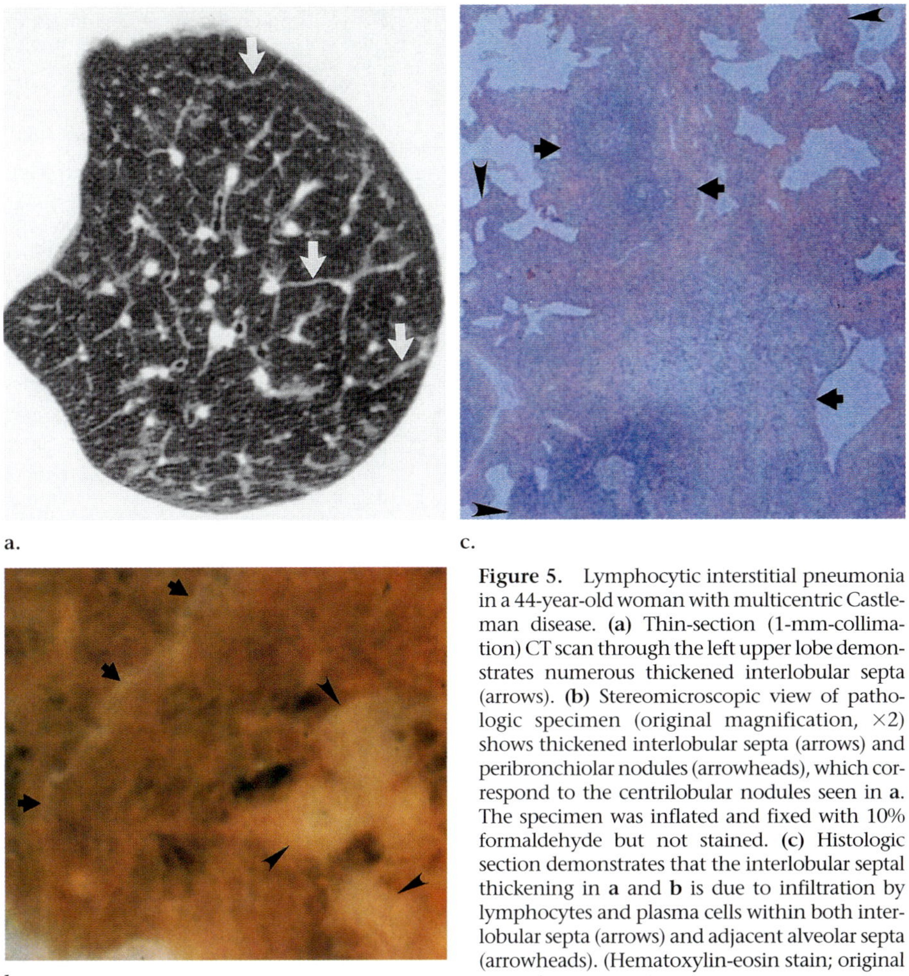

a. b. c.

Figure 5. Lymphocytic interstitial pneumonia in a 44-year-old woman with multicentric Castleman disease. **(a)** Thin-section (1-mm-collimation) CT scan through the left upper lobe demonstrates numerous thickened interlobular septa (arrows). **(b)** Stereomicroscopic view of pathologic specimen (original magnification, ×2) shows thickened interlobular septa (arrows) and peribronchiolar nodules (arrowheads), which correspond to the centrilobular nodules seen in **a**. The specimen was inflated and fixed with 10% formaldehyde but not stained. **(c)** Histologic section demonstrates that the interlobular septal thickening in **a** and **b** is due to infiltration by lymphocytes and plasma cells within both interlobular septa (arrows) and adjacent alveolar septa (arrowheads). (Hematoxylin-eosin stain; original magnification ×40.)

condition from lymphocytic interstitial pneumonia.

Lymphocytic interstitial pneumonia is seen with increased frequency in patients with AIDS (5). In patients with *Pneumocystis carinii* pneumonia and AIDS, cystic airspace formation is commonly seen (27,28). *P carinii* pneumonia may also cause small nodules and extensive areas of ground-glass attenuation. Distinguishing features of lymphocytic interstitial pneumonia include the presence of interlobular septal thickening and lymph node enlargement in patients with lymphocytic interstitial pneumonia. It may be difficult, however, to distinguish patients who have lymphocytic interstitial pneumonia from patients who have *P carinii* pneumonia, as well as from patients who have other AIDS-related complications such as tuberculosis. Moreover, it may be difficult to distinguish lymphocytic interstitial pneumonia from other lymphoproliferative disorders, particularly in patients with AIDS (7). Further studies are required to determine the value of thin-section CT in distinguishing lymphocytic interstitial pneumonia from other pulmonary disorders seen in nonimmunocompromised and immunocompromised patients.

Our study has several limitations. First, it is a descriptive, retrospective review of findings seen on CT scans obtained at five different institutions, which used different protocols.

Second, because open lung biopsy was performed in only 13 of the 22 patients and because the study was retrospective, it provides limited information about the correlation between the CT and the histologic findings. In particular, although 15 (68%) patients had cystic airspaces, in none of the patients was a cystic airspace included in the biopsy specimen.

Third, although similar to those in the study of Ichikawa et al (14), pathologic specimens in our study demonstrated peribronchovascular nodular infiltrates of lymphoid cells, and we found no definite evidence that these infiltrates resulted in distal air trapping and cystic airspace formation.

Last, the study findings do not allow conclusions to be drawn about the accuracy of thin-section CT in differentiating lymphocytic interstitial pneumonia from other disease entities. This would require a blind comparison of the thin-section CT findings in lymphocytic interstitial pneumonia with the findings in other diseases.

In conclusion, lymphocytic interstitial pneumonia is characterized by the presence of ground-glass attenuation, poorly defined centrilobular nodules, and thickening of perilymphatic interstitium. Lymph node enlargement is more common than previously recognized.

References

1. Liebow A, Charington C. Diffuse pulmonary hyporeticular infiltrations associated with dysproteinemia. Med Clin North Am 1973; 57:809–843.
2. Koss MN, Hochholzer L, Langloss JM, Wehunt WD, Lazarus AA. Lymphoid interstitial pneumonia: clinicopathological and immunopathological findings in 18 cases. Pathology 1987; 19:178–185.
3. Deheinzelin D, Capelozzi VL, Kairalla RA, et al. Interstitial lung disease in primary Sjögren syndrome: clinical-pathological evaluation and response to treatment. Am J Respir Crit Care Med 1996; 154:794–799.
4. Khardori R, Eagleton L, Soler N, McConnachie P. Lymphocytic interstitial pneumonitis in autoimmune thyroid disease. Am J Med 1991; 90:649–652.
5. Travis WD, Fox CH, Devaney KO, et al. Lymphoid pneumonitis in 50 adult patients infected with the human immunodeficiency virus: lymphocytic interstitial pneumonitis versus nonspecific interstitial pneumonitis. Hum Pathol 1992; 23: 529–541.
6. Carignan S, Staples CA, Müller NL. Intrathoracic lymphoproliferative disorders in the immunocompromised patient: CT findings. Radiology 1995; 197:53–58.
7. McGuinness G, Scholes JV, Jagirdar JS, et al. Unusual lymphoproliferative disorders in nine adults with HIV or AIDS: CT and pathologic findings. Radiology 1995; 197: 59–65.
8. Torii K, Ogawa K, Kawabata Y, Yokoi T, Takagi K, Miwa T. Lymphoid interstitial pneumonia as a pulmonary lesion of idiopathic plasmacytic lymphadenopathy with hyperimmunoglobulinemia. Intern Med 1994; 33:237–241.
9. Strimlan C, Isaacs H, Saxon A, et al. Lymphoid interstitial pneumonitis: review of 13 cases. Ann Intern Med 1978; 88:616–621.
10. Myers JL, Kurtin PJ. Lymphoid proliferative disorders of the lung. In: Thurlbeck WM, Churg AM, eds. Pathology of the lung. 2nd ed. New York, NY: Thieme, 1995; 553–587.
11. Julsrud PR, Brown LR, Li CY, Rosenow EC, Crowe JK. Pulmonary processes of mature-appearing lymphocytes: pseudolymphoma, well-differentiated lymphocytic

lymphoma, and lymphocytic interstitial pneumonia. Radiology 1978; 127:289–296.
12. Glickstein M, Kornstein MJ, Pictra GG, et al. Nonlymphomatous lymphoid disorders of the lung. AJR 1986; 147:227–237.
13. Kobayashi H, Matsuoka R, Kitamura S, Tsunoda N, Saito K. Sjögren syndrome with multiple bullae and pulmonary nodular amyloidosis. Chest 1988; 94:438–440.
14. Ichikawa Y, Kinoshita M, Koga T, Oizumi K, Fujimoto K, Hayabuchi N. Lung cyst formation in lymphocytic interstitial pneumonia: CT features. J Comput Assist Tomogr 1994; 18:745–748.
15. Desai SR, Nicholson AG, Stewart S, Twentyman OM, Flower CD, Hansell DM. Benign pulmonary lymphocytic infiltration and amyloidosis: computed tomographic and pathologic features in three cases. J Thorac Imaging 1997; 12:215–220.
16. Katzenstein AL. Primary lymphoid lung lesions. In: Katzenstein AL, Askin FB, eds. Katzenstein and Askin's surgical pathology of non-neoplastic lung disease. 3rd ed. Philadelphia, Pa: Saunders, 1995; 223–245.
17. Kradin RL, Mark EJ. Benign lymphoid disorders of the lung, with a theory regarding their development. Hum Pathol 1983; 14:857–867.
18. Colby TV, Swensen SJ. Anatomic distribution and histopathologic patterns in diffuse lung disease: correlation with HRCT. J Thorac Imaging 1996; 11:1–26.
19. Webb WR, Müller NL, Naidich DP. HRCT findings of lung disease. In: Webb WR, Müller NL, Naidich DP, eds. High-resolution CT of the lung. 2nd ed. Philadelphia, Pa: Lippincott-Raven, 1996; 41–108.
20. Feigin DS, Siegelman SS, Theros EG, et al. Nonmalignant lymphoid disorders of the chest. AJR 1977; 129:221–228.
21. Colby TV, Carrington CB. Lymphoreticular tumors and infiltrates of the lung. Pathol Annu 1983; 18:27–70.
22. Silver SF, Müller NL, Miller RR, Lefcoe MS. Hypersensitivity pneumonitis: evaluation with CT. Radiology 1989; 173:441–445.
23. Remy-Jardin M, Remy J, Wallaert B, Müller NL. Subacute and chronic hypersensitivity pneumonitis: sequential evaluation with CT and correlation with lung function tests and bronchoalveolar lavage. Radiology 1993; 198:111–118.
24. Moore AD, Godwin JD, Müller NL, et al. Pulmonary histiocytosis X: comparison of radiographic and CT findings. Radiology 1989; 172:249–254.
25. Brauner MW, Grenier P, Mouelhi MM, Mompoint D, Lenoir S. Pulmonary histiocytosis X: evaluation with high-resolution CT. Radiology 1989; 172:255–258.
26. Müller NL, Chiles C, Kullnig P. Pulmonary lymphangiomyomatosis: correlation of CT with radiographic and functional findings. Radiology 1990; 175:335–339.
27. Kuhlman JE, Knowles MC, Fishman EK, Siegelman SS. Premature bullous pulmonary damage in AIDS: CT diagnosis. Radiology 1989; 173:23–26.
28. Feuerstein I, Archer A, Pluda LM, et al. Thin-walled cavities, cysts, and pneumothorax in *Pneumocystis carinii* pneumonia: further observations with histopathologic correlation. Radiology 1990; 174:697–702.

Rossella Fattori, MD
Benedetta Descovich, MD
Paola Bertaccini, MD
Francesca Celletti, MD
Ilaria Caldarera, MD
Angelo Pierangeli, MD
Giampaolo Gavelli, MD

Index terms:
Aorta, grafts and prostheses, 56.1269, 941.1269
Aorta, MR, 56.121411, 56.121412, 56.12143, 941.129411, 941.129412, 941.12942

Radiology 1999; 212:573–577

[1] From the Institute of Radiology and Cardiovascular Surgery, Ospedale S Orsola, Via Massarenti 9, 40100 Bologna, Italy. Received March 10, 1998; revision requested May 12; revision received November 30; accepted March 16, 1999. **Address reprint requests to** R.F. (e-mail: *ross@med.unibo.it*).

Author contributions:
Guarantor of integrity of entire study, R.F.; study concepts, P.B.; study design, F.C.; definition of intellectual content, B.D.; clinical studies, I.C.; manuscript preparation, B.D.; manuscript editing, A.P.; manuscript review, G.G.

Composite Graft Replacement of the Ascending Aorta: Leakage Detection with Gadolinium-enhanced MR Imaging[1]

PURPOSE: To assess the value of magnetic resonance (MR) imaging in the detection of postoperative complications after composite valve graft replacement.

MATERIALS AND METHODS: Spin-echo and gradient-echo MR imaging was performed in 52 patients ½ to 200 months after composite graft replacement of the ascending aorta (22 for dissection, 30 for aneurysm). The prosthetic aortic segment, distal and proximal anastomoses, general morphologic characteristics, and diameter of the reimplanted coronary arteries were evaluated. In patients with abnormal perigraft thickening, additional spin-echo imaging was performed after injection of gadopentetate dimeglumine.

RESULTS: Normal postoperative perigraft thickening (≤10 mm) was observed in 42 patients. Ten patients had abnormal periprosthetic thickening of 15–52 mm. Gadolinium-enhanced MR imaging demonstrated leakage in five of those 10 patients. The lack of enhancement excluded the presence of bleeding in the remaining five patients (three with chronic hematomas, one with infection, and one with granulation tissue). These findings were confirmed at surgery or with subsequent follow-up MR examinations.

CONCLUSION: MR imaging was an optimal imaging modality for evaluating the morphologic characteristics of composite grafts and reimplanted coronary arteries. Gadolinium-enhanced MR imaging is a simple, accurate, and noninvasive method for detecting a leak, which necessitates urgent repeat surgery.

Advances in surgical techniques have substantially improved the survival rate in patients undergoing repair of the ascending aorta. Composite graft replacement of the ascending aorta and aortic valve, first described by Bentall and De Bono (1) (who used a Dacron tube with a prosthetic aortic valve sewn into one end), or their modification has become the procedure of choice in patients with annuloaortic ectasia or aortic dissection involving the aortic sinuses. Although this technique reduces the risk of recurrent aortic aneurysm, a relatively high frequency of early and late postoperative complications has been reported, justifying the need for close follow-up (2–4). Surgical replacement of the ascending aorta includes the risk of paravalvular leakage and false aneurysm formation as well as leakage or chronic partial dehiscence due to tension at the anastomosis of the coronary arteries. Postoperative assessment has been performed with angiography, echocardiography, and computed tomography, but magnetic resonance (MR) imaging has been shown to be the most effective procedure, providing multiplanar evaluation of the entire aorta and its surrounding structures (5–7).

The purpose of this study was to demonstrate the value of MR imaging in the depiction of postoperative anatomic details and complications after composite valve graft insertion.

MATERIALS AND METHODS

The study included 52 patients, 22 of whom underwent surgery for Stanford type A aortic dissection (14 in the acute phase and eight in the chronic phase) and 30 of whom

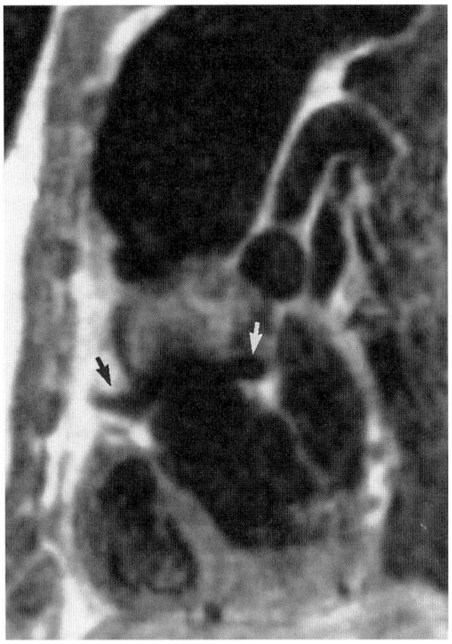

Figure 1. Sagittal oblique spin-echo MR image (20/650) of ascending aorta replaced with the Bentall technique (direct suture of coronary arteries [arrows] to the conduit).

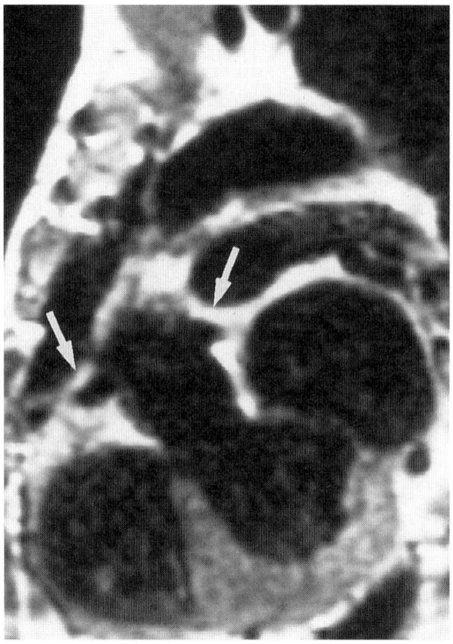

Figure 2. Sagittal oblique spin-echo MR image (20/830) of ascending aorta replaced with the button technique (reimplantation of coronary arteries [arrows] with a small button of surrounding tissue attached to the conduit).

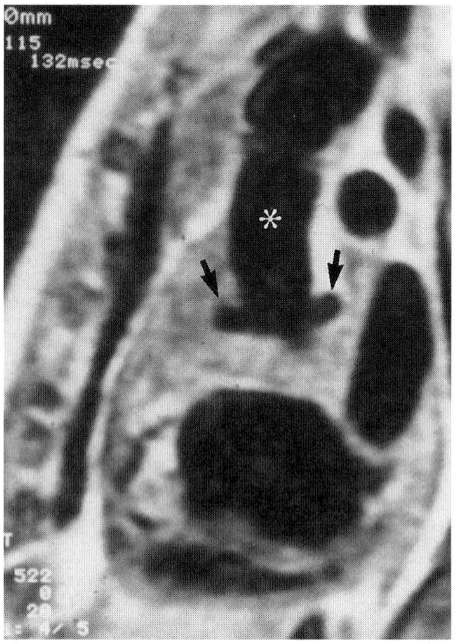

Figure 3. Sagittal oblique spin-echo MR image (20/600) of ascending aorta replaced with the Cabrol technique (interposition of Dacron T tubes [arrows] between coronary arteries and the main conduit [*]).

underwent surgery for aneurysm of the ascending aorta, annulus, or both between January 1982 and October 1996. Of the 22 patients with dissection, 20 were men and two were women; the mean age was 48.7 years ± 14 (SD), and the follow-up time ranged from ½ to 200 months after surgery. Of the 30 patients with aneurysm, 26 were men and four were women; the mean age was 43.2 years ± 16, and the follow-up time ranged from ½ to 120 months after surgery. The diagnosis of Marfan syndrome was established with clinical criteria (8) in 24 patients, six with aortic dissection and 18 with aortic aneurysm.

All patients underwent composite graft replacement of the ascending aorta. Among the 22 patients with aortic dissection, the Bentall technique (1) (direct suture of coronary arteries to the conduit and wrapping of the native aortic wall around the prosthetic conduit) (Fig 1) was used in nine (among them five without preclotting grafts), the button technique (9) (reimplantation of coronary arteries with a small button of surrounding tissue to the conduit, without wrapping) (Fig 2) was used in 10, and the Cabrol technique (10) (interposition of Dacron T tube between coronary arteries and the main conduit) (Fig 3) was used in three.

Among the 30 patients with aortic aneurysm disease, the Bentall technique associated with wrapping of the aneurysm wall around the aortic graft was used in 15. In two of the 15 patients, the Bentall operation was combined with coronary artery bypass graft replacement (left internal mammary artery on the descending anterior coronary artery and saphenous venous graft on the circumflex coronary artery) and replacement of the aortic arch. The remaining 15 patients underwent the button operation with an open technique (no wrapping).

Eighteen patients underwent surgery before January 1991, and they underwent a single MR examination at a variable time after surgery (range, 6–200 months). Thirty-four patients underwent surgery between January 1991 and December 1997. These patients were included in a follow-up program in which Institutional Review Board approval and informed consent were required and in which MR imaging was performed 15 days after surgery and, subsequently, if no major pathologic findings were present, at 6 months and once a year thereafter. The number of MR studies available for each patient ranged from two to nine.

In all patients, electrocardiographically gated multisection spin-echo imaging of the entire thoracic aorta was performed in the axial, sagittal oblique, and coronal planes. The repetition time was dependent on the R-R interval on the electrocardiograph. The echo time was 20 msec. The section thickness varied from 5 to 7 mm, and the matrix size ranged from 128 × 160 to 256 × 256. In addition, gradient-echo imaging (25/17 [repetition time msec/echo time msec]; flip angle, 35°) was performed in the sagittal oblique plane.

In each patient, the prosthetic aortic segment, along with surrounding structures, distal and proximal anastomoses, general morphologic characteristics, and diameter of reimplanted coronary arteries were evaluated by two authors (R.F., B.D.) together, who rendered a consensus opinion. The image quality was graded as good, fair, or inadequate. The diameter of reimplanted coronary arteries was measured with the spin-echo sequences, which are not influenced by the metallic artifacts of the prosthetic valve.

Special attention was directed to the identification of periprosthetic collections, and, according to findings of previous studies (11), a perigraft thickening greater than 10 mm was considered abnormal. In patients with perigraft thickening greater than 10 mm, to identify the presence of bleeding and the site of its origin, a multisection spin-echo sequence was performed in the coronal plane, transaxial plane, or both after manual intravenous bolus injection of gadopentetate dimeglumine (Magnevist; Schering, Ber-

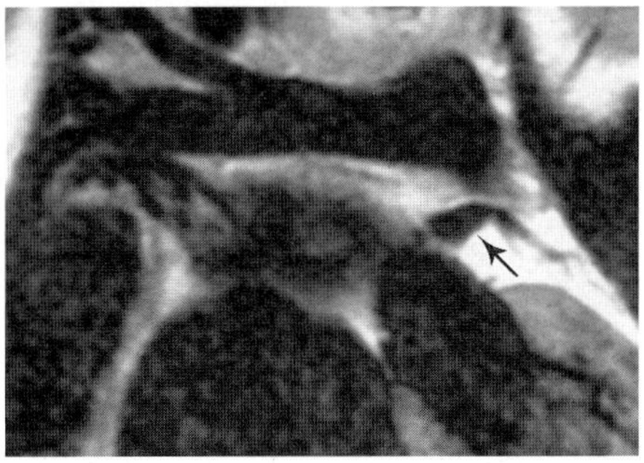

Figure 4. Coronal spin-echo MR image (20/720) in a patient with Marfan syndrome shows moderate dilatation (arrow) of the reimplanted left coronary artery ostium.

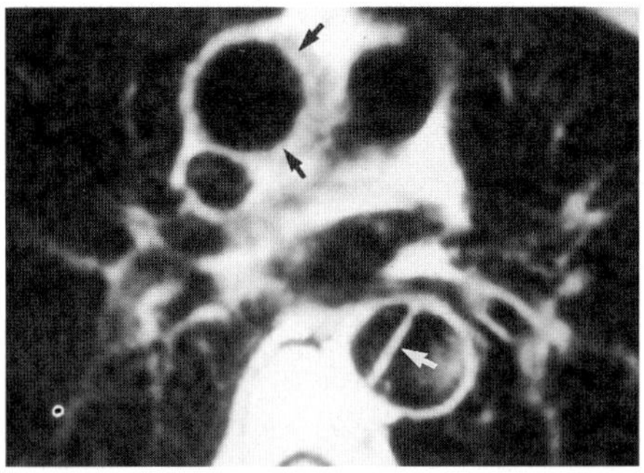

Figure 5. Axial spin-echo MR image (20/850) of ascending aorta and descending aorta. Normal perigraft thickening (black arrows), due to fibrosis and surrounding the prosthetic conduit of the ascending aorta, is visible. The perigraft thickening is less than 10 mm, and the signal intensity is intermediate compared to that of skeletal muscle. Residual dissection (white arrow) is present in the descending aorta.

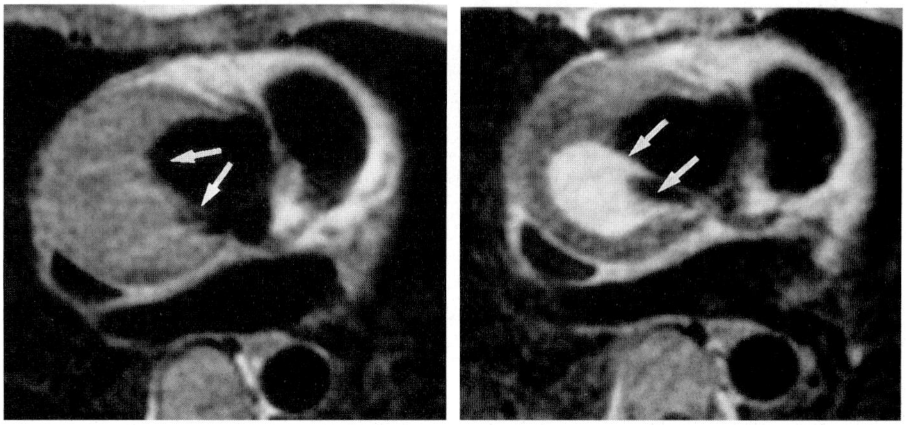

a. b.

Figure 6. **(a)** Nonenhanced and **(b)** contrast-enhanced axial spin-echo MR images (20/700) of ascending aorta and descending aorta at the anastomoses of the coronary arteries. **a** shows a wide perigraft collection (arrows) characterized by homogeneously low signal intensity. **b** shows high signal intensity at the site (arrows) of the left coronary arterial anastomosis, which helps identify the presence and origin of bleeding.

lin, Germany; 0.2 mmol per kilogram of body weight) via a catheter placed in a vein in the antecubital fossa.

RESULTS

In all patients, a fair to good image quality was achieved (43 good; nine, fair). The diameter of composite grafts ranged from 28 to 37 mm (mean, 32.2 mm ± 2.8 [SD]). No abnormality of the distal anastomosis was observed. The proximal segment of both coronary vessels was visualized in 48 patients; only one coronary artery was visualized in four patients. In 47 patients, the diameter of the coronary artery was normal (range, 6–10 mm). Slight to moderate dilatation of reimplanted coronary ostia (range, 11–16 mm) was observed with the classic Bentall technique in five patients with Marfan syndrome (Fig 4).

Forty-two patients had perigraft thickening of less than 10 mm. The area of perigraft thickening was isointense to skeletal muscle. As described in previous articles (6,11), perigraft thickening up to 10 mm, attributable to fibrosis, normal granulation tissue, or both, is the most common postoperative MR finding (Fig 5). Ten patients had perigraft thickening of more than 10 mm (range, 15–52 mm). On spin-echo images, the signal intensity of the thickening was homogeneously intermediate in eight patients, and the thickening was isointense but not homogeneous, with some areas of flow void, in the other two. After injection of gadopentetate dimeglumine, five of the 10 patients with abnormal perigraft thickening showed a marked increase in signal intensity. Enhancement was concentric around the graft in two patients. In the remaining three, enhancement appeared to be localized to the site of the reimplanted coronary arteries (Fig 6), which is indicative of bleeding that originates from the coronary ostial sutures. The lack of enhancement excluded the presence of bleeding in the remaining five patients (three with chronic hematomas, one with infection, and one with granulation tissue). Gradient-echo sequences did not conclusively demonstrate flow inside any of the collections owing to the artifact of the prosthetic valve.

Among patients who showed enhancement with gadopentetate dimeglumine, four underwent successful repeat surgery. One patient was unable to undergo surgery because his general clinical condition was poor. At surgery, the site of suture detachment (reimplanted coronary arteries in two patients and paravalvular suture lines causing a false aneurysm in the other two) was confirmed.

DISCUSSION

The underlying disease processes in patients referred for replacement of the ascending aorta represent a wide spectrum of conditions and acuity requiring different surgical strategies (10,12). Despite advances in surgical techniques that have substantially improved the survival rate over the years, follow-up data have documented the possible development of early and late complications (9). Most of the problems seen during long-term follow-up are due to the underlying disease process of the residual distal aorta, whereas early complications such as infection, suture dehiscence, or false aneurysm are mainly related to the prosthetic graft. Repeat surgery for bleeding at the site of repair has been reported in 8% of patients after 30 days and 4% of patients after 1 year.

The higher incidence of bleeding has been reported at the site of coronary arteries reimplanted according to classic Bentall technique (range, 4.2%–13.6%) (13–15). Moreover, aneurysmatic dilatation of the reimplanted coronary arteries may develop during long-term follow-up. For these reasons, this surgical procedure was modified (button technique) during the 1980s, particularly with regard to coronary arterial anastomosis to the prosthetic conduit, to avoid traction at the suture sites as a potential cause of bleeding.

There has also been controversy about the need to wrap the native aorta around the graft (2,9,16). Even though the wrapped wall may ensure better hemostasis and help avoid late sepsis, several reports describe a high incidence of false aneurysm formation. Our findings are in agreement with these data: False aneurysms were seen in two patients treated with the classic Bentall technique and none of the patients treated with button and Cabrol techniques (Fig 7). The largest surgical series (9) we know of that compares early and long-term survival among the most common methods used for composite valve graft replacement shows no substantial differences in perioperative bleeding, thus encouraging elimination of the wrapping procedure.

In our series, two patients treated with the button technique had a hematoma. In both cases, the suture detachment was not related to the surgical technique but was due to an inflammatory process (one patient had a Behçet aortitis and the other had a long-standing mediastinitis). The three cases of chronic hematoma were observed in patients treated with the Bentall technique before the introduction of the preclotting technique (the graft is impregnated with collagen or human serum albumin to control transgraft blood loss, therefore eliminating the need for inclusion techniques and their associated complications) (Fig 8) (17). This type of hematoma was reported in the first series of patients who underwent the Bentall operation but is not clinically relevant because it is not an evolving lesion.

Results of several studies have documented the superior performance of MR imaging in the evaluation of the thoracic aorta (5–7). This technique is able to provide multiplanar depiction of the aortic lumen and wall along with mediastinal structures; moreover, its reproducibility and noninvasive nature are optimal characteristics during the follow-up. In our series, spin-echo MR images enabled excellent visualization of the proximal portion of the reimplanted coronary arteries.

Dacron graft obstruction and thrombosis may be responsible for late sudden death observed during long-term follow-up after the Cabrol operation (9,18). In our three patients treated with the Cabrol technique, we did not detect any alteration in the anastomotic tube or in the proximal part of coronary arteries, whereas moderate dilatation of both reimplanted coronary arteries was present in five patients treated with the Bentall technique. Four of these five patients underwent three subsequent MR examinations at 1, 2, and 3 years: No substantial modification in diameters was visualized. Dilatation of the reimplanted coronary ostia after the classic Bentall operation has been reported (14), particularly in patients with Marfan syndrome, as a result of abnormal tension forces applied to a diseased wall. Even though this alteration does not seem to be clinically relevant, to our knowledge, results of imaging follow-up have not been reported. When we consider the young age of most of the patients undergoing composite valve graft replacement and the actual better survival rate, noninvasive monitoring of the reimplanted coronary arteries might be recommended.

Repeat surgery in patients with a composite valve graft has a high risk, and precise details, such as the identification of bleeding or the exact site of suture dehiscence, are necessary for a correct surgical approach. Nevertheless, the presence of a collection does not necessarily indicate bleeding. Perigraft thickening of less than 10 mm appears to be a normal postoperative appearance. Gaubert et al (11) analyzed the MR imaging aspect of 36 surgically treated aortic dissections and found perigraft thickening of less than 10 mm in 23 cases and perigraft thickening of up to 10 mm in 13 cases (nine false aneurysms). On MR images, normal granulation or fibrous tissue is hypo- to isointense compared with skeletal muscle. The distribution is usually uniform and concentric around the ascending aortic graft (11), whereas pathologic collections are often asymmetric (Fig 9).

Because of the possible different causes of perigraft thickening, it is important to differentiate this entity from other pathologic collections. On the basis of the signal intensity on spin-echo images, the differential diagnosis can be difficult because of the interaction of the different degradation compounds of hemoglobin that may result in variable signal intensity. Furthermore, in a periprosthetic hemorrhage collection, different aged foci can easily coexist.

Perigraft flow, outside the graft but contained within the wrapped aneurysmal sac, as in a false aneurysm, shows perigraft areas of signal void on spin-echo images or marked changes in signal intensity throughout the cardiac cycle on cine gradient-echo images. Gradient-echo sequences can enable visualization of moving blood between two different compartments, similar to angiography or Doppler echocardiography. Nevertheless, if the suture dehiscence is small, the flow could be too limited to be depicted with such techniques, as happened in three of our patients. Even though the bleeding was small in the five patients with bleeding in our study, a large, growing hematoma contained in the periaortic space was present and possibly evolved into graft compression and rupture. In our experience, gadolinium-enhanced MR imaging enabled us to diagnose suture detachment, which necessitated urgent repeat

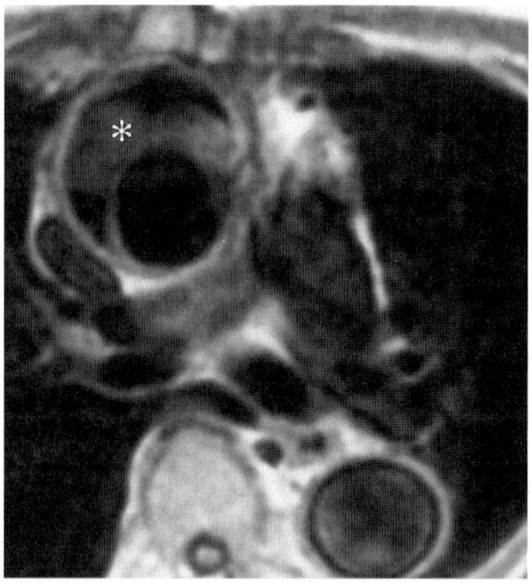

a.

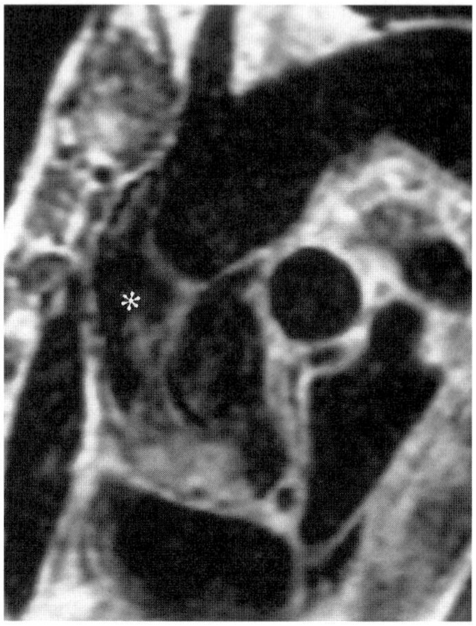

b.

Figure 7. **(a)** Axial spin-echo MR image (20/800) of ascending aorta replaced with the classic Bentall technique and wrapping of the native aortic wall. A false aneurysm (*) is seen surrounding the prosthetic ascending aorta. **(b)** Sagittal oblique spin-echo MR image (20/800) of the same case shows extension of the false aneurysm (*) to the distal anastomosis.

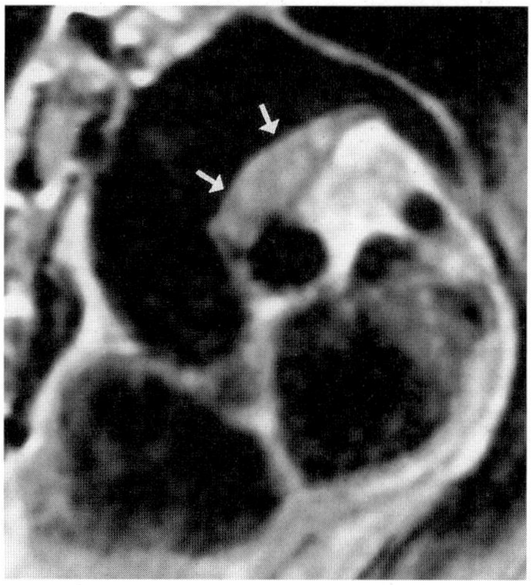

Figure 8. Sagittal spin-echo MR image (20/600) shows asymmetric perigraft thickening (arrows) with heterogeneous signal intensity due to chronic hematoma.

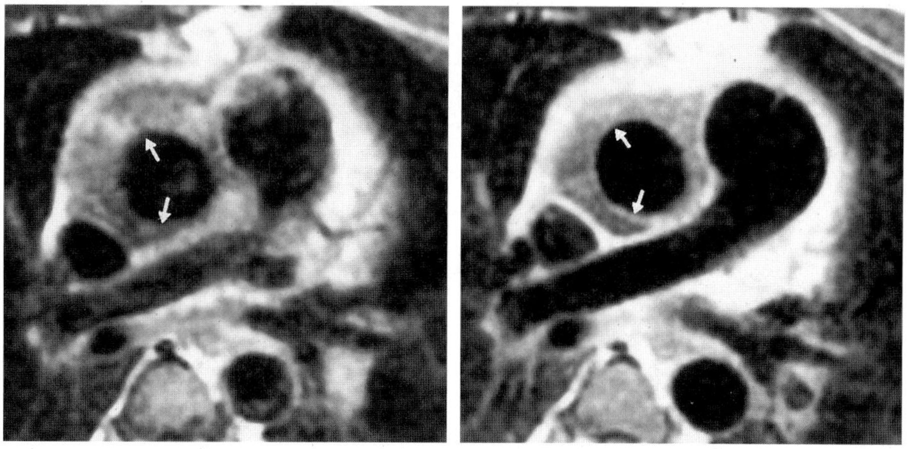

a. b.

Figure 9. **(a)** Axial nonenhanced spin-echo MR image (20/730) of the ascending aorta replaced with the button technique in a patient with a prosthetic collection (arrows), which is 18 mm thick. **(b)** Contrast-enhanced image demonstrates a minimal, insubstantial increase in signal intensity (arrows).

surgery. It clearly depicted the site of bleeding as an area of high signal intensity within the organized hematoma. Furthermore, it enabled us to define the bleeding site, clearly depicting the relationship with the reimplanted coronary artery.

In conclusion, routine follow-up studies with MR imaging should be recommended in all patients with composite graft replacement of the ascending aorta. MR imaging helped define the morphologic characteristics of the prosthetic graft and the anastomotic sites. The possibility of achieving a noninvasive evaluation of the proximal segment of reimplanted coronary arteries may be clinically relevant in long-term survival. Moreover, gadolinium-enhanced MR imaging can clearly help identify hemorrhagic complications, which represent a potential asymptomatic cause of death.

Acknowledgment: The authors are indebted to Albert de Roos, MD, for providing a critical review of the manuscript.

References

1. Bentall H, De Bono A. A technique for complete replacement of ascending aorta. Thorax 1968; 23:338–339.
2. Kouchoukos NT, Marshall WG, Wedige-Stecher TA. Eleven-year experience with composite graft replacement of the ascending aorta and aortic valve. Thorac Cardiovasc Surg 1986; 92:691–705.
3. Midulla PS, Ergin A, Galla J, et al. Three faces of the Bentall procedure. J Cardiovasc Surg 1994; 9:466–481.
4. Svensson LG. Approach to the insertion of composite valve graft. Ann Thorac Surg 1992; 54:376–378.
5. Nienaber CA, von Kodolitsch Y, Nicolas V, et al. The diagnosis of thoracic aortic dissection by noninvasive imaging procedures. N Engl J Med 1993; 328:1–9.
6. Lepore V, Lamm C, Bugge M, Larsson S. Magnetic resonance imaging in the follow-up of patients after aortic root reconstruction. Thorac Cardiovasc Surg 1996; 44:188–192.
7. Fattori R, Celletti F, Bertaccini P, et al. Delayed surgery of traumatic aortic rupture: role of magnetic resonance imaging. Circulation 1996; 94:2865–2870.
8. De Paepe A, Devereux RB, Dietz HC, Hannekam M, Pyeritz RE. Revised diagnostic criteria for the Marfan syndrome. Am J Med Genet 1996; 62:417–426.
9. Svensson LG, Crawford ES, Hess KR, et al. Composite graft replacement of the proximal aorta: comparison of techniques in 348 patients. Ann Thorac Surg 1992; 54: 427–439.
10. Cabrol C, Pavie A, Mesnildrey P, et al. Long-term result with total replacement of the ascending aorta and reimplantation of the coronary arteries. J Thorac Cardiovasc Surg 1986; 91:17–25.
11. Gaubert JY, Moulin G, Mesana T, et al. Type A dissection of the thoracic aorta: use of MR imaging for long-term follow-up. Radiology 1995; 196:363–369.
12. Bachet J, Termignon JL, Goudot B, et al. Aortic root replacement with a composite graft: factors influencing immediate and long-term results. Eur J Cardiothorac Surg 1996; 10:207–213.
13. Taniguchi K, Nakano S, Matsuda H, et al. Long-term survival and complication after composite graft replacement for ascending aortic aneurysm associated with aortic regurgitation. Circulation 1991; 84(suppl 3):31–39.
14. Svensson LG, Crawford ES, Coselli JS, Safi HJ, Hess KR. The impact of cardiovascular operation on survival in the Marfan patient. Circulation 1989; 80(suppl 1):233–242.
15. Coselli JS, Crawford ES. Composite valve graft replacement of aortic root using separate Dacron tube for coronary reattachment. Ann Thorac Surg 1989; 47:558–565.
16. Crawford ES, Svensson LG, Coselli JS, Safi HJ, Hess KR. Surgical treatment of aneurysm and/or dissection of the ascending aorta, transverse aortic arch, and ascending aorta and transverse aortic arch. J Thorac Cardiovasc Surg 1989; 98:659–674.
17. Savunen T, Inberg M, Niinikoski J, Rantakokko V, Vanttinen E. Composite graft in annulo-aortic ectasia: nineteen years' experience without graft inclusion. Eur J Cardiothorac Surg 1996; 10:428–432.
18. Sekine S, Tadaaki A, Keiji S, Shibata Y, Yamagishi I, Kamada M. Dacron coronary graft obstruction after composite graft replacement of aortic root. Ann Thorac Surg 1995; 60:1123–1126.

Matthias Stuber, PhD
René M. Botnar, PhD
Peter G. Danias, MD, PhD
Kraig V. Kissinger, BS, RT
Warren J. Manning, MD

Index terms:
Coronary vessels, MR, 54.121416, 54.12142
Heart, MR, 54.12142
Magnetic resonance (MR), motion correction
Magnetic resonance (MR), vascular studies, 54.121416, 54.12142

Radiology 1999; 212:579–587

Abbreviations:
CNR = contrast-to-noise ratio
LAD = left anterior descending coronary artery
LCX = left circumflex coronary artery
LM = left main coronary artery
LV = left ventricle
RCA = right coronary artery
SNR = signal-to-noise ratio
2D = two-dimensional
3D = three-dimensional

[1] From the Cardiovascular Division, Beth Israel Deaconess Medical Center and Harvard Medical School, 330 Brookline Ave, Boston, MA 02215 (M.S., R.M.B., P.G.D., K.V.K., W.J.M.), and Philips Medical Systems, Best, the Netherlands (M.S., R.M.B.). Received August 17, 1998; revision requested September 22; revision received October 19; accepted January 20, 1999. **Address reprint requests to** M.S. (e-mail: *mstuber@caregroup.harvard.edu*).

Author contributions:
Guarantor of integrity of entire study, W.J.M.; study concepts and design, M.S.; definition of intellectual content, M.S.; literature search, M.S.; experimental studies, M.S.; data acquisition, K.V.K.; data analysis, R.M.B.; statistical analysis, M.S.; manuscript preparation and editing, M.S.; manuscript review, P.G.D.

Submillimeter Three-dimensional Coronary MR Angiography with Real-time Navigator Correction: Comparison of Navigator Locations[1]

Three-dimensional free-breathing coronary magnetic resonance angiography was performed in eight healthy volunteers with use of real-time navigator technology. Images acquired with the navigator localized at the right hemidiaphragm and at the left ventricle were objectively compared. The diaphragmatic navigator was found to be superior for vessel delineation of middle to distal portions of the coronary arteries.

Coronary artery disease remains a leading cause of morbidity and mortality. As the majority of the clinically important stenoses are located in the proximal regions of the coronary arteries (1), an accurate noninvasive technique that allows assessment of these proximal segments would be of great value. Breath-hold two-dimensional (2D) coronary magnetic resonance (MR) angiography has been shown to be a promising approach (2–5). However, three-dimensional (3D) methods have inherent advantages (6–8). Unfortunately, high-spatial-resolution 3D coronary MR angiography is still methodologically and technically challenging due to prolonged acquisition times. A major limitation is compensation for the highly complex motion pattern of the heart related to normal respiration. If no motion-compensation strategies are applied, severe artifacts result in image degradation. Compensation for respiratory motion can be achieved with breath holding (4,9,10) or coached breathing patterns (11–13). Breath holds are limited in duration, substantial patient cooperation is required (14), and diaphragmatic drift is frequently observed during prolonged breath-hold periods. Therefore, approaches to prolong the breath-hold duration (14–16) are likely not practical for clinical use. Coached breathing patterns still require patient cooperation.

Removal of the time constraints of breath holding would allow 3D imaging and offer the option for improved spatial resolution (7,17–20) and enhanced clinical applicability. A very powerful method for this is the application of MR navigator techniques that allow signal sampling during free breathing (21–25). The real-time navigator motion-correction method has been shown to be useful for 2D techniques (21,26,27), but no 3D approaches have been reported, to our knowledge. Navigators with gating and real-time motion correction result in reduced partial volume effect, increased navigator efficiency, and therefore shortened imaging times when compared to those with gating-only methods (26,27).

The most obvious interface for navigator monitoring of the respiratory level is the lung and the right hemidiaphragm (23–31). However, diaphragmatic and coronary motion may not be linearly related (28). Therefore, a model that incorporates the relationship between diaphragmatic motion and coronary displacement may be used for real-time motion-correction techniques. For coronary MR angiography, positioning of the navigator at the base of the anterior wall of the left ventricle (LV) may therefore be advantageous, given the proximity of this region to the proximal coronary arteries. Although MR navigators that use interceptional planes suffer from the disadvantage that magnetization voids occur in the region of interest (31,32), navigators that use 2D selective-excitation pulses (33–36) allow use of a shallow flip angle without compromise of the magnetization for subsequent imaging. This approach allows a real-time 2D selective navigator to be applied for gating and correction directly at the base of the heart.

In the present study, a navigator for gating and real-time motion correction was extended with a high-spatial-resolution 3D sequence for free-breathing coronary MR angiography. Results obtained with the navigator at the basal LV free wall are compared to those with the more conventional approach, in which the navigator is positioned at the dome of the right hemidiaphragm. Quantitative assessment was performed of the sharpness of the vessel boundaries, signal-to-noise ratio (SNR), and contrast-to-noise ratio (CNR) on the coronary MR angiograms.

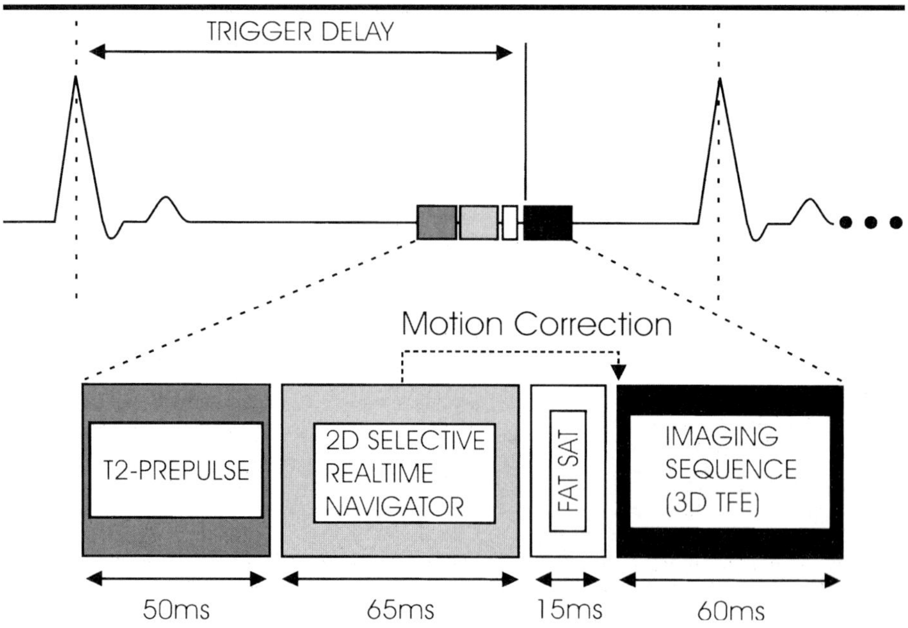

Figure 1. Schematic depicts the pulse sequence for 3D MR coronary angiography based on prospective navigator gating and real-time motion correction. The elements of the sequence (T2 prepulse, navigator, fat-saturation [*FAT SAT*] prepulse, and the 3D segmented-k-space gradient-echo [*TFE*] sequence) are shown in temporal relationship to the electrocardiogram and the trigger delay.

Materials and Methods

Subjects

Eight healthy adult volunteers (five men, three women; mean age, 25 years ± 10 [SD]) who were in sinus rhythm and did not have contradictions to MR imaging were studied. Written informed consent was obtained from all participants, and the research protocol was approved by the hospital committee on clinical investigation.

Sequence for 3D Coronary MR Angiography

Three-dimensional coronary MR angiography with real-time navigator gating and motion correction was implemented on a commercially available 1.5-T whole-body system (ACS-NT Gyroscan; Philips Medical Systems, Best, the Netherlands) equipped with a cardiac research patch software (CPR5) and a prototypic gradient system (PowerTrak 3000 [15 mT/m, 300-μsec rise time]) and six parallel digital receiver channels. For signal acquisition, a prototypic five-element cardiac phased-array coil with three rigid posterior elements and two flexible anterior elements was used. Each coil element is equipped with a separate preamplifier. The signals of the individual coil elements are combined as the square root of the sum of squares. A flow-insensitive T2 preparation sequence was applied (37–40) before the imaging part of the sequence. With this preparation of the magnetization, differences in the natural T2 of arterial blood (50 msec) and myocardial muscle (223 msec) can be used for contrast enhancement (38).

An electrocardiography-gated, fat-suppressed, 3D segmented-k-space gradient-echo sequence (Turbo Field Echo; Philips Medical Systems) with a repetition time of 7.4 msec and an echo time of 2.4 msec (7.4/2.4) was used. In Figure 1, the order of the sequence elements is displayed. The T2 preparation sequence (38) for contrast enhancement (echo time, 50 msec) is followed by the navigator excitation and postprocessing of the navigator data, the spectral-selective (chemical shift, 120° excitation) fat-saturation pulse, and the segmented-k-space gradient-echo sequence. The T2 preparation sequence involves a train of six nonselective composite radio-frequency pulses with corresponding radio-frequency pulse angles of 90°, 180°, 180°, −180°, −180°, and −90° (38). The excitation angle for the fat-saturation pulse was 110° to allow sampling of the center of k space at the zero crossing of the longitudinal magnetization, or M_z, of fat.

A reduction in flow artifacts on the images as induced by long echo times was achieved by means of partial Fourier sampling. Hereby, only 62.5% of the k space was sampled in the readout direction (partial echo). A 3-cm-thick 3D volume was imaged in the axial plane, with 20 3.0-mm-thick overlapping sections. During reconstruction, 20 1.5-mm-thick sections were calculated by means of interpolation. Hereby, through-plane zero filling was applied in the k space prior to the Fourier transform. A field of view of 360 mm and a matrix of 512 × 360 yielded an in-plane resolution of 0.7 × 1.0 mm. Eight phase-encoding steps were sampled during each cardiac cycle (acquisition window, 60 msec). The k space was sampled by means of centric ordering with priority for the low-k_y profiles. One signal was averaged, and no flow-compensating gradients were used. With a heart rate of 60 beats per minute, this would result in a total imaging time of 8 minutes 30 seconds.

The sequence was delayed with respect to the R wave of the electrocardiogram. The trigger delay (T_d) was adjusted to sample the low-k_y profiles in middle diastole and was defined according to the following equations (heart rate is measured in beats per minute): $t_{RR} = (1{,}000 \times 60)$/heart rate, and $T_d = [(t_{RR} - 350) \times 0.3] + 350$, where t_{RR} refers to the time delay between two subsequent R waves.

This definition takes advantage of the relatively constant duration of the systolic part of the cardiac cycle (~350 msec) (41).

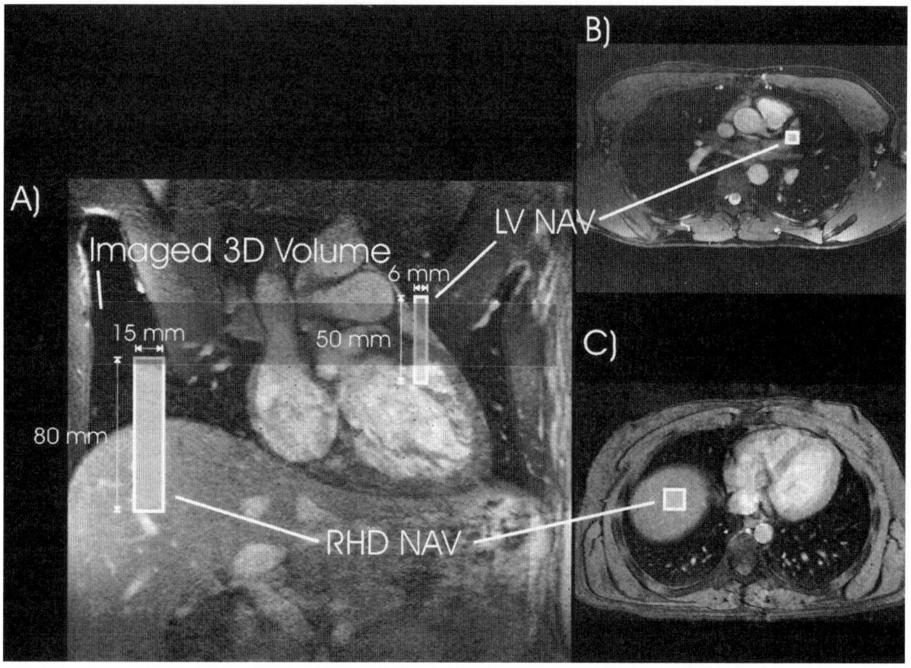

Figure 2. MR angiograms *A*, (coronal, 6.4/1.6) and *B* and *C*, (transverse, 11/1.8) depict planning of the position of the 3D volume, the navigator (kernel) at the dome of the right hemidiaphragm (*RHD NAV* in *A* and *C*) and the navigator at the free wall of the LV (*LV NAV* in *A* and *B*). All images were acquired with a segmented-k-space gradient-echo sequence.

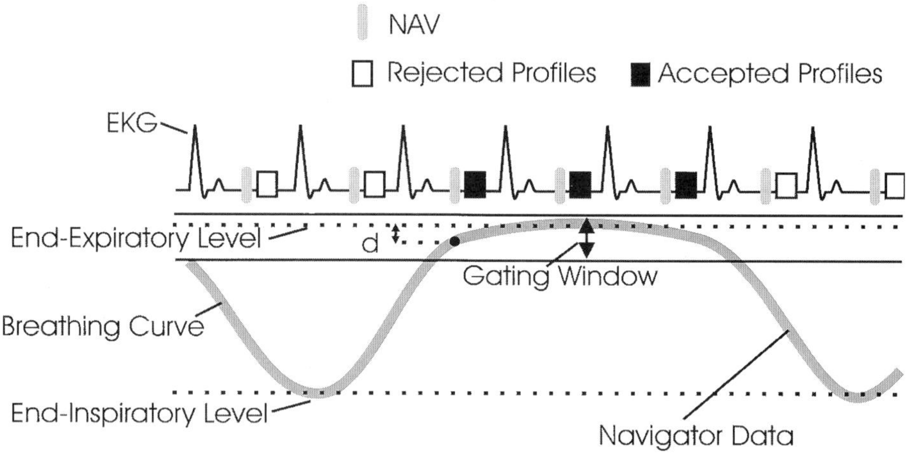

Figure 3. Schematic depicts navigator (*NAV*) gating and motion correction simultaneously with the electrocardiogram (*EKG*) and breathing curve. Profiles are accepted for reconstruction only if the position of the moving interface detected by the navigator is located within the gating window. Adaptation or correction of the measured volume is related to the distance (*d*) from the end-expiratory level (as defined by the reference kernel) to the detected interface position. Real-time motion correction is performed prospectively only if the position of the measured interface is within the gating window.

Navigator Technique

The navigator used a 2D selective excitation in which 256 data points were sampled along the longitudinal axis of the navigator beam with a spatial resolution of 1 mm. After the readout, the sampled signal was Fourier transformed and cross correlated with a reference navigator profile that was acquired at end expiration during the preparation steps of the sequence. A user-selected portion of this reference navigator (kernel) (Fig 2) was used for cross correlation. The peak position of the cross correlation helps localize the actual position of the detected interface (17). If this location is within a user-defined range or gating window (Fig 3), the subsequently acquired profiles are accepted. Otherwise, they are rejected, and the same set of profiles are sampled again.

In addition to navigator gating, adaptive real-time motion correction of the imaged volume position was performed. Dependent on the navigator-determined interface position (within the gating window) (*d* in Fig 3), the position of the imaged volume (Fig 1) is adapted on a real-time basis. The implementation allows correction of the position of the measured volume in all three spatial components of the measurement, phase-encoding, and section-selective coordinate system. In the section-selective direction, this correction is achieved by changing the frequency of the section-selective radio-frequency excitation pulse in the sequence. For the correction of the measured volume in the measurement and phase-encoding directions, the mixing frequency and mixing phase of the demodulator were modified in real time. Thus, the position of the imaged 3D volume can be adapted prospectively for all three spatial coordinates. In the current study, correction of the imaged volume was performed in only the superoinferior direction. For the left coronary artery system, transverse sections were acquired. Thus, correction was performed in the section-selective direction. However, for the oblique sagittal view of the right coronary artery system, correction was performed in only the measurement direction.

For navigator definition of the desired interface, the diameter of the navigator has to be relatively small with respect to the interface surface. Therefore, a navigator with a freely adjustable diameter was implemented on the system. The current implementation allowed a diameter adjustment of 4–100 mm. The real-time navigator for gating and motion correction was applied at two locations—at the dome of the right hemidiaphragm and at the basal anterior wall of the LV (Fig 2, *A* [coronal] and *B* and *C* [transverse]). For both navigator locations, a navigator excitation angle of 30° was applied. Signal acquisition for the navigator readout was performed with use of the body coil.

Right hemidiaphragm navigator.—For the localized vertical right hemidiaphragm navigator, a diameter of 15 mm with a kernel length of 80 mm was used (Fig 2, *A* [coronal]). The gating window for the diaphragm was 5 mm, and a relationship of 0.6 (correction factor) was used between the superoinferior position of the diaphragm and the superoinferior position of the proximal coronary arteries (28).

Anterior LV navigator.—For the vertically oriented LV navigator, a 6-mm diameter was used (Fig 2, *A* [coronal] and *B* [transverse]). Since the anatomic location of the detected heart-lung interface is close to the proximal coronary arteries, a correction factor of 1.0 was used for motion correction. At the heart, a reduced maximal superoinferior displacement is expected when compared to that with the diaphragm (28). Therefore, the kernel length was reduced to 50 mm for the LV navigator, and a gating window of 3 mm was used.

For both navigator locations, the reference kernel was acquired at an end-expiratory position. For all measurements, the imaging efficiency, defined as the number of excitations accepted divided by the total number of R waves detected during the measurement, was recorded. For example, an imaging efficiency of 50% refers to an acquisition in which on average, the k_y profiles of every other heartbeat are accepted.

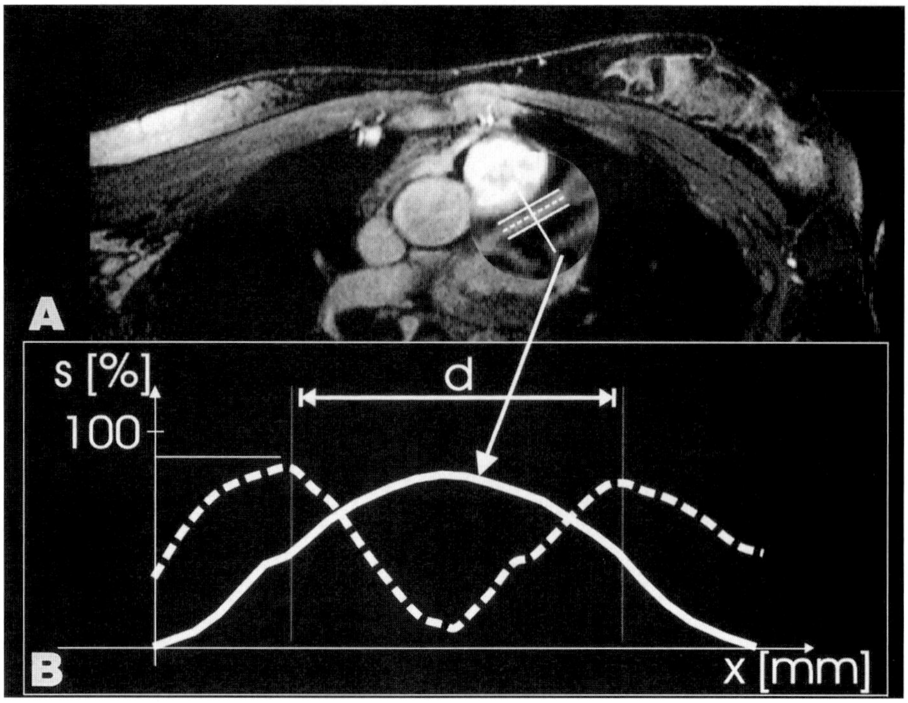

Figure 4. Semiautomatic evaluation of coronary segments. *A*, Transverse unfiltered MR angiogram (7.4/2.4) was acquired with a free-breathing, navigator-gated and motion-corrected, 3D T2 preparation, segmented-k-space gradient-echo sequence. *B*, Filtered image. The centerline on the vessel (dashed line in *A*) is defined by the user. The edges (solid lines) and vessel diameters (*d* in *B*) are automatically calculated by means of the Deriche algorithm. In *B*, local maximum values (dashed line) perpendicular to the centerlines define the sharpness (*s*) of the vessel walls.

Protocol

All subjects were examined in the supine position with electrocardiography leads on the anterior left hemithorax. All images (including the scout images) were acquired during free breathing. To localize the coronary arteries and position the navigator, two scout images were obtained. The first scout image (11/1.8) was an electrocardiography-triggered, non–fat-suppressed, multisection 2D segmented-k-space gradient-echo image with 10 transverse, 10 coronal, and 10 sagittal sections of the thorax, which allowed definition of the basal LV borders. Transverse, sagittal, and coronal sections were interleaved during acquisition of the same image. The field of view was 450 mm with a matrix of 256 data points. On these images, the navigator position at the base of the LV was planned for the second scout image.

For this second scout image (6.4/1.6), the data were acquired in diastole (2). Ten contiguous coronal 2D sections were acquired during free breathing by using a navigator-gated and motion-corrected, electrocardiography-triggered, non–fat-suppressed, segmented-k-space gradient-echo sequence. The field of view was 350 mm, and the image matrix included 256 data points in the measurement direction. Image data were acquired in the partial Fourier mode. The navigator for this second scout image was positioned at the anterior free wall of the LV. Navigator parameters included a 30° 2D selective excitation angle, a navigator diameter of 6 mm, a kernel length of 50 mm, a navigator window of 5.0 mm, and a superoinferior correction factor of 1.0 (28). In the second scout images, the dome of the right hemidiaphragm, the lateral free wall of the LV, and the left main coronary artery (LM) can be identified at an end-expiratory position (Fig 2, *A* [coronal]). The position of the LV navigator, the right hemidiaphragm navigator, and the location of the 3D volume for high-spatial-resolution coronary MR angiography were planned on the second scout images, with the center of the 3D volume positioned at the superoinferior position of the LM.

Coronary MR angiography of both right and left coronary arteries were acquired with (*a*) a navigator positioned at the dome of the right hemidiaphragm and (*b*) a navigator at the base of the LV free wall. For both navigator positions, transverse 3D volumes including the LM, the proximal and middle left anterior descending coronary artery (LAD), left circumflex coronary artery (LCX), and the proximal part of the right coronary artery (RCA) were imaged. For imaging of more distal parts of the RCA, another 3D image with a single oblique sagittal orientation was obtained for both navigator locations. This image was planned on the basis of findings on the transverse coronary MR angiograms. To avoid bias, the four images were obtained in random order.

Evaluation

For a quantitative assessment of image quality and contrast between the coronary segments and myocardial muscle or fat, an algorithm for edge detection as proposed by Deriche (42) was implemented on a personal computer (Red Hat 4.2; Linux, Durham, NC).

In a first step, the LAD, LCX, and RCA were manually identified by one author (M.S.) by drawing a centerline on the vessels (Fig 4, dashed line in *A*) of the unfiltered ×4 zoomed anatomic images. No adaptation of window or level was performed. In a second step, the Deriche algorithm, which combines low-pass filtering for noise reduction and high-pass filtering for edge detection, was applied

Results with Each Navigator Location

Coronary Artery Segment and Parameter	LV Navigator	Right Hemidiaphragm Navigator	Significance of Difference*
Sharpness (%)			
LAD	59.7 ± 2.6	63.2 ± 2.8	$P < .05$
RCA			
Proximal	53.3 ± 4.1	58.1 ± 4.1	NS
Distal	49.8 ± 2.4	57.3 ± 3.2	$P < .05$
LCX	53.1 ± 2.5	59.1 ± 3.0	NS
Diameter (mm)			
LAD	3.7 ± 0.1	3.5 ± 0.1	NS
RCA			
Proximal	3.8 ± 0.2	3.8 ± 0.2	NS
Distal	2.5 ± 0.1	2.3 ± 0.1	NS
LCX	2.4 ± 0.1	2.4 ± 0.1	NS
Parameter			
Imaging efficiency (%)	53.5 ± 5.7	57.3 ± 2.1	NS
SNR of blood at level of LM in ascending aorta	7.9 ± 0.2	7.7 ± 0.3	NS
SNR of myocardium of LV at level of proximal RCA	3.9 ± 0.2	3.6 ± 0.2	NS
SNR in front of chest at level of LM	1.1 ± 0.1	1.1 ± 0.1	NS
CNR between blood and myocardial muscle	4.8 ± 0.2	4.8 ± 0.2	NS

Note.—Data are the mean ± SEM.
* NS = not significant (Student *t* test).

to the zoomed images. On these edge-enhanced filtered images, maximum values near the centerline (constrained by full width at half maximum, or FWHM, of the raw images) were then automatically determined with the algorithm (Fig 4, *B*). These maximum values delineate the vessel borders and can be used to identify the vessel diameter (Fig 4). In addition, these values represent the sharpness of the vessel boundaries with respect to their environment. A sharpness of 100% refers to a maximum change in signal intensity in two adjacent pixels (full dynamic range on the image). This evaluation procedure was applied to all the acquired 3D data sets. Equal segments of the LAD, LCX, proximal RCA, and distal RCA were evaluated and compared for both navigator locations.

Image artifacts due to respiratory motion associated with chest wall motion as induced by unreliable navigator gating and correction can be identified as unexpected structures in front of the chest wall (in air). Therefore, the SNR is defined as SI_{mean}/SD_{mean}, where SI is signal intensity in the user-defined region of interest. The SNR was determined (at the level where the LM is best seen on the transverse images of the left coronary artery system) in front of the chest wall.

At the same level, the SNR was also quantified in the ascending aorta. The SNR of the muscle signal intensity was determined in the muscle of the LV anterolateral wall at the level of the proximal RCA. The CNR between blood and muscle was defined as $(SI_{blood} - SI_{muscle})/[0.5(SD_{muscle} + SD_{blood})]$, where all values are means.

For 3D reconstruction of the coronary arteries, the images were transferred to a commercially available workstation (EasyVision; Philips Medical Systems), on which three orthogonal sections through the 3D data set can be displayed. Interactively, the user navigates on these orthogonal planes through the entire 3D data set. The LM, LAD, LCX, and RCA were manually identified in all three displayed planes. The 3D pathway of the coronary arteries was then reformatted and depicted in one plane.

Statistical Analysis

All values are presented as the mean plus or minus SEM. Comparisons were made by means of a paired Student *t* test. In all cases, a two-tailed test was performed. *P* values of .05 or less were considered statistically significant.

Results

MR studies were completed without complications in all subjects. The LM could be reliably identified in all cases on the second scout image. For all of the 3D data sets, high values were measured for coronary artery sharpness (Table). For the LAD, LCX, and proximal RCA, sharpness of the vessel boundaries exceeded 50% for both navigator locations.

On images of the distal RCA acquired with the LV navigator, the sharpness was slightly less than 50% (differences not significant vs at other sites). For the LAD and the distal RCA, significantly sharper edges ($P < .05$) were found on the images acquired with the navigator at the right hemidiaphragm. No significant navigator-position–dependent difference was found for the proximal RCA and the LCX, although there was a trend for both to be more clearly depicted with the right hemidiaphragm navigator.

The vessel diameters for the LV navigator and the right hemidiaphragm navigator are shown in the Table. Navigator position resulted in no significant difference in diameter measurements for the proximal LAD, proximal LAD, distal RCA, or LCX.

For both navigator locations, the imaging efficiency of completed images exceeded 50% (Table) and was not significantly different. Average total imaging duration for both navigator locations was 16 minutes. In two cases, imaging was stopped due to the efficiency constraints given by the protocol. In the first case, with the navigator at the right hemidiaphragm, the imaging efficiency was below 20% for more than 3 minutes. In the second case, with the LV navigator, the patient moved and the detected interface between the lung and heart was no longer within the required window. In all completed images, there was excellent suppression of respiratory motion (Table, SNR in front of chest), and no evidence of image artifacts in the region of the LV navigator was seen on the images.

The SNR of muscle was markedly reduced when compared with that of the myocardium (CNR, ~5). This is a consequence of the T2 preparation sequence for contrast enhancement that additionally suppresses deoxygenated venous blood. No navigator-position–dependent change in SNR or CNR was found (Table).

In Figure 5, representative samples are shown from different transverse anatomic levels in different volunteers. The images in the top row were acquired with the LV navigator and in the bottom row with the right hemidiaphragm navigator. Consistent with the quantitative results, different parts of the coronary arteries were delineated equally well with both navigator locations. No navigator-position–dependent change in SNR or CNR was seen on the images, and respiratory artifacts were suppressed equally well.

In Figure 6, 3D off-line planar reformatted coronary arteries reconstructed from the acquired 3D volumes are shown. In the left

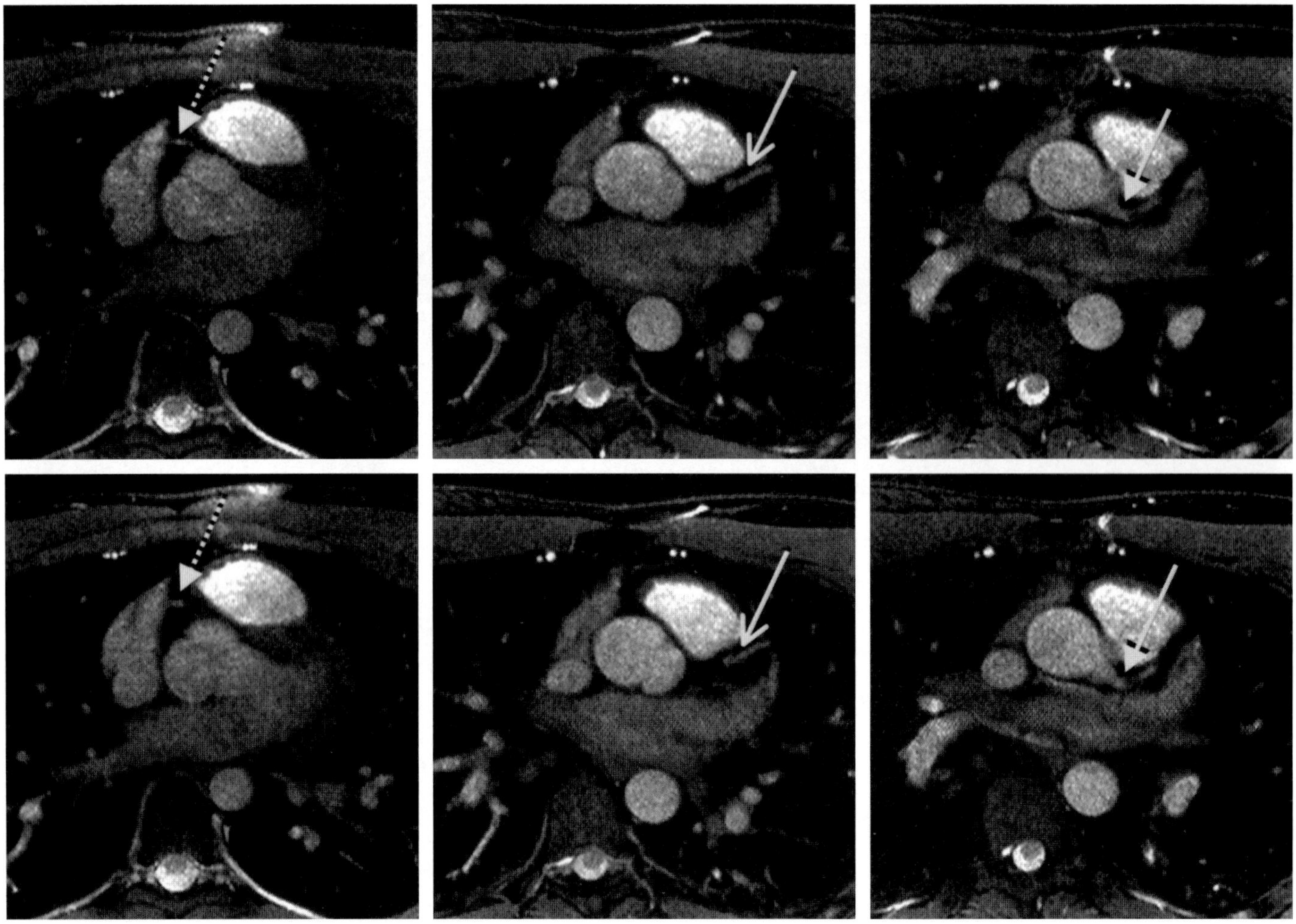

Figure 5. Sample transverse MR angiograms (7.4/2.4) were obtained in three volunteers, with a navigator at the LV free wall (top row) and at the dome of the right hemidiaphragm (bottom row). All images were acquired with a free-breathing, navigator-gated and motion corrected, 3D T2 preparation, segmented-k-space gradient-echo sequence. Left column, parts of the proximal RCA (arrow) are depicted. Middle column, a segment of the LAD (arrow) is present. Right column, the LM and a proximal segment of the LAD (arrow) can be seen.

column, images of the RCA obtained in the same volunteer with both navigator locations are compared. Long parts of the RCA are depicted on both images. In the middle column, a reformatted part of the LCX is displayed, and no major navigator-position–dependent differences are seen. In the right column, a long segment of the LAD is shown with similar image quality and anatomic information.

Discussion

Motion suppression with prospective real-time navigator gating and correction allows high-spatial-resolution 3D coronary MR angiography during free breathing. The sequence constraints given by patient cooperation or the limited duration of breath-hold intervals no longer apply. By removing the time constraints of breath holding, improved spatial resolution is allowed. Real-time adaptive correction also enables an increase in imaging efficiency, whereas image quality can be improved when compared to that with only gating (26,27). Blurring of stationary tissue may be expected as a result of the application of real-time motion correction. Still, minor blurring of sharp details in stationary tissue such as the anterior chest wall is seen on the images. This may be explained by the small superoinferior correction, which was only 3 mm for both navigator locations.

The use of a shallow flip angle and 2D selective navigator excitations is a distinct advantage, since they enabled positioning of the navigator at any arbitrary position. No magnetization in the region of interest was compromised, even though the navigator was positioned at the level of the imaged volume.

For both navigator locations, the objective measure for coronary artery sharpness exceeded 50%, indicating an excellent depiction of the coronary arteries in relation to myocardial muscle or epicardial fat. The relatively low SEM demonstrates a robust and reproducible image quality with either navigator location. This agrees with previously published results in 2D cases (43). In the case of the LV navigator position, geometric overlapping of the navigator and the imaged volume did not seem to affect the reliability of the navigator algorithm for suppression of respiratory motion. Imaging efficiency and, hence, imaging time were also not compromised by positioning the navigator at either location. It is important to note that use of the T2 preparation sequence (to suppress the signal of myocardial muscle and deoxygenated blood) (37,38) did not preclude use of this navigator technology.

Although navigator position close to

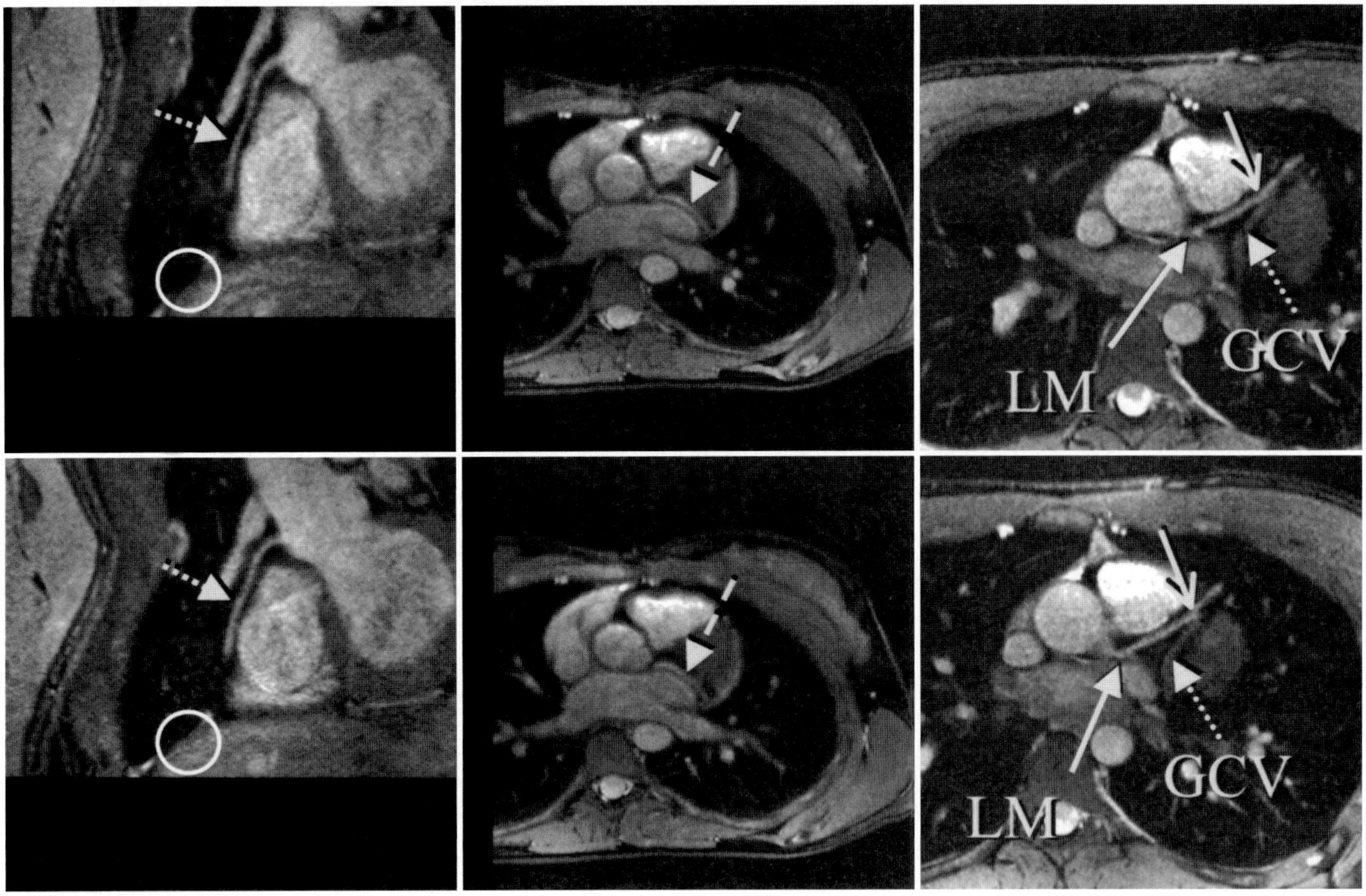

Figure 6. Three-dimensional reformatted segments of MR angiograms (7.4/2.4) acquired with a free-breathing, navigator-gated and motion-corrected, 3D T2 preparation, segmented-k-space gradient-echo sequence. Left column: Oblique sagittal images depict the RCA (arrow). Middle column: Transverse images depict the LCX (arrow). Right column: Transverse images depict the LM (long arrow), LAD (short arrow), and the great cardiac vein (*GCV*, dotted arrow). Top row: Images were acquired with an LV navigator. Bottom row: Images were acquired with a right hemidiaphragm navigator. A slight blurring of the lung-diaphragm interface (circle in left column) is seen with the LV navigator (top) as compared to depiction with the right hemidiaphragm navigator (bottom).

the coronary arteries is strategically appealing (no model function for correction has to be used), we found only minor quantitative differences in vessel sharpness, vessel diameter, CNR, SNR, or imaging time when comparing the right hemidiaphragm with the LV navigator positions. For the right hemidiaphragm navigator, vessel sharpness of the LAD and distal parts of the RCA was even slightly enhanced. The enhanced sharpness of the distal RCA may be related to the proximity of the right hemidiaphragm navigator to the distal part of the RCA. A basal LV navigator may not appropriately reflect breathing-induced motion of the distal RCA.

Considering the facilitated setup of the right hemidiaphragm navigator (navigator localization), our data suggest that a diaphragmatic navigator is preferable. These findings also confirm previously published results that suggest use of a constant correction factor of 0.6 for real-time motion correction (28). Even though this factor might be individually dependent, on average it seems to be a reliable value.

Future improvements in the LV navigator method may allow full advantage of the proximity to the coronary vessels. In the present study, a single vertically oriented navigator was applied, and only superoinferior correction of the imaged volume was performed. The breathing-induced anteroposterior, or left-right, displacement of the heart was neglected. Even though this displacement has been reported to be minor (28), further improvements may be expected with use of an oblique orientation of the cardiac navigator or multiple navigators that account for the breathing-induced 3D motion of the heart. But this remains to be studied. The SNR of the navigator signal is related to the diameter of the pencil beam that is excited. In the case of the LV navigator, the diameter of the beam needs to be small and, hence, a reduced SNR of the navigator signal results. This may have affected LV navigator performance.

In preparation for the present study, the sequences were optimized at imaging in a large number of healthy volunteers. It has turned out to be evident that plan imaging to position the navigator and the location of the imaged volume has to be performed under exactly the same conditions as the high-spatial-resolution 3D imaging; that is, plan imaging during free breathing with a consistent trigger delay and end-expiratory signal sampling is crucial. For the first scout image, no navigator gating or correction is possible since no image data for the localization of the lung-diaphragm or lung-heart interfaces is present. Thus, this first scout image needs to be obtained during free breathing. Despite some blurring of the lung-heart interface on the images, image quality in all cases was sufficient for appropriate localization of the navigator at the subsequent navigator-gated and motion-corrected coronal scout imaging.

By applying a short, 60-msec, acquisition window, cardiac-motion–induced blurring of the coronary arteries can be reduced to a minimum (40), the steady-state magnetization is potentially enhanced, and the T2 prepulses are more effective. In addition, a shortened acquisition window keeps the acquired profiles closer to the navigator, and therefore the sequence is less susceptible to residual breathing artifacts. Further improvements in SNR and CNR may be achieved by applying intravascular contrast agents (44), reordering the profiles in k space (45), or using alternative imaging strategies (6,46). Such approaches remain to be investigated further in combination with the present navigator technique.

In prior studies, visual comparisons, visual grading, or length and diameter determination have been applied successfully (7,10,18,31,47,48). However, such visual ratings may be of limited objectivity. The present computer-assisted image analysis allows objective assessment of vessel sharpness, diameter, SNR, and CNR. Thus, observer dependencies may be reduced, and the method is well suited for use in comparative studies in the field of coronary MR angiography.

In conclusion, free-breathing submillimeter 3D coronary MR angiography was successfully extended with real-time-navigator motion correction. The proximal and middle portions of the left and right native coronary artery system can be reliably depicted with both cardiac and diaphragmatic navigator locations, but the diaphragmatic navigator was objectively found to be superior for distal RCA visualization and LAD sharpness. Though an LV navigator may have theoretic advantages, the right hemidiaphragm navigator used for gating and real-time correction is at least as valuable as the LV navigator. Considering the easier setup for the right hemidiaphragm navigator (localization), we conclude that the use of a diaphragmatic navigator is currently preferred.

References

1. Zack PM, Chaitman BR, Davis KB, Kaiser GC, Wiens RD, Ng G. Survival patterns in clinical and angiographic subsets of medically treated patients with combined proximal left anterior descending and proximal left circumflex coronary artery disease (CASS). Am Heart J 1989; 118:220–227.
2. Manning WJ, Edelman RR. Magnetic resonance coronary angiography. Magn Reson Q 1993; 9:131–151.
3. Manning WJ, Li W, Boyle NG, Edelman RR. Fat-suppressed breath-hold magnetic resonance coronary angiography. Circulation 1993; 87:94–104.
4. Edelman RR, Manning WJ, Burstein D, Paulin S. Coronary arteries: breath-hold MR angiography. Radiology 1991; 181: 641–643.
5. Pennell DJ, Keegan J, Firmin DN, Gatehouse PD, Underwood SR, Longmore DB. Magnetic resonance imaging of coronary arteries: technique and preliminary results. Br Heart J 1993; 70:315–326.
6. Bornert P, Jensen D. Coronary artery imaging at 0.5 T using segmented 3D echo planar imaging. Magn Reson Med 1995; 34:779–785.
7. Li D, Kaushikkar S, Haacke EM, et al. Coronary arteries: three-dimensional MR imaging with retrospective respiratory gating. Radiology 1996; 201:857–863.
8. Wang Y, Rossman PJ, Grimm RC, Wilman AH, Riederer SJ, Ehman RL. 3D MR angiography of pulmonary arteries using real-time navigator gating and magnetization preparation. Magn Reson Med 1996; 36: 579–587.
9. Meyer CH, Hu BS, Nishimura DG, Macovski A. Fast spiral coronary artery imaging. Magn Reson Med 1992; 28:202–213.
10. Manning WJ, Li W, Edelman RR. A preliminary report comparing magnetic resonance coronary angiography with conventional angiography. N Engl J Med 1993; 328:828–832.
11. Doyle M, Scheidegger MB, de Graaf RG, Vermeulen J, Pohost GM. Coronary artery imaging in multiple 1-sec breath holds. Magn Reson Imaging 1993; 11:3–6.
12. Liu YL, Riederer SJ, Rossman PJ, Grimm RC, Debbins JP, Ehman RL. A monitoring, feedback, and triggering system for reproducible breath-hold MR imaging. Magn Reson Med 1993; 30:507–511.
13. Wang Y, Christy PS, Korosec FR, et al. Coronary MRI with a respiratory feedback monitor: the 2D imaging case. Magn Reson Med 1995; 33:116–121.
14. Gay SB, Sistrom CL, Holder CA, Suratt PM. Breath-holding capability of adults: implications for spiral computed tomography, fast-acquisition magnetic resonance imaging, and angiography. Invest Radiol 1994; 29:848–851.
15. Globits S, Sakuma H, Shimakawa A, Foo TK, Higgins CB. Measurement of coronary blood flow velocity during handgrip exercise using breath-hold velocity encoded cine magnetic resonance imaging. Am J Cardiol 1997; 79:234–237.
16. Goldfarb JW, Edelman RR. Coronary arteries: breath-hold, gadolinium-enhanced, three-dimensional MR angiography. Radiology 1998; 206:830–834.
17. Sachs TS, Meyer CH, Irarrazabal P, Hu BS, Nishimura DG, Macovski A. The diminishing variance algorithm for real-time reduction of motion artifacts in MRI. Magn Reson Med 1995; 34:412–422.
18. Hofman MB, Paschal CB, Li D, Haacke EM, van Rossum AC, Sprenger M. MRI of coronary arteries: 2D breath-hold vs 3D respiratory-gated acquisition. J Comput Assist Tomogr 1995; 19:56–62.
19. Post JC, van Rossum AC, Hofman MB, Valk J, Visser CA. Three-dimensional respiratory-gated MR angiography of coronary arteries: comparison with conventional coronary angiography. AJR 1996; 166: 1399–1404.
20. Muller MF, Fleisch M, Kroeker R, Chatterjee T, Meier B, Vock P. Proximal coronary artery stenosis: three-dimensional MRI with fat saturation and navigator echo. JMRI 1997; 7:644–651.
21. Ehman RL, Felmlee JP. Adaptive technique for high-definition MR imaging of moving structures. Radiology 1989; 173: 255–263.
22. Felmlee JP, Ehman RL, Riederer SJ, Korin HW. Adaptive motion compensation in MR imaging without use of navigator echoes. Radiology 1991; 179:139–142.
23. Sachs TS, Meyer CH, Hu BS, Kohli J, Nishimura DG, Macovski A. Real-time motion detection in spiral MRI using navigators. Magn Reson Med 1994; 32:639–645.
24. Fu ZW, Wang Y, Grimm RC, et al. Orbital navigator echoes for motion measurements in magnetic resonance imaging. Magn Reson Med 1995; 34:746–753.
25. Wang Y, Grimm RC, Felmlee JP, Riederer SJ, Ehman RL. Algorithms for extracting motion information from navigator echoes. Magn Reson Med 1996; 36:117–123.
26. McConnell MV, Khasgiwala VC, Savord BJ, et al. Prospective adaptive navigator correction for breath-hold MR coronary angiography. Magn Reson Med 1997; 37: 148–152.
27. Danias PG, McConnell MV, Khasgiwala VC, Chuang ML, Edelman RR, Manning WJ. Prospective navigator correction of image position for coronary MR angiography. Radiology 1997; 203:733–736.
28. Wang Y, Riederer SJ, Ehman RL. Respiratory motion of the heart: kinematics and the implications for the spatial resolution in coronary imaging. Magn Reson Med 1995; 33:713–719.
29. Danias PG, Stuber M, Kissinger KV. Relationship of cardiac and diaphragmatic respiratory motion assessed by real-time magnetic resonance imaging (abstr). In: Proceedings of the Sixth Meeting of the International Society for Magnetic Resonance in Medicine. Berkeley, Calif: International Society for Magnetic Resonance in Medicine, 1998; 721.
30. Taylor AM, Jhooti J, Firmin DN, Pennell DJ. Automated monitoring of diaphragm end-expiratory position for real-time navigator echo MR coronary angiography (abstr). In: Proceedings of the Sixth Meeting of the International Society for Magnetic Resonance in Medicine. Berkeley, Calif: International Society for Magnetic Resonance in Medicine, 1998; 21.
31. Wang Y, Rossman PJ, Grimm RC, Riederer SJ, Ehman RL. Navigator-echo-based real-time respiratory gating and triggering for reduction of respiration effects in three-dimensional coronary MR angiography. Radiology 1996; 198:55–60.
32. Haacke EM, Li D, Kaushikkar S. Cardiac MR imaging: principles and techniques. Top Magn Reson Imaging 1995; 7:200–217.
33. Hardy CJ, Pearlman JD, Moore JR, Roemer PB, Cline HE. Rapid NMR cardiography with a half-echo M-mode method. J Comput Assist Tomogr 1991; 15:868–874.
34. Hardy CJ, Darrow RD, Nieters EJ, et al. Real-time acquisition, display, and interactive graphic control of NMR cardiac pro-

files and images. Magn Reson Med 1993; 29:667–673.
35. Cline HE, Hardy CJ, Pearlman JD. Fast MR cardiac profiling with two-dimensional selective pulses. Magn Reson Med 1991; 17:390–401.
36. Takahashi A, Peters T. Compensation of multi-dimensional selective excitation pulses using measured k-space trajectories. Magn Reson Med 1995; 34:446–456.
37. Wright GA, Nishimura DG, Macovski A. Flow-independent magnetic resonance projection angiography. Magn Reson Med 1991; 17:126–140.
38. Brittain JH, Hu BS, Wright GA, Meyer CH, Macovski A, Nishimura DG. Coronary angiography with magnetization-prepared T2 contrast. Magn Reson Med 1995; 33: 689–696.
39. Brittain JH, Olcott EW, Szuba A, et al. Three-dimensional flow-independent peripheral angiography. Magn Reson Med 1997; 38:343–354.
40. Botnar RM, Stuber M, Kissinger KV, Danias PG, Manning WJ. T2 preparation prepulses for contrast enhancement in 3D-coronary MRA: implementation with real-time left ventricular navigator tracking (abstr). In: Proceedings of the Sixth Meeting of the International Society for Magnetic Resonance in Medicine. Berkeley, Calif: International Society for Magnetic Resonance in Medicine, 1998; 23.
41. Staffeld HF, Mertens HM, Gleichmann U. Influence of dynamic exercise and training on systolic time intervals in normals and patients with coronary heart disease. Z Kardiol 1978; 67:305–316. [German]
42. Deriche R. Fast algorithms for low-level vision. IEEE Trans Pattern Analysis Machine Intell 1990; 12:78–87.
43. McConnell MV, Khasgiwala VC, Savord BJ, et al. Comparison of respiratory suppression methods and navigator locations for MR coronary angiography. AJR 1997; 168:1369–1375.
44. Li D, Dolan RP, Walovitch RC, Lauffer RB. Three-dimensional MRI of coronary arteries using an intravascular contrast agent. Magn Reson Med 1998; 39:1014–1018.
45. Jhooti P, Keegan J, Gatehouse PD, et al. 3D coronary imaging with phase reordering for optimal scan efficiency (abstr). In: Proceedings of the Sixth Meeting of the International Society for Magnetic Resonance in Medicine. Berkeley, Calif: International Society for Magnetic Resonance in Medicine, 1998; 318.
46. Stuber M, Kissinger KV, Botnar RM, Danias PG, Manning WJ. Fast 3D coronary artery imaging using real time navigator tracking and breath holding (abstr). In: Proceedings of the Sixth Meeting of the International Society for Magnetic Resonance in Medicine. Berkeley, Calif: International Society for Magnetic Resonance in Medicine, 1998; 847.
47. Wang Y, Grimm RC, Rossman PJ, Debbins JP, Riederer SJ, Ehman RL. 3D coronary MR angiography in multiple breath-holds using a respiratory feedback monitor. Magn Reson Med 1995; 34:11–16.
48. Oshinski JN, Hofland L, Mukundan S Jr, Dixon WT, Parks WJ, Pettigrew RI. Two-dimensional coronary MR angiography without breath holding. Radiology 1996; 201:737–743.

Frederick R. Long, MD
Robert G. Castile, MD
Alan S. Brody, MD
Mark J. Hogan, MD
Robert L. Flucke, RTT
David A. Filbrun, RTT
Karen S. McCoy, MD

Index terms:
Children, respiratory system
Computed tomography (CT), in infants and children, 60.12118
Lung, CT, 60.12118
Lung, function

Radiology 1999; 212:588–593

[1] From the Children's Radiological Institute (F.R.L., M.J.H.) and the Department of Pulmonary Medicine (R.G.C., R.L.F., D.A.F., K.S.M.), Columbus Children's Hospital, 700 Children's Dr, Columbus, OH 43205-2696, and the Department of Radiology, Cincinnati Children's Medical Center, Ohio (A.S.B.). Received April 17, 1998; revision requested May 28; final revision received October 22; accepted January 6, 1999. Supported in part by grant R01HL-54062 from the National Heart, Lung, and Blood Institute. **Address reprint requests to** F.R.L. (e-mail: *flong@chi.osu.edu*).

Author contributions:
Guarantors of integrity of entire study, F.R.L., R.G.C.; study concepts, F.R.L., R.G.C., R.L.F., D.A.F.; study design, F.R.L., R.G.C.; definition of intellectual content, F.R.L., R.G.C., A.S.B.; literature research, F.R.L., R.G.C.; clinical studies, F.R.L., R.G.C., R.L.F., D.A.F., K.S.M.; data acquisition, F.R.L., R.G.C., R.L.F., D.A.F.; data analysis, F.R.L., R.G.C., M.J.H., A.S.B.; manuscript preparation and editing, F.R.L., R.G.C.; manuscript review, F.R.L., R.G.C., M.J.H., A.S.B.

Lungs in Infants and Young Children: Improved Thin-Section CT with a Noninvasive Controlled-Ventilation Technique—Initial Experience[1]

Three sedated young children underwent thin-section computed tomography (CT) of the chest while breathing and during controlled respiratory pauses induced by means of a step increase in positive-pressure ventilation applied via a face mask. Motion-free inspiratory and expiratory thin-section CT images were successfully acquired during 8–12-second respiratory pauses. This simple, reproducible technique produced thin-section CT images that were clearer and more clinically useful than those obtained during quiet tidal breathing.

Thin-section computed tomography (CT) of the chest is capable of providing anatomic detail similar to that available in pathologic sections of the lung (1). Thin-section CT with widely available conventional scanners requires voluntary breath holding in order to minimize motion-related artifacts, which are accentuated on thin-section CT scans (2,3). As performed in adults and older children, the technique also involves voluntary inspiration to nearly full lung inflation before breath holding, to minimize atelectasis and to distend and display the airways (1). In addition, expiratory thin-section CT scans are desirable to identify air trapping and differentiate causes for mosaic lung attenuation (4,5).

In infants and toddlers, who cannot cooperate with breath holding, thin-section CT has been limited due to motion artifacts (3). Ultrafast electron-beam CT scanners, which are capable of obtaining single sections of the chest in as little as 0.1 second, decrease problems related to patient cooperation (3,6). However, ultrafast scanners do not address the need to obtain images at nearly full lung inflation and deflation and are available at only a very limited number of centers.

At present, motion-free inspiratory and expiratory thin-section CT in infants and young children requires general anesthesia and intubation to provide the necessary control of respiration. Ideally, thin-section CT in these children should be performed less invasively. Four years ago in our infant pulmonary function laboratory, we developed a noninvasive method for measuring full maximum expiratory flow-volume curves in sedated infants and young children by inducing controlled pauses in spontaneous respiration with use of a positive-pressure ventilation device (7). The purpose of this study was to describe the application of this technique to thin-section CT of the lungs in infants and young children at full lung inflation and at resting end expiration and to compare thin-section CT images obtained during tidal breathing with those obtained during controlled respiratory pauses.

Materials and Methods

Three children younger than 3 years (two girls and one boy; age range, 10 months to 2 years 9 months; mean age, 1 year 9 months) underwent thin-section CT of the chest (1-mm section thickness, 1-second scan acquisition, 120 kVp, 200

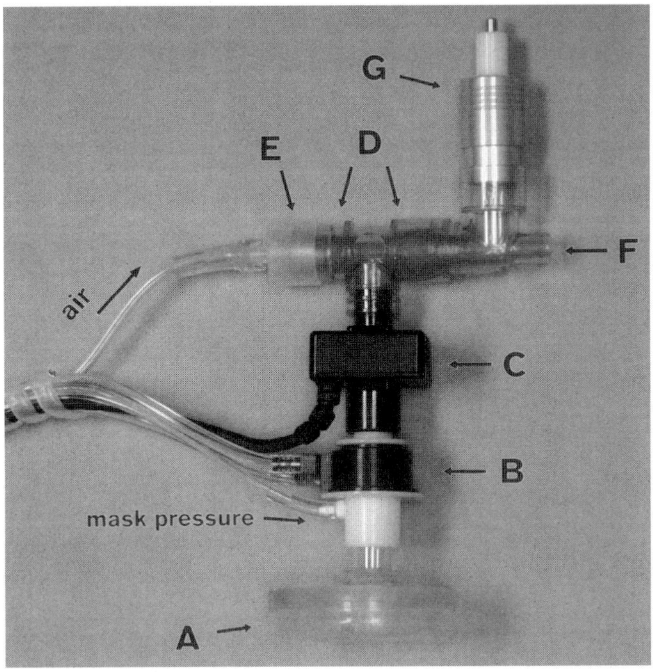

Figure 1. Positive-pressure ventilation device. Face mask (*A*) is attached to a pneumotachometer (*B*), carbon dioxide monitor (*C*), and bias flow apparatus (*D*), which has an inspiratory port (*E*) connected to a source supplying fresh air and an expiratory port (*F*). Pressure pop-off valve (*G*) is attached at top.

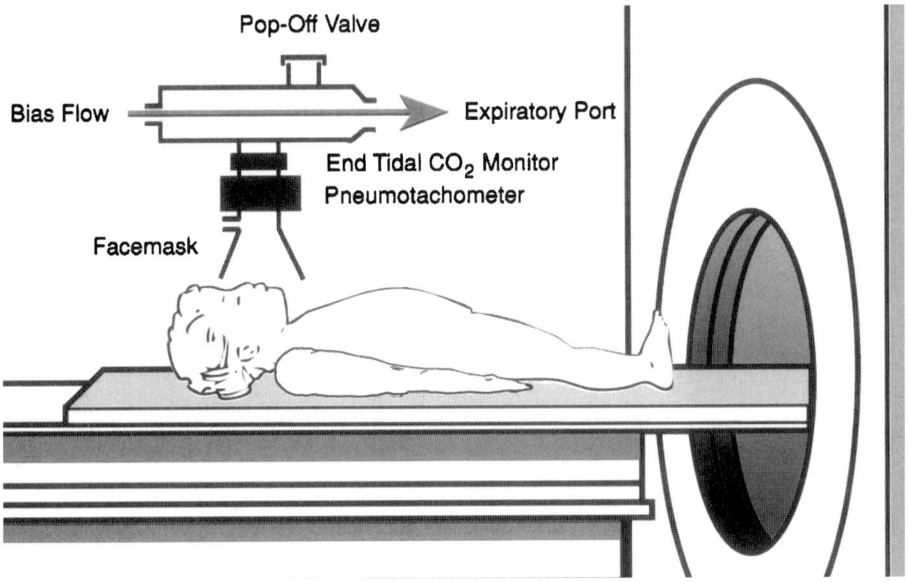

Figure 2. Schematic of child positioned supine, feetfirst on CT gantry table. While one person provides ventilation with positive pressure via the face mask, another applies gentle cricoid pressure, monitors vital signs, and signals to the CT technologist when a respiratory pause has been induced.

mA, high-frequency algorithm) for different clinical indications with use of a conventional CT scanner (CT HiSpeed Advantage; GE Medical Systems, Milwaukee, Wis). Thin-section CT was performed with deep sedation after mild sleep deprivation (oral chloral hydrate [50–100 mg per kilogram of body weight], Pharmaceutical Associates, Greenville SC, or intravenous pentobarbital [2–6 mg/kg], Wyeth Laboratories, Philadelphia, Pa) during quiet tidal breathing and with an institutional review board–approved controlled-ventilation technique, after informed consent was obtained.

Controlled-Ventilation Technique

The positive-pressure ventilation device (designed by R.G.C.) consists of a face mask attached to a pneumotachometer and bias-flow apparatus with an adjustable pressure pop-off valve (Fig 1). With this device, air flow, volume, mask pressure, and end-tidal carbon dioxide can be monitored. The face mask was placed over the nose and mouth (Fig 2) while fresh air was supplied continuously via the inspiratory port. Positive pressure was applied at the face mask by occluding the expiratory port at the downstream end with a thumb. The pressure applied was adjusted by changing the setting of the pressure pop-off valve. Respiratory pauses were induced by means of a step increase in ventilation combined with rapid lung inflation. An inflation pressure of 25 cm of water was given synchronously with spontaneous tidal inspiration by observing the child's breathing. Lung inflations were repeated approximately three to six times until a respiratory pause occurred. During lung inflations, gentle digital pressure was applied over the cricoid cartilage (the Sellick maneuver), to prevent air from passing down the esophagus into the stomach (8).

This controlled-ventilation procedure was practiced several times prior to CT to determine exactly how many lung inflations were required to produce reproducible pauses, which varied slightly between children. For CT at full lung inflation, the child was advanced into the CT gantry, and ventilation was augmented to produce a respiratory pause. During the pause, the child's lungs were inflated to nearly total lung capacity by occluding the expiratory limb with pop-off pressure set at 25 cm of water, and the positive pressure was held until the CT scan was completed or spontaneous respirations returned (Fig 3). For expiratory CT (Fig 4), ventilation was augmented in the same manner, but the expiratory occlusion was released (mask pressure, 0 cm of water), allowing the chest to deflate and remain deflated during the respiratory pause. The child was monitored over at least 60 seconds of normal breathing between controlled-ventilation maneuvers. Oxygen saturation, end-tidal carbon dioxide, and pulse were monitored throughout the procedure.

Image Analysis

In each case, thin-section CT images were obtained at a minimum of three anatomically defined positions: (*a*) upper lobes at the top of the aortic arch, (*b*) lung hilum at the level of the inferior pulmonary veins, and (*c*) lower lobes at a level approximately 2 cm above the diaphragm. Images obtained in these three patients during quiet tidal breathing and controlled ventilation were compared. Image quality was assessed at each of the three anatomic levels independently by three radiologists (F.R.L., A.S.B., M.J.H.) by using the following scoring system (score of 0–3 for each category [the higher score is superior]). (*a*) Sharply marginated pulmonary vessels: less than one-third of lung, 0; in one-third to two-thirds of lung, 1; in more than two-thirds of lung, 2; throughout the lung, 3. (*b*) Sharply defined bronchi (lumen with attenuation equal to or lower than that of normal parenchyma, well-defined interface between lumen and wall, well-defined wall): none, 0; at hilum, 1; central third of lung, 2; middle third of lung, 3. (*c*) Motion artifacts: affecting more than two-thirds of lung, 0; in one-third to two-thirds of lung, 1; in less than one-third of lung, 2; none, 3. (*d*) Overall assessment: poor quality, clinically unacceptable, 0; acceptable for gross diagnostic information, 1; good quality study but small lesions (<3 mm) could be missed, 2; excellent, similar to adult thin-section CT, 3. The scores of the three radiologists were averaged for each category.

Results

Case 1

This patient was a steroid-dependent 8-month-old boy with persistent dyspnea, tachypnea, wheezing, and hypoxemia.

Findings for infant pulmonary function tests, bronchoscopy with bronchoalveolar lavage, sweat testing, immunoglobulin measurements, and chest radiographs were nondiagnostic. A thin-section CT examination was requested to help detect and localize suspected small airway or interstitial lung disease before open lung biopsy.

With the infant sedated and breathing normally, a helical CT scan of the chest and three thin-section CT images at three levels were obtained. Controlled-ventilation thin-section CT images were then acquired at six anatomic levels with inflation pressures of 25 cm of water and at three levels at pressures of 7 cm of water.

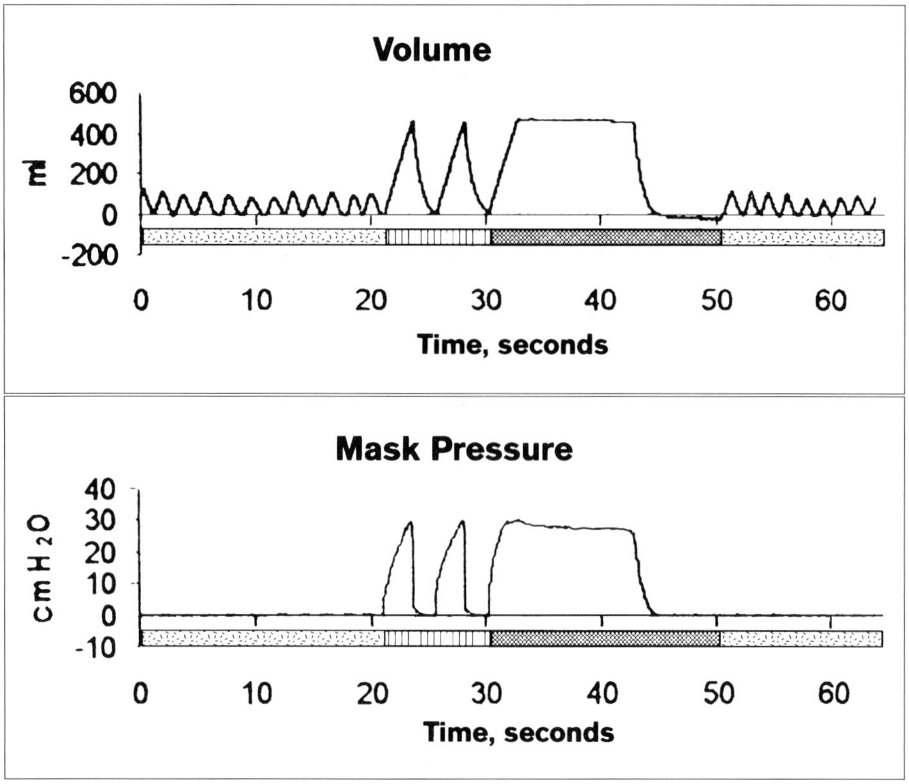

Figure 3. Graphs depict flow volume (top) and corresponding mask pressure (bottom) during a controlled-ventilation procedure at full lung inflation. In this case, the respiratory pause (crosshatch) lasted 20 seconds. Speckle = spontaneous tidal respirations, vertical lines = augmented breaths.

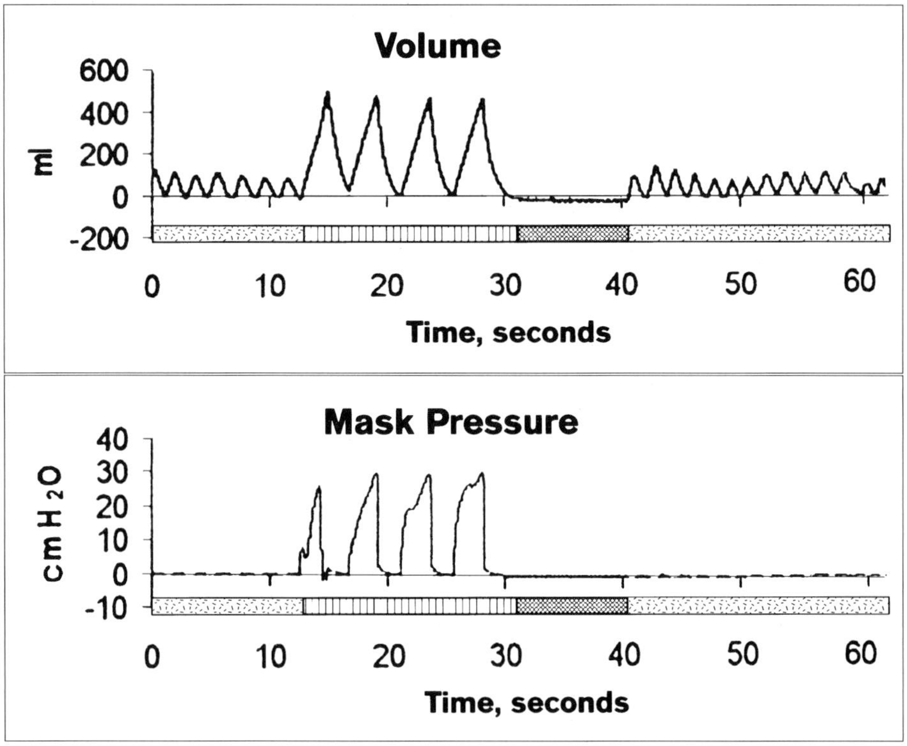

Figure 4. Graphs depict flow volume (top) and corresponding mask pressure (bottom) during controlled-ventilation procedure at end exhalation. In this case, the respiratory pause (crosshatch) lasted 10 seconds. Speckle = spontaneous tidal respirations, vertical lines = augmented breaths.

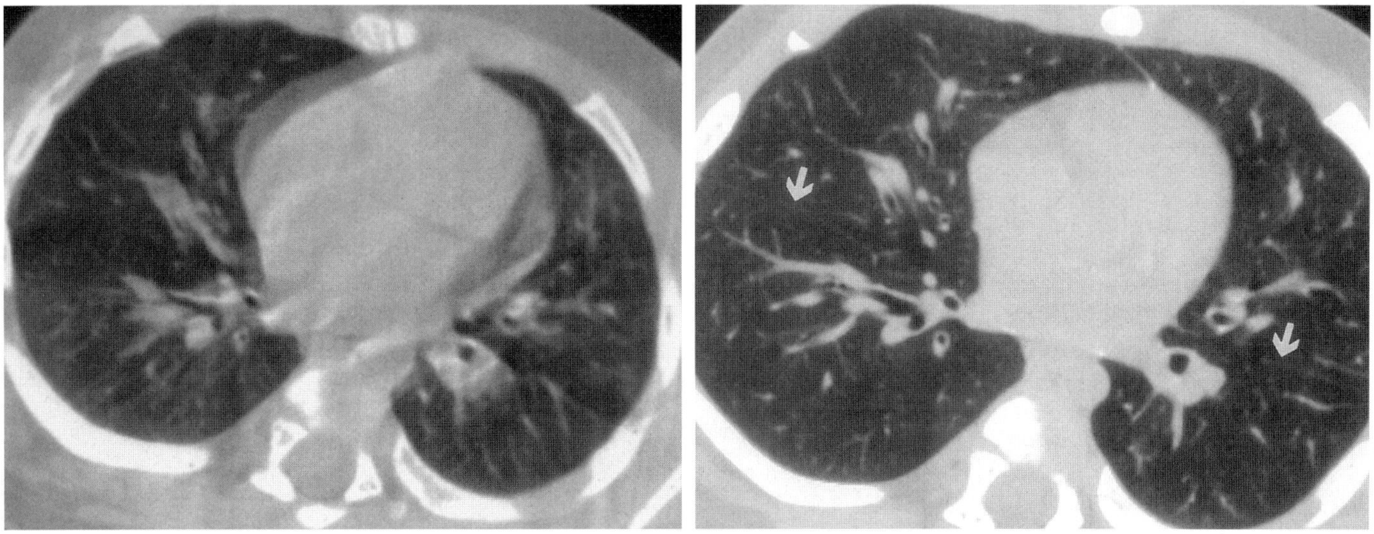

a. b.

Figure 5. Case 1. **(a)** Thin-section CT image of the lungs (window width, +1,900 HU; level, −650 HU) at the level of the inferior pulmonary veins during quiet tidal breathing depicts blurring of the bronchi and vessels and nonhomogeneous lung attenuation. The major fissures are indistinct as lines. **(b)** Thin-section CT image of the lungs (window width, +1,774 HU; level, −640 HU) at the same anatomic level was obtained during respiratory pause at full inflation (mask pressure, 25 cm of water). The bronchi and vessels are distinct from homogeneous normal low attenuation of the lungs. The major fissures (arrows) are visible as lines.

The induced respiratory pauses lasted approximately 10 seconds for the scans obtained at full inflation and end exhalation.

The thin-section CT images obtained during tidal breathing (Fig 5a) demonstrated multiple areas of increased and decreased lung parenchymal opacification that in this patient could be interpreted as areas of inhomogeneous aeration secondary to diffuse airways disease. The controlled-ventilation images (Fig 5b) revealed normal homogeneous lung attenuation and no evidence of airway or parenchymal disease. On the basis of the controlled-ventilation study, the biopsy was postponed, and the child is being followed up with a diagnosis of asthma.

Case 2

This patient was a steroid-dependent 18-month-old girl with chronic dyspnea after adenoviral pneumonia.

Infant pulmonary function tests revealed severe obstruction with moderate air trapping. An open lung biopsy revealed bronchiolitis obliterans. Findings at thin-section CT performed during quiet tidal breathing at the time of biopsy were consistent with the diagnosis (Fig 6a). Six months later, thin-section CT of the chest with controlled-ventilation technique was performed to further assess the extent of lung involvement. Full-inflation scans at mask pressure of 25 cm of water (Fig 6b) were acquired during respiratory pauses lasting approximately 12 seconds. Expiratory scans at mask pressure of 0 cm of water (Fig 6c) were obtained during pauses lasting approximately 8 seconds. The controlled-ventilation images (full inflation and end exhalation) revealed much more extensive central and peripheral airway damage (bronchiectasis and associated air trapping) secondary to adenoviral infection.

Case 3

This patient was a 2½-year-old girl with newly diagnosed cystic fibrosis.

The child presented with failure to thrive and no history of major respiratory disease or symptoms. Findings at physical examination and chest radiography were unremarkable. Infant pulmonary function testing revealed mild air trapping but no clear reduction in flows. Nitrogen washout studies revealed evidence of trapped gas and nonhomogeneous airway disease. A thin-section CT examination of the chest was performed to further assess the extent of pulmonary disease.

Thin-section CT images were obtained during quiet tidal breathing and controlled ventilation at full inflation (mask pressure, 25 cm of water) and end exhalation (mask pressure, 0 cm of water). The induced pauses lasted approximately 12 seconds at full inflation and at end exhalation. On the thin-section CT images obtained during quiet breathing, bronchiectasis was not evident, whereas bronchiectasis and peribronchial thickening were identified on the controlled-ventilation images obtained at full inflation. Areas of air trapping suggested on the tidal breathing images were more clearly defined on the end-exhalation images. On the images obtained during tidal breathing at the level of the inferior pulmonary veins, pseudobronchiectasis was seen. After the images were reviewed, the parents agreed to treatment with intravenous antibiotics.

Results of image quality scoring are summarized in the Table. For each of the three children, the average scores for the three levels were markedly better with the controlled-ventilation method. This was true for all categories and for controlled-ventilation images obtained at both full lung inflation and end exhalation.

Discussion

Combining the talents of the pulmonologist and the radiologist permits the collection of thin-section CT data in infants and very young children that are similar in quality to those obtainable in older children and adults who can voluntarily hold their breath at different lung volumes.

The physiologic basis for capturing ventilation depends on a combination of a step increase in ventilation, which pro-

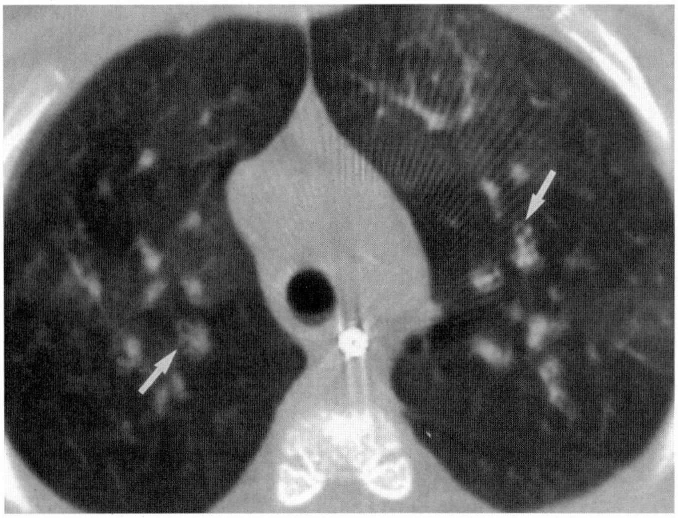

a.

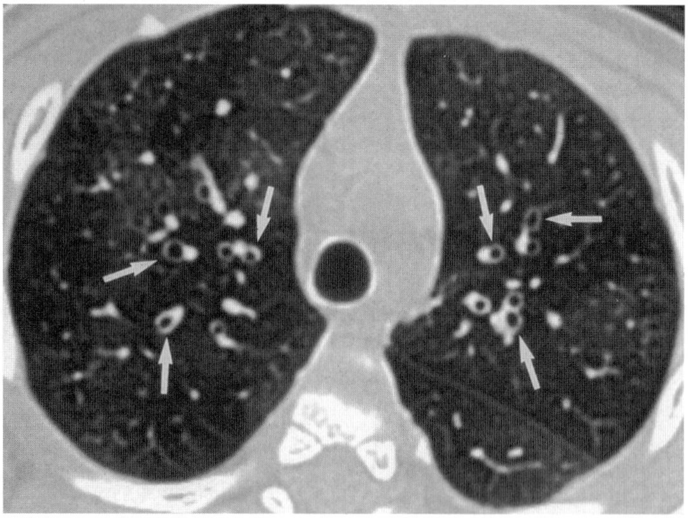

b.

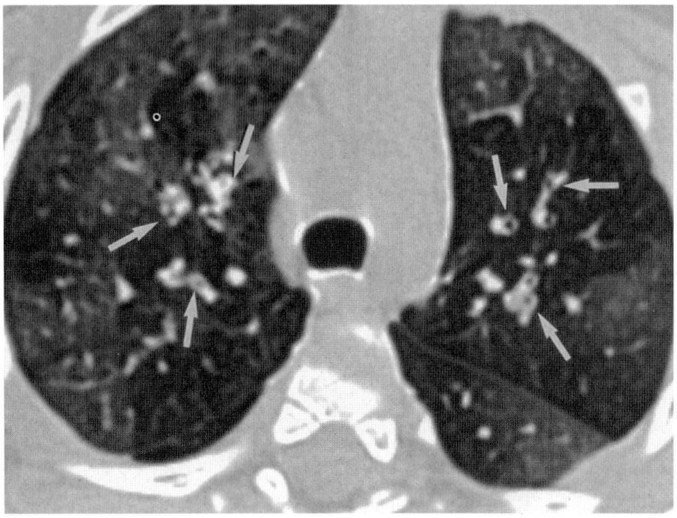

c.

Figure 6. Case 2. (a) Thin-section CT image of the lungs (window width, +1988 HU; level, −616 HU) at the level of the aortic arch depicts image blurring and a mosaic pattern of lung attenuation with probable mild bronchial dilatation (arrows). Note nasogastric tube in place. **(b)** Thin-section CT image of the lungs (window width, +1968 HU; level, −616 HU) near the same level during a respiratory pause at full inflation (mask pressure, 25 cm of water) depicts diffuse bronchiectasis (arrows) with peribronchial thickening and a mosaic pattern of lung attenuation. **(c)** Thin-section CT image of the lungs (window width, +1,988 HU; level −616 HU) during a respiratory pause at end exhalation (mask pressure, 0 cm of water) demonstrates that the mosaic pattern of lung attenuation is secondary to air trapping. Note the decreased luminal caliber of the bronchiectatic airways (arrows) at end exhalation.

duces mild hypocarbia and thus decreases respiratory drive (9), and rapid chest expansion, which produces a vagally mediated pause in spontaneous respiratory effort, the Hering-Breuer response (10,11). Over the past 4 years, we have applied this technique for obtaining pulmonary function tests in more than 500 children aged from 1 month to 4 years. We have been successful in producing controlled pauses in respiration in more than 98% of the other children tested and in the three children whose cases are presented herein. In newborns and children younger than 2 months, respiratory pauses are more difficult to induce because of their more rapid respiratory rates. We have not studied children older than 4 years.

The theoretic complications of the procedure relate to the known complications of sedation and to the potential problems associated with hyperventilation (hypocarbia, seizures) and lung inflation (air leaks). In our pulmonary function laboratory and clinical CT cases, we have not experienced any complications. During controlled-ventilation procedures, monitored oxygen saturation levels have remained in the normal range and monitored end-tidal carbon dioxide levels have dropped approximately 2–4 torr and remained constant during repeated deep inspirations. This small drop in carbon dioxide level is not known to have untoward effects. In addition, as pressures used for lung inflations are no greater than those that occur during normal crying or spontaneous sighing, air leaks are unlikely to occur.

We would not recommend this procedure in patients with a known seizure disorder or a known or potential air leak. None of our patients has experienced prolonged apnea after the procedure, and we would not expect this to occur as end-tidal carbon dioxide levels drop only 2–4 torr and do not drop further after repeated controlled-ventilation procedures. We have not studied patients with such severely compromised pulmonary reserve that the deep sedation required for the procedure would be contraindicated. Patients have undergone infant pulmonary function testing while receiving supplementary oxygen with a similar method. It should be reemphasized that this procedure is performed in a very controlled manner with a physician at the bedside already using ventilatory equipment and with continuous monitoring of vital signs.

Another potential complication is gastric air distention during positive-pressure ventilation, which is not likely to produce major consequences at mask pressures of less than or equal to 25 cm of water (12,13). Because gastric air distention could increase the risk of gastroesophageal reflux and aspiration, we recommend gentle cricoid pressure during lung

Image Quality Scores

Result	Patient 1		Patient 2		Patient 3*	
	Conventional†	Controlled Ventilation‡	Conventional†	Controlled Ventilation‡	Conventional†	Controlled Ventilation‡
Vessels	1.0	3.0	0.8	2.3	0.6	2.4 (2.1)
Bronchi	1.1	3.0	1.4	2.7	0.4	3.0 (2.7)
Motion artifacts	1.1	2.7	1.2	2.7	0.8	2.4 (2.1)
Overall quality	1.3	3.0	1.6	2.7	1.1	3.0 (2.8)
Total	1.1	2.9	1.2	2.6	0.7	2.7 (2.4)

Note.—Numbers are average scores (range, 0–3 [the higher score is superior]).
* Numbers in parentheses are average scores during end exhalation. Only patient 3 had end-exhalation images at levels matching full-inflation images and conventional images that could be scored.
† During tidal breathing.
‡ At full lung inflation.

inflations (the Sellick maneuver), to close the communication between the airway and esophagus. In one of our patients (case 3), mild gastric air distention occurred despite use of the Sellick maneuver, but this had no ill effect.

On the basis of our previous experience in the infant pulmonary function laboratory, the duration of spontaneously induced respiratory pauses varies between children but lasts approximately 5–15 seconds for full inflation and 3–10 seconds for end exhalation. In the three cases presented herein, pauses ranged from 8 to 12 seconds. This provides enough time for thin-section CT images to be acquired at three to six anatomic levels.

Findings in our three clinical cases demonstrate the improved image quality of thin-section CT of the lungs in infants and young children with the controlled-ventilation technique. This technique successfully eliminated or minimized blurring and artifacts related to breathing motion, which were widespread on thin-section CT images acquired during quiet tidal breathing. Artifacts included pseudobronchiectasis (case 3), which has been described as an imaging pitfall in the diagnosis of bronchiectasis (14).

The ability to acquire thin-section CT images at full lung inflation and end exhalation has considerable advantages. Images obtained during quiet tidal breathing in a sedated child are images of the lungs very near end exhalation (Fig 3, top). These images at low lung volume depict the effects of crowding of the pulmonary vessels and bronchi, as well as poor distention of the lumen of the airways (Figs 5a, 6a). With full lung inflation, the depiction of airways and vessels is improved so a true assessment of bronchial lumen diameter, bronchial wall thickness, and vessel size becomes possible. At low lung volumes, bronchiectasis can be obscured (Fig 6a), but it becomes obvious when the airways are inflated (Fig 6b).

On thin-section CT images acquired during tidal breathing, nonhomogeneous lung parenchymal opacification, which is probably secondary to low lung volumes and motion artifact (Fig 5a), cannot be differentiated from a mosaic pattern of lung attenuation secondary to parenchymal, vascular, or small airways disease. The end-exhalation images obtained during a respiratory pause (Fig 6c) allowed us to be confident that the mosaic pattern of lung attenuation was secondary to air trapping rather than vascular or lung parenchymal disease, as has been described by others in adult patients (4).

Because the equipment needed to produce controlled pauses in infant ventilation is inexpensive and easy to obtain, the controlled-ventilation method we describe should be transferable to the majority of centers in which children receive care. However, use of this method requires an additional investment in time and preparation, exposes the practitioner to a low level of radiation, and at first should be undertaken with the assistance of members of the pulmonary or anesthesia department, who are more experienced in providing patient ventilation. Although general acceptance of the technique awaits further studies with larger numbers of patients that demonstrate its clinical utility and applications, we believe that the controlled-ventilation technique, when applied in a selective manner, will prove valuable in infants and young children.

By applying physiologic responses to augmented ventilation, motion-free thin-section CT images of the chest can be acquired noninvasively in the sedated infant or young child at both full lung inflation and deflation. The technique is simple, reproducible, rapid, and safe.

Acknowledgment: We thank Brad Hoehne for his assistance with the illustrations for this article.

References

1. Webb RW. High-resolution CT of the lung parenchyma. Radiol Clin North Am 1989; 27:1085–1097.
2. Mayo JR. The high-resolution computed tomography technique. Semin Roentgenol 1991; 26:104–109.
3. Lynch DA, Brasch RC, Hardy KA, Webb RW. Pediatric pulmonary disease: assessment with high-resolution ultrafast CT. Radiology 1990; 176:243–248.
4. Arakawa H, Webb RW, McCowin M, Katsou G, Ki-Nam L, Seitz RF. Inhomogeneous lung attenuation at thin-section CT: diagnostic value of expiratory scans. Radiology 1998; 206:89–94.
5. Lucidarme O, Coche E, Cluzel P, Mourey-Gerosa I, Howarth N, Grenier P. Expiratory CT scans for chronic airway disease: correlation with pulmonary function test results. AJR 1998; 170:301–307.
6. Galvin JR, Gingrich RD, Hoffman E, Kao CS, Stern EJ, Stanford W. Ultrafast computed tomography of the chest. Radiol Clin North Am 1994; 32:775–793.
7. Feher A, Castile R, Kisling J, et al. Flow limitation in normal infants: a new method for forced expiratory maneuvers from raised lung volumes. J Appl Physiol 1996; 80:2019–2025.
8. Salem M, Wong A, Mani M, Sellick B. Efficacy of cricoid pressure in preventing gastric inflation during bag-mask ventilation in pediatric patients. Anesthesiology 1974; 40:96–98.
9. Henke KG, Arias A, Skatrud JB, Dempsey JA. Inhibition of inspiratory muscle activity during sleep: chemical and nonchemical influences. Am Rev Respir Dis 1988; 138:8–15.
10. Hering E, Breuer J. Die selbststeureung der atmung durch den nervus vagus. Sitzsungsberichte Akad Wissenschaft Wien 1868; 58:672–677
11. Hering E, Breuer J. Die selbststeureung der atmung durch den nervus vagus. Sitzsungsberichte Akad Wissenschaft Wien 1868; 58:909–937.
12. Brochard L, Isabey D, Piquet J, et al. Reversal of acute exacerbation of chronic obstructive lung disease by inspiratory assistance with a face mask. N Engl J Med 1990; 323:1523–1530.
13. Hillberg R, Johnson DC. Noninvasive ventilation. N Engl J Med 1997; 337:1746–1752.
14. McGuinness G, Naidich DP, Leitman BS, McCauley DI. Bronchiectasis: CT evaluation. AJR 1993; 160:253–259.

Gareth R. Tudor, FRCR
Peter M. Rodgers, FRCR
Kevin P. West, FRCPath

Index terms:
Biopsies, technology, 74.1261, 75.1261
Intestines, biopsy, 74.1261, 75.1261
Ultrasound (US), guidance, 74.1261, 75.1261, 74.12985, 75.12985

Radiology 1999; 212:594–597

Abbreviation:
HIV = human immunodeficiency virus

[1] From the Departments of Radiology (G.R.T., P.M.R.) and Histopathology (K.P.W.), Leicester Royal Infirmary NHS Trust, Infirmary Square, Leicester LE1 5WW, England, UK. Received March 10, 1998; revision requested May 7; final revision received November 30; accepted March 2, 1999. **Address reprint requests to** P.M.R.

Author contributions:
Guarantors of integrity of entire study, G.R.T., P.M.R.; study concepts and design, G.R.T., P.M.R.; definition of intellectual content, G.R.T., P.M.R.; literature research, G.R.T.; clinical studies, P.M.R., K.P.W.; data acquisition, G.R.T.; data analysis; manuscript preparation, editing, and review, G.R.T., P.M.R., K.P.W.

Bowel Lesions: Percutaneous US-guided 18-gauge Needle Biopsy—Preliminary Experience[1]

Ultrasonography-guided percutaneous biopsy was performed with local anesthesia and an 18-gauge needle in 10 patients with bowel-wall lesions. All patients underwent clinical review within 1 month. Biopsy was diagnostic in all patients. There were no complications, and all patients tolerated the procedure well. The technique appears to be safe and had an excellent diagnostic yield in our series.

Infiltration of the bowel wall by neoplastic or inflammatory cells may reveal the "target or pseudokidney appearance" at ultrasonography (US) (1–3). This appearance is nonspecific, and clinical management often requires histologic diagnosis. If the lesions are endoscopically inaccessible, patients may have to undergo laparoscopy or laparotomy to obtain a tissue diagnosis. Percutaneous US-guided fine-needle aspiration biopsy of bowel-wall lesions has been reported in several cases, which mostly involved gastric lesions (4–6). There can be problems when only cytologic examination is performed, however, particularly in reaching a definitive benign diagnosis (7–10). This study was performed to evaluate whether a diagnostic biopsy can be safely performed percutaneously with an 18-gauge biopsy needle to obtain a satisfactory sample for histologic examination in patients with bowel-wall lesions discovered at US.

Materials and Methods

US-guided percutaneous biopsy was performed in 10 patients (seven men and three women; age range, 30–77 years; mean age, 54 years) with bowel-wall lesions. Four of the patients had been treated for a primary malignancy, results in three were positive for human immunodeficiency virus (HIV), and three had no relevant medical history. The bowel-wall lesions were discovered at either US or computed tomography (CT), although one patient was found to have a thick-walled lesion at US after a stricture had been demonstrated at enteroclysis (Table). Each patient was believed to have high surgical risk for open biopsy. Informed consent was obtained individually after consultation on a case-by-case basis with the patient's physician and surgeon.

Platelet count, hemoglobin level, and coagulation screen (prothrombin time) were obtained prior to biopsy. Patients were restricted to nothing by mouth prior to the biopsy, and we did not use any bowel preparation or antibiotic prophylaxis. All biopsies were performed with a 3.5- or 5-MHz curvilinear probe (Masters Diasonics Sonotron, Milpitas, Calif). With color Doppler US, the route to the lesion and the target site were selected to avoid large vessels.

Percutaneous biopsy was performed by using standard aseptic technique with local anesthesia (5–10 mL of 1% lidocaine hydrochloride). The 18-gauge biopsy needle, with a throw of 1 cm, was mounted in an automated needle (Biopty Gun, Manan promag 2.2; Bard, Northbrook, Ill) that can be operated with one hand, which allowed US to be performed simultaneously. The biopsy needle was advanced until the lesion was seen to be indented, and then the trigger mechanism was fired and the needle was withdrawn. An average of two specimens were obtained for each patient. These specimens were fixed in formalin for histologic examination (n = 10) or sent fresh to the pathology department for microbiologic examination (n = 3). All patients were observed overnight and followed up clinically for possible complications.

Patient Data

Patient No.	History	Imaging and Finding	Biopsy Finding	Complication	Follow-up
1	None	US, CT; small-bowel–related mass	High-grade non-Hodgkin lymphoma	None	None
2	Melanoma, 1986	US, CT; small-bowel–related mass	Metastatic melanoma	None	Deceased
3	Dukes class C colon, 1994	US, CT; small-bowel–related mass	Adenocarcinoma	None	Deceased
4	None	US, mass involving terminal ileum	Malignant cells (nondiagnostic features)	None	Surgery, high-grade sarcoma
5	Breast carcinoma, 1987	US, thick-walled small bowel	Normal mucosa	Small hematoma discovered incidentally at laparotomy	Surgery, thick-walled small bowel; open biopsy, normal mucosa
6	HIV	US, bowel-related mass	High-grade non-Hodgkin lymphoma	None	Deceased
7	HIV	US, thick-walled small bowel; enteroclysis, strictures	Non-Hodgkin lymphoma	None	Deceased
8	HIV	US, CT; thick-walled small bowel	Acid-fast bacillus*	None	Deceased
9	None	US, CT; thick-walled small bowel	High-grade non-Hodgkin lymphoma	None	None
10	Ovarian carcinoma, 1994	US, CT; thick-walled cecum	Adenocarcinoma	None	None

* *Mycobacterium avium-intracellulare.*

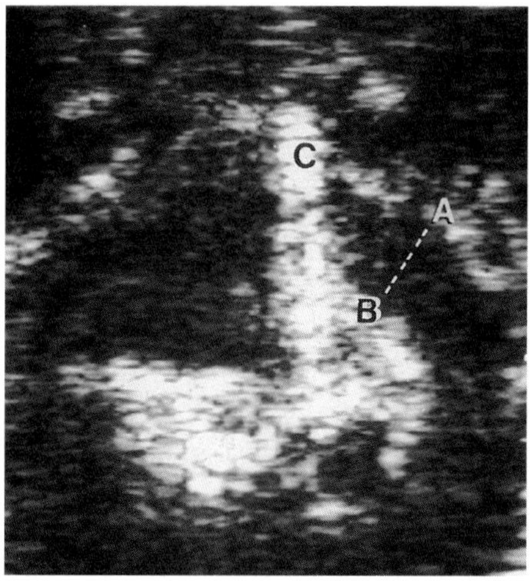

Figure 1. Patient 9. US image of thick-walled small bowel in a patient with non-Hodgkin lymphoma. The biopsy needle (*C*) can be seen in the thickened wall (*A--B*).

Results

Diagnostic biopsy samples were obtained in all patients. The lesions were all accessible to biopsy with US guidance, and no procedure was abandoned because of poor access. One of the biopsy specimens revealed malignant cells, the exact nature of which was unclear histologically. This patient later underwent small-bowel resection, and the histologic findings from this specimen showed high-grade histiocytoma. The Table shows the histologic findings in the biopsy specimens: high-grade non-Hodgkin lymphoma in four cases, adenocarcinoma in two cases, metastatic melanoma in one case, high-grade sarcoma in one case, and atypical tuberculosis (*Mycobacterium avium-intracellulare*) in one case. Histologic examination in one of the biopsy specimens showed normal mucosa although it was believed that abnormal bowel had been biopsied. This patient later underwent laparotomy and open biopsy of macroscopically abnormal small bowel, and histologic findings were again normal. No major complications occurred, but in one patient a small hematoma was discovered incidentally during laparotomy at the site of biopsy. This patient's abdominal symptoms resolved after 3 months, and she was followed up clinically for 2 years by her general practitioner without recurrence of symptoms. Some examples of the lesions sampled at biopsy together with the relevant histologic findings are shown in Figures 1–3.

Discussion

Although there have been advances in imaging techniques for the investigation of bowel-wall lesions, there is still a need in many cases to make a definitive diagnosis with histologic findings. Percutaneous US-guided biopsy with a fine (22-gauge) needle has been reported as safe (6). Percutaneous biopsy of other abdominal structures has also been shown to be a safe and cost-effective method of obtaining samples for histologic analysis with 18-gauge needles (11–13). The risks and costs of surgical biopsy and anesthesia can be avoided by using percutaneous biopsy methods. In our group of patients, surgical biopsy was avoided in eight of the 10 patients.

There has been some debate in the literature regarding the adequacy of sample material and complication rates with either 18-gauge or fine biopsy needles. Biopsy material must be of a sufficient quality to allow a correct diagnosis. Support has been given by many authors for the use of cutting needles, which generally provide adequate samples (14–17). The biopsy gun we use is a rapid firing system that reduces fragmentation and crush artifacts in the samples obtained. With 18-gauge needles, the percentage of inadequate samples obtained has been reported at 3%–10% (17–19). With fine needles, the percentage of insufficient samples has been reported at 20% and 24% (11,20). It would appear, therefore, that 18-gauge cutting needles acquire an acceptable specimen in more than 90% of biopsies. If there is close cooperation between the radiology and pathology departments, the adequacy of the biopsy specimen can be assessed at the time of the procedure. This may not be possible in all institutions because of staffing implications, but it should reduce the number of biopsy passes necessary to obtain an adequate sample.

It has been claimed that use of fine needles is the safest way to obtain tissue samples (21). Findings in several studies have shown that there is a marginally lower complication rate with 22-gauge compared with 18-gauge needles, but the differences were not statistically significant (22,23). In a review of the literature, however, Smith (21) found no evidence to support the suggestion that cutting needles less than 19 gauge cause more complications than do aspiration needles.

In our series, there was only one known complication, a very small hematoma noticed incidentally at the biopsy site in a patient who later underwent laparotomy.

There is little in the literature about percutaneous bowel-wall biopsy, and we know of no authors who have used 18-gauge cutting needles to obtain samples from the bowel wall. There are several references in the literature that claim no complications arise when bowel is traversed at biopsy of other abdominal masses.

We found that a diagnostic biopsy can be safely performed percutaneously with an 18-gauge biopsy needle to obtain a satisfactory sample for histologic examination in patients with bowel-wall lesions discovered at US. The role of this technique in bowel lesions has not been established. Although we realize this is a small series to determine a meaningful complication rate, there were no clinically important complications, and the diagnostic yield was excellent. We did not have to abandon any biopsy attempts because of poor access. The patients, because of their generally poor physical condition, were good candidates for US in most cases. None of the patients in this group had ascites, which might make performance of biopsy more difficult. In cases in which lesions are identified with US, this technique has the advantage over CT guidance because the operator is able to fix the bowel loop by means of compression with the US probe. The use of color flow Doppler US allows avoidance of larger mesenteric vessels. Laparotomy was obviated in eight of our 10 patients, in whom laparotomy was believed to be inappropriate or unacceptable risk.

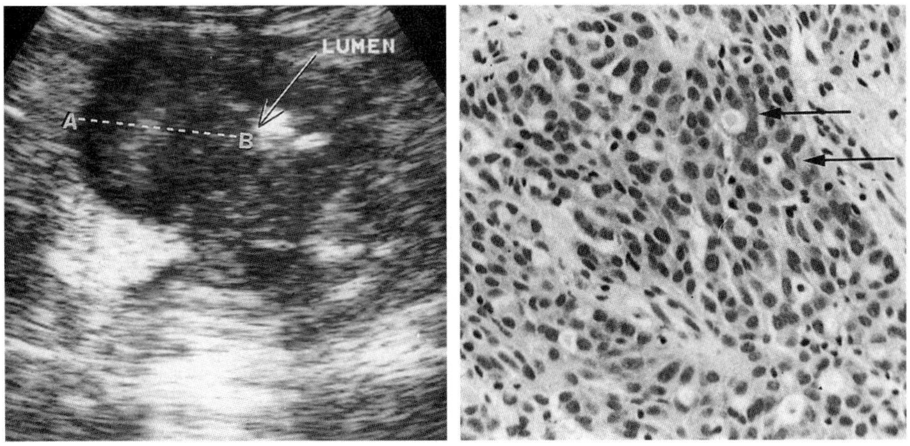

a. b.

Figure 2. Patient 10. **(a)** US image shows eccentric thickening (*A--B*) of the cecum. **(b)** Photomicrograph from the lesion in **a** shows sheets of malignant cells: adenocarcinoma-forming glandular structures (arrows). (Hematoxylin-eosin stain; original magnification, ×25.)

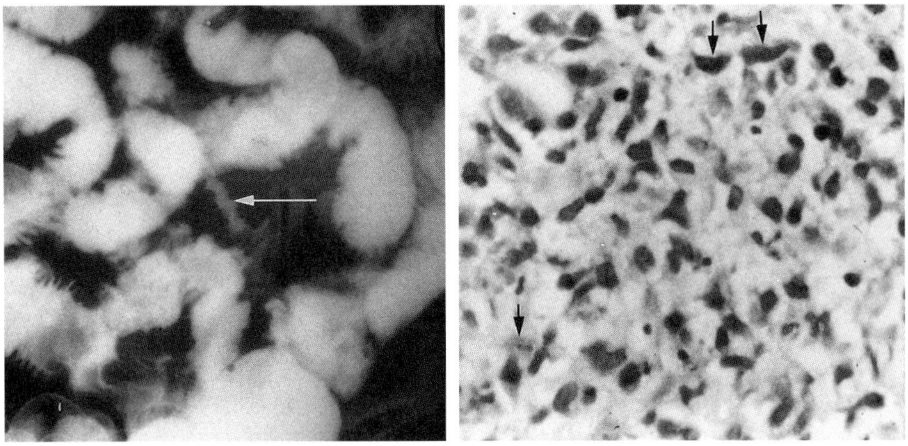

a. c.

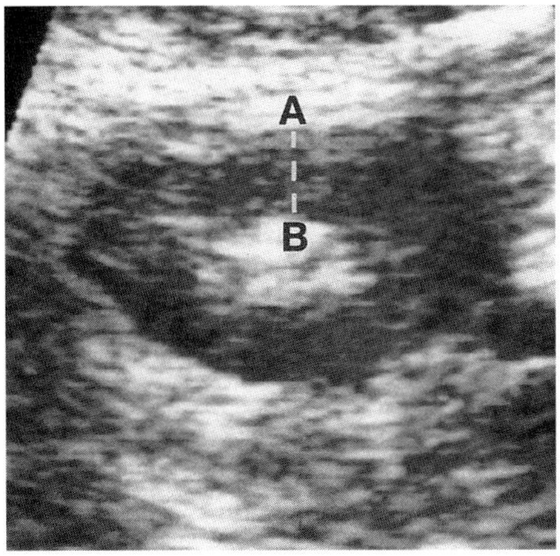

b.

Figure 3. Patient 7. **(a)** Image obtained during enteroclysis with barium and methylcellulose shows a stricture (arrow). **(b)** US scan shows thickened small-bowel wall (*A--B*) at the site of the stricture in **a**. **(c)** Photomicrograph from the lesion in **b** shows multiple small dysplastic cells (arrows), revealed to be non-Hodgkin lymphoma at immunocytochemical testing. (Hematoxylin-eosin stain; original magnification, ×25.)

References

1. Bluth EI, Merritt CR, Sullivan MA. Ultrasonic evaluation of the stomach, small bowel, and colon. Radiology 1979; 113:677–680.
2. Fakhry JR, Berk RN. The "target" pattern: characteristic sonographic feature of stomach and bowel abnormalities. AJR 1981; 137:969–972.
3. Morgan CL, Trought WS, Oddson TA, Clark WM, Rice RP. Ultrasound patterns of disorders affecting the gastrointestinal tract. Radiology 1980; 135:129–135.
4. Ennis MG, MacErlean DP. Biopsy of bowel wall pathology under ultrasound control. Gastrointest Radiol 1981; 6:17–20.
5. Green J, Katz S, Phillips G, et al. Percutaneous sonographic needle aspiration biopsy of endoscopically negative gastric carcinoma. Am J Gastroenterol 1988; 83:1150–1153.
6. Abbitt PL. Percutaneous fine needle aspiration of bowel wall abnormalities under ultrasonic guidance. J Clin Ultrasound 1991; 19:310–314.
7. Westcott JL. Percutaneous transhepatic needle biopsy. Radiology 1988; 169:593–601.
8. Perlmutt LM, Johnstone WW, Dunnick NR. Percutaneous transthoracic needle aspiration: a review. AJR 1989; 152:451–455.
9. Gazelle GS, Haaga JR. Guided percutane-

ous biopsy of intra-abdominal lesions. AJR 1989; 153:929–935.
10. Bocking A. Cytological vs histological evaluation of percutaneous biopsies. Cardiovasc Intervent Radiol 1991; 14:5–12.
11. Tikkakoski T, Paivansalo M, Siniluotu S, et al. Percutaneous ultrasound guided biopsy: fine needle biopsy, cutting needle biopsy, or both? Acta Radiol 1993; 34: 30–34.
12. Burbank F, Kaye K, Bellville J, Ekuan J, Blumenfeld M. Image-guided automated core biopsies of the breast, chest, abdomen and pelvis. Radiology 1994; 191:165–171.
13. Silverman SG, Lee BY, Mueller PR, Cibas ES, Seltzer SE. Impact of positive findings at image-guided biopsy of lymphoma on patient care: evaluation of clinical history, needle size, and pathological findings on biopsy performance. Radiology 1994; 190:759–764.
14. Elvin A, Andersson T, Sheibenpflug L, Lindgren PG. Biopsy of pancreas with biopsy gun. Radiology 1990; 176:677–679.
15. Jaeger HJ, Macfie J, Mitchell CJ, et al. Diagnosis of abdominal masses with percutaneous biopsy guided by ultrasound. BMJ 1990; 301:1188–1191.
16. Jennings PE, Coral A, Donald JJ, et al. Ultrasound-guided core biopsy. Lancet 1989; 1:1369–1371.
17. Parker SH, Hopper KD, Yakes WF, Gibson MD, Ownbey JL, Carter TE. Image-directed percutaneous biopsies with a biopsy gun. Radiology 1989; 171:663–669.
18. Bernardino M, Fernandez M, Neylan J, Hertzler G, Whelchel J, Olson R. Pancreatic transplants: CT-guided biopsy. Radiology 1990; 177:709–711.
19. Mitchell CJ, Wai D, Jackson AM, et al. Ultrasound guided percutaneous pancreatic biopsy. Br J Surg 1989; 76:706–708.
20. Dowlatshahi K, Yaremko ML, Kluskens LF, Jokich PM. Nonpalpable breast lesions: findings of stereotaxic needle-core biopsy and fine-needle aspiration cytology. Radiology 1991; 181:745–750.
21. Smith EH. Complications of percutaneous abdominal fine-needle biopsy: review. Radiology 1991; 178:253–258.
22. Welch TJ, Sheedy PF II, Johnson CD, Johnson CM, Stephens DH. CT-guided biopsy: prospective analysis of 1,000 procedures. Radiology 1989; 171:493–496.
23. Martino CR, Haaga JR, Bryan PJ, LiPuma JP, El Yousef SJ, Alfidi RJ. CT-guided liver biopsies: eight years' experience. Radiology 1984; 152:755–759.

Sanshin Hayashi, MD
Mitsue Miyazaki, PhD

Index terms:
Lymphography, 99.125
Thoracic duct, MR, 99.12942

Radiology 1999; 212:598–600

Abbreviations:
MIP = maximum intensity projection
3D = three-dimensional

[1] From the Department of Radiology, School of Medicine, Toho University, Tokyo, Japan (S.H.), and the MR Engineering Department, Toshiba Medical Engineering Center, 1385 Shimoishigami, Otawara, Tochigi, 324-8550 Japan (M.M.). Received June 29, 1998; revision requested July 27; final revision received December 28; accepted January 21, 1999. **Address reprint requests to** M.M. (e-mail: *miyazaki@mr.nasu.toshiba.co.jp*).

Author contributions:
Guarantor of integrity of entire study, S.H.; study concepts, S.H., M.M.; study design, M.M.; definition of intellectual content, S.H., M.M.; literature research, S.H., M.M.; clinical studies, S.H.; experimental studies, M.M.; data acquisition, M.M., S.H.; data analysis, S.H., M.M.; statistical analysis, S.H.; manuscript preparation and review, S.H., M.M.; manuscript editing, M.M.

Thoracic Duct: Visualization at Nonenhanced MR Lymphography—Initial Experience[1]

In six healthy volunteers, the thoracic duct was examined at magnetic resonance (MR) lymphography without contrast agent. With a 1.5-T clinical imager, a short echo spacing, three-dimensional, half-Fourier fast spin-echo sequence with electrocardiographic gating was employed to depict the thoracic duct along the thoracic aorta. The images clearly depicted the main duct in the region of the thoracic aorta in all six volunteers, drainage into the left subclavian region in four, and the cisterna chyli in one.

At present, x-ray lymphography with contrast agent is the only method available for examining the lymphatic vessels. However, x-ray lymphography is an invasive procedure with the drawbacks of contrast agent administration, patient discomfort, and a long examination time. To our knowledge, there have been no reports concerning visualization of the lymphatic vessels with magnetic resonance (MR) imaging. The thoracic duct is particularly difficult to image owing to its small size and the susceptibility effects in the lungs.

Recently, an MR angiographic technique has been reported for examining the pulmonary vessels with a half-Fourier fast spin-echo sequence, which is relatively resistant to susceptibility effects (1). To depict blood vessels containing fast and slow flow, electrocardiographic gating is employed to synchronize each section encoding with a three-dimensional (3D) half-Fourier fast spin-echo sequence (2).

The lymphatic system is an independent network for the circulation of fluid throughout the body. It is separate from the cardiovascular system and comprises relatively smaller vessels that contain slower flow. In this study, we evaluated depiction of the thoracic duct along the thoracic aorta at electrocardiography-gated MR imaging with a short echo spacing, 3D, half-Fourier fast spin-echo sequence.

Materials and Methods

MR lymphographic studies were performed on a 1.5-T clinical imager (Visart/Ex; Toshiba, Tokyo, Japan) in six healthy male volunteers (age range, 24–41 years; mean age, 30 years), according to a protocol approved by our institutional review board. Written informed consent was obtained from each volunteer.

A quadrature detection volume-array coil was employed to ensure a high signal-to-noise ratio and a uniform coil sensitivity (3). The sensitivity throughout the coil must be uniform, because the thoracic duct is located near the center of the body. To visualize both the thoracic duct and the thoracic aorta, late-diastolic electrocardiographic gating was used to trigger each section encoding in the 3D half-Fourier fast spin-echo sequence.

An intermittent breath-holding method was applied for each section encoding with use of gradient acoustic noise for biologic feedback. Each section encoding (or a single-shot acquisition window of 880 msec for a matrix size of 256 × 256) required a breath hold of less than 1 second, and normal breathing was permitted during the remainder of the repetition time. The effective temporal resolution of 880 msec is relatively long compared with the cardiac cycle. However, acquisition from near the center of k space, where the contrast is determined, allows fast flow in the thoracic aorta to be depicted with late-diastolic electrocardiographic gating (2). This was repeated for the number of section encodings in the

Visualization of Lymphatic System in Six Volunteers

Volunteer/Age (y)/Sex	Supraclavicular Part	Main Thoracic Duct	Cisterna Chyli
A/24/M	Visualized	Visualized	Visualized
B/32/M	Visualized	Visualized	Not visualized
C/41/M	Visualized	Visualized	Not visualized
D/27/M	Visualized	Visualized	Not visualized
E/25/M	Not visualized	Visualized	Not visualized
F/30/M	Not visualized	Visualized	Not visualized

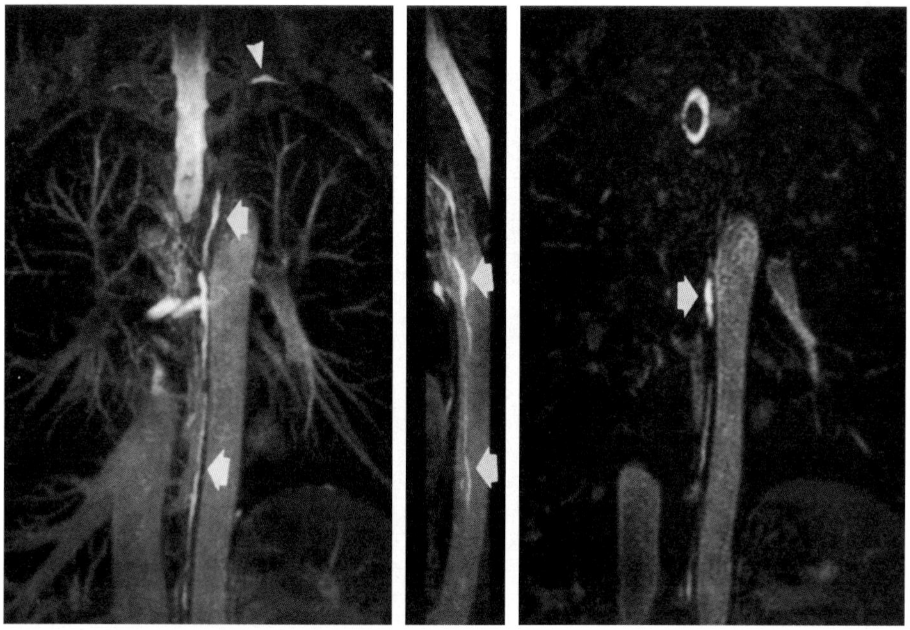

a. b. c.

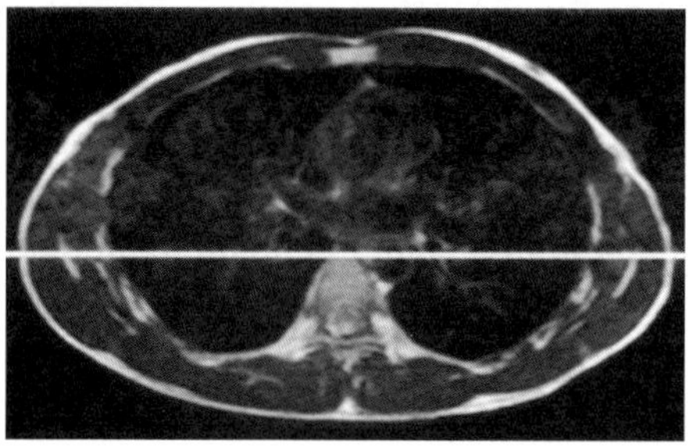

d.

Figure 1. Volunteer A. **(a)** Coronal MIP image (8,000/240 [effective]; echo spacing, 5 msec; matrix, 256 × 256; number of acquisitions, one; acquisition time, about 5 minutes) was obtained with an intermittent breath-hold technique. The main thoracic duct is indicated by arrows and drainage to the subclavian vein region by an arrowhead. **(b)** Sagittal MIP image generated from the same 3D data. The main thoracic duct is indicated by arrows. **(c)** Source image with the main thoracic duct indicated by an arrow. **(d)** Axial locator image.

3D acquisition. After acquisition, the 3D images underwent maximum intensity projection (MIP) processing.

Coronal in-plane imaging was performed with the following parameters: repetition time of 8,000 msec and effective echo time of 240 msec (8,000/240); echo spacing, 5 msec; matrix size, 256 × 256; 36 section partitions with a 1.4-mm section thickness; number of acquisitions, one; and field of view, 360 × 360 mm. To eliminate aliasing, a fat-suppression pulse was used, and phase-encoding saturation bands were applied in the superoinferior phase-encoding direction. The total acquisition time was about 5 minutes, depending on the heart rate.

All images were evaluated by a radiologist (S.H.) to assess depiction of the main thoracic duct, drainage into the left subclavian region, and the cisterna chyli.

Results

The Table summarizes visualization of the thoracic duct in the six volunteers. The main duct in the region of the thoracic aorta was consistently visualized in all six volunteers. Drainage in the region from the aortic arch to the left subclavian vein was visualized in four volunteers. In two volunteers, the region was outside the slab volume. The cisterna chyli was visualized in only volunteer A. This may be because the high signal intensity of gastric juice hinders visualization of the cisterna chyli.

Figure 1 shows coronal and sagittal MIP images obtained in volunteer A. The thoracic duct, with signal intensity somewhat higher than that of the blood vessels, is clearly visualized as an intermittent line along the thoracic aorta that runs toward the left supraclavicular region. Both the coronal and sagittal MIP images have high signal-to-noise ratio without artifacts or distortion, even at the thoracic region. To clarify the location, the source image is shown in Figure 1c and the axial locator image in Figure 1d. Figure 2 shows a partial MIP image (for only the thoracic region) for a better view of the cisterna chyli.

Figure 3 shows coronal and sagittal MIP images obtained in volunteer B. The main thoracic duct and drainage in the region of the left subclavian vein are clearly depicted. However, the diameter of the thoracic duct in the region of drainage into the subclavian vein is somewhat smaller than that of the main thoracic duct.

Discussion

The lymph-filled main thoracic duct was clearly depicted along the thoracic aorta with high spatial resolution in all six volunteers. The thoracic duct drains approximately three-quarters of the lymph in the body into the venous system. The duct originates from the cisterna chyli, which is usually located at the L1 to L2 level, enters the thoracic cavity via the aortic hiatus, and ascends between the aorta and the azygos vein. In the thorax, the thoracic duct crosses the mediastinum posteriorly and drains into the junction of the left subclavian and internal jugular veins. On the basis of x-ray lymphographic findings, the average diameter of the thoracic duct is approximately 1.3 mm (range, 0.5–2.0 mm) in the distal portion and 2.3 mm (range, 1.0–4.0 mm) in the proximal portion (4). The diameter of the thoracic duct in all our volunteers agreed with these values.

Our approach for depicting the thoracic duct employs 3D acquisition, which provided high spatial resolution in the section direction and permitted reformatting of the data for observation in any orientation. To ensure that the high signal intensity of lymph, which has long T1 and T2, was higher than that of blood, we used a long repetition time of 8,000 msec, which allowed full longitudinal recovery. In addition, a relatively long effective echo time of 240 msec gave a higher signal intensity for lymph because the shorter T2 of blood was attenuated.

The cerebrospinal fluid showed contrast similar to that of the lymph in the thoracic duct. Other pulmonary vessels in addition to the thoracic aorta were depicted in gray scale, which assisted identification of relative positions. The superoinferior phase-encoding direction was selected because of better blood signals in the phase-encoding direction (1). After interpolation in the section-encoding direction, the in-plane resolution was 1.4 × 1.4 mm, and the section thickness was 0.7 mm. Furthermore, distortion with the half-Fourier fast spin-echo sequence was lower than that at echo-planar imaging, even in the lungs, which show strong susceptibility effects. With electrocardiographic gating, the thoracic aorta and surrounding pulmonary vessels were clearly delineated, which also helped identification of the thoracic duct.

To our knowledge, this is the first report that MR lymphography with a short echo spacing, 3D, half-Fourier, fast spin-echo sequence can be used to visualize the thoracic duct without use of a contrast agent. With use of our technique, 3D data for the thoracic duct were easily acquired in a short time. This makes it possible to examine the lymphatic system while avoiding the problems associated with x-ray lymphography. Furthermore, this technique could also prove useful for the clinical diagnosis of chylothorax, traumatic chylous effusion, thoracic ductal abnormality, or megadolicholymphatics.

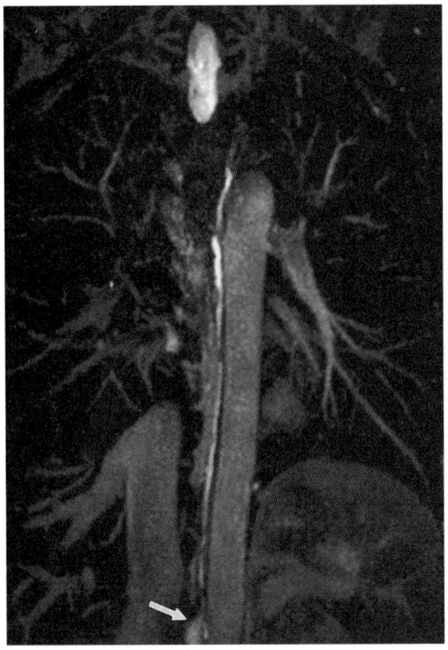

Figure 2. Volunteer A. Partial MIP image was processed in only the region of the thoracic duct, for a better view of the cisterna chyli (arrow).

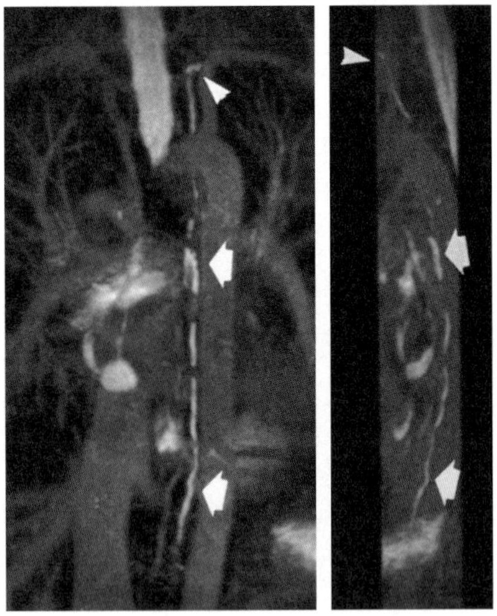

a. b.

Figure 3. Volunteer B. **(a)** Coronal and **(b)** sagittal MIP images were obtained with the same imaging parameters used for Figure 1. Both the main duct (arrows) and the region of drainage into the left subclavian vein (arrowhead) are depicted.

Acknowledgments: The authors thank Junichi Makita, BS, and Yoshimori Kassai, MS, of Toshiba Medical Engineering Center for their helpful discussion, and Karen Tanaka, BS, and David Spear, MD, of Toshiba Medical Systems Engineering for their assistance in manuscript preparation.

References

1. Miyazaki M, Ichinose N, Sugiura S, Kassai Y, Kanazawa H, Machida Y. A novel MR angiography technique: SPEED acquisition using half-Fourier RARE. JMRI 1998; 8:505–507.
2. Miyazaki M, Tateishi F, Sugiura S, Machida Y, Kassai Y, Abe H. Fresh blood imaging at 0.5-T: natural blood contrast 3D MRA within single breathhold (abstr). In: Proceedings of the Sixth Meeting of the International Society for Magnetic Resonance in Medicine. Berkeley, Calif: International Society for Magnetic Resonance in Medicine, 1998; 780.
3. Mori I, Hamamura Y, Kawamoto H. Recent problems of electromagnetic technology in MRI. IEICE Trans Commun 1995; E78-B: 809–817.
4. Wirth W, Frommhold H. Thoracicus und seine variationen: lymphographische studie. ROFO 1970; 112:450–459.

Letters to the Editor

MR Angiography in Acute Pulmonary Embolism

From:
Mathias Goyen, MD
Department of Radiology, University Hospital Essen
Hufelandstrasse 55, 45122 Essen, Germany
e-mail: *mathias@goyen.de*

Editor:
I read with great interest the excellent article by Dr Gupta and colleagues (1) in the February 1999 issue of *Radiology.* The authors show that three-dimensional pulmonary magnetic resonance (MR) angiography performed after injection of contrast material with high-performance gradients and echo times of 2 msec has overcome the problems of respiratory motion, cardiac pulsation, and susceptibility artifacts while still being able to depict small pulmonary arteries. This ability is comparable even with that of spiral computed tomographic angiography.

When one discusses imaging options for assessing acute pulmonary embolism (PE), it has to be considered that most patients with suspected PE are severely dyspneic and do not tolerate apnea for more than 15 seconds. This limits the application of three-dimensional contrast-enhanced MR angiography, which is performed with a single breath hold to eliminate the need for respiratory triggering, to those patients who are clinically able to suspend breathing. Dr Gupta and colleagues applied a steady-state gradient-recalled-echo sequence in a coronal volume with an echo time of 2 msec, a repetition time of 5 msec, and an acquisition time of 23 seconds. In their study, all patients tolerated the breath hold well. However, in the applied sequence, the breath hold could not be reduced without diminishing spatial resolution. Therefore, the collection of two separate sagittal acquisitions (with two injections of paramagnetic contrast material) may be an alternative approach. Because of a smaller field of view, images with a high spatial resolution can be obtained within a shorter breath hold. With the use of high-speed imaging gradients, images of a single lung can be achieved in less than 10 seconds (2).

References

1. Gupta A, Frazer CK, Ferguson JM, et al. Acute pulmonary embolism: diagnosis with MR angiography. Radiology 1999; 210:353–359.
2. Prince MR, Grist TM, Debatin JF. 3D contrast MR angiography. Berlin, Germany: Springer, 1999; 41–52.

Drs Gupta and Frazer respond:

We thank Dr Goyen for his interest in and comments on our article (1). Certainly, respiratory motion artifact was a limitation of the MR angiographic technique. Because of the constraints of the gradient hardware and pulse sequence that was commercially available at the time of the study, we had to reach a compromise between acquisition time and spatial resolution. Despite this constraint, there are ways to optimize image quality. Respiratory movement was minimized by good patient education, which included a description of the experience of undergoing an MR examination and the link between suspending respiration and image quality. In thin patients, a rectangular field of view was selected to reduce the acquisition time to 20 seconds. Also, patients were asked to hyperventilate for 30 seconds before suspending respiration in full expiration to minimize thoracic volume.

Our study group excluded patients with ventilation-perfusion scans that indicated a high probability of PE, and most patients were not severely dyspneic and tolerated the breath hold. If one were to perform MR angiography on patients with high-probability ventilation-perfusion scans, one may obtain better images by reducing acquisition time at the expense of spatial resolution.

Dr Goyen suggests performing two separate sagittal acquisitions with two injections of paramagnetic contrast material, thus reducing breath-hold time and increasing spatial resolution. This would, however, require double the dose of expensive contrast material and lengthen the examination time.

Newer, faster pulse sequences with shorter echo times and repetition times are becoming available, which will allow for shorter acquisition time and reduce breathing artifact problems in dyspneic patients.

Reference

1. Gupta A, Frazer CK, Ferguson JM, et al. Acute pulmonary embolism: diagnosis with MR angiography. Radiology 1999; 210:353–359.

Ashu Gupta, MBBS, and Christopher K. Frazer, FRACR
Department of Radiology, Sir Charles Gairdner Hospital
Hospital Avenue, Nedlands 6009, Western Australia, Australia

CT Reinterpretation

From:
Thomas J. White, Jr, MD
Department of Radiology (retired), University of Tennessee, Memphis
198 Greenbriar Drive, Memphis, TN 38117
e-mail: *twhite@utmem.edu*

Editor:
My thanks to Dr Gollub and colleagues for their article (1) in the January 1999 issue of *Radiology,* in which they demonstrated a willingness not only to review studies from other institutions but also to gather their results and attempt to assess their importance in the treatment of patients with cancer. I am aware that reinterpretations of studies have provided substantial value in patient care. The most obvious example is double or triple reading of mammograms for the detection of early breast cancer. Other second readings could be of similar value. However, I question the value of second interpretations of computed tomographic (CT) filmed images submitted to Dr Gollub and colleagues' department from referring radiologists' offices. Such hard copy is often a poor representation of CT images used for the original interpretation at the computer console with the flexibility in manipula-

tion available with digital information. Radiologists should use the information on the computer rather than rely on photographs. Filmed images are at best a compromise of images viewed on the computer.

Dr Gollub and colleagues say that a 3% effect on clinical treatment is substantial yet make no claim for the accuracy of the studies obtained or reinterpreted. Even if unintended by the radiologist, the reinterpretation of the images is regarded as correct by the clinician if it is being used to direct treatment.

I also question why a review of the original images cannot be performed without knowledge of the original interpretations. Bias could in that manner be reduced, if not eliminated. The best study design might not be best for patient care but should be considered in a research protocol.

Dr Gollub and colleagues could clarify the criteria they use to judge lymph node disease. It would also be interesting to know the circumstances of interpretation of the original CT studies, that is, before or after proof of malignancy.

Reference

1. Gollub MJ, Panicek DM, Bach AM, Penalver A, Castellino RA. Clinical importance of reinterpretation of body CT scans obtained elsewhere in patients referred for care at a tertiary cancer center. Radiology 1999; 210:109–112.

Dr Gollub and colleagues respond:

We thank Dr White for his interest in our article (1) and welcome the opportunity to respond to his questions and concerns.

When outside CT images are submitted to our department for official review (ie, a written report), we are given the hard-copy images and, for the past 5 years, a copy of the outside radiologist's interpretation. We agree that manipulation of images on a computer monitor (eg, to obtain region of interest measurements) is preferable, but this requires that all submitted CT scans be accompanied by laser disks. This is neither practical nor the standard of practice. With the advent of picture archiving and communication systems, such a mode of sending images to other institutions for reinterpretation may, in fact, become more common through either laser disks or Internet transmission. However, at the current time, the standard practice is to review hard-copy images, and this is reflected in our article.

Dr White misquotes our conclusion, which states that the effect on clinical treatment made a substantial difference in individual cases, such as that of the patient with a 3-cm melanoma mass in the groin that was not noted at the outside facility. It is a value judgment whether such an effect on 3% of the overall population is worthwhile.

We clearly stated that in our study we did not attempt to determine the accuracy of our interpretations in a comparison with interpretations by the outside radiologist. Our clinicians submitted scans for our reinterpretation to direct patient care. This occurs in other hospitals, as well, irrespective of the eventual accuracy of the subsequent second readings.

A research study could be designed to review the original images without knowledge of the original interpretation, as Dr White suggests. However, we believe it is irresponsible to ignore the outside radiologist's report in a clinical setting, since it is important to avoid the possibility of our overlooking a finding that was noted by the outside radiologist. As such, in the interest of patient care, we insist on receiving the outside report to review before issuing a final official reinterpretation. The reasons for this are discussed in the article by Castellino (2). We again emphasize that we did not attempt to assess the accuracy of either reading; in fact, knowledge of the outside reading gave us the advantage of preventing us from missing findings noted on the outside report.

For assessment of lymph node disease, we used standard criteria: nodes measuring 1 cm or larger in short-axis diameter (in most locations) or smaller in other locations (eg, left paratracheal, superior diaphragmatic) or, in certain disease states (such as testicular cancer), an increased number of normal-sized nodes clustered in sites where metastatic lymphadenopathy would be expected.

All the patients in our study had a biopsy-proved diagnosis of cancer, which was known to us when we reinterpreted the CT scans. This differs from other studies, such as that of Hricak et al (3), that include patients with a suspected but unproved malignancy in which the diagnosis for some patients eventually will be changed to benign, as first suggested by the reinterpretation. With respect to the original circumstances of interpretation of CT studies by the outside radiologist, we do not know whether there was proved malignancy at that time.

References

1. Gollub MJ, Panicek DM, Bach AM, Penalver A, Castellino RA. Clinical importance of reinterpretation of body CT scans obtained elsewhere in patients referred for care at a tertiary cancer center. Radiology 1999; 210:109–112.
2. Castellino RA. Official review of outside studies (opinion). Invest Radiol 1994; 1:80–81.
3. Hricak H, Kalbhen CL, Scheidler JE, et al. Value of expert interpretation in abdominal oncologic imaging: a multicenter study (abstr). Radiology 1997; 205(P):225.

Marc J. Gollub, MD, David M. Panicek, MD, Ariadne M. Bach, MD, and Ronald A. Castellino, MD
Department of Radiology, Memorial Sloan-Kettering Cancer Center
1275 York Avenue, New York, NY 10021

Abstracts of Current Literature

Cardiovascular System

The Brugada Syndrome: Clinical, Electrophysiologic and Genetic Aspects. Ihor Gussak, Charles Antzelevitch, Preben Bjerregaard, et al. *J Am Coll Cardiol* 1999; 33:5–15. (I.G., Department of Internal Medicine, Division of Cardiology, St Louis University Health Science Center, 1034 Brentwood Blvd, Suite 1550, St Louis, MO 63117)

This review deals with the clinical, basic and genetic aspects of a recently highlighted form of idiopathic ventricular fibrillation known as the Brugada syndrome. Our primary objective in this review is to identify the full scope of the syndrome and attempt to correlate the electrocardiographic manifestations of the Brugada syndrome with cellular and ionic heterogeneity known to exist within the heart under normal and pathophysiologic conditions so as to identify the cellular basis and thus potential diagnostic and therapeutic approaches. The available data suggest that the Brugada syndrome is a primary electrical disease resulting in abnormal electrophysiologic activity in right ventricular epicardium. Recent genetic data linking the Brugada syndrome to an ion channel gene mutation (SCN5A) provides further support for the hypothesis. The electrocardiographic manifestations of the Brugada syndrome show transient normalization in many patients, but can be unmasked using sodium channel blockers such as flecainide, ajmaline or procainamide, thus identifying patients at risk. The available data suggest that loss of the action potential dome in right ventricular epicardium but not endocardium underlies the ST segment elevation seen in the Brugada syndrome and that electrical heterogeneity within right ventricular epicardium leads to the development of closely coupled premature ventricular contractions via a phase 2 reentrant mechanism that then precipitates ventricular tachycardia/ventricular fibrillation (VT/VF). Currently, implantable cardiac defibrillator implantation is the only proven effective therapy in preventing sudden death in patients with the Brugada syndrome and is indicated in symptomatic patients and should be considered in asymptomatic patients in whom VT/VF is inducible at time of electrophysiologic study.
Authors' Abstract

Reasons for selecting abstract:
- New syndrome
- General medical background information

Selected by *Robert M. Steiner, MD*
New York Methodist Hospital–Weill Medical College of Cornell University, New York, NY

Coronary Calcification by Electron Beam Computed Tomography and Obstructive Coronary Artery Disease: A Model for Costs and Effectiveness of Diagnosis as Compared with Conventional Cardiac Testing Methods. John A. Rumberger, Thomas Behrenbeck, Jerome F. Breen, et al. *J Am Coll Cardiol* 1999; 33:453–462. (From the Department of Cardiovascular Diseases, Mayo Clinic and Foundation, Rochester, Minn)

Objectives: The purpose of this study was to determine if electron beam computed tomography (EBCT) has potential as a cost-effective approach to diagnosis of obstructive coronary disease. *Background:* Coronary calcification quantified by EBCT is closely related to the extent of atherosclerosis. *Methods:* A model based upon published sensitivities (Se)/specificities (Sp) for diagnosis in an ambulatory patient of obstructive coronary disease (≥50% stenosis) and population prevalence was tested for angiography alone, or treadmill exercise, stress echocardiography, stress thallium or predetermined EBCT calcium score outpoints, followed by angiography if indicated. *Results:* Total direct testing costs increased in proportion to disease prevalence whereas cost-effectiveness, direct costs/patient diagnosed correctly with disease, decreased as a function of prevalence. Using an EBCT calcium score of 168 (Se/Sp = 71%/90%) provided for the least costly and most cost-effective noninvasive pathway. Calcium scores of 80 (Se/Sp = 84%/84%) and 37 (Se/Sp = 90%/77%) were also cost-effective when prevalence of disease was ≤70%; but results for a >0 calcium score (Se/Sp = 95%/46%) cutpoint were not superior to conventional methods. Calcium score cutpoints of 37, 80 or 168 provided similar or superior overall negative and positive predictive values to conventional noninvasive testing pathways across all prevalence subgroups. *Conclusions:* In ambulatory patients evaluated for obstructive coronary disease, a testing pathway utilizing quantification of coronary calcium by EBCT as an initial noninvasive testing approach minimized direct costs, and maximized cost-effectiveness in population groups with low/moderate disease prevalence (≤70%); as expected, direct angiography as the first and only test proved most cost-effective in patients with a high prevalence (>70%) of disease.
Authors' Abstract

Reasons for selecting abstract:
- Efficacy study for EBCT
- Imaging modality
- Comparison with nonimaging testing

Selected by *Robert M. Steiner, MD*
New York Methodist Hospital–Weill Medical College of Cornell University, New York, NY

Echocardiographic Diagnosis Alone for the Complete Repair of Major Congenital Heart Defects. Wayne Tworetzky, Doff B. McElhinney, Michael M. Brook, et al. *J Am Coll Cardiol* 1999; 33:228–233. (Norman H. Silverman, Division of Pediatric Cardiology, University of California, San Francisco, 505 Parnassus Ave, M342A, San Francisco, CA 94143-0214)

Objectives: The study was done to determine the diagnostic accuracy of echocardiography alone in the preoperative diagnosis of children with major congenital heart defects undergoing primary complete repair. *Background:* Although echocardiography is well established as the first-line imaging technique for the diagnosis of all forms of congenital heart disease, most institutions continue to perform cardiac catheterization prior to complete repair of more complex defects. *Methods:* To determine the diagnostic accuracy of echocardiography alone and echocardiography plus catheterization, we reviewed the records of 503 children with major congenital heart defects who underwent primary complete repair at our institution between July 1992 and June 1997. We included children with transposition of the great arteries, tetralogy of Fallot, double-chamber right ventricle, interrupted aortic arch, aortic coarctation, atrioventricular septal defect, truncus arteriosus, aortopulmonary septal defect, and totally anomalous pulmonary venous return. We excluded children with less complex defects such as isolated shunt lesions, as well as those with the most complex defects that would require surgical palliation (e.g., functional univentricular heart). We defined major errors as those that increased the surgical risk and minor errors as those that did not. Errors in diagnosis were determined at surgery. *Results:* Eighty-two percent of children (412 of 503) underwent surgery after preoperative diagnosis by echocardiography alone. There were 9 major (2%) and 10 minor errors in the echocardiography alone group and 7 major and 5 minor errors in the echocardiography plus catheterization group. The most common type of error was misidentification of coronary artery anatomy in patients with transposition of the great arteries. No error in either group resulted in surgical morbidity or mortality. *Conclusions:* This study suggests that echocardiography alone is an accurate tool for the preoperative diagnosis of major congenital heart defects in most children undergoing primary complete repair, and may obviate the need for routine diagnostic catheterization.
Authors' Abstract

Reasons for selecting abstract:
- Imaging in congenital heart disease
- Algorithm for congenital heart disease

Selected by *Robert M. Steiner, MD*
New York Methodist Hospital–Weill Medical College of Cornell University, New York, NY

Ejection Fraction by Radionuclide Ventriculography and Contrast Left Ventriculogram: A Tale of Two Techniques. Pedro E. Ureña, Gervasio A. Lamas, Gary Mitchell, et al. *J Am Coll Cardiol* 1999; 33:180–185. (G.A.L., Division of Cardiology, Mount Sinai Medical Center, 4300 Alton Rd, Miami Beach, FL 33140)

Objectives: We assessed the abilities of two methods to measure ejection fraction (EF)—radionuclide ventriculography (RVG) and contrast left ventriculography (Cath-EFa) to predict cardiovascular events. *Background:* Both RVG and Cath-EFa are commonly used methods to measure left ventricular performance and assess prognosis. Their comparative abilities to predict clinical events have not been reported. *Methods:* Both RVG EF and Cath-EFa were measured within 16 days of myocardial infarction (MI) in 688 patients. The results

were divided into terciles. Prognosis by terciles was assessed for each technique. A multivariate analysis was performed to determine which EF measurement was a better predictor of prognosis. *Results:* Average RVG-EF was 32% ± 7, while Cath-EFa was 42% ± 10. Both RVG and Cath-EFa were poorly correlated ($R = 0.42$). Event rate declined across terciles with increasing EF for both techniques (events in lowest to highest tercile of Cath-EFa 40.7%, 25.9%, 11.6%, $p < 0.001$; and RVG-EF 39.9%, 26.1%, 15.6%, $p < 0.001$). There was concordance of terciles in 303 of 688 patients (44%). When patients in the highest RVG terciles were in the highest Cath-EFa tercile, the event rate was 7%. However, when patients in the highest RVG terciles were in the lowest Cath-EFa tercile, the event rate was 19%. Both Cath-EFa ($p < 0.001$) and RVG-EF ($p < 0.001$) were independent predictors of cardiovascular events. *Conclusions:* Ejection fraction measured by RVG or during catheterization is a valuable tool in the risk stratification of postinfarct patients. When disagreement is present between clinical impression and measurement by either method, the use of an alternative measurement is warranted and complementary.
Authors' Abstract
Reason for selecting abstract:
- Imaging comparison for an important cardiac physiologic parameter

Selected by *Robert M. Steiner, MD*
New York Methodist Hospital–Weill Medical College of Cornell University, New York, NY

Left Ventricular Pseudoaneurysm. Craig Frances, Anthony Romero, Deborah Grady. *J Am Coll Cardiol* 1998; 32:557–561. (C.F., Veterans Affairs Medical Center, 4150 Clement St, Rm 111A1, San Francisco, CA 94121)

Left ventricular (LV) pseudoaneurysms form when cardiac rupture is contained by adherent pericardium or scar tissue. Although LV pseudoaneurysms are not common, the diagnosis is difficult and they are prone to rupture. We evaluated the clinical presentation, diagnostic accuracy of imaging modalities, results of therapy and prognosis of 290 patients with LV pseudoaneurysms. Most cases of LV pseudoaneurysm were related to myocardial infarction (particularly inferior wall myocardial infarction) and cardiac surgery. Congestive heart failure, chest pain and dyspnea were the most frequently reported symptoms, but >10% of patients were asymptomatic. Physical examination revealed a murmur in 70% of patients. Almost all patients had electrocardiographic abnormalities, but these were usually nonspecific ST segment changes; only 20% of patients had ST segment elevation. Although radiographic findings were also usually nonspecific, the appearance of a mass was present in more than one half of patients and may be an important clue to the correct diagnosis. Left ventricular angiography was the most definitive test and can be useful in planning surgery since concomitant coronary angiography can be performed. Regardless of treatment, patients with LV pseudoaneurysms had a high mortality rate, especially those who did not undergo surgery. Because the symptoms, signs, electrocardiographic abnormalities and radiographic findings seen in patients with LV pseudoaneurysms can be indistinguishable from those in patients with coronary disease alone, a high clinical index of suspicion is needed to avoid missing the diagnosis.
Authors' Abstract
Reasons for selecting abstract:
- Important cardiac imaging problem
- Clinical care problem

Selected by *Robert M. Steiner, MD*
New York Methodist Hospital–Weill Medical College of Cornell University, New York, NY

Morphological Onset and Early Diagnosis in Apical Hypertrophic Cardiomyopathy: A Long Term Analysis with Nuclear Magnetic Resonance Imaging. Jun-ichi Suzuki, Ryoichi Shimamoto, Jun-ichi Nishikawa, et al. *J Am Coll Cardiol* 1999; 33:146–151. (J.S., Second Department of Internal Medicine, Faculty of Medicine, University of Tokyo, Hongo 7-3-1, Bunkyo-ku, Tokyo 1138655, Japan)

Objectives: A long-term follow-up study with nuclear magnetic resonance (NMR) imaging was undertaken to detect the morphological onset and to establish the early diagnosis in apical hypertrophic cardiomyopathy (HCM). *Background:* A spadelike configuration on left ventriculogram (LVG) is regarded as a diagnostic criterion for the classical apical HCM. There also exists a segmented hypertrophy at the apical level without indicating the spadelike features (a nonspade configuration). To detect the hypertrophied myocardium of the nonspade configuration, circumferential scrutiny of the apex is required. Although both configurations can be underlying causes of giant negative T waves, etiological relationship between the two is not clarified. *Methods:* The criteria for the spadelike configuration defined on left ventricular short-axis NMR images were as follows: (apical maximal thickness ≥15 mm), (apical anterior thickness over basal anterior thickness ≥1.3) and (apical posterior thickness over basal posterior thickness ≥1.3). Thirteen patients who had predominant hypertrophy (≥15 mm) at the apical level without the spadelike configuration underwent NMR imaging twice before and after 54 ± 10 months' follow-up. *Results:* Apical hypertrophy that had been confined to the lateral wall in four, the anterior-lateral wall in two, and the septal-anterior wall in one developed to become circumferential hypertrophy that fulfilled the criteria for the spadelike configuration after the follow-up period. *Conclusions:* The spadelike configuration can begin with the nonspade configuration and therefore, both can constitute a single disease entity of apical HCM. The early diagnosis of apical HCM can be achieved by identifying the hypertrophy frequently confined to the lateral wall at the apical level.
Authors' Abstract
Reason for selecting abstract:
- Indication for MR imaging

Selected by *Robert M. Steiner, MD*
New York Methodist Hospital–Weill Medical College of Cornell University, New York, NY

Noncardiac Surgery in Eisenmenger Syndrome. Naser M. Ammash, Heidi M. Connolly, Martin D. Abel, et al. *J Am Coll Cardiol* 1999; 33:222–227. (N.M.A., Division of Cardiovascular Diseases and Internal Medicine, Mayo Clinic, 200 First St SW, West 16B, Rochester, MN 55905)

Objectives: The purpose of this study was to evaluate the morbidity and mortality associated with noncardiac surgery (NCS) in patients (pts) with Eisenmenger syndrome. *Background:* Noncardiac surgery in pts with Eisenmenger syndrome is associated with increased cardiovascular complications. METHODS: Fifty-eight pts with Eisenmenger syndrome (17M, 41F aged 18 to 69 years (mean 41 years) who had been followed for up to 41.5 years (mean 9.3 years) were retrospectively evaluated for any NCS done at ≥17 years of age. *Results:* Twenty-four pts had a total of 28 NCSs at an age of 17 to 55 years (mean 29 years) including 9 tubal ligations, 3 neurosurgeries, 3 cholecystectomies, 3 hysterectomies, 3 vasectomies, and 1 each spinal fusion, appendectomy, eye enucleation, hernia repair, hand surgery, tonsillectomy and therapeutic abortion. There were two deaths (7%), one following spinal fusion and the other following appendectomy at another institution. Fourteen of these NCSs were performed at our institution, including 11 under general anesthesia. The duration of anesthesia varied from 75 to 525 min (mean 165 min). All pts remained in sinus rhythm. The lowest systolic blood pressure (BP) ranged from 78 to 125 mm Hg. Of those 11 pts, 9 were extubated immediately after surgery and 2 needed dopamine. Ten patients were discharged without any complications, including 3 within 1 day of surgery. One death occurred 10 days following spinal fusion. This pt had the longest anesthesia (525 min) and an intraoperative systolic BP as low as 78 mm Hg. She also needed the largest fluid administration (6,475 cc) in addition to postoperative mechanical ventilation and dopamine. *Conclusions:* Adult pts with Eisenmenger syndrome are at increased risk with NCS, but with current/modern techniques, the risk of death is less than previously thought. In the vast majority of cases, NCS can be undertaken without substantial morbidity, and early extubation is achievable. However, even with relatively minor surgery, significant complications, including death, can occur. Referral to major centers with expertise in the care of pts with Eisenmenger syndrome is advisable.
Authors' Abstract
Reasons for selecting abstract:
- Clinical observation
- Surgical patients are prone to complications

Selected by *Robert M. Steiner, MD*
New York Methodist Hospital–Weill Medical College of Cornell University, New York, NY

Classified Services

POLICY

As a service to its readers, *Radiology* accepts classified advertising, and every effort is made to ensure that the ads are relevant to the practice of radiology. Acceptable categories include positions available, positions sought, fellowships, announcements of postgraduate courses or symposia, practices for sale, medical facilities for rent or sale, used radiologic equipment and apparatus for sale, medical employment bureau advertising, academic posts to be filled, available posts for interns and residents, and malpractice insurance. We retain the right to refuse any advertisement considered not relevant, and respondents are advised to investigate each offer since we cannot assume responsibility for the offers or claims of advertisers.

RATES (per month, per insertion)

Line ads in *Radiology* (no agency commission)

50 words or less $100.00

51–100 words $145.00

Each word over 100—$1.00 per word.

Box Number—$30.00 additional per each insertion (this service is optional).

TERMS

Payment must accompany order.* Make checks payable to **Radiological Society of North America.** We accept American Express, VISA, Mastercard, and Diners Club for classified ads. Call for details. Send payment to:

RSNA, Radiology Classified Ad Department
Accounts Payable, 820 Jorie Boulevard
Oak Brook, IL 60523-2251 USA.

*Purchase Order Numbers are accepted with prior approval.

Please mark each issue:

❒ Jan ❒ Feb ❒ Mar ❒ Apr ❒ May ❒ June
❒ July ❒ Aug ❒ Sept ❒ Oct ❒ Nov ❒ Dec

Send invoice and tearsheet to:

____

____

____

____

Advertisers who cancel ads will not receive refunds.

DEADLINE

Copy must be received by the **20th of the second month preceding issue.** Please submit copy typed and double-spaced. Initials or abbreviations equal one word. Telephone numbers with area code equal one word.

CLASSIFIED DISPLAY ADVERTISING

Black and white frequency rates are based on the total number of insertions used within a 12-month period from date of first insertion.

Ad Space	Size	1X	6X	12X
1 page	7" x 9-1/2"	$2350	2270	2190
2/3 pg vert	4-1/2" x 9-1/2"	$2000	1930	1860
1/2 pg horzt	7" x 4-1/2"	$1550	1490	1430
1/2 pg vert	3-3/8" x 9-1/2"	$1550	1490	1430
1/2 pg island	4-1/4" x 7-1/2"	$1550	1490	1430
1/3 pg vert	2-1/4" x 9-1/2"	$1100	1050	1000
1/3 pg square	4-1/2" x 4-1/2"	$1100	1050	1000
1/4 page	3-3/8" x 4-1/2"	$ 900	860	820
1/6 page	2-1/4" x 4-1/2"	$ 650	630	610
1/9 page	2-1/4" x 3"	$ 450	430	410

Preferred materials are composite negatives, right-reading, emulsion side down. (Conversion materials such as positive film, repro proofs, and camera-ready artworks are acceptable; there may be an additional charge.)

Customer supplied negative: cost as noted
Customer supplied copy to be set and ad prepared: add 20%

Call Production Department for additional information. Address for correspondence, insertion orders, copy, proofs, box number, and payment:

Radiology **Advertising Production Office**
820 Jorie Boulevard
Oak Brook, IL 60523-2251

To respond to a box number ad, send your CV and/or any other information to the above address; on the front of the envelope, please indicate the appropriate box number.

For further information:
Patrick Williamson, *Advertising Coordinator*
630.571.7817
630.571.7837 (fax)

Positions Available

THE DEPARTMENT OF RADIOLOGY AT THE UNIVERSITY OF ALABAMA AT BIRMINGHAM—Is actively recruiting an interventional radiologist. The section of Vascular and Interventional Radiology provides services for 1,100-beds at the University and Veteran's Administration Hospitals and performs over 5,500 procedures per year. Currently there are three full-time faculty members. Facilities include a Siemens Multistar TOP and two Philips angio suites currently under construction. Applicants must be Board certified in diagnostic radiology, have a CAQ in vascular and interventional radiology (or eligible for a CAQ), and eligible for licensure in the state of Alabama. Duties include medical student and resident teaching, radiology service and clinical research. Academic rank and tenure status will depend upon qualifications and experience. Interested candidates should submit their CV to Robert J. Stanley, MD, Department of Radiology, University of Alabama at Birmingham, AL 35233. The University of Alabama at Birmingham is an affirmative action/equal opportunity employer.

THE UNIVERSITY OF KENTUCKY—Is seeking a full-time, tenured line, open rank academic thoracic radiologist. Must be Board eligible; certification preferred. Duties would also include interpretation of film for evaluation of occupational lung disease. Responsibilities include patient care, medical student and resident teaching, and regularly scheduled interdepartment conferences. Opportunity to pursue clinical research. Please mail or fax letter of interest and curriculum vitae to James C. Reed, MD, Chairman, Department of Radiology, HX304, UK Medical Center, Lexington, KY 40536-0084; fax 606-257-6014. UK is an equal opportunity employer.

ASHEVILLE, NC— A board certified radiologist is needed to help with night, weekend day, and holiday call coverage of 21 person group practice in major referral center. Partnership track available with excellent time off and benefits package in beautiful mountain vacation area. Send CV to Ms. Sue Spivey, P.O. Box 2959, Asheville, NC 28802

CROSS-SECTIONAL IMAGER (CT, ULTRASOUND AND MRI)—Northeastern PA partnership track position. Interventional skills a definite plus. Eight man group currently provides complete range of services for a busy commu-

Two hours to Atlantic or Gulf. Send CV to Dr Kelley P. Douglas, Tifton Radiology, PC, 1495 Kennedy Rd, Tifton, GA 31794 or fax to 912-386-4495.

WESTERN NORTH CAROLINA—Diagnostic radiologist needed to practice and live in Brevard, NC, a beautiful college town in the Smoky Mountains located 30 miles from Asheville. Individuals should have skills and interest in all phases of diagnostic radiology, including CT, NM, US, mammography and basic interventional/special procedures. This is a partnership track position within a 24-physician practice based in Asheville which will provide subspecialty backup, vacation coverage and after hours teleradiology. The individual selected for this position will rotate through the Asheville practice on a regular basis. Please contact Sue Spivey, PO Box 2959, Asheville, NC 28802.

THE DEPARTMENT OF REGIONAL RADIOLOGY AT THE CLEVELAND CLINIC FOUNDATION—Cleveland, Ohio, is in the process of recruiting ABR certified general diagnostic radiologists to practice in community hospitals and ambulatory care facilities, which are part of the Cleveland Clinic Health System. The department consists of 20 staff radiologists servicing four community hospitals and seven ambulatory care facilities/surgi centers. Approximately 278,000 examinations were performed at the sites in 1998. The hospital departments and outpatient facilities are fully networked (imaging and RIS) with the Cleveland Clinic Foundation main campus radiology department, which is staffed by 48 subspecialty radiologists. If this opportunity is appealing to you, please contact Gregory P. Borkowski, MD, FACR, Chairman, Regional Radiology Practice, The Cleveland Clinic Foundation, Department of Radiology, Hb-6, 9500 Euclid Ave, Cleveland, OH 44195; phone 216-444-6625, fax 216-445-4432, e-mail *borkowg @cesmtp.ccf.org.*

DIRECTOR OF BREAST IMAGING—Suburban LA hospital seeks breast imager to direct large breast imaging center affiliated with a 400-bed in-patient facility. Has screening, diagnostic mammography services, ultrasound, ABBI, mammotome, and access to MRI. Must be Board certified in radiology and capable of performing other routine radiographic studies. Please reply to Box R-107.

EVENING/WEEKEND DIAGNOSTIC RADIOLOGISTS—Midwest group seeking Board certified (eligible) individuals to rotate coverage. General, CT, US, nuclear medicine skills needed. Basic angio helpful. Salaried positions; 810-412-9944, ask for Judi.

MINNESOTA: BUSY MINNESOTA RADIOLOGY PRACTICE—Dakota Clinic, a 175-physician-owned multispecialty clinic based in Fargo, North Dakota, is seeking a BE/BC radiologist for our Thief River Falls, Minnesota division for the summer of 2000. Located in northwest Minnesota, this 16-physician group is looking to replace its retiring radiologist with an eager individual proficient in general, CT, MRI and nuclear radiology. Enjoy a new 50,000 square foot state-of-the-art clinic and modern hospital. We offer a competitive salary and benefits package with stockholdership available after two years. Thief River Falls, the home of Arctic Cat snowmobiles, is a growing community of 9,000 with a service area of 45,000. This family-oriented community offers excellent schools, low crime, hunting, fishing and easy access to Minnesota lakes. To learn more about this opportunity, mail, fax or e-mail your CV to Dick Reis, Physician Recruitment Manager, Dakota Clinic Ltd, 1702 S University Dr, Fargo, ND 58103. Fax 701-280-3229, e-mail *dreis @dakcl.com,* toll-free number 1-800-882-7310. Dakota Clinic: *www.dakotaclinic.com.*

NEURORADIOLOGIST—The University of Michigan at Ann Arbor is seeking an academic neuroradiologist. Call or e-mail Dr. Gebarski for details at 734-936-4484; *gebarski@umich.edu.*

VISITING FACULTY POSITION IN CLINICAL CT RESEARCH—The Department of Radiology at Indiana University School of Medicine has a research position for a radiologist with clinical research interest in multi-slice spiral CT. The researcher will help design and carry out clinical research studies in collaboration with faculty subspecialty radiologists in thoracic, abdominal, musculoskeletal and neuroradiology and write manuscripts for publication in peer-reviewed journals. There is excellent supporting infrastructure including research nurses, technologists, secretaries, statisticians, PACS, workstations, graphics/photographic equipment, and information systems. Rank and salary will be commensurate with experience and qualifications. Interested applicants should send their curriculum vitae to Dr Kenyon Kopecky, Department of Radiology, Indiana University Hospital Room 0279, 550 N University Blvd, Indianapolis, IN 46202-5253 or e-mail *kkopecky @iupui.edu*. Indiana University is an EO/AA employer.

WANTED: BOARD CERTIFIED RADIOLOGISTS IN NE PENNSYLVANIA—Radiological Consultants, Inc, has a demand for several radiologists secondary to both retiring members as well as an expanding service area. We are group of 17 radiologists in northeast Pennsylvania covering two hospitals in Scranton, one hospital in Wilkes Barre, one hospital in Nanticoke, as well as an MRI center which houses two 1.5 Tesla magnets as well as an open 0.3 Tesla magnet. We are currently targeting fellowship trained or an equivalent experienced radiologist. Competitive salary and benefits are being offered for this excellent opportunity. Reply to Radiological Consultants, Inc, c/o John J. Culliney, MD, 751 Keystone Industrial Park, Dunmore, PA 18512. Phone 717-346-8272 or fax CV to 717-346-4872.

MAMMOGRAPHER IN CENTRAL JERSEY—Group of five hospital-based private practice radiologists seeking fellowship trained mammographer for new state-of-the-art women's center including stereotactic biopsy. Partnership opportunity. Please contact Dr. McManus, 732-886-4445.

EXCELLENT PARTNERSHIP OPPORTUNITY IN LOUISIANA!—Growing, dynamic radiology group of nine is seeking two new partners to begin in June 2000. Group covers four hospitals performing 180k exams per year. Practice is located in northwest Louisiana in a beautiful community of 200k. Applicant should be Board certified and fellowship trained in interventional radiology or body imaging. Applicant should be competent in all areas of radiology. Please send your CV to J. Paul Price, MD, 939 Delaware St, Shreveport, LA 71106. Or via e-mail *Magnethead@msn.com.*

VASCULAR/INTERVENTIONAL—The University of Texas M.D. Anderson Cancer Center at Houston has an immediate opening for a full-time vascular and interventional radiologist. Applicants should be fellowship trained and ABR certified. The vascular and interventional section performs all non-coronary and non-neurologic vascular diagnostic and interventional procedures as well as the full range of non-vascular intervention. Applicants must be committed to patient care, teaching and research. Academic rank is dependent on qualifications. Interested candidates should submit a CV to Marshall E. Hicks, MD, UTMDACC, Diagnostic Radiology Box 57, 1515 Holcombe Blvd, Houston, TX 77030, Telephone 713-792-8295; fax 713-792-4098. U.T.M.D. Anderson Cancer Center is an equal opportunity employer. Women and minority candidates are encouraged to apply. Smoke-free environment.

GOSHEN, IN—Full-time position available beginning on July 12, 1999 for general radiologist in hospital-based three-person group. The position includes MRI, angio/intervention, mammography, CT, US, NM and general diagnostics. Partnership track. 1/3 year off. Good support from the hospital administration and board. Full benefits package available. For more information, contact John F. Maesaka, MD, at e-mail *john_anne .maesaka @ibm.net*, fax 219-533-2413, phone 219-535-2604, or send CV to John F. Maesaka, Dept of Radiology, Goshen General Hospital, 200 High Park, Goshen, IN 46526.

THE UNIVERSITY OF CINCINNATI, DEPARTMENT OF RADIOLOGY—Seeks qualified candidates for non-tenure track positions at the assistant or associate professor level, rank commensurate with experience. Opportunities are available for physicians with subspecialty interest in one or more of the following areas: general body imaging, abdominal, thoracic, breast imaging, body MRI, and angio/interventional. Fellowship training is preferred but not required. Must be ABR/AOBR certified and have, or be eligible for, an Ohio medical license. Applicants should be interested in pursuing a combined academic/clinical career. Responsibilities include clinical patient care and teaching/supervision of residents, fellows and students. Participation in basic and clinical research is supported. Letters of inquiry and CV should be forwarded to Ms Shira Karns, Radiology Business Office, 2600 Euclid Ave, Cincinnati, OH 45219. The University of Cincinnati is an AA/EOE/ADA employer. Women, minorities, persons with disabilities, Vietnam era and disabled veterans are encouraged to apply. UC is a smoke-free work environment.

PEORIA RADIOLOGY ASSOCIATES, PC—Is currently recruiting two general radiologists for one of our satellite institutions. This represents a unique career opportunity to join a large private subspecialty radiology group with close university affiliation. This is a partnership track offer. Peoria Radiology Associates, PC, is a 25-person, highly subspecialized group that has an active teaching program including radiology residents and fellowships in neuroradiology, breast imaging and interventional radiology. There is an excellent compensation and benefit package. Clinical responsibilities include all areas of medical imaging, including MRI and possibly some interventional radiology. All inquiries will be held confidential. Please indicate whether you wish to be contacted at home or at work. Please reply with CV to Kay Springer, Peoria Radiology Associates, PC, 530 NE Glen Oak Ave, Peoria, IL 61637, or fax 309-655-2951.

THE UNIVERSITY OF KENTUCKY MEDICAL CENTER—Is offering an unusual opportunity for an individual whose expertise and interest include adult and pediatric plain film, GI/GU, CT, ultrasound, nuclear medicine and mammography. Candidate must be certified by the American Board of Radiology. The opportunity presented is to live in a small, scenic, historical college town approximately 40 miles southeast of Lexington, be part of the University of Kentucky Department of Diagnostic Radiology faculty with regular participation in the teaching of residents and medical students. The position includes UK hospital privileges, as well as the local community hospital with an enlarged, newly renovated department, excellent equipment and technical staff. This opportunity offers UK benefits and open academic rank based on qualifications. If this unusual opportunity appeals to you, please send or fax your letter of interest and CV to James C. Reed, MD, Chairman, Department of Diagnostic Radiology, A110 KY Clinic, Lexington, KY 40536-0284; fax 606-257-6014. Position available immediately. The University of Kentucky is an equal opportunity employer.

MUSCULOSKELETAL RADIOLOGY STAFF POSITION—Available at the Cleveland Clinic Foundation. An opportunity exists for a Board-certified, fellowship-trained musculoskeletal radiologist to join a diverse, dynamic group of colleagues at one of the leading health care centers in the country. Our section works closely with the departments of orthopedics, rheumatology and endocrinology. Academic interests are encouraged. The section provides full musculoskeletal diagnostic and interventional services. Teaching within the department and in other departments is expected. The section performs over 100,000 studies per year in an atmosphere of cutting-edge technology. For further information or to forward your resume, please contact: Bradford J. Richmond, MD, Desk A-21, Cleveland Clinic Foundation, 9500 Euclid Ave, Cleveland, OH 44195; 216-444-3931.

DYNAMIC RADIOLOGY GROUP—In beautiful Pacific NW seeking a generalist with specialty expertise. 380+-bed, level II trauma center. Partnership track. Great community; affordable living; close to skiing, fishing, boating, wilderness. Qualified applicants please send CV to Ronald J. Cocchiarella, MD, 801 W 5th Ave, #205, Spokane, WA 99204 or fax 509-747-1180.

SEATTLE—Five-member group seeks ABR-certified diagnostic radiologist for partnership track position. MRI, mammography, and/or inter-ventional skills with fellowship training is desirable, but must be comfortable with all modalities. Both hospital- and outpatient-based practice with adjoining facilities in a growing community hospital. The hospital includes new Siemens angio suite and spiral CT. Outpatient practice has busy US, MRI, and mammography service. Competitive compensation package and partnership offered after 1 year. Flexible start date. Please send CV to Peter A. Ory, MD, Southwest Medical Imaging, 16259 Sylvester Road SW, Seattle, WA 98166. Phone: 206-248-8900, Fax: 206-248-8000

GENERAL DIAGNOSTIC RADIOLOGIST—Position available immediately for BC/BE general diagnostic radiologist skilled in CT, US, MRI and mammography. We are a 14-member radiology group in southern central Pennsylvania with hospital and private office practices. Telephone 717-652-5840, x130. Fax 717-652-2165, Attention: Paul DeLoia, Jr.

MAINE, DIAGNOSTIC RADIOLOGY—Private practice opportunity with full partnership after 1-year. Mammography, nuclear, MRI, CT, ultrasound. Join a successful B/C radiologist in a practice that does 30,000 annual exams. Live in a family-safe riverside community close to Maine's best ski resort and a beautiful lake region. Affiliate with a strong 90-bed community hospital. Escape traffic and gated communities. For more information, contact Lianne Harris, New England Health Search, 63 Forest Ave, Orono, ME 04473. Telephone 207-866-5680. Fax 207-866-5696.

DIAGNOSTIC RADIOLOGIST—Immediate opportunity for Board certified radiologist. Primary responsibilities include MR, CT, mammography, ultrasound and general diagnostics. Skills in routine angiography and additional training in cross-sectional imaging would be beneficial. Hospital is located in the Northwest suburbs of Chicago. Please fax CV to Dr Edwin Willgress, Good Shepherd Hospital, Barrington, IL 60010 at 847-842-4472.

NEURORADIOLOGIST—Radiology practice is seeking a Board certified, fellowship-trained radiologist for a full-time position. A strong background in neuroangiography, myelography, CT and MRI is required. Applicants should possess skills in general radiology, including fluoroscopy and ultrasound. Basic body angio skills are required. This is a dynamic group practice located in the Northwest suburbs of Chicago with an opportunity for partnership. Position available starting July 1, 1999. Please fax CV to Dr Edwin Willgress, Good Shepherd Hospital, Barrington, IL 60010 at 847-842-4472.

RADIOLOGIST—The Department of Veterans Affairs Medical Center, Fayetteville, Arkansas is seeking a Board certified radiologist, US citizen preferred. The position offers excellent benefits, liberal vacation, sick and educational leave, competitive salary with tenure incentives. No malpractice insurance required. The medical center is a 51-bed general medical and surgical facility providing acute health care for both inpatient and outpatient services. Fayetteville is located in beautiful Northwest Arkansas with abundant outdoor and community activities. Information on Fayetteville area available at *www.fayetevillear.com*. Inquiries should be addressed to Mark Enderle, Chief of Staff, VA Medical Center, 1100 N College, Fayetteville, AR 72703 or 501-444-5050. Equal opportunity employer.

PEDIATRIC RADIOLOGIST—Rainbow Babies and Children's Hospital of the University Hospitals of Cleveland, Case Western Reserve School of Medicine, is seeking a fellowship-trained academic pediatric radiologist at the assistant or associate professor level. Rainbow Babies is a 244-bed facility. The department performs approximately 43,000 exams/yr. The applicant will join five other pediatric radiologists. Candidates must be certified by the American Board of Radiology and must have or be eligible to sit for the certificate of added qualifications in pediatric radiology. Compensation and fringe benefits are competitive. Address inquiries to Carlos J. Sivit, MD, Director, Pediatric Radiology, Rainbow Babies and Children's Hospital, 11100 Euclid Ave, Cleveland, OH 44106-5056; 216-844-1172; fax 216-844-5474; e-mail *sivit@uhrad.com.*

MUSCULOSKELETAL RADIOLOGIST—Board certified and fellowship-trained musculoskeletal radiologist sought to join 14-member private radiology group in one of the most desirable and popular cities in the coastal Southeast. Interest in other modalities is necessary. This is a partnership tract with excellent benefits and compensation. Please reply to Charles Ferris, MD, Radiology Associates, 5223 Paulsen St, Savannah, GA 31405, phone 912-352-0731; fax 912-356-6954; e-mail *mmcrad@g-net.net.*

PEDIATRIC RADIOLOGIST—The Department of Radiology at Children's Hospital, Boston, is seeking a pediatric radiologist with special interest in cardiac MRI to join the full-time faculty at the academic rank of instructor or higher. Candidates must be certified in diagnostic radiology by the American Board of Radiology or its equivalent, must have completed a fellowship in pediatric radiology and must have passed the CAQ examination in pediatric radiology. Experience in pediatric

MRI and cardiac imaging are key. The cardiac MRI program is currently a combined effort between the departments of radiology and cardiology offering anatomic and functional imaging of patients with a variety of congenital heart diseases. Over 130 cardiac MRI examinations are performed each year on two 1.5Tesla GE MRI systems equipped with spectroscopy, MR angiography, as well as advanced clinical and experimental software. The successful candidate will be expected to take a leadership role in the continued development of this service. Responsibilities include performance and interpretation of cardiac MRI studies in collaboration with members of the department of cardiology, as well as non-cardiac MRI, CT, US studies and general diagnostic pediatric radiology. Children's Hospital is a 350-bed institution and performs over 122,000 radiological examinations annually in one of the largest pediatric medical centers in North America. The department has 24 faculty pediatric radiologists, 3 PhD research faculty, 1 physicist, 10 pediatric radiology fellows, 6 neuroradiology fellows, and many resident trainees. The department has an extremely active clinical service with state-of-the-art equipment as follows: two digital fluoroscopy rooms, five ultrasound units with Doppler and color-flow Doppler capabilities, planar and SPECT gamma cameras, two GE High-Speed Advantage Helical CT scanners and two vascular/interventional suites with digital imaging. The department provides extensive academic and research support including the Kresge Laboratory for Pediatric Imaging Research, the Stern Memorial Radiology Library and a departmental librarian. There are opportunities for collaborative research efforts at Children's Hospital, other Harvard teaching hospitals, Harvard Medical School and the Harvard School of Public Health. Children's Hospital and Harvard Medical School are affirmative action/equal opportunity employers. Address inquiry and curriculum vitae to Robert L. Leibowitz, MD, Acting Chairman, Department of Radiology, Children's Hospital, 300 Longwood Ave, Boston, MA 02115, 617-355-6305.

BODY IMAGING—Board certified/eligible radiologist opening with established private practice serving four hospitals and three outpatient facilities in Philadelphia, Bucks County, adjacent Central New Jersey. State-of-the-art, well developed practice with large volume, interesting and challenging cases. Excellent rapport/acceptance by clinical staff. Immediate availability. Send CV to L. Oliver, MD, Whitehorse Executive Center, Ste 514, 1255 Whitehorse-Mercerville Rd, Hamilton, NJ 08619.

MRI RADIOLOGIST—Established multi-hospital private practice seeks fellowship-trained radiologist with expertise in body/musculoskeletal and neuro MRI. Will also be responsible for all aspects of diagnostic radiology. Immediate availability. Send CV to L. Oliver, MD, Whitehorse Executive Center, Ste 514, 1255 Whitehorse-Mercerville Rd, Hamilton, NJ 08619.

VASCULAR/INTERVENTIONAL RADIOLOGIST—Portland, OR. Northwest Permanente, PC, a physician-managed multi-specialty group serving over 440,000 members of Kaiser Permanente in the Northwest has an excellent opportunity in the Portland area for a Board certified radiologist with fellowship training or extensive clinical experience in angiography or interventional radiology. Our practice includes opportunities to be involved in interpretation of neurological and peripheral vascular MRA and performances of TIPS, uterine artery embolizations, hepato-biliary and general body intervention and vascular stenting with an opportunity to develop a stent-graft program. Our program in Oregon and Washington offers a collegial and professionally stimulating environment in one of the most successful managed care systems in the country, plus a quality lifestyle in the Pacific Northwest. In addition, we provide a competitive salary and benefit package which includes a generous retirement program, sabbatical leave, professional liability coverage and more. Please forward CV to R.A. Clark, Director, Professional Resources, Northwest Permanente, PC, 500 NE Multnomah, Ste 100, Portland, OR 97232-2099. EOE.

INTERVENTIONAL RADIOLOGIST—Bay Imaging Consultants Medical Group, Inc, a large San Francisco Bay area private practice radiology group with multiple outpatient and hospital sites, is seeking a fellowship-trained interventional radiologist with experience in all general radiology modalities, as well as experience and interest in mammographic procedures. Must be Board certified. Partnership track. Competitive salary. Start date is around July 1999 or later. Please submit your CV, a cover letter and the names of three references to Human Resources, Attn: Jill Carley, 175 Lennon Lane, Suite 100, Walnut Creek, CA 94598. EOE.

SOUTH FLORIDA—Immediate openings. Desirable private practice with two hospitals in need of fellowship-trained MRI radiologist, fellowship-trained interventional radiologist, and fellowship-trained pediatric radiologist. The successful candidates must be willing to do general radiology as well. Excellent positions for excellent individuals. Please fax CVs to 561-488-8347.

CALIFORNIA CENTRAL COAST—Partnership track radiology position in challenging practice; 65-bed hospital three-man practice with new CT, MRI, and ultrasound and mammo equipment. Must be highly skilled in all modalities. No catheter angiography. Family oriented community of 40,000 plus. Please send inquiries and CV to David McAninch, MD, 1111 E Ocean Ave, Suite 2, Lompoc, CA 93436; fax 805-735-8540.

SALT LAKE CITY RADIOLOGY GROUP—Seeks Board certified radiologist, fellowship training desirable to join established five-member group starting immediately. Practice includes all modalities including angio/interventional. Send CV to Jonathan Naatz, MD, Valley Radiology, 632 W 7250 South, Midvale, UT 84047 or fax to 801-561-5520.

GENERAL RADIOLOGIST—Beautiful coastal community in central eastern Florida is seeking a radiologist with fellowship training preferably in MRI or musculoskeletal radiology. Partnership track position with excellent benefits. Send CV or contact Peter Joyce, MD, Vero Radiology Associates, Vero Beach, FL; 561-567-1942, fax 561-562-1505.

BOARD-CERTIFIED RADIOLOGIST—Wanted for hospital-based New Hampshire radiology practice (54 miles north of Boston). Must be competent in CT, US, MRI, mammography, and general radiology. Fellowship trained individual preferred. Generous salaried position. A 3-yr partnership track. For further information, contact G. Eric Geslien, MD, Department of Diagnostic Imaging, Exeter Hospital, PO Box 790, Exeter, NH 03833 or e-mail *RGESLIEN @EHR.ORG* or fax 603-778-6707.

NUCLEAR RADIOLOGY—The Penn State Geisinger Health System is currently seeking a fellowship trained and licensed nuclear radiologist to join the Geisinger Medical Center in Danville, PA. The practice will combine general and nuclear radiology. Background and experience in nuclear medicine, MRI, CT, ultrasound and general diagnostic radiology is preferred. Call coverage is on a rotational basis with 12 other diagnostic radiologists. The position will include both clinical and teaching responsibilities in a 458-bed tertiary care hospital and level 1 trauma center with its own radiology program. Geisinger Medical Center supports a 40-county area throughout northeastern and central Pennsylvania. We offer a competitive salary and excellent benefit package. For additional information regarding this opportunity please contact Kurt Scott, Penn State Geisinger Health System, Department of Professional Staffing and Credentialing (RAD-CT), 100 N Academy Ave, Danville, PA 17822-1528; phone 800-845-7112. CVs can be faxed to 800-622-2515. EOE, M/F/H/V.

COMMUNITY HOSPITAL, 180 BEDS—Near shore resorts in Delaware, seeks radiologist fellowship-trained in cross-sectional imaging or interventional radiology to join three-man group. Partnership track, a competitive salary, benefits and vacation. Contact E.J. Goldstein, MD, 8 Lexington Dr, Milford, DE 19963, phone after 6 pm 302-424-0613, e-mail *egoldstein@mmh .bayhealth.org.*

THE UNIVERSITY OF MISSISSIPPI MEDICAL CENTER—Department of Radiology is seeking an additional mammographer. The University of Mississippi Medical Center is among the fastest growing academic medical centers in the United States. The equipment is state-of-the-art. There is an opportunity to perform breast procedures on the General Electric interventional magnet. This magnet is one of 11 in the world. Salary is commensurate with training, experience and productivity. Interested parties should contact Dr Brent Harrison, Department of Radiology, 2500 N State St, Jackson, MS 39216, 601-984-2515, *RBHARRISON @email.MSN.com.* EOE, M/F/D/V.

NUCLEAR MEDICINE—Progressive subspecialized large private practice radiology group is seeking individual fellowship-trained in nuclear medicine. The practice is affiliated with a medical school and residency program, thereby offering the benefits of both private practice and the pursuit of academic interests. Position will include eventual directorship of nuclear medicine department. The practice is located on the Atlantic coastline with a mild climate and all water sports available. Interested persons should send a CV or contact Stephen Carr, MD, Director of Recruiting, Medical Center Radiologists, 6330 N Center Dr, Bldg 13, Ste 220, Norfolk, VA 23502; 757-466-0089 or fax 757-466-8017.

MUSCULOSKELETAL RADIOLOGIST—Progressive subspecialized large private practice radiology group is seeking individual with subspecialty training in musculoskeletal MR. The practice is affiliated with a medical school and residency program, thereby offering the benefits of both private practice and the pursuit of academic interests. The practice is located in coastal Virginia with a mild climate and many recreational activities available with the Chesapeake Bay and Atlantic Ocean nearby. Interested persons should send a CV or contact Stephen Carr, MD, Director of Recruiting, Medical Center Radiologists, 6330 N Center Dr, Bldg 13, Ste 220, Norfolk, VA 23502; 757-466-0089 or fax 757-466-8017.

GENERAL RADIOLOGIST—Progressive subspecialized large private practice radiology group is seeking a qualified body imaging radiologist comfortable with all modalities of diagnostic radiology except angiography and interventional. The practice is affiliated with a medical school and residency program, thereby offering the benefits of both private practice and the pursuit of academic interests. The practice is located on the Atlantic coastline with a mild climate and all water sports available. Interested persons should send a CV or contact Stephen Carr, MD, Director of Recruiting, Medical Center Radiologists, 6330 N Center Dr, Bldg 13, Ste 220, Norfolk, VA 23502; 757-466-0089 or fax 757-466-8017.

INTERVENTIONAL RADIOLOGIST—Progressive subspecialized large private practice radiology group is seeking an interventional radiologist. The practice is affiliated with a medical school and residency program, thereby offering the benefits of both private practice and the pursuit of academic interests. The practice is located in coastal Virginia with a mild climate and many recreational activities available with the Chesapeake Bay and Atlantic Ocean nearby. Interested persons should send a CV or contact Stephen Carr, MD, Director of Recruiting, Medical Center Radiologists, 6330 N Center Dr, Bldg 13, Ste 220, Norfolk, VA 23502; 757-466-0089 or fax 757-466-8017.

LAKE MICHIGAN SHORELINE COMMUNITY—Progressive six-member practice seeks Board-certified, preferably fellowship-trained radiologist for partnership track. Busy, rapidly expanding practice, with all modalities, including MRI and angiography/interventional. Candidate would be expected to cover all modalities. Generous compensation, benefit and vacation package. Community is in western Michigan, which offers low cost of living and abundant recreational activities, amongst other perks. Please reply to Box R-109.

FACULTY POSITION IN US AND CT, THOMAS JEFFERSON UNIVERSITY HOSPITAL—The Department of Radiology at Thomas Jefferson University Hospital in Philadelphia seeks a junior faculty member to join its very large practice in US and body CT. Jefferson performs 35,000 US exams of all types and 12,000 body CT exams per year on state-of-the-art equipment. The department has seven cross sectional imaging fellows per year, as well as 24 residents. We offer an abundance of interesting clinical and teaching material, numerous opportunities for research, and an excellent infrastructure to support clinical and research activities. Individuals just completing fellowship or scheduled to complete one in June 2000 are encouraged to apply. The position is available immediately but the start date can be delayed until July 2000 if necessary. Interested candidates should contact Barry B. Goldberg, MD, Director, Division of Diagnostic Ultrasound, Thomas Jefferson University Hospital, Philadelphia, PA 19107. Phone 215-955-6227, fax 215-955-8549.

BREAST IMAGING RADIOLOGIST—A 16-member group in North Florida seeking fellowship-trained mammographer or candidate with special interest in mammography for partnership position. Strong general radiology

member in diagnostic neuroradiology at the assistant professor level. The candidate must be Board certified in diagnostic radiology with completion of a minimum of 1 year of training in neuroradiology in an ACGME-accredited program and be CAQ certified or eligible. The candidate must be familiar with all aspects of neuroimaging, including CT, MRI/MRA, CT angiography, myelography and angiography. Candidates with some experience and a strong interest in functional MRI will be preferred. Occasional staffing of interventional neuroradiology will be required, as will be participation in teaching of residents and fellows. Imaging facilities include three recent GE helical CT scanners, one GE 1.5T MRI scanner and another one currently being installed with perfusion/diffusion imaging and spectroscopy capability, two standard angiography suites and a soon-to-be installed state-of-the-art biplane neurointerventional angiography suite. The candidate will be expected to participate in research in collaboration with other neuroscience services. Eligibility for Vermont medical licensure is required. Women and minority candidates are encouraged to apply. The deadline for receipt of applications is Tuesday, August 31, 1999. Interested applicants should forward their CV to and contact Lotfi Hacein-Bey, MD, Director, Diagnostic and Interventional Radiology, University of Vermont College of Medicine, FAHC-Patrick 107, 111 Colchester Ave, Burlington, VT 05401. Telephone 802-656-3592, fax 802-656-4822, e-mail *Lotfi.Hacein-Bey@vtmednet.org*. Fletcher Allen Health Care and the University of Vermont are equal opportunity/affirmative action employers.

WEST TEXAS-EXCELLENT RADIOLOGY OPPORTUNITY—Midland is a community of approximately 100,000 people in West Texas with a surrounding area of 150,000. Seven radiologists at two hospitals seek additional radiology support and expertise. We currently have three MR scanners, three helical CT scanners and two modern angio suites. There is an outpatient imaging facility and an established women's imaging center which includes on-site ultrasound and a stereotactic breast biopsy system. The women's imaging center, ultrasound practice and one MR scanner are ACR certified. We seek a body imaging fellowship-trained individual with a desire to complement our busy US/CT/MR practice and expand the mammography program. A second fellowship-trained interventionalist to assist with an established interventional radiology practice is also required. The group will consider a salaried or part-time position with no call responsibilities for an individual interested in mammography only. These are 2-year to partnership track positions with eight weeks vacation. Midland is a safe and clean community. There are good private schools, many church groups, warm climate and traffic is never a problem. There is a new, convenient airport with commercial jet service to anywhere in the country. Please contact us or forward your CV to Marlon D. Hughes, MD, 4 Dunblane, Midland, TX 79707, phone 915-685-1580 (work), 915-694-3150 (home), *mdhughesmd@msn.com.*

DEPARTMENT OF VETERANS AFFAIRS MEDICAL CENTER, ST. LOUIS, MO—Is seeking a part-time Board-certified diagnostic radiologist. The medical center is a 300-bed, dual division, tertiary care hospital with large outpatient department. Skills in general radiography, ultrasound, CT, neuroradiology and MRI with some angiography and interventional experience are desired. The VAMC offers good working conditions, competitive salary and excellent benefits in a moderately sized metropolitan area. Interested candidates should send CV to VAMC, Attn: Nancy Lauermann (O5JB), #1 Jefferson Barracks Dr, St. Louis, MO 63125. Phone 314-894-6620. EOE.

THE NEURORADIOLOGY SECTION AT THE UNIVERSITY OF ALABAMA AT BIRMINGHAM—Is recruiting two Board-certified neuroradiologists (CAQ certified) to join four neuroradiologists. Coverage for UAB Hospital, VAH and Kirklin Clinic includes 24,000 procedures annually, teaching house staff and research. The radiology department in the medical center has 4 GE CT/I helical scanners, and 4 MRI scanners: two GE Signa 1.5T, one Siemens Expert 1T and one GE Signa 1T; and one biplane Siemens Neurostar angiography

WELCOME TO THE WORLD OF

KAISER PERMANENTE

in Southern California

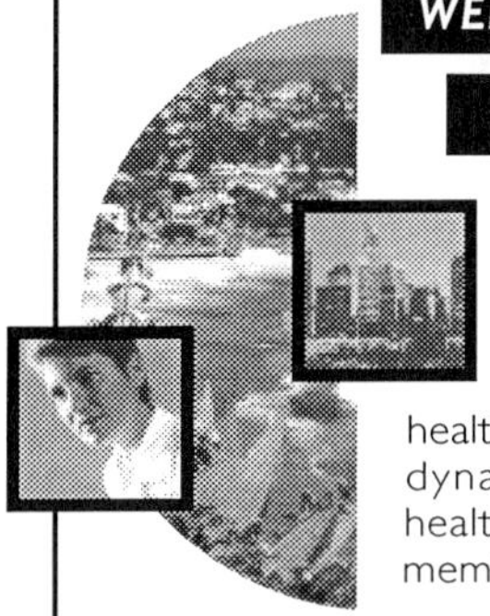

At **Kaiser Permanente**, the excellence of our physicians is reflected in the quality of our healthcare. At Kaiser, you'll be part of a dynamic medical group providing healthcare services to over 2.9 million members in Southern California.

We currently have outstanding opportunities at various locations within Southern California for Comprehensive Radiology, Interventional Radiology, Nuclear Medicine, Neuroradiology and Breast Imaging.

For more information regarding these opportunities, please mail/fax your CV to: **Kaiser Permanente, SCPMG, Dept.ADVE, Walnut Center, Pasadena, CA 91188-8013. FAX (626) 405-2675.**

Call 1-800-541-7946

KAISER PERMANENTE®
Southern California Permanente
Medical Group

National University Hospital Singapore

The National University Hospital (NUH) is a 900-bed multi-specialty tertiary hospital. We invite suitable qualified candidates to apply for the positions of:

CONSULTANT/SENIOR REGISTRAR/REGISTRAR
(DIAGNOSTIC IMAGING)

Applicants must hold a basic and postgraduate medical degree registrable with the Singapore Medical Council and any of the following postgraduate qualifications:

1. FRCR
2. FRACR
3. FRCP Canada
4. American Board Certified

Commencing salary will be competitive depending on qualifications and experience. Please give full personal particulars, pro-fessional qualifications, career history and expected salary together with medical testimonials, certificate of registration, recent photograph and telephone number to:

Chairman, Medical Board
Medical Affairs Department
National University Hospital
5 Lower Kent Ridge Road
Singapore 119074

Telefax: (65) 7756757
Website: http://www.nuh.com.sg
email: HoWY@nuh.com.sg
Closing date: 30 September 1999

room. Contact Dr Robert Stanley, Department of Radiology, University of Alabama at Birmingham, Birmingham, AL 35233; phone 205-934-9577, fax 205-934-8110. UAB is an equal opportunity employer.

RADIOLOGIST, PORTLAND, OR—Our well-established eight-member group has an immediate opening for a Board-certified radiologist with additional training in body imaging or interventional radiology. Other fellowship training considered. We anticipate the position to lead to partnership in 2 to 3 years. We practice at a major central city hospital with a large pediatric program and a Level I trauma center. Salary and benefits are competitive. Send CV to Blaine Kozak, MD, or fax to 503-413-2554. Call 503-413-4032 or e-mail *bkozak@lhs.org*.

SEEKING A BOARD CERTIFIED RADIOLOGIST—To join a progressive multi-hospital group practice in beautiful western Maryland. All modalities including '98 GE Horizon 1.5T MRI and Digital Siemens Angio Suite. Interventional training or experience preferred. Excellent compensation toward partnership. Contact Jong Kim, MD, Sacred Heart Hospital, Radiology Department, 900 Seton Dr, Cumberland, MD 21502, phone 301-723-5133.

FELLOWSHIP-TRAINED MUSCULOSKELETAL RADIOLOGIST—Sought for progressive, high-quality practice in the Pacific Northwest. Radia Medical Imaging is a 40+ radiologist group in the Seattle/Everett area which staffs several hospital systems and one multispecialty clinic. Our focus is on subspecialty practice. We also own and operate a series of well-established outpatient offices. The Seattle area is consistently rated as one of the top areas of the country to live and work, with an abundance of outdoor recreation, a progressive metropolitan area and a robust economy. If you are seeking an equitable group focused on the future, forward your CV to Mark Churchill, Radia Medical Imaging, 728 134th St SW, Ste #120, Everett, WA 98204. Fax 425-297-6250 or e-mail *mchurchill@radiax.com*. For more information on our practice, visit our website at *www.radiax.com*.

NUCLEAR MEDICINE—Portland, OR. Northwest Permanente, PC, a physician-managed multispecialty group serving over 440,000 members of Kaiser Permanente in the Northwest has an excellent opportunity in the Portland area for a radiologist, Board-certified or eligible in nuclear medicine. Our program in Oregon and Washington offers a collegial and professionally stimulating environment in one of the most successful managed care systems in the country, plus a quality lifestyle in the Northwest. In addition, we provide a competitive salary and benefit package which includes a generous retirement program, sabbatical leave, professional liability coverage and more. Please forward CV to N.M. Clark, Director, Professional Resources, Northwest Permanente, PC, 500 NE Multnomah, Ste 100, Portland, OR 97232-2099. EOE.

THE SECTION OF NEURORADIOLOGY IN THE DEPARTMENT OF RADIOLOGY AT THE CLEVELAND CLINIC FOUNDATION—Is offering 2 full-time staff positions due to rapid growth of their practice. Candidates should be Board-certified radiologists who have completed a fellowship, preferably two years, in an accredited neuroradiology program, and who are CAQ certified or eligible. A strong background in academic radiology, cerebral angiography, myelography, CT, MR and MR angiography is required. (Clinical interest in functional MR is particularly valuable.) The neuroradiology section provides a well-balanced team atmosphere with existing expertise in pediatric neuroradiology, interventional neuroradiology and three PhD level staff physicists and two (PhD and masters level) biostatisticians. A research center with a large commitment to vascular disease is available for basic investigations in interventional neuroradiology; clinical research protocols for all facets of neurointervention are already in place. Applications will be accepted until positions are filled. For more information, please contact Thomas J. Masaryk, MD, Section Head, Neuroradiology, Department of Radiology, Hb-6, 9500 Euclid Ave, Cleveland, OH 44195; e-mail *masaryk@ccisd2.ccf.org*. Equal opportunity/affirmative action employer.

ABDOMINAL RADIOLOGIST AT THE CLEVELAND CLINIC FOUNDATION—The section of abdominal imaging at the Cleveland Clinic Foundation has two openings starting immediately, one to fill an open position and another to meet expanding clinical demands. We are currently a seven-member section interpreting abdominal CT, ultrasound, vascular ultrasound, luminal GI studies, GU studies, abdominal MRI as well as performing common abdominal interventions, including biopsies and abscess drainages. The practice is busy, performing over 20,000 CTs, 18,000 ultrasounds, 500 abdominal MRs and 1,000 interventions last year. We serve a highly trained and sophisticated group of gastroenterologists, oncologists, and surgeons sub-specializing in colon and rectum, hepato-pancreatico-biliary surgery, urology and gynecology. Equipment is state-of-the-art CT, including a new multirow scanner, ultrasound and MRI. Cross-sectional imaging is fully networked and image interpretation is all work station based. The medical center is a multi-specialty group practice that is rapidly expanding on the main campus as well as in the community. Fellowship training in abdominal imaging and ABR certification is required. Salary and benefits are very competitive. Contact Mark E. Baker, MD, Head, Section of Abdominal Imaging, Division of Radiology/Hb6, The Cleveland Clinic Foundation, 9500 Euclid Ave, Cleveland, OH 44195; 216-444-6638.

INTERVENTIONAL RADIOLOGIST—Memorial Sloan-Kettering Cancer Center (MSKCC) has a faculty position open in the Vascular/Interventional section, which performs all types of vascular/interventional procedures related to the care of patients with cancer. This includes a very active role in hepatobiliary, genitourinary, and venous access procedures. The service is experiencing significant growth in ablative and minimally invasive methods of treating cancer, and excellent research opportunities exist at this Cornell University Medical College affiliate. Applicants should be Board certified with a CAQ in VIR. Appointment at Assistant or Associate level, commensurate with experience and accomplishments. Please send a curriculum vitae and letter of interest to Karen T. Brown, MD, Department of Radiology, Memorial Sloan-Kettering Cancer Center, 1275 York Ave, New York, NY 10021; fax 212-717-3325. MSKCC is an equal opportunity employer/affirmative action employer. Women and minorities are encouraged to apply; *www.mskcc.org*.

PEDIATRIC RADIOLOGIST—The Department of Radiology at the University of Rochester Medical Center/Strong Memorial Hospital has a full-time faculty position available for a fellowship-trained pediatric radiologist. Approximately 35,000 pediatric examinations are performed each year by three and one-half pediatric radiologists at The Children's Hospital at Strong. General imaging is performed as well as CT, ultrasound, and body MRI. Send cover letter and CV to Nina Klionsky, MD, 601 Elmwood Ave, Rochester, NY 14642, fax 716-758-8290, e-mail *nina_klionsky@urmc.rochester.edu*. The University of Rochester is an equal opportunity employer.

FELLOWSHIP IN IMAGING/ANGIO-INTERVENTIONAL—A 1-year fellowship program at Lehigh Valley Hospital in Allentown, PA is available beginning July 1, 2000. LVH is a 650-bed acute care, university affiliated hospital. The fellowship program offers training in CT (head and body), ultrasound, MR, angiography, and interventional radiology. For further information contact Elliot Shoemaker, MD, Department of Radiology, Lehigh Valley Hospital, PO Box 689, Allentown, PA 18105-1556 or telephone 610-402-8088 for fax 610-402-1023.

GENERAL RADIOLOGIST—Bassett Healthcare is seeking two BC/BE general radiologists. One of the candidates should be certified by the ABNM or ABR with special competency in nuclear medicine and would serve as Section Chief of Nuclear Medicine. Responsibilities for both will include general diagnostic radiology, mammography, MRI, CT, and US, along with student/resident teaching. Bassett Healthcare is a regional referral center and a teaching affiliate of Columbia University. It is located in a beautiful family-oriented mountain/lake region with an abundance of year-round recreational and cultural activities. We offer a competitive salary with incentives, paid malpractice, excellent benefits, and education/travel allowance. Please send CV and correspondence to Denise B. Harter, Medical Staff Recruiter, Bassett Healthcare, One Atwell Rd, Cooperstown, NY, 13326; fax 607-547-3844 or for more information, please call 607-547-6982.

WANT TO WORK—Full-time locums? Pick up extra hours? Explore positions leading to permanent placement? Linde HealthCare (*www.Lindehc.com*) provides competitive pay, malpractice, travel and lodging. Call us @ 800-588-4343, fax your CV to 314-843-2262, or send it to *Info@lindehc.com*

SOUTHERN OREGON—Opportunity for Board certified radiologists to join a group of five well-established radiologists. The practice includes two hospitals and outpatient facilities. Experience in all modalities and mammography certification necessary. Fellowship training is desired. Partnership track optional.

Excellent lifestyle with many outdoor activities from the Pacific coast to the Oregon Cascades. Great family environment. Send CV to Larry Strickland, Administrator, Roseburg Radiologists, PC, PO Box 1547, Roseburg, OR 97470.

NEURORADIOLOGIST/ASSISTANT PROFESSOR—Medical University of South Carolina Radiology Department: Opening for fellowship-trained neuroradiologist beginning Fall 1999, to complete group of three neuro faculty, one neuro fellow. There are four CT scanners (two multi-slice) and three up-to-date MRI scanners; 22 full-time radiologists, 26 residents and four fellows; includes College of Medicine appointment as assistant professor. The Neuro Division performs approximately 7,700 CT exams; 6,550 MR scans; 325 angiograms and 110 myelograms per year. Submit CV by August 30, 1999 to Jeremy W.R. Young, MD, Professor and Chairman, c/o Melanie Jackson, MUSC Radiology Department, 169 Ashley Ave, PO Box 250322, Charleston, SC 29425. MUSC is an equal opportunity employer.

MASSACHUSETTS—Immediate opening for Board-certified diagnostic radiologist to join progressive 14-person group just south of Boston. Partnership or per diem arrangement is possible. Strong interest in breast imaging preferred, but not essential. Please contact Peter H. Gordon, MD, Good Samaritan Medical Center, 235 N Pearl St, Brockton, MA 02301. *phgordon@massmed.org*

NUCLEAR MEDICINE/RADIOLOGIST—The Mount Auburn Hospital Department of Radiology has an opening for a staff radiologist to direct the Division of Nuclear Medicine. The hospital is a community teaching hospital affiliated with Harvard Medical School. The radiology department sponsors a fully accredited residency in diagnostic radiology. Requirements for position include Board certification, a fellowship in nuclear medicine, eligibility/certification for CAQ in nuclear medicine, and an interest in investigative nuclear medicine. Interested candidates should fax their curriculum vitae to Michael J. Shortsleeve, MD, Chairman, Department of Radiology, Mount Auburn Hospital, 330 Mount Auburn St, Cambridge, MA 02238; phone 617-499-5070, fax 617-499-5138.

SECTION HEAD-WOMEN'S IMAGING—The Department of Radiology at the SUNY Health Science Center at Syracuse seeks an individual to serve as Section Head of Women's Imaging. The SUNY Health Science Center is a 380-bed tertiary care academic health center in Syracuse, NY, a short drive from the Adirondack Mountains and Lake Ontario. Our 25-member subspecialized radiology group provides service to the main campus, one satellite office and three private imaging centers. Candidates must be Board certified with fellowship training in mammography, breast ultrasound, stereotactic biopsies, needle localizations and OB/GYN ultrasound. Responsibilities include teaching, research, publication and patient care. The level of faculty appointment and salary will depend upon the applicant's experience and academic productivity. Applicants should respond with a letter of interest and copy of their current CV to John F. Cardella, MD, Chairman, Department of Radiology, SUNY Health Science Center, 750 E Adams St, Syracuse, NY 13210 or *cardellj@mailbox.hscsyr.edu*. SUNY Health Science Center is a smoke-free campus, an equal opportunity/affirmative action employer and encourages minority and female applicants to apply.

THE UNIVERSITY OF KENTUCKY DEPARTMENT OF DIAGNOSTIC RADIOLOGY—Is recruiting a Board-certified radiologist, fellowship trained or comparable experience in breast imaging. Duties will include directing activities in comprehensive breast care center, developing a network of screening centers and a strong interest in education and research. Rank based on experience. This position also includes some general radiology to provide coverage of radiology network. Please send or fax letter of interest, along with curriculum vitae to James C. Reed, Chairman, Department of Diagnostic Radiology, A110 Kentucky Clinic, University of Kentucky Medical Center, Lexington, KY 40536-0284. Fax 606-257-6014. UK is an equal opportunity employer.

GENERAL RADIOLOGIST—The Department of Radiology at the University of Kansas Medical Center has an immediate opening for two or three Board-certified, general practice radiologists with emphasis in gastrointestinal radiology, breast imaging, nuclear medicine and computed body tomography. Salary, academic rank and excellent fringe package are commensurate with experience. Interested applicants should submit a curriculum vitae to Solomon Batnitzky, MD, Chairman, KUMC, 3901 Rainbow Blvd, Kansas City, KS 66160-7234; phone 913-588-6805, fax 913-588-7899. An EOE/AA employer.

THE RADIOLOGY DEPARTMENT AT THE UNIVERSITY OF PENNSYLVANIA MEDICAL CENTER—Has the following position available: a faculty appointment in the University of Pennsylvania at the assistant professor, associate professor or professor of radiology level. The position is in the ultrasound and computed body tomography sections. The level of the position will be determined by the applicant's experience and expertise. Applicants must be Board certified in radiology and have experience in ultrasound and computed tomography. The minimum experience needed is a US/CT fellowship. The University of Pennsylvania is an equal opportunity/affirmative action employer. Minority and women candidates are encouraged to apply. Please contact Beverly G. Coleman, MD, Director, Ultrasound Imaging, Radiology Department, University of Pennsylvania Medical Center, 3400 Spruce St, Philadelphia, PA 19104; phone 215-662-3466, fax 215-349-5627, e-mail *coleman@oasis.rad.upenn.edu.*

CHIEF OF RADIOLOGY/ARIZONA—Prosperous regional medical center seeks a director for radiology services that are expanding in volume and modalities. Department is equipped with the latest in technology. Imaging services include MRI, CT, nuclear, mammography, plain film and interventional studies. Location is a lake resort community of 45,000 in Arizona. Call David King (King Search, Inc) at 800-990-0780, 770-886-0780 or fax 770-886-9522. Send CV to King Search & Consulting, Inc, 1380 Zephyr Ct, Cumming, GA 30041. *Kingsearch@msn.com.*

THE UNIVERSITY OF TENNESSEE, MEMPHIS—Is actively recruiting for a mammographer. The radiology department provides services for 1600 adult and pediatric beds in an urban medical center which includes the Regional Medical Center at Memphis and its Level I trauma center, the tertiary UT/Bowld Hospital and its active renal, liver and pancreas transplant service, the Memphis VA Medical Center, the Le Bonheur Children's Hospital and the St. Jude Cancer Research Institute. Applicants must be Board certified or eligible in diagnostic radiology and eligible for licensure in the state of Tennessee. Subspecialty training is preferable but not required. Appointment will be commensurate with the successful candidate's experience and qualifications. Interested applicants should respond with a letter of interest, current curriculum vitae and the names and addresses of three references to Robert E. Gold, MD, Chair, Department of Radiology, Rm F150C Chandler, The University of Tennessee, Memphis, 800 Madison Ave, Memphis, TN 38163 or e-mail *rgold@utmem.edu.* The University of Tennessee is an equal opportunity/affirmative action/ Title IX/Section 504/ADA employer.

TWO RADIOLOGISTS NEEDED-TOLEDO, OH—Interventional radiologist and diagnostic radiologist. Premier seven-physician radiology group seeks two additional radiologists: one interventional and one diagnostic with a fellowship or a special interest in cross sectional ultrasound or MRI. The group practices out of a 350-bed facility with teleradiology and state-of-the-art equipment. Participate in a shared call arrangement of 1:8. Competitive starting guarantee with earnings in the top 25% and partnership opportunities. This vibrant Midwest city offers an abundance of cultural and recreational activities! For more information, contact Danise Cooper or Barb Kennington at 800-765-3055; fax 314-726-3009; e-mail *bkennington@cejka.com.* ID #6484RA. Visit our website at *www.cejka.com.*

PG-3-YEAR RADIOLOGY RESIDENT—Sought for opening at St Luke's Medical Center, Milwaukee, WI. Please direct your inquiry and send your curriculum vitae to David L. Olson, MD, Director, Radiology Residency, St Luke's Medical Center, 2900 W Oklahoma Ave, Milwaukee, WI 53215. 414-649-6298.

MULTIPLE RADIOLOGY OPPORTUNITIES, COASTAL CAROLINA AREA—Join a successful, expanding group in the beautiful coastal Carolina area. Board-certified radiologists are needed for the following positions: neuroradiologist, mammographer, general diagnostic, angiography and night radiologist. All positions offer excellent salary and compensation package. Please reply to Box R-111 and include a CV with letter of inquiry.

GENERAL RADIOLOGIST—The Department of Radiology at Indiana University School of Medicine seeks academically oriented general radiologist for faculty position in a small university-affiliated hospital. In addition to plain film, the hospital provides MRI, CT, nuclear medicine and US. Approximately 37,000 exams are performed annually. Tenure or clinical track dependent upon qualifications. Minimum requirements include MD with Board certification in radiology and eligibility for licensure in Indiana. Please reply with curriculum vitae to Mervyn D. Cohen, MD, Indiana University Hospital, Room UH 0663, 550 N University Blvd, Indianapolis, IN 46202-5253, or e-mail *jamriley@iupui.edu.* Indiana University is an equal opportunity/affirmative action employer.

NEURO AND MUSCULOSKELETAL RADIOLOGISTS—Excellent opportunity for well-trained BC/BE radiologists to join successful 10-member hospital-based group practice located in northeast Ohio. One full-time neuroradiologist and one full-time musculoskeletal radiologist are needed. There are partnership track positions with excellent salary and benefits. Please send CV to Trumbull Radiologists, Inc, c/o Marge Deley, Business Manager, 2588 Elm Rd, Cortland, OH 44410; 330-372-5859; fax 330-372-5901.

BREAST IMAGING RADIOLOGIST—The Department of Radiology at the Medical College of Georgia is seeking an ABR-eligible or -certified breast imaging radiologist for a full-time or part-time faculty position opening in July 1999. Fellowship training or extensive experience preferred but not mandatory. The successful candidate will direct and practice in a new, state-of-the-art breast center and will perform screening and diagnostic mammography, dedicated breast ultrasound, ultrasound procedures and stereotactic biopsies. A broad range of teaching and research opportunities is available. Appointment is anticipated at the assistant or associate professor level. For information, contact Eugene F. Binet, MD, Chairman, Department of Radiology, Medical College of Georgia, 1120 15th St, Augusta, GA 30912, 706-721-2464, fax 706-721-7319. The Medical College of Georgia is an equal opportunity/affirmative action employer.

VETERANS ADMINISTRATION SACRAMENTO MEDICAL CENTER AT MATHER—Has an immediate opening for an ABR-certified radiologist (or Board eligible, if newly trained) to join two other radiologists in a hospital-based practice. All modalities including MRI and state-of-the-art CT are available; nuclear medicine not required. Basic interventional skills are desirable. PACS (Cemax) is already in place for communication with the other clinics in the system. Cosmopolitan San Francisco (85 miles away) and Lake Tahoe recreation areas (80 miles away) are accessible via interstate highway. Salary commensurate with experience and qualifications; generous fringe and vacation package. Time off for meetings. Relocation expenses and recruitment bonuses are authorized. Please send your CV to Al Weinshelbaum, MD, Acting Chief, Radiology, VANCHCS (114A), 150 Muir Rd, Martinez, CA 94553 or contact John Livoni, MD, 916-843-7076, or Al Weinshelbaum, MD, 925-372-2191. A license in any state is required. The Veterans Administration is an affirmative action/equal opportunity employer. Women and minority candidates are encouraged to apply.

BREAST IMAGING RADIOLOGIST—Associated Radiologists of Oakland County, PC, is seeking a Board-certified radiologist with emphasis on mammography. Fellowship training or experience in mammography is preferred. Candidate will perform approximately 70% breast imaging in addition to general radiology. Prefer proficiency in all breast imaging procedures. Partnership track. Interested candidates should send CV to St. Joseph Mercy-Oakland, Department of Radiology H-56, Attn: Leah Creason, Office Coordinator, 900 Woodward Ave, Pontiac, MI 48341-2985.

WISCONSIN—Why not live where you vacation in the heart of one of the Midwest's favorite resort areas? Opportunity for a diagnostic radiologist to experience the unsurpassed North Woods lifestyle with a premier 44-member multi-specialty group. Surrounded by the beauty of a national forest and freshwater lakes, this setting provides a myriad of year-round recreation. Residents enjoy both a relaxed lifestyle and the conveniences of a metropolitan city. Join a well-established practice, which is connected to an advanced 99-bed hospital, with leading-edge equipment. For additional information, contact Jacki Brekke at 800-243-4353.

ANNISTON, AL—Due to practice growth and retiring partner, one or two BC/BE general diagnostic or fellowship-trained radiologists needed to join seven-member group located 60 miles east of Birmingham and 90 miles west of Atlanta. Group covers both Anniston hospitals (300 and 100 beds) and private office which generates greater than 135k procedures annually. Interest in all modalities preferred. Excellent salary and benefits package. State-of-the-art equipment includes ATL HC 13000 and Ultramark 9HD 1 Ultrasound, ADAC GENSYS with Pegasys Computer Nuclear Medicine Units, Siemens Digital Fluoroscopy, Siemens Somatom Plus-S Spiral CT, Second CT (Siemens Somaton Plus 4 with CT fluoro), replacement MRI (Siemens Symphony 1.5 short bore magnet), and ground-breaking OP diagnostic center scheduled Fall 1999. Positions available immediately or by July 1, 2000. Send CV to Robert Garner, MD, 230 E 10th St, Ste 108, Anniston, AL 36207-5790; telephone 256-236-3485, e-mail *ARGRB@aol.com*.

PITTSBURGH, PA—A five-member radiology group seeks BE/BC radiologist with competence in all modalities. Additional MRI or interventional experience is helpful but not necessary. Practice located in community hospital approximately 20 miles from Pittsburgh. Competitive salary and benefits with generous time off. Please reply to Box R-112.

DIAGNOSTIC RADIOLOGIST-WATERLOO, IA—Outstanding opportunity to join a busy five-person radiology group situated at the largest community hospital (300-beds) in the region. We are looking for a university-trained, Board-certified general diagnostic radiologist to join our practice due to an increasing volume. Short partnership track position with generous compensation and benefits. Family-oriented community of 100,000. Excellent technologist support, in part due to on-site school. Home teleradiology. 100,000+ exams yearly. Unique, enjoyable practice where no member has ever left, except for retirement. Send CV to Joseph Hooyman, MD, Radiology Department, Covenant Medical Center, 3421 W Ninth, Waterloo, IA 50702, or fax to 319-272-7105.

ABDOMINAL IMAGING-SECTION HEAD—The Georgetown University Medical Center Department of Radiology seeks a section head for its abdominal imaging group. The practice will be centered at Georgetown University Hospital in the District of Columbia, where there are excellent collaborative programs in surgery, gastroenterology, interventional radiology, as well as the Lombardi Cancer Center. The clinical practice includes MRI (Siemens Vision), CT (General Electric helical) and ultrasound. Integration with the Washington Veterans Administration Hospital began in February 1999. There are suburban offices in Washington, Virginia and Maryland. The successful candidate will join four other full-time faculty and three fellows in the section. The appointment will be at the associate or full professor level in the clinician educator track at Georgetown University. Please direct inquiries to Michael J. Pentecost, MD, Professor and Chairman, Department of Radiology, Georgetown University Medical Center, 3800 Reservoir Rd NW, Washington, DC 20007.

ACUTE STROKE MR PHYSICIST—The Neuroradiology Division at the Massachusetts General Hospital is seeking an experienced MR physicist to direct and manage the experimental and clinical application of advanced magnetic resonance imaging and spectroscopy methods in acute stroke. The successful candidate must have a PhD or equivalent in physics or engineering and seven years experience in operating clinical and experimental NMR instrumentation for both imaging and spectroscopy. A minimum of five years experience in the application of diffusion and perfusion MRI to stroke is required. It is essential that this experience include both human and animal studies. Expertise in this area of MR research should be demonstrated with a strong publication record. Applications from women and underrepresented minority groups are especially encouraged. Please send CV and names of three references to R. Gilberto Gonzalez, MD, PhD, Director of Neuroradiology, GRB 285, Massachusetts General Hospital, Fruit St, Boston, MA 02115.

GROWING PRACTICE—In a southwest suburb of Chicago has openings for two Board-certified radiologists. One requires fellowship training or experience in body imaging. This is a partnership track position with full benefits. The second position is for a general radiologist. This position requires no call. The hours and days/week are negotiable. Please reply to Box R-113.

VA MEDICAL CENTER, MILWAUKEE, WI—Has an immediate opening for a Board-certified radiologist to perform general and minor special procedure studies as well as interpret CTs, ultrasounds and MRIs. Knowledge of nuclear medicine is desirable but not required. Our medical center has extensive telemedicine capabilities with soft copy reading by our department for another VA facility. VA Milwaukee is a tertiary care facility affiliated with the Medical College of Wisconsin. The department is currently upgrading equipment in all areas. Inquiries may be directed to Charles J. Locher, MD, Lead Radiologist at 414-384-2000, x 2545. Submit CV and three references to VA Medical Center, Human Resources, Attn: John Polulach, 5000 W National Ave, Milwaukee, WI 53295 or fax to 414-382-5378. VA is an equal opportunity employer.

BEAUTIFUL SOUTHERN CALIFORNIA DESERT—Well-established eight-person radiology group in Southern California desert seeks Board-eligible, fellowship-trained radiologist for partnership track position. Candidate must have breast imaging and intervention experience as position includes back-up coverage for primary breast radiologist at high volume breast center. Group provides professional services at 350-bed regional medical center with all modalities. Interventional angio training is a plus. Contact David E. Conston, MD, Department of Radiology, Desert Regional Medical Center, 1150 N Indian Canyon Dr, Palm Springs, CA 92262. Phone 760-778-5948.

PALM SPRINGS, CA—An eight-physician radiology group seeks 2-year fellowship-trained neuroradiologist with CAQ or CAQ eligible for partnership track position. Must be willing to do his/her share of general radiology in group setting. Mammography experience a plus for back-up only. Please send CV to Christian H.

Neumann, MD, PO Box 2829, Palm Springs, CA 92263 or fax to 760-778-5999, e-mail at *chhneu-mann@msn.com.*

CHIEF, SECTION OF BODY IMAGING—The Department of Radiology at Northwestern Memorial Hospital, Chicago, IL is seeking a full-time faculty member to serve as chief of the Section of Body Imaging. The applicant must be a Board-certified radiologist who has experience in all aspects of cross-sectional body imaging and a strong background and interest in academic radiology. A demonstrated facility for research and teaching is highly desirable. The applicant must be able to qualify for appointment at the level of associate professor or professor of radiology at Northwestern University Medical School. Salaries and benefits are negotiable. The position is a continuing appointment which is available June 1, 1999. Northwestern Memorial Hospital is a 492-bed general hospital in the North Michigan Ave area of Chicago. Financially strong, NMH opened an entirely new Inpatient/Ambulatory Care Center in May 1999. The Section of Body Imaging at Northwestern is an active service, with nine faculty involved in sectional activities. Equipment includes five helical CT scanners (three GE Lightspeed, 1 Elscint, 1 GE CTi) with another (Siemens Somatom Plus 4) scheduled for installation, six state-of-the-art MR scanners (Siemens 1.5T Vision, Phillips 1.5T NT, four Siemens 1.5T Symphony) with another (Siemens .2T Open Viva) scheduled for installation and eight ultrasound machines. The department is greatly expanding its clinical and research MRI program. With the exception of ultrasonography, where a mini-PACS system is anticipated within the next few months, the imaging section operates in a filmless environment. Address inquiries and a current curriculum vitae to Albert A. Nemcek, Jr, MD, Northwestern Memorial Hospital, Department of Radiology, Feinberg Pavilion, 4-710T, 251 E Huron St, Chicago, IL 60611, phone 312-926-5302, fax 312-926-9029, e-mail *aan728@nwu .edu.* Northwestern University is an affirmative action/equal opportunity employer. Hiring is contingent upon eligibility to work in the United States and acquisition of a license to practice medicine in Illinois.

ABDOMINAL IMAGING—The Department of Radiology at the University of Washington is seeking a faculty member at the level of assistant or associate professor (WOT) to join the abdominal imaging section. The candidate will spend the majority of time in the ultrasound service area, with the remainder in computed tomography and MRI. Ultrasound is an active service that enjoys close relationships with all departments in the hospital and includes a large volume of material in high-risk obstetrical and transplantation patients. Responsibilities will include teaching of medical students, residents and fellows. Candidates for this position must be Board-certified in radiology and have a strong desire for a career in academic radiology. Address inquiries and current CV (please refer to #012999) to Albert A. Moss, MD, Professor and Chair, Department of Radiology, Box 357115, University of Washington, Seattle, WA 98195-7115. The University of Washington is an affirmative action/equal opportunity employer.

NORTH OF BOSTON—Dynamic growing practice seeking several additional Board-certified radiologists by 1/1/2000. Skill sets needed include generalists or fellowship-trained individuals in body section, ultrasound, and mammography. Angiographic skills helpful but not essential. Excellent salary and benefits. Send CV to Alan G. Pratt, Lawrence General Hospital, Lawrence, MA 01842.

FACULTY POSITION IN ULTRASOUND AND BODY CT, THOMAS JEFFERSON UNIVERSITY HOSPITAL—The Department of Radiology at Thomas Jefferson University Hospital seeks an academically oriented faculty member to join its active and highly respected ultrasound and body CT divisions. Jefferson has the largest clinical and research ultrasound facility in the country, with involvement in virtually every aspect of that discipline. There is also a major educational program at the residency, fellowship and continuing education levels. We operate five CT scanners and have very active clinical, teaching and research programs in this area as well. Research time is provided and there is an extensive infrastructure to support faculty research. Interested applicants should contact Barry Goldberg, MD, Director of Ultrasound, Department of Radiology, Thomas Jefferson University Hospital, Philadelphia, PA 19107. Phone 215-955-6227, fax 215-955-8549.

UNIVERSITY OF CHICAGO—Radiologist with emphasis in interventional/vascular radiology and abdominal imaging. Clinical research experience in the angio/interventional field and a strong interest and clinical experience in body MRA is preferred. Additional clinical duties will be in the section of abdominal imaging. Research experience in imaging reconstruction such as CTA and virtual colonography is desirable. The position requires teaching and training of both residents and fellows and there are vast research opportunities. Interested applicants should call or forward their CV to Dr Martin J. Lipton, Department of Radiology, 5841 S Maryland Ave, MC 2026, Chicago, IL 60637, fax 773-702-2523. The University of Chicago is an equal opportunity/affirmative action employer.

DIAGNOSTIC RADIOLOGIST—To join a strong, progressive, 12-member radiology group in southwestern Ontario, Canada. Interest in cross-sectional imaging (CT, MRI, US), GI radiology. Nonvascular interventional skills and breast imaging would be helpful. Fellowship preferred, but not required. Practice includes 400-bed tertiary care teaching hospital, three community hospitals and four private offices. State-of-the-art equipment. Please send CV to Dr R. Rozak, London X-Ray Associates, 104-450 Central Ave, London, Ontario, N6B 2E8.

ASSISTANT/ASSOCIATE PROFESSOR—The University of California, San Francisco is seeking a radiologist with expertise in mammography for San Francisco General Hospital, one of four core UCSF teaching hospitals. The candidate will be appointed at the level of assistant or associate professor in the residence or clinical series, depending upon experience. Responsibilities include mammography, teaching and research and may include general diagnostic radiology and/or ultrasound, teaching and research. The candidate will supervise and teach residents and a fellow in mammography and women's imaging techniques. Requirements include mammography expertise, including Board certification in diagnostic radiology and a California medical license. Recommended qualifications include fellowship training in mammography and experience in clinical research. UCSF is an affirmative action/equal opportunity employer. The University undertakes affirmative action to assure equal employment opportunity for underutilized minorities and women, for persons with disabilities, and for Vietnam-era veterans and special disabled veterans. Send CV and five professional references to Robert A. Halvorsen, MD, Chief, Department of Radiology, San Francisco General Hospital, 1001 Potrero Ave, Rm 1X55, San Francisco, CA 94110.

INTERVENTIONAL/VASCULAR RADIOLOGIST—The Department of Radiology of the University of Medicine and Dentistry of New Jersey is seeking an interventional and vascular fellowship-trained radiologist with nationally/internationally recognized research contributions in the field. Primary focus will be clinical, laboratory and animal research. ABR certification required. Academic rank open. UMDNJ-NJMS is an equal opportunity employer. Send CV to Dr Stephen Baker, MD, by fax 973-972-7429.

FELLOWSHIP-TRAINED INTERVENTIONAL RADIOLOGIST—A nine-physician diagnostic radiology group in a 450-bed tertiary care hospital, located in 125,000 populated city, 90 minutes from Pittsburgh, seeks a BC, capable, motivated radiologist qualified in all phases of diagnostic radiology but with fellowship training in interventional radiology to join our present interventionalist. Applicant should be CAQ eligible or certified. Generous starting salary and benefit package with partnership to follow. If interested, send CV to Lawrence McNiesh, MD, 600 Somerset Ave, Windber, PA 15963.

SAN DIEGO, CA—Fantastic opportunity to work with a premier radiation oncology practice in San Diego. Call 1:7, state-of-the-art equipment and facilities. Opportunity to develop niches in prostate brachytherapy, HDR brachytherapy, stereotactic radiosurgery, and head and neck brachytherapy. Enjoy everything San Diego has to offer, from 25 miles of ocean and beaches to cultural activities, plus much more. For more information, contact Anne Sheahan at 800-756-3055, x3478; fax CV to 314-726-0026; e-mail *asheahan@cejka.com.* ID# 6688RA. Visit our website at *www.cejka.com.*

FLORIDA GULF COAST—Interventional and general diagnostic radiologist needed to join department of eleven radiologists in premier 160+ physician multi-specialty group. Enjoy a four-day workweek with 1:6 call, state-of-the-art technology, competitive salary, full benefits and future partnership. Quality lifestyle in Pensacola with beautiful beaches, excellent schools and year-round recreational and cultural amenities. Call Kathy Jordan at 800-765-3055, fax 314-726-3009, e-mail *kjordan@cejka .com.* ID# 6699RE. Visit our website at *www .cejka.com.*

is desirable. Practice currently covers five hospitals and multiple imaging centers with state-of-the-art equipment. Send CV to John Walter, MD, 1500 Expo Pkwy, Sacramento, CA 95815, fax 916-920-4434, e-mail *jwalter@ns.net.*

IMMEDIATE OPENING—For a fellowship-trained radiologist to join large, subspecialized private practice. Partnership track. Majority of time to be spent in body cross-sectional imaging. Practice currently covers five hospitals and multiple imaging centers with state-of-the-art equipment. Send CV to John Walter, MD, 1500 Expo Pkwy, Sacramento, CA 95815, fax 916-920-4434, e-mail *jwalter@ns.net.*

SENIOR STAFF RADIOLOGIST—The Institute of Diagnostic Radiology at the University Hospital in Zurich is seeking an experienced MR scientist and clinician, who wishes to spend a sabbatical in the heart of Europe. For the time in Zurich, the individual, who should be a Board certified radiologist with extensive knowledge and experience in clinical and scientific magnetic resonance imaging, will serve in a senior staff position. The financial remuneration will be scaled accordingly. Please send application and CV to Professor B. Marincek, MD, Director, Institute of Diagnostic Radiology, University Hospital, CH-8091 Zurich, SWITZERLAND, phone +41-1-255-29-00, fax +41-1-255-44-43, e-mail *marincek@dmr.usz.ch.*

MUSCULOSKELETAL RADIOLOGIST—A six-member group in western Colorado seeking fellowship-trained MS radiologist. A 300-bed hospital serving 14 busy orthopedic surgeons. Partnership track with generous income and vacation. Growing community with lifestyle inherent to Rocky Mountain West. Respond to Reed Bumgarner, MD, 2530 N Eighth St, Ste#101, Grand Junction, CO 81501, 970-244-7067.

EXPANDING RADIOLOGY GROUP—Is in need of a diagnostic neuroradiologist, musculoskeletal radiologist and/or MRI radiologist to join us at a modern outpatient imaging center. We are fully equipped with both a high-field MRI and a new open MRI, CT, three US, two mammo, fluoro and plain film units. Plans are in place for upgrades and expansion, including a third MRI. This is a partnership opportunity, and there is currently no call requirement. We are located in northern California, within easy reach of San Francisco, Sacramento, and multiple Pacific coastal and Sierra destinations. Our thriving community is diverse, with good schools and abundant year-round activities. If you are interested in the California lifestyle and working in a cohesive group with progressive attitudes towards radiology and patient care, call or fax your curriculum vitae to 209-521-7949.

MEDICAL PHYSICIST SPECIALIZING IN DIAGNOSTIC IMAGING—The University of Texas Health Science Center at San Antonio, San Antonio, TX. The graduate program in Radiological Sciences at the University of Texas Health Science Center at San Antonio is seeking a medical physicist specializing in diagnostic imaging to serve as a core faculty member in the continuing development of the medical physics graduate program. The program is one of nine certified medical physics graduate programs in North America certified by CAMPEP (see web site for details *http://radscience.uthscsa.edu/*). The successful candidate will join a multidisciplinary faculty of 46. He/she will be responsible for teaching portions of two diagnostic physics courses (Fundamentals of Diagnostic Physics and Physics of Nuclear Imaging). In addition, the new junior faculty member will be expected to actively develop an independent research program in one of the existing imaging laboratories or clinics. Collaboration with existing projects in interventional cardiovascular imaging, nuclear imaging pharmacology, interventional tumor ablation, functional imaging-MRI and PET, and/or electronic imaging are encouraged. Imaging equipment for research is available in both research and clinical settings. Candidates must have a doctoral degree in medical physics, physics, biomedical engineering or other appropriate physical science. Experience with nuclear imaging, MR and electronic imaging methodologies are highly desirable. This position carries a tenure-track academic appointment in the Department of Radiology. Salary and academic rank commensurate with qualifications. Send curriculum vitae and references to Medical Physics Faculty Recruitment, c/o Gary D. Fullerton, PhD, Professor and Chief Radiological Sciences Division, University of Texas Health Science Center at San Antonio, Radiology Department, 7703 Floyd Curl Drive, San Antonio, TX 78284-7800. The UTHSCSA is an Equal Employment Opportunity/Affirmative Action Employer.

FACULTY POSITIONS IN BREAST RADIOLOGY—The Department of Radiology at the University of South Florida (USF) College of Medicine is seeking two breast imaging radiologists at the assistant/associate professor level and both positions may be tenure earning. These positions are based at the H. Lee Moffitt Cancer Center and Research Institute at USF, an NCI-designated cancer center. Clinical practice is divided between a multidisciplinary diagnostic breast center and a separate screening center. Breast imaging modalities include seven conventional mammography units, dedicated breast sonography, two stereotactic biopsy units, breast MRI, and investigational direct digital mammography. Both positions include clinical service, teaching of radiology residents and fellows, participation in clinical investigations, and other scholarly activities. Applicants should have an MD degree, be Board certified in diagnostic radiology, and have a minimum of 1 year fellowship training or practice experience in their subspeciality discipline, with expertise in all modalities of practice. Salary and rank are commensurate with qualifications and experience. A valid Florida medical license is required prior to beginning employment. One position will begin January 1, 2000 and the other starts on or after July 1, 2000. Applications or nominations for these positions should be addressed to Robert Clark, MD, Chairman, Department of Radiology, H. Lee Moffitt Cancer Center and Research Institute at USF, 12902 Magnolia Drive, Tampa, FL 33612. Phone 813-972-8425, fax 813-979-7231, e-mail *clark@moffitt.usf.edu.* Application deadline is October 29, 1999. USF is an Equal Opportunity/Affirmative Action/Equal Access Institution. For disability accommodations, contact Claudette Cigarran at 813-974-2538, TDD 974-2218, a minimum of five working days in advance.

Fellowships

THE DEPARTMENT OF RADIOLOGY OF THE BRIGHAM AND WOMEN'S HOSPITAL-HARVARD MEDICAL SCHOOL—Offers 1 or 2-year fellowship positions in the following areas: 1) cardiovascular and interventional, 2) neuroradiology, 3) abdominal, 4) abdominal interventional, 5) magnetic resonance, 6) women's imaging, 7) oncoradiology, 8) chest, 9) bone, 10) nuclear medicine, 11) computer science, 12) mammography, 13) EW. For more information please send curriculum vitae specifying your area of interest to Steven E. Seltzer, MD, Chairman, Department of Radiology, Brigham and Women's Hospital, 75 Francis St, Boston, MA 02115. Harvard Medical School and Brigham and Women's Hospital are equal opportunity, affirmative action employers.

INDIANA UNIVERSITY SCHOOL OF MEDICINE FELLOWSHIPS—The Department of Radiology at Indiana University in Indianapolis offers fellowships in abdominal imaging, breast imaging, chest imaging, musculoskeletal imaging, neuroradiology, nuclear medicine, pediatric radiology, and vascular and interventional radiology. Indiana has a 40-member teaching faculty, state-of-the-art equipment, a large clinical practice (over 400,000 patient examinations per year), and active research. For more information please visit our web site at *www.indyrad.iupui.edu.* Must obtain license to practice medicine in the state of Indiana. Grant (award) type/term/amount: competitive; 1-2-years. Department funding, contact Kathie Pedersen, Indiana University Hospital 0279, 550 N University Blvd, Indianapolis, IN 46202-5253; telephone 317-274-1840, fax 317-274-1848, e-mail *kmpeders@iupui.edu.* Deadlines: n.a. Key words: abdominal imaging, breast imaging, chest imaging, musculoskeletal imaging, neuroradiology, nuclear medicine, pediatric radiology, vascular and interventional radiology. Award amount key: n.a. Links: go to RFP/A.

NEURORADIOLOGY FELLOWSHIP POSITION FOR JULY 2000—A 1 or 2-year neuroradiology fellowship accredited by the ACGME. Training includes all aspects of neuroradiology, head and neck radiology and participation in interventional neuroradiology procedures. A one-month elective away is offered in pediatric neuroradiology or interventional for those in the 2nd-year. The hospital has state-of-the-art equipment: 1) three helical GE CT scanners, 2) two GE 1.5T Signa MR scanners, echospeed on one scanner and plans to upgrade to echospeed on the other, and 3) new biplane Toshiba neuroangiography unit. The outpatient center has an echospeed 1.5T Signa MR scanner with plans for addition of another MR scanner and helical CT scanner. There are five full-time neuroradiology, three PhD physicists and three visiting research faculty. The neuroradiology section conducts

ACCREDITED FELLOWSHIPS IN PEDIATRIC RADIOLOGY—The Department of Radiology, Children's Hospital and Harvard Medical School, Boston, MA offers a 2-year accredited (Residency Review Committee for Radiology of ACGME) fellowship in pediatric radiology beginning July 1, 2001. 1-year pediatric neuroradiology and pediatric vascular/interventional fellowship programs are also available. Children's Hospital is a 350-bed institution and performs over 125,000 radiological examinations annually in one of the largest pediatric medical centers in North America. The department has 24 faculty pediatric radiologists, three PhD research faculty, one physicist, 10 pediatric radiology fellows, six neuroradiology fellows and many resident trainees. Up to five pediatric radiology, one pediatric neuroradiology and one pediatric vascular/interventional fellowship positions are available annually. Training includes all aspects of pediatric imaging including neonatal radiology, neuroimaging, musculoskeletal radiology, cardiovascular and thoracic imaging, abdominal imaging, oncologic imaging, ultrasonography, nuclear medicine, computed tomography, MRI and vascular/interventional radiology. The department has a very active clinical service with state-of-the-art equipment as follows: two digital fluoroscopy rooms, five ultrasound units with Doppler and color-flow Doppler capabilities, planar and SPECT gamma cameras, two GE Hi-Lite CT scanners, two 1.5T GE MRI systems with spectroscopy and MR angiography, and two vascular/interventional suites with digital imaging. The department provides extensive academic support including the Stern Memorial Radiology Library and a departmental librarian as well as the Kresge Laboratory for Pediatric Imaging Research. The fellowship provides a broad clinical experience in pediatric radiology as well as numerous opportunities to participate in clinical, basic and health services research. There are opportunities for collaborative research efforts at Children's Hospital, other Harvard teaching hospitals, Harvard Medical School, and the Harvard School of Public Health. Candidates must be Board-certified or Board-qualified in diagnostic radiology and must obtain a Massachussetts medical license. Salary and fringe benefits are competitive. Applications are due no later than December 1, 1999. To receive more information about careers in pediatric radiology in general or the fellowships at Children's Hospital in particular, please contact Carlo Buonomo, MD, Director, Fellowship Program, Children's Hospital, Department of Radiology, 300 Longwood Ave, Boston, MA 02115, 617-355-6496. Children's Hospital and Harvard Medical School are affirmative action/equal opportunity employers.

THORACIC RADIOLOGY FELLOWSHIP AT NEW YORK UNIVERSITY—Fellowship position offered for July 2000 in a chest imaging section staffed by three full-time and two part-time chest radiologists, covering New York University Hospital and Bellevue Medical Center. Extensive clinical experience will include thoracic CT, plain film and digital chest radiography, and thoracic MR. Excellent opportunities for research are available. Interested candidates should send CV to Dr David P. Naidich, Director, Thoracic Imaging, Department of Radiology, New York University Medical Center, 560 First Ave, New York, NY 10016. New York University is an equal opportunity employer.

UNEXPECTED OPENING FOR FELLOWSHIP IN IMAGING/ANGIO-INTERVENTIONAL—A 1-year fellowship program at Lehigh Valley Hospital in Allentown, PA is available for 1999-2000. LVH is a 650-bed acute care, university-affiliated hospital. The fellowship program offers training in CT (head and body), ultrasound, MR, angiography and interventional radiology. For further information, contact Elliot Shoemaker, MD, Department of Radiology, Lehigh Valley Hospital, PO Box 689, Allentown, PA 18105-1556, telephone 610-402-8088 or fax 610-402-1023.

NEURORADIOLOGY FELLOWSHIP POSITION—The William Beaumont Hospital, Department of Diagnostic Radiology, Royal Oak, MI, is offering a 1-year accredited fellowship in neuro-radiology beginning July 1, 2000. The fellowship provides a broad clinical experience with training in all aspects of diagnostic and interventional neuroradiology, including computed tomography, MRI (including functional diffusion and perfusion MRI), MR spectroscopy, myelography, discography, cerebral arteriography, spine biopsy, GDC coil embolization for aneurysm and endovascular thrombolytic treatment for acute stroke as well as angioplasty/stent and other embolization procedures. The fellowship provides opportunities to participate in clinical research. The ACGME-accredited program is staffed by three full-time CAQ neuroradiologists and two part-time neuroradiologists, including one head and neck neuroradiologist and two interventional neuroradiologists. William Beaumont Hospital is a 929-bed tertiary care teaching hospital serving several large suburban communities in Oakland County, 13 miles north of Detroit, MI. The imaging facilities include five state-of-the-art CT scanners with helical and 3D capabilities, three Siemens 1.5T vision MR scanners, two up-to-date and one upcoming angiographic suites with state-of-the-art digital capabilities. For further information, please contact Ay-Ming Wang, MD, FACR, Chief, Division of Neuroradiology, Department of Diagnostic Radiology, William Beaumont Hospital, 3601 W Thirteen Mile Rd, Royal Oak, MI 48073. Phone 248-551-1005 or e-mail *amwang@beaumont.edu.*

FELLOWSHIPS AT YALE UNIVERSITY, 2001—The Department of Diagnostic Radiology at Yale University School of Medicine offer the following fellowships: abdominal imaging-four positions: balanced position CT/US/MR, CT focus, US focus, MR focus. Each focused position includes rotations through all three imaging services. Contact Shirley McCarthy, MD, PhD. Thoracic imaging: one position, includes plain film interpretation, lung biopsies, CT and MRI. Contact Ann McB. Curtis, MD. Breast imaging: one position, includes mammography, breast biopsies (stereotactic and ultrasound-guided), breast ultrasound, breast MRI and nuclear medicine breast imaging research opportunities. Contact Irena Tocino, MD. Neuroradiology: three 2-year positions offered each year. Contact Gordon Sze, MD. Vascular and interventional: three positions each year. Contact Jeffrey Pollak, MD. Pediatric radiology (ACGME-accredited): One position each year. Contact Mark S. Keller, MD. Interested applicants should send their CV and three letters of recommendation to the appropriate program director, at PO Box 20802 (333 Cedar St), New Haven, CT 06520.

Practice for Sale

EXCELLENT INCOME OPPORTUNITY—Radiology practice for sale in central California. Excellent location across from district hospital. Mammography, diagnostic imaging, MRI, CT and ultrasound. Terms available to qualified buyer. Call 970-259-3822 or mail letters of interest to PO Box 932, Sunset Beach, CA 90742.

RSNA®

RSNA Executive Offices • 820 Jorie Boulevard
Oak Brook, IL 60523 • (630) 571-2670

Bulletin Board

August 1999

✓ **RSNA '99 Registration Update**

✓ **Panelists Announced for Image Interpretation Session at RSNA '99**

✓ **Update on IHE Year 1 Symposium**

■ The 1999 RSNA Advance Registration and Housing brochure was sent to over 30,000 RSNA members in April with a second registration brochure sent to a broader audience including non-members in early June. Please remember hotel reservations are made on a first-come, first-serve basis. Hotels fill quickly, so the sooner you register the better your chance of booking the hotel of your choice.

Deadlines for Advance Registration and Housing are October 1, 1999, Non–North American, and October 29, 1999, for North American.

General Registration for nonmembers began June 14.

■ The panelists for the Image Interpretation Session to be held on Sunday, November 28, during the RSNA's Scientific Assembly and Annual Meeting have been announced. The panel, moderated by N. Reed Dunnick, MD, consists of the following: Denise R. Aberle, MD, C. Daniel Johnson, MD, Gabriel P. Krestin, MD, Daniel I. Rosenthal, MD, and Mutsumasa Takahashi, MD.

■ The IHE Year 1 Symposium at RSNA '99 will address the theme "Architecting Cost-effective, High-Quality, Patient-centered Care for the New Millennium." Scheduled to begin Wednesday, December 1, and run through Friday, December 3, the IHE Year 1 Symposium will function as a "Meeting within the Meeting" during RSNA '99. Noted experts and industry leaders will be brought in to provide perspective on current and upcoming changes in the technology, institutions, and methods used to deliver healthcare. The IHE Year 1 Symposium will be a distinct but concurrent event designed to broaden the concerns of the RSNA annual meeting, while capitalizing on the energy and attention focused on what has become the largest annual gathering of healthcare professionals in the world.

Attendees can register for the IHE Year 1 Symposium sessions only or incorporate a selection of these sessions as part of their overall program for RSNA '99.

■ The following is a list of applicants for RSNA membership, published as provided by the bylaws of the Society. Society members are asked to review these names. Should a member have a question concerning the eligibility of an applicant, within 30 days of the publication of this list, the member should request that the applicant's membership be withheld pending investigation and reconsideration by the Membership and Credentials Board. Please mark your signed letter of protest "Confidential" and address it to Secretary-Treasurer, RSNA, 820 Jorie Blvd, Oak Brook, IL 60523. Please note that listed here are only the locations in which the prospective members reside and the counselors for those areas.

ALABAMA
Counselor: Robert E. Koehler, MD
Jeffrey T. Marsch, MD, Birmingham

CALIFORNIA
Counselors: Deborah S. Ablin, MD
Kenneth W. Chin, MD
Nancy A. Ellerbroek, MD
Gary R. Hansen, MD
Eric W. Olcott, MD
Dolores H. Pretorius, MD
Curtis A. Cammarata, MD, Irvine
Robert D. Suh, MD, Fullerton
Robert M. Cothren, PhD, Walnut Creek
Karen Kinkel, MD, San Francisco
Souhil Zaim, MD, Paris
Roger S. Eng, Jr., MD, Lodi

CONNECTICUT
Counselor: Marc F. Glickstein, MD
Song Lai, PhD, Farmington

FLORIDA
Counselor: John A. Arrington, MD
Charles D. Lee, MD, Tampa

GEORGIA
Counselor: Norman B. Thomson III, MD
Janet T. Markle, MD, Martinez
Victor N. Mizrachi, MD, Fort Benning

IDAHO
Counselor: Stephen A. Sherman, MD
Reginald J. Gobel, MD, Boise

ILLINOIS
Counselors: Boyd E. Nelson, MD
Milton L. Paige, MD
Robert A. Marshall, MD, Berwyn

INDIANA
Counselor: Smari Thordarson, MD
David R. Martin, MD, Peru

KANSAS
Counselor: Peter E. Schloesser, MD
Pablo N. Delgado, MD, Fairway

MICHIGAN
Counselors: Judith M. Bender, MD
Walter W. Laidlaw, MD
Karen A. Hunt, MD, Plymouth
Norberto A. Sugayan, MD, Southfield

MISSISSIPPI
Counselor: Margaret T. Hatten, MD
Brian J. McCallie, MD, Biloxi

MISSOURI
Counselors: David P. Diemer, MD
G. David Dixon, MD
Jeffrey P. Turk, MD, Moberly
David R. Warden III, MD, Rolla

NEW JERSEY
Counselor: Karen L. Karlson, MD
Delilah M. Burrowes, MD, Asbury Park
Robert J. Graziano, MD, Cherry Hill
Darius P. Melisaratos, MD, Edgewater

NEW YORK
Counselors: Mario A. Grosso, MD
David M. Panicek, MD
Arthur J. Segal, MD
Michael O. Duhaney, MD, New York
Wen Y. Wang, MD, Forest Hills
Christopher J. Vaughn, MD

NORTH CAROLINA
Counselor: James A. Fagan, MD
Mark S. Zalaznik, MD, Fayetteville

OHIO
Counselors: Kimberly E. Applegate, MD
Jonathan S. Moulton, MD
Ronald A. Bailey, MD, Pepper Pike

OREGON
Counselor: Donald D. Sauser, MD
Randy H. Greene, MD, Lake Oswego

PENNSYLVANIA
Counselors: Nilima Dash, MD
Kathryn A. Evers, MD
John E. Madewell, MD
Elias S. Najem, MD, Clarks Summit

SOUTH CAROLINA
Counselor: Charles G. Hood, MD
Joseph A. Kavanagh, MD, Spartanburg

TEXAS
Counselors: Karl A. Glastad, MD
Chandra S. Katragadda, MD
Timothy W. Lillick, MD
George J. Abdo, MD, Houston

VIRGINIA
Counselors: Deborah A. Kuban, MD
Arnold J. Kuta, MD
Wesley L. Asbury, Jr, MD, Wytheville

WEST VIRGINIA
Counselor: Gary D. Marano, MD
Christopher A. Schlarb, MD, Charleston

WISCONSIN
Counselor: Thomas F. Berns, MD
Laura B. Ulmer, MD, Brookfield

NAVY
Counselor: Walter B. Goff II, DO
Kimberly M. McNeil, MD, FPO

MEXICO
Counselors: Jose H. Arredondo, MD
Manuel A. Cabal, MD
Jose M. Cardoso, MD
Miguel A. Carrillo, MD
Ramon R. Ponte, MD
Francisco J. Reynaga-Garcia, MD
Francisco Javier V. Solis, Jr, MD, Leon
Felipe S. Garza-Gracia, MD, Monterrey
Rocio Madrigal, MD, Monterrey

CANADA

QUEBEC
Counselors: Pierre M. Bourgouin, MD
Gilles J. Hudon, MD
Marie-Christine Roy, MD, Montreal

CORRESPONDING
Paulo J. Alvares, MD, Portugal
Maria Grazia Amorico, MD, Italy
Adriana Baca, MD, Colombia
Jeremy Berger, MBBS, MA, United Kingdom
Johannes L. Bester, MD, Australia
Sonja Borsky, MBBS, Australia
Ivan Drinkovic, Sr, MD, PhD, Croatia
Mohamed Z. El-Headik, MD, Saudi Arabia
Gulgun Engin, MD, Turkey
Luiz Augusto G. Gabure, MD, Brazil
Simon D. Grling, MBBS, BSc, United Kingdom
Claus P. Heussel, MD, Germany
Yoshinori Isobe, MD, Japan
Masayuki Kawanishi, MD, Japan
Toshiki Kazama, MD, Japan
Weijey Ko, MD, PhD, Japan
Satoshi Kobayashi, MD, Japan
Eugene B. Kots, MD, Israel
Francis Lau Sing Lee, MBBS, Malaysia
Geraldine A. Long, MBBS, Australia
Olivier Lucidarme, MD, France
Fumiko Nagahata, MD, Japan
Gloria Palazulloo, MD, Colombia
Anders Persson, MD, Sweden
Chaturbhuj L. Rajak, MD, India
Thomas Rettenbacher, MD, Austria
Harumi Sakahara, MD, Japan
Motohiro Sato, MD, PhD, Japan
Ichiro Tani, MD, Japan
Rana M. Tariq, MBBS, Norway
Andrzej S. Urbanik, PhD, MD, Poland
Alejandro Vara-Castrodeza, MD, Spain
Pier Carlo Villani, MD, Italy
Colin J. Walker, MBBS, Australia
Mariola Wierna, MBBS, Australia
Jorge D. Yamil, MD, Argentina

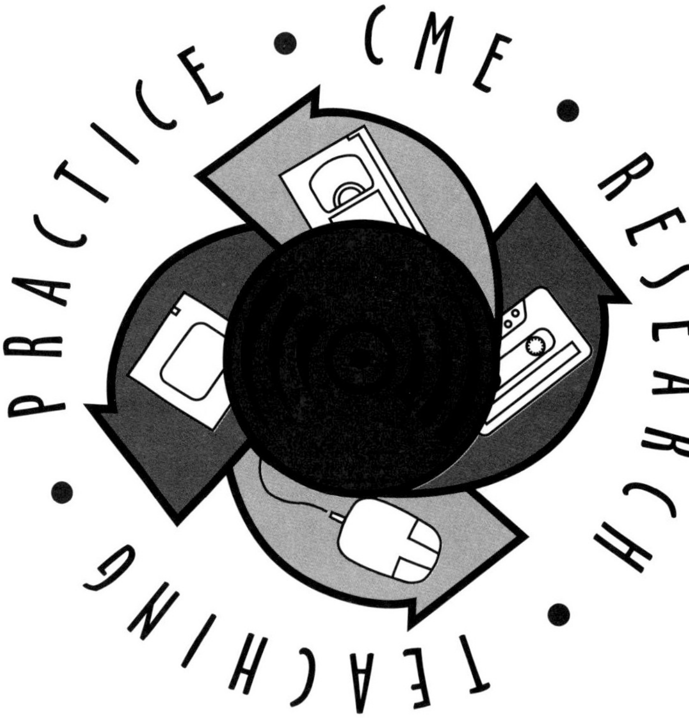

Pediatric

Learning Center Resources

August 1999

RSNA® | Radiological Society of North America
Founded in 1915

Featured Topics

- Urinary Tract Infection
- Pulmonary Infection
- Spinal Injuries
- Intracranial Injuries

New Service

The entire 1998–1999 Learning Center Resources Catalog is now available on the RSNA *Link*, the Web site of the Radiological Society of North America, on the Internet.

You can reach us through the World Wide Web (WWW) by entering the uniform resource locator: http://www.rsna.org

We invite you to browse through the catalog, search for specific courses of interest, then simply order via our fax or 800 phone number.

Detach and store for your future use.

The following 14 Pediatric titles and others are now available in the Learning Center Resources Library. All videotapes are available for purchase or rental (U.S., Canada, and Mexico). All video programs may be purchased in NTSC, PAL, and SECAM television standards. Slides and audiotapes are available for purchase only.

For more information, call or fax the RSNA Learning Center Resources at the numbers listed on the order form. To order by mail, use the form on the back.

NEW!

Posterior Fossa Tumors and Parameningeal Tumors in Children *RSP 720*

Gilbert Vezina, MD

The clinical and imaging findings of posterior fossa and parameningeal tumors that are common in or specific to childhood are presented along with management considerations. Such tumors include astrocytoma, medulloblastoma, ependymoma, brain-stem tumors, malformative tumors, tumor mimics, neuroblastoma, sarcomas, histiocytosis, plexiform neurofibroma, angiofibroma, and tumor seeding. *Learning objectives:* To review basic knowledge and skills and understand the latest advances in the imaging and management of vascular anomalies of the developing central nervous system and head and neck.

71 slides/audiotape *M$140, N$160*
VHS *M$140, N$160*

NEW!

Tumors about the Third Ventricle in Children *RSP 721*

Patrick D. Barnes, MD

The clinical and imaging findings of perisellar and pineal region tumors that are common in or specific to childhood are presented along with neuroendocrine and management considerations. Such tumors include optic/hypothalamic astrocytoma, craniopharyngioma, germ cell tumors, pineal cell tumors, pituitary tumors, malformative tumors, and tumor mimics. *Learning objectives:* To review basic knowledge and skills and understand the latest advances and approaches in the imaging and management of neuroendocrine disorders and tumors in the 3rd ventricle in childhood.

65 slides/audiotape *M$140, N$160*
VHS *M$140, N$160*

NEW!

Pediatric Congenital and Development Abnormalities: Dorsal and Ventral *RSP 722*

Neural Tube Defects

Marvin D. Nelson, Jr, MD

This presentation focuses on the imaging and neuropathologic features of malformations of the central nervous system that arise during the embryonic period. These include disorders of dorsal and ventral neurulation such as anencephaly, cephaloceles, dermal sinus, dermoid/epidermoid, Chiari malformations, holoprosencephalies, septum pellucidum anomalies, optic and olfactory defects, pituitary/hypothalamic anomalies, and hindbrain malformations (eg, Dandy-Walker, Lhermitte-Duclos). *Learning objectives:* To review basic knowledge and skills and understand the latest advances in imaging of anomalies of the developing central nervous system.

VHS *M$140, N$160*
Not available in slide/audiotape

NEW!

Migrational and Proliferative Disorders in Children *RSP 723*

Thomas P. Naidich, MD

The clinical, imaging, and neuropathologic features of malformations of cortical development are presented along with their embryologic and genetic correlates, particularly as they relate to the management of children with epilepsy and mental retardation. These include the focal, multifocal, and generalized cortical malformations resulting from abnormal neuronal and glial proliferation (eg, focal cortical dysplasia, hemimegalencephaly, tuberous sclerosis, focal transmantle dysplasia, DNET), abnormal neuronal migration (eg, lissencephalies, heterotopias), and abnormal cortical organization (eg, polymicrogyria, schizencephaly, microdysgenesis). *Learning objectives:* To review basic knowledge and skills and understand the latest advances in imaging and management of cortical malformations.

VHS *M$140, N$160*
Not available in slide/audiotape

M/N = Member/Nonmember prices
To order call (800) 272-2920 or FAX (630) 990-9958
(Outside U.S., phone (630) 990-9941)

NEW!

Pediatric Urinary Tract Infection: Multimodality Imaging *RSP 724*

Sara M. O'Hara, MD

This program emphasizes a multimodality approach to the work-up of urinary tract infections, building upon clinical decision-making and prior test results. While ultrasonography, nuclear imaging, and fluoroscopy remain the primary imaging tools, the adjuvant roles of urography, CT, and MR imaging are also discussed. *Learning objectives:* To develop imaging strategies for the evaluation of pediatric urinary tract infections based on current concepts of pathophysiology, clinical therapy, and common congenital anomalies.

VHS *M$140, N$160*

Not available in slide/audiotape

NEW!

Changing Patterns of Pulmonary Infection in Children *RSP 725*

Beverly P. Wood, MD

Because of new virulence factors, once uncomplicated and responsive infections of the respiratory system have become more complex and less predictable in course and outcome. Recognition of a complicated host response to infection is a key to proper management. This course reviews the changing patterns of respiratory infections related to the changing virulence of both old and new pathogens. *Learning objectives:* To describe the radiographic manifestations of pulmonary infections in children.

VHS *M$140, N$160*

Not available in slide/audiotape

NEW!

Spinal Injuries in Children: CT, MR Imaging *RSP 726*

Charles M. Glasier, MD

The applications of CT and MR imaging in acute spinal injury are presented, and their role in supplementing plain radiography is addressed. CT with multiplanar reconstruction allows precise localization of fracture fragments with respect to vital neurovascular structures and helps to characterize spinal injuries as stable or unstable. CT "scout views" and axial CT sections are essential for the accurate localization of injury levels, especially in preoperative planning. MR imaging is reserved for the examination of the child with known or suspected neurologic injury, especially in the presence of normal plain radiographs and abnormal findings at neurologic examination. *Learning objectives:* (1) To understand CT and MR findings of various spinal injuries in children. (2) To learn techniques of CT and MR imaging for spinal injuries.

VHS *M$140, N$160*

Not available in slide/audiotape

NEW!

Intracranial Injuries in Children *RSP 727*

Michele H. Johnson, MD

This program addresses the clinical and imaging spectrum of pediatric intracranial injuries caused by acute trauma. The role and timing of imaging and the appropriate selection of imaging tests in the emergent assessment of pediatric traumatic injuries are discussed. This program defines and illustrates imaging findings in direct parenchymal injuries, as well as the indirect consequences of pediatric cranial trauma. Features of intracranial injuries unique to childhood are discussed. *Learning objectives:* (1) To define the role of imaging techniques, including CT, MR imaging, and angiography in the diagnosis and management of pediatric cranial trauma. (2) To identify and describe features of cranial trauma unique to childhood. (3) To describe the physiologic, anatomic, and pathologic correlates of the imaging of pediatric cranial trauma.

VHS *M$140, N$160*

Not available in slide/audiotape

Color Doppler US: Pediatric Extracranial Applications *RSP 626*

Marta Hernanz-Schulman, MD

90 slides/audiotape *M$140, N$160*

VHS *M$140, N$160*

Pediatric Cervical Spine Trauma *RSP 627*

Leonard E. Swischuk, MD

Sharon E. Byrd, MD

198 slides/audiotape *M$205, N$225*

VHS *M$205, N$225*

The Subtleties of Pediatric Extremity Fractures *RSP 628*

Susan D. John, MD

115 slides/audiotape *M$140, N$160*

VHS *M$140, N$160*

Pediatric Spiral CT: Challenges of Childhood *RSP 594*

George S. Bisset III, MD

Marilyn J. Siegel, MD

Donald P. Frush, MD

144 slides/2 audiotapes *M$205, N$225*

VHS *M$205, N$225*

Obstetric US: Fetal CNS *RSP 540*

Alfred B. Kurtz, MD

42 slides/audiotape *M$140, N$160*

VHS *M$140, N$160*

Obstetric US: Growth Parameters and Growth Retardation *RSP 541*

Barbara S. Hertzberg, MD

53 slides/audiotape *M$140, N$160*

VHS *M$140, N$16*

We Offer Rentals! (Available for U.S., Canada, and Mexico)

All titles are available for rental. Single rentals are available for $50 each. For more information on annual subscriptions or to request a complete catalog, please contact RSNA Learning Center Resources.

Call today, (800) 272-2920, or fax (630) 990-9958. (Outside U.S., phone (630) 990-9941).

Place Stamp Here

TO: RSNA LEARNING CENTER RESOURCES
PO BOX 5316
OAK BROOK, IL 60522-5316
USA

FOLD HERE

PRACTICE • CME • RESEARCH • TEACHING

Order Form

You may mail or fax this form. To fax your order, dial 630-990-9958. Please print.

☐ *RSNA Member* ☐ *Nonmember*

NAME

RSNA MEMBER # (REQUIRED FOR MEMBER PRICING)

ADDRESS

CITY

STATE/COUNTRY

ZIP

PHONE

FAX

Order Information (for purchase and rentals)

Course Number	*Showing Date (Rental Only)*	*Format (Purchase Only)*	*Price*

FOLD HERE

Check one:

☐ *Rental*

☐ *Purchase*

Subtotal

Shipping & Handling

Total

Shipping Information

United States

1 program = $7

2 – 3 programs = $10

4 – 6 programs = $20

7 programs and up = $30

Rental

No charge for shipping to renter. Renter is responsible for return shipping charges.

Outside United States

1 program = $10

Each additional program = $5

All orders from outside the U.S. must be prepaid, either by MasterCard, VISA, AMEX or Diners Club or a check in U.S. dollars, drawn on a U.S. bank.

Payment Information

☐ Payment by check

☐ Payment by credit card: ☐ VISA ☐ MasterCard ☐ AMEX ☐ Diners Club

CARD NUMBER

SIGNATURE

EXP. DATE

For faster service, phone (800) 272-2920 or fax (630) 990-9958 (Outside U.S., phone (630) 990-9941).

TEAR HERE

Foto-Comm Corporation is the distributor of RSNA Learning Center Resources.

RAD 8.99

~~out~~sourcing?

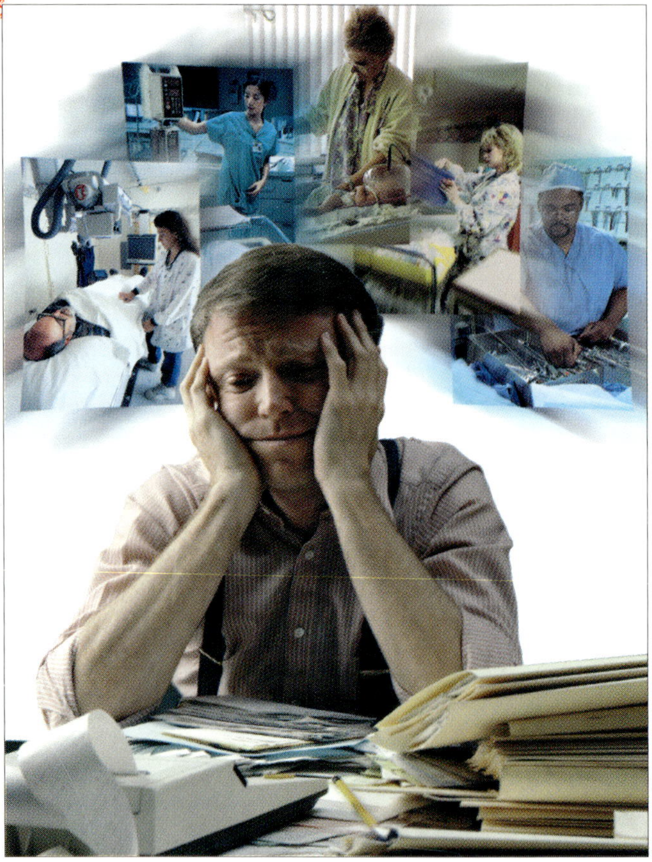

no, *re*sourcing

- Why do you suppose so many leading hospitals have chosen to off-load management of service for all their clinical equipment (biomedical as well as imaging, regardless of vendor) to a single source – GE's CompreCare?

  Because increasingly, customers are redefining "outsourcing" as "**re - sourcing**".

- **As demands grow, with revenue unpredictable,** clinical staff is stretched even thinner. With limited human resources, wise administrators have determined they'd rather have their people focus upon their core competencies where it counts most – in providing quality patient care.

- Wherever skilled and reliable help is available, customers tell us that it pays to eliminate distractions. Let GE handle infrastructure and support tasks.

- **In short, the key issue today is "Resourcing"... selective deployment of strategic resources – human and technological – to build the strongest team possible.** Isn't that what CompreCare provides?

And when you think re **~~ou~~tsourcing – think GE.**

Because CompreCare is only one of many resourceful solutions we can offer you to make your team unbeatable.

rethink. rework. *re*source.

GE Medical Systems

We bring good things to life.

September 1999
Volume 212 • Number 3
RADLAX 212 (3) 605–916

Radiology

From the Editor	605
Special Report	606
Special Communication	607
Editorial	609
State of the Art	615
Thoracic Imaging	637
Vascular and Interventional Radiology	655
Musculoskeletal	693
Diagnosis Please: Case 18	706
Case 14 Answer	708
Genitourinary Imaging	711
Experimental Studies	725
Radiation Oncology	755
Signs in Imaging	761
Neuroradiology	763
Nuclear Medicine	799
Computer Applications	811
Breast Imaging	829
Pediatric Imaging	837
Gastrointestinal Imaging	853
Technical Developments	885
Letters to the Editor	911
Erratum	912
In Memoriam	913
Revised Copyright and Certifications Agreement	44A
Revised Publication Information for Authors	45A
Revised Manuscript Categorization Terms	51A

THE RADIOLOGICAL SOCIETY OF NORTH AMERICA

RSNA®

85th Scientific Assembly and Annual Meeting
Chicago, November 28–December 3, 1999

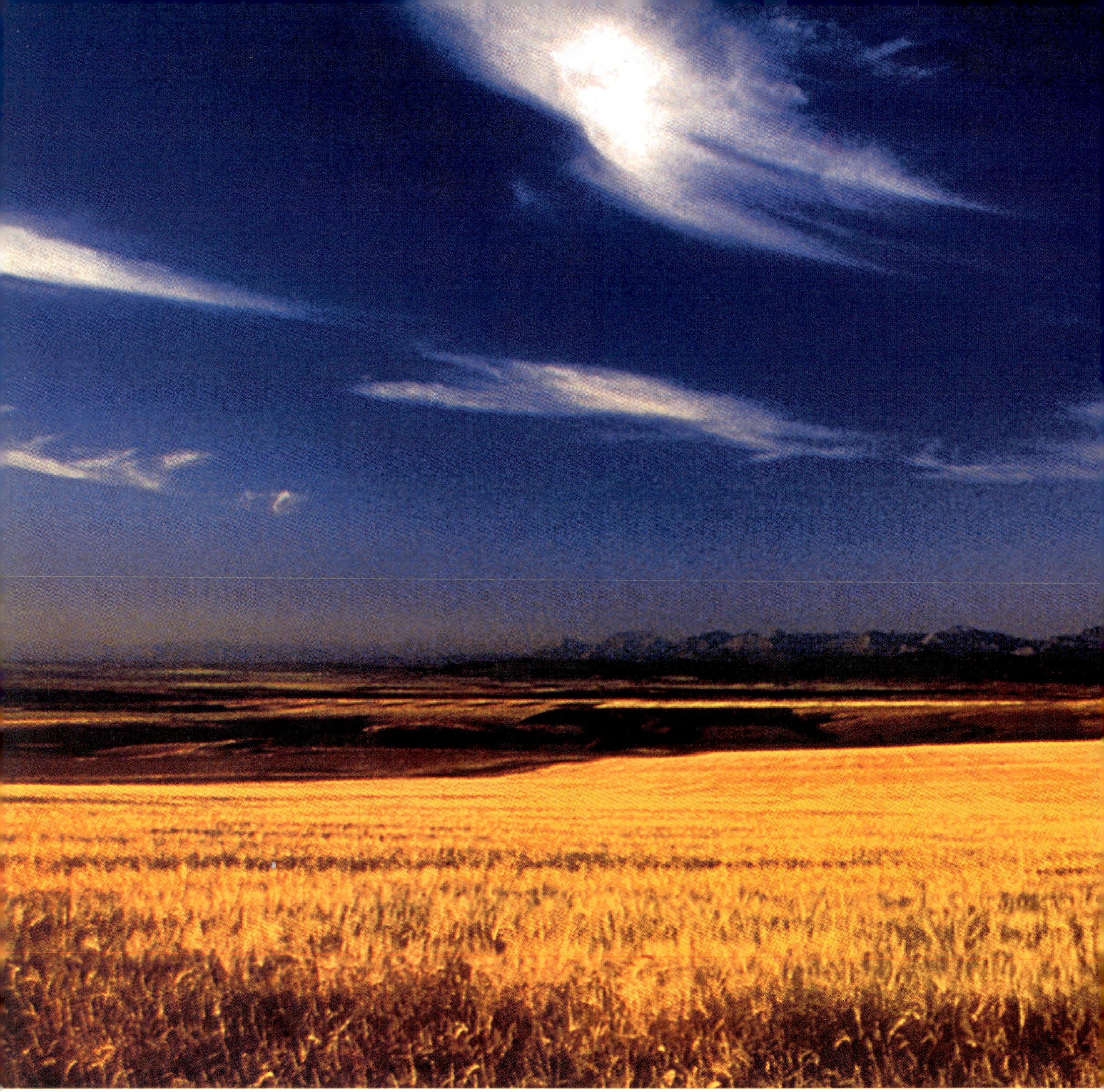

Introducing the FCR 5000 Series from Fuji.

RSNA® Radiological Society of North America Founded in 1915

2021 Spring Road, Suite 600
Oak Brook, Illinois 60523
630/571-2670
FAX: 630/571-7837

Quick Reference

RSNA PURPOSE

The purpose of the Radiological Society of North America is to promote and develop the highest standards of radiology and related sciences through education and research. The Society seeks to provide radiologists and allied health scientists with educational programs and materials of the highest quality, and to constantly improve the content and value of these educational activities. The Society seeks to foster closer fellowship among all radiologists and greater cooperation among radiologists and members of other branches of medicine and allied health care professionals.

RSNA OFFICERS FOR 1999

President, **Seymour H. Levitt, MD,** Minneapolis, MN

President-Elect, **C. Douglas Maynard, MD,** Winston-Salem, NC

First Vice-President, **William M. Thompson, MD,** Minneapolis, MN

Second Vice-President, **J. Frank Wilson, MD,** Milwaukee, WI

Third Vice-President, **Stephen Balter, PhD,** New York, NY

Secretary-Treasurer, **David H. Hussey, MD,** Iowa City, IA

Historian, **William R. Eyler, MD,** Beverly Hills, MI

RSNA BOARD OF DIRECTORS FOR 1999

Jerry P. Petasnick, MD, Chairman of the Board, Chicago, IL

David H. Hussey, MD, Secretary-Treasurer, Iowa City, IA

Brian C. Lentle, MD, Liaison for Education, Vancouver, BC

R. Nick Bryan, MD, PhD, Liaison for Publications and Educational Materials, Bethesda, MD

Peggy J. Fritzsche, MD, Liaison for Communications and Corporate Relations, Riverside, CA

Robert R. Hattery, MD, Liaison Designate for Publications and Educational Materials, Rochester, MN

Seymour H. Levitt, MD, President, Minneapolis, MN

C. Douglas Maynard, MD, President-Elect, Winston-Salem, NC

Delmar J. Stauffer, Executive Director

RSNA IMPORTANT TELEPHONE NUMBERS

MAIN TELEPHONE	(630) 571-2670	MEMBERSHIP	(630) 571-7873 e-mail: membersh@rsna.org
FAX	(630) 571-7837	RESEARCH DEVELOPMENT	(630) 368-3756
ACCOUNTING	(630) 571-7812	PROGRAM SERVICES	(630) 571-7874
EXECUTIVE	(630) 571-7866	RESEARCH & EDUCATION FOUNDATION	(630) 571-7816
EDUCATION CENTER	(630) 368-3753	ADVERTISING	(630) 571-7817
MARKETING COMMUNICATIONS	(630) 571-7830	CLASSIFIED ADVERTISING	(630) 571-7817
MEETINGS	(630) 571-7850	RSNA LINK	http://www.rsna.org
PERMISSIONS	(630) 571-7829	SUBSCRIPTIONS	(630) 571-7873 e-mail: subscrib@rsna.org

RSNA MEETING DATES AND LOCATIONS

1999 November 28 to December 3
McCormick Place, Chicago

2000 November 26 to December 1
McCormick Place, Chicago

2001 November 25 to November 30
McCormick Place, Chicago

RSNA YEAR-AT-A-GLANCE

October 1, 1999
Deadline for Non–North American Advance Registration for RSNA Scientific Assembly

October 29, 1999
Deadline for North American Advance Registration for RSNA Scientific Assembly

November 28 to December 3, 1999
RSNA 85th Scientific Assembly and Annual Meeting

January 1, 2000
Call for Scientific Papers, Scientific Exhibits, and *info*RAD Exhibits

January 8, 2000
Deadline for Receipt of all RSNA R&E Foundation Grant Materials

January 15, 2000
First Seed Grant Deadline

February 18–20, 2000
RSNA Board of Directors Meeting

March 1, 2000
Roentgen Centennial Fellow "Preliminary Letter of Interest" Deadline

April 12–13, 2000
R&E Foundation Trustee Meeting

April 15, 2000
Deadline for Submission of Scientific Paper, Scientific Exhibit, and *info*RAD Applications

May 1, 2000
Deadline for Receipt of Editorial Fellowship Applications

May 15, 2000
Second Seed Grant Deadline

June 8–10, 2000
RSNA Board of Directors Meeting

July 1, 2000
Deadline for Receipt of Derek Harwood-Nash Fellowship Application

July 1, 2000
Deadline for Receipt of International Visiting Scholar Application

September 15, 2000
Third Seed Grant Deadline

September 15–17, 2000
RSNA Board of Directors Meeting

Radiology

September 1999
Volume 212
Number 3

RSNA

A monthly journal devoted to clinical radiology and allied sciences, owned and published by THE RADIOLOGICAL SOCIETY OF NORTH AMERICA, INC.

http://www.rsna.org

I said, we want a CT system with speed so ***revolutionary*** it'll replace other technologies. They said,

get real.

So I got Toshiba.

Dr. Michael Vannier, Professor & Head, Department of Radiology, University of Iowa, Hospitals & Clinics

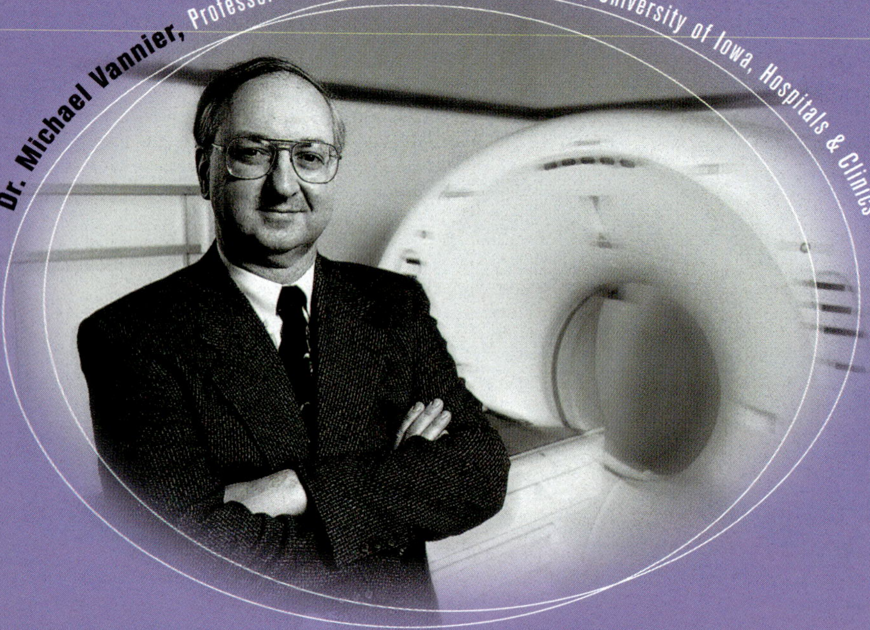

Yes, *you* can.

Defy the old CT standards. Broaden asset utilization with the speed to handle a whole new range of imaging studies on one CT system. Increase CT productivity by scanning faster, diagnosing and treating at the same time. Discover the vast potential of the new Aquilion™ with 1/2-second, full-rotation Helical scanning engineered for multi-slice.

Can you get a CT system that will carry you into the next millennium? *Yes. You Can.*

Visit our Web site today and get the real story on the University of Iowa and the benefits of the new Aquilion, or call (800) 421-1968 for more details.

TOSHIBA

www.medical.toshiba.com

September 1999
Volume 212 • Number 3

Radiology

A monthly journal devoted to clinical radiology and allied sciences, owned and published by the Radiological Society of North America, Inc.

RSNA

From the Editor

605 **Radiology 1999: Revised Publication Information for Authors**
Anthony V. Proto

Special Report

606 **Diagnosis Please Certificate of Recognition Awarded to Sergio Julio Moguillansky, MD**
Anthony V. Proto

Special Communication

607 **Radiology and Epcot Celebrate New Millennium with a Patient Education and Information Exhibit**
Jerry P. Petasnick and Peggy J. Fritzsche

Editorial

609 **Molecular Imaging: Exploring the Next Frontier**
Ralph Weissleder
The impact of the developing molecular imaging technology is an entire new universe that provides potential for earlier detection and characterization of disease, understanding of biology, and evaluation of treatment.

State of the Art

615 **Spiral CT Angiography of the Pulmonary Circulation**
Martine Remy-Jardin and Jacques Remy
The purpose of this article is to review the current clinical applications of spiral CT in the evaluation of a variety of congenital and acquired disorders of the pulmonary circulation, except the systemic arterial supply of the lung parenchyma.

Thoracic Imaging

637 **Follicular Bronchiolitis: Thin-Section CT and Histologic Findings**
Sarah J. Howling, David M. Hansell, Athol U. Wells, Andrew G. Nicholson, Julia D. A. Flint, and Nestor L. Müller
The cardinal signs of follicular bronchiolitis were a mixed pattern of small centrilobular nodules variably associated with patchy ground-glass opacity.

643 **Mucoepidermoid Carcinoma of the Tracheobronchial Tree: Radiographic and CT Findings in 12 Patients**
Tae Sung Kim, Kyung Soo Lee, Joungho Han, Jung-Gi Im, Joon Beom Seo, Joung Sook Kim, Hyae Young Kim, and Sang Wook Han
Mucoepidermoid carcinoma in the tracheobronchial tree is a rare airway tumor and is more common in the segmental bronchi than in the trachea or main bronchi.

649 **Electrocardiographically Gated Thin-Section CT of the Lung**
U. Joseph Schoepf, Christoph R. Becker, Roland D. Bruening, Thomas Helmberger, Axel Staebler, Patricia Leimeister, and Maximilian F. Reiser
Electrocardiographic gating improves image quality and reduces artifacts on thin-section CT scans of the lung, with little additional effort.

Vascular and Interventional Radiology

655 **Human Endothelium: Endovascular Biopsy and Molecular Analysis**
Lei Feng, David M. Stern, and John Pile-Spellman
Our data demonstrate that viable endothelial cells suitable for molecular analysis at the transcript and protein levels can be obtained during routine angiographic procedures.

665 **Hepatic Intraarterial ^{131}I Iodized Oil for Treatment of Hepatocellular Carcinoma in Patients with Impeded Portal Venous Flow**
Thierry de Baere, Patrice Taourel, Jean Michel Tubiana, Viseth Kuoch, Michel Ducreux, Jean Lumbroso, and Alain J. Roche
Owing to the complexity of and the poor tolerance for the procedure, the low response rate, and the doubtful gain in survival, hepatic intraarterial therapy with iodine 131 iodized oil cannot be considered a routine clinical treatment for hepatocellular carcinoma in patients with portal venous thrombosis.

669 **Multiple Fluid Collections: CT- or US-guided Aspiration— Evaluation of Microbiologic Results and Implications for Clinical Practice**
Joan P. Heneghan, Richard J. Everts, and Rendon C. Nelson
All intraabdominal fluid collections should be aspirated to optimize selection of antimicrobial therapy.

673 **CT Fluoroscopy–guided Abdominal Interventions: Techniques, Results, and Radiation Exposure**
Stuart G. Silverman, Kemal Tuncali, Douglass F. Adams, Richard D. Nawfel, Kelly H. Zou, and Philip F. Judy
Although CT fluoroscopy is a useful targeting technique, because significant radiation exposures may result, radiologists need to be aware of different methods of CT fluoroscopic guidance and the factors that contribute to radiation exposure.

682 **Primary Musculoskeletal Neoplasms: Effectiveness of Core-Needle Biopsy**
Lawrence Yao, Scott D. Nelson, Leanne L. Seeger, Jeffrey J. Eckardt, and Frederick R. Eilber
Our findings indicate that percutaneous core-needle biopsy results were highly effective for help in the diagnosis of masses suspected to be primary musculoskeletal neoplasms and appeared to be equally effective for evaluation of lesions of either bone or soft tissue.

687 **Osteoid Osteoma: CT-guided Percutaneous Resection and Follow-up in 38 Patients**
Nicolas Sans, Denise Galy-Fourcade, Jacques Assoun, Thierry Jarlaud, Hélène Chiavassa, Paul Bonnevialle, Nadine Railhac, Jacques Giron, Hélène Morera-Maupomé, and Jean-Jacques Railhac
The results of this study confirm the medium-term efficacy of CT-guided percutaneous resection of osteoid osteomas.

Musculoskeletal Imaging

693 **Liposclerosing Myxofibrous Tumor: A Radiologic-Pathologic–Distinct Fibro-osseous Lesion of Bone with a Marked Predilection for the Intertrochanteric Region of the Femur**
Mark J. Kransdorf, Mark D. Murphey, and Donald E. Sweet
Despite its histologic complexity, liposclerosing myxofibrous tumor has a relatively characteristic radiologic appearance and skeletal distribution, and, more important, it appears to be associated with an increased prevalence of malignant transformation compared with fibrous dysplasia and other benign fibro-osseous lesions; this factor underscores the need for close observation of this condition.

Continued—

Radiology is published monthly by the Radiological Society of North America, Inc, 820 Jorie Boulevard, Oak Brook, IL 60523-2251 (ISSN 0033-8419). Printed in USA. Periodical class postage paid at Oak Brook, Ill, and additional mailing offices. The nonmember subscription rate for the USA is $215.00 per year; for all other countries, $260.00 (includes postage). Information about subscription rates for residents is available on request. (Air freight is available; rates are furnished on request.) Single copies are $25.00 ($36.00 to a non-U.S. address). Notice of missing issues or change of address (include old mailing label and new address) should be sent to RSNA Subscriptions Department, 820 Jorie Boulevard, Oak Brook, IL 60523-2251. Inquiries via e-mail should be directed to *subscrib@rsna.org.* POSTMASTER: Send address correction "changes" to: *Radiology,* RSNA, 820 Jorie Boulevard, Oak Brook, IL 60523-2251.

Claims for copies lost in the mail are allowed within 90 days of the date of issue. Claims are not allowed for issues lost as a result of insufficient notice of change of address.

Membership in the Radiological Society of North America is by formal application. Membership information should be secured from the Executive Director, the Radiological Society of North America, Inc, 820 Jorie Boulevard, Oak Brook, IL 60523-2251. Dues are payable annually in January. In accordance with U.S. postal regulations, $107.50 of active membership dues is allocated to a subscription to *Radiology.*

699 **Glenohumeral Relationships during Physiologic Shoulder Motion and Stress Testing: Initial Experience with Open MR Imaging and Active Imaging-Plane Registration**
Christopher F. Beaulieu, Duncan K. Hodge, A. Gabrielle Bergman, Kim Butts, Bruce L. Daniel, Clay L. Napper, Robert D. Darrow, Charles L. Dumoulin, and Robert J. Herfkens
Our goal was to determine whether dynamic MR imaging can (*a*) be used to evaluate and define normal shoulder motion in active joint motion and muscle contraction and (*b*) be used in conjunction with physical examination.

Diagnosis Please

706 **Case 18**
Peter L. Choyke and John L. Doppman

708 **Case 14: Intramedullary Osteosclerosis**
Avinash R. A. Balkissoon and Curtis W. Hayes
The differential considerations for bone sclerosis are extensive, but the radiographic distribution in association with clinical and laboratory findings can substantially narrow the possibilities.

Genitourinary Imaging

711 **Radiologic Staging in Patients with Endometrial Cancer: A Meta-analysis**
Karen Kinkel, Yasushi Kaji, Kyle K. Yu, Mark R. Segal, Ying Lu, C. Bethan Powell, and Hedvig Hricak
In patients who require multifactorial assessment, contrast-enhanced MR imaging is the only modality that can be used to accurately evaluate myometrial, cervical, and nodal involvement.

719 **Three-dimensional US of the Prostate: Early Experience**
Ulrike M. Hamper, Victoria Trapanotto, M. Robert DeJong, Sheila Sheth, and Cynthia I. Caskey
Three-dimensional US has the potential to become a practical imaging technique for the evaluation of the prostate gland in a busy clinical environment.

Experimental Studies

725 **Renal Blood Flow in Pigs: Changes Depicted with Contrast-enhanced Harmonic Imaging during Acute Urinary Obstruction**
Michel Claudon, Carol E. Barnewolt, George A. Taylor, Patricia S. Dunning, Rita Gobet, and Abdel-Basset Badawy
Our data show that contrast-enhanced harmonic gray-scale US imaging shows potential for depicting changes in global renal blood flow in real time.

732 **Effect of Downstream Cross-sectional Area of an Arterial Bed on the Resistive Index and the Early Systolic Acceleration**
Ronald O. Bude and Jonathan M. Rubin
The increase in cross-sectional area that normally occurs as flow progresses through the arterial tree lowers both the early systolic acceleration and the resistive index independently of other factors such as vascular compliance and resistance.

739 **Simultaneous Noninvasive Determination of Regional Myocardial Perfusion and Oxygen Content in Rabbits: Toward Direct Measurement of Myocardial Oxygen Consumption at MR Imaging**
Scott B. Reeder, A. Alexander Holmes, Elliot R. McVeigh, and John R. Forder
By using a previously verified method of spin labeling and the principles of blood oxygenation level–dependent imaging, concomitant measurement of perfusion and oxygen content was performed in six to eight sections covering the entire left ventricle in less than 15 minutes.

748 **Brachytherapy for the Prevention of Stenosis in a Canine Hemodialysis Graft Model: Preliminary Observations**
Scott O. Trerotola, Timothy J. Carmody, Robert D. Timmerman, Kathleen Ann Bergan, R. Gerald Dreesen, Stephanie V. Frost, and Mitchell Forney
Our preliminary data with this animal model suggest that gamma brachytherapy can reduce in-stent restenosis in hemodialysis access.

Radiation Oncology

755 **Phases IB and II Multidose Trial of Gadolinium Texaphyrin, a Radiation Sensitizer Detectable at MR Imaging: Preliminary Results in Brain Metastases**
Juliette Viala, Daniel Vanel, Philippe Meingan, Eric Lartigau, Patrice Carde, and Markus Renschler
The accumulation of gadolinium texaphyrin in metastases over several months as revealed at brain MR studies should permit imaging of brain metastases after radiation therapy and, therefore, evaluation of response to the treatment.

Signs in Imaging

761 **The Radial Bands Sign**
Timothy A. Bernauer
The radial bands sign is believed by some authors to represent a manifestation of abnormal migration of dysplastic stem cells along the course of the radial glial-neuronal unit in patients with tuberous sclerosis.

Continued—

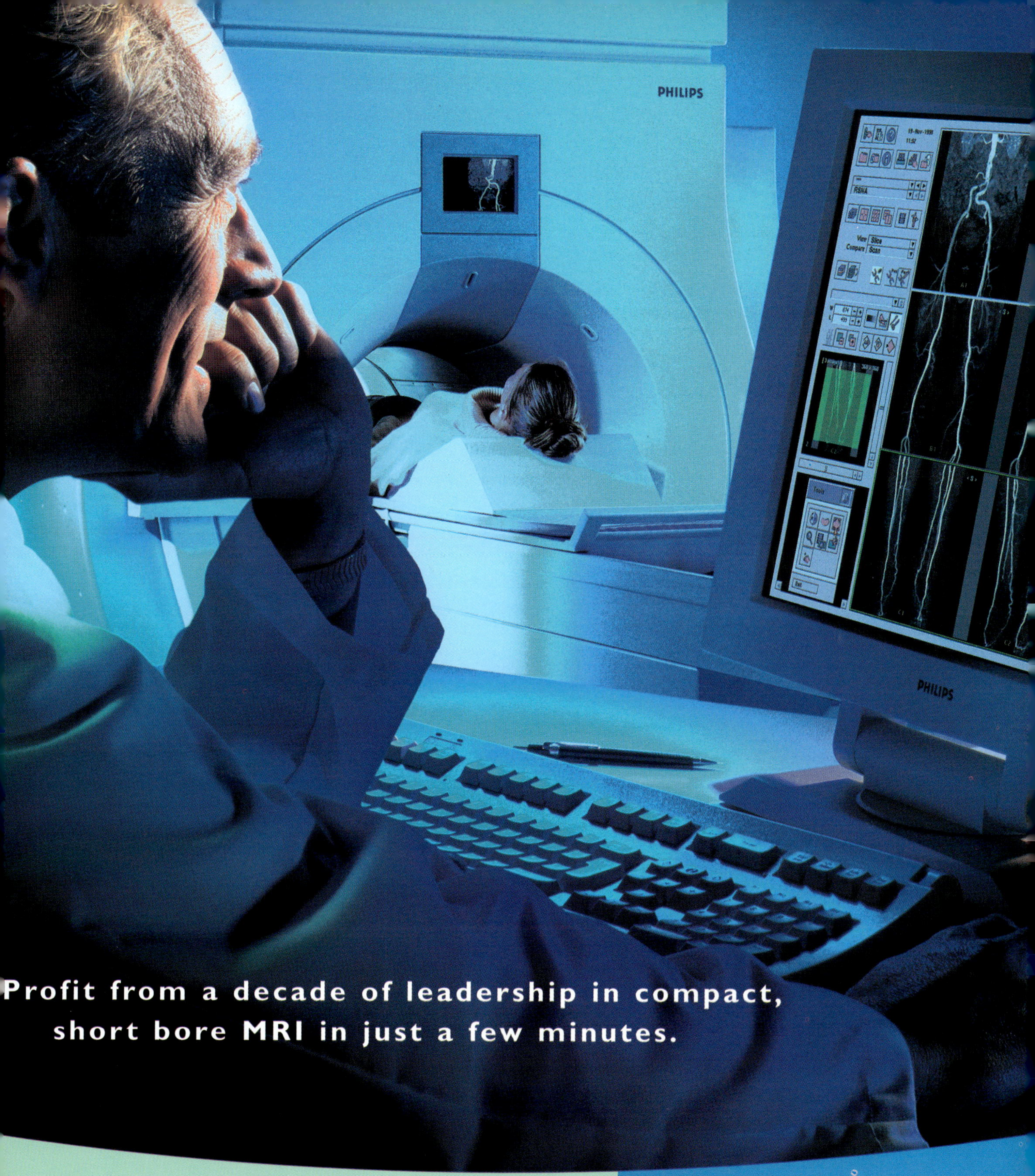
PHILIPS
PHILIPS
Profit from a decade of leadership in compact,
short bore MRI in just a few minutes.

Neuroradiology

763 **Motor Neuron Diseases: Comparison of Single-Voxel Proton MR Spectroscopy of the Motor Cortex with MR Imaging of the Brain**
Stephen Chan, Dikoma C. Shungu, Annette Douglas-Akinwande, Dale J. Lange, and Lewis P. Rowland
MR spectroscopy was more sensitive than MR imaging in the detection of an upper motor neuron abnormality in amyotrophic lateral sclerosis and primary lateral sclerosis.

770 **Quantitative Diffusion-Tensor Anisotropy Brain MR Imaging: Normative Human Data and Anatomic Analysis**
Joshua S. Shimony, Robert C. McKinstry, Erbil Akbudak, Joseph A. Aronovitz, Abraham Z. Snyder, Nicolas F. Lori, Thomas S. Cull, and Thomas E. Conturo
Anisotropy, or A_σ, images demonstrated white matter anatomy not typically seen on conventional MR images, with statistically significant A_σ differences in different histologic white matter classes that were ranked according to known resistance to edema spread, which is suggestive of a sensitivity to white matter microstructure.

785 **Human Acute Cerebral Ischemia: Detection of Changes in Water Diffusion Anisotropy by Using MR Imaging**
A. Gregory Sorensen, Ona Wu, William A. Copen, Timothy L. Davis, R. Gilberto Gonzalez, Walter J. Koroshetz, Timothy G. Reese, Bruce R. Rosen, Van J. Wedeen, and Robert M. Weisskoff
Human acute cerebral ischemia causes changes in the anisotropy or shape of the diffusion tensor in white matter.

793 **Brain Lesions: When Should Fluid-attenuated Inversion- Recovery Sequences Be Used in MR Evaluation?**
Tomoko Okuda, Yukunori Korogi, Yoshinori Shigematsu, Takeshi Sugahara, Toshinori Hirai, Ichiro Ikushima, Luxia Liang, and Mutsumasa Takahashi
It is important to recognize that lesions in the basal ganglia or brain stem may be missed with fluid-attenuated inversion-recovery sequences.

Nuclear Medicine

799 **Primary and Recurrent Early Stage Laryngeal Cancer: Preliminary Results of 2-[Fluorine 18]fluoro-2-deoxy-D-glucose PET Imaging**
Val J. Lowe, Han Kim, James H. Boyd, John F. Eisenbeis, Frank R. Dunphy, and James W. Fletcher
PET imaging can be used to identify primary or recurrent early stage laryngeal cancer.

803 **Staging Non–Small Cell Lung Cancer with Whole-Body PET**
Edith M. Marom, H. Page McAdams, Jeremy J. Erasmus, Philip C. Goodman, Donna K. Culhane, R. Edward Coleman, James E. Herndon, and Edward F. Patz, Jr
Whole-body PET is very useful in staging newly diagnosed lung cancer.

Computer Applications

811 **Brain Tumor Volume Measurement: Comparison of Manual and Semiautomated Methods**
Bonnie N. Joe, Melanie B. Fukui, Carolyn Cidis Meltzer, Qing-shou Huang, Roger S. Day, Phil J. Greer, and Michael E. Bozik
The tumor volume measurements calculated with standard manual tracing and a semiautomated computer program were comparable in interoperator reliability, but the semiautomated computer program was faster than manual tracing.

817 **Improvement of Radiologists' Characterization of Mammographic Masses by Using Computer-aided Diagnosis: An ROC Study**
Heang-Ping Chan, Berkman Sahiner, Mark A. Helvie, Nicholas Petrick, Marilyn A. Roubidoux, Todd E. Wilson, Dorit D. Adler, Chintana Paramagul, Joel S. Newman, and Sethumadavan Sanjay-Gopal
The improved separation between the confidence ratings of the malignant masses and those of the benign masses indicates the potential that computer-aided diagnosis may reduce the rate of biopsy of benign masses when decision thresholds are properly chosen by the radiologists.

Breast Imaging

829 **Local Tumor Recurrence following Breast-Conservation Therapy: Correlation of Histopathologic Findings with Detection Method and Mammographic Findings**
Catherine S. Giess, Delia M. Keating, Michael P. Osborne, and Ruth Rosenblatt
As microcalcifications were the only mammographic sign of local recurrence (three in situ, six invasive) in nine of 17 primary invasive carcinomas in our series, we believe that developing indeterminate microcalcifications at the lumpectomy site should be viewed with a high index of suspicion, regardless of whether the primary tumor was invasive or in situ and regardless of the appearance of the primary lesion.

Continued—

Pediatric Imaging

837 **Anterior Chest Wall: Frequency of Anatomic Variations in Children**
Lane F. Donnelly, Donald P. Frush, Joseph N. Foss, Sara M. O'Hara, and George S. Bisset III
Variations in the anterior chest wall are common, occurring in one-third of children, and should be considered normal.

841 **Soft-Tissue Venous Malformations in Pediatric and Young Adult Patients: Diagnosis with Doppler US**
Isabelle Trop, Josée Dubois, Laurent Guibaud, Andrée Grignon, Heidi Patriquin, Catherine McCuaig, and Laurent A. Garel
US can help in the diagnosis of clinically atypical venous malformations.

847 **Kyphomelic Dysplasia: Clinical and Radiologic Long-term Follow-up of One Case and Review of the Literature**
Rosanna Pallotta, Tamara Ehresmann, Mario Roggini, and Paola Fusilli
With long-term follow-up, we assessed the phenotypic, orthopedic, and radiologic progression of this syndrome [kyphomelic dysplasia].

Gastrointestinal Imaging

853 **Adult Intussusception Detected at CT or MR Imaging: Clinical-Imaging Correlation**
David M. Warshauer and Joseph K. T. Lee
Less than one-third of adult intussusceptions demonstrated at CT or MR imaging were caused by a neoplastic lead point.

861 **Tumorous Gastric Varices: Radiographic Findings in 10 Patients**
Laura R. Carucci, Marc S. Levine, Stephen E. Rubesin, and Igor Laufer
It is important to be aware of the characteristic features of tumorous gastric varices on double-contrast studies so that they are not mistaken for neoplastic lesions in the stomach.

866 **Hepatocellular Carcinoma and Intrahepatic Peripheral Cholangiocarcinoma: Enhancement Patterns with Quadruple Phase Helical CT—A Comparative Study**
Evelyne M. Loyer, Hsiao Chin, Ronelle A. DuBrow, Cynthia L. David, Farzin Eftekhari, and Chusilp Charnsangavej
The evolutions over time of the relative CT attenuation of hepatocellular carcinomas and peripheral cholangiocarcinomas differ sufficiently to be a differential diagnostic criterion.

876 **Abdominal MR Imaging with a Volumetric Interpolated Breath-hold Examination**
Neil M. Rofsky, Vivian S. Lee, Gerhard Laub, Michael A. Pollack, Glenn A. Krinsky, David Thomasson, Michael M. Ambrosino, and Jeffrey C. Weinreb
With volumetric interpolated breath-hold imaging, data sets that have nearly isotropic resolution in three dimensions (on the order of 2-mm voxel size) can be obtained while preserving adequate anatomic coverage and uniform fat saturation within a breath hold.

Technical Developments

885 **Cystic Fibrosis: Combined Hyperpolarized ^{3}He-enhanced and Conventional Proton MR Imaging in the Lung—Preliminary Observations**
Lane F. Donnelly, James R. MacFall, H. Page McAdams, J. Marc Majure, Jean Smith, Donald P. Frush, Paul Bogonad, H. Cecil Charles, and Carl E. Ravin
Because both functional and morphologic information concerning the pulmonary status of patients with cystic fibrosis can be generated on hyperpolarized helium 3 MR imaging studies in a safe, reproducible, and technically feasible manner and because radiation is not used, ^{3}He MR imaging may be an ideal way of serially evaluating patients with cystic fibrosis for progression of disease.

890 **Pulmonary Perfusion: Respiratory-triggered Three-dimensional MR Imaging with Arterial Spin Tagging—Preliminary Results in Healthy Volunteers**
David A. Roberts, Warren B. Gefter, Joshua A. Hirsch, Rahim R. Rizi, Lawrence Dougherty, Robert E. Lenkinski, John S. Leigh, Jr, and Mitchell D. Schnall
The arterial spin-tagging method may be used to obtain noninvasive images of pulmonary blood flow without the need for patient breath holding.

896 **Pulmonary Arterial Resistance: Noninvasive Measurement with Indexes of Pulmonary Flow Estimated at Velocity-encoded MR Imaging—Preliminary Experience**
Elie Mousseaux, Jean Pierre Tasu, Odile Jolivet, Gérard Simonneau, Jacques Bittoun, and Jean-Claude Gaux
This completely noninvasive approach should increase our understanding of the pathophysiologic changes affecting the pulmonary circulation of patients with various pulmonary diseases and should help in the follow-up of hemodynamic changes associated with medical therapies such as long-term vasodilator treatment in patients with primary pulmonary hypertension.

903 **Pulsed Magnetization Transfer Imaging: Evaluation of Technique**
Simon J. Graham and R. Mark Henkelman
Simulation results indicate that current use of magnetization transfer in imaging protocols is close to optimal for cerebral MR angiography, whereas neuroimaging protocols can likely be made more effective.

Continued—

Letters to the Editor

911 ROC Curve Analysis in the Evaluation of Contrast-enhanced Color Doppler US
Jonathan Winehouse, Michael Douek, and William Lees
Reply
Sabine Huber, Ivan Zuna, and Stefan Delorme

912 Erratum

In Memoriam

913 Harry W. Fischer, MD
John R. Thornbury, MD, and Helen C. Redman, MD

Book Reviews

724 Abdominal Plain Film with Correlative Imaging. 2nd ed.

760 Imaging in Oncology

810 Fog: A Collection of Backscatter

Interludes

836 Mousy Type of Calcification in a Breast Fibroadenoma

846 Gastrointestinal Tract Bug

Departments

915 Abstracts of Current Literature

16A Advertisers' Index

19A Announcements and Books, Audiovisual Materials, and Software Received

55A Classified Services

25A Continuing Medical Education

912 Erratum

38A *Radiology* Business Information

78A RSNA Bulletin Board

2A RSNA Quick Reference

22A Associated Sciences Workshop 1999

44A *Revised* Copyright and Certifications Agreement

45A *Revised* Publication Information for Authors

51A *Revised Radiology* Manuscript Categorization Terms

17A Request for Printed Copy of the January 2000 *RSNA Index to Imaging Literature*

Advertisers' Index

RSNA Advertising Policy

According to the advertising policy of the Radiological Society of North America, the information describing radiological equipment, products, and services offered by vendors in their advertisements should be ethical, educational, professional, of value in furthering the radiologic evaluation and treatment of patients and furthering the education of the radiologists and allied scientists. The guidelines below should be followed for advertising in RSNA journals.

- All advertising must be directed to radiologic diagnosis, therapy, research, communication and/or to the professional and managerial roles of radiologists and allied scientists. Advertising material should be consistent with the highest standards of professionalism.

- RSNA reserves the right to reject copy which, in its opinion, is not in good taste, is unprofessional, or is inappropriate for a radiology publication, or offers products or services not in the best interest of the patient or the Society. Advertisements that are constructed to resemble the journal's editorial pages will not be accepted in that form.

- Acceptance of advertising does not mean endorsement by RSNA of the products or services advertised, the advertisers, or the claims made.

For media kits and questions about advertising ONLY, contact:
Jim Drew, *Director of Advertising*
RSNA Publications
820 Jorie Boulevard
Oak Brook, IL 60523-2251
(630) 571-2670
FAX (630) 571-7837

For all other RSNA department telephone numbers, see "RSNA Quick Reference"; consult "Departments" in the Table of Contents for page.

Aloka 11A
American College of Radiology 25A

Beekley Corporation 35A–37A
Bioscan 61A
Brown University School of Medicine 61A

Click*View Corporation 19A
CompHealth 59A

Daniel & Yeager 57A
Diversified Diagnostic Products, Inc 24A, 32A
Duke University Health System 59A

Ethicon Endo-Surgery 39A

Fuji Medical Systems IFC–1A

GE Medical Systems OBC
Global Medical Staffing 71A
The Guthrie Clinic 65A

Hewlett-Packard 40A–41A, 43A
Hitachi Medical Systems America 20A–21A

Interim Physicians 74A

J & C Nationwide 68A

Kaiser Permanente 65A

Locum Medical Group 73A

Marshfield Clinic 67A
Monroe Clinic 63A
Mount Sinai School of Medicine 65A, 73A

Nihon Medi-Physics Co, Ltd 75A

Philips Medical Systems 9A
Picker International 30A–31A

RADX 29A
RSNA Associated Sciences 22A
RSNA Education Center 79A–82A
RSNA Index to Imaging Literature 17A–18A
RSNA ORD 28A, IBC
RSNA Resident Membership 53A–54A
RSNA Scientific Assembly and Annual Meeting 13A, 34A

Siemens Medical Systems, Inc 7A, 15A, 23A
SmartLight, Inc 26A–27A
The Society of Nuclear Medicine 19A
Staff Relief, Inc 71A
Staten Island University Hospital 25A
SUNY-Health Science Center at Brooklyn 69A
Synarc 33A

Team Health 74A
Toshiba 4A
Trex Medical Corporation 828

Vista Staffing Solutions 63A

Announcements and Books, Audiovisual Materials, and Software Received

Announcements

American Society of Neuroradiology Officer Elections

At its 37th annual meeting on May 22–28, 1999, the American Society of Neuroradiology announced its officers for 1999-2000. They are the following: Eric J. Russell, MD, FACR, president; William S. Ball, Jr, MD, president-elect; William P. Dillon, MD, vice president; Robert D. Zimmerman, MD, secretary; and Victor M. Haughton, MD, treasurer. For further information, contact Bonnie Mack, membership/society coordinator, American Society of Neuroradiology, 2210 Midwest Rd, Suite 207, Oak Brook, IL 60523-8205; telephone (630) 574-0220, ext 234; fax (630) 574-0661; e-mail *membership@asnr.org; http://www.asnr.org.*

French Society of Radiology

The French Society of Radiology (Société Française de Radiologie) will hold its annual meeting, "Journées Françaises de Radiologie," on October 25–29, 1999, at the Palais des Congrès, Paris, France. The program will feature scientific sessions, refresher courses, image interpretation, informatics, and technical exhibits. Topics include emergency and interventional radiology, cardiovascular and thoracic imaging, musculoskeletal and gastrointestinal radiology, neuroradiology, genitourinary and pediatric radiology, ultrasonography, and medicolegal issues. For further information, contact the Société Française de Radiologie, 20 avenue Rapp, F-75343 Paris Cedex 7, France; e-mail *SFRADIO@wanadoo.fr; http://www.sfr-radiologie.asso.fr/.*

15th Asia-Pacific Cancer Conference

The Cancer Institute of Chennai, under the auspices of the Asia and Pacific Federation of Organisations for Cancer Control and the International Union Against Cancer, is sponsoring the 15th Asia-Pacific Cancer Conference on December 12–15, 1999, in Chennai (Madras), India. For further information, contact the Congress Secretariat, XV Asia-Pacific Cancer Conference, Cancer Institute (W.I.A.), 18 Sardar Patel Rd, Chennai 600036, India; telephone 91 44 2350131 or 91 44 2350241; fax 91 44 4912085; e-mail *caninst@md2.vsnl.net.in.*

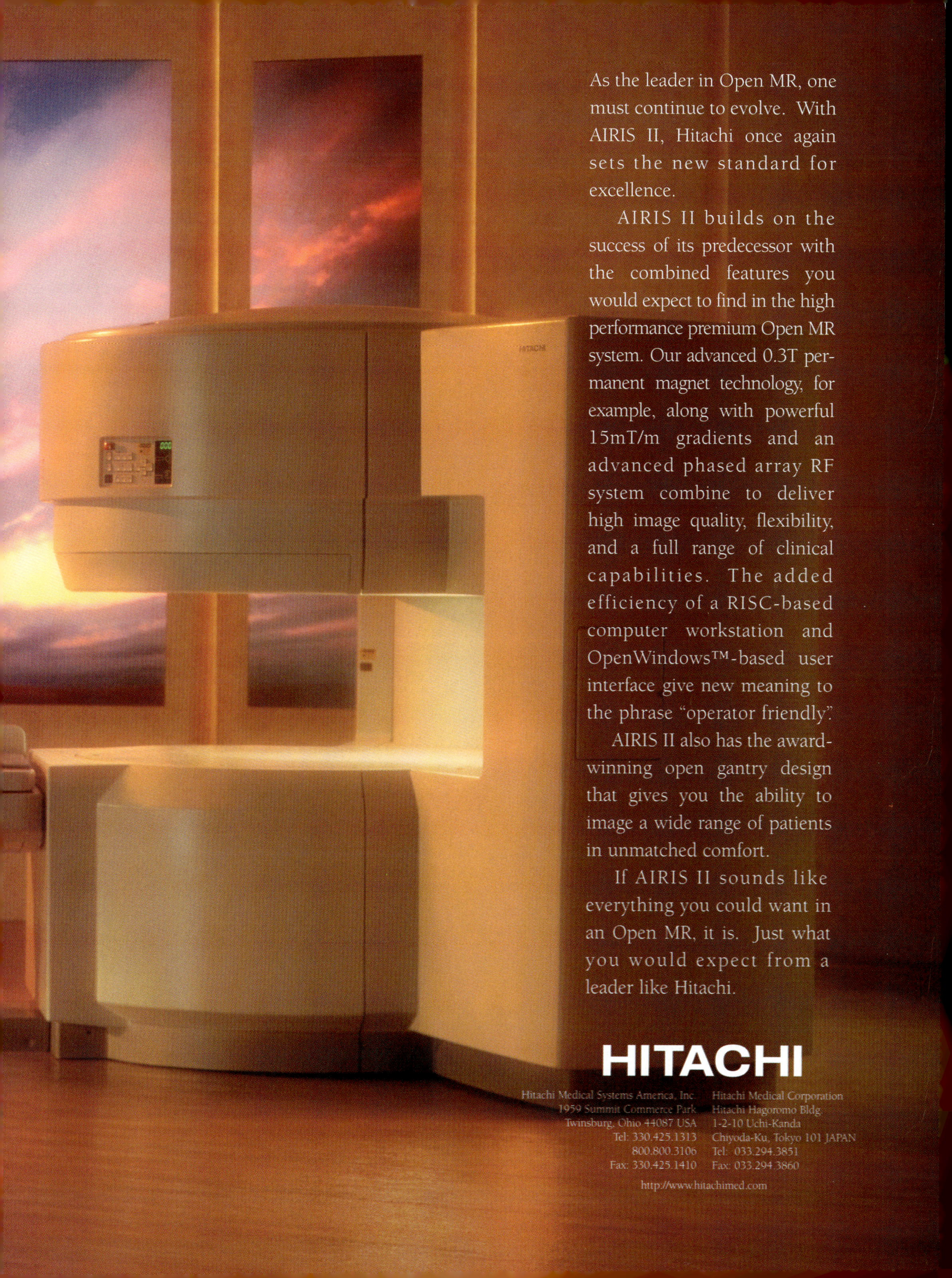

A CENTURY OF RESEARCH & EDUCATION
RSNA 1999

Radiological Society of North America
85th Scientific Assembly and Annual Meeting
November 28–December 3,1999
McCormick Place, Chicago

New Realities in Radiology: Multidisciplinary Strategies for Compliance

Associated Sciences Program at RSNA 1999

Workshop: Saturday, Nov. 27, 1999 10:15 am - 4:00 pm, McCormick Place South

Refresher Courses: Sunday, Nov. 28, through Friday, Dec 3, 1999

Credits: 5 hours

Welcome and Introduction
10:15 am
Samuel L. Hissong, MD, Chair, Associated Sciences Consortium and Committee
JoAnn Belanger, RN, CRN, Coordinator, Associated Sciences Consortium

Keynote Presentation
10:30 am - 11:50 am
Compliance, Audits and Radiology: The Art of Survival (AHRA)
Karol Handrahan RT(R)

Break
11:50 am - 12:10 pm

Special Luncheon Program
12:10 - 1:20 pm
Uncle Sam Strikes Back: Medicine in the Enforcement Age (RBMA)
Tom Hoffman

Break
1:20 - 1:30 pm

Panel Presentation
1:30 - 4:00 pm
(Break 2:45 pm - 3:00 pm)
Practicum (SROA)
Andrew Woods, Esq.
Gadi Weinreich, Esq.
Bruce Freid, Esq.

AAPM/RSNA Basic Physics Lecture for the Radiologic Technologists: Digital Imaging: What You Need to Know Now and What You Need to Know Next
Organized by
Gerald A. White, Jr., MS
3:00 - 4:30 pm
1½ hours credit

Refresher Courses

(Each Refresher Course is approved for 1½ hours credit)

Sunday RC 124
Organizational Culture and Health System Change
Sponsored by the Associated Sciences Consortium
Paula Maramonte, MEd, RT(R) (AERS) Coordinator
Cornelius J. Rater, MD (AERS)
Harry J. Granito, MS (RBMA)
Susan K. Snyder, BS, EdD (ASRT)

Monday RC 224
Asset Management for High-Technology Systems
Sponsored by the Associated Sciences Consortium
Chester T. Szerlag, MBA (SROA) Coordinator
Tim Guertin (SROA)
Sheila M. Sferrella (AHRA)
Dennis A. Bair, RT(R)(CV) (AVIR)

Monday RC 324
Economic Implications of Regulatory Change
Sponsored by the Associated Sciences Consortium
DuVonne Campbell (ASRT) Coordinator
Cherrill Farnsworth (AHRA)
Sherry Makely, PhD (ASRT, SNM)
Donna L. Wright, EdD, RT(R) (AERS)

Tuesday RC 424
Managing a Multisite Radiology Network
Sponsored by the Associated Sciences Consortium
Kathryn J. Canny, (RBMA) Coordinator
Larry A. Ranahan, MBA (RBMA) Moderator
Charles Deschamps RT(R)(MR) (SMRT)
Scott Seberg, MS (RBMA)
Chester T. Szerlag, MBA (RBMA)

Wednesday RC 524
Current Challenges in Radiology and Planning and Design
Sponsored by the Associated Sciences Consortium
Morris A. Stein (AIA-AAH) Coordinator
Bill Rostenberg (AIA-AAH)
Jerry W. Froelich, MD (AIA-AAH)
Eliot L. Siegel, MD (AIA-AAH)

Thursday RC 624
Specialized Accreditations: A Cost of Doing Business
Sponsored by the Associated Sciences Consortium
Luann J. Culbreth, MEd, RT(R) (SMRT) Moderator
John Kovelski, RT(R) (SMRT)
Karol Handrahan, RT(R) (SMRT)
Sandra Katanick, RN, RVT (SDMS)
Ronald F. Bernardi, BA, RT(R) (AHRA)

Thursday RC 724
Multidisciplinary Standards for the New Millennium
Sponsored by the Associated Sciences Consortium
Susan S. Weiss, CNMT (SNM-TS) Moderator
William R. Poller, MD (SNM-TS)
Michael R. Bloyd, RT(R), BSN (ASRT)
Sue M. Smith, RT(R)(CV)(M), FAVIR (AVIR)

Friday RC 824
Marketing Radiology: Getting the Message Out
Sponsored by the Associated Sciences Consortium
Ronald F. Bernardi, BA, RT(R) (AHRA) Moderator
Cherrill Farnsworth (AHRA)
Michael R. Favreau (AHRA)

Registration Information

Advance registration for the RSNA Scientific Assembly ends October 29. Onsite registration begins at 12:00 noon on Saturday, November 27, at McCormick Place. RSNA shuttle bus service to McCormick Place will be available beginning at 10:00 am on Saturday. Advance registration is not required for the Saturday workshop; however, to receive continuing education credit, you must register.

Advance registration information appears in the July issue of *Radiology.* Brochures are also available from your association or from the RSNA, 820 Jorie Boulevard, Oak Brook, IL 60523-1860. Phone: 630/571-7852.

Registration for the RSNA Scientific Assembly includes registration for the Associated Sciences Workshop. A box lunch will be available for purchase to facilitate your attendance at the workshop. These lunches must be purchased with your advance registration for the RSNA Meeting. **If you wish to purchase a box lunch, please check the appropriate box on the RSNA Advance Registration form and enclose your $11.50 payment.**

If you would like a copy of the published Associated Sciences Proceedings, please call 630/571-7874.

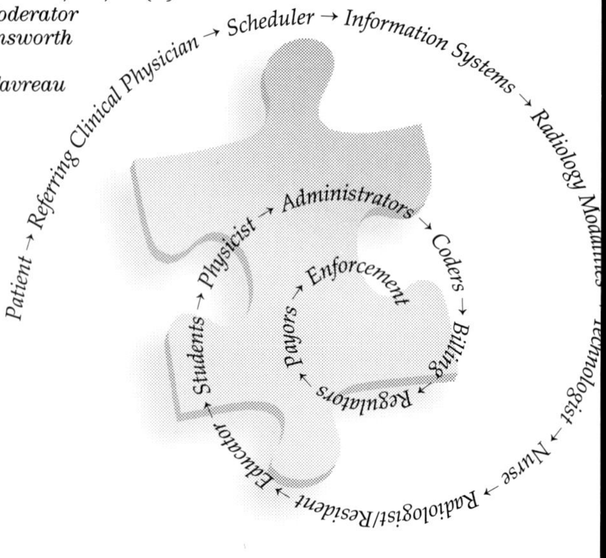

Sponsoring Organizations

- American Healthcare Radiology Administrators (AHRA)
- American Institute of Architects — Academy on Architecture for Health (AIA-AAH)
- American Radiological Nurses Association (ARNA)
- American Society of Radiologic Technologists (ASRT)
- Association of Educators in Radiological Sciences, Inc. (AERS)
- Association of Vascular and Interventional Radiographers (AVIR)
- Radiology Business Management Association (RBMA)
- Society for Radiation Oncology Administrators (SROA)
- Society of Diagnostic Medical Sonographers (SDMS)
- Section for Magnetic Resonance Technologists (SMRT-ISMRM)
- Society of Nuclear Medicine — Technologists Section (SNM-TS)

RSNA®
Radiological Society of North America
Founded in 1915

820 Jorie Boulevard
Oak Brook, Illinois 60523-1860
630/571-2670 FAX: 630/571-7837
www.rsna.org

Associated Sciences

Continuing Medical Education

Notices of continuing medical education programs will be accepted for publication in *Radiology* and *RadioGraphics* (*a*) if the program is directly relevant to radiologic imaging, practice, and oncology; and (*b*) if the course originates directly from and is organized by the radiology department of a medical school or medical center accredited for radiology residency training and approved to offer bona fide CME credit, or a radiologic organization that is a member of the Intersociety Commission of the American College of Radiology and approved to offer bona fide CME credit. Announcements of CME programs that do not meet these criteria will not be published. The RSNA assumes no responsibility for the content of CME programs appearing here.

Notices must include (*a*) the title of the course or meeting, (*b*) date and location, (*c*) listing of faculty, (*d*) fees, (*e*) number of category 1 credits available, (*f*) accredited sponsor of CME course, and (*g*) contact for further information. Notices should be submitted at least 4 months before the date of the meeting.

The opportunity to purchase classified and display ad space is also available.

Address announcements to Julie Pietryla, RSNA Publications, 820 Jorie Blvd, Oak Brook, IL 60523-2251.

Continuing medical education programs are listed according to diagnostic discipline; interdisciplinary programs are grouped under the predominant or first-listed specialty.

Breast Imaging

Breast Imaging Update 1999

"Breast Imaging Update 1999," a course cosponsored by the American Cancer Society and the North Carolina Breast and Cervical Cancer Control Program, will take place on October 21–24, 1999, at the Pinehurst Resort and Country Club, Pinehurst, NC. This course is designed to give the practicing radiologist a complete and updated overview of mammography. Topics include full-field digital mammography, ultrasonography (US), magnetic resonance imaging, interventional procedures, and quality control. In addition, hands-on training in stereotactic and US-guided core biopsy will be provided. Faculty: Braeuning, McLelland, Pisano, Rice, Shaw-de-Paredes. Fee: $500; 15 hours of category 1 credit will be available. For further information, contact Kerrie Kurgat, University of North Carolina, CB 7515, MRI Bldg, Mason Farm Rd, Chapel Hill, NC 27599-7515; telephone (919) 966-8067; fax (919) 966-2859; e-mail *kari_kurgat@med.unc.edu; http://www.cancer.org.*

Computed Tomography

Computed Body Tomography for the Technologist State of the Art 1999

"Computed Body Tomography for the Technologist State of the Art 1999," a course sponsored by the Department of Radiology, Johns Hopkins University School of Medicine, will be held on November 4–7, 1999, at the Peabody Orlando Hotel, Orlando, Fla. This course provides an integrated approach to the use of computed body tomography for technologists. The lectures are designed to address anatomic and pathologic anatomy with a specific emphasis on technique and technology. Presentations from leading imaging experts will provide a better understanding of scanner capabilities and future trends. Program director: Fishman. Fee: $475; 19.5 hours of category 1 credit will be available. For further information, contact the conference coordinator, Office of Continuing Medical Education, Johns Hopkins University School of Medicine, 720 Rutland Ave, Turner 20, Baltimore, MD 21205-2195; telephone (410) 955-2959; fax (410) 955-0807; e-mail *cmenet @jhmi.edu; http://www.med.jhu.edu/cme.*

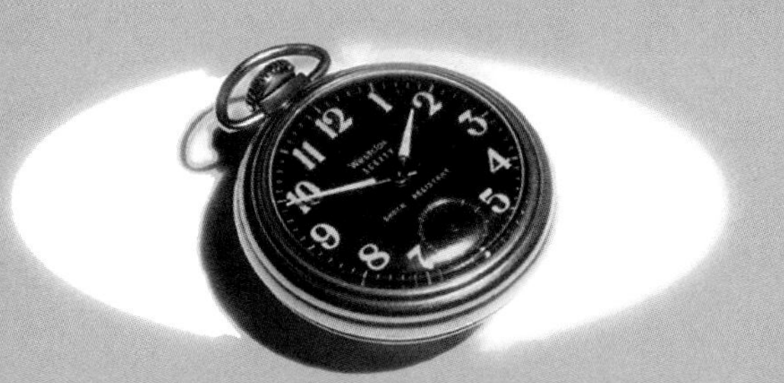

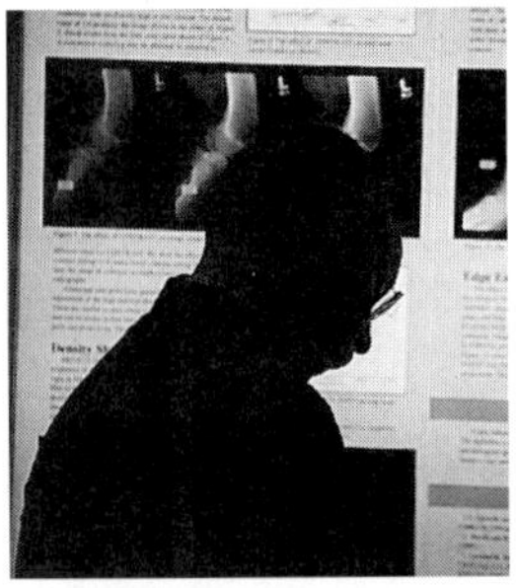

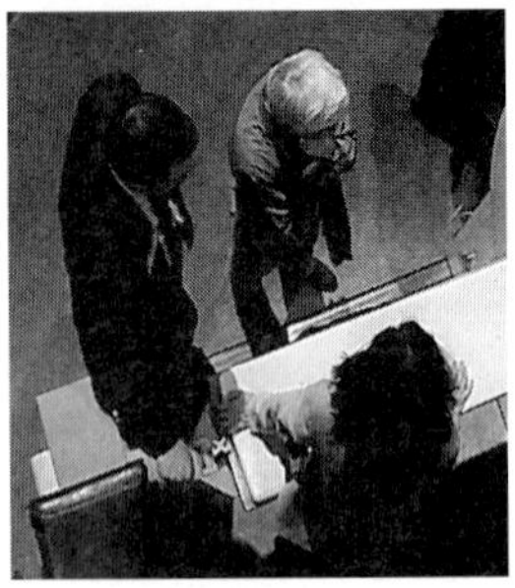

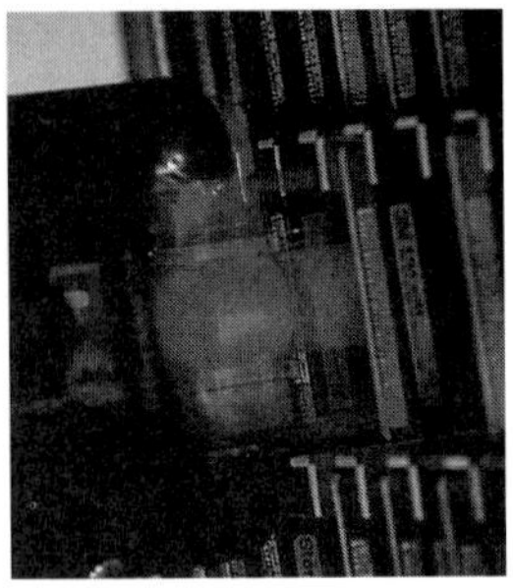

Radiology Business Information

Radiology, a monthly peer-reviewed journal devoted to clinical and other investigations relating to radiology and its allied sciences, is owned and published by

The Radiological Society of North America, Inc (RSNA)
820 Jorie Boulevard
Oak Brook, IL 60523-2251 USA
(630) 571-2670 • FAX (630) 571-7837
RSNA Link ***http://www.rsna.org***

Delmar J. Stauffer, *Executive Director and Business Manager for Publications*

■ JOURNAL BUSINESS

Send new manuscripts to the addresses given in the Publication Information for Authors.

Correspondence concerning accepted or published material should be addressed to

Anthony V. Proto, MD–Editor, *Radiology*
Radiology Editorial Office • 1001 East Broad Street
Suite 310 • Richmond, VA 23219
(804) 644-5667 FAX (804) 644-5672
e-mail: *radiolog@rsna.org*

■ COPYRIGHT AND PERMISSIONS

Material printed in *Radiology* is covered by copyright. No part of this publication may be reproduced or transmitted in any form without written permission from RSNA, except under circumstances within "fair use" as defined by U.S. copyright law. Requests for permission to use previously published material must be **in writing** and mailed or faxed to the Permissions Coordinator, RSNA Publications, 820 Jorie Blvd, Oak Brook, IL 60523-2251.

■ PHOTOCOPYING

Authorization to photocopy items for internal or personal use, or the internal or personal use of specific clients and educators, is granted by RSNA, provided that the appropriate fee is paid directly to Copyright Clearance Center, Inc (CCC), 222 Rosewood Dr, Danvers, MA 01923 (phone 978-750-8400; FAX 978-750-4744).

Consent for photocopying does not extend to copying for general distribution, resale, or advertising and promotional purposes, or for creating new collective works. Permission for the latter categories may be sought by writing to the Permissions Coordinator, RSNA Publications, 820 Jorie Blvd, Oak Brook, IL 60523-2251.

■ SUBSCRIPTION INFORMATION

The nonmember subscription rate for the USA is $215.00 per year; for outside USA, $260.00 (includes postage). (Air freight is available; rates are furnished on request.) Residents who are members of the RSNA may subscribe to **both** *Radiology* and *RadioGraphics* for a special rate of $80.00 (for North American addresses; residents from outside North America, add $60.00 for postage). Single copies are $25.00 (air freight, $11.00). Orders for subscriptions, remittances, and questions about subscriptions should be sent to

RSNA Subscriptions Department
820 Jorie Boulevard
Oak Brook, IL 60523-2251 USA
(630) 571-7873
FAX (630) 571-7837
e-mail: *subscrib@rsna.org*

The page containing advertising information (Advertisers' Index) may be located by consulting the Departments section in the Table of Contents.

■ CHANGE OF ADDRESS

The Post Office will not forward your journal to a new address. To avoid missing any issues, you must notify us of a change in address. At least 5 weeks before you move, please send (*a*) your **new address**, with zip code, and (*b*) your **current mailing label** showing your old address to the Subscriptions Department address given above.

■ MISSING ISSUES AND BACK COPIES

Claims for copies lost in the mail are allowed within 90 days of issue. Claims are not allowed for issues lost as a result of insufficient notice of change of address. To replace a missing issue or order a back copy contact RSNA Subscriptions Department at the address above. Back copies cost $25.00 (air freight, $11.00).

■ REPRINTS

The first footnote on the first page of each *Radiology* article contains the name and address of the author who answers requests for reprints. For reprint orders of 100 or more, place your order by using the address on the following page:

RSNA DEPARTMENT TELEPHONE NUMBERS

Accounting	(630) 571-7812
Advertising	(630) 571-7817
Copyrights and Permissions	(630) 571-7829
Executive	(630) 571-7866
Education Center	(630) 368-3753
Meetings	(630) 571-7850
Membership	(630) 571-7873
Office of Research	(630) 368-3756
Permissions	(630) 571-7829
Program	(630) 571-7874
Research and Education Foundation	(630) 571-7816
Reprints	(610) 250-7244
Subscriptions	(630) 571-7873
Syllabus sales	(800) 272-2920
Main telephone	(630) 571-2670
FAX	(630) 571-7837

Continued

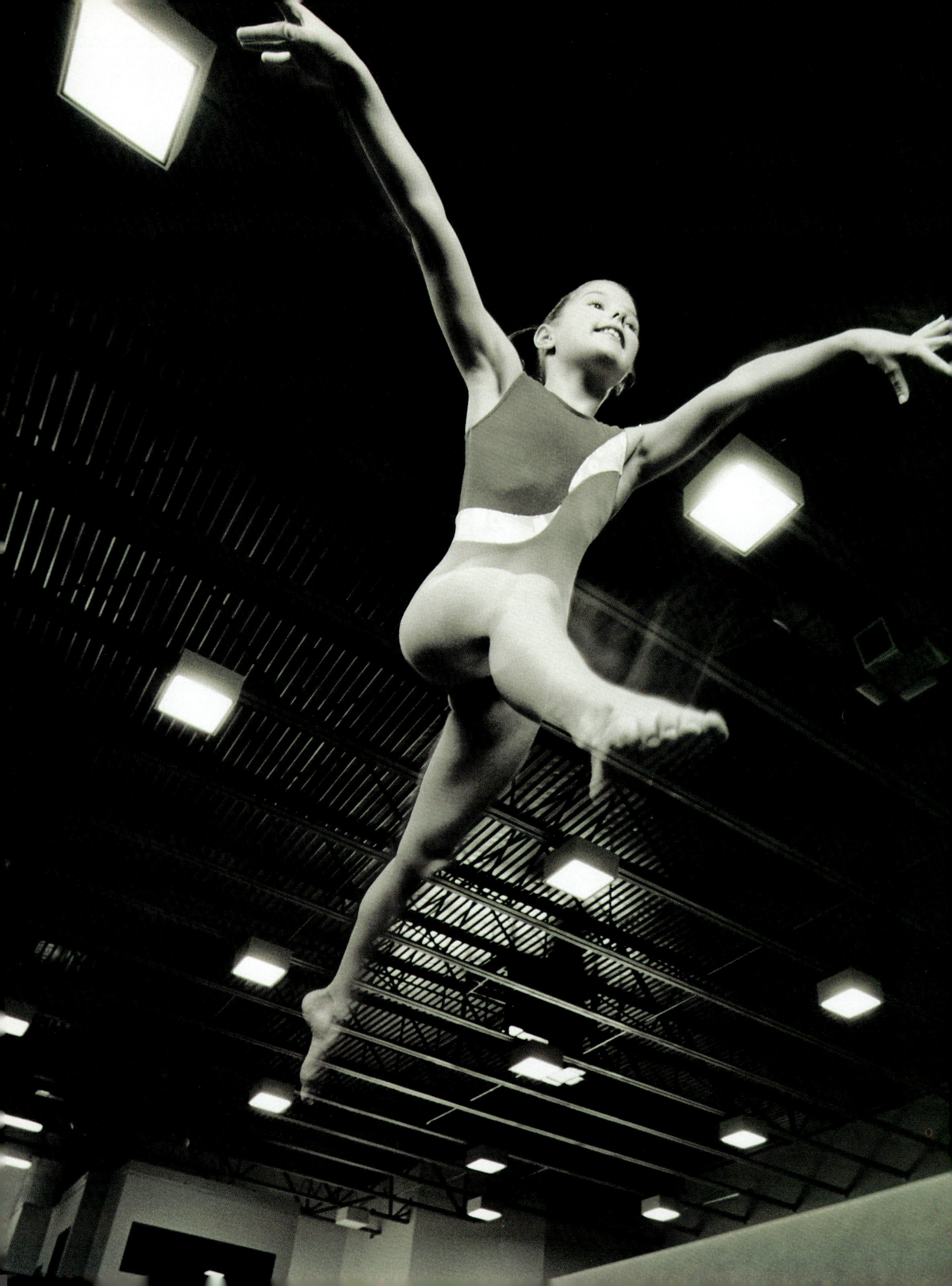

Radiology Reprints
1991 Northampton St
Easton, PA 18042-3189 USA
(610) 250-7244

For reprints of advertisements, contact the Advertising Production Manager (address under Advertising below).

■ MICROFORM

Radiology is available in microfilm and microfiche from

University Microforms International
300 N Zeeb Road
Ann Arbor, MI 48106 USA
(800) 521-3044

■ INDEXES

Radiology is included in the *RSNA Index to Imaging Literature,* a 3-year cumulative subject and author index of *Radiology* and approximately 40 radiologic journals, available for $35.00 per copy (air freight, $11.00). Subscribers to the Journal receive the index free of charge. *Radiology* is indexed in *Current Contents/Clinical Medicine,* available from the Institute for Scientific Information, and *Index Medicus,* available from the National Library of Medicine.

■ BOOK REVIEWERS AND BOOKS FOR REVIEW

Any person who would like to help in reviewing books for *Radiology* should contact

Richard A. Szucs, MD, Book Review Editor
Radiology Editorial Office
1001 E Broad St
Suite 310
Richmond, VA 23219

Publishers wishing to have books reviewed should send them to the same address.

■ PUBLISHERS' ROW

As a service to readers and colleagues in medical publishing, *Radiology* publishes a list of current imaging publications of interest to radiologists and allied scientists. Complete addresses and phone numbers of participating publishers are included. Publishers' Row is featured quarterly, in the March, June, September, and December issues. For information on publishing a list, contact Nancy Osborne at RSNA Publications at the Oak Brook address.

■ ADVERTISING

The advertising policy appears on the Advertisers' Index of each issue. Questions about advertising and billing, advertising contracts, and insertion orders and requests for media kits should be addressed to

James F. Drew, *Director of Advertising*
RSNA Publications
820 Jorie Boulevard
Oak Brook, IL 60523-2251 USA
(630) 571-7819
FAX (630) 571-7837

Questions about advertising production should be addressed to:

Pat Hollingsworth, *Advertising Production Manager*
RSNA Advertising Department
820 Jorie Boulevard
Oak Brook, IL 60523-2251 USA
(630) 571-7818
FAX (630) 571-7837

■ CLASSIFIED ADVERTISING

As a service to readers, *Radiology* accepts classified advertising, and every effort is made to ensure that the ads are relevant to the practice of radiology. For more details on the classified advertising policy and procedures, see the Classified Advertising section in each issue (consult the Departments section in the Table of Contents for page number) or contact the Advertising Production Manager (address under Advertising).

CHANGE OF ADDRESS FORM

Please allow 90 days for change to take effect

Name: ______________________ Address change effective as of ______________

Previous Address

Address: ______________________
____
____
City/State/Zip: ______________________

New Address

Address: ______________________
____
____
City/State/Zip: ______________________

Mail to:
RSNA Subscriptions Department • 820 Jorie Boulevard • Oak Brook, IL 60523-2251 USA **FAX:** (630) 571-7837

Transfer of Copyright and Certifications Agreement

Manuscript No. (for Editorial Office use only)______________________

Complete copyright to the article entitled:

____

____

is hereby transferred to the Radiological Society of North America (for **U.S. government employees:** to the extent transferable), effective if and when the article is accepted for publication in ***Radiology,*** printed or electronic format. In the case of authors who are officers or employees of the U.S. government, the Radiological Society of North America recognizes that works prepared by them as part of their official government duties are in the public domain.

Authors reserve the following rights:

1. Other than copyright, all proprietary rights including patent rights relating to the subject matter of the article.
2. The license for personal use in lectures, lecture notes, and exhibits.

Please return this form as soon as possible. The signed statement **must** be received by the Editor **before** the manuscript can be processed for publication.

A. All authors certify that this material or similar material has not been and will not be submitted by them or by colleagues in their institution to any other publication prior to its appearance in ***Radiology.***

B. All authors certify that they have read the Publication Information for Authors found in the most recently published issue of ***Radiology*** at the time the manuscript is submitted. They further certify their understanding of and compliance with the various requirements found therein, in particular those relating to authorship and redundant publication and potential sanctions for redundant publication.

C. All authors certify that they have submitted all required permissions and that all required statements have been inserted in the text where appropriate.

D. All authors certify that all individuals who have participated sufficiently in the conception and design of this work, in the analysis of the data, and in the writing of the manuscript have been listed as authors. All authors further certify that they have read the final version of the manuscript and approve it for submission for publication, agree with the author contributions listed on the Manuscript Categorization Terms form, and agree with the placement of authors in the author listing.

E. All authors certify that the Editor may correspond with the designated *corresponding author* regarding acceptance, rejection, revision of the manuscript and that the corresponding author is responsible for informing all other authors of the same.

F. All authors certify that responses, revisions received by the Editor from the designated *corresponding author* will be treated as if from all authors and that the corresponding author is responsible for informing all other authors of the same.

G. All authors certify that: **(must check one)** (Please see Publication Information for Authors for explanation.)

- ❐ they have no direct or indirect financial interest in the products under investigation or subject matter discussed in this manuscript, or
- ❐ one or more (please name) authors do have a direct or indirect financial interest in the products under investigation or subject matter discussed in this manuscript. A separate statement is attached that details this proprietary interest, and the authors hereby grant permission to publish this information or an appropriate summary thereof with the manuscript if the manuscript is published.

TO BE SIGNED BY ALL AUTHORS:

Name (print) (First) ____________________ Signature ____________________

Name (print) ____________________ Signature ____________________

Name (print) ____________________ Signature ____________________

Name (print) ____________________ Signature ____________________

Name (print) ____________________ Signature ____________________

Name (print) ____________________ Signature ____________________

This signed form (a photocopy is acceptable) must be submitted with all proffered works.

Radiology Publication Information for Authors

Radiology is a peer-reviewed journal that is published under the supervision of the Board of Directors of the Radiological Society of North America, Inc, which appoints the Editor who selects all material for publication, including advertisements. No responsibility is accepted by the Board of Directors or the Editor for the opinions expressed by the contributors. Please note that the instructions below are in accord with the *Uniform Requirements for Manuscripts Submitted to Biomedical Journals* (*Annals of Internal Medicine* 1997; 126:36-47). Although *Radiology* will receive material prepared and submitted according to these requirements, the right is reserved to introduce any changes necessary to make the contributions conform to the individual editorial standards of this Journal.

Manuscripts of original research, Technical Developments, and Case Reports should be addressed to:
Anthony V. Proto, MD—Editor, *Radiology*
Radiology Manuscripts • RSNA Publications
820 Jorie Boulevard • Oak Brook, IL 60523-2251 USA
FAX (630) 571-7837

All other submissions and correspondence concerning accepted or published material should be addressed to:
Anthony V. Proto, MD—Editor, *Radiology*
Radiology Editorial Office • 1001 East Broad Street
Suite 310 • Richmond, VA 23219
(804) 644-5667 FAX (804) 644-5672
e-mail: *radiolog@rsna.org*

Assistant to the Editor: Deborah L. Hogan
Office Coordinators: Tonya R. Emerson, Donna L. Schulze

Inquiries about manuscript status and preparation, as well as letters to the editor, can be directed to *radiolog@rsna.org*

The page containing advertising information (Advertisers' Index) may be located by consulting the Departments section in the Table of Contents.

■ TRANSFER OF COPYRIGHT AND CERTIFICATIONS AGREEMENT

Please send the copyright and certifications agreement with the initial submission of all proffered works. This may be accomplished by using a copy of the form that appears in this issue. **All** authors of any single composition must sign this agreement. In the case of officers or employees of the U.S. government, the Society recognizes that works prepared as part of their official government duties are in the public domain, but they must still sign the copyright and certifications agreement.

■ FINANCIAL INTEREST

Authors must describe any direct or indirect financial interest they may have in the subject matter of a submitted manuscript, and they must authorize the Society to publish this financial disclosure with the article if deemed appropriate by the editor. The Society's Financial Disclosure policy is as follows:

"Each author shall describe (*a*) any direct financial interest that author has in the subject matter discussed in the submitted manuscript, and (*b*) any affiliation or financial involvement that author has with or in any organization having a direct financial interest in the subject matter discussed in the submitted manuscript. Such information will be held in the confidence of the journal Editor during the review process. If necessary, in the Editor's view, this information may be shared with reviewers. The submission of a manuscript to *Radiology* grants permission for RSNA to publish the financial information described above, or an appropriate summary thereof, with the manuscript if the manuscript is accepted for publication."

Please note that financial interest also includes financial support of an author's study by any such organization.

■ REDUNDANT PUBLICATION

The Council of Biology Editors defines redundant publication as "... reporting (*publishing or attempting to publish*) substantially the same work more than once, without attribution of the original source(s) ..." [*CBE Views* 1996; 19(4):76–77]. Characteristics of reports that are substantially similar include (*a*) "at least one of the authors must be common to all reports (if there are no common authors, it is more likely plagiarism than redundant publication)"; (*b*) "the subject or study populations are often the same or similar"; (*c*) "the methodology is typically identical or nearly so"; and (*d*) "the results and their interpretation generally vary little, if at all." Please note that in addition to the foregoing, *Radiology* also includes as redundant publication (*a*) any work that has been previously published in a language other than English, unless the Editor agrees to publish and so identifies the material when it appears in *Radiology*, and (*b*) previously published abstracts substantially greater than 200–300 words.

If the Editor becomes aware of the possibility of redundant publication, he will ask the authors to provide a written explanation of their position regarding the same. As necessary, the Editor will seek the opinions of others (Deputy Editors, Associate Editors, Reviewers) to help him determine the presence of redundant publication. The authors will be informed of the editorial decision. If redundant publication is considered present, potential sanctions include (*a*) a ban on considering any other material presented by any of the involved authors for a period of 5 years, (*b*) notification of the other journal(s)

(continued)

to which the material has been submitted or in which it has been published, (*c*) notification of the authors' Department Chair(s), and (*d*) notification of the officials of the university or universities at which the authors reside.

Radiology accepts manuscripts of original research only with the understanding that they are contributed solely to this Journal. When submitting a manuscript, authors should send an accompanying letter informing the Editor of any potential overlap with other already published material or material being otherwise evaluated for publication. The provision of copies of such material is required and will aid the Editor in determining whether or not there is potential for redundant publication. The Editor, with help as necessary, will review the submission and the copies of other materials provided by the authors and will inform the authors of his decision to or not to proceed with peer review of the submission. Please see Sole Submission to *Radiology* regarding advertising media.

■ MANUSCRIPT CATEGORIZATION TERMS FORM

This form *must be submitted* before your manuscript can be evaluated. This may be accomplished by using a copy of the form that appears in this issue.

Terms: Please select as many terms as are appropriate to categorize the *major content* of your submission. It is important that you comply with this requirement since the terms you select are used to match your manuscript with the appropriate reviewers. Selection of inappropriate terms will result in sending your manuscript to inappropriate reviewers, who will return it to the Editorial Office, thereby resulting in substantial delays in the decision-making process.

Summary Statement: This single sentence taken from the text (not the Abstract) is to be included on the Manuscript Categorization Terms form. The page number on which the sentence appears is to be identified. The summary statement is the single sentence that best summarizes the message of your study or emphasizes an important point of the same. It will be printed in the Table of Contents and will serve as a kernel of information to help the reader in selecting articles of interest to read.

Author Contributions, Authorship: Authors are required to identify their manuscript contributions, for which they are responsible. The author(s) responsible for the integrity of the entire study should also be identified. To be listed as an author, an individual should have made substantial contributions to *all three* categories established by the International Committee of Medical Journal Editors (ICMJE): (*a*) "conception and design, or analysis and interpretation of data"; **and** (b) "drafting of the article or revising it critically for important intellectual content"; **and** (c) "final approval of the version to be published" (*Annals of Internal Medicine* 1997; 126:36–47). The ICMJE further states that "Participation solely in the acquisition of funding or the collection of data does not justify authorship. General supervision of the research group is not sufficient for authorship." *Radiology* asks that authors fulfill the ICMJE requirements to be so listed. Individuals who have not made substantial contributions in all three categories but who have made substantial contributions either to some of them or in other areas should be listed in Acknowledgments (see Acknowledgments below). Please note that the Manuscript Categorization Terms form should reflect the appropriate categories of contributions for authorship.

Once a manuscript has been received by *Radiology*, any changes in authorship will necessitate additional information: (*a*) The addition of an author requires that a letter be signed and submitted by all original authors indicating agreement with both the addition and the placement of the proposed author in the listing of authors. A Transfer of Copyright and Certifications Agreement form should be submitted after it has been signed by the additional author. The author contributions information should also be provided. (*b*) Deletion of an author requires that a letter be signed and submitted by the author to be deleted indicating his or her agreement to be deleted from the listing of authors and, if to be added to the Acknowledgments section, a mention in the letter by that author as to agreement with the same. (*c*) Rearrangement of the placement of authors in the listing of authors requires a letter from all authors agreeing to the same.

■ MANUSCRIPT ASSEMBLY

Manuscripts should be typewritten and **double-spaced (all pages)** on only one side of the paper with at least 3-cm margins and type size not smaller than 12 point. Each manuscript component should begin on a **new page** in this order: title pages, abstract, text, appendix, acknowledgments, references, tables (each on a separate page), captions for illustrations, and illustrations. The title pages and abstract page should not be numbered. Sequential numbering should begin with the text (Introduction). To ensure anonymity in the peer review process, authors' names should appear on only the full title page; names of authors, their initials, or the institution should **not** be given in the text or on the illustrations. Avoid language that reveals work previously published by you (eg, "as we have previously described," "continuing our former work," etc). **Three copies** of the manuscript and three complete sets of mounted illustrations should be submitted. The author should retain a complete copy of the manuscript because accepted manuscripts will not be returned and only the illustrations of rejected manuscripts will be returned. All manuscripts are acknowledged; please allow 2–3 weeks from the time you mailed the manuscript for receipt of an acknowledgment.

■ TITLE PAGES

Full Title Page: This page should include the title of the manuscript; the first and last names, middle initials, and degrees of all authors; the name and street address (not a postal box) of the institution from which the work originated; the telephone number, the FAX or Telex number, and the e-mail address of the **corresponding author**; and information concerning grants. The address for reprint requests should include the **complete** name, street address (not a postal box), and zip code. It is important to indicate on this title page whether your paper was presented at an RSNA meeting (please give year) or has been accepted for presentation at a future meeting. Lastly, indicate the type of manuscript you are submitting: original research; Technical Developments; Case Report; Signs in Imaging; Diagnosis Please; Letter to the Editor; Interlude; or solicited or unsolicited State of the Art, Review, Special Report, Special Review, Perspectives, Historical Perspectives, How I Do It, Viewpoint, or Editorial.

Abbreviated Title Page: This page should include only the title (at the top) and the type (see Full Title Page above) of manuscript (at the bottom) so as to allow for anonymity during the peer review process.

■ ABSTRACT, KEY WORDS

A structured abstract of 200 words or less must be submitted with each manuscript of original research. The abstract must be divided into four paragraphs with the following headings:

PURPOSE: State the hypothesis being tested or the procedure being evaluated.

MATERIALS AND METHODS: Briefly state what was done and what materials were used, including number of subjects. Also include the methods used to assess the data and to control bias.

RESULTS: Provide the findings of the study, including indicators of statistical significance. Include actual numbers, as well as percentages.

CONCLUSION: Summarize in one or two sentences the conclusion(s) made on the basis of the findings.

Below the abstract, please list three to six key words as derived from the terms used in the most recent 3-year *RSNA Index to Imaging Literature*.

An abstract of 60 words or less must be submitted for each Case Report or Technical Developments paper. The abstract must state (*a*) what was done, (*b*) what was found, and (*c*) what was concluded, but specific headings should not be included.

For State of the Art, Review, or other similar submissions, an abstract of 100–200 words should summarize the content of the submission, but specific headings should not be included.

■ TEXT

The text of original research and Technical Developments manuscripts is arranged in sections with the headings Introduction, Materials and Methods, Results, and Discussion. Lengthy papers may need subheadings within some sections to clarify their content, especially within the Materials and Methods and Results sections. Avoid idiosyncratic word usage, nonstandard terms or abbreviations, and self-evaluation of your work (eg, "new," "novel," "unique," "ground-breaking," "important"). Please spell out in full any acronym when first used, not only in the Abstract but also in the text. *We strongly recommend that authors for whom English is not their native language seek assistance from an English-speaking colleague to ensure that the words used convey the intended meaning both accurately and clearly. Failure to do so may delay the review of your manuscript.*

Introduction: Give only strictly pertinent background information and references that inform the reader as to why you undertook your study. Do not review the literature extensively. The final paragraph should clearly state the hypothesis or purpose of your study. Brevity and focus are important. Please note, *rarely should the Introduction exceed 1½ typewritten pages.*

Materials and Methods: For studies relating to humans, the first paragraph should indicate whether or not institutional review board approval and patient informed consent were obtained. If not, it should be clear that any studies performed were so performed for accepted clinical indications and that the studies themselves are considered acceptable for patient care. For animal experiments, please include instead a statement regarding approval by your institutional animal care committee or appropriate substitute. Please see Human and Animal Studies below for more information.

Describe clearly the number and selection of the subjects studied (patients or experimental animals, including controls). Identify the methods, instrumentation (trade names and manufacturer's name and location in parentheses), and procedures in sufficient detail to allow other workers to reproduce your study. It is *essential* that you state the manner by which studies were evaluated: independent readings, consensus readings, blinded or unblinded to other information, time sequencing between readings of several studies of the same patient or animal to eliminate recall bias, random ordering of studies. It should also be clear as to the retrospective or prospective nature of your study.

To ensure anonymity in the review process, do **not** include the name of the institution where the work was performed or authors' names or initials, either within the text or at the top of each manuscript page.

Give references to established methods, including statistical methods that have been published but are not well known; describe new or substantially modified methods and give reasons for using these techniques. Briefly state the statistical methods used to analyze your data. We *strongly recommend* that all authors seek statistical consultation before planning a study to ensure both the appropriate collection of data and the appropriate use of statistical tests to analyze those data. Similarly, studies relating to cost analysis or cost-effectiveness should also be discussed with individuals knowledgeable in these techniques. *Radiology* reserves the right to receive your raw data for use by our consultants should the need arise during their evaluation of your manuscript to recalculate your results. See below for information that should be placed in an Appendix. Make sure that the Materials and Methods section includes all items for which you present results in the Results section. Please note, *rarely should Materials and Methods exceed 4–5 typewritten pages.*

Results: Present the results in logical sequence in the text, along with tables and illustrations. Do not repeat in the text all the data in the tables and/or illustrations; summarize only important observations. Make sure to give results for all items evaluated as mentioned in the Materials and Methods. State the statistical significance of your findings. Numerators and denominators *must be provided* either in the text or the tables for all percentages given. The same applies to sensitivity, specificity, accuracy, and positive and negative predictive values. If you have used subheadings in Materials and Methods, it may be helpful to present the results in the same sequence using the same subheadings, if appropriate. Please note, *rarely should Results exceed 4 typewritten pages*, especially if tables have been included.

Discussion: Emphasize the advances in knowledge provided by your study and the conclusions that follow from them. Do not repeat in detail the data given in the Results section. Include in the Discussion the implications of the findings and their limitations, in particular with reference to the use of modified methods, statistical or otherwise. Relate the observations to other relevant studies. Link the conclusions with the goals of the study, but avoid unqualified statements and conclusions not supported completely by the data. Avoid claiming priority and alluding to or giving the results of your ongoing investigations that have not been completed or that are not part of your study. State new hypotheses when warranted, but clearly label them as such. Recommendations, when appropriate, may be included. Please note, *rarely should the Discussion exceed 4–5 typewritten pages.*

For Experimental Studies articles, please describe the importance of your conclusions as they relate to potential future practical applications. Please identify this paragraph, which should be the last, with the title "Practical Application(s)."

■ APPENDIX

When essential for the understanding of your study, detailed background information, mathematical derivations, statistical analyses, and the like, should be presented in one or more appendices. Include in the appropriate section of the text (eg, Materials and Methods, Results) a *brief* summary paragraph of the information contained in the Appendix and make reference to the Appendix.

■ ACKNOWLEDGMENTS

List here those who have contributed substantially to the work reported in the manuscript but who have not fulfilled the ICMJE requirements for authorship (see Author Contributions, Authorship in the Manuscript Categorization Terms Form section above). Authors are expected to obtain written permission of those acknowledged, and to submit the same, as readers might interpret that those acknowledged agree with the data and conclusions of the study.

■ REFERENCES

Number references consecutively in the order in which they are first mentioned in the manuscript. The abbreviations used for periodicals cited in the references should follow the style of *Index Medicus.* For journal articles, list surnames and initials of all authors when six or less, such as:

1. Stuart MJ, Elrad H, Graeber JE, Hakanson DO, Sunderji SG, Barvinchak MK. Increased synthesis of prostaglandin endoperoxides and platelet hyperfunction in infants of mothers with diabetes mellitus. J Lab Clin Med 1979; 94:12–26.

When seven or more authors are listed, only the first three names need to be identified, followed by "et al," such as:

1. Hibbard CT, Campbell S, Sabbagha RE, et al. Demonstration of tissue interfaces within the body by ultrasonic echo sounding. Br J Radiol 1961; 34:539–549.

Abstracts, editorials, and letters to the editor should be noted as such. In the case of books, the authors of a chapter, title of the chapter, editor(s), title of the book, edition, city and state, publisher, year, and specific pages must be provided.

1. Brown M, Gray L. Indications for hematology. In: Wintrobe MM, ed. Clinical hematology. 3rd ed. Philadelphia, Pa: Lea & Febiger, 1975; 1146–1167.

Please include the complete page numbers for the citation (eg, 1537–1544 rather than 1537–44). *It is the responsibility of the author(s) to ensure that all references are listed accurately.*

■ TABLES

Tables should be numbered in Arabic numerals and should have a title. All abbreviations used in the table should be explained in a footnote.

Tables should be presented in the style used in recent issues of the Journal. No vertical lines or shading should be included. Avoid excessive use of horizontal lines within the table. Either the text or the tables should include numerators and denominators for all percentages provided (see Results in the Text section above).

■ CAPTIONS FOR ILLUSTRATIONS

A caption must be supplied for each illustration, including drawings and graphs. It should not duplicate text material and should follow the style used in recent issues of the Journal. All captions should appear collectively on one or more pages separate from the text, and each caption should also appear below the corresponding illustration on the page to which the illustration is mounted (see Illustrations below). It is essential that the caption describes all labels placed on an illustration. The caption should include the type of image, its plane, whether or not contrast material was used, the pulse sequence information for MR images, and the features to be observed by the reader. For photomicrographs, please include the stain and original magnification. For drawings and graphs, it is *essential* that the caption state the important points you wish the reader to conclude by observing the same.

■ ILLUSTRATIONS

Illustrations should be limited to those required to show the essential features described in the manuscript. Space constraints prevent us from publishing redundant or excessive illustrations. Unretouched glossy prints no larger than 12.7 × 17.8 cm (5 × 7 inches) are desirable. Computer-generated prints are acceptable but must be in the correct format (see Illustrations File in the Electronic Submission of Accepted Manuscripts section below). Prints to be combined into one array, such as posteroanterior and lateral views, should be sized the same to facilitate reproduction. When several images of a given type (eg, CT, MR, US) are being shown, please reproduce each specific type at the same magnification. Prints should correspond in appearance to the tonal relations of the original radiograph (ie, showing the bones white on a dark background, with the patient's right to the observer's left; CT scans and MR images should employ the "view from below"). If an image has been enhanced electronically, explain the alterations that have been made and send an original image along with the enhanced one. Drawings and graphs should be rendered professionally in India ink on white paper. In computer-generated artwork, shading should be done in continuous tones (ie, solid black, solid gray, solid white): **Do not use dotted shadings or several shades of gray.** Vertical or horizontal lines and cross-hatching should be used for bar graphs only if additional distinctions are needed (first use black, white, gray). Whether for images, drawings, or graphs, we recommend that not greater than four components be used for a given figure (eg, a,b,c,d).

Since the size of the illustration printed in the Journal is typically smaller than that submitted by the author(s), it is essential that each submitted illustration show only the area(s) of interest with enough surrounding area for orientation purposes (eg, to illustrate a cavity at the right lung apex, show only that area with enough surrounding area for orientation, rather than the entire chest radiograph).

All illustrations must be numbered and "top" indicated on the back. For protection against loss or damage, each illustration should then be neatly attached to paper (one illustration per page), and the number and top should be reindicated on this page. For attachment, **avoid using glue, staples, folded tape, or corner mounts.** Because it holds the illustration securely to the page without damage, we recommend Scotch Removable Magic Tape (3M, St Paul, Minn) be placed at the periphery of the print. **Please** do not add letters or numbers to the **face** of the illustration to identify the figure component (such as 1a or 1b).

Please be sure to include on each page the appropriate caption for the illustration mounted on that page. *It is ESSENTIAL that you label all features described in the caption, using different labels for each feature.* See a recent issue of the Journal for the degree of labeling we require.

Arrows and other labels (do not use equilateral triangles for arrowheads) should be placed only on the final print, should be of professional quality, should be **removable**, and should touch the edge of the feature being labeled. Our professional artist service for such items is available to authors without charge. The desired labels may simply be indicated on a **transparent** overlay attached securely to the page either at the top or left side to allow the overlay to be lifted. For computer-generated prints, the labels may be part of the print rather than affixed to it provided they are clearly visible (eg, do not place a white region-of-interest circle on a white background).

Illustrations of accepted manuscripts become the property of the RSNA and will be stored for 2 years after publication. Illustrations will be returned only upon receipt of a written request from the corresponding author. We suggest that authors make and keep a set of illustrations in addition to the three sets submitted to the Journal.

Radiology strongly discourages the use of previously published illustrations unless absolutely essential and very few. Use of such illustrations is problematic because you may be asked by the publisher to pay a fee and some publishers will not provide permission for electronic publication, which precludes these illustrations from the online version of *Radiology*.

Note that color illustrations will be published only if the Editor concludes that color is essential to convey the message of these illustrations.

■ UNITS AND ABBREVIATIONS

Radiation measurements and laboratory values should be given in the *International System of Units (SI)* (resources: SI Units in Radiation Protection and Measurements, NCRP Report no. 82 [August 1985]; "Now Read This: The SI Units Are Here," *JAMA* 1986; 255:2329–2339). Abbreviations should be spelled out when first used in the text, such as "cerebrospinal fluid (CSF)," and the number used should be kept to a minimum. In general, only standard abbreviations will be used. Laboratory slang and clinical jargon should be avoided.

■ HUMAN AND ANIMAL STUDIES

Manuscripts reporting the results of experimental studies on human subjects must include a statement in the first paragraph of Materials and Methods to the effect that informed consent was obtained after the nature of the procedure(s) had been fully explained. In addition, a statement affirming approval of the appropriate institutional review board is required in the same paragraph of the Materials and Methods section. If a review board does not exist, then the Declaration of Helsinki principles should be followed and a statement affirming the same should be made in that paragraph (41st World Medical Assembly. Declaration of Helsinki: recommendations guiding physicians in biomedical research involving human subjects. *Bull Pan Am Health Organ* 1990; 24: 606–609).

The maintenance and care of experimental animals to provide humane treatment and to ensure reliable results are described in the National Institutes of Health guidelines for use of laboratory animals. Authors must affirm, in the first paragraph of the Materials and Methods section, their compliance with these guidelines or approval by the appropriate institutional review board or animal care committee.

■ RIGHTS AND PERMISSIONS

Written permission (we require a copy) must be granted by the publisher (and the author when applicable) to reproduce any previously published figures and tables. Any such material must be clearly noted and its source given in the manuscript.

A signed letter of permission must be included with your manuscript for any individual who might be identified due to written descriptions, photographs (masking the eyes in photographs is not sufficient protection of anonymity), or otherwise. Such permission, which requires that the individual be shown the manuscript, should be affirmed in the text or figure caption as appropriate.

If reference is made in the text to personal communication (oral or written) as a source of information, a signed statement of permission is required from each such source. The year of receipt of the personal communication should be provided in the text. Please see Acknowledgments above for additional required permissions.

■ SOLE SUBMISSION TO *RADIOLOGY*

Authors must be certain that a manuscript on the same or similar material has not already been published by them or has not been or will not be submitted to another journal by them or by colleagues at their institution before their work appears in *Radiology*. The submission by authors of similar material to advertising media must be indicated at the time *Radiology* receives the manuscript, and a copy of that material should be provided with your submission. Please see Redundant Publication for additional important information.

■ MANUSCRIPT REVISION

When you prepare a revised version of your manuscript, it is *essential* that you carefully follow the instructions given in the Editor's letter regarding preparation of the same, in particular preparation of the annotated copy. Failure to do so will cause a delay in the review of your revision and may result in return of the revision to you, without review, for proper preparation.

Revisions received more than 3 months after requested may be sent for another review cycle, at the Editor's discretion. If a revision is not received within 10 months after requested, copies of your manuscript retained by the Editorial Office will be returned to you and your file closed.

■ ELECTRONIC SUBMISSION OF ACCEPTED MANUSCRIPTS

Text File: Manuscripts that have been accepted for publication must be submitted on computer disk (required for text, desirable for illustrations). Submit text on a 3½-inch high-density disk prepared in WordPerfect or Microsoft Word format for Windows or Macintosh. *A hard copy should accompany the disk and should match the disk file exactly.* The disk should be labeled with its assigned manuscript number, the first author's last name, the word-processing program used, and the file name.

The entire article should be submitted as a single text file, with the elements in the standard order: title pages, abstract, text, appendix, acknowledgments, references, tables, captions.

Do not embed illustrations. Only the final version of the article should be on the submitted disk. Keep the text file as free from formatting codes as possible: Do not use boldface, italic, underlining, strange fonts, codes for centering, unnecessary line spacing, etc. Use the default settings of the word-processing program; *especially do not use right-justified margins*. Use tabs to indent at the beginnings of paragraphs, and insert only one space after end punctuation marks. Use hard returns only at the ends of paragraphs or between sections of the manuscript; do not insert them midparagraph. Do not insert tabs in references; use only one hard return at the end of each reference.

Illustrations File: Although not required, submission of illustrations on a 3½-inch disk, ZIP disk, or CD is acceptable. **All photographic images should be scanned as 300 dpi TIFs; all line-art images should be scanned as 800–1,200 dpi TIFs.** Any image saved as .bmp, .jpeg, .gif, a PowerPoint slide, or any other lower resolution file cannot be used. **Images embedded in word-processing programs will not be used.** Image mode for color photographic images should be CYMK; for black and white photographic images, it should be gray scale and bit map for line-art images. Image size should be submitted as close as possible to print size: 2¼ inches wide for 1 column, 3¼ inches wide for 1½ columns, and 4 inches wide for 2 columns.

Each image file should be named, and the following should be provided with the disk: a hard-copy inventory with specific information on the image, two sets of proofs obtained at 800–1,800 dpi, and one set of proofs obtained with a laser printer to be used as a reference set.

■ COPYEDITING

After final acceptance of your manuscript, it will be copyedited prior to publication to conform to *Radiology* style and usage, both of which are based on widely accepted conventions of grammar, the *American Medical Association Manual of Style,* and *Stedman's Medical Dictionary*. This editing *may* be substantive. It is the responsibility of the corresponding author to read the copyedited manuscript he or she will receive and to answer all queries fully. Because the production schedule for a monthly journal contains fixed deadlines, the copyedited manuscript and the figure proofs *must be returned by the date provided on the accompanying cover sheet*. Failure to do so may delay publication of your manuscript.

■ BOOK REVIEWERS

Any person who would like to help in reviewing books for *Radiology* should contact

Richard A. Szucs, MD, Book Review Editor
Radiology Editorial Office
1001 E Broad St
Suite 310
Richmond, VA 23219

■ BOOKS FOR REVIEW

Publishers wishing to have books reviewed should send them to the address above.

✔ Checklist of Requirements:

- ❑ 1. Send a completed copy of the Manuscript Categorization Terms form. Please remember to include the summary statement (see Summary Statement in the Manuscript Categorization Terms Form section).
- ❑ 2. Send copyright and certifications agreement with signatures of all authors (check one of the boxes in G).
- ❑ 3. Double space all parts of manuscript.
- ❑ 4. Send institutional affiliation for each author and the corresponding author's name, address, phone number, FAX or Telex number, and e-mail address.
- ❑ 5. Send 3 copies of manuscript and 3 copies of illustrations.
- ❑ 6. Mount each illustration on a separate page, 8½ × 11 inches. Indicate figure number and "top" on back of illustration and on face of page. Include appropriate caption on each page.
- ❑ 7. Digital images that do not meet the required dpi specifications will not be used (see Illustrations File in the Electronic Submission of Accepted Manuscripts section).
- ❑ 8. Send a **brief** abstract: 200 words or less or 60 words or less (see Abstract, Key Words).
- ❑ 9. Minimize the use of abbreviations and define each when first used both in the abstract and in the text.
- ❑ 10. Include information on institutional review board approval, informed consent, animal care committee approval.
- ❑ 11. Provide numerator and denominator for all percentages.
- ❑ 12. Give SI units for radiation measurements and laboratory values.
- ❑ 13. Send copy of letter giving permission to reprint any figure that was published previously or any other permissions (see Rights and Permissions).
- ❑ 14. Provide copies of any material for which there is overlap with your manuscript (see Redundant Publication).

Radiology Manuscript Categorization Terms

Please PRINT your name: ______________________________

Please print the title of your manuscript ______________________________

____

Please check one of the following items regarding the subject matter of your manuscript:

❑ Adults Only ❑ Pediatrics Only ❑ Adults and Pediatrics

For each section, please categorize your manuscript by checking off only those terms that reflect the ***major points*** of your manuscript.*

Modalities/Techniques
You must check at least one term in this section or the next (Procedures).

___ Absorptiometry/Bone Densitometry
___ Angiography
___ Arthrography
___ Conventional Radiography
___ CT
___ CT-Angiography
___ CT-Electron Beam
___ CT-High Resolution
___ CT-Spiral
___ Dacryocystography
___ Defecography
___ Digital Radiography
___ Echocardiography
___ Fluoroscopy
___ Gamma Knife
___ Hysterosalpingography
___ Image Manipulation/Reconstruction
___ Interventional
___ Lymphography
___ Mammography
___ MR-Angiography
___ MR-Diffusion/Perfusion
___ MR-Functional Imaging
___ MR-Imaging
___ MR-Spectroscopy
___ Neural Networks
___ PACS
___ PET
___ Radionuclide Studies
___ Sialography
___ SPECT
___ Ultrasound
___ Ultrasound-Color Doppler
___ Ultrasound-Doppler
___ Ultrasound-Power Doppler
___ Ultrasound-Spectral Doppler

Procedures
You must check at least one term in this section or the prior one (Modalities/Techniques).

___ Angioplasty
___ Angioscopy
___ Balloon Insertions
___ Biopsy
___ Drainage
___ Dilation
___ Embolization
___ Endoscopy
___ Filter Insertions
___ Intraoperative
___ Laser
___ Lithotripsy
___ Localization
___ Myelography
___ Percutaneous
___ Radiation Therapy/Oncology
___ Radionuclide Therapy
___ Shunts
___ Stents
___ Thrombolysis

Areas/Systems
You must check at least one term unless none apply.

___ Abdomen/GI
___ Biliary
___ Breast
___ Cardiac
___ CNS
___ Ear/Nose/Throat
___ Genital/Reproductive
___ Head/Neck
___ Hematologic
___ Lymphatic
___ Muscular
___ Nervous-Peripheral
___ Skeletal-Appendicular
___ Skeletal-Axial
___ Soft Tissues/Skin
___ Thorax
___ Urinary
___ Vascular

Structures
You must check at least one term unless none apply.

___ Adrenal
___ Ankle
___ Anus
___ Aorta
___ Appendix
___ Arteries
___ Bile Ducts
___ Bladder
___ Brain/Brain Stem
___ Breast
___ Cervix
___ Diaphragm
___ Duodenum
___ Ear
___ Elbow
___ Esophagus
___ Extremities
___ Eye
___ Face
___ Fallopian Tubes
___ Foot
___ Gallbladder
___ Hand
___ Heart
___ Hip
___ Jaw
___ Joints
___ Kidney
___ Knee
___ Lacrimal Glands
___ Large Bowel
___ Larynx
___ Ligaments
___ Liver
___ Long Bones
___ Lung
___ Marrow
___ Mediastinum
___ Meninges
___ Mesentery
___ Omentum
___ Orbit
___ Ovaries
___ Pancreas
___ Paranasal Sinuses
___ Parathyroid
___ Pelvis
___ Pelvicaliceal
___ Penis
___ Pericardium
___ Peritoneum
___ Pharynx
___ Pineal
___ Pituitary
___ Pleura
___ Prostate
___ Pylorus
___ Rectum
___ Retina
___ Retroperitoneum

***This form *must be* included with your manuscript submission.**

Continued

Structures, continued *You must check at least one term unless none apply.*

___ Ribs
___ Salivary Glands
___ Scrotum
___ Shoulder
___ Skull
___ Small Bowel
___ Spinal Cord
___ Spine
___ Spleen
___ Stomach
___ Tendons
___ Testes
___ Thymus
___ Thyroid
___ Tongue
___ Tracheobronchial Tree
___ Ureters
___ Urethra
___ Uterus
___ Vagina
___ Valves
___ Veins
___ Vena Cava
___ Wrist

Topics *You must check at least one term unless none apply.*

___ Abscess
___ Acceptance Testing
___ Acute
___ AIDS
___ Anatomy
___ Aneurysms
___ Animal Investigations
___ Arteriosclerosis
___ Arthritides
___ Artifacts
___ Atelectasis
___ Athletic Injuries
___ AVM
___ Axilla
___ Biological Effects
___ Blood
___ Calcifications/Calculi
___ Cardiac Assist Devices
___ Catheters
___ Cavitation
___ Cerebral Palsy
___ Chemistry
___ Chronic Obstructive Airways Disease
___ Cirrhosis
___ Comparative Studies
___ Complications
___ Computer Applications-3D
___ Computer Applications-Teleradiology
___ Computer Applications-Virtual Imaging
___ Computer Applications-General
___ Congenital
___ Connective Tissue Disorders
___ Contrast Agents-Intravenous
___ Contrast Agents-Oral
___ Contrast Agents-Other
___ Cost-effectiveness
___ CSF
___ Cysts
___ Dementia
___ Demineralization-Bone
___ Dilatation
___ Dissection
___ Diverticula
___ Dosimetry
___ Drugs/Reactions
___ Dysplasias
___ Eating Disorders
___ ECMO
___ Edema
___ Education
___ Efficacy Studies
___ Embolism/Thrombosis
___ Endocrine Disorders
___ Epidemiology
___ Equipment
___ Ethics
___ Experimental Investigations
___ Fetus
___ Fistula
___ Foreign Bodies
___ Forensics
___ Genetic Defects
___ Grafts
___ Health Policy and Practice
___ Hemangioma
___ Hematologic Diseases
___ Hemodynamics/Flow Dynamics
___ Hemorrhage
___ Hernia
___ History
___ Hyperplasia/Hypertrophy
___ Hypertension
___ Imaging Sequences
___ Infection
___ Inflammation
___ Instrumentation
___ Ischemia/Infarction
___ Laboratory Tests
___ Leukemia
___ Lymphoma
___ Medicolegal Issues
___ Metabolic Disorders
___ Metastases
___ Molecular Imaging
___ Monoclonal Antibodies
___ Motility
___ Neoplasms-Primary
___ Normal Variants
___ Observer Performance
___ Obstetrics
___ Obstruction/Occlusion
___ Occupational/Environmental Hazards
___ Outcomes Analysis
___ Parasites
___ Pathology
___ Perception Image
___ Physics
___ Physiological Studies
___ Pregnancy
___ Prostheses
___ QA/QC
___ Radiation Effects
___ Radiation Safety
___ Radiobiology
___ Safety
___ Screening
___ Sedation
___ Seizure Disorders
___ Socioeconomic Issues
___ Speech Disorders
___ Staging
___ Statistics
___ Surgery
___ Technical Aspects
___ Technology Assessments
___ Tissue Characterization
___ Transplantation
___ Trauma
___ Treatment Effects
___ Tropical Diseases
___ Varices
___ Volvulus

Print the *summary statement* here and provide the page no. from the text where this sentence appears (please see Publication Information for Authors for instructions).

____

____ page no. _______

Please provide author(s) initials for each *author contribution* category (use NA if not applicable). (Please see Publication Information for Authors for specific instructions regarding this item.)

________ Guarantor of integrity of entire study
________ Study concepts†
________ Study design†
________ Literature research
________ Clinical studies
________ Experimental studies
________ Data acquisition
________ Data analysis/interpretation†
________ Statistical analysis
________ Manuscript preparation†
________ Manuscript definition of intellectual content†
________ Manuscript editing
________ Manuscript revision/review†
________ Manuscript final version approval†

†These relate to the ICMJE categories for authorship. (Please read Publication Information for Authors before completing this section.)

Anthony V. Proto, MD

Radiology 1999: Revised Publication Information for Authors

Although the January 1998 issue of *Radiology* was my first as Editor, the transition of the editorship from the former Editor, Dr Stanley S. Siegelman, to me began in July of 1997. One of my self-assigned tasks at that time was to revise the Publication Information for Authors guidelines, which appear at the end of the front section of the "A" pages and just before the lead item in each issue of the Journal. Those revised guidelines were published in the August 1997 issue of *Radiology*.

With the September 1999 issue, we are publishing yet another extensive revision of these guidelines based on the experience of our Deputy Editors, that of our manuscript editors and production assistants in our Oak Brook office, and my own experience. In addition, our efforts to constantly improve and expedite the process of producing each issue of the Journal using modern techniques has mandated a number of changes.

These guidelines are meant for use by our authors. In addition to informing authors of the desired format for the submitted manuscript, the guidelines also inform authors of several of our policies and procedures regarding processing of their manuscripts. If authors follow these guidelines carefully, the processes of assigning the reviewers for a given manuscript, reviewer evaluation of that manuscript, decision by the Editor, manuscript revision(s), review by the Deputy Editors, final acceptance by the Editor, processing by the Editor for transmittal to our Oak Brook office, editing by our manuscript editors, processing of illustrations by our production staff, and approval of the edited manuscript by the authors will all be expedited. The additional layers of review that have been implemented in the *Radiology* Editorial Office in Richmond, Va, often uncover a number of items that require revision and thereby extend the process of manuscript evaluation. Many of these items are simply due to the authors not having followed the Publication Information for Authors guidelines.

The modifications and additions that compose the revised Publication Information for Authors appearing in this issue are numerous. Some of the major ones include the following:

1. Further clarification of financial interests
2. Addition of a section on redundant (duplicate) publication and potential sanctions for the same
3. Addition to and modifications of the Manuscript Categorization Terms form
4. Clarification of our guidelines for authorship
5. Expansion of the types of abstracts for different types of submissions
6. Guidelines for the length of each section of a manuscript of original research
7. Expanded information on the items to be included in each section of a manuscript of original research
8. Use of an Appendix
9. Expansion of the desired characteristics for illustrations and figure captions
10. Additional explanation of required items for human and animal studies
11. Addition of a section on manuscript revision
12. Modifications regarding electronic submissions of accepted manuscripts
13. Addition of a section on copyediting
14. Expansion of the Checklist of Requirements
15. Clarification of and additions to the Transfer of Copyright and Certifications Agreement form

We encourage our authors to follow these revised guidelines, so as to expedite the processing of their manuscripts.

Index terms:
Editorials
Radiology (journal)

Radiology 1999; 212:605

Anthony V. Proto, MD

Diagnosis Please Certificate of Recognition Awarded to Sergio Julio Moguillansky, MD

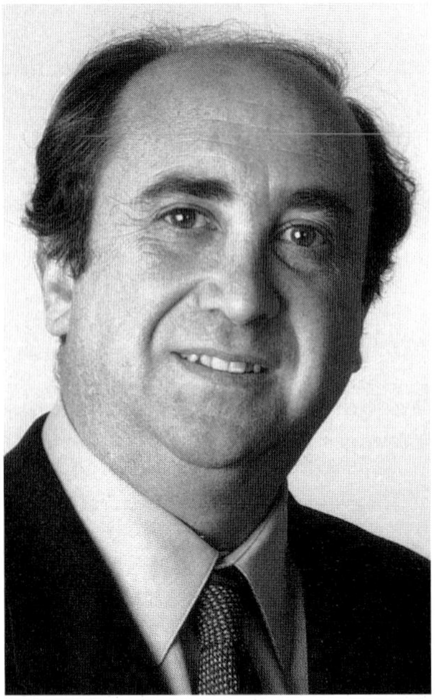

Sergio Julio Moguillansky, MD

In April 1998, we introduced a new feature in *Radiology*—Diagnosis Please (1). Each month, a challenging case is presented. Readers are asked to submit the most likely diagnosis based on the history and imaging findings provided. Four months later (to allow all of our international readers an opportunity to participate), the answer to the case is presented; this part includes a description of the imaging findings and a discussion of the differential diagnosis, indicating why the most likely diagnosis is indeed most likely.

Diagnosis Please has become a popular monthly feature; we receive hundreds of responses for each case and publish the names of those individuals who have submitted the most likely diagnosis. Several additional cases are now under preparation, and it is our plan to continue this feature as long as we have authors who are willing to prepare the cases. Each case is rigorously evaluated through our peer-review process.

Case 12 was presented in the March 1999 issue of *Radiology* and its answer in the July 1999 issue. We have now identified, for the 1st year of Diagnosis Please cases, one individual who submitted the highest number of correct answers—Sergio Julio Moguillansky, MD, from Cipolletti, Río Negro, Argentina.

Dr Moguillansky received his MD degree in 1977 from the School of Medicine of the Universidad de Buenos Aires in Argentina. He served as a resident in diagnostic radiology from 1978 to 1981 in the Medical Radiology Program directed by Pedro Moguillansky, MD. From 1983 to 1991, he served as chief of radiology of the Clínica Radiológica del Sur. Since 1991, he has held the position of chief of radiology at Medicina XXI, a radiology center located in the cities of Cipolletti and Neuquén. His practice includes general radiology, with a specialty focus in neuroradiology. In 1998, he joined the faculty of the School of Medicine of the Universidad Nacional del Comahue, where he directs the imaging section of theAnatomy and Normal Images course. Dr Moguillansky is certified in diagnostic radiology by the Board of Certification of Medical Professions of the Academia Nacional de Medicina and by the Recertification Committee of the Asociación Médica Argentina.

Dr Moguillansky has participated in numerous courses and meetings in both Argentina and the United States, including several visiting fellowships in the United States at Massachusetts General Hospital, Boston, and the Huntington Research Institutes, Pasadena, Calif. He has been and continues to be a popular speaker, in particular at the Congreso Argentino de Radiología and others. He has several publications to his credit and has been president of the Sociedad de Radiología y Medicina por Imágenes del Comahue and vice president of the Federación Argentina de Asociaciones de Radiología, Diagnóstico por Imágenes y Terapia Radiante.

In his letter to me, Dr Moguillansky stated his participation in Diagnosis Please was "... primarily based on the need to answer ... an intellectual challenge, check my knowledge in different areas, and learn more about differential diagnosis and clinical-radiological correlations." It is clear that he has the knowledge and has met the challenge. We extend our congratulations to him for his accomplishments! He will receive a certificate (pictured herein) in recognition of the same.

Reference

1. Proto AV. *Radiology* 1998—review and diagnosis please. Radiology 1998; 207:1.

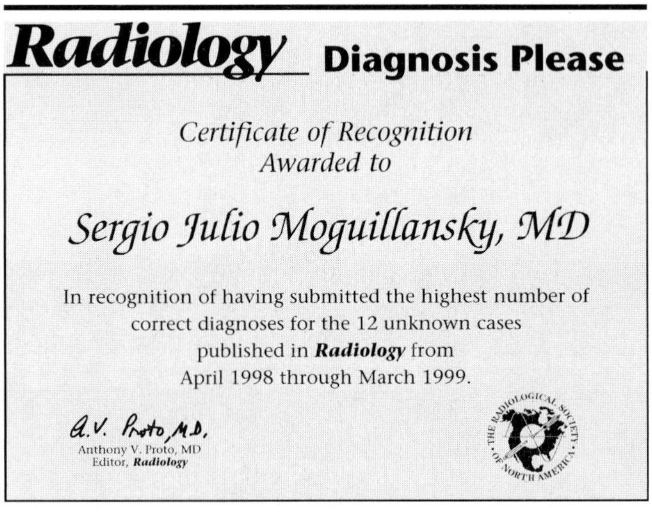

Radiology **Diagnosis Please**

Certificate of Recognition
Awarded to

Sergio Julio Moguillansky, MD

In recognition of having submitted the highest number of correct diagnoses for the 12 unknown cases published in ***Radiology*** from April 1998 through March 1999.

A.V. Proto, M.D.
Anthony V. Proto, MD
Editor, *Radiology*

THE RADIOLOGICAL SOCIETY OF NORTH AMERICA

Index terms:
Diagnosis please
Special reports

Radiology 1999; 212:606

Jerry P. Petasnick, MD, Chairman, Board of Directors
Peggy J. Fritzsche, MD, Liaison for Communications and Corporate Relations

Radiology and Epcot Celebrate New Millennium with a Patient Education and Information Exhibit[1]

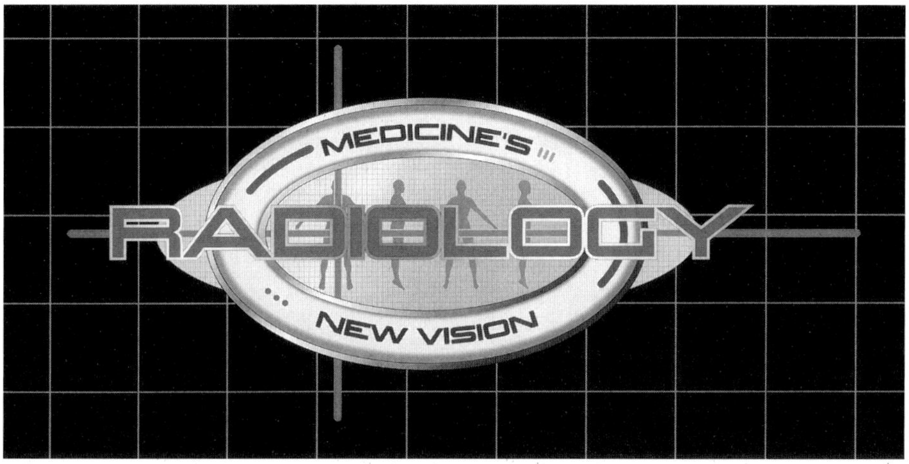

Recognizing that the public's interest in matters related to health care has increased over the past decade, and following a survey of a sample of RSNA members about public information and education materials, in 1998 the Board of Directors decided to expand the Society's public information and education program. The purpose of this expansion is to enhance the public's awareness of radiology and radiologists. Since the Board's decision, the Society has expanded its newsletter, *RSNA News*; developed a public information Web site, *Radiology Resource*; conducted annual campaigns of press releases on focused and timely topics; and issued monthly press releases on articles of general interest from the journal *Radiology*.

Index terms:
Radiological Society of North America
Special communications

Radiology 1999; 212:607–608

[1] From the Radiological Society of North America, 820 Jorie Boulevard, Oak Brook, IL 60523. **Address reprint requests to** J.P.P.

In the same year that the Board began this new public information program, there arose an opportunity to tell 12 million people per year about the contribution of radiology and radiologists to their health care. As part of its Millennium Celebration, the Disney Company planned to feature all new exhibits in the Epcot Innoventions Pavilions and was interested in an exhibit on health care. Through an intermediary, Disney and RSNA learned of their mutual interests—Disney's interest in telling the story of how medical technologies will improve peoples' lives in the new millennium, and the RSNA's particular interest in featuring those who develop and use diagnostic and therapeutic technology, radiologists. Following discussions in the fall of 1998, the RSNA Board of Directors decided to participate in a project with Disney's Epcot theme park to celebrate the millennium.

RSNA accepted the role as the primary sponsor of the exhibit that is designed to showcase radiology and radiologists, not the RSNA. The RSNA Board then appointed an ad hoc committee to oversee the development of the exhibit. The Board's Exhibit Committee includes Peggy J. Fritzsche, MD, as Chair, David B. Fraser, MD, Seymour H. Levitt, MD, and C. Douglas Maynard, MD. The Committee worked with the Epcot creative team, helping to educate them on the practice of radiology and providing direction for the creative development of the exhibit. The Epcot creative team then provided feedback and preliminary plans to the Committee.

The exhibit, tentatively titled, "Radiology: Medicine's New Vision" will occupy 3,002 square feet of space in an Epcot Innoventions exhibit hall. It will be the only exhibit featuring a medical topic. The entry to the exhibit will be similar to the opening of a giant magnetic resonance (MR) imaging machine, with the walkway resembling the carrier table and the entrance resembling the circular portal. Four etched-glass panels on either side of the entrance walkway will display stylized versions of the skeletal, circulatory, and nervous systems, as well as the musculature of the human body.

After passing through the MR portal, guests will enter an area called the Hall of Discovery and Exploration. There they will face a 72-inch video screen that will present a history of radiology and an overview of radiologic procedures and technology.

Following the presentation in the first Hall, the guests will be "pulsed" into a pathway to the 20-foot-high New Horizons Dome. Guests will view six 1½–2-

minute dramatizations of the role of radiologists in patient care. At the conclusion of these presentations, the guests will then exit out of the Dome space and enter the Exploration Zone.

The Exploration Zone will consist of four kiosks: one information kiosk and three interactive play stations. The information kiosk will provide guests the opportunity to visit *Radiology Resource*, the RSNA-ACR patient education Web site (though not in real time). The information kiosk will also be used to explain the training and certification of radiologists, acknowledge exhibit participants, and provide a list of radiologic societies and additional information. The three interactive play stations will feature three games that will convey to players the object of and technology involved in functional imaging of the brain, radiation oncology, and interventional radiology.

The exhibit will be staffed by hosts trained by RSNA and Epcot who will take part in the presentations, answer questions, and inform people about where they can obtain further information.

The cost of the exhibit during the initial year is projected to be $4.15 million. The exhibit will be maintained for an additional 2 years at an annual cost of $1 million. After the first 3 years, there is an option to revise and continue the exhibit for additional years. The RSNA Board has accepted the role as the primary sponsor of this public education/public information exhibit to improve public awareness of radiology and its impact on patient care. But the Board has invited other radiologic societies and commercial entities to participate. There are five levels of participation available: Major Sponsor, Sponsor, Donor, Contributor, and Endorser. A Major Sponsor contributes $1 million or more, a Sponsor contributes between $500,000 and $999,999, a Donor contributes between $100,000 and $499,000, and a Contributor contributes less than $100,000 to support the project. All levels will be acknowledged within the exhibit and in promotional efforts related to the exhibit.

Because the Board of Directors wants the exhibit to represent all of radiology, in order to make that possible for other societies unable to provide financial support, the Board has established the category of "Endorser." Simply, a society can endorse the concept of the Epcot Millennium Celebration Radiology Exhibit, and the society's endorsement will be acknowledged within the exhibit and in promotional efforts. Endorser status is available only to not-for-profit radiologic societies.

The RSNA Board of Directors is happy to announce that the American College of Radiology has become a Sponsor and the American Roentgen Ray Society has become a Contributor for the Radiology Exhibit.

The exhibit is scheduled to open in mid-September for a test run and then to officially open at the end of September 1999, in conjunction with the opening of the Disney Millennium Celebration. We encourage members of the radiology community to visit the exhibit.

Editorial

Ralph Weissleder, MD, PhD

Molecular Imaging: Exploring the Next Frontier[1]

Important developments in molecular sciences in the past decade have provided unprecedented opportunities in genome research (1), an understanding of the molecular mechanisms of disease, and the development of innovative therapies at the genetic level (2). These developments have been made possible, in part, because of automated and accelerated sequencing (3), progress in combinatorial drug development (4,5), the creative use of nonmammalian cells (insect, bacteria, phages, etc) to produce recombinant proteins or peptides, and the development of transgenic animal models (6). In parallel, imaging sciences have undergone remarkable advances over the past 2 decades. Image resolution is constantly improving for virtually all imaging modalities, and some experimental imaging systems already have microscopic-resolution capabilities (7,8). These advances have brought in vivo imaging to the basic sciences, and a flurry of program announcements from the National Institutes of Health (NIH) and other biomedical organizations reflect this progress.

Most traditional cross-sectional imaging techniques such as magnetic resonance (MR) imaging, computed tomography (CT), and ultrasonography (US) are reliant on physical (eg, absorption, scattering, proton density, relaxation rates) and physiologic (eg, blood flow) properties as the main source of contrast for the purposes of disease detection and characterization. Molecular imaging is built on these and other imaging techniques (nuclear, optical imaging) and is aimed at the exploitation of specific molecules as the source of image contrast. This paradigm shift from nonspecific physical to specific molecular sources is the underlying tenet for many of the current molecular imaging research efforts.

The impact of the developing molecular imaging technology is an entire new universe (9) that provides potential for earlier detection and characterization of disease, understanding of biology, and evaluation of treatment. For example, relatively gross parameters of disease (eg, in the case of cancer: tumor burden, anatomic location) could be improved by using more specific parameters (eg, detection of premalignant molecular abnormalities, growth kinetics, angiogenesis growth factors, tumor cell markers, or genetic alterations) (Fig 1). This imaging assessment, in combination with innovative targeted therapies, would allow assessment of therapeutic effectiveness at a molecular level, long before phenotypic changes occur. Molecular in vivo imaging could allow the study of pathogenesis in intact microenvironments of living systems. Finally, molecular imaging has the potential to provide three-dimensional information much faster than is currently possible with time-consuming, labor-intensive, invasive conventional techniques such as histologic analysis.

Overall, it has become clear that our specialty will play an increasingly important role as we develop and apply techniques to image genetic manipulations, to perform in vivo screening of novel drugs, and to understand functional molecular events in living organisms at the cellular and molecular levels (10,11). The aim of this communication is to summarize the prerequisites, recent accomplishments, and challenges in the development of molecular imaging techniques and to illustrate some of the potential applications.

Index terms:
Editorials
Genes and genetics
Magnetic resonance (MR), utilization, **.12149[2]
Radionuclide imaging, **.1217[2]

Radiology 1999; 212:609–614

[1] From the Center for the Molecular Imaging Research, Massachusetts General Hospital, 149 13th St, Charlestown, MA 02129. Received January 22, 1999; revision requested March 16; revision received March 18; accepted March 23. Supported in part by National Institutes of Health grants RO1CA54886, RO1NS35258, ROCA174424, and RO1CA59649. **Address reprint requests to** the author (e-mail: *weissleder@helix.mgh.harvard.edu*).

[2] **. Multiple body systems

Approaches to Molecular Imaging

The key elements (Fig 2) to sampling molecular information are (*a*) the use of special imaging probes with high specificity, (*b*) appropriate amplification strategies, and (*c*) sensitive systems capable of producing images with high resolution (12). For example, in vitro demonstration of messenger RNA requires the use of a complementary probe, an amplification method such as polymerase chain reaction (PCR), and detection systems (Fig 2). Likewise, demonstration of a given protein with immunohistologic methods requires a specific probe (usually an antibody), amplification (avidin-biotin, horseradish peroxidase, etc), and a visualization system such as a microscope. Acquisition of in vitro information has become relatively easy, because thousands of specialty reagents, ligands, protocols, and devices have been commercially developed over the past decade.

In vivo molecular imaging is more challenging than in vitro detection, primarily because of the need for probes to be biocompatible, the presence of additional delivery barriers, and the necessity for developing special in vivo amplification strategies. There are four broad areas in which considerable research efforts will thus be necessary: development of (*a*) suitable in vivo affinity ligands ("mo-

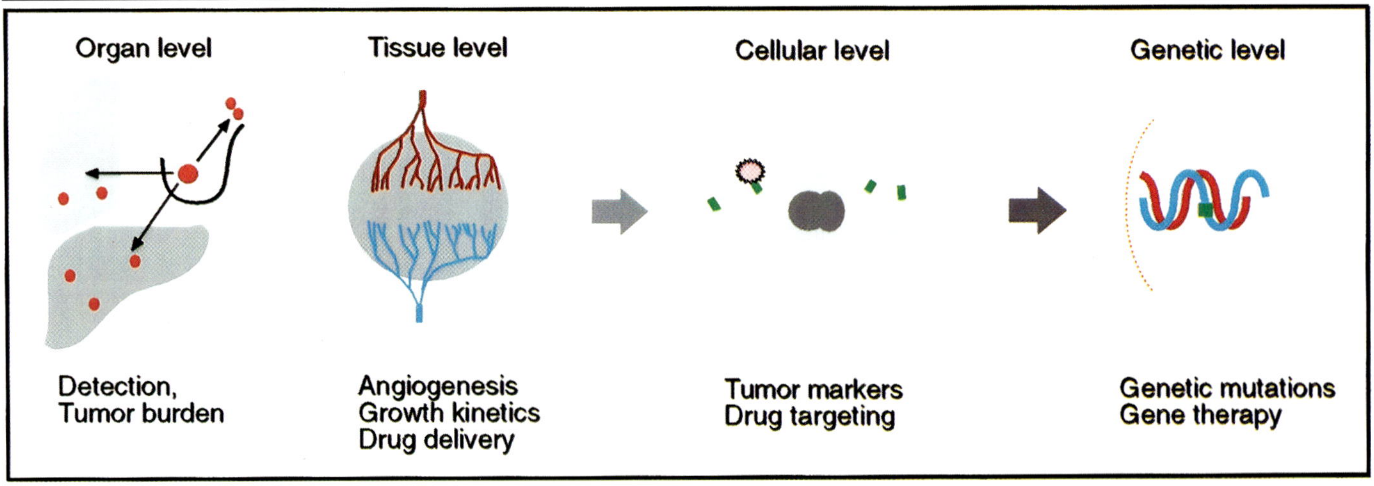

Figure 1. Diagrams show mechanisms for molecular imaging at the organ, tissue, cellular, and genetic levels.

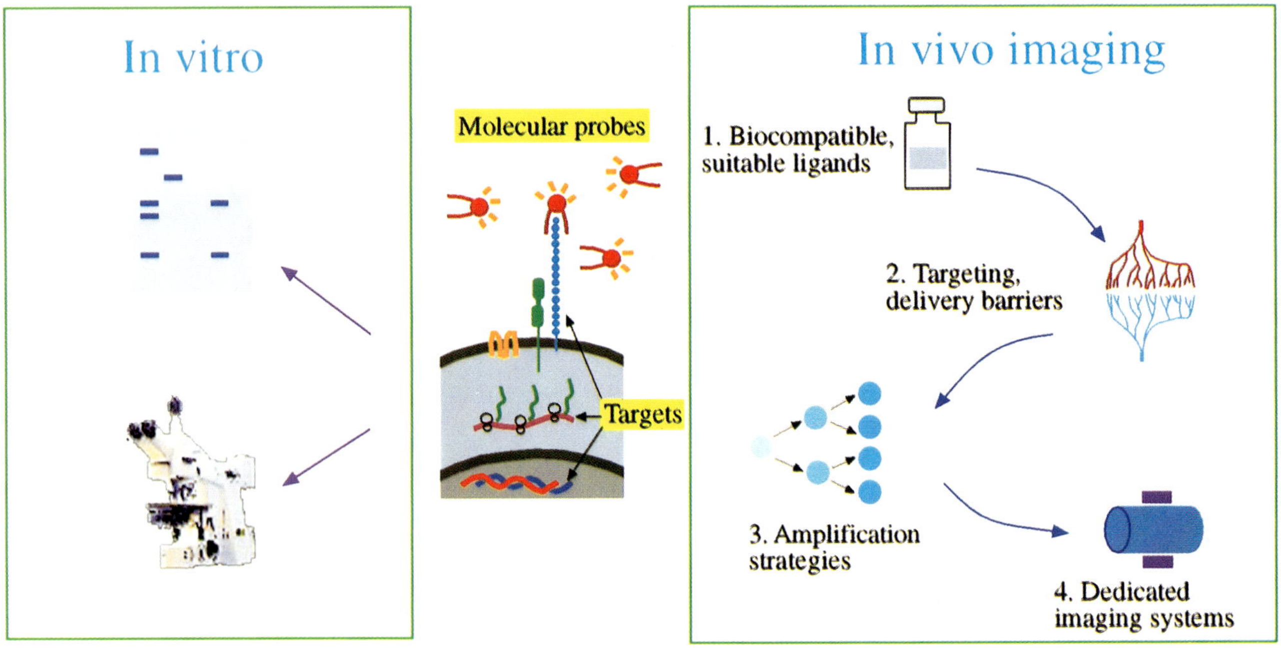

Figure 2. Diagrams show comparison of key elements for in vitro and in vivo molecular imaging.

lecular probes"); (*b*) efficient organ and intracellular targeting strategies; (*c*) amplification strategies, because typical target concentrations are in the pico- to nanomolar range; and (*d*) imaging systems with high spatial resolution and sensitivity (Fig 2). Since the recognition of these requirements (12), considerable developments already have occurred, and the NIH and other national funding agencies have made a considerable commitment to support innovative research in this field.

The most commonly used imaging techniques for extraction of molecular information are nuclear (13–19), MR (20-23), and optical techniques (24–26). Each of these techniques has its particular advantages and disadvantages, and use of one or another technique is mostly dependent on the specific research question and hypothesis to be tested. Positron emission tomography (PET) is frequently used when a substrate to a given target exists that can easily be labeled with a positron emitter, for example labeled 2′-fluoro-5-iodovinyl-1-β-D-arabinofuranosyl-uracil (FIAU) or ganciclovir for imaging of viral thymidine kinase gene expression (13,14,15,19,27). Nuclear imaging techniques also are especially suited to track small amounts of labeled therapeutic drugs (28) and to investigate multiple drug resistance (29,30) or delivery systems such as viral vectors (31).

MR imaging has two particular advantages over techniques that involve the use of isotopes: higher spatial resolution (micrometer rather than several millimeter) (7,32) and the fact that physiologic and anatomic information can be extracted simultaneously. Microscopic MR imaging, in particular, is expected to have a substantial influence in developmental biology, in imaging of transgenic animals, and in cell trafficking (33,34). In comparison with isotope techniques, however, MR imaging is several magnitudes less sensitive (millimolar rather than picomolar), which is why reliable signal ampli-

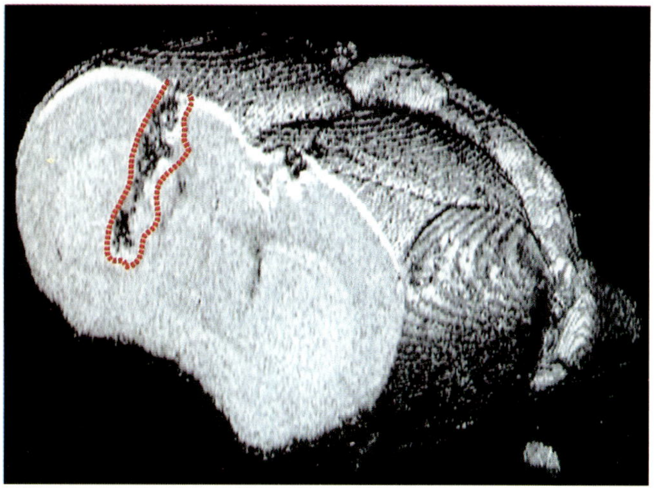

Figure 3. Three-dimensional T1-weighted gradient-echo MR imaging reconstruction (repetition time, 150 msec; echo time, 3.6 msec; flip angle, 34°; voxel size, 39 × 39 × 78 μm) shows tracking of immune cells with magnetically labeled lymphocytes homed to a human glioblastoma tumor (9L tumor model) xenograft in a mouse. Cell were labeled ex vivo by using a magnetic particle with membrane translocation signals (35). Approximately 10,000 cells are distributed throughout the elongated tumor (outlined in red) and cause low MR signal intensity, which is readily detectable. (Imaging was performed in collaboration with Helene Benveniste, MD, PhD, Center for In Vivo Microscopy, Duke Medical Center, Durham, NC.)

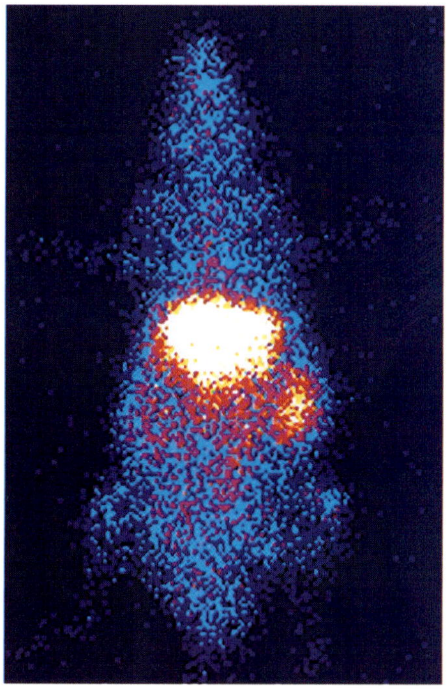

Figure 4. Viral gene delivery. Planar scintigraphic image of the whole-body distribution of a genetically engineered herpes simplex virus utilized for gene delivery in a rat. The indium 111–labeled replication-conditioned virus encoding for β-galactosidase was injected intravenously (150 μCi [5.6 MBq]). Image acquisition time was 5 minutes. Note the predominant viral distribution to liver (white and red areas), which should be useful for gene therapy in this organ (31).

fication strategies must be developed. Recently, cell labeling techniques have been developed (35) that will allow efficient in vivo tracking of stem cells, progenitor cells, or cell lines expressing transgenes (Fig 3), potentially at the single-cell level (33).

Finally, optical imaging techniques have already been developed for applications in molecular and cellular biology (eg, fluorescence microscopy) and in vivo surface imaging (25,36,37). Newer approaches have been advocated that may ultimately lead to the development of tomographic optical imaging systems in the near-infrared spectrum (38,39). One of the appealing advantages of near-infrared optical imaging is that quenched fluorescent labels that become brightly fluorescent after specific molecular interaction with their target can be used (26). Such "beacons" with molecular specificity would be suitable in applications to image enzymes, DNA and/or RNA targets (40), and a variety of other cellular and subcellular targets in vivo. Another notable advantage of optical techniques is the fact that multiple probes with different spectral characteristics can be used for multichannel imaging, similar to in vitro karyotyping (41).

Imaging of Gene Delivery and Expression

There are more than 250 ongoing clinical gene therapy trials in the United States. Radiologic techniques that can assist in such therapies include minimally invasive interventional help in delivering genetic material to its target, determination of the distribution of gene delivery, and imaging of gene expression in vivo (42–44).

Several investigators (43,45) have described the use of stereotactic delivery of viral vectors and subsequent anatomic changes after gene delivery. Direct imaging of gene delivery still is at an experimental level, but methods to label viral vectors such as replication-deficient herpes simplex virus (31) or adenovirus (46) have recently been described. Figure 4 is an example of the first in vivo image of a replication-conditioned herpes simplex virus encoding for β-galactosidase in an animal model. Viral labeling techniques are currently used to help estimate gene delivery to different target organs or cancers and to help evaluate treatment modifiers to improve gene delivery in vivo. Other techniques to track nonviral gene delivery systems also are under development (47).

Imaging of gene expression refers to the depiction of successfully expressed proteins in vivo. Several different types of imaging marker genes have been described and are summarized in the Table. Of all the different systems, the herpes simplex virus–thymidine kinase system has received the greatest attention and, at the time of this writing, is closest to being used in clinical trials (19). This system is based on the observation that intracellularly expressed viral thymidine kinase (but not endogenous mammalian thymidine kinase) acts to phosphorylate therapeutic (eg, ganciclovir) or imaging prodrugs (eg, FIAU labeled with fluorine 18, ^{18}F-ganciclovir), which are no longer cell membrane permeable and thus are "trapped" in cells (Fig 5). The intracellularly converted drugs are detectable with imaging assistance after elimination of precursors.

Similar strategies also are under development with other enzyme or substrate systems. Of particular interest is the enzyme tyrosinase, which is capable of therapeutic anticancer prodrug activation (55,56) and, at the same time, can be detected at MR imaging (20). Given the unique properties of tyrosinase, it should also be feasible to detect tyrosinase activity by means of scintigraphy (57,58), PET (59), or even optical imaging (60). Several other strategies have been proposed (17) to image gene expression with nuclear, MR imaging, and/or optical imaging techniques (Table).

Strategies for Imaging of Gene Expression

Marker Protein*	Imaging Method	Ligand or Substrate	Mechanism
Intracellular			
Thymidine kinase (13,15)	Nuclear	FIAU, ganciclovir	Phosphorylation of prodrug
Cytosine deaminase (48)	Nuclear	Cytosine	Deamination of prodrug
Tyrosinase (20)	Nuclear, MR imaging	Tyrosine, dopa	Oxidation of substrates into melanin or metal scavenging
β-galactosidase (49)	MR imaging	Galactosylated chelators	Cleavage of galactose residues changes relaxivity
Green fluorescent protein (50)	Optical	Not applicable	Fluorescence
Luciferase (25)	Optical	Luciferin	Bioluminescence
Cathepsin D (51)	Optical	Quenched near-infrared fluorescent fluorochromes	Fluorescence activation
Cell surface			
Gastrin-releasing peptide receptor (52)	Nuclear	Bombesin	Affinity binding
Somatostatin receptor (53)	Nuclear	Peptides	Affinity binding
Transferrin receptors (54)	MR imaging	Transferrin	Internalization
Fusion proteins (16)	Nuclear	Oxotechnetate	Transchelation

* Numbers in parentheses are reference numbers.

Imaging of Endogenous Gene Expression

In addition to imaging of transgenes expressed after gene therapy, there is general interest in the demonstration of expression of endogenous genes. Most of the current knowledge of endogenous gene expression and regulation in mammalian systems is limited to results from in vitro studies, which may or may not reflect the in vivo scenario. Such in vitro studies (Northern blot, Western blot, etc) usually require tissue sections, and time-course studies often are impractical. One of the goals in molecular imaging research, therefore, is the development and validation of universal "imaging genes." Such generic "reporters" could then be used to facilitate direct imaging of promoter activity over time.

One specific example of this type of research is in vivo imaging of vascular endothelial growth factor promoter activity "driving" green fluorescent protein expression and imaging of the latter by means of intravital microscopy (50). Recently, variants of green fluorescence protein have been developed that contain additional ligands to bind diagnostic labels such as technetium 99m, so that their expression could also be imaged by using nuclear techniques (16). It is expected that a number of approaches and transgenic animal models will ultimately be developed to assist in the study of key regulatory genes and their expression in vivo.

Early Detection and Molecular Characterization

An exciting application of molecular imaging is the potential to base disease detection on early molecular abnormalities, before diseases become obvious with traditional imaging techniques. Although enticing in concept, examples of this type of application currently are rare. One example however, is the early detection of small breast or prostate cancers on the basis of tumoral expression of tumor-associated enzymes (26). Key enzymes under current investigation are cathepsins, prostate-specific antigen (the interstitial fraction is a protease), and matrix metalloproteases (26). Unlike with traditional targeting approaches, where antibodies or other affinity molecules are used, enzymes offer the possibility to use specific imaging precursors that are not detectable unless they become activated. One of those activation strategies is shown in Figure 6, in which an optically quenched (not detectable), enzyme-specific substrate becomes detectable after enzyme activation in the tumor. In one specific example, it has been shown that breast cancer masses with a diameter of less than 0.3 mm are detectable in xenograft models (26,61). Extensive further research is needed to facilitate development and optimization of this imaging approach.

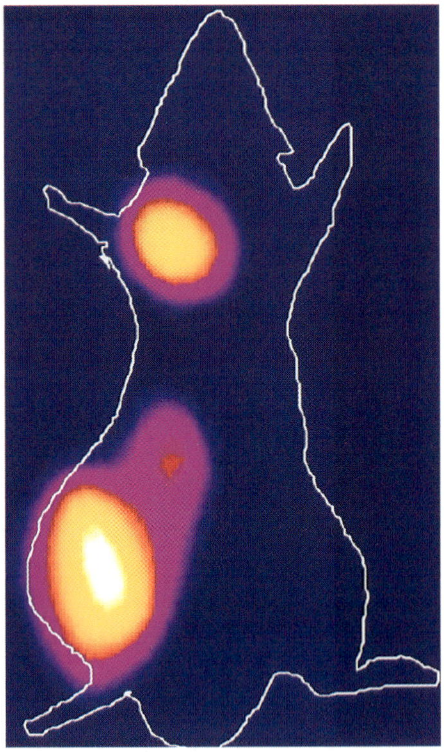

Figure 5. Gene expression. Summed coronal PET image of a rat injected with iodine 124–FIAU, a substrate for viral thymidine kinase. The tracer accumulates in the flank tumor (in vitro–transduced W256-Tk cells) and in the neck tumor (in vivo–transduced W256 tumor). (Reprinted, with permission, from reference 19.)

Imaging of Drug Therapy

Traditional therapeutic drug development has undergone considerable changes with the introduction of different combinatorial and other chemical library approaches. In vivo testing of drug effectiveness has thus become a major bottleneck in drug testing. The use of molecular imaging could be of considerable benefit (*a*) by helping determine the pharmacokinetics and pharmacodynamics of newly developed drugs and (*b*) by facilitating development of early and objective markers before phenotypic changes become obvious. In the ideal

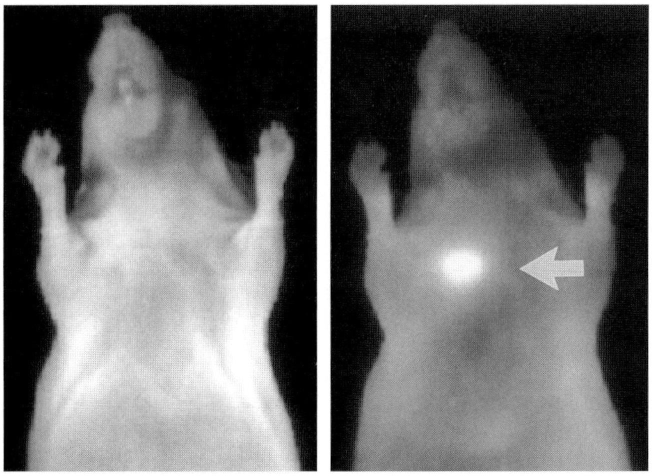

a. b.

Figure 6. Optical imaging of enzyme activity in a human LX1 tumor (2-mm diameter) xenografted into the mammary fat pad of a mouse. **(a)** Light image. **(b)** Raw near-infrared image. Note the bright tumor (arrow in **b**) in the chest. This appearance is due to enzymatic activation of the optically quenched cathepsin imaging probe. (For more information on this type of imaging, see reference 26.)

case, the imaging technique would be used to probe for the specific molecular target against which a therapeutic drug is directed—for example, enzymes, receptors, or signal transduction pathways. Another development in which imaging will have a major effect is the objective assessment of long-term and often expensive drug regimens. Imaging as a monitoring tool could help refine such treatments, potentially leading to reduced risks and cost savings. Finally, imaging has much to offer in terms of the understanding of delivery barriers for newly developed therapeutic agents, particularly large-molecular-weight, particulate, viral, or cellular systems (62).

It is clear that the foregoing is replete with "could," "would," and "potential." On the other hand, the results of successful innovation and feasibility studies are encouraging and give credibility to expectations and theories. The combined imaging possibilities probably were unimaginable 50 years ago and will certainly expand as we enter the new millennium.

Acknowledgments: The author expresses his gratitude to A. Bogdanov, PhD, and J. Wittenberg, MD, for review of the manuscript and colleagues at the Center for Molecular Imaging Research at Massachusetts General Hospital for many helpful discussions.

References

1. Pardee AB. Complete genome expression monitoring: the human race. Nat Biotechnol 1997; 15:1343–1344.
2. Herz JM, Thomsen WJ, Yarbrough GG. Molecular approaches to receptors as targets for drug discovery. J Recept Signal Transduct Res 1997; 17:671–776.
3. James P. Of genomes and proteomes. Biochem Biophys Res Commun 1997; 231: 1–6.
4. Lam KS. Application of combinatorial library methods in cancer research and drug discovery. Anticancer Drug Des 1997; 12:145–167.
5. Burbaum JJ, Sigal NH. New technologies for high-throughput screening. Curr Opin Chem Biol 1997; 1:72–78.
6. Wei LN. Transgenic animals as new approaches in pharmacological studies. Annu Rev Pharmacol Toxicol 1997; 37: 119–141.
7. Johnson GA, Benveniste H, Black RD, Hedlund LW, Maronpot RR, Smith BR. Histology by magnetic resonance microscopy. Magn Reson Q 1993; 9:1–30.
8. Jacobs R, Fraser S. Magnetic resonance microscopy of embryonic cell lineages and movements. Science 1994; 263:681–684.
9. Service RF. New probes open windows on gene expression, and more. Science 1998; 280:1010–1011.
10. Karp J, Broder S. Molecular foundations of cancer: new targets for intervention. Nat Med 1995; 1:309–320.
11. Larson S. Triumph over mischance: a role for nuclear medicine in gene therapy (editorial). J Nucl Med 1997; 38:1230–1233.
12. Weissleder R. Emerging new imaging techniques. Presented at the NCI Imaging Sciences Working Group Meeting, Rockville, Md, 1997.
13. Tjuvajev JG, Stockhammer G, Desai R, et al. Imaging the expression of transfected genes in vivo. Cancer Res 1995; 55:6126–6132.
14. Tjuvajev JG, Finn R, Watanabe K, et al. Noninvasive imaging of herpes virus thymidine kinase gene transfer and expression: a potential method for monitoring clinical gene therapy. Cancer Res 1996; 56:4087–4095.
15. Gambhir SS, Barrio JR, Wu L, et al. Imaging of adenoviral-directed herpes simplex virus type 1 thymidine kinase reporter gene expression in mice with radiolabeled ganciclovir. J Nucl Med 1998; 39:2003–2011.
16. Bogdanov A Jr, Simonova M, Weissleder R. Design of metal-binding green fluorescent protein variants. Biochim Biophys Acta 1998; 1397:56–64.
17. Bogdanov A, Weissleder R. The development of in vivo imaging systems to study gene expression. Trends Biotechnol 1998; 16:5–10.
18. Bogdanov A, Simonova M, Weissleder R. Towards imaging of gene expression: the engineering of metal binding sites. Nat Biotechnol 1997; 8:22.
19. Tjuvajev JG, Avril N, Oku T, et al. Imaging herpes virus thymidine kinase gene transfer and expression by positron emission tomography. Cancer Res 1998; 58:4333–4341.
20. Weissleder R, Simonova M, Bogdanova A, Bredow S, Enochs W, Bogdanov A. MR imaging and scintigraphy of gene expression through melanin induction. Radiology 1997; 204:425–429.
21. Koretsky A. NMR detection of the consequences of transgene expression. News Physiol Sci 1994; 9:197–202.
22. Koretsky A, Lin Y, Schorle H, Jaenisch R. Genetic control of MRI contrast by expression of the transferrin receptor (abstr). In: Proceedings of the Fourth Meeting of the International Society for Magnetic Resonance in Medicine. Berkeley, Calif: International Society for Magnetic Resonance in Medicine, 1996; 5471.
23. Weissleder R, Reimer P, Lee A, Wittenberg J, Brady T. MR receptor imaging: ultrasmall iron oxide particles targeted to asialoglycoprotein receptors. AJR 1990; 155:1161–1167.
24. Benaron D, Stevenson D. Optical time-of-flight and absorbance imaging of biologic media. Science 1993; 259:1463–1466.
25. Contag P, Olomu I, Stevenson D, Contag C. Bioluminescent indicators in living mammals. Nat Med 1998; 4:245–247.
26. Weissleder R, Tung C, Mahmood U, Bogdanov A. In vivo imaging of enzyme activity with activatable near infrared fluorescent probes. Nat Biotechnol 1999; 17: 375–378.
27. Silverman DH, Hoh CK, Seltzer MA, et al. Evaluating tumor biology and oncological disease with positron-emission tomography. Semin Radiat Oncol 1998; 8:183–196.
28. Marriott CJ, Cadorette JE, Lecomte R, Scasnar V, Rousseau J, van Lier JE. High-resolution PET imaging and quantitation of pharmaceutical biodistributions in a small animal using avalanche photodiode detectors. J Nucl Med 1994; 35:1390–1396.
29. Luker GD, Fracasso PM, Dobkin J, Piwnica-Worms D. Modulation of the multidrug resistance P-glycoprotein: detection with technetium-99m-sestamibi in vivo. J Nucl Med 1997; 38:369–372.
30. Crankshaw CL, Marmion M, Luker GD, et al. Novel technetium (III)-Q complexes for functional imaging of multidrug resistance (MDR1) P-glycoprotein. J Nucl Med 1998; 39:77–86.
31. Schellingerhout D, Bogdanov A, Marecos

E, Spear M, Breakefield X, Weissleder R. Mapping the in vivo distribution of herpes simplex virions. Hum Gene Ther 1998; 9:1543–1549.
32. Smith B, Johnson G, Groman E, Linney E. Magnetic resonance microscopy of mouse embryos. Proc Natl Acad Sci USA 1994; 91:3530–3533.
33. Dodd SJ, Williams M, Suhan JP, Williams DS, Korestky A, Ho C. Detection of single mammalian cells by high resolution magnetic resonance imaging. Biophys J 1999; 76:103–109.
34. Schoepf U, Marecos E, Melder R, Jain R, Weissleder R. Intracellular magnetic labeling of lymphocytes for in vivo trafficking studies. Biotechniques 1998; 24:642–651.
35. Josephson L, Tung C, Melder R, Moore A, Weissleder R. High efficiency magnetic cell labeling through Tat peptides. Bioconjug Chem 1999; 10:186–191.
36. Flotte TR, Beck SE, Chesnut K, Potter M, Poirier A, Zolotukhin S. A fluorescence video-endoscopy technique for detection of gene transfer and expression. Gene Ther 1998; 5:166–173.
37. Jain RK. The Eugene M. Landis Award Lecture 1996: delivery of molecular and cellular medicine to solid tumors. Microcirculation 1997; 4:1–23.
38. Wu J, Perelman L, Dasari RR, Feld MS. Fluorescence tomographic imaging in turbid media using early-arriving photons and Laplace transforms. Proc Natl Acad Sci USA 1997; 94:8783–8788.
39. Boas DA, O'Leary MA, Chance B, Yodh AG. Scattering of diffuse photon density waves by spherical inhomogeneities within turbid media: analytic solution and applications. Proc Natl Acad Sci USA 1994; 91:4887–4891.
40. Tyagi S, Kramer FR. Molecular beacons: probes that fluoresce upon hybridization. Nat Biotechnol 1996; 14:303–308.
41. Liyanage M, Coleman A, de Manoir S, et al. Multicolor spectral karyotyping of mouse chromosomes. Nat Genet 1996; 14:312–315.
42. Mulligan RC. The basic science of gene therapy. Science 1993; 260:926–932.
43. Thomas J, Kuo M, Chawla M, et al. Vascular gene therapy. RadioGraphics 1998; 18:1373–1394.
44. Voss S, Kruskal J. Gene therapy: a primer for radiologists. RadioGraphics 1998; 18: 1343–1372.
45. Boviatsis EJ, Chase M, Wei MX, et al. Gene transfer into experimental brain tumors mediated by adenovirus, herpes simplex virus, and retrovirus vectors. Hum Gene Ther 1994; 5:183–191.
46. Zinn KR, Douglas JT, Smyth CA, et al. Imaging and tissue biodistribution of 99mTc-labeled adenovirus knob (serotype 5). Gene Ther 1998; 5:798–808.
47. de Marco G, Bogdanov A, Marecos E, Moore A, Simonova M, Weissleder R. MR imaging of gene delivery to the central nervous system with an artificial vector. Radiology 1998; 208:65–71.
48. Haberkorn U, Oberdorfer F, Gebert J, et al. Monitoring gene therapy with cytosine deaminase: in vitro studies using tritiated-5-fluorocytosine. J Nucl Med 1996; 37:87–94.
49. Moats RA, Fraser SE, Meade TJ. A "smart" magnetic resonance imaging agent that reports on specific enzymatic activity. Angew Chem Int Ed Engl 1997; 36:726–731.
50. Fukumura D, Xavier R, Sugiura T, et al. Tumor induction of VEGF promoter activity in stromal cells. Cell 1998; 94:715–725.
51. Tung C, Mahmood U, Bredow S, Bogdanov A, Weissleder R. A cathepsin D sensitive near infrared fluorescence probe for in vivo imaging of enzyme activity. Bioconjug Chem (in press).
52. Rogers B, Rosenfeld M, Khazaeli M, et al. Localization of iodine-125-mIP-Des-Met14-bombesin (7-13)NH2 in ovarian carcinoma induced to express the gastrin releasing peptide receptor by adenoviral vector-mediated gene transfer. J Nucl Med 1997; 38:1221–1229.
53. Zinn K, Buchsbaum D, Mountz J, et al. Application of type 2 human somatostatin receptor (hSSTr2) as a reporter for imaging gene transfer. Presented at the Sixth International Conference of Anticancer Research, Kallithea, Greece, October 21–25, 1998.
54. Moore A, Basilion J, Chiocca A, Weissleder R. Measuring transferrin receptor gene expression by NMR imaging. Biochim Biophys Acta 1998; 1402:239–249.
55. Pankovich JM, Jimbow K, Ito S. 4-S-cysteaminylphenol and its analogues as substrates for tyrosinase and monoamine oxidase. Pigment Cell Res 1990; 3:146–149.
56. Jimbow K, Iwashina T, Alena F, Yamada K, Pankovich J, Umemura T. Exploitation of pigment biosynthesis pathway as a selective chemotherapeutic approach for malignant melanoma. J Invest Dermatol 1993; 100(suppl 2):231S–238S.
57. Enochs WS, Petherick P, Bogdanova A, Mohr U, Weissleder R. Paramagnetic metal scavenging by melanin: MR imaging. Radiology 1997; 204:417–423.
58. Agui T, Bryant G, Kebabian JW, et al. 125I-iodinated benzazepines bind to melanin: implications for the noninvasive localization of pigmented melanomas. Int J Rad Appl Instrum B 1987; 14:133–141.
59. van Langevelde A, van der Molen HD, Journee-de Korver JG, Paans AM, Pauwels EK, Vaalburg W. Potential radiopharmaceuticals for the detection of ocular melanoma. III. A study with 14C and 11C labelled tyrosine and dihydroxyphenylalanine. Eur J Nucl Med 1988; 14:382–387.
60. Rajadhyaksha M, Grossman M, Esterowitz D, Webb RH, Anderson RR. In vivo confocal scanning laser microscopy of human skin: melanin provides strong contrast. J Invest Dermatol 1995; 104:946–952.
61. Mahmood U, Tung C, Bogdanov A, Weissleder R. Near infrared optical imaging of protease activity allows tumor detection. Radiology (in press).
62. Jain R. Delivery of molecular medicine to solid tumors. Science 1996; 271:1079–1080.

Spiral CT Angiography of the Pulmonary Circulation[1]

Martine Remy-Jardin, MD, PhD
Jacques Remy, MD

Index terms:
Computed tomography (CT), angiography, 944.12916, 945.12916
Computed tomography (CT), helical, 944.12915, 945.12915
Computed tomography (CT), volume rendering, 944.12917, 945.12917
Embolism, pulmonary, 60.72, 944.77
Lung neoplasms, CT, 60.30
Pulmonary arteries, CT, 944.12916
Pulmonary veins, 945.12915
State-of-art reviews

Radiology 1999; 212:615–636

Abbreviations:
AVM = arteriovenous malformation
MIP = maximum intensity projection
MPR = multiplanar reformation
PE = pulmonary embolism
SSD = shaded surface display
STS = sliding thin slab
V-P = ventilation-perfusion
3D = three-dimensional

[1] From the Department of Radiology, Hospital Calmette, Boulevard Jules Leclerc, 59037 Lille, France. Received October 6, 1998; revision requested November 24; revision received January 5, 1999; accepted April 6. **Address reprint requests to** M.R.J. (e-mail: *mremy-jardin@chru-lille.fr*).

Spiral computed tomographic (CT) angiography of the pulmonary circulation has emerged recently as a potential useful diagnostic method for the evaluation of the pulmonary circulation. As a minimally invasive examination, this technique is becoming widely available and has progressively replaced conventional and digital pulmonary angiography as the standard diagnostic imaging modality of the pulmonary circulation. The purpose of this review is to capture the current state of the art of the technical aspects of spiral CT angiography, with special emphasis on the postprocessing techniques currently available. As CT is responsible for a considerable part of the medical radiation dose applied to the population, the current trends for dose saving will also be emphasized. With regard to the clinical applications of spiral CT angiography, its introduction into the diagnostic work-up of pulmonary embolism has considerably modified the diagnostic algorithms. Our 8-year review of the literature presented herein is expected to provide the readers with a basis for formulating an informed opinion on this topic. In addition, a large number of congenital and acquired disorders of the pulmonary circulation are also relevant to this technique, and these indications are discussed in the context of the corresponding therapeutic options. Owing to the multiple possibilities inherent to this technique, spiral CT has the potential for cost savings without reduction in image quality or diagnostic accuracy.

Several less-invasive modern technologies have largely replaced invasive procedures such as angiography for imaging of the pulmonary arteries. These techniques have the advantage of short exposure times and the ability to create three-dimensional (3D) data sets that have greater diagnostic possibilities than do standard projection angiographic images. Contrast material–enhanced spiral computed tomography (CT) provides these advantages. Since its introduction in the early 1990s, spiral CT angiography of the pulmonary circulation has progressively gained widespread acceptance, enabling one not only to obtain uniform and nearly constant opacification of pulmonary vessels down to 2–3 mm in diameter, but also to analyze the peripheral pulmonary vasculature with more precise anatomic details than those available with conventional angiographic studies.

The purpose of this article is to review the current clinical applications of spiral CT in the evaluation of a variety of congenital and acquired disorders of the pulmonary circulation, except the systemic arterial supply of the lung parenchyma. Although these disorders represent an increasing indication for spiral CT angiography in clinical practice, to our knowledge each specific indication has not been systematically evaluated in the literature. Therefore, in addition to a review of the available literature, several specific indications of this imaging modality will be suggested in the context of their expected clinical interest.

TECHNICAL APPROACH

Nonenhanced CT Examination

As reported for the evaluation of many vessels, spiral CT angiography of the pulmonary arteries results from a focal spiral CT examination that is usually preceded by nonenhanced CT scanning over the entire thorax. The value of this preliminary CT examination is threefold. First, it enables analysis of the lung parenchyma, pleura, and chest wall for associated abnormalities. Second, nonenhanced scans are helpful for identifying calcified lesions such as hilar lymph nodes (which could hamper analysis of contrast-enhanced CT scans) or calcified thrombi (which could be missed on contrast-enhanced images). Third, the preliminary CT examination enables an accurate localization of the anatomic volume of interest before spiral CT scanning. This preliminary CT examination can be performed with a conventional or spiral acquisition. When using the spiral mode, scanning with a low-dose technique is strongly recommended; this technique includes the selection of a pitch of 2 (especially when a subsecond scanning time is available), use of the lowest milliamperage available, and use of breast protection for young female patients. Although 180° interpolation and narrow beam collimation is ideal for a subsecond unit with the latest x-ray tube generating higher heat capacity, it should be emphasized that image noise in old spiral units with these parameters may substantially degrade the image.

Spiral CT Protocol

As recently reported by Fishman (1), the current challenges regarding CT angiography can be divided into three categories: data acquisition, data processing, and data display. For each step, several parameters have to be considered by the radiologist at the console to optimize the final display, as further detailed.

Acquisition Parameters

Scanning a distance of 10–12 cm (from the aortic arch to 2 cm below the level of the inferior pulmonary veins), enables imaging of central and peripheral pulmonary arteries of the upper, middle, and lower lobes during the CT sequence in every patient. This region-of-interest may be covered by scanning the patient in the craniocaudal direction or scanning in the caudocranial direction. In clinical practice, the direction of the table feed is not a major issue, as it does not influence the overall quality of the spiral CT examination. More important is the selection of the region to be surveyed in order to precisely include the target vasculature within the volume scanned.

The radiologist must select the collimation and the speed of the table feed with two imperatives in mind. The first is to find the optimal compromise between the patient's respiratory status and the breath-holding duration necessary for evaluation of the pulmonary vasculature in a single CT acquisition. The second objective is to scan the patient with the thinnest collimation possible, to reduce partial volume effects. This second point is of great concern for an accurate evaluation of the peripheral pulmonary arteries. During the past few years, modification of the interpolation algorithms and introduction of subsecond scanning times have considerably modified the spatial resolution of spiral CT. The older technique of scanning with 5-mm collimation and a pitch of 1 and reconstructing the images with a 360° linear interpolation algorithm resulted in an effective section thickness of 6.57 mm. Consequently, the main drawback was partial volume effects at the level of small vessels, thus limiting the evaluation of peripheral pulmonary abnormalities (2–5). With selection of a 180° linear interpolation algorithm and a subsecond scanning time, the effective section thickness is of 3.86 mm when scanning with 3-mm collimation and a pitch of 1.7; the effective section thickness is reduced to 2.65 mm with the use of 2-mm collimation and a pitch of 2. Applied to the evaluation of the pulmonary circulation, use of 3-mm collimation was found to improve spatial resolution at the level of segmental arteries as suggested by a lower number of peripheral arterial branches coded as nonanalyzable (6). The recent availability of subsecond scanning times has made it possible to select a thinner collimation and to scan with a pitch of 2 without any modification in the breath-hold duration or the anatomic coverage. This protocol was shown to allow marked improvement in the analysis of segmental and subsegmental pulmonary arteries (7).

It is strongly recommended that patients be scanned while they maintain strict apnea. Interpretable images might possibly be obtained while the patient is gently breathing, but this should be reserved for only those patients with severe lung impairment. However, this latter acquisition condition is associated with two main limitations: a confident evaluation of the pulmonary circulation limited to central vessels and the inability to generate high-quality multiplanar and/or 3D reformations. Whenever possible, patients should be scanned at total lung capacity owing to the direct relationship between the degree of arterial opacification and the level of pulmonary arterial resistance. Physiologic studies have demonstrated that pulmonary resistance increases at high states of lung inflation because lung inflation causes the small alveolar vessels to be compressed (8,9). The end result is an increase in the resistance to flow in all the vessels exposed to alveolar pressure, which facilitates high-quality arterial opacification. Obtaining a deep inspiration may be difficult for patients suspected of having PE. In such situations, several physiologic considerations suggest that the patient should stop breathing near end-expiration, which can also achieve high levels of pulmonary resistance and thus good arterial opacification (8,9). Intubated patients referred from intensive care units can benefit from a spiral CT evaluation of the pulmonary circulation. The overall quality of these examinations may be excellent as it is possible to manually suspend ventilation for 15–20 seconds in deep inspiration while the patient is sedated, thus avoiding motion artifacts.

Contrast Material Administration

The objective of the spiral protocol is to start scanning while the target vascular structures are opacified and to ensure a constant degree of pulmonary arterial opacification during the entire spiral sequence. An adequate examination of the pulmonary arteries requires the radiologist to select the most appropriate contrast agent and timing of injection, while carefully monitoring venous access. A power injection is mandatory for obtaining a homogeneous and constant level of arterial enhancement through the entire spiral examination. However, because of the rapid administration of contrast material, care must be taken to carefully adapt the rate of injection to the site of administration, especially when selecting high-flow protocols. In most spiral CT examinations, an 18- or 20-gauge catheter is inserted into a medially located antecubital vein, through which the bolus of contrast material is safely injected at a rate varying between 2 and 5 mL/sec. When an antecubital vein is not accessible, a more peripheral venous access can be used but care must be taken to avoid extravasation from a small and fragile peripheral vein. This requires reducing the rate of injection and increasing the start delay by 4–6 seconds. When a central venous access is available as frequently observed for patients referred from intensive care units, verifying the maximum rate of injection acceptable for a given catheter (often 4–5 mL/sec) is recommended. Because of the central location of the tip of the catheter, usually at the level of the superior vena cava, a shorter scanning delay is selected, which results in a shorter injection period.

The combination of an automated injection of contrast medium with the use of spiral CT enables an excellent quality of arterial opacification while using a smaller amount of iodine than previously recommended with sequential CT. Several approaches have been reported for the evaluation of pulmonary vessels with spiral CT, either selecting a low concentration–high flow protocol or a high concentration–low flow protocol. The low concentration–high flow protocol consists in injecting 150–240 mg/mL contrast agent at a rate of 4–5 mL/sec, whereas a high concentration–low flow protocol uses 300–350 mg/mL iodinated contrast agent administered at 2–3 mL/sec. In patients with normal right ventricular outflow, a 12–15-second scanning delay usually provides sufficient latitude so that the pulmonary arteries are almost always well opacified. For patients with right ventricular failure and patients with pulmonary hypertension, a longer scanning delay is required, varying from 15 to 18 seconds. In most cases, an empiric determination of the scanning delay is sufficient to obtain excellent arterial enhancement. An alternative is to monitor contrast enhancement visually or with densitometry during the early stages of contrast material injection. This method provides a mechanism by which the time of scanning initiation can be individualized on the basis of actual enhancement of anatomic structures. When a desired level of enhancement is reached for a particular structure, transition is made to a routine diagnostic spiral imaging series. This technique is mainly indicated for patients with pulmonary hypertension and/or right ventricular failure. Although back-to-back helical scans are available, the interval of time between the two acquisitions is not compatible with adequate intravascular levels of enhancement within pulmonary branches over time.

Image Reconstruction

A brief summary of the technical peculiarities of the postprocessing techniques currently applicable to the pulmonary circulation is presented below.

Transverse CT scans.—From each data set, transverse CT scans are systematically reconstructed. Creation of overlapping reconstructions is of major importance when scanning with a 5-mm collimation to avoid interpretive difficulties due to volume averaging effects. Owing to the considerable improvement in spatial resolution when scanning with a 2-mm collimation, reconstruction of contiguous sections is now widely accepted. An economic parameter (ie, the number of hard-copy films necessary to photograph overlapping images in a 2-mm collimation protocol) is the second major reason for generating contiguous images. Cost-reduction efforts regarding use of film by laser printers connected to spiral CT scanners are a challenge facing many medical centers. Consequently, reconstruction of overlapping sections from data sets acquired with thin collimation should be limited to the anatomic levels showing equivocal findings, namely, helping to distinguish an endoluminal clot from a partial volume effect with the arterial wall.

Multiplanar reformation.—This technique is most commonly used to obtain sagittal or coronal views of transverse CT data sets, but it also can be valuable to provide oblique or curvilinear views of CT data sets. Multiplanar reformation (MPR) images completely eliminate superimposition of pixels lying outside the selected plane, and all the attenuation values included in the reformatted plane are visualized. With most available software programs, reformation planes are defined by projecting a line on one of the transverse sections so that the resultant MPR images will be perpendicular to the transverse plane and parallel to the projected line. MPR may also be planned on frontal or profile scout views. These planar reformations, having a single obliquity relative to the x, y, and z axes, do not take into account the orientation of the more cranial and caudal parts of the structure to be imaged. Whenever the structure of interest is not strictly parallel to the chosen plane, its changing orientations will not be considered in the final image. Consequently, inaccurately selected MPR may lead to erroneous interpretations, either due to the omission of part of the lesion or to the creation of a pseudoabnormality. When a structure of interest requires optimal double oblique planar views, the adequate plane of reformation of this structure can be chosen on a 3D image. Another alternative is to determine the plane of reformation by a direct selection of the voxels located at the center of the vascular lumen.

Three-dimensional images.—Acquisition of the entire thorax within a single breath hold must be considered as a volumetric acquisition that offers multiple visualization techniques, which can be classified either according to their rendering, their projectional, or their computer-based image processing capabilities. As pointed out by Brink (10), a quality 3D image requires a combination of narrow section collimation and small intersection data reconstruction. As section thickness is a key factor, one should systematically envision the utility of a 3D reconstruction before selection of the acquisition protocol to be able to generate high-quality 3D images.

Until now, maximum intensity projection (MIP) has been the most popular method of obtaining 3D CT angiographic images (11,12). The MIP technique depicts the highest pixel value along the observer's line of sight and is particularly well suited for displaying small subvolumes in which superimposition of structures does not occur or is eliminated by editing procedures. However, several drawbacks have to be mentioned. The most important one is the inability to provide images of diagnostic quality when evaluating complex anatomic situations with superimposition of structures of interest. The depth information is absent unless a cine mode display with slightly varying viewing angles is used. According to the specificity of this technique for selection of voxels of interest, it is important to keep in mind that MIP does not enable the visualization of hypoattenuating intraluminal filling defects such as pulmonary emboli unless they are in close contact with the vessel wall.

The most frequently used 3D reconstruction of the pulmonary circulation is obtained with surface-rendering techniques. The shaded surface display (SSD) depicts the outer contour of the column of contrast material as an opaque surface. The main hallmark of SSD images is the thresholding segmentation that results in a binary classification of the voxels. Two categories of voxels are taken into account for the reformatted image: voxels higher than a user-selected single threshold or voxels included within a double-thresholding segmentation. For 3D SSD images of the pulmonary vasculature generated from nonenhanced data sets, the threshold values range from −600 to −700 HU. Should contrast medium be used, the thresholding segmentation has to be changed from −700 HU to +100 to 150 HU. Four categories of pitfalls can be encountered with this technique of reconstruction (13). The first group concerns the pitfalls related to the thresholding range, explaining why the stenosed part of a tubular structure can be artificially narrowed with too high a threshold or artificially minimized with too low a threshold. In such cases, an additional 3D display should be systematically performed with a lower or a higher thresholding segmentation, respectively, to avoid interpretive errors. However, low threshold values create a complex vascular background that may prevent optimal viewing of the vessel of interest, explaining why this kind of selection is usually obtained at second intention. The second group of pitfalls is related to the section thickness, either responsible for partial volume artifacts or stair-step artifacts. The third category of pitfalls may be caused by motion during data acquisition, either because of the patient's inability to maintain strict apnea or because of organ pulsation. The last group of pitfalls is related to contrast enhancement, which may be variable along the z axis.

The most recently introduced technique for creating angiographic-like images of the pulmonary vasculature is the volume-rendering technique. In this technique, classification of the voxels estimates the probability of a tissue type being homogeneously present in a voxel and attributes to this voxel a percentage corresponding to the amount of this tissue. This classification mode is called percentage classification or probabilistic classification, and a trapezoid is attributed to each tissue type (14). Several parameters have to be selected to generate volume-rendering technique reconstructions: (*a*) position of the trapezoid, which determines the attenuation of voxels incorporated into the image (this selection consists of defining a window width and a window level [15]); (*b*) shape of the trapezoid, corresponding to the intersections between the sides of the trapezoid and the top; (*c*) opacity value, which determines the relative transparency of the voxels incorporated into the image, and thus the degree of vascular transparency; and (*d*) shading option (not systematically available on volume-rendering programs), which modifies the vessel wall smoothness. Preliminary evaluation of the volume-rendering technique at the level of the pulmonary circulation has led to the selection of the following parameters: triangular trapezoid shape, selection of voxels from −750 to −450 HU for nonenhanced vessels and from 50 to 200 HU for enhanced vessels, 80% opacity value, and unshaded algorithm (authors' unpublished data, 1997). This selection was found to create diagnostically useful images of the pulmonary circulation, easily applicable in clinical practice. With continued advances in computer technology, interactive volume-rendering techniques soon will be widely available, an imperative for further evaluation of this technique at the level of the pulmonary circulation and rigorous comparison with alternative reconstruction techniques (16).

Slabs.—The delineation of peripheral pulmonary vessels is facilitated by the low attenuation of the surrounding lung parenchyma, explaining why their analysis does not systematically require injection of contrast medium. With regard to the technical particularities of a spiral CT evaluation of the peripheral vascular bed, one should mention the usefulness of generating slabs from nonenhanced focal spiral CT examinations. On cross-sectional images, a linear or tubular structure obliquely oriented or perpendicular to the plane of the CT section is segmented proportionally to the section thickness. Conversely, the stacking of several contiguous transverse images allows one to benefit from the advantages of the summation effect, thus enabling an easy identification of a pulmonary vessel in its entirety from the hilum to the periphery. Further anatomic details can be obtained when thin-slab MIP with or without automatic sliding in the acquired volume as well as targeted SSD images are obtained. The most frequently used technique is called sliding thin-slab (STS) MIP, which consists of an automatic sliding through the volume of interest (17). Because the selection of a narrow collimation is mandatory for high-quality reconstructions, care should be taken to precisely determine the volume to be scanned, usually limited to 2–3 cm.

Current Trends for Dose Saving

Because CT is responsible for a considerable part of the medical radiation dose applied to the population, concerted efforts are being made to minimize the dose required for a spiral CT examination without making compromises in image quality. To reach this goal at the level of the thorax, several recommendations can be made. First, a decreased kilovoltage can be easily applied to routine spiral CT angiography of the pulmonary circulation and the milliamperage setting can be individually selected. The use of subsecond scanning and the selection of a pitch of 2 are two additional efficient means of reducing the radiation dose. Moreover, dose modulation methods have been recently developed by manufacturers; these methods enable the tube current and hence the dose applied to be adjusted to the individual patient's geometry and patient's absorption during the acquisition. From preliminary evaluations, dose savings of up to 40% are obtained, depending on the patient and the examined region of the thorax (18). As recently proposed by Hopper et al (19), the use of thin layers of radiation absorbent material such as bismuth can provide breast radiation protection to women without affecting the quality of diagnostic CT images. These authors emphasized the seriousness of the dose administered to such a radiosensitive organ, reminding us that a woman's breast receives 2.0–3.5 rad (0.020–0.035 Gy) of radiation from a thoracic CT examination. To emphasize the importance of this radiation dose, one should keep in mind that delivery of 1 rad (0.01 Gy) of radiation to a woman's breasts before age 35 years fractionally increases her risk of breast cancer by 13.6% over the expected spontaneous rate for the general population.

CLINICAL INDICATIONS: ACQUIRED DISEASES

Pulmonary Embolism

Diagnosis of Acute Pulmonary Embolism

CT features and pitfalls.—Until the early 1990s, the standard diagnostic imaging procedures for evaluation of pulmonary embolism (PE) were ventilation-perfusion (V-P) scintigraphy and pulmonary angiography. During the past few years, there has been a progressive replacement of pulmonary angiography with spiral CT angiography, as the latter imaging procedure allows a noninvasive identification of intravascular clots. The CT criteria for acute PE are the tomographic equivalent of the classic angiographic signs of PE (ie, partial or complete filling defects and the "railway track" signs) (Figs 1, 2). In terms of contrast material administration, the drawbacks of the high concentration–low flow protocol argue for the use of the low concentration–high flow protocol in the evaluation of PE. The injection of a highly concentrated material usually results in streak artifacts at the level of the superior vena cava, which can substantially degrade quality in the adjacent right main pulmonary artery but also the right upper lobe pulmonary artery and its segmental branches. At the level of these branches, this may hamper detection of intraluminal changes. Although the low rate of injection recommended with this protocol is usually sufficient for depicting large emboli, it is not always compatible with the identification of emboli at the level of segmental arteries and precludes any detection of subsegmental emboli. The ideal concentration of contrast material for low concentration–high flow protocols has not yet been definitely determined, to our knowledge, but many users agree to consider a 150–200 mg/mL concentration.

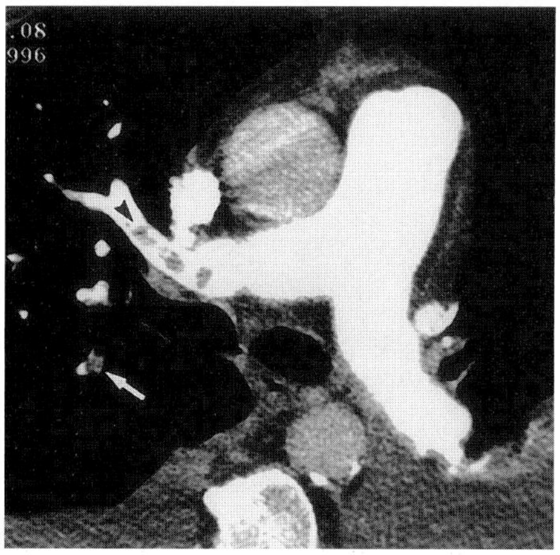

Figure 1. Spiral CT scan (2-mm collimation, pitch of 2, 24% iodinated contrast agent) obtained at the level of the right upper lobe in a 65-year-old patient with acute onset of dyspnea. There are multiple partial filling defects at the level of the anterior (arrowhead) and posterior (arrow) segmental arteries of the right upper lobe. Note the additional presence of bilateral pleural effusion.

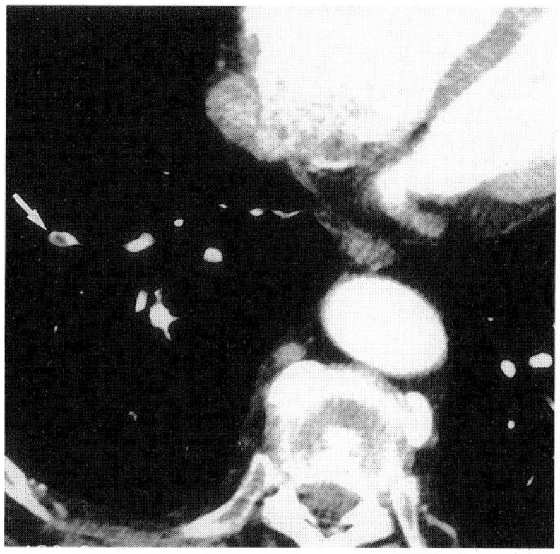

Figure 2. Spiral CT scan (2-mm collimation, pitch of 2, 24% iodinated contrast agent) obtained at the level of the lower lobes in a 70-year-old patient with a previous history of severe chronic obstructive pulmonary disease and acute dyspnea at the time of diagnosis. There is a partial filling defect (arrow) at the level of a subsegmental branch of the anterior segmental artery of the right lower lobe.

Two recent technical aspects of spiral CT angiography of PE are worth considering: the optimization of display window settings and the development of combined CT venography and pulmonary angiography. Although large thrombi are always easily detected on transverse CT scans, some partial-filling defects may be obscured by dense contrast material when standard mediastinal window settings are used. These practical difficulties have led Brink et al (20) to undertake an experimental study aimed at determining optimal display window settings for depiction of acute PE with spiral CT. These authors concluded that pulmonary emboli are best depicted as filling defects when displayed with a modified window referenced to the attenuation of the right and left main pulmonary arteries. As it is usually accepted that PE and venous thrombosis are different aspects of the same continuum, namely, thromboembolic disease, Loud et al (21) recently reported their experience with a CT protocol that examines the subdiaphragmatic deep venous system at the time of spiral CT angiography of the pulmonary circulation. Without additional contrast medium or separate venipuncture, the veins of the legs, pelvis, and abdomen are imaged with the venous opacification that follows the rapid infusion of contrast medium for the evaluation of the pulmonary circulation. Whereas previous studies have exclusively evaluated the vascular signs of acute PE, the value of lung parenchymal and pleural findings at contrast-enhanced spiral CT was only reported by Coche et al (22) in a study group of 88 patients with clinical suspicion of acute PE. The authors concluded that the ancillary signs of wedge-shaped pleural-based consolidation, linear bands, and dilated central or segmental pulmonary arteries were statistically significantly associated with PE. Consequently, identification of these features at CT may be useful to direct further investigations when there is suboptimal visualization of central or segmental vessels.

A number of interpretive pitfalls exist in assessing enhanced spiral CT images, but their recognition is less and less problematic as the radiologist gains experience with spiral CT of the pulmonary vasculature (23). Four main categories of technical or pathophysiologic factors may be responsible for pseudo–filling defects. In severely tachypneic patients, breathing artifacts may be observed at the level of obliquely oriented arteries due to the variable position of the vessel in the section width in two successive scans. Consequently, any abrupt decreased attenuation at the level of a given arterial section between two contiguous sections should not be mistaken for an arterial filling defect. The choice of the scanning delay may also influence the quality of arterial enhancement at the top or bottom of the scanned volume. If the scanning delay is too short, there is insufficient time to allow adequate opacification of the pulmonary arteries on the first images. On the other hand, if the scanning delay is too long, there is not enough material left at the bottom of the selected subvolume, which may hamper detection of intraluminal thrombi. Physiologic data must also be integrated in the spiral volumetric CT evaluation of vascular enhancement. Several cases of unilateral increased pulmonary vascular resistance due to extensive airspace consolidation have led to a false-positive diagnosis of PE (2,4). The asymmetric pulmonary vascular resistance results in asymmetry of arterial perfusion due to slow flow through the pulmonary arteries ipsilateral to the lung consolidation, with normally circulating contralateral pulmonary arteries. Any cause of unilateral increased vascular resistance may lead to asymmetry in pulmonary arterial opacification. The various causes of nonopacification or faint unilateral opacification of a pulmonary artery that have been previously described on conventional angiograms and lung V-P scans (24,25) can be summarized as follows: (*a*) "occult" pulmonary artery; (*b*) unilateral pulmonary artery obstruction of extrinsic, mural, or endoluminal origin; (*c*) unilateral increase in pulmonary vascular resistance secondary to proximal or distal bronchial obstruction, bronchiolar obstruction, parenchymal destruction, extensive airspace consolidation, pleural restrictive or expansive process, or conditions with elevated venous pressure; and (*d*) congenital and acquired hemithoracic shunting of blood from the systemic to the pulmonary circulation.

The best way to demonstrate on CT scans the patency of a unilateral faintly opacified pulmonary artery is to perform a second spiral CT acquisition with a longer scanning delay to suppress flow phenomena at the level of this vessel. There are acquired disorders that are associated with anatomic or surgical shunting from the systemic to pulmonary circulation and that are thus responsible for antegrade or retrograde left-to-right shunts. This situation results in regional or unilateral changes in pulmonary blood flow that is interrupted at the level of the anatomic communication between the systemic and pulmonary circulations. The most common clinical situation is represented by patients with severe chronic inflammatory disease, particularly those with bronchiectasis, in whom prominent bronchopulmonary collateral circulation may develop and produce a proximal retrograde flow. In these patients, nonvisualization of arteries or dilution de-

TABLE 1
Accuracy of Spiral CT in the Diagnosis of Acute PE

Study	Year	No. of Patients in Study	CT Protocols: Collimation (mm)	CT Protocols: Lower Anatomic Level of Interpretation	CT Protocols: Sensitivity (%)*	CT Protocols: Specificity (%)*	CT Protocols: κ Value*
Remy-Jardin et al (2)	1992	42	5	Segmental	100	96	NC
Goodman et al (4)	1995	20	5	Segmental	86	92	NC
Senac et al (26)	1995	45	5	Segmental	86	100	NC
Van Rossum et al (27)	1996	149	5	Segmental	82–90	93–96	0.774
Remy-Jardin et al (6)	1996	75	5, 3	Segmental	91	78	NC
Ferretti et al (28)	1997	164	5	Segmental	NC	NC	NC
Mayo et al (29)	1997	142	3	Segmental	87	95	0.85
Van Rossum et al (30)	1998	123	5	Segmental	75	90	NC
Drucker et al (31)	1998	47	5	Segmental	53–60	81–97	NC
Herold et al (32)†	1998	401	3	Subsegmental	88	94	0.72
Baghaie et al (33)‡	1998	370	3, 2	Subsegmental	96	100	0.87

* NC = not calculated in that study.
† European multicenter trial. This reference is an abstract.
‡ This reference is an abstract.

fects may simulate emboli (Fig 3), as previously reported on conventional pulmonary angiograms (24). In patients with a substantial regional variation in pulmonary blood flow, a long start delay (eg, 20 seconds) and selection of a high concentration–high flow protocol can help suppress the focal hypoattenuation in the pulmonary arterial bed related to retrograde left-to-right shunting. However, the difficulties in obtaining optimal enhancement of the pulmonary arterial vasculature on CT scans are similar to those encountered on unilateral angiograms on which poor opacification or pseudoamputation are commonly seen. In most cases, hyperselective catheterization of the lobar or segmental arteries of this region is required to demonstrate their patency. A transient or permanent increase in pulmonary arterial pressure may be responsible for a right-to-left shunt through a patent foramen ovale, which results in a lower degree of pulmonary arterial enhancement on CT scans. This situation is suspected when a massive and early enhancement of the aorta is observed in conjunction with a faint pulmonary arterial opacification.

Role of spiral CT in the management of acute PE.—Since the introduction of spiral CT in the clinical evaluation of patients suspected of having PE, several articles have reported high sensitivities and specificities in the identification of endoluminal thrombi down to the segmental level (Table 1). According to the specific advantages of spiral CT angiography over conventional or digital angiography, this technique is now considered as the first diagnostic procedure whenever direct imaging of endovascular clots is required. Van Erkel et al (34) have recently added economic clues to this diagnostic strategy, concluding that substituting spiral CT angiography for conventional angiography was likely to improve the mortality and cost-effectiveness in the diagnostic work-up of PE. It should be emphasized that spiral CT angiography and pulmonary angiography have a similar rate of suboptimal examinations, varying between 2% and 4% of cases with CT and reported in 3% of the angiograms of the prospective investigation of pulmonary embolism, or PIOPED, study (35). These technical failures have been observed in patients with severe dyspnea, which is mainly responsible for poor image quality (6,29,30,33). Winston et al (36) recently reported that contrast-enhanced helical CT depicted occult pulmonary emboli in 1% of patients scanned and resulted in the initiation of anticoagulation therapy in the majority of these patients. Detection is of great importance, since occult pulmonary emboli have high associated morbidity and mortality. Thorough evaluation of the pulmonary vasculature should be performed at all contrast-enhanced CT examinations, as clinical suspicion of this potentially life-threatening diagnosis may not exist (36,37).

Whereas the replacement of pulmonary angiography by spiral CT angiography has been increasingly accepted by clinicians known for their widespread reluctance to refer patients for pulmonary angiography (38), there remains a debate on the respective roles of spiral CT and V-P scintigraphy as noninvasive screening procedures. Correlative studies (6,29,30), including the European multicenter trial (32) that included 401 patients, have demonstrated that the sensitivity of spiral CT is greater than that of V-P scintigraphy, varying between 75%–92% and 36%–65% respectively (mean values, 85% vs 50%). The main advantage of spiral CT is the lower percentage of nondiagnostic examinations, because the lung parenchyma, mediastinum, and thoracic wall structures are also evaluated. Consequently, alternative causes of the clinical signs and symptoms may be identified, varying between 11% and 33% in the most recent studies (28,30,33). In addition, the agreement among readers of CT scans is better than that among readers of V-P scans. In the study of Mayo et al (29), the κ value was 0.85 with spiral CT angiography and 0.61 with V-P scanning. In the European multicentric trial (32), the agreement among CT scan readers was also better than that found among V-P scan readers (ie, 0.72 vs 0.39) (32). This study showed a considerable dependance of the interobserver agreement in CT angiography on the technical quality of the study, whereas interobserver agreement in V-P scintigraphy was neither dependent on study quality nor on the use of Biello or PIOPED criteria. These results explain why several authors suggest that spiral CT should be the initial imaging modality of choice, especially in the group of patients known to be associated with a high rate of indeterminate V-P scintigraphic studies (eg, all inpatients and patients with chronic obstructive pulmonary disease) (6,28,29,30,39). These conclusions are reinforced by the results

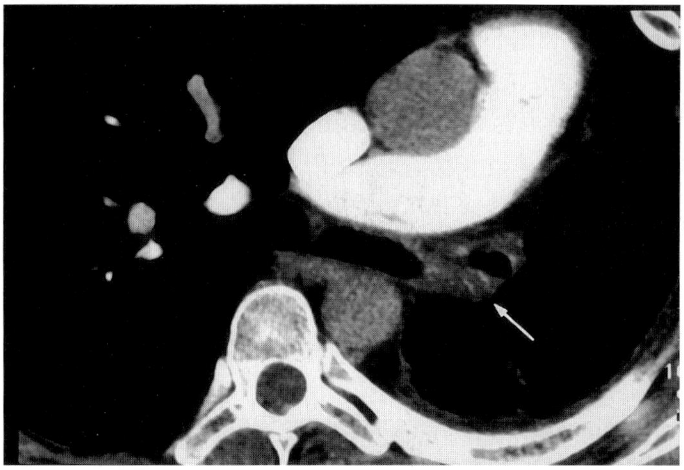

a.

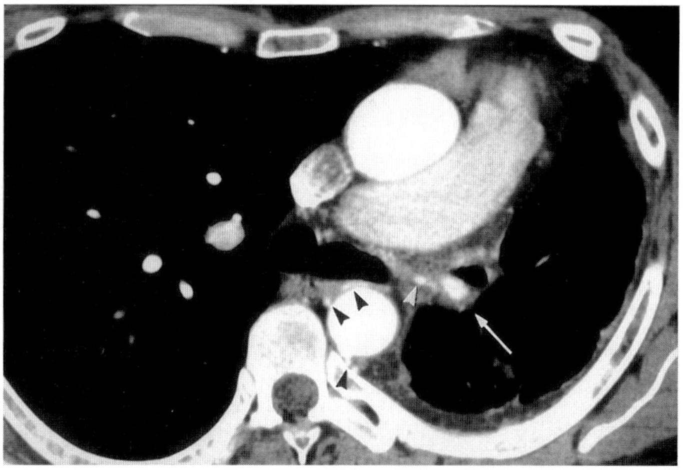

b.

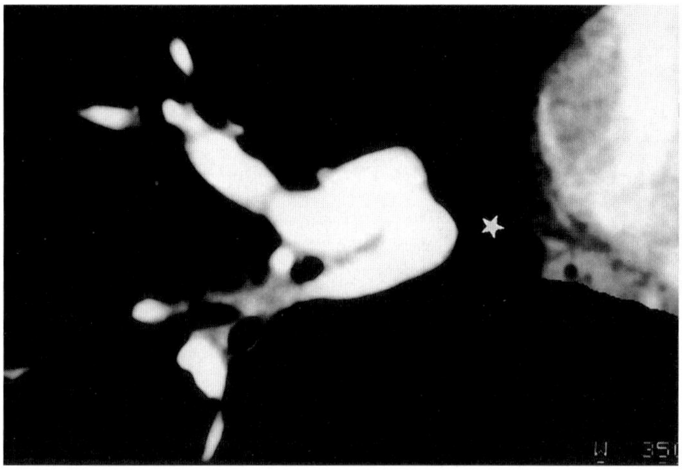

c.

Figure 3. Spiral CT scans obtained in a 41-year-old patient with previous history of recurrent left upper lobe hemoptysis. **(a)** Spiral CT scan (2-mm collimation, pitch of 2, 30% iodinated contrast agent, scanning delay of 15 seconds) obtained at the level of the left main bronchus shows the nonopacification of a small left interlobar pulmonary artery (arrow). Note the mediastinal shift to the left due to a small left lung. **(b)** Spiral CT scan obtained at the same level during the same session with a longer scanning delay (scanning delay, 22 seconds; other parameters same as in **a**). The opacification of the left interlobar pulmonary artery (arrow) at the systemic phase confirms that the focal hypoattenuation previously observed was related to retrograde left-to-right shunting, itself related to left pulmonary venous atresia. Note the enlargement of bronchial and intercostal arteries (arrowheads) and extensive left pleural thickening. **(c)** Stacking of eight 2-mm-thick sections of the right lower lobe from the same data set demonstrates an additional atresia of the right inferior pulmonary vein (☆).

of the cost-effectiveness analysis recently reported by Van Erkel et al (34). A limited number of patients could thus benefit from scintigraphy at first intention (ie, patients with low clinical suspicion of PE and no prior cardiopulmonary disease). An important question should then be considered: What are the remaining indications for pulmonary angiography? They should be reserved for patients in whom clinical suspicion for PE remains high despite normal results at spiral CT and duplex ultrasonography (US) of the legs. However, one should nuance the answer by considering the technical quality of the negative spiral CT angiogram. When the technical conditions of the latter examination limit the depiction of acute PE to central pulmonary arteries, pulmonary angiography should be reasonably indicated to search for thrombi at the level of the peripheral arterial bed. However, when a spiral CT angiogram is negative down to the subsegmental level, the clinical usefulness of pulmonary angiography is more debatable.

Recent improvement in scanner technology is leading the radiologists to reevaluate the role of spiral CT in the detection of subsegmental PE; the frequency of subsegmental PE as reported in the literature varies between 2% and 33% (4,6,33,34,40,41). Over the past few years, several studies have stressed that subsegmental pulmonary arteries are not accurately evaluated with spiral CT. This inability was the logical consequence of the scanning parameters chosen in early reports (ie, 5-mm collimation and 5 mm/sec table feed [pitch = 1]) responsible for partial volume effects at the level of small branches. Since then, selection of a 3-mm collimation and a 5 mm/sec table feed (pitch = 1.7) has improved evaluation of peripheral pulmonary arteries at routine CT examinations. As previously noted, a 2-mm collimation and a 4 mm/sec table feed (pitch = 2) are now available in routine clinical practice. In a study group of 370 patients, the percentage of the analyzable subsegmental arterial bed was statistically significantly higher when scanning the patients with a 2-mm collimation and a pitch of 2 than when scanning the patients with a 3-mm collimation and a pitch of 1.7 (65% vs 43%, respectively). A question often raised over the past few years is, what is the clinical relevance of peripheral emboli in acute PE? Several authors consider that tiny clots are from calf veins and do not require anticoagulation (4,42–45). However, occlusion of a few subsegmental branches perfusing the most "normal" part of the lung parenchyma has been reported to lead to respiratory failure in patients with preexistent bronchopulmonary disease (6,33).

Follow-up of Acute PE and Management of Chronic Thromboembolic Disease

In addition to facilitating the diagnosis of acute PE, spiral CT angiography may help us understand changes within central pulmonary arteries after acute PE. In a study group of 19 patients with acute PE initially identified with spiral CT, resolving clots were found in 13 of 19 patients (68%) at 6-week follow-up (46). Residual abnormalities consisted of eccentric, wall-adherent filling defects or filling defects with central contrast material, consistent with recanalized clots. In a study group of 62 patients, follow-up spiral CT angiograms over a mean period of 11 months showed an incomplete resolution of acute PE in 39% of cases and newly developed chronic PE in 13% of cases (47) (Fig 4). The morphologic changes directly available on spiral CT angiograms are expected to improve our knowledge of the evolution of acute PE toward chronic thromboembolic disease. To date, to our knowledge only a few scintigraphic studies have addressed this issue, and the development of chronic changes has been reported with a frequency varying between 2% and 18% of cases (48–50). The most conspicuous abnormality of chronic PE is the presence of complete filling defects at the level of stenosed pulmonary arteries. Several additional features are also suggestive of chronic PE, namely, eccentric thrombi, evidence of recanalization, and arterial stenosis or web. The creation of reformatted images through the longitudinal axis of obliquely oriented vessels can overcome some of the difficulties encountered with transverse sections in the identification of focal arterial stenosis (51). In addition, reformatted images provide a delineation of mural thrombi on a single image, which is usually considered a useful complement to pulmonary angiography whenever a surgical treatment is planned.

To date, only a few studies have evaluated the role of spiral CT in the management of chronic thromboembolic disease (52–54). As recently reported by Bergin et al (53), pulmonary angiography is the most widely used technique for definitive diagnosis and for determination, before surgery, of the extent of disease. Knowledge of the location and extent of disease helps in the selection of candidates for thromboendarterectomy. It is usually accepted that the presence of disease in central arteries virtually ensures surgical accessibility, but the proportion of central to peripheral disease that determines successful response after surgery is not clearly defined. In a study group of 55 patients, Bergin et al (53) evaluated the accuracy of spiral CT, magnetic resonance (MR) imaging, and conventional angiographic findings, with surgical findings as the reference standard. Central vessel disease was determined more accurately with spiral CT scans than with angiograms or with MR images. In addition, segmental vessel disease was also more accurately determined with CT scans than with MR images. These results led the authors to conclude that spiral CT is a useful alternative to conventional angiography for the diagnosis of chronic thromboembolic disease but that it may not be sufficient for selecting candidates for surgery in all cases.

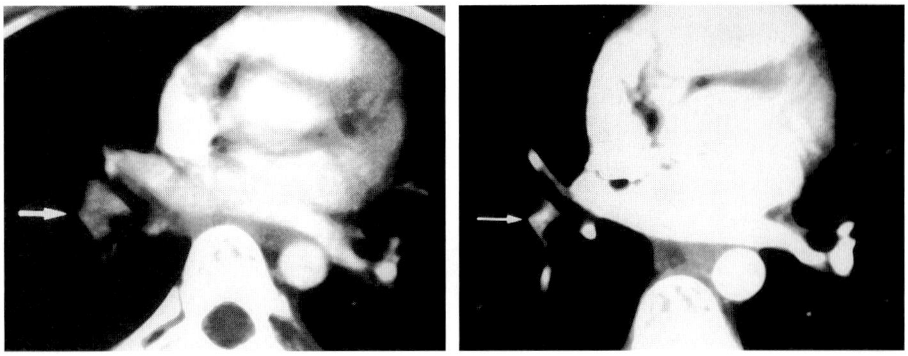

a. b.

Figure 4. Spiral CT scans obtained over 16 months in a 27-year-old woman with acute PE who presented with right-sided chest pain at the initial diagnosis. **(a)** Spiral CT scan (5-mm collimation, pitch of 1, 30% iodinated contrast agent) obtained at the level of the right bronchus intermedius at the time of initial diagnosis shows a complete obstruction of the right interlobar pulmonary artery (arrow). **(b)** Follow-up spiral CT scan (3-mm collimation, pitch of 1.7, 25% iodinated contrast agent) obtained at the same level as **a**, 16 months later, shows the dramatic reduction in diameter of the right interlobar pulmonary artery (arrow), partially recanalized.

CT can also depict changes at the level of the systemic arterial circulation, the collateral supply of the occluded pulmonary arterial bed. The most common findings on CT scans consist of dilated bronchial arteries, which can be detected as tortuous and/or dotted vascular sections in their mediastinal and/or hilar pathways (54,55). Enlargement of the internal mammary arteries is also easily detectable on CT scans, especially in cases of asymmetric or unilateral systemic supply. In addition, the possibility of identifying lung parenchymal abnormalities, such as areas of ground-glass attenuation and/or bronchial dilatation in cases of chronic PE, should be emphasized (56).

Pretherapeutic Management of Bronchial Carcinoma

Pulmonary Arterial Invasion from Bronchial Tumors

Precise staging is the key to rational management of bronchial tumors. Incremental CT has fallen short in predicting tumor extension in the mediastinum and the hilum, including vascular invasion. An improvement in CT-surgical correlations is expected with spiral CT with routine use of 2–5-mm thin sections (Fig 5). From clinical experience, we recommend performance of a contrast-enhanced spiral CT examination of the hila after analysis of the nonenhanced CT scans of the entire thorax. Careful interpretation of these sections helps determine the most appropriate injection protocol with special attention directed toward the target vasculature, the iodinated concentration, and the optimal start delay. The routine protocol for spiral CT angiography of the pulmonary circulation virtually guarantees an optimal opacification not only of the mediastinal and hilar pulmonary arteries but also of the venoatrial confluence and of the cardiac chambers. Strictly comparative performances of spiral CT acquisition are mandatory, before and after neoadjuvant chemotherapy, for a better estimation and, if needed, for a response quantification. This has to be taken into account as neoadjuvant chemotherapy has an initial response rate of approximately 50%, and subsequent resection rates in the responders may approach 80%.

Some specific indications for spiral CT angiography of the proximal pulmonary arterial tree can be reviewed in the light of therapeutic options (57). Central tumors may be resected by a sleeve lobectomy plus the excision of the adjacent part of the main stem bronchus, followed by a bronchial end-to-end anastomosis. Direct carcinomatous extension into the adjacent pulmonary artery may modify the initially planned surgical option, either requiring an additional angioplastic reconstruction or necessitating a pneumonectomy. Moreover, the potential postoperative complications of a pulmonary

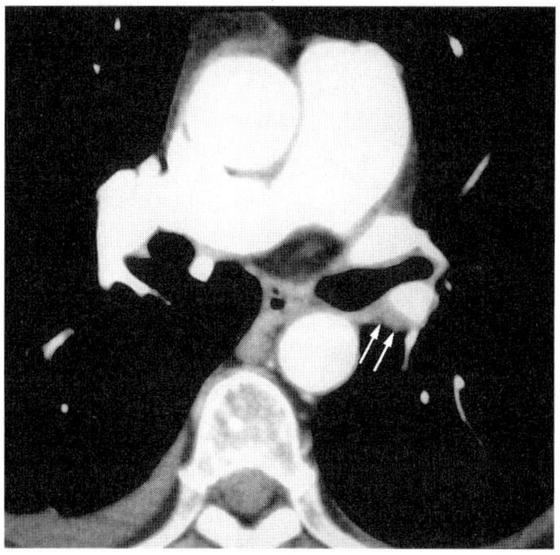

Figure 5. Spiral CT angiogram (2-mm collimation, pitch of 1, 30% iodinated contrast agent) obtained at the level of the left upper lobe bronchus in a 50-year-old woman with progressive dyspnea, 3 years after treatment of a breast carcinoma. There is a thick hypoattenuated area (arrows) around the medial border of the narrowed left interlobar pulmonary artery. An endoscopic biopsy of endobronchial abnormalities at the level of the posterior wall of the left upper lobe bronchus revealed left hilar invasion from adenocarcinoma.

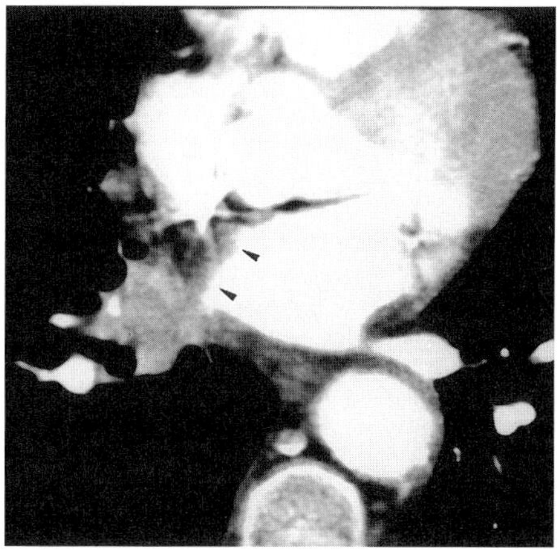

Figure 6. Preoperative spiral CT angiogram (3-mm collimation, pitch of 1.7, 30% iodinated contrast agent) obtained at the level of the lower lobes in a 63-year-old patient evaluated for right hilar carcinoma. There is tumoral invasion of the right venoatrial junction and of the right border (arrowheads) of the left atrium.

artery anastomosis, such as anastomotic strictures and bronchoarterial fistula, have to be accurately depicted. In the experience of Read et al (58), the arch of the left pulmonary artery, which is in close contact with the upper lobe bronchus, is compromised by 14.4% of lesions, otherwise suitable for left upper lobectomy. These data emphasize the imperative need to perfectly depict the left pulmonary arterial arch, which gives off from four to eight separate arteries to the left upper lobe. Most surgeons proceed to pneumonectomy once there is any vascular invasion, but others strongly recommend interposition grafting, excluding tangential angioplasty or resection-anastomosis (58). The expected consequence of such a conservative procedure is that the blood flow to the lower lobe can be postoperatively jeopardized by stenosis of an end-to-end anastomosis. Here again, spiral CT angiography of the proximal left pulmonary artery with use of MPR and simultaneous thresholding segmentation for renderings of both bronchial and vascular trees can play a role of the utmost importance postoperatively as well as preoperatively (59).

A hilar lymph node dissection can be influenced by the spiral CT findings. If an upper lobectomy is contemplated, lymph nodes smaller than 10 mm in diameter, outside the lobectomy field, can be discovered by their compression or invasion of the descending pulmonary artery. They run the risk of being unseen on an incremental CT study because they hardly modify the external pulmonary artery morphology. For the same reason, mediastinal lymph node imaging can also be improved by means of spiral CT angiography of the mediastinal vessels (60). Radiographically occult squamous cell carcinoma involving main stem bronchi and lobar bronchi can benefit from photodynamic therapy. These lesions may be extremely small and are very often beyond the ability of CT detection. But once they are endoscopically detected and pathologically proved, the two major problems are to determine whether the lesion is limited to the bronchial wall and to eliminate an N2 disease. Another point of interest is that, if there is an incomplete response after photodynamic therapy, the patient can undergo surgical resection. Spiral CT with thin sections and contrast medium can depict the peribronchial tissues and be used in the extrabronchial follow-up of the treated disease. Khanavkar et al (61) pointed out that centrally located squamous cell carcinomas represented a predisposing factor to hemorrhage and tried to identify patients at high risk of developing fatal hemoptysis after endobronchial brachytherapy. They emphasized the following anatomic factors: involvement of major arteries, considerable bronchial wall destruction, and mediastinal invasion. Posttreatment necrotic cavitation of a tumor located a few millimeters from a major vessel can also be considered as a potentially lethal situation. The preventive effect of spiral CT angiography should be seriously considered in the follow-up of this treatment, as well as after vasoocclusive therapy. Whereas bronchial carcinoids can be highly vascular lesions, they may only be depicted with a moderate homogeneous contrast enhancement on incremental CT scans (62). The transmural extension of this tumor can reach the peribronchial tissues and vessels, as well as the adjacent pulmonary parenchyma. If an endobronchial biopsy is anticipated, the highly vascular component should be demonstrated to prevent any further hemorrhagic complications. A sleeve resection can be performed depending on the peribronchial extent. Both findings can be searched for on pulmonary and systemic spiral CT angiograms.

Venoatrial Extension of Bronchial Carcinoma

In addition to invasion and obstruction of a pulmonary vein by a lung tumor, embolization into the left atrium may occur (Fig 6). The most common tumor able to invade the left atrium in this way is bronchogenic carcinoma. However, metastatic carcinoma and pulmonary sarcoma of the lung have also been reported with a similar extension. A preoperative diagnosis is imperative since the consequence of intraoperatively dislodging a macroscopic tumoral thrombus from the pulmonary vein can be multiple systemic tumor emboli and can be fatal in the short term (63). In patients with large central carcinomas in contact with one or several major pulmonary veins, a preoperative transthoracic or transesophageal echocardiogram and a spiral CT angiogram are recommended because a carcinomatous thrombus of a pulmonary vein may go unnoticed at surgery and become dislodged during surgical manipulations. The CT signs of venous invasion are those of a pulmonary veno-obstructive syndrome, including pulmonary edema and hemorrhage, pulmonary venous infarct, interlobular septal thickening, increased bronchial wall thickening, and pleural effusion (64). Spiral CT angiography can additionally show a massive enlargement in diameter of the invaded vein with an absence of opacification or a more or less notable filling defect of the adjacent part of the left atrium. The focal increase in pulmonary vascular resistance can also result in absent or delayed opacification of the pulmonary arteries in the area of venous obstruction, followed later by an unusual intense opacification of these pulmonary arteries due to pulmonary arterial stasis. On incremental CT scans, a space-occupying lesion in the left atrium could be easily missed on an insufficiently contrast-enhanced CT scan (65).

Postoperative Incidents, Accidents, and Follow-up

With precise knowledge of rearrangements of the pulmonary vascular pedicles after a lobectomy, CT follow-up of patients with normal results of bronchial endoscopy can be performed without administration of contrast material. However, after pneumonectomy, a contrast-enhanced study is systematically recommended since, although it is infrequently noticed, the presence of a clot in a pulmonary artery stump is not that exceptional (66) (Fig 7). This is partly because patients with carcinoma are at high risk for an associated state of hypercoagulability and partly because there are anatomic factors that can account for the stasis of blood flow in the stump. After pneumonectomy, a right-sided stump is longer than a left-sided one, thus explaining the higher frequency of stump clots after right pneumonectomy. In addition, the stump clot may enlarge over time and has to be differentiated from tumor recurrence (66). The main complication is a contralateral migration of endovascular clots, which may lead to acute respiratory failure, especially in patients with previous history of cardiopulmonary disease.

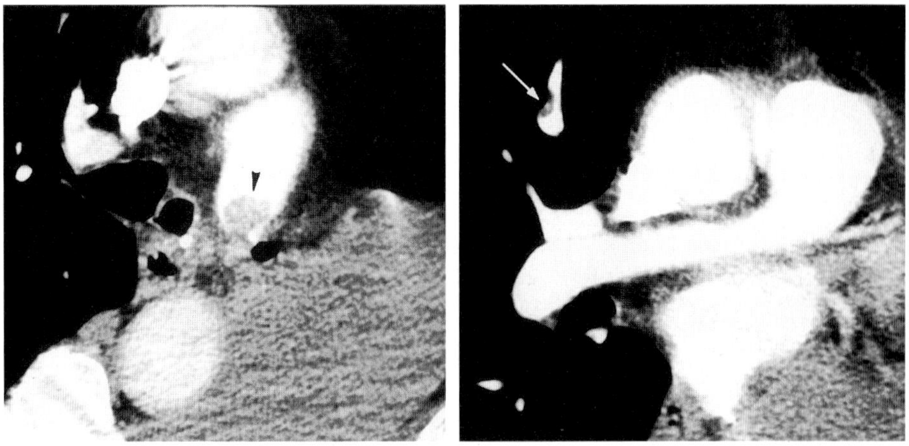

a. b.

Figure 7. Postoperative spiral CT angiography (2-mm collimation, pitch of 2, 24% iodinated contrast agent) performed in a 72-year-old patient treated by means of left pneumonectomy for lung carcinoma. **(a)** Spiral CT scan obtained at the level of the left pulmonary artery stump shows an endoluminal filling defect (arrowhead). **(b)** Spiral CT scan obtained at the level of the bronchus intermedius. Note the additional presence of a partial filling defect (arrow) at the level of a subsegmental branch of the anterior segmental artery of the right upper lobe.

Several additional postoperative complications can be assessed with a spiral CT angiogram. Among them, a postoperative right-to-left shunt between the inferior vena cava and the left atrium through a patent foramen ovale in the absence of pulmonary hypertension can be detected on spiral CT angiograms after injection of contrast material into the lower leg. One can also expect an earlier diagnosis of cardiac herniations or torsion with spiral CT angiography. Known to occur after intrapericardial pneumonectomy or after lobectomy including extensive pericardial resection, a cardiac torsion can be easily identified with spiral CT by means of the interventricular septal rotation. After lobectomy or bi-lobectomy, an acute episode of dyspnea with or without thoracic pain and hemoptysis, a complete consolidation of the remaining lobe, a drop in the hematocrit, and no flow on the lung perfusion scan can have two main causes: (*a*) lobar torsion or (*b*) pulmonary venous obstruction due to torsion, angulation, or thrombosis. These can be seen after a middle lobectomy alone or middle and lower lobectomy because ligation of the lowermost one or two branches of the superior pulmonary vein can traumatize this large remaining vein (67). Spiral CT angiography, performed after endobronchial endoscopy to exclude a lobar torsion, can obviate angiography and show the normal postoperative pulmonary artery anatomy and the absence of a venous phase. If the patient is not operated on for this complication, the development of a venous collateral bronchial and nonbronchial systemic supply to this persistent venous obstruction can be expected through the bronchial veins, the chest wall veins, and the azygos-hemiazygos system. Proximal pulmonary veno-occlusive disease has also been reported secondary to the reimplantation of pulmonary veins in the left atrium (64,68).

In the particular group of patients who have undergone lung transplantation, spiral CT can be helpful for the evaluation of anastomosis-related stenoses of the arteries and veins. The frequency of pulmonary artery stenosis has been recently estimated by Griffith et al (69) who observed obstructions in five of 60 single-lung transplant recipients and in none of 74 double-lung transplant recipients. In one case, obstruction was associated with an intraluminal thrombus. The association of systemic hypoxia, normal chest radiographic findings, and perfusion scan abnormalities represents an indication for spiral CT angiography whenever the patient is able to support breath holding for a few seconds. It is not easy to make the differential diagnosis between a true stenosis and a distorted or kinked anastomosis resulting from excessive lengths of donor and recipient artery cuff. The latter can spontaneously improve over a follow-up period, in contrast to a true stenosis, which leads to a surgical revision or to endovascular procedures. Owing to pulmonary-to-bronchial artery retrograde flow, pulmonary artery stenosis can compromise the bronchial anastomosis. In the absence of contraindications to contrast medium administration, a spiral CT study initially indicated for the follow-up of airway anastomosis can also allow evaluation of arterial and venous anastomoses. When the transplant recipient has to be treated with surgery, percutaneous angioplasty, and/or endoprosthesis (70), the precise shape, site, and length of the stenosis can be better appreciated with two-dimensional and 3D reformations because they permit unlimited viewing angles (Fig 8). Perfusion scanning and 3D spiral CT angiography can also avert the use of more invasive and repeated angiographic follow-up.

Pulmonary Hypertension

Pulmonary hypertension is a complicating feature of many cardiac and respiratory conditions, as well as of chronic liver disease. The causes of pulmonary hypertension are usually classified into four main categories: (*a*) hyperkinetic hypertension due to a left-to-right shunt secondary to congenital heart disease; (*b*) precapillary pulmonary hypertension,

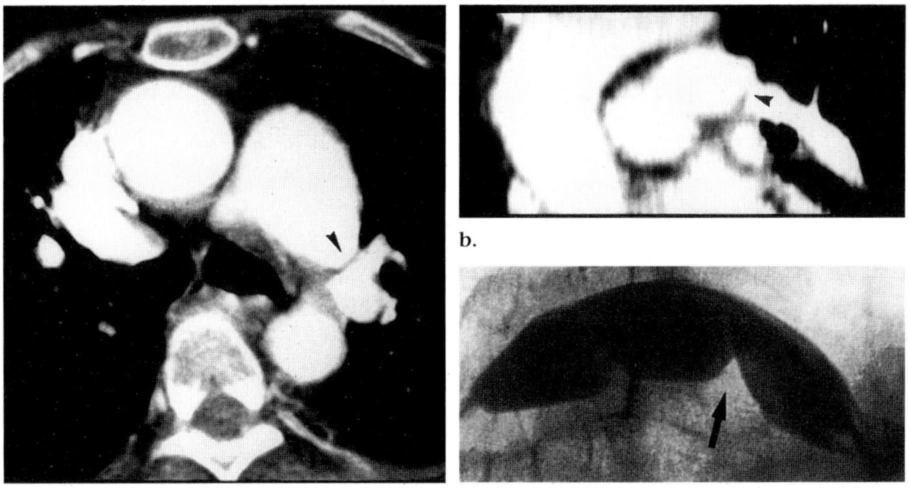

a. b. c.

Figure 8. Postoperative spiral CT angiography (3-mm collimation, pitch of 1.7, 24% iodinated contrast agent) performed in a 51-year-old patient, 10 days after left lung transplantation for idiopathic pulmonary fibrosis. **(a)** Spiral CT scan obtained at the level of the left main pulmonary artery suggests either an anastomotic stenosis or a postoperative kinking (arrowhead). **(b)** Oblique coronal reformation obtained along the main axis of the left pulmonary artery confirms the presence of an anastomotic stenosis (arrowhead). **(c)** Similar morphologic information to that shown in **b** is provided by means of the opacification of the balloon during the angioplasty procedure (the arrow points to the anastomotic stenosis).

including chronic thromboembolic pulmonary hypertension, primary pulmonary hypertension, and pulmonary capillary hemangiomatosis; (*c*) postcapillary pulmonary hypertension, secondary to left-sided heart diseases and pulmonary venous obstruction such as pulmonary veno-occlusive disease; and (*d*) rare causes, such as portopulmonary hypertension, a well-recognized complication of chronic liver disease, defined by the presence of pulmonary hypertension in combination with portal hypertension (71).

Imaging studies can contribute to the care of patients with pulmonary hypertension by helping to (*a*) detect its presence, (*b*) indicate possible causes, (*c*) grade its severity, and (*d*) evaluate the functional state of the right ventricle. Routine chest radiography, CT, MR imaging, pulmonary function studies, and echocardiography have all been studied with variable success in predicting the presence or severity of pulmonary hypertension in patients with underlying cardiopulmonary disease. More than 10 years ago, a main pulmonary artery diameter of 29 mm or greater on a CT scan was reported to have a sensitivity of 69% and a specificity of 100% for predicting pulmonary hypertension in patients with cardiac or intrinsic pulmonary vascular disease (72). Because CT of the chest is often used in the diagnosis and treatment of patients with parenchymal lung disease, Tan et al (73) undertook a retrospective study aimed at determining the diagnostic utility of CT-determined diameter of the main pulmonary artery for predicting pulmonary hypertension in this patient population. The diameter was measured at the widest portion of the main pulmonary artery within 3 cm of the bifurcation; in addition, the right pulmonary arterial diameter and left pulmonary arterial diameter were measured at the widest portions after bifurcation of the main pulmonary artery. The authors concluded that a main pulmonary artery diameter of 29 mm or greater enables identification of patients with even a mild degree of pulmonary hypertension and therefore should enable identification of those patients who may have the greatest pulmonary vascular limitation to exercise.

In addition to the enlargement of proximal pulmonary arterial branches, CT may help identify morphologic changes suggestive of pre- or postcapillary pulmonary hypertension. In favor of precapillary pulmonary hypertension, one may note small peripheral pulmonary arteries and veins with the concurrent presence of normal lung parenchyma and left atrium. Presence of postcapillary pulmonary hypertension is usually suggested by the identification of CT features of interstitial and/or alveolar edema, including septal lines and abnormal lung attenuation varying from ground-glass opacities to consolidation. These parenchymal abnormalities are observed with the concurrent presence of enlarged pulmonary veins, sometimes associated with pleural effusion.

During the past few years, several studies have shown that a mosaic pattern of lung attenuation can be seen in patients with pulmonary hypertension of various causes (74). In an attempt to determine whether infiltrative, airway, or vascular lung disease is the cause of mosaic attenuation on thin-section CT scans of the lung, one may pay attention to the size of the pulmonary vascular sections within the areas of ground-glass attenuation and search for air trapping. The areas of increased lung attenuation can be attributable to blood flow redistribution when the size and number of vessels in the areas of increased attenuation are increased compared with those in the areas with normal or decreased attenuation in the absence of air trapping (75–77). As recently demonstrated by Worthy et al (78), it should be emphasized that, whereas the diagnoses of infiltrative lung disease and airway disease are frequently correct and confident, vascular disease is more difficult to diagnose on thin-section CT scans as the cause of areas of ground-glass attenuation.

Primary Pulmonary Artery Sarcomas

Primary pulmonary artery sarcomas are infrequent tumors that are very often confused with acute and chronic thromboembolic disease. Apart from the particular endovascular development of the tumor, which can be seen as a floating mass resembling a endoluminal clot within the pulmonary artery trunk and/or its proximal branches, it should be emphasized that this tumor is often associated with thrombus formation. The absence of predisposing factors for PE, the absence of "thrombus" dissolution despite anticoagulation, and atypical distribution of the filling defects as seen at two-dimensional or Doppler US, pulmonary angiography, MR imaging or CT, and V-P scanning should alert the radiologist (79). Peripheral pulmonary infiltrates can correspond to pulmonary infarcts due to thrombi or embolization of tumor material from the original site.

The diagnosis can be strongly suspected when chest radiography, CT, or MR imaging shows a lobulated and heterogeneous hilar mass that originates from the pulmonary artery trunk or from the main right or left pulmonary arteries and expands the artery (80). Such polypoid

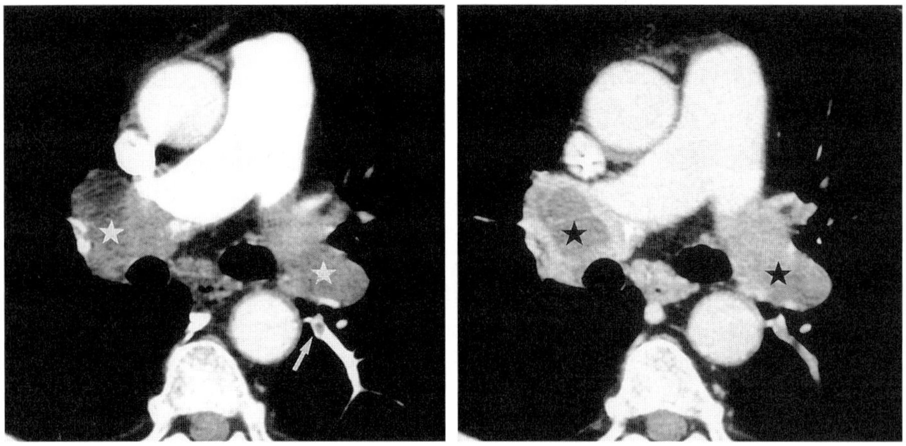

a. b.

Figure 9. Spiral CT angiography (2-mm collimation, pitch of 2, 24% iodinated contrast agent) performed in a 72-year-old patient. **(a)** Spiral CT scan obtained at the level of the right and left main pulmonary arteries shows bilateral endoluminal hypoattenuated areas (☆). Note the additional presence of a partial filling defect at the level of a subsegmental branch of the superior segmental artery (arrow) of the left lower lobe. **(b)** Spiral CT scan obtained at the same level as in **a**, 2 minutes after contrast material administration, shows heterogeneous enhancement of the right and left vascular regions (★) due to the presence of multicentric malignant histiocytofibroma (surgically confirmed).

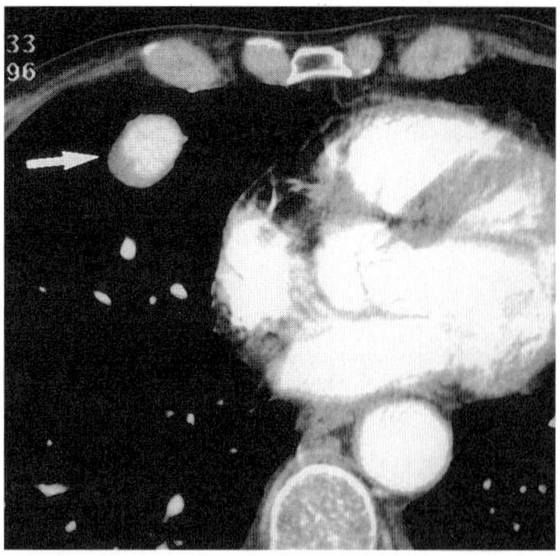

a.

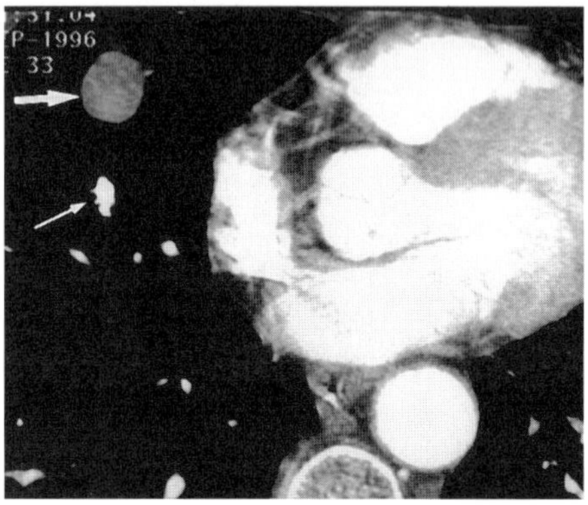

b.

Figure 10. Spiral CT angiography (2-mm collimation, pitch of 2, 24% iodinated contrast agent) performed in an asymptomatic 75-year-old patient This study was indicated for the evaluation of a right lung nodule incidentally identified on a postoperative chest radiograph. **(a)** Spiral CT scan obtained at the level of the right middle lobe shows a well-circumscribed enhancing nodule (arrow), corresponding to a false aneurysm of a right middle lobe peripheral artery induced by a Swan-Ganz catheter. **(b)** Spiral CT scan obtained at the same level after occlusion of a subsegmental branch of the medial segmental artery of the right middle lobe. There is absence of contrast enhancement at the level of the false aneurysm (thick arrow) after successful endovascular treatment (the thin arrow points to the deposited coils).

intraluminal masses can be partly hemorrhagic, necrotic, and hypervascularized with enhancement on spiral CT scans or after administration of gadopentetate dimeglumine on T1-weighted MR images. This finding helps eliminate a thrombus and indicates a neoplastic process (81,82–84). The pretherapeutic evaluation of this tumor can be performed with spiral CT, first during the passage of the contrast medium bolus, but also a few minutes later to search for contrast medium uptake by the tumor (Fig 9). In a minority of patients, the tumor arises from the right or left main pulmonary artery with or without contralateral spreading. Direct transmural growth in the hilum, the mediastinum, the lung parenchyma, and the pericardium can occur or it can be simultaneously multicentric. Such lesions can mimic a tumor from another origin, particularly a bronchial carcinoma invading the pulmonary artery. Extravascular infiltration and nodal invasion are also possible (85), and it should be noted that osteo-, chondro-, and carcinosarcomas may exhibit osteoid and bony components (79).

Pulmonary Artery Aneurysms

A pseudoaneurysm results from a tear or disruption of the layers of a vessel wall and when extravasated blood is held by a dilated adventitia, by clot, or by compressed surrounding tissues that form the wall of the pseudoaneurysm. Traumatic pulmonary artery pseudoaneurysms are most commonly encounter as a result of pulmonary artery perforation after improper placement of a Swan-Ganz catheter but have also been reported after blunt or penetrating trauma. Other causes include mycotic, syphilitic, or mycobacterial infection and vascular abnormalities such as cystic medial necrosis, Behçet disease, and Marfan syndrome. This arterial lesion may also be caused by septic emboli and neoplasms. In proper clinical settings, this lesion should be suspected either in a patient presenting with hemoptysis, resulting from leakage of blood into the bronchial tree, or when the chest radiograph shows a focal lung mass that remains stable or increases in size on subsequent studies. Diagnosing pseudoaneurysms before they rupture is essential. In a review of 28 catheter-induced pulmonary artery pseudoaneurysms, all patients treated before rupture survived, whereas the mortality rate was 100% if the aneurysm ruptured (86). As recently reported (87–89), the diagnosis can be easily made with spiral CT. With an appropriately timed bolus of iodinated contrast material, pulmonary artery pseudoaneurysms appear as enhancing, round lung masses that are isointense to the central pulmonary arteries (Fig 10). Apart from the diagnosis of the arterial lesion, spiral CT can also provide useful pretherapeutic information, especially prior to embolotherapy. In the latter situation, it is important to precisely identify the feeding vessel(s) prior to hyperselective catheterization and occlusion (90). In addition to transverse CT scans, 3D surface-rendering reconstruction and 3D MIP can help identify the relationships of the aneurysmal sac with the artery to be occluded, the number of aneurysms, and the spatial orientation and diameter of the arteries before catheterization (91).

In the specific context of Behçet disease, aneurysms and thrombotic complications can also occur at the site of venous or arterial puncture, leading one to avoid angiography whenever possible. To avoid a more invasive approach using conventional or digital angiography at largely higher risks than usual, spiral CT angiography can prove useful in the pretherapeutic evaluation and follow-up of pulmonary aneurysms and hemoptysis due to their rupture or fissuration. Additionally, MR angiography without injection of contrast material can avert the risk for thrombosis of a venous puncture. Spiral CT and/or MR angiography are also able to demonstrate involvement of other thoracic vessels, mainly the superior vena cava (92). Spiral CT is thus considered the noninvasive imaging modality of choice in the work-up of pulmonary artery aneurysms prior to therapeutic interventions.

Rounded Atelectasis

Any type of pleural inflammatory reaction can lead to round atelectasis. Asbestosis is the principal cause today and this diagnosis should be suspected when a peripheral nodule or mass is associated with signs of pleuritis and/or pleuroparenchymal changes related to asbestos. Usually, round atelectasis presents as a posterobasal, subpleural, round or lentiform lesion with some of the following features (93–95): (*a*) peripheral location, with the mass being incompletely surrounded by the lung; (*b*) increased attenuation value of the mass at its periphery; (*c*) pleural thickening in the vicinity of the mass; (*d*) curving of vessels and bronchi toward the mass; and (*e*) the presence of an air bronchogram within the mass. Correct diagnosis is very important, especially in asbestos-exposed patients owing to the increased incidence of mesothelioma and bronchogenic carcinoma in this population. Two main mechanisms are recognized to underlie round atelectasis: (*a*) pleural effusion or diffuse pleural thickening and (*b*) thickening of the visceral pleura with progressive wrinkling and folding of the subpleural lung (96). The lesion can be stable over time; however, it may progressively enlarge and then be confused with a malignant tumor (97).

The use of spiral CT angiography can be of particular interest, as a single data set can provide densitometric and morphologic clues to this diagnosis. On contrast-enhanced CT scans, an intense and homogeneous enhancement is usually observed at the level of a round atelectasis (98). This densitometric feature can help differentiate the atelectatic trapped lung from bronchial carcinoma or fibrosis in which enhancement is usually poor. Care should be taken to pay more attention to the degree of parenchymal enhancement rather than to the presence of the CT angiogram sign, that is, the ability to see normal pulmonary vasculature within parenchymal consolidations. As recently reported by Shah and Friedman (99), the CT angiogram sign is a common finding in lobar consolidations evaluated with contrast-enhanced CT whatever their cause. On thick horizontal sections or on thin interspaced sections, the internal architecture of this atelectatic pseudotumor is not easy to analyze. With spiral CT, thin overlapped sections can show a large curved tongue of the neighboring pleural cavity with fluid invaginating into the underlying lung parenchyma, in close correlation with the anatomic findings (100). Moreover, additional reconstructions may help identify a few additional criteria. The pulmonary vessels trapped in the atelectatic lung can be correctly opacified and enhanced by means of the MIP principle, unless the parenchyma is too highly vascularized. The distortion and regular bending of these vessels can provide another argument against suspected carcinoma.

By using MPR images from 3D SSD images, it is possible to acquire images in multiple planes parallel to the converging vessels and bronchi. According to Mc Hugh and Blaquiere (101), when it is possible to identify the previously cited criteria with conventional and spiral CT examinations, further diagnostic evaluation is unnecessary. If most of the criteria are absent, cautious follow-up or percutaneous needle biopsy is recommended.

Spiral CT Evaluation of Peripheral Vessels

STS MIP Appearance of Normal Peripheral Pulmonary Vasculature

Besides dichotomous branching, pulmonary vessels may display a disproportionate mode of division. Dichotomous branching is the division of a branch into two equal parts, both arising at an acute angle and having half the diameter of the original branch. The disproportionate mode occurs in small branches arising at nearly a right angle from the native vessel, the branches being of smaller diameter than in the case of the usual dichotomous mode of bifurcation (Fig 11). This asymmetric division mode, which was previously only seen with injections of autopsy specimens but not on angiograms, is now easily recognized on STS MIP images. This new morphologic aspect of the pulmonary circulation is expected to be further included in the description of disorders of the peripheral pulmonary circulation.

An additional advantage of analyzing peripheral vessels on STS MIP images is the ability to compare the respective diameters of pulmonary arteries and veins in the peripheral part of the lung. Consequently, analysis of the flow-diameter relationship on STS MIP images might represent an in vivo approach to several morphologic changes, in particular in pulmonary hypertension.

Clinical Applications of STS MIP

From the middle 1980s to the middle 1990s, thin-section CT was widely performed to evaluate respiratory symptoms or pulmonary function abnormalities suggestive of diffuse infiltrative lung disease. This technique has been shown to provide improved clarity of parenchymal abnormalities, thus enabling a better and more confident characterization of disease processes in even severely involved areas. However, a few limitations of this technique have been reported with regard to the detection of micronodular infiltration and in the assessment of arteriolocentric lesions. On thin sections, peripheral pulmonary arteries and veins are multifragmented and numerous vessels are not depicted in the nonacquired intervals of the lung. Conversely, on thick sections calculated with a high-spatial-frequency reconstruction kernel, the distal vessels are correctly depicted but tiny micronodules are masked by the high-amplitude volume averaging effect. An excellent compromise is the STS MIP technique because (*a*) it depicts submillimetric vessels over a longer length than on individual thin sections, (*b*) the contrast resolution is reinforced because of the MIP algorithm, (*c*) the background means is maintained at a minimal level, and (*d*) there is no background enhancement in the absence of injected contrast medium. The clinical value of this technique was evaluated in a study group of 81 patients with suspicion of mild micronodular patterns (102). In this study, the sensitivity of STS MIP was statistically significantly higher than that of conventional CT in the detection of lung micronodules. In addition, it helped recognize the peribronchovascular distribution of lung lesions, a feature indicative of infiltration of the peripheral compartment of lung interstitium. Similarly, the arteriolocentric distribution of micrometastases can be precisely demonstrated (103).

Another clinical application of STS MIP is the recognition of pulmonary

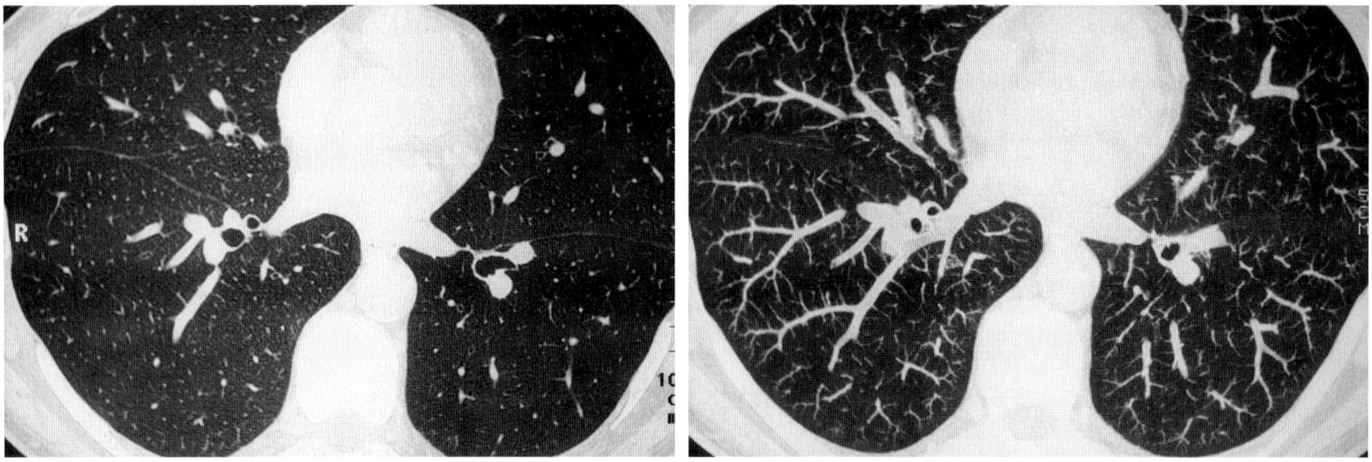

a. b.

Figure 11. Spiral CT scans of the lower lobes obtained in a 44-year-old asymptomatic volunteer. Note the striking difference in the identification of supernumerary vessels of normal pulmonary vasculature between **(a)** a 1-mm-thick section and **(b)** an 8-mm-thick slab generated from a focal spiral CT acquisition according to the STS MIP technique.

arteriovenous microfistulas (Fig 12). In congenital heart disease, a Glenn anastomosis, unifying the superior vena to the right descending pulmonary artery, has a reported incidence of pulmonary arteriovenous malformations (AVMs) of up to 25%. Other palliative surgical treatments, consisting of the diversion of the normal hepatic venous flow away from the pulmonary circulation, can also be responsible for the development of tiny pulmonary AVMs analogous to those described in chronic hepatopathies. Surgical channeling of hepatic venous blood flow in the pulmonary circulation is able to successfully remove pulmonary AVMs (104), but whether this resolution is transient or permanent is unknown. According to Srivastava et al (105) who conducted a pathologic study of two patients with pulmonary AVMs after cavopulmonary anastomosis, the distal pulmonary arteries at the level of the terminal and respiratory bronchioles are dilated and clusters of thin-walled vessels of indeterminate origin are also seen in the pleura. In close correlation to blood gases and angiographic findings, these tiny pulmonary AVMs can be identified on STS MIP images without using contrast medium (103). In chronic liver disease, Schraufnagel and Kay (106) described pulmonary artery–to–pulmonary vein anastomoses through pleural channels and arteriovenous channels within the lung parenchyma at intralobular, interlobular, and subpleural sites, ranging in size from 0.2 to 1.0 mm in diameter. These arteriovenous anastomoses, morphologically similar to those found in Rendu-Osler-Weber disease, can also be identified on STS MIP images without using contrast medium.

CLINICAL INDICATIONS: CONGENITAL DISEASES

Congenital Anomalies of the Pulmonary Artery

Left Pulmonary Artery Sling

Whereas most frequently diagnosed in symptomatic children, left pulmonary artery sling can be found in asymptomatic adults in whom it can mimic a mediastinal adenopathy (107). Until now, the need for surgical repair has necessitated sophisticated diagnostic evaluation that required bronchoscopy and tracheobronchography for identification of tracheal compression and associated abnormalities, barium swallow examination for depiction of an anterior esophageal indentation due to the intertracheoesophageal course of the aberrant left pulmonary artery, and pulmonary angiography for the definitive preoperative diagnosis. As recently emphasized, spiral CT angiography has the advantage of avoiding the above-mentioned invasive examinations because a precise diagnosis of both vascular and bronchial anomalies can be obtained with a single data set (108–110).

Whatever the patient's age and condition, the left pulmonary artery sling should be regarded as a multiplanar anomaly because it requires multiple planes of reformations for an optimal pretherapeutic evaluation. Transverse CT scans are particularly suited for depicting

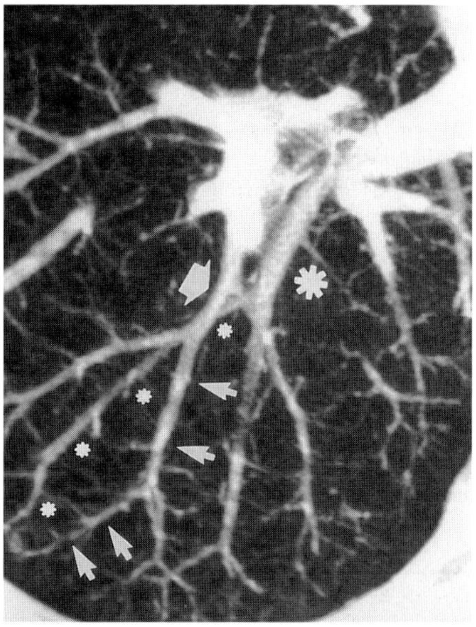

Figure 12. An 8-mm-thick slab of the right lower lobe generated from a focal spiral CT acquisition according to the STS MIP technique in a 29 year-old patient with Rendu-Osler-Weber disease. There are numerous pulmonary arteriovenous microfistulas in the periphery of the right lower lobe. On this STS MIP image, it is possible to demonstrate the vascular connections of the posterior microfistula, with a feeding artery (thin arrows) originating from the posterior segmental artery (thick arrow) and a draining vein (small asterisks) joining the superior segmental vein (large asterisk).

both the abnormal origin and the abnormal course of the left pulmonary artery. Owing to its orientation, the abnormal vessel can be completely hidden behind the proximal part of the right pulmonary artery on a frontal pulmonary angiogram, which explains some angiographic misinterpretations (108). Moreover, performance of spiral CT can avert endoscopy and tracheobronchography, which cannot be considered as safe procedures in patients with compromised ventilation. An overall understanding of the tracheobronchial tree can be obtained from the spiral CT data set either using 3D SSD and a double thresholding segmentation or bronchographic-like reconstructions generated with the volume-rendering technique (111). As recently emphasized by Lacrosse et al (112), MPR images or preferably 3D images can demonstrate the tracheal stenosis and the associated anomalies of the bronchial bifurcation.

Occult Pulmonary Artery

From a semantic viewpoint, it is preferable to use the term "occult pulmonary artery" rather than proximal "absence" of a pulmonary artery branch, because in the majority of cases, the so-called absent pulmonary artery does exit in the hilum and has to be identified for therapeutic purposes. When the occult pulmonary artery is not associated with congenital cardiac disease, the presence of a left occult pulmonary artery associated with a right aortic arch can be diagnosed late in life (113). In the majority of patients, spiral CT angiography should replace conventional or digital angiography as it enables a more complete evaluation of the malformations (114). First, it allows a noninvasive recognition of the pulmonary artery anomaly and helps detect its hilar postobstructive portion. Second, it permits estimation of the importance and variable origins of the systemic collateral supply, which develops from birth to adulthood and which may be responsible for massive hemoptysis.

Pulmonary AVMs

Conventional CT has already proved useful and highly sensitive for the detection of pulmonary AVMs (115), but it suffers from false-negative results due to variations in respiratory depth, partial volume averaging effects, and motion artifacts. It is now accepted that spiral CT of the entire thorax represents the method of choice for routine detection of pulmonary AVMs (116). In addition, this technique appears to be able to overcome the limitations of the most frequently recommended screening procedures. Contrast-enhanced two-dimensional echocardiography has proved to be an excellent technique for the identification of a right-to-left shunt (117). However, definite conclusions regarding the sensitivity of contrast-enhanced two-dimensional echocardiography cannot be drawn from previous investigations because pulmonary angiograms, until now the reference standard technique for the detection of pulmonary AVMs, are not always obtained in patients with hereditary hemorrhagic telangiectasia and negative results of echocardiography. In addition, this technique cannot determine the number of pulmonary AVMs, their location in the lung, and their size. It should also be pointed out that this technique is not devoid of complications in patients with pulmonary AVMs. A transitory cerebral accident may occur after an intravenous peripheral injection of agitated saline solution or of a mixture of saline solution and a small amount of air used as a microbubble contrast agent during echocardiography (98). Several articles have recently appeared concerning estimation of the anatomic intrapulmonary shunt by measurements of arterial oxygen saturation, or Sa_{O_2}, and measurements of arterial partial pressure of oxygen, or Pa_{O_2}, and hemoglobin after breathing 100% oxygen for 15 minutes, and intravenous injection of technetium 99m–labeled albumin macroaggregates or microspheres (118,119). Despite being able to detect and quantify a right-to-left shunt, these techniques suffer from the same drawbacks as those cited for echocardiography. Consequently, they can be routinely used in families with hereditary hemorrhagic telangiectasia for the detection of pulmonary AVMs (120), but not for the detection and the pretherapeutic evaluation of these malformations.

Apart from the detection of pulmonary AVMs, spiral CT is useful in the pretherapeutic evaluation of the angioarchitecture of a pulmonary AVM, namely, in the assessment of the number of vessels connected to the aneurysmal sac arteries. With regard to the embolization procedure, the number and orientation of the feeding arteries are the most important anatomic information that determines the technical difficulty and thus the duration of the embolization procedure (Fig 13). Contradictory results on the respective proportions of simple and complex pulmonary AVMs have been reported in the literature. According to White et al (121), 80% of the malformations have a simple angioarchitecture (ie, a single artery being connected to the aneurysmal sac), whereas this percentage decreased to 20% in the Haitjema et al series (122). After the nonenhanced spiral CT evaluation of the thorax aimed at determining the number of malformations, a selective acquisition of the pulmonary AVM to be treated is performed. This second acquisition is usually performed without administration of contrast medium, with selection of a volume of interest that includes the aneurysmal sac and the vascular pedicles. The main technical aspects of this focal spiral CT acquisition can be summarized as follows. The section collimation depends on the location of the malformation. Pulmonary AVMs with vertically oriented pedicles can require a z-axis coverage of up to 10 cm. These acquisitions can be obtained with a 3–5-mm collimation and a pitch of 2. When the vascular pedicles are horizontally oriented, 4–5 cm of the thorax is surveyed with a 2–3-mm collimation and a pitch of 2. Transverse CT scans of the volume of interest are systematically reconstructed, which can be completed by means of 3D reconstructions of the malformations to obtain an overall view of the malformation. For 3D SSD, the threshold values range from −500 to −700 HU to depict pulmonary AVMs from nonenhanced data sets. Whenever transverse CT scans suggest additional tiny arterial branches to be participating in the pulmonary AVM, an additional 3D display is systematically obtained with a lower thresholding segmentation (−850 HU). This lower threshold may allow identification of additional small feeding arteries but markedly increases the profusion of vessels in the volume, which may prevent optimal viewing of the malformation. This is the reason why such a reconstruction is not obtained at first intention. As previously pointed out, an MIP image can also be generated from the same data acquisition. Whereas the depth impression of a 3D SSD enables a clear understanding of the malformation with each viewing angle, analysis of MIP images may be confusing since crossing and looping vessels are not correctly identified, unless the cine loop technique is used.

A comparative study evaluated the respective values of 3D reconstructions and pulmonary angiography in the pretherapeutic management of pulmonary AVMs (123). As expected, it was found that unilateral and selective pulmonary angiography could still be considered the reference standard for the analysis of the angioarchitecture of a pulmonary AVM. However, this technique suffers from several drawbacks. Whatever the viewing angle chosen, unilateral angiography is often unable to depict tiny pulmonary AVMs owing to their superimposition on

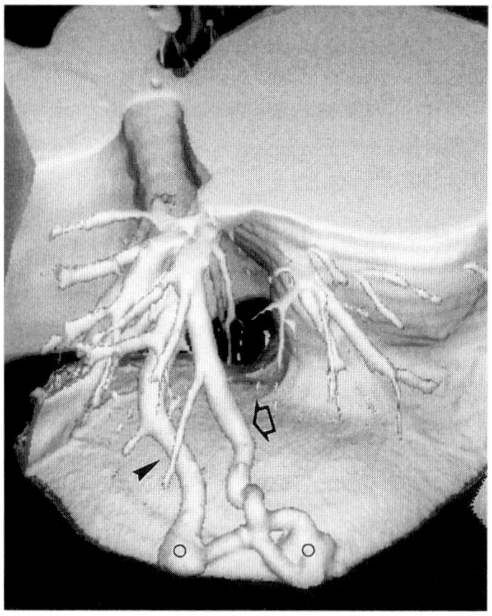

Figure 13. Three-dimensional SSD of a right lower lobe pulmonary AVM evaluated with nonenhanced spiral CT angiography (3-mm collimation, pitch of 1.3, threshold value of −520 HU). Demonstrated is the simple angioarchitecture of the AVM consisting of a single feeding artery (arrow) and a single draining vein (arrowhead), both connected to the aneurysmal sac (open circles).

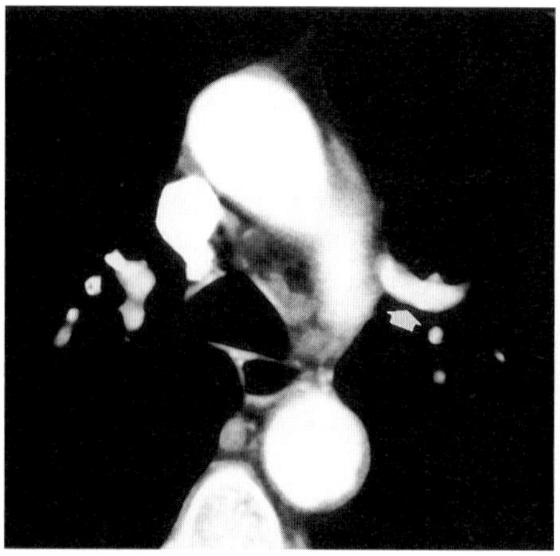

a.

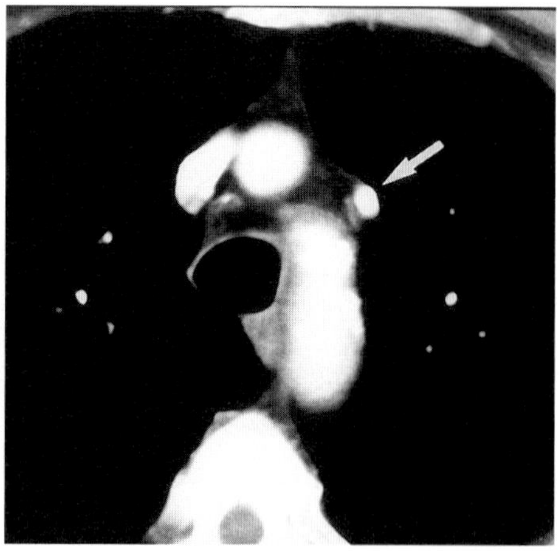

b.

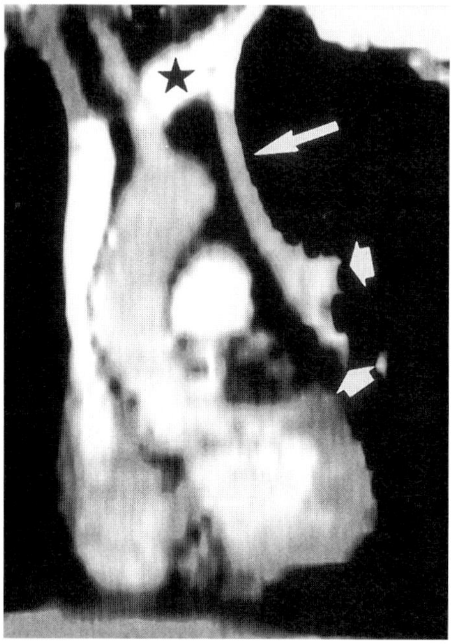

c.

Figure 14. Spiral CT angiography (5-mm collimation, pitch of 1, 30% iodinated contrast agent, inferosuperior acquisition) indicated for the suspicion of a left superior vena cava in a 76-year-old patient with obstructive airway disease. **(a, b)** Spiral CT scans show the partial anomalous pulmonary venous drainage of the left upper lobe (arrow in **a**) into a vertical vein (arrow in **b**). **(c)** Coronal reformation confirms the confluence of the left upper lobe pulmonary veins (short arrows) into the left vertical vein (long arrow), which drains into the left brachiocephalic vein (★).

larger vessels. Conversely, too selective an injection can omit an additional feeding artery or arteries. In the aforementioned study (123) with use of both spiral CT and unilateral selective pulmonary angiography as the reference standard, the angioarchitecture of the pulmonary AVM was confidently analyzed on 3D displays in 76% of cases, enabling correct recognition of 68% of simple and 8% of complex malformations. However, the accuracy of 3D spiral CT was considerably improved when cross-sectional images and 3D views, both from the same data acquisition, were concomitantly analyzed, enabling an accurate evaluation of pulmonary AVM angioarchitecture in 95% of cases. These results confirmed that transverse sections and 3D views provide complementary data, reducing their respective limitations in the analysis of the anatomy of a pulmonary AVM.

Congenital Anomalies of the Pulmonary Veins

Spiral CT is now the method of choice in the assessment of congenital anomalies of the pulmonary venous return. By means of a single data set, this technique enables a noninvasive assessment not only of pulmonary venous anomalies but also of the associated tracheobronchial and pulmonary arterial malformations. The congenital anomalies of the pulmonary venous return can be conveniently classified into one of the following categories: (*a*) anomalous pulmonary venous drainage with or without abnormal course in the lung, (*b*) anomalous pulmonary venous route without abnormal connection, or (*c*) abnormal venous diameters, including varices, stenoses, and atresia.

Partial Anomalous Pulmonary Venous Drainage without Abnormal Course in the Lung

Isolated anomalous drainage of the left superior pulmonary vein into the left brachiocephalic vein is reported to be one of the most common types of abnormal venous drainage. It runs the risk of being confounded with two other anomalies characterized by the presence of a vertical vein on the left border of the mediastinum (ie, a left superior vena cava ending in the coronary sinus, and a left superior vena cava draining into the left atrium). These differential diagnoses can be easily ruled out with spiral CT and specific injection techniques. In the case of a left superior vena cava draining into either the coronary sinus or the left atrium, the systemic venous flow is directed superoinferiorly, in the usual direction. Opacification of this abnormal vein is obtained with a very low concentration of iodinated contrast material, injected at a slow flow rate into the left arm positioned alongside the thorax to avoid the risk of obstruction at the thoracic inlet. An 8%–12% iodine concentration and a flow rate of 3 mL/sec are usually optimal technical parameters because the contrast medium is directed primarily toward the left superior vena cava owing to the absence or the small size of the left brachiocephalic vein. The start delay between injection and acquisition is short, usually 5 seconds.

In the case of partial anomalous venous return of the left upper lobe in a vertical vein, the blood flow is directed inferosuperiorly, partially draining the left upper lobe venous blood into the origin

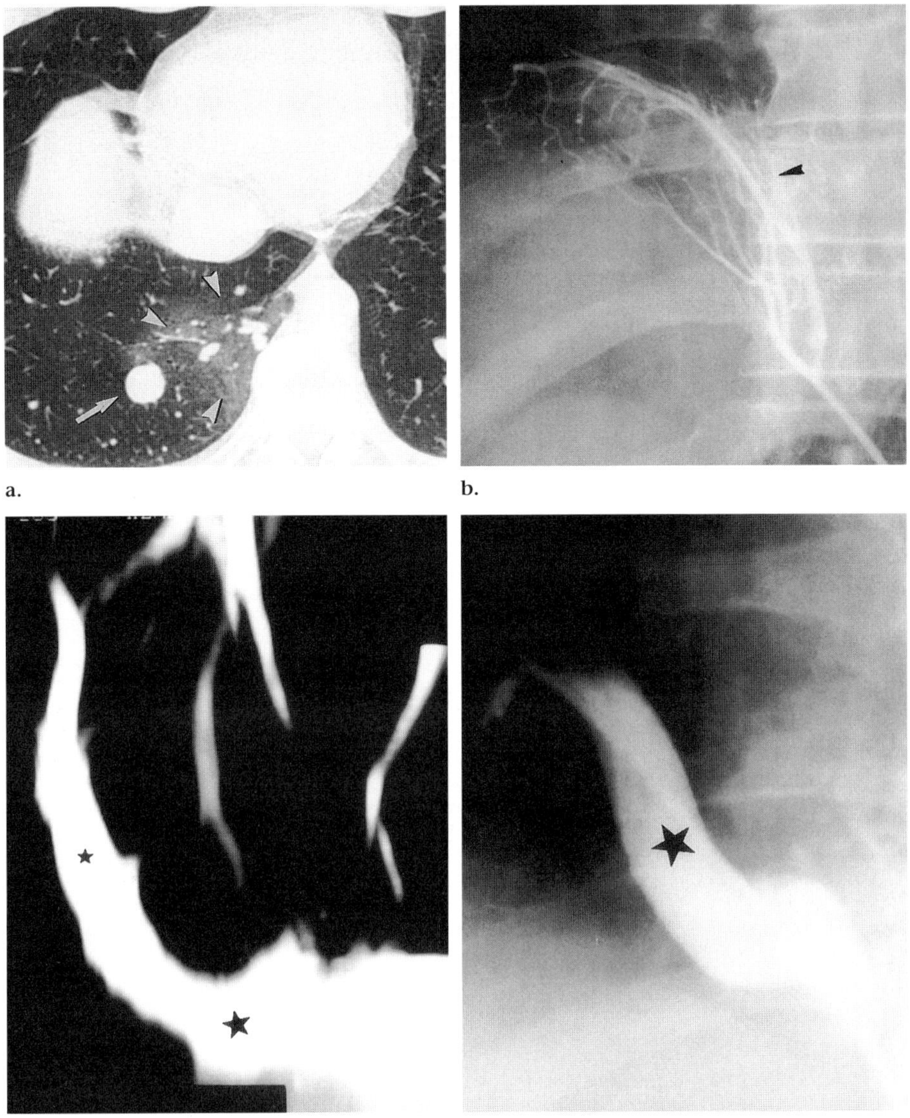

Figure 15. CT and conventional angiographic evaluation of a scimitar syndrome diagnosed in a 29-year-old patient who presented with hemoptysis originating from the right lower lobe. **(a)** Transverse thin-section CT scan obtained at the level of the lower lobes shows numerous and abnormally dilated vascular structures within an area of ground-glass attenuation (arrowheads) in the right posterobasal segment and a large vascular structure (arrow) corresponding to the scimitar vein. **(b)** Hyperselective catheterization of the right inferior phrenic artery, obtained prior to embolization, demonstrates the abnormal systemic arterial supply to the right posterobasal segment (arrowhead). **(c)** Frontal MIP image generated from a focal spiral CT angiogram (5-mm collimation, pitch of 1.4, 30% iodinated contrast agent) of the lower lung zones provides an overall analysis of the scimitar vein (small ★) draining into the inferior vena cava (large ★) without stenosis at its distal portion. **(d)** Selective catheterization (frontal angiogram obtained during the hemodynamic evaluation of the scimitar syndrome) of the scimitar vein (★) confirms the absence of stenosis of the abnormal pulmonary venous drainage.

TABLE 2
Pretherapeutic Assessment of Scimitar Spectrum

Anomalies	Invasive Assessment	Noninvasive Assessment
Systemic collateral supply to the right lung	Aortography	Spiral CT angiography of the aorta
Pulmonary artery anomalies and scimitar vein	Pulmonary angiography	Spiral CT angiography of the pulmonary circulation
Bronchial anomalies	Bronchography and/or bronchoscopy	Bronchographic-like volume-rendering technique
Left-to-right shunt from the scimitar vein to the right atrium	Measurement of right-to-left shunt	MR evaluation
Abnormal lobation of the right lung	None	Thin-section CT
Horseshoe lung	None	Thin-section CT

of the left brachiocephalic vein (Fig 14). Owing to the reversed flow, the vertical vein cannot be opacified by using the aforementioned technique because the small and slow bolus would be diluted in the left brachiocephalic vein. Consequently, the optimal injection technique employs a high iodine concentration (eg, 300 mg/mL, a flow rate of 5 mL/sec, and a minimum start delay of 12–15 seconds. As previously suggested, the most appropriate injection protocol can only be selected once the morphologic criteria are identified on nonenhanced scans. In the case of partial anomalous venous return in the vertical vein, its connection with the origin of the vertical vein is easily identified. Consequently, the rest of the normally positioned left superior pulmonary vein anterior to the left upper lobe bronchus is depicted as a small structure or is absent. The left brachiocephalic vein, which drains the left subclavian vein, the left internal jugular vein, and the vertical vein, is normal or slightly dilated. The coronary sinus is normal.

When it is associated with a septal defect, obstructive airway disease, or any other cause of restriction of the vascular bed, a left-to-right shunt due to the ectopic drainage of a part of the left upper lobe can be responsible for some dilatation of intraparenchymal vessels (124). If the left superior vena cava drains into the coronary sinus or the left atrium, the left brachiocephalic vein is absent or small, and the confluence of the left upper lobe pulmonary venous tributaries in the vertical vein does not exist. The left upper pulmonary vein has a normal size. If drainage is into the coronary sinus, the latter is dilated, whereas it is of normal size when drainage is into the left atrium.

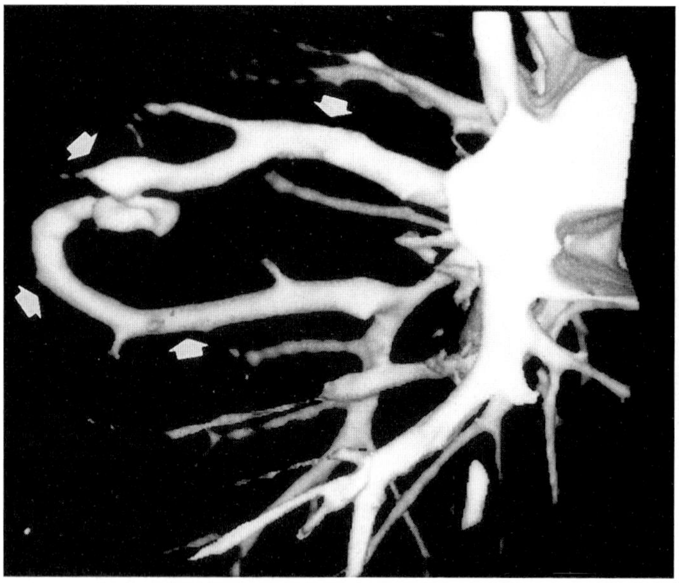

a.

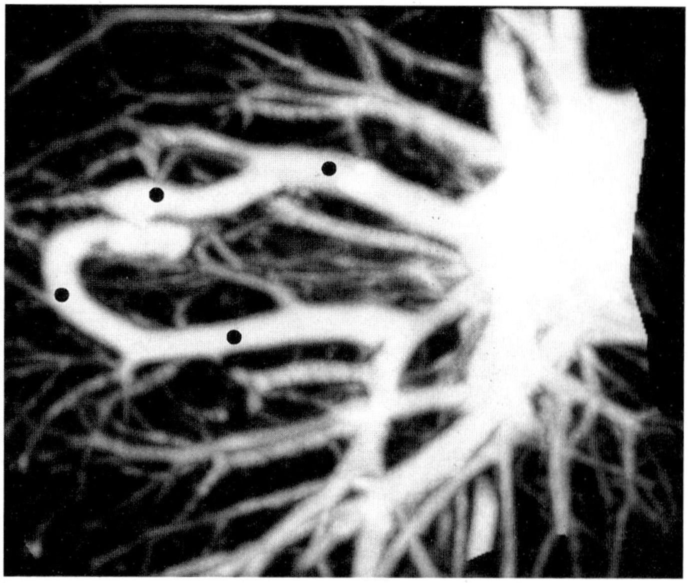

b.

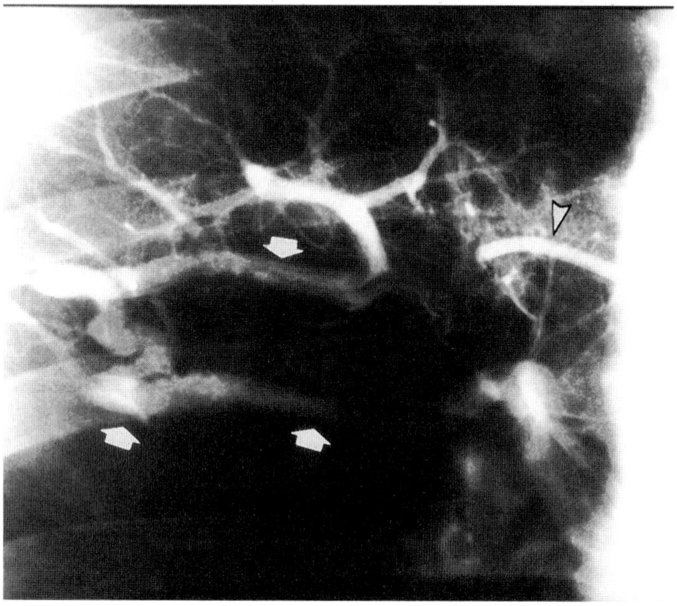

c.

Figure 16. Suspicion of a right upper lobe pulmonary AVM in a 60-year-old man. **(a)** Three-dimensional SSD (inferosuperior view, threshold of +150 HU) and **(b)** vertical MIP image, both generated from the same focal spiral CT angiogram (2-mm collimation, pitch of 1.5, 24% iodinated contrast agent), show the abnormal route of a right upper lobe pulmonary vein (arrows in **a**, ● in **b**), mimicking a pulmonary AVM. **(c)** The venous phase of the hyperselective right upper lobe angiogram (frontal view) confirms the abnormal route of the right upper lobe pulmonary vein (arrows) without abnormal connection (the arrowhead points to the tip of the catheter).

It is thus evident that precise analysis of relevant morphologic features on nonenhanced CT sections and physiologically adapted injection techniques constitute the state-of-the-art approach for these diagnoses. Moreover, MPR images and 3D images can elucidate further the course of the abnormal vessels.

When isolated, the degree of the left-to-right shunt is equal to or less than 25% of the cardiac output and is compatible with a normal life. However, this acceptable hemodynamic condition can decompensate after contralateral surgery and can become a major left-to-right shunt, almost 50% of the cardiac output, after a right pneumonectomy (125). Consequently, when routinely using preoperative CT of the thorax, it is important to bear in mind the surgical importance of an unsuspected partial anomalous venous drainage of the left superior pulmonary vein into the left brachiocephalic vein whenever the patient is a candidate for right lung surgery. Depending on the importance of the lung volume to be resected, the anomalous vein may be preventively reimplanted into the left atrial appendage.

The diagnosis of partial anomalous pulmonary venous return of the right upper lobe into the right superior vena cava or the azygos arch can be made on incremental CT scans (126,127). Cross-sectional images, without contrast material enhancement, show right dilated pulmonary veins in close contact with the superior vena cava and/or the terminal portion of the azygos arch. As previously pointed out with regard to the left superior pulmonary vein, the expected normal part in the hilum and near the left atrium is not found or is too small. The diagnosis is easily confirmed with spiral CT angiography, which can use 3D reconstructions with the aim of clarifying this anomaly (128). Optimally, however, contrast material should be injected into the inferior vena cava to avoid simultaneous opacification of the pulmonary venous return and the superior vena cava from an injection into the arm.

Abnormal Venous Drainage with Abnormal Route in the Lung

In the majority of patients, a partial or total pulmonary anomalous venous return of the right lung, usually into the inferior vena cava or the right atrium, is easily diagnosed on a chest radiograph provided that the right lung is not too

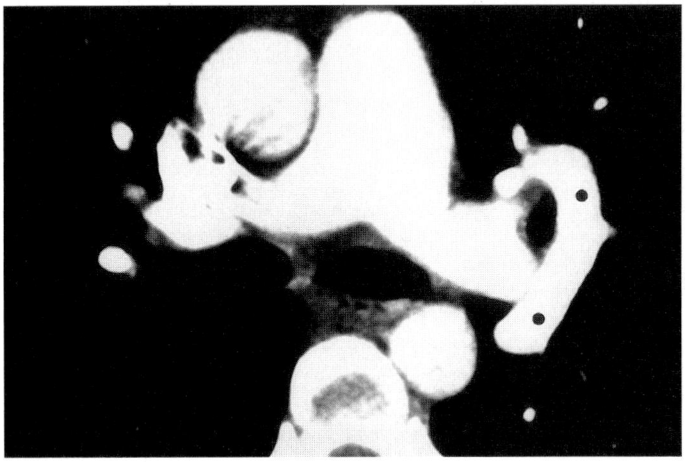
a.

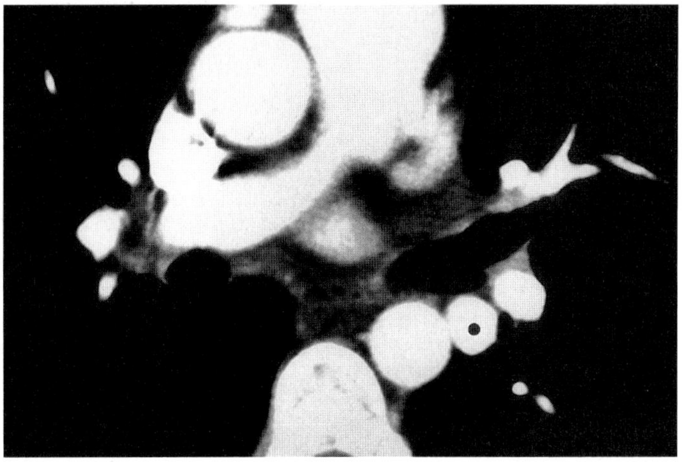
b.

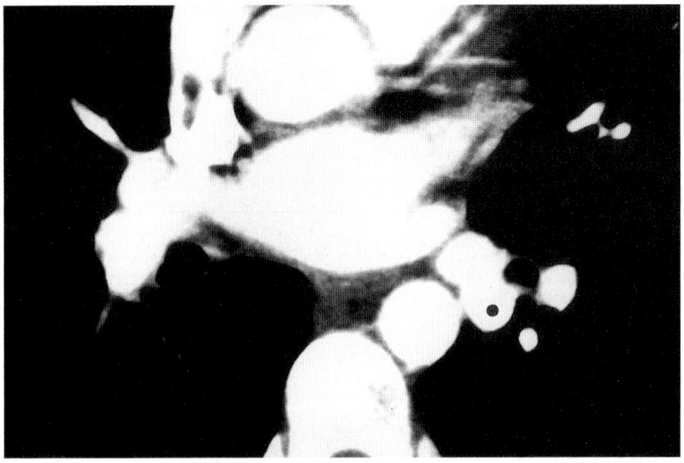
c.

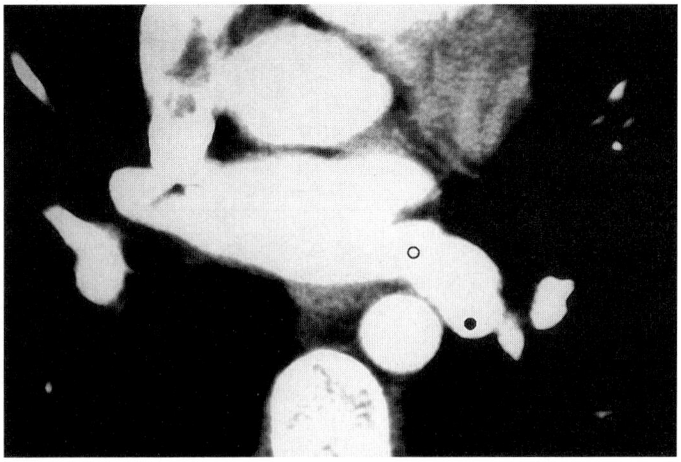
d.

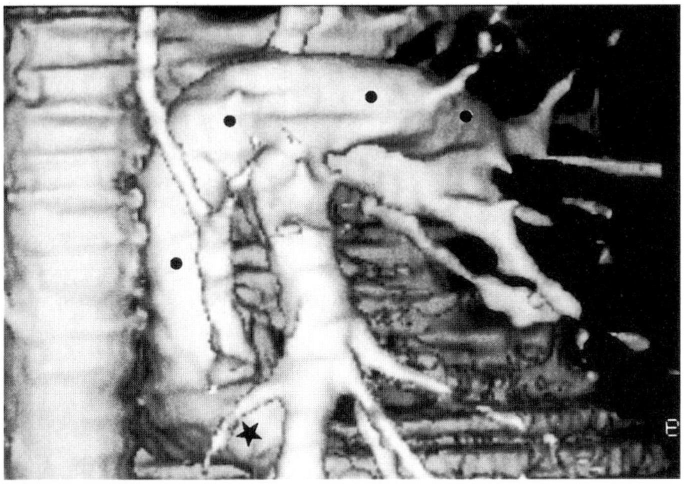
e.

Figure 17. Spiral CT angiography (5-mm collimation, pitch of 1.7, 30% iodinated contrast agent) performed in a 61-year-old patient evaluated for left hilar enlargement. **(a–d)** Spiral CT angiograms enable recognition of the abnormal juxtahilar route of a left upper lobe pulmonary vein (●) draining into the left inferior pulmonary vein (○ in **d**). **(e)** Three-dimensional SSD (lateral view, threshold of +150 HU) generated from the same data set provides an overall view of the sub- and retro-hilar route of the abnormal vein (●) and of its normal drainage into the left atrium (★).

hypoplastic. The abnormal vein can be an isolated finding or may be associated with other anomalies termed the "scimitar syndrome" or "scimitar spectrum." The abnormal right pulmonary vein drains the right lung or only one portion of it into the inferior vena cava just above or below the diaphragm, looking like a Turkish sword. It receives the abnormal systemic arterial supply of the right lung, which triggers an additional more or less severe left-to-right shunt. It can be stenosed at its implantation into the inferior vena cava. The scimitar syndrome can be considered as a multiplanar anomaly, particularly suited for a spiral CT angiographic evaluation. It requires 3D reformations with or without contrast medium to provide an overall view of the abnormal vein (Fig 15), while thin-section CT scans can depict septal lines when the abnormal pulmonary venous return is obstructed. In the context of a preoperative evaluation, depiction of the pseudofissural line corresponding to the close contact between the right lung herniated behind the heart (horseshoe lung) and the left lung also requires thin sections. Three-dimensional reformations of the tracheobronchial tree are useful for an easier description of the abnormal right bronchial tree and 3D reformations of the abnormal systemic artery or arteries require good opacification. These vessels can be identified by their spontaneous high contrast if the right lower lobe has a normal attenuation. But their subdiaphragmatic origin and course are only clearly seen after injection of contrast medium. When considering the abovementioned advantages of spiral CT in the recognition of the various anomalies observed in patients with scimitar syndrome (Table 2), one should strongly disagree with the conclusions of Schramel et al (129). In 1995, these authors stated that "angiography of the aorta, pulmonary arteries and veins, bronchoscopy, bronchography, spirometry, lung scintigraphy or bronchospirometry, and measurement of left/right shunt are essential in the management of patients with scimitar syndrome" (129). When surgery is needed, noninvasive follow-up after reimplantation of the abnormal vein in the left atrium can also require spiral CT angiography, especially when postoperative obstruction to the reimplanted abnormal pulmonary venous return in itself represents a further indication for pneumonectomy.

Abnormal Route without Abnormal Connection

Three-dimensional reconstructions with or without injection of contrast medium can help differentiate between some variants of the scimitar syndrome. In a first variation, the anomalous vein courses down to the diaphragm and drains simultaneously into the inferior vena cava and the left atrium. Surgical ligation of the part draining into the inferior vena cava may be required for rerouting of the venous return toward the left atrium. In another variant, despite a scimitar-like course in the lung, the vein normally enters the left atrium without any connection with the inferior vena cava, thus described as a "pseudo–scimitar syndrome" (130). However, there may be a more important overlap between the scimitar syndrome and the pseudo–scimitar syndrome as the latter can also include a hypoplastic right lung and an abnormal systemic arterial supply (131). Other ectopic venous routes can mimic a partial anomalous pulmonary venous return or pulmonary AVM (Fig 16) and can be associated with dextroposition of the heart and hypoplasia of the right lung (132). Whenever patients are asymptomatic without any cardiac hemodynamic alterations, pulmonary angiography must be considered disproportionate, and 3D CT angiography or MR angiography should be the first investigation to be considered. In rare cases of juxtahilar abnormal route, the venous anomaly can be an incidental finding on spiral CT angiograms (Fig 17).

Congenital Pulmonary Venous Stenosis or Atresia

Stenosis of the pulmonary veins at their junction with the left atrium is one cause of obstruction of pulmonary venous return. This disease is difficult to diagnose clinically, and in most of the published cases, the diagnosis was mainly made with surgical or anatomic postmortem studies. Before the introduction of spiral CT angiography, the definitive diagnosis of pulmonary venous stenosis was considered to be possible only with angiography, explaining the considerable delay in its recognition in the absence of high clinical suspicion. Whereas congenital pulmonary venous stenosis can be suspected on the basis of chest radiographic findings, this diagnosis can be assessed with thin-section CT of the lung parenchyma and spiral CT angiography on the basis of the identification of the following abnormalities: pleural thickening, absence of pulmonary venous reflux from the left atrium, discontinuity between the juxtaatrial part of the pulmonary veins and the left atrium, and retrograde systemic to pulmonary artery shunt (Fig 3).

CONCLUSION

Owing to the multiple possibilities inherent to this technique, spiral CT angiography has the potential for substantial cost savings without reduction in the quality of patient care or diagnostic accuracy. In addition, the concept of using spiral CT as a physiologic tool has just appeared. Advanced computer technology and image-processing techniques will allow automated volume segmentation as well as anatomy and physiology integration with present and future rendering techniques. Undoubtedly, these new technical possibilities are able to offer a large field of investigation. It is also very likely that simulation, treatment planning, and guidance of therapeutic or diagnostic interventions using 3D and multimodality imaging technologies will be routinely applied in the near future.

References

1. Fishman EK. High-resolution three-dimensional imaging from subsecond helical CT data sets: applications in vascular imaging. AJR 1997; 189:441–443.
2. Remy-Jardin M, Remy J, Wattinne L, Giraud F. Central pulmonary thromboembolism: diagnosis with spiral volumetric CT with the single-breath-hold technique—comparison with pulmonary angiography. Radiology 1992; 185:381–387.
3. Blum AG, Delafau F, Grignon B, et al. Spiral computed tomography versus pulmonary angiography in the diagnosis of acute massive pulmonary embolism. Am J Cardiol 1994; 74:96–98.
4. Goodman LR, Curtin JJ, Mewissen MW, et al. Detection of pulmonary embolism in patients with unresolved clinical and scintigraphic diagnosis: helical CT versus angiography. AJR 1995; 164:1369–1374.
5. Teigen CL, Maus TP, Sheedy PF II, Johnson CM, Stanson AW, Welch JJ. Pulmonary embolism: diagnosis with electron beam CT. Radiology 1993; 188:839–845.
6. Remy-Jardin M, Remy J, Deschildre F, et al. Diagnosis of acute pulmonary embolism with spiral CT: comparison with pulmonary angiography and scintigraphy. Radiology 1996; 200:699–706.
7. Remy-Jardin M, Remy J, Artaud D, Deschildre F, Duhamel A. Peripheral pulmonary arteries: optimization of the acquisition protocol. Radiology 1997; 204:157–163.
8. Green JF. Pressure-flow relationships of the pulmonary circulation. In: Green JF, ed. Mechanical concepts in cardiovascular and pulmonary physiology. Philadelphia, Pa: Lea & Febiger, 1977; 55–65.
9. Hughes JM, Glazier JB, Maloney JE, West JB. Effects of lung volume on the distribution of pulmonary blood flow in man. Respir Physiol 1968; 4:58–72.
10. Brink JA. Technical aspects of helical (spiral) CT. Radiol Clin North Am 1995; 33:825–841.
11. Heath DG, Soyer PA, Kuszyk BS, et al. Three-dimensional spiral CT during arterial portography: comparison of three rendering techniques. RadioGraphics 1995; 15:1001–1011.
12. Prokop M, Oh Shin H, Schanz A, Schaefer-Prokop CM. Use of maximum-intensity projections in CT angiography: a basic review. RadioGraphics 1997; 17:433–451.
13. Takahashi M, Ashtari M, Papp Z, et al. CT angiography of carotid bifurcation: artifacts and pitfalls in shaded-surface display. AJR 1997; 168:813–817.
14. Ney DR, Fishman EK, Magid D. Volumetric rendering of computed tomography data: principles and techniques. Comput Graph Applic 1990; 10:24–32.
15. Johnson PT, Heath DG, Kuszyk BS, Fishman EK. CT angiography with volume rendering: advantages and applications in splanchnic vascular imaging. Radiology 1996; 200:564–568.
16. Johnson PT, Heath DG, Kuszyk BS, Fishman EK. CT angiography: thoracic vascular imaging with interactive volume rendering technique. J Comput Assist Tomogr 1997; 21:110–114.
17. Napel S, Rubin GD, Jeffrey RB. STS-MIP: a new reconstruction technique for CT of the chest. J Comput Assist Tomogr 1993; 17:832–838.
18. Remy-Jardin M, Remy J, Pawlak S, et al. Reduction de dose en TDM haute-resolution du poumon (abstr). J Radiol 1998; 79:1109.
19. Hopper KD, King SH, Lobell ME, TenHave TR, Weaver JS. The breast: in-plane x-ray protection during diagnostic thoracic CT—shielding with bismuth radioprotective garments. Radiology 1997; 205:853–858.
20. Brink JA, Woodard PK, Horesh L, et al. Depiction of pulmonary emboli with spiral CT: optimization of display window settings

in a porcine model. Radiology 1997; 204: 703–708.
21. Loud PA, Grossman ZD, Klippenstein DL, Ray CE. Combined CT venography and pulmonary angiography: a new diagnostic technique for suspected thromboembolic disease. AJR 1998; 170:951–954.
22. Coche EE, Muller NL, Kim K, Wiggs BR, Mayo JR. Acute pulmonary embolism: ancillary findings at spiral CT. Radiology 1998; 207:753–758.
23. Remy-Jardin M, Remy J, Artaud D, Deschildre F, Fribourg M, Beregi JP. Spiral CT of pulmonary embolism: technical considerations and interpretive pitfalls. J Thorac Imaging 1997; 12:103–117.
24. Bookstein JJ, Silver TM. The angiographic differential diagnosis of acute pulmonary embolism. Radiology 1974; 110:25–33.
25. Sagel SS, Greenspan RH. Nonuniform pulmonary arterial perfusion: pulmonary embolism. Radiology 1970; 99:541–548.
26. Senac JP, Verhnet H, Bousquet C, et al. Embolie pulmonaire: apport de la tomodensitometrie helicoïdale. J Radiol 1995; 76:339–345.
27. Van Rossum AB, Pattynama PM, Tjin ER, et al. Pulmonary embolism: validation of spiral CT angiography in 149 patients. Radiology 1996; 201:467–470.
28. Ferretti GR, Bosson JL, Buffaz PD, et al. Acute pulmonary embolism: role of helical CT in 164 patients with intermediate probability at ventilation-perfusion scintigraphy and normal results at duplex US of the legs. Radiology 1997; 205:453–458.
29. Mayo JR, Remy-Jardin M, Muller NL, et al. Pulmonary embolism: prospective comparison of spiral CT and ventilation-perfusion scintigraphy. Radiology 1997; 205:447–452.
30. Van Rossum AB, Pattynama PM, Mallens WM, Hermans J, Heijerman HG. Can helical CT replace scintigraphy in the diagnostic process in suspected pulmonary embolism? A retrolective-prolective cohort study focusing on total diagnostic yield. Eur Radiol 1998; 8:90–96.
31. Drucker EA, Rivitz SM, Shepard JO, et al. Acute pulmonary embolism: assessment of helical CT for diagnosis. Radiology 1998; 209:235–241.
32. Herold C, Remy-Jardin M, Grenier PH, et al. Prospective evaluation of pulmonary embolism: initial results of the European Multicenter Trial (ESTIPEP) (abstr). Radiology 1998; 209(P):299.
33. Baghaie F, Remy-Jardin M, Remy J, Artaud D, Fribourg M, Duhamel A. Diagnosis of peripheral acute pulmonary emboli: optimization of the spiral CT acquisition protocol (abstr). Radiology 1998; 209(P): 299.
34. Van Erkel AR, van Rossum AB, Bloem J, Kievit J, Pattynama PM. Spiral CT angiography for suspected pulmonary embolism: a cost-effectiveness analysis. Radiology 1996; 201:29–36.
35. Stein PD, Athanasoulis C, Alavi A, et al. Complications and validity of pulmonary angiography in acute pulmonary embolism. Circulation 1992; 85:462–468.
36. Winston CB, Wechsler RJ, Salazar AM, Kurtz AB, Spirn PW. Incidental pulmonary emboli detected at helical CT: effect on patient care. Radiology 1996; 201:23–27.
37. Gouzien P, Chabierski M, Baccialone J, Jeanbourquin D. Embolie pulmonaire asymptomatique et thrombose veineuse des membres inferieurs. J Radiol 1996; 77:125–128.
38. Schluger N, Henschke C, King T, et al. Diagnosis of pulmonary embolism at a large teaching hospital. J Thorac Imaging 1994; 9:180–184.
39. Goodman LR, Lipchik RJ. Diagnosis of acute pulmonary embolism: time for a new approach. Radiology 1996; 199:25–27.
40. Oser RF, Zuckerman DA, Gutierrez FR, Brink JA. Anatomic distribution of pulmonary emboli at pulmonary angiography: implications for cross-sectional imaging. Radiology 1996; 199:31–35.
41. PIOPED Investigators. Value of the ventilation-perfusion scans in acute pulmonary embolism: result of the prospective investigation of pulmonary embolism diagnosis. JAMA 1990; 263:2753–2759.
42. Gurney JW. No fooling around: direct visualization of pulmonary embolism (editorial). Radiology 1993; 188:618–619.
43. Teigen CL, Maus TP, Sheedy PF II, et al. Pulmonary embolism: diagnosis with contrast-enhanced electron-beam CT and comparison with pulmonary angiography. Radiology 1995; 194:313–319.
44. Moser KM. Venous thromboembolism. Am Rev Respir Dis 1990; 141:235–249.
45. Dalen JE. When can treatment be withheld in patients with suspected pulmonary embolism? Arch Intern Med 1993; 153:1415–1418.
46. Van Rossum AB, Pattynama PM, Ton ET, Kieft G. Spiral CT appearance of resolving clots at 6 week follow-up after acute pulmonary embolism. J Comput Assist Tomogr 1998; 22:413–417.
47. Remy-Jardin M, Louvegny S, Remy J, et al. Acute central thromboembolic disease: posttherapeutic follow-up with spiral CT angiography. Radiology 1997; 203:173–180.
48. Paraskos JA, Aldenstein SJ, Smith RE, et al. Late prognosis of acute pulmonary embolism. N Engl J Med 1973; 289:55–58.
49. Hall RJ, Sutton GC, Kerr IH. Long-term prognosis of treated acute massive pulmonary embolism. Br J Med 1977; 39:1128–1134.
50. Sutton-Hall RJ, Kerr IH. Clinical course and late prognosis of treated subacute massive, acute minor and chronic thromboembolism. Br J Heart 1977; 39:1135–1142.
51. Remy-Jardin M, Remy J, Cauvain O, Petyt L, Wannebroucq J, Beregi J. Diagnosis of central pulmonary embolism with helical CT: role of two-dimensional multiplanar reformations. AJR 1995; 165:1131–1138.
52. Schwickert HC, Schweden FJ, Schild HH, et al. Pulmonary arteries and lung parenchyma in chronic pulmonary embolism: preoperative and postoperative CT findings. Radiology 1994; 191:351–357.
53. Bergin CJ, Sirlin CB, Hauschildt JP, et al. Chronic thromboembolism: diagnosis with helical CT and MR imaging with angiographic and surgical correlation. Radiology 1997; 204:695–702.
54. Roberts HC, Kauczor HU, Schweden F, Thelen M. Spiral CT of pulmonary hypertension and chronic thromboembolism. J Thorac Imaging 1997; 12:118–127.
55. Kauczor HU, Schwickert HC, Mayer E, Schweden F, Schild HH, Thelen M. Spiral CT of bronchial arteries in chronic thromboembolism. J Comput Assist Tomogr 1994; 1:855–861.
56. Remy-Jardin M, Remy J, Louvegny S, Artaud D, Deschildre F, Duhamel A. Airway changes in chronic pulmonary embolism: CT findings in 33 patients. Radiology 1997; 203: 355–360.
57. Shields TW. Surgical therapy for carcinoma of the lung. Clin Chest Med 1993; 14:121–147.
58. Read RC, Ziomek S, Ranval TJ, Eidt JF, Gocio JC, Schaefer RF. Pulmonary artery sleeve resection for abutting left upper lobe lesions. Ann Thorac Surg 1993; 55:850–854.
59. Maggi G, Casadio C, Pischedda F, Cianci R, Ruffini E, Filosso P. Bronchoplastic and angioplastic techniques in the treatment of bronchogenic carcinoma. Ann Thorac Surg 1993; 55:1501–1507.
60. Remy-Jardin M, Duyck PH, Remy J, et al. Hilar lymph nodes: identification with spiral CT and histologic correlation. Radiology 1995; 196:387–394.
61. Khanavkar B, Stern P, Alberti W, Nakhosteen JA. Complications associated with brachytherapy alone or with laser in lung cancer. Chest 1991; 99:1062–1065.
62. Aberle DR, Brown K, Young DA, Batra P, Steckel RJ. Imaging techniques in the evaluation of tracheobronchial neoplasms. Chest 1991; 99:211–215.
63. Spencer DD, Garza JL, Walker WA. Multiple tumor emboli after pneumonectomy. Ann Thorac Surg 1993; 55:169–171.
64. Matsumoto AH, Parker LA, Delany DJ. CT demonstration of central pulmonary venous and arterial occlusive diseases. J Comput Assist Tomogr 1987; 11:640–644.
65. Koo BC, Woldenberg LS, Kim KT. Pulmonary vein tumor thrombosis and left atrial extension in lung carcinoma. J Comput Tomogr 1984; 8:331–336.
66. Takahashi T, Yokoi K, Mori K, Miyazawa N. Clot in the pulmonary artery after pneumonectomy. AJR 1993; 161:1110.
67. Hovaguimian H, Morris JF, Gately HL, Floten HS. Pulmonary vein thrombosis following bilobectomy. Chest 1991; 99:1515–1516.
68. Van Son JA, Danielson GK, Puga FJ, Edwards WD, Driscoll DJ. Repair of congenital and acquired pulmonary vein stenosis. Ann Thorac Surg 1995; 60:144–150.
69. Griffith BP, Magee MJ, Gonzalez IF, et al. Anastomotic pitfalls in lung transplantation. J Thorac Cardiovasc Surg 1994; 107: 743–754.
70. Gaubert JY, Moulin G, Thomas P, Reynaud-Gaubert M, Noirclerc M, Bartoli JM. Anastomotic stenosis of the left pulmonary artery after lung transplantation: treatment by percutaneous placement of an endoprosthesis. AJR 1993; 161:947–949.
71. Kuo PC, Plotkin JS, Johnson LB, et al. Distinctive clinical features of portopulmonary hypertension. Chest 1997; 112:980–986.
72. Kuriyama K, Gamsu G, Stern RG, et al. CT-determined pulmonary artery diameters in predicting pulmonary hypertension. Invest Radiol 1984; 19:16–22.
73. Tan RT, Kuzo R, Goodman LR, Siegel R, Haasler GB, Presberg KW. Utility of CT scan evaluation for predicting pulmonary hypertension in patients with parenchymal lung disease. Chest 1998; 113:1250–1256.
74. Sheerick AD, Swensen SJ, Hartman TE. Mosaic pattern of lung attenuation on CT scans: frequency among patients with pulmonary artery hypertension of different causes. AJR 1997; 169:79–82.
75. Remy-Jardin M, Remy J, Giraud F, Wattine L, Gosselin B. Computed tomography assessment of ground glass opacity: semiology and significance. J Thorac Imaging 1993; 8:249–264.
76. Primack SL, Muller NL, Mayo JR, Remy-Jardin M, Remy J. Pulmonary parenchymal abnormalities of vascular origin: high-resolution CT findings. RadioGraphics 1994; 14:739–746.
77. Stern EJ, Muller NL, Swensen SJ, Hartman TE. CT mosaic pattern of lung attenuation: etiologies and terminology. J Thorac Imaging 1995; 10:294–297.
78. Worthy SA, Muller NL, Hartman TE, Swensen SJ, Padley SP, Hansell DM. Mosaic attenuation pattern on thin-section CT scans of the lung: differentiation among infiltrative lung, airway and vascular diseases as a cause. Radiology 1997; 205:465–470.
79. Eng J, Murday AJ. Leiomyosarcoma of the pulmonary artery. Ann Thorac Surg 1992; 53:905–906.

80. Delany SG, Doyle TC, Bunton RW, Hung NA, Joblin LU, Taylor DR. Pulmonary artery sarcoma mimicking pulmonary embolism. Chest 1993; 103:1631–1633.
81. Bressler EL, Nelson JM. Primary pulmonary artery sarcoma: diagnosis with CT, MR imaging, and transthoracic needle biopsy. AJR 1992; 159:702–704.
82. Cox JE, Chiles C, Aquino SL, Savage P, Oaks T. Pulmonary artery sarcomas: a review of clinical and radiologic features. J Comput Assist Tomogr 1997; 21:750–755.
83. Krinski G, Rofsky N, Sandler M, DeCorato D, Weinreb J. Dynamic breath-hold 3D gadolinium-enhanced MRI of intraarterial masses: findings in two patients. J Comput Assist Tomogr 1997; 21:631–634.
84. Parish JM, Rosenow EC, Swensen SJ, Crotty TB. Pulmonary artery sarcoma: clinical features. Chest 1996; 110:1480–1488.
85. Kauczor HU, Schwickert HC, Mayer E, Kerjes W, Moll R, Schweden F. Pulmonary artery sarcoma mimicking chronic thromboembolic disease: computed tomography and magnetic resonance imaging findings. Cardiovasc Intervent Radiol 1994; 17:185–189.
86. DeLima LG, Wynands JE, Bourke ME, Walley VM. Catheter-induced pulmonary artery false aneurysm and rupture: case report and review. J Cardiothorac Vasc Anesth 1994; 8:70–72.
87. Hubler B, Earls JP, Stevens K. Traumatic pulmonary arterial and venous pseudoaneurysms. AJR 1997; 169:1354.
88. Heussel CP, Kauczor HU, Heussel G, Mildenberger P, Dueber C. Aneurysms complicating inflammatory diseases in immunocompromised hosts: value of contrast-enhanced CT. Eur Radiol 1997; 7:316–319.
89. Iula G, Ziviello R, Vecchio WD. Aneurysms of proximal pulmonary arteries: CT diagnosis and preoperative assessment. Eur Radiol 1996; 6:730–733.
90. Feretti GR, Thony F, Link KM, et al. False aneurysm of the pulmonary artery induced by a Swan-Ganz catheter: clinical presentation and radiologic management. AJR 1996; 167:941–945.
91. Dondelinger RF, Vanderschelden P, Capasso P, Trotteur G. Spiral CT applied to interventional procedures. J Belge Radiol 1995; 78: 118–125.
92. Ahn JM, Im JG, Ryoo JW, et al. Thoracic manifestations of Behçet syndrome: radiographic and CT findings in nine patients. Radiology 1995; 194:199–203.
93. Taylor PM. Dynamic contrast enhancement of asbestos-related pulmonary pseudotumours. Br J Radiol 1988; 61:1070–1072.
94. O'Donovan PB, Schenk M, Lim K, Obuchowski N, Stoller JK. Evaluation of the reliability of computed tomographic criteria used in the diagnosis of round atelectasis. J Thorac Imaging 1997; 12:54–58.
95. Batra P, Brown K, Hayashi K, Mori M. Round atelectasis. J Thorac Imaging 1997; 11:187–197.
96. Hillerdal G. Rounded atelectasis: clinical experience with 74 patients. Chest 1989; 95:836–841.
97. Voisin CH, Fisekci F, Voisin-Saltiel S, Ameille J, Brochard P, Pairon JC. Asbestos-related rounded atelectasis: radiologic and mineralogic data in 23 cases. Chest 1995; 107:477–481.
98. Remy J, Remy-Jardin M. Spiral CT of pulmonary vessels. In: Remy-Jardin M, Remy J, eds. Spiral CT of the chest. Berlin, Germany: Springer-Verlag, 1996; 231–265.
99. Shah RM, Friedman AC. CT angiogram sign: incidence and significance in lobar consolidations evaluated by contrast-enhanced CT. AJR 1998; 170:719–721.
100. Ren H, Hruban RH, Kuhlman JE, et al. Computed tomography of rounded atelectasis. J Comput Assist Tomogr 1989; 12:1031–1034.
101. McHugh K, Blaquiere RM. CT features of rounded atelectasis. AJR 1988; 153:257–260.
102. Remy-Jardin M, Remy J, Artaud D, Deschildre F, Duhamel A. Diffuse infiltrative lung disease: clinical value of sliding-thin-slab maximum intensity projection CT scans in the detection of mild micronodular patterns. Radiology 1996; 200:333–339.
103. Remy J, Remy-Jardin M, Artaud D, Fribourg M. Multiplanar and three-dimensional reconstruction techniques in CT: impact on chest diseases. Eur Radiol 1998; 8:335–351.
104. Shah MJ, Rychik J, Fogel MA, Murphy JD, Jacobs ML. Pulmonary arteriovenous malformations after superior cavopulmonary connection: resolution after inclusion of hepatic veins in the pulmonary circulation. Ann Thorac Surg 1997; 63:960–963.
105. Srivastava D, Preminger T, Lock JE, et al. Hepatic venous blood and the development of pulmonary arteriovenous malformations in congenital heart disease. Circulation 1995; 92:1217–1222.
106. Schraufnagel DE, Kay JM. Structural and pathologic changes in the lung vasculature in chronic liver disease. Clin Chest Med 1996; 17:1–15.
107. Procacci C, Residori E, Bertocco M, Di Benedetto P, Andreis IA, D'Attoma N. Left pulmonary artery sling in the adult: case report and review of the literature. Cardiovasc Intervent Radiol 1993; 16:388–391.
108. Backer CL, Idriss FS, Holinger LD, Mavroudis C. Pulmonary artery sling: results of surgical repair in infancy. J Thorac Cardiovasc Surg 1992; 103:683–691.
109. Katz M, Konen E, Rozenman J, Szeinberg A, Itzchak Y. Spiral CT and 3D image reconstruction of vascular rings and associated tracheobronchial anomalies. J Comput Assist Tomogr 1995; 19:564–568.
110. Park HS, Im JG, Jung JW, Yeon KM. Anomalous left pulmonary artery with complete cartilaginous ring. J Comput Assist Tomogr 1997; 21:478–480.
111. Remy-Jardin M, Remy J, Artaud D, Fribourg M, Duhamel A. Volume rendering of the tracheobronchial tree: clinical evaluation of bronchographic images. Radiology 1998; 208:761–770.
112. Lacrosse M, Trigaux JP, Van Beers BE, Weynants P. 3D spiral CT of the tracheobronchial tree. J Comput Assist Tomogr 1995; 19:341–347.
113. Ko T, Gatz MG, Reisz GR. Congenital unilateral absence of a pulmonary artery: a report of two adult cases. Am Rev Respir Dis 1990; 141:795–798.
114. Catala FJ, Marti-Bonmati L, Morales-Marin P. Proximal absence of the right pulmonary artery in the adult: computed tomography and magnetic resonance findings. J Thorac Imaging 1993; 8:244–247.
115. Remy J, Remy-Jardin M, Wattinne L, Deffontaine C. Pulmonary arteriovenous malformations: evaluation with CT of the chest before and after treatment. Radiology 1992; 182:809–816.
116. Remy-Jardin M, Remy J, Giraud F, Marquette CH. Pulmonary nodules: detection with thick-section spiral CT versus conventional CT. Radiology 1993; 187:513–520.
117. Barzilai B, Waggoner AD, Spessert C, Picus D, Goodenberger D. Two-dimensional contrast echocardiography in the detection and follow-up of congenital pulmonary arteriovenous malformations. Am J Cardiol 1991; 68:1507–1510.
118. Ueki J, Hughes JM, Peters AM, et al. Oxygen and 99m Tc-MAA shunt estimations in patients with pulmonary arteriovenous malformations: effects of changes in posture and lung volume. Thorax 1994; 49:327–331.
119. Whyte MK, Peters AM, Hughes JM, et al. Quantification of right to left shunt at rest and during exercise in patients with pulmonary arteriovenous malformations. Thorax 1992; 47:790–796.
120. White RI. Pulmonary arteriovenous malformations: how do we diagnose them and why is it important to do so? Radiology 1992; 182:633–635.
121. White RI, Mitchell SE, Barth KH, et al. Angioarchitecture of pulmonary arteriovenous malformations: an important consideration before embolotherapy. AJR 1983; 140: 681–686.
122. Haitjema TJ, Overtoom TT, Westermann CJ, Lammers JW. Embolisation of pulmonary arteriovenous malformations: results and follow up in 32 patients. Thorax 1995; 50:719–723.
123. Remy J, Remy-Jardin M, Giraud F, Wattinne L. Angioarchitecture of pulmonary arteriovenous malformations: clinical utility of three-dimensional helical CT. Radiology 1994; 191:657–664.
124. Dillon EH, Camputaro C. Partial anomalous pulmonary venous drainage of the left upper lobe versus duplication of the superior vena cava: distinction based on CT findings. AJR 1993; 160:375–379.
125. Black MD, Shamji FM, Goldstein W, Sachs HJ. Pulmonary resection and controlateral anomalous venous drainage: a lethal combination. Ann Thorac Surg 1992; 53:689–691.
126. Posniak HV, Dudiak CM, Olson MC. Computed tomography diagnosis of partial anomalous pulmonary venous drainage. Cardiovasc Intervent Radiol 1993; 16:319–320.
127. Thorsen MK, Erickson SJ, Mewissen MW, Youker JE. CT and MR imaging of partial anomalous pulmonary venous return to the azygos vein. J Comput Assist Tomogr 1990; 14:1007–1009.
128. Zwetsch B, Wicky S, Meuli R, Schnyder P. Three-dimensional image reconstruction of partial anomalous pulmonary venous return to the superior vena cava. Chest 1995; 108:1743–1745.
129. Schramel FM, Westerman CJ, Knaepen PJ, Van Den Bosch JM. The scimitar syndrome: clinical spectrum and surgical treatment. Eur Respir J 1995; 8:196–201.
130. Takeda S, Imachi T, Arimitsu K, Minami M, Hayakawa M. Two cases of scimitar variant. Chest 1994; 105:292–293.
131. Cukier A, Kavakama J, Teixeira LR, Terra-Filho M, Vargas FS. Scimitar sign with normal pulmonary venous drainage and systemic arterial supply: scimitar syndrome or bronchopulmonary sequestration? Chest 1994; 105:294–295.
132. Rey C, Waksmann G, Francart CH. Anomalous unilateral single pulmonary vein mimicking partial anomalous pulmonary venous return. Cathet Cardiovasc Diagn 1986; 12:330–333.

Follicular Bronchiolitis: Thin-Section CT and Histologic Findings[1]

Sarah J. Howling, MB
David M. Hansell, MD
Athol U. Wells, MB
Andrew G. Nicholson, DM
Julia D. A. Flint, MD
Nestor L. Müller, MD, PhD

Index terms:
Bronchiolitis, 60.2191
Lung, CT, 60.12118
Lung, nodule, 60.281
Lymphatic system, hyperplasia, 996.826
Pneumonitis, lymphocytic interstitial, 60.213

Radiology 1999; 212:637–642

[1] From the Departments of Radiology (S.J.H., N.L.M.) and Pathology (J.D.A.F.), Vancouver Hospital and Health Sciences Centre, University of British Columbia, 855 W 12th Ave, Vancouver, BC, Canada V5Z 1M9; the Departments of Radiology (D.M.H.) and Pathology (A.G.N.), Royal Brompton National Heart and Lung Hospital, London, England; and the Department of Respiratory Medicine, Green Lane Hospital, Auckland, New Zealand (A.U.W.). Received September 10, 1998; revision requested November 2; revision received December 14; accepted March 26, 1999. **Address reprint requests to** N.L.M.

Author contributions:
Guarantors of integrity of entire study, S.J.H., N.L.M.; study concepts and design, D.M.H., N.L.M.; definition of intellectual content, S.J.H., A.U.W., N.L.M.; literature research, S.J.H., A.U.W., N.L.M.; clinical studies, D.M.H., A.U.W., A.G.N., J.D.A.F., N.L.M.; data acquisition, S.J.H., D.M.H., A.U.W., N.L.M.; data analysis, S.J.H., N.L.M.; statistical analysis, A.U.W.; manuscript preparation, S.J.H., N.L.M.; manuscript editing, S.J.H., D.M.H., A.U.W., N.L.M.; manuscript review, S.J.H., D.M.H., A.U.W., A.G.N., N.L.M.

PURPOSE: To evaluate the thin-section computed tomographic (CT) findings of follicular bronchiolitis and compare them with the histologic findings.

MATERIALS AND METHODS: Thin-section CT scans obtained in 12 patients (age range, 24–77 years; mean age, 47 years) with follicular bronchiolitis proved at open lung biopsy were reviewed by two observers. Underlying conditions included rheumatoid arthritis ($n = 8$), mixed collagen vascular disorders ($n = 2$), autoimmune disorder ($n = 1$), and acquired immunodeficiency syndrome ($n = 1$). All patients had thin-section CT scans (1.0–1.5-mm collimation, 11 patients; 3.0-mm collimation, one patient; high-spatial-frequency reconstruction algorithm) obtained at 10-mm intervals through the chest.

RESULTS: The main CT findings included bilateral centrilobular ($n = 12$) and peribronchial ($n = 5$) nodules. All 12 patients had nodules smaller than 3 mm in diameter; six patients also had nodules 3–12 mm in diameter. Areas of ground-glass opacity were present in nine (75%) patients. Histologically, all patients had lymphoid hyperplasia along the bronchioles; eight had peribronchiolar lymphocytic infiltration.

CONCLUSION: The cardinal CT feature of follicular bronchiolitis consists of small centrilobular nodules variably associated with peribronchial nodules and areas of ground-glass opacity.

Follicular bronchiolitis, defined as lymphoid hyperplasia of the bronchus-associated lymphoid tissue, is characterized histologically by the presence of hyperplastic lymphoid follicles with reactive germinal centers distributed along the bronchioles and, to a lesser extent, bronchi (1–3). Most cases are associated with collagen vascular diseases, immunodeficiency, or hypersensitivity reaction (2–5).

It has been postulated that follicular bronchiolitis accounts for the poorly defined centrilobular and subpleural nodules seen at computed tomography (CT) in 20%–70% of patients with collagen vascular disease (6,7). Limited information is available, however, about the correlation between the CT and histologic findings in follicular bronchiolitis (4,6,7). The aim of the present study was to review the CT findings in 12 patients with biopsy-proved follicular bronchiolitis and to compare the CT with the histologic findings.

MATERIALS AND METHODS

The thin-section CT scans obtained in 12 patients (five men, seven women; age range, 24–77 years; mean age, 47 years) with biopsy-proved follicular bronchiolitis were studied retrospectively. The study group included eight patients with rheumatoid arthritis, two with mixed collagen vascular diseases, one with a nonspecific autoimmune disorder, and another with acquired immunodeficiency syndrome. Two patients were current smokers, two were ex-smokers, and eight had never smoked. The 12 patients were all those with a diagnosis of follicular bronchiolitis who underwent CT at the authors' institutions between July 1987 and July 1997. Patients who had a histologic diagnosis of follicular bronchiolitis but did not have CT scans available for review were excluded from the study. A histologic

Main CT and Histopathologic Findings

Patient No./ Sex/ Age (y)	Underlying Disease	Main CT Findings: Centrilobular Nodules	Peribronchial Nodules	Nodule Size: <3 mm	3–10 mm	Ground-glass Opacity	Main Histologic Findings
1/M/31	Rheumatoid arthritis	Present	Absent	Present	Absent	Absent	Follicular bronchiolitis
2/F/53	Rheumatoid arthritis	Present	Present	Present	Present	Present	Follicular bronchiolitis and mild peribronchiolar interstitial inflammation
3/F/24	Rheumatoid arthritis	Present	Absent	Present	Absent	Present	Follicular bronchiolitis and mild peribronchiolar interstitial inflammation
4/M/73	Rheumatoid arthritis	Present	Absent	Present	Absent	Present	Follicular bronchiolitis and peribronchiolar interstitial inflammation
5/F/36	Rheumatoid arthritis	Present	Present	Present	Present	Present	Follicular bronchiolitis and mild diffuse interstitial inflammation
6/F/52	Collagen vascular disease	Present	Absent	Present	Present	Absent	Follicular bronchiolitis
7/M/61	Collagen vascular disease	Present	Absent	Present	Present	Present	Follicular bronchiolitis and mild peribronchiolar interstitial inflammation
8/F/54	Rheumatoid arthritis	Present	Absent	Present	Absent	Present	Follicular bronchiolitis
9/M/49	Acquired immunodeficiency syndrome	Present	Present	Present	Absent	Present	Follicular bronchiolitis and mild peribronchiolar interstitial inflammation
10/F/24	Rheumatoid arthritis	Present	Present	Present	Present	Present	Follicular bronchiolitis and peribronchiolar interstitial inflammation
11/F/28	Rheumatoid arthritis	Present	Present	Present	Absent	Present	Follicular bronchiolitis and peribronchiolar interstitial inflammation
12/M/77	Autoimmune disorder	Present	Absent	Present	Absent	Absent	Follicular bronchiolitis

diagnosis of follicular bronchiolitis characterized by prominent hyperplasia of lymphoid follicles around the airways was required for inclusion (1,3).

The study included only patients in whom follicular bronchiolitis was the predominant or the only abnormality seen histologically. Patients with lymphoid hyperplasia related to bronchiectasis or chronic pulmonary infection or in association with pulmonary neoplasms were excluded from the study.

CT scans were obtained with an electron-beam scanner (Imatron, San Francisco, Calif; n = 8), a model 9800 or Prospeed Sx Advantage scanner (GE Medical Systems, Milwaukee, Wis; n = 3), or a Somotom DR scanner (Siemens, Iselin, NJ; n = 1). Thin-collimation (1.0–1.5-mm-collimation, 11 patients; 3.0-mm-collimation, one patient) sections were obtained at 10-mm intervals from the lung apices to the bases, with the patient breath holding in full inspiration. Images were reconstructed by using a high-spatial-frequency algorithm and were printed with window settings appropriate for viewing the lungs (window width, 1,000–1,500 HU; window level, −700 to −600 HU). CT scans were interpreted simultaneously by two radiologists (S.J.H., N.L.M.), and conclusions were reached by consensus.

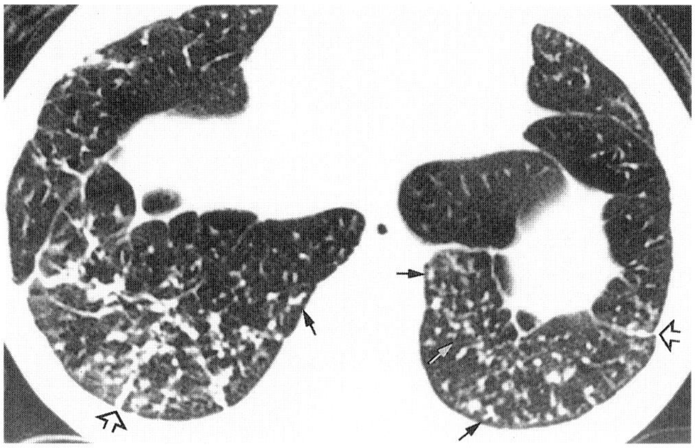

Figure 1. Follicular bronchiolitis. Thin-section (1.5-mm-collimation) CT scan through the lower zones in a 61-year-old man with a mixed collagen vascular disease demonstrates multiple well-defined nodules. Several nodules (solid arrows) are clustered and a few millimeters from the pleura or interlobular septa, which indicates centrilobular distribution. Mild interlobular septal thickening (open arrows) is also present.

The CT scans were assessed for the presence and distribution of ground-glass opacity, airspace consolidation, nodules, and peribronchial and interlobular septal thickening. The presence and extent of associated findings such as bronchial dilatation, emphysema, architectural distortion, honeycombing, mosaic perfusion, and pleural effusion were also assessed. "Ground-glass opacity" was defined as a hazy increase in lung opacity in which the bronchi and vessels remained visible,

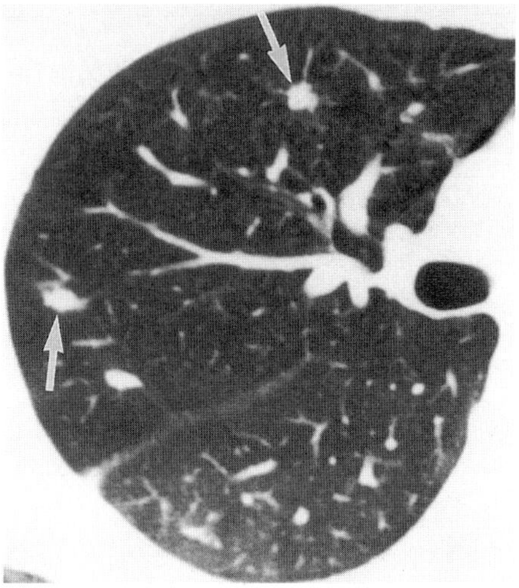

Figure 2. Follicular bronchiolitis. Thin-section (1.5-mm-collimation) CT scan in a 24-year-old woman with rheumatoid arthritis demonstrates nodules (arrows) in a peribronchovascular distribution. The nodules measure between 3 and 10 mm in diameter.

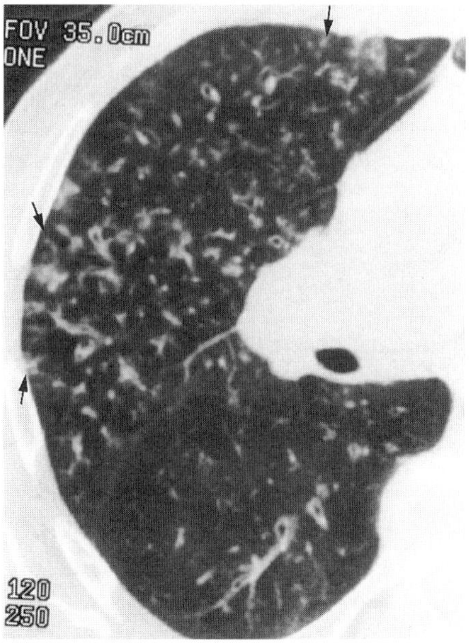

Figure 3. Follicular bronchiolitis. Thin-section (1-mm-collimation) CT scan in a 77-year-old man with an autoimmune disorder shows small centrilobular (arrows) and peribronchial nodules, peribronchial thickening, and small patchy areas of ground-glass opacity.

and "airspace consolidation" was defined as an area of increased attenuation with obscuration of bronchovascular structures. Bronchial dilatation was considered present when the internal diameter of a bronchus was greater than that of the adjacent pulmonary artery or when a bronchus was visualized within 1 cm of the costal pleura. The diagnosis of bronchial wall thickening was based on subjective assessment.

Parenchymal nodules were categorized according to size: smaller than 3 mm, between 3 and 10 mm, and larger than 10 mm. Distribution of parenchymal nodules was recorded as (*a*) centrilobular when nodules were identified around peripheral pulmonary arterial branches or 3–5 mm away from the pleura, interlobular septa, or pulmonary veins; (*b*) peribronchial when nodules were identified around lobar, segmental, or subsegmental bronchi; (*c*) subpleural if there was a predilection for the outer third of the lung in the transverse plane; and (*d*) indeterminate. The distribution of nodules was also assessed as being within areas of ground-glass opacity or away from areas of ground-glass opacity and as being greater in areas with ground-glass opacity or greater away from areas of ground-glass opacity. To determine the distribution of parenchymal abnormalities, each lung was divided into three zones: upper, or superior to the level of the tracheal carina; middle, or between the level of the carina and the level of the inferior pulmonary veins; and lower, or below the level of the inferior pulmonary veins. Each zone was evaluated separately.

Chest CT was performed within 15 days of histologic diagnosis in 11 patients and within 31 days in one patient (median, 8 days). In all patients, the diagnosis was proved at open lung biopsy. Lung biopsy specimens were obtained from at least two lobes at surgery in seven patients and from one lobe in five.

Statistical analysis was performed by using the Fisher exact test and the matched-pairs signed rank test.

RESULTS

CT Findings

The most common CT abnormalities consisted of parenchymal nodular opacities and areas of ground-glass opacity (Table).

Nodules were present in all 12 patients (Fig 1). They were bilateral in all patients and were diffuse ($n = 8$), involved mainly the lower zones ($n = 3$), or were equally distributed in the upper and lower zones ($n = 1$). Nodules less than 3 mm in diameter were observed in all 12 patients, with nodules between 3 and 10 mm in diameter identified in five (42%) patients (Fig 2). Nodules greater than 10 mm in diameter were seen in only one patient. A centrilobular distribution was observed in all 12 patients, with additional peribronchial nodules also present in five (42%) and subpleural nodules in three (25%) patients (Fig 2). There was no appreciable difference in the size, distribution, or profusion of nodules between patients with rheumatoid arthritis and patients with other collagen vascular diseases (Table).

The second most common finding, observed in nine (75%) of 12 patients, was the presence of areas of ground-glass opacity (Fig 3). In all but one patient, the areas of ground-glass opacity were bilateral and had a nonsegmental, patchy distribution.

The nodular profusion in areas of ground-glass opacity was compared with the nodular profusion in the remainder of the lung parenchyma. In seven of eight patients with a patchy ground-glass pattern, nodules were most profuse in the areas of ground-glass opacity ($P = .01$, matched-pairs signed rank test).

Less common CT findings included bronchial dilatation ($n = 4$), bronchial wall thickening ($n = 4$), emphysema ($n = 4$), architectural distortion ($n = 3$), mild interlobular septal thickening ($n = 2$), and peribronchovascular consolidation ($n = 1$). Mosaic perfusion was not seen in any of the patients. There were no pleural effusions or areas of honeycombing.

Histologic Findings

The histologic findings consisted of hyperplastic lymphoid follicles with reactive germinal centers distributed along the bronchioles and, to a lesser extent, bronchi (Fig 4). Eight (67%) patients also had a mild degree of lymphocytic interstitial infiltration, often more marked around the airways but also present to a lesser extent in the adjacent alveolar walls (Fig 5). Two patients showed slightly more extensive interstitial infiltration histologically (Fig 6). The infiltrate consisted of small lymphocytes, plasma cells, and histiocytes. Interstitial infiltrates were identified histologically in eight of the nine patients who had areas of ground-glass opacity at CT but not in the three patients who did not have areas of ground-glass opacity ($P < .005$, Fisher exact test).

DISCUSSION

In 1973, Bienenstock et al (8) detailed the normal anatomic distribution of lymphoid tissue in the lung as being along the bronchial tree and interlobular septa and within subpleural nodes. When

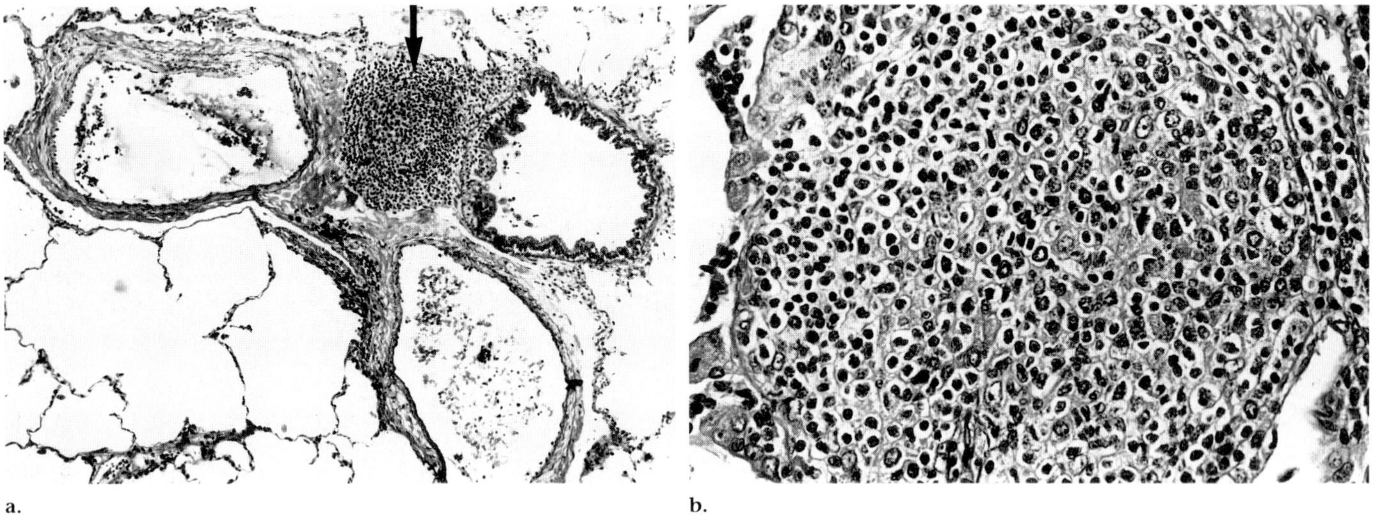

Figure 4. Follicular bronchiolitis in a 24-year-old woman with rheumatoid arthritis. **(a)** Histologic specimen shows mild hyperplasia of a lymphoid follicle (arrow). (Hematoxylin-eosin stain; original magnification, ×20.) **(b)** High-power view shows a benign hyperplastic germinal center. (Hematoxylin-eosin stain; original magnification, ×100.)

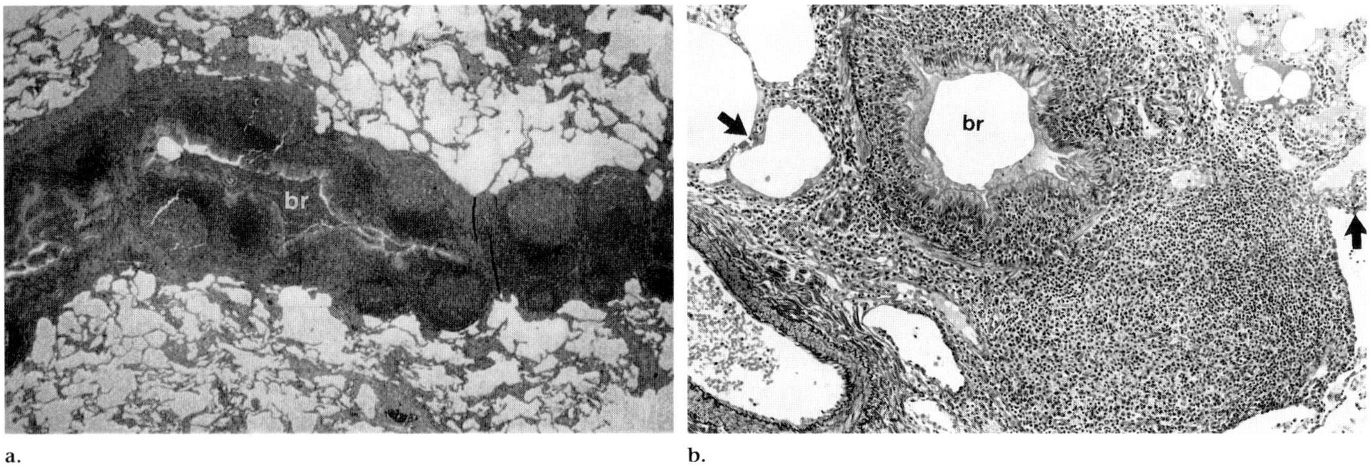

Figure 5. Follicular bronchiolitis. **(a)** Histologic specimen in a 36-year-old woman with rheumatoid arthritis shows that abundant lymphoid follicles are distributed along the bronchiole (*br*). This causes compression of the bronchiolar lumen, which contains an inflammatory exudate. There is only minimal peribronchiolar lymphocytic interstitial infiltration. (Hematoxylin-eosin stain; original magnification, ×20.) **(b)** Histologic specimen in a 49-year-old man with acquired immunodeficiency syndrome demonstrates marked lymphoid hyperplasia that expands the peribronchiolar tissue and encroaches on the bronchiolar wall (*br*). Also noted is infiltration into the adjacent alveolar walls (arrows). (Hematoxylin-eosin stain; original magnification, ×20.)

stimulation of the bronchus-associated lymphoid tissue results in a polyclonal hyperplasia of lymphoid follicles around the bronchioles, the term "follicular bronchiolitis" is used (1,2). Such reactive lymphoid follicles are situated between bronchioles and pulmonary arteries and frequently compress the bronchiolar lumen. Lymphoid hyperplasia of the lungs is a common phenomenon that frequently accompanies chronic infections and is often seen around tumors or abscesses (1,2). However, lymphoid hyperplasia in the absence of tumors or chronic inflammation is uncommon; the largest series we know of was reported by Yousem et al (2) and included only 19 cases.

There have been several recent studies describing the thin-section CT appearances in bronchial and bronchiolar diseases, but there has been little emphasis on the CT findings of follicular bronchiolitis (4,5,9). Remy-Jardin et al (6,7) reviewed the thin-section CT findings in patients with rheumatoid arthritis or progressive systemic sclerosis and found airway abnormalities in 23 (27%) of 84 patients with rheumatoid arthritis. Nodules less than 3 mm in diameter were identified in 17% of 84 patients with rheumatoid arthritis and 46% of 56 patients with systemic sclerosis. The authors suggested that these parenchymal micronodules presumably represented foci of follicular bronchiolitis, a frequent histologic feature in both conditions. Ground-glass opacities (in 54% of patients) and subpleural micronodules (in 85% of patients) were also observed in systemic sclerosis. The authors suggested that the subpleural micronodules might represent small lymphoid aggregates adjacent to the pleura (7).

In the present study, nodules were the most common finding at CT; they were

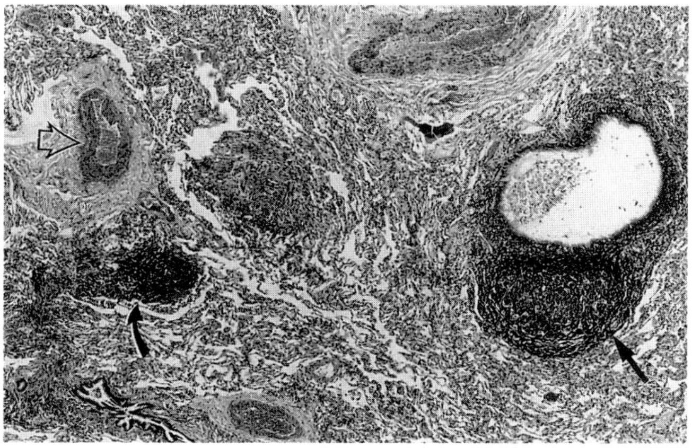

Figure 6. Follicular bronchiolitis in a 28-year-old woman with rheumatoid arthritis. Histologic specimen shows reactive peribronchial germinal center (straight solid arrow) and infiltration of the adjacent parenchyma by mononuclear cells, predominantly lymphocytes. A second focal collection of lymphocytes (curved arrow) obliterates the adjacent airway. The accompanying pulmonary artery (open arrow) can be seen.

observed in all 12 patients. Ranging in size from 1 to 12 mm, they were located predominantly in a centrilobular distribution, although additional peribronchial nodules were present in five (42%) patients. This CT pattern of nodular attenuation is not surprising considering that the predominant histologic findings were of peribronchiolar inflammation and coalescent germinal centers, which are frequently associated with an acute inflammatory exudate within the compressed bronchiolar lumen.

Bronchial dilatation is commonly seen in patients with bronchiolitis (10,11). It is, therefore, possible that the bronchiectasis seen in four patients in the current study was a secondary manifestation of the follicular bronchiolitis. Amorosa et al (12) also described the presence of bronchiectasis in children with lymphocytic interstitial pneumonia. They postulated that the bronchiectasis in lymphocytic interstitial pneumonia may be secondary to compression of the bronchiolar lumen by peribronchiolar infiltration, which may lead to atelectasis and bronchiectasis. The presence of interlobular septal thickening in two patients is difficult to explain on the basis of the histologic findings of follicular bronchiolitis and may have represented incidental, unrelated abnormalities.

The main differential diagnosis of follicular bronchiolitis is with lymphocytic interstitial pneumonia (1,13,14). Lymphocytic interstitial pneumonia shows several histologic features that are similar to those seen in follicular bronchiolitis and is also seen with increased frequency in patients with autoimmune disorders, particularly Sjögren syndrome and immunodeficiency states (13,15,16). The two conditions can be distinguished histologically by virtue of the extent of infiltration and expansion of the interstitium, which is predominantly peribronchial and peribronchiolar in follicular bronchiolitis but diffuse in lymphocytic interstitial pneumonia (1,13,14). Nevertheless, there may be considerable overlap between follicular bronchiolitis and lymphocytic interstitial pneumonia, which compose a spectrum of lymphoid hyperplasia within the lung, and the decision to allocate a specific diagnosis often rests on which component the pathologist believes to be dominant. Thus, although lymphocytic interstitial pneumonia and follicular bronchiolitis are part of the same spectrum of disease, a diagnosis of follicular bronchiolitis can be made when the mononuclear cell infiltration has a predominantly peribronchial and peribronchiolar distribution. This distribution and the focal nature of the infiltrates presumably account for the centrilobular and peribronchial distribution of nodules seen on CT.

Limited information is available about the CT findings in patients with lymphocytic interstitial pneumonia (17–21). The most common CT abnormality found in immunocompetent patients is bilateral areas of ground-glass opacity, which are infrequently associated with small nodules or cysts (17–19,21). In those adult patients with immunodeficiency states, small (2–4-mm) nodules are the predominant CT finding (20). Therefore it is reasonable to postulate that there is considerable overlap between the thin-section CT findings of lymphocytic interstitial pneumonia and those of follicular bronchiolitis.

A centrilobular distribution of abnormalities is by no means specific to follicular bronchiolitis and has been reported in a variety of diseases that predominantly affect the centrilobular bronchioles, pulmonary arteries, and lymphatic vessels (22). In the absence of a tree-in-bud sign, centrilobular nodules are most typical of bronchiolar diseases not associated with infection, including cystic fibrosis, bronchiectasis, panbronchiolitis, sarcoidosis, respiratory bronchiolitis, and extrinsic allergic alveolitis (23–25).

In three of our 12 patients, one of whom had rheumatoid arthritis, histologic examination also revealed a few airways with fibrous obliteration. Similar mixed findings have been reported in previous studies (4,26), and Wells and du Bois (27) speculated that follicular bronchiolitis and obliterative bronchiolitis might coexist. The exact relationship, if any, however, between these two lesions remains unclear. Furthermore, both conditions occur in isolation in rheumatoid arthritis, and thus an apparent relationship might be coincidental.

Our study has several limitations, including a relatively small number of patients, its retrospective nature, and a lack of direct correlation between the CT and the histologic findings. In particular, because the CT scans and histologic specimens were not obtained on the same day, it is conceivable that the areas of ground-glass opacity seen at CT may have been due to pulmonary edema or pneumonia. Furthermore, there may have been improvement or worsening of the interstitial lymphocytic infiltration in the interval between CT and lung biopsy.

In summary, we reviewed the CT scans of 12 patients who had biopsy-proved follicular bronchiolitis. The cardinal signs of follicular bronchiolitis were a mixed pattern of small centrilobular nodules variably associated with patchy ground-glass opacity. Additional peribronchial nodules were a frequent finding.

References

1. Myers JL, Kurtin PJ. Lymphoid proliferative disorders of the lung. In: Thurlbeck WM, Churg AM, eds. Pathology of the lung. 2nd ed. New York, NY: Thieme, 1995; 535–588.
2. Yousem SA, Colby TV, Carrington CB. Follicular bronchitis/bronchiolitis. Hum Pathol 1985; 16:700–706.
3. Fortoul TI, Cano-Valle F, Oliva E, Barrios R. Follicular bronchiolitis in association with connective tissue diseases. Lung 1985; 163:305–314.

4. Hayakawa H, Sato A, Imokawa S, Toyoshima M, Chida K, Iwata M. Bronchiolar disease in rheumatoid arthritis. Am J Respir Crit Care Med 1996; 154:1531–1536.
5. Kinoshita M, Higashi T, Tanaka C, Tokunaga N, Ichikawa Y, Oizumi K. Follicular bronchiolitis associated with rheumatoid arthritis. Intern Med 1992; 31:674–677.
6. Remy-Jardin M, Remy J, Cortet B, Mauri F, Declambre B. Lung changes in rheumatoid arthritis: CT findings. Radiology 1994; 193:375–382.
7. Remy-Jardin M, Remy J, Wallaert B, Bataille D, Hatron P. Pulmonary involvement in progressive systemic sclerosis: sequential evaluation with CT, pulmonary function tests, and bronchoalveolar lavage. Radiology 1993; 188:499–506.
8. Bienenstock J, Johnston N, Perey DYE. Bronchial lymphoid tissue. I. Morphologic characteristics. Lab Invest 1973; 28: 686–692.
9. Reittner P, Fotter R, Lindbichler F, et al. HRCT features in a 5-year-old child with follicular bronchiolitis. Pediatr Radiol 1997; 27:877–879.
10. Lentz D, Bergin CJ, Berry GJ, Stoehr C, Theodore J. Diagnosis of bronchiolitis obliterans in heart-lung transplantation patients: importance of bronchial dilatation on CT. AJR 1992; 159:463–467.
11. Müller NL, Miller RR. Diseases of the bronchioles: CT and histopathologic findings. Radiology 1995; 196:3–12.
12. Amorosa JK, Miller RW, Laraya-Cuasay L, et al. Bronchiectasis in children with lymphocytic interstitial pneumonia and acquired immune deficiency syndrome: plain film and CT observations. Pediatr Radiol 1992; 22:603–607.
13. Kradin RL, Mark EJ. Benign lymphoid disorders of the lung, with a theory regarding their development. Hum Pathol 1983; 14:857–867.
14. Nicholson AG, Wotherspoon AC, Diss TC, et al. Reactive pulmonary lymphoid disorders. Histopathology 1995; 26:405–412.
15. Strimlan CV, Rosenow EC, Divertie MB, et al. Pulmonary manifestations of Sjogren's syndrome. Chest 1976; 70:354–361.
16. White DN, Mattay RA. Non-infectious pulmonary complications of infection with the human immunodeficiency virus. Am Rev Respir Dis 1989; 140:1763–1787.
17. Fraser RG, Pare JAP, Pare PD, Fraser RS, Genereux GP. Diagnosis of diseases of the chest. 3rd ed. Philadelphia, Pa: Saunders, 1988; 1568–1573.
18. Ishikawa Y, Kinoshita M, Koga T, Oizumi K, Fujimoto K, Hayabuchi N. Lung cyst formation in lymphocytic interstitial pneumonia: CT features. J Comput Assist Tomogr 1994; 18:745–748.
19. Berdon WE, Mellins RB, Abramson SJ, Ruzal-Shapiro C. Pediatric HIV infection in its second decade: the changing pattern of lung involvement—clinical, plain film, and computed tomographic findings. Radiol Clin North Am 1993; 31:453–464.
20. McGuinness G, Scholes JV, Jagirdar JS, et al. Unusual lymphoproliferative disorders in nine patients with HIV or AIDS: CT and pathologic findings. Radiology 1995; 197: 59–65.
21. Desai SR, Nicholson AG, Stewart S, Twentyman OM, Flower DR, Hansell DM. Benign pulmonary lymphocytic infiltration and amyloidosis: computed tomographic and pathologic features in three cases. J Thorac Imaging 1997; 12:215–220.
22. Gruden JF, Webb WR, Warnock M. Centrilobular opacities in the lung on high-resolution CT: diagnostic considerations and pathologic correlation. AJR 1994; 162: 569–574.
23. Murata K, Itoh H, Todo G, et al. Centrilobular lesions of the lung: demonstration by high-resolution CT and pathologic correlation. Radiology 1986; 161:641–645.
24. Murata K, Khan A, Herman PG. Pulmonary parenchymal disease: evaluation with high-resolution CT. Radiology 1989; 172:467–471.
25. Gurney JW. Cross-section physiology of the lung. Radiology 1991; 178:1–10.
26. Epler GR, Snider GL, Gaensler EA, Cathcart ES, Fitzgerald MX, Carrington CB. Bronchiolitis and bronchitis in connective tissue disease: a possible relationship to the use of penicillamine. JAMA 1979; 242:528–532.
27. Wells AU, du Bois RM. Bronchiolitis in association with connective tissue disorders. Clin Chest Med 1993; 14:655–666.

Tae Sung Kim, MD
Kyung Soo Lee, MD
Joungho Han, MD
Jung-Gi Im, MD
Joon Beom Seo, MD
Joung Sook Kim, MD
Hyae Young Kim, MD
Sang Wook Han, MD

Index terms:
Bronchi, CT, 671.12111, 671.12112
Bronchi, neoplasms, 671.12111, 671.12112, 671.3113, 671.3115, 671.3116
Trachea, CT, 671.3113
Trachea, neoplasms, 671.12111, 671.12112, 671.3113

Radiology 1999; 212:643–648

[1] From the Departments of Radiology (T.S.K., K.S.L.) and Diagnostic Pathology (J.H.), Samsung Medical Center, College of Medicine, Sungkyunkwan University, 50, Ilwon-Dong, Kangnam-Ku, Seoul 135-710, Korea; the Department of Radiology, College of Medicine, Seoul National University, Korea (J.G.I., J.B.S.); the Department of Radiology, Sanggye Paik Hospital, Seoul, Korea (J.S.K.); the Department of Radiology, Asan Medical Center, College of Medicine, Ulsan University, Seoul, Korea (H.Y.K.); and the Department of Radiology, Kangdong Sungshim Hospital, Seoul, Korea (S.W.H.). Received August 5, 1998; revision requested September 25; final revision received December 17; accepted March 25, 1999. **Address reprint requests to** K.S.L. (e-mail: *kslee@smc.samsung.co.kr*).

Author contributions:
Guarantors of integrity of entire study, T.S.K., K.S.L.; study concepts, K.S.L.; study design, T.S.K., K.S.L.; definition of intellectual content, T.S.K., K.S.L.; literature research, T.S.K., K.S.L., J.H.; clinical studies, T.S.K., K.S.L.; data acquisition, T.S.K., K.S.L., J.G.I., J.B.S., J.S.K., H.Y.K., S.W.H.; data analysis, T.S.K., K.S.L., J.H.; manuscript preparation, T.S.K.; manuscript editing and review, T.S.K., K.S.L.

Mucoepidermoid Carcinoma of the Tracheobronchial Tree: Radiographic and CT Findings in 12 Patients[1]

PURPOSE: To determine the radiographic and computed tomographic (CT) findings and clinical features of mucoepidermoid carcinoma of the tracheobronchial tree.

MATERIALS AND METHODS: Chest radiographic and CT findings and clinical features of 12 histopathologically proved mucoepidermoid carcinomas in 12 consecutive patients (five male, seven female; age range, 9–72 years; mean age, 36 years) were reviewed retrospectively.

RESULTS: The tumors were located at the distal trachea (n = 1) or at a main (n = 2), lobar (n = 1), or segmental (n = 8) bronchus. On chest radiographs, the tumors appeared as central masses with postobstructive pneumonia or peripheral atelectasis in four patients and as solitary pulmonary or endotracheobronchial nodules in eight. At CT, the tumors were all smoothly oval (n = 6) or lobulated (n = 6) in shape (ranging 9–40 mm in diameter), adapting to the branching features of the airways. Punctate calcification within the tumor was seen in six patients. Neither metastasis nor recurrence was seen after the surgical resection (follow-up of 8–103 months; mean, 30 months).

CONCLUSION: Mucoepidermoid carcinoma of the tracheobronchial tree, usually located in a segmental bronchus, appears at CT as a smoothly oval or lobulated airway mass. It adapts to the branching features of the airways.

Mucoepidermoid carcinoma of the tracheobronchial tree is a rare airway tumor, composing only 0.1%–0.2% of the primary lung malignancies (1–5). The tumor is believed to originate from the minor salivary glands lining the tracheobronchial tree (6).

Reported radiographic findings of the bronchial mucoepidermoid carcinoma consist of a solitary nodule or a mass with or without findings of postobstructive pneumonia or atelectasis (6,7). Tracheal mucoepidermoid carcinoma may be seen as a localized endoluminal mass contrasting with the surrounding endoluminal air column.

Computed tomographic (CT) findings of the mucoepidermoid carcinoma of the tracheobronchial tree have been described in several case reports (8–10). Our study was aimed at determining the chest radiographic and CT findings and the clinical features of mucoepidermoid carcinoma in the tracheobronchial tree in 12 consecutive patients.

MATERIALS AND METHODS

Between January 1990 and September 1997, 12 cases of histopathologically proved mucoepidermoid carcinoma of the tracheobronchial tree in 12 consecutive patients were seen. The cases were collected from two tertiary referral hospitals of 1,100 and 1,200 beds. The patients were five male and seven female patients (age range, 9–72 years; mean, 36 years). We (T.S.K., K.S.L.) evaluated the initial symptoms of the patients and the long-term clinical status after the surgery.

Both the initial chest radiographs and CT scans were available in all patients and were obtained within 5 days of each other (mean, 2.9 days). The chest radiographs were obtained by using a standard posteroanterior projection with a high-kilovoltage technique (125 kVp, 5 mAs, 10–12:1 grid ratio). The CT scans were obtained with a variety of machines, but mainly with a model 9800 or CT HiSpeed Advantage scanner (GE Medical Systems, Milwaukee, Wis) or Somatom Plus S scanner (Siemens Medical Systems, Erlangen, Germany). The helical technique (7–10-mm collimation, pitch of 1) was used and covered the area from the lung apices to the middle portion of both kidneys. Additional thin-section (1.0-mm collimation) scans were obtained when the lesion was a solitary nodule. Contrast medium–enhanced (iopamidol [Iopamiron 300, Bracco, Milan, Italy]; 30-g injection; n = 12) and nonenhanced (n = 6) CT scans were obtained. The chest radiographs and CT scans were analyzed simultaneously, retrospectively, and jointly by two chest radiologists (T.S.K., K.S.L.), and the decisions on the findings were reached by a consensus.

The analysis of the chest radiographs included the location of the main tumor and examination for the presence of postobstructive pneumonia or atelectasis. When there was no evidence of associated postobstructive pneumonia or atelectasis, the lesion was regarded as a solitary nodule (less than 3 cm in diameter) or as a mass (3 cm or more in diameter).

The CT analysis included determination of the airway location, shape, and size and determination of the attenuation coefficient of the tumor. Tumors were subcategorized by location as tracheal or as main, lobar, segmental, or subsegmental bronchial. The tumors were also subcategorized according to shape as round, oval, or lobulated. Both the short and long diameters of the tumor were included in the measurement. When the tumors were located in a lobar or segmental bronchus and were oval or lobulated, the direction of the longest diameter of the tumor was compared with that of the branching airways (parallel or not).

Attenuation of the tumor was compared with that of the chest wall muscle before and after the injection of contrast medium. Presence of postobstructive pneumonia, bronchial dilatation, mucoid impaction, or atelectasis was also described. The presence and type of intratumoral calcification were also recorded. By reviewing additional expiratory thin-section CT scans (1–2-mm collimation, 3–5-mm intervals, and reconstruction with a bone algorithm) obtained in four patients, the presence of air trapping was evaluated by identifying the localized area of low attenuation and the small vessels within this area.

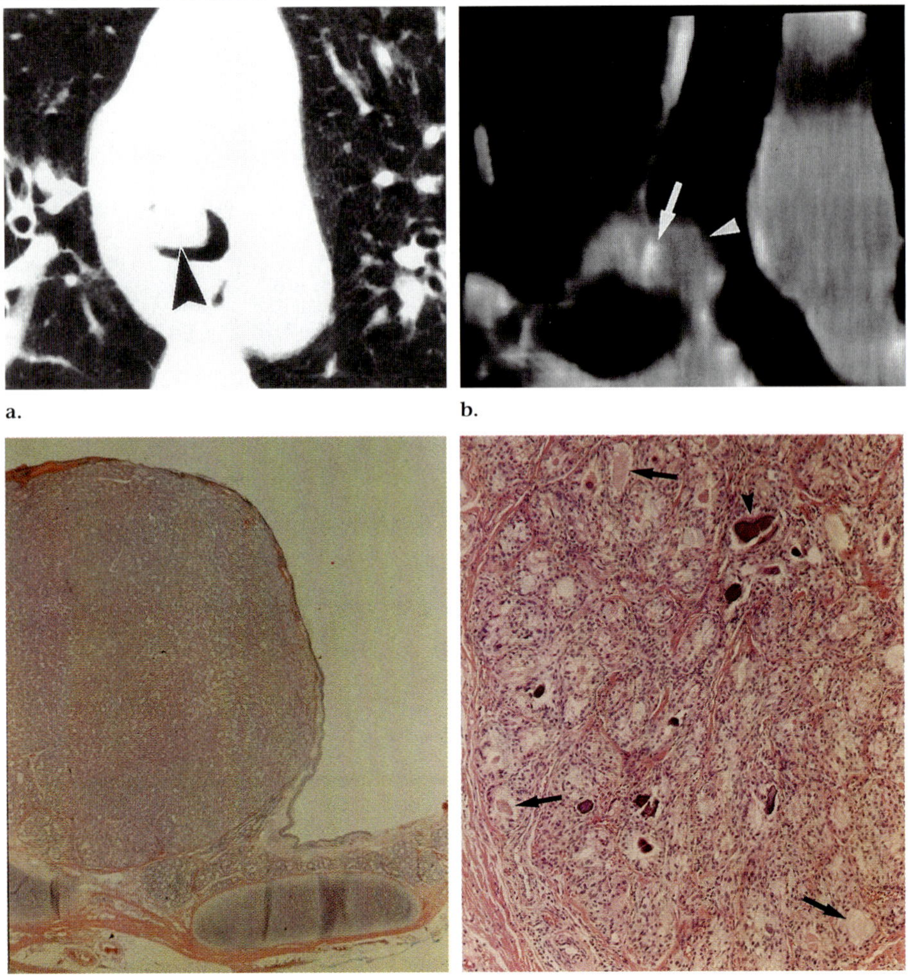

a. b. c. d.

Figure 1. Mucoepidermoid carcinoma in a 9-year-old boy. **(a)** Axial, lung-window, thin-section (1-mm-collimation) CT scan obtained at the distal tracheal level shows a 13-mm polypoid endotracheal mass (arrowhead). **(b)** Coronal reformation image shows the mass (arrowhead) with calcification (arrow). **(c)** Low-magnification photomicrograph of the histologic specimen obtained with segmental resection of the distal trachea shows a polypoid mass. (Hematoxylin-eosin stain; original magnification, ×12.) **(d)** High-magnification photomicrograph shows a low-grade mucoepidermoid carcinoma composed mainly of cystic areas (arrows). Cysts are lined with mucous cells, and lumina are filled with mucus and associated microcalcification (arrowhead). There is no evidence of necrosis or anaplasia. (Hematoxylin-eosin stain; original magnification, ×100.)

In all patients, the tumors were resected surgically, and histopathologic specimens were available. An experienced lung pathologist (J.H.) reviewed the specimens. At histopathologic examination, the histologic grade (low or high) (1–3,6) of the tumor and the presence of the intratumoral calcification, tumor necrosis, and extraluminal parenchymal component of the tumor were evaluated.

RESULTS

Clinical Findings

The symptoms of nine patients were cough (n = 6), dyspnea (n = 3), hemoptysis (n = 2), or chest pain (n = 2). Three patients (25%), in whom the tumor was detected incidentally, were asymptomatic. Lobectomy including sleeve resection was performed in 11 patients. The patient with the tumor in the distal part of the trachea underwent a resection anastomosis of the distal part of the trachea. Only one patient died, 4 years 4 months after the surgery, of a perforation of the sigmoid colon (not related to the previous mucoepidermoid carcinoma). The postoperative follow-up period for the remaining 11 patients ranged from 8 months to 8 years 7 months (mean, 30 months), and there was no evidence of tumor recurrence or metastasis.

Summary of Radiologic and Histopathologic Findings of Mucoepidermoid Carcinoma in 12 Patients

Patient No./Age (y)/Sex	Location*	Radiographic Findings	Size (mm)	Shape	CT Findings: Calcification	Obstructive Pneumonia	Bronchial Dilatation	Air Trapping	Subsegmental Atelectasis	Grade	Histopathologic Findings: Calcification	Bronchial Dilatation	Parenchymal Involvement
1/9/M	T, RMB	Polypoid endotracheal nodule	13 × 10	Ovoid	Yes	No	No	Yes	No	Low	Yes	No	No
2/43/F	RB_{10}	Round nodule	25 × 20	Lobulated	Yes	No	Yes	Yes	No	High	Yes	Yes	No
3/41/M	LB_{7+8}	Ovoid nodule	25 × 20	Ovoid	No	Yes	No	No	No	High	Yes	No	No
4/28/M	RB_6	Ovoid mass	35 × 30	Lobulated	Yes	Yes	No	No	No	High	Yes	No	Yes
5/37/M	LB_{10}	Ovoid mass within ectatic bronchus	30 × 20	Lobulated	Yes	No	Yes	No	Yes	Low	Yes	Yes	No
6/54/F	RB_9	Ovoid mass with segmental pneumonia	40 × 30	Lobulated	No	Yes	Yes	Yes	No	High	No	Yes	Yes
7/25/F	RB_8	Ovoid mass with distal cavitary lesion	33 × 25	Ovoid	No	No	Yes	No	No	Low	No	Yes	No
8/31/F	LMB	Polypoid endobronchial nodule	11 × 9	Ovoid	No	No	No	No	No	Low	No	No	No
9/72/F	RB_2	Lobulated mass	40 × 35	Lobulated	Yes	No	Yes	No	No	High	Yes	Yes	No
10/11/M	LB_3	Ovoid mass with distal pneumonia	30 × 25	Ovoid	Yes	Yes	No	No	No	Low	Yes	No	No
11/39/F	LMB	Polypoid endobronchial nodule	15 × 10	Ovoid	No	No	No	No	No	Low	No	No	No
12/38/F	RB_{4+5}	Ovoid nodule with subsegmental atelectasis	25 × 20	Lobulated	No	No	Yes	No	Yes	High	No	Yes	Yes

* LMB = left main bronchus, LB_3 = anterior segmental bronchus of left upper lobe, LB_{7+8} = anteromedial basal segmental bronchus of left lower lobe, LB_{10} = posterior basal segmental bronchus of left lower lobe, RMB = right main bronchus, RB_2 = posterior segmental bronchus of right upper lobe, RB_{4+5} = right middle lobar bronchus, RB_6 = superior segmental bronchus of right lower lobe, RB_8 = anterior basal segmental bronchus of right lower lobe, RB_9 = lateral basal segmental bronchus of right lower lobe, RB_{10} = posterior basal segmental bronchus of right lower lobe, T = trachea.

Radiographic Findings

The tumors were located in the distal part of the trachea (n = 1) (Fig 1) or in a main (n = 2), lobar (n = 1), or segmental (n = 8) bronchus (Table). On posteroanterior chest radiographs, the tumors were seen as an endotracheal or endobronchial nodule (n = 3), a solitary pulmonary nodule or mass (n = 5), a mass with postobstructive pneumonia or atelectasis (n = 3), or a mass with a distal cavitary lesion (n = 1).

CT Findings

The tumors ranged from 9 to 40 mm in diameter. The tumors were either smoothly oval (n = 6) or lobulated (n = 6). In all patients, the direction of the longest diameter of the oval or lobulated tumor in the lobar or segmental bronchus was parallel to that of the branching pattern in the corresponding airways containing the tumor.

In one patient, the tumor showed mild, diffuse areas of high attenuation (mean, 80 HU) in addition to punctate calcifications at nonenhanced CT. The tumor turned out to have diffuse microcalcification at the histologic examination. Punctate calcification within the tumor was seen in six of 12 patients (including the patient just described) at nonenhanced CT.

The tumors in all patients were homogeneous and showed mild enhancement after the administration of the contrast medium; the attenuation was slightly less than (n = 1), the same as (n = 10), or slightly more than (n = 1) that of the chest wall muscle.

The measurement of Hounsfield unit data was possible in three patients. The attenuations of these lesions at nonenhanced CT were 20, 20, and 80 HU. The lesions were mildly enhanced to 30, 45, and 90 HU, respectively. (The actual increments were 10, 25, and 10 HU, respectively.)

Associated CT findings suggestive of airway disease were seen in 10 patients and included distal bronchial dilatation with mucoid impaction (n = 6), postobstructive pneumonia (n = 4), air trapping (n = 3), and subsegmental atelectasis (n = 2) (Figs 2, 3). A peripheral area of hypoattenuation or a crescent of air was also noted around the tumor, which was suggestive of a residual lumen of an ectatic bronchus occupied by the endobronchial tumor (n = 2) (Figs 2, 3). No mediastinal or hilar lymph node enlargement was observed.

Histopathologic Findings

The patients had low- (n = 6) or high-grade (n = 6) mucoepidermoid carcinomas. In all patients, the tumors were mainly endoluminal, and they appeared as a polypoid gray, tan, or pink endobronchial nodule or mass. Histologically, three of six high-grade carcinomas showed focal parenchymal involvement (extraluminal component), which was not suggested at CT.

Intratumoral microscopic calcification was noted in seven patients. All six patients with punctate calcification on nonenhanced CT scans had histologic specimens that showed microscopic calcification. In the remaining patient with microcalcification, the nonenhanced CT scan did not reveal any gross calcification.

No tumor necrosis was observed. There was no metastatic regional lymphadenopathy. The detailed histopathologic record for sampled lymph nodes was available in four patients in whom eight to 30 regional lymph nodes all showed negative results when examined for malignancy.

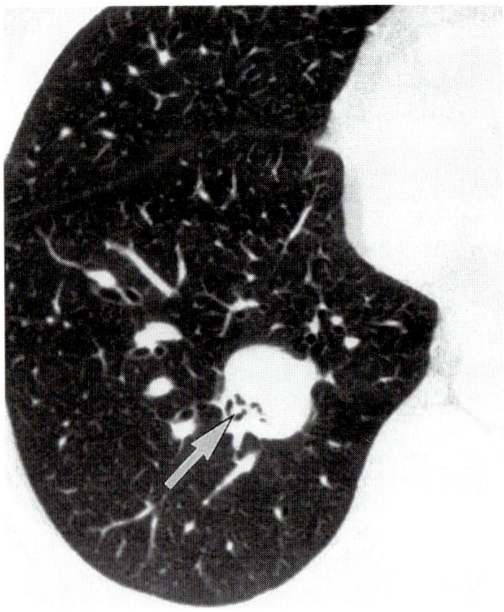

a.

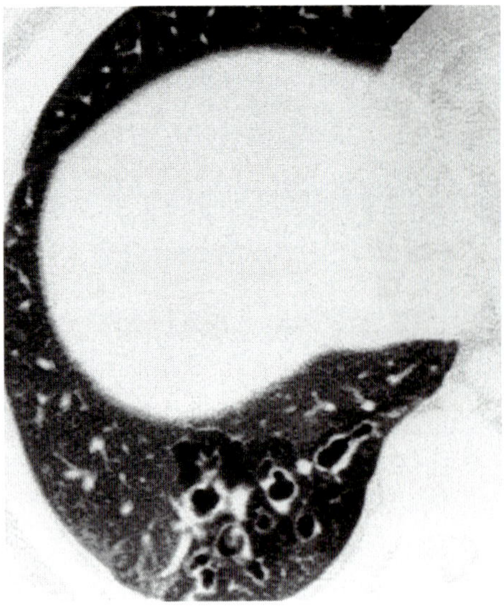

b.

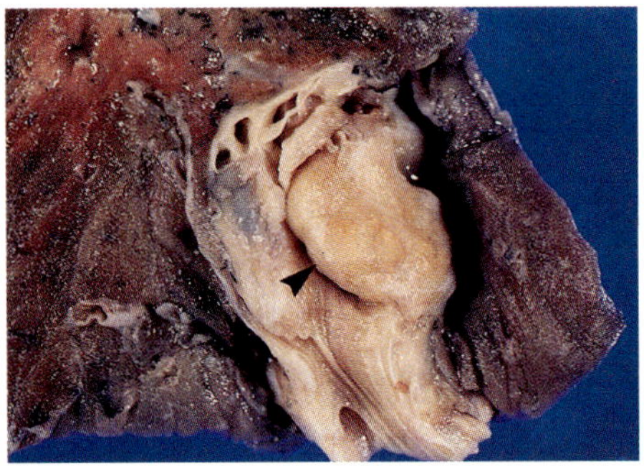

c.

Figure 2. Mucoepidermoid carcinoma in a 43-year-old woman. **(a)** Axial, lung-window, thin-section (1-mm-collimation) CT scan obtained at the atrial level shows a well-defined nodule in right lower lobe. Tiny areas of hypoattenuation (arrow) are noted in the peripheral portion of the nodule, which suggests ectatic bronchi. **(b)** Axial expiratory CT scan obtained at the level of the liver dome shows air trapping and bronchial dilatation localized in the posterobasal segment of right lower lobe. **(c)** Photograph of gross specimen obtained at right lower lobectomy shows an endobronchial polypoid nodule (arrowhead) in the ectatic posterior segmental bronchus of the right lower lobe.

DISCUSSION

The term "bronchial adenoma" has been used to describe a group of slow-growing neoplasms (many of which arise from the bronchial glands), including adenoid cystic carcinomas, mucoepidermoid carcinomas, mixed tumors, and carcinoid tumors (1). Since these tumors are usually low-grade malignancies rather than benign neoplasms, the term "bronchial adenoma" is a misnomer and should be discarded.

Histologically, mucoepidermoid carcinoma of the tracheobronchial tree consists of variable proportions of mucus-secreting cells, squamous cells, and so-called intermediate cells that show no particular differentiating characteristics (1). The tumor is histopathologically classified as a low- or high-grade malignancy. Mitoses, nuclear pleomorphism, and necrosis are usually absent or minimal (less than five mitoses per 50 high-power fields) in low-grade mucoepidermoid carcinomas (1,3). In high-grade tumors, mitoses are increased, averaging four per 10 high-power fields, and nuclear pleomorphism, hyperchromasia, and cellular necrosis are present (1,2,6,11). The tumor in the high-grade form invades the pulmonary parenchyma in nearly 46% (six of 13) of the cases (6). In our series, all low-grade mucoepidermoid carcinomas were well confined within the bronchial wall, and three of six (50%) high-grade tumors showed focal parenchymal involvement at pathologic examination.

It has been reported that patients with mucoepidermoid carcinoma range in age from 4 to 78 years, but nearly half are younger than 30 years (1,6,12). In our study, four of 12 patients were younger than 30 years (age range, 9–72 years; mean age, 36 years). Patients with mucoepidermoid carcinoma usually present with symptoms and signs of irritation in the large airways or obstruction (cough, hemoptysis, wheezing, and recurrent pneumonia), but 9%–28% are asymptomatic (1). In our study, three of 12 (25%) patients had no symptoms.

It is known that low-grade mucoepidermoid carcinomas grow slowly and are noninvasive and therefore rarely metastasize to regional lymph nodes or remote sites (1,2,6,13–15). In one study (6), only 2% (one of 45) of low-grade tumors and 15% (two of 13) of high-grade tumors metastasized to the regional lymph nodes. Completely resectable low-grade tumors generally have an excellent prognosis without recurrence or development of metastases (1,2,6).

The high-grade form is known to have better prognosis than that of the common bronchogenic carcinomas (6,7). In a study of 13 patients with the high-grade form of mucoepidermoid carcinoma (6), only three patients died of the disease (including two patients with regional lymph node metastases). In our series, there was no metastasis in the regional lymph node, even in patients with high-grade forms. In one patient with the high-grade form, in whom CT scans prior to admission were available, it took 23 months for the tumor to double its size. This finding demonstrates the slow growth rate. Findings of the overall follow-up examinations confirmed the excellent prognosis of the tumors in our study (no evidence of tumor recurrence or metastasis during the mean follow-up of 30 months).

Radiographic manifestations of 58 cases of tracheobronchial mucoepidermoid carcinoma reviewed by Yousem and Hochholzer (6) consisted of a solitary nodule or mass in 41 cases (71%) and "pneumonic consolidation" in 16 cases (28%) (one case showed no abnormality on chest

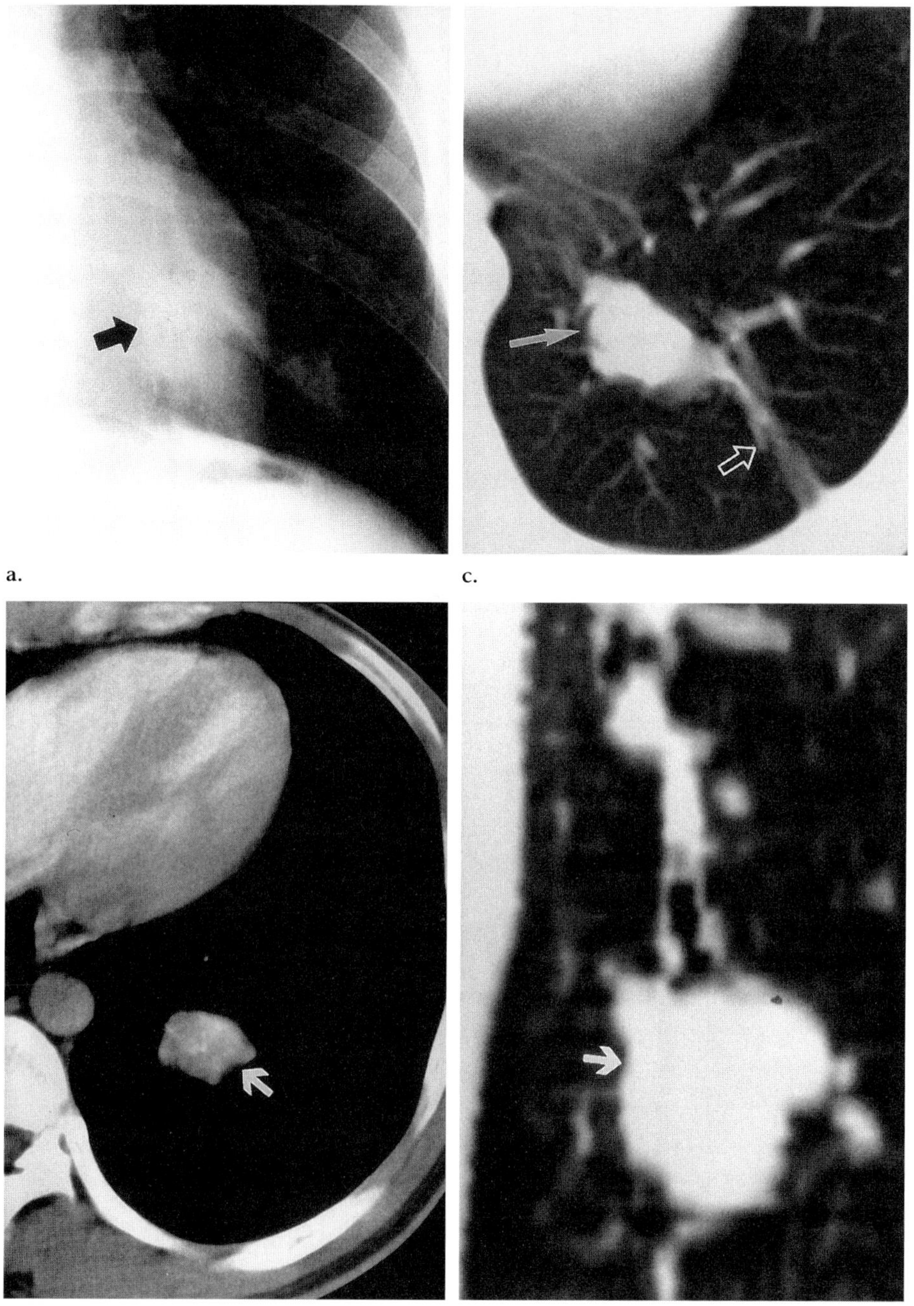

Figure 3. Mucoepidermoid carcinoma in a 37-year-old man. **(a)** Posteroanterior chest radiograph shows a retrocardiac mass (arrow). **(b)** Contrast-enhanced conventional 10-mm-thick axial CT scan obtained at the level of the left ventricle shows an oval mass (arrow) with punctate calcification in the left lower lobe. **(c)** Axial lung-window CT scan shows a well-defined oval mass with distal subsegmental atelectasis (open arrow). Solid arrow indicates a crescent of air, which is suggestive of an endobronchial lesion (see text). **(d)** Coronal reformation image shows an endobronchial lobulated mass (arrow) and the proximal segmental bronchus with some ectasia of the bronchus.

radiographs) (7). In our series, the prevalence (four of 12 patients [33%]) of postobstructive pneumonia or atelectasis on chest radiographs was similar to that in the study by Yousem and Hochholzer (6).

Mucoepidermoid carcinoma of the lung, an uncommon tracheobronchial tumor, manifests as a polypoid mass in the lumen of a main, lobar, or segmental bronchus. In our study, it was difficult to predict the exact endobronchial location of the tumors on chest radiographs, especially when they were present at the level of the segmental bronchus. When the tumor manifested as a solitary pulmonary nodule without any other associated findings, the radiographic finding was nonspecific and was not different from that of other benign and malignant nodules.

However, at CT, there were several clues that helped us to determine the endobronchial location of the tumors. With all tumors being nonspherical, the direction of the longest diameter of the tumor was parallel to the direction of the branching pattern in the corresponding airways containing the tumor. Associated findings of distal bronchial dilatation with mucoid impaction, postobstructive pneumonia, subsegmental atelectasis, or air trapping were suggestive of an endobronchial mass. Additional ancillary findings that indicated the endobronchial location of the tumors were areas of peripheral lucency or a crescent of air around the tumor. The findings were suggestive of a residual lumen of an ectatic bronchus that was occupied by the endobronchial tumor.

Foci of calcification or ossification have been reported to be present within the tumor (1). In our series, punctate calcification within the tumor was seen in six of 12 tumors (50%) on CT scans, whereas microscopic calcification was seen in seven of 12 tumors (58%) at histologic evaluation. The incidence of calcification in mucoepidermoid carcinoma of the lung was much higher than that of the more common forms of the pulmonary carcinomas (up to 14% [16]).

Mucoepidermoid carcinoma of the tracheobronchial tree shows CT findings similar to those of the bronchial carcinoid tumors. According to Zwiebel et al (17), bronchial carcinoid tumor also is associated with frequent postobstructive pneumonia or atelectasis, and the shape of the tumor is frequently nonspherical, with its long axis parallel to that of the nearest major bronchovascular bundle. The overall rate of intratumoral calcification of carcinoid tumor was 26% (eight of 31) (17). However, the tumor is known to be vascular, and marked enhancement of the tumor has been noted at CT (18,19), whereas mucoepidermoid carcinoma showed only mild enhancement in our series.

Adenoid cystic carcinoma, which is the second most common malignant tumor of the trachea and main bronchi (squamous cell carcinoma is the most common) and a kind of salivary gland–type airway tumor, can also be differentiated from mucoepidermoid carcinoma because of its frequent extraluminal extension. In a series of six cases of adenoid cystic carcinoma in the trachea (20), CT images demonstrated extratracheal extension in all cases. Moreover, adenoid cystic carcinomas usually arise in the lower trachea, main stem bronchi, or lobar bronchi. In our study, all mucoepidermoid carcinomas appeared as smoothly oval or lobulated intraluminal masses in the airways, and they were more likely to appear in the segmental bronchi.

In summary, mucoepidermoid carcinoma in the tracheobronchial tree is a rare airway tumor and is more common in the segmental bronchi than in the trachea or main bronchi. On chest radiographs, the tumor appears as a central mass with or without postobstructive pneumonia and/or peripheral atelectasis or as a solitary pulmonary nodule. Prediction of the endoluminal location of the tumor is plausible at CT, even when the tumor is located within a segmental bronchus. It appears as a sharply marginated oval or lobulated intraluminal mass adapting to the branching features of the airways. Postobstructive pneumonia or distal bronchial dilatation with mucoid impaction is frequently associated. Punctate calcification within the tumor is seen in about half of the patients. The tumor shows mild contrast medium enhancement. Metastasis to the regional lymph node is rare, and the prognosis is excellent.

References

1. Colby TV, Koss MN, Travis WD. Tumors of salivary gland type. In: Tumors of the lower respiratory tract: AFIP atlas of tumor pathology. 3rd series. Vol 13. Washington, DC: American Registry of Pathology, 1995; 65–89.
2. Heitmiller RF, Mathisen DJ, Ferry JA, Mark EJ, Grillo HC. Mucoepidermoid lung tumors. Ann Thorac Surg 1989; 47:394–399.
3. Leonardi HK, Jung-Legg Y, Legg MA, Neptune WB. Tracheobronchial mucoepidermoid carcinoma: clinicopathological features and results of treatment. J Thorac Cardiovasc Surg 1978; 76:431–438.
4. Miller DL, Allen MS. Rare pulmonary neoplasms. Mayo Clin Proc 1993; 68:492–498.
5. Turnbull AD, Huvos AG, Goodner JT, Foote FW Jr. Mucoepidermoid tumors of bronchial glands. Cancer 1971; 28:539–544.
6. Yousem SA, Hochholzer L. Mucoepidermoid tumors of the lung. Cancer 1987; 60:1346–1352.
7. Fraser RS, Paré JAP, Fraser RG, Paré PD. Neoplastic disease of the lungs. In: Synopsis of diseases of the chest. 2nd ed. Philadelphia, Pa: Saunders, 1994; 445–539.
8. Tsuchiya H, Nagashima K, Ohashi S, Takase Y. Childhood bronchial mucoepidermoid tumors. J Pediatr Surg 1997; 32:106–109.
9. Fisher DA, Mond DJ, Fuchs A, Khan A. Mucoepidermoid tumor of the lung: CT appearance. Comput Med Imaging Graph 1995; 19:339–342.
10. Deschildre A, Sardet A, Brouard J, et al. Bronchial mucoepidermoid carcinoma: apropos of 3 cases. Arch Pediatr 1996; 3:689–693. [French]
11. Klacsmann PG, Olson JL, Eggleston JC. Mucoepidermoid carcinoma of the bronchus: an electron microscopic study of the low grade and the high grade variants. Cancer 1979; 43:1720–1733.
12. Spencer H. Bronchial mucous gland tumours. Virchows Arch A Pathol Pathol Anat 1979; 383:101–115.
13. Barsky SH, Martin SE, Matthews M, Gazdar A, Costa JC. "Low grade" mucoepidermoid carcinoma of the bronchus with "high grade" biological behavior. Cancer 1983; 51:1505–1509.
14. Conlan AA, Payne WS, Woolner LB, Sanderson DR. Adenoid cystic carcinoma (cylindroma) and mucoepidermoid carcinoma of the bronchus: factors affecting survival. J Thorac Cardiovasc Surg 1978; 76:369–377.
15. Metcalf JS, Maize JC, Shaw EB. Bronchial mucoepidermoid carcinoma metastatic to skin: report of a case and review of the literature. Cancer 1986; 58:2556–2559.
16. O'Keefe NE, Good CA, McDonald JR. Calcification in solitary nodules of the lung. AJR 1957; 77:1023–1033.
17. Zwiebel BR, Austin JH, Grimes MM. Bronchial carcinoid tumors: assessment with CT of location and intratumoral calcification in 31 patients. Radiology 1991; 179: 483–486.
18. Aronchick JM, Wexler JA, Christen B, Miller W, Epstein D, Gefter WB. Computed tomography of bronchial carcinoid. J Comput Assist Tomogr 1986; 10: 71–74.
19. Davis SD, Zirn JR, Govoni AF, Yankelevitz DF. Peripheral carcinoid tumor of the lung: CT diagnosis. AJR 1990; 155:1185–1187.
20. Spizarny DL, Shepard JA, McLoud TC, Grillo HC, Dedrick CG. CT of adenoid cystic carcinoma of the trachea. AJR 1986; 146:1129–1132.

U. Joseph Schoepf, MD
Christoph R. Becker, MD
Roland D. Bruening, MD
Thomas Helmberger, MD
Axel Staebler, MD
Patricia Leimeister, RT
Maximilian F. Reiser, MD

Electrocardiographically Gated Thin-Section CT of the Lung[1]

PURPOSE: To determine whether electrocardiographic (ECG) gating improves image quality of thin-section computed tomographic (CT) scans of the lung obtained with a subsecond CT scanner.

MATERIALS AND METHODS: Thin-section CT was performed in 35 patients by using standard techniques. Three additional sections were obtained in each patient with prospective ECG gating at corresponding levels of the paracardiac lung parenchyma. Non–ECG-gated and ECG-gated sections were then rated in blinded fashion by three experienced radiologists for overall image quality, spatial resolution, and diagnostic value and for different types of respiratory and cardiac motion artifacts.

RESULTS: ECG gating helped significantly reduce artifacts caused by cardiac motion (ie, distortion of pulmonary vessels, double images, or blurring of the cardiac border) ($P < .05$). ECG gating did not reduce respiratory motion artifacts. In patients with heart rates of less than 76 beats per minute, ECG gating significantly improved overall image quality ($P = .041$). ECG gating was not perceived to increase the diagnostic value of thin-section CT scans.

CONCLUSION: ECG gating improves image quality of thin-section CT scans of the lung by reducing cardiac motion artifacts that may mimic disease. It must be established whether ECG gating can help increase the diagnostic accuracy of thin-section CT for the evaluation of subtle parenchymal disease.

Index terms:
Computed tomography (CT), technology, 60.12118
Computed tomography (CT), thin-section, 60.12118
Emphysema, 60.751
Fibrosis, cystic, 60.252
Lung, CT, 60.12111, 60.12118
Lung, infection, 60.2028. 60.2056, 60.2066, 60.213
Pneumonia, usual interstitial, 60.213

Radiology 1999; 212:649–654

Abbreviation:
ECG = electrocardiographic

[1] From the Department of Diagnostic Radiology, Klinikum Grosshadern, University of Munich, Marchioninistrasse 15, 81377 Munich, Germany. Received July 20, 1998; revision requested September 3; revision received December 16; accepted April 6, 1999. **Address reprint requests to** U.J.S. (e-mail: *schoepf@ikra.med.uni-muenchen.de*).

Thin-section computed tomography (CT) of the lung has become accepted as the method of choice for accurate demonstration of the pulmonary parenchyma. It has found widespread use in a number of clinical settings, including the assessment of interstitial pneumonitis, pulmonary fibrosis, emphysema, or bronchiectasis (1–6).

The quality of thin-section CT images, however, often is compromised because of respiratory or cardiac motion artifacts (6–9). Some of these artifacts mimic pathologic conditions and thus constitute a potential pitfall in the diagnosis of interstitial or bronchial disease (6,9–12). Whereas gross respiratory motion causes general blurring of the image, subtle movements due to transmitted cardiac pulsations may result in double images of pulmonary vessels (11) or fissures (12,13). The resultant double lines can be mistaken for the "tram-line" appearance of thickened bronchial walls (1,11). Curvilinear distortion of pulmonary vessels by means of cardiac movement results in a focal area of low attenuation adjacent to the vessel. This artifact may mimic the cystic appearance of bronchiectasis (7,9–11).

Despite of the advent of fast CT image acquisition techniques, these artifacts can still be observed with disturbing frequency (8,14). For effective suppression of motion artifacts on CT images, scanning times of less than 19.1 msec would be necessary (14). Even with increasingly faster CT technology, scanning times this short will not be accomplished in the near future.

Another potential way to reduce cardiac motion artifacts is to acquire images during the diastole of the cardiac cycle, when ventricular movement is at its minimum. Effective electrocardiographic (ECG) gating has so far been limited to use in electron-beam CT (15,16). However, prospective ECG gating, which allows the triggered acquisition of scans at a

Author contributions:
Guarantors of integrity of entire study, U.J.S., M.F.R.; study concepts, U.J.S.; study design, U.J.S., C.R.B.; definition of intellectual content, U.J.S., C.R.B., M.F.R.; literature research, U.J.S., C.R.B.; clinical studies, U.J.S., C.R.B., R.D.B., P.L.; data acquisition, U.J.S., C.R.B., P.L.; data analysis, U.J.S., R.D.B., T.H., A.S.; statistical analysis, U.J.S.; manuscript preparation and editing, U.J.S.; manuscript review, C.R.B., R.D.B., T.H., A.S., M.F.R.

predefined interval after the R wave of the electrocardiogram, has recently become commercially available for sequential scanning with conventional spiral CT systems (17). We performed a prospective study to determine whether transmitted cardiac motion artifacts are amenable to a CT protocol that involves prospective ECG gating with a subsecond CT scanner.

MATERIALS AND METHODS

Study Design

Sequential thin-section CT studies were obtained in 35 consecutive patients (21 men, 14 women; aged 19–68 years; mean age, 38 years) suspected of having a disease of the pulmonary parenchyma. CT studies were acquired by using a routine technique, as recommended by the manufacturer, and an alternative protocol that involved prospective ECG gating of scans. Double radiation exposure to the patient for the evaluation of prospective ECG gating at conventional CT was not considered to require approval by our internal review board, because the additional radiation dose did not exceed an effective dose of 0.86 mSv. Informed consent was obtained from each patient.

Indications for performance of thin-section CT in our patient population were pulmonary emphysema (n = 5), ambiguous findings on chest radiographs in healthy individuals (n = 4), aspergillosis after bone marrow transplantation (n = 4), evaluation for lung transplantation (n = 3), spontaneous pneumothorax (n = 3), usual interstitial pneumonitis (n = 2), cytomegalovirus infection after bone marrow transplantation (n = 2), cystic fibrosis (n = 2), interstitial pneumonia (n = 2), possible legionellosis after adult respiratory distress syndrome (n = 1), lymphangioleiomyomatosis (n = 1), allergic alveolitis (n = 1), hemoptysis (n = 1), drug-induced pulmonary fibrosis (n = 1), α1-antitrypsin deficiency (n = 1), graft rejection after lung transplantation (n = 1), and bronchiectasis after lung transplantation (n = 1).

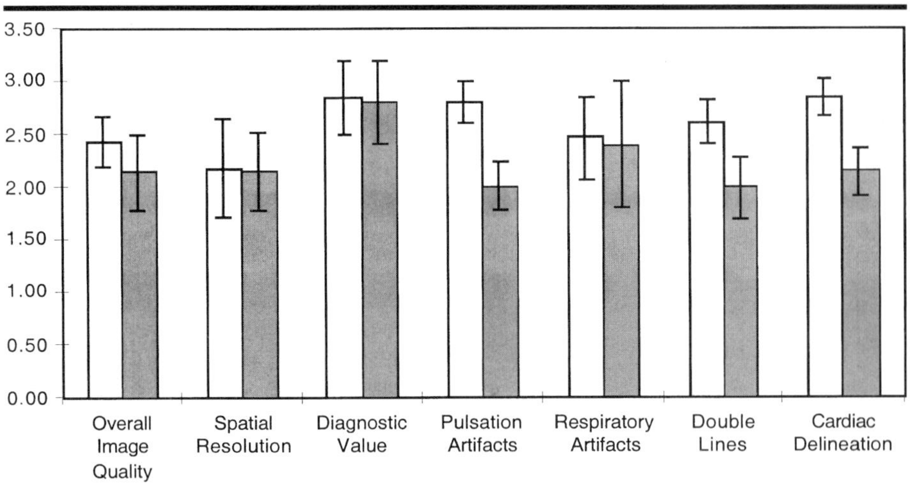

Figure 1. Bar graph shows mean scores from three readers for ECG-gated (white bars) and non–ECG-gated (gray bars) thin-section CT studies in 35 patients. Error bars = SD. ECG-gated studies were rated significantly superior to non–ECG-gated studies with regard to pulsation artifacts (P = .022), double images (P = .042), and cardiac delineation (P = .039).

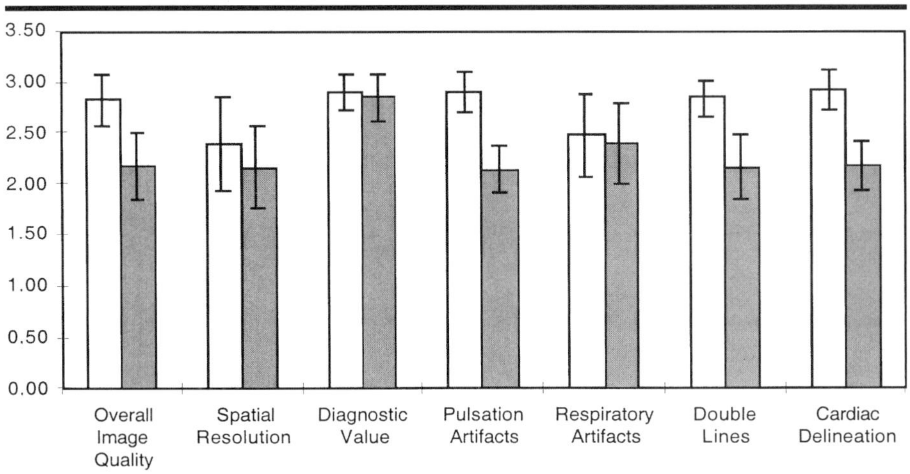

Figure 2. Bar graph shows mean scores from three readers for ECG-gated (white bars) and non–ECG-gated (gray bars) thin-section CT studies in 16 patients with a heart rate of less than 76 beats per minute. Error bars = SD. In addition to a significant reduction in cardiac motion artifacts, the overall image quality of ECG-gated studies was rated as significantly superior to that of non–ECG-gated studies.

Scanning Technique

Scanning was performed with a subsecond helical CT scanner (Somatom Plus 4A; Siemens Medical Systems, Erlangen, Germany), which is capable of prospective ECG-gating. In this setting, the ECG signal is detected by means of three ECG leads placed on the patient and an ECG monitor connected to the CT system. An update of the scanner software allowed identification of the R wave. Each scan acquisition was initiated by means of a trigger signal sent to the scanner after an operator-selected delay measured from the peak of the R wave. The ECG monitor was permanently connected to the scanner, and the ECG-gating protocol was stored in the protocol menu. Performance of ECG-gated versus non–ECG-gated CT, therefore, required an additional investment of less than 2 minutes to attach ECG electrodes to the patient.

By using this approach, a cluster of three ECG-gated scans with a 20-mm scan interval was acquired in each patient at three levels in the epiphrenic, paracardiac lung parenchyma. Pilot study results (not shown) had demonstrated that optimal image acquisition during the diastole of the heart can be achieved when scanning is initiated at 50% of the R-R interval. Therefore, scan acquisition was gated at this trigger interval by using 1-mm collimation at 120 kV, 170 mA, and 500 msec per 240° rotation (0.75 second per 360° rotation). To prevent artifacts from an insufficient number of projections acquired during the 500-msec scan acquisition time, images were reconstructed with a high-spatial-frequency algorithm ("AB82" [10.9 line pairs per cen-

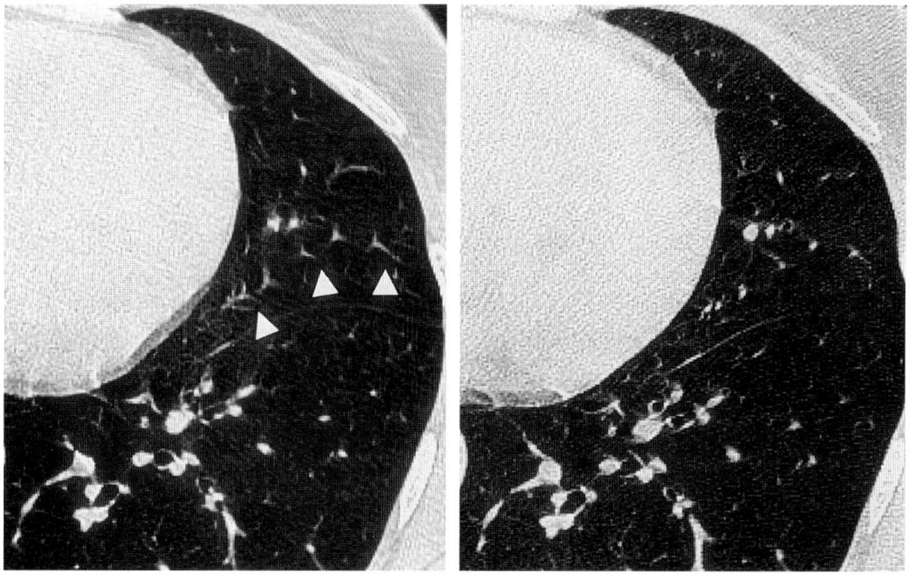

a. b.

Figure 3. (a) Non–ECG-gated and (b) ECG-gated thin-section CT scans in a 35-year-old woman with recurrent pneumothoraces. The "twinkling star" artifact (arrowheads), a motion artifact caused by distortion of pulmonary vessels due to cardiac motion is seen in the lingula of the left upper lobe in **a** but is less visible in **b**.

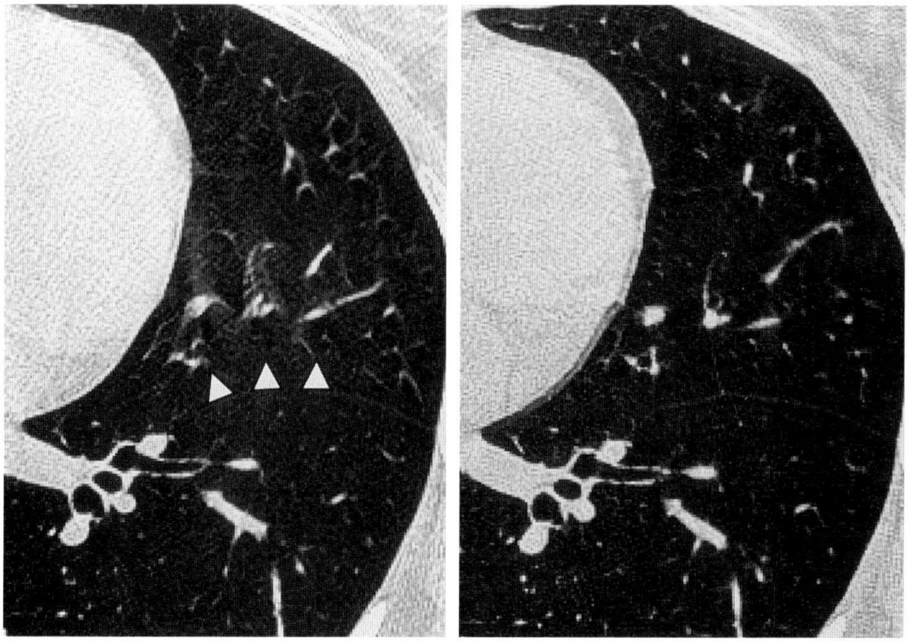

a. b.

Figure 4. (a) Non–ECG-gated and (b) ECG-gated thin-section CT scans in a 62-year-old man with hemoptysis of unknown etiology. Absence of ECG gating can allow cardiac motion to distort pulmonary vessels in the lingula into a U or Y shape and results in focal high-attenuating areas (arrowheads) next to the vessel, as in **a**. This artifact is sometimes misinterpreted as bronchiectasis and can be prevented by using ECG gating, as in **b**.

timeter at 2% modulation transfer function]; Siemens Medical Systems) instead of the very-high-frequency algorithm that was used for the standard technique.

On completion, each patient underwent scanning craniocaudally from the apex of the lung to the diaphragm by using two to three clusters of non–ECG-gated acquisitions with a scan interval of 10 mm and the standard thin-section CT techniques recommended by the manufacturer. One-millimeter collimation was again used at 120 kV, 90 mA, and 1,500-msec exposure per 360° rotation. Each cluster was acquired during one breath hold. Images were reconstructed by using a very-high-spatial-frequency algorithm ("AB91" [12.42 line pairs per centimeter at 2% modulation transfer function]; Siemens Medical Systems). The heart rate in each patient was documented.

Image Analysis

For each patient, the three ECG-gated scans were displayed at lung window settings (level, −400 HU; width, 1,400 HU) and were printed in four-on-one format without text. From the non–ECG-gated studies, the three scans of the paracardiac parenchyma that were acquired at levels closest to the table positions of the ECG-gated scans were chosen for comparison and were printed in the same manner as the ECG-gated scans.

The printed scans were presented in random order to three experienced radiologists (R.D.B., T.H., A.S.) in a way that did not allow direct comparison of ECG-gated and non–ECG-gated scans in an individual patient. Each reader reviewed the images individually and was blinded to the scanning technique. Studies were rated for general impression, spatial resolution, overall diagnostic value, and motion artifacts, by using a three-point scale, where the "best" value was 3. The criteria for motion artifacts included (*a*) double-imaged lung structures (bronchial walls, vessels, fissures), (*b*) doubling and blurring of the cardiac border, (*c*) pulsation artifacts attributable to cardiac motion (ie, distortion of vessels resulting in "star" artifacts or low-attenuating areas adjacent to the vessel), and (*d*) respiratory artifacts.

Statistical Analyses

Statistical analyses were performed by using commercially available software (Statview; Abacus Concepts, Berkeley, Calif). For each criterion and for each of the 35 patients, mean scores of the three readers were calculated for ECG-gated and non–ECG-gated studies and were tested to determine whether the scores were normally distributed. Mean scores were then tested for differences by using the paired Student *t* test. A *P* value of less than .05 was regarded as indicative of a

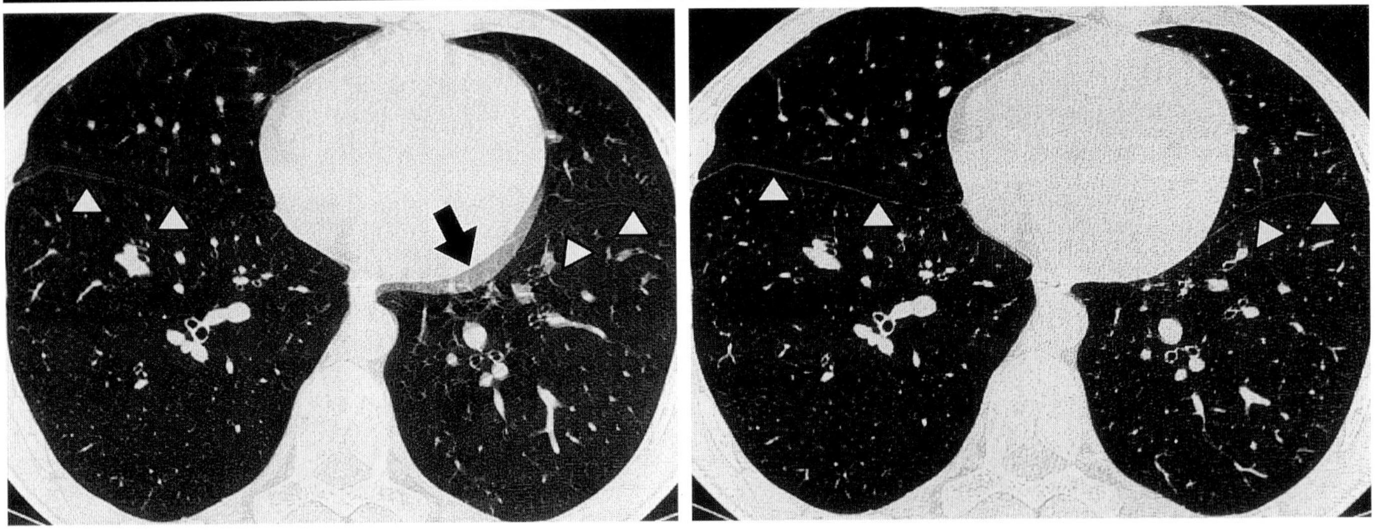

a. b.

Figure 5. (a) Non–ECG-gated and (b) ECG-gated thin-section CT scans obtained at the same level of the paracardiac parenchyma in a 25-year-old man with spontaneous pneumothorax. Note the clear delineation of the left ventricle in b versus the blurred cardiac border (arrow) in a. Both the right and left interlobar fissures (arrowheads) are seen as double lines in a but not in b.

statistically significant difference. Interobserver agreement was determined on the basis of total score values for all categories in each patient by calculating the product-moment correlation coefficient.

RESULTS

A total of 210 images were evaluated (two sets of three images each in 35 patients) by all three readers. The mean heart rate (± SD) was 80.5 beats per minute ± 12.0; 16 patients had a heart rate of 76 beats per minute or slower (mean, 71.5 beats per minute), and 19 had a heart rate faster than 76 beats per minute (mean, 88 beats per minute).

When all patients were considered, significant differences between ECG-gated and non–ECG-gated images were found for the presence of pulsation artifacts (P = .022) and double images (P = .042) and for delineation of the heart (P = .039). For these categories, the readers considered ECG-gated studies to be superior to non–ECG-gated studies (Fig 1). No differences between the two techniques were found for overall image quality, spatial resolution, diagnostic value, and respiratory artifacts (P > .05 for all).

When only patients with a slower heart rate were considered, scores for both ECG-gated and non–ECG-gated studies were slightly increased (Fig 2). The superiority of ECG-gated studies with respect to pulsation artifacts, double images, and cardiac delineation then became more pronounced (P = .020, .038, and .031, respectively) (Fig 2). In this group of patients, overall image quality of ECG-gated studies also was considered to be significantly superior (P = .041). Differences in spatial resolution, diagnostic value, and respiratory artifacts between the two techniques were not significant (P > .05).

Analysis of interobserver variation in total scores for all categories in each patient showed high correlations among the readers for ECG-gated (r = 0.82) and non–ECG-gated (r = 0.76) studies.

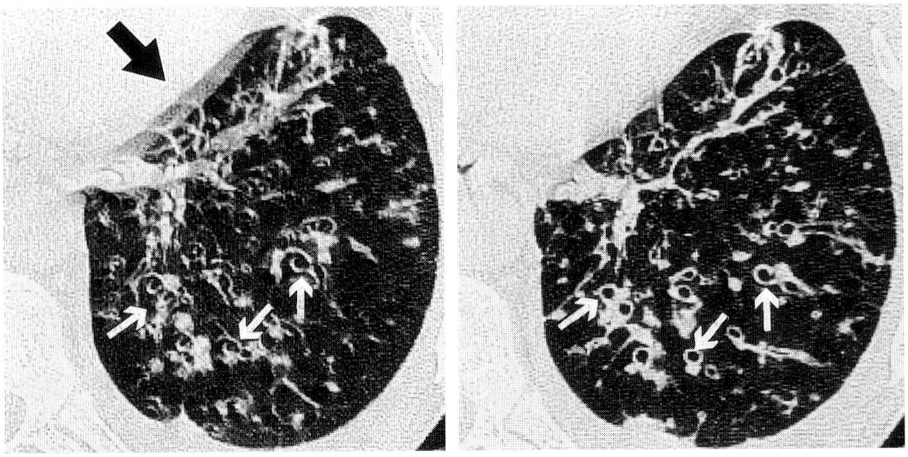

a. b.

Figure 6. (a) Non–ECG-gated and (b) ECG-gated thin-section CT scans obtained at the same level of the paracardiac parenchyma in a 24-year-old man who had undergone lung transplantation. Mild dilatation and bronchial wall thickening in the left lower lobe (white arrows) are better appreciated in b than in a. Also note the blurring of the cardiac border (black arrow) in a.

DISCUSSION

Thin-section CT is the method of choice for evaluation of the pulmonary parenchyma (6,18,19). The image quality of thin-section CT scans of the lung, however, is frequently degraded due to a variety of artifacts that can be confusing to an observer who is not familiar with them.

Fine streak artifacts radiating from bone, referred to as aliasing or correlated noise, are more evident on thin-section

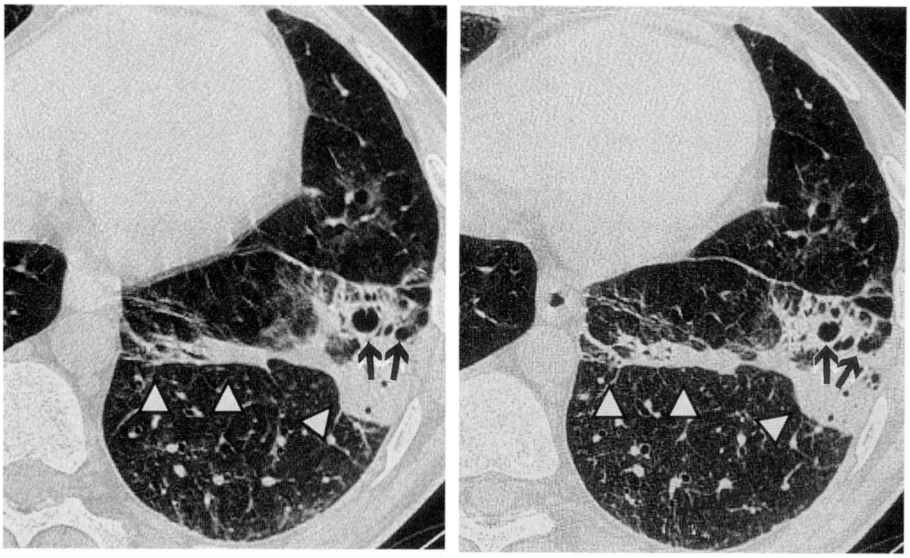

a. b.

Figure 7. (a) Non–ECG-gated and (b) ECG-gated thin-section CT scans in a 32-year-old man with fibrotic changes (arrowheads) in the left lower lobe after adult respiratory distress syndrome. The fibrotic areas are subject to cardiac motion in **a**. The degree of fibrosis and secondary bronchiectasis (arrows) are better appreciated in **b** than in **a**.

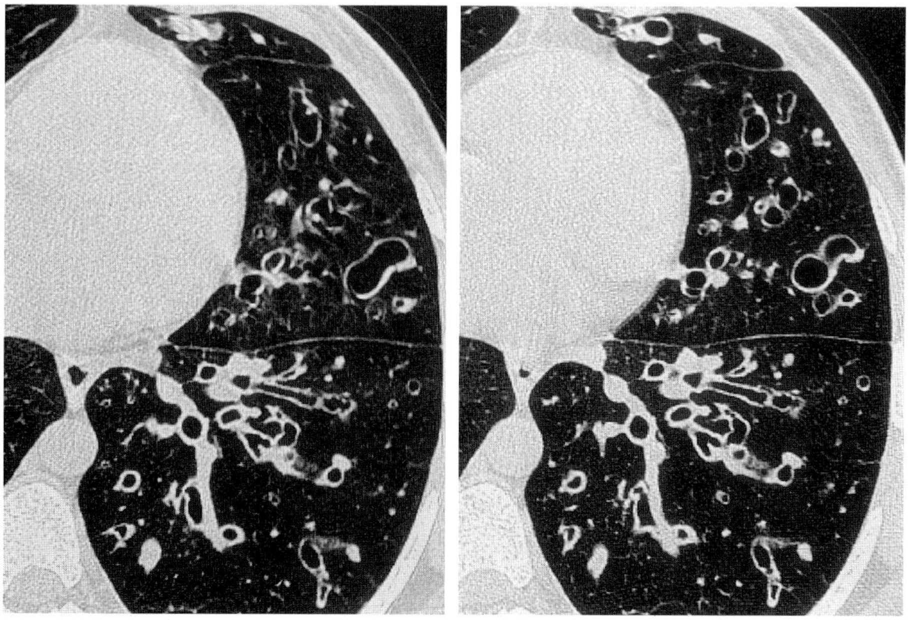

a. b.

Figure 8. (a) Non–ECG-gated and (b) ECG-gated thin-section CT scans obtained at the same level of the paracardiac parenchyma in a 21-year-old woman with cystic fibrosis. Note the clear delineation of dilated bronchi in the lingula of the left upper lobe in **b**. Cardiac motion results in blurring of the bronchi in **a**.

studies than on conventional studies (7). Motion artifacts can arise from respiratory motion or from transmitted cardiac pulsations (6,7,9): Gross motion results in general blurring of the image and can render single sections or an entire study nondiagnostic; slight motion, however, may result in artifacts that have long been recognized to mimic pathologic conditions. These artifacts are usually caused by transmitted cardiac pulsation and include curvilinear distortion of pulmonary vessels resulting in "starlike" streaks that radiate from the vessel, with focal low-attenuating areas between the streaks (Figs 3,4) (6,9–11). The low-attenuating areas, in particular, may be misinterpreted as dilated bronchi (Fig 4) (6,9,10). In addition, vessels, bronchi, and fissures in the vicinity of the heart may be in slightly different positions over the course of the study, which could result in double images on the reconstructed section (Fig 5) and thus mimic bronchiectasis (6,11,12).

One potential method to decrease motion artifacts due to cardiac pulsation is to acquire image data during the quiet diastolic phase of the cardiac cycle, when ventricular movement is minimal and only a little motion occurs due to atrial contraction. Effective use of ECG gating has so far been limited to electron-beam CT (14,15), where the low spatial resolution of 7 line pairs per centimeter does not suffice for the requirements of thin-section CT (6,7). Prospective ECG gating has now become available for conventional CT scanners (17). Our goal was to evaluate an ECG-gated image acquisition technique for the improvement of the quality of images obtained at thin-section CT relative to the quality of images obtained with a standard protocol.

Our results suggest that, besides the anticipated applications in cardiovascular CT (17), ECG gating may also prove to be beneficial in reducing cardiac motion artifacts at thin-section CT of the lung. ECG gating significantly reduced the types of artifact (distortion of pulmonary vessels, double images) that may be mistaken for disease by an observer who is less familiar with thin-section CT (Fig 1).

The ECG-gating protocol was better for reducing cardiac motion artifacts and improving overall image quality in patients with a slower heart rate than in those with a faster heart rate (Fig 2). In these patients, the scores for most criteria were higher than those in the total population, most likely because individuals with a normal heart rate usually are in less distress than patients experiencing tachycardia. More important, however, ECG gating partially loses its effectiveness when the heart rate is faster than 75–80 beats per minute, because the diastole of the heart becomes too short for a 500-msec data acquisition.

Although a scan acquisition time of 500 msec allows image acquisition during the diastole in patients with a normal heart rate, it does not generate the necessary number of projections for image reconstruction with a very-high-spatial-frequency algorithm. Reconstruction with a very-high-spatial-frequency algorithm still requires a 1,500-msec rotation for acquisition of a sufficient number of projections. However, effective reduction of cardiac motion artifacts cannot be achieved by using standard scanning times, which are longer than the diastole. To restrict image acquisition to the diastole, scanning time had to be decreased to 500 msec for ECG-gated acquisitions. To prevent artifacts because of an insufficient number of projections, we chose an algorithm with a somewhat lower spatial frequency for reconstruction with ECG-gated scans. This, however, evidently did not affect the quality of ECG-gated images as compared with that of non–ECG-gated images, which had been acquired during a 1,500-msec rotation (Figs 1, 2).

A possible limitation of our study that must be considered was that the influence of a 500-msec acquisition time without the use of ECG gating was not investigated. If the improvement in image quality was caused by the shorter acquisition time alone, however, differences in heart rate should not have influenced the results, and a reduction in the occurrence and severity of respiratory artifacts would also have been expected. Because this was not the case, ECG gating probably was the larger contributor to the improvement in image quality.

Differences between images obtained with ECG gating and those obtained without ECG gating might have been less pronounced had studies of the entire chest been considered. However, to evaluate the potential benefit of ECG gating, we intentionally focused on the paracardiac lung segments, because these regions are most likely to be subject to transmitted cardiac motion.

Three experienced interpreters of thin-section CT scans at our department volunteered as readers for this study. For these readers, ECG gating did not improve the diagnostic value of thin-section CT scans. This may partially result from the familiarity of these observers with the different types of artifacts that can degrade thin-section CT scans. It must be established whether ECG gating can help improve the diagnostic accuracy of thin-section CT for physicians who are less aware of diagnostic pitfalls. Furthermore, subtle and incipient changes in the parenchyma may be diagnosed earlier and more confidently on studies that are less subject to motion artifacts (Figs 6–8). Finally, ECG-gated CT with a variety of applications is likely to become more beneficial in a larger patient population with the advent of conventional CT scanners capable of even shorter scanning times.

We conclude that ECG gating improves image quality and reduces artifacts on thin-section CT scans of the lung, with little additional effort. Accordingly, ECG gating has become part of the routine thin-section CT protocol at our institution. However, it must be determined whether ECG gating can help improve the diagnostic sensitivity and accuracy of thin-section CT.

References

1. Naidich DP, McCauley DI, Khouri NF, Stitik FP, Siegelman SS. Computed tomography of bronchiectasis. J Comput Assist Tomogr 1982; 6:437–444.
2. Naidich DP, Zerhouni EA, Hutchins GM, Genieser NB, McCauley DI, Siegelman SS. Computed tomography of the pulmonary parenchyma. I. Distal air-space disease. J Thorac Imaging 1985; 1:39–53.
3. Zerhouni EA, Naidich DP, Stitik FP, Khouri NF, Siegelman SS. Computed tomography of the pulmonary parenchyma. II. Interstitial disease. J Thorac Imaging 1985; 1:54–64.
4. Grenier P, Maurice F, Musset D, Menu Y, Nahum H. Bronchiectasis: assessment by thin-section CT. Radiology 1986; 161: 95–99.
5. Murata K, Khan A, Herman PG. Pulmonary parenchymal disease: evaluation with high-resolution CT. Radiology 1989; 170: 629–635.
6. Webb WR, Müller NL, Naidich DP. High-resolution CT of the lung. 2nd ed. Philadelphia, Pa: Lippincott-Raven, 1996.
7. Mayo JR. High resolution computed tomography: technical aspects. Radiol Clin North Am 1991; 29:1043–1049.
8. Engeler CE, Tashjian JH, Engeler CM, Geise RA, Holm JC, Ritenour ER. Volumetric high-resolution CT in the diagnosis of interstitial lung disease and bronchiectasis: diagnostic accuracy and radiation dose. AJR 1994; 163:31–35.
9. McGuiness G, Naidich DP. Bronchiectasis: CT/clinical correlations. Semin Ultrasound CT MR 1995; 16:395–419.
10. Kuhns LR, Borlaza G. The "twinkling star" sign: an aid in differentiating pulmonary vessels from pulmonary nodules on computed tomograms. Radiology 1980; 135: 763–764.
11. Tarver RD, Conces DJ, Godwin JD. Motion artifacts on CT simulate bronchiectasis. AJR 1988; 151:1117–1119.
12. Mayo JR, Webb WR, Gould R, et al. High-resolution CT of the lungs: an optimal approach. Radiology 1987; 163:507–510.
13. Mayo JR, Müller NL, Henkelman RM. The double-fissure sign: a motion artifact on thin-section CT scans. Radiology 1987; 165:580–581.
14. Ritchie CJ, Godwin JD, Crawford CR, Stanford W, Anno H, Kim Y. Minimum scan speeds for suppression of motion artifacts in CT. Radiology 1992; 185:37–42.
15. Lynch DA, Brasch RC, Hardy KA, Webb WR. Pediatric pulmonary disease: assessment with high-resolution ultrafast CT. Radiology 1990; 176:243–248.
16. Stanford W, Rumberger JA, eds. Ultrafast computed tomography in cardiac imaging: principles and practice. Mount Kisco, NY: Futura, 1992.
17. Hayball MP, Coulden RA, Regn J, Fluhrer M, Clements L, Brown SJ. ECG triggered image acquisition on a sub-second CT system (abstr). Radiology 1998; 206:575.
18. Webb WR. High resolution CT of the lung parenchyma. Radiol Clin North Am 1989; 27:1085–1097.
19. Zerhouni E. Computed tomography of the pulmonary parenchyma: an overview. Chest 1989; 95:901–907.

Lei Feng, MD, PhD
David M. Stern, MD
John Pile-Spellman, MD

Index terms:
Arteries, biopsy, 9*.126, 9*.92[2]
Arteries, endothelium, 9*.92[2]
Arteries, iliac, 984.1261
Biopsies, technology
Carotid arteries, 90.1261
Molecular analysis, 9*.92[2]
Venae cavae, interventional procedure, 946.1261
Pulmonary arteries, 944.1261

Radiology 1999; 212:655–664

Abbreviations:
DiI = 1,1′-dilinoleyl-3,3,3′,3′-tetramethylindocarbocyanine perchlorate
GAPDH = glyceraldehyde-3-phosphate dehydrogenase
HUVEC = human umbilical vein endothelial cell
ICAM-1 = intercellular adhesion molecule 1
PCR = polymerase chain reaction
VCAM-1 = vascular cell adhesion molecule 1
vWF = von Willebrand factor

[1] From the Departments of Radiology (L.F., J.P.S.) and Surgery (D.M.S.), Columbia University, 177 Ft Washington Ave, New York, NY 10032. Received June 17, 1998; revision requested August 14; revision received September 23; accepted February 12, 1999. **Address reprint requests to** L.F. (e-mail: *lf66@columbia.edu*).

[2] 9*: Vascular system, location unspecified

Author contributions:
Guarantors of integrity of entire study, L.F., D.M.S., J.P.S.; study concepts, L.F., J.P.S.; study design, L.F., D.M.S.; definition of intellectual content, L.F., D.M.S., J.P.S.; literature research, L.F.; clinical studies, L.F., J.P.S.; experimental studies, L.F.; data acquisition, L.F.; data analysis, L.F., D.M.S.; statistical analysis, L.F., J.P.S.; manuscript preparation and editing, L.F., D.M.S.; manuscript review, J.P.S.

Human Endothelium: Endovascular Biopsy and Molecular Analysis[1]

PURPOSE: To develop a safe and reproducible method for harvesting viable vascular endothelium to analyze gene expression at sites of vascular lesions.

MATERIALS AND METHODS: Coaxial curved stainless-steel guide wires were used to obtain samples of endothelial cells from large arteries and veins in 29 patients undergoing routine endovascular procedures. Three immunocytochemical markers were used to identify cells as endothelial. Cellular viability was evaluated in terms of cell membrane integrity, energy-dependent uptake of acetylated low-density lipoprotein, and cellular response to lipopolysaccharide. Single-cell reverse transcription polymerase chain reaction (PCR) and immunocytochemistry were used to study endothelial gene expression.

RESULTS: Cells with endothelial morphology and immunoreactivity for von Willebrand factor, thrombomodulin, and angiotensin-converting enzyme were consistently obtained from iliac and carotid arteries and large veins (average yield [± standard error] from 26 iliac arteries, 262 endothelial cells ± 45, 20%–30% of which were viable). These cells displayed induction of E-selectin messenger RNA at PCR after exposure to lipopolysaccharide. Expression of vascular cell adhesion molecule 1 transcripts in endothelial cells increased with patient age ($P < .01$), whereas expression of intercellular adhesion molecule 1 did not.

CONCLUSION: Viable endothelium can be obtained during routine angiography. Immunocytochemical and reverse transcription PCR analyses of these cells allowed determination of transcripts and proteins expressed by endothelium at sites of vascular lesions. Such information could aid in understanding mechanisms of vascular diseases and in clinical decision making.

As the cells that form the tissue-blood interface, the endothelium has a critical role in the maintenance of vascular homeostasis. Endothelial regulation of the vascular microenvironment extends to many effector systems. In the coagulation pathway, quiescent endothelium promotes blood fluidity through expression of antithrombotic cofactors such as thrombomodulin (1,2) and CD39 (3); actively secretes tissue plasminogen activators (4), nitric oxide (5,6), and prostacyclins (7); and does not express the key procoagulant tissue factor (8). Similar multilayered, complex endothelial regulation of immune and inflammatory mechanisms (9), vasomotor tone (5), angiogenesis, and vessel wall proliferative activity also has been demonstrated.

Such a view of healthy endothelium as a participant in a myriad of physiologic processes has led to the hypothesis that endothelial dysfunction may, by way of analogy, orchestrate pathophysiologic perturbation of the vasculature in disease states. Induction of endothelial expression of inflammatory mediators such as cytokines (10) and cell adhesion molecules (11) in the earliest phases of the inflammatory response and at lesion-prone areas, with respect to atherogenesis, supports the potential of the endothelial monolayer to regulate processes within the luminal vascular space, as well as processes at sites of tissue injury.

Insights into the properties of the endothelium have come from several lines of inquiry. Results from tissue culture experiments have demonstrated potential endothelial activities that are relevant in vivo, such as expression of inducible cell adhesion molecules (12).

Authors of studies of vessel segments have emphasized particular properties of endothelialized versus deendothelialized vessels, as in the elaboration of nitric oxide (13). Investigators who have performed in vivo experiments with pathologic samples and, more recently, genetically manipulated mice have emphasized potentially pathogenic roles of key mediators such as vasoactive factors (14).

A critical missing link in the elucidation of endothelial mechanisms that contribute to vascular function in the normal and diseased vessel wall is the lack of information about the state of viable endothelial cells in situ; for example, their properties in healthy vessels and at the site of a lesion. Such a gap in our knowledge is due to the difficulty in obtaining viable endothelium from the vasculature in vivo.

These considerations led us to design a nondestructive method of in situ endothelial sampling by using an endovascular catheter. During endovascular procedures, catheters and guide wires inevitably come into contact with the vessel wall. We have found that endothelial cells become adherent to these vascular devices. A method was established to detach viable endothelial cells from the surface of the vascular device. These cells were analyzed with respect to messenger RNA and protein expression. By using immunocytochemical and single-cell reverse transcription polymerase chain reaction (PCR), we found that endothelial gene expression can be monitored. The methods we developed allow performance of endothelial biopsy and the opportunity to add a new dimension to our knowledge of vascular biology; namely, endothelial properties at the site of developing lesions. We hence introduce this technology. The purpose of this study was to demonstrate the feasibility of this technology and to explore possible applications.

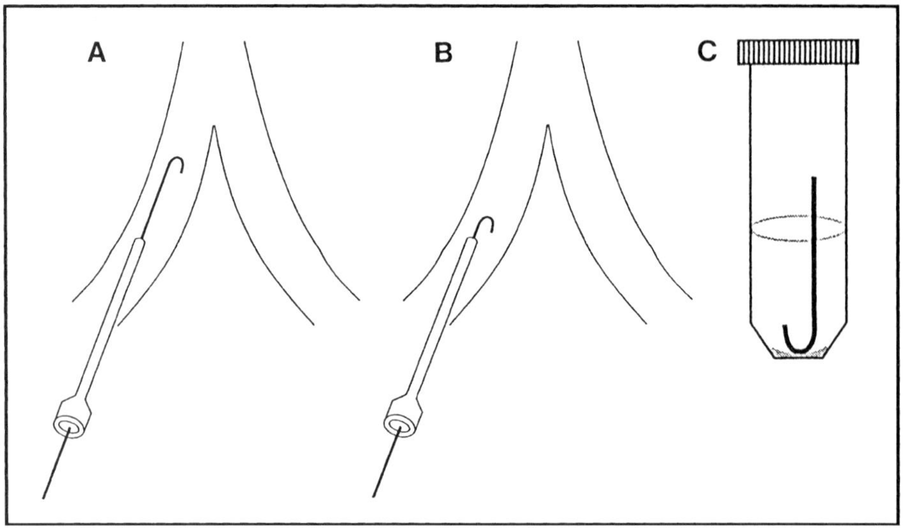

Figure 1. Schematic diagram of the endothelial biopsy method. *A,* The coaxial, curved, stainless-steel guide wire is inserted into an iliac artery. *B,* The wire is pulled back to sample the endothelium under the J-shaped tip. *C,* The tip of the wire is transferred to a test tube for dissociation of endothelial cells and further analysis.

MATERIALS AND METHODS

Patient Selection

A total of 29 patients (nine male patients, 20 female patients; mean age ± standard error, 49 years ± 4; age range, 15–84 years) were included in this study. Twenty-one patients who presented for cerebral angiography and/or embolization were recruited for biopsy with guide wires of the endothelium of iliac arteries. The diagnoses in these patients were arteriovenous malformation (n = 14), intracranial berry aneurysm (n = 5), meningioma (n = 1), and intracranial hemorrhage of unknown cause (n = 1). The patients included a consecutive series of 10 patients with arteriovenous malformation or aneurysm who were recruited for the study of association of endothelial activation with age. On several occasions, more than one endothelial sample was obtained in a patient.

To demonstrate that endothelial samples can be obtained from carotid arteries, four patients with carotid arterial stenosis who were undergoing angioplasty and stent placement were recruited. In addition, three patients with cancer who were undergoing percutaneous indwelling central catheter placement and one patient who was undergoing pulmonary angiography were recruited for the purpose of sampling the superior vena cava and pulmonary arteries, respectively.

General surgical consent, which allowed for performance of laboratory studies of tissues removed during the endovascular procedures, was obtained from each patient. Because the biopsy method involved only in vitro processing of existing guide wires that were used in routine fashion during the endovascular procedures, the institutional review board decided that no additional consent was required.

Biopsy and Isolation of Human Endothelial Cells

To perform biopsy (Fig 1) of iliac endothelium, a coaxial curved stainless steel wire with a 0.038-inch diameter, 3-mm curve radius, and heparin coating (J-wire; Cook, Bloomington, Ind) was inserted into the iliac artery through a Potts needle (Becton Dickinson, Franklin Lakes, NJ), and a femoral sheath (Cook) was advanced over the wire. The wire was then pulled back through the femoral sheath, and the tip of the wire was cut at about 3 inches (7.6 cm) and transferred in sterile fashion to a test tube or Petri dish that contained 25 mL of endothelial cell dissociation buffer (0.5% bovine serum albumin, 2 mmol/L ethylenediaminetetraacetic acid, and 100 µg/mL heparin in calcium- and magnesium-free phosphate-buffered saline solution), which was designed to inhibit adhesion of endothelial cells. After 15 minutes of incubation at room temperature and at least 10 rinses with endothelial dissociation buffer (performed with serologic pipets), cells were centrifuged and resuspended in Red Blood Cell Lysing Buffer (Sigma Chemical, St Louis, Mo) to remove contaminating red blood cells. The nonlysed cells were washed once with endothelial cell dissociation buffer and were resuspended in 50 µL of this buffer. A smear of 5 µL of the cell suspension was stained with a modified Wright stain kit (Leukostat; Fisher, Springfield, NJ). The yield of endothelial cells was estimated by counting cells that showed typical endothelial morphology at light microscopy.

To sample endothelial cells from the internal carotid artery in patients undergoing angioplasty, a guiding catheter (Ingenor; Nycomed, Paris, France) was placed in the common carotid artery. A Teflon-coated exchange wire of 0.038-

inch diameter and 3-mm curve radius (Roadrunner; Cook) was passed through the guiding catheter and advanced through the stenotic segment of the internal carotid artery. After a balloon catheter (Endeavor; Boston Scientific, Natick, Mass) was passed distal to the stenosis over the exchange wire, the wire was pulled back, and its tip was cut and processed as described earlier. In similar fashion, exchange wires were used to guide catheters to the superior vena cava and pulmonary arteries during percutaneous indwelling central catheter placement and pulmonary angiography, respectively. These wires were used to perform biopsy of endothelial cells from these sites in the same manner. Each guide wire was manipulated in routine fashion to ensure the safety of patients.

Culture of Control Endothelial Cells

Human umbilical vein endothelial cells (HUVECs), HUV-EC-C, ATCC CRL-1730, were obtained from the American Type Culture Collection (Rockville, Md). They were grown in either F12K medium (Life Technologies, Rockville, Md), as recommended by American Type Culture Collection, or EB medium (Clonetics, Walkersville, Md). These cells were used to demonstrate typical morphology of endothelial cells and as control cells for evaluation of cell viability and reverse transcription PCR assay results. To activate endothelial cells for reverse transcription PCR analysis of endothelial gene expression, HUVECs and patient-derived endothelial cells were treated with 50 ng/mL lipopolysaccharide at 37°C for 6 hours.

Immunocytochemical Confirmation of Endothelial Cell Type and Detection of Cell Adhesion Molecules

Immunocytochemical analysis is a technique for detection of cellular proteins by using antibodies that specifically recognize these proteins. Antibodies generated in different species can be applied together to localize two proteins at the same time. This technique was used to verify the endothelial identity of patient-derived cells. We double-labeled these cells with combinations of endothelial markers: rabbit anti–human von Willebrand factor (vWF) (Sigma Chemical); goat anti–angiotensin-converting enzyme, produced in the laboratory of one of the authors (D.M.S.); and mouse monoclonal antithrombomodulin (DAKO, Carpinteria, Calif). Antibodies to the leukocyte marker CD45 (also known as common leukocyte antigen) (Sigma Chemical) and to vascular smooth muscle α-actin (Sigma Chemical) were used as negative control markers.

Immunocytochemical analysis was also used to assess the activation state of patient-derived endothelial cells by using goat anti–human vascular cell adhesion molecule 1 (VCAM-1), goat anti–human intercellular adhesion molecule 1 (ICAM-1), or goat anti–human E-selectin (R&D, Minneapolis, Minn). Endothelial cells were identified on the basis of the presence of vWF.

Slides of isolated cells were prepared by using a cytocentrifuge and were fixed in 4% paraformaldehyde. Because treatment with Triton X-100 did not affect vWF staining but weakened the signal for membrane thrombomodulin, we did not pretreat the cells with Triton X-100. Sites of primary antibody binding were visualized with affinity-purified fluorescein- and rhodamine-labeled donkey antimouse, antigoat, and antirabbit antibodies (Jackson ImmunoResearch, West Grove, Pa).

Assays for Endothelial Cell Viability

We used two independent assays to evaluate the viability of patient-derived endothelial cells. The first assay was used to assess the membrane integrity of endothelial cells (LIVE/DEAD Viability/Cytotoxicity kit; Molecular Probes, Eugene, Ore); this kit contained two dyes: ethidium homodimer 1 and calcein AM. Ethidium homodimer 1 stains nuclear DNA red if the integrity of the cell membrane has been violated. Calcein AM is virtually nonfluorescent, but after passage through a cell membrane, it is converted to intensely fluorescent calcein by means of cellular esterase in the lysosomes (15). Therefore, a live cell will have speckled cytoplasmic staining, and a dead cell will show a collection of red fluorescence in the nucleus.

Patient-derived endothelial cells were resuspended in 200 µL of calcium- and magnesium-free phosphate-buffered saline solution with 0.5% bovine serum albumin and were plated in a well of an eight-well chamber slide (Lab Tek; Fisher) that had been coated with 0.1% gelatin. The cells were incubated with 2 mmol/L ethidium homodimer 1 and 4 mmol/L calcein AM for ½ hour before fixation in 4% paraformaldehyde. Endothelial cells were identified by observing their large size, and the numbers of live and dead cells were determined with the aid of a fluorescent microscope. HUVECs were processed in parallel as control cells. One-third of HUVECs were not exposed to dyes and served as negative control cells, whereas another one-third of HUVECs were permeabilized by means of incubation in 0.1% saponin for 10 minutes prior to staining to provide a positive control for dead cells.

The second assay, the incorporation of acetylated low-density lipoprotein labeled with 1,1′-dilinoleyl-3,3,3′,3′-tetramethylindocarbocyanine perchlorate (DiI), was used to test the metabolic function of endothelial cells. Acetylated low-density lipoprotein is taken up by endothelial cells through their scavenger receptors (16). This process is energy dependent and, thus, occurs only in metabolically active cells. The uptake of fluorescent DiI-labeled acetylated low-density lipoprotein also has been used to help identify endothelial cells (16).

After isolation, the number of patient-derived endothelial cells was determined by using a modified Wright stain. These cells were suspended in 200 µL of F12K medium that contained 10 mmol/L DiI-labeled acetylated low-density lipoprotein (Molecular Probes) and were plated on eight-well chamber slides (Lab Tek; Fisher). Cells were incubated for 4 hours before fixation in 4% paraformaldehyde. A similar number of HUVECs were processed at the same time as control cells. Endothelial cells were identified by observing their large size and were counter stained with anti–angiotensin-converting enzyme antibody.

Single-Cell Reverse Transcription PCR

Reverse transcription PCR is a standard molecular biologic technique that allows detection of tiny amounts of messenger RNA in cells and tissues. Specific segments of messenger RNA molecules are converted to complementary DNA molecules by means of reverse transcriptase and are amplified more than a millionfold by means of PCR so that these segments of complementary DNA can be detected with routine agarose gel electrophoresis.

Single-cell reverse transcription PCR was used to assess E-selectin gene expression in patient-derived cells to demonstrate the feasibility of detecting messenger RNA with this technique. This experiment was performed with four random samples of endothelial cells derived from iliac arteries. In each experiment, 20 individual endothelial cells were identified on the basis of size and shape by using an inverted–phase-contrast microscope. The cells were picked up with a micropipet and transferred to thin-walled PCR tubes that contained a detergent-based lysis buffer. Two rounds of nested PCR were used to examine gene expres-

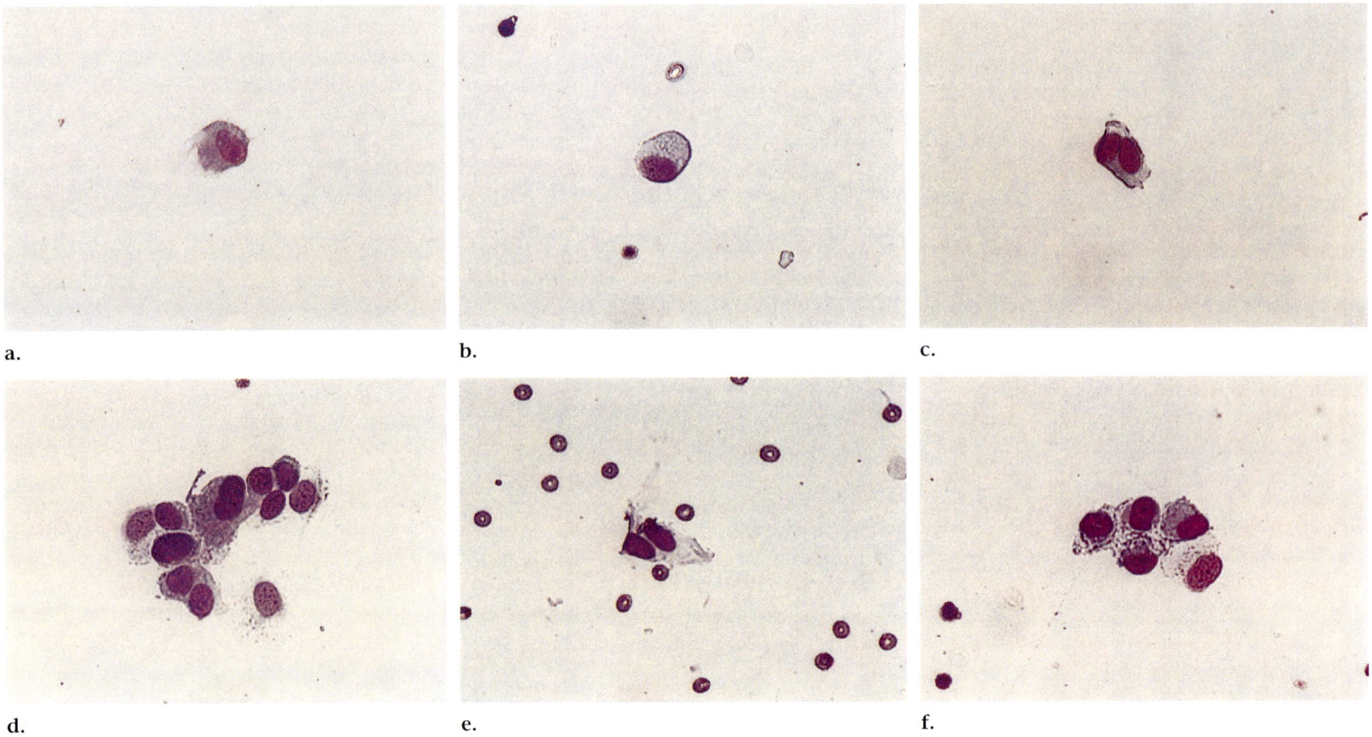

Figure 2. Photomicrographs of smears of patient-derived endothelial-like cells. (a) HUVEC obtained in suspension with dissociating buffer (same procedure used to detach patient-derived cells from curved guide wires). (b) Patient-derived endothelial-like cells (25 μm in diameter) from the iliac artery. (c, d) Sheets of patient-derived cells from the iliac vein. (e, f) Patient-derived cells from (e) the carotid artery and (f) the superior vena cava. (Modified Wright stain; original magnification, ×200.)

sion in endothelial cells. Three pairs of primers were simultaneously added to the PCR tubes: vWF, which served as an endothelial cell marker (17); glyceraldehyde-3-phosphate dehydrogenase (GAPDH) (18), which served as a positive control and internal standard; and E-selectin, which served as an indicator of endothelial activation (19). (See the Appendix for the sequences of the nested primers.) At least one set of the nested primers for each gene is located on a different exon.

A Titan reverse transcription PCR system (Boerhinger, Indianapolis, Ind) was used for reverse transcription PCR by following the manufacturer's instructions. In brief, cell lysis was carried out at 72°C, and reverse transcription was accomplished at 50°C for 30 minutes and at 60°C for 15 minutes. We used 20-μL volumes for 35 cycles of first-round PCR and 25 cycles of second-round PCR, which were performed with a thermocycler (GeneAmp 9600; Perkin-Elmer, Foster City, Calif). The PCR products were analyzed with electrophoresis on 2% agarose gel.

Endothelial Activation and Patient Age

To demonstrate the potential clinical application of endothelial biopsy, we studied the association of endothelial activation with patient age by using endothelial cells obtained from iliac arteries in 10 patients with arteriovenous malformation or aneurysm. The cells were subjected to immunocytochemical analyses with antibodies to E-selectin, ICAM-1, and VCAM-1. The total number of endothelial cells in the specimen was determined by means of double labeling with vWF. The number of endothelial cells that expressed the indicated cell adhesion molecules was determined, and the proportion of positive cells in the samples was calculated. The association of cell adhesion molecules with age was assessed with a linear regression model with logit transformation of the proportion of positive cells as the dependent variable. The effects of sex, diagnosis (aneurysm vs arteriovenous malformation), and hypertension were determined by means of multivariate logistic regression.

RESULTS

Biopsy of Endothelial Cells

We used 28 curved guide wires to sample iliac arteries in 21 patients. Two wires (one in each of two patients) yielded 5,000–6,000 cells, whereas the other 26 wires yielded a mean (± standard error) of 262 cells ± 45 (range, 30–880). Of the two patients in whom a high cell yield was achieved, one had a highly vascular meningioma and the other had a giant fusiform aneurysm of the internal carotid artery.

Salient features of the cell population dissociated from guide wires introduced into the iliac artery and that were initially identified as endothelial-like were revealed on Wright-stained smears: (*a*) Cells were more than 20 μm in diameter, which was considerably larger than leukocytes, the principal contaminating cell type; (*b*) on many occasions, cells were present in small aggregates (two to three cells) or sheets (five or more cells); and (*c*) individual cells were polygonal with a granular, faint blue cytoplasm, an oval nucleus with fine red-purple chromatin, and, sometimes, a nucleolus (Fig 2).

The overall appearance of endothelial cells detached from guide wires (Fig 2b–2f) was similar to that of cultured HUVECs incubated in dissociation buffer and obtained in suspension (Fig 2a) or of human aortic endothelial cells (not shown). The presence of sheets of endothelial cells suggested that the guide wire

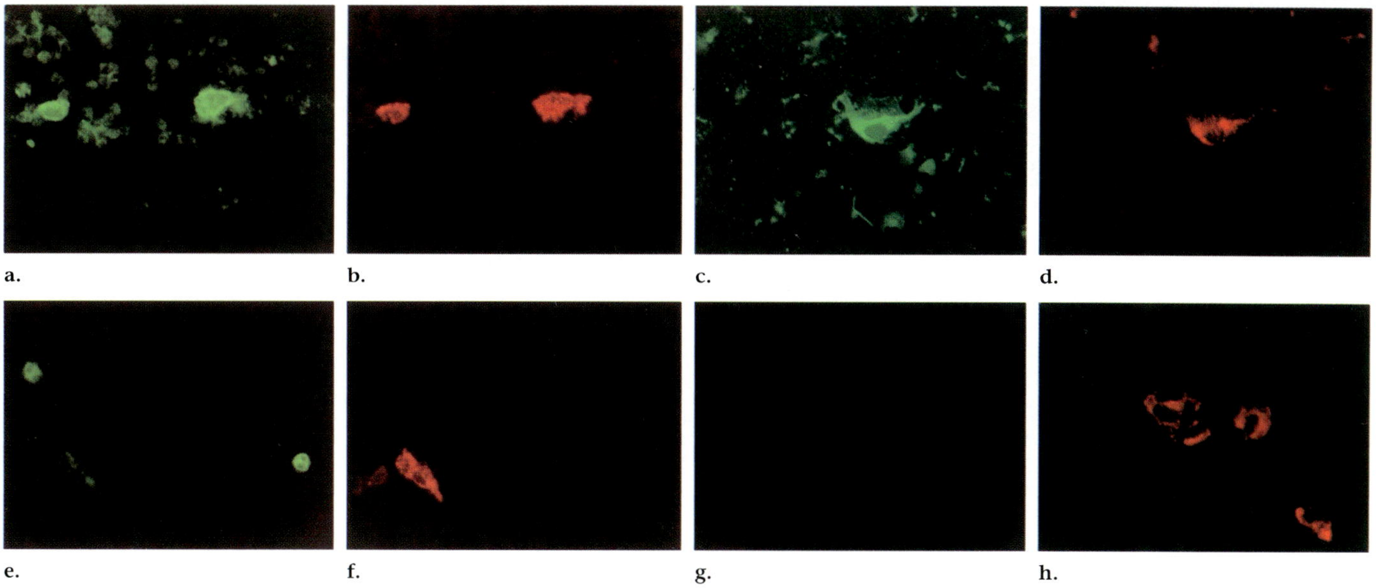

Figure 3. Photomicrographs of immunolabeled patient-derived cells dissociated from J wires. Dual immunofluorescence was used to visualize either **(a)** thrombomodulin and **(b)** vWF or **(c)** angiotensin-converting enzyme and **(d)** vWF in the same cells. Double staining of samples for **(e)** CD45 and **(f)** vWF did not show co-localization of the antigens. Similarly, there was no co-localization of **(g)** smooth muscle α-actin and **(h)** vWF. (Original magnification, ×200.)

had removed of a patch of endothelium, probably with underlying extracellular matrix material. On the basis of general morphologic appearance (absence of spindle-shaped cells of smooth muscle phenotype) and specific cell markers (absence of cells displaying smooth muscle α-actin), however, deeper layers of the blood vessel wall—namely, smooth muscle cells—were not present in preparations. Thus, it was unlikely that the guide wire penetrated more deeply than the endothelium and some of the contiguous matrix-associated material in the vessel wall. Taken together, the size, shape, and coloration of endothelial cells in these Wright-stained smears allowed us to distinguish them easily from other cells in peripheral blood.

Further characterization of cells putatively identified as endothelial was accomplished with antibodies to the endothelial markers angiotensin-converting enzyme (20), thrombomodulin (21), and vWF (22) (Fig 3). Dual-fluorescence microscopy demonstrated the presence of thrombomodulin (Fig 3a) and vWF (Fig 3b) in the same cells. Similarly, a cell positive for angiotensin-converting enzyme (Fig 3c) also was positive for vWF (Fig 3d). Whereas staining for vWF revealed a more punctate appearance, consistent with the presence of vWF in Weibel-Palade bodies, angiotensin-converting enzyme antigen was present more uniformly throughout the cytoplasm, which resulted in a ground-glass appearance, except for the absence of nuclear staining. Although none of these markers are exclusively endothelial (eg, vWF is expressed by both endothelial cells and platelets), only endothelial cells express all three markers.

Results of these immunocytochemical studies also confirmed the cell count obtained on Wright-stained smears. On the basis of the presence of CD45 (Fig 3e) and the absence of double staining for vWF (Fig 3f), certain cells dissociated from curved guide wires were leukocytes. Consistent with our impression from the Wright-stained smears, no cells positive for the smooth muscle α-actin were identified (Fig 3g), although the same field had cells that displayed the vWF antigen (Fig 3h). Thus, on the basis of general morphologic criteria and the presence of specific markers, endothelial cells could be distinguished from other nonendothelial contaminants in the cell population dissociated from curved guide wires.

Endothelial cells harvested with the same methods from large veins (four patients) had a similar appearance (Fig 2e) and number (mean, 245 cells ± 57). Comparable results were obtained from stenotic carotid arteries (four patients), although the mean number of cells was reduced (25 cells ± six). These data were suggestive of the potential for extrapolation of our method to particular vessels of interest and diverse lesion sites.

Viability of Patient-derived Endothelial Cells

Cell viability was most likely to be compromised during harvesting from the vessel wall and cell processing. Two independent methods, the viability assay (Fig 4b) and uptake of DiI-labeled acetylated low-density lipoprotein (Fig 4d, 4f), were used to evaluate cellular integrity in two random endothelial samples from iliac arteries. As a control for cell recovery, similar numbers of HUVECs were processed in parallel with cells dissociated from the guide wires. Green calcein-AM staining of live cells versus uptake of red ethidium homodimer 1 by dead cells was observed (Fig 4b). Uptake of DiI-labeled acetylated low-density lipoprotein in HUVECs (Fig 4d) resulted in a speckled appearance of the dye in a cellular distribution. Cells from the guide wires also displayed uptake of DiI-labeled acetylated low-density lipoprotein (Fig 4f).

Of the total number of endothelial cells derived from the curved guide wires, as determined at Wright staining, 20%–30% were in the adherent cell population evaluated for cell viability. Approximately 90% of these cells were viable and available as a starting point for molecular biologic studies such as single-cell reverse transcription PCR. Thus, of a total of 250 endothelial-like cells identified at Wright staining, 50 were viable and allowed for additional analysis.

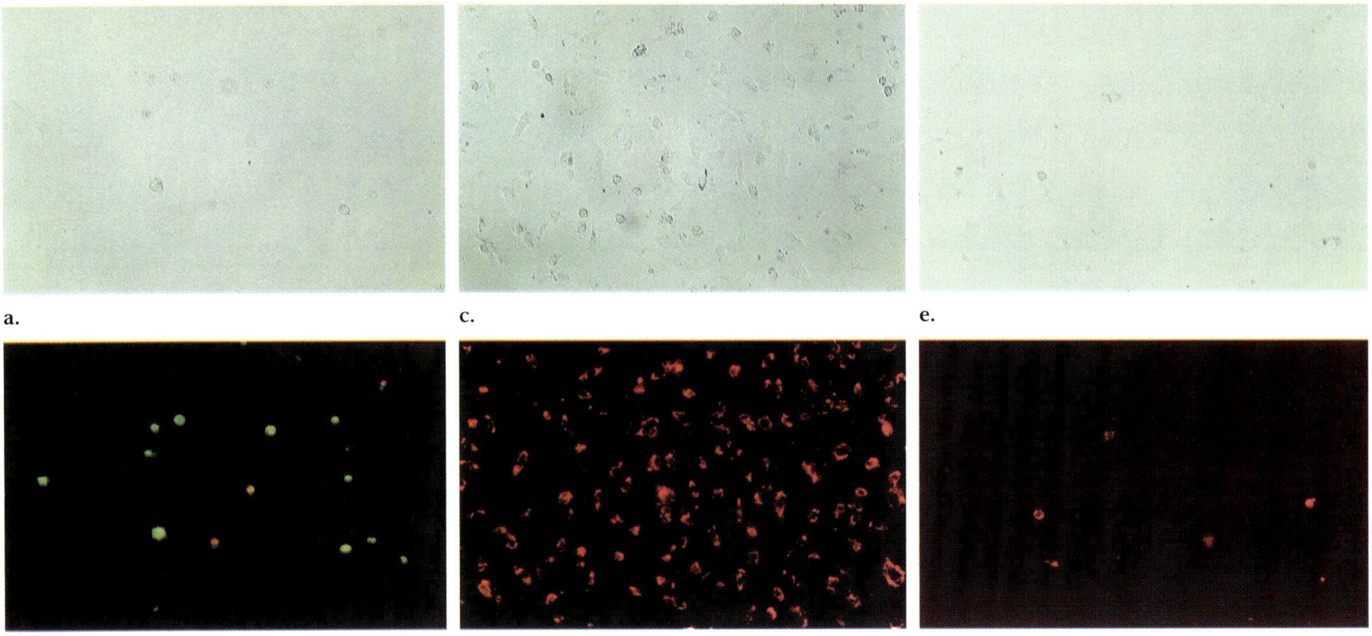

Figure 4. Viability of patient-derived endothelial cells. **(a, c, e)** Bright-field photomicrographs of endothelial-like cells. **(b)** Photomicrograph of cells shown in **a** after uptake of ethidium homodimer-1 and calcein AM for the membrane integrity assay. Dead cells appear red because of the uptake of ethidium homodimer 1; live cells appear green because of the uptake of calcein AM. **(d, f)** Photomicrographs of cells shown **(d)** in **c** and **(f)** in **e** after uptake of DiI-labeled acetylated low-density lipoprotein for the assay of metabolic function. (Original magnification, ×100.)

Reverse Transcription PCR Analysis of Transcripts in Endothelial Cells

The small final number of cells available for further study from patient samples (50 cells per sample, two patients) necessitated the use of sensitive molecular biologic techniques for analysis of cellular properties. For this reason, we developed a single-cell reverse transcription PCR method for simultaneous assessment of the expression of many genes in each cell.

After the cell isolation procedure, 20 cells with endothelial features were randomly selected from each sample for single-cell reverse transcription PCR by using primers for GAPDH and vWF (Fig 5). Approximately 20% of the cells (from five samples) yielded amplicons for GAPDH and vWF (Fig 5). This was consistent with the 25% viability of recovered endothelial cells as estimated with the viability and DiI-labeled acetylated low-density lipoprotein uptake assays. Control experiments with freshly prepared HUVECs, in which virtually all cells were viable, showed 100% of cells expressing transcripts for vWF (Fig 5).

Endothelial activation is characterized, in part, by the expression of inducible molecules such as the cell adhesion molecule E-selectin (23,24). In HUVECs, no transcripts for E-selectin were detected in quiescent cells, whereas after exposure to lipopolysaccharide, five of six cells displayed E-selectin messenger RNA (Fig 5). Endothelial cells were obtained from the iliac artery of a 15-year-old patient with arteriovenous malformation. Reverse transcription PCR demonstrated no E-selectin transcripts in any of the four cells incubated in buffer but did reveal three of five positive cells after lipopolysaccharide exposure (Fig 5). The ability of patient-derived endothelial cells to express inducible endothelial cell adhesion molecules is consistent with their viability, as revealed by the viability assay results.

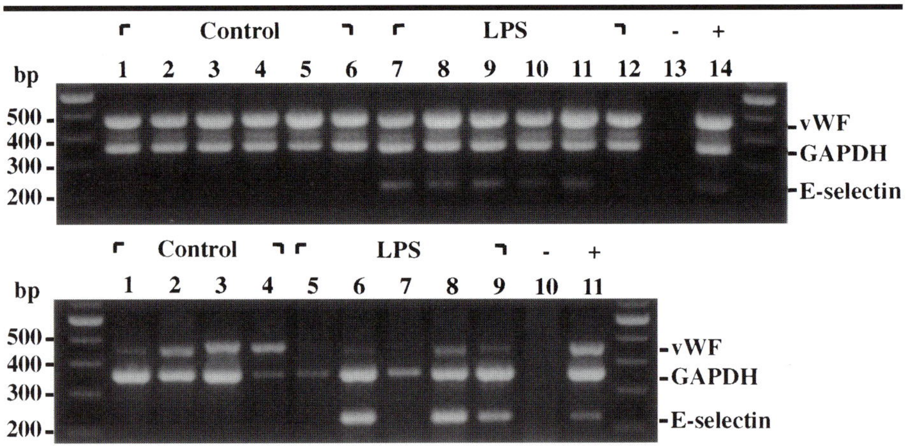

Figure 5. Ethidium bromide–stained agarose gels of results from single-cell reverse transcription PCR products show induction of E-selectin expression in the adherent endothelial cell population. Top: PCR product from HUVECs (control cells). Bottom: PCR product from patient-derived cells. Expression of amplicons for vWF, GAPDH, and E-selectin was studied in cells incubated in medium alone (top, lanes *1–6;* bottom, lane *1–4*) or after treatment with lipopolysaccharide (*LPS*) (top, lanes *7–12;* bottom, lanes *6–9*). For the negative control (−), we omitted reverse transcriptase; the positive control (+) consisted of purified total RNA from HUVECs.

Expression of Leukocyte Adhesion Molecules in Endothelial Cells

Endothelial cell expression of cell adhesion molecules, such as E-selectin,

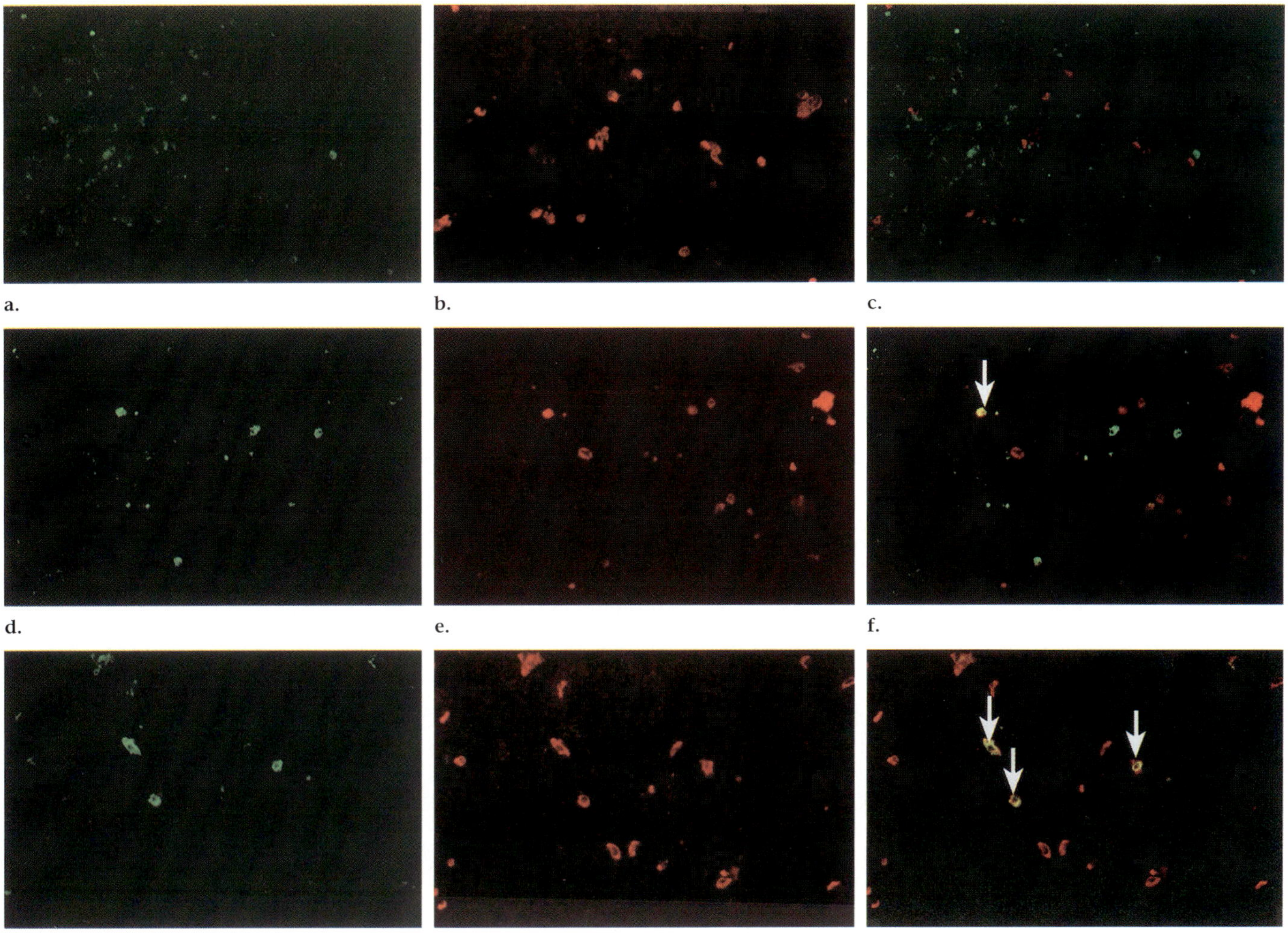

a. b. c. d. e. f. g. h. i.

Figure 6. Photomicrographs demonstrate expression of E-selectin, ICAM-1, and VCAM-1 antigens in the adherent endothelial cell population derived from one patient. Immunostaining for the indicated antigens **(a)** E-selectin, **(b)** vWF, **(c)** both E-selectin and vWF, **(d)** ICAM-1, **(e)** vWF, **(f)** both ICAM-1 and vWF, **(g)** VCAM-1, **(h)** vWF, and **(i)** both VCAM-1 and vWF. Arrows = double-labeled cells. E-selectin is not detected in endothelial cells. A subset of endothelial cells expresses ICAM-1 or VCAM-1. (Original magnification, ×100.)

ICAM-1, and VCAM-1, is altered with vascular perturbation (25). E-selectin has been most closely linked to acute inflammation and recruitment of leukocytes in postcapillary venules (26). Changes in ICAM-1 and VCAM-1 often are more sustained and associated with chronic conditions such as atherosclerosis (27). For example, VCAM-1 has been detected at the earliest stages of lesion development in genetically manipulated murine models of atherosclerosis (28), and increased levels of a soluble form of VCAM-1 have been noted (27,28) in cases of diabetes and other conditions associated with a high risk of vascular disease.

These considerations led us to analyze expression of these adhesion molecules in iliac arteries in 10 consecutive patients, four with a cerebral arterial aneurysm and six with arteriovenous malformation in the brain. The seven female and three male patients, four of whom were hypertensive, were 15–67 years of age. Figure 6 shows representative results from cells isolated from one patient. Immunostaining of patient-derived cells initially adherent to curved guide wires showed expression of E-selectin (Fig 6a) in a population of cells distinct from those with vWF (Fig 6b, 6c). Absence of E-selectin in endothelial cells harvested from patients was not due to methodological problems in cell isolation or to the detection procedure, because identically processed HUVECs treated with lipopolysaccharide showed strong E-selectin expression (data not shown).

ICAM-1 also was detected in the patient-derived cell population (Fig 6d) and, when compared with cells expressing vWF (Fig 6e), one cell in the field was observed to express both markers (Fig 6f). Similar studies performed with VCAM-1 revealed that VCAM-1 was expressed (Fig 6g) in a subpopulation of cells also positive for vWF (Fig 6h). The results of VCAM-1 and ICAM-1 expression are summarized in the Table. Linear regression analysis with age as the independent variable and logit transformations of the proportions of cells that were positive for ICAM-1 or VCAM-1 as the outcome variables showed a significant increase in VCAM-1 expression with age ($P < .007$; $r^2 = 0.624$). The expression of VCAM-1 was not associated with sex, presence of hypertension, or diagnosis, as determined with multivariate logistic regression in this small sample of patients. Further studies with larger numbers of patients are needed to rule out confounding variables and to assess the association of VCAM-1 expression with other risk factors for atherosclerosis. There also was a tendency toward an increased number of cells that express ICAM-1 with age, but this trend did not reach statistical significance ($P = .17$).

Expression of ICAM-1 and VCAM-1 in Endothelial Cells

Patient No./Age (y)/Sex	Diagnosis*	Hypertension	ICAM-1†	VCAM-1†
1/15/F	AVM	No	0.155 (168)	0.017 (118)
2/20/F	AVM	No	0.222 (18)	0.111 (9)
3/44/F	Aneurysm	No	0.143 (7)	0.067 (15)
4/46/M	AVM	No	0.273 (11)	0.125 (8)
5/54/M	AVM	Yes	0.188 (16)	0.158 (19)
6/58/F	Aneurysm	No	0.324 (37)	0.240 (25)
7/64/F	AVM	Yes	0.324 (37)	0.250 (28)
8/65/F	Aneurysm	No	0.171 (70)	0.172 (99)
9/66/F	Aneurysm	Yes	0.381 (21)	0.257 (35)
10/67/M	AVM	Yes	0.222 (9)	0.125 (8)

Note.—VCAM-1 expression was positively associated with age ($r^2 = 0.624$, $P < .007$), whereas there was no significant trend for ICAM-1 expression.

* AVM = arteriovenous malformation.

† Value is the proportion of positive endothelial cells. Value in parentheses is the number of cells examined. If no positive cells were observed, a hypothetic positive cell was added for comparison.

DISCUSSION

During routine endovascular procedures, catheters and guide wires come into contact with the vessel wall. Our results demonstrated that endothelial cells became adherent to the surface of a curved guide wire and, consequently, could be dissociated, purified, and provided in suitable form for detailed molecular analysis. This method of endothelial sampling is safe because it does not add any time to the endovascular procedure or risks to the patients.

These data emphasize the ease with which endothelial cells are dislodged during vascular procedures and are in keeping with previous electron microscopic studies (29) and observations of circulating endothelial cells after endovascular procedures (30,31). Even without the use of instrumentation, endothelial cells can become detached and circulate in blood (32). Especially in sickle cell disease, the authors of careful studies (32) have documented isolation of endothelial cells by using a monoclonal antibody and found that the number of circulating endothelial cells increases during crises. Thus, release of endothelial cells into the blood is likely to occur in many conditions and at an exaggerated rate during vascular perturbation.

Circulating and/or easily detached endothelial cells may also be considered a physiologic occurrence in two settings. Dividing endothelial cells display diminished adherence to the underlying substrate and, thus, are more likely to detach. Chen et al (33) showed an increase in the number of dividing cells at arterial bifurcations, which are sites of turbulent flow; this correlates with an increase in vascular permeability at these sites, which is consistent with a looser attachment of dividing endothelial cells to neighboring cells in the monolayer. In a pathologic context, tumor angiogenesis and other vascular responses that result in new vessel formation and/or remodeling also result in an increase in endothelial turnover and a looser association of endothelium with vessel wall (34,35).

Alternatively, circulating endothelial cells may represent endothelial progenitor cells ready to be incorporated into remodeling peripheral endothelium. Asahara and colleagues (36) have identified a population of circulating endothelial progenitor cells on the basis of the expression of CD34, vascular endothelial growth factor receptor 2, endothelial nitric oxide synthase, CD31, and tyrosine kinase that contains immunoglobulin-like loops and epidermal growth factor–like domains 2 (referred to as Tie-2).

In contrast to the process of angiogenesis, in which vessels were formed exclusively as an outgrowth of previously formed vasculature, the results reported by Asahara et al (36) have emphasized a contribution of vasculogenesis in new vessel formation. In vasculogenesis, circulating endothelial progenitor cells become adherent to the vessel wall and especially populate sites of ongoing new vessel formation. The source of endothelial progenitor cells is unknown at present, although the common expression of CD34 and vascular endothelial growth factor receptor 2 by endothelial progenitor cells and hematopoietic stem cells suggests that they may derive from bone marrow. The ease we experienced in detaching endothelial cells from peripheral vessels raises the possibility that endothelial progenitor cells may derive from peripheral vessels, especially in the presence of angiogenic stimuli.

The extraordinarily high yield of endothelial cells from a patient with a highly vascular meningioma may have been an incidental finding or may reflect pathologic changes in the endothelium. Under the influence of tumor angiogenesis, there may be increased proliferation in remote vessels, as well. Alternatively, more endothelial progenitor cells may be generated from peripheral vessels or incorporated in those vessels. The possibility of a relationship between angiogenesis and yield of endothelial cells appears to be an appropriate subject for further study.

After a typical endovascular procedure, about 250 cells dissociated from a curved guide wire displayed endothelial-like features on the basis of evaluation of Wright-stained smears. After our centrifugation and adherence procedure, which required 75 minutes, approximately 50 endothelial cells were available for further study. The morphology, viability, and reactivity of these cells to lipopolysaccharide suggested that these cells were random samples of the endothelium rather than sick cells that were ready to fall off. However, we cannot exclude the possibility that less adherent cells, such as dividing cells, were preferentially sampled. Because of the small number of cells obtained, we emphasized single-cell approaches to the analysis of patient-derived endothelium. Although it was a challenge, we showed that methods for analysis of single cells at the protein and messenger RNA levels are available and can be applied with our samples.

Because simultaneous visualization of up to three markers on the same cell is possible with the aid of immunocytochemical techniques, analysis with an accepted endothelial marker, such as vWF, and with two activation markers of interest certainly is feasible. This method would allow definitive characterization of the cell under study as endothelial in origin and would permit detection of additional antigens. Such other markers could include endothelial receptors for growth factors, developmental regulators and/or regulators of the blood coagulation mechanism, the presence of the TAT protein (37), or Bartonella-associated antigens (38) in patients suspected of having syndromes related to infection with the human immunodeficiency virus.

The most exciting implication of our results is the isolation of intact messenger RNA from patient-derived endothelial cells. By using single-cell reverse transcription PCR, transcripts in endothelial cells can be amplified, and, in the same sample, the presence of known markers can be detected. Furthermore, complementary DNA generated from the small amounts of messenger RNA in the cell samples provides the basis for construction of complementary DNA libraries to be used in the analysis of unexpected and unknown molecular species expressed by cells of the vessel wall. Thus, in the same cell, its endothelial origin can be ascertained by observing the presence of transcripts for vWF and potential activation markers, as well as previously unrecognized messenger RNA species, and these can be determined simultaneously.

There are caveats with respect to the use of reverse transcription PCR in such differential display strategies. For example, gene expression at the single-cell level may be variable, and selection bias must be carefully avoided. Our method will allow selection of multiple cells from any sample to serve as a starting point for comparisons with cells from the same individual harvested from a different location or with cells harvested from another patient.

In summary, our data demonstrate that viable endothelial cells suitable for molecular analysis at the transcript and protein levels can be obtained during routine angiographic procedures. Our initial results, which are based on a small sample, showed a trend toward an increase in VCAM-1 expression with increased age and the absence of the activation marker E-selectin in the endothelial cell population. Although further studies are needed to help strengthen these conclusions, patient-derived endothelial cells provide a useful tool for future analysis of vascular disease by using immunocytochemical and single-cell reverse transcription PCR methods.

Potential insights from the application of this technique to the comparison of endothelial cell gene expression from lesional or lesion-prone areas of the vessel wall in quiescent cells could be far-reaching. The same approach may also be applied to animal models of vascular diseases or be used to sample endothelial cells from various vascular segments in experimental animals such as nonhuman primates. The molecular techniques used in this study are standard and mature techniques that are routinely performed by molecular biologists, as well as by investigators in clinical laboratories.

Insights gained from the results of these studies offer promise for the stratification of disease, monitoring of therapeutic effects, and guidance for therapeutic interventions, including provision of targets for gene therapy. Nonetheless, it is essential to state that, as of yet, we have not obtained satisfactory numbers of endothelial cells from stenotic carotid arteries (an example of a vascular lesion) to allow molecular analysis. Modification of our procedure and the type of device used may be necessary at such sites, where high-velocity blood flow is in the opposite direction of wire retrieval. The results of the current study strongly suggest that efforts to pursue such an enhancement of the technique are warranted.

APPENDIX

The sequences for the vWF primers were 5′-TGCACCTGACTGCAGCCAGCC-3′ (5,145–5,165), 5′-TTGTGGAGGAAGGAA TTGCCC-3′ (5,708–5,688), 5′-ACGAGAT CCTTCTCCTGGATG-3′ (5,171–5,191), and 5′-TTCACCACGTTGGAGTCGCCT-3′ (5,648–5,628).

The sequences for the GAPDH primers were 5′-GGACCTGACCTGCCGTCTAGA- 3′ (730–750), 5′-GGTACATGACAAGGTGCGGCT-3′ (1,183–1,163), 5′-GGTGGTGAAGCAGGCGTCGGA-3′ (781–801), and 5′-GGTCTACATGGCAACTGTGAG-3′ (1,137–1,117).

The sequences for the E-selectin primers were 5′-CCTCTGACAGAAGAAGCCAAG-3′ (381–401), 5′-CTGCAAACCAGGCTTCCATGC-3′ (697–677), 5′-CAG GTGAACCCAACAATAGGC-3′ (412–432), and 5′-CACTTGAGTCCACTGAAGCCA-3′ (637–617).

Acknowledgments: We are indebted to Hoang Duong, MD, Karen Laffey, MD, Charles J. Prestigiacomo, MD, and Meng Vang, MD, who were instrumental in collecting guide wires and providing patient information. We thank Philip O. Alderson, MD, John H. M. Austin, MD, and William L. Young, MD, for critical review of the manuscript.

References

1. Grau GE, de Moerloose P, Bulla O, et al. Hemostatic properties of human pulmonary and cerebral microvascular endothelial cells. Thromb Haemost 1997; 77:585–590.
2. Wu KK, Thiagarajan P. Role of endothelium in thrombosis and hemostasis. Annu Rev Med 1996; 47:315–331.
3. Marcus AJ, Broekman MJ, Drosopoulos JH, et al. The endothelial cell ecto-ADPase responsible for inhibition of platelet function is CD39. J Clin Invest 1997; 99:1351–1360.
4. Lijnen HR, Collen D. Endothelium in hemostasis and thrombosis. Prog Cardiovasc Dis 1997; 39:343–350.
5. Vanhoutte PM, Mombouli JV. Vascular endothelium: vasoactive mediators. Prog Cardiovasc Dis 1996; 39:229–238.
6. Busse R, Fleming I. Regulation and functional consequences of endothelial nitric oxide. Ann Med 1995; 27:331–340.
7. Frolich JC. Prostacyclin in hypertension. J Hypertens Suppl 1990; 8:73–78.
8. Taubman MB, Fallon JT, Schecter AD, et al. Tissue factor in the pathogenesis of atherosclerosis. Thromb Haemost 1997; 78:200–204.
9. Gimbrone MA Jr, Bevilacqua MP, Cybulsky MI. Endothelial-dependent mechanisms of leukocyte adhesion in inflammation and atherosclerosis. Ann NY Acad Sci 1990; 598:77–85.
10. Wilcox JN, Nelken NA, Coughlin SR, Gordon D, Schall TJ. Local expression of inflammatory cytokines in human atherosclerotic plaques. J Atheroscler Thromb 1994; 1(suppl 1):S10–S13.
11. Richardson M, Kurowska EM, Carroll KK. Early lesion development in the aortas of rabbits fed low-fat, cholesterol-free, semi-purified casein diet. Atherosclerosis 1994; 107:165–178.
12. Chappey O, Wautier MP, Boval B, Wautier JL. Endothelial cells in culture: an experimental model for the study of vascular dysfunctions. Cell Biol Toxicol 1996; 12: 199–205.
13. Lloyd-Jones DM, Bloch KD. The vascular biology of nitric oxide and its role in atherogenesis. Annu Rev Med 1996; 47: 365–375.
14. Samdani AF, Dawson TM, Dawson VL. Nitric oxide synthase in models of focal ischemia. Stroke 1997; 28:1283–1288.
15. Wang XM, Terasaki PI, Rankin GW Jr, Chia D, Zhong HP, Hardy S. A new microcellular cytotoxicity test based on calcein AM release. Hum Immunol 1993; 37:264–270.
16. Kanda T, Yoshino H, Ariga T, Yamawaki M, Yu RK. Glycosphingolipid antigens in cultured microvascular bovine brain endothelial cells: sulfoglucuronosyl paragloboside as a target of monoclonal IgM in demyelinative neuropathy. J Cell Biol 1994; 126:235–246.
17. Bonthron D, Orr EC, Mitsock LM, Ginsburg D, Handin RI, Orkin SH. Nucleotide sequence of pre-pro-von Willebrand factor cDNA. Nucleic Acids Res 1986; 14: 7125–7127.
18. Allen RW, Trach KA, Hoch JA. Identification of the 37-kDa protein displaying a variable interaction with the erythroid cell membrane as glyceraldehyde-3-phosphate dehydrogenase. J Biol Chem 1987; 262:649–653.
19. Hession C, Osborn L, Goff D, et al. Endothelial leukocyte adhesion molecule 1: direct expression cloning and functional interactions. Proc Natl Acad Sci USA 1990; 87:1673–1677.

20. Matucci-Cerinic M, Jaffa A, Kahaleh B. Angiotensin converting enzyme: an in vivo and in vitro marker of endothelial injury. J Lab Clin Med 1992; 120:428–433.
21. DeBault LE, Esmon NL, Smith GP, Esmon CT. Localization of thrombomodulin antigen in rabbit endothelial cells in culture: an immunofluorescence and immunoelectron microscope study. Lab Invest 1986; 54:179–187.
22. Wagner DD, Bonfanti R. von Willebrand factor and the endothelium. Mayo Clin Proc 1991; 66:621–627.
23. Huang K, Fishwild DM, Wu HM, Dedrick RL. Lipopolysaccharide-induced E-selectin expression requires continuous presence of LPS and is inhibited by bactericidal/permeability-increasing protein. Inflammation 1995; 19:389–404.
24. Collins T, Read MA, Neish AS, Whitley MZ, Thanos D, Maniatis T. Transcriptional regulation of endothelial cell adhesion molecules: NF-kappa B and cytokine-inducible enhancers. FASEB J 1995; 9:899–909.
25. Abe Y, Sugisaki K, Dannenberg AM Jr. Rabbit vascular endothelial adhesion molecules: ELAM-1 is most elevated in acute inflammation, whereas VCAM-1 and ICAM-1 predominate in chronic inflammation. J Leukoc Biol 1996; 60:692–703.
26. Gurtner GC, Davis V, Li H, McCoy MJ, Sharpe A, Cybulsky MI. Targeted disruption of the murine VCAM1 gene: essential role of VCAM-1 in chorioallantoic fusion and placentation. Genes Dev 1995; 9:1–14.
27. De Caterina R, Basta G, Lazzerini G, et al. Soluble vascular cell adhesion molecule-1 as a biohumoral correlate of atherosclerosis. Arterioscler Thromb Vasc Biol 1997; 17:2646–2654.
28. Otsuki M, Hashimoto K, Morimoto Y, Kishimoto T, Kasayama S. Circulating vascular cell adhesion molecule-1 (VCAM-1) in atherosclerotic NIDDM patients. Diabetes 1997; 46:2096–2101.
29. Pap JM. Catheter-induced intimal injury during routine coronary catheterization in dogs. Cathet Cardiovasc Diagn 1987; 13:57–73.
30. George F, Brisson C, Poncelet P, et al. Rapid isolation of human endothelial cells from whole blood using S-Endo1 monoclonal antibody coupled to immunomagnetic beads: demonstration of endothelial injury after angioplasty. Thromb Haemost 1992; 67:147–153.
31. Sbarbati R, de Boer M, Marzilli M, Scarlattini M, Rossi G, van Mourik JA. Immunologic detection of endothelial cells in human whole blood. Blood 1991; 77:764–769.
32. Solovey A, Lin Y, Browne P, Choong S, Wayner E, Hebbel RP. Circulating activated endothelial cells in sickle cell anemia. N Engl J Med 1997; 337:1584–1590.
33. Chen YL, Jan KM, Lin HS, Chien S. Relationship between endothelial cell turnover and permeability to horseradish peroxidase. Atherosclerosis 1997; 133:7–14.
34. Provias J, Claffey K, delAguila L, Lau N, Feldkamp M, Guha A. Meningiomas: role of vascular endothelial growth factor/vascular permeability factor in angiogenesis and peritumoral edema. Neurosurgery 1997; 40:1016–1026.
35. Kalkanis SN, Carroll RS, Zhang J, Zamani AA, Black PM. Correlation of vascular endothelial growth factor messenger RNA expression with peritumoral vasogenic cerebral edema in meningiomas. J Neurosurg 1996; 85:1095–1101.
36. Asahara T, Murohara T, Sullivan A, et al. Isolation of putative progenitor endothelial cells for angiogenesis. Science 1997; 275:964–967.
37. Albini A, Soldi R, Giunciuglio D, et al. The angiogenesis induced by HIV-1 tat protein is mediated by the Flk-1/KDR receptor on vascular endothelial cells. Nat Med 1996; 2:1371–1375.
38. Schlupen EM, Schirren CG, Hoegl L, Schaller M, Volkenandt M. Molecular diagnosis of deep nodular bacillary angiomatosis and monitoring of therapeutic success. Br J Dermatol 1997; 136:747–751.

Hepatic Intraarterial ¹³¹I Iodized Oil for Treatment of Hepatocellular Carcinoma in Patients with Impeded Portal Venous Flow[1]

Thierry de Baere, MD
Patrice Taourel, MD
Jean Michel Tubiana, MD
Viseth Kuoch, MD
Michel Ducreux, MD
Jean Lumbroso, MD
Alain J. Roche, MD

Index terms:
Hepatic arteries, therapeutic blockade, 952.1266
Iodine and iodine compounds, radioactive, 761.1266
Liver neoplasms, chemotherapeutic infusion, 761.1266, 761.323
Portal vein, stenosis or obstruction, 957.751
Radionuclides, therapeutic, 761.1266, 761.323
Therapeutic radiology, 761.1266, 761.323

Radiology 1999; 212:665–668

[1] From the Departments of Interventional Radiology (T.d.B., V.K., A.J.R.), Medicine (M.D.), and Nuclear Medicine (J.L.), Institut Gustave Roussy, 94805 Villejuif, France; the Department of Medical Imaging, Saint Eloi Hospital, Montpellier, France (P.T.); and the Department of Medical Imaging, Hôpital Saint Antoine, Paris, France (J.M.T.). Received May 4, 1998; revision requested July 6; final revision received December 14; accepted March 26, 1999. **Address reprint requests to** T.d.B.

Author contributions:
Guarantors of integrity of entire study, P.T., J.M.T., A.J.R., T.d.B.; study concepts, J.L., T.d.B., M.D.; study design, J.L., T.d.B.; definition of intellectual content, J.L., P.T., J.M.T., T.d.B., M.D.; literature research, V.K., T.d.B.; clinical studies, J.L., J.M.T., A.J.R., M.D., P.T., V.K.; data acquisition, J.M.T., P.T., T.d.B.; data analysis, T.d.B., M.D.; statistical analysis, M.D.; manuscript preparation, T.d.B., P.T.; manuscript editing, T.d.B.; manuscript review, J.L., P.T., V.K.

PURPOSE: To evaluate the efficacy and safety of intraarterial hepatic iodine 131 iodized oil for treatment of hepatocellular carcinoma in patients with impeded portal venous flow.

MATERIALS AND METHODS: Twenty-four patients (mean age, 61 years) with hepatocellular carcinoma underwent 38 courses of ¹³¹I iodized oil (one to three per patient), with a mean dose of 2,146 MBq injected into the proper hepatic artery. Hepatocellular carcinoma manifested as single nodules (n = 8; mean, 7.75 cm), multiple nodules (n = 13; mean, 5.46 cm), or a mass (n = 3) occupying more than two hepatic segments. Portal venous thrombosis was complete (n = 10), right (n = 9), left (n = 2), or multisegmental (n = 1). Two patients had hepatofugal portal flow.

RESULTS: Among the 23 patients with evaluatable results, response to treatment was partial in three, and disease was stable in 12 and progressive in eight. Estimated actuarial survival rates were 70%, 33%, 12%, and 6% at 3, 6, 9, and 12 months, respectively, with two patients alive at 9 and 11 months. The median survival time was 147 days. Adverse events were the early death of one patient owing to hepatic failure and transient symptomatic hepatic failure after 12 courses in nine patients.

CONCLUSION: In this preliminary experience, intraarterial hepatic ¹³¹I iodized oil did not demonstrate high efficacy in the treatment of hepatocellular carcinoma in patients with portal venous thrombosis, as side effects were not rare.

Lipiodol Ultra-Fluide (Guerbet, Roissy, France) is an iodinated ethylic ester of poppy-seed oil. To our knowledge, iodized oil was first injected into the hepatic arteries in the early 1980s. Because of its capacity to target and remain fixed in tumors, iodized oil was first used as a diagnostic tool (1,2) and is still used in association with delayed computed tomography (CT) for the evaluation of disseminated hepatocellular carcinoma. Injection of iodized oil mixed with various drugs into hepatic arteries is widely used for the treatment of hepatic tumors and has been described frequently in the literature (3–6) during the past decade.

More recently, iodine 131 iodized oil (Lipiocis; Cis Bio International Laboratory, Gif sur Yvette, France) was injected into hepatic arteries for interstitial radiation therapy. Some clinical success has been reported with this method without the need for additional arterial embolization, notably in the treatment of hepatocellular carcinoma (7–11). The French Drug Agency recently approved ¹³¹I iodized oil for the treatment of inoperable hepatocellular carcinoma with portal venous thrombosis.

The aim of this study was to evaluate the efficacy and safety of hepatic intraarterial injection of ¹³¹I iodized oil in the treatment of hepatocellular carcinoma in patients with impaired portal venous flow.

MATERIALS AND METHODS

From October 1994 to January 1997, 24 patients (20 men, four women; age range, 52–75 years; mean age, 61 years ± 8 [SD]) with inoperable hepatocellular carcinoma entered the study at the authors' three institutions after the approval of the institutional review boards was obtained. After a full explanation of the nature of the treatment, patients gave their oral informed consent. No patients had undergone previous therapy, and the time between diagnosis and the initiation of ^{131}I iodized oil therapy was 3 days to 4 weeks (median, 13 days).

The diagnosis of hepatocellular carcinoma was made on the basis of either histologic examination results or an α-fetoprotein level exceeding 500 ng/mL (500 μg/L; normal value < 10 ng/mL [10 μg/L]) together with characteristic CT features. Eight patients had a single-nodule tumor 3–15 cm in diameter (mean, 7.75 cm ± 3.96), 13 patients had a multinodular tumor with the largest nodule 2–13 cm in diameter (mean, 5.46 ± 3.62), and three patients had a massive tumor occupying more than two hepatic segments.

In all patients, the tumor was inoperable because of either extensive disease or severe cirrhosis. All patients had disease confined to the liver except two who had lung or bone metastases. The cause of cirrhosis was alcohol (n = 10), virus (n = 9), or hemochromatosis (n = 1), or the cause was unknown (n = 4).

Because portal venous obstruction is a well-known risk factor for hepatic failure and infarction after hepatic arterial embolization (12), portal flow was considered insufficient to ensure safe embolization of the hepatic artery if two or more segmental branches feeding nontumorous liver were occluded in addition to the ones feeding tumorous segments. This insufficient portal flow was due to obstruction of the portal trunk (n = 10), the right branch (n = 9), the left branch (n = 2), or more than three segmental branches (n = 1), and portal flow was hepatofugal in two patients.

Before the first hepatic intraarterial injection of ^{131}I iodized oil was administered, the underlying hepatic disease, according to the Child classification, was as follows: Child A (n = 14), Child B (n = 8), and Child C (n = 2). Tumor stages according to the Okuda classification (13) were as follows: Okuda I (n = 10) and Okuda II (n = 14). Blood test results showed an increase in α-fetoprotein of 59–273,000 ng/mL (59–273,000 μg/L; normal value < 10 ng/mL [10 μg/L]) in 12 patients and a bilirubin value of 8–67 μmol/L (mean, 27 μmol/L ± 16; normal value < 17 μmol/L), a prothrombin time of 45%–100% (mean, 75% ± 14; normal value, 70%–100% [100% = 10–14 seconds]), and a serum albumin level of 25–54 g/L (mean, 35 g/L ± 9; normal value, 32–55 g/L) in all patients.

After iodized oil was labeled with an exchange isotopic reaction, ^{131}I iodized oil was produced. Labeling efficacy has been found to be greater than 99% with chromatography, and stability has been demonstrated without dehalogenation over a 3-month period (14). One to three hepatic intraarterial injections (mean, 1.6) were performed bimonthly, with a total of 38 courses. The dose injected for each treatment was 58 mCi ± 4.6 (2,146 MBq ± 170.2; range, 52–60 mCi [1,924–2,220 MBq]), except for one treatment that was performed with half the dose (ie, 30 mCi [1,110 MBq]). All the procedures were performed with local anesthesia.

After angiographic confirmation of insufficient portal flow for embolization, the proper hepatic artery was selectively catheterized, and 5–7 mL of ^{131}I iodized oil was injected without reflux, as fast as was allowed by arterial flow. No superselective injection of the ^{131}I iodized oil in tumorous segments was performed. In two patients, there was an additional replaced left hepatic artery, which prompted us to inject half of the dose of ^{131}I iodized oil into each hepatic artery.

After the injections, the patients were isolated for 7 days for radiation protection of other patients, and only short visits were authorized. The handling of all radioactive materials and the care of patients receiving radioisotope treatment were in accordance with local rules and recommendations of the French Organization for Protection against Ionizing Radiations.

Planar scintiscans of the liver and thorax were obtained 2–3 days later to allow quantification of the activity ratio of liver to lung plus liver. Tumor response was evaluated on CT scans 1 month after each course of treatment. Tumor size was appreciated by using the product of the two largest perpendicular diameters. A partial response was a decrease of at least 50% of this product, and progression was an increase of at least 25%. Survival was measured from initiation of ^{131}I iodized oil therapy by using the Kaplan-Meier method.

RESULTS

All hepatic arteries were catheterized successfully and injected with ^{131}I iodized oil, and no adverse event occurred during the procedure, except in one patient who had mild abdominal pain within a few seconds after the injection of 5 mL of ^{131}I iodized oil. The ratio of liver to lung plus liver after the first injection was higher than 75% in 13 patients, lower than 50% in one, intermediate in four, and not evaluated in six.

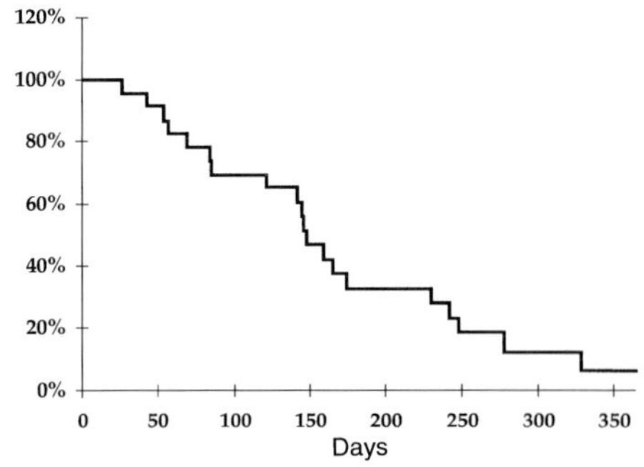

Graph shows the actuarial survival estimation with the Kaplan-Meier method in 23 patients with evaluatable results who were treated with intraarterial hepatic ^{131}I iodized oil. The patient lost to follow-up after 4 months has been excluded.

The tumor size was evaluated in 23 patients. One patient died before follow-up assessment of tumor size. After the first course, three (13%) of 23 patients had a partial response, 12 (52%) had stable disease, and eight had progressive disease. Among the three who responded, two died 69 and 145 days after the initiation of ^{131}I iodized oil therapy and received only one course of treatment, and one was still responding when lost to follow-up after 4 months and three courses of treatment.

Among the 12 patients with stable disease, six underwent only one course of treatment and died 85–230 days (mean, 154 days) after the initiation of ^{131}I iodized oil therapy. Six continued treatment, and disease remained stable at CT for 42–140 days (mean, 91 days) after the initiation of ^{131}I iodized oil therapy. Among these six patients, four underwent two courses of treatment and died after 142–329 days (mean, 189 days), and two patients who underwent three courses are still alive after 9 and 11 months. The eight patients with progressive disease died after 43–278 days (mean, 145 days) despite one course of treatment in four patients and two courses in the other four.

The median survival time was 147 days (mean, 137 days ± 83), with one patient lost to follow-up at 4 months and two patients alive after 9 and 11 months. The 3-, 6-, 9-, and 12-month estimations of actuarial survival with the Kaplan-Meier method (Fig) were 70%, 33%, 12%, and 6%, respectively.

Complications during the 1st month after treatment included one early death due to hepatic failure and transient symptomatic hepatic failure after 12 injections in nine patients. The early death occurred in a patient with Child A disease who developed jaundice, ascites, and encephalopathy 3–4 days after treatment and who died of hepatic insufficiency 28 days after the first course of treatment. Transient hepatic failure symptoms were ascites (n = 10), edema of the lower limb (n = 5), and jaundice (n = 6). These transient failures occurred in five patients with Child A disease, two with Child B, and two with Child C. Treatment was stopped in six patients owing to these adverse events, including in three patients who twice presented with symptomatic hepatic failure less than 2 weeks after injection of ^{131}I iodized oil.

DISCUSSION

Selective fixation of iodized oil in hepatic tumors is explained by its propensity to pass preferentially through tumor arteries and to embolize them temporarily (15), its ability to pass from the artery into the portal veins via the peribiliary plexus (16), the increased permeability of tumor vessels that allows the passage of iodized oil through their layers (17,18), the incorporation of iodized oil by tumor cells as vesicles by pinocytosis (19–21), and the low clearance of iodized oil by Kupffer cells in the tumor compared with clearance in healthy hepatic cells (16). The ratio of iodized oil fixation in tumors to that in healthy liver has been reported by various authors (22–25) to be roughly between five and 10, and this advantage has long been exploited for tumor targeting by mixing anticancer drugs with iodized oil. However, additional arterial embolization is needed to enhance the efficacy of drug targeting (26), which renders this technique inapplicable in patients with portal venous thrombosis.

More recently, iodized oil was labeled with a radioisotope, more often ^{131}I than rhenium 188 (24). This radiolabeled iodized oil allows the delivery of interstitial radiation therapy that targets tumors. Such treatment can be used in patients with portal venous thrombosis because additional embolization is not needed.

With this treatment, survival in our series is very similar to that reported for the group treated in the only randomized study published, to our knowledge, on hepatocellular carcinoma in patients with portal venous thrombosis, treated with ^{131}I iodized oil (27). Survival rates at 3, 6, and 9 months were 71%, 48%, 7% in the study by Raoul et al (27) and 70%, 33%, 12% in our series. These comparable survival rates were obtained in patients sharing, in both series, the same nationality and similar underlying hepatic disease and tumor stages.

Despite these similar survival rates, toxicity and tolerance were different in the two series. The response rate was 44% for Raoul et al (27) and 13% in our experience. Thus, response to treatment does not seem to have influenced survival to any notable extent, and in our experience survival was even slightly shorter for those who responded than for those who did not. Our median survival time is within the limits of the 2–7-month survival time usually reported in the literature (28–32) for all confounded untreated hepatocellular carcinoma. Moreover, the survival rates of 3, 6, and 9 months are very close to those of the untreated group of patients with hepatocellular carcinoma and portal venous thrombosis reported by Lee et al (33).

We had to deal with a high rate of treatment-induced hepatic failure. With the exception of one death, most cases of hepatic failure were reversible, but treatment had to be discontinued in six patients because of these side effects. Although intraarterial hepatic injections of ^{131}I iodized oil are reported by most authors (9, 10, 22, 27, 34) to be well tolerated, such frequent hepatic failure after treatment was reported by Bhattacharya et al (7) in a series of 26 patients with a 30-day mortality rate of 15%, despite the absence of portal venous thrombosis. Portal venous thrombosis alone is therefore not a valid explanation for these treatment-induced hepatic failures, nor is the severity of cirrhosis, because these side effects occurred both in patients with Child C disease and in patients with Child A disease.

We did not report adverse pulmonary events, such as chronic inflammatory interstitial infiltration and interstitial fibrosis, which have been reported in other studies (8,27) to occur 3–8 weeks after treatment. It occurred once in 27 patients of Raoul et al (27), and they used the same dose as was used in our study. It occurred in 57% of treated patients of Preketes et al (35), and they used a higher dose, although they subsequently reduced the dose injected for each session.

In other respects, hepatic therapy with intraarterial ^{131}I iodized oil is a relatively cumbersome therapy. First, appropriate isolation facilities are needed in which patients can spend several days. Second, radiation protection is difficult for the physicians who inject high-energy radioisotopes through a catheter, with fluoroscopic guidance, slowly enough to avoid reflux. Third, this treatment is relatively expensive because the cost of a dose of ^{131}I iodized oil is roughly eight- to 10-fold higher than that of the chemotherapy, iodized oil, and absorbable gelatin sponge (Gelfoam; Pharmacia and Upjohn, Portage, Mich) used for standard chemoembolization.

In spite of the disappointing results in our limited series, further studies are needed to reevaluate our findings in a larger series and also to refine the technique. This technique could be optimized in a number of ways. In an experimental model, we previously demonstrated that a fourfold lower lung passage of iodized oil could be achieved by using an appropriate emulsion of iodized oil with saline solution instead of pure iodized oil and, moreover, that the ratio between iodized oil fixation in tumor and nontumorous liver could be increased by a factor of two (25). Such emulsions, which seem appropriate in theory, potentially could maximize radiation doses to the tumor and minimize lung damage, a frequent side effect in at least one study (35). In addition, drugs emulsified with ^{131}I iodized oil could allow radiation therapy to be combined with administration of cytotoxic agents. However, use of such emulsions in clinical practice will be hampered by the mandatory radiation protection precautions required to prepare them.

Embolization after the intraarterial administration of ^{131}I iodized oil is an alternative that, to our knowledge, has never been tested experimentally or in clinical practice: Findings in a recently published article (11) by one of the teams most experienced in the use of ^{131}I iodized oil suggested using embolization to enhance the efficacy of ^{131}I iodized oil in patients without portal venous impediment.

Owing to the complexity of and the poor tolerance for the procedure, the low response rate, and the doubtful gain in survival, hepatic therapy with intraarterial ^{131}I iodized oil cannot be considered a routine clinical treatment for hepatocellular carcinoma in patients with portal venous thrombosis. Refinement of the technique by using an emulsion combined with cytotoxic agents or embolization should be evaluated.

Acknowledgment: We express our appreciation to Ms Lorna Saint Ange for her expert assistance in the linguistic revision of this manuscript.

References

1. Nakamura H, Hashimoto T, Oi H, Sawada S. Iodized oil in the portal vein after arterial embolization. Radiology 1988; 167:415–417.
2. Yumoto Y, Jinno K, Tokuyama K, et al. Hepatocellular carcinoma detected by iodized oil. Radiology 1985; 154:19–24.
3. Takayasu K, Shima Y, Muramatsu Y, et al. Hepatocellular carcinoma: treatment with intraarterial iodized oil with and without chemotherapeutic agents. Radiology 1987; 163:345–351.
4. Roche A. Chemoembolization of liver malignancies. In: Ferrucci JT, Mathieu D, eds. Advances in hepatobiliary radiology. St Louis, Mo: Mosby, 1990; 295–305.
5. Konno T, Maeda H, Iwai K, Maki S, Tashiro S, Uchida M. Selective targeting of anticancer drug and simultaneous image enhancement in solid tumors by arterially administered lipid contrast medium. Cancer 1984; 54:2367–2374.
6. Iwai K, Maeda H, Konno T. Tumor targeting by arterial administration of lipids: rabbit model with VX2 carcinoma in the liver. Anticancer Res 1987; 7:321–327.
7. Bhattacharya S, Novell JR, Dusheiko GM, Hilson AJ, Dick R, Hobbs KE. Epirubicin-Lipiodol chemotherapy versus 131 iodine-Lipiodol radiotherapy in the treatment of unresectable hepatocellular carcinoma. Cancer 1995; 76:2202–2210.
8. Raoul JL, Bretagne JF, Caucanas JP. Internal radiation therapy for hepatocellular carcinoma. Cancer 1992; 69:346–352.
9. Yoo HS, Park CH, Lee JT, et al. Small hepatocellular carcinoma: high dose internal radiation therapy with superselective intra-arterial injection of I-131-labeled Lipiodol. Cancer Chemother Pharmacol 1994; 33(suppl):S128–S133.
10. Leung WT, Lau WY, Ho S, et al. Selective internal radiation therapy with intra-arterial iodine-131-Lipiodol in inoperable hepatocellular carcinoma. J Nucl Med 1994; 35:1313–1318.
11. Raoul JL, Guyader D, Bretagne JF, et al. Prospective randomized trial of chemoembolization versus intra-arterial injection of 131 I-labeled-iodized oil in the treatment of hepatocellular carcinoma. Hepatology 1997; 26:1156–1161.
12. Chung J, Park J, Han J, et al. Hepatic tumors: predisposing factors for complications of transcatheter oily chemoembolization. Radiology 1996; 198:33–40.
13. Okuda K, Ohtsuki T, Obata H, et al. Natural history of hepatocellular carcinoma and prognosis in relation to treatment: study of 850 patients. Cancer 1985; 56: 918–928.
14. Madsen MT, Park CH, Thakur ML. Dosimetry of iodine-131 ethiodol in the treatment of hepatoma. J Nucl Med 1988; 29:1038–1044.
15. de Baere T, Dufaux J, Roche A, et al. Circulatory alterations induced by intra-arterial injection of iodized oil and emulsions of iodized oil and doxorubicin: experimental study. Radiology 1995; 194: 165–170.
16. Kan Z. Dynamic study of iodized oil in the liver and blood supply to hepatic tumors: an experimental investigation in several animal species. Acta Radiol 1996; 37(suppl):6–25.
17. Ackerman N, Hechmer P. Studies on the capillary permeability of experimental liver metastases. Surg Gynecol Obstet 1981; 152:262–267.
18. Jain RK. Transport of molecules across tumor vasculature. Cancer Metastasis Rev 1987; 6:559–593.
19. Chou FI, Fang KC, Chung C, et al. Lipiodol uptake and retention by human hepatoma cells. Nucl Med Biol 1995; 22: 379–386.
20. Bhattacharya S, Dhillon AP, Winslet MC, et al. Human liver cancer cells and endothelial cells incorporate iodised oil. Br J Cancer 1996; 73:877–881.
21. Miller DL, O'Leary T, Girton M. Distribution of iodized oil within the liver after hepatic arterial injection. Radiology 1987; 162:849–852.
22. Raoul JL, Bourguet P, Bretagne JF, et al. Hepatic artery injection of I-131–labeled Lipiodol. I. Biodistribution study results in patients with hepatocellular carcinoma and liver metastases. Radiology 1988; 168: 541–545.
23. Hind RE, Loizidou M, Fleming J, Batty V, Birch S, Taylor I. Biodistribution of lipiodol following hepatic arterial injection. Eur J Surg Oncol 1992; 18:162–167.
24. Wang SJ, Lin WY, Chen MN, et al. Biodistribution of rhenium-188 Lipiodol infused via the hepatic artery of rats with hepatic tumours. Eur J Nucl Med 1996; 23:13–17.
25. de Baere T, Zhang X, Aubert B, et al. Quantification of tumor uptake of iodized oils and emulsions of iodized oils: experimental study. Radiology 1996; 201:731–735.
26. Hatanaka Y, Yamashita Y, Takahashi M, et al. Unresectable hepatocellular carcinoma: analysis of prognostic factors in transcatheter management. Radiology 1995; 195: 747–752.
27. Raoul JL, Guyader D, Bretagne JF, et al. Randomized controlled trial for hepatocellular carcinoma with portal vein thrombosis: intra-arterial iodine-131-iodized oil versus medical support. J Nucl Med 1994; 35:1782–1787.
28. Nagasue N, Yukaya H, Hamada T, Hirose S, Kanashima R, Inokuchi D. The natural history of hepatocellular carcinoma. Cancer 1984; 54:1461–1465.
29. Razafimahaleo A, Burtin P, Joly JP, Dupas JL, Capron-Chivrac D, Capron JP. Prognostic factors of hepatocellular carcinoma: multifactorial analysis of 84 cases. Gastroenterol Clin Biol 1993; 17:564–569. [French]
30. Bayraktar Y, Balkanci F, Kayman B, et al. A comparison of chemoembolization with conventional and symptomatic treatment in cirrhotic patients with hepatocellular carcinoma. Hepatogastroenterology 1996; 43:681–687.
31. Castells L, Vargas V, Comas P, et al. Hepatocellular carcinoma: clinical aspects, diagnosis, and survival in 140 cases. Med Clin (Barc) 1993; 100:441–446. [Spanish]
32. Calvet X, Bruix J, Bru C, et al. Natural history of hepatocellular carcinoma in Spain: five year's experience in 249 cases. J Hepatol 1990; 10:311–317.
33. Lee H, Kim J, Choi I, Chung J, Park J, Kim C. The safety of transcatheter arterial chemoembolization in the treatment of patients with hepatocellular carcinoma and main portal vein obstruction. Cancer 1997; 79:2087–2093.
34. Novell JR, Hilson AJ. Iodine-131-Lipiodol for hepatocellular carcinoma: the benefits of targeting (editorial). J Nucl Med 1994; 35:1318–1320.
35. Preketes A, Boyd S, Cooper D, et al. Pulmonary toxicity following Lipiodol I-131 treatment for liver tumours. Reg Cancer Treatment 1996; 9:21–26.

Joan P. Heneghan, MD
Richard J. Everts, FRACP
Rendon C. Nelson, MD

Index terms:
Abdomen, abscess, 70.201, 70.202, 70.204, 70.21, 70.1262
Abscess, CT, 70.1211
Abscess, US, 70.12986
Pelvic organs, abscess, 80.201, 80.202, 80.204, 80.211, 80.1262

Radiology 1999; 212:669–672

[1] From the Department of Radiology (J.P.H., R.C.N.) and the Clinical Microbiology Laboratory (R.J.E.), Duke University Medical Center, Erwin Rd, Box 3808, Durham, NC 27710. From the 1998 RSNA scientific assembly. Received November 25, 1998; revision requested December 30; final revision received January 24, 1999; accepted March 1. **Address reprint requests to** J.P.H. (e-mail: *heneg002@mc.duke.edu*).

Author contributions:
Guarantor of integrity of entire study, J.P.H.; study concepts, J.P.H., R.J.E., R.C.N.; study design, J.P.H., R.J.E.; definition of intellectual content, J.P.H., R.J.E., R.C.N.; literature research, J.P.H.; clinical studies, J.P.H., R.J.E.; data acquisition, J.P.H., R.J.E.; data analysis, R.J.E.; manuscript preparation, J.P.H.; manuscript editing, J.P.H., R.J.E., R.C.N.; manuscript review, R.C.N.

Multiple Fluid Collections: CT- or US-guided Aspiration—Evaluation of Microbiologic Results and Implications for Clinical Practice[1]

PURPOSE: To determine if patients with multiple fluid collections need every collection aspirated and if cross-contamination is a risk if separate sterile procedures are not followed for each aspiration.

MATERIALS AND METHODS: Records from 1,076 imaging-guided percutaneous aspirations and drainages over 39 months were retrospectively reviewed; 124 patients had multiple fluid collections drained, which yielded 287 aspirates. The patients were divided into two groups: those (n = 82) with multiple collections aspirated on any 1 day, and those (n = 61) with multiple collections aspirated over 10 days. Nineteen patients were included in both groups. Gram stain microscopy and culture results were compared between sequential aspirates in each patient, and their potential effects on antimicrobial therapy and theoretic risk for cross-contamination were evaluated.

RESULTS: In 82 patients undergoing multiple aspirations on any 1 day, multiple microorganisms differed in 32 patients, which indicated a need for therapy change in 18 (22%) patients. In 61 patients undergoing aspiration on different days, microorganisms differed in 32 patients, which indicated a need for therapy change in 15 (25%) patients. Cross-contamination could have occurred in 28 of 93 (30%) aspirates from patients with a second or subsequent collection if separate sterile procedures had not been undertaken.

CONCLUSION: When multiple fluid collections are identified, aspirates from all collections should be obtained through separate sterile procedures to ensure optimal antimicrobial coverage and avoid cross-contamination.

Percutaneous drainage is the primary management option for intraabdominal or pelvic abscesses (1–3); aspiration and drainage of such collections under imaging guidance is routine in most radiology practices. For the most part, ultrasonographic (US) or computed tomographic (CT) guidance is employed. Often, patients have multiple fluid collections, which prompts a management question of whether to drain all collections immediately or initially drain the dominant collection and assume that other collections may be sympathetic or contain similar microorganisms. Furthermore, when multiple fluid collections are drained at one time, it is unknown how great the risk is of cross-contamination from an infected collection to another potentially sterile collection if separate sterile fields and separate sterile equipment are not used.

Management of abscesses has been repeatedly discussed in the surgery and radiology literature, particularly with regard to location, cause, and associated factors (carcinoma, enteric fistula, etc) (1–6). In addition, attention has been focused on management in terms of choice and number of catheters required for drainage, as well as the potential use of urokinase to facilitate drainage (7). However, to our knowledge, no study has specifically addressed the role of microbiologic data in determining the management of such collections.

In this study, we evaluated microbiologic data in patients whose multiple fluid collections were drained under US or CT guidance. Our specific purpose was to answer these questions: (*a*) Do multiple collections in an individual patient each require aspiration? (*b*) Is it necessary to create separate sterile fields and use separate equipment for each aspiration and drainage?

MATERIALS AND METHODS

We retrospectively reviewed the database of interventional procedures performed from November 1994 to January 1998 in the abdominal imaging section of our department. During this 39-month period, 1,076 aspirations and drainages of fluid collections were performed under CT or US guidance in 694 patients. Of these, 140 patients had two or more fluid collections aspirated within a 10-day period. We arbitrarily selected 10 days as a reasonable time in which to group sequential aspirates relating to the same episode of illness.

The results of Gram stain microscopy and culture were available for 287 aspirates obtained from the 124 patients who formed the study group. Data on the 16 remaining patients were incomplete; thus, they were excluded (although radiology reports indicated that two samples were obtained from each of these 16 patients, the microbiology laboratory received only one sample from each). Of the 124 patients who had multiple collections aspirated, 63 patients (51%) were postsurgical; 30 (24%) had pancreatitis; 10 (8%) had experienced trauma (motor vehicle accident or gunshot wound); and 21 (17%) had miscellaneous primary causes of infection, including diverticular disease and pelvic inflammatory disease. Ninety-two of 124 (74%) patients were in medical or surgical units, and the remaining 32 patients (26%) were in the intensive care unit.

Each procedure was performed by using a separate sterile biopsy tray, separate sterile equipment, and separate skin disinfection methods, even when multiple procedures were required in an individual patient at the same time. All but two patients had collections within the abdomen or pelvis (one patient had a collection in the thigh; the other had a collection in the chest wall).

Aspirated fluid was sent in an anaerobic transport container to the microbiology laboratory, examined by using Gram stain microscopy, and then cultured on the following media: tryptic soy agar with 5% sheep blood (Trypticase; Becton Dickinson Microbiology Systems, Sparks, Md), Columbia colistin-nalidixic acid agar with 5% sheep blood, MacConkey II agar, and, in nearly all cases, anaerobic *Brucella* blood agar and anaerobic laked blood agar with kanamycin and vancomycin (Becton Dickinson Microbiology Systems).

The 124 study patients were divided into two groups: those (n = 82) with two or more collections aspirated on 1 day and those (n = 61) with two or more collections aspirated on separate days over a 10-day period. There was an overlap of 19 patients between these two groups: These patients had multiple collections aspirated on any 1 day and underwent additional aspiration within 10 days. Our practice is to aspirate all fluid collections in a patient with sepsis (unless technically impossible; for example, a deep interloop abscess). Thus, patients who underwent procedures on separate days were those in whom a new collection was identified on a subsequent day and was duly drained. When multiple collections were present, we did not elect to aspirate some but not other collections on the basis of clinical or radiographic data. There was a mean of 4.9 days between aspiration of initial and subsequent collections.

The microbiologic results of different fluid collections in an individual patient were compared by a clinical microbiologist (R.J.E.); correlation of the interventional procedure report with the labeling of each specimen allowed for deduction of the order of aspirates (ie, first, second, etc). Then, the clinical microbiologist assessed whether a relevant change in antimicrobial therapy would have been indicated by the isolation of a different microorganism in a subsequent collection. A "relevant change" was defined as the need for introduction of a new antimicrobial agent. Cases in which different microorganisms were identified in subsequent fluid collections but in which therapy would not have been altered as a result were considered as "no change." Patient notes were not reviewed to determine whether such a change had actually taken place.

Finally, to assess the risk of cross-contamination, a second comparison was made by the microbiologist for the group of patients (n = 82) who underwent same-day aspirations. In each case, if microorganisms found in one collection were not present in subsequently aspirated collections, the latter collections were considered to be at risk for cross-contamination by microorganisms from the previous collection.

RESULTS

Of 124 patients who underwent multiple aspirations, 86 patients (69%) had microorganisms present in at least one aspirate, and 38 patients (31%) had fluid samples that were negative at Gram stain microscopy and culture. Of the 86 patients with infection, 34 patients had infections that involved a single microorganism, and 52 (60%) had infections that were polymicrobial. Overall, the following microorganisms were isolated: aerobic gram-positive bacteria, 55 patients (64%); aerobic gram-negative bacteria, 43 patients (50%); anaerobic bacteria, 30 patients (35%); and yeast, 30 patients (35%).

Of 82 patients who underwent multiple aspirations on any 1 day, 39 patients (48%) had first collections that were infected, and 43 patients (52%) had first collections that were sterile. The second aspirate was infected in 38 patients (46%) and sterile in 44 patients (54%). Microorganisms differed between sequential aspirates in 32 patients (39%). Detailed results of aspirations and implications for therapy are summarized in Table 1. In the group of patients who underwent multiple aspirations on any 1 day, a change in antimicrobial therapy was indicated by the results of the second aspiration in 18 of 82 patients (22%) (Figure). Nine patients had a third collection aspirated, and two had a fourth collection aspirated; none of these samples provided additional therapeutically relevant information.

Sixty-one patients underwent two or more aspirations on separate days, with no more than 10 days between the first and last aspirations. Of these, 46 patients (75%) had an infected first aspirate; 15 patients' (25%) first aspirates were sterile. The second collection aspirated was infected in 36 patients (59%) and was sterile in 25 patients (41%).

Microorganisms differed between sequential aspirates in 32 patients (52%). Detailed results of aspirations and potential effects on subsequent therapy are summarized in Table 2. Irrespective of the results of first and second aspirations, four samples from the 12 patients who provided a third sample, one sample from the seven patients who provided a fourth sample, and zero samples from the two patients who provided fifth samples provided new therapeutically relevant information. Overall, a change in antimicro-

TABLE 1
Results of Multiple Aspirations on Any 1 Day and Effect on Antimicrobial Therapy

First Collection	Second Collection	No. of Patients (n = 82)*	Change in Therapy
Sterile	Infected	13 (16)	Yes
	Sterile	30 (36)	No
Infected	Infected with different microorganisms	5 (6)	Yes
	Infected with same or therapeutically similar microorganisms	20 (24)	No
	Sterile	14 (17)	No

* Numbers in parentheses are percentages.

TABLE 2
Results of Multiple Aspirations Over 10 Days

First Collection	Second Collection	No. of Patients (n = 61)*	Change in Therapy
Sterile	Infected	4 (7)	Yes
	Sterile	11 (18)	No
Infected	Infected with different microorganisms	9 (15)	Yes
	Infected with same or therapeutically similar microorganisms	23 (37)	No
	Sterile	14 (23)	No

* Numbers in parentheses are percentages.

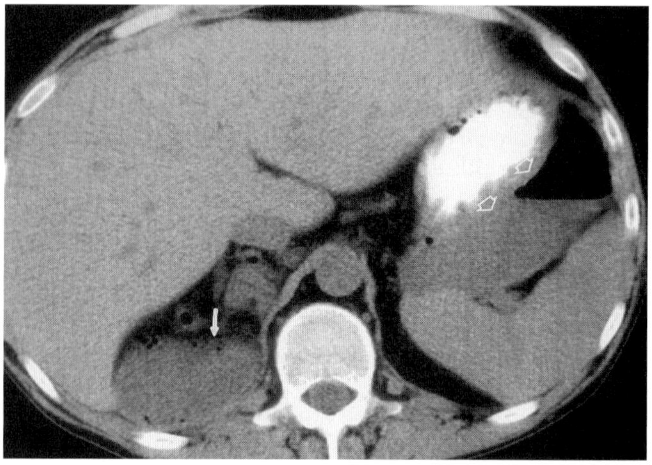

Nonenhanced axial CT image of the upper abdomen of a 29-year-old man with a history of Crohn disease demonstrates two air-containing fluid collections, one in the lesser sac (open arrows) and one in the right flank (solid arrow). *Morganella morganii* was isolated from the lesser sac collection; a single *Enterococcus* species was isolated from the right flank collection. These microorganisms had different antimicrobial susceptibility profiles.

bial therapy was indicated by the results of second or subsequent samples in 15 of 61 patients (25%) in this group.

With regard to the potential for cross-contamination, in the 82 patients in whom a second aspirate was obtained at the same session, 22 (27%) had microorganisms present in the first aspirate that were not present in the second; either the first collection was infected and the second was sterile or different microorganisms were present in the first and second collections.

Moreover, in the 82 patients in whom a second aspirate was obtained at the same session, microorganisms were present in previous aspirates that were not present in five of nine third aspirates and one of two fourth aspirates. Overall, 28 of 93 second or subsequent aspirates (30%) could have led to contamination of the sample or deep tissue if separate sterile procedures had not been followed for each aspiration.

DISCUSSION

Intraabdominal and pelvic abscesses develop as a result of localization of peritonitis, usually in the perihepatic spaces, pelvis, and paracolic gutters. An abscess may also develop near diseased organs, including the bowel, or as a complication of trauma or surgery. These infections tend to be polymicrobial, as was the case in our review for 60% of the 86 patients with infection. Previous investigators (8,9) have isolated anaerobic bacteria from 60% to 70% of patients; however, we found anaerobes in only 35% of patients with infected aspirates. This may reflect a relatively aggressive policy of aspirating and draining fluid collections that did not necessarily demonstrate classic features of anaerobic infection, such as the presence of air.

In addition, if fluid from an intraabdominal collection was mislabeled as having been collected from a drainage catheter rather than by direct aspiration, it was not cultured anaerobically in our clinical microbiology laboratory. We have found this to be a problem in our practice. Specimens sometimes are labeled with the patient's name by the radiologist or nurse at the time of the procedure, but clinical details on the microbiology laboratory request form are subsequently completed by staff members on the ward.

With regard to the need to aspirate multiple fluid collections in the same patient, we found that sampling a second collection resulted in information indicating a need for change in therapy in 22% of patients with multiple same-day aspirates and in 25% of patients with multiple subsequent-day aspirates. It is interesting that aspiration of a third collection yielded no new therapeutically relevant information in the same-day group but did indicate a need for alteration of therapy in one-third of patients in the subsequent-day group (albeit a very small number of patients; 12 underwent a third aspiration). Although these small numbers do not allow for meaningful comparison, it may be that patients who had a third collection aspirated over several days had chronic sepsis, which prompted repeat imaging and subsequent aspiration; the group undergoing a third aspiration on the same day had the third collection drained simply because it was present. Aspiration of fourth and fifth collections rarely provided new microbiologic information.

Patients with multiple or recurrent abscesses have been shown to have a greater mortality (6), and care must be taken to examine these patients for underlying anatomic defects (eg, fistula) that prevent resolution of the infected collection (1). Our study findings have demonstrated that these patients' complex conditions do need to be approached aggressively from the standpoint of aspirating multiple collections, as therapeutically important differences in microorganisms may be missed by aspirating fluid for culture only from a dominant collection. Indeed, untreated pathogens within unsampled fluid collections may contribute to the increased mortality seen in patients with multiple abscesses.

We also found that sterile collections frequently coexist with infected collections and that microorganisms requiring different therapy may be present in adjacent collections. For this reason, we advocate meticulous maintenance of separate sterile fields to prevent cross-contamination when aspirating or draining multiple collections at the same sitting. Most important, cross-contamination of deep tissues can, in theory, lead to the creation of a new abscess in a previously sterile collection. In addition, cross-contamination of samples sent for laboratory testing can lead to an inability to relate microbiologic results to a specific drainage site, which has implications for catheter management in terms of knowing whether an infected or sterile collection is being drained. Creation of a separate sterile field and use of separate sterile equipment does necessitate higher expense (for fresh sterile packs, guide wires, and dilators) and slightly longer procedure times.

We did not categorize collections by anatomic location or by complicating clinical features (fistula, compromised immune status, etc). These factors are of great importance in general management and prognosis and have been addressed in previous studies (1,9,10) but are not relevant to the purpose of this study.

Previous authors (3) have discussed the importance of adequately draining all foci of infection, as this follows the surgical axiom for achieving cure. Our findings complement this axiom. We are not aware of an analysis of microbiologic results in a similarly large study group. Our study was retrospective and was limited by the fact that data were incomplete for several patients ($n = 16$) with multiple collections aspirated and drained over the study time who were thus excluded from analysis. However, our results provide microbiologic support for the practice believed by the surgeons and radiologists in our institution to be correct; that is, aspiration of all collections in the patient who may have sepsis by using separate sterile procedures.

Initial surgery and radiology articles (2,11,12) suggested strict criteria for selecting patients for percutaneous drainage. These criteria specified that the collection should be unilocular and not associated with a fistula or communication, that there should be a clear access route, and that there should be surgical backup available. In the ensuing 15 or more years, these criteria have been abandoned, and percutaneous drainage is now considered to be the most appropriate initial treatment for almost all infected fluid collections, including those in critically ill patients in whom percutaneous drainage allows temporization prior to surgical treatment, if necessary (13). In light of the ever-increasing indication for percutaneous aspiration and drainage of fluid collections and the increasing complexity of diseases so managed, it is very important to consider microbiologic information in the decision-making process with regard to interventional procedures, not just in relation to antimicrobial therapy.

We conclude that all intraabdominal fluid collections should be aspirated to optimize selection of antimicrobial therapy. In addition, a rigorous separate sterile technique should be employed for each aspiration to prevent cross-contamination and the creation of a new abscess.

References

1. Lambiase RE, Deyoe L, Cronan JJ, Dorfman GS. Percutaneous drainage of 335 consecutive abscesses: results of primary drainage with 1-year follow-up. Radiology 1992; 184:167–179.
2. Aeder MI, Wellman JL, Haaga JR, Hau T. Role of surgical and percutaneous drainage in the treatment of abdominal abscesses. Arch Surg 1983; 118:273–280.
3. vanSonnenberg E, D'Agostino HB, Casola G, Halasz NA, Sanchez RB, Goodacre BW. Percutaneous abscess drainage: current concepts. Radiology 1991; 181:617–626.
4. Brolin RE, Leiman S, Greco RS. Percutaneous catheter versus open surgical drainage in the treatment of abdominal abscesses. Am Surg 1984; 50:102–108.
5. Pruett TL, Simmons RL. Status of percutaneous catheter drainage of abscesses. Surg Clin North Am 1988; 68:89–105.
6. Fry DE, Garrison RN, Heitsch RC, Calhoun K, Polk HC. Determinants of death in patients with intraabdominal abscess. Surgery 1980; 88:517–523.
7. Lahorra JM, Haaga JR, Stellato T, Flanigan T, Graham R. Safety of intracavitary urokinase with percutaneous abscess drainage. AJR 1993; 160:171–174.
8. Alttemeir WA, Culbertson WR, Fullen WD, et al. Intra-abdominal abscesses. Am J Surg 1973; 125:70–79.
9. Saini S, Kellum JM, O'Leary MP, et al. Improved localization and survival in patients with intra-abdominal abscesses. Am J Surg 1983; 145:136–142.
10. Levison MA. Percutaneous versus open operative drainage of intra-abdominal abscesses. Infect Dis Clin North Am 1992; 6:525–544.
11. Gerzof SG, Robbins AH, Johnson WC, Birkett DH, Nasbeth DC. Percutaneous catheter drainage of abdominal abscesses: a five year experience. N Engl J Med 1981; 305:637–641.
12. Haaga JR, Weinstein AJ. CT-guided percutaneous aspiration and drainage of abscesses. AJR 1980; 135:1187–1194.
13. vanSonnenberg E, Wing VW, Casola G, et al. Temporizing effect of percutaneous drainage of complicated abscesses in critically ill patients. AJR 1984; 142:821–826.

CT Fluoroscopy–guided Abdominal Interventions: Techniques, Results, and Radiation Exposure[1]

Stuart G. Silverman, MD
Kemal Tuncali, MD
Douglass F. Adams, MD
Richard D. Nawfel, MS
Kelly H. Zou, PhD
Philip F. Judy, PhD

Index terms:
Abdomen, interventional procedures, 70.126
Abscess, drainage, 70.1263
Biopsies, technology, 70.12119, 70.125
Computed tomography (CT), guidance, 70.12119, 70.125
Fluoroscopy, technology, 70.1261
Radiations, exposure to patients and personnel, 70.12119

Radiology 1999; 212:673–681

[1] From the Department of Radiology, Brigham and Women's Hospital, 75 Francis St, Boston, MA 02115 (S.G.S., K.T., D.F.A., R.D.N., K.H.Z., P.F.J.) and the Department of Health Care Policy, Harvard Medical School, Boston, Mass (K.H.Z.). From the 1998 RSNA scientific assembly. Received November 9, 1998; revision requested January 4, 1999; revision received February 12; accepted March 25. **Address reprint requests to** S.G.S. (e-mail: *silver@ulna.bwh.harvard.edu*).

PURPOSE: To evaluate the benefits of computed tomographic (CT) fluoroscopy–guided interventions and assess radiation exposures incurred with CT fluoroscopy.

MATERIALS AND METHODS: A 6-month period of use of CT fluoroscopy to guide abdominal biopsy procedures and catheter drainage was analyzed. Efficacy measures and needle placement and procedure room times were compared with those of the preceding 6 months during which conventional CT was used. CT fluoroscopic times and estimated radiation exposures were compared for two CT fluoroscopic methods.

RESULTS: The sensitivity and negative predictive values for biopsy procedures and the success rate for needle aspiration or catheter drainages for CT fluoroscopy—98%, 86%, and 100%, respectively—were not significantly different from those for conventional CT—95%, 80%, and 97%, respectively. Room time was not reduced significantly, but mean needle placement time for CT fluoroscopy (29 minutes; $n = 95$) was significantly lower than that for conventional CT (36 minutes; $n = 93$; $P < .005$). The mean patient dose index was 74 cGy. Limiting CT fluoroscopy to scanning the needle tip rather than scanning the entire needle pass significantly reduced the dose to the patient and the operator.

CONCLUSION: Although CT fluoroscopy is a useful targeting technique, significant radiation exposures may result. Therefore, radiologists need to be aware of different methods of CT fluoroscopic guidance and the factors that contribute to radiation exposure.

Computed tomography (CT) is commonly and successfully used for guiding percutaneous abdominal biopsy procedures and catheter drainage of fluid collections (1). However, compared with ultrasonography (US) and fluoroscopy, conventional (nonfluoroscopic) CT does not provide real-time guidance capability. Therefore, CT usually is associated with longer procedure times owing to the need to intermittently scan the region of interest each time needle or catheter location confirmation is required.

CT fluoroscopy was developed and reported on by Katada et al (2–7) and Kato et al (8,9). A slip-ring spiral (helical) CT scanner was modified by adding a high-speed array processor to increase the speed of image reconstruction. The system resulted in real-time reconstruction and display of CT images; it was possible to scan continuously and view a biopsy needle as it is advanced in real time on a display screen in the CT suite. Since its inception, CT fluoroscopy has been used to guide intracranial, chest, abdominal, and pelvic biopsy procedures and fluid collection drainage (2–17). While feasibility has been established, the benefits of CT fluoroscopy, particularly as compared with those of conventional CT, to our knowledge, have not been demonstrated. More important, the radiation exposure to patients and personnel incurred while conducting CT fluoroscopy during interventional procedures remains a concern.

CT fluoroscopy has the potential to improve the efficacy of CT-guided interventions, to reduce the time to place a needle into a lesion for performance of biopsy or drainage of fluid

Author contributions:
Guarantors of integrity of entire study, S.G.S., K.T.; study concepts, S.G.S., K.T., D.F.A, R.D.N., P.F.J.; study design, all authors; definition of intellectual content, all authors; literature research, S.G.S, K.T., R.D.N.; clinical studies, S.G.S, K.T., D.F.A.; data acquisition, K.T., R.D.N.; data analysis, K.T., R.D.N., K.H.Z.; statistical analysis, K.H.Z.; manuscript preparation, S.G.S., K.T., R.D.N.; manuscript editing and review, all authors

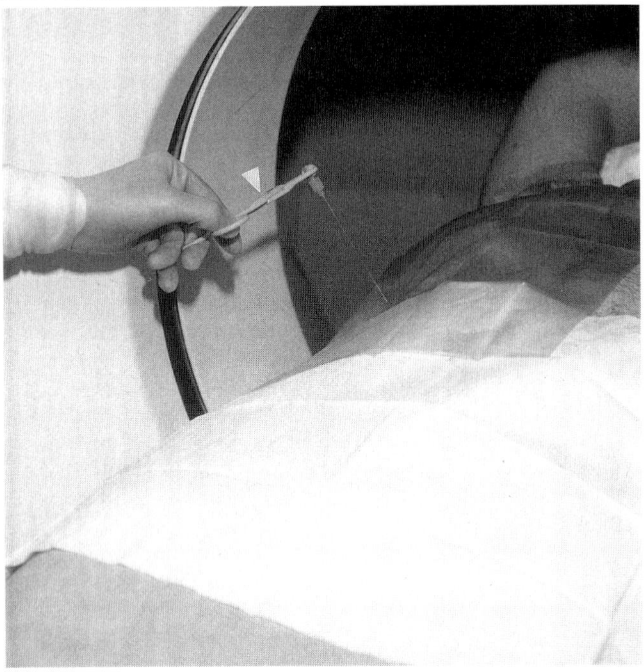

Figure 1. Photograph of needle holder used during CT fluoroscopy–guided abdominal intervention with use of the real-time method. A towel clamp (arrowhead) is affixed to the needle hub and can be used to direct a needle during real-time CT fluoroscopy such that the operator's hand is 10 cm from the primary x-ray beam.

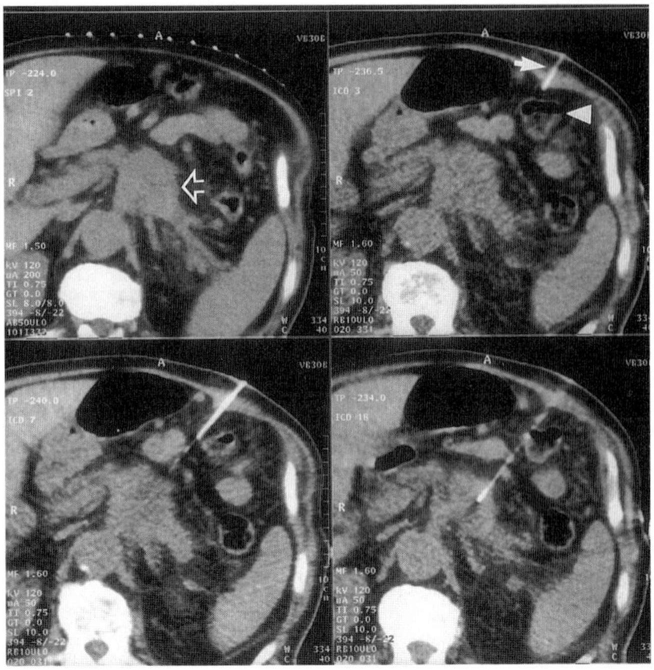

Figure 2. Images obtained during CT fluoroscopy–guided biopsy of pancreatic cancer (open arrow) with use of the real-time method. The initial nonfluoroscopic spiral CT scan (upper left) showed a bowel-free path to the target. When CT fluoroscopy began (upper right), the colon (arrowhead) was interposed between the needle (solid arrow) and the target. By using CT fluoroscopic guidance, the needle was placed to the right of the colon, and the colon was deflected to the left (lower left), which allowed the needle to be directed to the pancreatic mass without piercing the colon (lower right).

collections, and to reduce procedure times. We used a new CT fluoroscopic scanner to guide abdominal biopsy procedures and fluid collection drainage and evaluated whether using CT fluoroscopy would improve procedural efficacy and reduce procedural times compared with those of conventional CT. We assessed patient and personnel radiation exposures incurred with CT fluoroscopy and evaluated two CT fluoroscopic guidance methods.

MATERIALS AND METHODS

CT Fluoroscopic System

The system is a continuous rotation, fan-beam geometry CT unit modified by adding a high-speed array processor to increase image reconstruction speed and display images 3–6 frames per second (17). Images are displayed on an in-room monitor next to the CT table. Foot pedals alongside the CT table are used for controlling CT fluoroscopy and adjusting table position and height. The CT table can be moved in and out of the gantry during CT fluoroscopy by using a joystick anchored to the CT table. The components collectively are called "C.A.R.E.," or Combined Applications to Reduce Exposure, Vision CT, (Siemens Medical Systems, Forchheim, Germany). Reconstructed images are converted to standard television signals. A video recorder interface card connects a videocassette recorder for recording all of the images at CT fluoroscopy. The last image of the scan remains displayed on the monitor and is stored on the hard disk for photography.

Patients and Procedures

Of 143 cases referred for CT-guided interventions in the abdomen and pelvis during a 6-month period (August 15, 1997 to February 14, 1998), 107 procedures were performed with use of CT fluoroscopy. Conventional spiral CT was used in 36 procedures early in the study period mainly owing to unfamiliarity with the CT fluoroscopic system. Of the 107 procedures performed with use of CT fluoroscopy, 95 abdominal biopsy and needle or catheter drainage procedures (61 biopsies, 13 fluid aspirations, 21 catheter drainages) in 87 patients (43 women, 44 men; age range, 29–88 years; mean age, 55 years) were selected for study. Of the 107 procedures, 12 were excluded, seven owing to insufficient data and five because they were special procedures (celiac ganglion block, catheter manipulation, percutaneous gastrostomy), and our purpose was to study a homogeneous population of procedures.

All procedures were performed by both a staff abdominal radiologist and a fellow or resident. Radiologists and nurses wore protective lead aprons. All procedures began in the usual fashion with a spiral CT scan of the region of interest after a radiopaque surface grid was placed on the skin. This scan was used to plan the percutaneous approach to the lesion, and the skin was then marked. The operators then chose CT fluoroscopic parameters (ie, tube voltage, tube current, collimation) available on the scanner. The parameters available were the following: for 80 kVp, 75, 105, or 135 mA; for 120 kVp, 50, 70, or 90 mA; and for 140 kVp, 43, 60, or 77 mA. Available collimations were 1, 2, 3, 5, 8, and 10 mm. For all procedures, 6 frames per second was used. Images were acquired with a gantry rotation speed of 0.75 seconds per 360°. After sterile preparation, draping of the skin, and application of local anesthesia, the first needle,

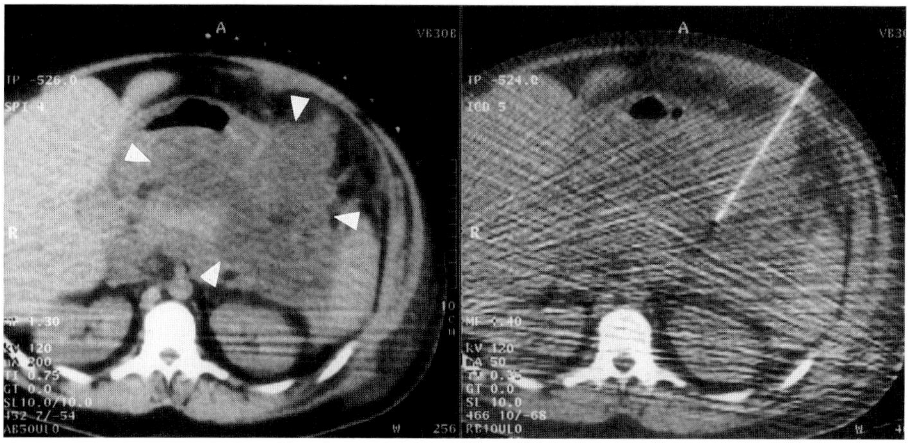

Figure 3. Images obtained during the performance of CT fluoroscopy–guided needle aspiration of a pancreatic fluid collection. Initial nonfluoroscopic spiral CT scan (left) showed a large superficial collection (arrowheads). By using the quick-check method, a 3-second scan (right) was used to visualize the needle tip (120 kVp, 50 mA, 10-mm collimation).

used as the guiding reference needle for subsequent needle or catheter placements, was placed by using one of two CT fluoroscopic guidance methods selected at the time of the procedure by the operator.

Real-time method.—The biopsy or aspiration needle was held by using a plastic clamp to keep the operator's hand approximately 10 cm outside of the primary beam (Fig 1). Needles were advanced during CT fluoroscopy. The radiologist stepped on the scanning foot pedal while adjusting the table position (and therefore the scanning plane) by using his or her free hand on the joystick to follow the needle tip. Once the needle tip was followed into the lesion, the foot pedal was released, and the last image was saved onto the hard disk and printed with other spiral CT images (Fig 2).

Quick-check method.—After the reference needle was placed by using the localizing spiral CT scan only as a guide, a short CT fluoroscopic examination was performed to locate the needle tip (Fig 3). As previously, the last image of the scan was printed. This technique also was used to confirm the position of a guide wire or a catheter. In all cases in which the quick-check method was used, only quick-check scans were used, but in some cases in which the real-time method was used quick-check scans were used in addition to real-time scans.

The group of 95 CT fluoroscopy–guided procedures performed during the study period were compared with the group of 94 conventional CT–guided abdominal and pelvic procedures (55 biopsies, 18 fluid aspirations, 21 catheter drainages) performed in 89 patients (46 women, 43 men; age range, 21–91 years; mean age, 57 years) during the prior 6 months by using a Somatom Plus S (Siemens Medical Systems). Of the 100 cases referred for CT-guided interventions during this period, six were excluded, five owing to insufficient data and one because it was a celiac ganglion block. Conventional CT–guided procedures, performed by a staff abdominal radiologist and a fellow or resident, also began with a localizing spiral CT scan with a surface-marking grid placed over the region of interest. Needles were placed in the conventional fashion by using the initial scan to plan the needle placement (18). Needle tip localizations were confirmed by using spiral CT scans obtained intermittently between needle manipulations (19).

Diagnostic test characteristics (sensitivity and negative predictive value of biopsy results, success rate of fluid collection drainage), mean needle placement times, mean CT procedure room times, and mean target sizes (ie, mass or fluid collection) were determined for both CT fluoroscopy– and conventional CT–guided groups. Needle placement time, defined as the time elapsed between the start of the initial localizing spiral CT scan and the start of the scan showing the needle tip in the target, was determined retrospectively by using images obtained during the procedure. Room time, representing the total time the patient was in the CT procedure room, was logged by CT technologists for all cases in each group. In addition to the procedure time, this time included monitor hookup and removal and in some cases, intravenous catheter placement. When a biopsy was performed, the time required for the cytopathology team to examine initial specimens for adequacy was included. Some fluid aspiration and drainage procedures included the time needed to obtain a Gram stain result. Catheter drainage procedures also included time spent securing the catheter to the skin site.

All patients provided written informed consent prior to entering the room. Statistical comparisons were performed by using two-sample Student *t* tests of the times described. Logarithmic transformation was used to offset skewed distributions in the data for procedure times and lesion sizes. Sex, mean patient age, and mean target size were compared.

For the 95 procedures in which CT fluoroscopy was used, total CT fluoroscopy times were obtained retrospectively. Per departmental policy, they were recorded by technologists for each case. The real-time method (ie, scanning that depicted the entire needle pass) was used in 75 procedures, and the quick-check method (ie, short scanning of the needle tip) was used in 20. Total CT fluoroscopy times represented the total time used during CT fluoroscopy for each procedure, and in some instances it consisted of several individual CT fluoroscopic scans. The two methods were compared by using two-sample Student *t* tests for their mean CT fluoroscopy times, and mean target sizes were compared by using a logarithmic transformation of the available data. The two methods also were compared with the data stratified according to target size, again by using Student *t* tests of logarithmically transformed data.

The CT parameters (ie, tube voltage, tube current, collimation) chosen by the operators during the 95 CT fluoroscopy–guided procedures were recorded. Assessments of patient doses were calculated by multiplying the CT fluoroscopy time for each procedure by the CT dose index rate in a 20-cm Plexiglas phantom for each technique used (20). This product was called the "patient dose index." If one wishes to imagine the patient dose index as a patient skin dose, it is the upper bound of the maximum skin dose to a patient of size comparable to the Plexiglas phantom. The upper bound means that the maximum skin dose to such a patient will not exceed the patient skin dose. The CT dose index was estimated at a 2-cm depth from the surface in the Plexiglas phantom by using a 10-cm pencil ionization chamber for a 10-second CT fluoroscopy time (20). The CT dose index rates were 3.1–13.8 mGy/sec.

The patient dose index values provide an overestimation of the patient skin dose because the same patient tissue is not always within the section thickness. The mean patient dose index for all procedures was calculated by averaging the patient dose index for each procedure. The mean patient dose indexes in the real-time and quick-check method groups also were compared by using a two-sample Student *t* test. The real-time and quick-check methods were compared for the frequency of use of different exposure techniques by using a Fisher exact test. A *P* value less than .05 was considered to indicate a statistically significant difference.

Estimates of personnel exposure at the level of the operator's hand and neck or body were obtained by multiplying the CT fluoroscopy times by the scatter exposure rates obtained from phantom measurements at 10 cm from the x-ray beam, as an approximation of the position of the operator's hand, and at 100 cm, as an approximation of the position of the operator's neck or body, by using 120 kVp, 50 mA, and 10-mm collimation (20). Estimates of exposure to the operator's hand were obtained by using only the cases (n = 39) in which the real-time method and 120 kVp, 50 mA, and 10-mm collimation were used, which were the parameters for which scatter rate phantom experiment data were available. This estimation of exposure to the hands was based on the assumption that the hands were at 10 cm, the approximate distance when holding the towel clamp attached to the needle, for the entire CT fluoroscopy time. Because quick-check scans were used in some of the real-time cases, this estimate is a maximum.

Hand exposures were not assessed for the cases in which only the quick-check method was used because the hands do not manipulate the needle during quick-check scanning. Estimates of exposure to the operator's neck or body were obtained for all cases in which 120 kVp, 50 mA, and a 10-mm section thickness were used (n = 49). Mean personnel exposure was calculated by averaging the estimates of personnel exposure per procedure.

RESULTS

For the group of patients undergoing procedures guided with CT fluoroscopy (n = 95), biopsy sensitivity was 98% (42 of 43), the negative predictive value of biopsy was 86% (six of seven), and the success rate of needle aspiration or catheter drainage was 100% (34 of 34). These results were not significantly different from those for procedures guided by conventional CT (n = 94), in which biopsy sensitivity was 95% (40 of 42), the negative predictive value of biopsy was 80% (eight of 10), and the success rate of needle aspiration or catheter drainages was 97% (38 of 39). All positive biopsy results (n = 82) were considered true-positive. The cases of false-negative results were proved by means of surgical biopsy results in one, repeat biopsy results in one, and 9 months of imaging follow-up in the other. True-negative results were verified by means of surgical biopsy results (n = 3) and imaging follow-up (n = 7; range, 4–19 months of follow-up).

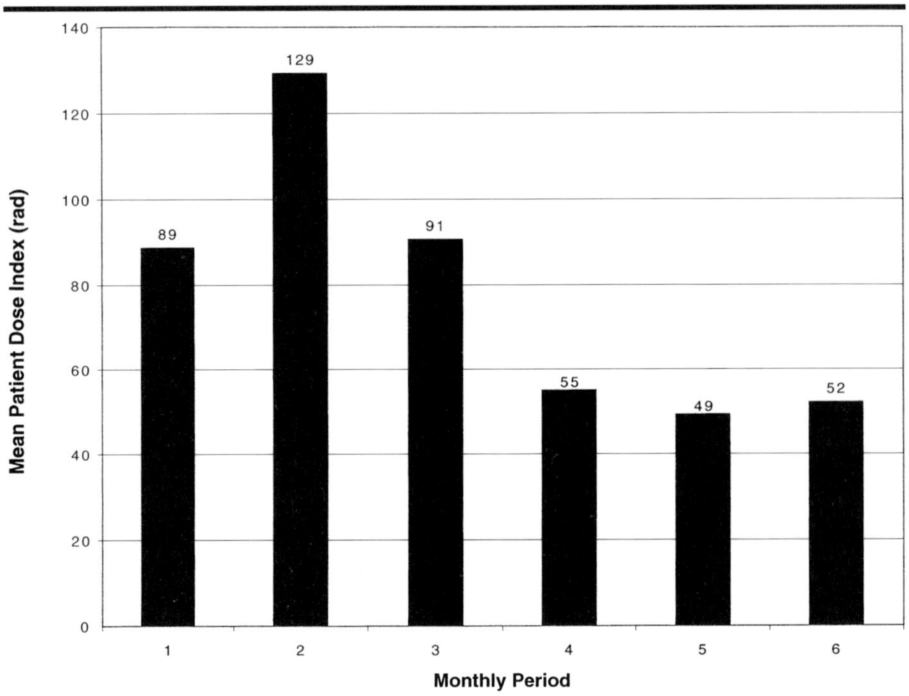

Figure 4. Graph shows that the mean patient doses for each of the 6 monthly periods decreased during the study. To convert rad to SI units (gray), divide by 100.

All aspirations and drainages were successful, except in one case in the conventional CT group in which the collection was considered inaccessible. There were three self-limited small hematomas in each group and one mild vasovagal reaction in the conventional CT group. There were no significant complications in either group. The mean needle placement time for CT fluoroscopy–guided procedures (29 minutes; standard error = 1.1; range, 6–67 minutes; n = 95) was significantly shorter than the mean needle placement time for conventional CT (36 minutes; standard error = 1.6; range, 17–100 minutes; n = 93; $P < .005$) and was independent of target size. The one case of an unsuccessful attempt at fluid aspiration by using conventional CT could not be analyzed for mean needle placement time or room time.

There was no significant difference in mean target size between CT fluoroscopy–guided (5.2 cm; standard error = 0.38; range, 1.2–15.0 cm; n = 95) and conventional CT–guided (6.0 cm; standard error = 0.28; range, 0.8–25.0 cm; n = 93) groups. The mean room time for CT fluoroscopy–guided procedures (87 minutes; standard error = 3.4; range, 31–260 minutes; n = 95) was not significantly different from the mean room time for procedures guided with conventional CT (90 minutes; standard error = 3.0; range, 48–190 minutes; n = 93). There was no significant difference in patient demographics (age, sex) between the two groups.

The overall mean CT fluoroscopy time was 79 seconds (range, 8–546 seconds). A CT fluoroscopy time of 546 seconds was used during a difficult procedure involving two catheter drainages and two needle aspirations of four separate fluid collections in the same patient. The mean CT fluoroscopy time was significantly shorter with use of the quick-check method (41 seconds; standard error = 7.4; n = 20) than with use of the real-time method (90 seconds; standard error = 12.2; n = 75; $P < .005$). The mean target size was significantly smaller in the latter group (4.9 cm; standard error = 0.3; range, 1.2–15.0 cm; n = 75 vs 6.1 cm; standard error = 0.5; range, 3.0–10.0 cm; n = 20; P = .02).

Stratified analysis indicated that radiologists chose real-time more often than quick-check when performing biopsies in masses smaller than 5 cm. Moreover, when biopsies were performed in masses smaller than 5 cm or collections smaller than 5 cm were drained, the mean size of the target when the real-time method was chosen (2.9 cm; standard error = 0.1; n = 40) was smaller than the mean target size when the quick-check method was chosen (3.8 cm; standard error = 0.2; n = 6; P = .02). In contrast, when targets 5 cm or larger were encountered, we did not find a significant difference in target size between the group in which the real-time method was used (7.3 cm; standard error = 0.4; n = 35) and the group in which the quick-check method was used (7.1 cm; standard error = 0.4; n = 14).

The most commonly chosen CT parameters, or tube voltage and tube current, were 120 kVp and 50 mA (n = 50), 120 kVp and 90 mA (n = 26), and 80 kVp and 135 mA (n = 10). In a minority of cases, 80 kVp and 75 mA (n = 4), 120 kVp and 70 mA (n = 3), 80 kVp and 105 mA (n = 1), and 140 kVp and 43 mA (n = 1) were used. Collimation was 10 mm for all but seven cases in which a 5-mm collimation was used. The mean patient dose index (n = 95) was 74 cGy (range, 3–494 cGy) and decreased during the 6-month study period (Fig 4). In the case with a resultant mean patient dose index of 494 cGy, 546 seconds of CT fluoroscopy time was used. There was an initial increase and then a modest monthly decrease in mean CT fluoroscopy times (Fig 5). There was a progressive decrease in the use of relatively higher CT parameters (eg, 120 kVp and 90 mA) and more frequent use of lower parameters (eg, 120 kVp and 50 mA) during the study period (Fig 6).

The mean patient dose index was lower in the group in which the quick-check method (30 cGy) was used compared with that in the group in which the real-time method (85 cGy) was used (P < .005). However, real-time and quick-check methods were significantly different for the frequency of use of different exposure parameters (P = .05). In particular, the relatively higher dose exposure parameter of 120 kVp and 90 mA was more likely to be used in cases in which the real-time method was used. The relatively lower dose parameters of 80 kVp and 75 mA or 80 kVp and 135 mA were more likely to be used with the quick-check method.

The estimated maximal mean personnel hand exposure was 78.6 µC/kg (305 mR) (n = 39) with use of the real-time method at 120 kVp, 50 mA, and 10-mm section thickness. Estimated maximal operator neck or body exposure for all cases with use of 120 kVp, 50 mA, and 10-mm collimation was 2.6 µC/kg (10 mR) (n = 49).

DISCUSSION

CT fluoroscopy represents a substantial technologic advance. Since the first CT-guided intervention, to our knowledge, was proposed in 1976 (21), viewing of the needle while it is advanced into the body was not possible until CT fluoroscopy was developed. However, benefits and the optimal use of this technology need to be determined, particularly with respect to the radiation exposure that results with CT fluoroscopy, and the more than 20-year excellent record with conventional CT.

Compared with results obtained with conventional CT, our study results show the successful use of CT fluoroscopy to guide abdominal biopsy procedures and drainage, but we could not demonstrate an increase in efficacy or a reduction in room time. Test characteristics of CT-guided biopsy and catheter drainage were so good that they were difficult to improve. Needle placement time was reduced, however. This is probably because CT fluoroscopy helped target more effectively. CT fluoroscopy likely helped avoid errors in targeting owing to patient movement or breathing.

The inability to reduce room time was in part because room time at our institution included many aspects of the procedure unrelated to needle placement, which was the only aspect of the procedure affected by this new technology. Although we were able to demonstrate a significantly shorter needle placement time with use of CT fluoroscopy, the reduction was only 7 minutes, and its effect on room time was lessened by the fact that our room times averaged approximately 90 minutes.

There are two major factors that contributed to the length of our room times. First, intraprocedural time was used to teach trainees. Second, cytologists rendered a preliminary interpretation of all biopsy results. This process added approximately 10–20 minutes.

Because the study was performed within weeks of the equipment's installation, there was probably a start-up or learning factor that prolonged needle placement time, as well as the entire procedure. It is possible that with more experience, needle placement time could be shortened further. Also, our needle placement time included acquisition of the initial localizing spiral CT scan. With CT fluoroscopy, targeting could have begun by placing the needle over the patient and scanning the region to determine the puncture site. This method may have resulted in shorter needle placement time but probably would have required more CT fluoroscopy and therefore more radiation exposure to personnel.

CT fluoroscopy has been reported to reduce procedure times (17). Although the absolute reduction in procedure time reported by others was similar to ours, it was considered significant because their definition of procedure time did not include the entire time the patient was in the procedure room (17). It is difficult to compare procedure times between studies because the definition of procedure time (eg, start time, end time, included components of the procedure) differs. Furthermore, procedure times are a result of numerous factors, including procedure type, level of difficulty of the procedure, operator experience, and whether and how much time is used to train residents and fellows.

Our study results demonstrated the potential for high dose. The mean patient dose index was 74 cGy. As a comparison, the CT dose index during two needle-tip localizing spiral abdominal CT scans (120 kVp, 240 mA, 10-mm collimation, pitch of 1, 6 seconds) would be approximately 6 cGy delivered to 6 cm of tissue. Our mean CT fluoroscopy time with use of the real-time method (90 seconds) is comparable to the scanning times reported by others (9,10,12,14,16). The patient dose during CT fluoroscopy could have been reduced with shorter CT fluoroscopy times and lower CT dose parameters (ie, lower tube voltage, lower tube current, and thinner collimation).

During our initial 6-month experience, the patient dose decreased progressively as the use of lower CT parameters was adopted (Figs 4, 6). We now believe that the lower CT parameters (80 kVp and 135 mA) would be qualitatively satisfactory in most upper abdominal cases in which the arms can be raised cephalad to the imaging plane (Fig 7). The higher CT parameters of 120 kVp and 50 mA would be satisfactory in the remainder of cases

(Fig 8). Currently, when a tube voltage of 120 kVp is used, we no longer use tube currents of 70 and 90 mA; we begin by using settings of 80 kVp and 135 mA, and sometimes lower, and a tube voltage of 120 kVp and a tube current of 50 mA only when necessary. Thinner collimation may be used if the increased noise that results from thinner sections does not prevent the ability to target the lesion.

Our study results demonstrated that our personnel likely received high exposures. The estimated mean personnel exposures per procedure at 10 cm for the hand and 100 cm for the neck or body of 78.6 µC/kg (305 mR) and 2.6 µC/kg (10 mR), respectively, are comparable with the personnel exposures reported during cardiac catheterization (22). At a maximal permissible dose of 500 mSv (50 rem) to the hands per year, 164 CT fluoroscopic procedures would be allowed. Similarly, at a maximal permissible dose of 50 mSv (5 rem) to the body per year, 481 procedures would be allowed.

There are ways to reduce radiation exposure to personnel by using needle holders that remove the hands from the beam. One such needle holder removes the hands 4 cm from the beam (9). In our method, we used a towel clamp that removed the hands approximately 10 cm from the beam. We found this method effective and inexpensive for holding and guiding the needle. However, there were times when the needle became dislodged from the clamp, and at other times it was difficult to exert sufficient inward force. Further research in needle holder development is warranted, with the goal of removing the hands as much as possible while maximizing tactile feedback and the ability to maneuver the needle (9,15).

Although we did not use it during the study, we currently are using a lead drape positioned over the patient immediately caudad to the cutaneous access site because it has been shown to reduce scatter exposure to personnel significantly (20). The patient radiation dose and potential exposure to the CT fluoroscopist that we report are considerably lower than those previously reported with use of the same model scanner (17). However, our phantom-derived dose rates are consistent with the manufacturer's specifications.

Our report describes two basic guidance methods of using CT fluoroscopy and their implications for radiation exposure. Others have used methods similar to our real-time method (2–17). Because of the possibility of high radiation exposures when using CT fluoroscopy to either continuously or intermittently view an advancing needle, we developed and evaluated the quick-check method to reduce radiation exposure. The quick-check method, which uses less CT fluoroscopy time, used less radiation than the real-time method but was used in slightly

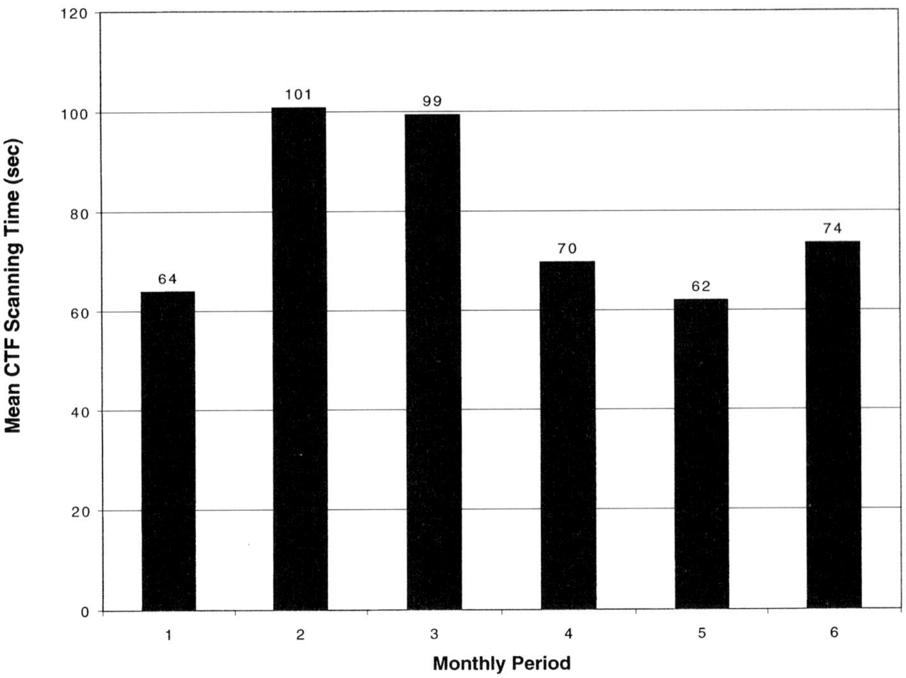

Figure 5. Graph shows that the mean CT fluoroscopy times for each of the 6 monthly periods decreased only slightly after an initial increase. *CTF* = CT fluoroscopy.

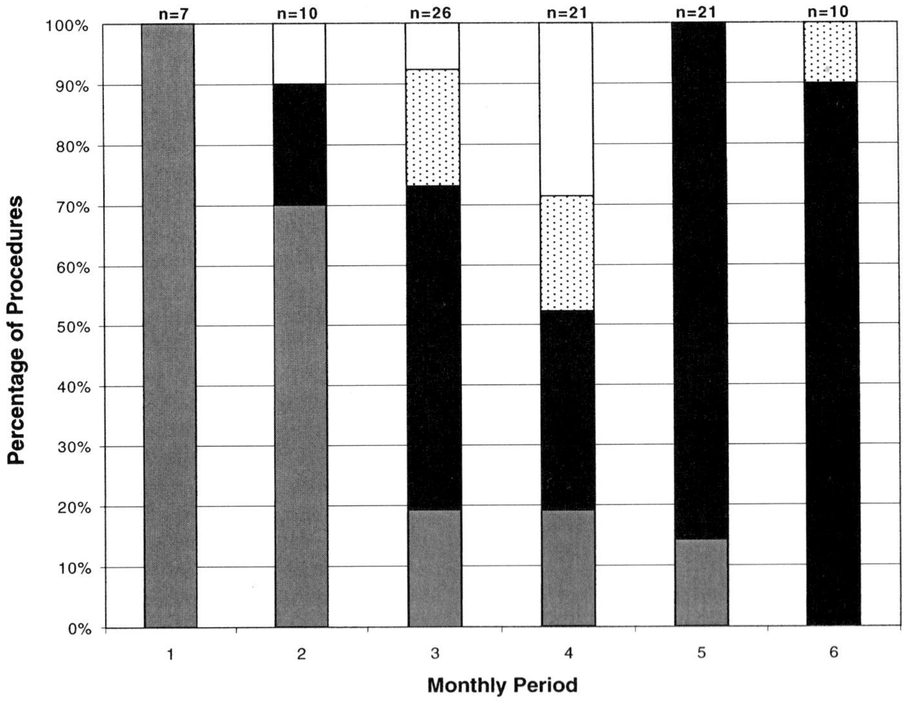

Figure 6. Graph demonstrates the relative distribution of chosen CT parameters for each of the 6 monthly periods and shows the gradual decrease in the use of the higher dose parameter of 120 kVp and 90 mA and the increase in the use of the relatively lower dose parameter of 120 kVp and 50 mA. Black bar = 120 kVp and 50 mA, dotted bar = 80 kVp and 135 mA, gray bar = 120 kVp and 90 mA, and white bar = 80 kVp and 75 mA, 80 kVp and 105 mA, 120 kVp and 70 mA, and 140 kVp and 43 mA.

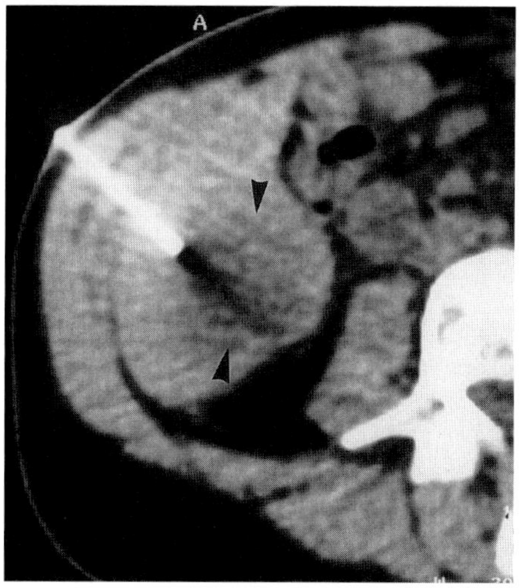

Figure 7. Image obtained during CT fluoroscopy–guided biopsy of a liver metastasis with use of the quick-check method. The liver lesion (arrowheads) is visualized well enough to be targeted with use of 80 kVp, 135 mA, and 5-mm collimation.

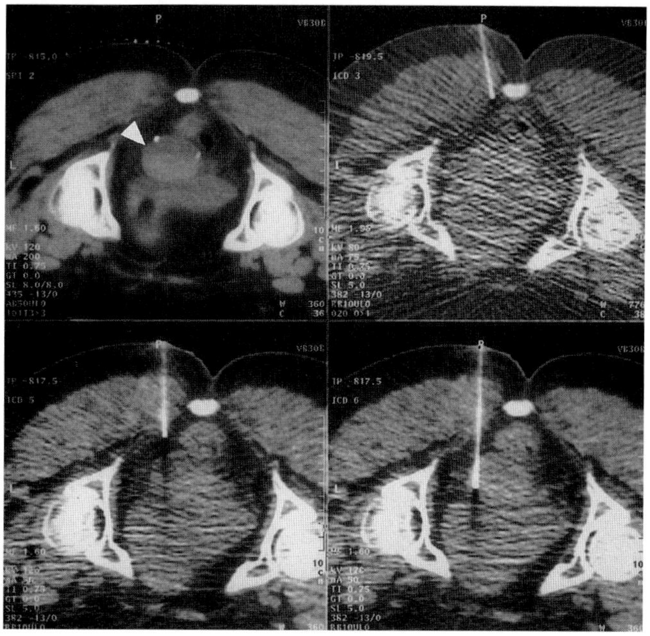

Figure 8. Images obtained during CT fluoroscopy–guided needle aspiration of a pelvic hematoma. Initial nonfluoroscopic spiral CT scan (upper left) shows the hematoma (arrowhead) well. However, with use of CT fluoroscopy, the artifact of the pelvic bones prevented adequate visualization of the target at 80 kVp, 75 mA, and 5-mm collimation (upper right). The lesion was targeted successfully with 120 kVp, 50 mA, and 5-mm collimation (lower left and lower right).

larger targets. Another factor contributing to the lower mean dose in the quick-check group may be that the relatively lower dose exposure parameters of 80 kVp and 75 mA or 80 kVp and 135 mA were more likely to be used with this method, and the higher dose parameters of 120 kVp and 90 mA were more likely to be used with the real-time method. Radiologists may have preferred the parameters of 120 kVp and 90 mA when using the real-time method because the lesions were smaller in this group.

The same targeting methods are used with the quick-check method as with conventional CT, but needle-tip location can be more easily and quickly checked with a short CT fluoroscopic scan and the in-room monitor (Fig 3). Large targets also afford the use of lower CT dose parameters because, given a fixed target-to-background contrast-to-noise ratio, they are easier to visualize. It is possible in some cases to use the quick-check method to view the position of a drainage catheter with the stiffening cannula in place when entering anteriorly, or posteriorly in a patient in the prone position (Fig 9). This is not possible with many CT systems, as there is not enough space to fit the catheter in the gantry, particularly with side entries. The quick-check method can be used to image the catheter after the stiffening cannula has been removed and during catheter placement with use of the Seldinger technique (Fig 10).

We found the real-time method advantageous for small or deep targets because the operator can view the needle insertion throughout and make adjustments en route to redirect toward the target or to avoid intervening structures (Fig 2). We preferred this method when targeting small (less than 5 cm) targets. We also found the real-time technique helpful in cases in which an out-of-plane, angled approach to the lesion was required. When the needle is angled, the tip may be followed by using the joystick to position the table, and therefore the scanning plane, at the tip and move the table to follow the tip as it is advanced. In addition, the gantry may be angled during CT fluoroscopy. As expected with the real-time method, however, longer CT fluoroscopy times (mean, 90 seconds), or a mean patient dose of 85 cGy and a mean personnel hand exposure as high as 78.6 μC/kg (305 mR), were used. The long CT fluoroscopy times were likely due to more difficult cases. Therefore, the cost of using the real-time method was significantly higher radiation exposure to both patients and personnel.

Our patient dose index and personnel exposure values are reference doses, that is, they represent maximal values and provide a basis for comparisons between devices or protocols. The actual patient doses were lower because the CT fluoroscopic table is moved about the needle, and therefore CT fluoroscopy did not occur always at the same location. The case in which the highest mean patient dose index was estimated is an overestimation because four different body regions were scanned. We have no information regarding patient location during CT fluoroscopy and could not estimate the magnitude of dose reduction. More accurate estimates of patient dose could be provided by obtaining a record of patient locations during CT fluoroscopy or by estimating skin exposures by using thermoluminescent dosimetry, or TLD, measurements. To further evaluate personnel exposure, we now wear ring radiation badges from which we can measure radiation exposure.

To optimize the use of CT fluoroscopy for this initial evaluation, we chose conservative estimates of patient dose and personnel exposure. Also, as noted earlier, our study was conducted soon after the arrival of the equipment. These factors would tend to increase CT fluoroscopy times, and hence radiation exposures, and room times. The learning curve associated with new technology also likely affected the choice of CT dose parameters during the procedures, with higher doses used more often initially.

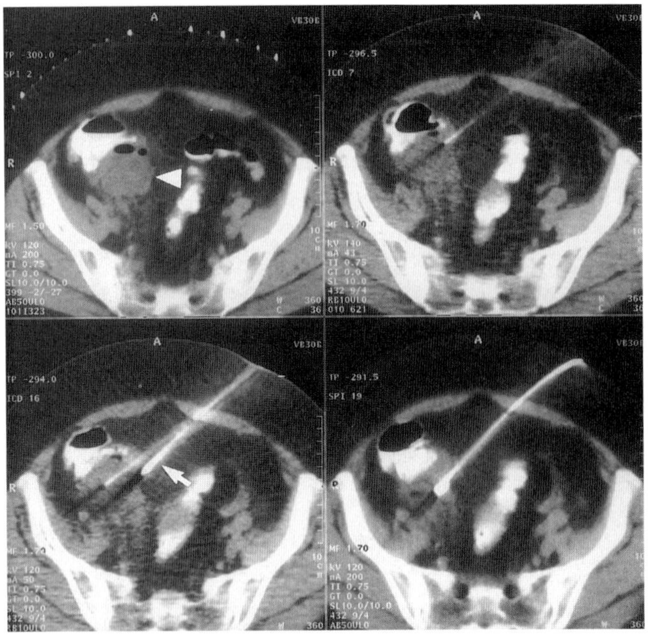

Figure 9. Images obtained during CT fluoroscopy–guided catheter drainage of a pelvic abscess with use of the trocar technique. Initial nonfluoroscopic spiral CT scan (upper left) shows the abscess (arrowhead). With use of CT fluoroscopy, the real-time method (upper right) was used to place the needle, and the quick-check method (lower left) was used to image the catheter (arrow) with the stiffening cannula. Spiral CT scan (lower right) shows complete drainage of the collection.

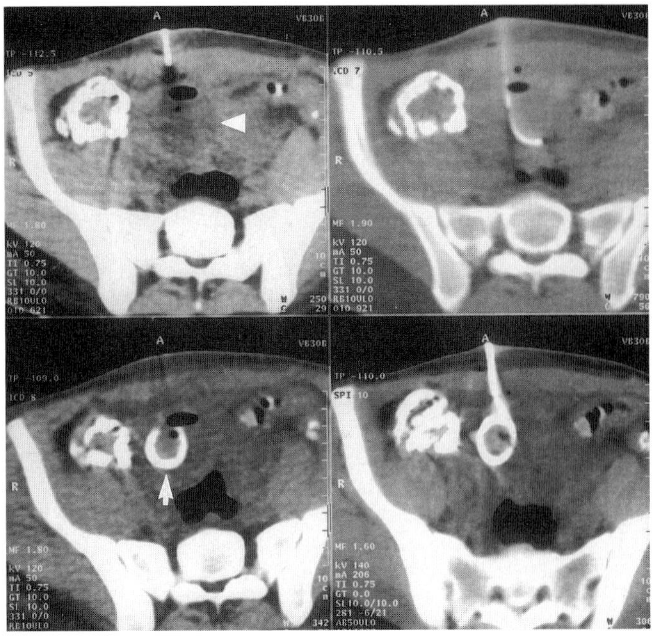

Figure 10. Images obtained during CT fluoroscopy–guided catheter drainage of an abscess with use of the Seldinger technique. The quick-check method was used to direct the needle into the abscess (arrowhead; upper left) and confirm appropriate needle, guide wire (upper right, shown with a wider window setting), and catheter (arrow; lower left position). Spiral CT scan (lower right) documents complete drainage.

The comparison of the quick-check and real-time methods may have been affected by selection bias. Radiologists chose the real-time method when targeting small masses, as shown by results of statistical comparison of lesion sizes in both groups, and they probably chose the real-time method when performing technically difficult procedures. These factors tended to increase CT fluoroscopy times in the real-time group.

In conclusion, use of CT fluoroscopy reduced the time required to target abdominal masses and fluid collections. While it did not reduce the CT procedure room time or improve the already high efficacy of conventional CT–guided biopsy, it has been embraced enthusiastically by our interventional team because of its ease of use and because it facilitates the performance of difficult abdominal interventions. Although CT fluoroscopy is a useful targeting technique, because significant radiation exposures may result, radiologists need to be aware of different methods of CT fluoroscopic guidance and the factors that contribute to radiation exposure.

Because radiation exposures to both patient and personnel were high in our study, we now recommend use of CT fluoroscopy in selected cases and use of the quick-check method whenever possible. However, the real-time method is a useful way to target small or deep targets. In this case, the lowest possible CT parameters necessary to view the target should be used. A comprehensive educational program of the potentially high patient and personnel exposures should be implemented to teach radiologists, nurses, and technologists. Use of lead drapes on the patient (20) or needle holders (9,15) and development of ways to reduce radiation exposure at the time of image acquisition (23) are warranted.

Acknowledgments: The authors thank Claudia Scherf and John Sandstrom of Siemens Medical Systems for their editorial assistance and Susan McLaughlin for manuscript preparation.

References

1. Mueller PR, vanSonnenberg E. Interventional radiology in the chest and abdomen. N Engl J Med 1990; 322:1364–1374.
2. Katada K, Anno H, Koga S, et al. Initial trial with CT fluoroscopy (abstr). Radiology 1994; 190(P):662.
3. Katada K, Anno H, Ogura Y, et al. Early clinical experience with real-time CT fluoroscopy (abstr). Radiology 1994; 193(P):339.
4. Katada K, Anno H, Takeshita G, et al. Development of real-time CT fluoroscopy. Nippon Acta Radiol 1994; 54:1172–1174.
5. Katada K, Anno H, Ogura Y, et al. Development and early trials of real-time CT fluoroscopy. Neuroradiology 1995; 37(suppl): 587–588.
6. Katada K, Anno H, Ogura Y, Koga S, Nonomura K, Kanno T. Puncture and drainage of intracranial lesions with CT: fluoroscopic guidance (abstr). Radiology 1995; 197(P):494.
7. Katada K, Kato R, Anno H, et al. Guidance with real-time CT fluoroscopy: early clinical experience. Radiology 1996; 200:851–856.
8. Kato R, Katada K, Anno H, Ida Y, Suetsugu S, Koga S. Transthoracic needle biopsy with real-time CT fluoroscopy (abstr). Radiology 1995; 197(P):529.
9. Kato R, Katada K, Anno H. Radiation dosimetry at CT fluoroscopy: physician's hand dose and development of needle holders. Radiology 1996; 201:576–578.
10. Daly BD, Krebs TL, Wong-You-Cheong JJ, Hastings GS, Pais SO. Therapeutic percutaneous interventional procedures of the gastrointestinal tract guided by continuous CT fluoroscopy (abstr). Radiology 1997; 205(P):374.
11. Seibel RM, Sehnert C, Plassmann J, Schmidt AM. First 318 interventional procedures with real-time CT (abstr). Radiology 1997; 205(P):383.
12. Gianfelice D, Lepanto L. CT-fluoroscopy: an important technological development facilitating CT-guided interventional procedures (abstr). AJR 1998; 170(suppl):80.
13. White CS, Templeton PA, Hasday JD. CT-assisted transbronchial needle aspiration:

usefulness of CT fluoroscopy. AJR 1998; 169:393–394.
14. Meyer CA, White CS, Wu J, Futterer SF, Templeton PA. Real time CT fluoroscopy: usefulness in thoracic drainage. AJR 1998; 171:1097–1101.
15. Mori M, Nitta N, Murata K, Sakamoto T, Morita R. A newly-developed equipment for biopsy under CT fluoroscopy (abstr). AJR 1998; 170(suppl):128.
16. Sonin AH, Penrod B, Owens-Brown E. CT-fluoroscopic guidance of sacroiliac joint injection (abstr). AJR 1998; 170(suppl):38.
17. Froelich JJ, Saar B, Hoppe M, et al. Real-time CT-fluoroscopy for guidance of percutaneous drainage procedures. JVIR 1998; 9:735–740.
18. Gazelle GS, Haaga JR. Guided percutaneous biopsy of intraabdominal lesions. AJR 1989; 153:929–935.
19. Silverman SG, Bloom DA, Seltzer SE, Tempany CM, Adams DF. Needle-tip localization during CT-guided abdominal biopsy: comparison of conventional and spiral CT. AJR 1992; 159:1095–1097.
20. Nawfel RD, Judy PF, Silverman SG, Hooton S, Tuncali K, Adams DF. Patient and personnel exposure during CT fluoroscopy (abstr). Med Phys 1998; 25:156.
21. Haaga JR, Alfidi RJ. Precise biopsy localization by computed tomography. Radiology 1976; 118:603–607.
22. Renaud L. A 5-y follow-up of the radiation exposure to in-room personnel during cardiac catheterization. Health Phys 1992; 62:10–15.
23. Kalender WA, Wolf H, Suess C, et al. Dose reduction in CT by anatomically adapted tube current modulation: experimental results and first patient studies (abstr). Radiology 1997; 205(P):471.

Primary Musculoskeletal Neoplasms: Effectiveness of Core-Needle Biopsy[1]

Lawrence Yao, MD
Scott D. Nelson, MD
Leanne L. Seeger, MD
Jeffrey J. Eckardt, MD
Frederick R. Eilber, MD

Index terms:
Biopsies, **.1261[2]
Desmoid, 49.3132
Lipoma and lipomatosis, **.31[2]
Liposarcoma, 40.371
Lung neoplasms, 60.31, 60.32, 60.33
Lymphoma, 60.34

Radiology 1999; 212:682–686

[1] From the Department of Radiology, Georgetown University Medical Center, MRI, 2nd Fl, CCC Bldg, 3800 Reservoir Rd, NW, Washington, DC 20007 (L.Y.) and the Departments of Pathology (S.D.N.), Radiological Sciences (L.L.S.), Orthopaedic Surgery (J.J.E.), and General Surgery (F.R.E.), UCLA Center for the Health Sciences University of California, Los Angeles. Received October 15, 1998; revision requested November 11; revision received December 15; accepted April 22, 1999. **Address reprint requests to** L.Y. (e-mail: *yaol@gunet.georgetown.edu*).

[2] **. Multiple body systems

PURPOSE: To analyze the effectiveness of core-needle biopsy for evaluation of possible primary musculoskeletal neoplasms, which often are evaluated with open biopsy.

MATERIALS AND METHODS: Core-needle biopsy was performed at a tertiary care institution in 141 patients suspected of having a mesenchymal neoplasm. In 85 patients, the lesion was in soft tissue; in 56 patients, the lesion was in bone. Eighty-nine patients had a malignant lesion, and 52 had a benign lesion. Twenty-eight patients had undergone previous surgery.

RESULTS: In 105 (74%) patients, core-needle biopsy results were concordant with results from specimens subsequently obtained at surgery with respect to tumor histologic features and grade, or they provided sufficient diagnostic information to obviate surgery. In 36 (26%) patients, inaccurate core-needle biopsy results were obtained: In nine, results were imprecise about exact histologic features; in three, results were correct about histologic features but incorrect about tumor grade. In 25 (18%) patients, open biopsy was performed after core-needle biopsy. The accuracy and rate of performance of open biopsy for soft-tissue lesions were not significantly different from those for bone lesions.

CONCLUSION: Percutaneous core-needle biopsy can be an effective alternative to open biopsy in the evaluation of possible mesenchymal neoplasms of either bone or soft tissue. Needle biopsy of such lesions, however, is best performed as part of a multidisciplinary team approach to tumor management.

In the management of mesenchymal tumors, treatment decisions and prognosis are dependent not only on a diagnosis of malignancy or benignity but also on the histologic features and grade of the tumor. Immunohistochemistry and, occasionally, ultrastructural studies may be necessary for specific diagnosis. Furthermore, these tumors often are spatially heterogeneous with respect to tumor grade and histologic features, and tumor necrosis may be widespread. For these reasons, the limited sampling that is possible at needle biopsy may be a source of problems or may limit confidence in diagnosis. Hence, patients with masses suspected to be primary neoplasms of the bone or soft tissue are often referred directly for open biopsy.

In contradistinction to fine-needle aspiration biopsy, larger-gauge percutaneous cutting-needle or core-needle biopsy yields solid specimens that are amenable to histologic analysis. In one series (1), core-needle biopsy of soft-tissue sarcoma was successful in allowing establishment of a histologically accurate diagnosis in 70% (42 of 60) of cases. The accuracy of core-needle biopsy in terms of correct histologic features in another combined series (2) of soft-tissue and bone tumors was 84% (52 of 62). Some authors (2,3) have suggested that core-needle biopsy may be more effective for evaluation of primary tumors of bone than for evaluation of tumors of the soft tissue. In one early series (4), however, the success rate of large-gauge trephine core biopsy of 16 primary bone tumors was only 44%.

In this study, we analyzed the effectiveness of imaging-guided core-needle biopsy of possible mesenchymal neoplasms of bone and soft tissue in patients examined at a tertiary care center specializing in orthopedic oncology.

Author contributions:
Guarantor of integrity of entire study, L.Y.; study concepts, L.Y., S.D.N., J.J.E., F.R.E.; study design, L.Y., S.D.N.; definition of intellectual content, L.Y.; literature research, L.Y.; clinical studies, all authors; data acquisition, L.Y., S.D.N., L.L.S.; data analysis, L.Y.; statistical analysis, L.Y.; manuscript preparation, L.Y.; manuscript editing, L.Y., S.D.N.; manuscript review, L.Y., S.D.N., L.L.S.

TABLE 1
Histologic Results in 56 Patients with Bone Lesion

Diagnosis	No. of Patients
Giant cell tumor	11
Osteosarcoma	10
Lymphoma	9
Plasmacytoma	4
Ewing tumor	3
Chondroblastoma	2
Chondrosarcoma	3
Metastasis	2
Osteomyelitis	2
Aneurysmal bone cyst	1
Enchondroma	1
Fibrous dysplasia	1
Fibrosarcoma	1
Hemangioma	1
High-grade undifferentiated sarcoma	1
Kaposi sarcoma	1
Malignant fibrous histiocytoma	1
Osteofibrous dysplasia	1
Paget sarcoma	1

TABLE 2
Histologic Results in 85 Patients with Soft-Tissue Lesion

Diagnosis	No. of Patients
Liposarcoma	20
Malignant fibrous histiocytoma	8
Lipoma or lipoma variant	6
Lymphoma	6
Desmoid	5
Hemangioma	5
Pigmented villonodular synovitis	4
Leiomyosarcoma	3
Metastatic carcinoma	3
Synovial sarcoma	3
Ganglion	2
Mesenchymal chondrosarcoma	2
Myositis ossificans	2
Myxoid chondrosarcoma	1
Elastofibroma dorsi	1
Extraskeletal Ewing tumor	1
Fat necrosis	1
Fibroma	1
Hemangioendothelioma	1
Angiosarcoma	1
Dermatofibrosarcoma protuberans	1
Lymphocele	1
Muscle injury	1
Myxoma	1
Neurofibroma	1
Neurofibrosarcoma	1
Osteosarcoma	1
Schwannoma	1
Treatment-related fibrosis	1

MATERIALS AND METHODS

This study included 141 patients (80 male and 61 female patients) who underwent percutaneous core-needle biopsy of a soft-tissue or bone lesion in whom the putative diagnosis was a mesenchymal neoplasm. Patients were excluded in whom the diagnosis prior to biopsy was metastatic carcinoma and who had a history of a known primary carcinoma with high metastatic potential or multifocal skeletal disease as demonstrated at bone scintigraphy. Also excluded were patients in whom the diagnosis was infection, which was determined on the basis of clinical, physical, and laboratory findings.

Patients were consecutively encountered during 6 years at a single tertiary care institution. The mean age of the patients was 44 years (range, 9–83 years). In 89 patients, the lesion was malignant; in 52, the lesion was benign. In 85 patients, the lesion arose in soft tissue; in 56, the lesion arose in bone. In 28 patients, the lesions had been previously resected, and these patients were suspected of having recurrent disease. The final histologic diagnoses are presented in Tables 1 and 2. The anatomic distribution of lesions is presented in Table 3.

One of two musculoskeletal radiologists (L.Y., L.L.S.) performed all needle biopsies after obtaining informed consent for the procedure from the patient. The biopsy approach was chosen after review of imaging studies obtained at outside institutions, which often included magnetic resonance (MR) images, and in consultation with the referring orthopedic oncologist, such that the biopsy track would not compromise the anticipated surgical approach to the lesion. All procedures were performed with administration of local anesthesia alone, without conscious sedation. In all but 19 patients, the biopsy was performed with computed tomographic (CT) or combined CT and fluoroscopic guidance (in a CT- and fluoroscopy-capable interventional radiology suite). Among the patients who underwent biopsy without CT guidance, the bone lesion in 13 was sampled with fluoroscopic guidance alone, the soft-tissue lesion in four was sampled with ultrasonographic guidance, and the superficial soft-tissue lesion in two was sampled without imaging guidance.

For soft-tissue lesions, three to eight biopsy specimens were routinely obtained by using an automated 14-gauge cutting needle (Quickcore, Cook, Bloomington, Ind; or Temno, Bauer Medical, Clearwater, Fla) or a 16-gauge suction-coring biopsy needle (Surecut; TSK Laboratory, Tochigi City, Japan). For lesions that were more than 1 cm below the surface of the skin, multiple biopsy samples were obtained through a single puncture site by using a 12-gauge blunt introducer (Hawkins; MD Tech, Gainesville, Fla) and a coaxial technique. For soft-tissue lesions suspected of being vascular in origin, a 17-gauge introducer (Cook or Bauer Medical) and an 18-gauge automated cutting needle (Cook or Bauer Medical) were used. For bone biopsies in which the cortex was intact, intralesional needle placement was facilitated with either a 12-gauge Ackerman needle (Cook) or a Craig vertebral body biopsy set (Baxter International, Deerfield, Ill) (which yields 3.5-mm-diameter core samples). Multiple samples were then obtained coaxially by using either a trephine (Ackerman needle, Cook; or Craig biopsy set, Baxter International) or a 14-gauge automated cutting needle (Cook or Bauer Medical), depending on the degree of lesion mineralization. Specimens were sent in buffered formalin and, in cases of possible lymphoma, saline solution for histologic analysis. Aspirates were not routinely sent for cytologic examination.

Follow-up data on study subjects were obtained by one of the authors (L.Y., S.D.N., L.L.S.) from the computerized hospital and radiology information systems, as well as from the weekly management conference notes of the multidisciplinary musculoskeletal oncology group. For each patient, tumor histologic features and tumor grade (high or low) were recorded for the percutaneous biopsy results and were compared with subsequent results from pathologic examination of surgical specimens. Examination of pathologic specimens was performed by one of two pathologists (including S.D.N.) experienced in musculoskeletal tumor analysis. The number of patients who required open biopsy after percutaneous biopsy was tabulated. In 30 patients, treatment decisions were made on the basis of percutaneous biopsy results, and no surgery was performed. The diagnoses in this group included lymphoma in 10 patients, plasmacytoma in four, metastasis in two, desmoid tumor in two, and other in 12.

On the basis of follow-up clinical and pathologic information, needle biopsy results were classified by consensus (L.Y., S.D.N.) as diagnostically accurate or inaccurate. Accurate needle biopsy results were in agreement with subsequent pathologic examination results of surgical specimens with respect to both tumor histologic features and grade, or they provided adequate information to indicate treatment without surgery. Clinical follow-up in untreated patients was 6–52 months. For purposes of determining accuracy, tumor grade was considered to be either high (grade II–III out of III) or low (grade I out of III). Inaccurate needle biopsy results differed from subsequent surgical pathologic results with regard to detection of malignancy, tumor grade, or specific histologic features.

Needle biopsy results were further classified as effective or ineffective. Effective needle biopsy results were accurate with respect to malignancy and grade but not necessarily with respect to exact histologic features and formed the basis for appropriate treatment decision making while obviating open biopsy. Any needle biopsy that was followed by open biopsy was classified as ineffective. Furthermore, any needle biopsy that resulted in incorrect histologic features that could potentially prompt inappropriate management was considered to be ineffective, even if no harm was actually done.

An analysis of the accuracy and effectiveness of needle biopsy results was performed according to patient subgroups, to examine possible determinants of effectiveness: soft-tissue versus skeletal origin, benign versus malignant lesion, and whether there was prior surgical treatment of the lesion. These differences in rates were tested by using the χ^2 statistic with continuity correction or, when appropriate, the Fisher exact test.

RESULTS

Accuracy of Needle Biopsy

According to the definition given in the Materials and Methods, the results of core-needle biopsy in 105 (74%) of 141 patients were accurate, and the results in 36 (26%) were inaccurate. The histologic diagnoses for patients in whom needle biopsy results were inaccurate are given in Table 4. In 36 patients with inaccurate biopsy results, adequate information regarding the benign or malignant nature of the lesion was obtained in nine, but the results were imprecise with regard to exact histologic features. In three of the 36 patients with inaccurate biopsy results, the findings were correct with regard to tumor histologic features but were incorrect with regard to tumor grade. If these findings are included as conditional true-positives, the accuracy for needle biopsy would be 83% (117 of 141). In only one patient did the biopsy yield results that were falsely positive for malignancy: a case of chronic osteomyelitis of the clavicle that was interpreted as possible lymphoma at both needle and open biopsy.

No infections resulted from needle biopsy. There also were no hematomas that required transfusion or evacuation or that altered subsequent surgical management.

TABLE 3
Lesion Location

Location	No. of Patients
Soft-tissue lesions	
Thigh	37
Forequarter*	15
Leg or foot	15
Buttock	10
Retroperitoneum	4
Pelvis	2
Chest	1
Neck	1
Bone lesions	
Lower extremity	26
Pelvis	13
Upper extremity	10
Spine or sacrum	6
Rib	1

* Forequarter is the upper extremity, including the scapula and shoulder girdle musculature.

Rate of Performance of Open Biopsy

Twenty-five (18%) patients underwent open biopsy after core-needle biopsy. In two of these patients, open biopsy was performed when the results of the needle biopsy were consistent with the final diagnosis but the level of confidence achieved with the material from needle biopsy was insufficient. One of these patients had an unusual parosteal lipoma of the ilium with associated cortical perforation and marrow edema; the other had a hemangioendothelioma of the calf that was thought to represent synovial sarcoma.

The results of open biopsy in four patients were concordant with the results of needle biopsy but were at variance with the final diagnoses after definitive surgical excision. These included the hemangioendothelioma of the leg mentioned in the preceding paragraph; a chondroblastic osteosarcoma of the sacrum, which was interpreted as a mesenchymal chondrosarcoma; an osteosarcoma of the femur, which was interpreted as aneurysmal bone cyst; and the chronic osteomyelitis of the clavicle mentioned earlier.

Open biopsy results in one patient were discordant with the final diagnosis with respect to tumor grade. A high-grade fibrosarcoma of the femur was interpreted as low grade at open biopsy, which was performed after the needle biopsy results were interpreted as indicative of benign histiocytoma.

Open biopsy results in two patients were inaccurate, although subsequent needle biopsy results were diagnostic: A sclerotic lesion of the ischium was inter-

TABLE 4
Final Diagnoses for 36 Inaccurate Biopsy Results

Diagnosis	No. of Patients
Histologic result	
Malignant fibrous histiocytoma	2
Osteosarcoma*	2
Chondroblastoma*	1
Chronic osteomyelitis*	1
Elastofibroma dorsi	1
Fibrosarcoma*	1
Hemangioendothelioma*	1
Hemangioma	1
Lipoma	1
Liposarcoma	1
Plantar fibroma	1
Synovial sarcoma	1
Grade	
Liposarcoma	2
Chondrosarcoma	1
Nondiagnostic biopsy result	
Non-Hodgkin lymphoma	3
Liposarcoma	2
Metastatic carcinoma	2
Malignant fibrous histiocytoma	2
Osteosarcoma	2
Pigmented villonodular synovitis	2
Ewing tumor	1
Ganglion	1
Giant cell tumor	1
Hemangioma	1
Mesenchymal chondrosarcoma	1
Paget sarcoma	1

* Open biopsy results also were inaccurate.

TABLE 5
Final Diagnoses for 25 Needle Biopsies Followed by Open Biopsy

Diagnosis	No. of Patients
Non-Hodgkin lymphoma	3
Malignant fibrous histiocytoma	3
Liposarcoma	2
Mesenchymal chondrosarcoma*	2
Metastatic carcinoma	2
Pigmented villonodular synovitis	2
Osteosarcoma*	2
Chondroblastoma*	1
Chronic osteomyelitis*	1
Fibrosarcoma*	1
Ganglion	1
Giant cell tumor	1
Hemangioendothelioma†	1
Hemangioma	1
Parosteal lipoma‡	1
Paget sarcoma	1

* Open biopsy results were inaccurate.
† Needle biopsy diagnosis proved to be accurate.
‡ Open biopsy results were inaccurate, but needle biopsy diagnosis proved to be accurate.

TABLE 6
Outcome of Needle Biopsy by Patient Subgroups

Subgroup	Accurate*	Effective*	Open Biopsy Performed	Total
Benign	39 (75)	43 (83)	8 (15)	52
Malignant	66 (74)	69 (78)	17 (19)	89
Prior surgery	20 (71)	22 (79)	4 (14)	28
No prior surgery	85 (75)	90 (80)	21 (19)	113
Bone lesion	41 (73)	42 (75)	12 (21)	56
Soft-tissue lesion	64 (75)	70 (82)	13 (15)	85
All cases	105 (75)	112 (79)	25 (18)	141

Note.—Number in parentheses is the percentage.
* Term defined in Materials and Methods.

TABLE 7
Distribution of Cases by Subgroups

Subgroup	Bone Lesion	Soft-Tissue Lesion	Total
Benign	20 (36)	32 (38)	52
Malignant	36 (64)	53 (62)	89
Prior surgery	8 (14)	20 (24)	28
No prior surgery	48 (86)	65 (76)	113
All cases	56	85	141

Note.—Number in parentheses is the percentage.

preted as Paget disease but proved to be B-cell lymphoma, and a recurrent liposarcoma of the proximal thigh was negative for malignancy at open biopsy but positive at CT-guided needle biopsy.

Given these seven diagnostic errors, the accuracy of open biopsy in this series was 72% (18 of 25). The histologic diagnoses for patients in whom open biopsy was performed are given in Table 5.

Effectiveness of Needle Biopsy

By using the definitions outlined in the Materials and Methods, where a needle biopsy followed by an open biopsy was considered to be ineffective regardless of the accuracy or results and where inaccurate needle biopsy results were considered to be effective if they were adequate to guide treatment, needle biopsy results were effective in 112 (79%) patients and ineffective in 29 (21%).

For the inaccurate biopsy results in 12 of 36 patients, treatment decisions were determined without performance of open biopsy. The effectiveness in these 12 patients was classified as follows: In nine patients, the results were classified as effective. In seven of these nine patients, needle biopsy results were correct with regard to malignancy, but there was a minor discordance with regard to specific histologic features. Appropriate excisions (of an angiolipoma and an elastofibroma) were performed in two of these seven patients, and appropriate wide resections were performed in the other five (lipoma-like liposarcoma, hemangioma of bone, high-grade liposarcoma, synovial sarcoma, and plantar fibroma). In two of the nine patients, there was concordance between biopsy results and histologic features but discordance with respect to tumor grade. In these patients, the treatment plan was unaltered: A large recurrent chondrosarcoma was diagnosed as low grade at needle biopsy but showed a focal grade II–III tumor after internal hemipelvectomy; a large, recurrent, fatty tumor of the thigh showed possible lipoma-like liposarcoma at needle biopsy, but, after wide resection, the final diagnosis was intermuscular lipoma with occasional atypical cells.

In three of the 12 patients who underwent needle biopsy but did not undergo subsequent open biopsy, the results were classified as ineffective. One patient had myxoid liposarcoma that was interpreted as low-grade myxoid liposarcoma at needle biopsy but showed focal grade II–III elements after wide excision; no chemotherapy was administered. A second patient had a large osteosarcoma of the pelvis and acetabulum, with osteoblastoma-like features at imaging. This lesion was misdiagnosed as osteoblastoma on the basis of needle biopsy results, and the patient underwent hemipelvectomy without preoperative chemotherapy. Finally, a third patient had a presumed recurrent Ewing tumor of the pelvis. This patient, who was in frail medical condition and was a poor surgical candidate, underwent palliative treatment with radiation therapy alone after nondiagnostic needle biopsy results were obtained.

Patient Subgroups

In the 56 patients with bone tumor, the results of core-needle biopsy were accurate in 41 (73%) and effective in 42 (75%). In the 85 patients with soft-tissue tumor, the results of core-needle biopsy were accurate in 64 (75%) and effective in 70 (82%). Open biopsy was performed in 12 (21%) patients after needle biopsy of bone tumor and in 13 (15%) after needle biopsy of soft-tissue tumor. There were no significant differences between soft-tissue and bone tumors in terms of accuracy (P = .94) and effectiveness (P = .40) of needle biopsy results and the rate of open biopsy (P = .48).

From the perspective of accuracy, effectiveness, and rate of performance of open biopsy, there were no significant differences between patients who did or did not undergo prior surgery (P = .87, $P >$ .99, and P = .78, respectively) or between benign and malignant lesions ($P >$ .99, P = .61, and P = .74, respectively). These results are summarized in Table 6.

Of the 28 patients who had undergone previous surgery, eight had a benign lesion, and 20 had a malignant lesion. The distribution according to subgroups (surgery vs no surgery, benign vs malignant) is given in Table 7. There were no significant associations between the site of tumor origin and the frequency of prior surgery (P = .26) or malignancy ($P >$ .99).

DISCUSSION

Our findings indicate that percutaneous core-needle biopsy results were highly effective for help in the diagnosis of masses suspected to be primary musculoskeletal neoplasms and appeared to be equally effective for evaluation of lesions of either bone or soft tissue. In our series, core biopsy results were accurate in 74% of patients and effective in 79%. This accuracy reflects concordance for both histologic features and tumor grade. The effectiveness of core-needle biopsy was not significantly different for benign versus malignant lesions or for recurrent versus nonrecurrent lesions.

These accuracies for core-needle biopsy are comparable to those of similar studies. In the multicenter survey by Mankin et al (5) of bone and soft-tissue tumors in patients referred to major treatment centers, the accuracy of core-needle biopsy was 69% (43 of 62). In the experience of Heslin et al (1), core-needle biopsy findings resulted in the correct histologic diagnosis in 70% (42 of 60) of soft-tissue masses. In a combined series of suspected mesenchymal tumors of soft tissue and bone reported by Skrzynski et al (2), the accuracy of core-needle biopsy results for correct histologic features and tumor grade was 77% (48 of 62).

Our results reflect the effectiveness of

core-needle biopsy in the setting of an integrated, multidisciplinary, musculoskeletal tumor practice. The contribution of such an approach to improved outcomes is supported by results reported in the literature (5). An appropriate biopsy approach should be consistent with the anticipated surgical approach to the lesion. There is a small but well-documented risk of seeding the biopsy track with tumor cells that can compromise the success of definitive treatment, and the biopsy track should optimally be included in any surgical resection.

If the confidence in a needle biopsy–based diagnosis is not sufficiently high to facilitate the often difficult management decisions posed in cases of suspected mesenchymal neoplasm, performance of open biopsy may be warranted even when the needle biopsy result is correct. For this reason, the effectiveness of percutaneous needle biopsy should account for the rate of subsequent open biopsy. Open biopsy after core-needle biopsy was necessary in 18% of the patients in our series. This rate was slightly but not significantly higher for tumors that involved bone, as compared with those that involved soft tissue (21% and 15%, respectively). This overall rate of the performance of open biopsy could be biased. Although the results of needle biopsy may obviate open biopsy, lingering uncertainty in diagnosis may prompt the evaluation of frozen sections during a subsequent excisional procedure. Such "conditional excisions" were not considered to be open biopsies in our analysis. These procedures usually constituted the definitive treatment for typically benign but clinically problematic masses, and needle biopsy was of assistance in treatment decision making in such cases.

According to the criteria we used for needle biopsy, the results of open biopsy had a surprisingly low accuracy (72%) in our series. Open biopsy, when used as a front-line diagnostic strategy, yields results with a reported (2) accuracy of 96% (48 of 50). This difference undoubtedly reflects selection bias, because only those patients with problematic or confusing needle biopsy results underwent open biopsy in our series. Nevertheless, an accuracy of 100% for open biopsy is likely too high in theoretic analyses of cost-effectiveness (6).

Some authors (2) have suggested that percutaneous needle biopsies are more effective for bone tumors than for soft-tissue tumors. The more specific manifestation of bone tumors on radiographs may narrow the differential diagnosis for the pathologist. However, MR imaging now provides greater specificity in the evaluation of soft-tissue masses prior to biopsy. From our perspective, technical factors probably are the most critical to the outcome of needle biopsy. Large-gauge core-needle biopsy, performed with a coaxial technique, of soft-tissue masses can yield a generous quantity of tissue quickly and with little morbidity. The ability to obtain multiple biopsy specimens is intrinsically more limited with bone lesions, especially those that are sclerotic, even when a large-gauge coaxial tool is used. An equivalent specimen yield may necessitate additional cortical approaches, something we routinely avoid to minimize procedure time and patient discomfort.

Although fine-needle aspiration biopsy of suspected bone metastases (6,7) yields accurate results and is cost-effective, the utility of cytologic diagnosis for primary mesenchymal tumors is more questionable. Published data are difficult to interpret, because studies often differ in their definitions of effectiveness. A diagnostic accuracy as high as 76% (51 of 67) has been reported (3) for the fine-needle aspiration biopsy diagnosis of primary bone tumor. In the same report, however, a large but unspecified proportion of fine-needle aspiration biopsies were followed by open surgical biopsies. Such needle biopsies would be considered ineffective according to our criteria. The diagnostic accuracy of fine-needle aspiration biopsy in another series (8) of 101 primary bone tumors was 61%, but the effective accuracy was 41%. In a series (9) of 117 soft-tissue tumors, fine-needle aspiration biopsy results were diagnostically adequate in 63%. However, in another series (10) of 52 sarcomas (46 soft-tissue and six bone lesions), fine-needle aspiration biopsy resulted in a correct histologic diagnosis in only 21% of cases. A prospective and paired analysis (11) of soft-tissue tumors confirmed a higher accuracy for core-needle biopsy results than for fine-needle aspiration biopsy results. Hence, as an evaluation method for possible primary musculoskeletal tumors, fine-needle aspiration biopsy might be cost-effective only if performed without imaging guidance, perhaps as part of the initial office examination.

In the evaluation of primary musculoskeletal neoplasms, the cost-benefit ratio of core-needle biopsy appears to be favorable (2,6). A needle biopsy can be performed expeditiously, and, in cases of a large mass, imaging guidance may not be essential (2). Our preference has been to use CT guidance. In conjunction with preprocedural MR imaging, CT facilitates appropriate sampling of heterogeneous lesions and helps select a trajectory that is safe and consistent with the anticipated surgical approach. With the confidence in approach and localization afforded by CT, large-gauge needle biopsy can be performed quickly and without the use of sedation, factors that further reduce costs.

In summary, our experience indicates that percutaneous core-needle biopsy is effective for the diagnostic evaluation of suspected primary musculoskeletal neoplasms, whether of bone or soft tissue. Open biopsy can be obviated in the majority of cases. Although percutaneous core-needle biopsy of a suspected primary musculoskeletal neoplasm is potentially safe, accurate, and cost-efficient, it is still less accurate and more demanding than needle biopsy of a suspected metastasis. Biopsy of a suspected primary musculoskeletal mass should be used judiciously and preferably as part of a multidisciplinary team approach to orthopedic tumor management.

Acknowledgments: We thank Cecilia Yap, BS, for her dedicated assistance in data collection and organization and Xin Li, MS, for his innovative integration of the computer information systems that were used in retrieval of patient data.

References

1. Heslin MJ, Lewis JJ, Woodruss JM, Brennan MF. Core needle biopsy for diagnosis of extremity soft tissue sarcoma. Ann Surg Oncol 1997; 4:425–431.
2. Skrzynski C, Biermann JS, Montag A, Simon MA. Diagnostic accuracy and charge-savings of outpatient core needle biopsy compared with open biopsy of musculoskeletal tumors. J Bone Joint Surg [Am] 1996; 78:644–649.
3. Kreichbergs A, Bauer HCF, Brosio O, Lindholm J, Skoog L, Soderlund V. Cytological diagnosis of bone tumors. J Bone Joint Surg [Br] 1996; 78:258–263.
4. Tehranzadeh J, Freiberger RH, Ghelman B. Closed skeletal needle biopsy: review of 120 cases. AJR 1983; 140:113–115.
5. Mankin HJ, Mankin CJ, Simon MA. The hazards of the biopsy, revisited: members of the Musculoskeletal Tumor Society. J Bone Joint Surg [Am] 1996; 78:656–663.
6. Fraser-Hill MA, Renfrew DL, Hilsenrath PE. Percutaneous needle biopsy of musculoskeletal lesions. II. Cost-effectiveness. AJR 1992; 158:813–818.
7. Fraser-Hill MA, Renfrew DL. Percutaneous needle biopsy of musculoskeletal lesions. I. Effective accuracy and diagnostic utility. AJR 1992; 158:809–812.
8. Layfield LJ, Armstrong K, Zaleski S, Eckardt J. Diagnostic accuracy and clinical utility of fine-needle aspiration cytology in the diagnosis of clinically primary bone lesions. Diagn Cytopathol 1993; 9:168–173.
9. Bennert KW, Abdul-Karim FW. Fine needle aspiration cytology versus needle core biopsy of soft tissue tumors: a comparison. Acta Cytol 1994; 38:381–384.
10. Costa MJ, Campman SC, Davis RL, Howell LP. Fine-needle aspiration cytology of sarcoma: retrospective review of diagnostic utility and specificity. Diagn Cytopathol 1996; 15:23–32.
11. Barth RJ Jr, Merino MJ, Solomon D, Yang JC, Baker AR. A prospective study of the value of core needle biopsy and fine needle aspiration in the diagnosis of soft tissue masses. Surgery 1992; 112:536–543.

Osteoid Osteoma: CT-guided Percutaneous Resection and Follow-up in 38 Patients[1]

Nicolas Sans, MD
Denise Galy-Fourcade, MD
Jacques Assoun, MD
Thierry Jarlaud, MD
Hélène Chiavassa, MD
Paul Bonnevialle, MD
Nadine Railhac, MD
Jacques Giron, MD
Hélène Morera-Maupomé, MD
Jean-Jacques Railhac, MD

Index terms:
Computed tomography (CT), guidance, 40.12119
Interventional procedures, 40.12119, 40.1267
Osteoma, 40.3122

Radiology 1999; 212:687–692

[1] From the Central Medical Imaging Service, Centre Hospitalier Universitaire Purpan, Place du Docteur Baylac, F-31059 Toulouse, France. Received July 21, 1998; revision requested August 13; final revision received December 3; accepted March 16, 1999. **Address reprint requests to** N.S. (e-mail: *sans.n@chu-toulouse.fr*).

Author contributions:
Guarantors of integrity of entire study, N.S., J.J.R.; study concepts, N.S., D.G.F., J.A., J.J.R., P.B., N.R.; study design, N.S., J.J.R.; definition of intellectual content, N.S., J.J.R.; literature research, N.S., J.J.R., T.J., H.C., J.G.; clinical studies, N.S., D.G.F., J.A., H.M.M., J.J.R.; experimental studies, N.S., H.M.M., J.J.R.; data acquisition, N.S., H.M.M., J.J.R.; data analysis, N.S.; manuscript preparation and editing, N.S., T.J., H.C., J.G.; manuscript review, N.S., J.G.

PURPOSE: To reevaluate at medium term the results of computed tomography (CT)-guided percutaneous resection of osteoid osteomas.

MATERIALS AND METHODS: Thirty-eight patients who had undergone treatment by means of this technique were reexamined with a mean follow-up of 3.7 years. The short- and medium-term clinical course and histologic features of the resection specimens were analyzed.

RESULTS: The bone fragment could be analyzed in all cases, and the diagnosis of osteoid osteoma was confirmed in 28 patients (74%). A different diagnosis was made in six patients: mucoid cyst, subchondral arthritic geode, fibrous dysplastic lesion, focal osteochondritis, or focal chronic osteomyelitis. Cure was obtained in 32 patients (84%), whatever the cause. Complications, generally minor and transient, were observed in nine patients (24%). The most severe complications were two femoral fractures and one focal chronic osteomyelitis due to *Staphylococcus aureus* infection.

CONCLUSION: The results of this study confirm the efficacy of percutaneous resection of osteoid osteomas and the possibility of using this method for successful treatment of other small bone lesions.

The treatment of osteoid osteomas long consisted of en bloc excision, which is damaging and disproportionate to the size of the lesion. Alternatives recently have been proposed that use computed tomographic (CT) guidance, in particular percutaneous excision, described by Voto et al (1) and Kohler et al (2) and developed since 1989 at our institution. Percutaneous resection of osteoid osteomas is a technique of interventional radiology that is becoming more commonly used. We report our experience with this technique in 38 patients to evaluate the medium-term outcome of this technique of percutaneous resection.

MATERIALS AND METHODS

Population

From March 1989 to December 1995, lesions suggestive of osteoid osteoma were resected percutaneously in 41 patients. The diagnosis was oriented by a range of clinical and radiologic features. The treatment option and decision were proposed to the patient after multidisciplinary discussions between surgeons and radiologists. The course was thus followed in 38 patients, three being lost to follow-up in the intervening period. The population in our study comprised nine women and 29 men (sex ratio, 3:2; mean age, 23.4 years; age range, 5–64 years). The lesions were located in the leg (n = 32), the arm (n = 2), the spine (n = 2), and the pelvic girdle (n = 2).

Methods

Resection technique.—Percutaneous resection (1–6) required coaxial instruments (Aesculap, Tuttlingen, Germany) comprising a guide wire, a trocar, an 11-mm-diameter external sheath, a toothed drill (7- or 10-mm diameter), and a 9-mm diameter drill (Figs 1, 2). Resection was performed in the CT room with sterile surgical conditions. The procedure

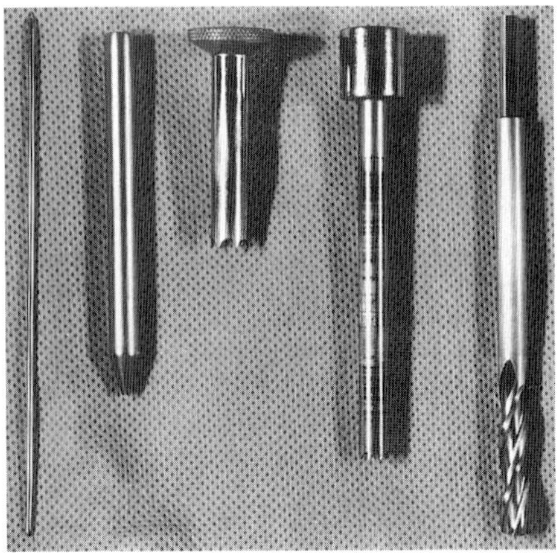

Figure 1. Photograph of the drill resection system shows (left to right) guide wire, trocar, 11-mm-diameter external sheath, 9-mm-diameter toothed drill, and 9-mm-diameter drill.

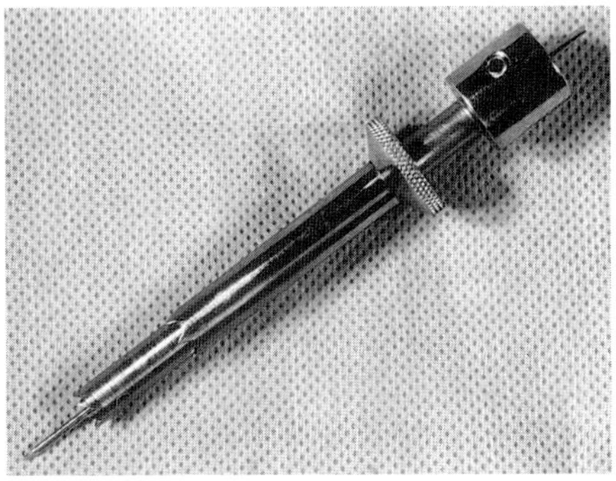

Figure 2. Photograph of the coaxial system assembled for resection.

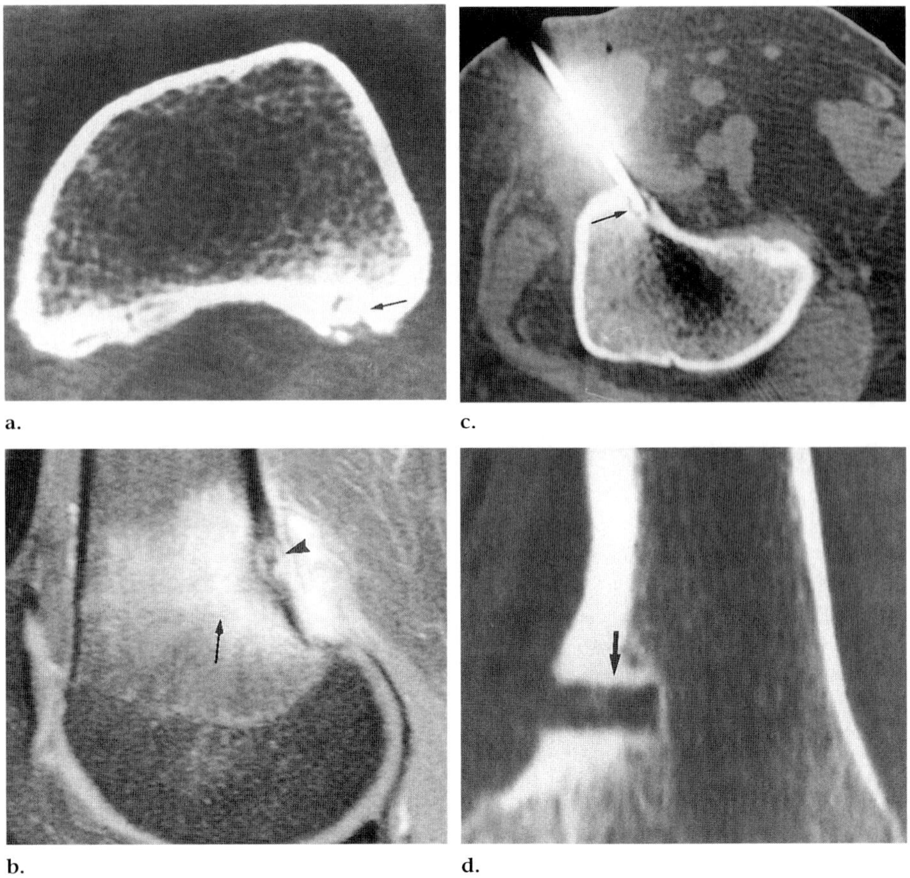

Figure 3. Images obtained in a 21-year-old woman. **(a)** Axial CT scan obtained with contiguous 2-mm sections demonstrates a typical 5-mm-diameter calcified nidus (arrow) of osteoid osteoma of the distal femur. **(b)** Sagittal T1-weighted fat-saturated magnetic resonance image (repetition time, 642 msec; echo time, 12 msec) with contrast enhancement shows localized enhancement and demonstrates the inflammatory reaction (arrow) near the osteoid osteoma (arrowhead). **(c)** Axial CT scan obtained with the patient in the prone position shows the guide wire being inserted into the nidus (arrow). **(d)** Postprocedural reformatted two-dimensional sagittal CT image shows complete excision (arrow) of the nidus.

was performed with local-regional (four cases) or general (34 cases) anesthesia. The latter made the procedure easier by lessening patient discomfort due to a prolonged period on the table and also ensured perfect immobility.

The lesion was localized by using 2-mm-thick contiguous sections (Fig 3a–3c) to plan the ballistic course. The lesion was then extracted by using the toothed drill or a Laredo trocar, a small trocar 3 mm in diameter, for smaller lesions. At the end of the procedure, additional scans were obtained to confirm complete or partial excision of the lesion. If excision was partial, a second drilling procedure could be attempted. In certain cases, curettage was performed to remove any residual nidus fragments.

Follow-up of the course.—Thirty-eight patients were examined by the radiologic and surgical teams during the first 6 months of 1997. All patients were examined after a minimal postoperative period of 1 year (mean follow-up, 3.7 years; range, 1.0–6.6 years). For each patient, retrospective and prospective data were collected, including the result of histologic examination of the resected specimen, the immediate postoperative and longer term clinical course, and any complications. Cure was evidenced by rapid and definitive disappearance of pain and in certain cases by means of follow-up radiographs or CT scans (Somatom Plus 4; Siemens, Erlangen, Germany) obtained with a delay of at least 1 year after the procedure. Informed consent was always obtained from the patients. No invasive procedure was performed subsequently.

RESULTS

Clinical Data

Clinical data for all the patients are provided in Table 1. In agreement with the data in the literature (1–3), the prevalence of osteoid osteoma was higher in the second and third decades of life. The initial presentation of the lesion generally was classic. Pain, greater at night, was present in 30 of 38 patients (79%) and responded well to acetylsalicylic acid in 25 patients (66%). The mean interval before diagnosis was about 1.6 years, with a minimum of 46 days and a maximum of 9 years.

Technique

Resection was performed with a toothed drill in 33 cases and with a Laredo trocar in three cases. In two cases, excision with a toothed drill was completed by means of curettage. Resection was considered radiologically complete (Fig 3d) in 31 cases (82%) and partial in seven (18%).

TABLE 1
Symptoms, Localization, and Clinical Course

Patient No./Age (y)/ Sex	Pain Accentuated at Night	Pain Relief with Acetylsalicylic Acid	Local Swelling	Local Inflammation	Restricted Motion	Muscle Atrophy	Localization	Histologic Finding*	Clinical Course*
1/23/M	Yes	Yes	No	No	No	No	Femur	Nidus found	R + S
2/65/F	Yes	No	Yes	No	No	No	Tibia	Benign fibromatous tumor	R
3/20/M	No	No	Yes	No	No	No	Tibia	Intraosseous mucoid cyst	Cure
4/16/M	Yes	No	No	No	No	No	Femur	Nidus found	Cure
5/15/M	Yes	Yes	No	No	No	No	Femur	Nidus found	Cure
6/12/F	No	No	Yes	Yes	No	No	Tibia	Intraosseous mucoid cyst	R
7/21/M	Yes	Yes	Yes	Yes	No	No	Talus	Nidus found	Cure
8/44/M	Yes	No	Yes	Yes	No	No	Tibia	Nidus found	Cure
9/22/M	No	No	No	No	No	No	Patella	Osteochondritis	Cure
10/19/F	No	Yes	No	No	No	No	Tibia	Nidus found	Cure
11/11/M	Yes	No	No	No	No	No	Femur	Nidus found	Cure
12/41/F	Yes	Yes	No	No	No	No	Femur	Nidus found	Cure
13/24/M	Yes	No	No	No	No	No	Iliac wing	Nidus not found	Cure
14/21/M	Yes	No	No	No	No	No	Femur	Nidus not found	Cure
15/32/M	Yes	Yes	No	No	Yes	No	Femur	Nidus found	Cure
16/20/M	Yes	No	No	No	No	No	Femur	Nidus found	Cure
17/24/F	No	No	No	Yes	No	No	Tibia	Nidus found	Cure
18/31/M	Yes	Yes	No	No	No	No	Femur	Nidus found	Cure
19/13/F	Yes	Yes	No	No	No	No	Femur	Nidus found	Cure
20/20/M	Yes	Yes	No	No	No	No	Femur	Nidus found	Cure
21/23/M	Yes	Yes	Yes	No	No	No	Femur	Nidus found	Cure
22/6/M	Yes	No	No	No	No	Yes	Tibia	Nidus not found	Cure
23/15/M	Yes	No	No	No	No	No	Tibia	Nidus found	Cure
24/24/F	No	No	Yes	No	No	No	S1	Nidus found	R + S
25/46/M	Yes	Yes	Yes	No	No	No	Femur	Osteomyelitis	Cure
26/49/F	No	No	No	No	Yes	No	Acetabulum	Degenerative geode	Cure
27/15/M	Yes	No	Yes	No	Yes	No	Femur	Nidus found	Cure
28/19/M	Yes	No	No	Yes	Yes	No	Femur	Nidus found	Cure
29/12/M	Yes	No	Yes	No	No	No	Tibia	Nidus not found	Cure
30/23/M	Yes	No	Yes	Yes	No	No	Femur	Nidus fragmented	Cure
31/25/M	Yes	No	Yes	No	No	Yes	Radius	Nidus found	Cure
32/22/M	Yes	No	Yes	No	No	No	Fibula	Nidus found	Cure
33/13/M	Yes	Yes	Yes	No	No	No	Tibia	Nidus found	Cure
34/37/M	Yes	Yes	No	No	No	No	Femur	Nidus fragmented	Cure
35/16/M	Yes	No	No	No	No	No	L2	Nidus found	R + 2
36/19/F	Yes	No	Yes	Yes	No	No	Tibia	Nidus fragmented	R + S
37/19/M	Yes	Yes	Yes	Yes	No	No	Tibia	Nidus found	Cure
38/13/M	No	No	No	Yes	Yes	No	Ulna	Nidus fragmented	Cure

* Patients with nidus found, not found, or fragmented had osteoid osteoma. R = recurrence, R + S = recurrence and surgery, R + 2 = recurrence and second resection.

Histology

The bone fragment sampled could be analyzed in all cases. If the nidus appeared fragmented, histologic confirmation of the diagnosis was certain or very probable in 28 cases (74%). Complete excision of the lesion was confirmed in 21 cases (55%). However, at histologic examination no nidus was found in the excised specimen in four cases (11%). In addition, at histologic analysis the diagnosis of osteoid osteoma was eliminated formally in six cases (16%), and a different type of bone involvement was revealed. These lesions were two intraosseous mucoid cysts, one subchondral geode of degenerative arthritic type, one benign fibromatous tumor, one focal osteochondritis, and one focal chronic osteomyelitis (Table 2).

Among patients who were cured, four distinct groups were defined at histopathologic analysis. In group 1, the nidus was present and complete. In group 2, the nidus was present, but it was not possible to conclude as to the totality of excision. In group 3, no lesion that appeared to be an osteoid osteoma was found. In group 4, histologic examination revealed a lesion of a different type.

Clinical Course

Pain disappeared durably and completely in 32 of the 38 patients treated. This was the equivalent of a cure rate of 84% for a mean follow-up of 3.7 years. If we excluded the patients whose histologic finding was not osteoid osteoma, the cure rate was about 88% (28 of 32). In most cases (68% [26 of 38]), pain relief was obtained as soon as the patient awakened from anesthesia.

Hospitalization lasted a mean of 4.8 days (range, 2–21 days), and patients were able to use or to bear weight on the extremity at a mean of 30 days. In our series, the patients treated surgically had a much longer hospital stay, but this is not comparable as these cases were therapeutic failures after percutaneous resection. Sporting activities were resumed completely after a mean of 112 days (range, 15 days to 1 year), a period which varied markedly according to the area initially involved.

Treatment failed in four cases, with the return of pain similar in nature and intensity to the pain before the procedure. The interval before the reappearance of pain varied: early in two cases (3 and 7 days) and later in two other cases (6 and 18 months). A curative surgical procedure was performed in three cases; in the fourth case, a second percutaneous excision was performed, which completely and durably eliminated clinical symptoms.

Other Diagnoses

Six bone lesions of a different nature were revealed, and these lesions followed two different courses. Either pain persisted with intensity similar to that of the pain before percutaneous resection (n = 2), or there was clinical cure with complete elimination of pain. Four lesions followed this favorable course: one intraosseous mucoid cyst, one focal osteochondritis, one focal chronic osteomyelitis, and one arthritic geode.

Complications

Nine patients (24%) presented with complications (Table 3). The mean duration before occurrence of complications was 40 days (range, 1–150 days). We differentiated early complications (five cases), which occurred within 2 weeks after the procedure, from later complications (four cases). The early complications were usually local and resolved rapidly, and they were mainly skin burns around the entry site of the resection instruments. In a single case, in a 6-year-old child, superficial thermal damage deepened and became secondarily infected, requiring daily local care for 2 months. Five years after the procedure, the child had no sequelae except an extensive scar on the tibia where the lesion was resected.

Muscular hematomas occurred during the course of excision in two cases. In the first case, secondary surgical evacuation was necessary owing to hematoma of the quadriceps muscle during resection of an osteoid osteoma of the femoral shaft. In the second case, a hematoma of the psoas muscle after resection of a spinal lesion resolved spontaneously.

Later complications were often more severe. A case of focal chronic osteomyelitis due to *S aureus* occurred 25 days postoperatively. A fracture of the femoral shaft occurred 2 months postoperatively, and a stress fracture of the femoral neck occurred 5 months postoperatively. The last complication was a late but more benign case of dysesthesia along the course of the femoral cutaneous nerve.

DISCUSSION

Osteoid osteoma is a benign tumor in the young adult. It is located preferentially in the shaft of the long bones near the metaphyseal junctions, with a predilection for the lower limbs (5). The clinical manifestations are generally typical—nocturnal pain that prevents sleep and that is relieved with acetylsalicylic acid. Conventional radiolographs and CT scans generally suffice to establish the diagnosis, which is already strongly suggested by the clinical picture.

CT has led to a marked advance in the rapidity and reliability of diagnosis after the first clinical signs. It also provides precise localization of the lesion and indication of the size of the nidus. These parameters orient the therapeutic strategy: either surgical excision or excision and percutaneous destruction with CT guidance. When the approach to the osteoma is not without risk, in particular near the course of vessels and nerves, we merely localize it precisely, perhaps by inserting a small-diameter pin, and the tumor is secondarily resected surgically.

While these various imaging techniques allow precise diagnosis, the interval before diagnosis is still astonishingly long (a mean of 1.6 years in our series) and does not seem to have notably decreased in comparison with that in other series in the literature (1,2,5). Every possible means thus must be used to find the osteoma at the slightest clinical suspicion.

Although this tumor may regress spontaneously after some years (7,8), excision is often necessary to relieve the patient and is justified by the necessity of obtaining histologic confirmation. En bloc resection was long the only surgical technique enabling resection of the entire nidus and complete cure. This mode of resection is not always necessary, but it is important to note the difficulties of the surgery or even the damage it can cause in certain locations such as the deep posterior acetabulum.

In spite of the various methods used to localize the nidus during the procedure, this may be difficult and require wide bone excision disproportionate to the small size of the lesion and sometimes is followed by osteosynthesis and bone grafting.

The development of CT-guided percutaneous treatment techniques, associated if necessary with scintigraphic localization (9), has profoundly modified the treatment of osteoid osteoma. Leaving aside the contraindications related to anesthesia and coagulation disorders, the contraindications seem to be nonindications. These are large lesions (>15 mm in diameter) or lesions that cannot be reached without jeopardizing vessels or nerves. In such cases, we merely localize the nidus and perhaps insert a pin.

On the other hand, in the majority of cases (>90% [35 of 38]) the osteoid osteoma was in a superficial or cortical location. A tumor that is endosteal or within the marrow cavity is in no way an obstacle to percutaneous resection. In most cases, percutaneous ablation will remove both the superficial and deep cortical bone (Fig 3d).

Successful Treatments

Treatment by means of CT-guided percutaneous resection appears to be effective. Clinical cure was obtained in 84% of patients and in 88% if patients whose lesion was not an osteoid osteoma are excluded. Four patients were not cured with the first resection and required either a second resection or surgical removal of the lesion.

Among the patients who were cured, four distinct groups were defined at histologic analysis. In group 1, the nidus was present and complete at histologic examination. Cure was complete and the risk of recurrence is nil. This was the case in 21 patients in our series.

In group 2, the nidus was present at histologic examination, but it was not possible to conclude as to the totality of excision because the nidus appeared fragmented or incomplete. Although these patients (three in our series) have been free of symptoms since excision, risk of recurrence in this type of patient cannot be neglected.

In group 3, no lesion was found that appeared to be an osteoid osteoma at histologic examination. This was the case in four patients in our series. These patients presented with clinical and radiologic signs strongly suggestive of osteoid osteoma; in two, pain disappeared immediately after awakening from anesthesia. In the third patient, pain progressively lessened and disappeared about 1 month after treatment. At the present time, these four patients are completely free of symptoms. This leads us to think that in these cases the nidus was probably excised but was not found at histologic examination.

Several hypotheses may explain this phenomenon (10). First, the nidus may

TABLE 2
Differential Diagnosis at Histologic Analysis

Patient No.	Patient Age (y)	Localization	Radiologic Resection*	Clinical Course	Histologic Diagnosis
2	65	Tibia	Complete	Recurrence	Benign fibromatous tumor
3	20	Tibia	Partial	Cure	Intraosseous mucoid cyst
6	12	Tibia	Complete	Recurrence	Intraosseous mucoid cyst
9	22	Patella	Partial	Cure	Focal osteochondritis
25	46	Femur	Complete	Cure	Osteomyelitis
26	49	Acetabulum	Partial	Cure	Degenerative geode

* All resections were performed with a toothed drill.

TABLE 3
Short- and Long-Term Complications

Patient No.	Gravity of Complication	Interval (d)	Complication
6	Serious	25	*Staphylococcus aureus* osteomyelitis
11	Minor	60	Femorocutaneous dysesthesia
12	Serious	150	Stress fracture of femoral neck
17	Minor	7	Skin infection
22	Serious	45	Skin necrosis
23	Minor	2	Skin burn
27	Minor	15	Muscular hematoma
34	Serious	60	Femoral fracture
35	Minor	1	Muscular hematoma

have been fragmented during excision, which would make histologic study difficult or impossible.

Second, the nidus was present and not fragmented within the material sent to the laboratory but was not found during examination. When the nidus is very small, only very thin serial sections allow its identification by the pathologist.

Third, the nidus was not resected. In this case, clinical cure may be explained by the theory of Jackson et al (11). According to these authors, surgical treatment may cause traumatic thrombosis of the vessels of the nidus, and this thrombosis may then be responsible for infarction of the lesion and lead to clinical cure. It could be suggested that, like surgery, percutaneous resection may cause lesional trauma. This would explain the fact that the pain decreases progressively and then disappears.

Fourth, it is possible that the nidus was not resected and not infarcted. In this case, the relief from pain could be a result of the decompression that occurs when the lesion is opened; this decrease in intralesional pressure then provides temporary elimination of pain. Progressive regrowth of the lesion accounts for the return of pain in the short or medium term. The risk of recurrence appears to be greatest in such a context.

Last, in the absence of histologic certainty, the possibility cannot be excluded that these three patients had a histologically different lesion, like the patients of group 4.

In group 4, histologic examination revealed a lesion of a different type. Of the six patients who did not have an osteoid osteoma, four obtained durable relief after percutaneous resection (one old focal chronic osteomyelitis, two intraosseous mucoid cysts, and one osteochondritis). Certain authors (12) have raised the hypothesis that if histologic examination cannot lead to a conclusion of osteoid osteoma, the clinical features, imaging findings, and above all the notion of immediate cure after the procedure, will establish the diagnosis. These four examples suggest that a lesion that is cured by means of percutaneous resection and that presents the radiologic and clinical characteristics of an osteoid osteoma may in fact be a bone lesion of a different nature, and a definite diagnosis can be reached only at histologic study.

In the six cases in which the diagnosis of osteoid osteoma had been presumed erroneously, retrospective analysis of the records always revealed an atypical element, whether in clinical, scintigraphic, radiologic, or CT findings. Moreover, the diagnosis of osteoid osteoma is rare after the age of 45 years and exceptional after 65 years. More advanced age is an atypical factor, which we found in patients 2, 25, and 26 in our study; a differential diagnosis of osteoid osteoma was made at histologic examination. The relative simplicity of the resection procedure and its low morbidity rate have contributed to the increase in the number of indications for this method of treatment. Moreover, the fact that the biopsy procedure and the therapeutic procedure are indissociably linked also indirectly increases the number of indications; if the lesion is small, percutaneous resection allows not only good quality histologic analysis but also total excision.

These diagnostic errors emphasize the necessity for histologic confirmation, even when clinical examination and medical imaging results appear typical (8). This incites us to remain prudent and to weigh carefully the indications for treatments that do not permit histologic confirmation: laser photocoagulation (13), alcoholization (14), and simple trituration or ablation with radio-frequency electrodes (15).

Unsuccessful Treatments

Treatment has failed if pain persists or recurs after excision (16), and this reflects incomplete ablation of the nidus. The number of recurrences decreases with time, but recurrences may occur very late—up to 10 years later in one case in the literature (17). In our series, the failure rate seems acceptable (16% [six of 38]), taking into account the simplicity of application and performance of the technique. The main source of failure seems to be the large size of the lesion, and this is one of the limitations of the technique. Thus, in two cases, resection was incomplete because the size of the lesion (21 and 25 mm) was disproportionate to the size of the material excised with a Kohler toothed drill with a 9-mm outer diameter (Fig 1). The follow-up CT scan performed at the end of the procedure showed that in these two cases the nidus had not been removed completely. However, resection had to be interrupted because of the risk of fracture.

To our knowledge, there are no objective criteria for assessing fracture risk at the time of or during percutaneous resection. According to Caillieret et al (12), the risk is high when resection includes the deep cortex of a long bone shaft, and osteosynthesis is desirable in such cases. From our experience, a lesion larger than 15 mm appears difficult to extract, extraction is often incomplete, and repeated resections are required. The occurrence of fracture, in particular in long bones, also seems correlated with the amount of cortical bone resected. In such cases, removal of the osteoid osteoma should be performed by means of directed surgery after placing a pin in the nidus with CT guidance.

Preventive osteosynthesis is performed according to the location and volume of resection. In such cases, primary surgical treatment seems preferable so that osteosynthesis can be performed if necessary in the course of the same procedure. However, as it is difficult to localize the nidus during surgery, some teams continue to use percutaneous resection in large lesions and associate it at the end of the procedure with destruction of the nidus by means of trituration or alcoholization.

According to the theory of McLeod et al (18), lesions more than 15 mm in diameter may be potentially malignant osteoblastomas. In such cases, treatment must always be surgical and oncologically satisfactory (19).

Complications

The complications we observed were in general early and minor. Skin burns occurred immediately after the procedure at the entry site of the resection instruments; they were due to the heat caused by the high rotation speed of the toothed drill. These minor complications most frequently observed in our series usually required only treatment of symptoms and resolved without sequelae. When we were aware of this complication, we were able to decrease its frequency by means of constant surveillance of the state of the skin during resection.

Irritation of the femoral cutaneous nerve occurred twice during resection of osteoid osteomas of the femoral neck. The femoral cutaneous nerve gives rise to a femoral branch that runs in the superficial planes of the lateral inguinofemoral region, which it innervates. Planning the course of resection on the initial CT scan makes it possible to avoid only the major nerve and vascular trunks. Patients who had this complication still had hypoesthesia in the territory of the affected nerve up to 3 years after the procedure.

Hematomas were unpredictable and seemed to be unavoidable. They were generally of moderate size and regressed spontaneously, only exceptionally requiring secondary surgical evacuation.

Major complications mainly were femoral fractures. Bone resection in these two cases was not extensive—the bone defect was less than 10 mm in diameter—but these fractures appeared to be related to resumption of professional or sporting activities too early and against medical advice.

We had one patient with focal chronic osteomyelitis due to *S aureus*, which occurred 25 days after the procedure. This emphasizes the necessity for strict surgical asepsis in the CT room throughout any resection procedure.

The results of this study confirm the medium-term efficacy of CT-guided percutaneous resection of osteoid osteomas. This technique allows minimal and generally complete bone resection owing to precise and reliable localization. Hospital stay is reduced to 2 or 3 days, and weight-bearing and physical activity can be resumed at an early date. In comparison with other treatment methods that are being developed, with this method histologic confirmation of the lesion is obtained in the majority of cases, and we believe this is indispensable. These varied reasons tend to widen the indications for percutaneous resection, which we believe should be considered as first-line therapy if it seems technically possible. However, it would seem permissible to resect only lesions with a diameter of less than 10 mm. This study also shows that percutaneous resection may be useful in treating other small localized bone lesions.

References

1. Voto SJ, Cook AJ, Weiner DS, Ewing JW, Arrington LE. Treatment of osteoid osteoma by computed tomography guided excision in the pediatric patient. J Pediatr Orthop 1990; 10:510–513.
2. Kohler R, Mazoyer JF, Besse JL, Bascoulergue Y. Treatment of osteoid osteoma with percutaneous resection under computerized tomography control: apropos of 5 cases. Rev Chir Orthop Réparatrice Appar Mot 1990; 76:284–287. [French]
3. Poey C, Clement JL, Baunin C, et al. Percutaneous extraction of an osteoid osteoma of the lumbar spine under CT guidance. J Comput Assist Tomogr 1991; 15:1056–1058.
4. Poey J, Assoun J, Duparc B, et al. Percutaneous extraction of osteoid osteoma. Semin Intervent Radiol 1993; 10:308–315.
5. Assoun J, Railhac JJ, Bonnevialle P, et al. Osteoid osteoma: percutaneous resection with CT guidance. Radiology 1993; 188: 541–547.
6. Baunin C, Puget C, Assoun J, et al. Percutaneous resection of osteoid osteoma under CT guidance in eight children. Pediatr Radiol 1994; 24:185–188.
7. Moberg E. The natural course of osteoid osteoma. J Bone Joint Surg 1951; 33:166.
8. Sim FH, Dahlin CD, Beabout JW. Osteoid osteoma: diagnostic problems. J Bone Joint Surg [Am] 1975; 57:154–158.
9. Roger B, Bellin MF, Wioland M, Grenier P. Osteoid osteoma: CT-guided percutaneous excision confirmed with immediate follow-up scintigraphy in 16 outpatients. Radiology 1996; 201:239–242.
10. Ward WG, Eckardt JJ, Shayestehfar S, et al. Osteoid osteoma diagnosis and management with low morbidity. Clin Orthop 1993; 291:229–235.
11. Jackson RP, Reckling FW, Mantz FA. Osteoid osteoma and osteoblastoma. Clin Orthop 1977; 128:303–313.
12. Caillieret J, Fontaine C, Ducloux M, Letendart J, Duquennoy A. Ostéomes ostéoïdes de l'extrémité supérieure du fémur. Rev Chir Orthop 1985; 72(suppl 2):101–103.
13. Gangi A, Dietemann JL, Gasser B, et al. Interstitial laser photocoagulation of osteoid osteomas with use of CT guidance. Radiology 1997; 203:843–848.
14. Sanhaji L, Gharbaoui IS, Hassani RE, et al. Un nouveau traitement de l'ostéome ostéoïde: la sclérose percutanée à l'éthanol sous guidage scanographique. J Radiol 1996; 77:37–40.
15. Rosenthal DI, Alexander A, Rosenberg AE, Springfield D. Ablation of osteoid osteomas with a percutaneously placed electrode: a new procedure. Radiology 1992; 183:29–33.
16. Railhac JJ, Assoun J, Poey C, et al. Ablation percutanée des ostéomes osteoïdes sous contrôle tomodensitométrique. Rev Imagerie Med 1992; 4:463–470.
17. Regan MW, Galey JP, Oakeshott RD. Recurrent osteoid osteoma: case report with a ten-year asymptomatic interval. Clin Orthop 1990; 253:221–224.
18. McLeod RA, Dahlin DC, Beabout JW. The spectrum of osteoblastoma. AJR 1976; 126: 321–335.
19. Gitelis S, Schajowicz F. Osteoid osteoma and osteoblastoma. Orthop Clin North Am 1989; 20:313–325.

Liposclerosing Myxofibrous Tumor: A Radiologic-Pathologic–Distinct Fibro-osseous Lesion of Bone with a Marked Predilection for the Intertrochanteric Region of the Femur[1]

Mark J. Kransdorf, MD
Mark D. Murphey, MD
Donald E. Sweet, MD

Index terms:
Bone neoplasms, 40.3219
Bones, CT, 40.1211
Bones, diseases, 40.3139
Bones, MR, 40.121411, 40.121413

Radiology 1999; 212:693–698

Abbreviations:
LSMFT = liposclerosing myxofibrous tumor
MDP = methylene diphosphonate

[1] From the Department of Radiology, Saint Mary's Hospital, 5801 Bremo Rd, Richmond, VA 23226 (M.J.K.); the Departments of Radiologic Pathology (M.J.K., M.D.M.) and Orthopedic Pathology (D.E.S.), Armed Forces Institute of Pathology, Washington, DC; the Department of Radiology and Nuclear Medicine, Uniformed Services University of the Health Sciences, Bethesda, Md (M.D.M.); and the Department of Radiology, University of Maryland School of Medicine, Baltimore (M.D.M.). Received February 4, 1998; revision requested April 14; final revision received November 24; accepted March 29, 1999. **Address reprint requests to** M.J.K.

The opinions or assertions contained herein are the private views of the authors and are not to be construed as official or as reflecting the views of the Department of the Army or the Department of Defense.

Author contributions:
Guarantor of integrity of entire study, M.J.K.; study concepts, M.J.K., M.D.M., D.E.S.; study design, M.J.K., M.D.M., D.E.S.; definition of intellectual content, M.J.K., M.D.M., D.E.S.; literature research, M.J.K., D.E.S.; clinical and experimental studies, M.J.K.; data acquisition and analysis, M.J.K.; manuscript preparation, editing, and review, M.J.K., M.D.M., D.E.S.

PURPOSE: To describe the characteristic features of liposclerosing myxofibrous tumor (LSMFT) of bone.

MATERIALS AND METHODS: The radiographs and clinical histories of 39 patients (21 male, 18 female; mean age, 42 years; age range, 15–69 years) with histologically verified LSMFT of bone were retrospectively studied.

RESULTS: LSMFT had a predilection for the proximal femur; more than 90% (30 of 33) of the femoral lesions were in the intertrochanteric region. Radiographs showed an indolent growth pattern with a well-defined and often extensively sclerotic margin. The bone contour either was normal or showed mild expansile remodeling. Mineralization within the lesion was not uncommon. Scintigrams showed mild to moderate focal tracer accumulation. Findings at computed tomography reflected those at radiography, whereas magnetic resonance imaging findings were nonspecific. Four (10%) patients had evidence of malignant transformation.

CONCLUSION: The radiologic appearance of LSMFT in the intertrochanteric region of the femur is characteristic. The substantial prevalence of malignant transformation associated with LSMFT underscores the need for close observation of this lesion.

Liposclerosing myxofibrous tumor (LSMFT) of bone is a benign fibro-osseous lesion that is characterized by a complex mixture of histologic elements, which may include lipoma, fibroxanthoma, myxoma, myxofibroma, fibrous dysplasia–like features, cyst formation, fat necrosis, ischemic ossification, and, rarely, cartilage (1–3). The lesion has also been referred to as "polymorphic fibrocystic disease of bone" and "polymorphic fibro-osseous lesion of bone"; however, the descriptive designation, "liposclerosing myxofibrous tumor of bone" is preferred (2).

Despite its histologic complexity, LSMFT has a relatively characteristic radiologic appearance and skeletal distribution, and, more important, it appears to be associated with an increased prevalence of malignant transformation compared with fibrous dysplasia and other benign fibro-osseous lesions; this factor underscores the need for close observation of this condition. Herein, we report our experience with the radiologic and histologic appearances of 39 cases of histologically proved LSMFT of bone in a retrospective study conducted to define the characteristic features of this condition.

MATERIALS AND METHODS

We retrospectively reviewed the radiologic and clinical parameters of 39 patients (21 male, 18 female; mean age, 42 years; age range, 15–69 years) who had histologically verified

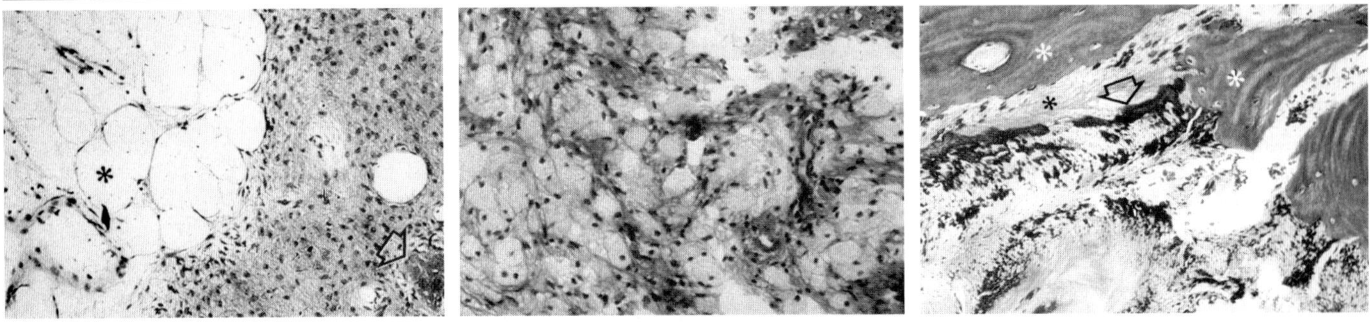

a. b. c.

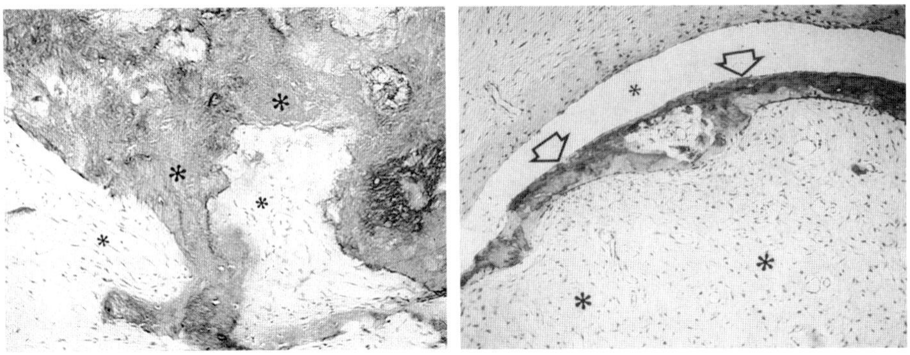

d. e.

Figure 1. **(a–e)** High-power composite photomicrographs demonstrate the complex admixture of solid benign histologic patterns typically encountered in LSMFT of bone, including **(a)** hypertrophic fat (*) with early trophic features and fibrous change with focal osseous metaplasia (arrow); **(b)** xanthoma (foam) cell modulation; **(c)** dystrophic mineralization (arrow) within degenerated myxoid tissue (black *) adjacent to remodeling trabecular bone (white *); **(d)** atypical bone formation (ischemic ossification) (large *) within a myxofibrous background (small *); and **(e)** metaplastic woven bone (arrows) emerging from the myxofibrous stroma (large *). The metaplastic woven bone is indistinguishable from fibrous dysplasia. The cleft (small *) is an artifact of the tissue preparation. (Hematoxylin-eosin stain; original magnification, ×125–200.)

LSMFT of bone. The patients were selected from a computer-generated database that contained the diagnoses of all cases seen in consultation at the Armed Forces Institute of Pathology since 1970. The diagnosis of LSMFT of bone was made in accordance with previously published criteria after a review of the patients' histologic biopsy material (Fig 1) (1–3).

The radiologic findings assessed included the bone involved, location of lesion (ie, epiphysis, metaphysis, metadiaphysis, or diaphysis), type of margin, size of lesion, presence or absence of bone remodeling ("expansile remodeling") and periosteal reaction, and pathologic fracture. Bone scintigrams were reviewed for intensity of tracer accumulation; computed tomographic (CT) scans were reviewed for the margin, matrix, and tissue attenuation; and magnetic resonance (MR) images were reviewed for the margin, signal intensity, and associated marrow or soft-tissue signal intensity abnormalities. Additional clinical data that were reviewed included presenting symptoms, age at presentation, and sex of patient.

Radiographs were available for review in all cases, bone scintigrams were available in 11 cases (one with flow and blood pool images), CT scans were available in nine cases, and MR images were available in six cases. Owing to the consultative nature of the cases, the MR images were obtained with a variety of magnets. These images included T1- (repetition time range msec/echo time range msec, 600–994/16–38) and T2-weighted (2,000–2,600/80–100) spin-echo studies obtained in multiple planes. Inversion-recovery MR images also were available in one case, and conventional tomographic images also were available in two cases.

RESULTS

LSMFT of bone was found most commonly in the femur; 33 (85%) of the 39 lesions were in this location. Approximately 91% (30 of 33) of the femoral lesions were located proximally in the intertrochanteric region. The remaining three femoral lesions were in the shaft. The six nonfemoral lesions were located in the ilium ($n = 3$), humerus ($n = 2$), and second rib ($n = 1$).

Pain, the most common presenting clinical symptom, was present in 14 (48%) of the 29 patients in whom presenting clinical data were available. The duration of pain varied from a few weeks to 10 years. The lesion was an incidental finding in 12 (41%) of these 29 patients; in 10 patients, it was identified on radiographs, and in two, it was found on scintigrams. Three (10%) of these patients presented with pathologic fracture.

The radiographs showed a well-defined, geographic lytic lesion with a sclerotic margin; these findings were suggestive of an indolent pattern of growth. Marginal sclerosis was always present, but the amount of sclerosis was variable; it was mild in four (10%), moderate in 23 (59%), and extensive in 12 (31%) of 39 cases (Figs 2–5). The bone contour was normal in 25 (64%) cases and demonstrated mild expansile remodeling in 11 (28%) cases (Fig 5). Expansile remodeling was moderate in two (5%) cases and marked in one (3%) case. Mineralized matrix was present in 28 (72%) of the 39 cases and absent in four (10%). In the remaining seven (18%) cases, the identification of matrix was inconclusive because of extensive marginal sclerosis. The matrices demonstrated mixed patterns of opacification, which included globular and linear areas of intense opacity as well as regions with small rounded and arclike configurations (Figs 2–6).

The CT scan findings in nine cases reflected the radiographic findings and were very useful in further characterizing the nature and extent of marginal sclerosis and mineralized matrix. At CT, the mineralized matrix was globular and irregular, and it often extended to the margin of the lesion (Figs 3, 5). The surrounding sclerosis was relatively uniskeletal muscle (Fig 2). On the T2-weighted images, the lesion was mildly to moderately heterogeneous, with a signal intensity equal to or greater than that of fat. Areas of matrix had decreased signal intensity (Figs 2, 4, 5). The inversion-recovery MR images that were available in one case showed markedly increased signal intensity. No lesions demonstrated a signal intensity similar to that of fat.

The bone scintigrams that were available in 11 cases showed focal radionuclide accumulation within the lesion. Increased tracer activity varied; it was mild in three (27%), moderate in six (54%), and marked in two (18%) cases. The flow and blood pool images that were available in a single case showed minimally increased tracer accumulation.

Malignant transformation was identified in four (10%) patients; osteosarcoma was identified in two patients, malignant fibrous histiocytoma was identified in one patient, and low-grade malignant change was identified in one patient. These neoplasms occurred in the femur in three patients, and two of the femoral lesions were in the intertrochanteric region. The final case occurred in the humerus. In the cases of malignant transformation, the radiographs showed evidence of areas of aggressive biologic behavior within a preexistent benign process, with areas of focal bone destruction and an associated soft-tissue mass (Fig 6).

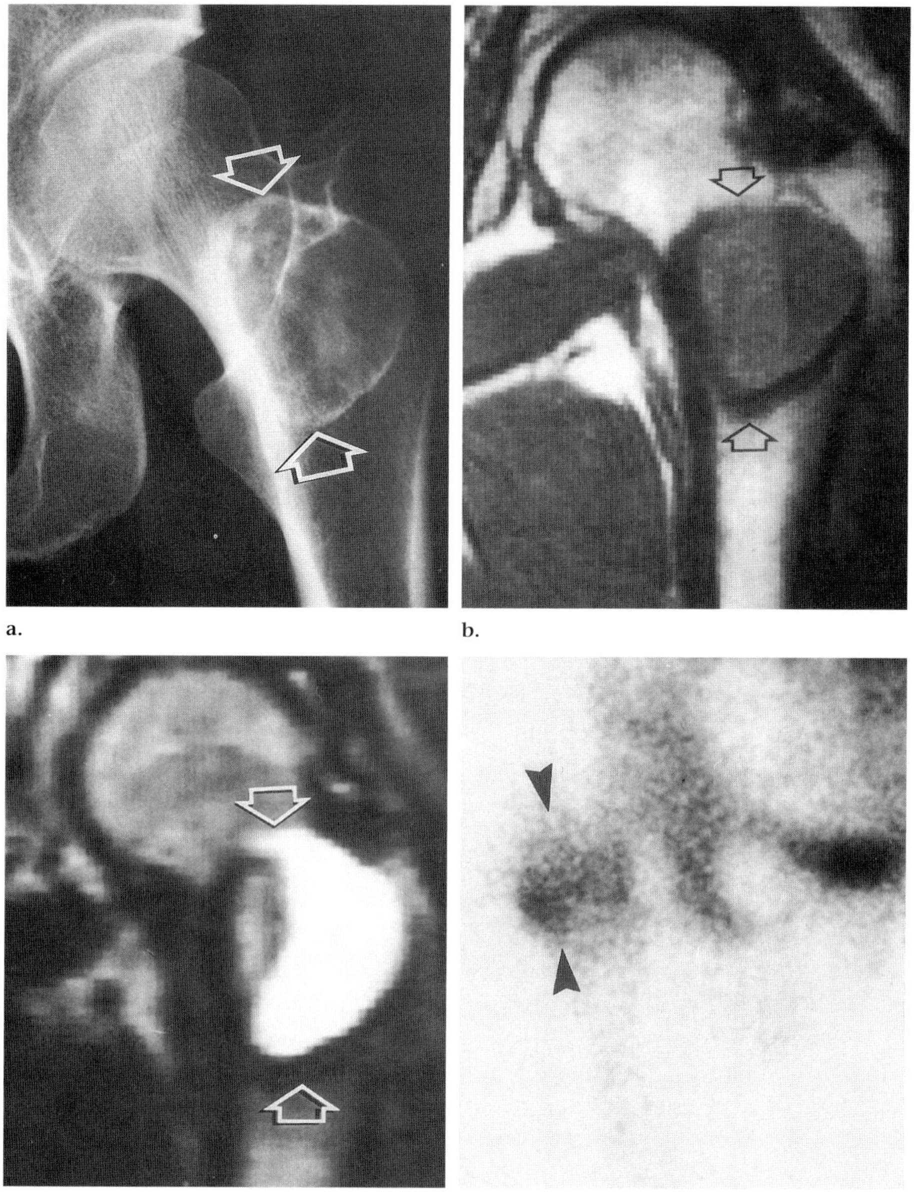

a. b. c. d.

Figure 2. LSMFT of bone in a 39-year-old man. **(a)** Anteroposterior radiograph of the hip shows a geographic lesion (arrows) with a thin, well-defined sclerotic margin in the intertrochanteric region of the femur. There is globular amorphous mineralized matrix in the middle lower portion of the lesion, with more extensively mineralized globular matrix in the upper aspect. **(b)** Coronal T1-weighted (700/33) spin-echo MR image shows the lesion (arrows) to have a signal intensity similar to that of skeletal muscle. The relatively vertical septation is due to wrap artifact. **(c)** Corresponding coronal T2-weighted (2,000/100) spin-echo image shows the lesion (arrows) to be moderately heterogeneous, with a well-defined margin and areas of high and intermediate signal intensity. **(d)** Posterior technetium 99m methylene diphosphonate (MDP) bone scan of the pelvis shows a mild focal increase of tracer accumulation in the lesion (arrowheads).

form in thickness. The attenuation of the lesion was difficult to establish, especially in small lesions and in those with extensive matrix. The attenuation of the nonmineralized portions of the lesions was lower than that of skeletal muscle and higher than that of fat (Fig 5). No areas with tissue attenuation similar to that of fat were identified.

The MR images that were available in six cases showed the lesion to be well-defined, with a variable-thickness peripheral rind of low signal intensity that corresponded to the sclerosis seen on the radiographs. On the T1-weighted images, the lesion was relatively homogeneous, with a signal intensity similar to that of

DISCUSSION

LSMFT of bone, a benign fibro-osseous lesion, is characterized by a complex mixture of histologic elements. These include lipoma, fibroxanthoma, myxoma, myxofibroma, fibrous dysplasia–like features, cyst formation, fat necrosis, ischemic ossification, and, rarely, cartilage (1–3). The descriptive term "liposclerosing myxofibrous tumor" has been advocated for this lesion. The designation of "sclerosing" refers to the intralesional bone formed or mineralized within altered fat; this bone is distinct relative to the reactive surrounding sclerosis and usually a combination of lamellar, pseudopaget (mosaic), woven, and ischemic bone. The term "myxofibrous" refers to the fibrous or myxofibrous areas that may demonstrate metaplastic curvilinear or circular woven bone ossicles and/or dystrophic mineralization in necrotic fat.

These tissue components are seen in varying proportions, and although they all are mentioned in the description of fibrous dysplasia by Lichtenstein and Jaffe

(4), the histologic pattern of LSMFT goes beyond the current description of this entity (5). One may hypothesize that these histologic patterns are ultimately derived from intramedullary fat, because there are clear histologic and radiologic similarities between LSMFT and the involuting (stage 3) variant of intraosseous lipoma (6–9). The concept that intraosseous lipomas are not static masses of mature fat was advanced by Milgram (6–9), who demonstrated that these lesions undergo involutional changes that include fat necrosis, calcification, variable degrees of cyst formation, and reactive woven bone formation.

The origin of LSMFT is not clear, but we suspect that it is a combination of changes in the altered fat of a partially involuted lipoma or lipogenic lesion of bone with superimposed proliferative change. This proliferative change includes myxomatous, myxolipomatous, myxofibrous, fibrous, and fibro-osseous features. Despite its histologic similarities to involuting lipoma, when there is differentiation or modulation of fat to proliferating myxofibrous and/or fibro-osseous tissue, the designation of LSMFT seems more appropriate.

The radiologic appearance of LSMFT is often quite characteristic. LSMFT has a striking predilection for the femur: In the present study, approximately 85% of the lesions were at this site, and 91% of the femoral lesions were in the intertrochanteric region. Radiographs typically showed a geographic lesion with a well-defined, often extensively sclerotic margin; such findings indicate an indolent pattern of growth. The bone contour was normal or showed mild expansile remodeling. Mineralization within the lesion was not uncommon.

Despite its name, lipomatous tissue was not identified on CT and MR imaging studies, probably because of the small amount of fat present and the admixture of fat with the more prominent myxofibrous and/or fibro-osseous tissue. It is the presence of this myxoid tissue that accounted for the decreased attenuation seen in portions of the lesions on the CT scans and for the high signal intensity seen on the T2-weighted MR images. LSMFT can be readily distinguished from intraosseous lipoma on CT scans or MR images by the identification of fat within a lipoma. Intraosseous lipomas do occur in the proximal femur, and the differentiation between LSMFT and intraosseous lipoma with involutional change may not be possible on imaging studies. Similarly, in some cases, differentiation between infarct and myxoma may not be possible.

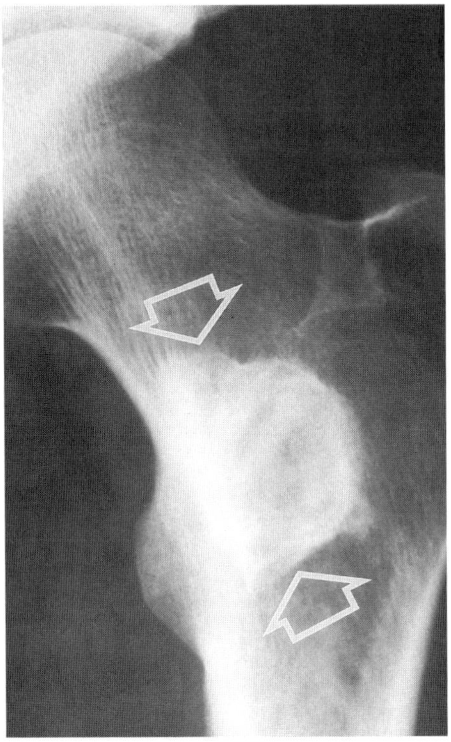

a.

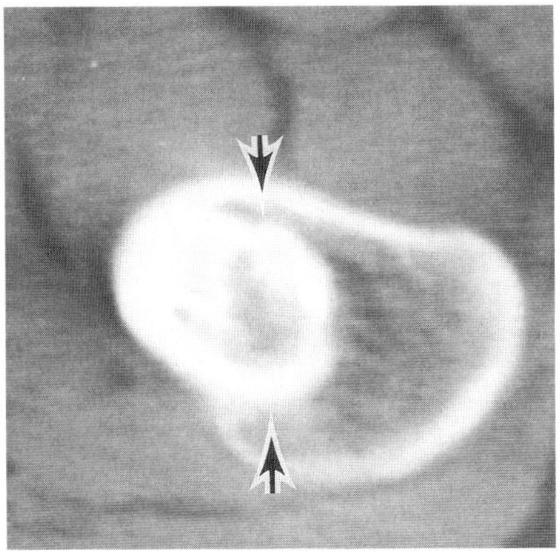

b.

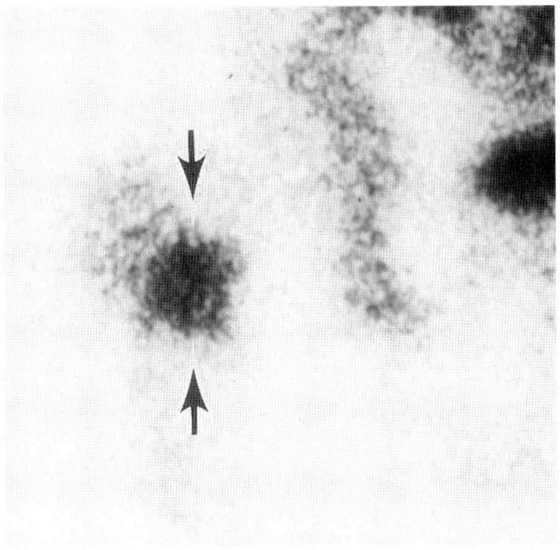

c.

Figure 3. LSMFT of bone in a 30-year-old man with an asymptomatic lesion found during the evaluation for low back pain. **(a)** Anteroposterior radiograph of the hip shows a geographic lesion (arrows) with a thin, well-defined sclerotic margin in the intertrochanteric region of the femur. Extensive amorphous cloudlike areas of mineralized matrix are seen in this lesion. **(b)** Axial CT scan through the middle portion of the lesion (arrows) shows the globular nature of the mineralized matrix. The attenuation of the lesion, although difficult to assess, is greater than that of marrow fat and less than that of skeletal muscle. The surrounding sclerosis appears to be more pronounced than that in **a**. **(c)** Posterior ^{99m}Tc MDP bone scan of the pelvis shows a moderate focal increase of tracer accumulation in the lesion (arrows).

Malignant transformation in lipomatous lesions has been well documented (10). Milgram (10) reported four cases and noted that three (75%) of them occurred in lesions with secondary involutional changes that included necrotic fat with secondary calcification and reactive ossification with ischemic woven bone. He speculated that the malignant transformation arises in the reactive border of the ischemic bone marrow (10). The prevalence of malignant transformation in LSMFT has been previously reported to be 10%–16% (1,2). The increased propensity of LSMFT for malignant transformation is likely to be secondary to its extensive involutional and ischemic change, with the associated sarcoma arising from areas of ischemic ossification within the lesion or from progressive in situ atypism of the altered lipomatous elements (5).

The malignant transformation in 10% of the cases in this series is consistent with previously reported rates (1,2); however, this percentage must be viewed with caution. One could speculate that this percentage is an underestimation of the true rate of malignant transformation, because we included only those cases of malignancy in which there was histologic

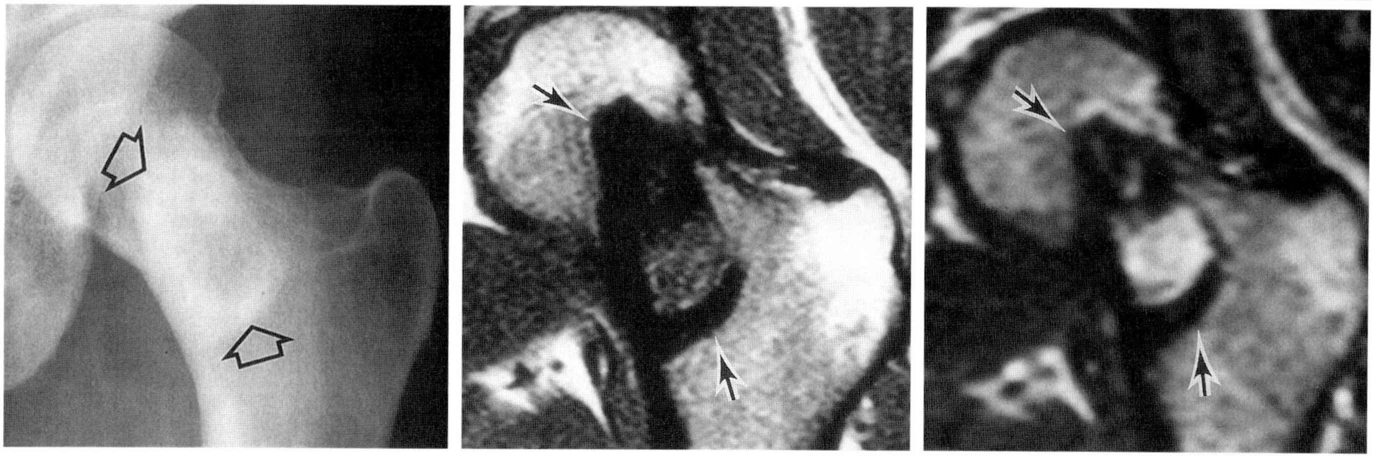

a. b. c.

Figure 4. LSMFT of bone in a 38-year-old woman with vague hip pain. **(a)** Anteroposterior radiograph of the hip shows a geographic lesion (arrows) with a thick, well-defined sclerotic margin in the intertrochanteric region of the femur. **(b, c)** Corresponding coronal **(b)** T1-weighted (600/16) and **(c)** T2-weighted (2,500/80) spin-echo MR images show the lesion (arrows) to be moderately heterogeneous, with nonspecific signal intensity. The sclerotic rind has no signal intensity.

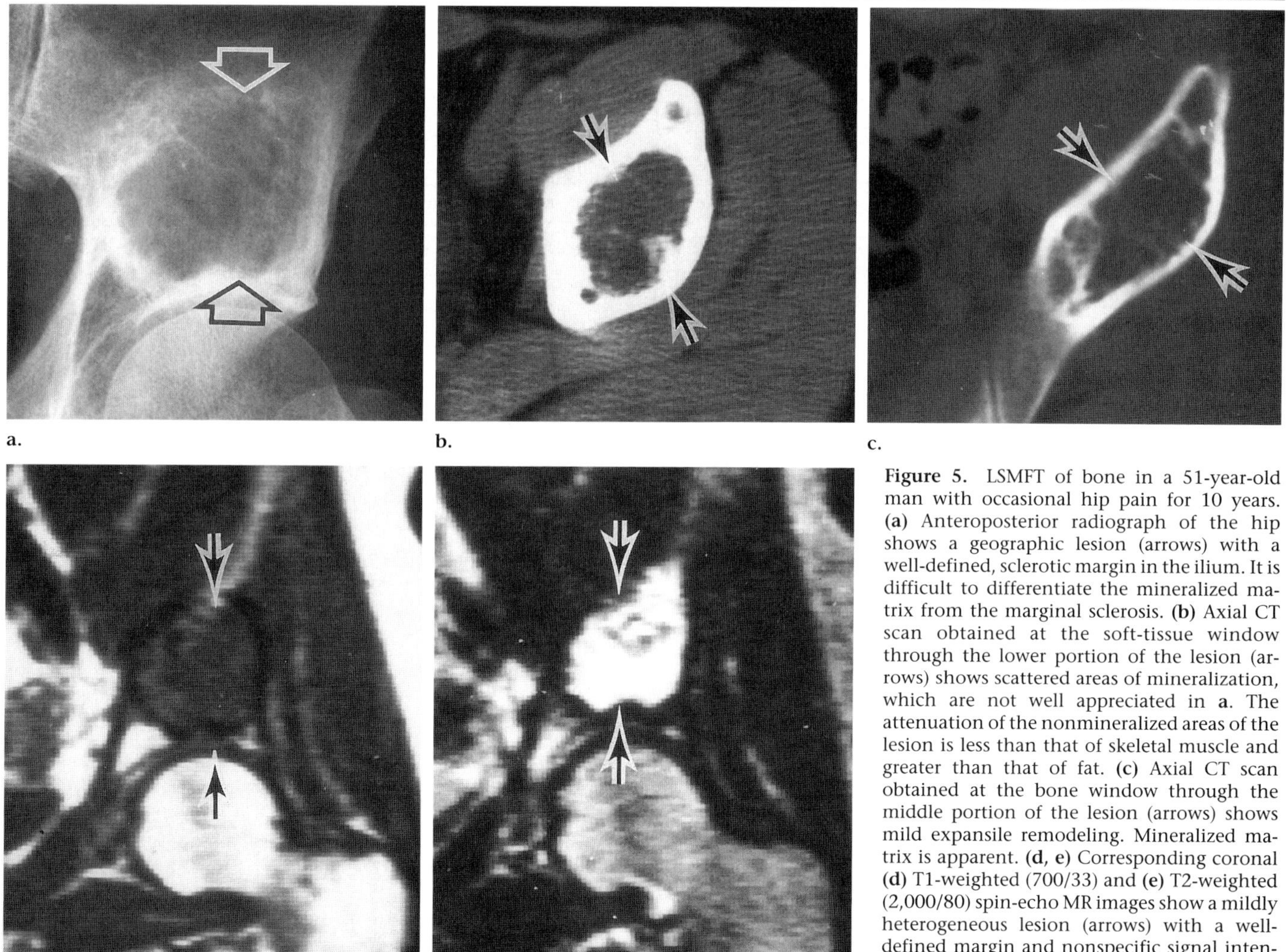

a. b. c. d. e.

Figure 5. LSMFT of bone in a 51-year-old man with occasional hip pain for 10 years. **(a)** Anteroposterior radiograph of the hip shows a geographic lesion (arrows) with a well-defined, sclerotic margin in the ilium. It is difficult to differentiate the mineralized matrix from the marginal sclerosis. **(b)** Axial CT scan obtained at the soft-tissue window through the lower portion of the lesion (arrows) shows scattered areas of mineralization, which are not well appreciated in **a**. The attenuation of the nonmineralized areas of the lesion is less than that of skeletal muscle and greater than that of fat. **(c)** Axial CT scan obtained at the bone window through the middle portion of the lesion (arrows) shows mild expansile remodeling. Mineralized matrix is apparent. **(d, e)** Corresponding coronal **(d)** T1-weighted (700/33) and **(e)** T2-weighted (2,000/80) spin-echo MR images show a mildly heterogeneous lesion (arrows) with a well-defined margin and nonspecific signal intensity. There are no areas with a signal intensity suggestive of fat.

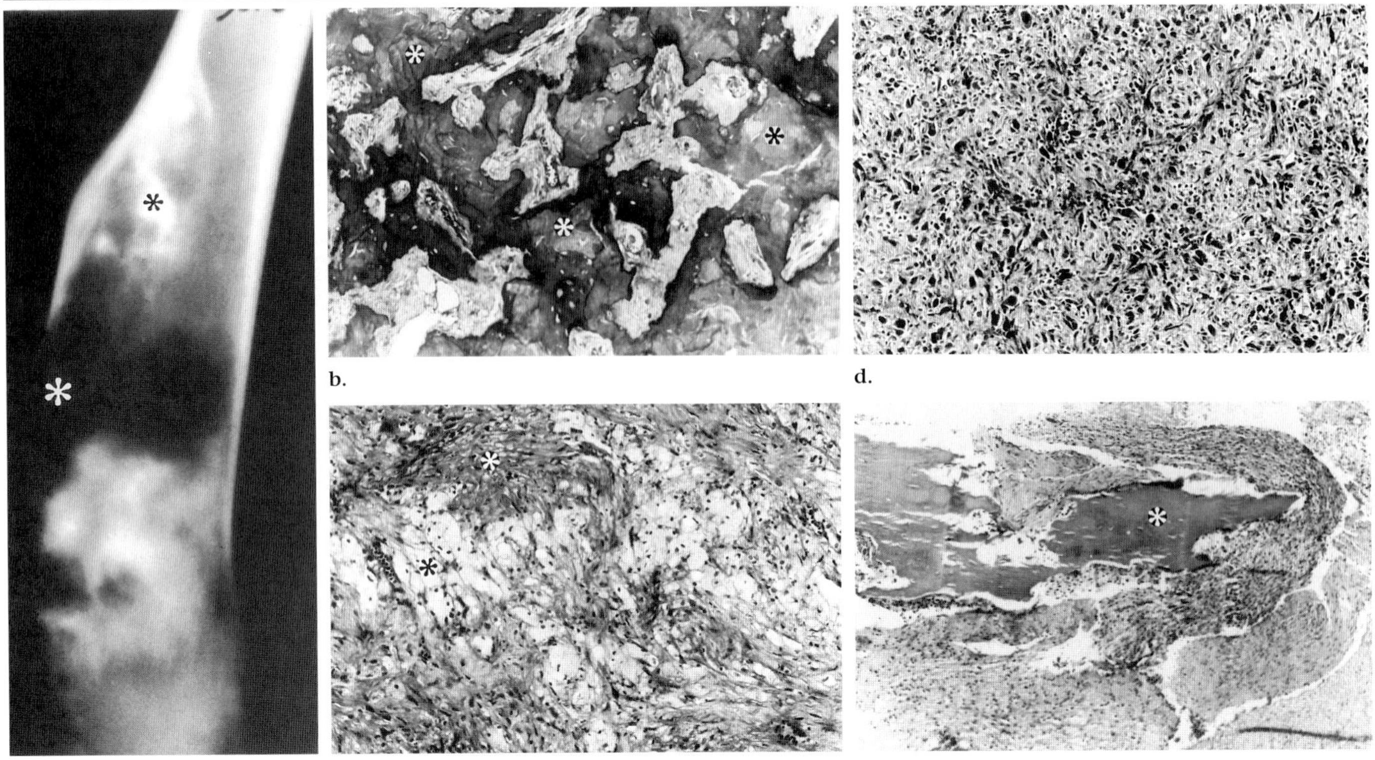

a. b. c. d. e.

Figure 6. Malignant fibrous histiocytoma in preexistent LSMFT of bone in a 54-year-old man. **(a)** Conventional anteroposterior tomogram of the distal femur shows a poorly defined area of lysis (white *), which represents a high-grade sarcoma. Note the extensive mineralized matrix within the LSMFT (black *). **(b, c)** Photomicrographs of the underlying LSMFT show **(b)** ischemic ossification (black and white *) and **(c)** fibroxanthomatous areas (black * marks the xanthomatous area and white * marks the area of spindle cells). (Hematoxylin-eosin stain; original magnification, ×75.) **(d, e)** Photomicrographs of the area of malignant transformation show **(d)** a high-grade sarcoma with atypical spindle cells in a storiform or pinwheel pattern, with **(e)** fragments of bone (white *) encased by tumor. (Hematoxylin-eosin stain; original magnification, ×75–150.)

evidence of preexistent LSMFT. Cases in which there was only radiologic evidence of a preexistent LSMFT were not included. This referral bias probably accounts for the two cases of diaphyseal malignant transformation. Conversely, the prevalence of malignant transformation may be considerably lower, because the lesion is often an incidental finding and its benign appearance does not indicate the need for biopsy. Among those patients in whom biopsy is performed, the consultative nature of the Armed Forces Institute of Pathology probably introduces a bias toward the difficult cases and the cases in which there is malignant transformation.

About half of the patients in this review study presented with pain. There was great variability in symptom duration, which varied from a few weeks to 10 years. We speculate that this pain was probably due to mechanical weakening of the bone secondary to osseous replacement by the lesion. Three patients had a pathologic fracture.

In summary, we present the radiologic features of LSMFT of bone—a lesion characterized by a complex admixture of histologic patterns. Although LSMFT is not unique in terms of histogenesis, it is distinctive in terms of its morphologic and characteristic radiologic appearances and skeletal distribution. The apparent increased risk of malignant transformation associated with LSMFT underscores the need for close observation of this condition.

References

1. Ragsdale BD, Sweet DE. Bone. In: Henson DE, Albores-Saavedra J, eds. The pathology of incipient neoplasia. Philadelphia, Pa: Saunders, 1986; 381–423.
2. Ragsdale BD. Polymorphic fibro-osseous lesions of bone: an almost site-specific diagnostic problem in the proximal femur. Hum Pathol 1993; 24:505–512.
3. Gilkey FW. Liposclerosing myxofibrous tumor of bone (letter). Hum Pathol 1993; 24:1264.
4. Lichtenstein L, Jaffe HL. Fibrous dysplasia of bone. Arch Pathol 1942; 33:777–816.
5. Ragsdale BD, Sweet DE, Vinh TN. Radiology as gross pathology in evaluating chondroid lesions. Hum Pathol 1989; 20:930–951.
6. Milgram JW. Involuted intraosseous lipoma of the sacrum. Spine 1991; 16:243–245.
7. Milgram JW. Introsseous lipomas with reactive ossification in the proximal femur. Skeletal Radiol 1981; 7:1–13.
8. Milgram JW. Intraosseous lipomas: radiologic and pathologic manifestations. Radiology 1988; 167:155–160.
9. Milgram JW. Intraosseous lipomas: a clinicopathologic study of 66 cases. Clin Orthop 1988; 231:277–302.
10. Milgram JW. Malignant transformation in bone lipomas. Skeletal Radiol 1990; 19:347–352.

Glenohumeral Relationships during Physiologic Shoulder Motion and Stress Testing: Initial Experience with Open MR Imaging and Active Imaging-Plane Registration[1]

Christopher F. Beaulieu, MD, PhD
Duncan K. Hodge, BA
A. Gabrielle Bergman, MD
Kim Butts, PhD
Bruce L. Daniel, MD
Clay L. Napper, MD
Robert D. Darrow, MS
Charles L. Dumoulin, PhD
Robert J. Herfkens, MD

Index terms:
Magnetic resonance (MR), motion studies, 414.121412
Shoulder, MR, 414.1214

Radiology 1999; 212:699–705

Abbreviation:
RF = radio frequency

[1] From the Department of Radiology (C.F.B., A.G.B., K.B., B.L.D., C.L.N., R.J.H.) and the School of Medicine (D.K.H.), Stanford University Medical Center, Rm S-056, 300 Pasteur Dr, Stanford, CA 94305; and the GE Corporate Research and Development Center, Schenectady, NY (R.D.D., C.L.D.). Received July 7, 1998; revision requested September 11; final revision received, October 27; accepted March 29, 1999. C.F.B. supported in part by a 1997 RSNA Scholar Award. A.G.B. supported in part by a 1997 Toshiba America/RSNA (1) Seed Grant. **Address reprint requests to** C.F.B.

PURPOSE: To test the hypotheses that open dynamic magnetic resonance (MR) imaging can (*a*) be used to evaluate and define normal shoulder motion in active joint motion and muscle contraction and (*b*) be used in conjunction with physical examination.

MATERIALS AND METHODS: With an open-configuration, 0.5-T MR imaging system and active image-plane tracking, 10 shoulders were studied in five asymptomatic subjects to establish normal patterns of glenohumeral motion during abduction and adduction and internal and external rotation. Preliminary studies of physical examination during MR imaging, in which a physician examiner applied mechanical force to the humeral head, were also performed.

RESULTS: During abduction and adduction and internal and external rotation maneuvers with active subject muscle contraction, the humeral head remained precisely centered on the glenoid fossa in all asymptomatic subjects, which is in agreement with findings of previous radiographic studies. Application of force to the humeral head by an examiner was associated with as much as 6 mm of anterior translation and 13 mm of posterior translation.

CONCLUSION: Dynamic MR imaging of the glenohumeral joint is possible over a wide range of physiologic motion in vertically open systems. Use of an MR tracking coil enabled accurate tracking of the anatomy of interest. These preliminary measurements of normal glenohumeral motion patterns begin to establish normal ranges of motion and constitute a necessary first step in characterizing pathologic motion in patients with common clinical problems such as instability and impingement.

Author contributions:
Guarantor of integrity of entire study, C.F.B.; study concepts, C.F.B., A.G.B., D.K.H., R.J.H.; study design, C.F.B., A.G.B., D.K.H.; definition of intellectual content, C.F.B., A.G.B., D.K.H.; literature research, C.F.B.; clinical studies, C.F.B., D.K.H., B.L.D., K.B., C.L.N.; data acquisition, C.F.B., D.K.H., B.L.D., K.B., C.L.N.; data analysis, C.F.B., D.K.H.; manuscript preparation, C.F.B., D.K.H.; manuscript editing, A.G.B., K.B., B.L.D., C.L.N., R.D.D., C.L.D.; manuscript review, all authors.

Glenohumeral instability, defined as unwanted translation of the humeral head on the glenoid, is associated with pain and functional impairment in a large number of individuals (1). Accurate clinical diagnosis of instability remains difficult, even for experienced orthopedic surgeons. Newer open magnetic resonance (MR) imaging devices, originally designed for interventional procedures, permit rapid multiplanar imaging of the shoulder over a broad range of physiologic motion and allow direct patient contact by an examiner during the MR image acquisition (2). We hypothesized that this practice should allow valuable characterization of dynamic articular relationships during active muscle contraction and stress maneuvers performed by the patient or a physician examiner. Our goal was to determine whether dynamic MR imaging can (*a*) be used to evaluate and define normal shoulder motion in active joint motion and muscle contraction and (*b*) be used in conjunction with physical examination.

MATERIALS AND METHODS

We imaged 10 shoulders in five asymptomatic individuals (three men, two women; age range, 22–36 years; mean age, 28 years) by using a vertically open-configuration, 0.5-T MR imager (Signa SP; GE Medical Systems, Milwaukee, Wis). All subjects gave signed informed consent, and their shoulders were imaged by following protocols approved by the medical human subjects panel of the university.

Subjects were evaluated in an upright, seated position with a flexible transmit-receive, circular large-crown radio-frequency (RF) coil (GE Medical Systems) placed around the shoulder. A fast gradient-echo sequence was used: 19.8/7.2 (repetition time msec/echo time msec); flip angle, 30°–40°; 256 × 128 matrix; field of view, 24–30 cm; section thickness, 7 mm; one signal acquired. Sequential single-plane images were acquired at a rate of approximately 2.5 seconds per image. Total examination time was 10–20 minutes per shoulder. The imaging parameters as listed were chosen to provide the fastest possible acquisition of diagnostic-quality images and were based on findings of pilot studies in asymptomatic volunteers. In this context, diagnostic-quality images were defined as images that depicted the anatomy of interest and demonstrated sufficient contrast to allow reproducible measurements of spatial relationships between relevant osseous structures. Such images could not be substantially degraded by motion or other MR artifacts.

In preliminary imaging of the shoulder without the use of a device for maintaining a consistent image plane, we found it extremely difficult to maintain structures of interest in the image. We therefore applied the method of active image-plane tracking (3) to the shoulder. This practice placed additional constraints on the choice of imaging parameters, as there are limited options for manipulating imaging parameters in the software coupled to the active image-plane device.

Imaging planes were determined by two factors: (*a*) interactive subject positioning in the magnet by an examiner and (*b*) active image-plane registration (MR tracking) (3). These factors are closely related because, in its initial implementation, MR tracking was limited to image planes either parallel or perpendicular to the constant magnetic induction field, B_0; images could not be prescribed in an oblique plane.

On the basis of the constrained choices among three orthogonal imaging planes, imaging-plane obliqueness to the subject's shoulder was instead achieved by rotating or shifting the subject into an oblique orientation relative to the magnet. Careful positioning was necessary to ensure that the humeral head and glenoid would both be captured on the same image, so spatial relationships could be measured. For abduction, an imaging plane oblique-coronal to the body and parallel to the supraspinatus tendon and scapula was chosen, which is analogous to choosing the plane used for oblique coronal imaging in static MR. For evaluation of internal and external rotation, an axial image plane transverse to the shoulder was used. To obtain this plane, it was necessary to try to maintain both shoulders relatively parallel to the floor, as excessive lateral leaning of the subject created oblique axial sections that frequently did not include both the humeral head and glenoid. Transaxial images were also used for evaluations of applied glenohumeral force.

MR tracking uses a specialized hardware and software configuration that includes a miniature RF coil for spatial localization of the imaging plane (3,4). In our initial implementation, a 7-mm-diameter loop of copper wire surrounded a 2-mL plastic cuvet containing dilute gadopentetate dimeglumine (Magnevist; Berlex Laboratories, Wayne, NJ) (1:200 ratio with water). The system uses a four-excitation Hadamard pulse sequence to calculate the position of the protons within the sensitive volume of the small RF coil. When run in an interleaved sequence alternating with an image acquisition, MR tracking interactively provides control over the position of the image section.

In the shoulder studies, the same examiner (C.F.B., D.K.H.) that positioned the subject in the imager adjusted the position of the MR tracking coil to capture the anatomy of interest, then taped the coil to the subject. Direct visual feedback was available via image display on LCD monitors inside the imager. The MR tracking coil was placed on the skin overlying the anterolateral aspect of the acromion for abduction and adduction maneuvers and anterior to the coracoid process for the internal and external rotation and stress maneuvers.

We adapted measurement methods initially developed for projection radiographic studies (5,6) for quantifying the relationship of the humeral head to the glenoid fossa. Initially, measurements on five shoulders were made with the imager

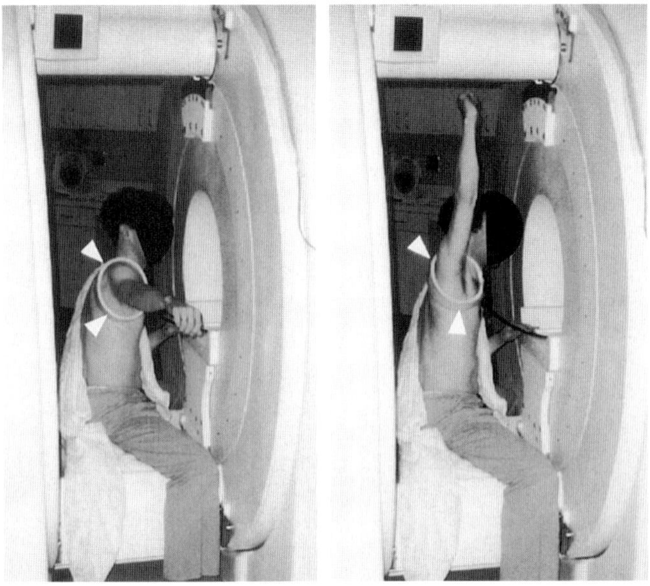

a. b.

Figure 1. Photographs demonstrate subject positioning in the vertically open MR imager. Subject sits between two doughnut-shaped magnet components, straddling the lower connector. Loop RF coil (arrowheads) is placed around the shoulder such that its magnetic field is perpendicular to the B_0 direction (left to right in these photographs). Arm position **(a)** with approximately 80° glenohumeral abduction and **(b)** with 140° abduction.

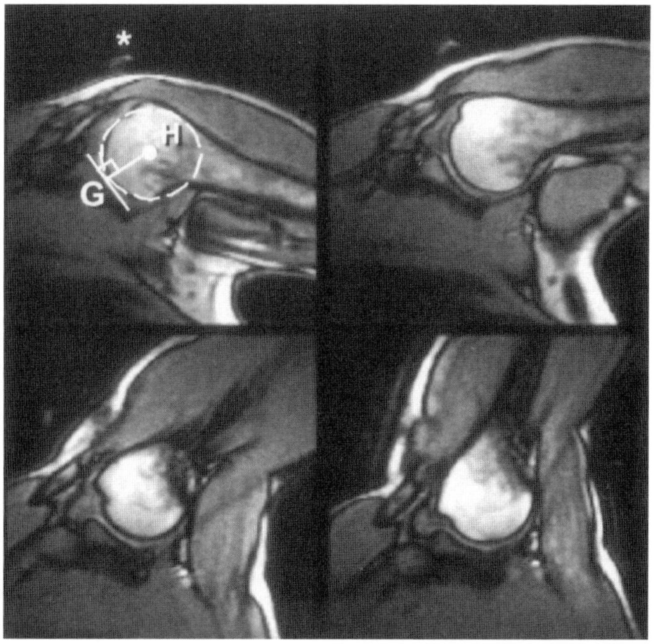

Figure 2. Representative oblique coronal fast gradient-echo dynamic MR images (19.8/7.2; flip angle, 30°) of the glenohumeral joint during abduction in an asymptomatic 26-year-old man. In the top left image, * marks the location of the MR tracking coil. Images show top left, 40°; top right, 68°; bottom left, 104°; and bottom right, 127° of total abduction. Measurement techniques are illustrated at top left, in which a circle is prescribed along the articular surface of the humeral head (*H*) to determine its geometric center (white dot). A line between the superior and inferior margins of the glenoid (*G*) is used to define its center. A perpendicular line from the humeral head center to the glenoid line allows measurement of translation in humeral head position relative to the glenoid center point. The degree of glenoid (scapular) and humeral elevation relative to the fully adducted position is determined by measuring and following the angles of the glenoid and a line prescribed along the humeral shaft (not shown) relative to the vertical axis of the image.

operating console by using standard geometric constructions and measurement tools. Because this process was tedious and because we wanted an offline system for analysis, subsequent measurements were made with macros written for NIH IMAGE software (National Institutes of Health, Bethesda, Md) operating on Macintosh desktop computers (Apple Computers, Cupertino, Calif). Most of the measurements reported were performed by one author (D.K.H.), with some completed by another (C.F.B.). No systematic studies of intra- or interobserver variability in the measurements have been done.

The humeral head center was determined by prescribing a circle on the humeral articular surface. The center of the circle was then defined as the center of the head. This method has been validated in earlier studies and relies on the uniformity of the radius of curvature or the relative sphericity of the humeral articular surface (6). The margins of the glenoid were used to construct a line along and parallel to the glenoid fossa; the geometric center of this line determined the center of the glenoid. To do this, care was taken to not include the glenoid labrum or portions of the joint capsule in the line.

Humeral head centering on the glenoid was determined by constructing a perpendicular line from the humeral head center to the glenoid line. By measuring the position of intersection of this perpendicular line with the glenoid line, a linear position of the humeral head along the glenoid was established for any shoulder position. During imaging, we used active image-plane tracking to maintain the midglenoid in the image plane. Findings of preliminary studies showed that the humeral head remained centered on the glenoid whether measured in axial or oblique coronal sections to the glenoid. Given this and the symmetry of the glenoid, we did not observe systematic changes in measurements of humeral position when images were not obtained precisely through the glenoid center.

Another parameter needed to characterize the glenohumeral motion pattern was the position of the long axis of the humerus relative to the subject's body. For abduction and adduction, imaging started with the subject in the position of maximum adduction; this point was defined as 0° abduction. During normal abduction, overall humeral elevation occurs as a result of two coupled mechanisms—the glenohumeral and scapulothoracic components of abduction (6). The glenohumeral component is a result of humeral rotation on the glenoid. The scapulothoracic component is a result of scapular rotation on the thorax. Initially, abduction is primarily a result of glenohumeral motion, with scapulothoracic motion composing the latter stages.

In MR imaging in the coronal oblique plane, glenohumeral motion primarily changes the angle of the humeral shaft with respect to an external reference (as long as the subject's body maintains a similar position), and scapulothoracic motion primarily changes the angle of the glenoid face relative to the external reference. We measured each of these components separately; however, for this report, their combined effect, or the net change in humeral angle relative to baseline, was recorded for each increment of motion.

For internal and external rotation maneuvers, imaging began with the patient's shoulder in a position of maximum internal rotation. Degree of humeral rotation was determined by measuring the angle between the center of the humeral head and the bicipital groove. By using a convention established by Davis and colleagues (7), we defined 0° of rotation as the point where a line connecting the humeral head center and the bicipital groove was parallel to the glenoid face.

Measurements of glenohumeral translation with stress applied to the humeral head were analogous to those of internal and external rotation motions performed by the patient. The humerus was kept in a position of neutral (0°) rotation and adduction during these maneuvers.

In an attempt to apply reproducible stress to each of the subjects, the maneuvers were performed by a single examiner (C.F.B.), and subjects were asked to relax their muscles during the test. Despite this practice, it was difficult to ensure that the same amount of stress was applied to each subject; the results should be viewed with this potential lack of reproducibility in mind.

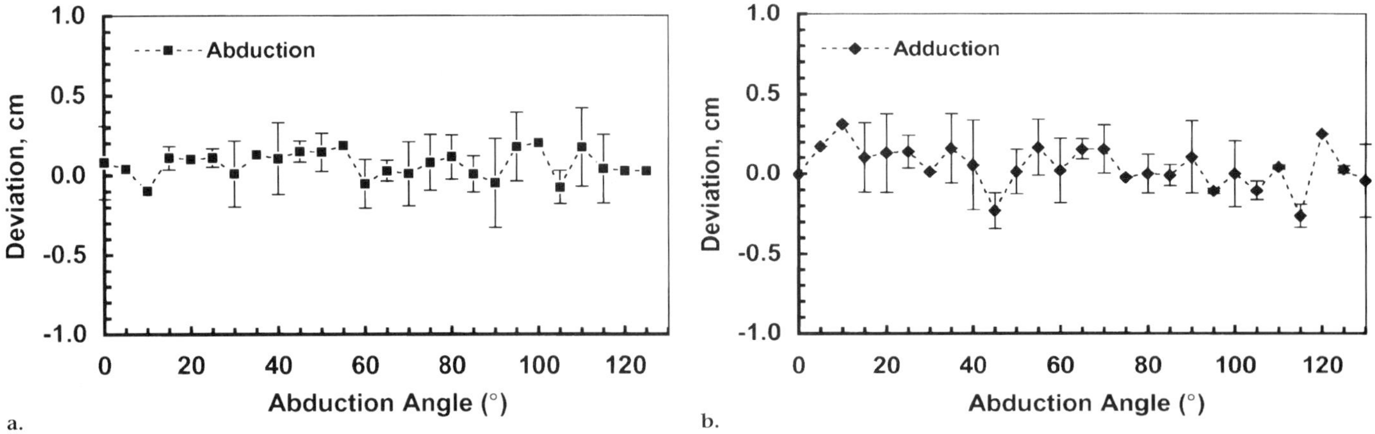

Figure 3. Graphs demonstrate glenohumeral motion patterns with **(a)** abduction and **(b)** adduction. For both abduction and adduction, the humeral head remained well centered on the glenoid, with fluctuations in position on the same order of magnitude as SDs of the measurements. Measurements of humeral head position relative to the center of the glenoid were made on serial oblique coronal images acquired during abduction and adduction motion in 10 asymptomatic shoulders. The glenoid center point is represented by 0 cm on the y axis. Positive translations from 0 cm indicate superior shifting of the humeral head, and negative values indicate inferior shifting. Data for different volunteers were pooled by breaking the abduction or adduction motion into 5° intervals and determining the mean humeral head position across patients within each angular increment. Individual data points represent, on average, three measurements within the increment of abduction or adduction (mean, 3.0 measurements ± 1.9; range, one to seven measurements). Vertical bars show the SD of the mean for each point.

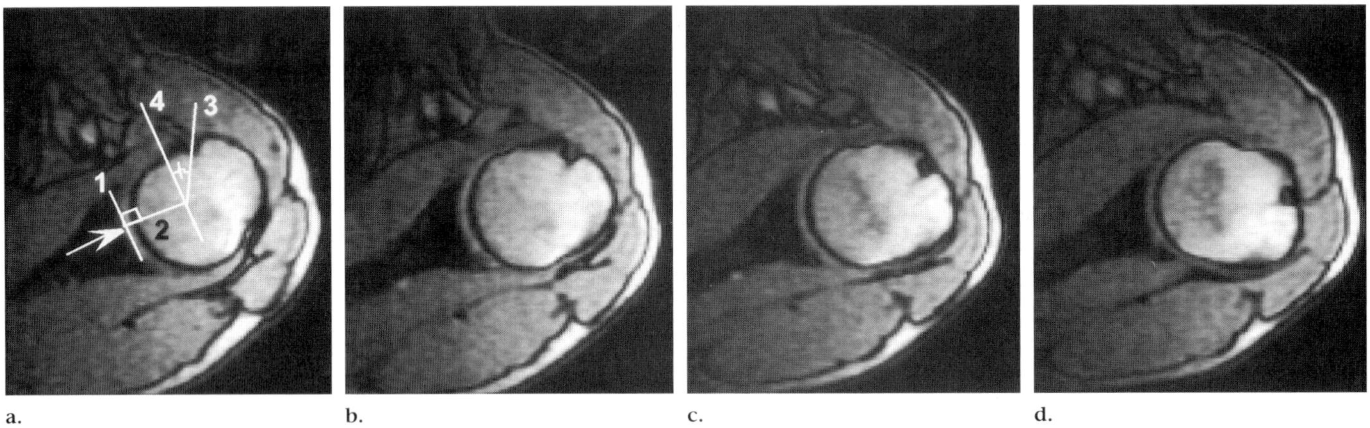

Figure 4. Transaxial fast gradient-echo dynamic MR images (19.8/7.2; flip angle, 30°) obtained through the center of the glenohumeral joint during internal and external rotation. Images show **(a)** 24°, **(b)** 48°, **(c)** 61°, and **(d)** 99° of external rotation. Measurement techniques are illustrated in **a**, in which a line defined by the anterior and posterior margins of the glenoid (*1*) determines its center point (arrow); another line perpendicular to the line through the humeral head defines the humeral head centering on the glenoid for different degrees of internal or external rotation (*2*). By using a line from the humeral head center through the bicipital groove (*3*), the rotation angle is determined relative to a line parallel to the glenoid face (*4*), identified as 0° rotation (6).

RESULTS

Abduction and Adduction

Subjects were positioned in the imager as shown in Figure 1. The torso was rotated from the position illustrated to obtain images directly coronal to the glenohumeral joint. The MR tracking device was applied to the anterior aspect of the acromion. Sequential MR images were rapidly obtained (15–20 images each for abduction and adduction) while the subjects slowly but continuously abducted or adducted the arm. Figure 2 presents selected images illustrating 40°–105° of abduction in one subject.

For each shoulder, a subset of images was analyzed quantitatively for humeral head position relative to the glenoid center by using methods described earlier and illustrated in Figure 2, top left image. Some images were unsuitable for measurement because of motion artifacts; others were unsuitable because they did not simultaneously display the humeral head and both superior and inferior margins of the glenoid.

For the 10 shoulders studied, the mean number of images per shoulder analyzed during abduction was 10.9 ± 3.1 (SD), with a range of seven to 17 images; during adduction, the mean was 9.1 images ± 2.2, with a range of six to 11 images.

By plotting humeral head position on the glenoid as a function of the total abduction angle (including both glenohumeral and scapulothoracic components), one obtains graphs such as those in Figure 3a for abduction and Figure 3b for adduction. Notice that, over the full range of motion, the humeral head remained centered on the glenoid, deviating from

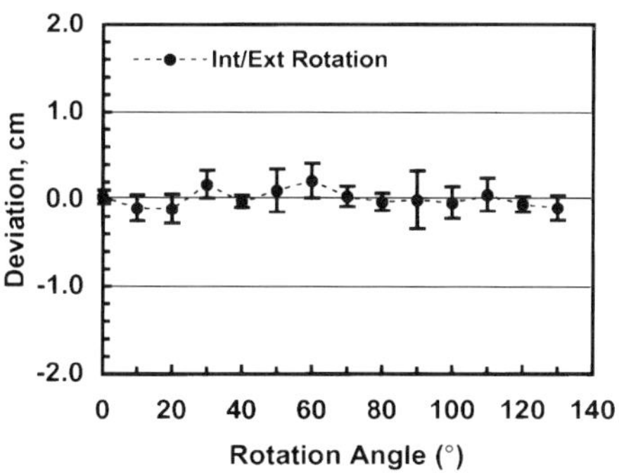

Figure 5. Graph demonstrates glenohumeral motion patterns with internal and external (*Int/Ext*) rotation. Deviation in humeral head centering relative to the glenoid center is plotted as a function of the rotation angle. Measurements for the 10 shoulders were pooled by dividing the rotation motion into 10° increments; the mean was calculated by averaging across patients within each rotation increment. Each data point represents the mean of three to five individual measurements on a given shoulder. Vertical bars indicate SD from the mean for each value. Note that for these normal shoulders, the humeral head remained well centered on the glenoid during internal and external rotation.

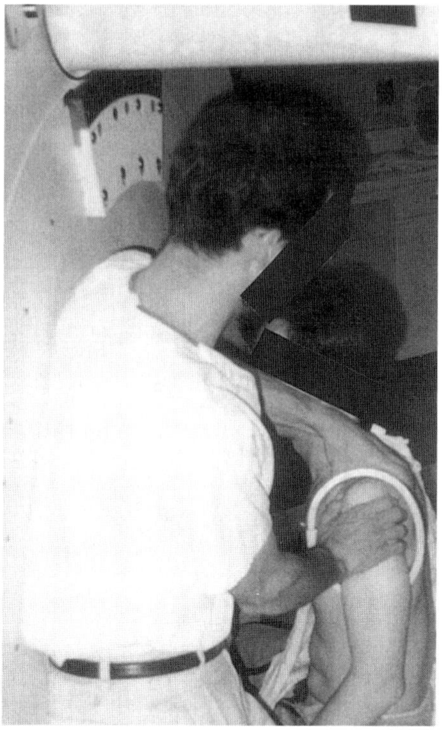

Figure 6. Photograph obtained at physical examination during MR imaging. Subject is seated with left shoulder toward the examiner. Examiner uses one hand to stabilize the scapula while the other applies anteroposterior or posteroanterior force to the humeral head.

the glenoid center point, on average, less than 0.3 cm over the entire motion. Minor fluctuations in humeral head centering were within the range of the SD of the measurements, as shown in the graphs. For the 10 shoulders, the mean amount of maximal abduction was 119° ± 19, with a range of 95°–155°.

Internal and External Rotation

Active internal and external rotation of the humerus was performed in the adducted position while successive axial images were acquired. The MR tracking coil was applied to the skin overlying the coracoid process at an image level simultaneously depicting the anterior and posterior margins of the glenoid fossa and the humeral head at a level showing the bicipital groove. Ten to 15 images were acquired for each shoulder during external rotation, followed by a similar number of images during internal rotation. Figure 4 shows representative images in one shoulder, illustrating from 24° to 99° of external rotation, with 0°, or neutral, rotation defined as the point where the line through the bicipital groove is parallel to the glenoid (7).

For the 10 shoulders studied, the graph in Figure 5 plots the humeral head position on the glenoid as a function of the rotation angle for the external rotation maneuver. Results for internal rotation were similar. As with abduction and adduction, the humeral head remained precisely centered on the glenoid during the entire range of motion, deviating, on average, less than 0.4 cm from the glenoid center. In the shoulders studied, the mean maximum amount of external rotation was 115° ± 13, with a range of 100°–140°.

Stress Testing

Physical examination during MR imaging was performed by a physician who applied a direct manual force to the subject's humeral head in an anteroposterior followed by posteroanterior direction during sequential imaging, as illustrated in Figure 6. Subjects had the arm adducted and in neutral rotation. In the early phases of these studies, it was difficult to coordinate direct physical manipulation with MR imaging. This was largely due to the logistic challenges of applying an appropriately directed force to the humeral head while stabilizing the subject's scapula with the opposite hand and maintaining the imaging plane of interest.

Figure 7 shows axial images obtained without applied force and images then obtained with the examiner applying anteroposterior or posteroanterior force to the humeral head. In the subject, an asymptomatic 28-year-old woman, application of anteroposterior force resulted in 6 mm of posterior humeral translation; application of posteroanterior force resulted in 4 mm of anterior translation.

Figure 8 summarizes the results of stress testing for nine of the 10 shoulders studied. In the 10th shoulder, image review showed that the examiner's hands were not appropriately positioned to apply adequate stress; thus, data for that shoulder were excluded. It is evident from Figure 8 that application of external force to the relatively relaxed shoulder caused measurable translation of the humerus on the glenoid. However, the SDs of the measurements were large, as indicated by the error bars. For anteroposterior force, the mean posterior translation was 4.6 mm ± 5.6, with a range of 0.1–13.4 mm. For posteroanterior force, the mean anterior translation was 4.5 mm ± 2.5, with a range of 1.0–6.0 mm.

DISCUSSION

Instability of the glenohumeral joint is a common condition that leads to pain and functional impairment in a large number of individuals (1). While static MR imaging and MR arthrography can routinely provide detailed anatomic images (8), direct correlation of imaging findings with a specific patient's symptoms is difficult. Some useful information on glenohumeral motion has been derived from radiographic studies (5,6,9). However, there has been no direct means of dynamically evaluating shoulder motion on cross-sectional images that simultaneously display osseous and soft-tissue structures.

We hypothesize that MR imaging of the shoulder during active joint motion, in which normal structures are engaged in their intended functions to restrain glenohumeral translation, will provide relatively direct insight into glenohumeral biomechanics. While ultimately the goal is to better understand the relationship between specific anatomic lesions and pathologic motion patterns, normal baselines with which to compare abnormal findings must be established.

The results of this study show that a vertically open MR system was capable of allowing dynamic joint evaluation over a wide range of physiologic motion. We have established imaging protocols and methods for quantitative assessment of glenohumeral relationships. In addition, we have begun to practice a form of joint assessment—physical examination during MR imaging.

In studies of abduction and adduction (Figs 1–3), the humeral head remained precisely centered in the glenoid fossa over a wide range of motion. These results concur with those of radiographic studies, although little directly comparable information is available (5,6). Investigators in reported series utilized incremental motion and static radiographs, which may not be appropriate comparisons to the slow but continuous motion we employed.

An additional facet of shoulder motion that can eventually be derived from dynamic MR studies is the relative contributions of the glenohumeral and scapulothoracic components of abduction. This report combines these two components into a net abduction. Separating the components, particularly with regard to differences between subjects and those with altered shoulder mechanics such as large rotator cuff tears (10), will be of interest in the future.

In studies of internal and external rotation of the humerus, the humeral head remained precisely centered in the glenoid over the full range of physiologic motion (Figs 4, 5). This result is similar to that of a static radiographic study by Howell and colleagues (5) of glenohumeral motion in the axial plane.

Use of conventional narrow-bore MR systems in so-called kinematic MR imaging of the shoulder has been reported for asymptomatic subjects. The kinematic technique refers to simulation of dynamic motion by playing multiple static images in a cine loop. These studies may not be directly comparable with ours, because in kinematic studies the muscle groups are typically relaxed. Sans and colleagues (11) performed kinematic MR imaging on 39 shoulders during internal and external rotation and characterized the shape and signal intensity of the labrum and labral position. Imaging time was 32 seconds per position. No quantitative measures of humeral head position on the glenoid were reported. Similar qualitative features were reported by Cardinal and colleagues (12) and by Bonutti and colleagues (13), but again, no quantitation of glenohumeral position was reported.

Whereas previous studies have emphasized morphologic assessments, our work focuses on quantitation of motion patterns during slow but continuous motion initiated and maintained by the subject without the use of a positioning device or restraint. Ideally, further studies will allow integration of morphologic, signal intensity, and quantitative observations together and lead to a comprehensive assessment. Along these lines, it is worth pointing out that a full understanding of dynamic joint motion may require image display and review in a dynamic fashion to appreciate subtle motion features.

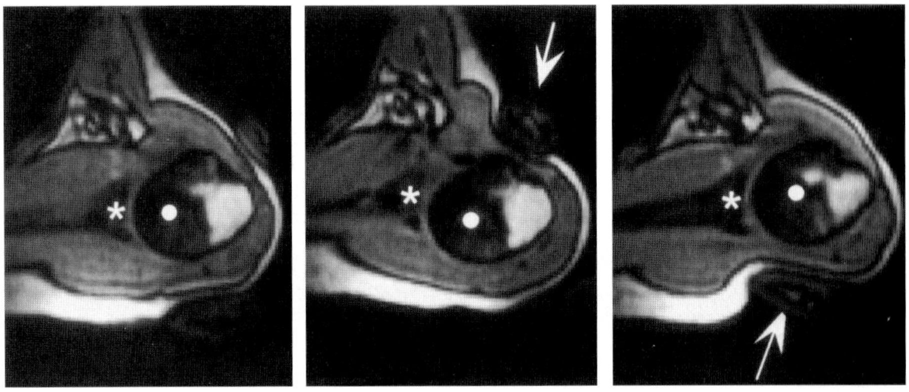

a. b. c.

Figure 7. Transaxial fast gradient-echo dynamic MR images (19.8/7.2; flip angle, 30°) of the glenohumeral joint obtained during application of force to the humeral head by a physician examiner. The subject was an asymptomatic 28-year-old woman. Images obtained with **(a)** no external force applied, **(b)** anteroposterior force on the humeral head (arrow), and **(c)** posteroanterior force on the humeral head (arrow). The center of the humeral head is indicated by a dot and the glenoid center by *. Measurement methods analogous to those used to obtain Figure 2 were used to quantify glenohumeral relationships. In **b**, the center of the humerus shifted 6 mm posteriorly relative to the glenoid center. In **c**, the center of the humeral head shifted 4 mm anteriorly relative to the glenoid center.

We report on dynamic MR imaging of the glenohumeral joint during actual physical manipulation by a physician examiner. This is an exciting aspect of open MR imaging that may have broad potential applications. In principle, the addition of objective anatomic and dynamic information to physical examination maneuvers can provide insights into clinical signs and maneuvers whose exact anatomic basis has only been inferred.

Initial attempts at application of anteroposterior or posteroanterior force to the humeral head to evaluate translation were encouraging, although the maneuvers were initially challenging to perform. As our experience has increased, physical examination and manipulation during MR imaging appears to be routinely feasible. Unquestionably, a learning process is involved, much like learning physical examination or patient-interactive imaging such as ultrasonography.

It is important to point out that it is unknown whether application of force to a relatively relaxed shoulder provides clinically relevant information, as individuals may exhibit joint laxity but not suffer from the clinical problem of instability (14). Further studies on the reproducibility of stress testing in asymptomatic and symptomatic subjects, as well as between examining physicians, will be necessary, as the large SDs in Figure 8 most likely reflect inherent variability in the maneuvers.

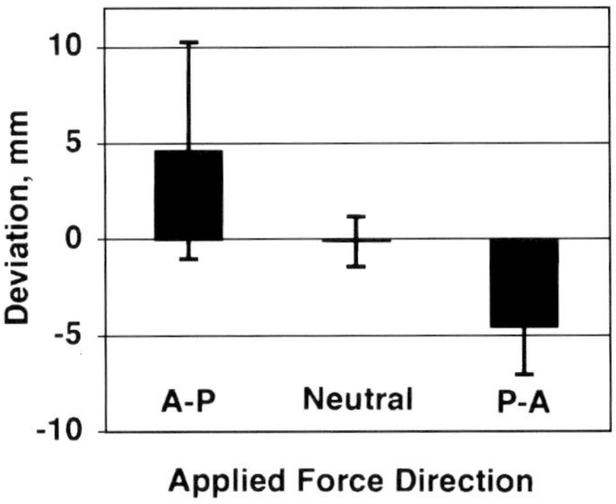

Figure 8. Bar graph demonstrates glenohumeral deviation with stress testing. Mean values for humeral head deviation from the center of the glenoid were determined by averaging measurements across nine shoulders. Vertical bars indicate SD for the measurements. Note that a mean of approximately 4.5 mm deviation from the center was observed for both anteroposterior and posteroanterior forces. SDs, however, were relatively large, reflecting individual subject variations or differences in the amount of stress applied by the examiner. *A-P* = anteroposteriorly directed force, as illustrated in Figure 7b; *Neutral* = no force applied; *P-A* = posteroanteriorly directed force, as illustrated in Figure 7c.

Key advantages of open MR imaging with rapid imaging time include the ability for patients to undergo a wide range of active joint motion and physical examination during MR imaging. With fast imaging, one pays a price of diminished signal-to-noise ratio and spatial resolution relative to longer-duration images in higher field strength magnets. In addition, the image contrast is currently limited, which produces images with T1 or spin-density weighting in the very short repetition time and echo time regime.

Advances in pulse programming, such as the introduction of preparation pulses, may help overcome current imaging contrast limitations. Another notable technical development that enabled the performance of the current study is the use of active image-plane MR tracking (3,4). This permits placement of an MR tracking coil on the patient's skin, with spatial localization of the coil by RF pulses used to define the position of an axial, sagittal, or coronal plane.

At the time the current study was performed, the software coupled to this tracking device was limited in that only imaging planes parallel or perpendicular to the constant magnetic induction field, B_0, of the magnet could be obtained. More recent versions of the tracking software enable use of oblique imaging and multiple tracking devices, which will aid in patient positioning and selection of imaging axes (Dumoulin CL, personal communication, 1999). The interactive MR examination is currently a demanding undertaking in which an examiner actively positions the patient to obtain a desired image plane relative to the body and manipulates the MR tracking device to select a specific level of interest. Also, transferring the images to a separate computer and performing the measurements is tedious and time-consuming. With further experience, it is hoped that a comprehensive examination can be performed in a reasonable amount of time.

Our study had a number of limitations. First, the results reported were for a small number of subjects in a young age group and included both female and male volunteers. Age, sex, and dominance of the extremity may influence glenohumeral motion patterns and need to be studied further.

Second, the motions studied were confined to single-plane motions that do not entirely mimic everyday shoulder motion. Measurements were also confined to the planes of motion, such that for abduction and adduction we measured the superoinferior centering of the humerus on the glenoid but did not test for possible shifts in the anteroposterior plane.

Third, while we were able to obtain images during continuous movement, the motion was slow relative to the dynamic and ballistic movements that may give rise to pain in the shoulder in patients, particularly in athletes (15). As always, faster imaging is desirable, as long as crucial anatomic and signal intensity information is not sacrificed. Along these lines, preliminary results with "fluoroscopic" MR sequences are encouraging (16).

Finally, the measurements reported have not been evaluated for intra- or interobserver variability. We plan to continue to characterize normal motion patterns and validate the measurement methods described in this preliminary work.

In conclusion, our preliminary experience with dynamic, physiologic MR imaging during glenohumeral motion is very encouraging. Further experience with asymptomatic and symptomatic subjects will be necessary to prove that the techniques are clinically relevant. Technologic advances in the form of more flexible MR tracking devices and optimized MR pulse sequences will be helpful. We are optimistic that open MR imaging can provide useful insights into not only normal joint function but also altered mechanics in patients with instability. As we begin to examine symptomatic individuals, having a clear idea of motion patterns in asymptomatic subjects will be a requisite.

Acknowledgments: Some of the initial imaging was performed at L'Hôpital St François d'Assise, Quebec City, Canada, and our accommodation, especially by Jean-Marie Moutquin, MD, and Marie Dufour, MD, is gratefully acknowledged. The excellent technical assistance of Claudia Cooper, RT, is sincerely appreciated. Thanks to Andrew Pearle, MD, for helping to develop the tip-tracking apparatus. In addition, we acknowledge infrastructure support from the Packard Foundation (Los Altos, Calif), the Lucas Foundation (Menlo Park, Calif), and the Phil N. Allen Trust (Menlo Park, Calif).

References

1. Matsen FA, Harryman DT, Sidles JA. Mechanics of glenohumeral instability. Clin Sports Med 1991; 10:783–788.
2. Jolesz FA. Image-guided procedures and the operating room of the future. Radiology 1997; 204:601–612.
3. Dumoulin CL, Souza SP, Darrow RD. Real time position monitoring of invasive devices using magnetic resonance. Magn Reson Med 1993; 29:411–415.
4. Daniel BL, Norbash AM, Butts K, et al. Active scan plane registration during dynamic musculoskeletal MR-imaging using an external MR-tracking coil (abstr). In: Proceedings of the Fifth Meeting of the International Society for Magnetic Resonance in Medicine. Berkeley, Calif: International Society for Magnetic Resonance in Medicine, 1997; 1927.
5. Howell SM, Galinat BJ, Renzi AJ, Marone PJ. Normal and abnormal mechanics of the glenohumeral joint in the horizontal plane. J Bone Joint Surg [Am] 1988; 70: 227–232.
6. Poppen NK, Walker PS. Normal and abnormal motion of the shoulder. J Bone Joint Surg [Am] 1976; 58:195–201.
7. Davis SJ, Teresi LM, Bradley WG, Ressler JA, Eto RT. Effect of arm rotation on MR imaging of the rotator cuff. Radiology 1991; 181:265–268.
8. Palmer WE, Brown JH, Rosenthal DI. Labral-ligamentous complex of the shoulder: evaluation with MR arthrography. Radiology 1994; 190:645–651.
9. Ozaki J. Glenohumeral movements of the involuntary inferior and multidirectional instability. Clin Orthop 1989; 238:107–111.
10. Burkhart SS. Fluoroscopic comparison of kinematic patterns in massive rotator cuff tears: a suspension bridge model. Clin Orthop 1991; 284:144–152.
11. Sans N, Richardi G, Railhac JJ, et al. Kinematic MR imaging of the shoulder: normal patterns. AJR 1996; 167:1517–1522.
12. Cardinal E, Buckwalter KA, Braunstein EM. Kinematic magnetic resonance imaging of the normal shoulder: assessment of the labrum and capsule. Can Assoc Radiol J 1996; 47:44–50.
13. Bonutti PM, Norfray JF, Friedman RJ, Genez BM. Kinematic MRI of the shoulder. J Comput Assist Tomogr 1993; 17:666–669.
14. Harryman DT, Sidles JA, Clark JM, McQuade KJ, Gibb TD, Matsen FA. Translation of the humeral head on the glenoid with passive glenohumeral motion. J Bone Joint Surg [Am] 1990; 72:1334–1443.
15. Bonci CM, Hensal FJ, Torg JS. A preliminary study on the measurement of static and dynamic motion at the glenohumeral joint. Am J Sports Med 1986; 14: 12–17.
16. Butts RK, Pauly JM, Kerr AB, Bergman AG, Beaulieu CF. Real-time MR imaging of joint motion on an open MR imaging scanner (abstr). Radiology 1997; 205(P): 387.

Diagnosis Please

Peter L. Choyke, MD
John L. Doppman, MD

Case 18[1]

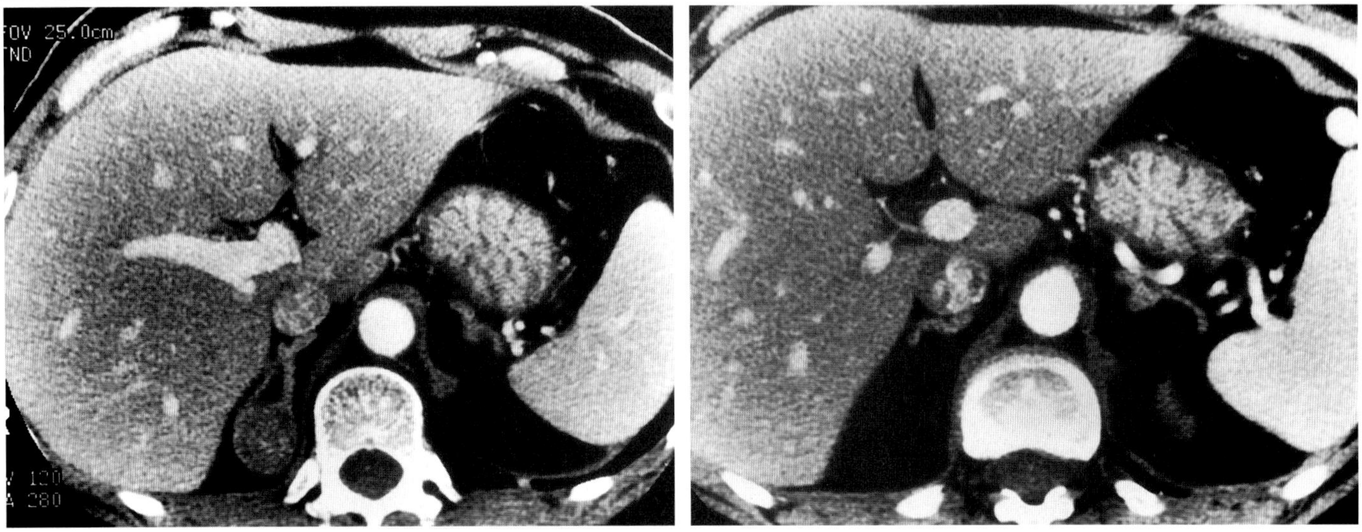

a. b.

Figure 1. Contrast material–enhanced CT scans of the abdomen at two levels.

HISTORY

A 45-year-old woman presented with a history of central obesity and blood pressure of 160/105 mm Hg. Computed tomographic (CT) scans of the abdomen (Fig 1) and a magnetic resonance (MR) image of the pituitary gland (Fig 2) were obtained.

(continued)

Index term:
Diagnosis please

Radiology 1999; 212:706–707

[1] From the Department of Diagnostic Radiology, Imaging Sciences Program, Clinical Center, National Institutes of Health, Bldg 10, Rm 1C660, 10 Center Dr, MSC 1182, Bethesda, MD 20892-1182. Received August 28, 1998; revision requested September 25; revision received October 26; accepted April 6, 1999. **Address reprint requests to** P.L.C. (e-mail: *pchoyke@nih.gov*).

E-mail the most likely diagnosis to *dxplease@rsna.org* (use ***only*** for submission of diagnosis). Include case number, your name (as you would want it to appear in the journal), address, phone and fax numbers. Only one case, one name, and one diagnosis per e-mail submission. Multiple diagnoses, multiple submissions, submissions without a case number will not be considered. ***Deadline***: November 15, 1999. Answer will appear in the January 2000 issue. Authors wishing to submit cases for Diagnosis Please should first write to the Editor to obtain approval for the case and further information.

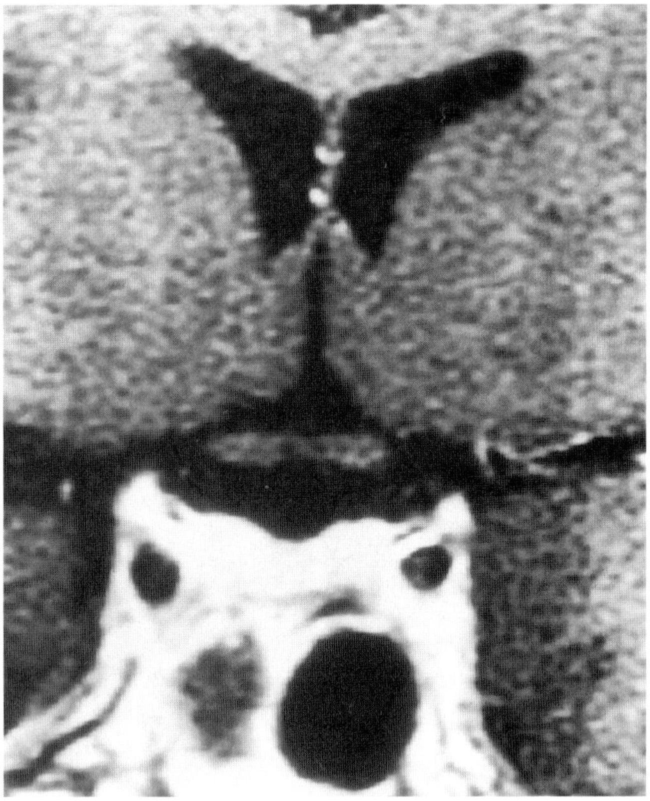

Figure 2. Gadolinium-enhanced coronal T1-weighted (repetition time, 400 msec; echo time, 11 msec) MR image.

Avinash R. A. Balkissoon, MB, BS, FRCR
Curtis W. Hayes, MD

Case 14: Intramedullary Osteosclerosis[1]

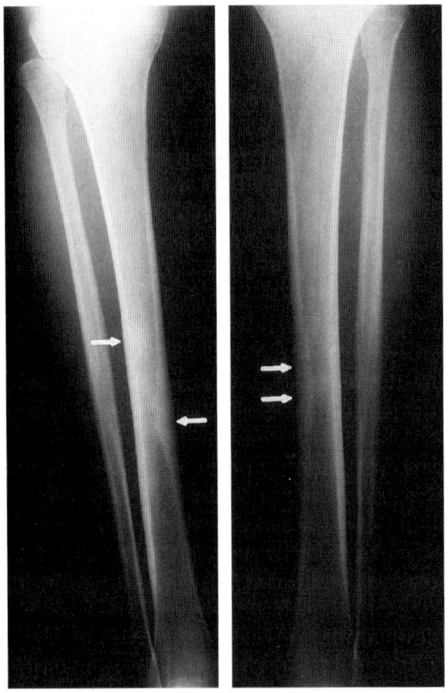

a. b.

Figure 1. Frontal radiographs of the **(a)** right and **(b)** left legs demonstrate bilateral asymmetric midtibial shaft scleroses (arrows), predominantly endosteal, more marked on the right side.

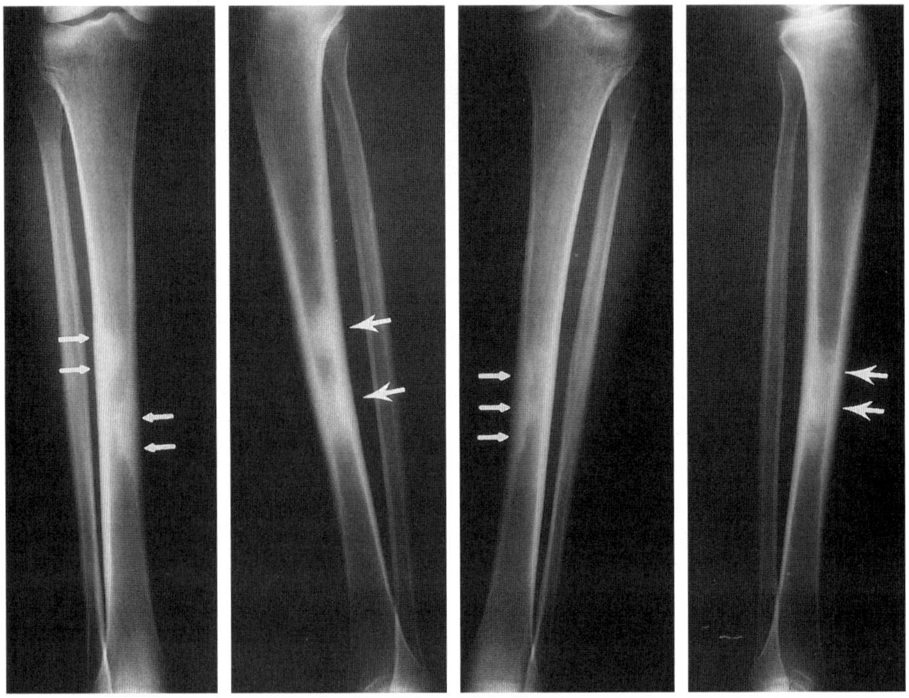

a. b. c. d.

Figure 2. **(a)** Frontal and **(b)** lateral radiographs of the right leg and **(c)** frontal and **(d)** lateral radiographs of the left leg obtained 1 year after the radiographs in Figure 1 demonstrate bilateral increase in the midtibial undulating endosteal scleroses (arrows). The lesions remain confined to the diaphyses.

Index terms:
Bones, sclerosis, 45.155, 45.599
Diagnosis please
Tibia, 45.599

Radiology 1999; 212:708–710

[1] From the Department of Radiology, Medical College of Virginia of Virginia Commonwealth University, 401 N 12th St, Richmond, VA 23298-0615. Received May 7, 1998; revision requested June 17; revision received July 28; accepted December 16. **Address reprint requests to** A.R.A.B. (e-mail: *avirb@yahoo.com*).

HISTORY

A 39-year-old woman experienced intermittent severe pain in both lower legs for several years. The pain alternated from side to side and had been worsening over the past 6 months. The woman was otherwise healthy; results of all laboratory tests were normal. In terms of activity, the woman was an avid "power walker," although she had to curtail this activity owing to pain. There was no relevant past medical or family history.

Radiographs of both lower legs were obtained 1 year apart. Findings on a radionuclide bone scan, not shown here, were positive only in the areas of abnormality seen on the radiographs.

IMAGING FINDINGS

The initial radiographs demonstrated bilateral asymmetric midtibial and minimal fibular shaft endosteal cortical scleroses

(Fig 1). There was no substantial soft-tissue abnormality. There was no focal area of lysis and no extension to the metaphyses.

Radiographs obtained 1 year later show progression of the endosteal scleroses with partial obliteration of the medullary space and mild progression along the diaphyses (Fig 2).

DISCUSSION

The differential considerations for bone sclerosis are extensive, but the radiographic distribution in association with clinical and laboratory findings can substantially narrow the possibilities (1). In view of the history of power walking, stress fractures would be a major consideration. However, the continued progression of endosteal sclerosis and extensive involvement along the shaft of the bone would be extremely unusual. The bilateral nature of the process and the benign nature of the cortical thickening would make a malignancy such as lymphoma or osteosarcoma highly unlikely. Multifocal osteoid osteomas have been reported but are extremely rare. The absence of a focal area of lysis and the circumferential pattern of bone formation would make this possibility very unlikely. Chronic multifocal sclerosing osteomyelitis would be highly unusual in a healthy adult with no abnormal laboratory test results, such as elevated erythrocyte sedimentation rate or white blood cell count. This condition is more common in children and adolescents and tends to involve the metaphysis of tubular bones with recurrent attacks of pain and swelling.

Metabolic and endocrine disorders that require consideration include renal osteodystrophy, hypervitaminosis A, pseudohypoparathyroidism, and pseudopseudohypoparathyroidism. Renal osteodystrophy usually causes diffuse sclerosis along with the usual gamut of other bone and soft-tissue changes. Normal laboratory and clinical features virtually exclude this disease. Hypervitaminosis A is characterized by periosteal new bone deposition in contrast to the mainly endosteal deposition seen in this patient. Other characteristic features of hypervitaminosis A include soft-tissue nodules and swollen tender limbs, not present in this patient. Pseudohypoparathyroidism and pseudopseudohypoparathyroidism manifest in childhood and are associated with characteristic shortening of the metacarpals, as well as areas of soft-tissue calcification and a more diffuse sclerosis. Pseudohypoparathyroidism is associated with hypocalcemia, whereas the serum calcium is normal in psuedopsuedohypoparathyroidism.

Congenital or developmental diseases to consider include Chester-Erdheim disease, a lipogranulomatous disorder characterized by reactive diffuse, symmetric new bone formation. Unlike in this patient, this disease affects the metaphysis and the diaphysis. Familial hyperphosphatasemia is characterized by diffuse sclerosis of the cortical surfaces of long bones with wide, coarse medullary cavities. Bowing deformities and fractures are common. The appearance may mimic Paget disease in a young patient and is characterized by sustained elevation of serum alkaline phosphatase.

The sclerosing bone dysplasias are a poorly understood group of developmental anomalies, much of the cause of which is still obscure. The conditions constituting this group are enostosis (bone island), osteopoikilosis, osteopathia striata (Voorhoeve disease), osteopetrosis (Albers-Schönberg disease), pyknodysostosis (Maroteaux-Lamy disease), progressive diaphyseal dysplasia (Camurati-Engelmann disease), hereditary multiple diaphyseal dysplasia (Ribbing disease), intramedullary osteosclerosis, hyperostosis corticalis generalisata (van Buchem syndrome), metaphyseal dysplasia (Pyle disease), craniometaphyseal dysplasia, melorheostosis (Leri-Weill disease), craniodiaphyseal dysplasia, and sclerosteosis.

Of this list, enostosis, osteopoikilosis, and osteopathia striata can be excluded easily on the basis of radiographic appearance. Osteopetrosis is invariably more diffuse with common involvement of the axial skeleton and the tendency for Erlenmeyer flask deformities and a bone-in-bone appearance. Pyknodysostosis manifests in childhood with dwarfism and generalized osteosclerosis, wormian bones, small facial bones, and obtuse mandibular angle. Van Buchem syndrome, a rare autosomal recessive abnormality, has been described in both adults and children and simulates acromegaly. It is characterized by diffuse medullary and cortical sclerosis with sparing of the spine. In addition, there is an elevation of alkaline phosphatase levels. In melorheostosis, dense new bone is deposited on long bones, with a tendency for sclerotome distribution, and is almost always monomelic.

Pyle disease and craniometaphyseal dysplasia may simulate osteopetrosis at birth, but in the adult there is a tendency for constriction of the diaphysis and flaring (Erlenmeyer flask deformity) of the metaphysis. The spine may demonstrate platyspondylia with central vertebral body sclerosis and varying amounts of face and skull sclerosis and vault thickening. In craniodiaphyseal dysplasia, there is marked sclerosis of the skull and facial bones with diaphyseal expansion of tubular bones, ribs, and the clavicle. The patients are mentally retarded, and inheritance is autosomal recessive. Osteosclerosis is an autosomal dominant condition with bone changes similar to those seen with van Buchem syndrome but with normal alkaline phosphatase levels. In sclerosteosis, there is general bone overgrowth of the skull, mandible, pelvis, and spine in addition to the long and short bones.

In this patient, the three main differential considerations would be hereditary multiple diaphyseal dysplasia (Ribbing disease), progressive diaphyseal dysplasia (Camurati-Engelmann disease), and intramedullary osteosclerosis. Both dysplasias are characterized by endosteal and periosteal new bone formation along the diaphysis of long bones, most commonly involving the lower extremities. The conditions can be distinguished on clinical grounds.

Camurati-Engelmann disease (2–4), an autosomal dominant disorder, manifests during childhood; is bilateral and symmetric; and is characterized by pain, progressive muscle weakness, and a waddling gait. Also, because the disease affects bones formed by intramembranous ossification, the skull is often affected in the later stages. The disease begins in the diaphysis of long bones but may eventually spread to the metaphysis. Bone biopsy results demonstrate trabecular thickening and both osteoblasts and osteoclasts. In view of the limited sites of involvement, normal gait, and older age of appearance, this would be unlikely.

Ribbing disease (5–7) manifests in middle age as a unilateral or bilateral and asymmetric asymptomatic to moderately painful condition, usually of the lower extremity. Pain when present is usually unresponsive to nonsteroidal antiinflammatory drugs. The inheritance is probably autosomal recessive, and other family members are usually affected. Laboratory test results, including erythrocyte sedimentation rate, complete blood cell count, and serum alkaline phosphatase level, are within normal limits. Histopathologic findings of bone biopsy are nonspecific and demonstrate only osteoblastic activity and progressive obstruction of the haversian canals.

In 1988, a condition termed "intramedullary osteosclerosis" was described (8). This condition is characterized by mild to moderate pain in the legs, which increases with physical activity. As with Ribbing disease and Camurati-Englemann disease, laboratory values are within normal limits. The radiographic appearance is almost identical to that of Ribbing disease, with intramedullary sclerosis within the middle or distal portions of the tibia and the fibula (9). This condition may be unilateral or bilateral and can manifest at any age. There is, however, no substantial periosteal reaction, and most useful in the differentiation from Ribbing disease is a lack of family history, because this is a nonhereditary idiopathic condition.

On the basis of the radiographic appearance alone, hereditary multiple diaphyseal dysplasia and intramedullary osteosclerosis may be identical. However, the lack of a family history to support the hereditary nature of the disease makes the former condition less likely, and intramedullary osteosclerosis is thus the most likely diagnosis.

References

1. Jacobson HG. Dense bone—too much bone: radiological considerations and differential diagnosis. Skeletal Radiol 1985; 13:1–20.
2. Hild JR. Progressive diaphyseal dysplasia (Engelmann's disease). Radiology 1956; 67:233–240.
3. Sparkes RS, Graham CB. Camurati-Englemann disease: genetics and clinical manifestations with a review of the literature. J Med Genet 1972; 9:73–85.
4. Kaftori JK, Kleinhaus U, Naveh Y. Progressive diaphyseal dysplasia (Camurati-Englemann): radiographic follow-up and CT findings. Radiology 1987; 164:777–782.
5. Seeger LL, Hewel KC, Yao L, et al. Ribbing disease (multiple diaphyseal sclerosis): imaging and differential diagnosis. AJR 1996; 167:689–694.
6. Ribbing S. Hereditary, multiple diaphyseal sclerosis. Acta Radiol 1949; 31:522–536.
7. Paul LW. Hereditary multiple diaphyseal sclerosis (Ribbing). Radiology 1953; 60:412–416.
8. Abdul-Karim FW, Carter JR, Makley JT, et al. Intramedullary osteosclerosis: report of the clinicopathologic features of five cases. Orthopedics 1988; 11:1667–1675.
9. Resnick D. Diagnosis of bone and joint disorders. Philadelphia, Pa: Saunders, 1995; 4416–4421.

Our congratulations to the four individuals who submitted the most likely diagnosis (intramedullary osteosclerosis) for Diagnosis Please, Case 14. The names and locations of the individuals, as submitted, are as follows:

Jaemin Cho, *Seoul, South Korea*
Seyed A. Emamian, MD, PhD, *Washington, DC*
Lorenz (Larry) Ramseyer, MD, *Enid, Okla*
H. Wouter van Es, MD, *Nieuwegein, the Netherlands*

Radiologic Staging in Patients with Endometrial Cancer: A Meta-analysis[1]

Karen Kinkel, MD
Yasushi Kaji, MD
Kyle K. Yu, MD
Mark R. Segal, PhD
Ying Lu, PhD
C. Bethan Powell, MD
Hedvig Hricak, MD, PhD

Index terms:
Computed tomography (CT), comparative studies, 854.12111
Lymphatic system, neoplasms, 99.33
Magnetic resonance (MR), comparative studies, 854.1214
Pelvic organs, CT, 854.12111
Pelvic organs, MR, 854.1214, 854.12143
Pelvic organs, US, 854.1298
Ultrasound (US), comparative studies, 854.1298
Uterine neoplasms, 854.32
Uterus, endometrium, 854.32

Radiology 1999; 212:711–718

Abbreviations:
FIGO = International Federation of Gynecology and Obstetrics
Q* = point on the summary receiver operating characteristic curve where sensitivity and specificity are equal
ROC = receiver operating characteristic

[1] From the Departments of Radiology (K.K., H.H., Y.K., K.K.Y., Y.L.), Biostatistics (M.R.S.), and Gynecologic Oncology (C.B.P.), University of California-San Francisco, Box 0628, 505 Parnassus Ave, San Francisco, CA 94143-0628. Received September 9, 1998; revision requested October 26; revision received November 25; accepted April 16, 1999. K.K. supported in part by a grant from the French Society of Radiology. K.K.Y. supported in part by a GE-AUR Radiology Research Associate Fellowship. **Address reprint requests to** H.H. (e-mail: *Hedvig.Hricak@radiology.ucsf.edu*).

Author contributions:
Guarantors of integrity of entire study, K.K., H.H.; study concepts, K.K., H.H.; study design, K.K., K.K.Y.; definition of intellectual content, K.K., K.K.Y., H.H.; literature research, K.K., Y.K.; data acquisition, K.K., Y.K.; data analysis, K.K., K.K.Y.; H.H., M.R.S., Y.L.; statistical analysis, M.R.S.; manuscript preparation, K.K.; manuscript editing, H.H., C.B.P., K.K.Y.; manuscript review, K.K.Y., H.H., M.R.S.

PURPOSE: To apply a meta-analysis to compare the utility of computed tomography (CT), ultrasonography (US), and magnetic resonance (MR) imaging in staging endometrial cancer.

MATERIALS AND METHODS: Data were obtained from a MEDLINE literature search and from manual reviews of article bibliographies. Articles were selected that included results in patients with proved endometrial cancer and imaging-histopathologic correlation and that presented data that allowed calculation of contingency tables. Data for the imaging evaluation of myometrial and cervical invasion were abstracted independently by two authors. Data on year of publication, International Federation of Gynecology and Obstetrics (FIGO) stage distribution, and methodologic quality were also collected. A subgroup analysis was performed to compare contrast medium–enhanced MR imaging with nonenhanced MR imaging, US, and CT.

RESULTS: Six studies met the inclusion criteria for CT; 16, for US; and 25, for MR imaging. Summary receiver operating characteristic analysis showed no significant differences in the overall performance of CT, US, and MR imaging. In the assessment of myometrial invasion, however, contrast-enhanced MR imaging performed significantly better than did nonenhanced MR imaging or US ($P < .002$) and demonstrated a trend toward better results, as compared with CT. The lack of data on the assessment of cervical invasion at CT or US prevented meta-analytic comparison with data obtained at MR imaging. Results were not influenced by year of publication, FIGO stage distribution, or methodologic quality.

CONCLUSION: Although US, CT, or MR imaging can be used in the pretreatment evaluation of endometrial cancer, contrast-enhanced MR imaging offers "one-stop" examination with the highest efficacy.

Treatment and prognosis of endometrial carcinoma is influenced by tumor morphologic prognostic factors that include depth of myometrial invasion, cervical extension, and lymph node metastasis (1–4). As clinical staging carries an overall understaging rate of 13%–22%, routine surgical staging has been recommended by the International Federation of Gynecology and Obstetrics (FIGO) since 1988 (5). Lymphadenectomy and pre- or postoperative radiation therapy are indicated in patients at high risk of extrauterine disease or lymph node metastasis. Since the probability of extrauterine disease and lymph node metastasis correlates with the depth of myometrial invasion, preoperative knowledge of myometrial invasion directly influences the choice of treatment (6). Furthermore, tumor extension into the cervix affects the type of surgery, and parametrial invasion requires irradiation as the first treatment or a more radical surgical approach.

The diagnostic performance of magnetic resonance (MR) imaging, computed tomography (CT), and ultrasonography (US) in assessing myometrial invasion and cervical extension has been extensively evaluated. Results from studies (7,8) in which MR imaging was compared with CT suggest MR imaging is more accurate than CT. Investigators (9,10) who have compared MR imaging with endovaginal US have reported similar performances for both techniques. However, to our knowledge, only one group of investigators (11) has compared the three techniques in the same patient population ($n = 26$). In addition, when taken individually, each of these studies lacks the statistical power to determine whether differences between the techniques are significant or represent merely random variation.

Meta-analysis is a statistical method that allows the results of individual studies to be combined and that allows the literature to be reviewed systematically (12,13). We undertook a meta-analysis to compare the three modalities and to define evidence-based imaging guidelines for staging endometrial cancer.

TABLE 1
Results of MEDLINE Search and Study Selection for Radiologic Staging of Endometrial Cancer

Articles	CT	US	MR Imaging	Total
Retrieved	24	27	33	84
Reasons for exclusion	17	11	9	37
Incomplete or inconclusive data	13	8	4	25
Imaging before radiation therapy	0	1	2	3
No surgical staging with histopathologic results	3	0	0	3
Results from patients published twice	1	2	0	3
Readers not blinded to histopathologic results	0	0	2	2
Patient selection based on imaging quality	0	0	1	1
Included	6	16	25	47
Myometrial invasion data	6	16	20	42
Cervical invasion data	2	2	10	14
Extrauterine disease data	2	1	3	6
Lymph node metastasis data	1	0	0	1

Note.—Data are the number of articles. Each article may have included data on subresults concerning myometrial invasion and/or cervical invasion and/or extrauterine disease and/or lymph node assessment.

MATERIALS AND METHODS

Data Sources

A comprehensive search of abstracts of English-language articles on studies in human subjects was performed by using the following key words on the MEDLINE database: uterine neoplasms or endometrial carcinoma with CT, MR imaging, or US. Considering the time of clinical introduction of each modality, we conducted the searches from January 1980 to September 1997 for US and CT and from January 1985 to September 1997 for MR imaging. Review articles, letters, comments, and articles that did not present raw data were excluded.

To identify additional relevant references, the reference lists of the articles retrieved were checked manually. Unpublished data were not included. A total of 84 articles were found: Sixty-eight were published in English; seven, in Japanese; four, in French; three, in Italian; and two, in German.

Study Selection

The studies included in the meta-analysis met the following inclusion criteria: (*a*) the patients had a histologic diagnosis of endometrial carcinoma; (*b*) the standard of reference was surgical staging with histopathologic results; (*c*) the presented data were obtained by observers who were blinded to the pathologic results; (*d*) the presented data allowed for the calculation of true-positive, true-negative, false-positive, and false-negative results for imaging tests; and (*e*) the data or a subset of the data was not published more than once.

Forty-seven of 84 references fulfilled the inclusion criteria (Table 1). Thirty-seven of 84 references were excluded. Reasons for exclusion were incomplete or inconclusive data ($n = 25$), presurgical radiation therapy after imaging ($n = 3$), lack of surgical staging with histopathologic results ($n = 3$), results presented in two publications ($n = 3$), imaging interpretation with knowledge of pathologic results ($n = 2$), and patient selection based on imaging quality (selection bias, $n = 1$).

Data Extraction

Articles published in Japanese, Italian, French, or German were translated into English. Two readers (K.K., Y.K.) abstracted the data from each article. When disagreement occurred, a third reader reviewed the article, and the disagreement was resolved in conference. The readers were not blinded to the authors, journal, or year of publication.

The following data were recorded for each article: (*a*) sample size; (*b*) stage distribution, by using FIGO staging guidelines (Table 2); (*c*) imaging modality (CT, US, MR imaging) and technique (helical vs nonhelical CT, transabdominal vs combined transabdominal and transvaginal US, frequency of US transducer, contrast medium–enhanced vs nonenhanced MR imaging, magnetic field strength [in tesla] of MR imaging equipment); (*d*) design of imaging interpretation (prospective, retrospective, not specified); (*e*) diagnostic criteria used for image interpretation; and (*f*) true-positive, true-negative, false-positive, and false-negative study results for the staging elements of myometrial invasion, cervical invasion, presence of extrauterine disease, and presence of lymph node metastasis.

Articles were included if they contained results for only one staging element (such as myometrial invasion) or if only a subgroup of patients fulfilled the inclusion criteria. If an article presented data on more than one staging element, inclusion and exclusion criteria were checked for each discrete data set.

TABLE 2
Revised Surgical FIGO Staging of Endometrial Carcinoma

Stage	Definition
0	Carcinoma in situ
I	Tumor confined to corpus
A	Tumor limited to endometrium
B	Invasion of greater than 50% of the thickness of the myometrium
C	Invasion of less than 50% of the thickness of the myometrium
II	Tumor invades cervix but does not extend beyond uterus
A	Invasion of endocervix
B	Cervical stromal invasion
III	Tumor extends beyond uterus but not outside of pelvis
A	Invasion of serosa and/or adnexa or positive peritoneal cytologic findings
B	Invasion of vagina
C	Pelvic and/or paraaortic lymphadenopathy
IV	Tumor extends outside pelvis or invades bladder or rectal mucosa
A	Invasion of bladder or rectal mucosa
B	Distant metastasis (includes intraabdominal or inguinal lymphadenopathy)

Methodologic Quality Rating

The methodologic quality rating was based on four criteria, as follows: (*a*) ad-

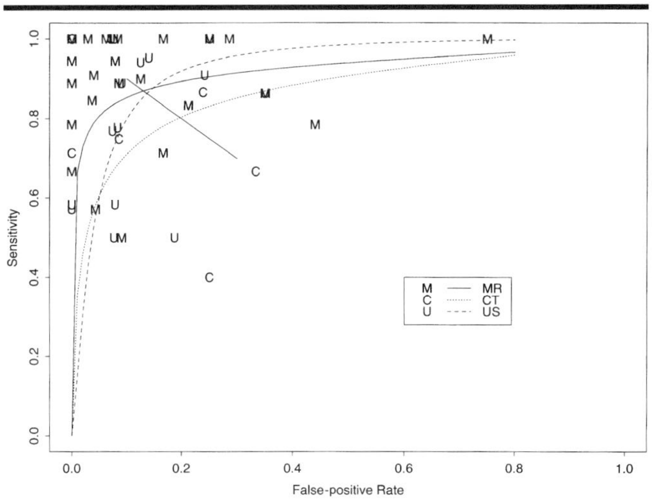

Figure 1. Summary ROC curves for CT, US, and MR imaging for overall staging (myometrial and cervical assessment). MR imaging curve is positioned above and crosses the US curve immediately above the Q* point (where sensitivity equals specificity), as indicated by the diagonal line. CT curve has the lowest position. Differences in overall staging performance are not significant.

equate description of the study group (selection criteria were defined, and patient characteristics were presented), (*b*) adequate description of diagnostic criteria (imaging staging criteria were defined, and staging results were presented accordingly), (*c*) no potential work-up bias (results of imaging did not influence the decision to perform surgery), and (*d*) congruence of presented data.

Studies were classified as "high quality" if they met all methodologic requirements, "medium quality" if they met three methodologic requirements, "fair quality" if they met two methodologic requirements, and "not acceptable" if they met only one methodologic requirement.

Data Analysis

The meta-analytic method used in our study was based on summary receiver operating characteristic (ROC) curves (14,15). Sensitivity and specificity were recalculated for each reference study by using the conventional corrections for zero counts (16). Because of the interdependence of sensitivity and specificity (Pearson correlation coefficients of 0.5 for CT, −0.22 for US, and −0.23 for MR imaging), quantitative integration of data by means of standard meta-analytic methods for the comparison of CT, US, and MR imaging was considered inappropriate.

To compare the three imaging modalities, we used summary ROC analysis, which accounts for the interdependence between sensitivity and specificity. Summary ROC, a mathematic transformation of sensitivity and specificity, has been described by Moses et al (14). In addition, transformed data of all studies were combined through a robust regression (Huber M-regression) analysis (17) in a regression line. The robust regression analysis reduces the effect of heterogeneity among studies by attributing appropriate weights to each study according to its deviation from the normal distribution. The regression line is then back-transformed into a summary ROC curve. By combining the data from all studies, summary ROC curves were independent of the diagnostic thresholds that were used to diagnose deep myometrial invasion.

Following the guidelines for fitting summary ROC curves, we obtained corresponding single-number summaries. These were the points on the summary ROC curve where sensitivity and specificity are equal (Q* values). Testing for differences between CT, US, and MR imaging was based on Q* values and on their associated standard errors.

Covariate Adjustment

To determine whether imaging results were significantly affected by heterogeneity in the studies, we extracted covariates, including the severity of disease (FIGO stage distribution in the study population), year of publication, results of methodologic quality rating, and subtype of imaging technique (contrast-enhanced vs nonenhanced MR imaging, transabdominal vs combined transabdominal and transvaginal US). Covariate adjustment analysis was performed by applying a series of statistical tests that followed the method described by Moses et al (14).

RESULTS

Literature Search

Among the 47 studies included, only one group of investigators (11) compared CT with US and MR imaging, two groups (9,10) compared MR imaging with US, and two groups (7,8) compared MR imaging with CT. Data were collected from six groups (7,8,11,18–20) that evaluated CT, from 16 groups (9–11,21–33) that evaluated US, and from 25 groups (7–11,34–53) that evaluated MR imaging (Table 1). Two authors presented MR imaging results from the same population twice, but the second results were obtained by using different imaging techniques. Data from both of these studies were combined and were presented as one study with two subgroups.

Subsets of data were obtained for the assessment of myometrial invasion in 42 studies, of cervical invasion in 14 studies, of extrauterine disease in six studies, and of lymph node metastasis in one study. Because of the limited number of investigators who evaluated extrauterine disease and lymph node metastasis, meta-analytic comparison between imaging modalities for these staging elements was not possible, and these data sets were, therefore, excluded from the analysis. Studies were performed prospectively (n = 19) or retrospectively (n = 3), or the method of data collection was not specified (n = 25).

Overall Performance

Data sets on myometrial invasion and cervical involvement were combined for the evaluation of overall staging performance for each imaging modality. Because of the interdependence of sensitivity and specificity, we used summary ROC analysis to compare the three imaging modalities. Summary ROC analysis revealed no statistically significant differences in the performance of CT, US, and MR imaging (Fig 1). Q* values were 0.80 (95% CI: 0.62, 0.98) for CT, 0.86 (95% CI: 0.81, 0.91) for US, and 0.87 (95% CI: 0.85, 0.89) for MR imaging.

To test the validity of the results, a covariate analysis, which took into account the separate, potentially significant covariates, was performed. This analysis showed imaging results were not influenced by year of publication, stage distribution, or methodologic quality rating.

Myometrial Invasion

Data on myometrial invasion met the inclusion criteria for meta-analysis in six of six studies with CT (203 patients, articles published between 1982 and 1995), in 16 of 16 studies with US (611 patients, articles published between 1987 and 1996), and in 20 of 25 studies with MR imaging (742 patients, articles published between 1987 and 1997) (Table 3). All studies of CT included the use of iodinated contrast media administered intravenously; none of the studies included use of helical CT.

Among the 16 articles on US, 14 data sets were obtained with and two data sets were obtained without the use of an endovaginal probe. The small number of data sets that were obtained without the use of an endovaginal probe precluded a meta-analytic comparison among US techniques. Frequencies of endovaginal US transducers were 5.0 MHz (n = 6), 6.5 MHz (n = 1), 5.0–6.5 MHz (n = 1), and 5.0–7.5 MHz (n = 6).

Among the 20 articles on MR imaging, nine data sets with and 18 data sets without the use of intravenous contrast media were available for meta-analytic comparison. Magnetic field strength was 1.5 T (n = 12); 1.0 T (n = 1); 0.5 T (n = 5); 0.35 T (n = 2); 0.02 T (n = 1); unknown (n = 4); or varied from 0.15 to 1.5 T because the study was multiinstitutional (n = 2).

Q* values were 0.79 (95% CI: 0.61, 0.96) for CT, 0.85 (95% CI: 0.81, 0.88) for US, 0.86 (95% CI: 0.83, 0.89) for MR imaging, 0.83 (95% CI: 0.79, 0.87) for nonenhanced MR imaging, and 0.91 (95% CI: 0.89, 0.92) for contrast-enhanced MR imaging.

Summary ROC curves were obtained for the comparison among CT, US, and MR imaging (Fig 2); between contrast-enhanced MR imaging and nonenhanced MR imaging (Fig 3); and among CT, US, and contrast-enhanced MR imaging (Fig 4). For the comparison among CT, US, and MR imaging, the summary ROC curves were of similar shape and showed no significant differences in performance (Fig 2). Comparison between MR imaging techniques showed significantly better results for contrast-enhanced versus nonenhanced MR imaging ($P < .001$) (Fig 3). Differences in Q* values did reach statistical significance when contrast-enhanced MR imaging was compared with US (P = .002). The summary ROC curves also showed a trend toward higher diagnostic accuracy for contrast-enhanced MR imaging than for CT (P = .18) (Fig 4).

TABLE 3
Assessment of Myometrial Invasion at CT, US, and MR Imaging

Technique	Author and Year	No. of Patients	Sensitivity (%)	Specificity (%)
CT	Hasumi et al, 1982 (18)	20	100	100
CT	Takahashi, 1983 (19)	19	71.4	100
CT	Varpula et al, 1993 (8)	39	66.7	66.7
CT	Dore et al, 1987 (20)	63	75	91.4
CT	Takahashi et al, 1995 (7)	36	86.7	76.2
CT	Kim et al, 1995 (11)	26	40	75
US, ev−	Fleischer et al, 1987 (21)	20	100	75
US, ev−	Cacciatore et al, 1989 (22)	77	83.3	79.3
US, ev+	Cacciatore et al, 1989 (23)	21	77.8	91.7
US, ev+	Gordon et al, 1990 (24)	25	94.1	87.5
US, ev+	Conte et al, 1990 (25)	20	88.9	90.9
US, ev+	Sahakian et al, 1991 (26)	18	100	92.3
US, ev+	Garzetti et al, 1992 (27)	34	57.1	100
US, ev+	Shipley et al, 1992 (28)	50	58.3	92.1
US, ev+	Artner et al, 1994 (29)	69	100	100
US, ev+	DelMaschio et al, 1993 (9)	42	86.4	65
US, ev+	Yamashita et al, 1993 (10)	40	76.9	92.6
US, ev+	Lehtovirta et al, 1994 (30)	78	95.2	85.9
US, ev+	Prompeler et al, 1994 (31)	51	90.9	75.9
US, ev+	Kim et al, 1995 (11)	26	50	81.2
US, ev+	Kochli et al, 1995 (32)	25	58.3	100
US, ev+	Teefey et al, 1996 (33)	15	100	92.9
MR, c−	Hricak et al, 1987 (34)	39	100	97
MR, c−	Yazigi et al, 1989 (35)	15	50	90.9
MR, c−	Harrill et al, 1990 (36)	24	71.4	83.3
MR, c−	Belloni et al, 1990 (37)	30	57.1	95.7
MR, c−	Chen et al, 1990 (38)	50	94.4	100
MR, c−	Karube, 1991 (39)	10	100	25
MR, c−	Hricak et al, 1991 (40)	88	83.3	97.4
MR, c−	Hricak et al, 1991 (41)	18	100	75
MR, c−	Hirano et al, 1992 (42)	53	88.9	88.6
MR, c−	Sironi et al, 1992 (43)	65	88.2	85.4
MR, c−	Varpula et al, 1993 (8)	39	83.3	78.8
MR, c−	Yamashita et al, 1993 (10)	40	76.9	88.9
MR, c−	DelMaschio et al, 1993 (9)	42	86.4	65
MR, c−	Ito et al, 1994 (44)	22	100	58.3
MR, c−	Atsukawa et al, 1994 (45)	39	78.6	56
MR, c−	Takahashi et al, 1995 (7)	25	100	75
MR, c−	Joja et al, 1996 (46)	46	88.9	78.6
MR, c−	Seki et al, 1997 (47)	40	78.6	88.5
MR, c+	Hricak et al, 1991 (41)	18	100	91.7
MR, c+	Sironi et al, 1992 (48)	56	94.4	92.1
MR, c+	Hirano et al, 1992 (42)	53	88.9	91.4
MR, c+	Yamashita et al, 1993 (10)	40	84.6	96.3
MR, c+	Ito K et al, 1994 (44)	22	100	83.3
MR, c+	Kim et al, 1995 (11)	26	90	87.5
MR, c+	Minderhoud-Bassie et al, 1995 (49)	31	100	71.4
MR, c+	Joja et al, 1996 (46)	46	88.9	100
MR, c+	Seki et al, 1997 (47)	40	78.6	100

Note.—Reference numbers are in parentheses. c− = nonenhanced, c+ = contrast-enhanced, ev− = without endovaginal probe, ev+ = with endovaginal probe.

Cervical Involvement

Only two of six studies of CT (published in 1982 or 1995) with data on 56 patients, two of 16 studies of US (published in 1989 or 1994) with data on 162 patients, and 10 of 25 studies of MR imaging (published between 1987 and 1996) with data on 318 patients had sufficient data to be included in this subgroup (Table 4). Q* values could be calculated only for MR imaging (0.92; 95% CI: 0.87, 0.95).

DISCUSSION

Endometrial cancer is the most common gynecologic malignancy, with an esti-

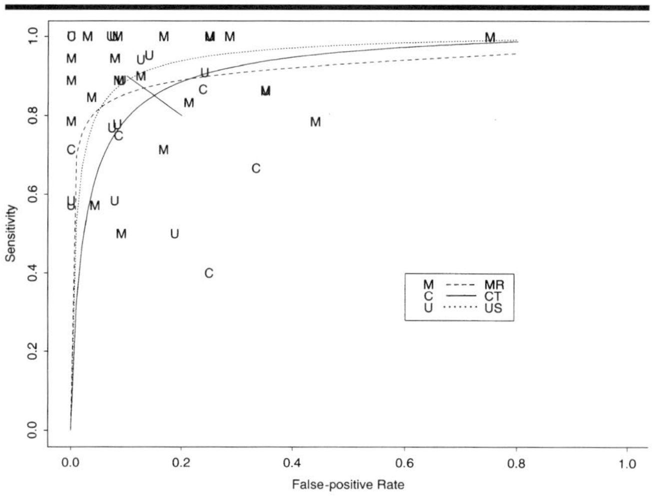

Figure 2. Summary ROC curves for CT, US, and MR imaging for the evaluation of myometrial invasion. MR imaging curve, which combines contrast-enhanced with nonenhanced studies, crosses the US curve slightly below the Q* point. Q* point on the CT curve is below the other curves, which demonstrates the lowest, but not a significantly different, performance.

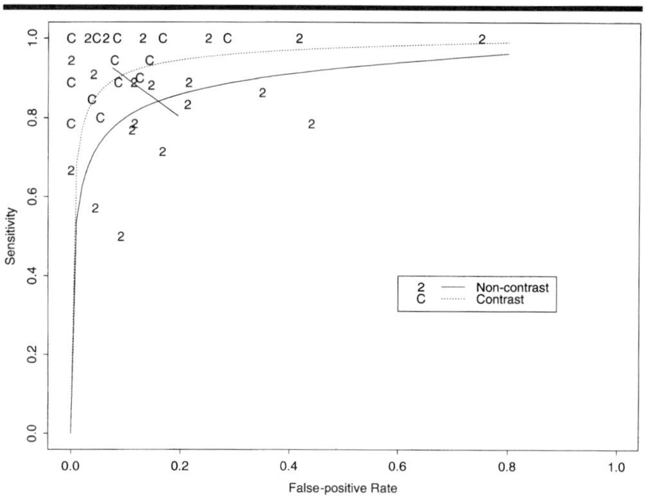

Figure 3. Summary ROC curves for contrast-enhanced and nonenhanced MR imaging for the evaluation of myometrial invasion. Contrast-enhanced MR imaging curve was positioned above the nonenhanced MR imaging curve at every point, which indicates significantly better performance ($P < .001$) in depicting myometrial invasion.

mated 34,900 cases newly diagnosed per year (54). The improved survival rate of patients with endometrial cancer over the past 20 years (28% decrease in mortality rate) is mostly the result of earlier diagnosis (2). Further improvement may be achieved through better pretreatment assessment of prognostic factors, which would allow for the optimal choice of primary treatment and decreased morbidity and mortality. For example, if a patient undergoes a simple hysterectomy, but surgical-histologic findings reveal deep myometrial or cervical invasion, the patient will be referred to a gynecologic oncologist and will require a second operation for lymph node dissection.

As well-established "primary treatment in a cancer patient gives the best opportunity for cure" (55), preoperative knowledge of local-regional tumor extent may indirectly affect patient survival. Therefore, gaining knowledge of morphologic prognostic factors of cancer and of their inclusion in treatment planning could be an important step in further improving prognosis. Prognostic factors that influence the choice of treatment are patient factors (age, health), tumor extent (depth of myometrial invasion, cervical invasion, and lymph node invasion), and histologic factors (tumor grade, histologic type, lymphatic vascular space invasion) (2).

Histologic factors are related to depth of myometrial invasion, endocervical extension, and lymph node metastasis. A higher tumor grade correlates with lower survival rates and higher rates of myometrial invasion (eg, the incidence of deep myometrial invasion is about 7% for grade I tumors versus 46% for grade III tumors) (1). For grade II tumors with deep myometrial invasion and for all grade III tumors, the lymph node invasion rate is about 31% for pelvic lymph nodes and 23% for paraaortic lymph nodes (2).

Gross evaluation of myometrial invasion becomes less reliable with increasing tumor grade (gross inspection has 80% reliability vs 94% reliability for frozen-section analysis) (56,57). The 5-year mortality rates of 51% for clear cell carcinoma and of 21% for papillary serous carcinoma are worse than the 6% 5-year mortality rate for the more common adenocarcinomas (58). The worse outcome of these histologic types also correlates with a higher incidence of lymph node metastasis and myometrial invasion (eg, 50% of patients with clinical stage I papillary serous carcinoma have deep myometrial invasion) (59). Invasion of the cervical stroma (FIGO stage IIB) and of the lymph nodes (FIGO stage IIIC) are well-known adverse prognostic factors that are strongly correlated with myometrial invasion and tumor grade (1,60). However, diagnosis of cervical invasion by means of endocervical curettage is unreliable because of false-positive rates of up to 25% and false-negative rates of up to 10% (61).

In 1988, the inadequacies of pretreatment diagnostic assessment of endometrial cancer led to recommendations for routine surgical staging (5). However, since the introduction of surgical staging in 1988, the technology for diagnostic radiology has markedly advanced with the improvement of spatial resolution of CT and with the development of endovaginal US, MR imaging, and MR contrast media. Accurate pretreatment assessment of endometrial cancer at imaging can potentially optimize surgical and nonsurgical treatment. Pretreatment knowledge of myometrial or cervical invasion affects the performance and extent of lymphadenectomy (3,62,63). Presence of cervical invasion alters the type of hysterectomy that is performed (64), and the poor outcome of associated parametrial invasion (65) indicates irradiation, rather than immediate surgery, is the best treatment in these patients (2).

Despite the breadth of information provided with modern imaging methods, no imaging guidelines or algorithms are available for the use of imaging in the pretreatment assessment of endometrial cancer. In part, this is due to the lack of multimodality studies with adequate sample size and statistical power in which state-of-the-art imaging techniques are compared. When a single imaging modality is evaluated, the investigator tends to overestimate its value because of a variety of biases. This meta-analysis was undertaken to address some of the shortcomings in the existing literature.

In our meta-analysis of 10–15 years of literature, we attempted to minimize some of the well-known limitations of meta-analysis. If primary studies suffer from inadequate scientific quality, combining them in a meta-analytic comparison will yield only poor results. We attempted to minimize this problem by applying strict inclusion and exclusion criteria to every study and by taking into account a methodologic quality rating. To avoid confounding due to the use of different thresholds for the diagnosis of myometrial invasion, we used the summary ROC method rather than the pooling method that combines the patient populations to determine a combined value of sensitivity and specificity.

Another potential pitfall of meta-analysis is that differences in patients may preclude application of the results of a meta-analysis to the target population. We attempted to avoid this pitfall by assessing the severity of the disease and by performing a covariate analysis, which demonstrated no differences in results when the FIGO stage distribution of each study population was considered.

By including only published data, we did not exclude publication bias, which tends to cause overestimation of diagnostic performance because of the greater likelihood of publication of positive rather than negative results. Although meta-analysis does not replace large prospective studies, the results from a meta-analysis in which results of smaller trials are combined may not differ significantly from the results of larger prospective trials (13).

Findings of this study showed that, in the evaluation of myometrial invasion, contrast-enhanced MR imaging performed significantly better than nonenhanced MR imaging and US ($P < .002$) and showed a trend toward better results when compared with CT ($P = .18$).

Although commonly used in clinical settings, to our knowledge there have not been sufficient published data evaluating the performance of CT in endometrial cancer staging. Due to the lack of published data on helical CT in staging endometrial cancer, the performance of CT may be underestimated in this meta-analysis.

Comparison of US studies that use the transabdominal approach and studies that use the endovaginal approach was not possible because of insufficient data on US studies that use only the transabdominal approach. As 88% of the included US studies combined the transabdominal approach with the endovaginal approach, this combination appeared to represent the recommended standard technique in the published literature. Compared with CT, US has a significantly lower sensitivity for paraaortic and pelvic lymph node detection (66,67).

Recently, a meta-analysis in which the use of MR imaging, CT, and lymphography in patients with cervical cancer was compared showed a trend toward better performance with MR imaging than with CT or lymphography in the diagnosis of pelvic lymphadenopathy (68). Although the meta-analysis included only patients with cervical cancer, these results might still apply to patients with endometrial cancer. Therefore, in patients with a large uterine mass and a resultant higher probability of lymph node metastasis, MR imaging or CT, and not US, should be used as the primary imaging modality. Incomplete data on lymph node status in patients with endometrial cancer precluded meta-analytic comparison.

Although six studies compared contrast-enhanced with nonenhanced MR imaging (10,41,42,44,46,48), the difference in accuracy between these techniques reached statistical significance in only one study (10). This meta-analysis increased the statistical significance (from $P = .03$ in Yamashita's study [10] to $P < .001$ in this analysis) and therefore confirmed, with higher confidence, the previously published superiority of contrast-enhanced over nonenhanced MR imaging. Staging of endometrial cancer at MR imaging should, therefore, include the use of intravenous contrast media.

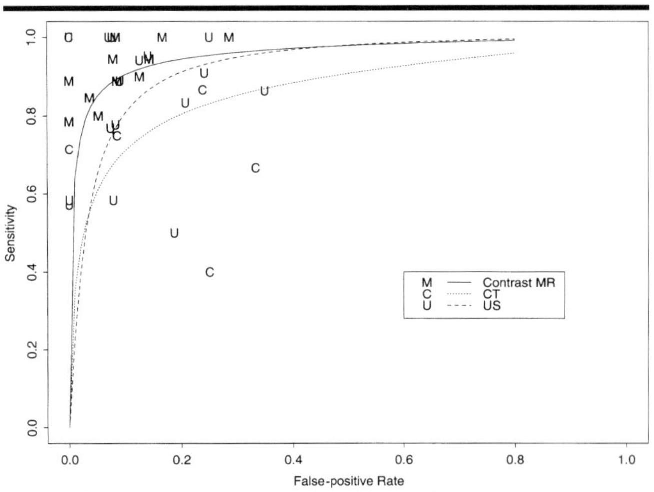

Figure 4. Summary ROC curves for contrast-enhanced MR imaging versus CT and US for the evaluation of myometrial invasion. Curves have similar shapes. Higher position of the contrast-enhanced MR imaging curve indicates a significantly better performance ($P = .002$) than US. Comparison between CT and contrast-enhanced MR imaging reveals a trend toward better results for contrast-enhanced MR imaging ($P = .18$).

TABLE 4
Assessment of Cervical Invasion

Technique	Author and Year	No. of Patients	Sensitivity (%)	Specificity (%)
CT	Hasumi et al, 1982 (18)	20	71.4	100
CT	Takahashi et al, 1995 (7)	36	40	100
US	Cacciatore et al, 1989 (22)	93	80	95.2
US	Artner et al, 1994 (29)	69	66.7	100
MR	Hricak et al, 1987 (34)	44	100	97.4
MR	Kaketa et al, 1989 (50)	21	100	93.8
MR	Posniak et al, 1990 (51)	13	66.7	100
MR	Belloni et al, 1990 (37)	30	83.3	94.4
MR	Karube, 1991 (39)	20	71.4	92.3
MR	Atsukawa et al, 1994 (45)	39	83.3	92.6
MR	Minderhoud et al, 1995 (49)	31	55.6	100
MR	Murakami et al, 1995 (52)	27	100	100
MR	Takahashi et al, 1995 (7)	32	66.7	96.2
MR	Matsushita et al, 1996 (53)	61	90.9	96

Note.—Reference numbers are in parentheses.

The lack of reported data on the assessment of cervical invasion at CT and US may be related to diagnostic difficulties with these imaging modalities. Results of MR imaging for this indication ranged from 66% to 100% (mean, 86%) for sensitivity; from 92% to 100% (mean, 97%) for specificity; and from 87% to 95% for the CIs for the Q* value.

Among 10 articles that included assessment of cervical invasion at MR imaging, the authors of only one article (49) differentiated cervical stromal invasion (the only cervical prognostic factor) from superficial cervical invasion (not a prognostic factor). The authors demonstrated an increase in sensitivity from 56% to 100% and no change in specificity if only cervical stromal invasion was considered a positive sign of cervical invasion. The meta-analytic results for the assessment of cervical invasion at MR imaging could not reflect this differentiation and might, therefore, underestimate the real sensitivity of MR imaging. If the patient is at high risk for cervical invasion, on the basis of findings at clinical examination, contrast-enhanced MR imaging might represent the appropriate cost-effective solution for evaluating myometrial, cervical, and lymph node involvement.

Although the algorithmic approach to diagnostic tests offers the potential for evidence-based assessment, guidelines need to be adopted. Imaging should be used because it offers an important adjunct to treatment decision making. The choice of the primary imaging modality should be tailored to local expertise; to the patient's pretest probability for myometrial, cervical, or lymph node disease; and to the patient's habitus.

For endometrial cancer staging, the choice of an imaging modality depends on tumor grade, histologic type, and findings at clinical examination.

On the basis of our meta-analysis of imaging findings and well-established prognostic factors that are assessed at endometrial biopsy, endocervical curettage, and clinical examination, the following clinical practice guidelines can be formulated for staging endometrial cancer. (*a*) No imaging is required for patients with grade I tumors and a nonenlarged uterus at physical examination because the pretest probability of myometrial, cervical, or nodal involvement is low. If results from the physical examination are inconclusive or if there is concomitant pelvic disease, US, CT, or MR imaging can be used at the initial radiologic investigation. (*b*) Patients with high-grade papillary or clear cell tumors should undergo CT or MR imaging because there is a high pretest probability of nodal involvement. (*c*) Patients with possible cervical involvement at physical examination or with positive or inconclusive results from endocervical curettage should undergo MR imaging, since this is the only modality that has been shown to accurately depict cervical invasion. (*d*) In patients who require multifactorial assessment, contrast-enhanced MR imaging is the only modality that can be used to accurately evaluate myometrial, cervical, and nodal involvement.

References

1. Boronow RC, Morrow CP, Creasman WT, et al. Surgical staging in endometrial cancer: clinical-pathologic findings of a prospective study. Obstet Gynecol 1984; 63: 825–832.
2. Morrow CP, Curtin JP, Townsend DG. Tumors of the endometrium. In: Morrow CP, Curtin JP, eds. Synopsis of gynecologic oncology. 5th ed. New York, NY: Churchill Livingstone, 1998; 151–185.
3. Larson DM, Connor GP, Broste SK, Krawisz BR, Johnson KK. Prognostic significance of gross myometrial invasion with endometrial cancer. Obstet Gynecol 1996; 88:394–398.
4. Kodama S, Kase H, Tanaka K, Matsui K. Multivariate analysis of prognostic factors in patients with endometrial cancer. Int J Gynaecol Obstet 1996; 53:23–30.
5. Shepherd JH. Revised FIGO staging for gynaecological cancer. Br J Obstet Gynaecol 1989; 96:889–892. [Erratum: Br J Obstet Gynaecol 1992; 99:440.]
6. Creasman WT, Morrow CP, Bundy BN, Homesley HD, Graham JE, Heller PB. Surgical pathologic spread patterns of endometrial cancer: a Gynecologic Oncology Group study. Cancer 1987; 60:2035–2041.
7. Takahashi K, Yoshioka M, Kosuge H, et al. The accuracy of computed tomography and magnetic resonance imaging in evaluating the extent of endometrial carcinoma. Nippon Sanka Fujinka Gakkai Zasshi 1995; 47:647–654. [Japanese]
8. Varpula MJ, Klemi PJ. Staging of uterine endometrial carcinoma with ultra-low field (0.02 T) MRI: a comparative study with CT. J Comput Assist Tomogr 1993; 17:641–647.
9. DelMaschio A, Vanzulli A, Sironi S, et al. Estimating the depth of myometrial involvement by endometrial carcinoma: efficacy of transvaginal sonography vs MR imaging. AJR 1993; 160:533–538.
10. Yamashita Y, Mizutani H, Torashima M, et al. Assessment of myometrial invasion by endometrial carcinoma: transvaginal sonography vs contrast-enhanced MR imaging. AJR 1993; 161:595–599.
11. Kim SH, Kim HD, Song YS, Kang SB, Lee HP. Detection of deep myometrial invasion in endometrial carcinoma: comparison of transvaginal ultrasound, CT, and MRI. J Comput Assist Tomogr 1995; 19: 766–772.
12. Irwig L, Tosteson AN, Gatsonis C, et al. Guidelines for meta-analyses evaluating diagnostic tests. Ann Intern Med 1994; 120:667–676.
13. Cappelleri JC, Ioannidis JP, Schmid CH, et al. Large trials vs meta-analysis of smaller trials: how do their results compare? JAMA 1996; 276:1332–1338.
14. Moses LE, Shapiro D, Littenberg B. Combining independent studies of a diagnostic test into a summary ROC curve: data-analytic approaches and some additional considerations. Stat Med 1993; 12:1293–1316.
15. Midget AS, Stoxil TA, Littenberg B. A meta-analytic method for summarizing diagnostic test performances: receiver-operating-characteristic-summary point estimates. Med Decis Making 1993; 13: 253–257.
16. Haldane JB. The estimation and significance of the logarithm of a ratio of frequencies. Ann Hum Genet 1955; 20:309–314.
17. Venables WN, Ripley BD. Robust statistics. In: Venable WR, Ripley BD. Modern applied statistics with S-Plus. 2nd ed. New York, NY: Springer, 1997; 247–266.
18. Hasami K, Matsuzawa M, Chen HF, Takahashi M, Sakura M. Computed tomography in the evaluation and treatment of endometrial carcinoma. Cancer 1982; 50: 904–908.
19. Takahashi K. Role of x-ray CT in diagnosis and therapy of endometrial carcinoma. Nippon Sanka Fujinka Gakkai Zasshi 1983; 35:683–690. [Japanese]
20. Dore R, Moro G, D'Andrea F, La Fianza A, Franchi M, Bolis PF. CT evaluation of myometrium invasion in endometrial carcinoma. J Comput Assist Tomogr 1987; 11:282–289.
21. Fleischer AC, Dudley BS, Entman SS, Baxter JW, Kalemeris GC, James AE Jr. Myometrial invasion by endometrial carcinoma: sonographic assessment. Radiology 1987; 162:307–310.
22. Cacciatore B, Lehtovirta P, Wahlstrom T, Ylostalo P. Preoperative sonographic evaluation of endometrial cancer. Am J Obstet Gynecol 1989; 160:133–137.
23. Cacciatore B, Lehtovirta P, Wahlstrom T, Ylanen K, Ylostalo P. Contribution of vaginal scanning to sonographic evaluation of endometrial cancer invasion. Acta Oncol 1989; 28:585–588.
24. Gordon AN, Fleischer AC, Reed GW. Depth of myometrial invasion in endometrial cancer: preoperative assessment by transvaginal ultrasonography. Gynecol Oncol 1990; 39:321–327.
25. Conte M, Guariglia L, Benedetti Panici P, Scambia G, Cento R, Mancuso S. Transvaginal ultrasound evaluation of myometrial invasion in endometrial carcinoma. Gynecol Obstet Invest 1990; 29:224–226.
26. Sahakian V, Syrop C, Turner D. Endometrial carcinoma: transvaginal ultrasonography prediction of depth of myometrial invasion. Gynecol Oncol 1991; 43:217–219.
27. Garzetti GG, Ciavattini A, Cignitti M, et al. Transvaginal echography in the evaluation of the grade of myometrial invasion in locally advanced endometrial carcinoma. Ann Ostet Ginecol Med Perinat 1992; 113:114–118. [Italian]
28. Shipley CF III, Smith ST, Dennis EJ III, Nelson GH. Evaluation of pretreatment transvaginal ultrasonography in the management of patients with endometrial carcinoma. Am J Obstet Gynecol 1992; 167: 406–411.

29. Artner A, Bosze P, Gonda G. The value of ultrasound in preoperative assessment of the myometrial and cervical invasion in endometrial carcinoma. Gynecol Oncol 1994; 54:147–151.
30. Lehtovirta P, Cacciatore B, Ylostalo P. Serum CA 125 levels and sonography in the pre-operative assessment of myometrial invasion of endometrial cancer. Br J Obstet Gynaecol 1994; 101:532–535.
31. Prompeler HJ, Madjar H, du Bois A, et al. Transvaginal sonography of myometrial invasion depth in endometrial cancer. Acta Obstet Gynecol Scand 1994; 73:343–346.
32. Kochli OR, Bajka M, Schar G, Schmidt D, Haller U. Measuring the depth of invasion of endometrial carcinoma: preoperative transvaginal ultrasound and correlation with intraoperative and histopathologic findings—a prospective study. Ultraschall Med 1995; 16:8–11. [German]
33. Teefey SA, Stahl JA, Middleton WD, et al. Local staging of endometrial carcinoma: comparison of transvaginal and intraoperative sonography and gross visual inspection. AJR 1996; 166:547–552.
34. Hricak H, Stern JL, Fisher MR, Shapeero LG, Winkler ML, Lacey CG. Endometrial carcinoma staging by MR imaging. Radiology 1987; 162:297–305.
35. Yazigi R, Cohen J, Munoz AK, Sandstad J. Magnetic resonance imaging determination of myometrial invasion in endometrial carcinoma. Gynecol Oncol 1989; 34: 94–97.
36. Harrill CD, Kopecky KK, Weaver SR, Sutton GP. Magnetic resonance imaging in the preoperative assessment of clinical stage I endometrial carcinoma. Comput Med Imaging Graph 1990; 14:191–195.
37. Belloni C, Vigano R, del Maschio A, Sironi S, Taccagni GL, Vignali M. Magnetic resonance imaging in endometrial carcinoma staging. Gynecol Oncol 1990; 37:172–177.
38. Chen SS, Rumancik WM, Spiegel G. Magnetic resonance imaging in stage I endometrial carcinoma. Obstet Gynecol 1990; 75:274–277.
39. Karube M. Role of magnetic resonance imaging (MRI) in evaluation of the extension of endometrial carcinoma. Nippon Sanka Fujinka Gakkai Zasshi 1991; 43:101–108. [Japanese]
40. Hricak H, Rubinstein LV, Gherman GM, Karstaedt N. MR imaging evaluation of endometrial carcinoma: results of an NCI cooperative study. Radiology 1991; 179: 829–832.
41. Hricak H, Hamm B, Semelka RC, et al. Carcinoma of the uterus: use of gadopentetate dimeglumine in MR imaging. Radiology 1991; 181:95–106.
42. Hirano Y, Kubo K, Hirai Y, et al. Preliminary experience with gadolinium-enhanced dynamic MR imaging for uterine neoplasms. RadioGraphics 1992; 12:243–256.
43. Sironi S, Taccagni G, Garancini P, Belloni C, DelMaschio A. Myometrial invasion by endometrial carcinoma: assessment by MR imaging. AJR 1992; 158:565–569.
44. Ito K, Matsumoto T, Nakada T, Nakanishi T, Fujita N, Yamashita H. Assessing myometrial invasion by endometrial carcinoma with dynamic MRI. J Comput Assist Tomogr 1994; 18:77–86.
45. Atsukawa H, Sasaki H, Tada S. A multivariate analysis of assessment of myometrial invasion of endometrial carcinoma by magnetic resonance imaging. Gynecol Oncol 1994; 54:298–306.
46. Joja I, Asakawa M, Asakawa T, et al. Endometrial carcinoma: dynamic MRI with turbo-FLASH technique. J Comput Assist Tomogr 1996; 20:878–887.
47. Seki H, Kimura M, Sakai K. Myometrial invasion of endometrial carcinoma: assessment with dynamic MR and contrast-enhanced T1-weighted images. Clin Radiol 1997; 52:18–23.
48. Sironi S, Colombo E, Villa G, et al. Myometrial invasion by endometrial carcinoma: assessment with plain and gadolinium-enhanced MR imaging. Radiology 1992; 185:207–212.
49. Minderhoud-Bassie W, Treurniet FE, Koops W, Chadha-Ajwani S, Hage JC, Huikeshoven FJ. Magnetic resonance imaging (MRI) in endometrial carcinoma: preoperative estimation of depth of myometrial invasion. Acta Obstet Gynecol Scand 1995; 74:827–831.
50. Kaketa M, Takemoto O, Akamine M, Iwasaki H, Takamizawa H. MRI in evaluation of myometrial invasion and staging of endometrial carcinoma. Nippon Sanka Fujinka Gakkai Zasshi 1989; 41:859–866. [Japanese]
51. Posniak HV, Olson MC, Dudiak CM, et al. MR imaging of uterine carcinoma: correlation with clinical and pathologic findings. RadioGraphics 1990; 10:15–27.
52. Murakami T, Kurachi H, Nakamura H, et al. Cervical invasion of endometrial carcinoma: evaluation by parasagittal MR imaging. Acta Radiol 1995; 36:248–253.
53. Matsushita H, Kodama S, Kase H, Kurata H, Tanaka K. Usefulness of magnetic resonance imaging in the determination of cervical involvement in endometrial cancer. Nippon Sanka Fujinka Gakkai Zasshi 1996; 48:821–826. [Japanese]
54. American Cancer Society. Cancer facts and figures. Atlanta, Ga: American Cancer Society, 1997.
55. Rutledge FN, Freedman RS, Gershenson DM. Gynecologic cancer: diagnosis and treatment strategies. Austin, Tex: University of Texas Press, 1987; 3.
56. Noumoff JS, Menzin A, Mikuta J, Lusk EJ, Morgan M, LiVolsi VA. The ability to evaluate prognostic variables on frozen section in hysterectomies performed for endometrial carcinoma. Gynecol Oncol 1991; 42:202–208.
57. Goff BA, Rice LW. Assessment of depth of myometrial invasion in endometrial adenocarcinoma. Gynecol Oncol 1990; 38:46–48.
58. Christopherson WM, Connelly PJ, Alberhasky RC. Carcinoma of the endometrium. V. An analysis of prognosticators in patients with favorable subtypes and stage I disease. Cancer 1983; 51:1705–1709.
59. Hendrickson M, Ross J, Eifel PJ, Cox RS, Martinez A, Kempson R. Adenocarcinoma of the endometrium: analysis of 256 cases with carcinoma limited to the uterine corpus—pathology review and analysis of prognostic variables. Gynecol Oncol 1982; 13:373–392.
60. Kinsella TJ, Bloomer WD, Lavin PT, Knapp RC. Stage II endometrial carcinoma: 10-year follow-up of combined radiation and surgical treatment. Gynecol Oncol 1980; 10:290–297.
61. Chen SS, Lee L. Reappraisal of endocervical curettage in predicting cervical involvement by endometrial carcinoma. J Reprod Med 1986; 31:50–52.
62. Eltabbakh GH, Piver MS, Hempling RE, Shin KH. Excellent long-term survival and absence of vaginal recurrences in 332 patients with low-risk stage I endometrial adenocarcinoma treated with hysterectomy and vaginal brachytherapy without formal staging lymph node sampling: report of a prospective trial. Int J Radiat Oncol Biol Phys 1997; 38:373–380.
63. Yokoyama Y, Maruyama H, Sato S, Saito Y. Indispensability of pelvic and paraaortic lymphadenectomy in endometrial cancers. Gynecol Oncol 1997; 64:411–417.
64. Rubin SC, Hoskins WJ, Saigo PE, et al. Management of endometrial adenocarcinoma with cervical involvement. Gynecol Oncol 1992; 45:294–298.
65. Yura Y, Tauchi K, Koshiyama M, et al. Parametrial involvement in endometrial carcinomas: its incidence and correlation with other histological parameters. Gynecol Oncol 1996; 63:114–119.
66. Mamsen A, Ledertoug S, Horlyck A, et al. The possible role of ultrasound in early cervical cancer. Gynecol Oncol 1995; 56: 187–190.
67. Munker R, Stengel A, Stabler A, Hiller E, Brehm G. Diagnostic accuracy of ultrasound and computed tomography in the staging of Hodgkin's disease: verification by laparotomy in 100 cases. Cancer 1995; 76:1460–1466.
68. Scheidler J, Hricak H, Yu KK, Subak L, Segal MR. Radiological evaluation of lymph node metastases in patients with cervical cancer: a meta-analysis. JAMA 1997; 278:1096–1101.

Ulrike M. Hamper, MD
Victoria Trapanotto, DO, MS
M. Robert DeJong, RDMS, RDCS, RVT
Sheila Sheth, MD
Cynthia I. Caskey, MD

Three-dimensional US of the Prostate: Early Experience[1]

PURPOSE: To assess the feasibility of using a three-dimensional (3D) endorectal transducer at ultrasonography (US) in the prostate gland in a clinical setting.

MATERIALS AND METHODS: Sixteen patients underwent 3D imaging of the prostate gland with a 3D endorectal probe following conventional two-dimensional (2D) US and prior to prostatic biopsy. Image acquisition was performed as a volume of data with nearly immediate reconstruction and simultaneous display of sectional anatomy in three orthogonal planes—sagittal plane, transverse or coronal plane, or any arbitrary oblique plane. Images were evaluated for presence of focal lesions, glandular volume, visualization of lateral and anterior portions of the gland, and extraglandular extension of tumor.

RESULTS: Three-dimensional US allowed better visualization of the gland and focal lesions, especially on the coronally reconstructed images, which were judged superior to the sagittally or transversely reconstructed images for interpretation in 50% of the patients. Prostatic volumes obtained from 3D US were consistently smaller than volumes obtained from 2D US (20% difference, $P = .006$). Three-dimensional US was superior to 2D US in depicting tumor presence (nine of 10 right hemispheres, three of eight left hemispheres) and extraglandular extent of disease (three of five hemispheres).

CONCLUSION: Three-dimensional endorectal prostatic US appears to be clinically feasible and easy to perform. Added anatomic information from the coronal plane may allow better depiction of tumors and extraglandular spread than is possible with current 2D techniques.

Index terms:
Prostate, neoplasms, 844.30
Prostate, US, 844.12987, 844.12989
Ultrasound (US), technology, 844.12987, 844.12989
Ultrasound (US), three-dimensional, 844.12987, 844.12989

Radiology 1999; 212:719–723

Abbreviations:
PSA = prostate-specific antigen
2D = two-dimensional
3D = three-dimensional

[1] From the Department of Radiology, Ultrasound Section, Johns Hopkins Hospital, 600 N Wolfe St, Baltimore, MD 21287 (U.M.H., V.T., M.R.D.J., S.S., C.I.C.); and the Department of Radiology, University of Texas at Houston, Lyndon B. Johnson General Hospital (C.I.C.). Received February 5, 1998; revision requested April 14; final revision received November 25; accepted March 29, 1999. **Address reprint requests to** U.M.H. (e-mail: *umhamper@rad.jhu.edu*).

Author contributions:
Guarantor of integrity of entire study, U.M.H.; study concepts and design, U.M.H., V.T., C.I.C.; definition of intellectual content, U.M.H., V.T., C.I.C.; literature research, U.M.H., V.T.; clinical studies, U.M.H., V.T., M.R.D.J.; data acquisition, U.M.H., V.T., M.R.D.J.; data analysis, U.M.H., V.T., S.S.; statistical analysis, U.M.H., V.T., S.S.; manuscript preparation, U.M.H., V.T., M.R.D.J., C.I.C.; manuscript editing and review, all authors.

Three-dimensional (3D) ultrasonography (US) has recently gained much attention in the evaluation of a variety of clinical, primarily obstetric, applications (1–7). Limited abdominal, pelvic, cardiac, ocular, or vascular applications have also been described (7–10). Reports of the use of endocavitary 3D US to image the prostate, urethra, or rectum have likewise been scant (11–20).

The purpose of this study was to assess the feasibility of using a 3D endorectal transducer in a clinical setting and to present our preliminary experience with 3D US of the prostate gland. To our knowledge, this may be the first clinical series in which 3D endorectal US was used prior to endorectal US–guided biopsy in a select patient population, with correlation at histopathologic examination.

MATERIALS AND METHODS

Sixteen consecutive patients scheduled for endorectal US and US-guided endorectal prostatic biopsy were examined with 3D US following conventional 2D US and prior to biopsy.

Indications for the original studies included the following: elevated prostate-specific antigen (PSA) level ($n = 11$), abnormal digital rectal examination findings alone ($n = 2$), abnormal digital rectal examination findings and elevated PSA level ($n = 2$), and abnormal endorectal US findings with normal digital rectal examination findings and PSA level ($n = 1$). The level of PSA in our population ranged from 2.9 to 40.0 ng/mL. Three patients had a PSA level less than or equal to 4.0 ng/mL, seven patients had levels between 4 and 10 ng/mL, four patients had levels between 10 and 20 ng/mL, and two patients had levels above 20 ng/mL.

All patients were examined with an experimental 7.5-MHz mechanically driven bifocal volume transducer coupled to a commercially available US unit (Combison 530; Medison America, Pleasanton, Calif) (Fig 1a). The age range of our patient population was 59–76 years, with a mean age of 66 years. Approval by the institutional review board was granted for the performance of the 3D examination. Informed consent was obtained from all patients prior to performance of the 3D endorectal US and biopsy procedure.

Correlation with histopathologic results was obtained in all patients with either endorectal biopsy findings ($n = 15$) or radical retropubic prostatectomy findings ($n = 1$). Image acquisition was performed as a complete block or volume of data for a total of two to five volumes (mean, 3.8 volumes) per patient. The time to acquire a volume of data ranged from 5 to 10 seconds.

Automatic volume scanning allowed nearly immediate reconstruction and simultaneous display of sectional anatomy in three orthogonal planes—sagittal plane, transverse or coronal plane, or any arbitrary oblique plane—or in a plane parallel to the transducer surface (Figs 1b, 2). The individual planes could be manipulated in the volume in real time, which allowed measurements—dual linear, area, volume—to be performed in all planes. Total examination time was 20–30 minutes, including time for patient and machine preparation, data acquisition, and patient discharge.

In addition, transparent volume or surface-rendered imaging was performed at a later time, which required 2–5 minutes for image reconstruction, depending on the area of interest chosen or reconstruction parameters (Fig 2d). Images were evaluated by two independent observers (U.M.H., V.T.) with special expertise in US and 3D imaging for the presence of focal lesions, size and volume of the entire gland or focal lesions, and extent of extraglandular spread. In cases of nonagreement between the observers, a consensus was reached. Assessment criteria were superior, equal, or inferior visualization of the gland or focal lesions when 3D US was compared with 2D US. In addition, a binomial (yes or no) decision as to the presence of capsular extension was made independently by the two observers.

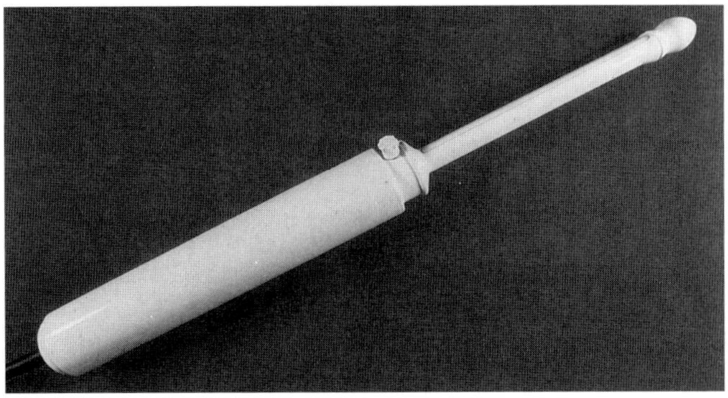

a.

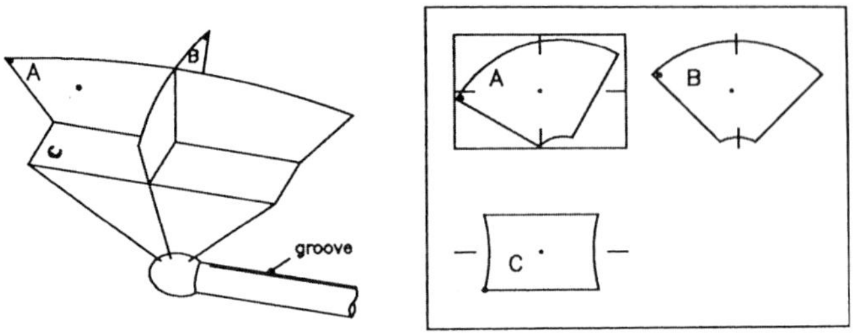

b.

Figure 1. **(a)** Photograph of 3D endorectal volume transducer. **(b)** Schematic drawing of the acquired volume and planimetric display of orthogonal planes.

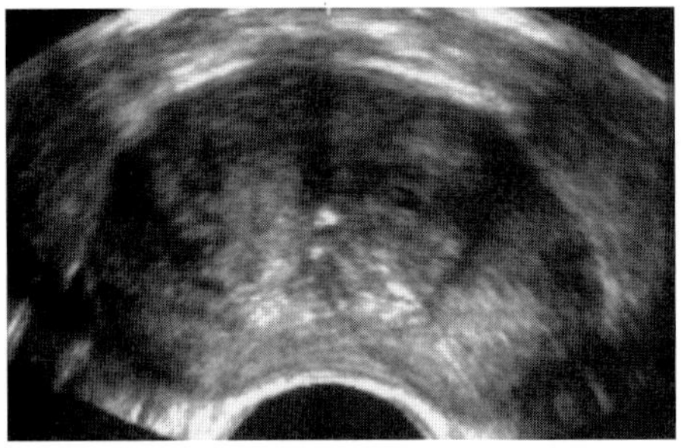

a.

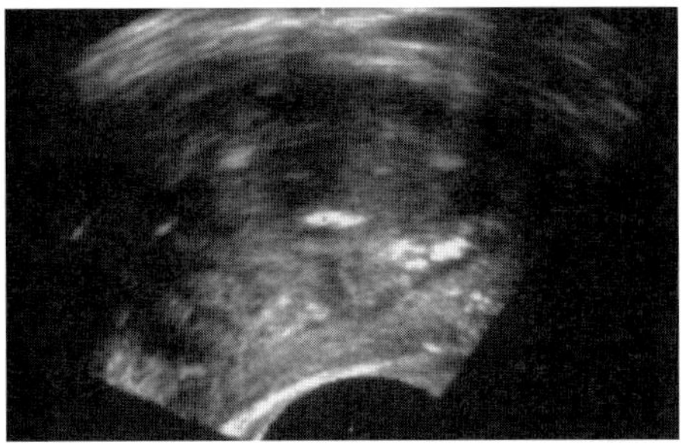

b.

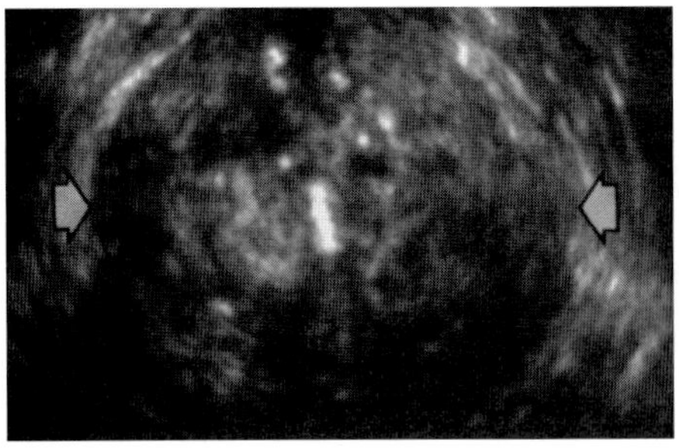

c.

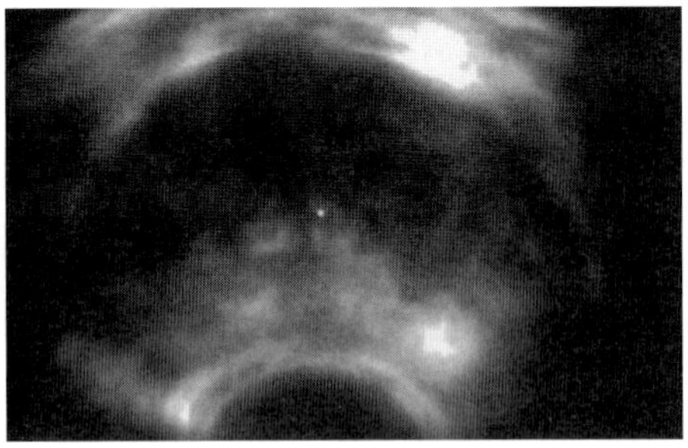

d.

Figure 2. Three-dimensional US planimetric images of the prostate gland. **(a)** Transverse image, initial acquisition. **(b)** Sagittal reconstruction image, with the patient's head to the left. **(c)** Coronal reconstruction image allows excellent demonstration of the lateral borders (arrows) of the gland. **(d)** Surface-rendered volumetric image.

Volume measurements were calculated on the 2D images by measuring glandular size in longitudinal, anteroposterior, and transverse dimensions. By using the formula for an ellipse, length (in centimeters) × height (in centimeters) × width (in centimeters) × 0.523, volumes were determined from the 2D images and were compared with 3D volume measurements calculated from a summation of individual areas measured on parallel sections (mean, five to six sections) and the distance between the individual sections.

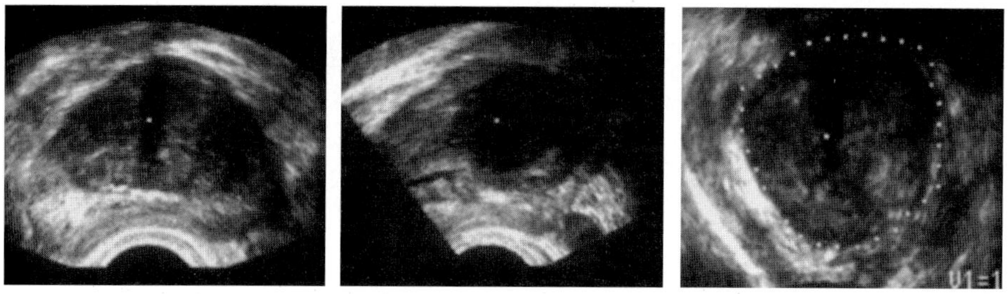

a. b. c.

Figure 3. Three-dimensional US planimetric images of a prostate with central benign prostatic hyperplasia. **(a)** Transverse image, initial acquisition. **(b)** Sagittal reconstruction image, with patient's head to the left. **(c)** Coronal image. Volume of the benign prostatic hyperplasia (dotted circle) was measured by summing area measurements from multiple contiguous sections.

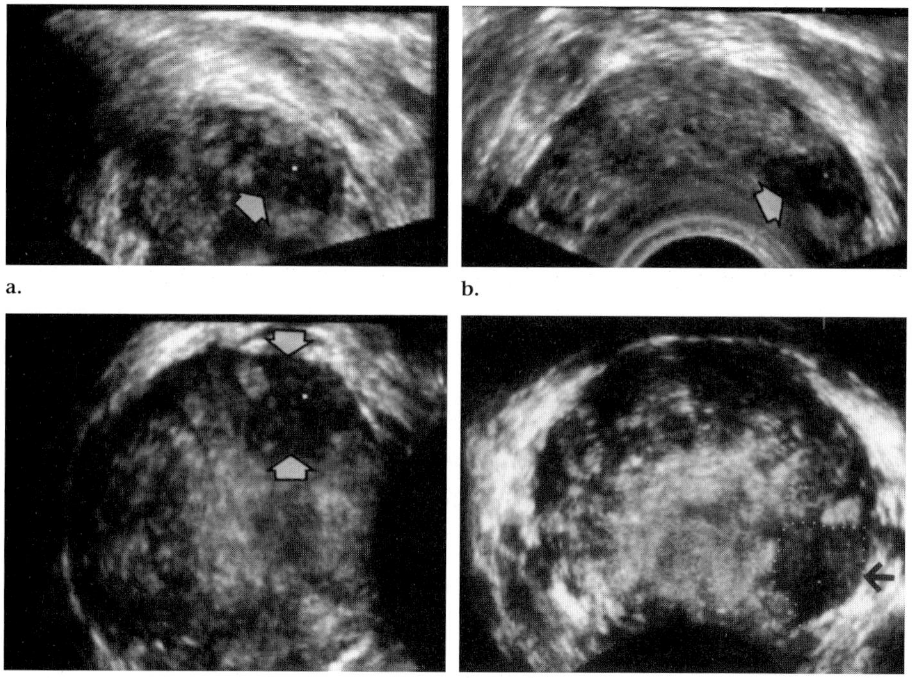

a. b. c. d.

Figure 4. Three-dimensional US images of a left-sided hypoechoic nodule (arrow in **a** and **b**, arrows in **c**), which was proved at biopsy to be prostatic cancer. **(a)** Sagittal image, initial acquisition. The patient's head is visible to the left. **(b)** Transverse image. **(c)** Coronal reconstruction image. Note how the lesion is best seen on this image. **(d)** Same image as in **c**, from the same patient as in **a–c**, but rotated for better anatomic appreciation of the coronal plane. Lesion (dotted outline) has a volumetric assessment of 0.88 mL. Note how the lateral contour (arrow) of the gland in the region of the nodule is smooth, indicating confinement of the tumor to the gland. This was confirmed at histopathologic examination.

Data were recorded on hard-copy images or were digitally stored on removable media (cartridge; SyQuest Technology, Fremont, Calif) for later offline review. Statistical analysis was performed (by U.M.H., V.T., S.S.) by using the paired Student *t* test.

Endorectal US–guided core biopsy was performed (by U.M.H., S.S.) as a systematic "sextant" biopsy. If a focal hypoechoic nodule was identified at endorectal US, one to two passes through the lesions were performed in addition to the routine sextant biopsy. No staging biopsy into the neurovascular bundle or seminal vesicles was performed. Correlation of the US findings with the sextant biopsy results was performed at histopathologic examination.

The correlate for positive and negative findings at the biopsies was the hemisphere since gray-scale US alone was used, and not color Doppler US, which would warrant a correlate for each biopsy site.

RESULTS

Three-dimensional US was easily performed and was well tolerated by all patients. It enabled display of the prostate gland in planes usually not obtainable at conventional 2D US. The region of interest (entire gland) was seen in 16 patients (100%) on the transversely and coronally reconstructed images and in 12 patients (75%) on the sagittally reconstructed images. Visualization of focal lesions at 3D US was judged superior to that at 2D US in four patients (25%) and equal to that at 2D US in eight patients (50%). In four patients (25%), no lesions were identified at either 2D or 3D US. Coronal images were judged superior to and easier to interpret than the sagittal or transverse images in eight patients (50%) (Figs 2, 3). Prostatic volume measurements, as obtained from the 2D images by using the formula for the prostatic ellipse, yielded a mean volume of 55 mL (range, 34–148 mL).

The volume obtained from summing multiple parallel planes on the 3D images yielded a consistently smaller volume, with a mean volume of 44 mL (range, 26–104 mL). This 22% difference in volume was statistically significant (P = .006, paired Student t test). The inner gland could be differentiated from the outer gland in all 16 patients in the coronal view. Volume measurements of the central gland to assess the volume of benign prostatic hyperplasia could be performed easily on the coronal 3D images (Fig 3).

Histopathologic evaluation of 32 prostatic hemispheres in 16 patients revealed tumor in the right hemisphere of the gland in 10 patients and in the left hemisphere in eight patients. Two-dimensional US and 3D US correctly depicted tumor as a hypoechoic lesion in the right hemisphere in nine of 10 patients (Figs 4, 5). Two-dimensional US images demonstrated tumor in the left hemisphere in only one of eight glands, whereas 3D US images correctly depicted three of eight of the histopathologically proved tumors in the left hemisphere (Table 1).

Extraglandular extent of disease was present at histopathologic evaluation in five hemispheres in four patients. Two-dimensional US images depicted extraglandular extent of disease in only one hemisphere in one patient, whereas extraglandular spread was depicted on 3D US images in three hemispheres in two patients (Table 2), with histopathologically proved extracapsular disease best seen on the coronal 3D images (Figs 4, 5).

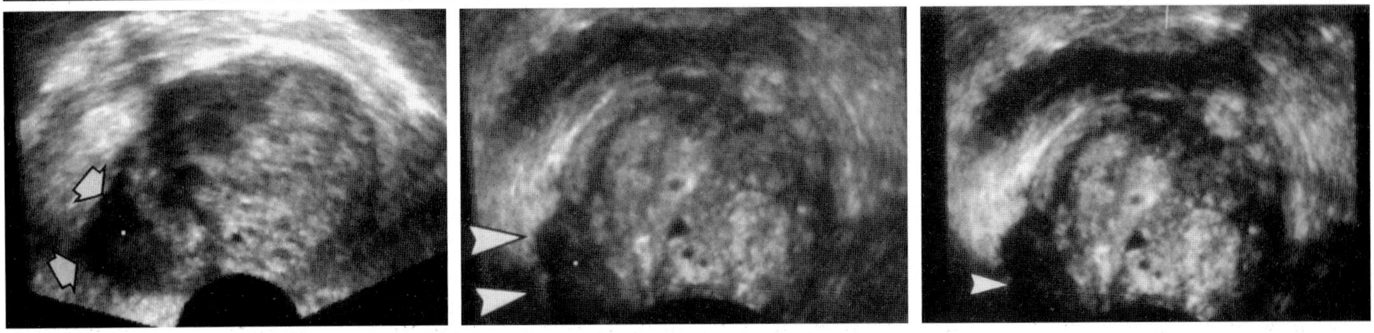

a. c. e.

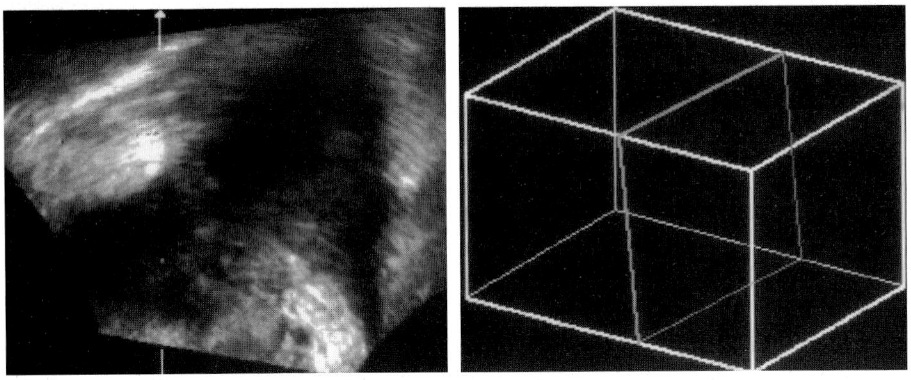

b. d.

Figure 5. (a–c, e) Three-dimensional US images of a right-sided lobulated hypoechoic tumor. (a) Transverse image of the tumor (arrows). (b) Sagittal image. (c) Coronal image. Contour of the gland is irregular and bulging, indicating extraglandular spread of the tumor (arrowheads), which is best seen in the coronal plane. This spread was confirmed at histopathologic examination. (d) Schematic representation of the imaging plane in **a** in the 3D volume. (e) Image from the same patient as in **a–d** in coronal view for better visualization of the irregular contour of the gland (arrowhead).

TABLE 1
Presence of Tumor in 32 Hemispheres

Examination	Right	Left	Total
Histopathologic	10	8	18
2D US	9	1	10
3D US	9	3	12

Note.—Data are number of hemispheres.

TABLE 2
Extraglandular Extent of Carcinoma

Examination	No. of Patients	No. of Hemispheres
Histopathologic	4	5
2D US	1	1
3D US	2	3

DISCUSSION

Endorectal US, introduced by Watanabe et al (21) in 1971, has become the dominant imaging modality for the evaluation of prostatic disease, especially as the guidance modality for prostatic biopsy. Two-dimensional endorectal US examinations, however, are limited primarily by the subjectivity and expertise of the examiner. In addition, the examiner must interpret multiple 2D images and must mentally integrate this information to develop a 3D impression of anatomic or pathologic structures. With a 3D US system, transducer motion is mechanically controlled and standardized, and the 3D integration is achieved by means of a computer system (8,19). Although each examiner must gain experience with the operation of the system and with the interpretation of 3D volumes, the computer-generated image acquisition and display aids the examiner by decreasing subjectivity and by giving the examiner an unlimited opportunity to view findings in multiple planes, thereby increasing his or her certainty of findings or diagnosis.

Another advantage of 3D US is the data are stored on a hard drive for subsequent retrieval, which keeps examination times short and keeps patient discomfort at a minimum. In addition, it allows for later detection of lesions or findings that may have been missed on the original 2D scans.

Volume determination of the prostate gland or focal lesions is clinically important. It is used in conjunction with interpretations of the PSA level to identify patients at risk for prostatic cancer through calculation of PSA density (PSA level/volume), to help with treatment planning, or to evaluate response to therapy for benign prostatic hypertrophy (22–24). Volume determinations of the prostate gland or individual lesions at 3D US may in the future be performed with greater accuracy than is currently possible at 2D US.

Findings from a previous article (13) have shown that ellipsoid volume calculations in the prostate gland had errors of about 20%. Recent study findings by Elliot et al (19) showed 3D US images accurately reflect true prostatic volumes measured in vitro. Our in vivo results seem to agree with findings in this study.

Although no exact volume correlation could be performed with prostatectomy specimens in our study, the measurement of prostatic volumes as obtained at 3D US, when compared with 2D US, showed a statistically significant difference of 20%. Although it is generally accepted that an inaccuracy rate of 20% is acceptable for the evaluation of conservative therapy for prostatic cancer or hypertrophy, this degree of volume difference is not acceptable for calculating PSA densities and for assessing the size of prostatic cancer (13). Therefore, more accurate means of determining prostatic volumes at 3D US may be important for a more accurate determination of the PSA density measurement and of the selection criteria for patients to undergo a prostatic biopsy, especially when PSA elevations are in the "gray zone" between 4 and 10 mg/mL.

In our initial experience, 3D US of the prostate gland appears to be a clinically feasible and useful adjunct to 2D US. The short time needed for the initial acquisition and immediate multidimensional reconstruction, with unlimited off-site review of images, may, in the future, allow for increased efficiency and may maximize the patient's, the sonographer's, and the sonologist's time. Added information from the coronal or oblique planes enables better evaluation of the lateral, anterior, superior, and inferior aspects of the gland. This, in turn, allows better assessment of the extraglandular spread of disease, as seen in our small series. Future developments of 3D color flow imaging may allow targeting of isoechoic yet hypervascular lesions with greater accuracy than is possible with 2D US, thus further increasing diagnostic yield.

Limitations of our study include the small number of patients examined. In addition, although the patients represented a consecutive group of men, they were part of a select group of patients, of whom a relatively high proportion had abnormal results at digital rectal examination and had high PSA levels. This selection bias may also partially explain the greater number of hemispheres with positive findings and hypoechoic lesions in our series compared with the number in most populations of men who undergo prostatic biopsy.

Likewise, although the study is based on findings in 16 consecutive patients and therefore does not demonstrate an exclusion bias, the fact that the 3D examination was always performed after the 2D examination may lead to other biases. The patient may be more amenable to one rather than two endorectal examinations, therefore limiting the results of one technique. Patient cooperation theoretically could decrease for the 3D examination because of fatigue and discomfort, which may hamper the results of the 3D examinations.

On the other hand, since the investigators were not blinded to the findings on 2D scans, they may have been biased by the 2D results, thus improving the results of the 3D study. Some of these biases, however, could not be eliminated since the clinically requested 2D endorectal US examination had to be performed initially for patient care and management decisions prior to any experimental 3D examinations.

Transparent rendered images were subjectively judged difficult to interpret and were not found to be useful for lesion detection. Last, histopathologic correlation was performed in most patients with only biopsy specimens and not with prostatectomy specimens.

Further large-scale studies are needed, preferably studies in which 3D US findings are correlated with findings from histopathologic specimens obtained from radical retropubic prostatectomy for exact histopathologic correlation, and further clinical experience is needed to realize the full clinical potential of 3D US of the prostate.

In summary, our preliminary data suggest 3D US has the potential to become a practical imaging technique for the evaluation of the prostate gland in a busy clinical environment. Three-dimensional US may become a valuable clinical tool and an adjunct to 2D US, allowing depiction of normal and abnormal structures in previously unattainable planes. This facilitates clinical diagnoses, increases the operator's diagnostic confidence, and yields increased efficiency by allowing unlimited off-site review of previously acquired volume data. Further work, however, is needed before the use of this technique can become routine practice and accepted not only as a research tool but as a clinically valuable and cost-effective measure for the evaluation of men with prostatic problems.

References

1. Kelly IM, Gardener JE, Brett AD, Richards R, Lees WR. Three-dimensional US of the fetus: work in progress. Radiology 1994; 192:253–259.
2. Riccabona M, Johnson D, Pretorius DH, Nelson TR. Three-dimensional ultrasound: display modalities in the fetal spine and thorax. Eur J Radiol 1996; 22:141–145.
3. Mueller GM, Weiner CP, Yankowitz J. Three-dimensional ultrasound in the evaluation of fetal head and spine anomalies. Obstet Gynecol 1996; 88:372–378.
4. Pretorius DH, Nelson TR. Fetal face visualization using three-dimensional ultrasonography. J Ultrasound Med 1995; 14:349–356.
5. Merz E, Bahlmann F, Weber G, Macchiella D. Three-dimensional ultrasonography in prenatal diagnosis. J Perinat Med 1995; 23:213–222.
6. Chan L, Uerpairojkit B, Reece EA. Diagnosis of congenital malformations using two-dimensional and three-dimensional ultrasonography. Obstet Gynecol Clin North Am 1977; 24:49–69.
7. Hamper UM, Trapanotto V, Sheth S, DeJong MR, Caskey CI. Three-dimensional US: preliminary clinical experience. Radiology 1994; 191:397–401.
8. Rankin RN, Fenster A, Downey DB, Munk PL, Levin MF, Vellet AD. Three-dimensional sonographic reconstruction: techniques and diagnostic applications. AJR 1993; 161:695–702.
9. Downey DB, Fenster A. Vascular imaging with a three-dimensional power Doppler system. AJR 1995; 165:665–668.
10. Downey DB, Nicolle D, Levin M, Fenster A. Three-dimensional ultrasound imaging of the eye. Eye 1996; 10:75–81.
11. Richard WD, Grimmel CK, Bedigian K, Frank KJ. A method for three-dimensional prostate imaging using transrectal ultrasound. Comput Med Imaging Graph 1993; 17:73–79.
12. Ng KJ, Gardener JE, Rickards D, Lees WR, Milroy EJ. Three-dimensional imaging of the prostatic urethra: an exciting new tool. Br J Urol 1994; 74:604–608.
13. Kimura A, Kurooka Y, Hirasawa K, Kitamura T, Kawabe K. Accuracy of prostatic volume calculation in transrectal ultrasonography. Int J Urol 1995; 2:252–256.
14. Aarnink RG, Huynen AL, Giesen RJ, de la Rosette JJ, Debruyne FM, Wijkstra H. Automated prostate volume determination with ultrasonographic imaging. J Urol 1995; 153:1549–1554.
15. Tong S, Downey DB, Cardinal HN, Fenster A. A three-dimensional ultrasound prostate imaging system. Ultrasound Med Biol 1996; 22:735–746.
16. Downey DB, Fenster A. Three-dimensional power Doppler detection of prostatic cancer. AJR 1995; 165:741.
17. Chin JL, Downey DB, Onik G, Fenster A. Three-dimensional prostate ultrasound and its application to cryosurgery. Tech Urol 1996; 2:187–193.
18. Downey DB, Fenster A. Three-dimensional power Doppler detection of prostatic cancer. AJR 1995; 165:741.
19. Elliot TL, Downey DB, Tong S, McLean CA, Fenster A. Accuracy of prostate volume measurements in vitro using three-dimensional ultrasound. Acad Radiol 1996; 3:401–406.
20. Ivanov KD, Diacov CD. Three-dimensional endoluminal ultrasound. Dis Colon Rectum 1997; 40:47–50.
21. Watanabe H, Kaiho H, Terasawa Y. Diagnostic application of ultrasonotomography to the prostate. Invest Urol 1971; 8:548–549.
22. Benson MC, Whang IS, Pantuck A, et al. Prostate specific antigen density: a means of distinguishing benign prostatic hypertrophy and prostate cancer. J Urol 1992; 147:815–816.
23. Benson MC, Whang IS, Olsson CA, McMahon DJ, Cooner WH. The use of prostate specific antigen density to enhance the predictive value of intermediate levels of serum prostate specific antigen. J Urol 1992; 147:817–821.
24. Rahmouni A, Yang A, Tempany CM, et al. Accuracy of in-vivo assessment of prostatic volume by MRI and transrectal ultrasonography. J Comput Assist Tomogr 1992; 16:935–940.

Book Review

Abdominal Plain Film with Correlative Imaging. 2nd ed.

Steven R. Baker, MD, and Kyunghee C. Cho, MD
Stamford, Conn: Appleton & Lange, 1998. ISBN 0-8385-0275-X.
Hardcover, $165.00; pp 664; 958 figures; tables.

Dr Cho has joined Dr Baker to produce the extensively revised and expanded second edition of this textbook. Both are well-known gastrointestinal radiologists. Although conventional "plain film" radiography is not as glamorous and may not receive as much attention as newer cross-sectional imaging techniques, it remains an important part of diagnostic imaging. As the authors point out in the preface, after chest and extremity views, conventional radiography of the abdomen remains the third most commonly performed radiographic study. It is widely ordered by referring physicians and performed in outpatient clinics, physician offices, urgent care centers, and the emergency department, as well as within the hospital.

The first edition of this book was well received and filled a void as the first single comprehensive treatise on the interpretation of conventional abdominal radiographs. As the title suggests, the second edition has been expanded to include correlative imaging, which consists primarily of computed tomographic (CT) and to a lesser degree barium contrast studies. The basic organizational structure of the book remains the same, but the new edition has been expanded by almost 200 pages.

The first two chapters discuss uses, limitations, technical considerations, and general principles of obtaining and interpreting conventional abdominal radiographs. Chapter 3 discusses radiography of the peritoneal and retroperitoneal spaces. Subsequent chapters follow an organ system approach, and there are chapters on the stomach and duodenum; the intestines and appendix; the liver, bile ducts, and spleen; the pancreas and adrenal glands; the urinary tract; and the female and male genital tracts. The final chapter is a brief overview of radiopaque surgical materials and other extraneous "radiodensities."

As the authors point out in the first chapter, many conditions are not amenable to diagnosis on conventional radiographs. Suspected intestinal obstruction and perforated hollow viscus remain two of the most common indications for conventional abdominal radiographs. Since the first edition, a number of new radiographic signs of pneumoperitoneum have been described. Chapter 3 is an excellent discussion of radiographic findings of free intraperitoneal air. Recognition of some of the subtle signs of free air on the supine radiograph is often critical to making this diagnosis. The information in this chapter should be required reading for anyone who interprets conventional abdominal radiographs.

Throughout the book, the inclusion of CT scout images (essentially digital abdominal images) emphasizes the important information that can be gained from this sometimes overlooked portion of the CT examination, a point we often stress to residents in training. The final chapter on radiology of opaque surgical material is not designed to be comprehensive and discusses primarily clip and staple placement associated with some of the more common surgical procedures. There is not very much discussion or illustration of radiopaque surgical drains, tubes, and devices. Reading this chapter cannot replace the responsibility of each radiologist to become familiar with the many surgical devices in use at his or her own institution. The addition of correlative imaging helps to show how radiographic findings are displayed and confirmed by other modalities.

The quality of the paper, printing, and binding is excellent. The images are of good quality, although many do not seem to reproduce as well in the second edition as they did in the first. The changes in this second edition ensure that this book will remain the indispensable standard of reference for anyone involved in the interpretation of conventional abdominal radiographs. The book should be on the reference shelf of any department, imaging center, or office where these studies are performed and interpreted.

Reviewed by Richard Szucs, MD

Michel Claudon, MD
Carol E. Barnewolt, MD
George A. Taylor, MD
Patricia S. Dunning, RT
Rita Gobet, MD
Abdel-Basset Badawy, MD

Index terms:
Kidney, stenosis or obstruction, 81.145, 81.84
Kidney, US, 81.12981, 81.12982, 81.12984, 81.12988
Renal arteries, US, 963.12981, 963.12982, 963.12984, 963.12988, 963.762
Ultrasound (US), Doppler studies, 963.12984
Ultrasound (US), harmonic study
Ureter, stenosis or obstruction, 82.145, 82.84

Radiology 1999; 212:725–731

Abbreviations:
ANOVA = analysis of variance
RI = resistive index

[1] From the Departments of Radiology (M.C., C.E.B., G.A.T., P.S.D.) and Urology (R.G., A.B.B.), Children's Hospital and Harvard Medical School, 300 Longwood Ave, Boston, MA 02115. Received August 26, 1998; revision requested September 23; final revision received November 23; accepted March 29, 1999. G.A.T. supported in part by Alliance Pharmaceutical, San Diego, Calif, and Acuson, Mountain View, Calif. **Address reprint requests to** G.A.T. (e-mail: *taylor_g@a1.tch.harvard.edu*).

Author contributions:
Guarantor of integrity of entire study, G.A.T.; study concepts, M.C., G.A.T.; study design, M.C., C.E.B., G.A.T., P.S.D., R.G.; definition of intellectual content, M.C., G.A.T.; literature research, M.C., G.A.T.; experimental studies, all authors; data acquisition, all authors; data analysis, M.C., C.E.B., G.A.T.; statistical analysis, M.C., G.A.T.; manuscript preparation, M.C., G.A.T.; manuscript editing, M.C., C.E.B., G.A.T., P.S.D.; manuscript review, all authors

This paper received the Caffey Award for Best Basic Science Research at the 1999 Annual Meeting of the Society for Pediatric Radiology.

Renal Blood Flow in Pigs: Changes Depicted with Contrast-enhanced Harmonic US Imaging during Acute Urinary Obstruction[1]

PURPOSE: To evaluate contrast agent–enhanced harmonic ultrasonographic (US) imaging and Doppler hemodynamics during acute urinary obstruction.

MATERIALS AND METHODS: In 12 piglets, the distal ureter was obstructed for 60 minutes, followed by intravenous injection of furosemide. In six piglets, ureteral pressure was further elevated to mean arterial pressure, and in six other piglets ureteral obstruction was released. Contrast-enhanced harmonic imaging was performed, and interlobar resistive index (RI) and renal blood flow were determined at baseline and during each experimental condition. A bolus injection curve was constructed by plotting mean pixel intensity versus time, and the area under this normalized curve was compared with renal blood flow values.

RESULTS: Ureteral obstruction and high ureteral pressure reduced cortical renal blood flow to 88% and 66%, respectively, of baseline values. Administration of contrast agent resulted in marked homogeneous enhancement of the renal cortex. The area under the curve diminished during ureteral obstruction and correlated well with mean cortical blood flow. RI correlated well with renal perfusion pressure but poorly with changes in renal blood flow.

CONCLUSION: Contrast-enhanced harmonic US imaging depicts changes in renal blood flow during acute obstruction. Interlobar RI is a good predictor of renal perfusion pressure but not of changes in renal blood flow.

Harmonic ultrasonography (US) is an imaging modality that takes advantage of the nonlinear properties of microbubble-based contrast agents. By transmitting at the fundamental frequency and receiving at the second harmonic frequency, backscatter from contrast agents is much greater than tissue backscatter (1). As a result, signal-to-noise ratio is greatly increased. In the evaluation of tissue blood flow, this technique has several theoretic advantages over conventional Doppler methods (2,3). There is no blooming artifact, shadowing artifacts are lessened, temporal resolution is better, sensitivity to flow in blood vessels at or near 90° from the transducer face is not diminished, and gray-scale pixel brightness calculations do not rely on angle-dependent frequency shift estimates (3). Thus, it is possible that contrast agent–enhanced gray-scale harmonic imaging will be able to depict tissue blood flow by allowing backscatter from capillary blood flow to be separated from tissue clutter.

Results from previous animal and human studies (4–6) have shown that occlusion of the ureter is associated with a reduction in global renal blood flow by up to 45%. Results of several studies (7–9) have suggested that this vasoconstrictive response could be identified by using the Doppler criteria of intrarenal resistive index (RI) of 0.70 or greater or an increased difference between the RI of the obstructed and contralateral kidney of 0.08–0.10 or greater. Intravenous administration of furosemide and a bolus of normal saline solution also has been reported to increase the differences in RI between the kidneys by causing the RI to increase in the obstructed kidney and decrease in the nonobstructed kidney (10–12). However, other authors (13–16) have shown a lack of sensitivity of renal Doppler US to acute obstruction. Because of this uncertainty, an alternative or complementary noninvasive method to detect early hemodynamic changes in the obstructed kidney might be desirable. The aims of this study were therefore to assess the feasibility of contrast-enhanced gray-scale harmonic US imaging and to compare it with Doppler hemodynamics for the evaluation of renal blood flow during acute ureteral obstruction.

MATERIALS AND METHODS

Surgical Procedure

Anesthesia was induced in 12 Yorkshire pigs (weight, 4.5–15 kg) by means of intramuscular injection of 11–15 mg of ketamine hydrochloride (Ketalar; Parke-Davis, Morris Plains, NJ) per kilogram of body weight and 1.1 mg/kg xylazine hydrochloride (Rompun; Miles, Shawnee, Kan). Inhalation of 1%–2% isoflurane (Enflurane; Wyeth-Ayerst Laboratories, Wayne, Pa) and intramuscular injection of 0.2 mg/kg butorphanol tartrate (Torbugesic; Fort Dodge Laboratories, Ft Dodge, Iowa) were used to maintain anesthesia. Ventilation was controlled via an oral endotracheal tube throughout the experiment. Polyvinyl chloride catheters were placed in the left ventricle via the right femoral artery for microsphere injections, the right femoral vein for injection of the US contrast agent, the left femoral artery for arterial blood pressure monitoring, and the left femoral vein for intravenous fluid administration.

A cystotomy was performed, and a 4-F balloon catheter (Cook, Bloomington, Ind) was placed in the orifice of the right ureter. The balloon was inflated with fluoroscopic guidance, and the catheter was connected to a pressure transducer. The positions of the cardiac and ureteral catheters were confirmed fluoroscopically. Arterial, left ventricular, and ureteral pressure and the core temperature were monitored continuously with a physiologic monitoring system (model 76; Hewlett-Packard, Andover, Mass). Arterial P_{O_2}, P_{CO_2}, pH, and hematocrit levels were measured intermittently throughout the experiment.

Imaging Protocol

The right kidney was imaged in situ by using a curved transducer (Sequoia Systems; Acuson, Mountain View, Calif) transmitting at 4.0 MHz and receiving at 8.0 MHz and held in place by an articulated mechanical holder during the entire experiment. Linear image pre- and postprocessing, or input-output conversion, curves were used. The mechanical index was set at 0.5 units, the gray-scale gain was set at 0 dB, and no persistence was used. These imaging parameters were held constant during the entire experiment.

The contrast agent, AF0150 (Imagent; Alliance Pharmaceutical, San Diego, Calif), was reconstituted according to the manufacturer's directions and yielded a dispersion of surfactant-coated perfluorohexane nitrogen-containing microbubbles with a volume-weighted median diameter of approximately 5 μm. Elimination from the blood is accomplished by evaporation through the lungs (17). The contrast agent was administered at a dose of 0.1 mL/kg. Each dose was injected intravenously over an interval of 1–2 seconds. At least 15 minutes elapsed between injections. The catheter and stopcock were flushed with saline solution by using three times the catheter volume after each dose to clear any residual contrast agent.

The transducer-to-kidney surface distance was 1.5–2.0 cm in each animal. Serial harmonic gray-scale images of the kidney were obtained in sagittal projection before, during, and after the injection of contrast agent. The renal pelvis diameter was measured in the anteroposterior dimension, and at least three interlobar arteries were interrogated with pulsed Doppler US at every experimental point. Waveforms lasting at least 3 seconds were selected, and an RI was measured electronically. The mean of these three values was used for analyses.

Image Processing

A continuous digital movie clip of the kidney was started at the onset of the intravenous injection of contrast agent. Images were captured electronically every 0.3 second for a total of 60 seconds by using a digital image processing unit (Sequoia Systems, Acuson) and were saved in an 8-bit tag image file format, or TIFF. Images were then transferred onto a computer (G3 MacIntosh; Apple Computer, Cupertino, Calif) and analyzed by using OPEN LAB (Improvision, Coventry, UK). Each digital movie clip was saved as a serial image stack.

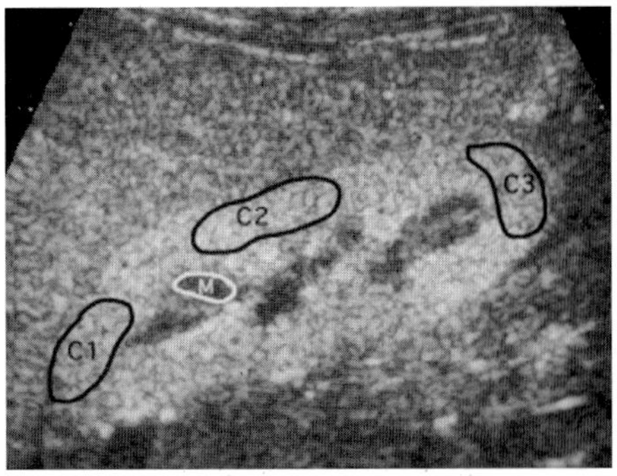

Figure 1. Sagittal contrast-enhanced harmonic US image of the right kidney shows regions of interest used for upper-pole (*C1*), middle (*C2*), and lower-pole (*C3*) cortex and for medulla (*M*) to derive time-intensity curves for the kidney.

Three separate regions of interest of similar size were drawn over the cortex and medulla in the upper, middle, and lower portions of the kidney (Fig 1). These regions of interest were identified on images obtained before the administration of contrast agent and electronically superimposed on subsequent anatomically registered images obtained after the administration of contrast agent. Thus, the same region of interest was used for the determination of mean pixel intensity in each area of the kidney so that differences in intensity reflected changes in mean pixel value and not variations in the size and location of the area measured. The number of pixels and mean pixel value were calculated for each region of interest by using the program's measurement and results functions. Mean pixel intensity was measured on a scale with equal increments from 0 for black to 255 for white and was expressed as the mean intensity per number of pixels in the region of interest.

Time-intensity curves were plotted as the mean pixel intensity per unit area versus time (seconds). The pixel intensity values before the appearance of contrast agent were averaged, and the curve was normalized by subtracting the mean from each point along the curve. The area in pixels under the normalized curve and the peak enhancement ratio, defined as the mean pixel intensity at maximum contrast enhancement minus the precontrast mean pixel intensity divided by the precontrast mean pixel intensity multiplied by 100, were calculated and used for further analyses.

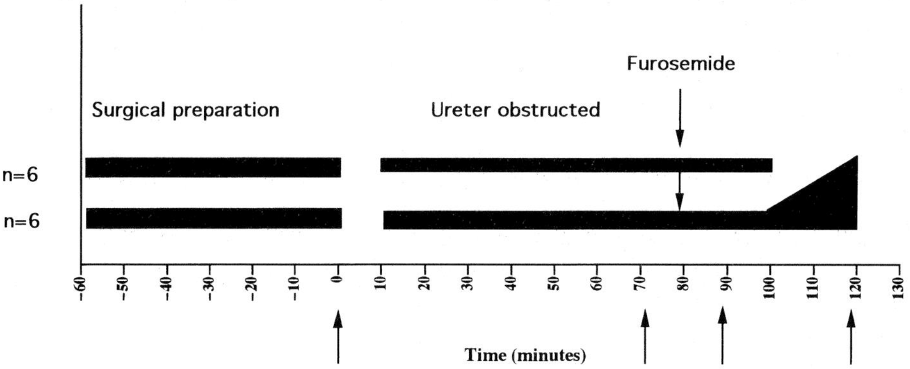

Figure 2. Timeline shows sequence and duration of experimental protocols. In six animals (top bar), the ureter was obstructed for 90 minutes and released. In six additional animals (lower bar), the ureteral pressure was sequentially increased to mean arterial pressure. Upward arrows denote the timing of injections of microspheres and US contrast agent. Downward arrows denote the timing of furosemide injection.

Regional Renal Blood Flow Determinations

Renal blood flow was determined for both kidneys in every animal by using the reference-sample radiolabeled-microsphere technique (18). We used microspheres of 16 μm ± 0.5 (SD) labeled with four separate isotopes: cerium 141, tin 113, ruthenium 103, and scandium 46 (Dupont-New England Nuclear Products, Boston, Mass). Each of these isotopes has a different photon energy and therefore can be measured independently. For each blood flow determination, a volume containing 1.5×10^6 microspheres labeled with one of these isotopes was injected into the left ventricle and flushed with 5 mL of saline solution for 20 seconds to distribute the spheres throughout the body according to regional blood flow. A reference blood sample was withdrawn from a femoral catheter at a rate of 2 mL/min beginning 30 seconds before microsphere injection and continued for 90 seconds after completion of the saline solution flush. Microsphere injection did not alter the mean arterial blood pressure.

At the end of each experiment, the animals were killed with an intravenous injection (2 mL/kg) of pentobarbital and potassium chloride. Both kidneys were resected and immediately sectioned to determine regional renal blood flow, or r-RBF, to the cortical regions identified on the US images. After sectioning, each tissue sample was weighed and placed in a 15-mL vial for analysis in an autogamma scintillation spectrometer (Cobra II Gamma Counter; Packard Instruments, Meriden, Conn). Blood flow was determined by comparing counts for each radiolabel in each tissue sample to counts in the reference blood samples. All counts were corrected for isotope decay. Cortical blood flow was expressed in milliliters per minute per gram of tissue by normalizing for tissue weight. The medullary vascular bed is unique in that venous outflow is consistently higher than arterial inflow. The radiolabeled microsphere method relies on the assessment of inflow and, as a result, it is likely to cause underestimation of medullary blood flow (19). Therefore, only cortical blood flows were used for analysis.

Experimental Protocol

Contrast-enhanced US images, interlobar arterial RIs, and renal blood flow determinations in the right kidney were obtained at baseline, 60 minutes after ureteral occlusion, and 10 minutes after the intravenous administration of 1 mg/kg furosemide (Lasix; American Regent Laboratories, Shirley, NY). In six animals, the ureteral obstruction was relieved by removing the balloon catheter. In the other six animals, a bag of saline solution was connected to the ureteral catheter, and its height was adjusted to increase ureteral pressure in increments of 10 mm Hg approximately to mean arterial pressure (65–80 mm Hg). US evaluation and microsphere injections were performed 10 minutes after the release of ureteral obstruction in the first six animals and at maximal ureteral pressure in the other six. An experimental timeline is shown in Figure 2.

Data Analysis

For each kidney imaged, the area under the curve and the peak enhancement ratio for the renal cortex were compared with the regional cortical flow in milliliters per minute per gram of tissue by means of linear regression. The changes in continuous variables for each experimental condition were compared by means of analysis of variance (ANOVA) techniques or by means of the Student *t* test, where appropriate. Renal perfusion pressure, or the mean arterial pressure minus the mean ureteral pressure, and renal vascular resistance, or the renal perfusion pressure divided by the renal blood flow (20), were calculated at each interval. All results were expressed as the mean plus or minus the SEM. A *P* value less than .05 was considered to indicate a statistically significant difference.

This study was approved by our institutional animal care and use committee and complied with the guidelines of the National Institutes of Health for the care and handling of animals.

RESULTS

The Table shows the effect of each experimental condition on the obstructed kidney. Acute ureteral obstruction with and that without high ureteral pressure reduced cortical renal blood flow to 88% and 66%, respectively, of baseline values ($P < .001$, ANOVA). Compared with baseline values, renal blood flow was not significantly changed during administration of furosemide and during subsequent release of ureteral obstruction. However, compared with blood flow during obstruction, blood flow after the administration of furosemide increased by approximately 30% ($P < .05$).

Furosemide, compared with obstruction alone, did not significantly increase RI or ureteral pressure ($P > .05$, ANOVA). There were no significant differences in regional blood flow to the upper-pole, middle, or lower-pole cortices in the obstructed kidney during any experimental condition. In the contralateral kidney, in which no surgery was performed, obstruction resulted in no significant change in renal blood flow. However, furosemide and high right ureteral pressure increased renal blood flow to 134% and 136%, respectively, of baseline values ($P < .001$). Mean ureteral pressure progressively increased from a mean of 8.4 mm Hg at baseline to a mean of 34.3 mm Hg during obstruction and 38.4 mm Hg during subsequent diuresis ($P < .001$). Mean arterial blood pressure also significantly increased after furosemide administration, and during high ureteral pressure, and dropped to below baseline levels after release of

Effects of Experimental Conditions on Obstructed Kidneys

Condition	Mean Arterial Pressure (mm Hg)	Renal Blood Flow (mL/min/g)	Ureteral Pressure (mm Hg)	Area under the Curve (pixels)	Peak Enhancement Ratio (%)	RI	Renal Pelvis Diameter (mm)
Baseline (n = 12)	74 ± 2	2.9 ± 0.2	8.4 ± 0.4	2,778 ± 141	129 ± 13	0.61 ± 0.8	2.1 ± 0.3
Obstruction (n = 12)	79 ± 2	1.9 ± 0.2*	34.3 ± 1.9*	2,105 ± 141*	101 ± 9*	0.72 ± 1.5*	6.2 ± 0.3*
Furosemide (n = 12)	82 ± 2*	2.5 ± 0.1	38.4 ± 2.1*	1,788 ± 114*	75 ± 6*	0.74 ± 1.4*	5.7 ± 0.4*
High pressure (n = 6)	80 ± 3*	2.3 ± 0.3*	69.7 ± 1.6*	1,842 ± 109*	64 ± 6*	0.83 ± 0.9*	6.5 ± 0.3*
Release of obstruction (n = 6)	71 ± 2	2.6 ± 0.1	NA†	2,128 ± 269*	104 ± 23	0.56 ± 1.0*	3.8 ± 0.5

* $P < .05$ compared with baseline values.
† NA = Not applicable. Ureteral pressure was not measured during release because the catheter was withdrawn.

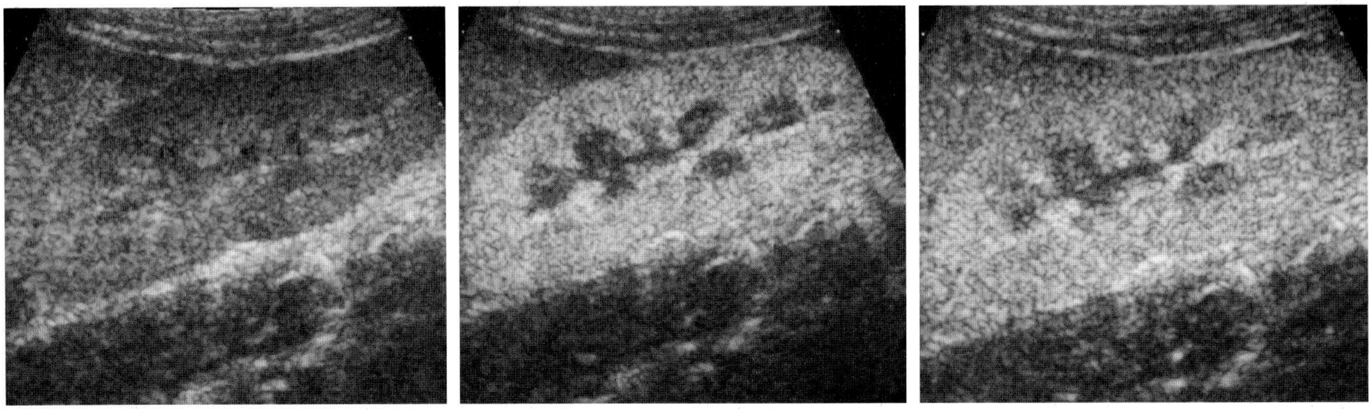

a. b. c.

Figure 3. Sagittal harmonic US images of the right kidney before ureteral obstruction, obtained **(a)** before the administration of contrast agent, **(b)** during peak cortical contrast enhancement, and **(c)** during peak medullary enhancement, show marked homogeneous cortical enhancement. Cortical mean pixel intensity increased from 85 intensity units before the administration of contrast agent to 162 intensity units at the peak effect of the contrast agent. Medullary enhancement is later and less intense than cortical enhancement. Mean medullary pixel intensity increased from 90 intensity units before the administration of contrast agent to 143 intensity units at the peak effect of the contrast agent.

obstruction ($P < .004$, overall ANOVA model).

Distention of the renal pelvis was present almost immediately after the placement of the ureteral catheter and correlated strongly with changes in ureteral pressure ($r = 0.63$, $P = .001$; linear regression). The pelvis was largest at peak ureteral pressures and became smaller with release. Perinephric fluid collections 1–4 mm thick developed in six animals: after furosemide administration in two animals and during maximal ureteral pressure in four animals.

Before obstruction, administration of contrast agent resulted in marked homogeneous enhancement of the renal cortex (Fig 3). The mean cortical pixel intensity increased from 67.8 intensity units ± 5 before the injection of contrast agent to 138.6 intensity units ± 5 at the peak effect of the contrast agent ($P < .001$). The percentage of enhancement, expressed as the peak enhancement ratio, was significantly less in the upper pole of the kidney (85% ± 11) compared with the middle (153% ± 11) and lower-pole (150% ± 21) regions of the kidney ($P < .04$).

Only seven kidneys had medullary pyramids that were clearly visible without obvious partial volume averaging with overlying cortex. As a result, medullary pyramid enhancement data were collected from only this subset of animals. The mean medullary pixel intensity increased from 58 intensity units ± 4 before the administration of contrast agent to 98 intensity units ± 5 at the peak effect of the contrast agent ($P < .001$). The peak medullary enhancement was later and was significantly less ($P < .001$) than peak cortical enhancement (Fig 3).

Both peak cortical enhancement and measures of the area under the curve diminished during acute ureteral obstruction. They were further reduced by furosemide and high ureteral pressures ($P < .001$) (Table, Fig 4). The release of ureteral obstruction resulted in only a minimal increase in enhancement values. These differences did not reach statistical significance. There was a weak but significant correlation between the area under the curve during the administration of contrast agent and the mean cortical blood flow averaged from all three regions of the kidney ($r = 0.43$, $P < .001$; linear regression) (Fig 5). The area under the curve also correlated with ureteral pressure ($r = 0.37$, $P < .001$).

RI was affected by ureteral obstruction. There was a pattern of progressively increasing RI with obstruction, furosemide administration, and high ureteral pressure, with a marked diminution in RI during the release of obstruction compared with the baseline RI (Table). However, administration of furosemide during obstruction did not significantly increase RI compared with RI during obstruction without furosemide ($P > .05$, ANOVA). There was a strong and significant correlation between interlobar arterial RI and ureteral pressure ($r = 0.792$, $P < .001$) and renal perfusion pressure ($r = 0.721$, $P < .001$) (Fig 6a). However, RI was a poor predictor of changes in renal

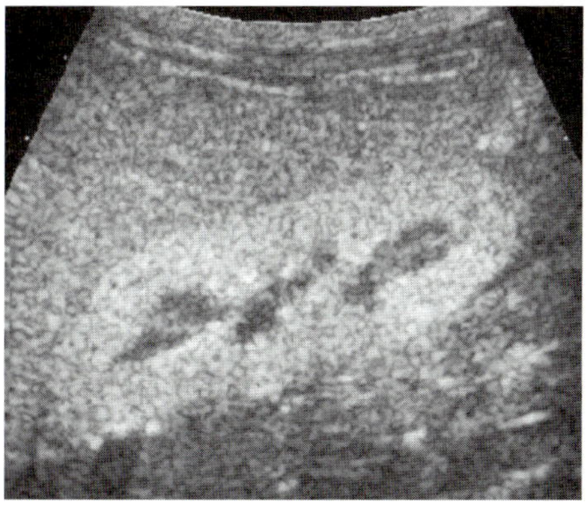

a.

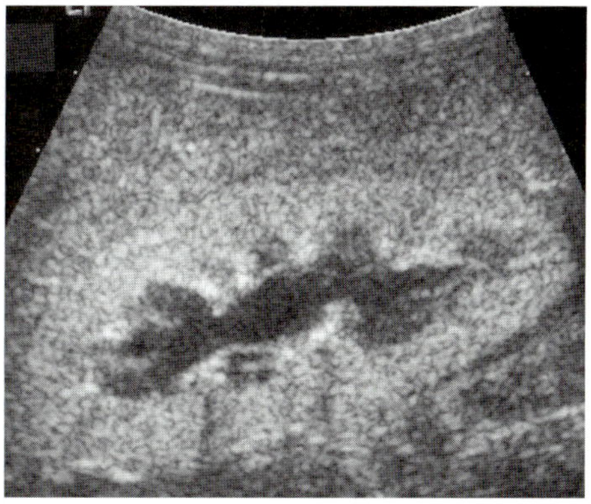

b.

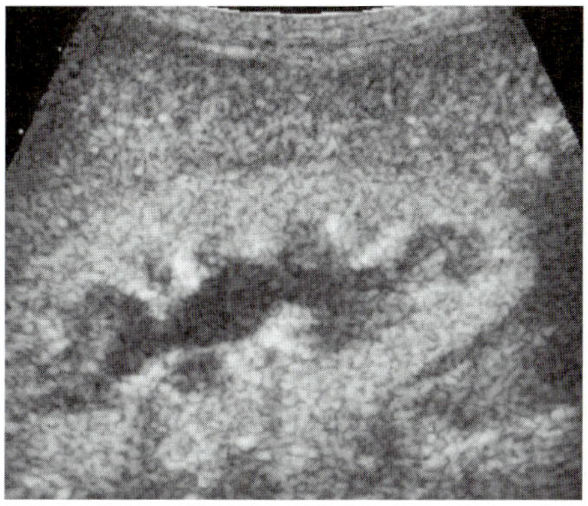

c.

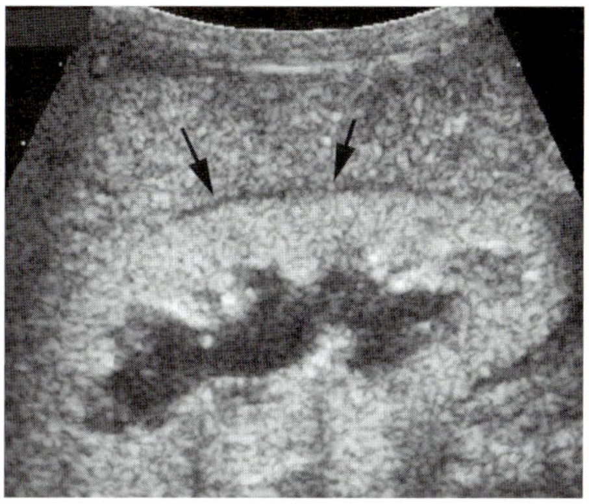

d.

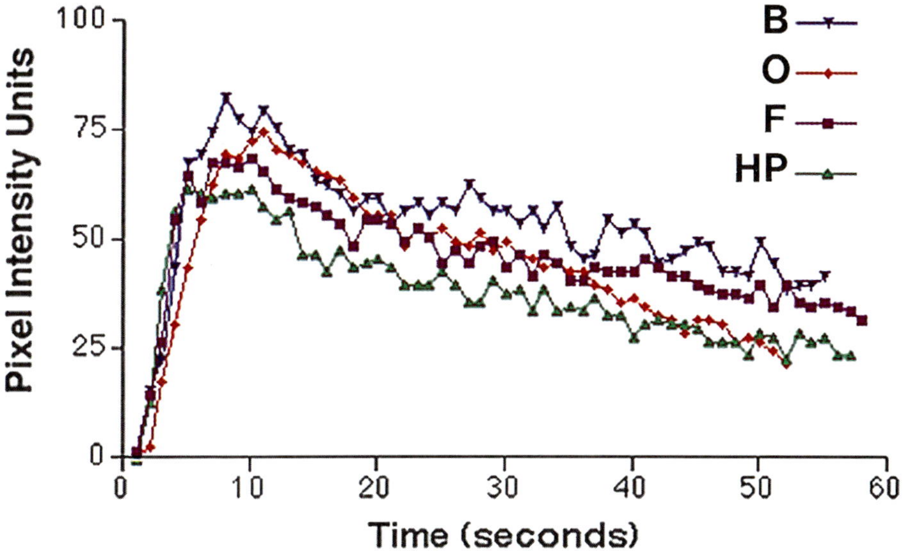

e.

Figure 4. Sagittal harmonic US images of the right kidney obtained **(a)** during peak cortical enhancement at baseline (190 intensity units), **(b)** during acute obstruction (168 intensity units), **(c)** 10 minutes after the intravenous injection of furosemide (163 intensity units), and **(d)** during peak ureteral pressure of 64 mm Hg (160 intensity units) show reduction in peak cortical enhancement during obstruction compared with baseline values. Note the small perinephric fluid collection (arrows) present at high ureteral pressure. **(e)** Graph of cortical time-intensity curves from the middle of the kidney shows changes in peak enhancement and the area under the curve. The mean pixel intensity refers to mean pixel intensity per number of pixels in the region of interest. *B* = baseline, *F* = furosemide, *HP* = high pressure, *O* = obstruction.

cortical blood flow ($r = 0.13$, $P = .15$) (Fig 6b) and only a weak predictor of renal vascular resistance ($r = 0.38$, $P < .001$) (Fig 6c).

RI and ureteral pressure were analyzed separately for the subset of six animals that developed perinephric fluid collections. There was no change in either ureteral pressure or RI in two animals. In the remaining four animals, small but significant changes in RI and ureteral pressure were observed; with the detection of fluid, mean RI decreased from 86% ± 2 to 82% ± 2 ($P < .01$, paired Student t test), and mean ureteral pressure decreased from 63 mm Hg ± 5 to 59 mm Hg ± 4 ($P = .05$).

DISCUSSION

The main findings in this study are that contrast-enhanced harmonic US imaging can depict global changes in renal blood flow and that interlobar RI values are strong predictors of ureteral pressure but not of renal blood flow during acute renal obstruction.

Blood flow to the normal, nonobstructed kidney is characterized by large differences in flow to the cortex and medulla. Cortical blood flow is approximately 15- to 20-fold greater than blood flow to the medulla (21). Contrast-enhanced harmonic imaging of the normal kidney depicted these normal regional differences in blood flow. Enhancement was bright and homogeneous throughout the renal cortex and was proportionately lower in medullary pyramids. This differential enhancement is consistent with enhancement results obtained by other authors (22).

During occlusion of the ureter, a consistent reduction in ipsilateral renal blood flow and glomerular filtration rate has been shown in a variety of experimental animals (4,5). In animals with multipapillary kidneys, such as the pig or rat, this reduction occurs immediately after the onset of acute obstruction and appears to be effected primarily by prostaglandin mediators (5,20). The renal resistance to blood flow follows these changes and correlates strongly with intrarenal pressure (5). Blood flow to the contralateral kidney may or may not be elevated depending on how elevated intrarenal pressure is on the obstructed side (5,20).

In this study, alterations in renal hemodynamics during obstruction were evident on contrast-enhanced harmonic images. Compared with baseline values, the peak enhancement ratio and the area under the curve decreased during obstruction. Both measures were further reduced after furosemide administration and during high ureteral pressure. After release of

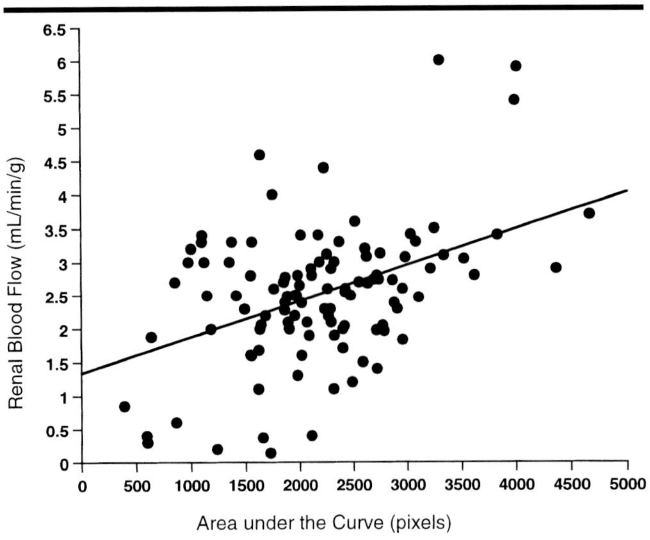

Figure 5. Graph shows weak but significant correlation between the area under the curve and cortical blood flow ($r = 0.43$, $P < .001$; linear regression).

ureteral obstruction, cortical enhancement did not return to baseline levels. We postulate that this was owing to mild residual obstruction related to ureteral edema after prolonged instrumentation. Although there was a highly significant correlation between cortical blood flow and the area under the curve, there was considerable variability about the regression line, and the relationship was relatively weak.

Contrast-enhanced power Doppler US images have shown markedly reduced enhancement of peripheral portions of cortex during hemorrhagic shock while enhancement of deeper cortical areas is preserved (23). We hypothesized that similar regional redistribution of blood flow might be seen during ureteral obstruction, particularly at higher pressure levels. As shown in Figure 3, there was homogeneous cortical enhancement throughout the entire thickness of the renal cortex during obstruction. Unlike the kidney imaged during shock, there was no visual evidence of diminished enhancement of the peripheral cortex.

Findings of the current study confirm that the RI increases in the setting of acute ureteral occlusion and that there is a strong correlation between RI and ureteral pressure in the obstructed kidney (24). Our data also show that RI is a poor predictor of changes in renal blood flow and only a weak predictor of renal vascular resistance. Administration of furosemide during obstruction did not increase RI or ureteral pressure significantly compared with obstruction without furosemide.

These data may help us understand the variability in clinical results reported for Doppler US in acute renal obstruction. According to Platt (25), marked elevations of pressure in the collecting system occur quickly with the onset of acute urinary occlusion, with the rate of increase dependent on the rate of urine flow at the onset of obstruction. With urinary occlusion, there may be a return of renal pelvic pressure to normal levels soon after the onset of obstruction (25,26). As shown in this study, the RI is strongly dependent on intrarenal pressure. Thus, if intrarenal pressure is not high, the RI may not be elevated at certain times during renal occlusion, despite the presence of diminished renal blood flow.

An additional factor that may dampen the intrarenal RI during occlusion is the development of small perforations of the upper urinary tract, probably at the fornix of a calix. These tears have been described in association with distal obstruction and may result in urinomas or ascites (27). In this study, we observed the development of similar perinephric fluid collections in six animals during obstruction and the administration of furosemide or under conditions of high ureteral pressure. Although these collections were associated with only small reductions in RI and ureteral pressure, it is likely that tears resulting in larger fluid collections may have larger reductions in intrarenal pressure and RI.

There are several technical problems that may limit the utility of contrast-enhanced harmonic imaging. First, peak enhancement of the upper-pole cortex

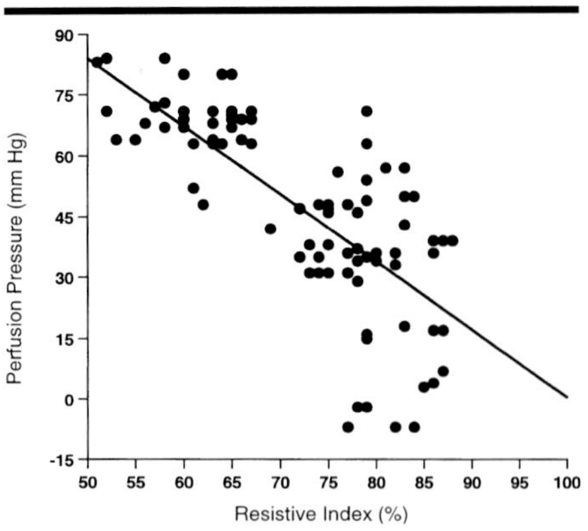

a.

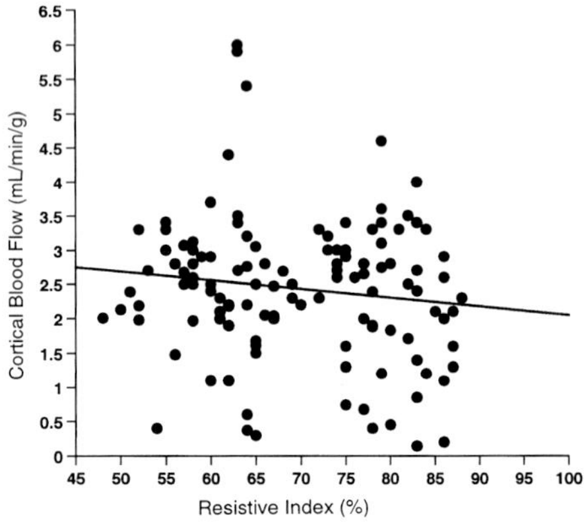

b.

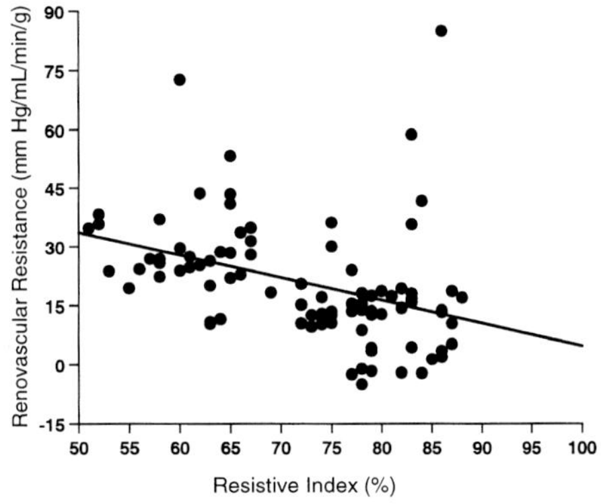

c.

Figure 6. Graphs show the correlation between interlobar RI and renal hemodynamics. **(a)** There is a strong correlation between RI and renal perfusion pressure ($r = 0.721$, $P < .001$; linear regression). RI is **(b)** a poor predictor of cortical blood flow ($r = 0.13$, $P = .15$) and **(c)** only a weak predictor of renovascular resistance ($r = 0.38$, $P < .001$).

was less than that observed in other regions of the kidney, without an associated reduction in the area under the curve or renal blood flow. This diminished enhancement may be due to differences in the destruction of contrast agent by US energy experienced by bubbles of contrast agent near the focal zone of the transducer or possibly due to relative shadowing by echogenic contrast agent in the liver overlying the upper renal pole.

Second, the correlation between the degree of cortical enhancement and renal blood flow was significant but not strong ($P < .05$). According to Ophir and Parker (28), when stable contrast agents are used, the peak time and mean transit time are related directly to the flow rate. However, the properties of the time-intensity curves may be affected substantially by the attenuation and instability of microbubble-based contrast agents within the vascular bed. Nonetheless, our data show that contrast-enhanced harmonic gray-scale US imaging shows potential for depicting changes in global renal blood flow in real time.

Practical application: Harmonic imaging techniques might be a useful adjunct for serial bedside evaluation of abnormalities in renal cortical perfusion without the use of radioactive agents. This would have important applications in children in whom respiratory and voluntary motion are more difficult to control and in large adults in whom Doppler and gray-scale signal intensity from renal parenchyma can be attenuated markedly by distance and fat. However, further work is needed before this technique is used for clinical assessment of renal blood flow.

The identification of urinary obstruction still remains a challenge, especially in young children in whom an intrarenal RI of 70 or more may be normal and in patients with obstruction without elevated intrarenal pressure.

Acnowledgments: The authors thank Christopher Contois, BA, for help with manuscript preparation, Arthur Nedder, DVM, for help with animal care and anesthesia, and N. Thorne Griscome, MD, for editorial review and advice.

References

1. Schrope B, Newhouse VL, Uhlendorf V. Simulated capillary blood flow measurement using a nonlinear ultrasonic contrast agent. Ultrason Imaging 1992; 14:134–158.
2. Burns PN. Harmonic imaging with ultrasound contrast agents. Clin Radiol 1996; 51(suppl 1):50–55.
3. Forsberg F, Goldberg BB, Liu JB, Merton DA, Rawool NM. On the feasibility of real-time, in vivo harmonic imaging with proteinaceous microspheres. J Ultrasound Med 1996; 15:853–860.
4. Provoost AP, Van Aken M, Molenaar JC. Sequential renography and renal function in Brown-Norway rats with congenital hydronephrosis. J Urol 1991; 146:588–591.
5. Hvistendahl JJ, Pedersen TS, Jorgensen HH, Rehling M, Frokiaer J. Renal hemodynamic response to gradated ureter obstruction in the pig. Nephron 1996; 74:168–174.
6. Platt JF. Urinary obstruction. Radiol Clin North Am 1996; 34:1113–1129.
7. Platt JF, Rubin JM, Ellis JH, DiPietro MA. Duplex Doppler US of the kidney: differentiation of obstructive from nonobstructive dilatation. Radiology 1989; 171:515–517.
8. Sauvain JL, Bourscheid D, Pierrat V, et al. Duplex Doppler ultrasonography of renal parenchyma arteries: normal and pathological aspects. Ann Radiol 1991; 34:237–247.
9. Gilbert R, Gara B, Gibbons MD. Renal duplex Doppler ultrasound: an adjunct in the evaluation of hydronephrosis in the child. J Urol 1993; 150:1192–1194.
10. Shokier AA, Nijman RJ, El-Azab M, Provoost AP. Partial ureteral obstruction: effect of intravenous normal saline and furosemide upon the renal resistive index. J Urol 1997; 157:1074–1077.
11. Bude RO, DiPietro MA, Platt JF, Rubin JM. Effect of furosemide and intravenous normal saline fluid load upon the renal resistive index in nonobstructed kidneys in children. J Urol 1994; 151:438–441.
12. Piepsz A, Ham HR, Collier F, et al. Sensitivity of cortical transit and furosemide response in the diagnosis of renal obstruction: an experimental model. Uremia Invest 1985–1986; 9:245–252.
13. Palmer JM, Lindfors KK, Ordorica RC, Marder DM. Diuretic Doppler sonography in postnatal hydronephrosis. J Urol 1991; 146:605–608.
14. Cronan JJ, Tublin ME. Role of the resistive index in the evaluation of acute renal obstruction (editorial). AJR 1995; 164:377–378.
15. Tublin ME, Dodd GD III, Verdile VP. Acute renal colic: diagnosis with Duplex Doppler US. Radiology 1994; 193:697–701.
16. Coley BD, Arellano RS, Talner LB, Baker KG, Mattrey RF. Renal resistive index in experimental partial and complete ureteral obstruction. Acad Radiol 1995; 2:373–378.
17. Goldberg BB, Liu JB, Forsberg F. Ultrasound contrast agents: a review. Ultrasound Med Biol 1994; 20:319–333.
18. Heymann MA, Payne BD, Hoffman JI, Rudolph AM. Blood flow measurements with radionuclide-labeled particles. Prog Cardiovasc Dis 1977; 20:55–79.
19. Strick DM, Fiksen-Olsen MJ, Lockhart JC, Roman RJ, Romero JC. Direct measurement of renal medullary blood flow in the dog. Am J Physiol 1994; 267:R253–R259.
20. Frokiaer J, Nielsen AS, Knudsen L, Djurhuus JC, Pedersen EB. The effect of indomethacin infusion on renal hemodynamics and on the renin-angiotensin system during unilateral ureteral obstruction of the pig. J Urol 1993; 150:1557–1563.
21. Hollenberg NK. The physiology of the renal circulation. In: Black D, Jones NF, eds. Renal disease. Oxford, England: Blackwell Scientific Publications, 1979; 30–63.
22. Mattrey RF, Steinbach G, Lee Y, Wilkening W, Lazenby J. High-resolution harmonic gray-scale imaging of normal and abnormal vessels and tissues in animals. Acad Radiol 1998; 5(suppl 1):S63–S65.
23. Taylor GA, Barnewolt CE, Adler BH, Dunning PS. Renal cortical ischemia in rabbits revealed by contrast-enhanced power Doppler sonography. AJR 1998; 170:417–422.
24. Fung LC, Steckler RE, Khoury AE, McLorie GA, Chait PG, Churchill BM. Intrarenal resistive index correlates with renal pelvis pressure. J Urol 1994; 52:607–611.
25. Platt JF. Urinary obstruction. Radiol Clin North Am 1996; 34:1113–1129.
26. Klahr S. New insights into the consequences and mechanisms of renal impairment in obstructive nephropathy. Am J Kidney Dis 1991; 18:689–699.
27. Barnewolt CE, Paltiel HJ, Lebowitz RL, Kirks DR. Genitourinary tract. In: Kirks DR, ed. Practical pediatric imaging: diagnostic radiology of infants and children. 3rd ed. Philadelphia, Pa: Lippincott-Raven, 1998; 1009–1170.
28. Ophir J, Parker KJ. Contrast agents in diagnostic ultrasound. Ultrasound Med Biol 1989; 15:319–333.

Effect of Downstream Cross-sectional Area of an Arterial Bed on the Resistive Index and the Early Systolic Acceleration[1]

Ronald O. Bude, MD
Jonathan M. Rubin, MD, PhD

Index terms:
Blood, flow dynamics, 9∗.1312, 9∗.133, 9∗.91, 9∗.92
Phantoms, 9∗.12984, 9∗.131, 9∗.133, 9∗.91, 9∗.92
Ultrasound (US), Doppler studies, 9∗.12984

Radiology 1999; 212:732–738

Abbreviations:
ESA = early systolic acceleration
RI = resistive index

[1] From the Department of Radiology, University of Michigan Medical Center, TC 2910K, 1500 E Medical Center Dr, Ann Arbor, MI 48109-0326. From the 1996 RSNA scientific assembly. Received July 17, 1998; revision requested August 13; revision received November 30; accepted March 26, 1999. **Address reprint requests to** R.O.B. (e-mail: *ronbude@umich.edu*).

[2]9∗. Vascular system, location unspecified

PURPOSE: To evaluate the effect of the increase in total cross-sectional area of arteries as they branch beyond the main trunks on the resistive index (RI) and early systolic acceleration (ESA).

MATERIALS AND METHODS: An essentially noncompliant in vitro model that used a pulsatile pump, blood-mimicking fluid, and a branching tubing network that could be configured to produce a downstream cross-sectional area one, two, four, or eight times that of the feeding vessel was used to investigate the relationship, if any, between arterial bed cross-sectional area and the RI and ESA.

RESULTS: The mean ESA in the branching network was inversely proportional to cross-sectional area, decreasing by approximately a factor of two for every doubling of the cross-sectional area. The mean RI in the branching network decreased with increasing cross-sectional area, but not as greatly as the ESA did; the mean RI in the bed with eight times the upstream cross-sectional area had an RI that was approximately three-fourths the upstream RI. These relationships are real, as the slopes of the plots (ESA vs cross-sectional area, $P = .001$; RI vs cross-sectional area, $P < .02$) are significantly different from zero.

CONCLUSION: RI and ESA decrease as a result of increasing downstream cross-sectional diameter of the arterial bed.

Arterial Doppler ultrasonography (US) has been extensively investigated in the detection and categorization of pathophysiologic conditions and disease. One of the most common parameters used to characterize the Doppler waveform is the resistive index (RI). Another parameter that has more recently been investigated is the early systolic acceleration (ESA), which is the slope of a tangent of the initial systolic upsweep of the arterial waveform (1). Less than stellar results of studies in which these parameters were used to detect disease have led investigators to begin to delineate the factors responsible for alteration of the arterial waveform (and therefore the RI and ESA) in the hope that a better understanding of the underlying mechanisms may improve the accuracy of future study findings. To our knowledge, most of the attention so far has been directed to the roles of vascular resistance, compliance, and impedance (1–4).

The total cross-sectional area of an arterial bed progressively increases as the arteries branch beyond the main trunks (5). We speculated that the cross-sectional area of a vascular bed affects the arterial waveform and therefore the RI and ESA. We designed an in vitro model and performed experiments with it to evaluate the effect of the cross-sectional area of a vascular bed on the arterial waveform.

MATERIALS AND METHODS

The phantom (Fig 1) was constructed to study, independently of vascular compliance, the effect of the normal increase in an organ's arterial bed cross-sectional area that occurs as

Author contributions:
Guarantor of integrity of entire study, R.O.B.; study concepts and design, R.O.B.; definition of intellectual content, R.O.B., J.M.R.; literature research, R.O.B.; experimental studies, R.O.B.; data acquisition, R.O.B.; data analysis, R.O.B., J.M.R.; statistical analysis, R.O.B.; manuscript preparation, R.O.B.; manuscript editing and review, R.O.B., J.M.R.

TABLE 1
Reynolds Numbers

No. of Network Branches	Reynolds Number		
	Input	Output	Mean Branch
1	$(1.75 \pm 0.03) \times 10^3$	$(2.10 \pm 0.02) \times 10^3$	$(2.00 \pm 0.01) \times 10^3$
2	$(1.99 \pm 0.02) \times 10^3$	$(2.08 \pm 0.02) \times 10^3$	$(1.15 \pm 0.04) \times 10^3$
4	$(2.04 \pm 0.02) \times 10^3$	$(2.14 \pm 0.01) \times 10^3$	$(6.54 \pm 0.3) \times 10^2$
8	$(1.91 \pm 0.03) \times 10^3$	$(1.96 \pm 0.02) \times 10^3$	$(3.41 \pm 0.3) \times 10^2$

Note.—Data are the mean ± SD.

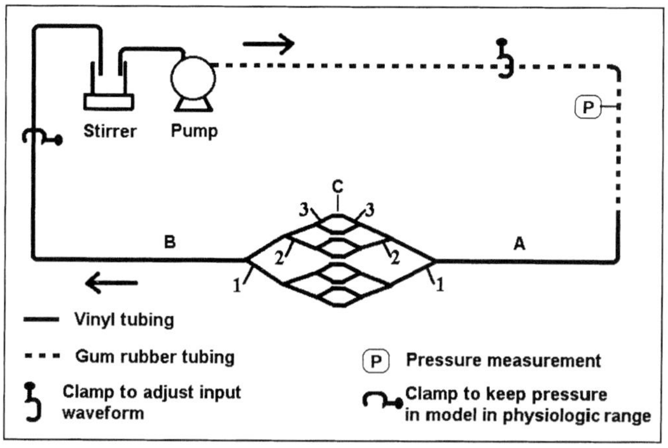

Figure 1. Schematic diagram of the model. Appropriate placement or removal of clamps at *1, 2,* and/or *3* as described in the text produced the appropriate number of branches. *A* and *B* are US sites and also are reference points regarding the direction of fluid flow (Discussion). *C* is where US was performed in the branching model.

flow progresses from the feeding artery to the arterioles on the early systolic acceleration, and on the RI. The phantom was composed of three main components, as follows: (*a*) a pump and tubing assembly to supply pulsatile flow to the branching vascular network, (*b*) a noncompliant branching vascular network of progressively increasing cross-sectional area, and (*c*) a blood-mimicking fluid.

Flow Phantom

Pump and tubing assembly.—A pump (model 1421; Harvard Apparatus, Holliston, Mass) supplied pulsatile flow to the branching tubing network through gum rubber tubing (Fig 1). A variable clamp on the rubber tubing allowed the pulsatility, and therefore the RI, of the flow to be altered as needed by varying the degree of tightness of the clamp (the compliant rubber tubing and clamp functioned as the fluid-flow analogue of a resistive-capacitive circuit [2]).

Pressure was measured in the rubber tubing with a pressure transducer (Transpac IV; Abbott Laboratories, Hospital Products, North Chicago, Ill) connected to a pressure monitor (model 78354A; Hewlett-Packard, Bad Homburg, Germany). Flow returned to a reservoir that resupplied the pump, with the reservoir fluid level held constant at approximately 30 cm above the model. The reservoir was situated on top of a magnetic stirrer (Magnestir; A.S. Aloe, St Louis, Mo), which kept the scatterers suspended. A variable clamp downstream of the downstream US site was used to ensure that pressure in the model was within the physiologic range.

The pump settings were constant through the whole experiment, as follows: 30% phase ratio (amount of the "cardiac" cycle occupied by systole), 36 beats per minute, and 20 mL per stroke. To ensure that flow was laminar at all measurement sites throughout the experiment, Reynolds numbers for each experimental trial were calculated. The peak systolic velocity was used for this determination as it was the highest velocity that occurred at each measurement site, which ensured that the largest Reynolds number was calculated. These data are displayed in Table 1. Since flow makes the transition from laminar to turbulent at a Reynolds number of about 2,300 (6), flow was considered to be laminar if the Reynolds number was less than this value (the largest Reynolds number was 2,100).

Branching vascular network.—The network, including the input and output segments, consisted of vinyl tubing (0.95-cm [3/8-inch] outer diameter, 0.64-cm [1/4-inch] inner diameter) and was configured as shown in the schematic diagram (Fig 1). Y-type plastic connectors (Nalgene, Nalge Nunc International, Rochester, NY) connected end-to-end through three orders of branching resulted both in expansion from one vessel to a network of eight branches and in reconstitution of flow to a single exit vessel. US was performed upstream and downstream (at *A* and *B*, respectively, in Fig 1) to the network and within the network in stable regions of flow, as defined later (in "Inlet Lengths of Tubing").

Blood-mimicking fluid.—The model was filled with 1,500 mL of a solution with the mean viscosity of blood (2.5 centipoise [7]) at 20°C that was composed of a mixture of glycerol and water in the following proportions: 35 mL of glycerol for every 100 mL of water (8). One gram of microparticles (Sephadex G-50; Sigma Chemical, St Louis, Mo) was added as ultrasound scatterers and produced adequate Doppler signals from the branched network that was set up with one, two, or four branches. With eight branches, however, it was necessary to add an additional gram of scatterers for adequate Doppler US because of the relatively slow flow in each branch.

Inlet lengths of tubing.—A flow perturbation (bifurcation, stenosis, tight turn, etc) transiently alters the flow profile for a variable distance, up to a maximum length known as the inlet length (9, pp 38–43). Since the nonpulsatile, laminar flow inlet length is longer than the inlet lengths for other types of flow, it was used to ensure our Doppler measurements were performed in areas of stable flow, with all measurements performed at least one inlet length from any flow perturbation.

The nonpulsatile, laminar flow inlet length is defined as follows: $L = 2kVr^2/\upsilon$, where L is inlet length in centimeters, k is an experimentally derived constant with a value of 0.08, V is mean velocity in centimeters per second, r is tube radius in centimeters, and υ is kinematic viscosity in stokes (centimeters squared per second) (9, pp 38–43). The inlet length for the input and output regions for all experimental trials and also for the branch in the one-branch mode was 26.2 cm. The inlet lengths for the branches in the two-, four-, and eight-branch modes were, respectively, 13.1, 6.6, and 3.3 cm.

Doppler US

A freestanding aluminum framework above the model supported the US transducer and allowed it to be moved among all insonation sites with ease. Doppler waveforms were obtained at 4.0 MHz with a 5.0-MHz curvilinear transducer (Spectra; Diasonics Vingmed Ultrasound, Santa Clara, Calif) at the following settings: At the input region upstream and the output region downstream to the branching vascular network, the wall filter was 75 or 105 Hz; pulse repetition frequency, 2.9 or 4.0 kHz; and Doppler angle, 51° or 53°. At the branches of the network, the wall filter was 35 or 105 Hz; pulse repetition frequency, 1.4 or 4.0 kHz; and Doppler angle, 45°–53°.

The Doppler sample volume included the entire vessel lumen. Doppler gains were optimized by scanning at gains just below those at which background noise first became apparent. Water-filled plastic bags coupled with US gel to the transducer and tubing facilitated US. A sound-absorbent material (SOAB [MKI] nonresonant acoustic absorber; B.F. Goodrich, Richfield, Ohio) interposed between the tubing and the tabletop reduced ultrasound reverberations.

Waveform RIs were calculated by using measurements taken by hand with calipers (Absolute Digimatic; Mitutoyo, Tokyo, Japan) according to the following formula: RI = $(S - D)/S$, where S is the height of the systolic peak and D is the height of the end-diastolic trough. All reported RIs are the means of four waveform RIs, with the waveform sweep speed set at four waveforms per waveform strip for RI measurement.

ESAs were calculated by using measurements taken with calipers as the slope of a tangent of the initial systolic upsweep (1), with the waveform sweep speed set at two waveforms per waveform strip. All reported ESAs are the means of four waveform ESAs. For both RIs and ESAs, the Doppler velocity scale that gave the largest possible waveforms without aliasing was used to decrease measurement error.

Validaton That the Model Had Extremely Low and Essentially Zero Compliance

To determine if our model had appreciable compliance, the input RI proximal to and the output RI distal to the branching segments for each mode of the experiment were determined. The rationale for this is described in "Discussion."

TABLE 2
RI Data

No. of Network Branches	RI Input	RI Mean Branch	RI Output	RI Normalized Mean Branch*
1	0.62 ± 0.02	0.60 ± 0.01	0.58 ± 0.01	1.00 ± 0.02
2	0.63 ± 0.01	0.59 ± 0.02	0.62 ± 0.01	0.94 ± 0.03
4	0.63 ± 0.01	0.55 ± 0.03	0.63 ± 0.01	0.87 ± 0.05
8	0.60 ± 0.01	0.46 ± 0.03	0.60 ± 0.01	0.77 ± 0.05

Note.—Data are the mean ± SD.
* Normalized to the mean of the input and output RIs.

TABLE 3
ESA Data

No. of Network Branches	ESA Input (cm/sec²)	ESA Mean Branch (cm/sec²)	ESA Output (cm/sec²)	ESA Normalized Mean Branch*	ESA Theoretic Normalized Mean Branch
1	238 ± 21	314 ± 32	305 ± 38	1.15 ± 0.12	1.00
2	265 ± 17	146 ± 34	349 ± 56	0.48 ± 0.11	0.50
4	301 ± 4	84 ± 16	402 ± 25	0.24 ± 0.05	0.25
8	229 ± 13	22 ± 3	230 ± 19	0.10 ± 0.01	0.13

Note.—Data are the mean ± SD, except for theoretic normalized mean branch.
* Normalized to the mean of the input and output ESAs.

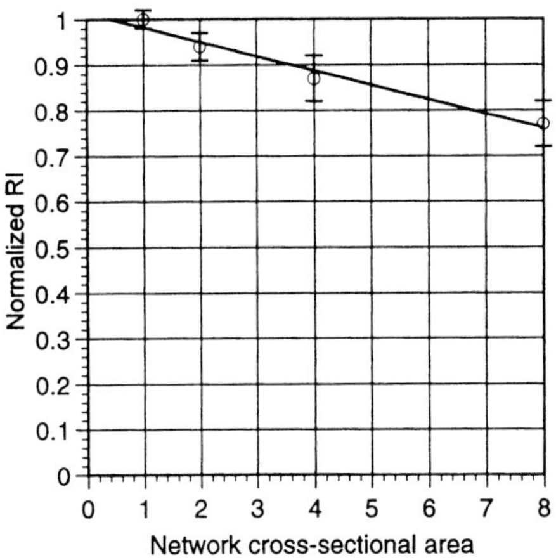

Figure 2. Plot of normalized RI versus cross-sectional area with a linear least-squares fit of the data. Mean RI of each branch of the network decreased with increasing cross-sectional area. Short vertical and horizontal bars about the data points are error bars (± 1 SD).

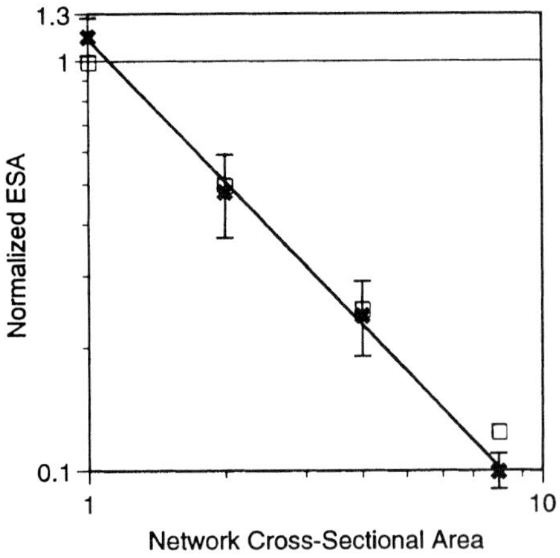

Figure 3. Log-log plot of the mean branch ESA as a function of cross-sectional area, with a linear least-squares fit of the data. ESA decreases with increasing cross-sectional area, closely matching the theoretically predicted values. Short vertical and horizontal bars about the data points are error bars (± 1 SD). × = experimental data, □ = values predicted by using theory (Appendix).

Experimental Trials

Experimental trials were performed by using one, two, four, or eight branches of the network, by appropriately placing or removing the clamps at sites 1, 2, and/or 3 in the model (Fig 1). Placement of clamps at sites 1, 2, and 3 produced a model without branching; placement of clamps at sites 1 and 2 produced two

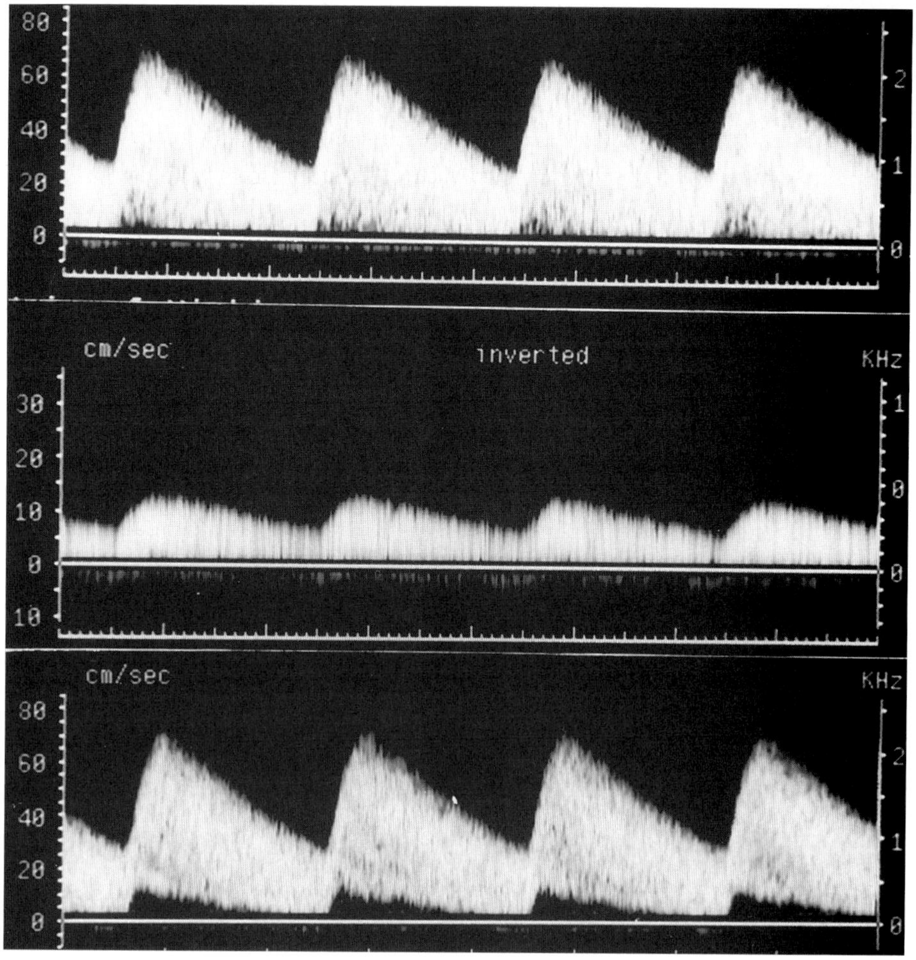

Figure 4. Illustrative waveforms, with the model configured with the network cross-sectional area eight times that of the input cross-sectional area. Top waveform is the input waveform. Middle waveform is that from one of the eight branches. Bottom waveform is the output waveform. Note the output waveform is essentially indistinguishable from the input waveform. RI and ESA of the branch waveform were less than those of the input or output waveform (Tables 2, 3).

branches; placement of clamps at site 1 produced four branches; and absence of clamps produced eight branches.

In this way, since the tubes had the same diameter, cross-sectional areas of the vascular network of one, two, four, and eight times that of the input were obtained. (Cross-sectional areas of three, five, six, and seven times that of the input were not studied because this would have resulted in different orders of branching at some parts of the model compared with others, which would have altered the distribution of flow so that it was no longer symmetric.)

Doppler waveforms were obtained at the input, at each branch of the network (RIs and ESAs were averaged to obtain means for all branches for each trial), and at the output. For all trials, the input RI was set at 0.6 (a "generic" in vivo organ RI), as measured on the display screen by using machine calipers; subsequent caliper measurement taken by hand from the film hard-copy images showed the input RIs varied slightly (see Results). Pressures were within the physiologic range, with mean pressures ranging from 9.9×10^3 to 1.2×10^4 Pa (74–87 mm Hg) for all trials.

Data Analysis

To analyze the mean branch RI data and to compare it from trial to trial, it was necessary to compensate for the slight variability of the input RIs. To accomplish this, we wished to normalize the mean branch RIs to the input RI for each trial. However, because the input and output RIs for two of the four trials were not the same, we decided to first average the input and output RIs and then to normalize the mean branch RIs of any trial to the mean of the input and output RIs. An analogous procedure was performed for the ESAs.

Because the velocity of flow decreases as the cross-sectional area of a tube increases, it seemed that the acceleration should also decrease with increasing cross-sectional area. A theoretic derivation of the relationship between cross-sectional area and acceleration was performed (Appendix) to see if the experimental results agreed with the theoretic results.

RI data were plotted with Cartesian coordinates. ESA data were plotted in log-log coordinates to obtain a linear plot. Linear least-square fits were performed for both RI and ESA data. To determine if there were functional relationships between RI and cross-sectional area and between ESA and cross-sectional area, (ie, to show that the slopes of the plots of RI or ESA vs cross-sectional area were not zero), regression analyses (analysis of variance) of the slopes of the plots were performed. The 95% CIs of the slopes were calculated to determine if they included zero. A P value less than .05 was considered to indicate a statistically significant difference.

RESULTS

The data are displayed numerically (Tables 2, 3) and graphically (Figs 2, 3). Sample waveforms are also illustrated (Fig 4).

As shown in Table 2, the input and output RIs were the same for two of the trials. In the other two trials, the input and output RIs varied slightly, with the difference (input RI minus output RI) measuring 0.01 and 0.04. The importance of this is discussed in "Discussion."

The mean ESA of a vascular bed branch was inversely proportional to cross-sectional area, decreasing by approximately a factor of two for every doubling of the cross-sectional area (Table 3, Fig 3). The mean RI of a vascular bed branch also decreased with increasing cross-sectional area of the vascular bed (Table 2, Fig 2), but the decrease was not as great as the decrease in ESA.

The following data applied to the RI versus cross-sectional area relationship. The R^2 value of the linear-curve fit of the data was 0.972. The slope of the linear-curve fit of the data was −0.0315 (P = .014; 95% CI of the slope: −0.0153, −0.0477).

The following data applied to the ESA versus cross-sectional area relationship. The R^2 value of the linear curve fit of the data was 0.998. The slope of the linear curve fit of the data was −1.16 (P = .001; 95% CI of the slope: −1.00, −1.32).

DISCUSSION

The total cross-sectional area of an arterial bed progressively increases as the arteries branch beyond the main trunks because the fact that the vessels become progressively smaller is outweighed by the increasing numbers of branches. However, many factors interact to make it difficult to know the exact extent of this increase (5). These factors include interspecies and intraspecies variation, the difficulty in performing accurate in vivo measurements, and the difficulty in achieving an accurate and representative distending pressure in postmortem specimens (5;9, pp 30–35). Therefore, the exact increase in cross-sectional area that occurs in the human from the feeding artery of an organ to arterioles of a certain size is unknown.

In the dog, the total cross-sectional area increases approximately 3–5 times from arteries approximately 4 mm in diameter to arterioles approximately 100 µm in diameter and increases approximately 11 times from arteries approximately 4 mm in diameter to arterioles approximately 50 µm in diameter. For vessels that branch dichotomously (most do), the mean total cross-sectional area of the branches is 1.26 times that of the feeding artery (5). It has been inferred that similar increases occur in humans.

Our model was designed to achieve an increase in cross-sectional area similar to that just described, with incremental increases up to eight times the cross-sectional area of the feeding artery evaluated. Since it is currently possible to obtain power Doppler images and spectral Doppler waveforms from very small arteries (the renal interlobular arteries are seen with power Doppler US, especially in transplants), we believe this is a reasonable range of cross-sectional area to study, especially since technologic advances may allow the future study of smaller and smaller arteries.

Because vascular compliance is one of the factors that alters waveform pulsatility and morphology (1,2) and because we desired to study only the effect of cross-sectional area on the waveforms, it was necessary for our model to possess a compliance so low that it would not substantially affect the waveforms. Vascular compliance, however, is a dynamic phenomenon that we could not measure directly. Therefore, we used the following indirect method to determine if our model had appreciable compliance.

Vascular compliance, in conjunction with vascular resistance, progressively damps waveform pulsatility as flow progresses from the highly pulsatile central arteries to the essentially nonpulsatile capillaries (1,10–12), which have an RI of essentially zero. Therefore, our model can be assumed to have a very low compliance if the pulsatility is not substantially damped, as would be manifested with an output RI equal to or very nearly the same as the input RI. The input and output RIs in each mode of our experiment varied from 0.00 to 0.04 (Table 2).

The upstream measurements were not independent of each other. The downstream measurements were also not independent of each other. Therefore, it was impossible to prove statistically that the upstream and downstream RIs were not significantly different. However, the minute RI changes just described indicate the compliance of our model was very low, and for these experiments, it was considered to be essentially zero.

Our results show the ESA decreased with increasing cross-sectional area of an arterial bed, independently of vascular compliance and resistance (Table 3, Fig 3), by a factor of approximately two for every doubling of the cross-sectional area. (Since the P value for the slope indicates a significant difference and the 95% CIs for the slope do not intersect zero, this relationship is real.) This agrees with theoretic results (Appendix).

Thus, the ESA measured in the feeding artery of an organ is likely to be substantially different than the ESA in an arteriole owing to cross-sectional area alone. This is independent of other factors such as vascular compliance, which also considerably affects the ESA (1,2) since the difference in cross-sectional area between these two sites is as much as a factor of 10, as described earlier. These results corresponded to the results of Halpern et al (1) from a study in the human kidney in which they noted the ESA decreases from the central arteries to more peripheral ones. Thus, our results provide a basis for understanding why ESA criteria developed from more central arteries to detect disease may not apply to ESAs obtained from arteries substantially downstream from these central arteries.

Of additional interest is that the RI is dependent on cross-sectional area (Table 2, Fig 2), independent of the effects of vascular resistance and compliance, which also alter the RI (3,4,13–17). (Since the P value for the slope indicates a significant difference and the 95% CIs for the slope do not intersect zero, this relationship also is real.) This helps explain why the RI varies with the site of measurement in the normal renal arterial tree (decreasing centrally to peripherally), as shown by Knapp et al (18). Thus, as with ESA, on the basis of cross-sectional area alone, RI criteria developed in one region of the arterial tree may not necessarily apply to substantially different regions of the arterial tree.

The cause for the RI dependence on cross-sectional area is unknown. We presumed that an essentially incompressible fluid flowing through an essentially noncompliant system would proportionately transfer the velocities downstream at each time increment, with these velocities scaled by the ratio of the upstream cross-sectional area to the cross-sectional area at the site of measurement downstream, as happens with acceleration (Eq [A4], Appendix). If so, the ratio would be present in both the numerator and denominator of the RI expression and would cancel out, leaving the RI unchanged.

We speculate the RI dependence on cross-sectional area may be due to the effects of velocity and pulsatility on laminar flow. Steady laminar flow produces a parabolic flow profile, with flow absent at the wall and maximal at the center of the vessel. When laminar flow is pulsatile, a true parabolic flow profile is no longer present, and the flow profile alters with time as a function of pulsatility (9, pp 35–38). As the cross-sectional area increases and as the bulk flow rate slows, the laminar flow profile may alter, changing the relationship between peak systole and end diastole. Further experimentation is required to evaluate this hypothesis.

The following are potential limitations of our study. First, the ESA of the reconstituted flow waveforms (at B in Fig 1) was higher than the ESA of the input waveforms (at A in Fig 1), although the effect was not great (Table 3). If cross-sectional area is the only factor affecting the waveform, the reconstituted downstream ESA should equal the upstream ESA. To counteract this effect, we normalized the mean branch ESAs to the mean of both the upstream and downstream ESAs. This was done on the assumption that the effect of this factor on the branch ESAs, which were obtained at a site essentially halfway between the input and output waveform measurement sites, is likely nullified by normalizing the mean branch ESAs to the mean of the input and output ESAs.

We speculate the factor responsible for this effect is wave reflection. Wave reflection occurs at changes in vascular impedance and increases with increasing impedance (19). In our model, the clamp downstream of the branching network had a very large impedance analogous to peripheral vascular resistance in vivo. In vivo, peripheral resistance causes a pressure wave that reflects back to the heart. In healthy elderly individuals whose vessels are less compliant than those of younger individuals, this reflected wave returns to the heart during systole, which increases systolic pressure. This is one of the reasons for the increased systolic pressures of healthy older individuals (20,21).

In our essentially noncompliant model, such a reflected wave traveled much more quickly than it would have in vivo because of the lower compliance of our model (the lower the compliance, the faster the transmission of reflected waves) (21). It may, therefore, augment flow velocity earlier in systole downstream (*B* in Fig 1) than it does upstream (*A* in Fig 1) ("downstream" and "upstream" refer to the actual direction of fluid flow, not the direction of the reflected waves) and thus may augment the downstream ESA more than the upstream ESA. Further experimentation is required to test this hypothesis. This factor did not affect the RIs, as they were essentially the same upstream as downstream (Table 2).

Second, we did not study turbulent flow, which can occur in vivo and which alters the flow profile differently than laminar flow does.

Third, it may never be possible to determine vascular bed cross-sectional area noninvasively. If so, it will not be possible to correct for this factor when analyzing arterial waveforms, and the results of our study may be limited only to helping explain why disease detection based on analysis of intrarenal arterial waveforms is limited by cross-sectional area without the ability to correct for cross-sectional area.

In summary, the increase in cross-sectional area that normally occurs as flow progresses through the arterial tree lowers both the ESA and the RI independently of other factors such as vascular compliance and resistance. Therefore, our results help explain why ESA and RI criteria developed for disease detection in one site do not necessarily apply to disease detection at another substantially different site in the arterial tree. Since vascular compliance and resistance also alter the arterial waveform, the waveform changes that occur as a consequence of disease are a function of a very complex set of phenomena. Unless these factors can be taken into account, it may not be possible to use Doppler US with arterial waveform analysis to detect disease any better than has currently been shown, and it may be fortuitous that it works as well as it does.

Practical application: A greater understanding of the role of cross-sectional area in altering the Doppler arterial waveform may enable future studies in which this effect is taken into account to better depict pathologic conditions. This may be especially important when intrarenal ESA or RI measurements are used to detect renal arterial stenosis.

APPENDIX

We assumed that flow is pulsatile, the fluid is incompressible, the tubing is noncompliant, the cross-sectional areas of all the branches are equal, and the volume flows in all the branches are equal (Fig A1); therefore, the volume flow into the model equaled the volume flow out of the model, as follows: $V_{in} = V_{out}$ and $V_{out} = nV_b$, where V_{in} and V_{out} are volume flow in and out of the model, respectively, n is the number of branches in the arterial bed, and V_b is the branch volume flow. Therefore,

$$V_{in} = nV_b. \quad \text{(A1)}$$

Differentiating Equation (A1) with respect to time t gives $dV_{in}/dt = n(dV_b/dt)$. Since $V/A = v$, where V is volume flow, A is cross-sectional area, and v is velocity, Av can be substituted for V, giving

$$A_{in}(dv_{in}/dt) = (nA_b)(dv_b/dt), \quad \text{(A2)}$$

where A_{in} and A_b are constants and are the input cross-sectional area and cross-sectional area in each branch, respectively, and where v_b is the velocity in each branch.

Since dv/dt equals acceleration a, Equation (A2) reduces to $A_{in}a_{in} = nA_ba_b$, where a_{in} and a_b are the input and branch accelerations, respectively. Rearranging terms gives

$$a_b/a_{in} = A_{in}/(nA_b). \quad \text{(A3)}$$

Since nA_b equals the total cross-sectional area of the bed A_{bed}, Equation (A3) can be rearranged to

$$a_b = a_{in}(A_{in}/A_{bed}). \quad \text{(A4)}$$

Thus, at any instant in time, the acceleration in any branch of the network of equal-size branches is the acceleration of the input branch multiplied by the ratio of the cross-sectional area of the input vessel divided by the total cross-sectional area of the branch vessels.

This theoretic explanation must be regarded as a first approximation only. This is because the distribution of velocities across the diameter of a vessel lumen in pulsatile laminar flow is not constant but changes with time and is influenced by factors including the cross-sectional area of the vessel (9, pp 35–38). Thus, in vivo, it is possible this dependence might further influence the acceleration as calculated from the maximum velocity envelope differently than the ratio of cross-sectional areas does.

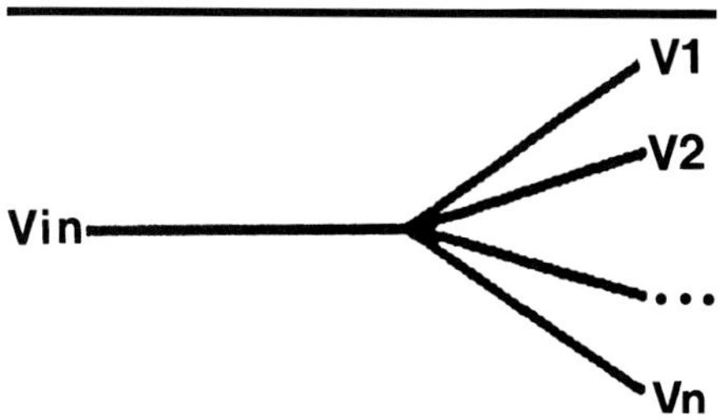

Figure A1. Schematic diagram of a branching vascular network. V = volume flow. Volume flows in branches are equal.

References

1. Halpern EJ, Deane CR, Needleman L, Merton DA, East SA. Normal renal artery spectral Doppler waveform: a closer look. Radiology 1995; 196:667–673.
2. Bude RO, Rubin JM, Platt JF, Fechner KP, Adler RS. Pulsus tardus: its cause and potential limitations in detection of arterial stenosis. Radiology 1994; 190:779–784.
3. Halpern EJ, Merton DA, Forsberg F. Effect of distal resistance on Doppler US flow patterns. Radiology 1998; 206:761–766.
4. Saunders HM, Burns PN, Needleman L, et al. Hemodynamic factors affecting uterine artery Doppler waveform pulsatility in sheep. J Ultrasound Med 1998; 17:357–368.
5. Milnor WR. Steady flow. In: Milnor WR, ed. Hemodynamics. 2nd ed. Baltimore, Md: Williams & Wilkins, 1989; 41–47.
6. Nichols WW, O'Rourke MF. Turbulent blood flow and its relation to cardiovascular pathophysiology. In: Nichols WW, O'Rourke MF, eds. McDonald's blood flow in arteries: theoretical, experimental and clinical principles. 3rd ed. Philadelphia, Pa: Lea & Febiger, 1990; 54.
7. Duck FA. Mechanical properties of tissue. In: Physical properties of tissue. San Diego, Calif: Academic Press, 1990; 161.
8. Weast RC. General chemical. In: Weast RC, ed. Handbook of chemistry and physics: a ready-reference book of chemical and physical data. 52nd ed. Cleveland, Ohio: Chemical Rubber, 1971; D191–D192.
9. Nichols WW, O'Rourke MF. The nature of flow of a fluid. In: Nichols WW, O'Rourke MF, eds. McDonald's blood flow in arteries: theoretical, experimental and clinical principles. 3rd ed. Philadelphia, Pa: Lea & Febiger, 1990; 30–43.
10. Nichols WW, O'Rourke MF. Introduction. In: Nichols WW, O'Rourke MF, eds. McDonald's blood flow in arteries: theoretical, experimental and clinical principles.

4th ed. New York, NY: Oxford University Press, 1998; 3.

11. Nichols WW, O'Rourke MF. Coupling of the left ventricle with the systemic circulation: implications to cardiac failure. In: Nichols WW, O'Rourke MF, eds. McDonald's blood flow in arteries: theoretical, experimental and clinical principles. 4th ed. New York, NY: Oxford University Press, 1998; 295–296.
12. McDonald DA, Taylor MG. The hydrodynamics of the arterial circulation. Prog Biophys Chem 1959; 9:107–173.
13. Spencer JAD, Giussani DA, Moore PJ, Hanson MA. In vitro validation of Doppler indices using blood and water. J Ultrasound Med 1991; 10:305–308.
14. Norris CS, Pfeiffer JS, Rittgers SE, Barnes RW. Noninvasive evaluation of renal artery stenosis and renovascular resistance. J Vasc Surg 1984; 1:192–201.
15. Norris CS, Barnes RW. Renal artery flow velocity analysis: a sensitive measure of experimental and clinical renovascular resistance. J Surg Res 1984; 36:230–236.
16. Adamson SL, Morrow RJ, Langille BL, Bull SB, Ritchie WK. Site-dependent effects of increases in placental vascular resistance on the umbilical arterial velocity waveform in fetal sheep. Ultrasound Med Biol 1990; 16:19–27.
17. Morrow RJ, Adamson SL, Bull SB, Ritchie JW. Effect of placental embolization on the umbilical arterial velocity waveform in fetal sheep. Am J Obstet Gynecol 1989; 161:1055–1060.
18. Knapp R, Plotzeneder A, Frauscher F, et al. Variability of Doppler parameters in the healthy kidney: an anatomic-physiologic correlation. J Ultrasound Med 1995; 14: 427–429.
19. Nichols WW, O'Rourke MF. Wave reflections. In: Nichols WW, O'Rourke MF, eds. McDonald's blood flow in arteries: theoretical, experimental and clinical principles. 3rd ed. Philadelphia, Pa: Lea & Febiger, 1990; 251–269.
20. Marchais SJ, Guerin AP, Pannier B, Delavaud G, London GM. Arterial compliance and blood pressure. Drugs 1993; 46(suppl 2):82–87.
21. O'Rourke M. Arterial stiffness, systolic blood pressure, and logical treatment of arterial hypertension. Hypertension 1990; 15:339–347.

Simultaneous Noninvasive Determination of Regional Myocardial Perfusion and Oxygen Content in Rabbits: Toward Direct Measurement of Myocardial Oxygen Consumption at MR Imaging[1]

Scott B. Reeder, MD, PhD
A. Alexander Holmes, MSE
Elliot R. McVeigh, PhD
John R. Forder, PhD

Index terms:
Animals
Heart, MR, 511.121411, 511.91
Magnetic resonance (MR), experimental studies, 511.121411
Magnetic resonance (MR), perfusion study, 511.121411
Magnetic resonance (MR), technology, 511.121411
Myocardium, blood supply, 511.91

Radiology 1999; 212:739–747

Abbreviations:
BOLD = blood oxygenation level–dependent
SE = spin echo
τ_{180} = time between refocusing pulses

[1] From the Departments of Biomedical Engineering (S.B.R., A.A.H., E.R.M.) and Radiology (E.R.M., J.R.F.), Johns Hopkins University School of Medicine, Baltimore, Md. Received September 12, 1997; revision requested November 24; final revision received December 12, 1998; accepted February 15, 1999. J.R.F. is supported by a grant from the Whitaker Foundation. S.B.R. is supported by a Medical Scientist Training Program Fellowship. **Address reprint requests to** J.R.F., Department of Medicine, Division of Cardiovascular Disease, University of Alabama at Birmingham, CMRL Bldg, 828 8th Ct S, Birmingham, AL 35294-4470.

Author contributions:
Guarantors of integrity of entire study, all authors; study concepts and design, all authors; definition of intellectual content, all authors; literature research, all authors; experimental studies, all authors; data acquisition and analysis, all authors; statistical analysis, all authors; manuscript preparation, editing, and review, all authors.

PURPOSE: To determine whether myocardial arterial perfusion and oxygen concentration can be quantified simultaneously from the same images by using spin labeling and the blood oxygenation level–dependent (BOLD) effect with fast spin-echo (SE) imaging.

MATERIALS AND METHODS: A T2-weighted fast SE pulse sequence was written to image isolated, arrested, blood-perfused rabbit hearts (n = 6) at 4.7 T. Perfusion images with intensity in units of milliliters per minute per gram that covered the entire left ventricle with 0.39 × 0.39 × 3.00-mm resolution were obtained in less than 15 minutes with a 32-fold reduction in imaging time from that of a previous study. Estimates of oxygen concentration were made from the same images acquired for calculation of perfusion images.

RESULTS: Estimates of regional myocardial oxygen content could be made from the perfusion images; this demonstrated the feasibility of three-dimensional calculation of regional oxygen consumption, which requires concomitant measurement of both oxygen content and flow. Fast SE imaging was shown to be as sensitive to hemoglobin desaturation as standard SE imaging. Perfusion abnormalities and oxygen deficits were easily identified and verified qualitatively with gadopentetate dimeglumine on both perfusion and BOLD images obtained after coronary arterial ligation.

CONCLUSION: T2-weighted fast SE imaging combined with perfusion-sensitive spin labeling can be used to measure myocardial arterial perfusion and oxygen concentration. This provides the groundwork for calculation of regional myocardial oxygen consumption.

Cardiovascular disease remains the leading cause of death in the United States (1). In vivo measurement of regional myocardial oxygen consumption remains an important goal toward the assessment of myocardial viability, since cardiac function is critically dependent on the ability of the myocardium to consume oxygen. Traditionally, total organ oxygen consumption has been estimated from total flow through the organ and from arteriovenous differences in blood oxygen levels. This method, however, does not account for tissue heterogeneity in either oxygen delivery or metabolic activity.

Current methods for determining regional oxygen consumption and perfusion that are compatible with clinical application include phosphorus 31 or carbon 13 nuclear magnetic resonance (MR) spectroscopy (2–6); positron emission tomography with carbon 1 to carbon 11, nitrogen 14, oxygen 17, rubidium 82, or fluorine 18 isotopes (7–11); and single photon emission computed tomography (CT) with thallium 201 or technetium 99 (12). These techniques, although they are valuable, require ionizing radiation and are limited by poor spatial and temporal resolution. Coronary catheterization techniques with radiopaque dyes can provide information about flow, but they are projection techniques that offer no depth information.

In recent years, developments in cardiac MR imaging (7,9,13) and CT (7,14–16) have relied on the use of exogenous contrast agents. Their mechanisms of signal modulation in vivo are poorly understood, however, which makes perfusion quantification difficult.

More recently, several noninvasive MR spin-labeling methods to estimate tissue perfusion have been introduced. These methods are used to detect flow enhancement by using selective radio-frequency pulses to alter the magnetization of flowing or static spins. The adiabatic fast-passage spin-labeling method proposed by Williams et al (17) has been demonstrated to estimate arterial myocardial perfusion quantitatively. This technique, however, has been demonstrated only at superphysiologic perfusion (5–22 mL/min/g) and requires a long inflow track that precludes in vivo application. The echo-planar MR imaging and signal targeting with alternating radio-frequency, or EPISTAR, method has been applied to measure perfusion qualitatively in the brain (18) and is related to time-of-flight MR angiography (19). Kwong et al (20,21) and Kim (22) applied a nonselective/selective inversion method in the brain, although no distinction can be made between arterial and venous flows, and perfusion estimates obtained by using this method are qualitative. We recently introduced a spin-labeling method that provides noninvasive quantitative estimates of myocardial arterial perfusion (23) and avoids many of the problems of the above techniques.

We previously exploited the blood oxygenation level–dependent (BOLD) effect with T2-weighted spin-echo (SE) imaging to estimate regional oxygen content in both arrested and beating, isolated, blood-perfused rabbit hearts (24–26). Wendland et al (27) observed decreases in image intensity from in vivo rat myocardium during episodes of apnea by using T2*-weighted echo-planar imaging. In addition, Niemi et al (28) used echo-planar imaging to measure enhancement of signal intensity from human myocardium during infusion with dipyridamole. Dipyridamole decreases the concentration of deoxyhemoglobin through increases in perfusion caused by coronary vasodilation. Other groups have also done similar work with animal models (29,30) and in vivo (31).

Measurement of regional oxygen consumption in tissue can be determined by measuring regional oxygen content and tissue perfusion. In this work, we determine the feasibility of combining spin labeling and T2-weighted BOLD imaging to measure arterial perfusion and oxygen content simultaneously from the same images.

MATERIALS AND METHODS

Perfusion Imaging with MR Spin Labeling: T1 Weighting

We developed a noninvasive spin-labeling method that provides quantitative estimates of coronary arterial perfusion as previously described (23). This technique relies on the unique geometry of the coronary vasculature in which arterial blood flows predominantly from the base to the apex (32,33). Coronary arteries descend from the root of the aorta along the epicardial surface and then dive into the myocardium toward the endocardium, while venous drainage runs parallel with the arteries, but flow is in the opposite direction.

Selective inversion of the magnetization in the short-axis section of interest along with all myocardium on its apical side renders any flow-induced enhancement of signal intensity insensitive to venous flow, ensuring that only unlabeled arterial spins can act to enhance tissue signal intensity. The behavior of longitudinal magnetization after selective preinversion in the myocardium and in regions of low and high flow is shown in Figure 1. Calculation of perfusion images is described in the Appendix.

BOLD Imaging: T2 Weighting

The BOLD effect has been used extensively in the evaluation of oxygenation in the brain (34–36) and myocardium (24–28). The approach relies on the fact that deoxyhemoglobin unlike oxyhemoglobin is paramagnetic (37). Hemoglobin is concentrated in erythrocytes, which are in turn confined to the intravascular space. This compartmentalization in concert with the paramagnetism of deoxyhemoglobin generates spatially dependent susceptibility gradients when oxygen tension is low. These gradients enhance transverse magnetization dephasing (T2*), which manifests as reduced signal intensity on gradient-echo T2*-weighted images.

Although SE imaging will refocus static inhomogeneities generated by deoxyhemoglobin, it remains sensitive to the dephasing of spins caused by the diffusion of spins through these local gradients. Also, Boxerman et al (38) have shown that SE imaging is most sensitive to compartmentalization of deoxyhemoglobin in capillary-sized vessels, implying that T2-weighted SE imaging is sensitive to the oxygen tension in myocardial capillary beds. Last, a linear relationship between normalized signal intensity and hemoglobin saturation has been demonstrated previously at SE imaging in rabbit myocardium (26).

The modulation of T2 with hemoglobin saturation is strongly dependent on the time between refocusing pulses (τ_{180}). According to the measurements by Wright et al (39) and the numeric predictions by Bandettini et al (40), however, the modulation of T2 should be only moderately affected for the τ_{180} used with the fast SE sequence in these experiments (8.4 msec, see Discussion). The Appendix contains further elaboration on this subject and also includes a discussion of the construction of calibration curves for calculation of tissue oxygenation from signal intensities.

Isolation and Perfusion of the Rabbit Heart

Isolation, attachment, and perfusion of hearts from New Zealand White male rabbits (2–4 kg, $n = 6$) has been previously described in detail (23–26). In all hearts, a snare occluder was placed on the left anterior descending coronary artery for ligation near the conclusion of the experiment, as previously described (23,26).

The height of a perfusate reservoir was varied to adjust coronary flow that was measured from a cannula in the pulmonary artery by using an MR-compatible flow meter (Transonics, Ithaca, NY). Heart preparations that failed to maintain stable coronary flow were not used. The heart preparations were maintained at 39°C, as previously described (23), since T1 is temperature dependent (41).

Perfusate Composition

A modified Krebs-Henseleit buffer was used as the initial perfusate during the attachment of the heart to the Langendorff apparatus. This buffer contained the following: NaCl, 118.0 mmol/L; KH_2PO_4, 1.2 mmol/L; $MgSO_4$, 1.0 mmol/L; $NaHCO_3$,

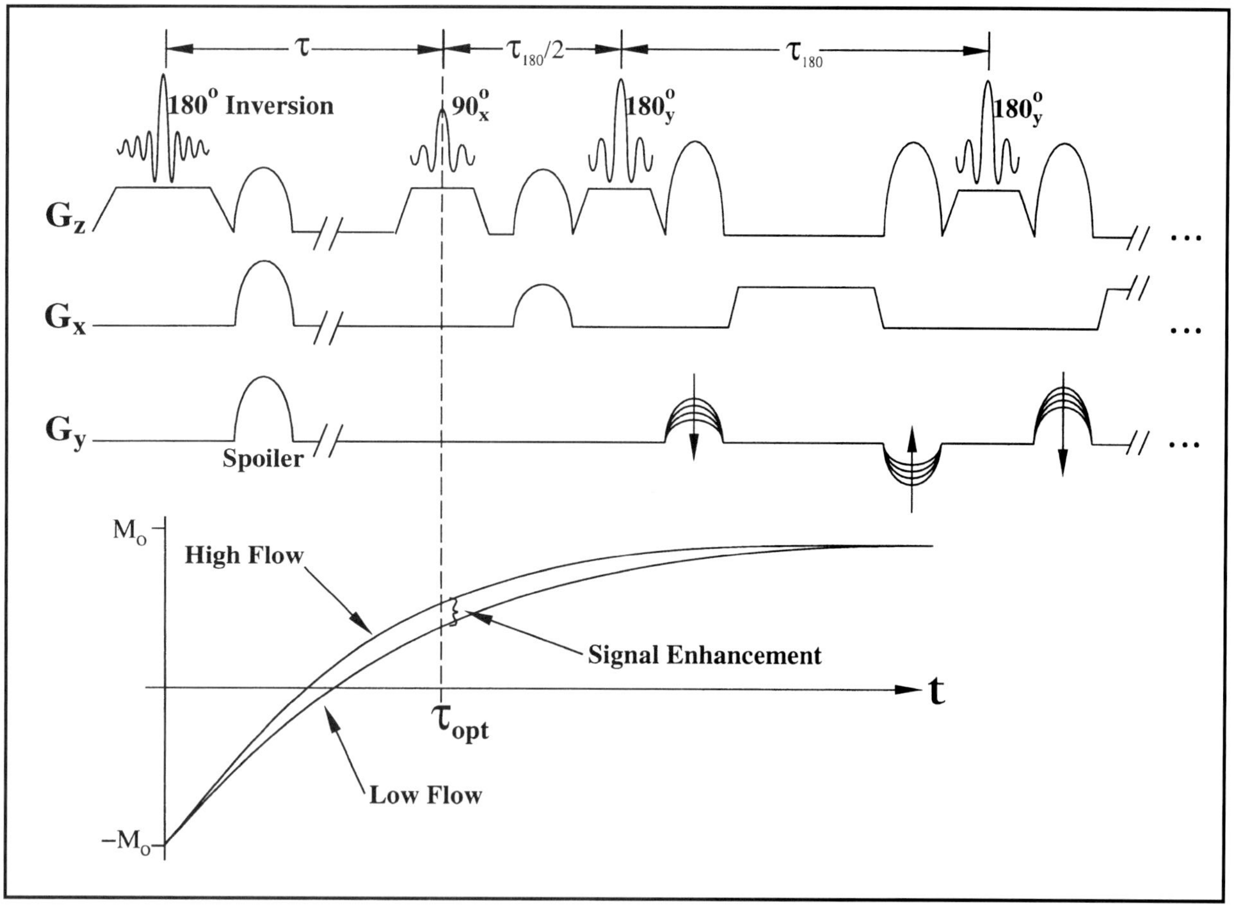

Figure 1. Diagram depicts pulse sequence timing. Fast SE imaging is preceded by slab inversion and a delay τ. The inversion radio-frequency sinc spans 8π radians to create a selective inversion with a sharp transition and high inversion efficiency. Two T1 recovery curves show the differential enhancement seen between regions of high and low arterial perfusion. M_0 = without preinversion, τ_{opt} = optimal time between refocusing pulses.

25.0 mmol/L; KCl, 4.8 mmol/L; $CaCl_2$, 2.5 mmol/L; and dextrose, 5.0 mmol/L. The buffer was not recirculated and was saturated with 95% O_2 and 5% CO_2 (39°C, pH 7.4) with a low-volume membrane oxygenator (42). Bovine serum albumin (3% weight by volume) was added to prevent formation of edema in the myocardium. Bovine serum albumin was dialyzed for 24 hours (10,000–molecular weight dialysis tubing; Sigma Chemical, St Louis, Mo) against 20 volumes of a NaCl (118 mmol/L) and $CaCl_2$ (2.5 mmol/L) solution to remove low-molecular-weight contaminants. Dialysis also saturated the albumin calcium binding sites to help maintain a physiologic concentration of calcium in the final perfusate.

After attachment, the perfusate was switched to a cardioplegic solution (modified St Thomas Hospital solution [43]) containing the following: NaCl, 110.0 mmol/L; $NaHCO_3$, 10.0 mmol/L; KCl, 16.0 mmol/L; $MgCl_2$, 16.0 mmol/L; $CaCl_2$, 1.2 mmol/L; and dextrose, 5.0 mmol/L. Bovine serum albumin (3% weight by volume) was added to prevent tissue edema (see previous paragraph). Washed sheep red blood cells (HemoStat Laboratories, Dixon, Calif) obtained 1 day after venipuncture and processing were resuspended in the cardioplegic solution to a final hematocrit level of 32%–36%. The red blood cell perfusate was oxygenated with the same membrane oxygenator described previously. (Throughout the remainder of the article, "blood" will be used in place of "red blood cell perfusate." The authors acknowledge the obvious distinction between real blood and the perfusate used in these experiments.)

Two gas lines—one carrying 95% O_2 and 5% CO_2 and the second carrying 95% N_2 and 5% CO_2—were connected to the oxygenator. The relative flows of the two lines were changed to vary the partial pressure of the oxygen in the perfusate and hence the hemoglobin saturation. Leukocyte adhesion filters (Pall filters; KOL Biomedical Instruments, Chantilly, Va) were used to prevent coronary embolization caused by particulate matter and/or microaggregates in the red blood cell perfusate. This perfusate was recirculated.

Animal Care Guidelines

All animals in this study received humane care in compliance with the guidelines set forth in "Principles of Laboratory Animal Care" formulated by the National Society for Medical Research and the "Guide for the Care and Use of Laboratory Animals" prepared by the Institute of Laboratory Animal Resources, Commission on Life Sciences, National Research Council and published by the National Academy of Sciences for the National Institutes of Health (44).

Imaging Examinations

All imaging was performed on an Omega CSI 4.7-T nuclear MR spectrometer (GE Medical Systems, Milwaukee,

Wis) equipped with shielded gradients (S-150 Accustar). This gradient set has maximum gradient strengths of approximately 19 G/cm (0.19 T/m) and slew rates of 27 G/cm/msec (270 T/m/sec). A home-built loop-gap radio-frequency coil (31-mm diameter) tuned to 200.08 MHz (proton resonance) was used for imaging. The coil was wrapped around a closed-end, cylindric, acrylic bathing chamber in which the heart was suspended.

Interleaved fast SE (45) and standard SE sequences were used for all imaging; the fast SE sequence is shown in Figure 1. The echo train length was 32; conventional phase encoding was used for fast SE, in which the phase-encoding gradient was rewound after each readout gradient (45,46). T2 weighting was achieved by means of encoding central lines of k space at later echoes in the echo train (46). A 90° phase shift between the initial 90° excitation and subsequent 180° refocusing pulses was used to align all SEs. This $90_x:180_y:180_y:180_y$ . . . scheme gave constructive alignment of SEs and stimulated echoes, as described by Plewes and Bishop (47). Small hardware phase errors can necessitate the need for phase correction algorithms (48), although such algorithms were not found to be necessary with these experiments, as ghost artifacts were negligible.

Inversion of myocardial water spins in the imaging section along with all myocardium on its apical side was achieved with a 2-msec selective 180° pulse (Fig 1). High uniformity of the inversion slab was achieved by using a symmetric sinc radio-frequency pulse spanning 8π radians. The large number of sinc lobes created a sharp transition between the inverted and noninverted myocardium, reduced side-lobe excitation, and improved inversion efficiency.

Experimental Protocol and Data Acquisition

Following isolation and attachment of the heart, the apparatus was inserted into the magnet and a stack of six to eight left ventricular short-axis images was prescribed from SE scout images. The inversion slab was prescribed and its shape and tip angle were optimized by using a long-axis profile that contained mostly myocardium. This procedure was performed in all hearts studied ($n = 6$).

In all hearts, two images were acquired sequentially for each section. The first was a four-shot fast SE image (echo-train length, 32) preceded by one shot that was discarded to ensure that magnetization was in a steady state (49). Each shot was preceded with a selective inversion pulse and a 2.1-second delay and was followed by a 10-second delay for T1 recovery (repetition time, 12,100 msec; τ_{180}, 8.4 msec). Section thickness was 3 mm, field of view was 50 mm, and pixel resolution was 128 × 128, which gave voxel dimensions of 0.39 × 0.39 × 3.00 mm. Bandwidth was ±50 kHz. The central line of k space was positioned at the fifth echo, producing an effective echo time of 42 msec. The second image was an additional fast SE image, identical to the first, but obtained without the preinversion pulse and the 2.1-second delay.

Last, in four of the six hearts, an additional standard T2-weighted SE image was acquired with the same imaging parameters as for the previous fast SE image, but the repetition time for this image was 1,000 msec. Each T2-weighted SE image was acquired immediately after each fast SE image without preinversion to ensure that the tissue oxygenation status was identical in the event of fluctuations in oxygen content. No averaging was performed for any image, and 12–20 sets of images were acquired in this manner for each heart at different flows and oxygen concentrations.

The total imaging time for each fast SE image was approximately 1 minute, and the imaging time for T2-weighted SE images was 2 minutes. With eight sections and including the image reconstruction time, the total imaging time for all sections for one oxygenation and flow level was approximately 30 minutes. When only fast SE images were acquired, total imaging time was reduced to approximately 15 minutes. This represents a 32-fold reduction in imaging time from that of previous perfusion imaging with SE pulse sequences (23).

Experiments were conducted within 3 hours to ensure myocardial viability, although it has been shown that this preparation can remain viable for as long as 6 hours (50). This allowed the procedure describe previously to be repeated at three to five oxygenation levels and two to four coronary flow rates. Following each change in oxygenation, 15 minutes was allowed for equilibration prior to imaging. Oxygenation measurements were taken after each section was acquired by withdrawing blood samples from the pulmonary arterial cannula. Hemoglobin saturation was calculated by using an algorithm for sheep hemoglobin based on blood gases and by using pH (51) measured with a blood-gas analyzer (ABL-3; Radiometer, Copenhagen, Denmark).

In all experiments, the left anterior descending coronary artery was occluded following acquisition of data sets at different oxygenation levels. Fast SE images with or without preinversion were acquired immediately after ligation, with no change in perfusion pressure.

Finally, a series of 16-shot fast SE images (repetition time, 400 msec; echo time, 42 msec) were acquired over all sections after administration of a 25-mL bolus injection of 20 mmol/L gadopentetate dimeglumine into the perfusate line. These images were used to delineate qualitatively regions of perfusion deficit. The images were acquired sequentially from base to apex, and imaging was repeated for several minutes.

RESULTS

Perfusion Images

A panel of 18 images is shown in Figure 2. Values for inversion efficiency and T1 were taken as the measured values of 0.81 and 2.25 seconds, which were typical and highly reproducible (23). No masking was performed in these calculations since perfusion images delineated the heart anatomy as well as and sometimes better than the fast SE images. The septum in these images appeared collapsed because the left ventricle was vented to atmospheric pressure, whereas right ventricular circulation remained closed as the perfusate in the right ventricle exited through the pulmonary arterial cannula.

Mean pixel intensities in septal and free wall regions in different sections in the perfusion images in Figure 2 were approximately 2.0 mL/min/g, with notable and expected heterogeneity, as observed by King et al (52) and predicted by Bassingthwaighte et al (53). The total coronary flow from this 10.0-g heart was 18 mL/min (measured from a pulmonary arterial cannula with a flow meter), which made the mean perfusion through the myocardium 1.8 mL/min/g, which was in close agreement with that seen in the perfusion images. Bright regions in the right and left ventricular cavities were due to the movement of bulk flow in the perfusion chamber down through the imaging section.

Perfusion images were calculated in all hearts ($n = 6$) at different flow levels. Figure 3 is a plot of the coronary flow (in milliliter per minute per gram) estimated from perfusion images against the mean total coronary flow, which was determined by dividing the total coronary flow measured from the pulmonary arterial cannula by the wet weight of the

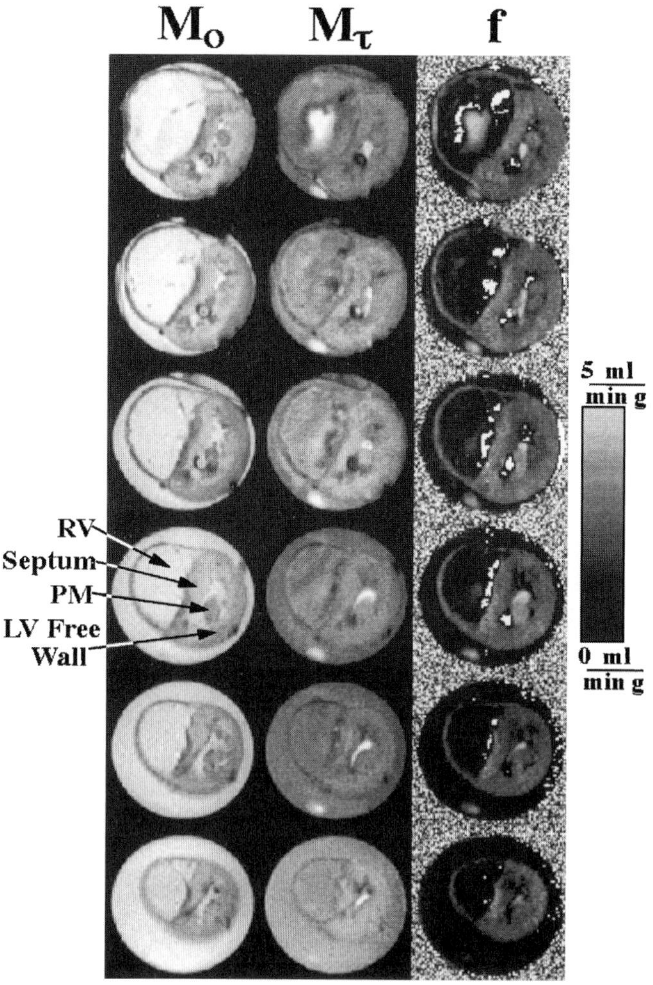

Figure 2. Typical fast SE images acquired in six of eight sections covering the left ventricle include images acquired without preinversion (M_0), images with preinversion (M_τ), and perfusion (f) images calculated (Eq [A1]) on a pixel-by-pixel basis from the images with and without preinversion. Image signal intensity of perfusion images is in units of milliliter per minute per gram, and an intensity scale is shown to map pixel intensity to perfusion values. *LV* = left ventricular, *PM* = papillary muscle, *RV* = right ventricle, *Septum* = interventricular septum.

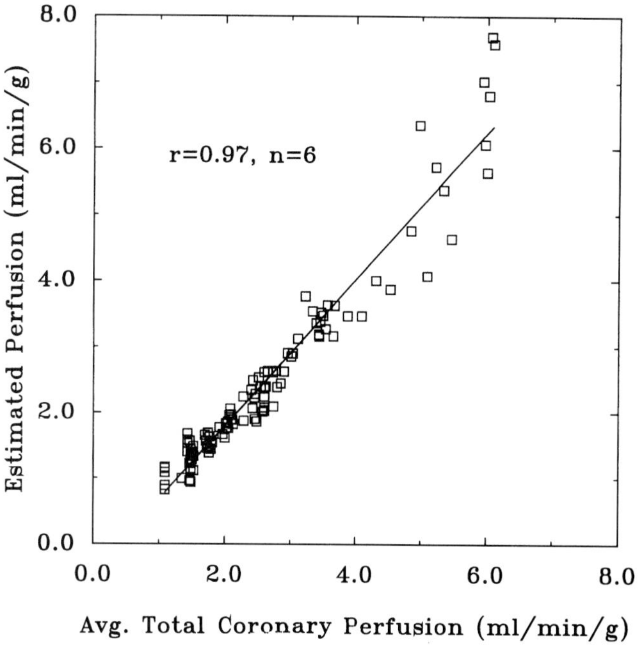

Figure 3. Plot of estimated perfusion from images (f_{images}) against mean total coronary perfusion (f_{avg}) from six hearts at different flows. Mean total coronary flow was determined by dividing the total coronary flow (in milliliters per minute) measured from the pulmonary arterial cannula by the wet weight of the heart (in grams).

heart. Estimates of mean coronary flow were made from images by averaging pixel intensities in regions of interest confined to the left ventricular wall. The right ventricular wall was excluded from these estimates because of concern for partial voluming effects. Exclusion of the right ventricular wall from mean perfusion estimates was expected to introduce little error, however, since the proportion of total flow to the right ventricular wall is small, and the mean coronary perfusion of left and right ventricular myocardia is similar (54–56).

A strong correlation (r = 0.97, n = 6) was found between the estimated mean perfusion (measured from images) and the total mean coronary flow (measured from the pulmonary arterial cannula). The slope and intercept of a linear least-squares fit of these data were 1.11 ± 0.03 (mean ± SD) and −0.43 ± 0.08, respectively. The deviation from a slope of 1.0 and an intercept of 0.0 was consistent with thebesian venous losses not measured at the pulmonary arterial cannula.

Typical signal-to-noise ratios in images with preinversion were 25–35, and signal-to-noise ratios in images without preinversion were greater than 60. According to previous analysis (23), the minimum perfusion difference Δf that can be detected with 95% certainty, or perfusion resolution, is

$$\Delta f_{(P<.05)} \geq \frac{\lambda e^{\tau/T1}}{\tau W(\mathrm{SNR})\sqrt{N}}, \qquad (1)$$

where λ is the blood-tissue water partition coefficient in units of milliliters of water per gram of myocardium, τ is the inversion delay, T1 is the spin-lattice relaxation time, W is the inversion efficiency, SNR is the signal-to-noise ratio, and N is the number of pixels averaged in a region. For an SNR of 30, a T1 of 2.25 seconds, a τ of 2.1 seconds, a W of 0.81, and a 10 × 10 region of interest, minimum perfusion differences of 0.2 mL/min/g were discernible.

Figure 4 shows calculated perfusion images from three of eight sections in a different heart from that shown in Figure 3 that were acquired immediately before and after occlusion of the left anterior descending coronary artery. Mean total coronary perfusion was 1.6 mL/min/g before occlusion, and the perfusion pressure was held constant. After occlusion, the total mean perfusion decreased to 1.1 mL/min/g. The mean total perfusion determined from perfusion images across the left ventricular wall in all sections was 1.8 mL/min/g before the occlusion and 1.2 mL/min/g after the occlusion, which was in close agreement with the mean total perfusion.

Regions of perfusion deficit in the region of the left ventricular free wall were seen easily and were verified qualitatively with early and late gadolinium-enhanced images. Early gadolinium-enhanced images were acquired with low concentrations of gadopentetate dimeglumine, and enhancement was governed primarily by changes in T1. Late gadolinium-enhanced images were acquired at relatively high concentrations of gadopentetate dimeglumine, and normal regions were heavily T2 weighted.

Perfusion measured in the occluded region of the perfusion images, delineated by the gadolinium-enhanced images, was approximately 0 mL/min/g. A scale is shown to map signal intensity to perfusion values (Fig 4).

Oxygenation Measurements

A marked decrease in signal intensity was observed on T2-weighted fast SE images as hemoglobin saturation decreased. Figure 5 shows three T2-weighted fast SE images without preinversion pulses. Hemoglobin saturations of the images in Figure 5a and 5b are 50.5% and 100%, respectively, which resulted in a 31% difference in signal intensity averaged over the entire left ventricular wall. Figure 5c was acquired 14 minutes after ligation of the left anterior descending coronary artery, with 100%-saturated arterial blood. The occluded region was expected to be at 0% saturation since 14 minutes is sufficient time to allow complete desaturation of occluded regions in arrested hearts (26). The mean signal intensity in the occluded region was 52% lower than in that in the septum.

These images are the same images (without preinversion) used to calculate the perfusion images shown in Figure 4 (third section). The occluded region in Figure 4 overlaps substantially with the region of oxygen deficit seen in Figure 5c.

In four of the six hearts studied, standard T2-weighted SE images were acquired in addition to the two fast SE images needed for perfusion measurements. For images acquired at different oxygenation levels, Figure 6 is a plot of the signal intensity of SE images against the signal intensity of the fast SE image acquired immediately after this image and at the same section location. For each SE–fast SE image pair, a region of interest was chosen to include all of the left ventricular myocardium. Values from SE images were normalized to the intensity of the left ventricular wall from the 100% oxygen-saturated SE images, and, similarly, values from fast SE images were normalized to the 100% oxygen-saturated fast SE images to remove the effects of gain and T1 saturation of SE images. The effects of T1 saturation will be removed since T1 does not depend on blood oxygenation (25). The relationship between these values was found to be highly linear, with a correlation coefficient r of 0.93. The linear equation describing this line was as follows: $S_{SE} = (1.15 \pm 0.08)S_{FSE} - (0.16 \pm 0.06)$, where S_{SE} is the SE image signal intensity and S_{FSE} is the fast SE image intensity.

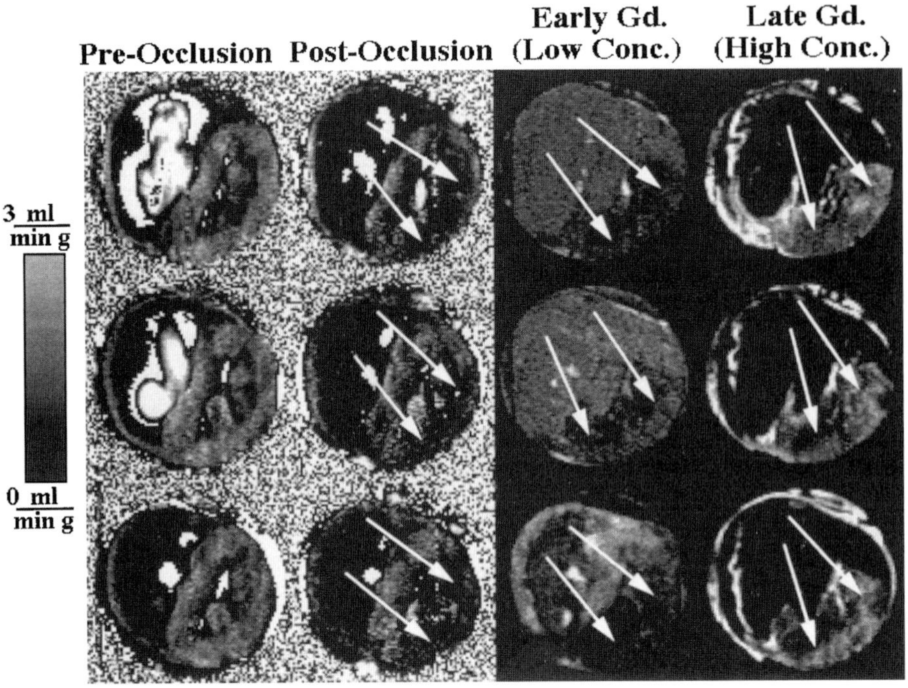

Figure 4. Perfusion images calculated before (*Pre-Occlusion*) and after (*Post-Occlusion*) occlusion in three of eight sections spanning the entire left ventricle. Regions of perfusion deficit are visible in the left ventricular free wall (arrows) and are also delineated on early and late gadolinium-enhanced images (*Early Gd. [Low Conc.]* and *Late Gd. [High Conc.]*). Flow in the occluded region was approximately 0 mL/min/g. Scale for image intensity in late images is not the same as that for early images.

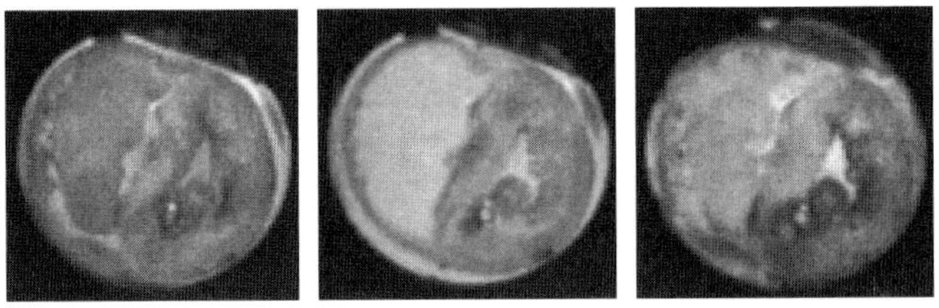

a. b. c.

Figure 5. Three T2-weighted fast SE images without preinversion acquired at **(a)** 50.5% **(b)** 100%, **(c)** 100% hemoglobin saturation. **c** was acquired 14 minutes after occlusion of the left anterior descending coronary artery. These images demonstrate the BOLD signal intensity modulation as oxygenation levels in the myocardium are adjusted and were also used in the generation of the perfusion images in Figure 4 (third section).

Figure 7 is a plot of the normalized T2-weighted fast SE signal intensity against hemoglobin saturation from one heart preparation. Least-squares linear regression yielded the following relationship: $S_{FSE} = (8.3 \pm 0.6) \times 10^{-3}$ (hemoglobin saturation) $+ (1.6 \pm 0.5) \times 10^{-1}$, with an r of 0.99. This graph demonstrates how signal intensity can then be used to map signal intensity to oxygenation levels in the tissue for a given heart. Similar work has been done previously by Atalay et al with T2*-weighted gradient-echo imaging (24) and T2-weighted SE imaging (26).

DISCUSSION

Summary of Results

A method for simultaneous noninvasive measurement of myocardial arterial

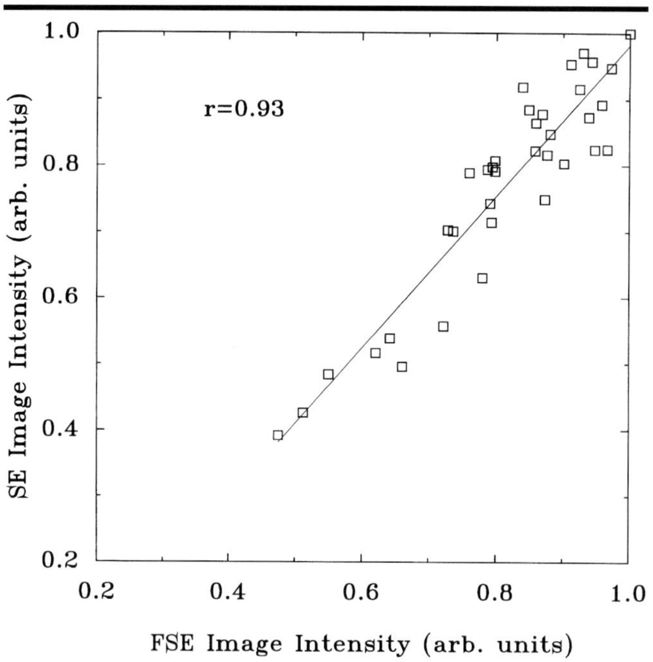

Figure 6. Plot of normalized SE image signal intensity against normalized fast SE (*FSE*) image signal intensity from images acquired in four hearts at the same section location, temporally adjacent, and at different hemoglobin saturations. Regions of interest covered the entire myocardium of the left ventricle and the same region of interest was used for an SE–fast SE image pair. *arb.* = arbitrary.

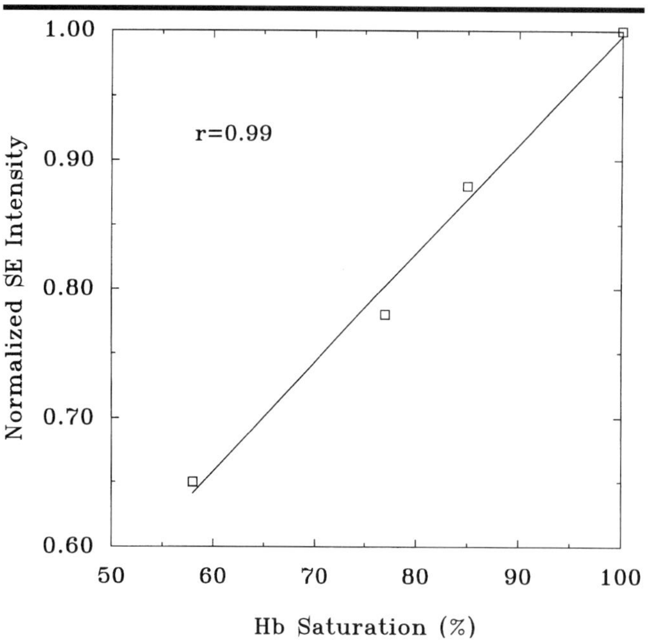

Figure 7. Plot of normalized T2-weighted SE image signal intensity against hemoglobin (*Hb*) saturation at four oxygenation levels is an example of an oxygenation calibration curve from a typical heart preparation.

perfusion and myocardial oxygen content has been presented in the isolated, blood-perfused, arrested rabbit heart. By using a previously verified method of spin labeling and the principles of BOLD imaging, concomitant measurement of perfusion and oxygen content was performed in six to eight sections covering the entire left ventricle in less than 15 minutes. The primary advantages of simultaneous acquisition of perfusion and oxygenation information is a reduction in the total acquisition time and improved image registration between oxygen concentration images and perfusion images.

Myocardial perfusion measurements were performed by using a selective slab that inverted all spins in the imaging section and those apical to that section and by relying on the unique geometry of the coronary vasculature to ensure that enhancement of signal intensity resulted from arterial perfusion. Acquisition of a second image without preinversion enabled the calculation of a perfusion image whose signal intensity was a direct measure of arterial perfusion in units of milliliters per minute per gram.

Excellent registration between images with or without preinversion resulting from reduced imaging times of the fast SE sequence permitted direct calculation of perfusion images on a pixel-by-pixel basis.

Perfusion defects created by ligation of the left anterior descending coronary artery were easily detected with this method and were highly correlated with images acquired after bolus injection of gadopentetate dimeglumine. Signal intensities measured in the core of perfusion deficit regions were found to be approximately 0 mL/min/g. The low perfusion measurements could not be a result of decreased T2 or spin density, since these effects are identical on the images with and without inversion and cancel out in the perfusion calculation (Eq [A1]).

The implementation of fast SE in conjunction with the spin-labeling method provided a 32-fold reduction in imaging time by increasing the number of k_y lines acquired during one excitation from one to 32. This permitted an improvement in image resolution from previous work (23) and complete coverage of the entire left ventricle with six to eight sections.

All images required for perfusion calculations were also T2-weighted. This meant that the images acquired without selective preinversion could be used also for estimation of oxygen content. The signal intensities from these images were found to have excellent linear correlation with those of the standard SE images acquired in the same locations and at the same oxygen tension (r = 0.93). Since we have previously shown that signal intensity on T2-weighted SE images obeys a linear relationship with hemoglobin saturation (26), these results demonstrate that normalized fast SE signal intensity also demonstrates a linear relationship with hemoglobin saturation and therefore can be used in the determination of oxygen content. The equation describing the relationship between SE and fast SE image signal intensity is as follows: $S_{SE} = (1.15 \pm 0.08)S_{FSE} - (0.16 \pm 0.06)$. The slope of this relationship is not significantly different from 1, which implies that fast SE imaging is equally sensitive to hemoglobin saturation as SE imaging.

It may have been expected that SE imaging would be slightly more sensitive than fast SE to hemoglobin saturation since the observed T2 depends on τ_{180}. This dependence has been measured by Wright et al (39) and has been predicted by Bandettini et al (40). Their results show that the observed T2 decreases with increasing τ_{180} at lower hemoglobin saturations, while the T2 at 100% saturation is unaffected by τ_{180}.

Construction of calibration curves for normalized signal intensity with changes in hemoglobin saturation must be performed for a particular τ_{180} since there is a strong dependence of observed T2 on τ_{180}. Normalization to the 100% hemoglobin saturation for the calibration curve is also important to remove the effects of regional differences in blood volume (24).

Similarly, good image registration would, in principle, allow for calculation of calibration images. Blood volume, oxygen consumption, and perfusion are the relevant parameters affected most under pathologic conditions.

An advantage of the perfusion imaging scheme described previously is that information about both perfusion and oxygen content can be collected simultaneously by T2 weighting both images acquired for estimates of perfusion (M_τ, M_0). The perfusion information is T1 encoded and oxygen content is T2 encoded; these effects are separable. Since the same T2 weighting exists in both images, this effect is exactly canceled on division as part of the perfusion image calculation (Eq [A1]).

Although T2 weighting the perfusion images allows for simultaneous acquisition of perfusion and oxygen content information, it has drawbacks. The primary disadvantage is that the image signal-to-noise ratio will decrease, which reduces perfusion resolution (23), especially in regions of oxygen deficit. As was seen in Figure 5, for example, signal intensity can decrease by as much as 50% in ischemic regions, which reduces the perfusion resolution by 50%. This is because the images acquired with preinversion must also be T2-weighted to cancel the T2 weighting of the image acquired without perfusion in the perfusion calculation.

Clearly, optimization of the imaging parameters can be performed to enhance our ability to measure regional perfusion and oxygen content simultaneously at MR imaging. We have previously described methods for optimizing echo time for T2-weighted SE imaging in the estimation of oxygen content (25). An optimization for T2-weighted fast SE imaging for measuring oxygen content also needs to take into account the effect of τ_{180}. Also, the optimum echo time for measuring oxygen content may be suboptimal for perfusion sensitivity, which decreases in regions with low oxygen content.

Toward Combination of Perfusion and Oxygen Content into Regional Oxygen Consumption Measurements

All measurements necessary for oxygen consumption were available for the hearts studied. Oxygen consumption was not calculated in these experiments, however, because of the low metabolic rate that accompanies cardioplegic arrest. As a result, there were no detectable differences in transcoronary hemoglobin saturation under these conditions. In situations in which oxygen consumption is appreciable, oxygen consumption can be calculated as follows.

By using the perfusion image f and the oxygen content image $[O_2]_{tiss}$, oxygen consumption MVO_2 can be calculated as the product of the oxygen extraction (arterial oxygen concentration minus the tissue oxygen concentration) and the arterial perfusion as follows: $MVO_2 = ([O_2]_{art} - [O_2]_{tiss}) \times f$, where $[O_2]_{art}$ is the oxygen concentration measured at the arterial input line and $[O_2]_{tiss}$ is oxygen concentration determined from T2-weighted fast SE images, a fast SE image at 100% oxygen saturation, and a calibration curve.

A method for noninvasively measuring regional myocardial perfusion and regional myocardial oxygen content by using arterial spin labeling and the BOLD effect has been presented. This provides a foundation for laboratory and clinical measurement of regional myocardial oxygen consumption.

Practical applications: The advent of imaging techniques that can be used to measure metabolic processes, if they are successful, promises to revolutionize diagnostic and prognostic procedures that are currently in practice. The ability to estimate noninvasively the rate of oxygen consumption in the heart would provide the clinician with a tool to examine basic energy metabolism and the relationship of oxygen consumption to mechanical function. Conceivably, increased sensitivity to detection of mild ischemia, reversibly damaged myocardium, and perfused and viable but noncontracting tissue may have a profound influence on future therapeutic interventions and treatments.

The additional information available with the successful clinical implementation of these techniques includes estimations of regional flow with high spatial and/or temporal resolution, regional oxygen extraction, and regional oxygen consumption. Continued improvements in fast imaging techniques and new cardiac-gating strategies have provided substantial promise for the use of these tools in laboratory investigations and may provide for their eventual clinical application.

APPENDIX

Calculation of Perfusion Images

Arterial perfusion can be determined from two images by acquiring one image with preinversion at a fixed delay τ (M_τ) and a second image without preinversion (M_0) as previously shown (23), as follows:

$$f = \frac{\lambda}{2\tau W e^{-\tau/T1}}\left(\frac{M_\tau}{M_0} + 2We^{-\tau/T1} - 1\right), \quad (A1)$$

where W is 1.0 for perfect inversion and 0.5 for 90° saturation. The value of λ is relatively constant across mammalian species and is approximately 0.78 mL/g (58). This value of λ was used for all calculations in this study.

Maximal sensitivity to perfusion is achieved when W is 1.0 and τ is optimized. The optimal time between refocusing pulses τ_{opt} is approximately the T1 of the tissue (23). During this period, inflowing arterial magnetization mixes with tissue magnetization, which enhances the apparent T1 recovery.

Equation (A1) allows direct perfusion calculations from the normalized signal intensity and can be used to construct a perfusion image in units of milliliters per minute per gram if adequate registration exists between the images with M_τ or without M_0 selective preinversion.

BOLD Signal Intensity Dependence and Fast SE

The signal intensity S for a T2-weighted fast SE image is related as follows:

$$S \propto M_0 e^{-|TE_{eff}/[T2(\%HbO_2,\tau_{180})]|}, \quad (A2)$$

where TE_{eff} is the effective echo time determined by the acquisition timing of the central lines of k space and $T2(\%HbO_2,\tau_{180})$ is the spin-spin relaxation time T2 of the tissue as a function of the oxygen status of capillary vessel beds, myocardial vascular volume, and τ_{180}.

Thus, by constructing an oxygen calibration curve from the normalized signal intensity on images acquired at known oxygen levels, the oxygen tension in the myocardium can be determined (26). Changes in τ_{180} require the measurement of a new calibration curve because of its dependence on T2. With fast SE imaging, however, TE_{eff} can be adjusted by changing the k-space ordering alone (47), unlike with SE imaging, and in this case a new calibration curve is not required. With a calibration curve, images of myocardial oxygen content $[O_2]_{tiss}$ can be generated under a variety of conditions, such as ischemia, infarction, reperfusion, vasodilation, and inotropic stimulation.

Acknowledgment: We gratefully acknowledge the assistance of Rong Xue, MS, with the experimental protocol.

References

1. American Heart Association. Heart and stroke facts. Dallas, Tex: American Heart Association, 1993.
2. Evanochko WT, Pohost GM. Myocardial nuclear magnetic resonance spectroscopy. In: Frontiers in cardiovascular imaging. New York, NY: Raven, 1993.

3. Bottomley PA, Hardy CJ, Roemer PB, Mueller OM. Proton-decoupled, Overhauser-enhanced, spatially localized carbon-13 spectroscopy in humans. Magn Reson Med 1989; 12:348–363.
4. Weiss RG, Gloth ST, Kalil-Filho R, Chacko VP, Stern MD, Gerstenblith G. Indexing tricarboxylic acid cycle flux in intact hearts by carbon-13 nuclear magnetic resonance. Circ Res 1992; 70:392–408.
5. Chatham JC, Forder JR, Glickson JD, Chance EM. Calculation of absolute metabolic flux and the elucidation of the pathways of glutamate labeling in perfused rat heart by 13C NMR spectroscopy and nonlinear least squares analysis. J Biol Chem 1995; 270:7999–8008.
6. Xu X, White LT, Doumen C, Damico LA, et al. Kinetic analysis of dynamic 13C NMR spectra: metabolic flux, regulation, and compartmentation in hearts. Biophys J 1995; 69:2090–2102.
7. Marcus M, Schelbert HR, Skorton DS, Wolf GL. Cardiac imaging: a companion to Braunwald's heart disease. Philadelphia, Pa: Saunders, 1991; 634–1256.
8. Go RT, MacIntyre WJ, Chen EQ, Cook SA, Neumann DR, Saha GB. Current status of the clinical applications of cardiac positron emission tomography. Radiol Clin North Am 1994; 32:501–519.
9. Hartiala J, Knuuti J. Imaging of the heart by MRI and PET. Ann Med 1995; 27:35–45.
10. Watson NE Jr, Cowan RJ, Ball JD. Conventional radionuclide cardiac imaging. Radiol Clin North Am 1994; 32:477–500.
11. Gould KL. Management of coronary artery disease with positron emission tomography. In: Frontiers in cardiovascular imaging. New York, NY: Raven, 1993.
12. Wackers FJT. Single photon emission computer tomography. In: Frontiers in cardiovascular imaging. New York, NY: Raven, 1993.
13. Robles HB, Lawson MA, Johnson LL. Role of imaging in assessment of ischemic heart disease. Curr Opin Cardiol 1994; 9:435–447.
14. Thompson BH, Stanford W. Evaluation of cardiac function with ultrafast computed tomography. Radiol Clin North Am 1994; 32:537–551.
15. McCollough CH, Morin RL. The technical design and performance of ultrafast computed tomography. Radiol Clin North Am 1994; 32:521–536.
16. Brundage BH. Myocardial imaging with ultrafast computed tomography. In: Frontiers in cardiovascular imaging. New York, NY: Raven, 1993; 80.
17. Williams DS, Grandis DJ, Zhang W, Koretsky AP. Magnetic resonance imaging of perfusion in the isolated rat heart using spin inversion of arterial water. Magn Reson Med 1993; 30:361–365.
18. Edelman RR, Siewert B, Darby DG, et al. Qualitative mapping of cerebral blood flow and functional localization with echo-planar MR imaging and signal targeting with alternating radio frequency. Radiology 1994; 192:513–520.
19. Nishimura DG, Macovski A, Pauly JM, Conolly SM. MR angiography by selective inversion recovery. Magn Reson Med 1987; 4:193–202.
20. Kwong KK, Chesler DA, Weisskopf BR, Rosen BR. Perfusion MR imaging (abstr). In: Proceedings of the Second Meeting of the Society of Magnetic Resonance. Berkeley, Calif: Society of Magnetic Resonance, 1994; 1005.
21. Kwong KK, Chesler DA, Weisskopf RM, et al. MR perfusion studies with T1-weighted echo planar imaging. Magn Reson Med 1995; 34:878–887.
22. Kim SG. Quantification of relative cerebral blood flow change by flow-sensitive alternating inversion recovery. Magn Reson Med 1995; 34:293–301.
23. Reeder SB, Atalay MK, McVeigh ER, Zerhouni EA, Forder JR. Quantitative cardiac perfusion: a non-invasive spin-labeling method that exploits coronary vessel geometry. Radiology 1996; 200:177–184.
24. Atalay MK, Forder JR, Chacko VP, Kawamoto S, Zerhouni EA. Oxygenation in the rabbit myocardium: assessment with susceptibility-dependent MR imaging. Radiology 1993; 189:759–764.
25. Atalay MK, Reeder SB, Zerhouni EA, Forder JR. Blood oxygenation dependence of T1 and T2 in the isolated, perfused rabbit heart at 4.7T. Magn Reson Med 1995; 34:623–627.
26. Atalay MK, Zerhouni EA, Forder JR. Relationship between regional oxygen content and MRI signal intensity in the perfused rabbit heart: assessment in the setting of regional ischemia (abstr). Circulation 1994; 90:I–468.
27. Wendland MF, Saeed M, Lauerma K, de Crespigny A, Moseley ME, Higgins CB. Endogenous susceptibility contrast in myocardium during apnea measured using gradient recalled echo planar imaging. Magn Reson Med 1993; 29:273–276.
28. Niemi P, Poncelet BP, Kwong KK, et al. Myocardial intensity changes associated with flow stimulation in blood oxygenation sensitive magnetic resonance imaging. Magn Reson Med 1996; 36:78–82.
29. Balaban RS, Taylor JF, Turner R. Effect of cardiac flow on gradient recalled echo images of the canine heart. NMR Biomed 1994; 7:89–95.
30. Stillman AE, Wilke N, Jerosch-Herold M, et al. BOLD contrast of the heart during occlusion and reperfusion (abstr). In: Proceedings of the First Meeting of the Society of Magnetic Resonance. Berkeley, Calif: Society of Magnetic Resonance, 1994; S24.
31. Li D, Dhawale P, Rubin PJ, Haacke EM, Gropler RJ. Myocardial signal response to dipyridamole and dobutamine: demonstration of the BOLD effect using a double-echo gradient echo sequence. Magn Reson Med 1996; 36:16–20.
32. Bassingthwaighte JB, Yipintsoi T, Harvey RB. Microvasculature of the dog left ventricular myocardium. Microvasc Res 1974; 7:229–249.
33. Grayson J, Davidson JW, Fitzgerald-Finch A, Scott C. The functional morphology of the coronary microcirculation in the dog. Microvasc Res 1974; 8:20–43.
34. Ogawa S, Tank DW, Menon R, et al. Intrinsic signal changes accompanying sensory stimulation: functional brain mapping with magnetic resonance imaging. Proc Natl Acad Sci USA 1992; 89:5951–5955.
35. Turner R, Le Bihan D, Moonen CT, Despres D, Frank J. Echo-planar time course MRI of cat brain oxygenation changes. Magn Reson Med 1991; 22:169–166.
36. Kwong KK, Belliveau JW, Chesler DA, et al. Dynamic magnetic resonance imaging of human brain activity during primary sensory stimulation. Proc Natl Acad Sci USA 1992; 89:5675–5679.
37. Pauling L, Coryell C. The magnetic properties and structure of the hemochromogens and related substances. Proc Natl Acad Sci USA 1936; 22:159–163.
38. Boxerman JL, Hamberg LM, Rosen BR, Weisskoff RM. MR contrast due to intravascular magnetic susceptibility perturbations. Magn Reson Med 1995; 34:555–566.
39. Wright GA, Hu BS, Macovski A. Estimating oxygen saturation of blood in vivo with MR imaging at 1.5 T. JMRI 1991; 1:275–283.
40. Bandettini PA, Boxerman JL, Davis TL, Wong EC, Weisskoff RM, Rosen BR. Numerical simulations of the oxygenation dependence of the T2 and T2* of whole blood using a deterministic diffusion model (abstr). In: Proceedings of the Third Meeting of the International Society for Magnetic Resonance in Medicine. Berkeley, Calif: International Society for Magnetic Resonance in Medicine, 1995; 456.
41. Glasel JA. Nuclear magnetic resonance studies on water and ice. In: Frank F, ed. His water: a comprehensive treatise. Vol 1, The physics and physical chemistry of water. New York, NY: Plenum, 1972; 238.
42. Gamcsik MP, Forder JR, Millis KK, McGovern KA. A versatile oxygenator and perfusion system for magnetic resonance studies. Biotechnol Bioeng 1996; 49:348–354.
43. Yamamoto F, Braimbridge MV, Hearse DJ. Calcium and cardioplegia: the optimal calcium content for the St. Thomas' Hospital cardioplegic solution. J Thorac Cardiovasc Surg 1984; 87:908–912.
44. Institute of Laboratory Animal Resources, Commission on Life Sciences, National Research Council. Guide for the Care and Use of Laboratory Animals. National Institutes of Health publication 93-23. Washington, DC: U.S. National Academy of Sciences; 1996.
45. Henning J, Nauerth A, Friedburg H. RARE imaging: a fast imaging method for clinical MR. Mag Reson Med 1986; 3:823–833.
46. Mulkern RV, Wong ST, Winalski C, Jolesz FA. Contrast manipulation and artifact assessment of 2D and 3D RARE sequences. Magn Reson Imaging 1990; 8:557–566.
47. Plewes DB, Bishop H. Spin-echo MR imaging. In: Sprawls P, Bronskill MJ, eds. The physics of MRI: 1992 AAPM Summer School. Woodbury, NY: American Institute of Physics, 1993; 170–171.
48. Hinks RS, Kohli J, Washburn S. Fast spin echo prescan for artifact reduction (abstr). In: Proceedings of the Third Meeting of the International Society for Magnetic Resonance in Medicine. Berkeley, Calif: International Society for Magnetic Resonance in Medicine, 1995; 634.
49. Reeder SB, McVeigh ER. Tag contrast in breath-hold CINE cardiac MRI. Magn Reson Med 1994; 31:521–525.
50. Segel LD, Ensunsa JL, Boyle WA III. Prolonged support of working rabbit hearts using Fluosol-43 or erythrocyte media. Am J Physiol 1987; 252:H349–H359.
51. Sharan M, Popel AS. Algorithm for computing oxygen dissociation curve with pH, PCO2, and CO in sheep blood. J Biomed Eng 1989; 11:48–52.
52. King RB, Bassingthwaighte JB, Hales JR, Rowell LB. Stability of heterogeneity of myocardial blood flow in normal awake baboons. Circ Res 1985; 57:285–295.
53. Bassingthwaighte JB, King RB, Roger SA. Fractal nature of regional myocardial blood flow heterogeneity. Circ Res 1989; 65:578–590.
54. Schlant RC, Sonnenblick EH, Katz AM. Normal physiology of the cardiovascular system. In: Alexander RW, Schlant RC, Fuster V, O'Rourke RA, Roberts R, Sonnenblick EH, eds. Hurst's the heart, arteries, and veins. Vol 1. New York, NY: McGraw-Hill Health Professions, 1998.
55. Klocke FJ, Frank MW. Principles of myocardial perfusion. In: Skorton DS, Schelbert HR, Wolf GL, Brundage BH, eds. Marcus cardiac imaging: a companion to Braunwald's heart disease. 2nd ed. Vol 1. Philadelphia, Pa: Saunders, 1996; 8–19.
56. Hendry PJ, Nathan H, Rajagopalan K. Right ventricular blood flow during left ventricular support in an experimental porcine model. Ann Thorac Surg 1996; 61:1199–1204.
57. Altman PL, Dittmer DS, eds. Respiration and circulation. Bethesda, Md: Federation of American Societies for Experimental Biology, 1971; 264.

Scott O. Trerotola, MD
Timothy J. Carmody, MD
Robert D. Timmerman, MD
Kathleen Ann Bergan, MS
R. Gerald Dreesen, RT
Stephanie V. Frost, MS
Mitchell Forney

Brachytherapy for the Prevention of Stenosis in a Canine Hemodialysis Graft Model: Preliminary Observations[1]

Index terms:
Animals
Dialysis, shunts, 80.42, 92.457, 93.457
Grafts, interventional procedures, 92.1268, 93.1268
Grafts, stenosis or thrombosis, 92.1268, 92.458, 93.1268, 93.458
Iridium, radioactive

Radiology 1999; 212:748–754

[1] From the Departments of Radiology (S.O.T., T.J.C., R.G.D.), Radiation Oncology (R.D.T., S.V.F.), Medicine (K.A.B.), and Surgery (M.F.), Indiana University Medical Center, UH0279, 550 N University Blvd, Indianapolis, IN 46202-5253. From the 1998 RSNA scientific assembly. Received July 8, 1998; revision requested August 6; revision received November 23; accepted February 16, 1999. **Address reprint requests to** S.O.T. (e-mail: *streroto@iupui.edu*).

PURPOSE: To determine whether gamma brachytherapy can prevent in-stent stenosis in hemodialysis grafts.

MATERIALS AND METHODS: Six-millimeter polytetrafluoroethylene arteriovenous grafts were created bilaterally in six dogs. After 1 month, Wallstents spanning the venous anastomosis were placed to accelerate restenosis. Gamma irradiation (12 Gy) was delivered endoluminally to one of the two grafts by using an iridium 192 source; thus, each animal served as its own control. Fistulography was performed monthly for 10 months or until graft thrombosis, with measurement of stenosis at each time point. At the conclusion of the study period, the treated area was examined histologically, and a computer model was used to calculate the volume of intimal hyperplasia.

RESULTS: Delayed stent migration resulted in exclusion of one dog. In the remaining five dogs, maximum stenosis across all time intervals was less for the treated side ($P < .04$), and the volume of intimal hyperplasia was less for the treated side ($P < .045$). In one animal studied at 1 year, this trend reversed in terms of percentage stenosis but not total neointimal volume.

CONCLUSION: Brachytherapy with ^{192}Ir (gamma) delivered at the time of stent placement reduces restenosis in this hemodialysis graft model, but, depending on the parameter evaluated (stenosis vs total volume of neointima), the benefit may wane or even reverse with time.

Patients undergoing chronic hemodialysis rely heavily on their vascular access. This access, either in the form of synthetic conduits or native fistulas, is, unfortunately, prone to repeated episodes of venous stenosis that eventually lead to thrombosis and failure of the access. Venous stenosis in hemodialysis access is the result of intimal hyperplasia, a firm rubbery relatively acellular substance thought to occur in response to turbulence and shear stress (1). While there have been efforts at preventing intimal hyperplasia with drugs in hemodialysis access, to date none has been successful clinically (2).

Over the past 15 years, balloon angioplasty has become an accepted, approved treatment alternative to traditional surgical revision of hemodialysis-related venous stenosis (3–6). Balloon angioplasty is thought by many to be preferable to surgical revision because of its lower cost, because it is an outpatient procedure, because it can be easily repeated when restenosis occurs, and, most important, because it results in preservation of other veins for future access. Using percutaneous transluminal angioplasty, investigators have documented decreased graft thrombosis rates and prolonged access life (6–8). Despite its numerous advantages, venous angioplasty does have a number of drawbacks—most important, restenosis. Recurrence rates following balloon angioplasty are high, reportedly 37%–62% at 6 months (3–6,9). To our knowledge, efforts at controlling restenosis with stents (10–12) have been unsuccessful to date.

Brachytherapy, the endovascular delivery of radiation therapy, has been introduced as a

Author contributions:
Guarantor of integrity of entire study, S.O.T.; study concepts, S.O.T.; study design, S.O.T., T.J.C., R.D.T.; definition of intellectual content, S.O.T., T.J.C., R.D.T.; literature research, T.J.C., S.O.T., R.D.T.; experimental studies, T.J.C., S.O.T., R.D.T., R.G.D., S.V.F., M.F.; data acquisition, T.J.C., R.D.T., S.O.T., S.V.F., R.G.D.; data analysis, K.A.B., S.O.T., R.D.T.; statistical analysis, K.A.B.; manuscript preparation, S.O.T., R.D.T.; manuscript editing, S.O.T., R.D.T., T.J.C., R.G.D.; manuscript review, S.O.T., T.J.C., R.D.T., R.G.D., K.A.B., S.V.F.

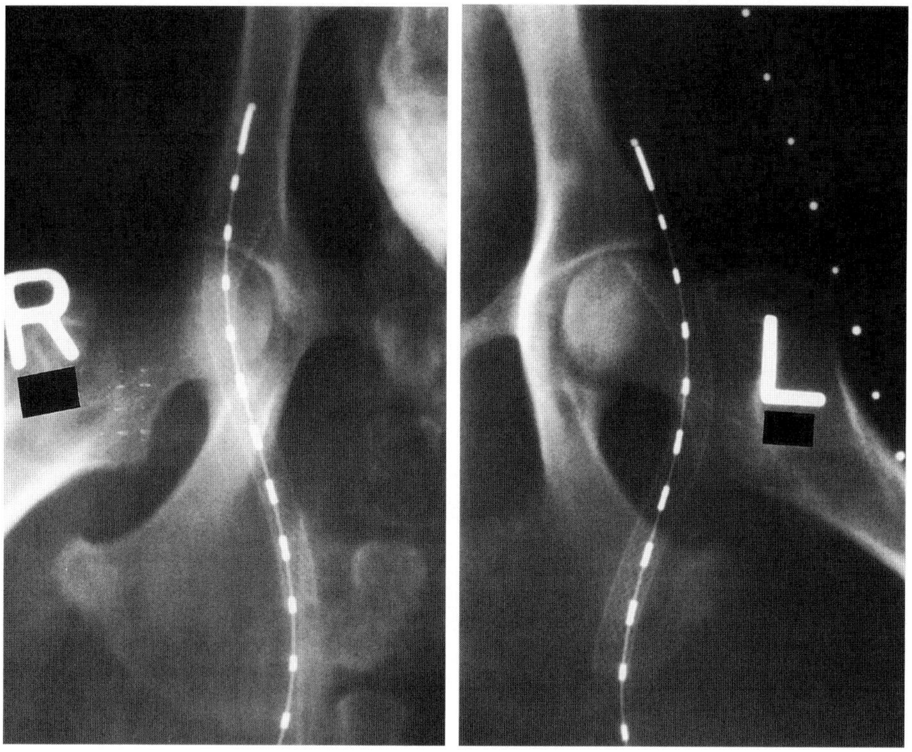

a. b.

Figure 1. Brachytherapy planning procedure. Spot radiographs of the **(a)** right (*R*) and **(b)** left (*L*) grafts following Wallstent placement, with dummy seeds in place within the stent-treated segment. Radiopaque seeds allow proper positioning of the radiolucent carrier catheter prior to treatment. Metallic markers to the animal's left represent 1-cm increments.

possible means of controlling restenosis in coronary arteries (13–19) and peripheral arteries (20,21) following percutaneous treatments for stenosis, including percutaneous transluminal angioplasty and stent placement. To our knowledge, few data are available concerning the effects of brachytherapy on venous restenosis (22,23); however, the basic restenotic process of smooth muscle cell hyperplasia and proliferation is similar in arterial and venous lesions (1). The purpose of this study was to determine whether iridium 192 brachytherapy could be used to prevent in-stent stenosis in a canine hemodialysis graft model.

MATERIALS AND METHODS

All aspects of handling and caring for the animals in this study, including anesthesia, analgesia, and euthanasia, adhered to the recommendations of the National Institutes of Health's "Guide for the Care and Use of Laboratory Animals," as well as state and institutional guidelines.

Twelve femoral artery–to–femoral vein arteriovenous grafts were created (M.F.) according to the method of Fillinger et al (24–27) in six adult mongrel dogs weighing 20–30 kg. The animals fasted for 12 hours prior to surgery or any percutaneous procedure, as required for anesthesia. Prophylactic cefazolin (1 g; Kefzol; Marsam Pharmaceuticals, Cherry Hill, NJ) was administered intramuscularly. Anesthesia was induced with thiopental sodium (Pentothal; Abbott Laboratories, North Chicago, Ill; 20–30 mg per kilogram of body weight). An endotracheal tube was inserted, and inhalation anesthesia (isoflurane [Isoflo]; Rhone-Poulenc Chemicals, Avonmouth, Bristol, UK) was administered to effect.

A transverse incision was made in each groin 3 cm below the inguinal ligament. The femoral artery and vein were mobilized. By using nontapered 6-mm reinforced expanded polytetrafluoroethylene (Gore-Tex; W.L. Gore, Flagstaff, Ariz) graft material, a 25-cm loop-type arteriovenous shunt was created by means of end-to-side anastomosis with a running 7-0 expanded polytetrafluoroethylene suture. The grafts were tunneled subcutaneously. Intraoperative medication consisted of only a flush solution containing heparin. The wounds were closed in layers by using polyglycolic acid suture (Dexon; Davis-Feck, Manati, Puerto Rico). After surgery, 500 mg of cefadroxil (Cefa-Tabs; Fort Dodge Laboratories, Fort Dodge, Iowa) was given orally daily for 5 days. The shunts were palpated daily to assess patency.

After 4 weeks of graft maturation, the animals were returned to the radiology research laboratory for stent placement (T.J.C., S.O.T.) and brachytherapy (R.D.T.). Anesthesia and preprocedural medication were identical to those described earlier. By using a sterile technique, access to the grafts was obtained by direct percutaneous puncture, and a 7-F sheath (Pinnacle; manufactured by Terumo and distributed by Boston Scientific, Natick, Mass) was placed in each graft directed toward the venous anastomosis.

After initial fistulography to determine the exact location of the venous anastomosis, 10-mL-diameter, 42-mm-long Wallstents (Schneider, Minneapolis, Minn) were placed percutaneously to span the venous anastomosis and were centered on the anastomosis. Stents were used as a part of the experimental model; previous work using this model had indicated that the most reliable way of producing stenosis in this model was to place Wallstents in this position, and the intimal hyperplasia produced was indistinguishable from that seen in hemodialysis access-related stenoses with or without stents (28). Angioplasty was not performed before or after stent placement. During stent placement, iodinated contrast material (iohexol [Omnipaque 350]; Nycomed, Princeton, NJ) and a flush solution containing heparin were used as needed. Post–stent placement baseline fistulography was performed by using spot radiography.

After stent placement, one graft in each animal was randomly assigned to receive brachytherapy; in this way, each animal served as its own control. Identical 6-F carrier catheters (Nucleotron, Columbia, Md) were placed through each stent via the 7-F sheath and were positioned by using a dummy seed cable (Nucleotron) under fluoroscopic guidance so that the radiation dose would be delivered to the area with the stent and to the vein 2.5 mm central to the stent, with a total length of radiation delivery of 7.5 cm (Fig 1). The carrier catheters on the untreated side served as a control for the manipulation involved in the delivery of brachytherapy.

After positioning the carrier catheters, the animal was transported to a remotely controlled high-dose radiation therapy suite, where endovascular gamma irradia-

Percentage Stenosis Measured Angiographically at Each Time Interval

Animal	Side	Months after Treatment												Volume of Neointimal Hyperplasia (cm^3)
		1	2	3	4	5	6	7	8	9	10	11	12	
1	Irradiated	4	17	NA	17	NA	18	23	27	31	Sacrificed	Sacrificed	Sacrificed	0.37
	Control	23	35	NA	32	NA	35	36	37	36	Sacrificed	Sacrificed	Sacrificed	0.45
2	Irradiated	NA	6	NA	5	13	14	11	18	14	Sacrificed	Sacrificed	Sacrificed	0.12
	Control	NA	17	NA	19	22	25	33	31	36	Sacrificed	Sacrificed	Sacrificed	0.25
3	Irradiated	NA	12	NA	14	16	15	17	18	22	NA	NA	28	0.44
	Control	NA	15	NA	22	20	21	20	19	15	NA	NA	16	0.49
4	Irradiated	4	NA	14	15	NA	17	13	NA	22	Sacrificed	Sacrificed	Sacrificed	0.23
	Control	27	NA	34	42	NA	46	40	NA	45	Sacrificed	Sacrificed	Sacrificed	0.34
5	Irradiated	7	NA	28	48	Occluded	Occluded	Occluded	Occluded	Occluded	Occluded	Occluded	Occluded	0.44
	Control	13	NA	49	82	Occluded	Occluded	Occluded	Occluded	Occluded	Occluded	Occluded	Occluded	0.76

Note.—NA = Data points not obtained due to scheduling difficulties.

tion was delivered to the treatment side by using a ^{192}Ir source (Microselectron-HDR; Nucleotron). A dose of 12 Gy was prescribed at a distance of 3.75 mm from the linear central axis of the carrier catheter. Total dosing time was approximately 200 seconds. Following brachytherapy, the carrier catheters and hemostatic sheaths were removed, and hemostasis was achieved with manual compression. After recovery, the animals were returned to their cages, and the grafts were palpated daily. Cefadroxil was given orally (500 mg/d) for 5 days.

The grafts were examined by using contrast material fistulography (T.J.C.) at 1-month intervals following brachytherapy to assess development of neointimal hyperplasia and/or stenosis. Note that scheduling conflicts precluded performance of several of the interval fistulographic examinations (Table).

The end point of the study for each graft was 10 months after creation of the graft or thrombosis (defined as absence of a thrill or pulse in the graft), whichever came first. At the study end point, the grafts, stents, and draining vein were excised en bloc for histopathologic examination. If one graft clotted prior to the contralateral graft or at the study end point, the animal was killed and both grafts were removed.

Measurements

Measurement of intimal hyperplasia and stenoses was performed by direct measurement on the spot radiographs by using a micrometer (S.O.T.). Because relative measurements were used, correction for magnification was unnecessary. Measurements were obtained at the site of maximum stenosis within the treatment area by using the stent diameter as a reference. Percentage stenosis was calculated as follows: percentage = $(1 - MLD/S) \times 100$, where MLD is the measured minimum lumen diameter and S is the stent diameter measurement. Measurements were made at a time remote from the performance of fistulography by an investigator who did not participate in the brachytherapy delivery and who was blinded to the side of irradiation.

Histologic Examination

Excised grafts, stents, and veins were fixed in formalin. Gross photographs of each sample were taken. Prior to sectioning, a silk suture was threaded within the outer (adventitial) fibrous layer through the entire length of each explant. This allowed proper orientation of each section with respect to adjacent sections for computer modeling (see earlier). Transverse sections were made in 5-mm increments extending 2 cm proximal to and 2 cm distal to the venous anastomosis or to the end of the stent. When cutting through the portions of the vein or graft with the stent, a razor blade was used to first cut through the soft tissue and then a wire cutter was used to cut each of the stent wires. A gross photograph was taken of each section. Magnified gross photographs were taken by using a dissecting microscope with a camera attachment.

Stent wires were individually removed by using fine forceps under the dissecting microscope. All sections were processed through paraffin, and three 5-µm sections were cut from each block. The sections were stained with hematoxylin-eosin. Neointimal thickness was approximated by using an ocular micrometer on the microscope.

Blinded analysis of the histologic sections was performed by a pathologist with extensive experience in stent histologic analysis.

Computer Modeling

Computer modeling based on the histologic specimens was also used to determine an estimated volume of intimal hyperplasia. This was used to try to overcome variations in the degree of neointima from point to point in the graft that have been seen in previous experiments (28). Since marked variations in intimal thickness may be encountered with this model, sampling error might be high if histologic sections are used for comparison. These variations occur in cross-section as well as longitudinally.

The computer modeling and interpretation were done in a blinded fashion. Hematoxylin-eosin–stained slides of the axial sections were input via a flatbed scanner (ScanJet 3c; Hewlett Packard, Palo Alto, Calif) and were enhanced by using a commercial graphics software package (Microsoft Imager 1.0; Microsoft, Seattle, Wash). The images were then digitized into a commercial three-dimensional radiation therapy treatment planning system (Render Plan 3-D; Precision Therapy International, North Miami Beach, Fla), where the vessels were virtually reconstructed in three dimensions. By using the computer model, the volume of remaining lumen could be calculated and subtracted from that of the bare stent lumen, which allowed calculation of the volume of neointimal hyperplasia present. This technique is an extension of planimetry used widely in studies of neointimal hyperplasia, in which three-dimensional rendering techniques similar to those used for computed tomography are applied.

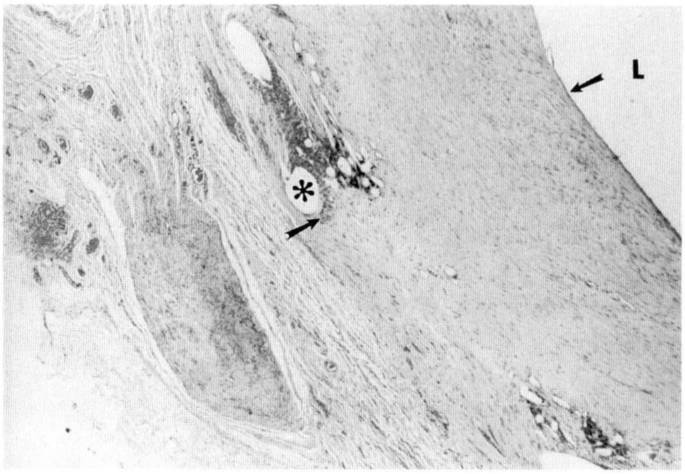

a.

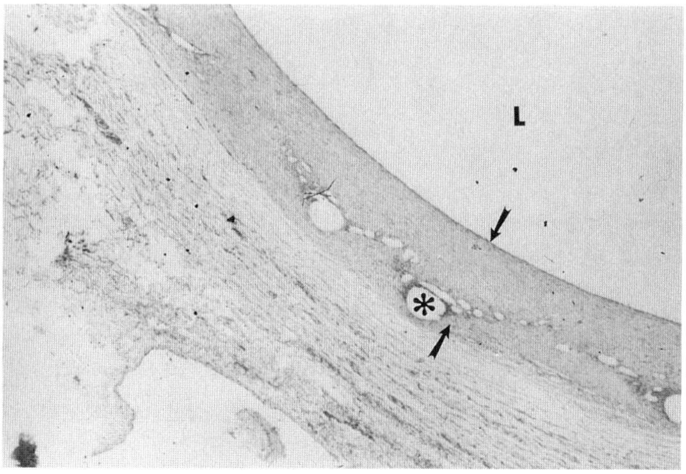

b.

Figure 2. Photomicrographs of the **(a)** control and **(b)** treated grafts 1.5 cm central to the anastomosis. Note the greater neointimal thickness (arrows) in **a** than in **b** and the artifacts (*) from the stent wire removal. *L* = lumen. (Hematoxylin-eosin stain; original magnification, ×20.)

Statistical Evaluation

The two-tailed paired Student *t* test was used to compare the volume of neointima between the treated and untreated legs. The difference in percentage stenosis between the two legs was plotted against the number of days since surgery for each dog to identify changes over time. In looking at the difference in percentage stenosis between the two legs, one dog had both grafts thrombose within 1 day of each other at 118 days after brachytherapy. To not possibly bias the results toward the alternative hypothesis, four new data points at months 6, 7, 8, and 9 were added, with a difference in percentage stenosis of 0 between the two legs. Four new points were added to make this dog have the same number of measurements as the mean number of 7 for the other four dogs. A weighted paired *t* test was used to compare the mean difference in percentage stenosis between the two legs across all times for each dog. The test was weighted by the number of times the measurements were made. The number of days since surgery was grouped into monthly categories, which were based on 30 days in a month plus or minus 15 days. A weighted paired *t* test was also used to compare the mean difference in percentage stenosis between the two legs of each dog during the time intervals. The test was weighted by the number of measurements in each dog during the time interval. In only one case did a dog have two measurements made within the same month. Differences were considered statistically significant if *P* was less than .05.

RESULTS

Stent migration occurred in one animal at the first postbrachytherapy follow-up. The stent had migrated out of the graft into the common femoral vein. The procedure in this animal was considered a failure of the experimental model and was thus killed and excluded from evaluation. Of the remaining five dogs, four had patent grafts at the study end point (mean, 294 days after brachytherapy; range, 258–359 days; note that one animal was examined beyond the planned end point). In one animal, both grafts thrombosed within 1 day of each other at 118 days after brachytherapy. The Table summarizes the graft survival, percentage stenosis at each interval, and volume of neointima at completion of the study.

The mean volume of neointima determined with computer modeling was higher in the untreated legs (0.32 cm^3 ± 0.14 vs 0.46 cm^3 ± 0.19, $P < .045$). In all five dogs, the neointimal volume was greater in the untreated leg than in the treated leg. Across all time intervals, the percentage stenosis was higher for untreated legs ($P < .04$). When looking at each of the time intervals, the untreated leg showed a significantly greater percentage stenosis during the third ($P < .02$), fourth ($P < .015$), and seventh ($P < .05$) months. There was no significant difference between the treated and untreated legs during the first ($P = .09$), second ($P = .12$), fifth ($P = .28$), sixth ($P = .13$), eighth ($P = .38$), or ninth ($P = .27$) months. There was only one observation in the 10th and 12th months. Note that in all but one animal, the percentage stenosis was always higher in the control group. In this animal, this effect was reversed beginning at the 9-month point and persisting at 1 year.

All sections showed varying amounts of neointima consisting of mature fibrous connective tissue. Figure 2 shows representative sections from each group. Even within individual sections, there was marked variation in neointimal thickness, ranging from 0 to 1,950 µm, as has been demonstrated in prior studies by using this model (28). Focal chronic inflammation was seen in two specimens, both in the treatment arm, but was immediately adjacent to microperforations due to stent wires and was not thought to be due to the brachytherapy. Similar inflammation has been seen previously in nonirradiated specimens by using this model (28).

DISCUSSION

Endovascular radiation therapy, or brachytherapy, is a recent addition to the growing list of devices and drugs under evaluation for the prevention or abatement of restenosis. To our knowledge, most studies to date have examined the use of brachytherapy in the arterial system, including the superficial femoral (20,21) and coronary (13–18) arteries. Several different approaches have been used, including gamma and beta emitters delivered to an angioplasty or stent site and placement of radioactive stents (29–31). Early results indicate that, regardless of the technique used, brachytherapy can diminish restenosis in the arterial system, and large-scale clinical trials are currently under way, with a probability of U.S. Food and Drug Administration approval within the next year or so.

Relatively little is known about the effects of brachytherapy in the venous system and hemodialysis circuits. A clinical trial of gamma brachytherapy in patients with failing hemodialysis grafts is reportedly under way (32), but results of this trial are not yet available. Smith et al (22) reported a trend toward reduction of intimal hyperplasia at 1 month in a sheep arteriovenous graft model with a rhenium 186–filled balloon (a beta emitter). Waksman et al (23) reported results of a pilot study in failing human hemodialysis grafts. They used ^{192}Ir following balloon angioplasty at a dose of 14 Gy in 18 grafts in 11 patients. At a mean follow-up of 44 weeks, 11 of 18 sites remained patent. These preliminary human data are not particularly promising, although the authors indicated they believed suboptimal centering accounted for the poor results.

Nowhere is a feasible approach to the reduction of restenosis needed more than in hemodialysis access. Even the best results of balloon angioplasty in hemodialysis-related venous stenosis are measured in months, with a 38%–63% 6-month primary patency rate reported in several large series (3–6). Currently available vascular stents appear to be no better than balloon angioplasty, as determined in three prospective randomized trials (10–12). Medical treatments designed to reduce restenosis in hemodialysis access have been equally disappointing (2).

The results of our study suggest a possible role for brachytherapy in hemodialysis access–related stenosis. Gamma brachytherapy in this established animal model yielded significant reductions in in-stent restenosis, as measured as maximum percentage stenosis measurements at multiple time points during the study, with a consistent trend toward reduction even when statistical significance was not achieved. This effect was confirmed by volumetric computer modeling, which we believe more accurately conveys the difference in volume of intimal hyperplasia as opposed to stenosis at a single site. However, in the single animal followed up for 1 year, the treated side became the more stenotic side at 9 months. It should be noted that this late reversal could conceivably indicate a delayed detrimental effect of brachytherapy, which will need even longer-term studies to evaluate. Since this represents only a single observation, one must be vary cautious when trying to interpret it. The possible waning or even late detrimental benefit of brachytherapy in this dialysis graft model suggests that to obtain a durable result, treatment might need to be repeated at intervals after the initial intervention. This will need to be studied with further animal experiments and/or human clinical trials.

The animal model used here is an established model of hemodialysis access. This model has been shown to result in intimal hyperplasia indistinguishable from that seen in human dialysis grafts (24–28). Two downsides of this model are that it is inconsistent in its production of intimal hyperplasia and, in the natural state (ie, without stents), tends to develop stenosis at a relatively slow pace. Further, there tends to be greater accumulation of intimal hyperplasia within the graft as opposed to within the vein, which makes it slightly different from human grafts. Since we were studying in-stent restenosis as opposed to graft-vein anastomotic stenosis, this consideration may be less important. In a study in which the same model was used, Trerotola et al (28) showed that when Wallstents were placed across the venous anastomosis in this model, restenosis occurred at an accelerated rate: By 5 months, five of six grafts treated with Wallstents had thrombosis as compared with four of six untreated grafts and three of six grafts treated with Gianturco stents. Further, the mean percent stenosis in the Wallstent group was consistently higher at all time intervals. Thus, to create a more consistent and accelerated model, grafts with Wallstents in place served as the experimental model. Hence, the results obtained here can be directly applied only to the reduction of in-stent restenosis, although we believe they would apply to lesions treated with angioplasty alone as well, since such lesions are histologically indistinguishable from in-stent restenosis. Similar studies in coronary arteries have shown reductions in in-stent restenosis following brachytherapy (19–21) or when radioactive stents were used (29–31).

It is interesting that, despite the use of Wallstents as part of the model, only one of five dogs developed intimal hyperplasia at the rate seen by Trerotola et al, and the remaining four dogs' grafts remained patent for up to 1 year. The explanation for this disparity is unclear. Unlike in prior trials (24–28), aspirin was not administered to the animals on a daily basis. We chose not to use aspirin in this study to eliminate a potentially confounding variable. Conflicting data exist with regard to the role of aspirin in hemodialysis access failure; however, findings of at least one trial have suggested that aspirin worsens graft survival (33). If this is true, the discrepancy in neointimal hyperplasia between this and prior studies by using this model might be explained on this basis.

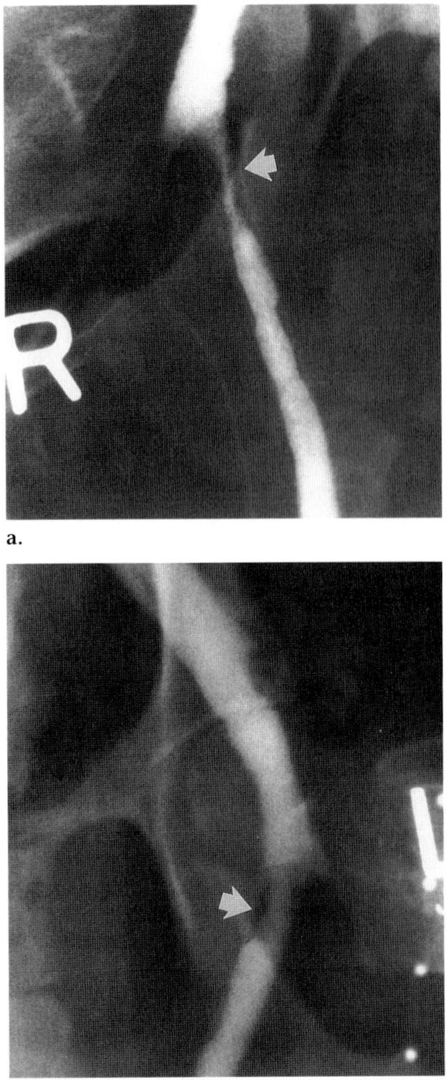

a.

b.

Figure 3. Spot radiographs obtained during contrast material injection into grafts at 2 months after radiation therapy in the **(a)** control side and **(b)** radiated side. **a** shows greater stenosis (arrow) and greater overall volume of intimal hyperplasia than does **b**. *R* = right.

Due to the small number of animals in the study, we were able to perform histologic analysis at only a single data point. Many studies of brachytherapy in coronary arteries have used shorter end points, usually in the 1-month range. By sampling at the 9-month time point, it is possible that we missed greater differences in neointimal volume occurring at an earlier time point. We chose to follow the grafts for a longer time to determine whether any late detrimental effects of brachytherapy might be evident, as well as to determine whether the effect of a single treatment with brachytherapy would be durable. While no detrimental effects were observed histologically, the late reversal of results seen in a single animal suggests that further observations at this time point should be made before universally accepting the concept of brachytherapy on the basis of findings of shorter-term studies.

The mechanism of action of brachytherapy in the arterial system is thought to be inhibition of smooth muscle cell proliferation (14,16,17,29,30). Studies have shown that despite inhibition of smooth muscle cells, endothelial regrowth is not inhibited (15,17,30). Since restenosis in hemodialysis access appears to be due to mechanisms similar to those in arteries (1,27), the mechanism of action of brachytherapy in veins is likely similar. The exact dosing regimen and timing of brachytherapy have yet to be determined, as has the ideal source. Theoretically, applying the dose several days after the intervention would be ideal, as this is when smooth muscle cells are most actively proliferating: Waksman et al (17) found greater inhibition or intimal hyperplasia when brachytherapy was given 48 hours after instead of immediately after intervention. For practical reasons, timing of brachytherapy must by necessity coincide with the intervention; to our knowledge, this has been the approach taken by most investigators. In dialysis access grafts, however, due to the superficial nature of the lesion, it would be possibly to apply external beam therapy at a time remote from the intervention; more work is needed in this area. External beam therapy has been shown to reduce restenosis in animal arterial models (34,35).

The doses used in most studies to date that we know of have ranged from 7 to 56 Gy, with doses of 12–14 Gy being the most commonly used (13–21). Findings of one study (18) showed increasing benefit in the coronary arteries up to but not beyond 28 Gy; however, for safety reasons, lower doses have been advocated. Bottcher et al (20), in human superficial femoral arteries, used gamma brachytherapy with an ^{192}Ir source to prevent restenosis in stents used to treat atherosclerotic lesions, with excellent results at follow-up from 3 to 27 months; the dose used was 12 Gy. In the clinical study by Teirstein et al (13) of coronary brachytherapy, the dose was calculated at between 8 and 30 Gy, depending on the distance from the source.

We chose to use 12 Gy, as it was the dose most commonly used in preclinical studies and clinical studies. It should be noted, however, that no centering device was used; thus, the delivered dose varied depending on the course of the catheter in the treated area (Fig 1). The maximum dose delivered could not be reliably determined, while the minimum dose was 6 Gy. Whether centering the source within the vessel lumen would have improved results will require further study.

Finally, with respect to the choice of radiation source, both gamma and beta emitters have been used. Beta emitters have the advantage of less exposure to the operator and do not require the use of an afterloader (18,36). However, longer treatment times are required if beta emitters are used, although this can be reduced by using liquid beta emitting sources in balloons (36). Use of beta-emitting stents obviates this problem (29–31). Gamma emitters have the advantage of being readily available, as they are used clinically for such indications as treatment of keloids and prevention of heterotopic bone and pterygia. Further, the delivery of the dose takes only a matter of seconds. We chose to use a ^{192}Ir source in this study because it was readily available. Because of dosing and radiation protection issues, it is likely that beta emitters will be the preferred sources for brachytherapy in clinical applications (36).

Many investigators have used maximum intimal thickness as the primary determinant of efficacy (14–19,29–31). While this may be applicable to the coronary acute balloon injury model, we did not think it applied to the present model because of the wide variations in intimal thickness observed. We believe the computer model allows a more meaningful description of the extent of the restenotic process, as it allows determination of the total volume of neointimal hyperplasia and is less affected by variations in neointimal thickness. The importance of the model can be seen in Figure 3: Clearly, there is a much greater volume of intimal hyperplasia in the untreated graft, yet this is poorly conveyed by measurement of percent stenosis or in a single histologic section. The model allows us to quantify this visual impression. There is an important limitation to the model, however: It makes assumptions about data points between actual sections; the more sections obtained, the less this limitation. We chose to section at 5-mm intervals; below this would be prohibitively expensive. Nonetheless, we believe the data from the model are representative of the actual neointimal volumes. A potential improvement for further study might be the application of this model to intravascular ultrasonographic (US) data, thus allowing a greater number of data points. However, findings of one recent study (37) showed that under experimental conditions, angiography and intravascular US were equivalent in determining in-stent stenosis; thus, we believe our use of angiographic measurements in this experiment is valid.

Besides the limitations discussed above, several other limitations to our study should be noted. As with any animal model, one should exercise caution when extrapolating these data to humans. However, we believe that since this is a well-established model proved to mimic the behavior of human dialysis grafts, the results seen here will apply to humans as well. The number of observations in this study is relatively small, and the differences between study and control groups were not always statistically significant. However, with the exception of the single crossover at 1 year, the percentage stenosis and neointimal volume were always higher in the control group, and we believe that further studies will validate these preliminary observations. The reversal in percentage stenosis with long-term observation in one animal indicates that further long-term studies are needed to determine whether there is a late detrimental effect of brachytherapy in hemodialysis access.

Practical applications: Our preliminary data with this animal model suggest that gamma brachytherapy can reduce in-stent restenosis in hemodialysis access. We believe the results are sufficiently compelling to warrant further animal study; however, the long-term (>1-year) effects and optimal dosing of brachytherapy remain to be determined.

Acknowledgments: We thank Schneider for supplying the stents and funding the histologic analysis and W. L. Gore and Associates for providing the graft material used in this study. We thank Kathleen Pedersen, MA, for her secretarial assistance. We also thank Luke Brennecke, DVM, DACVP, at Pathology Associates for performing the histologic analysis.

References

1. Swedberg S, Brown B, Sigley R, Wight T, Gordon D, Nicholls S. Intimal fibromuscular hyperplasia at the venous anastomosis of PTFE grafts in hemodialysis patients: clinical, immunocytochemical, light and electron microscopic assessment. Circulation 1989; 80:1726–1736.

2. Diskin CJ, Stakes TJ, Pennell AT. Pharmacologic intervention to prevent intimal hyperplasia. In: Ferguson RM, Henry ML, eds. Vascular access for hemodialysis III. Chicago, Ill: Precept Press, 1993; 41–73.
3. Beathard GA. Percutaneous transvenous angioplasty in the treatment of vascular access stenosis. Kidney Int 1992; 42:1390–1397.
4. Glanz S, Gordon D, Butt K, Hong J, Lipkowitz G. The role of percutaneous angioplasty in the management of chronic hemodialysis fistulas. Ann Surg 1987; 206:777–781.
5. Kanterman RY, Vesely TM, Pilgram TK, Guy BW, Windus DW, Picus D. Dialysis access grafts: anatomic location of venous stenosis and results of angioplasty. Radiology 1995; 195:135–139.
6. Safa AA, Valji K, Roberts AC, Ziegler TW, Hye RJ, Oglevie SB. Detection and treatment of dysfunctional hemodialysis access grafts: effect of a surveillance program on graft patency and the incidence of thrombosis. Radiology 1996; 199:653–657.
7. Schwab S, Raymond J, Saeed M, Newman G, Dennis P, Bollinger R. Prevention of hemodialysis fistula thrombosis: early detection of venous stenoses. Kidney Int 1989; 36:707–711.
8. Besarab A, Sullivan KL, Ross RP, Moritz MJ. Utility of intra-access pressure monitoring in detecting and correcting venous outlet stenoses prior to thrombosis. Kidney Int 1995; 47:1364–1373.
9. Turmel-Rodrigues L, Pengloan J, Blanchier D, et al. Insufficient dialysis shunts: improved long-term patency rates with close hemodynamic monitoring, repeated percutaneous balloon angioplasty, and stent placement. Radiology 1993; 187:273–278.
10. Beathard GA. Gianturco self-expanding stent in the treatment of stenosis in dialysis access grafts. Kidney Int 1993; 43:872–877.
11. Quinn SF, Schuman ES, Demlow TA, et al. Percutaneous transluminal angioplasty versus endovascular stent placement in the treatment of patients undergoing hemodialysis: intermediate results. JVIR 1995; 6:851–855.
12. Hoffer EK, Sultan S, Herskowitz MM, Daniels ID, Sclafani S. Prospective randomized trial of a metallic intravascular stent in hemodialysis graft maintenance. JVIR 1997; 8:965–973.
13. Teirstein PS, Massullo V, Jani S. Catheter-based radiotherapy to inhibit restenosis after coronary stenting. N Engl J Med 1997; 336:1697–1703.
14. Verin V, Popowski Y, Urban P, et al. Intra-arterial beta irradiation prevents neointimal hyperplasia in a hypercholesterolemic rabbit restenosis model. Circulation 1995; 92:2284–2290.
15. Sarac TP, Riggs PN, Williams JP, et al. The effects of low-dose radiation on neointimal hyperplasia. J Vasc Surg 1995; 22:17–24.
16. Wiedermann JG, Marboe C, Amols H, Schwartz A, Weinberger J. Intracoronary irradiation markedly reduces restenosis after balloon angioplasty in a porcine model. J Am Coll Cardiol 1994; 23:1491–1498.
17. Waksman R, Robinson KA, Crocker IR, Gravanis MB, Cipolla GD, King SB. Endovascular low-dose irradiation inhibits neointima formation after coronary artery balloon injury in swine. Circulation 1995; 91:1533–1539.
18. Waksman R, Robinson KA, Crocker IR, et al. Intracoronary low-dose β-irradiation inhibits neointima formation after coronary artery balloon injury in the swine restenosis model. Circulation 1995; 92:3025–3031.
19. Waksman R, Robinson KA, Crocker IR, et al. Intracoronary radiation before stent implantation inhibits neointima formation in stented porcine coronary arteries. Circulation 1995; 92:1383–1386.
20. Bottcher HD, Schopohl B, Liermann D, Kollath J, Adamietz IA. Endovascular irradiation: a new method to avoid recurrent stenosis after stent implantation in peripheral arteries—technique and preliminary results. Int J Radiat Oncol Biol Phys 1994; 29:183–186.
21. Liermann D, Bottcher HD, Kollath J, et al. Prophylactic endovascular radiotherapy to prevent intimal hyperplasia after stent implantation in femoropopliteal arteries. Cardiovasc Intervent Radiol 1994; 17:12–16.
22. Smith III EF, Pipes D, Konijnenberg M, Ferguson MS, Kirkman T. Efficacy of a Re-186 filled PTCA balloon system to prevent restenosis of peripheral vessels in swine and AV grafts in sheep. Presented at Advances in Cardiovascular Radiation Therapy, Washington, DC, 1997.
23. Waksman R, Crocker IR, Lumsden AB, MacDonald JM, Kikeri D, Martin LG. Long term results of endovascular radiation therapy for prevention of restenosis in the peripheral vascular system (abstr). Circulation 1996; 94:I–300.
24. Fillinger MF, Kerns DB, Bruch D, Reinitz ER, Schwartz, RA. Does the end-to-end venous anastomosis offer a functional advantage over the end-to-side venous anastomosis in high-output arteriovenous grafts? J Vasc Surg 1990; 12:676–690.
25. Fillinger MF, Reinitz ER, Schwartz RA, et al. Beneficial effects of banding on venous intimal-medial hyperplasia in arteriovenous loop grafts. Am J Surg 1989; 158:87–94.
26. Fillinger MF, Reinitz ER, Schwartz RA, et al. Graft geometry and venous intimal-medial hyperplasia in arteriovenous loop grafts. J Vasc Surg 1990; 11:556–566.
27. Sottiurai VS. Biogenesis and etiology in distal anastomotic intimal hyperplasia. Int Angiol 1990; 9:59–69.
28. Trerotola SO, Fair JH, Davidson D, Samphilipo MA, Magee CA. Comparison of Gianturco Z stents and Wallstents in a hemodialysis graft animal model. JVIR 1995; 6:387–396.
29. Hehrlein C, Gollan C, Donges K, et al. Low-dose radioactive endovascular stents prevent smooth muscle cell proliferation and neointimal hyperplasia in rabbits. Circulation 1995; 92:1570–1575.
30. Laird JR, Carter AJ, Kufs WM, et al. Inhibition of neointimal proliferation with low-dose irradiation from a β-particle-emitting stent. Circulation 1996; 93:529–536.
31. Fischell TA, Kharma BK, Fishchell DR, et al. Low-dose, β-particle emission from "stent" wire results in complete, localized inhibition of smooth muscle cell proliferation. Circulation 1994; 90:2956–2963.
32. Nori D, Parikh S, Moni J. Management of peripheral vascular disease: innovative approaches using radiation therapy. Int J Radiat Oncol Biol Phys 1996; 36:847–856.
33. Sreedhara R, Himmelfarb J, Lazarus JM, Hakim RM. Anti-platelet therapy in graft thrombosis: results of a prospective, randomized, double-blind study. Kidney Int 1994; 45:1477–1483.
34. Schwartz RS, Koval TM, Edwards WK, et al. Effect of external beam irradiation on neointimal hyperplasia after experimental coronary artery injury. J Am Coll Cardiol 1992; 19:1106–1112.
35. Shimotakahara S, Mayberg MR. Gamma irradiation inhibits neointimal hyperplasia in rats after arterial injury. Stroke 1994; 25:424–428.
36. Diamond DA, Vesely TM. The role of radiation therapy in the management of vascular restenosis. II. Radiation techniques and results. JVIR 1998; 9:389–400.
37. Schurmann K, Vorwerk D, Uppenkamp R, Klosterhalfen B, Bucker A, Gunther RW. Determination of stent stenosis: an in vivo experimental comparison of intravascular ultrasound and angiography with histology. Cardiovasc Intervent Radiol 1998; 21:189–198.

Juliette Viala, MD
Daniel Vanel, MD
Philippe Meingan, MD
Eric Lartigau, MD
Patrice Carde, MD
Markus Renschler, MD

Index terms:
Brain neoplasms, MR, 10.121412, 10.30
Brain neoplasms, secondary, 10.33
Brain neoplasms, therapeutic radiology, 10.1299, 10.33
Contrast media , 10.12143, 10.1299
Texaphyrins, 10.33, 10.1299

Radiology 1999; 212:755–759

[1] From the Departments of Radiology (J.V., D.V., P.M.) and Medicine (E.L., P.C.), Institut Gustave-Roussy, 39 rue Camille Desmoulins, 94805 Villejuif, France; and Pharmacyclics, Sunnyvale, Calif (M.R.). From the 1997 RSNA scientific assembly. Received May 27, 1998; revision requested July 30; final revision received December 30; accepted March 26, 1999. Supported by Pharmacyclics. **Address reprint requests to** J.V. (e-mail: *vanel@igr.fr*).

Dr Carde and Dr Renschler each has a financial interest through ownership of stock or stock options in the company developing gadolinium texaphyrin, Pharmacyclics. Dr Carde also serves as a consultant to the company. Dr Renschler is the senior director of clinical research and is an employee of the company.

Author contributions:
Guarantor of integrity of entire study, D.V.; study concepts, M.R.; study design, P.C.; definition of intellectual content, D.V.; literature research, J.V.; clinical studies, E.L.; data acquisition and analysis, P.M., J.V.; manuscript preparation and editing, J.V.; manuscript review, D.V.

Phases IB and II Multidose Trial of Gadolinium Texaphyrin, a Radiation Sensitizer Detectable at MR Imaging: Preliminary Results in Brain Metastases[1]

PURPOSE: To evaluate magnetic resonance (MR) imaging results after administration of gadolinium texaphyrin, a tumor-selective radiation sensitizer that is detectable at MR imaging, and to determine an appropriate intravenous dose of gadolinium texaphyrin for repeated injections during radiation therapy, the dose-limiting toxicity of reiterated doses of gadolinium texaphyrin, the maximal tolerated dose, the biolocalization of gadolinium texaphyrin (as assessed at MR examinations), and the response to treatment.

MATERIALS AND METHODS: Ten daily intravenous injections of gadolinium texaphyrin, each followed by whole-brain radiation therapy (total of 10 fractions, 30 Gy), were administered to patients with brain metastases in a multicenter study. At the study institution, 11 patients underwent MR imaging before and after the first injection, after the 10th injection, and 8 weeks after entry into the study.

RESULTS: MR imaging revealed selective drug uptake in metastases, without enhancement of normal brain tissue. In 10 patients, tumor uptake was higher after the 10th injection than after the first injection, which indicated accumulation of gadolinium texaphyrin in metastases. One lesion was visible only after the 10th injection and not at the pretherapeutic MR examination with injection of conventional gadolinium-based contrast material. Response to treatment was defined as a reduction in the size of the metastases between the preinjection MR study and the last MR study; seven patients achieved partial remission with tumor regression exceeding 50% of the initial size, and four achieved a minor response with less than 50% tumor regression.

CONCLUSION: These preliminary results indicate that gadolinium texaphyrin is tumor selective and that brain metastases can be depicted at MR imaging long after the administration of gadolinium texaphyrin.

Radiation therapy is an important treatment for localized cancers. Unfortunately, the radiation dose is often too limited because of injury to normal surrounding tissue. A radiation-sensitizing agent capable of maximizing the cytotoxic effect of radiation delivered to the tumor while minimizing exposure of surrounding tissue would improve the chances of achieving local control.

Gadolinium texaphyrin is the prototype of a new class of compounds, the texaphyrins, which are expanded porphyrins. Several models have been used to demonstrate the radiation-sensitizing effect of gadolinium texaphyrin in studies carried out with HT29 cells in vitro and experimentally in single and multifraction irradiation studies with a murine model (mammary carcinoma) in vivo (1). Findings from a phase IA study, in which 38

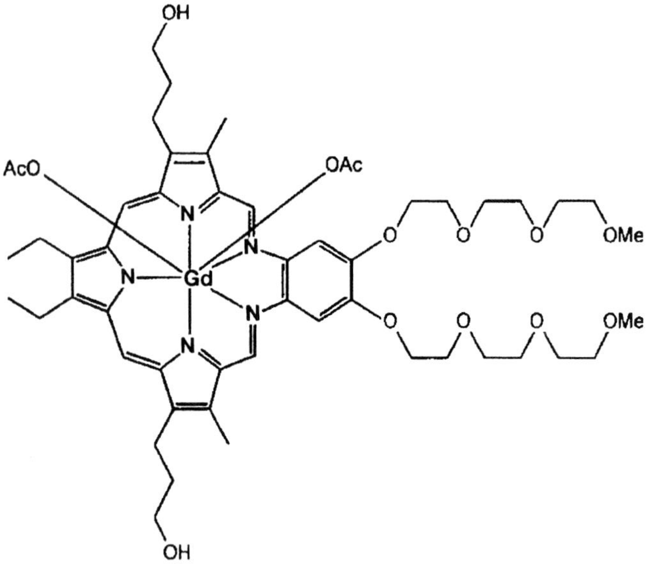

Figure 1. Diagram of the gadolinium texaphyrin molecule. *Ac* = acetyl, *Gd* = gadolinium, *H* = hydrogen, *Me* = methyl, *N* = nitrogen, *O* = oxygen.

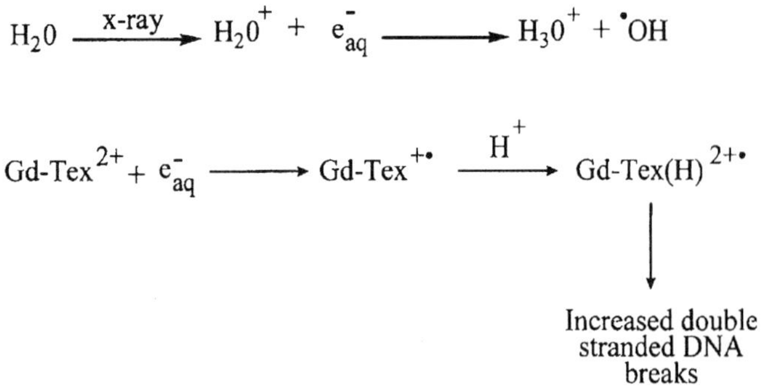

Figure 2. Diagram demonstrates the mechanism of action of gadolinium texaphyrin (*Gd-Tex*).

patients were enrolled, demonstrated very good tolerance and a maximal tolerated dose of 19.4 μmol per kilogram of body weight in a single bolus (2).

The present study is part of a multicenter phase IB study (establishment of the maximal tolerated dose in patients with brain metastases requiring palliative therapy) in which gadolinium texaphyrin and standard radiation therapy are being used in patients with brain metastases. Magnetic resonance (MR) imaging was used exclusively for the follow-up of these patients in our institution, Institut Gustave-Roussy. We report the preliminary results of our participation in the phase IB study in which MR imaging is being used.

The primary objectives of the multicenter phase IB study were to determine an appropriate intravenous dose of gadolinium texaphyrin for repeated injections during radiation therapy, the dose-limiting toxicity of reiterated doses of gadolinium texaphyrin, the maximal tolerated dose, the biolocalization of gadolinium texaphyrin (as assessed at MR examinations), and the response to treatment.

Texaphyrins are expanded porphyrins that are capable of binding lanthanide metals such as lutetium or gadolinium (Fig 1) (3). Gadolinium texaphyrin captures x rays that are delivered in radiation treatment and can be activated by radiofrequency pulses, such as those used in MR imaging (Fig 2) (4).

Gadolinium texaphyrin is water soluble and kinetically stable and is not dependent on tumor oxygenation or on cell-cycle phases. The radiation-sensitizing property of texaphyrins is not dependent on the inserted metal and is exclusively a function of the ligand. Porphyrins localize selectively in tumors; this prompted the simultaneous use of gadolinium texaphyrin as a selective radiosensitizer and as a contrast agent for MR imaging.

MATERIALS AND METHODS

This phase IB and II study, initiated in September 1996 and ended in May 1998, is a multidose trial. The study protocol was approved by the institutional review board of the University of Bicelie, Paris, France.

All patients older than 18 years with brain metastases requiring palliative radiation therapy were eligible, providing the following other criteria were met: a baseline World Health Organization (5) performance status of 0–2 (ambulatory and capable of all self-care but unable to carry out any work activities, ambulatory more than 50% of waking hours); neurologic function less than 2 (able to carry out normal activities with minimal difficulties, neurologic impairment does not require nursing care or hospitalization); and a life expectancy of at least 2 months.

Patients had a hematologic profile with a white blood cell count greater than 3,000 per cubic millimeter (0.003×10^9 per liter), an absolute granulocyte count greater than 1,500 per cubic millimeter (0.0015×10^9 per liter), platelets greater than 100,000 per cubic millimeter (0.1×10^9 per liter); hepatic and renal functions with bilirubin level less than 2 mg/dL (34.2 μmol/L); aspartate aminotransferase, alanine aminotransferase, and alkaline phosphatase levels less than 2 times the upper normal limit; prothrombin time and activated partial thromboplastin time less than 1.5 times the upper normal limit; and serum creatinine level less than 1.5 mg/dL (132.6 μmol/L).

Patients had no concomitant chemotherapy during the 14-day follow-up observation period after the end of treatment; no prior surgical resection of metastases; and no medical or psychiatric condition likely to compromise their ability to give informed consent. They were fully informed of the type of disease diagnosed, the objectives, and the experimental nature of the study and were able to return to the study site for treatment and follow-up visits, as defined in the protocol.

Eleven patients (six women, five men), aged 41–82 years, were enrolled in this study. Ten patients had already undergone treatment for a tumor: three for breast cancer, five for lung cancer, one for thyroid cancer, and one for skin cancer (melanoma). One patient had brain metastases, which revealed a lung cancer.

Each patient received 10 daily intravenous injections of gadolinium texaphyrin (Xcytrin; Pharmacyclics, Sunnyvale, Calif), except during weekends and on public holidays, followed within 2–5 hours with whole-brain radiation therapy. Radiation therapy was delivered in 10 fractions of 3 Gy, for a total of 30 Gy.

The gadolinium texaphyrin doses injected were as follows: 0.25 μmol/kg (no patients), 0.50 μmol/kg (one patient), 0.80 μmol/kg (one patient), 1.30 μmol/kg (two patients), 1.80 μmol/kg (one patient), 2.30 μmol/kg (one patient), 3.10 μmol/kg

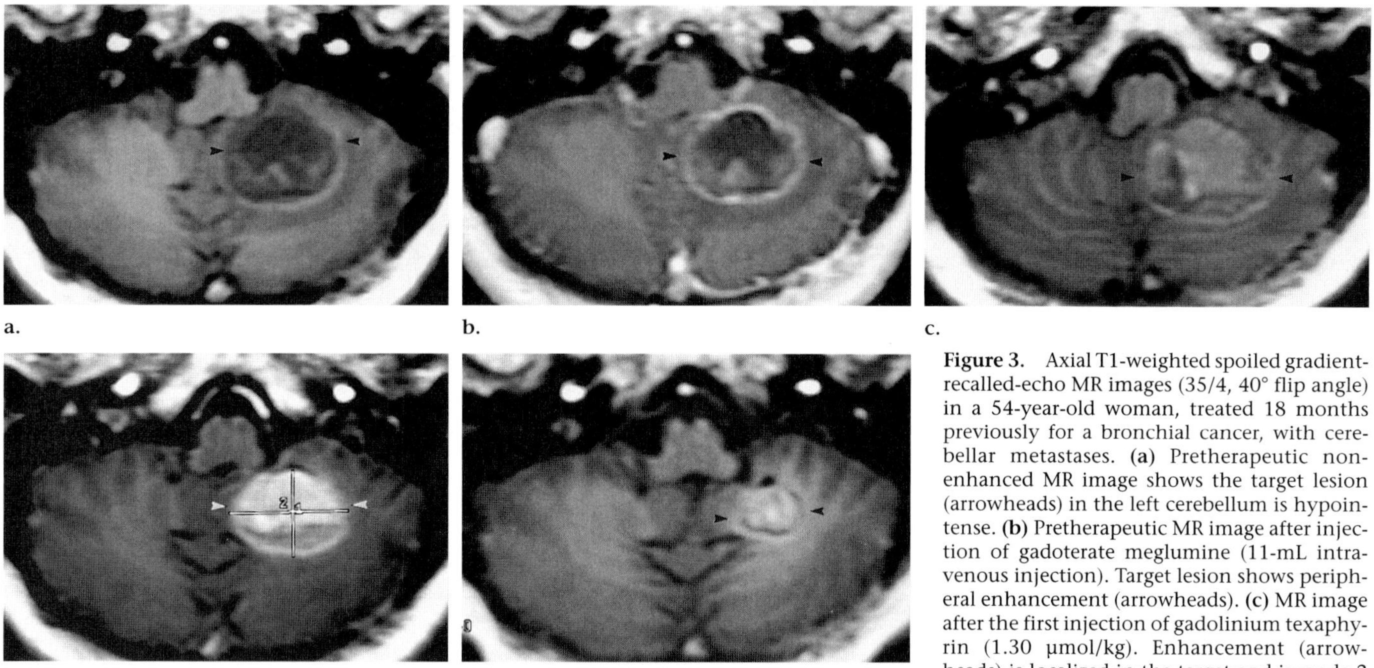

a. b. c. d. e.

Figure 3. Axial T1-weighted spoiled gradient-recalled-echo MR images (35/4, 40° flip angle) in a 54-year-old woman, treated 18 months previously for a bronchial cancer, with cerebellar metastases. **(a)** Pretherapeutic nonenhanced MR image shows the target lesion (arrowheads) in the left cerebellum is hypointense. **(b)** Pretherapeutic MR image after injection of gadoterate meglumine (11-mL intravenous injection). Target lesion shows peripheral enhancement (arrowheads). **(c)** MR image after the first injection of gadolinium texaphyrin (1.30 μmol/kg). Enhancement (arrowheads) is localized in the target and is grade 2 (completely visible enhancement). **(d)** MR image after the 10th injection of gadolinium texaphyrin. Enhancement (arrowheads) is higher and is grade 3 (high enhancement). *1* and *2* are the two largest perpendicular diameters of the lesion. **(e)** MR image 56 days after the first gadolinium texaphyrin injection, without injection of contrast agent. Enhancement (arrowheads) is still well visible and is grade 2. Tumor decreased to 65% of initial size.

Dose of Gadolinium Texaphyrin Injection

Group	Dose	Increase above Preceding Dose (%)	Actual Dose (μmol/kg)
1	. . .	. . .	0.25
2	2.0 × group 1 dose	100	0.50
3	3.3 × group 1 dose	67	0.80
4	5.0 × group 1 dose	50	1.30
5	7.0 × group 1 dose	40	1.80
6	9.3 × group 1 dose	33	2.30
7	12.4 × group 1 dose	33	3.10
8	16.5 × group 1 dose	33	4.10

(three patients), and 4.10 μmol/kg (two patients).

A modified Fibonacci system (with modifications imposed by the manufacturer) was used for dose escalation of gadolinium texaphyrin injections in subsequent cohorts of treated patients (Table).

Three patients were evaluated at each nontoxic dose. The second patient in a cohort must have completed a 7-day follow-up period (after the last injection and irradiation), and the third patient in a cohort must have completed at least the 10-day therapy course before the next cohort was initiated.

If the maximal tolerated dose was not reached by group 8, additional cohorts of three patients were to have been enrolled and were to have received incremental increases of 33% in relation to the previous dose level until the maximal tolerated dose was reached. Three patients were required per cohort, which could have been increased to five patients if grade 3 or 4 toxic reactions had been observed. Data in patients with toxic reactions attributable to radiation therapy were excluded from the determination of the maximal tolerated dose (no patients in our institution, Institut Gustave-Roussy).

Timing of MR Studies

In our institution, Institut Gustave-Roussy, each patient underwent at least four brain MR imaging examinations. The first MR study was performed before the first injection (pretherapeutic) without or with intravenous injection of gadoterate meglumine (0.1 mmol per kilogram of body weight; Dotarem; Guerbet, Roissy, France). The second study was performed after the first injection of gadolinium texaphyrin and before radiation therapy. The third study was performed after the last injection of gadolinium texaphyrin and before the last radiation therapy session, and the fourth was performed 56 days after the beginning of the treatment. Two patients underwent an extra MR examination 3–4 months after the beginning of the treatment. One patient underwent two additional MR examinations 6 and 9 months after the beginning of the treatment.

A 1.5-T magnet (Signa; GE Medical Systems, Milwaukee, Wis) and a T1-weighted spoiled gradient-recalled-echo pulse sequence (35/4 [repetition time msec/echo time msec], 40° flip angle) were used. Images were acquired in axial, coronal, and sagittal planes. A maximum of three studies were graded for each patient per target lesion. Two radiologists (J.V., D.V.) evaluated together, by consensus, enhancement of signal intensity after the first and last injections and 56 days later. This enhancement was graded 0–3, where 0 was no enhancement, 1 was moderate enhancement, 2 was fully visible enhancement, and 3 was high enhancement.

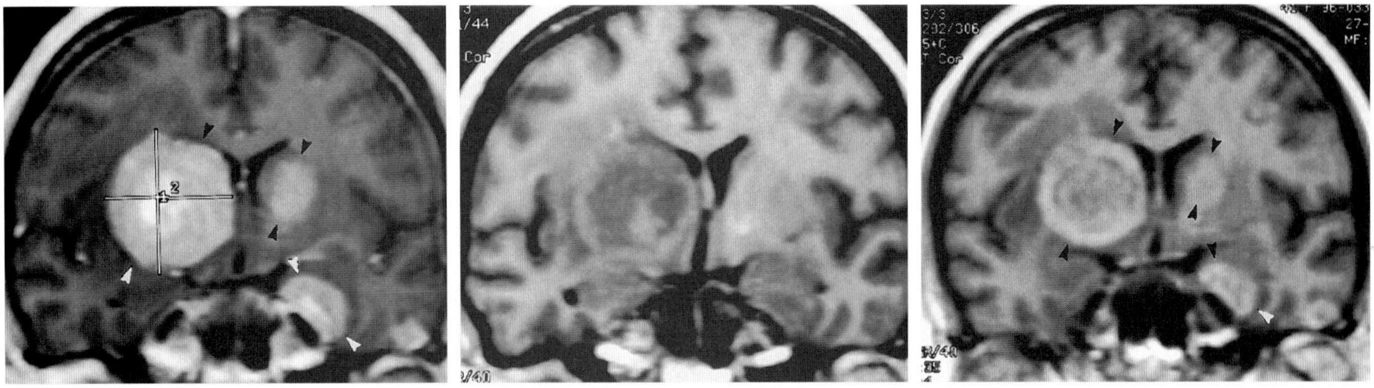

a. b. c.

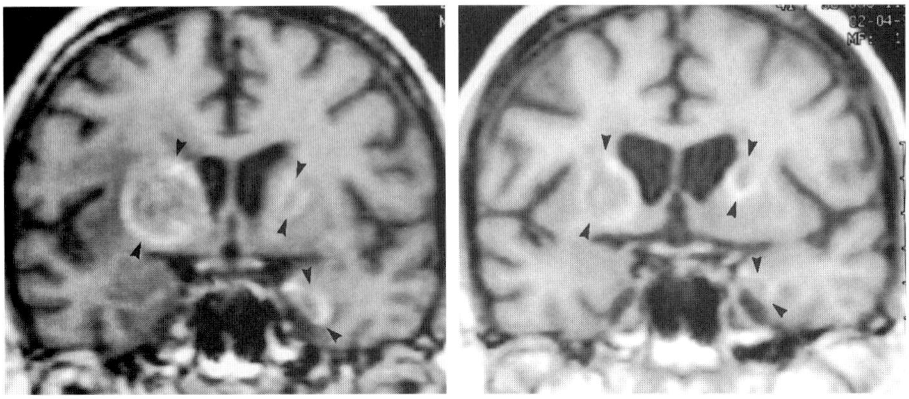

d. e.

Figure 4. Coronal T1-weighted spoiled gradient-recalled-echo MR images (35/4, 40° flip angle) in a 41-year-old woman with brain metastases from a breast cancer. **(a)** Pretherapeutic MR image after injection of 16 mL of gadoterate meglumine. Target lesions (arrowheads) localized in the caudate nucleus show fully visible signal intensity enhancement. *1* and *2* are the two largest perpendicular diameters of the lesion. **(b)** MR image after the first injection of gadolinium texaphyrin (2.30 μmol/kg). No enhancement in the target lesions. **(c)** MR image after the 10th injection of gadolinium texaphyrin. Enhancement is localized in the target lesions (arrowheads) and is grade 3 (high enhancement). **(d)** MR image 56 days after the first gadolinium texaphyrin injection. Enhancement (arrowheads) is still visible and is grade 3. Tumor decreased to 68% of initial size. **(e)** MR image 16 weeks after the first gadolinium texaphyrin injection. Enhancement (arrowheads) is still visible and is grade 1 (moderate enhancement).

Evaluation of Response

Response to the treatment was assessed between the pretherapeutic MR study and the MR study performed 56 days after the beginning of the treatment. Response was based on World Health Organization criteria (the product of the two largest perpendicular diameters of measurable lesions).

RESULTS

Treatment was very well tolerated. There was no nausea or vomiting after administration of gadolinium texaphyrin. A single incident of considerably increased intracranial pressure occurred in one patient on the day of the first injection and treatment. Gradual yellow-green discoloration of urine was noted from the fourth dose level (1.30 μmol/kg) upward, and discoloration of skin was noted by the seventh level (3.10 μmol/kg). Biologic functions, in particular, liver or kidney functions, were normal.

During the months following treatment, five patients died; one died of massive pulmonary embolism, one died of septic shock (which was probably pulmonary in origin), and three died of tumor progression. The maximal tolerated dose had not been reached in our center.

Results of Brain MR Examinations

Enhancement of signal intensity.—In the patient with a melanoma, signal intensity was high in brain metastases before injection of any contrast agent; this patient was excluded from the evaluation of enhancement. Therefore, signal intensity was evaluated in 10 patients (Figs 3, 4).

On MR images acquired after the first injection, enhanced signal intensity was visible in five patients. No enhancement was observed when the dose injected was below or equal to 0.80 μmol/kg. On MR images obtained after the last injection, enhanced signal intensity was visible in nine patients. The patient with no enhancement had received a dose of 0.80 μmol/kg. The patient who had received a dose of 0.50 μmol/kg per injection had no enhancement of signal intensity in the target lesion on the MR image obtained after the first injection of gadolinium texaphyrin. However, after the 10th injection, there was enhanced signal intensity, which was grade 2. One lesion was visible on the MR study acquired after the 10th injection of gadolinium texaphyrin (1.80 μmol/kg per injection), but it had not been visible on the first MR image obtained after injection with conventional gadolinium-based contrast material.

MR images obtained 56 days after the beginning of treatment showed persistent enhancement of signal intensity in seven patients. The patient who had received the dose of 0.80 μmol/kg per injection had images that showed enhanced signal intensity in the three grade 1 target lesions that had become visible only on the fourth MR study.

Additional MR studies were obtained in two patients 3–4 months after the beginning of treatment; the high level of signal intensity was still visible and was of a magnitude comparable to that of the fourth MR studies.

In a patient who received a dose of 1.30 μmol/kg per injection, the MR images acquired after the beginning of treatment showed enhancement of signal intensity, which had been grade 3 on the fourth MR image and was still fully visible at 6 months (grade 2) and moderate at 9 months (grade 1).

Localization of enhanced signal intensity.—Enhancement of signal intensity was noted only in target lesions, never in normal brain tissue or the mucous membrane.

Appearance of enhanced signal intensity.—There was no remarkable modification in the appearance of the signal intensity noted on successive MR images, which means enhancement was not due to hemorrhage in metastases.

Response to Treatment

Response was evaluated according to World Health Organization criteria. Seven patients achieved a partial remission, with tumor regression greater than or equal to 50%. One patient achieved a minor response with a tumor regression of 25%–49% of the initial size, and in three patients the disease stabilized, with tumor regression of 1%–24% of the initial size. One patient had new brain metastases 2 months after the end of the treatment.

DISCUSSION

Radiation therapy is an important treatment for localized cancers. Unfortunately, the radiation dose is often too limited because of injury to normal surrounding tissue. An ideal radiosensitizer would exert its effect only when administered in the appropriate sequence with radiation therapy, with no direct toxic reaction.

Metronidazole, which was used as a radiation sensitizer in the treatment of supratentorial glioblastomas 20 years ago, achieved a notable positive effect (6). A few years later, nimorazole was used as a hypoxic radiation sensitizer in the treatment of supraglottic laryngeal and pharyngeal carcinoma; the study findings (7) revealed an apparent independent and additive relationship between the hemoglobin concentration and the use of the hypoxic radiosensitizer, and the tumor response was better in patients randomly assigned to the nimorazole group than in patients in the placebo group.

Unfortunately, most radiation sensitizers do not show any differential therapeutic index between tumor and surrounding normal tissues. The use of a tumor-selective radiation sensitizer could help maximize tumor exposure to ionizing radiation and could help improve the chances of obtaining tumor control. Furthermore, a tumor-selective radiation sensitizer that is detectable at MR imaging could help in the appreciation of response to radiation therapy. Such was the case with gadolinium texaphyrin, the prototype of a new class of compounds.

These preliminary results based on limited findings in 11 patients indicate that gadolinium texaphyrin is safe and tumor selective, since enhancement of signal intensity was detected only in target lesions and never in normal brain tissue. Uptake in target lesions was higher after 10 daily injections of gadolinium texaphyrin than after the first one, which indicated the accumulation of gadolinium texaphyrin in brain metastases and its persistence several months later in metastases, as revealed at additional MR examinations. The lesion that was visible only after the 10th injection of gadolinium texaphyrin was either a new metastasis or a lesion that was undetectable with conventional gadolinium-based contrast material.

It is possible not only to depict brain metastases at MR imaging with gadolinium texaphyrin but also to evaluate response to treatment at successive MR imaging examinations, since gadolinium texaphyrin remains in tumors for several months. Injection of a paramagnetic contrast agent for the follow-up MR examinations would be redundant.

These preliminary results do not reflect the radiation-sensitizing effect of gadolinium texaphyrin, which requires further investigation.

Findings of this phase IB and phase II study indicate that gadolinium texaphyrin is tumor selective. The accumulation of gadolinium texaphyrin in metastases over several months as revealed at brain MR studies should permit imaging of brain metastases after radiation therapy and, therefore, evaluation of response to the treatment. A further study in more patients is necessary to appreciate the radiation-sensitizing effect of gadolinium texaphyrin.

References

1. Young S, Qing F, Harriman A, et al. Gadolinium(III) texaphyrin: a tumor selective radiation sensitizer that is detectable by MRI. Proc Natl Acad Sci USA 1996; 93:6610–6615.
2. Rosenthal DI, Nurenberg P, Becerra CR, et al. A phase I single-dose trial of gadolinium texaphyrin (Gd-Tex), a tumor selective radiation sensitizer detectable by magnetic resonance imaging. Clin Cancer Res 1999; 5:739–745.
3. Young SW, Sidhu MK, Qing F, et al. Preclinical evaluation of gadolinium (III) texaphyrin complex: a new paramagnetic contrast agent for magnetic resonance imaging. Invest Radiol 1994; 29:330–338.
4. Sessler JL, Hemmi G, Mody TD, Murai T, Burrell A, Young SA. Texaphyrins: synthesis and applications. Accounts Chem Res 1994; 27:43–50.
5. Borgelt B, Gelber R, Kramer S, et al. The palliation of brain metastases: final results of the first two studies by the Radiation Therapy Oncology Group. Int J Rad Oncol Biol Phys 1980; 6:1–9.
6. Urtasun R, Band P, Chapman JD, Feldstein ML, Mielke B, Fryer C. Radiation and high-dose metronidazole in supratentorial glioblastomas. N Engl J Med 1976; 294:1364–1367.
7. Overgaard J, Sand Hansen H, Lindelov B, et al. Nimorazole as a hypoxic radiosensitizer in the treatment of supraglottic larynx and pharynx carcinoma: first report from the Danish Head and Neck Cancer Study (DAHANCA) protocol 5-85. Radiother Oncol 1991; (suppl 1):143–149.

Book Review

Imaging in Oncology

Edited by Walter L. Curati, MD, FRCR, David O. Cosgrove, MA, MSc, FRCP, FRCR, Martin J. Lipton, MD, and David J. Allison, BSc, MD, FRCR, FRCP
London, England: Greenwich Medical Media, 1998. ISBN 1-9001-5103-0. Softcover, $57.50; pp 230; 137 figures; tables.

The editors of this book seek to provide a concise, integrative resource of modern imaging techniques as applied to the diagnosis and staging of cancer. The book is intended for medical students and physicians at all levels of clinical practice. In their introduction, the editors acknowledge the value of efficiency in cancer imaging, where factors of available technology, clinical expertise, radiation exposure, and cost must be balanced. They advocate and provide an algorithmic approach that directs the clinician to the most appropriate radiologic evaluation for initial diagnosis and more advanced diagnostic and staging procedures. The editors and many contributors include an international group of experts in imaging and several nonradiologic specialties.

The book is arranged by organ systems. Topics include the central nervous system; head and neck; chest; breast; upper gastrointestinal tract; colon and rectum; liver, biliary tract, and pancreas; kidney and male reproductive system; endocrine system; female reproductive system; lymphatic system; bone and soft tissue; and cardiovascular system. Each chapter is organized along anatomic or histologic lines as best suits that organ system. For example, the chapter on the central nervous system considers intraaxial, extraaxial, pituitary, pineal, skull base, and spinal tumors, while the chapter on the colon and rectum discusses colorectal cancer, carcinoid tumors, lymphoma, Kaposi sarcoma, and leiomyosarcoma.

Within each section, a concise clinical discussion of epidemiology, common presenting features, and histologic classification is presented. The principles of staging are detailed in conjunction with critical questions and the diagnostic modality best suited to answer them. Screening, initial evaluation, definitive staging, and imaging follow-up of treated patients are discussed in turn. Clear, easy-to-understand algorithms describe the overall work-up and which radiologic tests are most appropriate. These tests include conventional radiography, ultrasonography, computed tomography, magnetic resonance (MR) imaging, nuclear medicine, and positron emission tomography. Newer and more advanced studies such as functional MR imaging and single photon emission computed tomography are mentioned as well. The benefits of intravascular contrast agents are discussed when needed. The generous illustrations provide clear, well-annotated examples of the major radiologic findings discussed.

This small book is well organized and clear; a surprising amount of information is included. It is very easy to read, and it makes excellent use of illustrations and diagrams. The quality of the printing and illustrations is high. For its nominal cost, this book should be of great value to all physicians who treat patients with cancer. It provides a much-needed guide to all that modern radiology has to offer these patients; at the same time, it promotes a logical, cost-conscious approach.

Reviewed by David Michael Cohen, MD

Timothy A. Bernauer, MD

The Radial Bands Sign[1]

APPEARANCE

The radial bands sign is a finding that is sometimes seen on magnetic resonance (MR) images of the brain (1). Images with this finding show linear or curvilinear areas of abnormal signal intensity that extend in a radial fashion from the periventricular to subcortical regions of the cerebral hemispheres (Figs 1, 2).

EXPLANATION

The radial bands sign is believed by some authors to represent a manifestation of abnormal migration of dysplastic stem cells along the course of the radial glial-neuronal unit in patients with tuberous sclerosis (1–3). This finding has also been called migration tracts or linear abnormalities (2,4). The abnormal signal intensity of the white matter in the radial bands sign represents clusters of giant cells with varying neuronal differentiation, astrocytic differentiation, and cells that are not easily classified (1,5,6). The same giant cell can differ in classification with different histologic techniques. This suggests that tuberous sclerosis may be the product of a dysgenetic event that occurs early in development and results in cells with aberrant or incomplete astrocytic or neuronal differentiation.

Similar histopathologic features are found in the other major intracranial manifestations of tuberous sclerosis (1). The abnormal signal intensity of the white matter lesions presumably relates to a lack of normal myelination and to differences in cellular or interstitial fluid content compared with these findings in the normal brain parenchyma.

Index terms:
Brain, diseases, 13.1832, 30.1832
Brain, MR, 13.121411, 13.121413, 13.121417
Nervous system, diseases, 13.1832, 30.1832
Signs in Imaging, 13.1832

Radiology 1999; 212:761–762

[1] From the Department of Radiology, Indiana University Medical Center, Indianapolis. Received March 30, 1998; revision requested May 6; revision received July 22; accepted January 7, 1999. **Address reprint requests to** the author, 16 Southbrooke Place, Mt Zion, IL 62549.

DISCUSSION

Tuberous sclerosis was described by von Recklinghausen (7). Bourneville (8), who provided a detailed report of the neurologic symptoms and gross cerebral pathologic features of tuberous sclerosis, identified it as a distinct clinical syndrome. Tuberous sclerosis is now recognized as the second most frequently occurring neurocutaneous syndrome after neurofibromatosis type 1 (9) and is characterized by dysplasias and neoplasias of organs derived from all three embryonic germ layers (1). The clinical diagnosis of this disease in the past typically depended on the identification of the characteristic cutaneous manifestations of tuberous sclerosis and the classic triad of seizures, mental retardation, and facial angiofibromas. The advent of diagnostic radiology and subsequent improvements in imaging technology have since altered the approach to diagnosing tuberous sclerosis.

The four major intracranial manifestations of tuberous sclerosis are subependymal nodules, subependymal giant cell astrocytomas, cortical tubers, and white matter abnormalities (1). Before the use of cross-sectional imaging, only the periventricular manifestations could be discerned radiologically. Conventional radiographs showed the calcifications within subependymal nodules in a minority of cases. Pneumoencephalography demonstrated the characteristic "candle wax" appearance of periventricular lesions, but this procedure was invasive. Computed tomography (CT) and MR imaging have revolutionized the radiologic evaluation of this disorder in the past few decades; these modalities now enable confident diagnosis in virtually all cases (6).

Numerous white matter abnormalities have been identified by using cross-sectional imaging. These include wedge-shaped, tumefactive, and linear or curvilinear (ie, radial band) lesions in the cerebral hemispheres and multiple linear bands extending from a conglomerate focus near the fourth ventricle into the cerebellar hemispheres (1). Migration tracts may be seen connecting with cortical tubers, subependymal nodules, or both (4). The migration tracts are almost always hypointense to isointense on T1-weighted images and hyperintense on T2-weighted images in adults. In neonates and young children, they are hyperintense to premyelinated white matter on T1-weighted images and isointense to hypointense compared with premyelinated white matter on T2-weighted images (1). For unknown reasons, enhancement after contrast material administration is seen in a minority of cases.

White matter abnormalities are commonly seen at CT, but they are generally more numerous and conspicuous at MR imaging (4,9). Magnetization transfer and fluid-attenuated

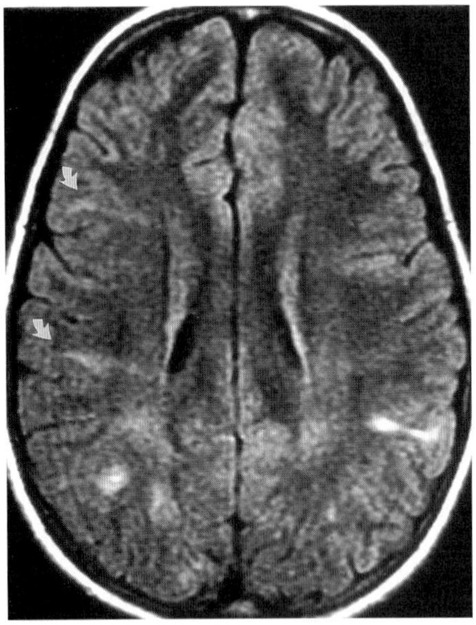

Figure 1. Radial bands sign. Axial fluid-attenuated inversion-recovery MR image (repetition time msec/echo time msec/inversion time msec, 10,002/148/2,200) through the upper lateral ventricles shows linear areas of abnormal white matter with high signal intensity (arrows) extending from the periventricular to subcortical regions of the cerebral hemispheres.

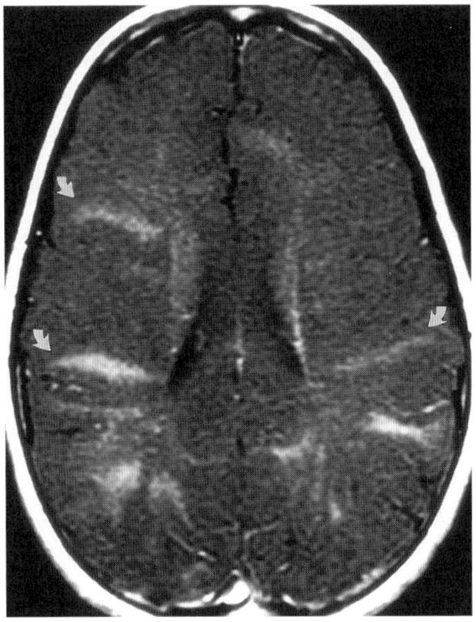

Figure 2. Radial bands sign. Axial, T1-weighted magnetization transfer image (repetition time msec/echo time msec, 500/9) obtained in the same patient as in Figure 1 after administration of a gadolinium-based contrast material, shows the same radiating linear white matter lesions (arrows) as those in Figure 1.

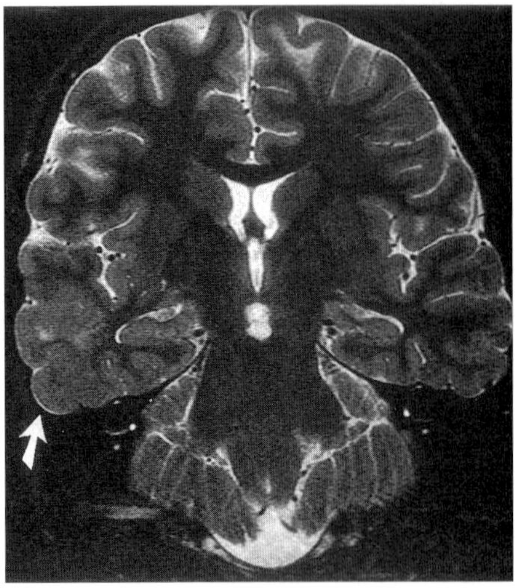

Figure 3. Coronal T2-weighted fast multiplanar inversion-recovery image (5,000/108/120) obtained in the same patient as in Figures 1 and 2 shows a cortical tuber (arrow) in the right temporal lobe. A few small (2–3-mm) subependymal nodules (not shown) also were present.

inversion-recovery images are particularly sensitive to these abnormalities; these modalities have shown substantially more lesions than has CT or other MR images in previous studies (10,11). Consequently, MR imaging findings may be dominated by white matter changes in some patients with tuberous sclerosis. Visualization of radial bands, which appear to be specific to tuberous sclerosis (1), may be helpful in distinguishing this disease from other possible entities such as demyelinating or dysmyelinating processes, infection, tumor, or ischemic changes. This is particularly true when subependymal nodules and cortical tubers are inconspicuous, and visualization of the radial bands should lead the observer to review the imaging study closely for these findings (Fig 3).

At pathologic examination, the white matter lesions of tuberous sclerosis show clusters of giant cells that characteristically align in rows that appear to follow the path of neuronal migration tracts (1). This distribution closely resembles the patterns of heterotopic gray matter distribution and thus suggests that the cerebral manifestations of tuberous sclerosis may be due to abnormal migration of dysplastic cells from the germinal zone (1). In theory, the dysplastic stem cells give rise to dysplastic glia and neurons that are unable to differentiate, migrate, or organize properly (2). It is hoped that future clinical and laboratory studies will substantiate this hypothesis and lead to a better understanding of the pathogenesis of the cerebral abnormalities in tuberous sclerosis.

References

1. Braffman BH, Bilaniuk LT, Naidich TP, et al. MR imaging of tuberous sclerosis: pathogenesis of this phakomatosis, use of gadopentetate dimeglumine, and literature review. Radiology 1992; 183:227–238.
2. Barkovich AJ. Pediatric neuroimaging. 2nd ed. New York, NY: Raven, 1995; 296–304.
3. Steffanson K, Wollmann R, Huttenlocher P. Lineages of cells in the central nervous system. In: Gomez MR, ed. Tuberous sclerosis. 2nd ed. New York, NY: Raven, 1989; 75–87.
4. Iwasaki S, Nakagawa H, Kichikawa K, et al. MR and CT of tuberous sclerosis: linear abnormalities in the cerebral white matter. AJNR 1990; 11:1029–1034.
5. Barkovich AJ, Gressens P, Evrard P. Formation, maturation and disorders of brain neocortex. AJNR 1992; 13:423–446.
6. Seidenwurm DJ, Barkovich AJ. Understanding tuberous sclerosis. Radiology 1992; 183:23–24.
7. Altman NR, Purser RK, Post MJ. Tuberous sclerosis: characteristics at CT and MR imaging. Radiology 1988; 167:527–532.
8. Bourneville DM. Contribution a l'etude de l'idiote. Arch Neurol 1882; 1:81–91.
9. Menor F, Marti-Bonmati L, Mulas F, et al. Neuroimaging in tuberous sclerosis: a clinicoradiological evaluation in pediatric patients. Pediatr Radiol 1992; 22:485–489.
10. Jeong M, Chung T, Coe C, et al. Application of magnetization transfer imaging for intracranial lesions of tuberous sclerosis. J Comput Assist Tomogr 1997; 21:8–14.
11. Takanashi J, Sugita K, Fujii K, Niimi H. MR evaluation of tuberous sclerosis: increased sensitivity with fluid-attenuated inversion recovery and relation to severity of seizures and mental retardation. AJNR 1995; 16:1923–1928.

Motor Neuron Diseases: Comparison of Single-Voxel Proton MR Spectroscopy of the Motor Cortex with MR Imaging of the Brain[1]

Stephen Chan, MD
Dikoma C. Shungu, PhDM
Annette Douglas-Akinwande, MD
Dale J. Lange, MD
Lewis P. Rowland, MD

Index terms:
Amyotrophic lateral sclerosis, 13.89
Brain, cortex, 13.89
Brain, diseases, 13.89
Brain, MR, 13.121411, 13.121412, 13.121416, 13.12145
Magnetic resonance (MR), comparative studies, 13.121411, 13.121412, 13.121416, 13.12145
Magnetic resonance (MR), spectroscopy, 13.12145

Radiology 1999; 212:763–769

Abbreviations:
ALS = amyotrophic lateral sclerosis
Cr = creatine
NAA = *N*-acetylaspartate
PLS = primary lateral sclerosis
SE = spin echo

[1] From the Departments of Radiology (S.C., D.C.S., A.D.A.) and Neurology (D.J.L., L.P.R.), Neurological Institute of New York, Columbia University, Milstein Hospital Bldg, 3rd Floor, 177 Fort Washington Ave, New York, NY 10032. Received July 16, 1998; revision requested August 12; revision received November 17; accepted January 27, 1999. S.C. supported by an RSNA Scholars Award and a General Electric-AUR Radiology Research Academic Fellowship. D.C.S. supported by an R-29 award from the National Institute of Neurological Disorders and Stroke (National Institutes of Health). **Address reprint requests to** S.C.

Author contributions:
Guarantors of integrity of entire study, S.C., L.P.R.; study concepts, S.C., D.C.S., L.P.R.; study design, S.C., L.P.R.; definition of intellectual content, S.C., D.C.S., L.P.R.; literature research, S.C., D.C.S., A.D.A., L.P.R.; clinical studies, S.C., D.J.L., L.P.R.; data acquisition, S.C., D.C.S., A.D.A.; data analysis, S.C., D.C.S.; statistical analysis, S.C., D.C.S.; manuscript preparation, S.C.; manuscript editing and review, all authors.

PURPOSE: To evaluate single-voxel proton magnetic resonance (MR) spectroscopy in detection of abnormality of the upper motor neuron in patients with motor neuron diseases.

MATERIALS AND METHODS: In 43 of 50 patients with motor neuron disease and 14 of 14 control subjects, matching sets of MR spectra were obtained in the left and right motor cortex. The ratio of *N*-acetylaspartate (NAA) to creatine (Cr) was derived from peak area measurements. Mean ratios were calculated for control subjects and several patient groups, including patients with amyotrophic lateral sclerosis (ALS) or primary lateral sclerosis (PLS). MR images were evaluated for corticospinal tract hyperintensity and central sulcus dilatation.

RESULTS: Mean NAA/Cr values were significantly different between control subjects and the ALS or PLS groups ($P < .05$). With an optimal cutoff of 2.5, NAA/Cr values were abnormal in 15 (79%) of 19 patients with ALS, 12 (67%) of 18 patients with PLS, and one (7%) of 14 control subjects. Corticospinal tract hyperintensity, central sulcus enlargement, or both were found in 43% of the ALS group, 24% of the PLS group, and 7% of the control group.

CONCLUSION: NAA/Cr values determined at single-voxel proton MR spectroscopy are more sensitive than are standard findings at MR imaging in the detection of upper motor neuron disease.

Proton magnetic resonance (MR) spectroscopy can help detection of focal neuronal loss in brain diseases, including epilepsy, Alzheimer disease, and stroke. This is achieved by measuring the ratio of *N*-acetylaspartate (NAA) to creatine (Cr) (hereafter, NAA/Cr). NAA is presumed to be found only within neurons and not within glia (1,2). With multivoxel proton MR spectroscopy, Pioro et al (3) found a statistically significant focal decrease in NAA/Cr within the motor and sensory cortex in patients with amyotrophic lateral sclerosis (ALS) compared to that in control subjects. They concluded that MR spectroscopy is useful in the detection of upper motor neuron lesions. Findings in several preliminary studies with single-voxel MR spectroscopy suggest that decreased NAA may be found in the motor cortex region in patients with ALS (4–6). Findings in more recent studies corroborate the decrease in NAA in the motor cortex, but only grouped analyses were performed (7,8).

In single-voxel MR spectroscopy, a specific region of the brain must be targeted for study. The motor cortex is usually affected in ALS, so targeting of the motor cortex at single-voxel MR spectroscopy should yield relevant clinical information. Although single-voxel MR spectroscopy does not have the spatial resolution of MR spectroscopic imaging, it is now widely available on commercial MR imagers, is fully automated after voxel placement, and requires only 7–15 minutes of additional imaging time. Therefore, single-voxel MR spectroscopy may be implemented as part of a clinical MR imaging study with no increase in patient discomfort or cost. In this study, we evaluated use of single-voxel MR spectroscopy to help distinguish patients with disorders involving the upper motor neuron, such as ALS, from those with non–upper motor neuron disorders.

MATERIALS AND METHODS

Study Population

Over a 24-month period from March 1995 to March 1997, 52 consecutive patients suspected of having motor neuron disease were referred for a specialized MR imaging and MR spectroscopic protocol approved by the institutional review board. All participants gave their written informed consent.

The patient population comprised 28 men and 24 women with motor neuron disease (age range, 31–78 years; mean age, 60.5 years; SD, 10.7 years). The clinical diagnoses were based on institutional criteria for four broad groups: (*a*) ALS; (*b*) ALS with probable upper motor neuron signs; (*c*) primary lateral sclerosis (PLS); and (*d*) non–upper motor neuron disorders, which included pure lower motor neuron disorders (such as progressive spinal muscular atrophy or multifocal motor neuropathy) and focal spinal cord disorders, including the myelopathy of multiple sclerosis or spinal cord trauma.

Control subjects comprised eight men and six women (age range, 45–77 years; mean age, 56.8 years; SD, 10.7 years) who were recruited by means of an advertisement. People were excluded who were younger than 45 years or who had a known neurologic disease.

Institutional Criteria

Patients with motor neuron disease were divided into five diagnostic categories on the basis of the presence or absence of lower motor neuron signs or upper motor neuron signs, respectively. Lower motor neuron signs include focal weakness and wasting and is often accompanied by overt fasciculation. Upper motor neuron signs include Hoffmann sign, Babinski sign, clonus, snout reflex, or jaw jerk, any one of which was considered an unequivocal sign of upper motor neuron disease. The presence of brisk tendon reflexes (hyperreflexia) was considered a "probable" sign of upper motor neuron disease.

ALS is a progressive disorder denoted by the presence of both lower and upper motor neuron signs.

ALS with probable upper motor neuron signs is a progressive disorder denoted by the presence of brisk tendon reflexes in limbs with unequivocal lower motor neuron signs and the absence of unequivocal upper motor neuron signs.

Adult-onset progressive spinal muscular atrophy is a progressive disorder characterized by the presence of lower motor neuron signs and the absence of tendon reflexes and upper motor neuron signs. Electromyography reveals no conduction abnormality.

Multifocal motor neuropathy is a clinical syndrome similar to progressive spinal muscular atrophy except for the presence of conduction block or slowing at electromyography.

PLS is a syndrome with slowly progressive gait disturbance and only upper motor neuron signs. The diagnosis is one of exclusion after consideration of multiple sclerosis, spinal cord trauma, compression of the cervical spinal cord, syringomyelia, bilateral strokes, and other conditions. Electromyography reveals no conduction abnormality.

MR Studies

All MR studies were conducted with a 1.5-T MR imager (Signa; GE Medical Systems, Milwaukee, Wis). For all patients, a standard brain MR imaging protocol included the following: (*a*) scout T1-weighted spin-echo (SE) sagittal imaging (repetition time msec/echo time msec = 500/14–16 with one signal acquired); (*b*) high-spatial-resolution, intermediate-weighted, fast SE axial imaging (2,500/21; echo train length, four; field of view, 20 cm; two signals acquired; imaging matrix, 256 × 256; section thickness, 5 mm with 1.5-mm gap; flow compensation; imaging time, 5.5 minutes); and (*c*) standard T2-weighted fast SE axial and coronal imaging (4,000/96; echo train length, eight; field of view, 22 cm at 75% field of view; one or two signals acquired; imaging matrix, 192 × 256; section thickness, 5 mm with 1.5-mm gap; flow compensation; imaging time, 2–3 minutes). The brain MR imaging study was followed by the brain MR spectroscopic study. Finally, in 35 of the 52 patients, an adequate MR imaging study of the cervical spine was obtained, which included high-spatial-resolution axial imaging of the cervical cord (4,000/92; echo train length, eight; field of view, 16 cm; four signals acquired; imaging matrix, 256 × 256; section thickness, 5 mm with 1.5-mm gap; imaging time, 8.5 minutes).

Because of limited availability of the MR imager, the control subjects underwent abbreviated MR imaging and MR spectroscopic studies of the brain. These consisted mainly of T1-weighted SE sagittal imaging (500/14–16 with one signal acquired) and single-echo T2-weighted fast SE axial imaging (4,000/96 with one or two signals acquired) followed by proton MR spectroscopy. Intermediate-weighted axial imaging was omitted, as was the MR imaging study of the cervical spine.

The single-voxel proton MR spectroscopic studies were performed with a point-resolved spectroscopic sequence, or PRESS, supplied by the manufacturer (2,000/272 [SE delay] with 96 signals acquired). A single 8-cm^3 voxel (2 × 2 × 2 cm) was placed over the motor cortex (Fig 1a, 1b), first on the right side and then on the left side. In all cases, correct and reproducible voxel placement was achieved by first locating the central sulcus in the most superior sections on the T2-weighted axial images (9) and then tracing it down to the axial section located about 1 cm above the top of the lateral ventricles (defined as the "plan section"). The voxel was then centered on the precentral gyrus. To ensure maximal sampling of brain parenchyma within the boundaries of the voxel, the location of the voxel was adjusted to fulfill the following three conditions: (*a*) the posterior edge of the voxel intersected or came within 2 mm of the obliquely oriented central sulcus at some point in the plan section, (*b*) the medial edge of the voxel did not include the lateral ventricle in the section 1 cm inferior to the plan section (the section that included the top of the lateral ventricles), and (*c*) the lateral edge of the voxel did not overlap the bone marrow of the calvarium in the axial section 1 cm superior to the plan section. Preimaging required about 3 minutes, and imaging required 4 minutes 24 seconds, or about 7.5 minutes to obtain each MR spectrum of the motor cortex. The entire MR spectroscopic examination required about 15 minutes.

MR spectra were analyzed by one observer (D.C.S.), who was blinded to the patient's condition, with use of a spectroscopic analysis program (SOSNMR) he developed (10). This program uses the Simpson method, which consists of a set of classic function integration formulas for equally spaced abscissas, to compute the area under each metabolite peak (11). (This approach is appropriate for the present study since the long echo time spectra recorded exhibit a good frequency separation between the resonances of interest and a relatively flat baseline.) The peaks corresponding to NAA and Cr were integrated digitally to obtain the area under each metabolite resonance for both right

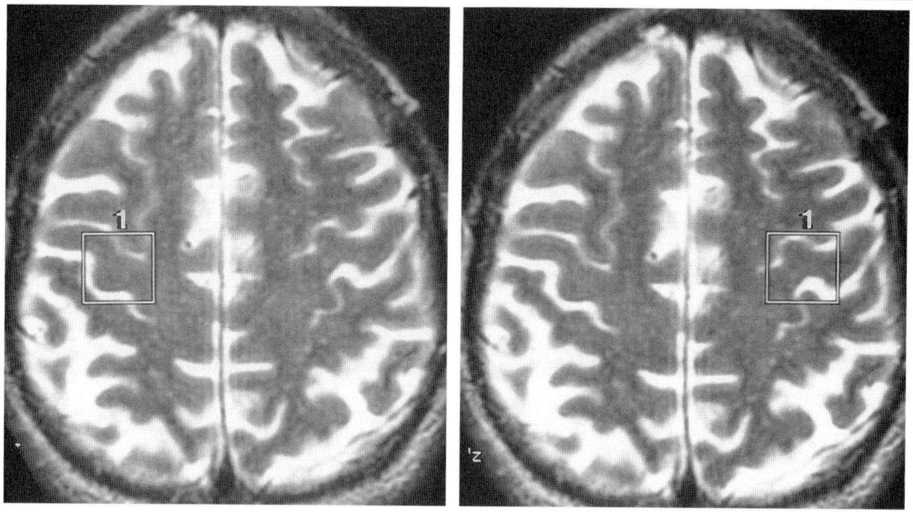

a. b.

Figure 1. MR spectroscopy of the right and left motor cortex in a patient with ALS. **(a, b)** Axial T2-weighted fast SE MR images (4,000/96 with one signal acquired) were obtained about 1 cm above the superior margin of the lateral ventricles. They demonstrate placement of the $2 \times 2 \times 2$ cm voxel (*1*) in the right and left posterior frontal lobes, respectively. Each voxel is centered on the precentral gyrus. **(c, d)** Point-resolved spectroscopic proton MR (2,000/270) spectra from **(c)** the right motor cortex (NAA/Cr = 2.5) and **(d)** the left motor cortex (NAA/Cr = 2.6). They demonstrate peaks of NAA at 2.02 ppm, Cr at 3.0 ppm, and choline (*Cho*) at 3.2 ppm.

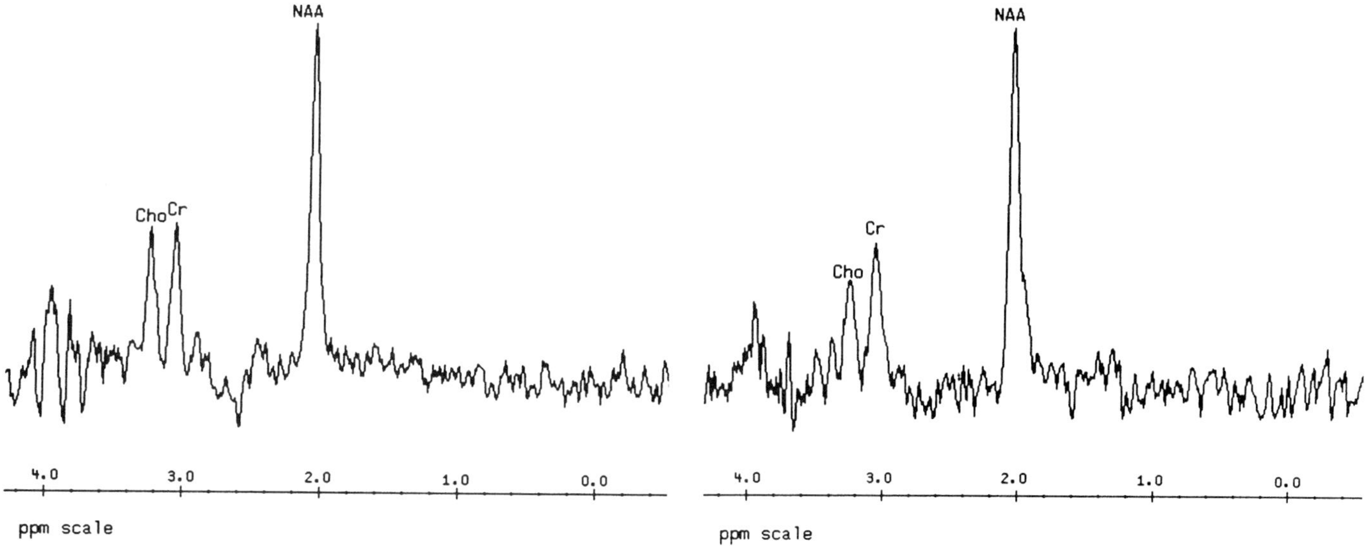

c. d.

and left motor cortex. Ratios of NAA to Cr peak areas were computed, tabulated, and printed onto each spectrum (Fig 1c, 1d). These ratios were cross-referenced with each patient's clinical diagnosis at the conclusion of the data collection period. Mean values for NAA/Cr in the right motor cortex, left motor cortex, and both right and left motor cortices were calculated for the groups with ALS alone, ALS with probable upper motor neuron signs, PLS, and non–upper motor neuron disorders, and the control group. The statistical significance of differences between mean NAA/Cr values in the patient groups was determined by means of one-way analysis of variance with the Scheffe multiple range test and the F statistic. (One-way analysis of variance is a more stringent method than is the Student *t* test for performing multiple comparisons of means.)

Sensitivity and specificity analyses were performed for a range of NAA/Cr values to generate a receiver operating characteristic curve (12) and to determine the optimal cutoff of NAA/Cr for the detection of upper motor neuron abnormality. The optimal cutoff point was defined as the NAA/Cr value at which the sum of the sensitivity and the specificity was maximized (13). An MR spectroscopic study was considered abnormal if the NAA/Cr value was lower than the cutoff in the right motor cortex, the left motor cortex, or both. For the purpose of identifying an optimal cutoff point for each patient group, we defined the disease groups as the combined group, with ALS alone and ALS with probable upper motor neuron signs, or the PLS group, and the nondisease group as the control group. Spectroscopic data from the groups with PLS or non–upper motor neuron disorders were analyzed separately because, in comparison to ALS alone and ALS with probable upper motor neuron signs, less is known about the severity and pathologic extent of upper motor neuron involvement in PLS or lower motor neuron disorders.

The high-spatial-resolution MR images were interpreted prospectively by one neuroradiologist (S.C.), who was blinded to clinical diagnosis. He evaluated the MR images for the following signs: (*a*) focal increased signal intensity on intermediate-weighted axial images within the corticospinal tracts in the posterior limb of the internal capsule (Fig 2) (14), (*b*) disproportionate enlargement of the central sulcus on T1-weighted sagittal images (Fig 3) (15), and (*c*) focally increased signal intensity in the lateral columns of the

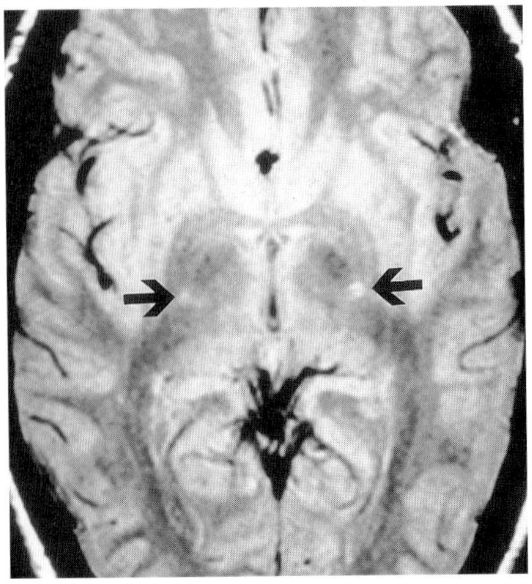

Figure 2. Axial intermediate-weighted fast SE MR image (2,500/21 with two signals acquired) in a 31-year-old man with ALS. At the level of the anterior commissure, abnormal increased signal intensity (arrows) is depicted within the right and left corticospinal tracts (within the posterior limbs of both internal capsules).

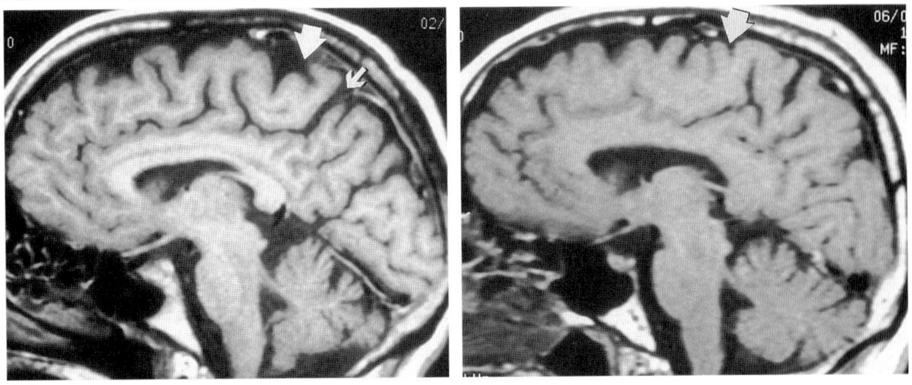

a. b.

Figure 3. **(a)** Sagittal T1-weighted SE MR image (500/14 with one signal acquired) in a 57-year-old woman with PLS shows marked enlargement of the central sulcus (large arrow). The marginal ramus of the cingulate sulcus (small arrow) is identified as the sulcus immediately posterior to the central sulcus. **(b)** Sagittal T1-weighted MR image (500/16 with one signal acquired) in a control subject was obtained at the same level as **a**. The central sulcus (arrow) is not enlarged.

cervical cord on T2-weighted axial images (16). For purposes of reliability, a second blinded neuroradiologist (A.D.A.) retrospectively reviewed the 52 MR studies of the brain to determine the presence or absence of each of the first two findings. The retrospective readings were then compared with the prospective readings; disagreement among readings was resolved by means of consensus review. Interrater reliability was determined with the κ statistic (17). Sensitivity and specificity analyses were performed of the cerebral MR imaging findings; comparative receiver operating characteristic data were generated by using the corticospinal tract finding alone or the combination of the corticospinal tract and the central sulcus findings. No retrospective reading was performed of the 35 MR studies of the cervical spine because (*a*) the initial prospective readings indicated a low sensitivity for detection of corticospinal tract abnormalities within the cord ($n = 2$) and (*b*) the main focus of the study was the comparison of MR spectroscopy of the motor cortex with MR imaging of the brain.

Two patients were excluded from the study because (*a*) the correct MR imaging and MR spectroscopic study protocol was not performed ($n = 1$) or (*b*) the suspected clinical diagnosis was multiple sclerosis, not motor neuron disease ($n = 1$). Patients were not excluded from the study on the basis of failure to complete the MR spectroscopic study.

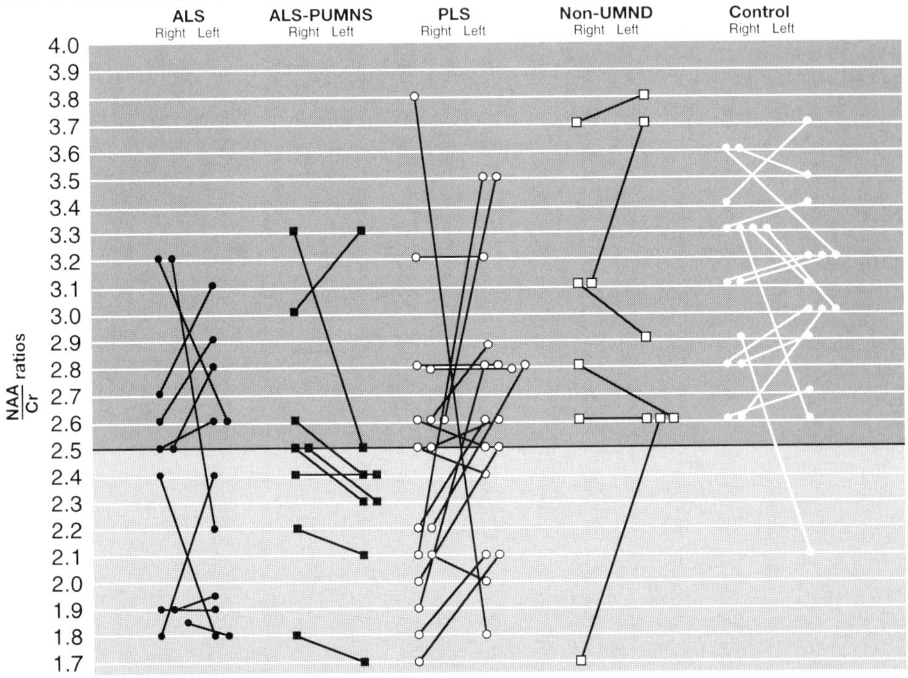

Figure 4. Scatterplot demonstrates the paired data sets of NAA/Cr values derived for each of the 43 patients in whom single-voxel MR spectroscopy of the right and left motor cortex was successfully completed. Each data set is displayed in the column that corresponds to the clinical diagnosis for each patient. The dark horizontal line at the NAA/Cr value of 2.5 indicates the level at or below which abnormality of the upper motor neuron is indicated. Note that for most of the patients with ALS alone (*ALS*) or ALS with probable upper motor neuron signs (*ALS-PUMNS*), one or both NAA/Cr values is 2.5 or less, whereas data in the group with non–upper motor neuron disorders (*Non-UMND*) and the control group are rarely associated with an NAA/Cr of 2.5 or less.

RESULTS

MR Spectroscopy

Satisfactory MR spectroscopic studies were obtained in 43 of the 50 patients (Fig 4). Patient motion and technical difficulties resulted in inadequate MR spectroscopic studies in seven patients. Among these 43 patients, 11 had ALS, eight had ALS with probable upper motor neuron signs, 18 had PLS, and six had non–upper motor neuron disorders, including "pure" lower motor neuron disorders ($n = 4$) and focal pathologic conditions of the cord

TABLE 1
Mean NAA/Cr Values

Group and Motor Cortex	No. of Patients	Mean	SD	SEM	*P* Value*
Control					
Right	14	3.12	.34	.09	NA
Left	14	3.04	.40	.11	NA
Combined	14	3.08	.32	.09	NA
ALS					
Right	11	2.42	.50	.15	<.05
Left	11	2.37	.46	.14	<.05
Combined	11	2.40	.42	.13	<.05
ALS with probable upper motor neuron signs					
Right	8	2.54	.46	.16	NS
Left	8	2.38	.45	.16	<.05
Combined	8	2.44	.41	.15	<.05
PLS					
Right	18	2.46	.53	.13	<.05
Left	18	2.68	.50	.12	NS
Combined	18	2.57	.38	.09	<.05
Non–upper motor neuron disorders					
Right	6	2.83	.67	.27	NS
Left	6	3.03	.57	.23	NS
Combined	6	2.93	.58	.24	NS

* For comparison with the control group. NA = not applicable, NS = not significant.

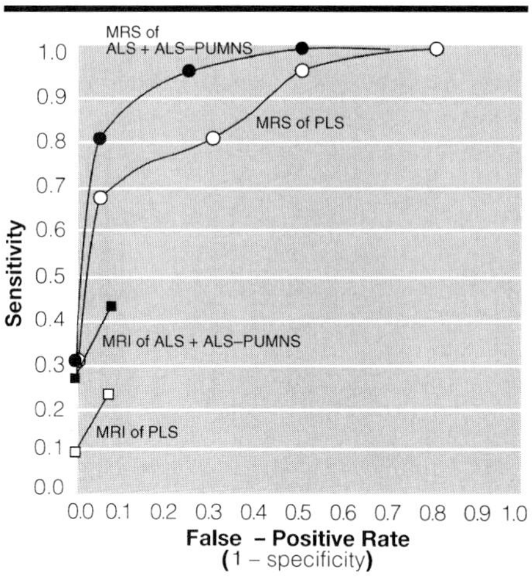

Figure 5. Receiver operating characteristic curves for MR spectroscopic (*MRS*) and MR imaging (*MRI*) data obtained in the combined group with ALS alone (*ALS*) and ALS with probable upper motor neuron signs (*ALS-PUMNS*) and the PLS group. The curves demonstrate that MR spectroscopy has greater accuracy in detection of upper motor neuron abnormality in the former than in the latter. Note also that at the specificity rates of 93% and 100%, MR spectroscopy is more sensitive than MR imaging in detection of upper motor neuron abnormality in both groups.

attributable to cord trauma (n = 1) or demyelinating plaque (n = 1). MR spectroscopy was completed successfully in all 14 control subjects (Fig 4). Differences in mean NAA/Cr were significant between the ALS and control groups for the right or left motor cortex or both motor cortices (Table 1). Statistically significant differences in mean NAA/Cr were found between the group with ALS with probable upper motor neuron signs and the control group for the left motor cortex alone and both motor cortices combined. Statistically significant differences in mean NAA/Cr were found between the PLS and control groups for the right motor cortex alone and both motor cortices combined. Relatively large differences in mean NAA/Cr were found between the group with ALS with probable upper motor neuron signs and the control group for the right motor cortex and between the PLS and control groups for the left motor cortex, but the differences did not meet a 95% level of statistical significance.

The receiver operating characteristic curve for the combined group with ALS alone and ALS with probable upper motor neuron signs compared to that for the PLS group illustrates that MR spectroscopy has greater accuracy in the detection of upper motor neuron abnormality in the combined group than in the PLS group (Fig 5). Sensitivity and specificity analysis of the NAA/Cr values with respect to the combined group relative to the control group showed maximal combined sensitivity and specificity for the detection of upper motor neuron diseases with a cutoff of 2.5; that is, ratios of 2.5 or less were deemed abnormal (Fig 5). The optimal cutoff value for PLS was also 2.5. With use of this criterion, eight of 11 patients with ALS, seven of eight patients with ALS with probable upper motor neuron signs, 12 of 18 patients with PLS, and one of six patients with non–upper motor neuron disorders were deemed to have an abnormal single-voxel MR spectroscopic study of the sensorimotor cortex. NAA/Cr was abnormally decreased in one of the 14 control subjects. With this cutoff, the sensitivity for detection of upper motor neuron involvement in the combined group was 79% and in the PLS group was 67%. The combined sensitivity for upper motor neuron abnormality in the groups with ALS alone, ALS with probable upper motor neuron signs, and PLS was 73%. With the cutoff of 2.5, the specificity was 93% on the basis of findings in the control group alone (and 90% for the control group combined with the group with non–upper motor neuron disorders).

MR Imaging

Satisfactory MR imaging studies of the brain were obtained in all 50 patients. In the 13 ALS patients, brain MR abnormalities included hyperintensity of the corticospinal tracts in five and enlargement of the central sulcus in three. In the eight patients with ALS with probable upper motor neuron signs, hyperintensity of the corticospinal tracts and enlargement of the central sulcus were each seen in one. Nine (43%) of the 21 patients with ALS alone or ALS with probable upper motor neuron signs had one or both MR imaging abnormalities. In the 21 patients with PLS, abnormalities included hyperintensity of the corticospinal tracts in two and enlargement of the central sulcus in three. Five (24%) of the 21 patients with PLS had at least one of these MR imaging findings. Hyperintensity of the corticospinal tracts was found in none of the eight patients with non–upper motor neuron disorders, but enlargement of the central sulcus was seen in three, all of whom had pure lower motor neuron disorders (two with adult-onset progressive spinal muscular atrophy). Only one patient had both hyperintensity of the corticospinal tract and enlargement of the central sulcus, with both findings on only the left side; that patient had ALS. The signal intensity of the corticospinal tracts could not be evaluated formally in the 14 control subjects because we did not obtain high-spatial-resolution intermediate-weighted fast SE axial images. Focal enlargement of the central sulcus was seen in one of 14 control subjects. For the purposes of comparing MR imaging with MR spectroscopy in the receiver operating characteristic analyses, we assumed that the false-positive rate of corticospinal tract hyperintensity on intermediate-weighted images was 0%; this assumption is supported by evidence from another study (18).

The sensitivity of specific MR imaging abnormalities for upper motor neuron disease was compared with that of abnormal NAA/Cr at single-voxel MR spectroscopy (Table 2). Interrater reliability measurements for brain MR image readings yielded the following: corticospinal tract hyperintensity, κ = 0.66; central sulcus enlargement, κ = 0.57; overall, κ = 0.62. A κ value of 0.61–0.81 is taken as good interrater agreement and of 0.41–0.60 as moderate agreement (17).

TABLE 2
Sensitivity of MR Imaging and MR Spectroscopy

Group	No. Who Underwent MR Imaging	No. Who Underwent MR Spectroscopy	Corticospinal Tract Hyperintensity (n = 50)	Widening of Central Sulcus (n = 50)	Decreased NAA/Cr (n = 43)
ALS	13	11	38%	23%	73%
ALS with probable upper motor neuron signs	8	8	12%	12%	88%
PLS	21	18	10%	14%	67%
Non–upper motor neuron disorders	8	6	0%	38%	17%
Control	14	14	NA	7%	7%

Note.—NA = not applicable.

Cervical cord MR imaging was successfully completed in 35 patients. We did not see focally increased signal intensity in the anterolateral columns of the cervical cord on T2-weighted axial images in patients with ALS alone, ALS with probable upper motor neuron signs, or non–upper motor neuron disorders. Focal signal intensity abnormality, limited to the anterolateral columns of the cervical cord, was found in two of 15 patients with PLS. More extensive cord abnormalities were identified in two patients with non–upper motor neuron disorders, one of whom had a history of spinal trauma. However, each of these cord abnormalities involved an area much larger than the anterolateral columns of the cervical cord and were ultimately attributed to origins other than motor neuron disease (specifically, trauma and demyelinating plaque).

DISCUSSION

Neuronal loss in ALS may affect the precentral gyri and other gyri subserving motor activity and anterior horn cells. Axonal degeneration of the corticospinal tracts follows loss of upper motor neurons. In the proton MR spectroscopic study by Pioro et al (3) of the frontal lobe in patients with ALS, neuronal loss was focal with the most severe involvement within the precentral gyrus itself. NAA is a putative marker of neurons (1,2); loss of NAA (with respect to Cr) is considered an indicator of neuronal loss. However, several caveats should be noted. (*a*) NAA is found within both gray and white matter, and, in one study (19), NAA levels decreased after experimental axonal transection. Therefore, the decrease in NAA/Cr within one 8-cm^3 voxel could be a result of either axonal degeneration or focal loss of neuronal cell bodies in the sensorimotor cortex. (*b*) Enlargement of the central sulcus could spuriously decrease NAA/Cr because of partial volume effects stemming from inclusion of an increased proportion of cerebrospinal fluid within the voxel. However, that possibility could not apply to our data because the central sulcus was enlarged in only four of 21 patients with ALS or ALS with probable upper motor neuron signs and in three of 21 patients with PLS. (*c*) We assumed that Cr levels in the motor cortex would remain stable in all participants—both patients and control subjects. This assumption can be verified only by measuring absolute metabolite concentrations, a time-consuming spectroscopic procedure that is not routinely available for clinical work.

The MR spectroscopic decision criterion involved detection of an abnormality within the motor cortex of either one or both cerebral hemispheres. With this criterion, the MR spectroscopic findings in 79% (15 of 19) of patients with ALS alone and ALS with probable upper motor neuron signs and 67% (12 of 18) of patients with PLS were deemed abnormal. These percentages compare favorably to those associated with both MR imaging abnormalities, either corticospinal tract hyperintensity or central sulcus enlargement: 43% (nine of 21) for ALS alone and ALS with probable upper motor neuron signs and 24% (five of 21) for PLS. With the same criterion, a false-positive MR spectroscopic diagnosis was seen in 7% (one of 14) of control subjects and 17% (one of six) of patients with non–upper motor neuron disorders. We note that it is likely that some false-positive findings of non–upper motor neuron disorders were clinically occult upper motor neuron disease; in autopsy examination of patients with motor neuron disease without upper motor neuron signs (including adult-onset progressive spinal muscular atrophy), more than half (17 of 25 patients) had degeneration of the corticospinal tracts (20,21). In fact, postmortem examination of one of our patients with non–upper motor neuron disorders (who had clinically diagnosed spinal muscular atrophy) revealed degeneration of the corticospinal tracts. This pathologic result correlates well with the antemortem findings at MR spectroscopy (NAA/Cr = 1.7) and MR imaging that were indicative of upper motor neuron disease.

The spectroscopic abnormality was unilateral in five of 15 patients with ALS alone or ALS with probable upper motor neuron signs and in seven of 12 PLS patients. This could arise from asymmetric loss of motor neurons in the two cerebral hemispheres. In one patient with ALS who had both left-sided corticospinal tract involvement and left central sulcus enlargement, NAA/Cr was significantly lower in the left (1.8) than in the right (2.4) motor cortex. However, as the full extent of variation in NAA/Cr in the motor cortex is not known, more data are needed to ascertain the importance of cerebral asymmetries seen at MR imaging and MR spectroscopy.

Several types of MR abnormalities have been found in patients with ALS or PLS. First, the corticospinal tract can be identified readily on intermediate- and T2-weighted images in the posterior third of the posterior limb of the internal capsule (22). In one MR imaging study in patients with ALS (14), hyperintensity of the corticospinal tract was identified primarily at the level of the posterior limb of the internal capsule, but, in some cases, high signal intensity extended up to the cortex or down through the cerebral peduncle and brainstem. Findings in another study suggested that this abnormality, when present, is characteristic of ALS but is not sensitive for the diagnosis of ALS (18).

This abnormality was also reported in one case of PLS (23). Second, atrophy of the precentral gyrus may be identified indirectly as enlargement of the adjacent central sulcus (15). Although this was initially described in cases of PLS, we also found the abnormality in patients with either ALS or lower motor neuron disease. Third, cortical signal intensity may be decreased in the precentral gyrus on T2-weighted conventional SE axial images (24,25). We did not evaluate this finding because we used fast SE imaging, which is known to be less sensitive to magnetic susceptibility effects than is conventional SE imaging (26). The use of multiple "refocusing" 180° pulses in fast SE pulse sequences results in attenuation of the effects of T2*-weighted signal decay and, therefore, of magnetic susceptibility effects. This abnormality has also been seen in the motor cortex of healthy elderly subjects (27), which suggests that this finding may be less characteristic of motor neuron disease than was previously believed.

Our MR imaging data included two noteworthy findings. First, we did not confirm the findings of Pringle et al (15) that enlargement of the central sulcus is seen in cases of PLS but not ALS. By using qualitative visual assessments of the central sulcus, we may have failed to detect central sulcus enlargement in some cases of PLS in which an abnormality might have been identified with the quantitative approach of Pringle et al. However, our qualitative approach sufficed to help identify central sulcus enlargement in cases of ALS. Second, we found marked corticospinal tract hyperintensity in two patients with clinically diagnosed PLS, similar to that reported in another case of PLS (23). However, in both of our PLS cases, MR spectroscopy of the motor cortex indicated a nonsignificant decrease in NAA/Cr (2.8 in both cases) compared with the decrease in the control group (mean, 3.1). (With our cutoff criterion of NAA/Cr of 2.5 or less, these two cases would be considered normal.) This suggests that the upper motor neuron disorder in some patients with PLS may arise in the corticospinal tracts or in subcortical neurons.

Single-voxel MR spectroscopy of the motor cortex will be made even easier by the introduction of automated spectral quantitation for rapid calculation of NAA, choline, and myo-inositol levels (relative to Cr) during diagnostic MR examinations. These techniques became available to us only after we concluded the study. After 1996, preliminary data implied good correlation between the NAA/Cr values generated with autoquantitation and by our spectroscopist; the largest discrepancy was about 10% (Shungu DC, unpublished data). We are currently using the autoquantitative technique to perform single-voxel MR spectroscopy of the motor cortex, and we are further delineating the sensitivity and specificity of this refinement of the method.

In conclusion, our data indicate that MR spectroscopy of the motor cortex is useful in the detection of abnormality of the upper motor neuron. MR spectroscopy was more sensitive than MR imaging in the detection of an upper motor neuron abnormality in ALS and PLS. We recommend further exploration of this technique in evaluation of motor neuron disease. A reliable measure of upper motor neuron dysfunction could offer the following clinical advances: (*a*) provide a useful diagnostic tool for monitoring therapy of ALS and other motor neuron diseases; (*b*) help identify cases of adult-onset progressive spinal muscular atrophy that are, in fact, ALS; and (*c*) help ascertain the clinical diagnosis of PLS.

References

1. Urenjak J, Williams SR, Gadian DG, Noble M. Proton nuclear magnetic resonance spectroscopy unambiguously identifies different cell types. J Neurosci 1993; 13: 981–989.
2. Simmons ML, Frondoza CG, Coyle JT. Immunocytochemical localization of *N*-acetyl-aspartate with monoclonal antibodies. Neuroscience 1991; 45:37–45.
3. Pioro EP, Antel JP, Cashman NR, Arnold DL. Detection of cortical neuron loss in motor neuron disease by proton magnetic resonance spectroscopic imaging in vivo. Neurology 1994; 44:1933–1938.
4. Jones AP, Gunawardena WJ, Coutinho CM, Gatt JA, Shaw IC, Mitchell JD. Preliminary results of proton magnetic resonance spectroscopy in motor neuron disease (amyotrophic lateral sclerosis). J Neurol Sci 1995; 129(suppl):85–89.
5. Giroud M, Walker P, Bernard D, et al. Reduced brain *N*-acetylaspartate in frontal lobes suggests neuronal loss in patients with amyotrophic lateral sclerosis. Neurol Res 1996; 18:241–243.
6. Gredal O, Rosenbaum S, Topp S, Karlsborg M, Strange P, Werdelin L. Quantification of brain metabolites in amyotrophic lateral sclerosis by localized proton magnetic resonance spectroscopy. Neurology 1997; 48:878–881.
7. Block W, Karitsky J, Traber F, et al. Proton magnetic resonance spectroscopy of the primary motor cortex in patients with motor neuron disease. Arch Neurol 1998; 55:931–936.
8. Rooney WD, Miller RG, Gelinas D, Schuff N, Maudsley AA, Weiner MW. Decreased *N*-acetylaspartate in motor cortex and corticospinal tract in ALS. Neurology 1998; 50:1800–1805.
9. Berger MS, Cohen WA, Ojemann GA. Correlation of motor cortex brain mapping data with magnetic resonance imaging. J Neurosurg 1990; 72:383–387.
10. Shungu DC, Bhujwalla ZM, Li SJ, Rose LM, Wehrle JP, Glickson JD. Determination of absolute phosphate metabolite concentrations in RIF-1 tumors in vivo by ^{31}P-^{1}H-^{2}H NMR spectroscopy using water as an internal intensity reference. Magn Reson Med 1992; 28:105–121.
11. Press WH, Flannery BP, Teukolsy SA, Vetterling WT. Integration of functions. In: Numerical recipes in C: the art of scientific computing. New York, NY: Cambridge University Press, 1988; 111–141.
12. Metz CE. Basic principles of ROC analysis. Semin Nucl Med 1978; 8:283–298.
13. Desmond DW, Tatemichi TK, Hanzawa L. The telephone interview for cognitive status (TICS): reliability and validity in a stroke sample. Int J Geriatr Psychiatry 1994; 9:803–807.
14. Cheung G, Gawal MJ, Cooper PW, Farb RI, Ang LC. Amyotrophic lateral sclerosis: correlation of clinical and MR imaging findings. Radiology 1995; 194:263–270.
15. Pringle CE, Hudson AJ, Munoz DG, Kiernan JA, Brown WF, Ebers GC. Primary lateral sclerosis. Brain 1992; 115:495–520.
16. Friedman DP, Tartaglino LM. Amyotrophic lateral sclerosis: hyperintensity of the corticospinal tracts on MR images of the spinal cord. AJR 1993; 160:604–606.
17. Landis JR, Koch GG. The measurement of observer agreement for categorical data. Biometrics 1977; 30:159–174.
18. Hofmann E, Ochs G, Petzl A, Warmuth-Metz M. The corticospinal tract in amyotrophic lateral sclerosis: an MRI study. Neuroradiology 1998; 40:71–75.
19. Rango M, Spagnoli D, Tomei G, Bamonti F, Scarlato G, Zetta L. Central nervous system trans-synaptic effects of acute axonal injury: a H-1 magnetic resonance spectroscopy study. Magn Reson Med 1995; 33:595–600.
20. Brownell B, Oppenheimer DR, Hughes JT. Central nervous system in motor neuron disease. J Neurol Neurosurg Psychiatry 1970; 33:338–357.
21. Lawyer T, Netsky MG. Amyotrophic lateral sclerosis: clinicoanatomic study of 53 cases. Arch Neurol Psychiatry 1953; 69: 171–192.
22. Yagashita A, Nakano I, Oda M, et al. Location of the corticospinal tract in the internal capsule at MR imaging. Radiology 1994; 191:455–460.
23. Marti-Fabregas J, Pujol J. Selective involvement of the pyramidal tract on magnetic resonance imaging in primary lateral sclerosis. Neurology 1990; 40:1799–1800.
24. Ishikawa K, Nagura H, Yokota T, Yamanouchi H. Signal loss in the motor cortex on magnetic resonance images in amyotrophic lateral sclerosis. Ann Neurol 1993; 33:218–222.
25. Oba H, Araki T, Ohtomo K, et al. Amyotrophic lateral sclerosis: T2 shortening in motor cortex at MR imaging. Radiology 1993; 189:843–846.
26. Norbash AM, Glover GH, Enzmann DR. Intracerebral lesion contrast with spin-echo and fast spin-echo pulse sequences. Radiology 1992; 185:661–665.
27. Imon Y, Yamaguchi S, Katayama S, et al. A decrease in cerebral cortex intensity on T2-weighted images with aging of normal subjects. Neuroradiology 1998; 40:76–80.

Quantitative Diffusion-Tensor Anisotropy Brain MR Imaging: Normative Human Data and Anatomic Analysis[1]

Joshua S. Shimony, MD, PhD
Robert C. McKinstry, MD, PhD
Erbil Akbudak, PhD
Joseph A. Aronovitz, MD, PhD
Abraham Z. Snyder, PhD, MD
Nicolas F. Lori, BS
Thomas S. Cull, PhD
Thomas E. Conturo, MD, PhD

Index terms:
Brain, diffusion, 10.99
Brain, gray matter, 10.92
Brain, MR, 10.121411, 10.121416, 10.12144
Brain, white matter, 10.92
Magnetic resonance (MR), diffusion study, 10.12144

Radiology 1999; 212:770–784

Abbreviations:
A_{major} = anisotropy variation in ellipsoid shape along major axis
A_{minor} = anisotropy variation in ellipsoid shape along minor axis
A_σ = total anisotropy
AW_{ortho} = orthogonal anisotropy-weighted index
AW_{tet} = tetrahedral anisotropy-weighted index
f_{ortho} = fraction of anisotropy in AW_{ortho}
f_{tet} = fraction of anisotropy in AW_{tet}
GM = gray matter
ROI = region of interest
SNR = signal-to-noise ratio
WM = white matter

[1] From the Mallinckrodt Institute of Radiology (J.S.S., R.C.M., E.A., J.A.A., A.Z.S., T.S.C.) and Dept of Physics (N.F.L., T.E.C.), Washington University Medical Center, 510 S Kingshighway Blvd, St Louis, MO 63110. Received Jul 20, 1998; revision requested Aug 19; revision received Nov 10; accepted Jan 15, 1999. Supported in part by grants from Major Grants Program of McDonnell Center for Higher Brain Function, National Multiple Sclerosis Society Pilot Research Award, Charles A. Dana Foundation Consortium on Neuroimaging Leadership Training, and PRAXIS III Fellowship from the Portuguese government. J.S.S. supported by RSNA Research and Education Foundation Research Resident Grant. **Address reprint requests to** J.S.S. (e-mail: *shimonyj@npg.wustl.edu*).

Author contributions:
Guarantors of integrity of entire study, J.S.S., T.E.C.; study concepts, T.E.C., R.C.M.; study design, T.E.C., R.C.M., J.S.S.; definition of intellectual content, all authors; literature research, J.S.S., T.E.C.; experimental studies, R.C.M., T.E.C., J.S.S.; data acquisition, R.C.M., E.A., J.S.S., T.E.C.; data analysis, J.S.S., A.Z.S., J.A.A., T.S.C., N.F.L., R.C.M., T.E.C.; statistical analysis, J.S.S., T.E.C.; manuscript preparation and review, J.S.S., T.E.C.; manuscript editing, T.E.C., J.S.S., R.C.M.

PURPOSE: To obtain normative human cerebral data and evaluate the anatomtomic information in quantitative diffusion anisotropy magnetic resonance (MR) imaging.

MATERIALS AND METHODS: Quantitative diffusion anisotropy MR images were obtained in 13 healthy adults by using single-shot echo-planar MR imaging and a combination of tetrahedral and orthogonal gradient encoding (whole-brain coverage in about 1 minute). White matter (WM) anatomy was assessed at visual inspection, and values were measured in various brain regions. Different anisotropy measures, including total anisotropy (A_σ), were compared on the basis of information content, rotational invariance, and susceptibility to noise. Partial volume and noise effects were simulated.

RESULTS: Anisotropy MR images depicted WM features not typically seen on conventional MR images (eg, external capsule, thalamic substructures, basal ganglia, occipital WM, thickness of the internal capsule). Statistically significant anisotropy differences occurred across brain regions, which were reproducible within and across subjects. A_σ was highest in commissural WM and progressively lower in projection and association WM. This order paralleled that of known resistance to spread of vasogenic edema, which suggested that anisotropy may be sensitive to WM histologic structure. Gray matter (GM) A_σ data were consistent with zero anisotropy, and partial volume WM-GM effects were approximately linear. A_σ image quality could be effectively improved by means of averaging.

CONCLUSION: Quantitative diffusion anisotropy images can be obtained rapidly and demonstrate subtle WM anatomy. Different histologic types of WM have significant and reproducible anisotropy differences.

Random diffusive motion of water along the direction of a strong field gradient will cause spin dephasing in magnetic resonance (MR). As shown by Stejskal and Tanner (1), quantitative diffusion coefficients can be measured with MR by encoding diffusion with balanced gradients applied before and after a spin-echo refocusing pulse and comparing this signal loss to a reference signal acquired with no diffusion encoding. The amount of diffusion sensitivity is indicated by the b factor, which is dependent on the timing and strength of the diffusion-encoding gradients.

MR imaging of diffusion effects with a combination of spin-echo imaging and Stejskal-Tanner gradients was used by Le Bihan and colleagues (2,3) and by Taylor and Bushell (4). The technique of echo-planar MR imaging (5) has been particularly useful for acquisition of diffusion information, as demonstrated by Avram and Crooks (6), Turner and colleagues (7,8), and McKinstry et al (9).

In early human diffusion MR imaging studies (10,11), it was realized that water diffusion is anisotropic in many biologic media such as white matter (WM) and muscle (ie, the rate of water diffusion varies with direction). Anisotropic diffusion can, in general, be represented by a symmetric 3×3 diffusion tensor $\mathbf{D}$ at each position in space (12,13) and can be modeled as ellipsoidal water displacements (12), as was suggested by Basser et al (14) for modeling of MR image data. Anisotropy is a quantitative parameter that represents the degree to which diffusion varies in different directions. The authors of more recent studies (15,16) have demonstrated the benefit of removal of anisotropic diffusion effects by creating a directionally averaged diffusivity. However, anisotropic diffusion effects provide anatomic information in regions of WM (11,17–19) and may provide diagnostic information for certain WM diseases (20), including multiple sclerosis (21–23). Unlike averaged diffusivity, measures of anisotropy in humans have been shown to be different in various regions of the normal adult brain (17,19) and to vary with gestational age in neonates (24) and with postnatal age in the first several months of life (25).

A number of anisotropy measures have been proposed in the literature (16,26–29). The theoretic basis and advantages of several of these will be discussed. In our study, quantitative anisotropy images were computed from echo-planar MR imaging data (30) that sampled the diffusion tensor along four tetrahedral directions (26) and three coordinate axes. Anatomic findings and anisotropy values are presented from different regions of interest (ROIs) in the normal human brain. The purpose of our study was to obtain normative human cerebral data and evaluate the anatomic information in quantitative diffusion anisotropy MR imaging.

MATERIALS AND METHODS

Theory

In the general case of homogeneous anisotropic media, the diffusion tensor can be represented by a 3 × 3 matrix. For Gaussian diffusion, the matrix is symmetric (12) and is completely characterized by six scalars: three diagonal elements, D_{xx}, D_{yy}, D_{zz}, and three off-diagonal elements, D_{xy}, D_{xz}, D_{yz}. An ellipsoid, whose surface represents the root mean square diffusive displacement, provides a convenient pictorial representation of anisotropic diffusion in a voxel (14,26,27). Measurement of the diffusion tensor is then equivalent to sampling of enough discrete points on the ellipsoid surface so that the ellipsoid can be uniquely defined (31). Individual elements of the diffusion tensor are not rotationally invariant and, as markers of brain pathologic conditions, have been shown to be misleading in comparison with invariant measures (15,29). In contrast, the trace of the diffusion tensor is invariant under rotations of the coordinate system and is the basis for the directionally averaged diffusivity $\overline{D} = (D_{xx} + D_{yy} + D_{zz})/3$.

Each voxel has a unique principal ellipsoid coordinate system (x', y', z') that, in general, is rotated with respect to the laboratory coordinate system (27). This principal coordinate system lies along the major and minor axes of the diffusion ellipsoid, and, in this rotated system, the diffusion tensor is diagonal. The diagonal matrix elements are the principal diffusivities of the rotated coordinate system $\lambda_{x'}$, $\lambda_{y'}$, and $\lambda_{z'}$ and are the eigenvalues of the diffusion tensor. In the laboratory, the six scalars that represent the diffusion tensor can be expressed in terms of the three eigenvalues ($\lambda_{x'}$, $\lambda_{y'}$, and $\lambda_{z'}$) that are rotationally invariant and the three Euler angles (ϕ, θ, ψ) that describe the relative rotation between the principal and laboratory coordinates (26).

Multiple measures of tissue anisotropy have been proposed (16,26–29). An ideal measure of anisotropy should be quantitative and rotationally invariant. It is desirable that it be a function of the directly measured diffusion coefficients, because any diagonalization of the diffusion tensor and evaluation of its eigenvalues may introduce additional noise. Furthermore, it is advantageous to use anisotropy calculations that are not dependent on sorting of the eigenvalues according to size, because this can introduce additional uncertainty (29), especially in regions with low anisotropy or a low signal-to-noise ratio (SNR). Finally, to facilitate comparison across sequences, institutions, and clinical and basic science disciplines, it would be preferable if anisotropy measures were on an absolute anisotropy scale.

The natural choices for anisotropy measures are A_{major} and A_{minor} (26), which describe the variation in ellipsoid shape along the major and minor axes, respectively. These are obtained by decomposing the diffusion tensor into isotropic and anisotropic components in the x', y', z' ellipsoid coordinate system (26):

$$A_{\mathrm{major}} = \frac{1}{3\overline{\lambda}}\left[\lambda_{z'} - \frac{\lambda_{x'} + \lambda_{y'}}{2}\right], \tag{1}$$

and

$$A_{\mathrm{minor}} = \frac{\lambda_{x'} - \lambda_{y'}}{2\overline{\lambda}}, \tag{2}$$

where $\overline{\lambda}$ is the average of the eigenvalues (equivalent to averaged diffusivity $\overline{D}$), z' is the axis of greatest symmetry, and $\lambda_{x'}$ is greater than or equal to $\lambda_{y'}$. The parameter A_{major} ranges from −0.5 to 1.0, where the sign contains shape information. An A_{major} value that is greater than 0 indicates a prolate ("cigar-shaped") diffusion ellipsoid where $\lambda_{z'}$ is the largest eigenvalue. An A_{major} value that is less than 0 indicates an oblate ("pancake-shaped") diffusion ellipsoid where $\lambda_{z'}$ is the smallest eigenvalue. These measures may be useful but require that one solve for and sort the eigenvalues.

An alternative anisotropy measure is a coefficient of variation determined on the basis of the second moment (variance) of **D** (26):

$$A_{\sigma} = \frac{1}{\sqrt{6}\,\overline{D}} \times \sqrt{\sum_{i=x,y,z} (D_{ii} - \overline{D})^2 + 2(D_{xy}^2 + D_{xz}^2 + D_{yz}^2)}, \tag{3}$$

with $\overline{D}$ as already given. A_{σ} represents total anisotropy, irrespective of ellipsoid shape; it is on an absolute anisotropy scale and has a value between 0 and 1. A_{σ} is an invariant quantitative measure of anisotropy that does not require diagonalization of the diffusion tensor and is independent of the order of the eigenvalues. A_{σ} was derived to correspond in range and meaning to the spectroscopic definition of anisotropy used in the physical sciences (32). This is most easily seen in the axisymmetric approximation (26), where A_{minor} is 0, A_{σ} is the absolute value of A_{major} and

$$A_{\mathrm{major}} = \frac{D_{\parallel} - D_{\perp}}{\overline{D}} = \frac{D_{\parallel} - D_{\perp}}{D_{\parallel} + 2D_{\perp}}, \tag{4}$$

with $D_{\parallel} = \lambda_{z'}$ and $D_{\perp} = \lambda_{x'} = \lambda_{y'}$. The parameter A_{σ} is similar to the relative anisotropy defined by Basser and Pierpaoli (28,29) except for a scaling factor of $2^{-1/2}$ contained in Equation 3 (also see factor of $2^{-1/2}$ in Eq [A1] in the Appendix) that places A_{σ} on an absolute anisotropy scale. A_{σ} also can be written in terms of A_{major} and A_{minor} (see Appendix, Eq [A2]).

The diffusion tensor is completely determined by measuring its six scalar components. This can also be viewed as sampling of sufficient points on the surface of the diffusion ellipsoid to constrain the ellipsoid size (ie, averaged diffusivity), shape (ie, A_{major}, A_{minor}), and orientation (ie, ϕ, θ, ψ). To reduce the effects of noise on the measurements, the diffusion ellipsoid should be sampled with strong gradients at points widely spaced over its surface while avoiding sampling of points related by inversion symmetry.

The tetrahedral gradient-encoding method (26) uses maximal simultaneous application of all three orthogonal gradients to construct each of the four noncolinear tetrahedral gradient vectors. This method has an inherently high SNR for measurements of averaged diffusivity (18,30), because the tetrahedral gradients have a strength that is $3^{1/2}$ times larger than the orthogonal gradient-encoding method. Accordingly, the tetrahedral method also is expected to have favorable noise properties for A_σ measurement, particularly because of the wide uniform sampling of coordinate space (31). Linear combinations of the tetrahedral diffusion measurements D_1, D_2, D_3, and D_4 are used to evaluate the off-diagonal elements of the diffusion tensor (26). In cases of axisymmetric diffusion ($A_{minor} = 0$), these measurements describe the entire diffusion tensor. In more general cases, the individual diagonal elements of the diffusion tensor must be determined by means of additional sampling along other directions, such as the orthogonal x, y, and z magnet coordinate system. Combined tetrahedral-orthogonal encoding was chosen because the tetrahedral and orthogonal gradient vectors are complementary in terms of sampling of the diffusion tensor, since each set of vectors bisects the others to achieve wide coverage of the ellipsoid surface.

The diagonal element information is contained in the orthogonal gradient-encoded data, whereas the off-diagonal information is contained in the tetrahedral gradient-encoded data. Accordingly, A_σ as expressed in Equation (3) can be decomposed into two partial, noninvariant, anisotropy-weighted measures AW_{ortho} and AW_{tet}, which are dependent, respectively, on the orthogonal and tetrahedral measurements (see Appendix, Eqq [A4,A5]). The fractional amount of anisotropy contained in each of these measures can be expressed as $f_{tet} = AW_{tet}/A_\sigma$ and $f_{ortho} = AW_{ortho}/A_\sigma$ (see Appendix, Eqq [A7,A8]).

Data Acquisition

Approval for this study was obtained from the human studies committee at our institution. Quantitative diffusion-tensor MR imaging was performed in 13 neurologically healthy adults (11 men, two women; mean age, 31 years; age range, 23–47 years) recruited from the population at our institution. Informed consent was obtained from all subjects after the nature of the experiment was fully explained.

All examinations were performed with a 1.5-T system (Magnetom Vision; Siemens Medical Systems, Erlangen, Germany) equipped with a standard, circularly polarized clinical radio-frequency head coil. Custom single-shot spin-echo echo-planar MR pulse sequences with Stejskal-Tanner gradients were used. In each subject, diffusion-tensor information was collected by using a combination of tetrahedral (26) and orthogonal gradient-encoded diffusion-weighted images, together with reference signal intensity data. This tetrahedral-orthogonal configuration of diffusion-encoding directions was chosen because it was found to provide a high SNR for both averaged diffusivity and A_σ (simulations not shown). This configuration contains tetrahedral gradient vectors that are of maximal strength and spatial separation and three orthogonal vectors that bisect the tetrahedral vectors to provide sufficient measurements for overdetermined estimation of the full tensor, with wide angular coverage. Both angular coverage and gradient strength are important in anisotropy measurement (31). Other configurations for tensor measurement have been used, such as a three-dimensional hexagonal array (17,33,34), where all diffusion-weighted images can have the same diffusion-encoding strength (b factor) and echo time but where gradient strengths are weaker than those of tetrahedral encoding.

Quantitative diffusion-tensor data were acquired first under conditions optimized for accuracy for reporting of normative values. For this purpose, a peripherally gated single-section echo-planar MR imaging sequence (sequence A) was implemented with a nonselective 180° pulse and no cross terms. Axial MR images were acquired at the level of the basal ganglia in a subset of the subjects (nine men, two women; mean age 31 years; age range, 23–47 years). Each acquisition was repeated once under the same conditions to provide two identical data sets for noise calculation (35) and statistical testing (described later). Sequence A was used for measurement of all normative values reported herein.

To assess the performance of quantitative diffusion-tensor and anisotropy MR imaging under more clinically practical conditions, axial MR images were then acquired in six of the subjects (five men, one woman; mean age, 31 years; age range, 28–39 years) by using sequence B, a nongated multisection version of sequence A. Four of the six subjects (three men, one woman; mean age, 29 years; age range, 23–39 years) in the sequence B group underwent imaging with tetrahedral-only encoding and were also in the sequence A group. These data were used for statistical comparison between the single-section (sequence A) and multisection (sequence B) results. For the remaining two subjects (two men, aged 32 and 39 years) in the sequence B group, combined tetrahedral-orthogonal, whole-brain, multisection encoding was used. In one of these subjects, sequence B was used with additional repetitions to assess the effect of averaging of repeated image acquisitions.

For both sequences, the compensating lobes of the readout and phase-encoding gradients were applied after the diffusion-encoding gradients, and the section-selective gradient for the 90° radio-frequency pulse was refocused immediately to prevent cross terms between the diffusion and imaging gradients (31).

For sequence A, cross terms between the diffusion gradients and the imaging section–selective gradients were reduced further by using nonselective refocusing with a composite (one-two-one) 180° radio-frequency pulse. Thus, for sequence A, all phase shifts induced by imaging gradients were zero when the diffusion gradients were applied, and all cross terms with the diffusion gradients were zero. The composite nonselective 180° pulse was chosen to increase the uniformity of the 180° radio-frequency pulse, which potentially reduces the effect of radio-frequency inhomogeneities on diffusion encoding.

For sequence B, the only nonzero cross term was between the section-selective and the diffusion-encoding gradients, and this cross term (δ_{12}) contributed a diffusion coefficient error of less than 0.5% (31). For both sequences, navigator echo gradient pulses were present for all acquisitions, but the navigator echo of the reference image was used to correct all the diffusion-encoded acquisitions, because this procedure was found to reduce the severity of artifacts. The effect from the navigator echo gradient pulses and the readout and phase-encoding gradient pulses occurring during the echo-planar readout can contribute additional self and cross terms, but these are negligible in clinical echo-planar MR imaging (36).

When possible, diffusion-weighted MR images were acquired with a b value of approximately 1,000 sec/mm^2 in each encoding direction in conjunction with image data with a b value of approximately 0 sec/mm^2, to provide a high SNR per unit time (31,37). For the sequence A tetrahedral acquisitions, the input Cartesian gradients were 20.0 mT/m, and the echo time was 106 msec with a b value of 1,022 sec/mm^2 (diffusion-encoding durations δ of 17.0 msec and a time Δ between gradient onsets of 46.85 msec). For the orthogonal acquisitions, the echo time and the diffusion-encoding timings δ and Δ were lengthened to an echo time of 121

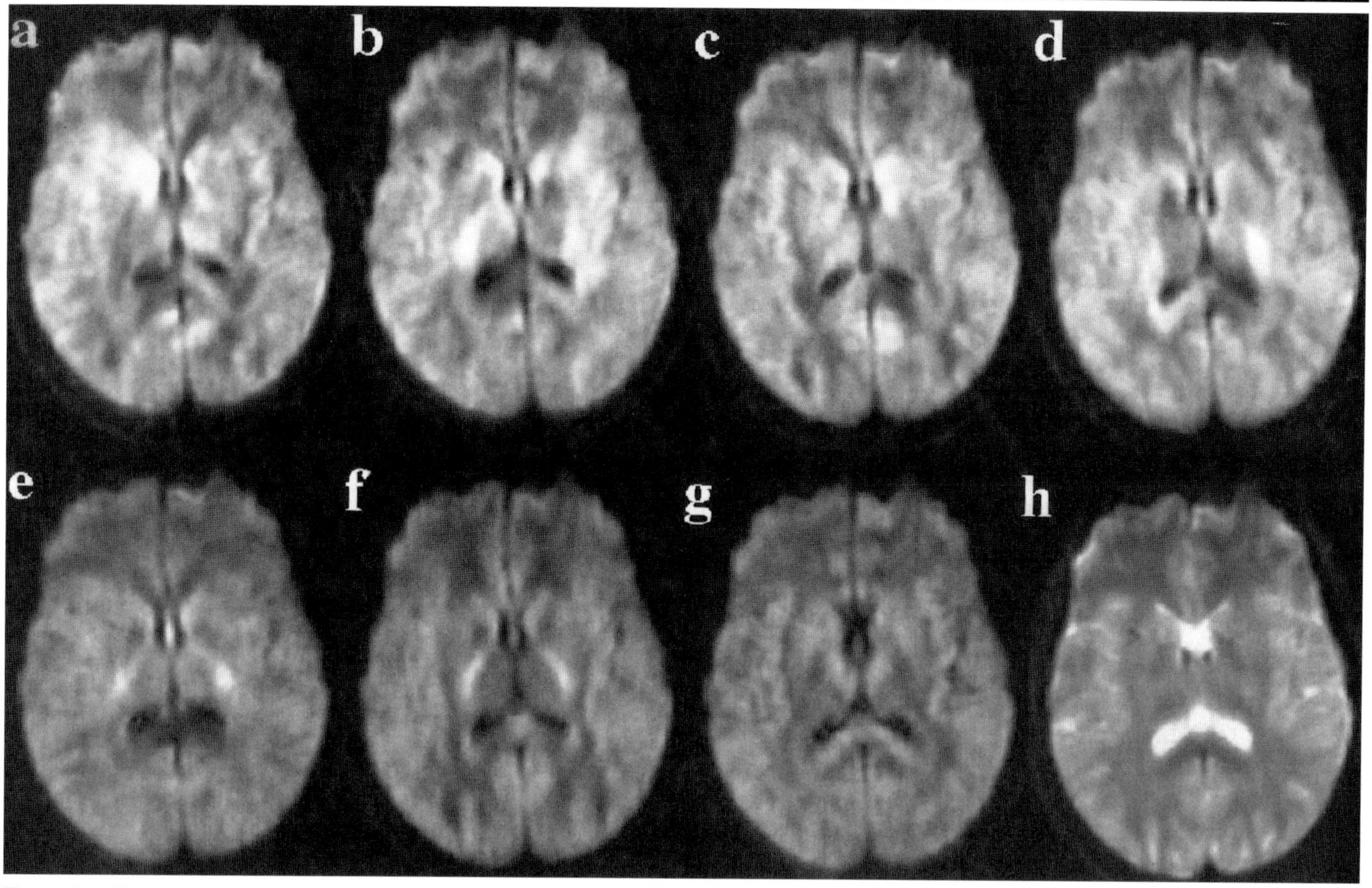

Figure 1. Characteristic axial single-section MR images (echo time = 106 msec, repetition time > 8,000 msec) obtained from a single acquisition of combined tetrahedral-orthogonal gradient encoding. *a–d,* Diffusion-weighted MR images encoded along tetrahedral directions one (*a*), two (*b*), three (*c*), and four (*d*) (26) by using a *b* value of 1,022 sec/mm². *e–g,* Diffusion-weighted MR images encoded along orthogonal directions x (*e*), y (*f*), and z (*g*) by using a *b* value of 999 sec/mm². *h,* One of the seven T2-weighted reference images acquired with very weak diffusion encoding (b = 12 sec/mm²) for each encoding direction. Voxel sizes were 2.11 × 2.11 × 5.00 mm, and the imaging time was approximately 26 seconds per encoding direction (approximately 3 minutes total). All diffusion-weighted images are from a single acquisition and are displayed with the same window width and center, which are one-third the window width and center of *h.* Note the different WM contrasts in *a–g,* which encode anisotropic diffusion.

msec, δ of 27 msec, and Δ of 56.85 msec, to yield a *b* value of 999 sec/mm².

Data for each of the seven encoding directions were acquired with a separate pulse sequence, each with its own reference acquisition. Each reference acquisition had weak diffusion encoding (b = 12 sec/mm²) along the same direction as the strong diffusion encoding, to spoil residual spurious free induction decay signals arising from imperfections in the nonselective 180° radio-frequency pulse. For sequence B, all diffusion-weighted images in the tetrahedral-only (four subjects) and tetrahedral-orthogonal (two subjects) cases were acquired with a combined pulse sequence that included one reference acquisition (b = 0 sec/mm²). Weak diffusion encoding in the reference acquisition was found to be unnecessary in sequence B, because spurious free induction decay signals were reduced by means of the volume selectivity of the 180° radio-frequency pulse and the spoiling caused by the 180° section-selective gradient. For the tetrahedral-only sequence B case, the echo time, input gradient strength, and diffusion-weighted *b* factors were the same as those for sequence A. For the tetrahedral-orthogonal sequence B case, the input diffusion-encoding gradient strength was increased to 22.0 mT/m, and the echo time was reduced to 97 msec, which yielded a *b* value of 1,003.3 sec/mm² for tetrahedral encoding (δ = 15.75 msec, Δ = 44.80 msec). For the orthogonal encodings in this sequence, echo time and diffusion timings were the same as those in the tetrahedral encodings, with a *b* value of 334.3 sec/mm². The same timings were chosen for pulse sequence simplicity. Although this sequence has different diffusion-weighted *b* factors for tetrahedral and orthogonal encoding, this was not expected to contribute systematic error, on the basis of results from an initial study (not shown) that established that the same averaged diffusivity was measured with orthogonal encoding at *b* values of approximately 300 and 1,000 sec/mm².

In addition, for typical *b* factors and diffusion times used in clinical imaging, different groups (38,39) have found a lack of multiexponential dependence of brain signal intensity on the *b* factor, as well as a lack of explicit dependence of the brain diffusion coefficient on diffusion time at a constant *b* factor. Although multiple intravoxel tissue components can potentially lead to multiexponential dependence on the *b* factor, these results suggest that this effect is small, due possibly to the similarity in averaged diffusivity between gray matter (GM) and WM. Intravoxel averaging of multiple anisotropic components could lead to complex effects on diffusion-weighted images that are not completely described with one tensor. Such partial volume effects were considered in simulations to be described subsequently.

To limit the effects of physiologic motion (eg, cerebrospinal fluid pulsatility), sequence A was gated so that the 90° pulse was applied 500 msec after the peak signal from the peripheral pulse oximeter, which corresponds to brain diastole (30,40). To reduce effects from heart rate variability in the presence of partial saturation of cerebrospinal fluid, the pulse sequence repetition time was set to a minimum of 8,000 msec. One warm-up step was programmed to ensure that cerebrospinal fluid signals were at steady state. The overall acquisition time was thus approximately 26 seconds to encode each direction with a small and a large b factor (approximately 3 minutes for one acquisition of all seven encoding directions).

Sequence B was performed with a repetition time of 3,050–3,500 msec without gating and with three warm-up steps. A 15-section axial set of tetrahedral-orthogonal brain data, including warm-up steps, was acquired in 33 seconds. This sequence was performed twice with gaps that were 100% of the section thickness, with the second acquisition offset by a section thickness. Thus, contiguous whole brain data were collected during 66 seconds, for an overall acquisition time of approximately 1½ minutes, including setup and tuning.

For qualitative assessment of the effectiveness of averaging acquisitions, three interleaved multisection data sets were acquired with 200% gaps in one subject, and these acquisitions were repeated to produce a total of 10 thin-section whole-brain data sets for averaging (total acquisition time, 16 minutes 40 seconds). For both sequences A and B, a sinusoidal readout gradient, a constant phase-encoding gradient, and linear time sampling were used to yield a raw data matrix of 96 × 200, which was interpolated to a rectilinear k-space matrix of 96 × 128 by using a gridding procedure. The field of view ranged from 180 × 240 mm to 210 × 280 mm (in-plane voxel size range, 1.88 × 1.88 mm to 2.19 × 2.19 mm). The section thickness was 5.0 mm in all cases except the triple-interleaved acquisition for sequence B, where the section thickness was 3.3 mm.

Data Analysis

Images were sinc interpolated to a 192 × 256 image matrix (0.94 × 0.94 × 5.00 mm pixels in sequence A) to facilitate selection of ROIs. In some cases, the rectilinear matrix produced after k-space gridding was zero filled prior to reconstruction; in the other cases, the interpolation was performed after reconstruction.

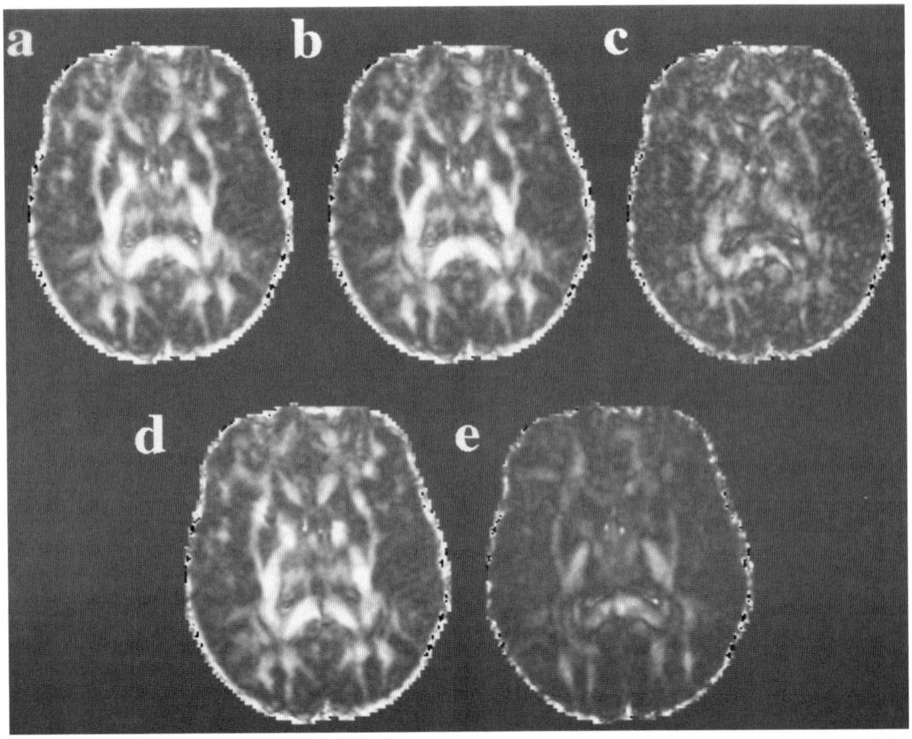

Figure 2. Axial anisotropy (*a–c*) and anisotropy-weighted (*d, e*) MR images computed at the level of the basal ganglia by using the data in Figure 1. A_σ (*a*), A_{major} (*b*), and A_{minor} (*c*) images were obtained from a single acquisition of combined tetrahedral-orthogonal encoding. *d,* AW_{tet} image was obtained from the tetrahedral encodings. *e,* AW_{ortho} image was obtained from the orthogonal encodings. All images have the same window width and center. Note the high sensitivity to WM depiction in *a,* with delineation of the external capsule, the peripheral occipital WM projections, the thalamic heterogeneity, and the width of the internal capsule. Note also the structural heterogeneity of WM in *a* (eg, dark bands between the internal capsule, corpus callosum, and adjacent WM) and the heterogeneity in the thalamus, which is not seen on T2-weighted MR images (see Fig 1, *h*). Visible differences in anisotropy strength exist between WM classes, where the image intensity in *a* and *b* can be ranked, from highest to lowest, as follows: commissural WM, projection WM, and association WM. In comparison with *a,* the anisotropy-weighted component images in *d* and *e* show a loss of intensity in the splenium and genu of the corpus callosum, respectively, and there generally is less intensity in *e,* as compared with that in *d.*

All images were realigned in two dimensions to the reference images to correct for two-dimensional displacements and linear distortions (ie, stretch and shear) caused by eddy currents. These linear distortions have been found to constitute the major eddy-current effects in echo-planar diffusion MR imaging (41), which also was supported by cine visual inspection of the realigned images in the present study. The realignment algorithm used a combination of intramodality (42) and cross-modality affine realignment procedures; the cross-modality procedure was used for realignment of image pairs with substantial contrast differences. We routinely use these intra- and cross-modality realignment procedures for functional MR imaging (43). Because all realignments were to the reference echo-planar MR image, the realignment was specifically targeted to low-order eddy-current–induced distortions, which must be corrected to bring the reference and diffusion-weighted images into register for tensor computation (described subsequently). Higher-order distortions also were typically present on the echo-planar MR images (in comparison with those on anatomic spin-echo MR images), but these need not necessarily be corrected for the diffusion computation because the distortions are constant on all diffusion-weighted and reference images. Eddy-current effects also were specifically targeted by performing the realignments in two dimensions, because the principal eddy-current effects are in plane. The realignment procedure additionally corrects for in-plane subject motion, although typical in-plane and through-plane motion effects are estimated to be very small in comparison with the eddy-current effects at these acquisition times.

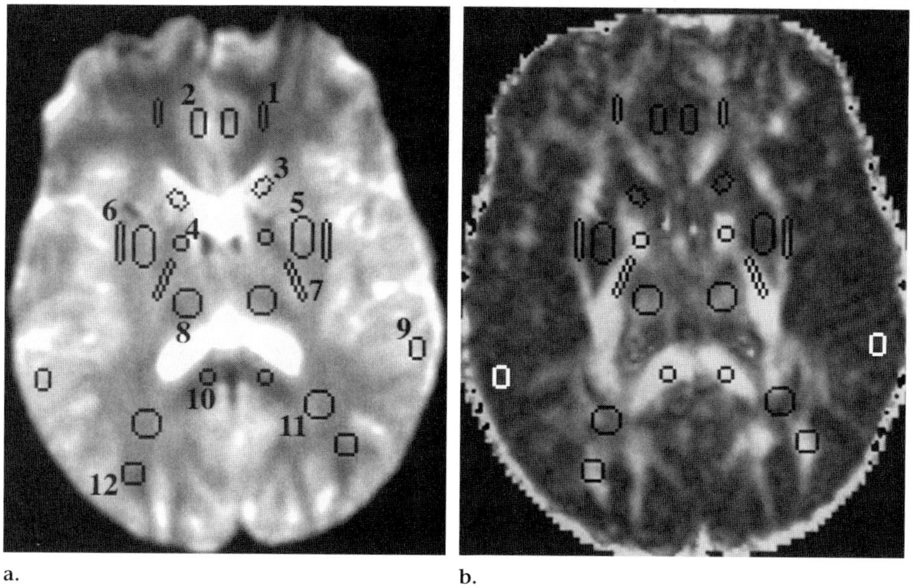

Figure 3. ROIs used in data analysis are superimposed on **(a)** axial T2-weighted reference MR image (echo time = 106 msec, repetition time > 8,000 msec) (same image as Fig 1, *h*) and **(b)** axial A_σ MR image (same image as Fig 2, *a*). *1* = frontal WM, *2* = frontal GM, *3* = head of the caudate nucleus, *4* = genu of the internal capsule, *5* = putamen, *6* = external capsule, *7* = posterior limb of internal capsule, *8* = thalamus, *9* = occipital-temporal GM, *10* = splenium of the corpus callosum, *11* = occipital WM, and *12* = optic radiations. The location of the ROI for occipital-temporal GM varied across subjects. ROI sizes and shapes were kept constant across hemispheres but varied across subjects.

Tetrahedral and orthogonal diffusion-weighted images were obtained. The intensities are functions of the *b* factors and the elements of the diffusion tensor, weighted by the direction of the diffusion gradient used (27,31). The logarithm of these intensities was computed to create a set of linear equations that were solved by using standard weighted least-squares techniques (13,14,44). The six diffusion tensor elements were determined with global analysis (see Appendix) of all eight tetrahedral-orthogonal log intensities, and averaged diffusivity $\overline{D}$ and A_σ were then computed directly from the diffusion-tensor elements according to Equation (3) (see Appendix, Eq [A1]). Images were computed on a pixel-by-pixel basis, without spatial filtering.

From the estimated diffusion tensor, the principal axes and eigenvalues were then computed by using standard matrix procedures. The eigenvalues were sorted according to size and symmetry ($\lambda_{z'} > \lambda_{x'} > \lambda_{y'}$ for the prolate case, $\lambda_{x'} > \lambda_{y'} > \lambda_{z'}$ for the oblate case), and A_{major} and A_{minor} were calculated by using Equations (1,2). In addition, by using only the tetrahedral or orthogonal data, anisotropy-weighted images were calculated (see Appendix, Eqq [A4,A5]) by means of direct computation of D_1, D_2, D_3, and D_4, or D_{xx}, D_{yy}, and D_{zz}, from log intensity ratios. In the one sequence B case where the acquisition was repeated multiple times for the purpose of averaging, the diffusion-weighted images and reference image were arithmetically averaged prior to the log intensity computation. Averaging was performed at this stage, as opposed to averaging of computed A_σ images, to minimize anisotropy bias caused by input noise (discussed subsequently). The fraction of total anisotropy contained in the anisotropy-weighted measures also was computed for arbitrary orientations and was displayed with MATLAB software (MathWorks, Natick, Mass) by using Equations (A7,A8) in the Appendix.

Elliptical ROIs were positioned on each subject data set by using interactive software (ANALYZE; Mayo Foundation, Rochester, Minn) for evaluation of anisotropy in different anatomic areas of the brain. The ROI calculations were performed by using a custom program that partially weights edge voxels according to the fraction of the voxel that lies inside the ROI, as determined with analytic ellipse expressions. This procedure was performed instead of more standard routines that sample only voxels that are completely inside the ROI. This procedure is equivalent to obtaining ROI measurements on highly interpolated images (but without large memory or disk requirements).

Normative data were measured from ROIs of 12 brain regions in the 11 subjects examined with sequence A. The ROIs were placed in equivalent structures in each hemisphere for averaging and analysis of hemispheric differences. In each subject, the ROIs were initially located by using the T2-weighted reference images (echo time = 106 msec, repetition time > 8,000 msec), and ROI sizes and positions were refined by means of overlay onto the A_σ images. Mean ROI values were measured for all 12 regions in each hemisphere, for each of the two acquisitions, and for each subject. Statistical variations across these factors were assessed with the two-tailed Student *t* test of the mean ROI values. The random (thermal) noise properties of images also were estimated in individual subjects by subtracting the two images acquired under identical experimental conditions (35). The thermal noise of a single acquisition was taken as $2^{-1/2}$ times the single-pixel SD measured from the subtraction image by using the ROIs. The SNR was estimated as the mean of the two acquisitions divided by the thermal noise value. The subtraction images were also inspected visually for artifacts, especially in the locations of the ROIs. No ROI positions were changed, and all data were included in the measurements and statistical analyses.

Computer Simulations

Computer simulations were performed to evaluate the effects of noise and partial volume averaging on the measurement of anisotropy. In a noise-free isotropic region, the true A_σ is 0. In the presence of noise, the measured A_σ is greater than 0 even in isotropic regions, because, according to Equation (3), noise causes variance in the diffusion measurements that elevates A_σ. This low-level anisotropy is expected to be strongly dependent on the SNR of the measurement.

To evaluate the baseline isotropic level of A_σ at different noise levels, a Monte Carlo program was written that generated voxel intensity data for an idealized tissue having the same averaged diffusivity as the brain ROI under consideration but with the assumption of zero anisotropy ($A_\sigma = 0$). The signal intensities that would be observed in isotropic tissues in a tetrahedral-orthogonal diffusion experiment were simulated by calculating the ideal signal intensity and adding Gaussian random noise. The ideal signal intensity was calculated by assuming (*a*) that *b* equalled 1,000 sec/mm² for all seven diffusion-weighted images and (*b*) that all diffusion-weighted images and the reference T2-weighted image had the same echo time.

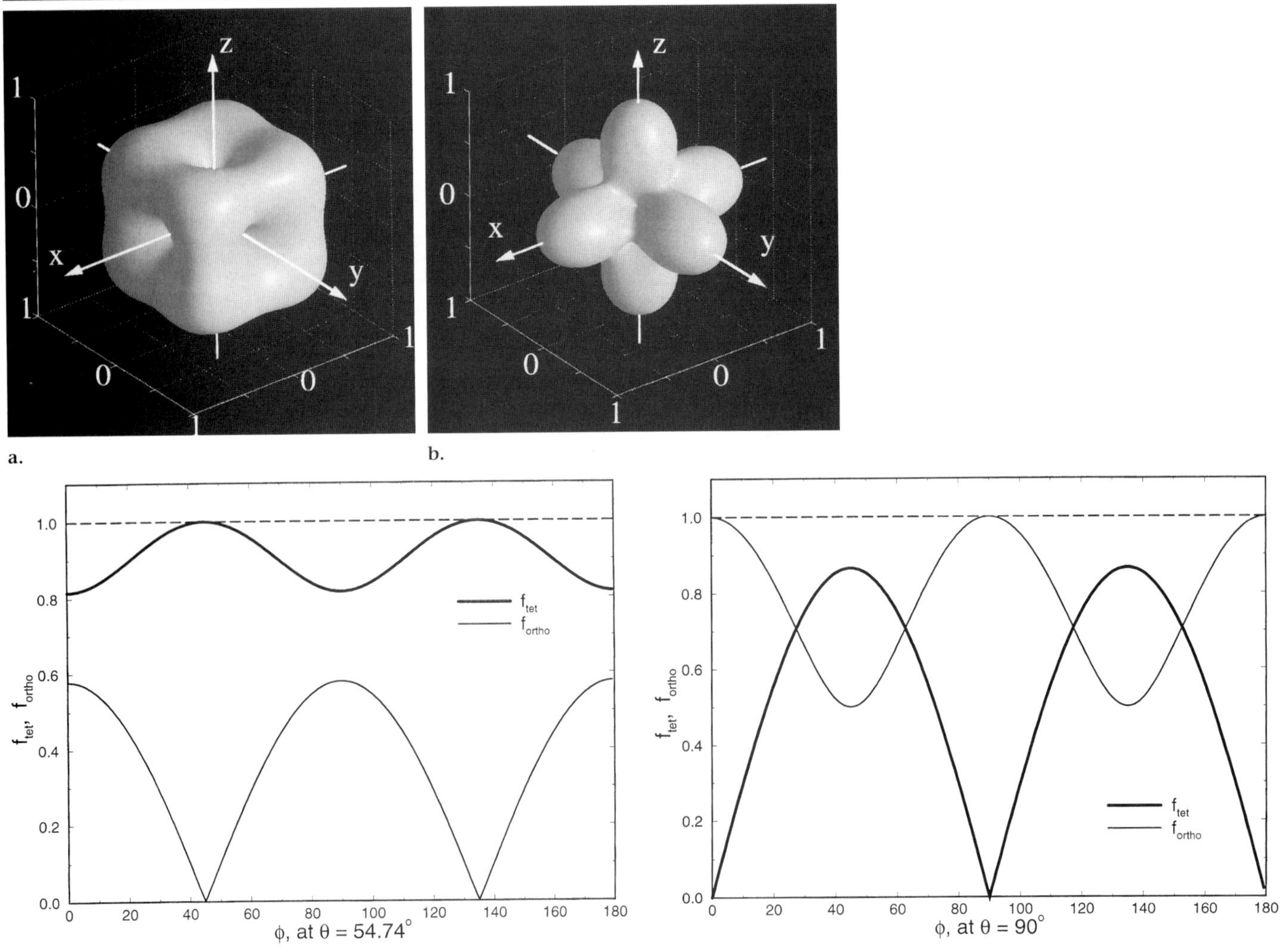

a. b. c. d.

Figure 4. Ratio of tetrahedral and orthogonal anisotropy-weighted indexes (AW_{tet} and AW_{ortho}) to total anisotropy (A_σ) as a function of θ and ϕ. Three-dimensional displays of the ratios **(a)** f_{tet} and **(b)** f_{ortho} were computed by using Equations (A7) and (A8) (see Appendix), respectively. These ratios are displayed as the radial distance of a surface in a spherical coordinate system as a function of the directional angles θ and ϕ. **(c, d)** Graphs that show profiles of the data when **(c)** θ is 54.74° and **(d)** θ is 90° indicate the orientation of the maxima and minima. The recovery of A_σ generally is higher for the AW_{tet} measurement than for the AW_{ortho} measurement. Thus, the majority of the anisotropy information is in the tetrahedral measurements (ie, the majority of anisotropy information is contained in the off-diagonal tensor elements). Note the extent to which the surfaces in **a** and **b** approach the ideal case of a sphere (ie, a true A_σ measurement, also indicated by the approach of the solid curves to the dashed lines in **c** and **d**). Note also that the surfaces in **a** and **b** are complementary, with AW_{tet} insensitive in the orthogonal directions and AW_{ortho} insensitive in the tetrahedral directions.

Gaussian noise was added to real and imaginary channels at various reference image SNR levels. A constant level of uncorrelated noise was assumed for the diffusion-weighted and reference images. The A_σ value was calculated from these simulated intensities by using Equation (3), and A_σ statistics were determined from 16,000 sets of simulated tetrahedral-orthogonal diffusion experiments. The mean and SD of the computed A_σ values were compared with the experimentally determined, average ROI A_σ value within subjects.

The second simulation was performed to evaluate the effect of partial volume averaging on the measurement of A_σ. This is especially important in transition zones between regions of high anisotropy and those of low anisotropy, such as the borders between GM and WM and in areas of WM with fibers that cross in different directions. Anisotropy measurements in voxels located at GM-WM interfaces were simulated by assuming a mixture of idealized WM and GM tissue components on the basis of ROI measurements in homogeneous areas of GM and WM. The WM tissue component was modeled to have the same $\overline{D}$ and A_σ values as the splenium of the corpus callosum ($\overline{D} = 0.72 \times 10^{-3}$ mm²/sec, A_σ = 0.5), but with zero minor-axis anisotropy (A_{minor} = 0) to represent an idealized axisymmetric case imaged at high spatial resolution. The GM component was chosen to be representative of the putamen ($\overline{D} = 0.72 \times 10^{-3}$ mm²/sec), but with zero anisotropy ($A_\sigma = 0$). Noise-free signal intensities were calculated separately for GM and WM and were combined at various partial volume weightings, from which A_σ was calculated by using Equation (3).

In the third simulation, we evaluated the case of WM regions with crossing fibers. Anisotropy measurements were simulated for WM tracts that crossed at variable angular separations within the

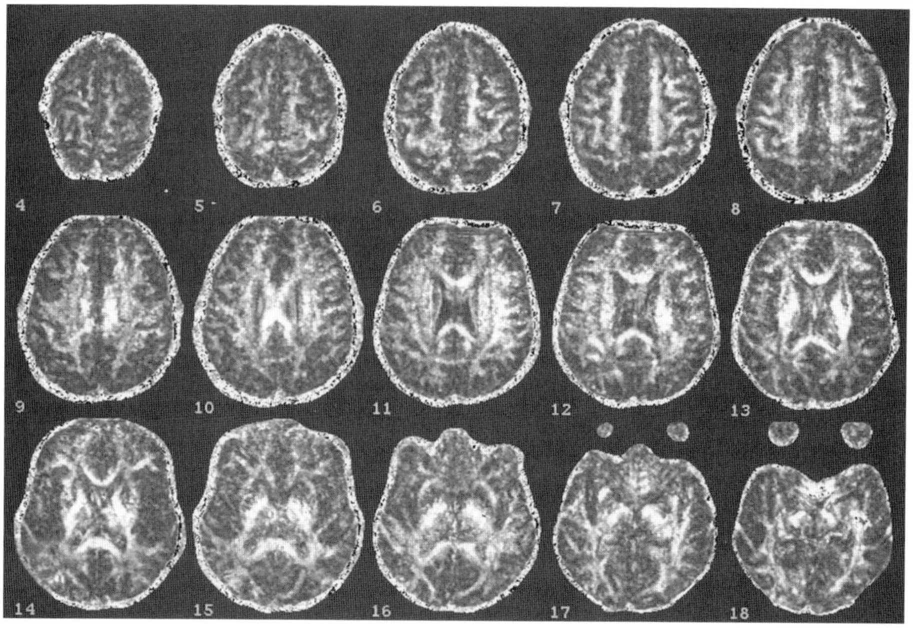

a.

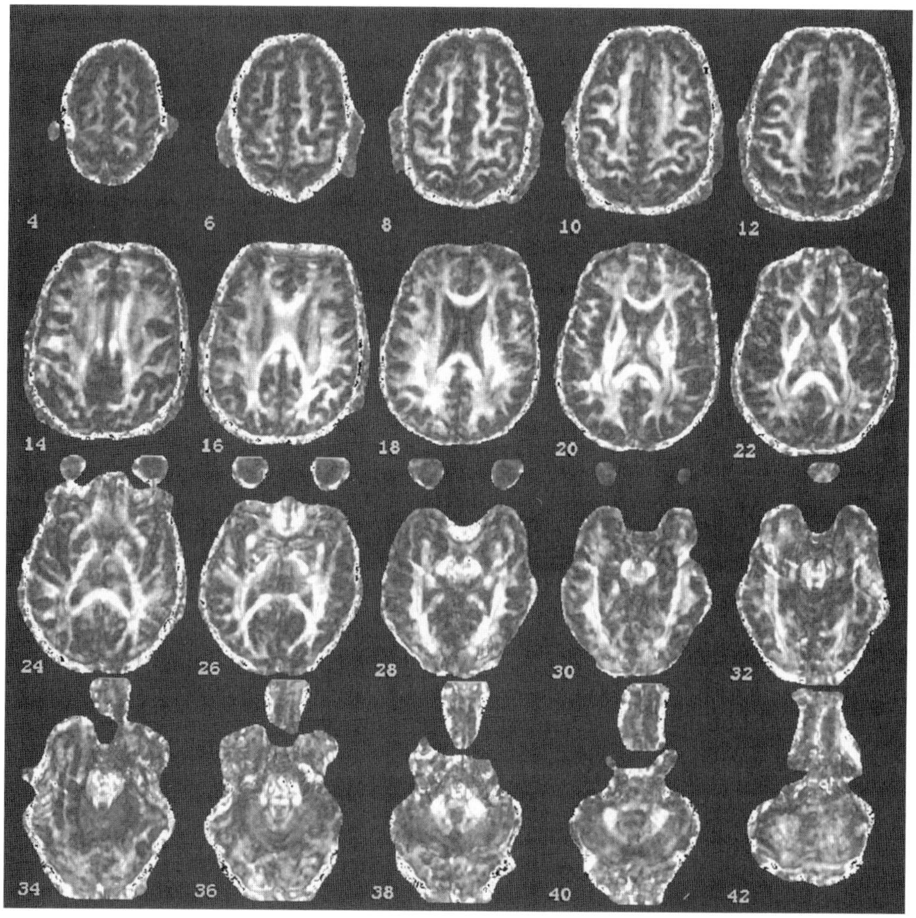

b.

Figure 5. Axial multisection MR imaging demonstration of A_σ obtained **(a)** without and **(b)** with data averaging. Numbers indicate the section numbers. Combined tetrahedral-orthogonal multisection data were acquired with one axial T2-weighted reference MR image obtained with a single sequence (echo time = 97 msec, repetition time = 3,100 msec), with b of 1,003.3 sec/mm^2 for tetrahedral data, b of 334.4 sec/mm^2 for orthogonal data, and b of 0 sec/mm^2 for reference data. In **a**, only one image was acquired per encoding direction (one shot per image; total acquisition time, 66 seconds), with a voxel size of 1.88 × 1.88 × 5.00 mm. In **b**, the pulse sequence used in **a** was repeated a total of 10 times in a different subject (total acquisition time, 16 minutes 40 seconds) but with a section thickness of 3.3 mm. In **b**, the source image data as depicted in Figure 1 were averaged, followed by computation of the diffusion tensor. In both **a** and **b**, A_σ was computed from the estimated diffusion tensor according to Equation (3). Note the sensitive demonstration of WM structures throughout the brain, including subcortical U fibers. In addition to the findings shown in Figure 2, note the detection of other WM structures such as cerebral peduncles (section *18* in **a** and section *30* in **b**) and the cerebellar peduncles (sections *38* and *40* in **b**), as well as heterogeneity in the thalamus, basal ganglia, and occipital WM (eg, in **b**, note band of anisotropy in the region of the globus pallidus in sections *24* and *26* and ridges of low anisotropy along the optic radiations in sections *20–32*). Comparison of **a** and **b** indicates that A_σ image quality can be improved by increasing the number of signals acquired and obtaining thinner sections.

plane of a transverse image. Signal intensities were calculated for two tissue components, each modeled as for the idealized WM tissue in the second simulation and each containing fibers oriented in the plane ($\theta = 90°$). The signals were added at equal weightings for varying in-plane angles (one component with $\phi = 0°$, the other with $-90° < \phi \leq +90°$). The A_σ value of the combined voxel was calculated with Equation (3) and compared with the two component values.

RESULTS

Figure 1 presents a complete set of characteristic single-section diffusion-weighted MR images obtained from one of the subjects (sequence A): four tetrahedral diffusion-weighted images (Fig 1, *a–d*), three orthogonal diffusion-weighted images (Fig 1, *e–g*), and the baseline T2-weighted reference image (Fig 1, *h*). Different levels of brightness in the diffusion-weighted images are due to the anisotropy of WM fiber tracts that were sampled along different directions.

Figure 2 presents the anisotropy images computed from the data in Figure 1. Images of the various anisotropy measures have a wide range of intensities in the brain, in contrast to the typically uniform appearance of the adult brain on averaged diffusivity images (17,18). Areas of high A_σ in Figure 2, *a*, are seen in the corpus callosum, internal capsule, and

TABLE 1
Mean Anisotropy Measures from Brain ROIs in 11 Human Subjects: Single-Section Data

ROI	A_σ	A_{major}	A_{minor}	AW_{tet}	AW_{ortho}	RA/$2^{1/2}$*
Commissural WM						
Splenium of corpus callosum	0.50 (0.02)	0.49 (0.02)	0.16 (0.01)	0.45 (0.01)	0.21 (0.02)	0.46 (0.02)
Projection WM						
Genu of internal capsule	0.45 (0.02)	0.43 (0.02)	0.21 (0.01)	0.44 (0.02)	0.07 (0.01)	0.37 (0.01)
Posterior limb of internal capsule	0.39 (0.02)	0.38 (0.02)	0.13 (0.01)	0.30 (0.02)	0.24 (0.01)	0.42 (0.02)
Optic radiations	0.31 (0.02)	0.30 (0.02)	0.13 (0.01)	0.29 (0.02)	0.11 (0.01)	No data
Association WM						
Frontal WM	0.26 (0.01)	0.23 (0.01)	0.18 (0.02)	0.22 (0.02)	0.12 (0.01)	0.22 (0.02)
External capsule	0.23 (0.02)	0.21 (0.02)	0.13 (0.01)	0.21 (0.02)	0.08 (0.01)	No data
Occipital WM	0.21 (0.01)	0.19 (0.01)	0.12 (0.01)	0.16 (0.01)	0.11 (0.01)	No data
Thalamus	0.19 (0.01)	0.16 (0.01)	0.15 (0.01)	0.17 (0.01)	0.05 (0.005)	No data
GM						
Head of caudate nucleus	0.10 (0.01)	0.09 (0.01)	0.08 (0.005)	0.09 (0.01)	0.04 (0.01)	0.11 (0.004)
Frontal GM	0.09 (0.01)	0.08 (0.01)	0.07 (0.01)	0.08 (0.01)	0.04 (0.01)	No data
Putamen	0.08 (0.01)	0.07 (0.01)	0.07 (0.004)	0.07 (0.01)	0.03 (0.003)	0.11 (0.01)
Occipital-temporal GM	0.05 (0.003)	0.05 (0.003)	0.04 (0.003)	0.05 (0.003)	0.02 (0.002)	0.13 (0.01)

Note.—Data based on computed anisotropy and anisotropy-weighted MR images obtained with sequence A (single-section method; Fig 2). Means are derived from ROI measurements (Fig 3) of both hemispheres from two equivalent sections, averaged across subjects, and weighted by the ROI area. Number in parentheses is the SEM weighted by ROI area, unless otherwise noted. SEM was calculated as SD of mean values from each subject, divided by the square root of the number of subjects.

* Data are results in six monkeys reported by Pierpaoli and Basser (29) expressed in terms of A_σ. Number in parentheses is the SEM. RA = relative anisotropy.

optic radiations. The external capsule also is well depicted. The ROIs were located on the reference image and were confirmed with A_σ images, as shown in Figure 3. Comparison of A_σ values between the matched left and right ROIs demonstrated no statistically significant differences on the basis of measured within-subject thermal noise levels and the results of a two-tailed pairwise Student t test at the 95% confidence level. Comparison of A_σ ROIs between the first and second acquisition in each volunteer similarly demonstrated no significant differences from thermal noise at the 95% confidence level.

Figure 2, *b* and *c*, are images of A_{major} and A_{minor}, respectively. A_{major} and A_σ are similar in appearance and, when diffusion is axisymmetric, equal in magnitude. Figure 2, *d* and *e*, are images of AW_{tet} and AW_{ortho}, respectively. In general, the intensity of AW_{tet} is larger than that of AW_{ortho}. Artifactual loss of intensity is seen in AW_{tet} in the midline of the splenium of the corpus callosum and in AW_{ortho} in the genu of the corpus callosum owing to fiber direction. The fraction of anisotropy recovered by separate tetrahedral and orthogonal anisotropy-weighted indexes is displayed in Figure 4 for different orientations by using Equations (A7,A8), in the Appendix.

Figure 5a presents A_σ in the 66-second multisection experiment (sequence B). Comparison of ROI A_σ values between single-section and multisection acquisitions at the same level demonstrated no significant differences within subjects on the basis of measured thermal noise and the results of a two-tailed pairwise Student t test at the 95% confidence level. Figure 5b demonstrates the ability to average A_σ. These data were acquired as an average of 10 66-second multisection acquisitions. In Figure 5, high anisotropy is present in WM tracts throughout the brain, such as the centrum semiovale, the subcortical U fibers, and the cerebral and cerebellar peduncles.

TABLE 2
Mean Principal Diffusion Coefficients (Eigenvalues) for Various ROIs

ROI	$\lambda_{z'}$	$\lambda_{x'}$	$\lambda_{y'}$
Commissural WM			
Splenium of corpus callosum	1.43 (0.08)	0.49 (0.04)	0.25 (0.03)
Projection WM			
Genu of internal capsule	1.33 (0.05)	0.57 (0.04)	0.26 (0.03)
Posterior limb of internal capsule	1.23 (0.05)	0.52 (0.03)	0.34 (0.02)
Optic radiations	1.18 (0.06)	0.61 (0.03)	0.43 (0.03)
Association WM			
Frontal WM	1.17 (0.06)	0.75 (0.03)	0.47 (0.03)
External capsule	1.14 (0.05)	0.73 (0.04)	0.52 (0.03)
Occipital WM	1.07 (0.04)	0.73 (0.03)	0.54 (0.03)
Thalamus	0.94 (0.04)	0.72 (0.03)	0.50 (0.03)
GM			
Head of caudate nucleus	0.94 (0.03)	0.79 (0.02)	0.66 (0.03)
Frontal GM	1.02 (0.04)	0.88 (0.03)	0.75 (0.03)
Putamen	0.84 (0.03)	0.73 (0.02)	0.63 (0.02)
Occipital-temporal GM	1.02 (0.04)	0.93 (0.04)	0.85 (0.04)

Note.—ROI data were measured on the basis of eigenvalue images computed from single-section (sequence A) source images shown in Figure 1. Number in parentheses is the SEM, which was calculated as for Table 1.

Table 1 presents values for several anisotropy measures in the brain ROIs demonstrated in Figure 3. These include A_σ, A_{major}, and A_{minor}, as in Figure 2, *a–c*. The ROIs are sorted in order of decreasing A_σ value and demonstrate the variability of anisotropy between different types of WM and GM. Additional columns in Table 1 show the comparison of A_σ with its noninvariant components and with AW_{tet} and AW_{ortho}, which were obtained separately by using the tetrahedral and orthogonal techniques, respectively. The larger anisotropy contribution contained in the tetrahedral component as compared with that in the orthogonal measure is again demonstrated. Also, our human A_σ results are compared with the relative anisotropy

TABLE 3
Comparison of Differences among A_σ Values in Various Brain ROIs

	ROI											
ROI	CCS	ICG	ICP	OR	FWM	EC	OWM	Th	HC	FGM	Pu	OTGM
CCS		T	T									
ICG	T		T	T								
ICP	T	T		T	T							
OR		T	T		T	T	T	T				
FWM			T	T		T	T	T				
EC				T	T		T	T				
OWM				T	T	T		T				
Th				T	T	T	T					
HC										T	T	
FGM									T		T	T
Pu									T	T		T
OTGM										T	T	

Note.—CCS = splenium of corpus callosum, EC = external capsule, FGM = frontal GM, FWM = frontal WM, HC = head of caudate nucleus, ICG = genu of internal capsule, ICP = posterior limb of internal capsule, OR = optic radiations, OTGM = occipital-temporal GM, OWM = occipital WM, Pu = putamen, T = "true" null hypothesis (A_σ values not significantly different, per student *t* test and 95% confidence level), Th = thalamus.

divided by $2^{1/2}$, as evaluated in monkeys by Pierpaoli and Basser (29). This comparison was made because relative anisotropy is the anisotropy measure mentioned in the MR imaging literature that is most closely related to A_σ. There is general agreement between A_σ and relative anisotropy divided by $2^{1/2}$. The A_σ SNR averaged across subjects in the reported WM structures ranged from 5.1 to 15.6. The measured thermal noise levels in A_σ, A_{major} and A_{minor} (0.0118, 0.0112, and 0.0121, respectively) were similar to one another.

Table 2 presents characteristic values of sorted eigenvalues obtained from the same ROIs as those in Table 1. Table 3 presents results of the pairwise Student *t* test comparison of A_σ between different ROIs. The null hypothesis was that there is no significant difference in A_σ between ROIs at the 95% confidence level. Table 3 indicates ROI comparisons for which the null hypothesis was true, that is, ROIs that were not significantly different from each other at the 95% confidence level. If anisotropy were uniform across the brain, the null hypothesis would have been true for all comparisons. If all ROIs differed from one another, only the diagonal elements of Table 3 would have been filled. The actual results in Table 3 resemble a block-diagonal structure, in which A_σ is significantly similar within tissue groups (ie, blocks) and significantly different across groups.

The simulation results for noise and partial volume effects on measurement of A_σ are given in Figures 6 and 7, respectively. In Figure 6a, the measurement bias in the A_σ of isotropic tissues caused by noise is graphed versus the SNR on the reference T2-weighted image for tetrahedral-orthogonal encoding with a *b* value of 1,000 sec/mm^2 for all encodings. The results of this simulation demonstrate that the values measured in GM and the basal ganglia are consistent with zero anisotropy ($A_\sigma = 0$) at the reference T2-weighted SNR levels present in the experiment (reference SNR of approximately 40–60).

In Figure 6b, the A_σ measurement bias is graphed versus true anisotropy for anisotropic tissues at various SNR levels for the same tetrahedral-orthogonal encoding. The results of this simulation demonstrate that the anisotropy values measured in the thalamus ($A_\sigma = 0.19$) and in other WM areas in Table 1 are consistent with an A_σ value that is greater than 0 at the experimental SNR levels. The results of this simulation also indicate that the noise in A_σ was not stationary but instead increased as A_σ increased (see error bars in Fig 6b).

A simulation of the partial volume effects on A_σ in border regions between GM and WM is presented in Figure 7a. The results of this simulation demonstrate that a combination of signals from anisotropic and isotropic diffusion elements within a voxel generally caused reduction in the measured A_σ proportional to the relative amount of isotropic tissue (given the assumption that the components have similar T1 and T2 weightings). The partial volume effects of averaging between two groups of WM fibers with equal anisotropy is simulated in Figure 7b as a function of angular separation. In this case, the measured A_σ value was reduced by an amount that was dependent on the degree of angular separation between the component tensors.

DISCUSSION

Quantitative images of different anisotropy measures were obtained by means of a combination of measurements with tetrahedral and orthogonal gradient encoding (Figs 2, 5). This combination provides wide spatial coverage of the diffusion ellipsoid surface at high gradient strength. The tetrahedral encodings represent the most widely spaced set of four encoding directions (and are at the maximum gradient strength), whereas the orthogonal encodings are in directions that bisect the angular gaps of the tetrahedral encodings. The invariant anisotropy measure A_σ has multiple advantages, including an absolute anisotropy scale and direct calculation from the diffusion-tensor elements without matrix diagonalization or eigenvalue sorting.

The A_σ MR images shown in Figure 2, *a*, and Figure 5 demonstrate anatomic detail that is not typically evident on conventional T1- and T2-weighted MR images. This detail includes depiction of the peripheral extensions of the densely myelinated optic radiation and the posterior limb of the internal capsule. In particular, the posterior limb of the internal capsule appeared wider on A_σ MR images than on conventional MR images, which is compatible with the appearance on gross anatomic sections (eg, see figs 8 and 13 in DeArmond et al [45]). The anterior limb of the internal capsule appeared thinner than the posterior limb and tapered anteriorly, which again is compatible with the appearance on gross anatomic sections (figs 13 and 14 in DeArmond et al). As a consequence, ROI measurements are not reported for the anterior limb of the internal capsule, because this structure was too thin to yield reliable results. The thin external capsule was well defined, which helped demarcate the lateral extent of the putamen.

Strong anisotropy also was present in the centrum semiovale, the peripheral U fibers, and the cerebral and cerebellar peduncles. The anisotropy MR images provided evidence for substructures in the thalamus and in the occipital WM, which otherwise appear homogeneous on conventional T1- and T2-weighted MR images. This high sensitivity to WM structure presumably is due to suppression of adjacent GM, which has zero anisotropy (confirmed by the simulation results shown in Fig 6a), and to the straightforward, nearly linear partial volume effects at GM-WM interfaces (confirmed by the simulation results in Fig 7a). This phenomenon is similar to the improvement of small vessel detection in MR angiography due to suppression of the signal from adjacent tissue.

Signal averaging was effective at improving the sensitivity to WM structures, as seen by comparing Figure 5a with Figure 5b. Figure 5 also demonstrates other regions of structural heterogeneity in WM, such as the "ridged" appearance of decreased anisotropy adjacent to the optic radiations and splenium of the corpus callosum on sections 20 and 22 in Figure 5b. The simulation results shown in Figure 7b indicate that partial volume averaging between WM fiber tracts can lead to a decrease of more than 50% in measured anisotropy, which may be a possible cause of this appearance. Another example is heterogeneity in the basal ganglia, seen in the region of the globus pallidus, which may be due to structures such as the ansa lenticularis (section 24 in Fig 5b). Further investigation is needed to assess the relevance of these findings for clinical anisotropy MR imaging.

The results in Tables 1 and 2 indicate that consistent A_σ values and principal diffusion coefficients can be measured across subjects for different brain regions, as indicated by the small SEMs in Tables 1 and 2. This consistency across subjects indicates that there generally are characteristic values for A_σ in different brain structures in healthy adults. The results also indicate that there are significant differences in A_σ across brain regions, as was also found by Pierpaoli and colleagues (17,29). The general correspondence between A_σ in humans and relative anisotropy divided by $2^{1/2}$ in monkeys (29) also is suggestive that these characteristics may extend across species. The consistency of data across human subjects

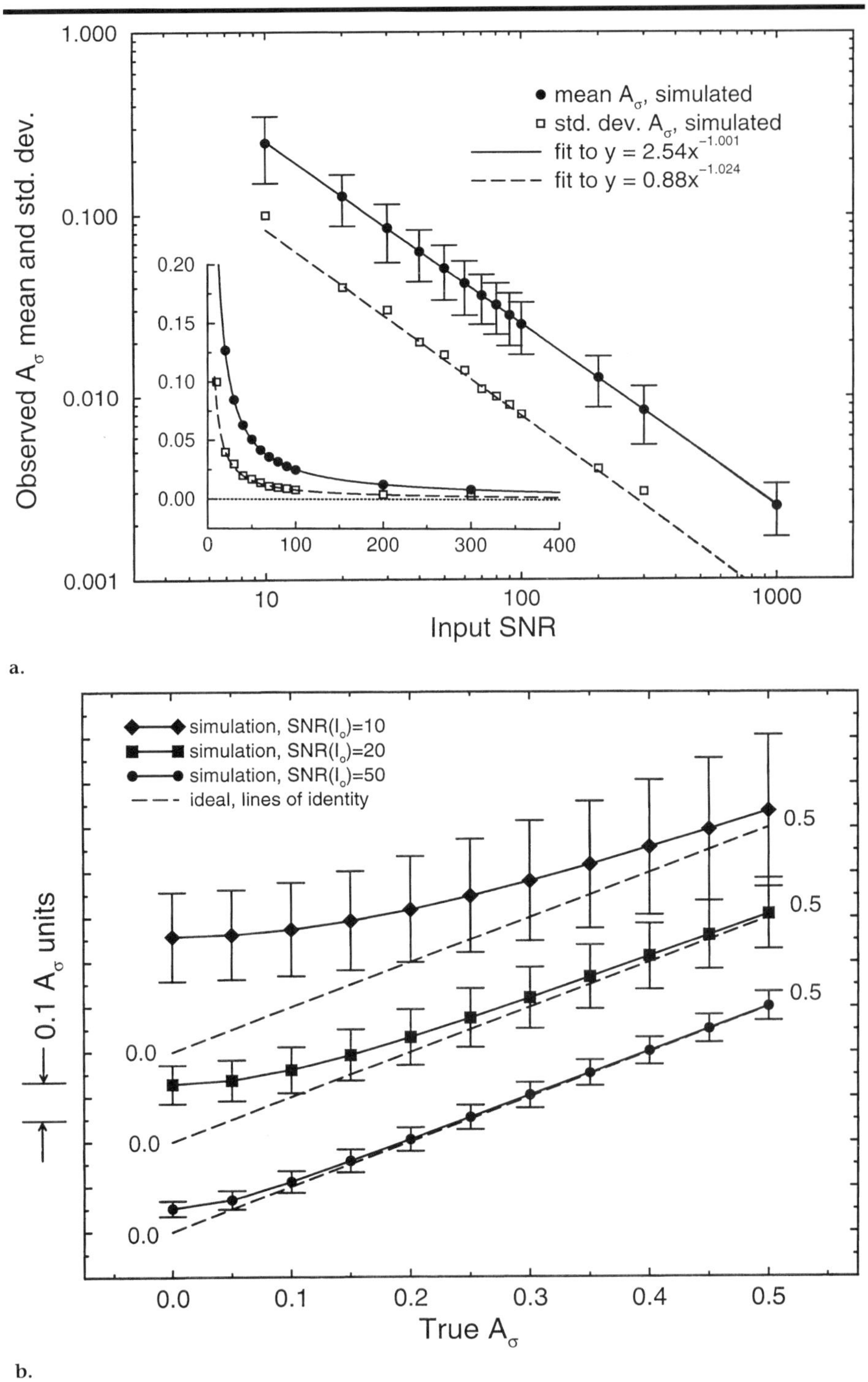

Figure 6. Graphs show results of simulation of the effect of noise on the accuracy and precision of A_σ measurements for **(a)** isotropic tissues and **(b)** axisymmetric anisotropic tissues. **(a)** Bias and random noise in the observed A_σ are graphed on linear (inset) and log-log scales versus the input SNR on the T2-weighted reference image. The bias and random noise are calculated as the mean and SD (*std. dev.*) of multiple experimental simulations as described in Materials and Methods. The simulation in **a** is for an ideal isotropic GM tissue that has the averaged diffusivity value of the putamen ($\overline{D} = 0.72 \times 10^{-3}$ mm²/sec). The mean and SD in A_σ are fit to the expression $y = Ax^B$, where A is the value at an SNR of 1 and B is the power of the dependence on SNR. **(b)** Bias and random noise in the observed A_σ are graphed as a function of A_σ at different reference image (I_0) SNR levels for an ideal axisymmetric WM tissue that has the same averaged diffusivity value as in **a**, similar to the averaged diffusivity value of the splenium of the corpus callosum. The simulations are for an A_σ value that ranges from 0.0 to 0.5, to represent the range for tissues shown in Table 1. Three reference SNR levels indicative of a range of MR imaging hardware are simulated, and the results are offset on the vertical axis for clarity. The SNR for the data acquired for Table 1 was approximately 40–60.

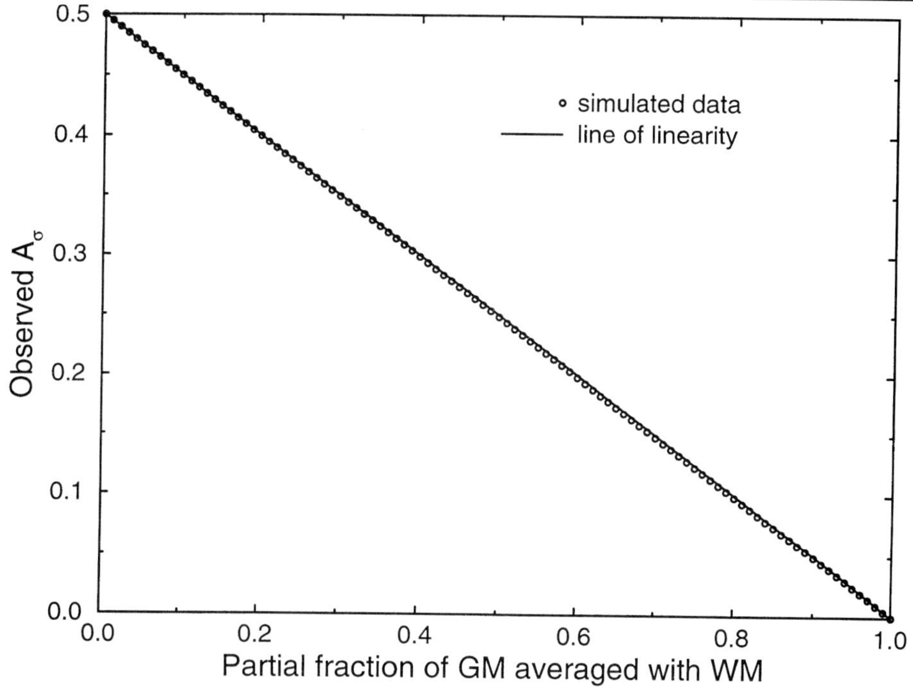

a.

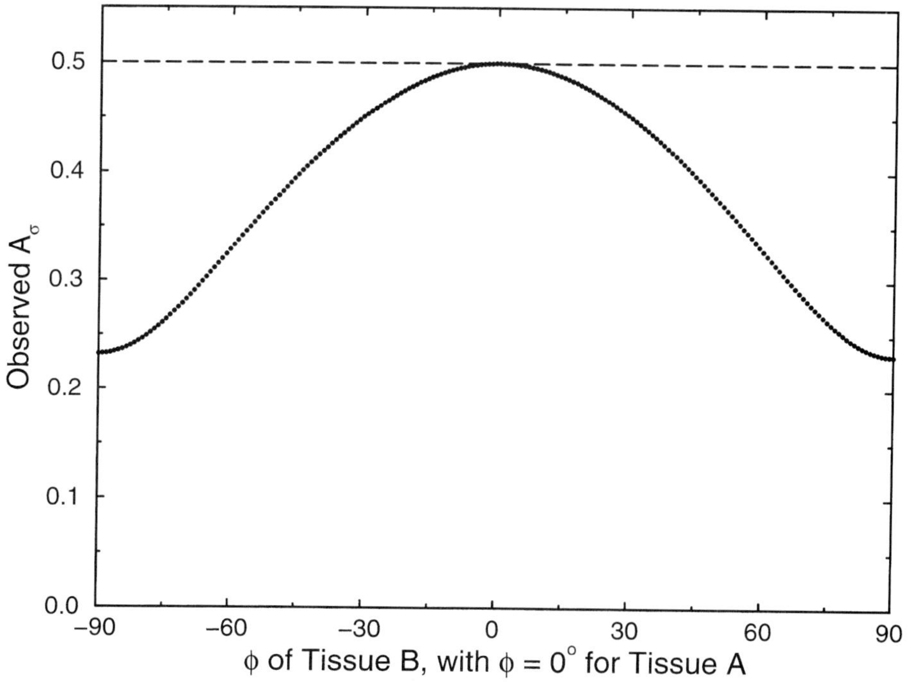

b.

Figure 7. Graphs shows the results of simulation of partial volume effects on measurement of A_σ for **(a)** intravoxel averaging of GM and WM and **(b)** averaging of two WM tissues with unaligned fiber orientations. **(a)** Ideal GM and WM were modeled after the putamen and splenium of the corpus callosum ($\overline{D} = 0.72 \times 10^{-3}$ mm^2/sec for GM and WM, $A_\sigma = 0$ for GM, $A_\sigma = 0.5$ and $A_{minor} = 0$ for WM, and arbitrary settings of $\phi = 20°$ and $\theta = 30°$ for WM). Note the nearly exact linear partial volume effect of GM on WM measurements. **(b)** Two WM tissues, each with the same WM averaged diffusivity ($\overline{D}$) and A_σ values as in **a** and with fibers lying in the transverse imaging plane ($\theta = 0°$), were averaged at different in-plane angular separations (ϕ). Note that angular separations of 90° result in a decrease of more than 50% in the observed A_σ. Dashed line = ideal measurement with no partial volume effect.

and across species is indicative that the data in Tables 1 and 2 can serve as a baseline for comparison with data from diseased brain.

Sorting of the ROIs according to A_σ value (Table 1) reveals a hierarchy of tissue types. The largest A_σ value was seen in the corpus callosum, which belongs to the commissural class of WM. The next largest group of values was seen in the internal capsule and the optic radiations, which belong to the projection class of WM. The association fibers seen in subcortical WM and the external capsule have a still lower set of anisotropy values. This grouping of A_σ values also is suggested in Table 3, where block-diagonal groups of tissue with statistically similar A_σ values generally segregated into these functional tissue classes.

It is interesting that the clinically observed spread of vasogenic edema into these tissue classes has a known similar order of preference, with distribution into association fibers in mild cases and into commissural fibers only in severe cases (46,47). This observation suggests that A_σ may be correlated with resistance to vasogenic fluid spread, possibly owing to dependence on common histologic structural features of WM. The A_σ value and other anisotropy measures may thus be indexes of microscopic architectural characteristics, such as fiber packing density, myelination, order, and/or directional coherence. The sensitivity of A_σ to WM class suggests that, in general, A_σ may be sensitive to changes and abnormalities in WM structure and organization. This sensitivity is supported by results from recent studies of human brain maturation (24,25) and multiple sclerosis (21–23) and other myelination abnormalities (20). The time (approximately 1½ minutes) needed to obtain these data with full brain coverage makes this method practical for clinical applications.

The GM tissues listed in Table 1 (basal ganglia and cortical GM), which are composed mainly of cell bodies, demonstrate an A_σ value consistent with 0 at the SNR levels used in this study. This conclusion is based on the simulation results shown in Figure 6a. Among the ROIs in Table 1 that are consistent with nonzero anisotropy, the thalamus has the smallest A_σ value (see also the simulation results in Fig 6b). Structured anisotropy patterns were present in the thalamus (Figs 2, 5) and likely affected the ROI measurements (Fig 3); thus, the thalamic values should be considered only an average of tissue substructures (eg, nuclei and WM tracts).

The simulation results shown in Figure 6a demonstrate that the bias and noise in GM A_σ values will both be reduced by increasing the SNR of the acquired images (graphed as the SNR of the reference T2-weighted image). Specifically, the A_σ bias and noise are inversely proportional to the reference SNR (Fig 6a); that is, the SNR and signal-to-bias ratios of A_σ are proportional to the reference SNR. The inverse proportionality between bias and reference SNR is a direct result of the definition of A_σ, where A_σ is, in effect, a measure of the SD of diffusivity measurements in different directions (see Appendix, Eq [A1]). Because the SD of a scalar diffusivity measurement generally is inversely proportional to the reference SNR at typical clinical SNR levels (26,48), there is an overall inverse proportionality between A_σ and the reference SNR.

The simulation results shown in Figure 6b indicate that A_σ bias can also occur in WM measurements and can be reduced by increasing the reference SNR. At a reference SNR of approximately 40–60 (as used in this study), bias becomes significant (ie, greater than the SD of the random noise) for anisotropy measurements of less than 0.05. For the lower input SNRs of 20 and 10, A_σ measurements of less than 0.1 and 0.2, respectively, were predicted to contain significant bias. The curves in Figure 6 can serve as calibrations to adjust WM A_σ measurements on the basis of the input SNR.

The simulation results shown in Figure 6 suggest that acquisition of data with an increased SNR (eg, by means of signal averaging, as in Fig 5) will likely improve the statistical characterization of tissue types, owing to a reduction in A_σ noise and bias. Reduction in bias is particularly relevant to characterization of tissues across institutions and equipment, where SNR levels may differ.

However, the improvements in tissue characterization that can be gained by increases in the SNR may be limited by two factors: (*a*) practical limitations in the number of signals acquired, and (*b*) biologic variability across subjects. The first factor is demonstrated in Figure 6a, which indicates that reductions in A_σ noise and bias that could be achieved by means of averaging would be modest when the input SNR already is high (eg, >50). For example, with a reference T2-weighted MR image SNR of 50:1 without averaging, approximately four signals would need to be acquired and averaged to reduce the bias by a factor of two, from 0.05 to 0.025, and approximately 16 signals would need to be acquired and averaged to reduce the bias by a factor of four to 0.0126. The A_σ noise would be reduced by similar relative amounts. As a corollary, extensive signal acquisition would be necessary to enable detection of low-level GM anisotropy below the detectable level in this study. Such extensive signal acquisition may not be practical in the clinical setting.

The second practical limitation in tissue characterization is variability across subjects. Further analysis of the raw ROI data that contributed to the results given in Table 1 (not shown) indicated that the variation in ROI A_σ values of GM across subjects was dominated by thermal MR noise, with an overall observed SD that was only 1.1–1.7 times that predicted on the basis of thermal MR noise alone. In contrast, for the WM tissues listed in Table 1, the overall SD, across subjects, was 1.5–4.0 times that predicted on the basis of thermal noise alone.

Such variations in measurement that are beyond the thermal noise limit may be due to two factors: biologic variability across subjects and variability in ROI sampling of spatially heterogeneous or small structures. GM measurement variability was near the thermal noise limit, likely because of the spatial homogeneity (Fig 3) and zero anisotropy of the regions, which led to accurate sampling and low biologic variation, respectively. In contrast, the higher variability in WM measurements likely was due to the spatial inhomogeneity and small size of the measured WM structures (Fig 3), which would contribute to sampling errors, and the nonzero anisotropy values, which may be sensitive to biologic differences between subjects. Because the variation in WM A_σ values across subjects was due to factors in addition to thermal noise, increases in the reference SNR alone may have a limited effect on statistical tissue characterization across subjects. If a major component of the WM variability is due to region sampling rather than to biologic differences, measurement variability across subjects may be reduced by trading off a higher SNR for higher spatial resolution.

The images of A_{major} (Fig 2, *b*) have an appearance and noise level similar to those of A_σ (Fig 2, *a*). The rank order of A_{major} across tissue was identical to that of A_σ, both being correlated with WM class (Table 1). In contrast, A_{minor} (Fig 2, *c*) had a different appearance than A_σ and did not correlate well with WM class (Table 1). Regions of higher A_{minor} (eg, genu of the internal capsule) deviated from axisymmetry, possibly because of inhomogeneous fiber orientation and/or spacing. It is possible that the appearance of A_{minor} may be dependent on spatial resolution due to partial volume effects (see Fig 7b). The principal diffusion coefficients $\lambda_{x'}$, $\lambda_{y'}$, and $\lambda_{z'}$ given in Table 2 generally had a ranking that could be correlated with WM tissue class, but the ranking was less characteristic for the thalamus and GM. Also shown in Table 2 is the wide range of values (nearly sixfold) in the principal diffusion coefficients in tissue with high A_σ such as the splenium of the corpus callosum.

Evaluation of partial anisotropy-weighted MR measures (see Appendix, Eqq [A4,A5]) demonstrates their qualitative utility and limitations in cases where the full diffusion tensor is not available. A larger component of the anisotropy resides in the tetrahedral gradient encoding as compared with orthogonal gradient encoding. This is shown qualitatively in Figure 2, *d* and *e*, and quantitatively by comparing the two anisotropy-weighted components in Table 1. The average value of the ratio of AW_{tet} to AW_{ortho} is 2.56, as computed with the data in Table 1. An example of the orientation-dependent deficits predicted earlier (see "Theory" in Materials and Methods) for the anisotropy-weighted components is the focal AW_{tet} deficit in the splenium of the corpus callosum (Fig 2, *d*), which was consistent across subjects. The direction of the fibers in this tract is aligned with the y axis ($\theta = 90°$, $\phi = 90°$), a direction in which anisotropy is not expected to be effectively recovered by AW_{tet} on the basis of Figure 4 and Equation (A7) in the Appendix. This focal deficit can, in principle, be partially corrected in the case of a tetrahedral-only acquisition by dividing AW_{tet} by f_{tet} in Equation (A7) in the Appendix, where f_{tet} is computed by using θ and ϕ derived from the tetrahedral data (26). This procedure would be equivalent to generation of the entire diffusion tensor from the tetrahedral data, given the axisymmetric assumption, and then by computing A_σ from Equation (3).

Noticeable deficits also were present on AW_{ortho} MR images, such as the marked reduction in intensity in the lateral genu of the corpus callosum (Fig 2, *e*), where the fibers are oriented toward the tetrahedral directions. However, AW_{ortho} cannot be corrected by dividing by f_{ortho}, in the case of orthogonal-only acquisition, because the data are not sufficient to determine θ and ϕ.

In summary, high-SNR MR diffusion-tensor data were analyzed, and quantitative anisotropy was measured in 13 neurologically healthy adults. Anisotropy, or A_σ, images demonstrated WM anatomy not typically seen on conventional MR images, with statistically significant A_σ differences in different histologic WM classes that were ranked according to known resistance to edema spread, which is suggestive of a sensitivity to WM microstructure. Images of A_σ demonstrated the external capsule; the thickness of the internal capsule; and substructures of the thalamus, basal ganglia, and occipital white matter, which are not readily seen on conventional MR images. The rotationally invariant A_σ can be calculated directly from the diffusion tensor elements or, as an alternative, directly from the seven diffusion coefficients measured with tetrahedral and orthogonal diffusion encoding. Unlike other anisotropy measures, determination of A_σ does not require diagonalization of the diffusion tensor or sorting of eigenvalues and is on an absolute anisotropy scale of 0–1. Statistically significant differences were found between A_σ values in different histologic classes of WM: From highest to lowest A_σ value, these were commissural WM, projection WM, association WM, and the thalamus. This anisotropy rank was correlated with the known resistance of WM to the spread of vasogenic edema as seen radiologically. Anisotropy measured in the basal ganglia and the cortical GM was consistent with an A_σ value of 0. The ability to distinguish among different histologic classes of cerebral tissue by using anisotropy measurement is suggestive of a sensitivity to microscopic WM fiber structure and may presage the ability to use A_σ to identify WM disease.

APPENDIX

Theory and Computation of Diffusion-Tensor Anisotropy

The A_σ value is a measure of diffusion variation derived from the second moment (variance) of the diffusion tensor **D**:

$$A_\sigma = \frac{1}{\sqrt{2}}\frac{\sigma(\mathbf{D})}{\overline{D}} = \frac{1}{\sqrt{6}}\frac{\sqrt{Tr[(\mathbf{D}-\overline{D}\mathbf{I})^2]}}{\overline{D}}, \quad \text{(A1)}$$

where **I** is the unit matrix; *Tr* is the trace of the matrix specified in the brackets, which is given by the sum of its diagonal elements; and $\sigma(\mathbf{D})$ represents the SD of diffusion coefficients that would be obtained with multiple measurements in different directions. Equation (A1) can be expanded to

$$A_\sigma = \frac{1}{\sqrt{6}\overline{D}}\sqrt{\sum_{i,j=x,y,z}(D_{ij}-\overline{D}\delta_{ij})^2}$$

$$= \sqrt{A^2_{major} + \frac{1}{3}A^2_{minor}}, \quad \text{(A2)}$$

with δ_{ij} representing the Kronecker delta value. The first part of Equation (A2) yields Equation (3). The last part of Equation (A2) is derived by decomposing the diffusion tensor into axisymmetric and nonaxisymmetric parts (26) and expresses A_σ in terms of the major and minor anisotropy values, A_{major} and A_{minor}.

The A_σ value in Equation (A2) can be written as a function of the seven diffusion coefficients measured in the combined tetrahedral-orthogonal approach:

$$A_\sigma = \frac{1}{\sqrt{6}\overline{D}} \times \sqrt{\sum_{i=x,y,z}(D_{ii}-\overline{D})^2 + \frac{9}{8}\sum_{j=1-4}(D_j-\overline{D})^2}, \quad \text{(A3)}$$

where D_1, D_2, D_3, and D_4 are the diffusion coefficients in the tetrahedral directions (26). To assess the anisotropy information contained in the data, A_σ can then be decomposed into partial, noninvariant anisotropy-weighted component measures. Anisotropy weighting can be obtained from the SD of the diagonal elements measured from orthogonal encoding, as proposed by van Gelderen et al (16):

$$AW_{ortho} = \frac{1}{\sqrt{6}\overline{D}}\sqrt{\sum_{i=x,y,z}(D_{ii}-\overline{D})^2}. \quad \text{(A4)}$$

In similar fashion, anisotropy weighting can be obtained from the SD of the off-diagonal elements contained in Equation (3) and expressed in terms of the tetrahedral diffusion measurements in Equation (A3):

$$AW_{tet} = \frac{\sqrt{3}}{4\overline{D}}\sqrt{\sum_{j=1-4}(D_j-\overline{D})^2}. \quad \text{(A5)}$$

The full, invariant anisotropy A_σ is obtained by adding the two-component anisotropy-weighted measures in quadrature:

$$A_\sigma = \sqrt{AW^2_{tet} + AW^2_{ortho}}. \quad \text{(A6)}$$

In general, A_σ can be computed from Equation (3) by using values of the diffusion-tensor elements that have been globally fit to the entire data set. As an alternative, A_σ can be computed from Equation (A3) by using the diffusion coefficients directly measured at separate orthogonal and tetrahedral experiments. In comparison with the latter approach, the former global analysis procedure constrains the analysis in this overdetermined case (ie, seven diffusion-weighted images that encode seven diffusion coefficients D_1, D_2, D_3, D_4, D_{xx}, D_{yy}, and D_{zz} used to estimate six unknown diffusion-tensor elements). Separate calculation of the diagonal and off-diagonal elements from the orthogonal and tetrahedral data, respectively, would not take advantage of the additional constraint that both methods should yield the same averaged diffusivity (ie, $\overline{D} = ⅓[D_{xx} + D_{yy} + D_{zz}] = ¼[D_1 + D_2 + D_3 + D_4]$).

Information Content of Anisotropy-weighted Indexes

Certain WM regions may exhibit symmetry that can simplify the evaluation of the diffusion tensor and provide insight about the information contained in anisotropy-weighted indexes in Equations (A4,A5). Voxels composed of muscle or WM fibers with uniform packing and direction may demonstrate axial or cylindric symmetry. In this approximation, the diffusion ellipsoid is prolate, with diffusivity parallel to the tract that is larger than the diffusivity perpendicular to the tract. Furthermore, the two perpendicular diffusivities would be equal ($A_{minor} = 0$ and $A_\sigma = |A_{major}|$); therefore, the rotation angle around the major axis can be set to 0° with no loss of generality. In the axisymmetric approximation, only four scalars are needed to represent the diffusion tensor: the parallel and perpendicular diffusivity and two rotation angles (26,49). In this case, the tetrahedral gradient-encoding method, which is used to acquire diffusion data in four diffusion directions for each voxel, can be used to completely determine the diffusion tensor.

Under conditions of axisymmetry, a direct expression can be written relating A_σ to the off-diagonal diffusion-tensor elements by using equations (16,27c) in Conturo et al (26). However, computation of A_σ with this expression may, in some cases, be unstable, due to division by small off-diagonal elements (data not shown). In contrast, computations of the in-plane angle ϕ and the through-plane angle θ by using equations (27a,27b) in Conturo et al are stable for imaging in humans (30) because of the favorable properties of the arc-tangent function. Thus, a more stable procedure for computation of A_σ from tetrahedral measurements can be devised as follows in the case of axisymmetric diffusion: The A_σ value can be expressed as a function of its anisotropy-weighted tetrahedral component in Equation (A5) and of the angles θ and ϕ, computed with the arc-tangent function. We derive expressions for the fractional recovery of anisotropy contained in the anisotropy-weighted tetrahedral ($f_{tet}[\theta,\phi]$) and orthogonal ($f_{ortho}[\theta,\phi]$) components as a ratio of the full A_σ. These ratios are only functions of θ and ϕ:

$$f^2_{tet}(\theta,\phi) = \frac{AW^2_{tet}}{A^2_\sigma} = \frac{3}{4}(\sin^4\theta\sin^2 2\phi + \sin^2 2\theta), \quad \text{(A7)}$$

and

$$f^2_{ortho}(\theta,\phi) = \frac{AW^2_{ortho}}{A^2_\sigma} = 1 - f^2_{tet}(\theta,\phi). \quad \text{(A8)}$$

The ratios f_{tet} and f_{ortho} indicate how much of A_σ is recovered in the anisotropy-weighted measures. The expressions in Equations (A7,A8) are specific to the axisymmetric case. Because AW_{tet} can be calculated directly from the tetrahedral diffusion coefficient measurements by using Equation (A5), and θ and ϕ can be calculated under the axisymmetric assumption (26), A_σ can be obtained with Equation (A7) in the axisymmetric case.

Because the averaged diffusivity can be obtained from the tetrahedral or orthogonal gradient-encoding data alone, either encoding method can have clinical applications in cases such as cerebral ischemia. It is thus desirable to analyze what anisotropy-weighted information can be obtained in those cases. The ratios in Equations (A7,A8) are estimates of how much of the total anisotropy A_σ is contained in the separate anisotropy-weighted measurements; that is, in the on- and off-diagonal elements. If the axes of the diffusion ellipsoid are aligned along the coordinate axes, all four tetrahedral measurements are equivalent, and the full anisotropy is contained in AW_{ortho}. In similar fashion, if the ellipsoid axes are aligned with the tetrahedral directions, the full anisotropy is contained in AW_{tet}.

For axisymmetric diffusion, only the major axis must be aligned for these conditions to be met. Specifically, it can be shown from Equation (A7), in the axisymmetric case, that f_{tet} is 0 at θ values of 0° and 180° (along the z axis) and at θ values of 90° when φ is 0°, 90°, 180°, and 270° (along the x or y axis) (see Fig 4a, 4d). Likewise, it can be shown from Equation (A8) that f_{ortho} is 0 at a θ of 54.74° (half the tetrahedral angle) when φ is ±45°, ±135° and at θ of 125.26° (180° − 54.74°) when φ is ±45°, ±135° (see Fig 4b, 4c). For intermediate alignments, the anisotropy is distributed between the two anisotropy-weighted components, which add in quadrature to yield the full anisotropy value.

References

1. Stejskal EO, Tanner JE. Spin diffusion measurements: spin echoes in the presence of a time dependent field gradient. J Chem Phys 1965; 42:288–292.
2. Le Bihan D, Breton E. Imagerie de diffusion in vivo par résonance magnètique nucléaire. CR Acad Sci Paris 1985; 301:1109–1112.
3. Le Bihan D, Breton E, Lallemand D, Grenier P, Cabanis E, Laval-Jeantet M. MR imaging of intravoxel incoherent motions: application to diffusion and perfusion in neurologic disorders. Radiology 1986; 161:401–407.
4. Taylor DG, Bushell MC. The spatial mapping of translational diffusion coefficients by the NMR imaging technique. Phys Med Biol 1985; 30:345–349.
5. Mansfield P. Multi-planar imaging using NMR spin-echoes. J Phys [C] 1977; 10:L55–L58.
6. Avram H, Crooks L. Effect of self-diffusion on echoplanar imaging (abstr). In: Book of abstracts: Society of Magnetic Resonance in Medicine 1988. Berkeley, Calif: Society of Magnetic Resonance in Medicine, 1988; 980.
7. Turner R, Le Bihan D, Maier J, Vavrek R, Hedges LK, Pekar J. Echo-planar imaging of intravoxel incoherent motion. Radiology 1990; 177:407–414.
8. Turner R, Le Bihan D. Single-shot diffusion imaging at 2.0 Tesla. J Magn Reson 1990; 86:445–452.
9. McKinstry RC, Weisskoff RM, Cohen MS, et al. Instant MR diffusion/perfusion imaging (abstr). In: Book of abstracts: Society of Magnetic Resonance in Medicine 1990. Berkeley, Calif: Society of Magnetic Resonance in Medicine, 1990; 401.
10. Moseley ME, Cohen Y, Kucharczyk J, et al. Diffusion-weighted MR imaging of anisotropic water diffusion in cat central nervous system. Radiology 1990; 176:439–445.
11. Doran M, Hajnal JV, Van Bruggen N, King MD, Young IR, Bydder GM. Normal and abnormal white matter tracts shown by MR imaging using directional diffusion weighted sequences. J Comput Assist Tomogr 1990; 14:865–873.
12. Crank J. The mathematics of diffusion. Oxford, England: Clarendon, 1975.
13. Basser PJ, Mattiello J, Le Bihan D. Estimation of the effective self-diffusion tensor from the NMR spin echo. J Magn Reson B 1994; 103:247–254.
14. Basser PJ, Mattiello J, Le Bihan D. MR diffusion tensor spectroscopy and imaging. Biophys J 1994; 66:259–267.
15. Sorensen AG, Buonanno FS, Gonzalez RG, et al. Hyperacute stroke: evaluation with combined multisection diffusion-weighted and hemodynamically weighted echo-planar MR imaging. Radiology 1996; 199:391–401.
16. van Gelderen P, de Vleeschouwer MH, DesPres D, Pekar J, van Zijl PC, Moonen CT. Water diffusion and acute stroke. Magn Reson Med 1994; 31:154–163.
17. Pierpaoli C, Jezzard P, Basser PJ, Barnett A, Di Chiro G. Diffusion tensor MR imaging of the human brain. Radiology 1996; 201:637–648.
18. Shimony JS, McKinstry RC, Akbudak E, Snyder AZ, Aronovitz JA, Conturo TE. Cerebral diffusion tensor imaging: normative data, signal to noise measurements, and anatomical findings (abstr). In: Proceedings of the Fifth Meeting of the International Society for Magnetic Resonance in Medicine. Berkeley, Calif: International Society for Magnetic Resonance in Medicine, 1997; 225.
19. Shimony JS, McKinstry RC, Akbudak E, Aronovitz JA, Snyder AZ, Conturo TE. Quantitative diffusion tensor anisotropy imaging: normative human cerebral data (abstr). In: Proceedings of the Sixth Meeting of the International Society for Magnetic Resonance in Medicine. Berkeley, Calif: International Society for Magnetic Resonance in Medicine, 1998; 1241.
20. Ono J, Harada K, Mano T, Sakurai K, Okada S. Differentiation of dys- and demyelination using diffusional anisotropy. Pediatr Neurol 1997; 16:63–66.
21. Werring DJ, Clark CA, Barker GJ, et al. The structural properties of multiple sclerosis lesions demonstrated by diffusion tensor imaging (abstr). In: Proceedings of the Sixth Meeting of the International Society for Magnetic Resonance in Medicine. Berkeley, Calif: International Society for Magnetic Resonance in Medicine, 1998; 119.
22. Zhong J, Graham GD, Guarnaccia JB, Hadeishi Y, Gore JC. Quantitative apparent diffusion coefficient and diffusion anisotropy analysis of multiple sclerosis plaques (abstr). In: Proceedings of the Sixth Meeting of the International Society for Magnetic Resonance in Medicine. Berkeley, Calif: International Society for Magnetic Resonance in Medicine, 1998; 1324.
23. Shimony JS, Akbudak E, McKinstry RC, Lori N, Cull TS, Conturo TE. Quantitative diffusion anisotropy imaging: normal values, anatomical findings, and results in relapsing remitting multiple sclerosis (abstr). Radiology 1998; 209(P):240.
24. Neil JJ, Shiran SI, McKinstry RC, et al. Normal brain in human newborns: apparent diffusion and diffusion anisotropy measured by using diffusion tensor MR imaging. Radiology 1998; 209:57–66.
25. Takeda K, Nomura Y, Sakuma H, Tagami T, Okuda Y, Nakagawa T. MR assessment of normal brain development in neonates and infants: comparative study of T1- and diffusion weighted images. J Comput Assist Tomogr 1997; 21:1–7.
26. Conturo TE, McKinstry RC, Akbudak E, Robinson BH. Encoding of anisotropic diffusion with tetrahedral gradients: a general mathematical diffusion formalism and experimental results. Magn Reson Med 1996; 35:399–412.
27. Basser PJ. Inferring microstructural features and the physiological state of tissues from diffusion-weighted images. NMR Biomed 1995; 8:333–344.
28. Basser PJ, Pierpaoli C. Microstructural and physiological features of tissues elucidated by quantitative-diffusion-tensor MRI. J Magn Reson B 1996; 111:209–219.
29. Pierpaoli C, Basser PJ. Toward a quantitative assessment of diffusion anisotropy. Magn Reson Med 1996; 36:893–906.
30. McKinstry RC, Akbudak E, Snyder AZ, Aronovitz JA, Conturo TE. Echo planar human diffusion tensor imaging with tetrahedral encoding (abstr). In: Proceedings of the Fourth Meeting of the International Society for Magnetic Resonance in Medicine. Berkeley, Calif: International Society for Magnetic Resonance in Medicine, 1996; 192.
31. Conturo TE, McKinstry RC, Aronovitz JA, Neil JJ. Diffusion MRI: precision, accuracy and flow effects. NMR Biomed 1995; 8:307–332.
32. Cantor CR, Shimmel PR. Biophysical chemistry part II: techniques for the study of biological structure and function. San Francisco, Calif: Freeman, 1980; 457–458.
33. Reese TG, Weisskoff RM, Smith RN, Rosen BR, Dinsmore RE, Wedeen VJ. Imaging myocardial fiber architecture in vivo with magnetic resonance. Magn Reson Med 1995; 34: 786–791.
34. Basser PJ, Pierpaoli CA. A simplified method to measure the diffusion tensor from seven MR images. Magn Reson Med 1998; 39:928–934.
35. National Electrical Manufacturers Association. Determination of SNR in diagnostic magnetic resonance images. Washington, DC: National Electrical Manufacturers Association, 1988.
36. Mattiello J, Basser PJ, Le Bihan D. The b matrix in diffusion tensor echo-planar imaging. Magn Reson Med 1997; 37:292–300.
37. Le Bihan D. Diffusion and perfusion magnetic resonance imaging: applications to functional MRI. New York, NY: Raven, 1995.
38. Moonen CT, Pekar J, de Vleeschouwer MH, van Gelderen P, van Zijl PC, DesPres D. Restricted and anisotropic displacement of water in healthy cat brain and in stroke studied by NMR diffusion imaging. Magn Reson Med 1991; 19:327–332.
39. Norris DG, Niendorf T, Hoehn-Berlage M, et al. Incidence of apparent restricted diffusion in three different models of cerebral infarction. Magn Reson Imaging 1994; 12:1175–1182.
40. McKinstry RC, Weiskoff RM, Belliveau JW, et al. Ultrafast MR imaging of water mobility: animal models of altered cerebral perfusion. JMRI 1992; 2:377–384.
41. Haselgrove JC, Moore JR. Correction for distortion of echo-planar images used to calculate the apparent diffusion coefficient. Magn Reson Med 1996; 36:960–964.
42. Snyder AZ. Difference image vs ratio image error function forms in PET-PET realignment. In: Myers R, Cunningham V, Bailey D, Jones T, eds. Quantification of brain function using PET. San Diego, Calif: Academic Press, 1995; 131–137.
43. Ojemann JG, Buckner RL, Akbudak E, et al. Functional MRI studies of word stem completion: reliability across laboratories and comparison to blood flow imaging with PET. Hum Brain Mapp 1998; 6:203–215.
44. Bevington P. Data reduction and error analysis for the physical sciences. New York, NY: McGraw-Hill, 1969.
45. DeArmond SJ, Fusco MM, Dewey MM. Structure of the human brain: a photographic atlas. New York, NY: Oxford University Press, 1989.
46. Cowley AR. Dyke award: influence of fiber tracts on the CT appearance of cerebral edema—anatomic-pathologic correlation. AJNR 1983; 4:915–925.
47. Moody DM, Bell MA, Challa VR. The corpus callosum, a unique white-matter tract: anatomic features that may explain sparing in Binswanger disease and resistance to flow of fluid masses. AJNR 1988; 9:1051–1059.
48. Chien D, Buxton RB, Kwong KK, Brady TJ, Rosen BR. MR diffusion imaging of the human brain. J Comput Assist Tomogr 1990; 14:514–520.
49. Hsu EW, Mori S. Analytical expressions for the NMR apparent diffusion coefficients in an anisotropic system and a simplified method for determining fiber orientation. Magn Reson Med 1995; 34:194–200.

A. Gregory Sorensen, MD
Ona Wu, MS
William A. Copen, AM
Timothy L. Davis, PhD
R. Gilberto Gonzalez, MD, PhD
Walter J. Koroshetz, MD
Timothy G. Reese, PhD
Bruce R. Rosen, MD, PhD
Van J. Wedeen, MD
Robert M. Weisskoff, PhD

Index terms:
Anisotropy
Brain, diffusion, 10.12144, 10.92
Brain, infarction, 10.78
Brain, ischemia, 10.781
Brain, MR, 10.121411, 10.12144
Diffusion tensor
Magnetic resonance (MR), diffusion study, 10.12144, 10.92
Magnetic resonance (MR), echo planar, 10.121412, 10.12144

Radiology 1999; 212:785–792

Abbreviations:
ADC = apparent diffusion coefficient
CNR = contrast-to-noise ratio
ROI = region of interest
SNR = signal-to-noise ratio

[1] From the Departments of Radiology (A.G.S., O.W., W.A.C., T.L.D., R.G.G., T.G.R., B.R.R., V.J.W., R.M.W.) and Neurology (W.J.K.), Massachusetts General Hospital and Harvard Medical School, Neuroradiology Section and MGH-NMR Center, Mailcode CNY 149-2301, Boston, MA 02119. Received April 13, 1998; revision requested June 30; revision received November 24; accepted March 29, 1999. **Address reprint requests to** A.G.S. (e-mail: *sorensen@nmr.mgh.harvard.edu*).

Author contributions:
Guarantor of integrity of entire study, A.G.S.; study concepts and design, A.G.S., O.W., B.R.R., R.M.W.; definition of intellectual content, A.G.S., O.W., T.L.D., T.G.R., B.R.R., V.J.W., R.M.W.; literature research, A.G.S., O.W.; clinical studies, A.G.S., R.G.G., W.J.K.; experimental studies, A.G.S., O.W., T.L.D., T.G.R., B.R.R., V.J.W., R.M.W.; data acquisition, A.G.S., R.G.G., W.J.K.; data analysis, A.G.S., O.W., W.A.C., T.L.D., B.R.R., R.M.W.; statistical analysis, A.G.S., O.W., W.A.C., B.R.R., R.M.W.; manuscript preparation, A.G.S., O.W., T.L.D.; manuscript editing and review, all authors.

Human Acute Cerebral Ischemia: Detection of Changes in Water Diffusion Anisotropy by Using MR Imaging[1]

PURPOSE: To (*a*) determine the optimal choice of a scalar metric of anisotropy and (*b*) determine by means of magnetic resonance imaging if changes in diffusion anisotropy occurred in acute human ischemic stroke.

MATERIALS AND METHODS: The full diffusion tensor over the entire brain was measured. To optimize the choice of a scalar anisotropy metric, the performances of scalar indices in simulated models and in a healthy volunteer were analyzed. The anisotropy, trace apparent diffusion coefficient (ADC), and eigenvalues of the diffusion tensor in lesions and contralateral normal brain were compared in 50 patients with stroke.

RESULTS: Changes in anisotropy in patients were quantified by using fractional anisotropy because it provided the best performance in terms of contrast-to-noise ratio as a function of signal-to-noise ratio in simulations. The anisotropy of ischemic white matter decreased ($P = .01$). Changes in anisotropy in ischemic gray matter were not significant ($P = .63$). The trace ADC decreased for ischemic gray matter and white matter ($P < .001$). The first and second eigenvalues decreased in both ischemic gray and ischemic white matter ($P < .001$). The third eigenvalue decreased in ischemic gray ($P = .001$) and white matter ($P = .03$).

CONCLUSION: Gray matter is mildly anisotropic in normal and early ischemic states. However, early white matter ischemia is associated with not only changes in trace ADC values but also significant changes in the anisotropy, or shape, of the water self-diffusion tensor.

Magnetic resonance (MR) imaging has excelled at depicting the macroscopic anatomy of the human brain. However, many normal cellular functions and disease processes that occur at the microscopic level do not affect conventional MR relaxation parameters. As a result, certain disease processes such as early acute cerebral ischemia are poorly assessed with conventional MR imaging. Routine diagnosis could be improved if MR imaging could be used to investigate events at the microscopic level; this has been shown to be possible with acute ischemic stroke, for which diffusion- and perfusion-weighted MR imaging have been used to document abnormalities, even when conventional MR imaging shows no abnormality (1–3).

To date, most diffusion imaging of humans in a clinical environment has been used to measure either a single direction of the diffusion tensor (1,2,4–12) or the trace of the diffusion tensor (1,3,13–18). Several studies (19–24) have documented marked anisotropy in the normal human brain, particularly in regions of white matter. However, to our knowledge, in only a few studies (25,26) has the full diffusion tensor been measured. Studies (26,27) sampling the full diffusion tensor in patients with chronic stroke have found changes in anisotropy values in infarcted tissue compared with those for normal contralateral tissue. In addition, with use of the full diffusion tensor, chronic changes in tensor orientation were measured in a patient who had an embolic infarct (27).

On the basis of evidence of changes in anisotropy in patients with chronic stroke, we hypothesize that changes in anisotropy will also occur in cases of acute cerebral ischemia, particularly in white matter. Measuring the entire diffusion tensor during ischemia may thus provide insight regarding the mechanisms involved in acute ischemia and could improve diagnosis. In two earlier studies (28,29) in which middle cerebral arterial occlusion in cats was used, changes in anisotropy were not detected 15 hours after occlusion. However, in one study (30) in which middle cerebral arterial occlusion in rats was used, a reduction in anisotropy 24–48 hours after occlusion was measured. In none of these studies was the full diffusion tensor sampled. We sought to investigate changes in anisotropy in white matter and gray matter in human acute cerebral ischemia. We hypothesize that acute ischemic tissue, in particular areas normally anisotropic, such as white matter, will show changes in anisotropy compared with tissue in its normal state.

The diffusion tensor has six independent components, and therefore, the choice of the optimal way to view changes in the shape of the tensor is not obvious. Furthermore, if changes are to be measured and quantified, some type of metric, preferably a scalar metric rather than a vector or tensor metric, must be used. To visualize and to quantify changes in anisotropy during ischemia, we chose to evaluate and use scalar metrics. Because measurement of diffusion anisotropy can be complicated by the presence of noise (31), we first used Monte Carlo simulations and data from a healthy human volunteer to validate our metrics. We then applied our metrics to investigate changes during ischemia.

The Materials and Methods section of this article is divided into two parts. In the first section, Technical Development, we describe our implementation of diffusion tensor imaging and our evaluation of scalar metrics of anisotropy. In the second section, Human Acute Cerebral Ischemia, we describe the application of full-tensor imaging to human acute cerebral ischemia.

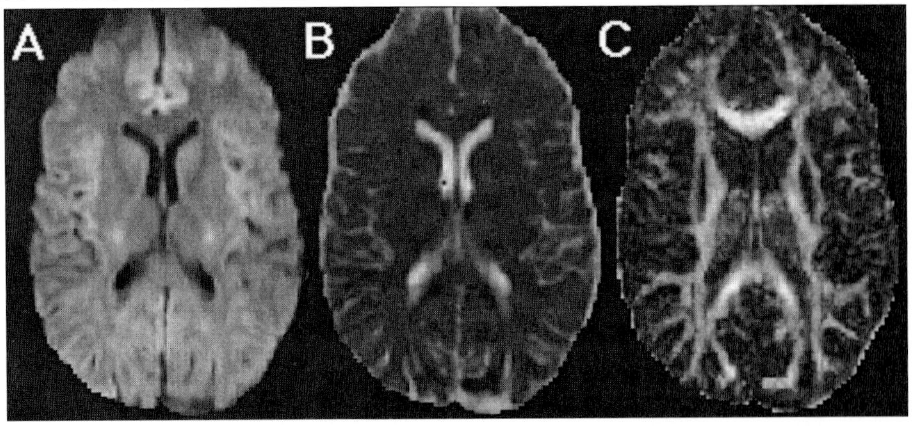

Figure 1. Images obtained axially in the healthy volunteer with use of 30 repetitions that resulted in an estimated SNR of 65. The SNR of our typical full-head diffusion tensor data set is 20. The imaging parameters were 6,000/118 (repetition time msec/echo time msec) with a b value of 1,221 sec/mm². *A*, Isotropic (trace) diffusion-weighted image. *B*, Mean trace ADC map. *C*, Fractional anisotropy map.

MATERIALS AND METHODS

Institutional review board approval and informed consent were obtained for our study.

Technical Development

Diffusion is the random translational motion of molecules owing to thermal energy. The diffusion process in three-dimensional space can be characterized by a symmetric tensor because its rate is direction-dependent and symmetric. This tensor has six degrees of freedom and thus can be represented by **D**, a 3 × 3 symmetric matrix (vector and tensor quantities are denoted in boldface). In isotropic media, **D** reduces to an identity matrix scaled by a constant, D, because the rate of diffusion is independent of direction, meaning that the probability that a particle moves to another point follows the behavior of a spherically symmetric Gaussian function (32). However, in the case of restricted diffusion, the diffusing particles encounter barriers that are direction dependent. The probability that a particle will move to another point then becomes a function of the geometry of the diffusion barriers (33) and results in diffusion coefficients that are anisotropic or direction dependent.

To measure the full diffusion tensor on a voxel-by-voxel basis, we used the pulsed field gradient method described by Stejskal and Tanner (34) by using seven measurements. The tensor was sampled by using a T2-weighted one-shot echo-planar imaging technique (35) repeated in seven different directions, which is the minimum required for solving for the diffusion coefficients that characterizes the diffusion tensor (36–39). Imaging was performed on a 1.5-T MR instrument with 5.4.2 software (Signa; GE Medical Systems, Milwaukee, Wis) and echo-planar imaging capabilities by means of a hardware upgrade (ANMR, Wilmington, Mass), including the "catch and hold" modification. We used T2-weighted single-shot pulsed field gradient spin-echo sequences that consisted of diffusion encoding pulses of a duration (∂) of 47 msec, with an interpulse temporal offset (Δ) of 52 msec, placed symmetrically about the 180° radio-frequency pulse. With catch-and-hold enabled, the echo time was 118 msec. We used a repetition time of 6,000 msec and obtained up to 20 axial sections with a 6-mm section thickness and a 1-mm spacing between sections. A fixed field of view of 40 × 20 cm and an acquisition matrix of 256 × 128 pixels were used. A single complete tensor acquisition required 42 seconds for imaging all sections.

Three full-head diffusion tensor samples typically were acquired and then averaged with a resultant signal-to-noise ratio (SNR) of approximately 20 in a total acquisition time of 126 seconds. The SNR was estimated from nondiffusion-weighted images after averaging by calculating the ratio of the mean signal intensity of a 5 × 5 region of interest (ROI) in the thalamus to the SD of the noise measured in background areas outside the head that were artifact free. A healthy 34-year-old man underwent imaging with an estimated SNR of 65 by using 30 full diffusion tensor samples for one axial section, with a total acquisition time of 21 minutes.

Diffusion gradients were applied in turn at $\mathbf{r_o} = (x,y,z) = (0.05, 0.05, 0.0)$ (a finite low b value rather than a b value of zero was used to avoid image artifacts) and the six $\mathbf{r_i} = \{(1,1,0), (1,-1,0), (0,1,1), (0,-1,1), (1,0,1), (-1,0,1)\}$ G/cm, which corresponded to the centers of the nonopposed edges of a cube. The approximate b value, where b is a measure of diffusion weighting (4), was 1,221 sec/mm² for each of the six directions and 3

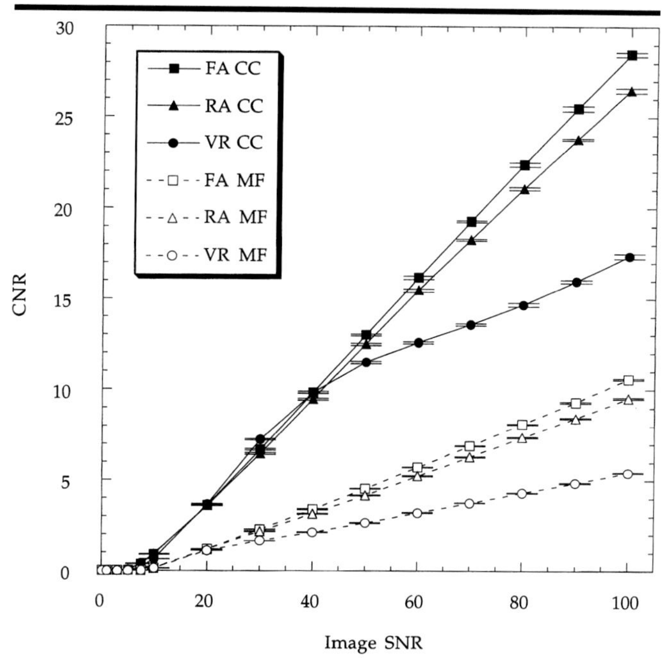

Figure 2. Graph shows CNR as a function of SNR for fractional anisotropy (*FA*), relative anisotropy (*RA*), and volume ratio (*VR*) indices computed from Monte Carlo simulations of two tissue types with different levels of anisotropy. The eigenvalues for the two tissue types were based on in vivo measurements of the splenium of the corpus callosum (*CC*) and the left forceps major (*MF*) in the healthy volunteer who underwent imaging with 30 repetitions instead of three and whose data are shown in Figure 1. The corpus callosum had eigenvalues of 1.7, 0.3, and 0.1 × 10^{-3} mm^2/sec, and the left forceps major had eigenvalues of 1.2, 0.9, and 0.3 × 10^{-3} mm^2/sec. The error bars represent the SD in computed CNR over 10 different simulations.

sec/mm^2 for the image obtained with a low *b* value. A unique solution for **D** can be obtained provided the 3 × 3 symmetric matrices, $\{\mathbf{r_i}\ \mathbf{r_i}^T\}$, $i = 1, \ldots, 6$, are linearly independent. In our calculations, we also included the effects of the imaging gradients in which techniques were used similar to those previously described (32–34). In addition, we corrected for eddy-current warping artifacts.

Once the diffusion tensor coefficients were computed, the diffusion tensor's eigenvalues, λ_i, and eigenvectors were calculated. The eigenvectors of the symmetric diffusion tensor, a set of orthogonal vectors, defined the orientation of the principal axes of the diffusion tensor ellipsoid in space. Their corresponding eigenvalues represent the lengths of the axes. These quantities therefore defined the size and shape of the ellipsoids of **D** and are independent of its orientation in its frame of measurement. From these eigenvalues, coordinate independent scalar functions of **D** were constructed that measured its degree of anisotropy.

A challenge to measuring anisotropy from the computed eigenvalues arises from noise contamination (31). For example, even in an isotropic sample, noise will make the computed eigenvalues unequal, with the resultant implication of some anisotropy. For anisotropy metrics that rely on sorting of the eigenvalues, a bias and a variance that depend on the diffusion properties of the tissue have been demonstrated (31). Therefore, in this study, we limited our evaluation of anisotropy metrics to intravoxel scalar indices (25,31,40) that did not require the sorting of eigenvalues.

We computed maps of fractional anisotropy, relative anisotropy, and volume ratio indices. Fractional anisotropy (FA), the ratio of the anisotropic component of the diffusion tensor to the whole diffusion tensor, is defined (40) as

$$\mathrm{FA}(\mathbf{D}) = \sqrt{\frac{3}{2}}\,\frac{\sqrt{\begin{array}{l}(\lambda_1 - \langle D\rangle)^2 + (\lambda_2 - \langle D\rangle)^2\\ \quad + (\lambda_3 - \langle D\rangle)^2\end{array}}}{\sqrt{\lambda_1^2 + \lambda_2^2 + \lambda_3^2}},$$

with $\langle D\rangle = ⅓(\lambda_1 + \lambda_2 + \lambda_3)$, which is the trace apparent diffusion coefficient (ADC), or mean diffusivity. Relative anisotropy (RA), the ratio of the variance of the computed eigenvalues to their mean, is defined (40) to be

$$\mathrm{RA}(\mathbf{D}) = \sqrt{\frac{1}{3}}\,\frac{\sqrt{\begin{array}{l}(\lambda_1 - \langle D\rangle)^2 + (\lambda_2 - \langle D\rangle)^2\\ \quad + (\lambda_3 - \langle D\rangle)^2\end{array}}}{\langle D\rangle}.$$

Volume ratio (VR), the ratio of the volume of the diffusion tensor ellipsoid to the volume of a sphere in which the radius is the mean diffusivity, is defined (31) as

$$\mathrm{VR}(\mathbf{D}) = 1 - \frac{\lambda_1\lambda_2\lambda_3}{\langle D\rangle^3}.$$

We compared these scalar diffusion anisotropy metrics by using Monte Carlo methods to simulate diffusion-weighted images over a range of SNRs of 0.1–100. Anisotropy maps were generated by using the three metrics described, and the contrast-to-noise ratio (CNR) between the anisotropic and isotropic region was computed. The CNR was defined as

$$\mathrm{CNR} = \frac{|\bar{x} - \bar{y}|}{\sqrt{\sigma_x^2 + \sigma_y^2}},$$

where *x* and *y* are computed anisotropy values for anisotropic and isotropic media, respectively, and σ_x and σ_y are their SDs.

The diffusion-weighted images were simulated by using eigenvalues measured in a healthy volunteer. The mean of 30 diffusion tensor data sets was used to increase the SNR of the acquired diffusion images to approximately 65. We outlined 2 × 2 ROIs in two homogeneous white matter regions—the splenium of the corpus callosum and the left forceps major. The measured mean eigenvalues, 1.7, 0.3, and 0.1 × 10^{-3} mm^2/sec in the corpus callosum and 1.2, 0.9, and 0.3 × 10^{-3} mm^2/sec in the left forceps major were used in Monte Carlo simulations to synthesize diffusion-weighted images. The simulated diffusion-weighted images consisted of 128 × 128-pixel regions of anisotropic white matter media and 128 × 128-pixel regions of isotropic media. For the isotropic media, eigenvalues of 0.8, 0.8, and 0.8 × 10^{-3} mm^2/sec were used because they were representative of values measured in cortical gray matter and also matched values reported by another group (31). The mean and SD of each anisotropy measure as a function of image SNR were then calculated.

The CNR between the white matter regions and the isotropic regions was computed for SNR levels of 0.1–100.0. The

SNR was varied by changing the statistical characteristics of the noise added to the real and imaginary components of the noise-free diffusion-weighted images (31,41). These random noise values were normally distributed with a mean of zero and different variances, depending on the desired SNR. The simulated acquired signal was taken to be the magnitude of the complex images. These steps were repeated 10 times to assess the variability of results between different simulations. In addition, Monte Carlo simulations were used to estimate the contribution of noise bias and variance to the computed eigenvalues.

To investigate the variability of ADC and anisotropy metrics between different imaging sessions in the same subject, the same healthy 34-year-old male volunteer underwent imaging three times in three separate sessions, with a resultant total of nine full-head tensor data sets. The trace ADC values, anisotropy index values, and eigenvalues were calculated by using 2 × 2 ROIs. The mean and SD of ADC and anisotropy values in ROIs placed in deep gray matter, or thalamus; deep white matter, or corpus callosum; and cerebrospinal fluid, or atrium of the right lateral ventricle, were calculated.

TABLE 1
Stability of Mean of the ADC, Fractional Anisotropy, and Eigenvalue Measurements

Measurement*	Thalamus	Splenium	Cerebrospinal Fluid
ADC	0.72 (0.05)	0.62 (0.07)	2.46 (0.08)
FA	0.37 (0.04)	0.84 (0.04)	0.19 (0.03)
λ_1	1.00 (0.08)	1.43 (0.13)	2.94 (0.14)
λ_2	0.70 (0.06)	0.30 (0.08)	2.41 (0.11)
λ_3	0.45 (0.05)	0.12 (0.04)	2.03 (0.07)

Note.—Stability of gray and white matter measurements of the ADC, fractional anisotropy, and eigenvalues in nine separate scanning sessions in the same volunteer at three imaging acquisitions at three different dates; 2 × 2 ROIs were placed for each study in the thalamus, the splenium of the corpus callosum, and the cerebrospinal fluid (atrium of the right lateral ventricle). Data are the mean of the ROIs for the nine images. Numbers in parentheses are the SD.

* FA = fractional anisotropy. The units of ADC, λ_1, λ_2, and λ_3 are in 10^{-3} mm²/sec. Fractional anisotropy values are unitless.

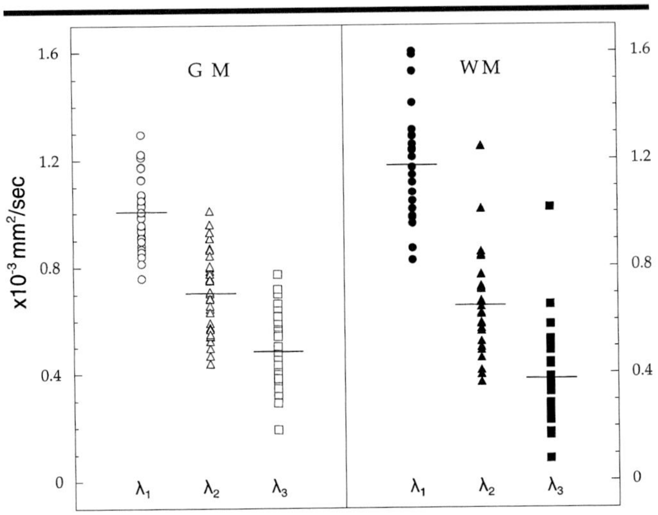

Figure 3. Graph shows eigenvalues in normal contralateral regions of the brain in patients with acute ischemia. The horizontal lines indicate the sample means. Normal mean λ_1, λ_2, and λ_3 values are all significantly different from each other for both gray matter (*GM*) and white matter (*WM*) ($P < .001$).

Human Acute Cerebral Ischemia

Patient recruitment.—Patients who presented with symptoms of acute cerebral ischemia underwent imaging with an acute stroke protocol similar to published techniques (3). The protocol included evaluation by the hospital stroke service, computed tomographic scanning, and MR imaging, which may involve both diffusion- and, at the radiologist's and neurologist's discretion, perfusion-weighted functional MR imaging. For this study, patients were selected at random from patients with acute stroke who underwent full diffusion tensor imaging. This study included only patients who underwent imaging less than 24 hours after they were last known to be asymptomatic.

All patients underwent full diffusion tensor imaging averaged over three data sets for a total acquisition time of 126 seconds. Isotropic diffusion-weighted images were calculated by taking the geometric mean of the six images obtained with a b value of 1,221 sec/mm². No head restraints or navigator echoes were used to control or correct for patient motion. Patients were excluded if the data contained image artifacts due to motion or other technical reasons. Patients were excluded if their isotropic diffusion-weighted image was normal. Patients were also excluded if the time of onset of symptoms was not available or determinable to be less than 24 hours or if follow-up imaging to confirm the infarct was not available. Fifty patients (33 men, 17 women; age distribution, 62.9 years ± 21 [mean ± SD]) met our selection criteria, and there were 25 white matter infarcts and 35 gray matter infarcts. Ten patients had lesions in both gray and white matter. The mean time and SD to imaging from the time the patient was last seen to be healthy was 7.8 hours ± 3.7.

Data analysis.—For the purpose of this work, the ischemic focus was defined as the area of hyperintensity on the initial trace diffusion-weighted images and was confirmed by comparison with follow-up images. We placed the following 2 × 2 ROIs: ischemic gray matter, contralateral normal-appearing gray matter, ischemic white matter, and contralateral normal-appearing white matter. In the ischemic regions, the ROIs were placed in the geometric center. Care was taken that the same type of gray or white matter (eg, deep or cortical) was chosen in the contralateral hemisphere as in the ischemic focus. If the lesion did not involve both gray and white matter as determined by the neuroradiologist (A.G.S.), then only the appropriate ROI and its corresponding contralateral ROI were placed. The areas chosen as normal were also confirmed to be normal at follow-up examinations. The mean and SD for trace ADC and anisotropy values were obtained for each ROI.

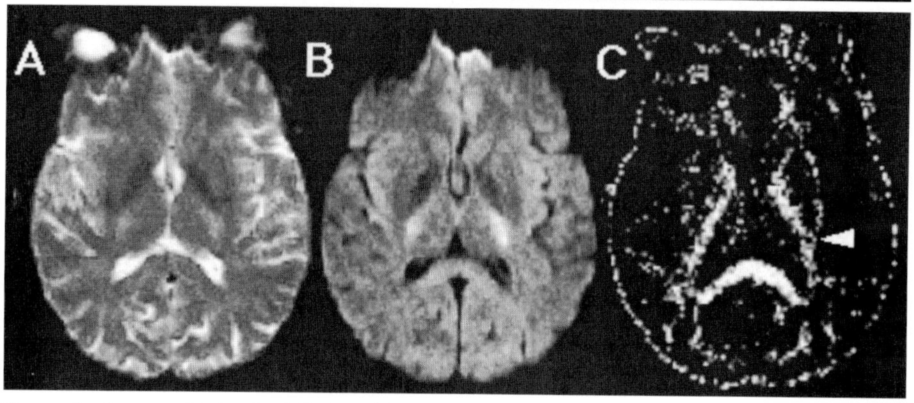

Figure 4. Images obtained axially in a 42-year-old woman 9.5 hours after the onset of symptoms. The imaging parameters were 6,000/118 with a b value of 1,221 sec/mm^2. *A*, T2-weighted echo-planar image (the image obtained with low b value). *B*, Isotropic diffusion-weighted image. *C*, Fractional anisotropy map. The conspicuity of the ischemic zone is greatest in *B* owing to the homogeneity of the background. In *C*, the white matter in the area of ischemia (arrowhead) shows a decrease in fractional anisotropy.

TABLE 2
Changes in ADC and Fractional Anisotropy in Normal and Ischemic Gray Matter and White Matter

A: Mean (SD) Values of 2 × 2 ROIs

Measurement	Normal GM	Ischemic GM	Normal WM	Ischemic WM
ADC	0.73 (0.12)	0.46 (0.13)	0.74 (0.17)	0.54 (0.21)
FA	0.35 (0.12)	0.36 (0.12)	0.52 (0.14)	0.45 (0.15)

B: Significance between Populations

	Normal Differences	Ischemic Differences	
Measurement	GM vs WM	GM vs GM Infarct	WM vs WM Infarct
ADC	.89	<.001	<.001
FA	<.001	.63	.01

Note.—FA = fractional anisotropy, GM = gray matter, WM = white matter.

The statistical analysis was either nonparametric two-tailed Wilcoxon signed rank tests for paired comparisons or Student t tests, assuming heteroscedasticity for nonpaired comparisons. Wilcoxon signed rank tests were used for comparing differences in anisotropy, eigenvalues, and ADC between ipsilateral and contralateral hemispheres. Student t tests were used for computing the statistical significance of differences in fractional anisotropy, eigenvalues, and ADC values between normal white and gray matter and cerebrospinal fluid. A one-way analysis of variance was performed followed by a two-tailed Student t test, assuming heteroscedasticity to compare group differences between λ_1, λ_2, and λ_3. An F test was performed to compare variances between gray and white matter eigenvalues. A P value less than .05 was considered to indicate a statistically significant difference.

RESULTS

Figure 1 displays a representative isotropic diffusion-weighted image, an ADC image, and a fractional anisotropy image for the healthy volunteer who underwent imaging with use of 30 signals acquired for one section. The white matter has a higher degree of fractional anisotropy than the gray matter.

The mean of the eigenvalues measured from ROIs placed in the splenium of the corpus callosum and left forceps major in Figure 1 were used for the Monte Carlo simulations. The results of the Monte Carlo simulations are shown in Figure 2. The corpus callosum had a higher level of anisotropy than the left forceps major, with a resultant higher CNR when the simulated corpus callosum tissue was compared with simulated isotropic tissue. On the basis of empiric measurements, we estimated an SNR of 20 for our clinically acquired diffusion data. At our SNR, these three metrics performed approximately the same. However, at a higher SNR, volume ratio has poorer performance than the other two metrics. To be consistent, we chose to use fractional anisotropy for measuring changes in anisotropy because it provided the highest CNR of the metrics studied in both the corpus callosum and the left forceps major (Fig 2).

Table 1 summarizes the trace ADC values, fractional anisotropy index values, and eigenvalues measured in the healthy volunteer in 2 × 2 ROIs. ADC values in gray matter, white matter, and cerebrospinal fluid are stable at repeated measures. Moving from cerebrospinal fluid to normal gray matter to normal white matter, a stepwise increase in anisotropy is observed. While white matter is much more anisotropic than gray matter or cerebrospinal fluid, deep gray matter voxels are not completely isotropic. Gray matter has twice the fractional anisotropy value of isotropic cerebrospinal fluid (Table 1), a significant difference ($P < .001$). The difference between gray matter and white matter fractional anisotropy values was significant ($P < .001$). For ADC, the difference between gray matter and white matter was also significant ($P = .003$).

Figure 3 shows the eigenvalues of the normal contralateral regions in the patients with acute stroke. Using a one-way analysis of variance, we found that the eigenvalues were all significantly different ($P < .001$) from each other in both normal gray matter and normal white matter. Performing a two-tailed heteroscedastic Student t test further demonstrated a significant difference between all pairs of eigenvalues ($P < .001$). However, this difference may be due to noise-related bias and variance (25). Monte Carlo simulations predicted that given the SNR of 20 and assuming true eigenvalues of 1.0, 0.7, and 0.7 × 10^{-3} mm^2/sec, differences in the second and third eigenvalues greater than 0.5 were needed to substantiate nonaxisymmetry. Consistent with previous reports (25), eigenvalues from normal white matter have slightly larger variability than those from normal gray matter. However, the differences in variances between gray and white matter for our data set were not significant, except for λ_1 (F test for λ_1, $P = .006$; λ_2, $P = .08$; and λ_3, $P = .08$).

Figure 4 displays T2-weighted, diffusion-weighted, and fractional anisotropy images acquired at an SNR of 20 in a representative case of acute ischemic

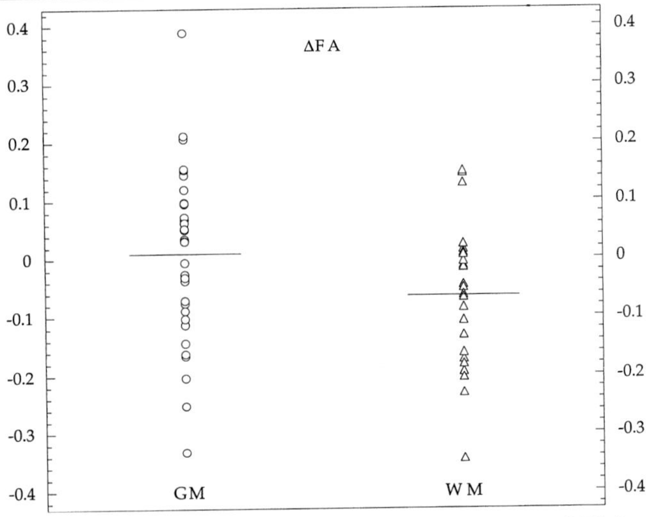

Figure 5. Graph shows fractional anisotropic differences (Δ*FA*) between ischemic gray matter (*GM*) and ischemic white matter (*WM*) and normal contralateral regions. Regions that were abnormal on initial diffusion-weighted images and infarcted at follow-up examination and their contralateral regions were selected. The values plotted are the difference between the abnormal and contralateral values in unitless dimensions. The change in white matter was significant (P = .01). The horizontal lines indicate the sample means.

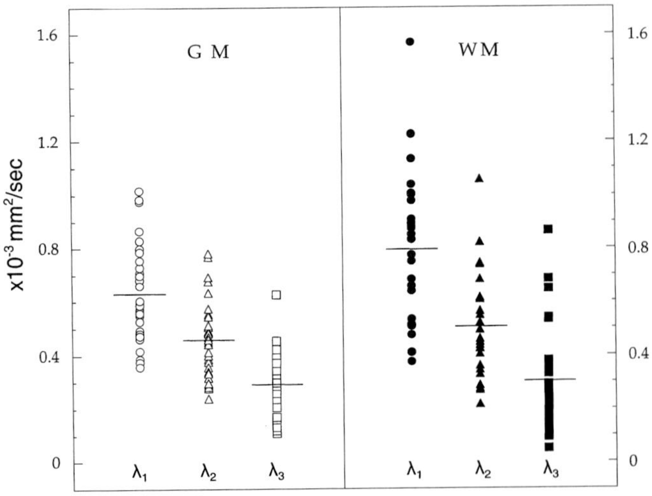

Figure 6. Graph shows eigenvalues in abnormal regions in patients with acute ischemia. The horizontal lines indicate the sample means. Abnormal mean λ_1, λ_2, and λ_3 values are still significantly different from each other in both gray matter (*GM*) and white matter (*WM*). With the exception of the significance between λ_2 and λ_3 in white matter, the level of significance between the other eigenvalues is P less than .001 as determined by using heteroscedastic Student t tests. In the case of λ_2 and λ_3 for white matter, the differences are significant at P equals .001.

stroke. Consistent with expectations from results of Monte Carlo simulations (Fig 2), a higher CNR was seen in the high-SNR brain image from the healthy volunteer (Fig 1) than in the ischemic brain image (Fig 4). Nonetheless, even at an SNR of 20, the decreased anisotropy in the region of decreased ADC was clearly evident as an area of hypointensity.

Table 2 summarizes the results from patients presenting with acute ischemic stroke. There was a significant decrease in ADC between ischemic brain and normal brain, for both white and gray matter ischemia ($P < .001$). A significant decrease in fractional anisotropy ($P = .01$) between the contralateral and ipsilateral hemispheres was detected in only white matter and not in gray matter ($P = .63$). Figure 5 displays the differences between abnormal and contralateral fractional anisotropy values for all of the patients. Figure 6 shows the eigenvalues measured in the abnormal ischemic ROIs. F tests comparing the observed variabilities between gray matter and white matter ischemic tissue yielded P values of .005 for λ_1, .06 for λ_2, and .003 for λ_3.

In Figure 7, the difference in eigenvalues between the ischemic and normal contralateral hemispheres is plotted. A significant decrease for the first ($P < .001$ for both gray and white matter) and second ($P < .001$ for gray matter and P = .001 for white matter) eigenvalues was found. A significant decrease in the third eigenvalue (λ_3) was found in gray matter ($P < .001$) and in white matter ($P = .03$).

DISCUSSION

While the focus of recent clinical studies (1,2,7,10,11,15–17) appropriately has been on the decrease in the trace or single-direction ADC in acute cerebral ischemia, our results confirm those of earlier reports of changes in anisotropy in animal models of cerebral ischemia (30) and in patients with chronic stroke (26,27). Our data extend previous work by documenting acute changes in the eigenvalues of white and gray matters, thus demonstrating that measurement of the full tensor can provide additional microanatomic information in human tissue.

Our results also confirm the results of earlier work (25,31,40) on the choice of scalar metric and extend this work by identifying fractional anisotropy as the metric with the best performance characteristics over the range of SNRs available to us. We now use fractional anisotropy as our anisotropy metric of choice for investigation of changes in anisotropy.

As Tables 1 and 2 and Figures 1 and 4 demonstrate, anisotropy maps can be used to differentiate clearly between gray and white matter. The distance scale to which our sequence is sensitive can be derived from the Einstein relation, which states that the time scale (Δ) is sensitive to diffusion on the length scale, $L = (2D\Delta)^{1/2}$. For our implementation, L = 11 µm, assuming $D = 1.2 \times 10^{-3}$ mm²/sec, the average λ_1 measured in the white matter in the normal hemisphere for the patient population in our study. This distance scale is comparable to typical neuroglial cell soma diameters of 7–15 µm (42). The resultant images are different from those obtained with conventional MR imaging in that they are based on microscopic diffusion properties rather than on relaxation properties.

The exact mechanisms underlying the ADC changes in ischemic brain remain controversial. Anisotropy has not been a major component of the proposed models to date. However, such information may prove useful as the models used to understand the ADC changes in early cerebral ischemia are refined. For example, the ADC decrease in ischemic white matter was largest in λ_1, the direction of which has been shown to align with white matter tracts (27). One thus can speculate that ADC decreases might be along the long axis of the white matter fiber tracts.

Our data with a high SNR of 65 demonstrated a significant difference between λ_2 and λ_3 in nonischemic gray matter (P = .001) and nonischemic white matter (P =

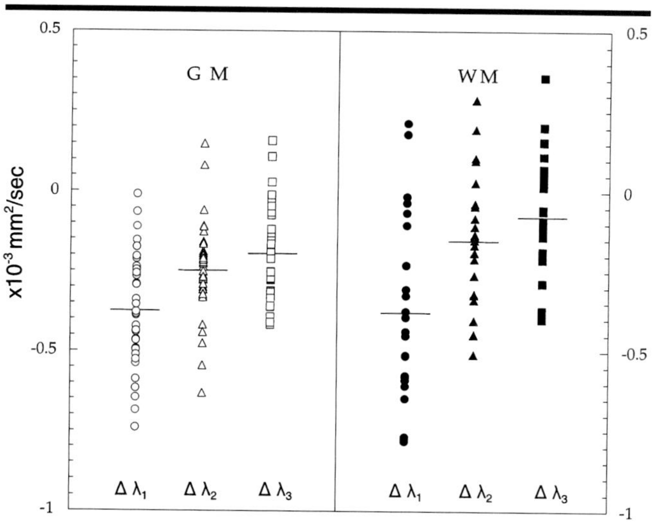

Figure 7. Graph shows changes in λ_1, λ_2, and λ_3 during ischemia in gray matter (*GM*) and white matter (*WM*). The horizontal lines indicate the sample means. All eigenvalues have significant changes ($P \leq .001$), with the exception of λ_3 in white matter ($P = .03$) as determined by using a Wilcoxon signed rank test. The plotted data points are the difference between eigenvalues measured in the ipsilateral and contralateral hemispheres.

.01). These findings of nonaxisymmetry have also been detected by other groups (25). Furthermore, our data indicate that during ischemia, λ_2 and λ_3 may behave differently, which suggests that the assumption of axisymmetry may prevent an accurate description of water diffusion behavior in acute cerebral ischemia. Therefore, it may be prudent to acquire the full six diffusion directions in tensor studies.

As can be seen in Figure 6, the variance in the ischemic white matter ROIs is quite high, which suggests that there may be some biologic heterogeneity. The changes we see in anisotropy may occur to a different degree in different white matter locations; further subset analyses await collection of additional data. While the anisotropy maps were sensitive to changes in white matter anisotropy, we found the visual conspicuity of early ischemia is still highest on the trace diffusion-weighted images. These images normally have little or no gray-white contrast. In addition, on the basis of our Monte Carlo simulations, fluctuations in noise had greater effects on anisotropy metrics than they do on ADC values.

Anisotropy maps provide useful information not captured in ADC values. One example is the ability to differentiate between white and gray matter in cases in which the biology of ischemic injury may well differ. Water can diffuse into the neuronal cell bodies that make up gray matter through neurotransmitter-gated ion channels, synapses, and a concentration of voltage-gated ion channels not found in white matter. The dense arrays of parallel white matter tracts create a structured extracellular space that differs substantially from that found in the meshwork of gray matter. It may be that diffusion tensor changes in shape are more evident in white matter than in gray matter owing to the greater structure and hence anisotropy present in normal white matter as compared with normal gray matter.

Nonetheless, careful evaluation of anisotropy metrics is needed. There are at least three causes for variability: (*a*) anisotropy metrics, themselves, are sensitive to noise contamination (Fig 2); (*b*) anisotropy itself is quite variable throughout white matter (Fig 1); (*c*) just as ADC values first decrease and later pseudonormalize, anisotropy values may also vary in different stages of stroke. These many causes of variability may contribute to the fractional anisotropy changes in our sample size. With such high variability, even conspicuous changes reach only moderate significance ($P = .01$). Changes in anisotropy and the eigenvalues that characterize the full diffusion tensor therefore need further investigation.

In conclusion, our data demonstrate that full-tensor imaging is feasible in the clinical setting of stroke imaging. Even at the low SNR available clinically, useful maps of anisotropy metrics can be generated. Most important, human acute cerebral ischemia causes changes in the anisotropy or shape of the diffusion tensor in white matter. Further investigation into such changes may help clarify the nature of the biophysical changes in acute cerebral ischemia and eventually shed further light on the pathophysiology of this leading cause of morbidity and mortality.

References

1. Warach S, Chien D, Li W, Ronthal M, Edelman RR. Fast magnetic resonance diffusion-weighted imaging of acute human stroke. Neurology 1992; 42:1717–1723.
2. Warach S, Gaa J, Siewert B, Wielopolski P, Edelman R. Acute human stroke studied by whole brain echo planar diffusion-weighted magnetic resonance imaging. Ann Neurol 1995; 37:231–241.
3. Sorensen AG, Buonanno FS, Gonzalez RG, et al. Hyperacute stroke: evaluation with combined multisection diffusion-weighted and hemodynamically weighted echo-planar MR imaging. Radiology 1996; 199:391–401.
4. Le Bihan D, Breton E, Lallemand D, Grenier P, Cabanis E, Laval-Jeantet M. MR imaging of intravoxel incoherent motions: application to diffusion and perfusion in neurologic disorders. Radiology 1986; 161:401–407.
5. Thomsen C, Henriksen O, Ring P. In vivo measurement of water self-diffusion in the human brain by magnetic resonance imaging. Acta Radiol 1987; 28:353–361.
6. Le Bihan D, Breton E, Lallemand D, Aubin ML, Vignaud J, Laval-Jeantet M. Separation of diffusion and perfusion in intravoxel incoherent motion MR imaging. Radiology 1988; 168:497–505.
7. Hajnal J, Doran M, Hall A, et al. MR imaging of anisotropically restricted diffusion of water in the nervous system: technical, anatomic, and pathologic considerations. J Comput Assist Tomogr 1991; 15:1–18.
8. Tsuruda JS, Chew WM, Moseley ME, Norman D. Diffusion-weighted MR imaging of extraaxial tumors. Magn Reson Med 1991; 19:316–320.
9. Chien D, Kwong KK, Gress DR, Buonanno FS, Buxton RB, Rosen BR. MR diffusion imaging of cerebral infarction in humans. AJNR 1992; 13:1097–1102.
10. Welch K, Windham J, Knight R, et al. A model to predict the histopathology of human stroke using diffusion and T2-weighted magnetic resonance imaging. Stroke 1995; 26:1983–1989.
11. Lutsep HL, Albers GW, De Crespigny A, Kamat GN, Marks MP, Moseley ME. Clinical utility of diffusion-weighted magnetic resonance imaging in the assessment of ischemic stroke. Ann Neurol 1997; 41:574–580.
12. Takeda K, Nomura Y, Sakuma H, Tagami T, Okuda Y, Nakagawa T. MR assessment of normal brain development in neonates and infants: comparative study of T1- and diffusion-weighted images. J Comput Assist Tomogr 1997; 21:1–7.
13. Brunberg JA, Chenevert TL, McKeever PE, et al. In vivo MR determination of water diffusion coefficients and diffusion anisotropy: correlation with structural alter-

ation in gliomas of the cerebral hemispheres. AJNR 1995; 16:361–371.
14. de Crespigny AJ, Marks MP, Enzmann DR, Moseley ME. Navigated diffusion imaging of normal and ischemic human brain. Magn Reson Med 1995; 33:720–728.
15. Baird AE, Benfield A, Schlaug G, et al. Enlargement of human cerebral ischemic lesion volumes measured by diffusion-weighted magnetic resonance imaging. Ann Neurol 1997; 41:581–589.
16. Lovblad KO, Baird AE, Schlaug G, et al. Ischemic lesion volumes in acute stroke by diffusion-weighted magnetic resonance imaging correlate with clinical outcome. Ann Neurol 1997; 42:164–170.
17. Schlaug G, Siewert B, Benfield A, Edelman RR, Warach S. Time course of the apparent diffusion coefficient (ADC) abnormality in human stroke. Neurology 1997; 49:113–119.
18. Ulug AM, Beauchamp N, Bryan RN, van Zijl PCM. Absolute quantitation of diffusion constants in human stroke. Stroke 1997; 28:483–490.
19. Chien D, Buxton RB, Kwong KK, Rosen BR. MR diffusion imaging of the human brain. J Comput Assist Tomogr 1990; 14: 514–520.
20. Chenevert TL, Brunberg JA, Pipe JG. Anisotropic diffusion in human white matter: demonstration with MR techniques in vivo. Radiology 1990; 177:401–405.
21. Douek P, Turner R, Pekar J, Patronas N, Le Bihan D. MR color mapping of myelin fiber orientation. J Comput Assist Tomogr 1991; 15:923–929.
22. Sakuma H, Nomura Y, Takeda K, et al. Adult and neonatal human brain: diffusional anisotropy and myelination with diffusion-weighted MR imaging. Radiology 1991; 180:229–233.
23. Coremans J, Luypaert R, Verhelle F, Stadnik T, Osteaux M. A method for myelin fiber orientation mapping using diffusion-weighted MR images. Magn Reson Imaging 1994; 12:443–454.
24. Nomura Y, Sakuma H, Takeda K, Tagami T, Okuda Y, Nakagawa T. Diffusional anisotropy of the human brain assessed with diffusion-weighted MR: relation with normal brain development and aging. AJNR 1994; 15:231–238.
25. Pierpaoli C, Jezzard P, Basser PJ, Barnett A, Di Chiro G. Diffusion tensor MR imaging of the human brain. Radiology 1996; 201: 637–648.
26. Pierpaoli C, Penix L, De Graba T, Basser PJ, Di Chiro G. Identification of fiber degeneration and organized gliosis in stroke patients by diffusion tensor MRI (abstr). In: Proceedings of the Fourth Meeting of the International Society for Magnetic Resonance in Medicine. Berkeley, Calif: International Society for Magnetic Resonance in Medicine, 1996; 563.
27. Makris N, Worth AJ, Sorensen AG, et al. Morphometry of in vivo human white matter association pathways with diffusion-weighted magnetic resonance imaging. Ann Neurol 1997; 42:951–962.
28. van Gelderen P, de Vleeschouwer MHM, Des Pres D, Pekar J, van Zijl PCM, Moonen CTW. Water diffusion and acute stroke. Magn Reson Med 1994; 31:154–163.
29. Moonen CT, Pekar J, de Vleeschouwer MH, van Gelderen P, van Zijl PC, Des Pres D. Restricted and anisotropic displacement of water in healthy cat brain and in stroke studied by NMR diffusion imaging. Magn Reson Med 1991; 19:327–332.
30. Kajima T, Azuma K, Itoh K, et al. Diffusion anisotropy of cerebral ischemia. Acta Neurochir Suppl (Wien) 1994; 60:216–219.
31. Pierpaoli C, Basser PJ. Toward a quantitative assessment of diffusion anisotropy. Magn Reson Med 1996; 36:893–906.
32. Einstein A. Investigations on the theory of the Brownian movement. New York, NY: Dover Publications, 1956.
33. Tanner JE, Stejskal EO. Restricted self-diffusion of protons in colloidal systems by the pulsed-gradient, spin-echo method. J Chem Phys 1968; 49:1768–1777.
34. Stejskal E, Tanner J. Spin diffusion measurements: spin echoes in the presence of a time-dependent field gradient. J Chem Phys 1965; 42:288–292.
35. McKinstry RC, Weiskoff RM, Belliveau JW, et al. Ultrafast MR imaging of water mobility: animal models of altered cerebral perfusion. JMRI 1992; 2:377–384.
36. Basser PJ, Mattiello J, Le Bihan D. MR diffusion tensor spectroscopy and imaging. Biophys J 1994; 66:259–267.
37. Mattiello J, Basser PJ, Le Bihan D. Analytical expressions for the *b* matrix in NMR diffusion imaging and spectroscopy. J Magn Reson 1994; 108:131–141.
38. Basser PJ, Mattiello J, Le Bihan D. Estimation of the effective self-diffusion tensor from the NMR spin echo. J Magn Reson 1994; 103:247–254.
39. Mattiello J, Basser PJ, Le Bihan D. The *b* matrix in diffusion tensor echo-planar imaging. Magn Reson Med 1997; 37:292–300.
40. Basser PJ, Pierpaoli C. Microstructural and physiological features of tissues elucidated by quantitative-diffusion tensor MRI. J Magn Reson 1996; 111:209–219.
41. Henkelman RM. Measurement of signal intensities in the presence of noise in MR images. Med Phys 1985; 12:232–233.
42. Gray H. Anatomy of the human body. 37th ed. Edinburgh, UK: Longman, 1989; 875.

Brain Lesions: When Should Fluid-attenuated Inversion-Recovery Sequences Be Used in MR Evaluation?[1]

Tomoko Okuda, MD
Yukunori Korogi, MD
Yoshinori Shigematsu, MD
Takeshi Sugahara, MD
Toshinori Hirai, MD
Ichiro Ikushima, MD
Luxia Liang, MD
Mutsumasa Takahashi, MD

Index terms:
Basal ganglia, MR, 14.121411, 14.121413, 15.121416
Brain, diseases, 14.30, 14.76, 14.871, 15.30, 15.76, 15.871
Brain, ischemia, 14.76, 15.76
Brain, neoplasms, 14.30, 15.30
Brain stem, MR, 15.121411, 15.121413, 15.121416
Magnetic resonance (MR), pulse sequences, 18.121411, 18.121413, 18.121416
Sclerosis, multiple, 18.871

Radiology 1999; 212:793–798

Abbreviations:
CNR = contrast-to-noise ratio
CSF = cerebrospinal fluid
FLAIR = fluid-attenuated inversion recovery
MS = multiple sclerosis
SE = spin echo
SI = signal intensity

[1] From the Department of Radiology, Kumamoto University School of Medicine, 1-1-1 Honjo, Kumamoto 860, Japan. From the 1997 RSNA scientific assembly. Received February 13, 1998; revision requested April 15; final revision received December 16; accepted March 16, 1999. **Address reprint requests to** T.O.

Author contributions:
Guarantor of integrity of entire study, Y.K.; study concepts and design, T.O., Y.K.; definition of intellectual content, T.O., Y.K.; literature research, T.O.; clinical studies, L.L., I.I., T.H., T.S., Y.S.; data acquisition and analysis, T.O.; statistical analysis, T.O.; manuscript preparation, T.O.; manuscript editing and review, Y.K., M.T.

PURPOSE: To compare qualitatively and quantitatively the contrast of brain lesions detected with fluid-attenuated inversion-recovery (FLAIR) and intermediate-weighted sequences at magnetic resonance (MR) imaging.

MATERIALS AND METHODS: In this prospective study, 47 patients suspected of having a brain lesion underwent MR imaging with FLAIR, intermediate-weighted, and T2-weighted sequences. Qualitative assessment was performed of lesion conspicuity, detection, overall image artifact, and additional clinical information. Contrast and contrast-to-noise ratio (CNR) were calculated between lesions and the normal brain or cerebrospinal fluid (CSF).

RESULTS: FLAIR images were equal to intermediate-weighted images for overall lesion conspicuity and detection but were associated more often with image artifacts. Lesion-to-background contrast was significantly higher on FLAIR than on intermediate-weighted images. FLAIR images failed to demonstrate multiple sclerosis (MS) plaques located in the basal ganglia and brain stem.

CONCLUSION: Although FLAIR images provided additional information in some cases, they did not have distinct advantages over intermediate-weighted images. When cases of MS are evaluated, intermediate-weighted images are preferable to FLAIR images. Except in cases of MS, either FLAIR or intermediate-weighted sequences should be added to T2-weighted sequences at MR imaging.

Fluid-attenuated inversion-recovery (FLAIR) sequences have been developed that null the signals from cerebrospinal fluid (CSF) and yield heavily T2-weighted images. The usefulness of FLAIR sequences has been reported in central nervous system diseases, including infarction, multiple sclerosis (MS), subarachnoid hemorrhage, head injury, and others (1–14). Most of these reports confirm the superiority of FLAIR over spin-echo (SE) magnetic resonance (MR) imaging, and some reports suggest the possibility of replacing SE with FLAIR technique (1,2), although other investigators have recently pointed out disadvantages of FLAIR sequences (3,4,15–17).

At present, FLAIR images are usually obtained in addition to T1- and T2-weighted images, since they are expected to give additional useful information. There is some similarity between intermediate-weighted and FLAIR imaging in regard to suppression of the signal of CSF. However, the number of examinations with intermediate-weighted sequences has tended to decrease with the development of the fast SE sequence. In the previously mentioned reports about the usefulness of FLAIR images, however, they were compared with T2-weighted, short inversion time inversion-recovery, or STIR, or gadolinium-enhanced T1-weighted images (1–17). Only a few of these articles reported a direct comparison between FLAIR and intermediate-weighted sequences.

The purpose of this study was to compare qualitatively and quantitatively the image contrast of brain lesions detected on FLAIR images and intermediate-weighted images and to document which is more suitable as an additional sequence in routine MR examinations.

MATERIALS AND METHODS

In this prospective study, 47 patients (23 male and 24 female; age range, 0–76 years; mean age, 37.6 years) suspected of having brain lesions on the basis of clinical history or neurologic findings underwent MR imaging at 1.5 T (Magnetom-Vision; Siemens Medical Systems, Erlangen, Germany) with FLAIR, intermediate-weighted, and T2-weighted pulse sequences.

All images were obtained in the axial plane (5-mm section thickness with 1-mm section gap). In all patients, T2-weighted imaging was performed with the following sequences and parameters: T2-weighted fast SE (repetition time msec/effective echo time msec = 4,500/96, one signal acquired, 19 sections, echo train length of seven) or T2-weighted SE (2,400/90, one signal acquired, 19 sections). In all patients, intermediate-weighted fast SE imaging was performed with a single-echo sequence (2,400/15, two signals acquired, 19 sections, echo train length of seven). In all patients, FLAIR imaging (8,000/119/2,000 [inversion time msec]) was performed with two signals acquired, acquisition time of 4 minutes 24 seconds for 15 sections, echo train length of seven, 180–224 × 256 matrix, and field of view of 150–220 mm. In all patients, nonenhanced T1-weighted images (670/14) were obtained with one signal acquired. As proof of existence of a lesion on the MR images, two neuroradiologists (T.O., Y.K.) carefully reviewed the nonenhanced T1-weighted, T2-weighted, and gadolinium-enhanced T1-weighted images (if available) by consensus.

FLAIR images were compared with intermediate-weighted images qualitatively and quantitatively. Qualitative evaluations were performed independently by two neuroradiologists (T.S., Y.S.) with knowledge of the patient's clinical diagnosis. FLAIR and intermediate-weighted images were presented at the same time as were the T2-weighted images. Four qualitative evaluations were performed: the value of additional clinical information, image artifacts, lesion conspicuity, and lesion detection.

The value of additional clinical information was defined on the basis of the following grading system: +2, FLAIR or intermediate-weighted images contributed to clinical diagnosis or treatment; +1, FLAIR or intermediate-weighted images contributed to lesion detection or visualization; 0, FLAIR or intermediate-weighted images added no information to T2-weighted images; −1, FLAIR or intermediate-weighted images caused misdiagnosis. The statistical significance of differences with this criterion was determined with the paired *t* test.

TABLE 1
Additional Clinical Information: FLAIR versus Intermediate-weighted Images

	FLAIR Images		Intermediate-weighted Images	
Grade*	Radiologist 1	Radiologist 2	Radiologist 1	Radiologist 2
+2	2	3	1	3
+1	14	15	11	14
0	40	38	44	39
−1	0	0	0	0

Note.—Data are the number of studies.
* +2, FLAIR or intermediate-weighted images contributed to clinical diagnosis or treatment; +1, FLAIR or intermediate-weighted images contributed to lesion detection or visualization; 0, FLAIR or intermediate-weighted images added no information to T2-weighted images; −1, FLAIR or intermediate-weighted images caused misdiagnosis.

The following three-point grading system was used to evaluate the criteria of overall image artifacts, lesion conspicuity (defined as ease of lesion visualization), and lesion detection (defined as the presence or absence of lesions): +1, FLAIR images were superior to intermediate-weighted images; 0, FLAIR and intermediate-weighted images were equal; −1, FLAIR images were inferior to intermediate-weighted images. All studies were evaluated for overall image artifact, and studies with pathologic conditions were evaluated for lesion conspicuity and lesion detection. The statistical significance of differences with these three qualitative criteria was determined with the signed rank test.

FLAIR and intermediate-weighted images were also compared quantitatively by one neuroradiologist (T.O.). The quantitative criteria were lesion-to-background contrast and contrast-to-noise ratio (CNR) and lesion-to-CSF contrast and CNR. "Background" was defined as the normal brain parenchyma adjacent to the lesion. For each patient, contrast and CNR were measured and compared for a maximum of two representative lesions, which were chosen randomly from the group of lesions visualized equally well with both sequences. Mean lesion signal intensity (SI) was measured in regions of interest placed within similar uniform areas of the lesion. Mean background SI was measured in areas immediately surrounding the lesion. The SDs of noise were measured on the image along the phase-encoding direction in space outside the head. With these measurements, contrast and CNR for each lesion were calculated as follows: contrast = $(SI_{lesion} - SI_{B\ or\ CSF})/SI_{B\ or\ CSF}$ and CNR = $(SI_{lesion} - SI_{B\ or\ CSF})/SD\ SI_{noise}$, where B is background. Paired *t* tests were performed to evaluate the statistical significance of differences with these quantitative data.

TABLE 2
Overall Assessment of Artifacts: FLAIR versus Intermediate-weighted Images

Artifact Grade*	Radiologist 1	Radiologist 2
+1	0	10
0	14	12
−1	33	25
Mean ± SD	−0.72 ± 0.81†	−0.32 ± 0.90‡

Note.—Data are the number of patients.
*+1, FLAIR images have fewer artifacts than do intermediate-weighted images; 0, FLAIR and intermediate-weighted images have artifacts equally; −1, FLAIR images have more artifacts than do intermediate-weighted images.
† $P < .001$.
‡ $P < .05$.

RESULTS

No lesions were seen on the MR images of seven of the 47 patients. Two different types of lesions were observed in nine of the 47 patients. Therefore, a total of 49 different lesions or groups of lesions were identified and evaluated. The final clinical diagnoses included MS (n = 12), ischemia or infarction (n = 9), brain tumor (n = 12), or miscellaneous other conditions (three, tuberous sclerosis; three, white matter lesions; three, basal ganglia lesions of uncertain pathogenesis; two, edema; one, parenchymal hemorrhage; one, subdural fluid collection; one, acquired immunodeficiency syndrome, or AIDS-related lesions; one, dilated Virchow-Robin space; and one, laminar necrosis).

The 12 brain tumors were extraaxial (five, arachnoid cyst or other cysts; two, epidermoid; one, meningioma; one, chon-

TABLE 3
Lesion Conspicuity and Lesion Detection: FLAIR versus Intermediate-weighted Images

Criterion, Grade*, Lesion, and No. of Studies	Radiologist 1	Radiologist 2
Conspicuity		
+1	19	17
0	16	14
−1	14	18
Mean (n = 49)	0.10 ± 0.70	−0.04 ± 0.75
MS (n = 12)	−0.41 ± 0.79	−0.50 ± 0.90
Ischemia or infarction (n = 9)	0.55 ± 0.72	0.56 ± 0.73
Tumor (n = 12)	0.16 ± 0.58	−0.08 ± 0.90
Miscellaneous ion (n = 16)	0.19 ± 0.91	0.00 ± 0.82
Detection		
+1	7	5
0	33	32
−1	9	12
Mean (n = 49)	−0.04 ± 0.57	−0.14 ± 0.58
MS (n = 12)	−0.33 ± 0.65	−0.58 ± 0.51
Ischemia or infarction (n = 9)	0.22 ± 0.44	0.33 ± 0.50
Tumor (n = 12)	−0.08 ± 0.29	−0.17 ± 0.39
Miscellaneous (n = 16)	0.06 ± 0.68	−0.06 ± 0.57

Note.—Data are the number of studies or the mean grade ± SD.
* +1, FLAIR images superior to intermediate-weighted images; 0, FLAIR images equal to intermediate-weighted images; −1, FLAIR images inferior to intermediate-weighted images.

TABLE 4
Lesion Conspicuity and Lesion Detection in the 12 Patients with MS

Criterion and Grade*	Supratentorial Lesions		Infratentorial Lesions	
	Radiologist 1	Radiologist 2	Radiologist 1	Radiologist 2
Conspicuity				
+1	5	3	0	0
0	4	4	1	0
−1	3	5	6	7
Mean	0.16 ± 0.83	−0.16 ± 0.83	−0.85 ± 0.37*	−1 ± 0†
Detection				
+1	1	0	0	0
0	10	10	2	1
−1	1	2	5	6
Mean	0 ± 0.42	−0.16 ± 0.38	−0.71 ± 0.48	−0.85 ± 0.37†

Note.—Data are the number of studies or the mean grade ± SD.
* +1, FLAIR images superior to intermediate-weighted images; 0, FLAIR images equal to intermediate-weighted images; −1, FLAIR images inferior to intermediate-weighted images.
† $P < .05$.

droma) or intraaxial (one, lymphoma; two, glioma). Diagnoses of the brain tumors were proved histopathologically except for the arachnoid cyst and other cysts.

In cases without verification by means of biopsy, diagnoses were based on clinical history, clinical presentation, and findings on nonenhanced T1- and T2- weighted images and gadolinium-enhanced T1-weighted images (if available). MS, ischemia or infarction, and tumor were evaluated as separate entities. Because of the small number of cases, the remaining 16 lesions were evaluated together as miscellaneous lesions.

Results of the qualitative comparison of FLAIR and intermediate-weighted images are summarized in Tables 1–4. Additional clinical information based on FLAIR and intermediate-weighted images was evaluated in 56 studies (49 with pathologic conditions and seven without lesions). Radiologists 1 and 2, respectively, evaluated as useful (grades +1 or +2) 16 (29%) and 18 (32%) FLAIR studies and 12 (21%) and 17 (30%) intermediate-weighted studies. There were no significant differences between FLAIR and intermediate-weighted images (Table 1). For overall image artifact, radiologists 1 and 2 evaluated FLAIR studies as inferior to intermediate-weighted studies in 33 (70%) and 25 (53%) of 47 patients, respectively. FLAIR images received an overall score of −0.72 ± 0.81 (mean ± SD) (radiologist 1) and −0.32 ± 0.90 (radiologist 2), and they were rated as significantly inferior to intermediate-weighted images ($P < .001$, $P < .05$, respectively) (Table 2). Artifacts tended to occur in areas of prominent CSF pulsatility, such as inferiorly located sections and areas near the foramen of Monro.

For lesion conspicuity and detection, FLAIR studies were rated as roughly equivalent to intermediate-weighted studies. MS plaques, however, were demonstrated less clearly on FLAIR than on intermediate-weighted images (Table 3). When the locations of the MS plaques were separated into supra- and infratentorial regions, both radiologists graded FLAIR studies as inferior to intermediate-weighted studies for infratentorial lesions (Table 4). In particular, lesion contrast was insufficient at the brain stem (Fig 1). For supratentorial lesions, both radiologists graded FLAIR studies as roughly equivalent to intermediate-weighted studies, although grades for conspicuity and detection of basal ganglia lesions were lower for FLAIR than for intermediate-weighted studies. In one case of MS, a basal ganglia lesion had low SI on FLAIR images and was difficult to identify, but it had high SI on intermediate- and T2-weighted images (Fig 2). Lesions of the cerebral white matter appeared to be more extensive on FLAIR images.

In most of the cases of ischemia or infarction, conspicuity was better on FLAIR than on intermediate-weighted studies. In one case of infarction, the lesion of the middle cerebellar peduncle had low SI on FLAIR images. For extraaxial tumors, there were no differences in conspicuity or detection between the FLAIR and intermediate-weighted studies, whereas FLAIR studies were graded as slightly superior to intermediate-weighted studies for the intraaxial tumors. In cases of tuberous sclerosis, some cortical tuber lesions not detected on the FLAIR images were detected on the intermediate-weighted images (Fig 3).

Results of the quantitative evaluation are shown in Table 5. Lesion-to-CSF and lesion-to-background contrast were significantly superior on FLAIR compared with intermediate-weighted studies. Lesion-to-background CNR was significantly superior on intermediate-weighted studies, but differences in lesion-to-CSF CNR were not significant.

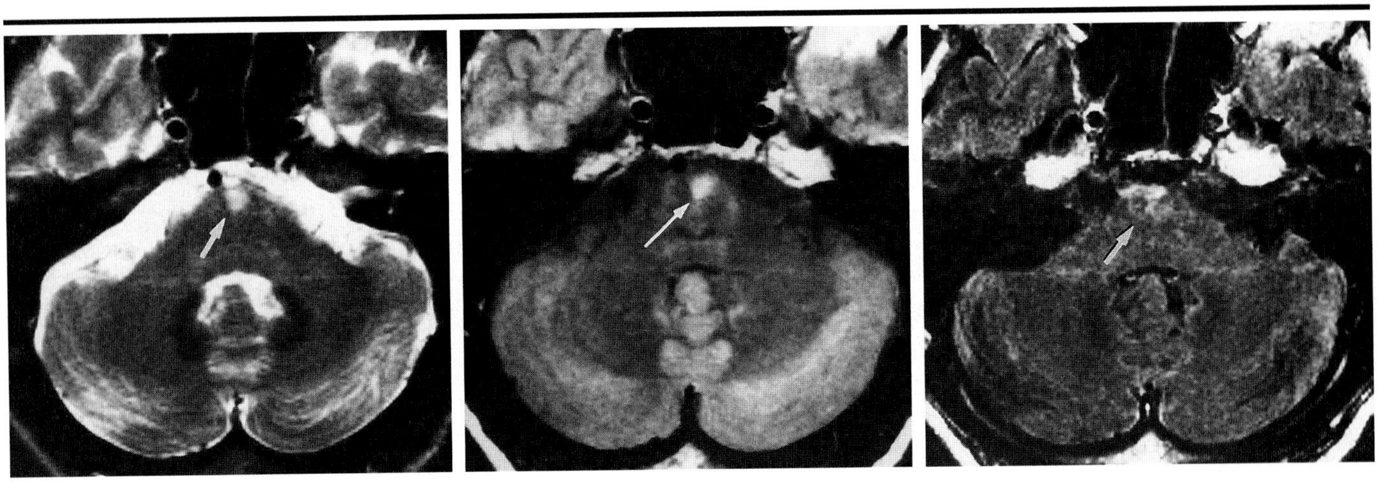

a. b. c.

Figure 1. Axial MR images in a 53-year-old man with MS. **(a)** T2-weighted image (4,500/96). **(b)** Intermediate-weighted image (2,400/15). **(c)** FLAIR image (8,000/119/2,000). MS plaque in the pons (arrow), which is clearly depicted in **a** and **b**, is difficult to identify in **c** because of insufficient contrast.

DISCUSSION

FLAIR imaging is a relatively new technique with a long inversion time and a long echo time that can null the signals from CSF and produce heavily T2-weighted studies. This type of sequence is particularly useful in the detection of subtle changes at the periphery of the hemispheres and in the periventricular region close to CSF. Although advantages with intermediate-weighted sequences are similar to those with FLAIR sequences in regard to suppression of the signal of CSF, intermediate-weighted studies have insufficient contrast owing to a short echo time, and the number of intermediate-weighted examinations has decreased with the development of the fast SE sequence. The usefulness of FLAIR sequences has been evaluated in diseases of the central nervous system such as infarction, MS, subarachnoid hemorrhage, head injuries, and others (1–14). The authors of most of these reports have concluded that FLAIR sequences are superior to intermediate- and T2-weighted sequences, and some suggest a possibility of replacing the SE technique with FLAIR (1,2). However, a few investigators have recently pointed out disadvantages of FLAIR sequences (3,4,15–17). It is now necessary to evaluate which pulse sequence is more useful for the imaging of brain abnormalities.

Since a long acquisition time is needed with conventional FLAIR sequences, a faster FLAIR sequence is now routinely used with multiple echoes per repetition time that is based on rapid acquisition with relaxation enhancement, or RARE, and fast SE sequences (1–7). Although the current technique represents an improvement over previous methods, another problem with FLAIR sequences remains. Incomplete nulling of CSF signals due to CSF inflow effects has been reported to produce imaging artifacts (1,3,5). These artifacts occurred in areas of prominent CSF pulsatility, such as inferiorly located sections and those containing foramina of the CSF ventricular system. In this study, we also encountered similar CSF flow-related artifacts on FLAIR images, which contributed to failure to detect lesions located in the brain stem.

TABLE 5
Lesion-to-Background and Lesion-to-CSF Contrast and CNR: FLAIR versus Intermediate-weighted Images

Ratio, Lesion, and No. of Studies	No. of Lesions	Contrast: FLAIR Images	Contrast: Intermediate-weighted Images	CNR: FLAIR Images	CNR: Intermediate-weighted Images
Lesion-to-background ratio					
MS (n = 12)	21	0.65 ± 0.24	0.26 ± 0.11	15.35 ± 5.82	28.11 ± 11.96
Ischemia or infarction (n = 9)	13	0.94 ± 0.54	0.29 ± 0.11	22.04 ± 14.33	27.13 ± 9.34
Tumor (n = 12)	14	0.67 ± 0.34	0.21 ± 0.18	15.12 ± 5.87	22.62 ± 20.48
Miscellaneous (n = 9)	14	0.68 ± 0.27	0.26 ± 0.12	16.92 ± 6.60	29.08 ± 14.66
Total (n = 42)	63	0.72 ± 0.36*	0.25 ± 0.13*	17.06 ± 8.71*	26.85 ± 14.31*
Lesion-to-CSF ratio					
MS (n = 12)	21	6.64 ± 3.32	0.26 ± 0.11	31.62 ± 8.50	27.96 ± 12.09
Ischemia or infarction (n = 9)	13	7.24 ± 4.98	0.31 ± 0.09	36.96 ± 19.33	30.00 ± 12.68
Tumor (n = 12)	14	3.26 ± 3.67	0.22 ± 0.18	19.12 ± 14.70	24.25 ± 21.34
Miscellaneous (n = 9)	14	5.53 ± 5.65	0.29 ± 0.08	29.18 ± 13.77	30.37 ± 10.44
Total (n = 42)	63	5.76 ± 4.49*	0.27 ± 0.12*	29.37 ± 14.91	28.06 ± 14.38

Note.—Data are the mean value ± SD.
* $P < .001$.

In addition to the appearance of CSF flow-related artifacts, poor lesion contrast may be another drawback with FLAIR sequences. For lesion conspicuity and detection of MS plaques, FLAIR studies received a lower grade and were judged inferior to intermediate-weighted studies, particularly in the posterior fossa and basal ganglia. Flow-related artifacts may not be the sole contributing factor to poor lesion conspicuity and detection. Although the cause is not clear, there are some possible explanations for the poor contrast on FLAIR images. One possible

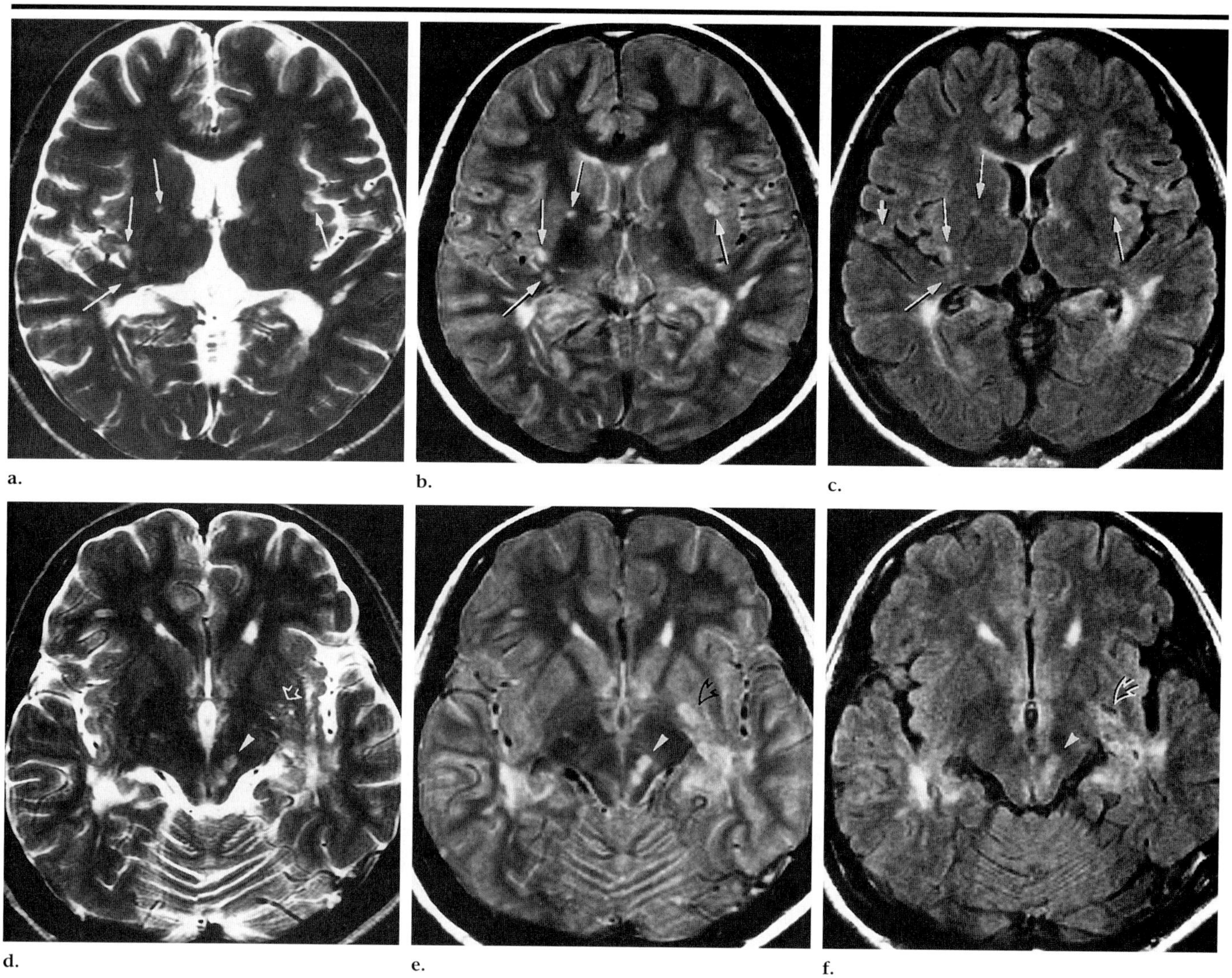

Figure 2. (a–f) Axial MR images in a 20-year-old woman with MS. (a, d) T2-weighted images (4,500/96). (b, e) Intermediate-weighted images (2,400/15). (c, f) FLAIR images (8,000/119/2,000). (a–c) MS plaques in the basal ganglia (long arrows) were slightly hyperintense in a and were clearly depicted in b but have insufficient contrast in c. However, another MS plaque (short arrow) in the frontal lobe lateral to the Sylvian fissure is clearly seen in c but not in a or b. (d–f) Images were obtained at a level slightly inferior to that in a–c. MS plaque in the left basal ganglia (open arrow) has high SI in d and e but low SI in f. Another MS plaque in the midbrain (arrowhead) is seen more clearly in e than in f.

explanation is that the MS plaques in the brain stem or basal ganglia may have different T2 characteristics (15). Hittmair et al (3) reported limitations of FLAIR sequences in patients with MS of the spinal cord. With only slightly prolonged T2, characteristic of inactive MS plaques, the signals of the normal cord and pathologic lesions have already decreased at a long echo time. In these cases, use of shorter echo times can produce a higher contrast between the normal cord and pathologic lesions. Since the fast FLAIR sequence consists of an inversion pulse followed by a heavily T2-weighted fast SE sequence, the long echo time and echo train length in fast FLAIR studies may explain the poor plaque contrast (3,15). In addition, the inversion pulse in FLAIR sequences introduces considerable T1 weighting, which acts antagonistically to the T2 contrast (3). The brain stem and basal ganglia have a structure different from that of white matter. In these regions, MS plaques may have relaxation times similar to those of adjacent brain parenchyma.

In chronic infarctions, some lesions with high SI on T2-weighted images are depicted with low SI or isointensity on FLAIR images and are difficult to identify (2,4). It is presumed that these foci may be liquefied or gliotic and, therefore, their SI matches that of CSF and is nulled with FLAIR sequences. This opens the possibility that FLAIR images can help differentiate acute from chronic infarctions on the basis of their SI. However, it should be noted that FLAIR studies sometimes could not help identification of lesions with low SI or isointensity. In our study, MS plaques depicted with low SI were also observed on FLAIR images, and they were deemed chronic lesions.

There are several limitations in this study. First, many different kinds of disease were evaluated as one group. For example, miscellaneous lesions included nine kinds of diseases, and the number of these lesions was insufficient to enable definitive conclusions. Also, we did not differentiate acute MS plaques or infarctions from chronic lesions. Evaluation of a large number of each type of lesion may

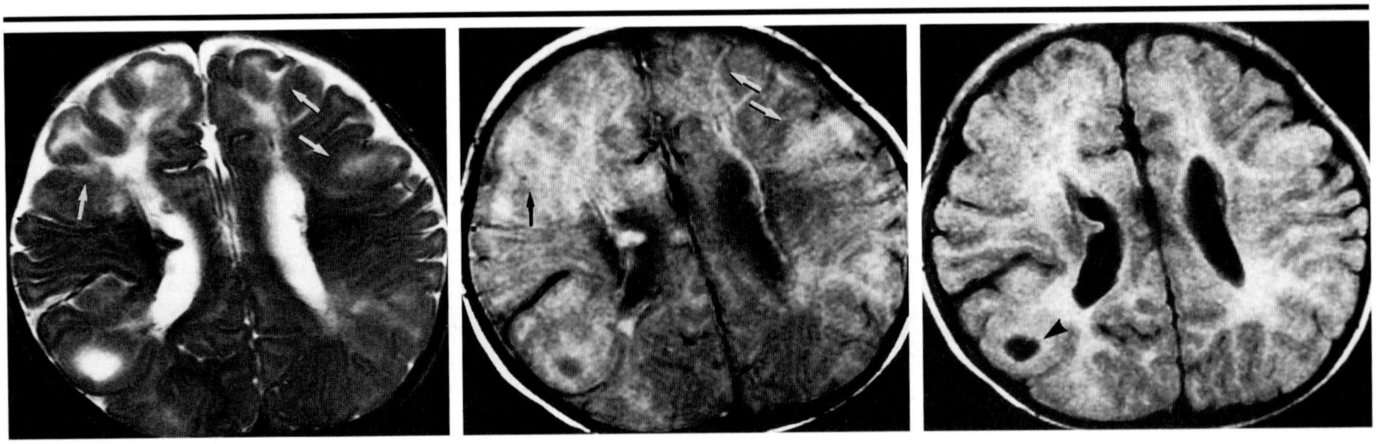

a. b. c.

Figure 3. Axial MR images of cortical tubers in a 5-month-old infant with tuberous sclerosis. **(a)** T2-weighted image (4,500/96). **(b)** Intermediate-weighted image (2,400/15). **(c)** FLAIR image (8,000/119/2,000). Multiple cortical tubers (arrows in **a** and **b**) are depicted most clearly in **a**, followed by **b**. Most of these lesions are not depicted in **c**, but the subcortical lesion (arrowhead in **c**) in the right parietal area is clearly depicted in **c** as cystic.

be more effective to choose the optimum sequence. Furthermore, use of an optimum pulse sequence suitable for each disease may be necessary. Second, two different T2-weighted sequences were used. Since examinations with each sequence included a variety of lesions, comparison of the two sequences was impossible. Third, the presence of CSF flow-related artifacts on FLAIR images, which contributed to failure to demonstrate lesions located in the brain stem, may be directly related to the pulse sequence design and its implementation. CSF signals would be completely nulled if the pulse sequence were further optimized. Fourth, the subjective part of the study was somewhat biased. The reviewers could identify which was the FLAIR image, they evaluated the images side by side rather than separately and independently, and the grading criteria were subjective. We included seven patients who had no lesions and evaluated additional clinical information and image artifacts on their studies. The subjective nature of the criteria regarding additional information may also be a source of potential bias.

In some cases, the FLAIR studies offered useful clinical information as an adjunct to T2-weighted images, particularly in the detection of subtle changes in the region contiguous to CSF. The FLAIR studies also helped differentiate cystic lesions on the basis of their SI, whereas T2-weighted images depicted almost all lesions as hyperintense areas (2,4–7). Intermediate-weighted studies were equivalent to FLAIR studies, however, in their ability to provide useful clinical information. FLAIR studies had some pitfalls, such as CSF flow-related artifacts, insufficient lesion contrast in the basal ganglia and posterior fossa (particularly MS plaques), and the inability to clearly depict cystic lesions.

In summary, FLAIR sequences have advantages and disadvantages in the demonstration of central nervous system diseases and cannot replace T2-weighted sequences. It is important to recognize that lesions in the basal ganglia or brain stem may be missed with FLAIR sequences. Intermediate-weighted images should be obtained in patients with MS, but the FLAIR sequence may be omitted from the MR evaluation. Except in cases of MS, FLAIR images provided additional information compared with T2-weighted images and offered higher lesion contrast than did intermediate-weighted images, and we recommend routine use of FLAIR sequences in addition to T2-weighted sequences. Intermediate-weighted images can substitute for FLAIR images.

References

1. Hashemi RH, Bradley WG Jr, Chen DY, et al. Suspected multiple sclerosis: MR imaging with a thin-section fast FLAIR pulse sequence. Radiology 1995; 196:505–510.
2. Alexander JA, Sheppard S, Davis PC, Salverda P. Adult cerebrovascular disease: role of modified rapid fluid-attenuated inversion recovery sequences. AJNR 1996; 17:1507–1513.
3. Hittmair K, Mallek R, Prayer D, Schindler EG, Kollegger H. Spinal cord lesions in patients with multiple sclerosis: comparison of MR pulse sequences. AJNR 1996; 17:1555–1565.
4. Shiono T, Teshima Y, Iwasaki N. Advantages and disadvantages of fast fluid-attenuated inversion recovery sequences in the evaluation of brain infarction. Nippon Igaku Hoshasen Gakkai Zasshi 1996; 56:625–628.
5. Rydberg JN, Hammond CA, Grimm MS, et al. Initial clinical experience in MR imaging of the brain with a fast fluid-attenuated inversion-recovery pulse sequence. Radiology 1994; 193:173–180.
6. Hajnal JV, Bryant DJ, Kasuboski L, et al. Use of fluid attenuated inversion recovery (FLAIR) pulse sequence in MRI of the brain. J Comput Assist Tomogr 1992; 16:841–844.
7. Coene BD, Hajnal JV, Gatehouse P, et al. MR of the brain using fluid-attenuated inversion recovery (FLAIR) pulse sequence. AJNR 1992; 13:1555–1564.
8. Coene BD, Hajnal JV, Pennock JM, Bydder GM. MRI of the brain stem using fluid-attenuated inversion recovery pulse sequence. Neuroradiology 1993; 35:327–331.
9. Noguchi K, Ogawa T, Inugami A, et al. Acute subarachnoid hemorrhage: MR imaging with fluid attenuated inversion recovery pulse sequences. Radiology 1995; 196:773–777.
10. Bergin PS, Fish DR, Shorvon SD, Oatridge A, deSouza NM, Bydder GM. Magnetic resonance imaging in partial epilepsy: additional abnormalities shown with the fluid attenuated inversion recovery (FLAIR) pulse sequence. J Neurol Neurosurg Psychiatry 1995; 58:439–443.
11. Murata T, Itoh S, Koshino Y, et al. Serial cerebral MRI with FLAIR sequences in acute carbon monoxide poisoning. J Comput Assist Tomogr 1995; 19:631–634.
12. Baratti C, Barkhof F, Hoogenraad F, Valk J. Partially saturated fluid attenuated inversion recovery (FLAIR) sequence in multiple sclerosis with fully relaxed FLAIR and conventional spin-echo. Magn Reson Imaging 1995; 13: 513–521.
13. Ashikaga R. Clinical utility of MR FLAIR imaging for head injury. Nippon Igaku Hoshasen Gakkai Zasshi 1996; 56:1045–1049.
14. Tsuchiya K, Inaoka S, Mizutani Y, Hachiya J. Fast fluid-attenuated inversion-recovery MR of intracranial infections. AJNR 1997; 18:909–913.
15. Bastianello S, Bozzao A, Paolillo A, et al. Fast spin-echo and fast fluid-attenuated inversion-recovery versus conventional spin-echo sequences for MR quantification of multiple sclerosis lesions. AJNR 1997; 18:699–704.
16. Yousry TA, Filippi M, Becker C, Horsfield MA, Voltz R. Comparison of MR pulse sequences in the detection of multiple sclerosis lesions. AJNR 1997; 18:959–963.
17. Keiper MD, Grossman RI, Brunson JC, Schnall MD. The low sensitivity of fluid-attenuated inversion-recovery MR in the detection of multiple sclerosis of the spinal cord. AJNR 1997; 18:1035–1039.

Primary and Recurrent Early Stage Laryngeal Cancer: Preliminary Results of 2-[Fluorine 18]fluoro-2-deoxy-D-glucose PET Imaging[1]

Val J. Lowe, MD
Han Kim, MD
James H. Boyd, MD
John F. Eisenbeis, MD
Frank R. Dunphy, MD
James W. Fletcher, MD

Index terms:
Emission CT (ECT), comparative studies, 27.12163
Fluorine, radioactive
Head and neck neoplasms, CT, 27.12115, 27.37
Head and neck neoplasms, emission CT (ECT), 27.12163, 27.37
Larynx, neoplasms, 27.37

Radiology 1999; 212:799–802

Abbreviation:
FDG = 2-[fluorine 18]fluoro-2-deoxy-D-glucose

[1] From the Departments of Nuclear Medicine (V.J.L., J.W.F.), Radiation Oncology (H.K.), Otolaryngology-Head and Neck Surgery (J.H.B., J.F.E.), and Hematology/Oncology (F.R.D.), PET Imaging Facility, St Louis University Health Sciences Center, 3635 Vista Ave at Grand Blvd, St Louis, MO 63110-0250. From the 1997 RSNA scientific assembly. Received April 15, 1998; revision requested May 29; final revision received December 16; accepted March 16, 1999. **Address reprint requests to** V.J.L. (e-mail: *lowe@nucmed.slu.edu*).

V.J.L. is on the speaker's bureau for and has received honoraria from ADAC Laboratories, CTI, GE Medical Systems, and P.E.T. Net.

Author contributions:
Guarantor of integrity of entire study, V.J.L.; study concepts and design, H.K., V.J.L., J.H.B., J.F.E., F.R.D.; definition of intellectual content, H.K., V.J.L., J.H.B., J.F.E., F.R.D.; literature research, V.J.L.; clinical studies, V.J.L.; data acquisition and analysis, V.J.L.; manuscript preparation, V.J.L.; manuscript editing and review, H.K., J.H.B., J.F.E., F.R.D., J.W.F.

PURPOSE: To evaluate the effectiveness of 2-[fluorine 18]fluoro-2-deoxy-D-glucose (FDG) positron emission tomography (PET) in the identification of early stage (T1–T2) primary and recurrent laryngeal cancer.

MATERIALS AND METHODS: Twelve patients with T1 or T2 laryngeal cancer underwent imaging prospectively with PET. Seven patients had new disease, and five had recurrent disease. All patients underwent imaging prior to planned therapy and tissue biopsy. PET images were evaluated by using standardized uptake ratios and visual analysis.

RESULTS: Histopathologic evidence of early stage cancer was documented in the 12 patients. One had a carcinoma in situ, nine had T1 tumors, and two had T2 tumors. Of the 12 patients, 10 had vocal cord tumors, one had a hypopharyngeal tumor, and one had a preepiglottic tumor. Eleven (92%) patients with early stage cancer had standardized uptake ratios indicative of malignancy (mean, 4.6; SD, 1.8; 95% CI, 1.2; range, 2.8–7.6). One had false-negative results (standardized uptake ratio = 2.3). Nine underwent CT, and results in the larynx were normal in seven and abnormal in two.

CONCLUSION: FDG PET can be used to identify primary and recurrent early stage laryngeal cancer. It may be useful for follow-up after therapy.

Early stage laryngeal cancer (T1–T2; T1, one [a] or both [b] vocal cords involved, with normal vocal cord mobility; T2, extension either above or below the vocal cords, with or without limitation of mobility, and no vocal cord fixation) can be treated with good success by using radiation therapy or surgery. Anatomic computed tomography (CT) is unable to depict the majority of early stage laryngeal lesions, and most lesions are identified with direct visualization. This difficulty in imaging is related to normal variations in the symmetry of the vocal cords, small size of the tumors, oral secretions, and movement. For these reasons, CT is not generally recommended for T1 lesions (1–3). If used, CT is more commonly performed to assess lymph node status in such patients. Moreover, clinical follow-up after therapy can be challenging. Radiation effects such as edema or scarring can make both physical examination and CT difficult.

Cancer cells have increased metabolism and rapid cell proliferation. In the 1930s, malignant cells were shown to have increased glucose metabolism (4). Their increased metabolism can, in part, be related to increased levels of glucose transport protein messenger RNA and glucose transport proteins (5). Because 2-[fluorine 18]fluoro-2-deoxy-D-glucose (FDG) is an analogue of glucose, FDG accumulates at increased rates in highly metabolic, malignant cells (6). After phosphorylation, FDG-6-phosphate does not proceed further in the metabolic pathway and for the most part remains trapped within cells, which allows for positron emission tomographic (PET) imaging. High FDG accumulation is thereby a marker of high metabolic activity.

PET can be used to accurately identify recurrent disease after therapy of advanced stage laryngeal cancer (7–9), but these results may not be applicable to early stage tumors. The small size of T1 or T2 tumors may well make PET imaging challenging in regard to these lesions. If PET can be used to identify early stage laryngeal cancer, PET may be able to provide an accurate means of assessing recurrent or residual disease. We, therefore, evaluated the ability of FDG PET to depict primary or recurrent early stage (T1–T2) laryngeal cancer in this prospective trial in patients with documented early stage disease.

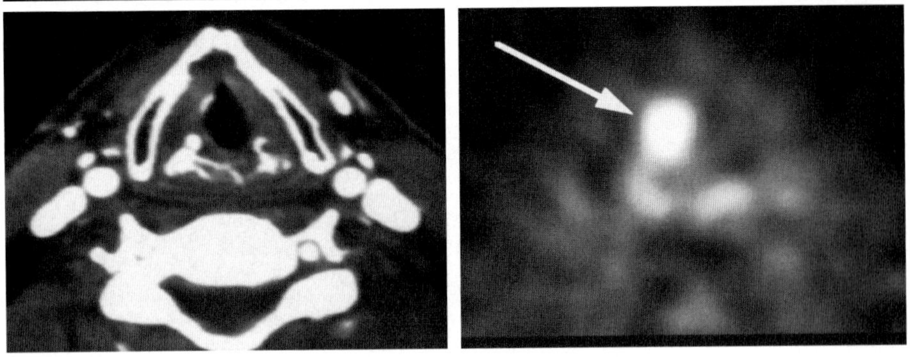

a. b.

Figure 1. (a) Axial CT and (b) axial PET scans obtained at the same level in a 55-year-old male patient with a T1a squamous cell cancer in the right vocal cord that was a new diagnosis. The CT scan was reported as normal. The PET scan demonstrates hypermetabolism (arrow) indicative of active tumor (standardized uptake ratio = 4.4).

MATERIALS AND METHODS

Patients

Twelve patients (11 men, one woman; age range, 20–77 years; mean age, 52 years ± 16 [SD]) with documented T1 or T2 laryngeal cancer were examined prospectively. Seven patients had new disease, and five had recurrent disease. Of the patients with recurrent disease, the time from the completion of initial radiation therapy until recurrence was between 5 months and 5 years (mean, 21 months). All patients underwent imaging prior to planned therapy. Tissue biopsies of all lesions were performed by means of direct laryngoscopic visualization 6–30 days before PET. CT scans were obtained in most patients (nine of 12) and were also obtained after biopsy was performed (1–27 days). All patients gave informed consent to participate in this protocol. The protocol had been approved by our institutional review board. All patients fasted before the PET study, and a serum glucose value was obtained in each patient.

PET Imaging

FDG PET imaging was performed with use of an ECAT 951/31 PET scanner (Siemens Medical Systems, Hoffman Estates, Ill). This scanner has an axial field of view of 10.8 cm that is composed of 16 bismuth germanate rings that produce 31 transaxial in-plane and cross-plane images. It has an axial resolution of 5.7 mm full width at half maximum from a point source at a 10.0-cm radius from the center and an axial resolution of 4.5 mm full width at half maximum at the center. The scanner has whole-body imaging capability.

The fluorine 18 fluoride was produced with use of an RDS 112 cyclotron (Siemens Medical Systems) that is on-site. The ^{18}F fluoride ions were transferred to an automated system for synthesis of FDG by means of the Hamacher method. The FDG was tested for sterility, pyrogenicity, and radiochemical purity at each production run. No problems with sterility, pyrogenicity, or radiochemical purity occurred.

Transmission scans were obtained in all patients by using a germanium 68 ring source prior to the injection of FDG at 7 minutes per position. Emission images of two bed positions at 10 minutes per position to include the area from the inferior orbit to the upper lung fields were obtained 50 minutes after the intravenous injection of 370 MBq of FDG.

Transmission images were reconstructed with filtered backprojection smoothed by using a Hann filter with a cutoff frequency of 7.0 mm. Emission images were reconstructed with filtered backprojection by using a Hann filter with a cutoff frequency of 5.0 mm. Emission data were corrected for scatter, random events, and dead time losses by using the manufacturer's software.

CT Imaging

CT scans of the neck were obtained with use of a CT/i HiSpeed scanner (GE Medical Systems, Milwaukee, Wis) to include the area from the malar arch to the aortic arch. Iohexol (Omnipaque 350 [100 mL]; Nycomed Amersham, Princeton, NJ) was injected intravenously, and helical imaging was started 30 seconds thereafter with use of 5-mm collimation.

Data Analysis

PET images were evaluated by using the standardized uptake ratio as well as visual interpretation. One circular region of interest was placed on a single image over the region of greatest activity by an experienced nuclear medicine physician (V.J.L.). The regions of interest were placed in abnormalities that were visually apparent on the PET scan in the region of the larynx but that could not be explained by normal uptake. The region of interest was placed in the region of highest uptake and within the borders of the abnormality. As a check of placement and size, the region-of-interest mean activity measurement was confirmed to be about 80% of the maximum activity measurement in the region of interest (10).

Activity concentrations in megabecquerels per milliliter were measured as mean pixel values in the regions of interest. After correction for radioactive decay, the standardized uptake ratio was computed for each lesion identified on the PET scan according to the following formula: standardized uptake ratio equals the average pixel values of region-of-interest activity in megabecquerels per milliliter divided by the injected dose in megabecquerels divided by body weight in grams.

Analysis was performed without knowledge of histopathologic data and the location of the tumor. A standardized uptake ratio greater than 2.5 was considered positive for malignancy (11).

For visual interpretation, the findings considered to be positive for malignancy were focally increased FDG accumulation in the larynx clearly more intense than the background activity in the neck, asymmetry of the abnormality if bilateral, and presence on two adjacent axial image sections. These readings were performed by an experienced nuclear medicine physician (V.J.L.) without knowledge of other clinical or imaging data.

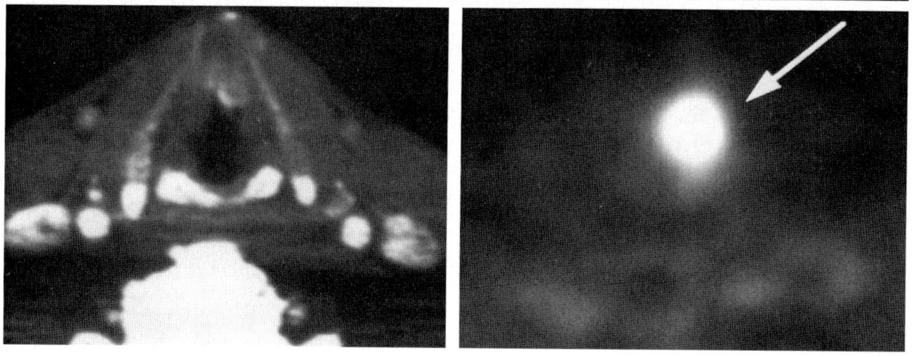

a. b.

Figure 2. (a) Axial CT and (b) axial PET scans obtained at the same level in a 58-year-old male patient with a T2 squamous cell cancer in the left anterior vocal cord that was a new diagnosis. The CT scan was reported as normal, although in retrospect, there appears to be some asymmetry of the vocal cords in the region of the PET abnormality shown in **b**. This region may have been thought to be a normal variation on the axial CT scan. The PET scan demonstrates hypermetabolism (arrow) indicative of active tumor (standardized uptake ratio = 7.1).

The CT scans were interpreted independently from the PET images, and the dictated impressions as reported were extracted as the results for this study. The interpreting radiologists were not blinded to clinical information. CT images that did not indicate tumor were thereafter re-reviewed by an experienced radiologist in light of the PET and surgical findings.

RESULTS

Histopathologic evidence of early stage cancer was documented in the 12 patients. One patient had a carcinoma in situ, nine had T1 tumors, and two had T2 tumors. Ten patients had vocal cord tumors, one had a hypopharyngeal tumor, and one had a preepiglottic tumor. Eleven (92%) patients with early stage cancer had standardized uptake ratios indicative of malignancy (mean, 4.6; SD, 1.8; 95% CI, 1.2; range, 2.8–7.6). One patient of five with recurrent disease had false-negative results (standardized uptake ratio = 2.3). Visual interpretation yielded the same results, with the scans considered positive for tumor in 11 patients. The same patient who had the standardized uptake ratio of 2.3 had scans visually interpreted as normal. Examples of T1 and T2 tumors demonstrated at PET are shown in Figures 1 and 2.

Nine patients underwent CT, and the results were normal in the larynx in seven. Six of these seven patients with normal CT scans had T1 lesions, and one had a T2 lesion. Two patients had abnormal CT scans. One of these had a T1b right vocal cord tumor and had a CT scan that showed a thickened right cord. The other patient had a T2 left vocal cord lesion that was seen as a mass at CT. Both of these CT scans were in patients with new disease. Retrospective review of the CT scans that did not indicate tumor was performed in light of the histopathologic results and the PET findings. Six of the seven CT scans were available for review. On one of the CT scans in one of the six patients with recurrent disease, fullness was seen in the region of the PET abnormality (Fig 2). In one other patient with new disease, fullness of the right cord was thought to be present. In this patient, the PET scan was negative, and the patient had a left vocal cord tumor. On the four remaining CT scans, no correlative abnormality could be found.

DISCUSSION

Some 20% of primary early stage laryngeal cancers will fail standard treatment. Early detection of these recurrences is difficult owing to the inherent difficulties in assessing disease with physical examination after therapy. CT does not have good accuracy in depiction of these lesions and is often used to evaluate the possibility of any neck nodal involvement. This is especially true of T1 lesions. A higher percentage of T2 lesions may be identified on CT scans, and some authors (12) advocate the use of CT for pretherapy staging of T2 lesions as some evidence has shown that CT may depict a more advanced stage.

PET imaging has been shown to be sensitive for the detection of head and neck cancer (7–9). We postulated that because there is a smaller volume of soft tissue in the neck as compared with that in the torso, and because laryngeal lesions are central in location, the optimum situation should exist for maximizing PET imaging capabilities. This should allow detection of small lesions in this area. Therefore, in this study we evaluated the ability of PET to depict small, early stage laryngeal cancer.

With this protocol, we studied primary or recurrent early stage laryngeal cancer to determine if PET could depict these lesions. Although other authors have described the use of PET to detect disease in more advanced head and neck cancer, to our knowledge, no work to date has described the use of PET in such small, early stage lesions. In the article by Bailet et al (7), only two patients had laryngeal cancer, and only one of these had early stage disease (T1N0). Anzai et al (8) described 12 patients with head and neck cancer, four of whom had laryngeal cancer, and three of these had undergone prior laryngectomy (ie, not early stage). Austin et al (9) discussed 10 patients with laryngeal cancer who had undergone an organ-salvage protocol of chemotherapy and radiation therapy and likely had stage III or IV disease. Another article (13) describes detection of recurrent laryngeal cancer by means of PET and includes T1–T4 disease.

We thought that data regarding PET detection of primary or recurrent early stage laryngeal cancer would be important. It could lead to future trials of PET in assessing recurrent early stage disease. Such trials could include performance of biopsy and be undertaken even when there may be no other indication to perform biopsy of these small lesions. Because performance of biopsy of the larynx after treatment can result in necrosis, we believed that it would be unethical to subject patients to a potentially harmful biopsy procedure without evidence to support the findings of PET in early stage disease. We, therefore, assessed the use of PET in detecting small primary or recurrent laryngeal lesions in a group that had not undergone therapy or had not undergone recent therapy. In the group studied, PET depicted 92% (11 of 12) of the lesions. One of the lesions was not detected and had a standardized uptake ratio of 2.3, which did not meet the criteria for malignancy.

In comparison, a group of nine of these patients underwent CT imaging, and CT did not depict seven of the nine lesions. Six of the seven were T1 lesions. In retrospect, one of the negative CT scans demonstrated some fullness in the area of the PET abnormality, and this was a T2 lesion (Fig 2).

These data demonstrate for the first time, to our knowledge, that primary or recurrent early stage laryngeal cancers can be detected by means of FDG PET with high sensitivity. Because no patients with benign disease were included in the study, we were not able to determine the specificity of PET for early stage cancer. One could implicate bias in the visual interpretations of the study owing to the fact that patients were referred because they all had documented cancer. For this reason, standardized uptake ratios were also used in the analysis. Further work in pretreatment and posttreatment groups that include patients with benign lesions will need to be performed to assess the accuracy of PET in distinguishing benign from malignant laryngeal disease. Our data show that such work is promising.

All patients underwent biopsy 6–30 days before the PET scans were obtained. It is possible, although we think it unlikely, that performance of biopsy without any complications may cause substantial hypermetabolism. We have subsequently obtained negative PET scans in a few patients after biopsy of the larynx, and in one patient biopsy was performed 3 days before PET. Nevertheless, hypermetabolism from recent performance of biopsy cannot be completely excluded given the methods in our study, and future studies with a healthy control group will need to be performed.

Some published data (14) on posttherapy PET scans have demonstrated substantial hypermetabolism in association with treatment-related inflammatory changes without the presence of residual tumor. Other authors (15) have described relatively few changes with radiation therapy. This issue would need to be considered in any future project concerning the accuracy of PET in assessing the larynx after therapy in cases of early stage cancer.

The findings from this study indicate that PET imaging can be used to identify primary or recurrent early stage laryngeal cancer. This may be helpful in the assessment of primary laryngeal cancer. PET imaging may aid in biopsy guidance when the initial tissue sample is negative. PET may also be useful for differentiating benign from malignant laryngeal lesions, but further work will be needed to document the accuracy of PET in distinguishing benign from malignant disease. PET likely will be unable to aid in further staging of the tumor, as soft-tissue or cartilage invasion will not be factors that PET can be used to assess.

PET may be most useful in assessing the larynx for any residual or recurrent disease after therapy in people with early stage tumors. Prior work performed at our institution has shown that posttherapy PET can be of aid in advanced stage lesions (16). More data will be needed to evaluate the utility of PET in the posttreatment period, but the present study of early stage lesions demonstrates that it has promise: FDG PET can be used to identify primary and recurrent early stage laryngeal cancer and may be useful for follow-up after therapy.

Acknowledgments: The authors wish to thank Penny Yost, CNMT, Sue Paulik, CNMT, Ranajit Bera, PhD, and Rita Gentilcore, MS, of the St Louis University PET Imaging Center for their contributions in performance of the PET imaging and PET radiopharmaceutical production for this study.

References

1. Thabet HM, Sessions DG, Gado MH, Gnepp DA, Harvey JE, Talaat M. Comparison of clinical evaluation and computed tomographic diagnostic accuracy for tumors of the larynx and hypopharynx. Laryngoscope 1996; 106:589–594.
2. Charlin B, Brazeau LL, Guerrier B, Leduc C. Assessment of laryngeal cancer: CT scan versus endoscopy. J Otolaryngol 1989; 18:283–288.
3. Kolbenstvedt A, Charania B, Natvig K, Tausjo J. Computed tomography in T1 carcinoma of the larynx. Acta Radiol 1989; 30:467–469.
4. Warburg O. The metabolism of tumors. New York, NY: Smith, 1931; 129.
5. Flier JS, Mueckler MM, Usher P, Lodish HF. Elevated levels of glucose transport and transporter messenger RNA are induced by ras or src oncogenes. Science 1987; 235:1492–1495.
6. Gallagher BM, Fowler JS, Gutterson NI, MacGregor RR, Wan CN, Wolf AP. Metabolic trapping as a principle of radiopharmaceutical design: some factors responsible for the biodistribution of [18F] 2-deoxy-2-fluoro-D-glucose. J Nucl Med 1978; 19:1154–1161.
7. Bailet JW, Sercarz JA, Abemayor E, Anzai Y, Lufkin RB, Hoh CK. The use of positron emission tomography for early detection of recurrent head and neck squamous cell carcinoma in postradiotherapy patients. Laryngoscope 1995; 105:135–139.
8. Anzai Y, Carroll WR, Quint DJ, et al. Recurrence of head and neck cancer after surgery or irradiation: prospective comparison of 2-deoxy-2-[F-18]fluoro-D-glucose PET and MR imaging diagnoses. Radiology 1996; 200:135–141.
9. Austin JR, Wong FC, Kim EE. Positron emission tomography in the detection of residual laryngeal carcinoma. Otolaryngol Head Neck Surg 1995; 113:404–407.
10. Lowe VJ, DeLong DM, Hoffman JM, Coleman RE. Optimum scanning protocol for FDG-PET evaluation of pulmonary malignancy. J Nucl Med 1995; 36:883–887.
11. Lowe VJ, Duhaylongsod FG, Patz EF, et al. Pulmonary abnormalities and PET data analysis: a retrospective study. Radiology 1997; 202:435–439.
12. Mukherji SK, Mancuso AA, Mendenhall W, Kotzur IM, Kubilis P. Can pretreatment CT predict local control of T2 glottic carcinomas treated with radiation therapy alone? AJNR 1995; 16:655–662.
13. Greven KM, Williams DW, Keyes JJ, McGuirt WF, Watson NJ, Case LD. Can positron emission tomography distinguish tumor recurrence from irradiation sequelae in patients treated for larynx cancer? Cancer J Sci Am 1997; 3:353–357.
14. Lowe VJ, Hebert ME, Hawk TC, Anscher MS, Coleman RE. Chest wall FDG accumulation in serial FDG-PET images in patients being treated for bronchogenic carcinoma with radiation (abstr). J Nucl Med 1994; 35:76P.
15. Rege SD, Chaiken L, Hoh CK, et al. Change induced by radiation therapy in FDG uptake in normal and malignant structures of the head and neck: quantitation with PET. Radiology 1993; 189:807–812.
16. Lowe V, Dunphy F, Varvares M, et al. Evaluation of chemotherapy response in patients with advanced head and neck cancer using FDG-PET. Head Neck 1997; 19:666–674.

Edith M. Marom, MD
H. Page McAdams, MD
Jeremy J. Erasmus, MD
Philip C. Goodman, MD
Donna K. Culhane, MD
R. Edward Coleman, MD
James E. Herndon, MD
Edward F. Patz, Jr, MD

Index terms:
Bronchi, neoplasms, 60.3211, 60.3212, 60.3214, 60.3216, 60.3217
Lung neoplasms, emission CT (ECT), 60.12163
Lung neoplasms, staging, 60.3211, 60.3212, 60.3214, 60.3216, 60.3217

Radiology 1999; 212:803–809

Abbreviation:
FDG = 2-[fluorine 18]fluoro-2-deoxy-D-glucose

[1] From the Departments of Radiology (E.M.M., H.P.M., J.J.E., P.C.G., R.E.C., E.F.P.) and Medicine (J.E.H.), Duke University Medical Center, Box 3808, Durham, NC 27710; and the Department of Radiology, Veterans Affairs Medical Center, Durham, NC (D.K.C.). Received July 27, 1998; revision requested September 24; final revision received December 9; accepted March 29, 1999. **Address reprint requests to** E.F.P.

Author contributions:
Guarantors of integrity of entire study, E.M.M., J.J.E., P.C.G.; study concepts, R.E.C., E.F.P., J.J.E., H.P.M., P.C.G.; study design, E.F.P.; definition of intellectual content, J.J.E., H.P.M., P.C.G., E.F.P.; literature research, E.M.M., E.F.P.; clinical studies, all authors; data acquisition and analysis, E.M.M., D.K.C., E.F.P.; statistical analysis, J.E.H.; manuscript preparation, editing, and review, all authors

Staging Non–Small Cell Lung Cancer with Whole-Body PET[1]

PURPOSE: To compare the accuracies of whole-body 2-[fluorine 18]fluoro-2-deoxy-D-glucose (FDG) positron emission tomography (PET) and conventional imaging (thoracic computed tomography [CT], bone scintigraphy, and brain CT or magnetic resonance [MR] imaging) in staging bronchogenic carcinoma.

MATERIALS AND METHODS: Within 20 months, 100 patients with newly diagnosed bronchogenic carcinoma underwent whole-body FDG PET and chest CT. Ninety of these patients underwent radionuclide bone scintigraphy, and 70 patients underwent brain CT or MR imaging. For each patient, all examinations were completed within 1 month. A radiologic stage was assigned by using PET and conventional imaging independently and was compared with the pathologic stage. The accuracy, sensitivity, specificity, and negative and positive predictive values were calculated.

RESULTS: PET staging was accurate in 83 (83%) patients; conventional imaging staging was accurate in 65 (65%) patients ($P < .005$). Staging with mediastinal lymph nodes was correct by using PET in 67 (85%) patients and by using CT in 46 (58%) patients ($P < .001$). Nine (9%) patients had metastases demonstrated by using PET that were not found with conventional imaging, whereas 10 (10%) patients suspected of having metastases because of conventional imaging findings were correctly shown with PET to not have metastases.

CONCLUSION: Whole-body PET was more accurate than thoracic CT, bone scintigraphy, and brain CT or MR imaging in staging bronchogenic carcinoma.

Bronchogenic carcinoma is the leading cause of cancer-related death in the Western world (1). Accurate staging is essential, as it provides prognostic information and influences treatment options. Currently, radiologic staging is pursued by using a combination of studies, which usually include contrast material–enhanced thoracic computed tomography (CT) through the liver, radionuclide bone scintigraphy, and brain CT or magnetic resonance (MR) imaging. No single modality provides all of the requisite information (2).

Positron emission tomography (PET) by using 2-[fluorine 18]fluoro-2-deoxy-D-glucose (FDG) has been shown to be an accurate imaging modality that complements conventional studies in evaluating patients with bronchogenic carcinoma. Previous studies have examined the utility of PET for imaging the primary tumor, regional lymph nodes, and distant disease (3–8). The purpose of this study was to compare the accuracy of whole-body FDG PET imaging to the accuracies of other routine conventional imaging studies used in staging newly diagnosed bronchogenic carcinoma.

MATERIALS AND METHODS

Patient Selection

From November 1995 to July 1997, 139 consecutive patients who had newly diagnosed lung cancer or who were strongly suspected because of radiologic studies to have lung cancer were prospectively examined. Thirty-nine patients were subsequently excluded because of equivocal diagnoses at biopsy ($n = 12$), nonbronchogenic neoplasms ($n = 10$), small cell lung cancer ($n = 9$), inability to retrieve outside chest CT scans ($n = 7$), and poor-quality PET scans because of prior insulin injection ($n = 1$). Thus, 100 patients were included in the study group.

Radiologic Staging

One hundred patients (58 men, 42 women; mean age, 63 years; age range, 25–83 years) underwent whole-body PET and thoracic CT. Ninety of the 100 patients underwent radionuclide bone scintigraphy, and 78 patients underwent brain CT or MR imaging. All studies were completed within 1 month of the diagnosis and before treatment.

PET Imaging

All 100 patients underwent whole-body FDG PET, as requested for staging of newly diagnosed lung cancer at our institution. Studies were performed with an Advance (GE Medical Systems, Milwaukee, Wis) PET scanner (9). Patients fasted for at least 4 hours before receiving the intravenous administration of 145 μCi/kg (5,365 kBq/kg; maximum, 20 mCi [740 MBq]) FDG. Thirty minutes following the injection, a 4-minute acquisition in the brain was performed by using the three-dimensional acquisition mode (9). The system was switched to the two-dimensional acquisition mode, and non–attenuation-corrected scans were obtained for 4 minutes per bed position from the level of the base of the brain through the middle of the thighs. A two–bed-position, attenuation-corrected regional chest scan was then obtained by using 8 minutes for emission scanning and 10 minutes for transmission scanning at each bed position. The emission brain scan was corrected for attenuation by using a calculated attenuation correction (10). The images were reconstructed by using a Hann filter, with a cutoff of 0.71/cm. Reconstructed images were displayed in a 128 × 128 matrix with 35 sections, which contained 3.5 × 3.5 × 4.25-mm voxels.

Standardized uptake values were obtained by placing a circular region of interest within the visible margin of the lesion in an area of abnormal FDG accumulation on the attenuation-corrected PET images in the axial plane that best showed the lung abnormality to include the most intense area of FDG accumulation (11). Activity concentration was averaged over the circular region of interest. After correction for radioactive decay, the standardized uptake value was calculated by dividing the mean activity in the lesion by the administered FDG dose per kilogram of body weight (11).

All PET studies were interpreted independently on film hard copy in combination with an interactive video display by two experienced nuclear medicine physicians. Disagreements in interpretation were resolved by consensus. Images were correlated with the chest CT scans. Bone and brain images were not available for comparison.

PET images were read as positive or negative at the primary site (T status), regional lymph nodes (N status), and distant metastases (M status). Lung lesions were considered positive when uptake was greater than the mediastinal blood pool activity. If visual uptake in the lung lesion was similar to that in the mediastinal blood pool, a standardized uptake value was obtained; the lesion was considered malignant if the value obtained was greater than 2.5 (11). Areas of accumulations greater than that in the surrounding normal tissue were considered abnormal for regions outside of the lungs. A PET stage based on the TNM status was assigned according to the revised International System for Staging Lung Cancer (12).

TABLE 1
Correlation of Conventional Imaging, PET, and Clinical-Pathologic Stages

PET Stage	Conventional Imaging Stage: IA	IB	IIA	IIB	IIIA	IIIB	IV
IA	pIA: 10	0	0	pIIB: 1	0	0	pIA: 4
IB	0	pIB: 3	0	0	0	pIIIA: 1	pIV: 2
IIA	0	0	0	0	pIIIB: 1	0	pIIA: 1 pIV: 1
IIB	0	0	0	pIIIA: 1	0	pIIB: 1 pIIIB: 1	0
IIIA	pIA: 1	pIIIA: 1	pIIIB: 1	pIIIA: 1	pIIIA: 3 pIIIB: 1	0	pIIIA: 2
IIIB	pIIIA: 1 pIIIB: 2	pIIIB: 1	0	0	pIIIB: 3	pIIIB: 9	pIB: 1 pIIIB: 2 pIV: 1
IV	pIA: 2	pIV: 1	pIIIB: 1	pIV: 1	pIV: 3	pIV: 4	pIV: 31

Note.—The final clinical-pathologic stage is designated in each box as a p stage. The data are numbers of patients.

CT Imaging

Sixty-one patients underwent chest CT at our institution with a model 9800 CT HiSpeed Advantage scanner (GE Medical Systems) by using 10-mm collimation (pitch = 1) from the lung apex through the liver. The remaining 39 patients underwent examinations (n = 39) outside our institution with a variety of scanners and either 7- or 10-mm collimation (pitch = 1) from the lung apices through the liver. Intravenous contrast material was administered in 72 patients (72%).

All contrast-enhanced and nonenhanced chest CT scans were interpreted independently by at least two experienced thoracic radiologists (E.M.M., H.P.M., J.J.E., P.C.G., D.K.C., E.F.P.), and a CT stage was assigned by using TNM descriptors according to the revised International System for Staging Lung Cancer (12,13). We did not make a distinction between contrast-enhanced and nonenhanced scans in view of our prior experience (13). Disagreements in interpretation were resolved by consensus. Lymph nodes greater than 1 cm in the short axis were considered positive. The bone scintigrams and PET scans were not available at the time of interpretation.

Brain CT and MR Imaging

Seventy-eight (78%) patients underwent conventional imaging of the brain as routine staging for newly diagnosed lung cancer at our institution: 58 patients, brain CT; 15 patients, brain MR imaging; and five patients, brain CT and MR imaging. Brain CT examinations were performed with contrast material (100 mL of iopamidol [Isovue 300; Bracco Diagnostics, Princeton, NJ]) and a model 9800 CT HiSpeed Advantage scanner (GE Medical Systems) by using 5-mm collimation (pitch = 1) through the posterior fossa and 10-mm collimation (pitch = 1) through the rest of the brain.

Axial T1-weighted nonenhanced (500/20) and gadolinium-enhanced (500/20; Magnevist [gadopentetate dimeglumine]; Berlex, Wayne, NJ; dose, 0.1 mmol per kg of body weight), T2-weighted (2,500/80), and intermediate-weighted (2,500/30) MR images and coronal gadolinium-enhanced T1-weighted MR images (500/20) were obtained with a 1.5-T imager (GE Medical Systems; Signa 5X platform).

All brain studies were interpreted by an experienced neuroradiologist, and sites of

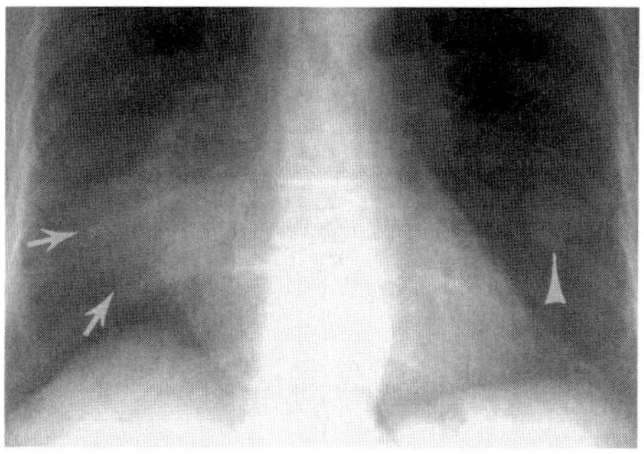

a.

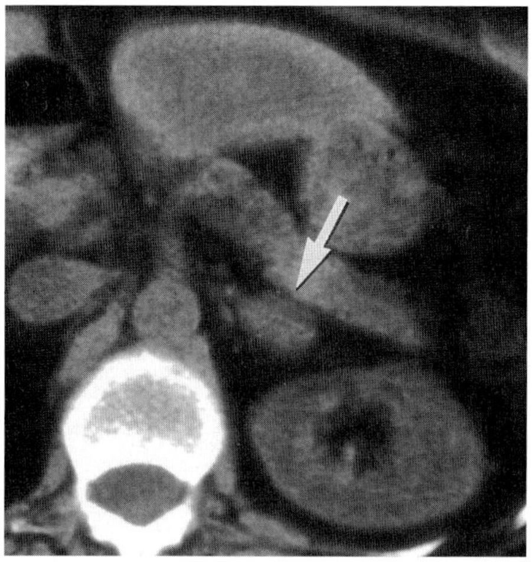

b.

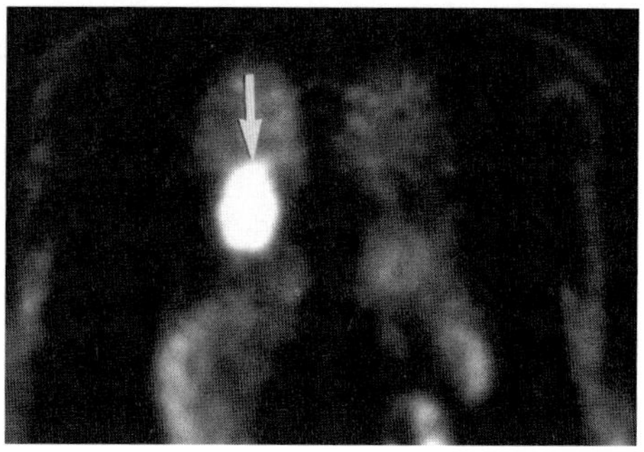

c.

Figure 1. Images obtained in a 56-year-old woman with a 4-month history of dry cough. **(a)** Posteroanterior chest radiograph shows right middle lobe lung mass (arrows) with right hilar adenopathy and a 2.5-cm left middle lobe lung nodule (arrowhead). **(b)** Axial CT scan shows a 30-HU, 2-cm left adrenal mass (arrow). **(c)** Coronal PET scan shows increased uptake consistent with malignancy in a right lung mass (arrow), with no uptake in a left lung nodule or adrenal mass, which is consistent with a benign process. Biopsy of the right lung mass showed adenocarcinoma, and comparison with prior studies demonstrated stability of the left lung nodule over 8 years. Follow-up CT at 20 months showed the adrenal gland to be stable.

metastatic disease were recorded. The PET scans were not available at the time of interpretation.

Bone Scintigraphy

Ninety (90%) patients underwent radionuclide bone scintigraphy as routine staging for newly diagnosed lung cancer at our institution. Whole-body images were obtained in the anterior and posterior projections starting 2–3 hours following the intravenous injection of 430 μCi/kg (15,910 kBq/kg; 30.0 mCi [1,110 MBq] maximum) of technetium 99m methylene diphosphonate. Either a Bodyscan (Nuclear Medicine Group, Siemens Medical Systems, Hoffman Estates, Ill) or a T-22 Twin Detector Nuclear Imaging System (SMV, Twinsburg, Ohio) was used for the radionuclide bone imaging studies.

Bone scintigrams were interpreted by two nuclear medicine physicians, and sites of metastatic disease were recorded. The PET scans were not available at the time of interpretation.

Clinical-Pathologic Correlation

All 100 patients had histologic confirmation of lung cancer. Transbronchial needle biopsy (n = 41), transthoracic needle biopsy (n = 38), mediastinoscopy (n = 26), thoracotomy (n = 41), or video-assisted thoracoscopic biopsy (n = 1) was performed. In 47 patients, histologic confirmation of lung cancer was obtained by using more than one of these methods.

Of the 100 patients, 79 patients had clinical-pathologic lymph node status assigned following biopsy (n = 48) or imaging follow-up with CT (n = 31) for a mean of 12.8 months (range, 1–49 months). Those patients with clinical follow-up had lymph nodes recorded as pathologic if there was a substantial change in size (>5 mm) at follow-up examinations relative to the baseline size. Twenty-one patients did not undergo nodal sampling or did not have sufficient follow-up because of distant metastatic disease or T4 lesions. Fourteen patients with metastases suggested on imaging studies underwent biopsy of distant sites.

Biopsy specimens from outside institutions were reviewed by an experienced pulmonary pathologist at our institution. A final pathologic stage was assigned after correlation of the radiologic findings and biopsy specimens.

Patients were followed up by reviewing their medical charts and radiologic studies for a mean of 10.7 months ± 7.4 (SD; range, 1–49 months). Radiologic follow-up intervals and imaging varied according to staging and treatment, but follow-up included a combination of chest or abdominal CT, radionuclide bone scintigraphy, brain CT or MR imaging, and chest or musculoskeletal radiography.

Statistical Analysis

The McNemar test was used to compare the accuracies of PET with those of conventional imaging modalities for nodal disease, M status, and site-specific metastases to the brain, bone, adrenal glands, liver, and lungs. Sensitivity, specificity, and positive and negative predictive values were calculated for PET, chest CT, bone scintigraphy, and brain CT and MR imaging for mediastinal nodal staging and staging of metastases by sites.

RESULTS

Forty-one patients (41%) had adenocarcinoma (including four [4%] with bronchoalveolar carcinoma), 33 (33%) had squamous cell carcinoma, seven (7%) had large cell carcinoma, 18 (18%) had unspecified non–small cell carcinoma, and one (1%) had sarcomatoid carcinoma.

PET staging was correct in 83 patients (83%), as compared with correct conventional imaging staging in 65 patients (65%; $P < .005$). PET correctly indicated that disease was unresectable in 12 (12%) patients in whom disease had been understaged and considered resectable at conventional imaging. Conventional imaging indicated that disease was unresectable in four (4%) patients in whom disease had been understaged and considered resectable at PET. PET correctly indicated disease was resectable in 11 (11%) patients in whom disease had been overstaged and considered unresectable at conventional imaging (Fig 1), whereas conventional imaging indicated disease was resectable in only two (2%) patients in whom disease had been overstaged and considered unresectable at PET. The distribution and correlation of the conventional imaging stages, PET stages, and clinical-pathologic stages are shown in Table 1.

Primary Tumor Status

CT demonstrated the primary tumor in all 100 patients. There were 38 patients (38%) with a T1 lesion, 31 patients (31%) with a T2 lesion, 12 patients (12%) with a T3 lesion, and 19 patients (19%) with a T4 lesion. PET correctly indicated malignancy at the primary site in all 100 patients (100%).

Lymph Node Status

PET correctly indicated the N status in 67 patients (85%), and CT correctly indicated the N status in 46 patients (58%; $P < .001$). Most important, for differentiation of surgical and nonsurgical candidates with N3 disease, the sensitivity of PET was 92% and that of CT was 25%; the specificity of PET was 93% and that of CT was 98% ($P = .005$). The distribution and correlation of lymph node status according to CT findings, PET findings, and clinical-pathologic confirmations are shown in Table 2.

TABLE 2
Correlation of Conventional Imaging, PET, and Clinical-Pathologic Nodal Stages

PET Nodal Status	CT Nodal Status: N0	N1	N2	N3
N0	pN0: 24 pN2: 1	pN0: 1	pN0: 2	pN0: 1
N1	pN1: 1 pN2: 1	pN1: 2 pN3: 1	pN2: 1	0
N2	pN0: 1 pN2: 3	pN0: 1 pN2: 1	pN0: 1 pN2: 10 pN3: 1	0
N3	pN2: 1 pN3: 10	0	pN2: 2 pN3: 6	pN0: 1 pN3: 6

Note.—The final clinical-pathologic nodal status is designated in each box as a pN stage.

Metastasis Status

PET correctly indicated the M status in 40 (91%) of 44 patients with metastatic disease, while conventional imaging correctly indicated the M status in 35 (80%) of the 44 patients with metastatic disease (Fig 2). In nine patients (9%) not suspected at conventional imaging of having metastases, PET showed lesions suggestive of metastases; these were confirmed with biopsy ($n = 1$) or imaging follow-up ($n = 8$). Only four patients (4%) not suspected of having metastases at PET had lesions suggestive of metastases at conventional imaging that were proved with biopsy ($n = 1$) or imaging follow-up ($n = 3$).

Eleven (11%) patients thought to have metastases at conventional imaging had normal PET findings; these cases were confirmed not to be metastases at biopsy ($n = 1$) or imaging follow-up ($n = 10$). Only two (2%) patients thought to have metastases at PET were confirmed not to have metastases at follow-up conventional imaging. Therefore, the overall accuracy of PET for M staging was 94%, and that of conventional imaging was 80% ($P < .011$).

Brain Imaging

Five of the 78 patients who underwent conventional imaging of the brain had metastases at presentation that were confirmed with biopsy ($n = 2$) or with progression on follow-up CT scans ($n = 3$; mean follow-up, 3 months; range of follow-up, 1–6 months). PET showed brain metastases in three of the five patients with brain metastases. The other two patients had normal PET studies and had understaged disease; one proved to have a 5-mm lesion in the pons and the other had leptomeningeal disease. One patient had disease overstaged with PET, as increased uptake in the junction between gray matter and white matter was interpreted as metastatic disease, but no disease was found at initial and 8-month-follow-up brain MR imaging. The accuracy of PET for brain M staging was 96% ($n = 75$) and that of conventional imaging was 100% ($n = 78$; $P = .248$). The sensitivity, specificity, and positive and negative predictive values of PET for brain metastases were 60%, 99%, 75%, and 97%, respectively, and those of conventional imaging were 100%, 100%, 100%, and 100%, respectively.

TABLE 3
Radionuclide Bone Scintigraphic versus Histopathologic Findings

Histopathologic Findings	Bone Scintigraphic Findings: Positive	Negative
Positive	6	6
Negative	6	72

TABLE 4
PET versus Histopathologic Findings of Bone Metastasis

Histopathologic Findings	PET Findings: Positive	Negative
Positive	11	1
Negative	1	77

Bone Imaging

Twelve patients had bone metastases at presentation proved with biopsy ($n = 4$) or clinical follow-up ($n = 8$) that showed progression on bone scintigrams obtained at a mean follow-up of 3 months (range, 1–8 months). Staging was correct with PET in 88 of the 90 patients who underwent bone scintigraphy, with an accuracy of 98%. Bone metastases were correctly identified with PET in 11 (92%) patients with bone metastases. One patient had disease that was understaged and had a metastasis to the distal femur, a region not included in the whole-body PET study, confirmed with biopsy. One patient had disease overstaged with PET, which demonstrated a focal thoracic vertebral body abnormality. There was no abnormality on CT scans, bone scintigrams, or conventional radiographs at the time of diagnosis, and 23 months after resection, the patient had no evidence of disease.

Bone metastases were correctly staged with bone scintigraphy in 78 of the 90 patients who underwent bone scintigraphy, with an accuracy of 87%. Bone metastases were correctly identified with bone scintigraphy in six of the 12 patients who had bone metastases, although disease was understaged in six patients, as the bone scintigrams were interpreted as normal. Six patients had disease that was overstaged or had equivocal bone scintigrams for metastatic disease, which was confirmed with a mean of 12 months of bone scintigraphic and/or radiographic follow-up (range, 9–15 months). PET was significantly more accurate than bone scintigraphy ($P = .016$). The sensitivity, specificity, and positive and negative predictive values of PET were 92%, 99%, 92%, and 99%, respectively, and those of bone scintigraphy were 50%, 92%, 50%, and 92%, respectively (Tables 3, 4).

Adrenal Gland Imaging

Six patients had adrenal metastases at presentation that were confirmed with biopsy ($n = 1$) or a mean CT follow-up of 4.6 months ($n = 5$; range, 3–7 months), which revealed interval growth of the masses. All six adrenal metastases (100%) were identified with PET, with no under- or overstaging. CT helped identify all six

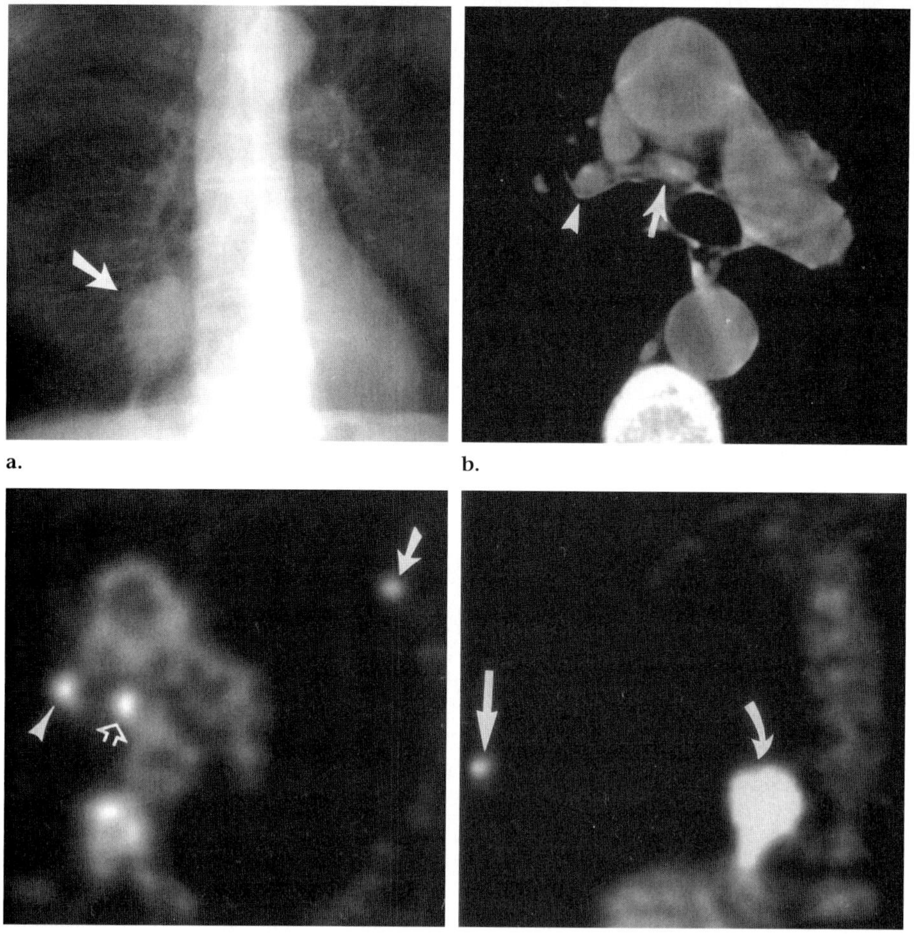

a. b. c. d.

Figure 2. Images obtained in a 65-year-old man with a 2-month history of cough. **(a)** Posteroanterior chest radiograph shows a 2.5-cm right lower lobe lung mass (arrow). **(b)** Axial CT scan obtained at the level of the carina shows a small precarinal (arrow) and a right hilar (arrowhead) lymph node. The ribs appear normal. **(c)** Axial PET image obtained at the same level as **b** shows increased uptake consistent with malignancy in the precarinal (open arrow) and right hilar (arrowhead) lymph nodes and in the left lateral rib (solid arrow). The lymph nodes had increased in size at 3-month follow-up CT; this is consistent with metastasis. **(d)** Coronal PET image shows increased uptake in a right lung mass (curved arrow) and the right humerus (straight arrow), which is consistent with malignancy. Biopsy of the lung mass showed large cell carcinoma, and bone metastases had progressed by 7-month bone scintigraphy.

patients with proved adrenal metastases (100%). Seven additional patients had masses on CT scans that did not meet the criteria for a benign abnormality (14), although none proved to be malignant according to CT follow-up (mean, 15.4 months; range, 6–24 months) findings. Therefore, adrenal M staging with CT was correct in 93 of the 100 patients, for a 93% accuracy in comparison to a 100% accuracy of PET. PET was significantly more accurate than CT for adrenal imaging ($P = .023$). The sensitivity, specificity, and positive and negative predictive values of PET for adrenal metastases detection were 100%, 100%, 100%, and 100%, respectively; those of CT were 100%, 93%, 46%, and 100%, respectively.

Liver Imaging

Six patients had liver metastases at presentation that were confirmed with CT follow-up, which showed interval growth over a mean of 6.8 months (range, 3–17 months). All hepatic lesions (100%) were correctly identified with PET. There were no false-positive liver lesions seen at PET. All six patients with liver metastases were correctly identified with CT. With CT, however, five benign liver lesions were overstaged as metastases, which was confirmed with CT follow-up (mean, 11.8 months; range, 4–18 months). Therefore, CT liver M staging was accurate in 95 (95%) patients in comparison to 100 (100%) patients with PET ($P < .074$). On follow-up CT scans, three additional patients developed new liver metastases. All had known distant metastases at other sites at the time of staging. One developed the metastases 14 months after staging, and the remaining two had liver metastases diagnosed at 9 and 15 months; however, each had a CT scan 3 months prior to development of the metastases that was negative. In two of the six patients with liver metastases at presentation, there were no other distant metastases at the time of presentation. The diameter ranged from 8 to 50 mm (mean ± SD, 18.7 mm ± 4.4). The sensitivity, specificity, and positive and negative predictive values of PET for liver metastases detection were 100%, 100%, 100%, and 100%, respectively; those of CT were 100%, 95%, 55%, and 100%, respectively.

Lung Imaging

Eighteen patients had lung metastasis proved with biopsy ($n = 2$) or had conventional imaging follow-up findings ($n = 16$) of interval growth during a mean of 3.5 months (range, 1–8 months). PET staging of the lung for metastases was correct in 98 (98%) of the 100 patients. PET helped identify 17 of the 18 patients with lung metastases (94%) at presentation. PET findings resulted in underestimation of disease in one patient (1%) with lymphangitic spread that had progressed in the 4-month conventional imaging follow-up interval and in overestimation of disease as metastatic in one (1%) patient whose region of FDG uptake was retrospectively thought to represent inflammation, as it had resolved on the follow-up 5-month PET scan and CT scan, while sites of metastatic disease showed progression. Lung metastases were correctly staged with CT in 91 (91%) of the 100 patients ($P = .070$). Fourteen (78%) of the 18 patients with lung metastases at presentation were identified at CT, with underestimation in the remaining four patients, which was proved by interval growth on CT follow-up scans (mean follow-up, 5.5 months; range, 4–8 months), and overstaging in five additional patients, which was proved by the stability of indeterminate lung nodules at CT over a mean of 8.5 months (range, 7–10 months). The sensitivity, specificity, and positive and negative predictive values of PET for lung metastases detection were 94%, 99%, 94%, and 99%, respectively, and those of CT were 78%, 94%, 74%, and 95%, respectively.

DISCUSSION

Tumor staging is an essential part of cancer management, as it determines treatment options and prognosis. While conventional imaging provides anatomic and morphologic information, it does not always allow accurate assessment of the extent of disease. More recently, FDG PET has been used to address some of the problems of diagnosing, staging, and following up patients with lung cancer, because it exploits fundamental biochemical differences between normal and neoplastic cells for imaging purposes. This study was initiated to determine if whole-body PET was more accurate in staging newly diagnosed lung cancer than the series of conventional imaging studies.

The new staging system and the TNM descriptors were designed for conventional imaging. They were constructed to reflect size and sites of disease, and this anatomic information is not always relevant for PET imaging. Describing the conventional T status is more problematic with PET than CT because of spatial resolution. As seen in this study, however, PET is adequate, and rare changes in the T status did not have a substantial effect on overall stage.

PET clearly demonstrates an advantage over CT in determining the N status. In a recent study, CT had only a 63% sensitivity and 57% specificity for mediastinal lymph node metastases, and 24% of normally sized nodes contained metastases (15). Thoracic CT provides only presumptive, not definitive, evidence for nodal disease. Its current utility is as a road map for guiding lymph node sampling, as small nodes may harbor tumor and large nodes may be reactive.

As conventional imaging is less than optimal, most thoracic surgeons still perform cervical mediastinoscopy (15), although this procedure alone cannot always be used to sample all pertinent lymph node groups. The addition of scalene lymph node biopsy has routinely been abandoned; however, in a recent study, Lee and Ginsberg (16) demonstrated that 15% of patients with N2-staged lung cancer harbored occult nonpalpable supraclavicular disease, which upstaged disease to N3 and resulted in an alteration in treatment. Evaluation of other nodal stations, including prevascular or paraesophageal stations, requires an additional procedure (17).

PET could have a substantial effect on nodal sampling. Whole-body studies demonstrate all lymph node stations and in some cases obviate mediastinoscopy. Because the negative predictive value of PET for N3 disease is identical to that of mediastinoscopy, which is 96% (15), patients with negative mediastinal PET findings could go directly to surgical resection of the primary lesion. Patients with a positive PET study in the mediastinum could undergo a single procedure guided by areas of abnormal FDG uptake.

PET also has an advantage over the combination of other routine studies required to determine the M status. Forty percent of patients with newly diagnosed lung cancer have distant metastases at presentation (1), although clinical and laboratory indicators for metastases are nonspecific, with an accuracy of only approximately 50% (18,19). Conventional imaging with thoracic CT, bone scintigraphy, or brain CT or MR is also less than optimal.

Overall, PET showed greater accuracy than conventional imaging in the detection of distant metastases. In nine patients (9%) not suspected of having metastases at conventional imaging, PET showed metastases. This result is similar to those of other studies (1,5).

When evaluating metastases by site, PET was almost uniformly superior to other conventional imaging modalities. PET was 92% sensitive and 99% specific for bone metastasis as compared to bone scintigraphy, with 50% sensitivity and 92% specificity. The whole-body PET study can eliminate the need for staging bone scintigraphy, as PET findings resulted in overstaging in only one patient and in understaging in one patient (98% accuracy). Understaging of a bone metastasis at PET may have been avoided by inclusion of the whole leg within the scanning plane, as the distal femur metastasis was not imaged with PET and therefore was missed.

Approximately two-thirds of the adrenal masses detected with conventional imaging in patients with lung cancer are reported to be benign (20,21). Our findings are in agreement with those of prior studies, as eight (57%) of 14 adrenal masses indeterminate at conventional imaging were benign. This low positive predictive value (43% in this study) leads to unnecessary adrenal biopsy, which is not without risk and is not always diagnostic. In a review of 83 adrenal biopsies, Mody et al (22) reported an 8.4% rate of complications, including pneumothorax, pain, perinephric hemorrhage, intrahepatic hematoma, and hepatic needle-track metastasis. The rate of false-negative percutaneous biopsy findings ranges from 2% to 8.6% (23–26).

In this study, the positive predictive value of PET for adrenal metastases detection was 100%. The high specificity (100%) in this study, when compared to that in a prior PET adrenal study (80%) (27), may be due to sampling error in the prior study's percutaneous biopsies because those patients with "false-positive" PET findings died shortly after the study, with no prior or follow-up imaging for comparison.

The normal brain has substantial glucose uptake, and a focal area of abnormal accumulation in the brain due to metastasis may be difficult to detect with PET. The low sensitivity (60%) is problematic when staging lung carcinoma, as the brain is a common site of metastatic disease; 5.5%–16.3% of patients with brain metastases are asymptomatic (28,29). Although brain imaging in whole-body PET lengthens the examination by 4 minutes, it is probably unnecessary because of PET's low sensitivity. Abnormalities likely to influence clinical management prospectively were not identified with PET (7), and PET should not replace conventional imaging for routine staging in the brain.

In this limited series, PET proved useful for hepatic metastases, as it showed no false-positive or, to our knowledge, false-negative liver lesions. This is in comparison with eight indeterminate abnormalities at CT. The true sensitivity and specificity still need to be evaluated further in a detailed study that would compare PET with a dedicated contrast-enhanced liver CT examination with sequential follow-up; however, preliminary study findings have shown PET to be superior to conventional imaging in the detection of liver metastases (30–34). Findings of this study suggest that the whole-body PET examination appears to complement conventional imaging in the liver, particularly when lesions are indeterminate.

From a clinical and radiologic perspective, one of the most important decisions is to determine if the patient is a surgical candidate. Disease that is stage IIIa or less is potentially resectable, while disease that is stage IIIB or higher is not. In this study, PET findings indicated that 12% of patients had disease mistakenly understaged and considered resectable at conventional imaging, whereas conventional imaging findings indicated that only 4% of the study patients considered surgical candidates at PET had disease understaged.

The cost-effectiveness of FDG PET in staging lung cancer has been studied in comparison to only that of chest CT. FDG

PET, combining improved patient care with reduced treatment cost, has been found to be decisively more cost-effective than CT (35,36). When PET was considered as an addition to conventional staging procedures, the ratio of savings to cost was greater than 2:1. When PET was considered as replacing CT and bone scintigraphy, the ratio was greater than 3:1. PET was effective in reducing management costs even when it was an add-on procedure (35).

In conclusion, we believe whole-body PET is very useful in staging newly diagnosed lung cancer. There is marked improvement in staging the thorax with PET than with CT, with a predicted reduction in the morbidity rate and cost associated with unnecessary interventional procedures. PET appears to be more accurate than other modalities in differentiating resectable from nonresectable disease. Radionuclide bone scintigraphy may be eliminated, although brain imaging is still required if clinically indicated.

References

1. Landis SH, Murray T, Bolden S, Wingo PA. Cancer statistics, 1998. CA Cancer J Clin 1998; 48:6–29.
2. Bragg DG. Current applications of imaging procedures in the patient with lung cancer. Int J Radiat Oncol Biol Phys 1991; 21:847–885.
3. Steinert H, et al. Non-small cell lung cancer: nodal staging with FDG PET versus CT with correlative lymph node mapping and sampling. Radiology 1997; 202:441–446.
4. Bury T, Dowalti A, Paulus P, et al. Whole-body 18FDG positron emission tomography in the staging of non-small cell lung cancer. Eur Respir J 1997; 10:2529–2534.
5. Valk PE, Pounds TR, Hopkins DM, et al. Staging non-small cell lung cancer by whole-body positron emission tomographic imaging. Ann Thorac Surg 1995; 60:1573–1582.
6. Lewis P, Griffin S, Marsden P, et al. Whole-body ^{18}F-fluorodeoxyglucose positron emission tomography in preoperative evaluation of lung cancer. Lancet 1994; 344:1265–1266.
7. Larcos G, Maisey MN. FDG-PET screening for cerebral metastases in patients with suspected malignancy. Nucl Med Commun 1996; 17:197–198.
8. Lowe VJ, Fletcher JW, Gobar L, et al. Prospective investigation of PET in lung nodules (PIOPILN). J Clin Oncol 1998; 16:1075–1084.
9. DeGrado TR, Turkington TG, Williams JJ, Stearns CW, Hoffman JM, Coleman RE. Performance characteristics of a whole-body PET scanner. J Nucl Med 1994; 35: 1398–1406.
10. Coleman RE, Hoffman JM, Hanson MW, Sostman HD, Schold SC. Clinical application of PET for the evaluation of brain tumors. J Nucl Med 1991; 32:616–622.
11. Patz EF, Lowe VJ, Hoffman JM, et al. Focal pulmonary abnormalities: evaluation with F-18 fluorodeoxyglucose PET scanning. Radiology 1993; 188:487–490.
12. Mountain CF. Revisions in the International System for Staging Lung Cancer. Chest 1997; 111:1710–1717.
13. Patz Jr EF, Erasmus JJ, McAdams HP, et al. Lung cancer staging and management: comparison of contrast-enhanced and nonenhanced helical CT of the thorax. Radiology 1999; 212:56–60.
14. Korobkin M, Brodeur FJ, Yutzy GG, et al. Differentiation of adrenal adenomas from nonadenomas using CT attenuation values. AJR 1996; 166:531–536.
15. Gdeedo A, Van Schill P, Corthouts B, Van Mieghem F, Van Meerbeek J, Van Mark E. Prospective evaluation of computed tomography and mediastinoscopy in mediastinal lymph node staging. Eur Respir J 1997; 10:1547–1551.
16. Lee JD, Ginsberg RJ. Lung cancer staging: the value of ipsilateral scalene lymph node biopsy performed at mediastinoscopy. Ann Thorac Surg 1996; 62:338–341.
17. Nakanishi R, Yasumoto K. Combined thoracoscopy and mediastinoscopy for mediastinal lymph node staging of lung cancer. Int Surg 1996; 81:359–361.
18. Salvatierra A, Baamonde C, Llamas JM, Cruz F, Lopez-Pujol J. Extrathoracic staging of bronchogenic carcinoma. Chest 1990; 97:1052–1058.
19. Quinn DL, Ostrow LB, Porter DK, Shelton DK Jr, Jackson DE Jr. Staging of non-small cell bronchogenic carcinoma. Chest 1986; 89:270–275.
20. Reinig JW, Doppman JL, Dwyer AJ, Johnson AR, Knop RH. Adrenal masses differentiated by MR. Radiology 1986; 158:81–84.
21. Oliver TW Jr, Bernardino ME, Miller JI, Mansour K, Greene D, Davis WA. Isolated adrenal masses in nonsmall-cell bronchogenic carcinoma. Radiology 1984; 153: 217–218.
22. Mody MK, Kazerooni EA, Korobkin M. Percutaneous CT-guided biopsy of adrenal masses: immediate and delayed complications. J Comput Assist Tomogr 1995; 19:434–439.
23. Caldironi MW, Boccato P, Maifredini CS, et al. Cyto-assisted, ultrasound-guided biopsy in the diagnosis of focal disease of the abdomen. Tumori 1991; 77:65–69.
24. Jaeger HJ, MacFie J, Mitchel CJ, Couse N, Wai D. Diagnosis of abdominal masses with percutaneous biopsy guided by ultrasound. BMJ 1990; 301:1188–1191.
25. vanSonnenberg E, Wittenberg J, Ferruci JT Jr, Mueller PR, Simone JF. Triangulation method for percutaneous needle guidance: the angled approach to upper abdominal masses. AJR 1981; 137:757–761.
26. Bernardino ME, Walther MM, Phillips VM, et al. CT-guided adrenal biopsy: accuracy, safety, and indications. AJR 1985; 144: 67–69.
27. Erasmus JJ, Patz EF, McAdams HP, et al. Evaluation of adrenal masses in patients with bronchogenic carcinoma by using 18F-fluorodeoxyglucose positron emission tomography. AJR 1997; 168:1357–1360.
28. Tarver RD, Richmond BD, Klatte EC. Cerebral metastases from lung carcinoma: neurological and CT correlation. Radiology 1984; 153:689–692.
29. Yokoi K, Miyazawa N, Arai T. Brain metastasis in resected lung cancer: value of intensive follow-up with computed tomography. Ann Thorac Surg 1996; 61:546–551.
30. Hustinx R, Paulus P, Jacquet N, Jerusalem G, Bury T, Rigo P. Clinical evaluation of whole-body 18F-fluorodeoxyglucose positron emission tomography in the detection of liver metastases. Ann Oncol 1998; 9:397–401.
31. Abdel-Nabi H, Doerr RJ, Lamonica DM, et al. Staging of primary colorectal carcinomas with fluorine-18 fluorodeoxyglucose whole-body PET: correlation with histopathologic and CT findings. Radiology 1998; 206:755–560.
32. Delbeke D, Martin WH, Sandler MP, Chapman WC, Wright JK, Pinson CW. Evaluation of benign vs malignant hepatic lesions with positron emission tomography. Arch Surg 1998; 133:510–515.
33. Schiepers C, Penninckx F, De Vadder N, et al. Contribution of PET in the diagnosis of recurrent colorectal cancer: comparison with conventional imaging. Eur J Surg Oncol 1995; 21:517–522.
34. Ogunbiyi OA, Flanagan FL, Dehdashti F, et al. Detection of recurrent and metastatic colorectal cancer: comparison of positron emission tomography and computed tomography. Ann Surg Oncol 1997; 4:613–620.
35. Valk PE, Pounds TR, Tesa RD, Hopkins DM, Haseman MK. Cost-effectiveness of PET imaging in clinical oncology. Nucl Med Biol 1996; 23:737–743.
36. Gambhir SS, Hoh CK, Phelps ME, Madar I, Maddahi J. Decision tree sensitivity analysis for cost-effectiveness of FDG-PET in the staging and management of non-small-cell lung carcinoma. J Nucl Med 1996; 37:1428–1436.

Book Review

Fog: A Collection of Backscatter

Brad Tipler, MD

Waynesboro, Va: Evil Humours Press, 1998. ISBN 0-9666738-0-8. Softcover, $16.00; pp 125.

Dr Tipler, a radiologist in private practice in Roanoke, Va, is well known to readers of *Diagnostic Imaging*. He has been writing a column entitled "Backscatter" for the past 5 years, and this book is a collection of essays originally published in that journal.

In this book, the author finds humor in the everyday experiences in a busy radiology department, including patients waiting in halls, whining radiologists, over- and underexposed films, and hospital paging systems. Changes in health care (including the advent of health maintenance organizations), medical meetings (including the RSNA annual meeting), and the exponential growth of continuing medical education courses are also targets of his pen. Occasionally, our referring colleagues are the objects of his wit. I found his column on the sometimes seemingly unreasonable demands from the emergency department particularly amusing. However, apparently not all emergency department physicians did, since the author admits in a later column that he received "some spicy faxes from humor impaired ER docs around the country."

As a gastrointestinal radiologist, I was particularly pleased that the first chapter is entitled "We Have Met the Barium Enemy and It Is Us." In this essay, Dr Tipler reminds us that we are dealing with a person, not a colon. What is routine for us is often foreign and sometimes frightening for a patient. It is important to empathize with our patients and help them through the sometimes intimidating experiences they confront in the radiology department. Another essay speaks of the healing value in the caring touch of a physician. In fact, an underlying theme throughout the book is that although our work is important, people are more important. This includes our co-workers as well as our patients.

Another chapter reminds us that our technologists need to be appreciated all year long, not just for 1 week. It is easy to become so busy that we don't take time for one another. "The Good, the Bad, and the Ugly of Everyday Practice" is a chapter that encourages us not to take ourselves too seriously—to laugh at the bad and the ugly and be thankful for the good.

I recommend this affordably priced book without hesitation. We all face the uncertainties and anxieties of health care reform and the changing practice of medicine. We all face the challenges and frustrations of keeping up with the latest scientific advances in the midst of the busy everyday practice of radiology. This book allows one to sit back for a few moments and look at some of these things from a little less serious and more humorous perspective. Sometimes laughter is good medicine.

Reviewed by Richard Szucs, MD

Bonnie N. Joe, MD, PhD
Melanie B. Fukui, MD
Carolyn Cidis Meltzer, MD
Qing-shou Huang, MS
Roger S. Day, ScD
Phil J. Greer, BS
Michael E. Bozik, MD

Index terms:
Brain neoplasms, 10.363, 10.3634
Brain neoplasms, MR, 10.12141, 10.12143
Magnetic resonance (MR), volume measurement, 10.12141, 10.12143
Technology assessment

Radiology 1999; 212:811–816

[1] From the Departments of Radiology, Division of Neuroradiology (B.N.J., M.B.F., C.C.M., P.J.G.), Psychiatry (C.C.M.), Neurosurgery (M.E.B.), Neurology (M.E.B.), and Medicine (M.E.B.), and the Pittsburgh Cancer Institute (Q.H., R.S.D.), University of Pittsburgh Medical Center, Pittsburgh, Pa. Received May 29, 1998; revision requested July 22; revision received November 11; accepted March 29, 1999. **Address reprint requests to** M.B.F., Department of Radiology, Presbyterian University Hospital, Rm D-132, 200 Lothrop St, Pittsburgh, PA 15213-2582 (e-mail: *fukuimb@radserv.arad.upmc.edu*).

Author contributions:
Guarantors of integrity of entire study, B.N.J., M.B.F., C.C.M.; study concepts, B.N.J., M.B.F., C.C.M., R.S.D., M.E.B.; study design, B.N.J., M.B.F., C.C.M., R.S.D.; definition of intellectual content, B.N.J., M.B.F., C.C.M.; literature research, B.N.J., M.B.F., C.C.M.; clinical studies, M.E.B.; experimental studies, M.B.F., B.N.J., C.C.M., P.J.G.; data acquisition, M.B.F., B.N.J., P.J.G., C.C.M.; data analysis, B.N.J., M.B.F., C.C.M., P.J.G., Q.H., R.S.D.; statistical analysis, B.N.J., Q.H., R.S.D.; manuscript preparation, B.N.J.; manuscript editing, B.N.J., M.B.F., C.C.M.; manuscript review, all authors.

Brain Tumor Volume Measurement: Comparison of Manual and Semiautomated Methods[1]

PURPOSE: To compare the reliability of two approaches to measuring enhancing brain tumor volumes—the conventional manual trace method and a threshold-based, semiautomated computer software method.

MATERIALS AND METHODS: Two operators rated contrast material–enhanced, T1-weighted axial magnetic resonance (MR) image data sets from 16 patients aged 21–71 years with high-grade gliomas. Each MR data set was rated twice by using manual tracing and twice by using the semiautomated method. The semiautomated measurement method involved a thresholding algorithm based on mixture modeling. The data collection time for each method was recorded. Reliability was measured by using inter- and intraoperator agreement indexes.

RESULTS: Mean intraoperator agreement indexes (± SD) were 0.90 ± 0.09 (operator 1) and 0.83 ± 0.15 (operator 2) for the manual trace method and 0.83 ± 0.17 (operator 1) and 0.84 ± 0.16 (operator 2) for the semiautomated measurement method. The mean interoperator agreement was 0.85 ± 0.14 for the manual method and 0.82 ± 0.18 for the semiautomated method. The semiautomated method was faster than the manual trace method by an average of 4.6 minutes per patient.

CONCLUSION: The semiautomated computer method of measuring tumor volume was faster than the manual trace method. Semiautomated computer approaches offer an alternative to manual tracing for measuring serial tumor volumes in patients with high-grade brain neoplasms.

Brain tumor volumes measured from diameters on computed tomographic (CT) and magnetic resonance (MR) images have been commonly used in the evaluation of intracerebral tumors and have implications for patient prognosis and treatment. Tracing the enhancing margin could potentially provide a more representative measurement of tumor size and has been used in clinical trials to assess treatment response (1). At many institutions, brain tumor volume measurements are obtained by the MR technologist, who manually traces the enhancing tissue on each image by using widely available imaging software. This approach is potentially subjective and prone to large variations in intra- and interoperator performance. Such variations affect the validity of serial measurements used in the planning of therapy, because a single technologist does not necessarily perform all tumor volume measurements in a given patient. Variability in serial volume measurements and inconsistency between observers have been noted by others (2–5) in studies involving tumor volume measurement methods used to follow tumor response to treatment or to plan treatment. Although previous studies (2,3) have involved limited evaluations of the reliability of tumor volumetrics, detailed comparisons of alternative semiautomated methods versus the conventional manual trace method have not been performed. To our knowledge, the reliability of manual tracing has not been considered in the more extensive studies (6,7) of inter- and intraoperator reliability of tumor volume measurement methods.

In this study, we quantitatively compared two methods of measuring enhancing tumor volumes from MR image data—the conventional manual trace method and a threshold-based semiautomated computer segmentation method. To compare the inter-and intraoperator reliability of the two methods, two operators performed tumor volume determinations twice with each method in the same subjects. Our hypotheses were that (*a*) the manual trace method would be more user dependent—that is, have low interoperator reliability, and (*b*) the semiautomated method would provide more reproducible measurements—that is, have high intraoperator reliability.

MATERIALS AND METHODS

Patient Population

The study group consisted of 16 adult patients (13 men, three women; mean age, 53 years; age range, 22–71 years) with histologically proved, unresected high-grade gliomas, who were randomly selected from an ongoing treatment protocol conducted by the University of Pittsburgh Medical Center Neuro-Oncology Service. The inclusion criterion was the presence of an enhancing tumor on more than one MR image obtained by using routine imaging parameters.

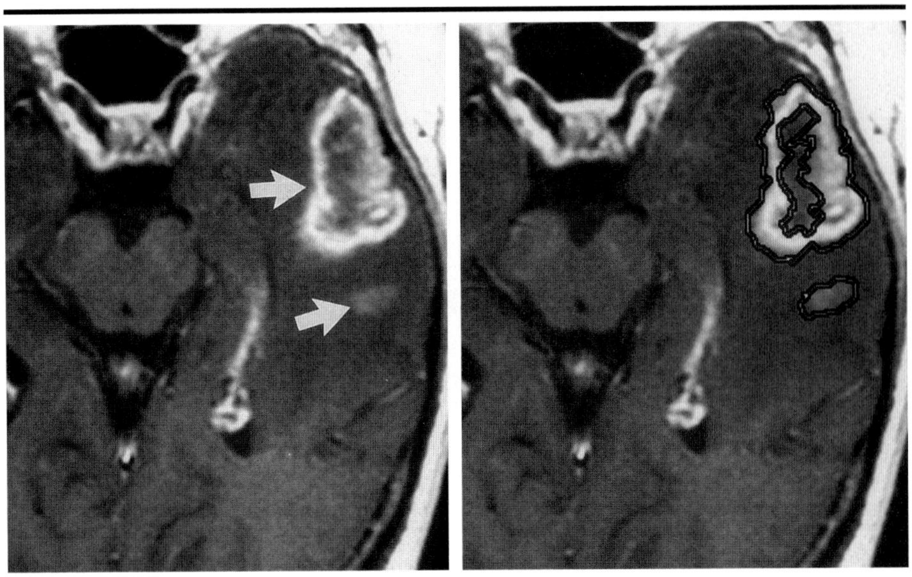

a. b.

Figure 1. **(a, b)** Axial T1-weighted MR images (repetition time msec/echo time msec, 466/11) demonstrate the manual trace method in two areas of tumor enhancement (arrows in **a**) in the left temporal lobe of a patient with glioblastoma multiforme. In **b**, the contours generated by manually tracing the enhancing portions of the tumor are shown.

MR Image Acquisition

From images obtained by using the routine clinical imaging protocol performed with a Signa 1.5-T imaging unit (GE Medical Systems, Milwaukee, Wis), we selected the contrast material–enhanced (0.1 mmol/kg gadoteridol [Prohance; Bracco Diagnostics, Princeton, NJ] or gadopentetate dimeglumine [Magnevist; Berlex Laboratories, Wayne, NJ]), T1-weighted axial MR series for the tumor volume measurements. The following parameters were used to obtain the T1-weighted images: 450–650/16–35 (repetition time range msec/echo time range msec), 256 × 192 matrix, 24-cm field of view, 5-mm section thickness with a 1-mm intersection gap, and one signal acquired.

Tumor Volume Measurement

Two nonradiologists (B.N.J., who was a medical student at the time of the study, and P.J.G., a research assistant in our positron emission tomography [PET] center) independently rated each MR image twice by using each of the two measurement methods—that is, manual tracing and semiautomated segmentation. Operator 1 followed the order ABBA, whereas operator 2 followed the order ABAB, where method A was the semiautomated segmentation method and method B was the manual trace method. The images obtained in all 16 subjects were rated in one batch for each manual or semiautomated measurement trial. The rationale for using the two nonradiologists in this study was that tumor volume measurements are typically performed by MR technologists rather than radiologists in our radiology department. To compare inter- and intraoperator reliability, we needed two individuals who were available to perform the repetitive measurements. Because our technologists were not available to obtain these measurements, we chose a medical student and a PET research assistant, because their familiarity with imaging approached that of an imaging technologist but not that of a radiologist.

The image processing time for both methods was recorded by both operators during the second trial. In each patient, the total processing time included two components—the time required to generate tumor contours and the time required to load and save image data.

For both methods, only the enhancing portions of the tumor were included in the volume calculation. The nonenhancing portions within the tumor (ie, areas of tumor necrosis) were traced, and their volumes were excluded from the total tumor volume.

Manual trace method.—Tumor volume measurements were determined by manually outlining, with a track ball, the enhancing portion of the mass on each image by using standard software on the imager console (GE Medical Systems). Nonenhancing regions within the tumor also were outlined and subtracted so that only the enhancing tumor area was measured. An example of manual tracing is shown in Figure 1. The area measurements were automatically calculated and multiplied by the MR image section thickness plus the intersection gap to calculate a per-section tumor volume. The total tumor volume was obtained by summing the volume calculations for all sections. Each image, along with its traced contours, was saved by using the "screen save" function on the console and then stored on optical disks.

Semiautomated segmentation method.—For the semiautomated segmentation method, threshold-based segmentation software (Morph; Silicon Graphics, Mountain View, Calif) was used. This software, which has not yet been released for general use (Thulborn K., personal communication, September 1998) (8), was operated on an SGI workstation (Silicon Graphics). For each image, the operator selected a point just within the enhancing border of the mass (Fig 2a) and a point just outside the enhancing border of the mass (Fig 2b). These two points defined the threshold used to generate the contour surrounding the enhancing area (Fig 2c). Similarly, nonenhancing regions within the tumor were excluded by choosing a point inside the nonenhancing (ne-

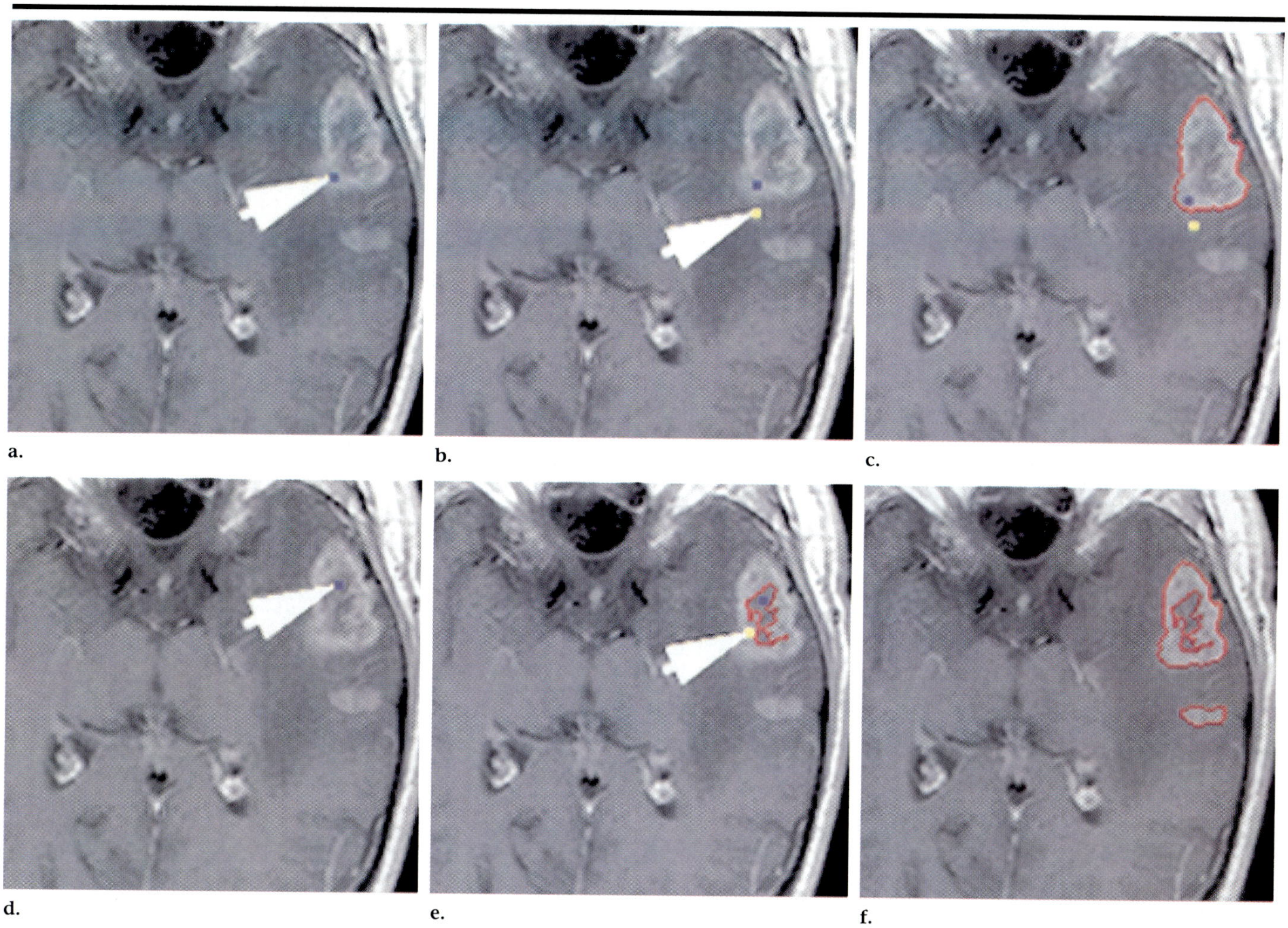

Figure 2. **(a-d)** Axial T1-weighted MR images (466/11) obtained in the same patient and same image section as those in Figure 1 illustrate the semiautomated computer tracing method. **(a–c)** First, a point just inside the enhancing border (blue dot at tip of arrow in **a**) is selected. **(b, c)** Next, a point just outside the enhancing border (yellow dot at tip of arrow in **b**) is selected. In **c**, the enhancing area is automatically outlined (shown in red). **(d, e)** By selecting a point inside the nonenhancing (necrotic) region (blue dot at tip of arrow in **d**) and a point outside the nonenhancing region (yellow dot at tip of arrow in **e**), the contour surrounding the nonenhancing area (outlined in red in **e**) is generated and excluded from the final tumor volume measurement. (In **a–e**, all dots have been increased from 1 pixel to 4 pixels in width for clarity of reproduction.) **(f)** The final result after all enhancing areas have been segmented is shown.

crotic) region (Fig 2d) and a point outside the nonenhancing region (Fig 2e) to generate the contour surrounding the nonenhancing area. Figure 2f shows the result after all enhancing areas have been segmented. As with the manual trace method, the calculated tumor volume reflects the enhancing area only. A similar method, which involves the same mixture modeling algorithm for contour derivation, was previously validated for volume measurements in a phantom, with errors of 4%–6% (9). With the semiautomated method, the contours were linked to the original images, and only the contour information plus the linking information was stored.

Each operator underwent a training and validation exercise before beginning the tumor volume measurements. This involved using the semiautomated method to measure the volume of a cadaverous brain hemisphere that was imaged with a volumetric spoiled gradient-recalled-echo sequence (25/5, 40° flip angle, one signal acquired, 256 × 192 matrix, 1.5-mm section thickness, 24-cm field of view). Both operators obtained measurements within 2% of the actual brain volume (as measured by the displacement of water by a brain fixed in a preservative substance) before proceeding with the tumor volume measurement study (8).

Statistical Considerations and Data Analyses

To compare the intra- and interoperator reliability of the two measurement methods, we used the following agreement index, AI, equation (10):

$$\mathrm{AI} = 1 - \frac{|x_a - x_b|}{(x_a + x_b)/2}.$$

For interoperator agreement calculations, x_a was the measurement obtained by operator 1 and x_b, the measurement obtained by operator 2 with the same technique on the same image. For intraoperator agreement calculations, x_a was the measurement made during the first trial, and x_b, the measurement made during the second trial by the same operator with the same technique on the same image.

Intraoperator and interoperator agreement indexes were calculated for each image, because the tumor contours were generated on a section-by-section basis and represented independent observations. Making the agreement comparisons on a section-by-section basis also increased the statistical power of the study, because the tumors in the 16 patients spanned about 100 sections in total and consequently provided about 100 comparison data points.

An agreement index was calculated for each instance in which both volume measurements (ie, x_a and x_b) were greater than 0. (There were instances at the extreme inferior and superior tumor margins on the axial images in which very small contours [generally representing 2%–5% of the total tumor volume] were generated by one observer and not the other. The results of statistical analyses of these instances by means of the McNemar test showed no significant difference between the semiautomated method and manual trace method and no significant difference between operators in terms of the tendency to find tumor in a particular section.) A value of 1.0 indicated perfect agreement, and a value of 0 indicated no agreement. The measurements made by each operator during the second trial were used in the interoperator agreement calculations. A paired Student t test was used to evaluate differences in interoperator agreement between the semiautomated and manual trace methods. Intraoperator reliability was similarly assessed by evaluating the intraoperator agreement between operators and between methods. Statistical significance was determined by a P value of less than .05. A paired Student t test was also used to look for systematic bias in volume measurements between the two approaches.

RESULTS

Tumor Volume Measurements

A total of 384 axial images obtained in the 16 patients were evaluated; approximately 100 of these images demonstrated enhancing tumor. Tumor enhancement was seen on approximately four to 10 (mean, 6.2) images per patient. The range of tumor volume measurements is presented in Table 1. In 49 (77%) of 64 volume measurements, the volume measurement obtained with the semiautomated method was lower (mean difference ± SD, 12.1% ± 11.6) than that obtained with the manual method (P = .001).

Intraoperator Agreement

The intraoperator agreement indexes for the two operators who used the two tumor volume measurement methods are summarized in Table 2. The difference in mean intraoperator agreement between the manual and semiautomated methods was significant for operator 1 (P = .003) but not for operator 2 (P = .74). Scatterplots of the intraoperator agreement indexes for the manual trace method versus the semiautomated segmentation method illustrate the superior reliability of operator 1 with the manual trace method compared with the reliability of this operator with the semiautomated method (Fig 3a). In contrast, for operator 2, there was no significant difference in intraoperator reliability between the two methods (Fig 3b). There was a significant difference in intraoperator reliability between operators when they used the manual trace method (P = .001), whereas there was no significant difference in intraoperator reliability between operators when they used the semiautomated method (P = .60).

Interoperator Agreement

There was no significant difference (P = .20) in interoperator reliability between the two tumor volume measurement methods (Fig 4). The mean interoperator agreement index (± SD) was 0.85 ± 0.14 for the manual trace method and 0.82 ± 0.18 for the semiautomated segmentation method.

Time Considerations

The mean time required to generate contours and the total tumor measurement time—that is, the time required to generate contours plus the time required to load and save image data—by using the two measurement methods are presented in Table 3. There was no significant difference in the average time required to generate contours between the manual trace method and the semiautomated segmentation method (P = .24). However, a significant difference in the total processing time between the two methods was found; the semiautomated method required an average of 4.6 minutes less per patient than did the manual trace method (P = .001). A significant difference in the total processing time per image section also was found between the two methods; the semiautomated method required an average of 0.6 minutes less per image than did the manual trace method (P = .008).

TABLE 1
Range of Tumor Volume Measurements per Patient

Tumor Volume	Manual Trace Measurement	Semi-automated Threshold-based Measurement
Minimum	2,616	2,501
Maximum	35,064	32,340
Mean ± SD	18,381 ± 7,199	17,109 ± 7,188

Note.—All measurements are in cubic millimeters.

TABLE 2
Mean Intraoperator Agreement Indexes

Operator	Manual Trace Measurement	Semiautomated Threshold-based Measurement
1	0.90 ± 0.09	0.83 ± 0.17
2	0.83 ± 0.15	0.84 ± 0.16

Note.—Data are the mean agreement index ± SD.

DISCUSSION

In a study conducted by the Brain Tumor Cooperative Group (11), the tumor size at CT, as measured by using diameters, was determined to be of prognostic importance, independent of other known prognostic variables. In addition, Blankenberg et al (12) suggested that MR imaging– or CT-determined volumetric tumor doubling time is superior to histologic grade in predicting the survival of patients with intracranial astrocytomas. Currently, MR imaging is considered to be superior to CT in determining the extent of tumor infiltration, although histologic evidence of malignancy may extend beyond the margin of enhancement (13–15). In addition, surgery, steroids, and radiation therapy may substantially alter the enhancement characteristics of the tumor bed (16,17). Despite this, the extent of tumor enhancement at MR imaging or CT is routinely used to guide radiation therapy, and recent attention has been given to improving the accuracy of in vivo brain tumor volume measurements that are obtained with MR imaging and used in patient treatment and prognostic determinations (1,3,7,18).

In our study of the reliability of brain tumor volume measurements, we quantitatively compared the conventional manual trace method with a semiautomated computer segmentation method. We hypothesized that the semiautomated method would provide more reproduc-

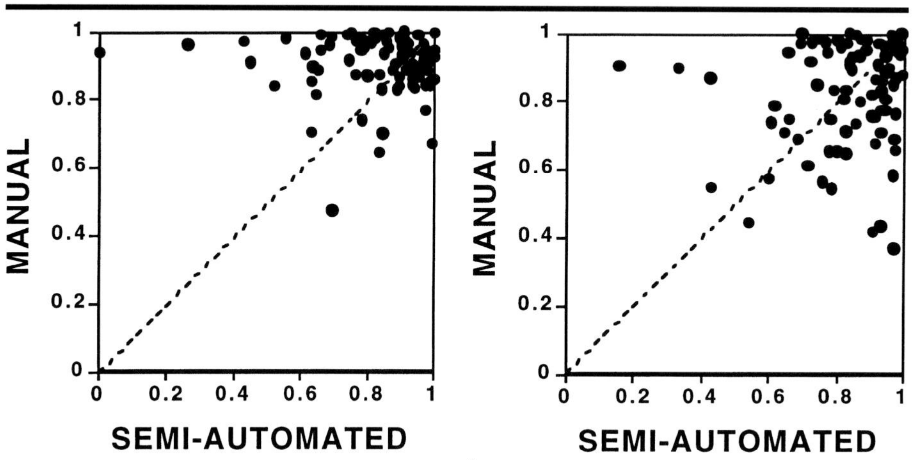

a. b.

Figure 3. Scatterplots of intraoperator agreement indexes for the manual versus semiautomated segmentation method. The dotted line is the line of equality, along which the agreement indexes for the manual and semiautomated methods are equal. Each data point represents one image. **(a)** Agreement indexes for operator 1. Note that there are more points clustered toward the manual axis; this indicates that operator 1 had better reliability with the manual trace method. **(b)** Agreement indexes for operator 2. In this case, the points are evenly distributed on both sides of the equality line; this indicates that operator 2 had comparable reliability with the two measurement methods.

TABLE 3
Mean Tumor Volume Measurement Times

Time	Manual Trace Measurement	Semiautomated Threshold-based Measurement
Tracing	11.2 ± 3.3	12.5 ± 5.5
Total*	21.2 ± 3.7	16.6 ± 5.8

Note.—Data are the mean number of minutes required to obtain the measurement per patient ± SD.

* Total time includes the time required to generate tumor contours and to load and save image data.

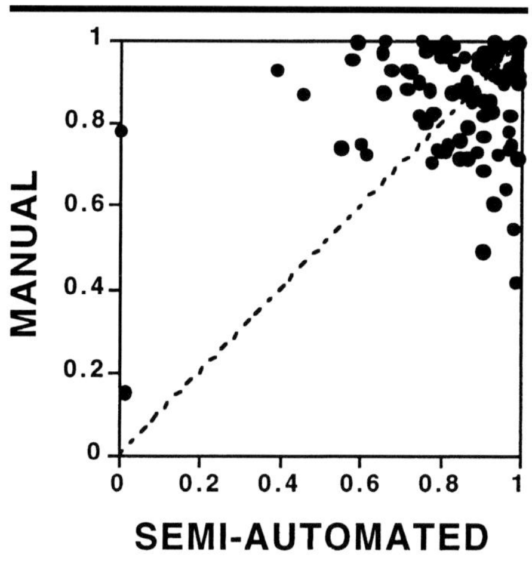

Figure 4. Scatterplot of interoperator agreement indexes for the manual versus semiautomated segmentation method. The agreement indexes for the manual and semiautomated methods are equal along the dotted line. The points are evenly distributed on both sides of the equality line; this indicates similar interoperator reliability between the two measurement methods.

ible measurements—that is, have high inter- and intraoperator reliability—whereas the manual trace method would be more user dependent and have low interoperator reliability. As expected, we found no significant difference in intraoperator reliability between operator 1 and 2 (mean agreement index, 0.83) when they used the semiautomated measurement method. In addition, interoperator reliability (agreement index, 0.82) was comparable to intraoperator reliability when the semiautomated method was used. However, the manual trace method was more user dependent in that operator 1 had better intraoperator reliability (agreement index, 0.90) than did operator 2 (agreement index, 0.83). When we compared the interoperator reliability of the two methods, we found no significant difference between the manual and semiautomated measurement methods (agreement index, 0.85 vs 0.82, respectively).

There was a highly significant difference in absolute volume measurements between the two methods; the semiautomated method resulted in lower volume measurements than did the manual tracing method 77% (49 of 64 measurements) of the time. We postulate that this may have resulted from the ability of the semiautomated method to provide a more detailed outline of the irregular edges of the tumor, whereas the manual trace method tends to approximate the tumor border with a smooth curve. Because the true histologic extent of these tumors is not delineated with contrast enhancement, it is impossible to determine which of the tumor volume measurement methods is more accurate (13–15). Given the systematic differences, all serial volume measurements that are typically used to follow tumor response to treatment should be performed with the same method.

In some studies (19), attempts to correlate survival with volume of abnormal tissue at T2-weighted imaging have been made. The semiautomated method used in this study would be impractical to apply to T2-weighted images because of the lack of contrast and the inability to discern a complete border between the tumor-related signal intensity abnormality and the cerebrospinal fluid. However, the semiautomated method potentially could be used for volume measurement of abnormal signal intensity at T2-weighted imaging with fluid-attenuated inversion recovery sequences, because the contrast between tumor and cerebrospinal fluid would be increased and thus allow appropriate segmentation. Morph software is currently being used to measure white matter signal intensity abnormalities on fluid-attenuated inversion recovery images in an ongoing study (C.C.M., personal communication, September 1998).

The semiautomated method required less time to generate tumor volume measurements than did the manual trace method. This difference reflects the decreased time required to load and save image data with the semiautomated measurement method. In addition, the semiautomated method required less storage space than did the manual trace method.

The differences between the two measurement methods that were difficult to quantify included qualitative "ease of use" factors. Both operators subjectively believed that the manual trace method was highly labor intensive and required more concentration to do well than did the semiautomated method. Because editing functions were not available with the manual trace method, an image had to be completely retraced if a mistake was made. Also, the outputs of the manual trace method were area measurements, which then had to be multiplied by the section thickness to generate volume measurements. The semiautomated method enabled tumor volumes to be calculated automatically and allowed basic editing functions.

The tumor volume measurements calculated with standard manual tracing and a semiautomated computer program were comparable in interoperator reliability, but the semiautomated computer program was faster than manual tracing. The reliability of MR imaging–determined tumor volume measurements potentially may be improved with decreased reliance on subjective image interpretation. Although the semiautomated method used in this study still requires an operator to choose the points that determine the threshold value used to outline the area of enhancement, generation of the tumor contour is based on consistent objective criteria. Several automated methods of MR image segmentation based on texture analysis (20), clustering techniques (eg, unsupervised fuzzy c-means) (21,22), or vector decomposition and probability techniques (23) have been reported on. These alternative approaches to MR image segmentation remain under development and retain problems with misclassification. Ultimately, by improving the reliability of MR imaging–based tumor volume measurements, these types of analyses may be used to follow tumor response to therapy and thus potentially influence patient care and treatment planning.

Acknowledgment: We thank Keith Thulborn for supplying the Morph software before its completion.

References

1. Grossman S, Wharam M, Sheidler V, et al. Phase II study of continuous infusion carmustine and cisplatin followed by cranial irradiation in adults with newly diagnosed high-grade astrocytoma. J Clin Oncol 1997; 15:2596–2603.
2. Zijlstra EJ, Taphoorn MJ, Barkhof F, Hoogenraad FG, Heimans JJ, Valk J. Radiotherapy response of cerebral metastases quantified by serial MR imaging. J Neurooncol 1994; 21:171–176.
3. Ten Haken RK, Thornton AF Jr, Sandler HM, et al. A quantitative assessment of the addition of MRI to CT-based, 3-D treatment planning of brain tumors. Radiother Oncol 1992; 25:121–133.
4. Pan DH, Guo WY, Chung WY, Shiau CY, Liu RS, Lee LS. Early effects of Gamma Knife surgery on malignant and benign intracranial tumors. Stereotact Funct Neurosurg 1995; 64(suppl 1):19–31.
5. Clarke LP, Velthuizen RP, Camacho MA, et al. MRI segmentation: methods and applications. Magn Reson Imaging 1995; 13: 343–368.
6. Vaidyanathan M, Clarke LP, Hall LO, et al. Monitoring brain tumor response to therapy using MRI segmentation. Magn Reson Imaging 1997; 15:323–334.
7. Vaidyanathan M, Clarke LP, Velthuizen RP, et al. Comparison of supervised MRI segmentation methods for tumor volume determination during therapy. Magn Reson Imaging 1995; 13:719–728.
8. Uttecht S, Betancourt C, Thulborn K. Evaluation of semi-automated border recognition software from quantitative brain morphometry and topology from high-resolution MRI (abstr). In: Proceedings of the Sixth Meeting of the International Society for Magnetic Resonance in Medicine. Berkeley, Calif: International Society for Magnetic Resonance in Medicine, 1998; 2075.
9. Johnson LA, Pearlman JD, Miller CA, Young TI, Thulborn KR. MR quantification of cerebral ventricular volume using a semiautomated algorithm. AJNR 1993; 14:1373–1478.
10. Filippi M, Horsfield MA, Bressi S, et al. Intra- and inter-observer agreement of brain MRI lesion volume measurements in multiple sclerosis: a comparison of techniques. Brain 1995; 118:1593–1600.
11. Wood JR, Green SB, Shapiro WR. The prognostic importance of tumor size in malignant gliomas: a computed tomographic scan study by the Brain Tumor Cooperative Group. J Clin Oncol 1988; 6:338–343.
12. Blankenberg FG, Teplitz RL, Ellis W, et al. The influence of volumetric tumor doubling time, DNA ploidy, and histologic grade on the survival of patients with intracranial astrocytomas. AJNR 1995; 16: 1001–1012.
13. Greene GM, Hitchon PW, Schelper RL, Yuh W, Dyste GN. Diagnostic yield in CT-guided stereotactic biopsy of gliomas. J Neurosurg 1989; 71:494–497.
14. Johnson PC, Hunt SJ, Drayer BP. Human cerebral gliomas: correlation of postmortem MR imaging and neuropathologic findings. Radiology 1989; 170:211–217.
15. Earnest IV F, Kelly PJ, Scheithauer BW, et al. Cerebral astrocytomas: histopathologic correlation of MR and CT contrast enhancement with stereotactic biopsy. Radiology 1988; 166:823–827.
16. Hatam A, Bergstrom M, Yu ZY, Granholm L, Berggren BM. Effect of dexamethasone treatment on volume and contrast enhancement of intracranial neoplasms. J Comput Assist Tomogr 1983; 7:295–300.
17. Jeffries BF, Kishore PRS, Singh KS, Ghatak NR, Krempa J. Contrast enhancement in the postoperative brain. Radiology 1981; 139:409–413.
18. Thornton Jr AF, Sandler HM, Ten Haken RK, et al. The clinical utility of magnetic resonance imaging in 3-dimensional treatment planning of brain neoplasms. Int J Radiat Oncol Biol Phys 1992; 24:767–775.
19. Brunberg JA, Eldevik OP, Junck L, et al. Gliomas: correlation of MR imaging findings, patient age and pathologic grade with duration of patient survival (abstr). In: Proceedings of the 34th Annual Meeting of the American Society of Neuroradiology. Seattle, Wash: American Society of Neuroradiology, 1996; 151.
20. Schad LR, Bluml S, Zuna I. MR tissue characterization of intracranial tumors by means of texture analysis. Magn Reson Imaging 1993; 11:889–896.
21. Velthuizen RP, Clarke LP, Phuphanich S, et al. Unsupervised measurement of brain tumor volume on MR images. JMRI 1995; 5:594–605.
22. Phillips WE, Velthuizen RP, Phuphanich S, Hall LO, Clarke LP, Silbiger ML. Application of fuzzy c-means segmentation technique for tissue differentiation in MR images of a hemorrhagic glioblastoma multiforme. Magn Reson Imaging 1995; 13:277–290.
23. Kao YH, Sorenson JA, Bahn MM, Winkler SS. Dual-echo MRI segmentation using vector decomposition and probability techniques: a two-tissue model. Magn Reson Med 1994; 32:342–357.

Heang-Ping Chan, PhD
Berkman Sahiner, PhD
Mark A. Helvie, MD
Nicholas Petrick, PhD
Marilyn A. Roubidoux, MD
Todd E. Wilson, MD
Dorit D. Adler, MD
Chintana Paramagul, MD
Joel S. Newman, MD
Sethumadavan Sanjay-Gopal, PhD

Index terms:
Breast neoplasms, 00.31, 00.32
Breast neoplasms, radiography, 00.111, 00.119
Breast radiography, 00.111, 00.119
Computers, diagnostic aid
Receiver operating characteristic curve (ROC)

Radiology 1999; 212:817–827

Abbreviations:
CAD = computer-aided diagnosis
PPV = positive predictive value
ROC = receiver operating characteristic

[1] From the Department of Radiology, University of Michigan Hospital, UH B1F510, 1500 E Medical Center Dr, Ann Arbor, MI 48109-0030. From the 1997 RSNA scientific assembly. Received August 10, 1998; revision requested September 8; revision received November 30; accepted January 21, 1999. Supported in part by United States Public Health Service grant CA 48129 and by U.S. Army Medical Research and Materiel Command grant DAMD 17-96-1-6254. B.S. supported by Career Development award DAMD 17-96-1-6012 from the U.S. Army Medical Research and Materiel Command. N.P. supported by a grant from the Whitaker Foundation. **Address reprint requests to** H.P.C. (e-mail: *chanhp@umich.edu*).

The content of this article does not necessarily reflect the position of the funding agencies, and no official endorsement of any equipment or product of any companies mentioned in this article should be inferred.

Author contributions:
Guarantor of integrity of entire study, H.P.C.; study concepts and design, H.P.C., M.A.H., B.S., N.P.; literature research, H.P.C., M.A.H.; experimental studies, M.A.H., M.A.R., T.E.W., D.D.A., C.P., J.S.N.; data acquisition, all authors; data analysis, H.P.C., B.S., N.P.; statistical analysis, H.P.C.; manuscript preparation, editing, and review, H.P.C., B.S., M.A.H., N.P., M.A.R., T.E.W., D.D.A., C.P., J.S.N.

Improvement of Radiologists' Characterization of Mammographic Masses by Using Computer-aided Diagnosis: An ROC Study[1]

PURPOSE: To evaluate the effects of computer-aided diagnosis (CAD) on radiologists' classification of malignant and benign masses seen on mammograms.

MATERIALS AND METHODS: The authors previously developed an automated computer program for estimation of the relative malignancy rating of masses. In the present study, the authors conducted observer performance experiments with receiver operating characteristic (ROC) methodology to evaluate the effects of computer estimates on radiologists' confidence ratings. Six radiologists assessed biopsy-proved masses with and without CAD. Two experiments, one with a single view and the other with two views, were conducted. The classification accuracy was quantified by using the area under the ROC curve, A_z.

RESULTS: For the reading of 238 images, the A_z value for the computer classifier was 0.92. The radiologists' A_z values ranged from 0.79 to 0.92 without CAD and improved to 0.87–0.96 with CAD. For the reading of a subset of 76 paired views, the radiologists' A_z values ranged from 0.88 to 0.95 without CAD and improved to 0.93–0.97 with CAD. Improvements in the reading of the two sets of images were statistically significant (P = .022 and .007, respectively). An improved positive predictive value as a function of the false-negative fraction was predicted from the improved ROC curves.

CONCLUSION: CAD may be useful for assisting radiologists in classification of masses and thereby potentially help reduce unnecessary biopsies.

Breast cancer is the most prevalent non–skin cancer in women; 178,700 new cases are estimated to have occurred in 1998 (1). The mortality of breast cancer is the second highest among all cancer deaths in women (1). At present, there is no effective method to prevent breast cancer. The best approach to reducing the breast cancer mortality rate is early detection and treatment. Because the mammographic features of early-stage breast cancers are not very specific, the need for high detection sensitivity leads to biopsy of many low-suspicion lesions. The positive predictive values (PPVs) of mammographic signs are, therefore, often below 30% (2,3).

Computer-aided diagnosis (CAD) is considered to be one of the approaches that may improve the efficacy of mammography (4). With CAD, a computerized detection algorithm alerts a radiologist to the location of the suspicious lesions, and/or a trained computer classifier provides the radiologist with an estimate of the likelihood of malignancy of a lesion. The radiologist takes into consideration the information provided by the computer before making a decision. This "second opinion" may improve the diagnostic accuracy because it serves as a form of double reading (5). Furthermore, a computer evaluation is often more consistent and reproducible than a human decision maker (6).

Considerable research has been devoted to the development of computerized schemes for the detection and classification of mammographic abnormalities. These efforts have advanced the CAD technology such that clinical application appears to be possible in the

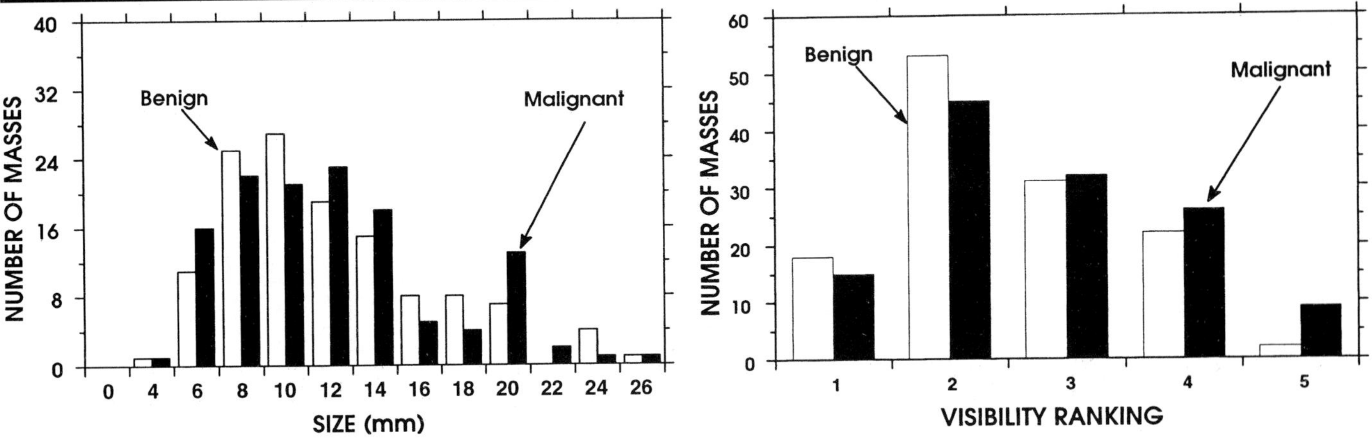

a. b.

Figure 1. Histograms illustrate the distributions of **(a)** size (ie, length of the long axis) and **(b)** visibility ranking (1 = obvious, 5 = subtle) of the 253 masses included in the data set. Because classification accuracy depends on the case mix, these distributions provided some information on the masses in the data set.

near future. It is, therefore, necessary to evaluate the effects of CAD on radiologists' detection and diagnosis of mammographic lesions. In a previous receiver operating characteristic (ROC) study, we demonstrated that CAD could improve radiologists' accuracy in the detection of subtle microcalcifications on mammograms (7). Kegelmeyer et al (8) also reported an improvement in radiologists' sensitivity for the detection of spiculated masses with use of a computer aid. For the classification of mammographic lesions, it has been shown that a computer classifier that estimated the likelihood of malignancy on the basis of mammographic features extracted by radiologists could improve radiologists' accuracy in distinguishing malignant from benign lesions (9–11).

We previously conducted ROC studies to compare the performance of radiologists with that of the computer (12) and to compare radiologists' ability to classify masses with and without CAD (13). Jiang et al (14) also performed an ROC study of the effect of CAD on radiologists' performance in classifying microcalcifications. The results of all of these observer performance studies indicate the potential to improve mammographic interpretation with a computer aid.

We have developed an automated method to analyze masses seen on mammograms (15–17). A mass is segmented from its surrounding breast tissue, and an image transformation technique is used to transform the mass margin from the polar coordinate system to the Cartesian coordinate system. A linear discriminant classifier then extracts the useful texture features from the transformed image and merges them into a relative malignancy rating. Our approach is different from others that use a trained classifier to merge radiologist-extracted image features or feature codes by using the American College of Radiology Breast Imaging Reporting and Database System lexicon (9–11). Our fully automated method has the advantage that, unlike a human reader, it does not have variability in feature recognition and coding. In addition, the computer may be able to extract some information, such as texture features, that may not be readily perceived by human eyes. We conducted an ROC study to evaluate whether this computer aid can improve radiologists' performance in the classification of mammographic masses (13). The results of our observer performance study are described in this article.

Other investigators also have reported on automated algorithms for the classification of mammographic masses (18–21). The methods used in these algorithms varied, and their accuracy in classification cannot be compared directly because of the differences in the data sets. However, the effects of CAD on radiologists' performance are not expected to depend strongly on the specific algorithm if different computer aids of comparable accuracy are used. Therefore, the applications of the findings of this study should not be limited to our computerized classification aid.

MATERIALS AND METHODS

Data Set

The data set for this study consisted of 253 mammograms obtained in 103 patients. Each image contained a biopsy-proved mass that was evaluated in this study. Some cases involved multiple views or images from multiple examinations. The cases were randomly selected from patient files from the breast imaging division of a National Cancer Institute–designated national cancer center with the approval of the Institutional Review Board. The PPV of masses recommended for biopsy at this center is about 25%–30%, but an approximately equal number of malignant and benign masses (127 and 126, respectively) were chosen to enhance the statistical power in this observer performance study. Any images that were judged to be technically poor were excluded.

The mammograms were acquired with a contact technique. The dedicated mammographic systems had a molybdenum anode and molybdenum filter, a 0.3-mm nominal focal spot, and a reciprocating grid. MinR/MinR-E screen-film systems (Eastman-Kodak, Rochester, NY) were used with these units. Sixty-two of the malignant masses and six of the benign masses were judged to be spiculated by a radiologist (M.A.H.) experienced in mammography. The radiologist also measured the size (ie, longest dimension) and ranked the visibility of the masses on a scale of 1 (obvious) to 5 (subtle) relative to the range of visibility of masses encountered in clinical practice. For a description of the masses included in the data set, histograms of the size and visibility of the masses are shown in Figures 1a and 1b, respectively.

For the computer analysis, the selected mammograms were digitized with a laser

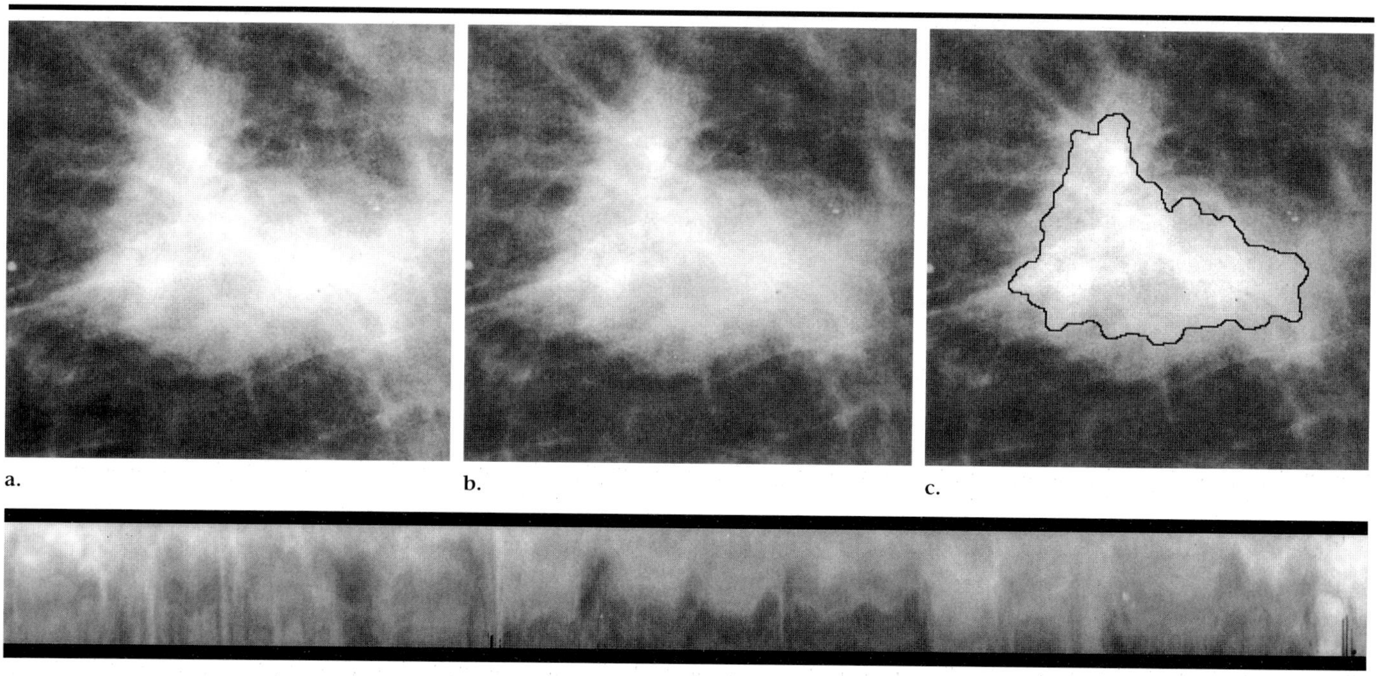

Figure 2. Example of rubber-band-straightening transform for extraction of texture features in the margin region surrounding a mass. (a) Original and (b) background-corrected images showing the region of interest with the mass, (c) mammogram showing an outline of the segmented mass, and (d) rubber-band-straightening–transformed image of a 40-pixel-wide region surrounding the segmented mass.

imager (Lumisys DIS-1000, Los Altos, Calif) at a pixel size of 0.1 × 0.1 mm and 12-bit gray levels. This imager has an optical density range of about 0.0–3.5. The optical density on the film was digitized linearly to pixel value at a calibration of 0.001 optical density unit/pixel value in the optical density range of about 0.0–2.8. The digitizer deviated from a linear response at an optical density higher than 2.8.

For the observer experiments, we used laser-printed images of the digitized mammograms for all readings. The images were printed with a 969HQ laser imager (Imation, Oakdale, Minn) that was connected to a Macintosh computer (Apple Computer, Cupertino, Calif) through a special digital interface. The interface provided a 12-bit in, 10-bit out look-up table and allowed images to be scaled to different factors with 15 interpolation methods. Because this laser imager has a pixel size of about 0.085 mm, we enlarged the images by about 18% during printing to maintain them at the same size as the original mammograms. One of the interpolation methods was chosen by an experienced radiologist (M.A.H.), who inspected the printed images with a magnifier and evaluated the sharpness of the spicules and mass boundaries. Because of the small pixel size used for both digitization and printing, basically no noticeable blurring of the masses could be seen with the chosen interpolation method. The images were also inspected for the potential contouring effect of 10-bit output images, but no noticeable artifacts could be found. A linear pixel value–to–output optical density calibration curve of the laser imager was used for the printing. All images were printed with the same settings.

Computerized Classification of Masses

Our computerized method of classifying mammographic masses has been described in detail previously (15–17). The method is summarized as follows: A region of interest that contained the biopsy-proved mass was identified on the mammogram by the radiologist. Background correction based on a distance-weighted estimation method was applied to the region of interest to reduce the low-frequency density variation in the region. A median-filtered smoothed image and two high-frequency enhanced images were generated from the background-corrected region of interest. The smoothed and enhanced gray-level values at each pixel were used as features in a k-means clustering algorithm to classify the pixels into two clusters; one was the mass, and the other was the surrounding breast tissue background. By choosing an appropriate criterion, a mass region slightly smaller than the actual mass that was visible on the image was segmented.

The boundary of the segmented region was smoothed by morphologic filtering. A new image transformation technique, referred to as the rubber-band-straightening transform, was used to transform a 40-pixel-wide region that surrounded the segmented mass boundary into a rectangular region. After transformation, the mass margin became approximately parallel, and any spicules that were radiating from the mass became approximately perpendicular, to the long dimension of the rectangular region. The rubber-band-straightening transform enabled the spicules to be aligned approximately in a uniform direction and thus facilitated the extraction of texture features from the margin of the mass. An example of a rubber-band-straightening–transformed image is shown in Figure 2.

Two types of texture features were found to be useful for classification. The first set of features included eight texture measures derived from the spatial gray-level dependence matrices of the rubber-band-straightening–transformed image. A spatial gray-level dependence matrix ele-

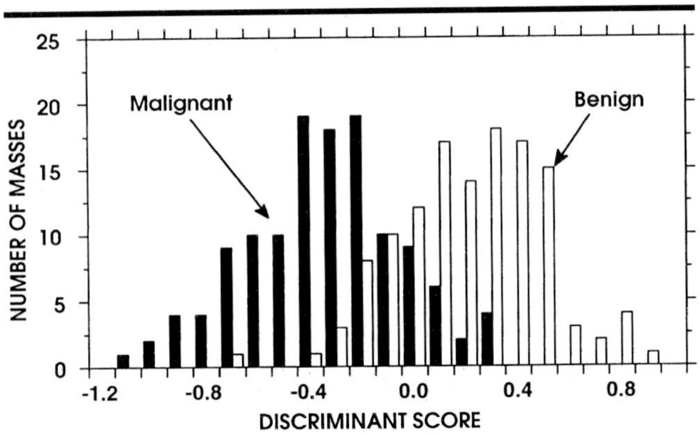

Figure 3. Histogram of the test discriminant scores of the 253 masses obtained from the linear discriminant classifier by using a "leave one case out" training and test resampling scheme. For this classifier, a smaller discriminant score corresponded to a higher likelihood of malignancy. The discriminant scores were used as the decision variable in the ROC analysis of classification performance.

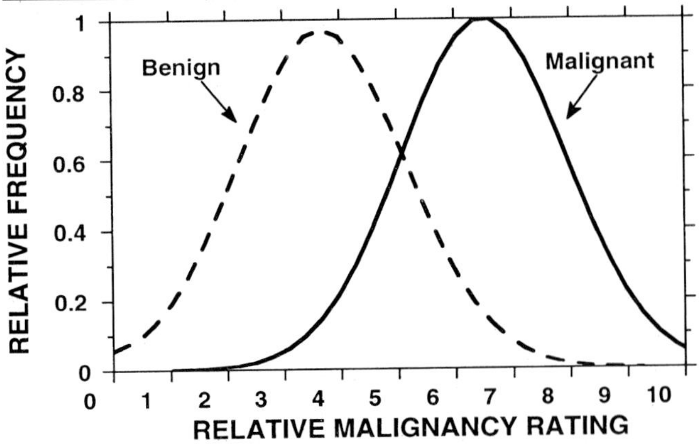

Figure 4. Binormal distribution fitted to the histogram of the discriminant scores of the malignant and benign masses. The discriminant scores were linearly transformed into a relative malignancy rating ranging from 1 to 10, where 1 corresponded to the most benign rating and 10 corresponded to the most malignant rating. This binormal distribution was shown to the observers during the training session to explain the rating scale of the computer classifier.

ment $p_{\theta,d}(i,j)$ is the joint probability of the occurrence of gray levels i and j for pixel pairs that are separated by a distance d and at a direction θ (22). For analysis of the masses, the spatial gray-level dependence matrices were constructed for 10 pixel distances (d = 1, 2, 3, 4, 6, 8, 10, 12, 16, 20 pixels) and in four directions (0°, 45°, 90°, 135°) relative to the mass boundary. Therefore, a total of 320 spatial gray-level dependence texture features were extracted.

The second set of texture features was derived from the run length statistics matrices of the horizontal and vertical gradient images of the rubber-band-straightening–transformed margin region. Five texture measures were extracted from the run length statistics matrix in each of the two directions (0° or 90°) on each gradient image. A total of 20 run length statistics texture features were thus obtained. Therefore, we had a total of 340 features from the two types of texture measures.

A stepwise linear discriminant feature selection procedure (23) was used to select the most effective features from the available feature set. A total of 41 features were selected. The selected features were input into the Fischer linear discriminant classifier (24) as predictor variables. A "leave one case out" resampling scheme was used to train and test the classifier. A histogram illustrating the test discriminant scores of the 253 masses is shown in Figure 3. For this classifier, a smaller discriminant score corresponded to a higher likelihood of malignancy. By using the test discriminant score as the decision variable, the performance of the computer classifier could be evaluated by using ROC analysis (17,25,26) and compared with that of the radiologists, as described later.

Relative Malignancy Rating of the Masses

For the observer performance study, we provided a relative malignancy rating of each mass to the observer during the reading session with CAD. The relative malignancy rating was obtained by taking a linear transformation of the computer classifier's decision variable to a range of 1–10 and rounding the value to the nearest integer. The transformation also reversed the relative magnitude of the decision variables so that 1 corresponded to the highest benignity rating, and 10 corresponded to the highest malignancy rating.

The purpose of the transformation was to provide a simple and intuitive relative scale for the observer. Because the transformation was linear and monotonic, the distributions of the normal and abnormal samples, as well as their ROC curves, were not affected, with the exception of a small error caused by making the decision variables discrete. Furthermore, the slope a and intercept b parameters that were fitted to the transformed discriminant scores for the normal and abnormal samples by using the LABROC program (26) were used to generate a binormal distribution. The fitted binormal distribution with the relative malignancy rating on a 1–10 scale (Fig 4), together with the computer's ROC curve, were shown and explained to the observers during a training session.

Observer Performance Study

Two ROC experiments (27) were conducted: The masses were evaluated from a single view in the first experiment and from two views in the second experiment. The location of the biopsy-proved mass was marked on each image so that the correct mass was evaluated by all observers. The observers were instructed to ignore any other possible masses on the images. Six radiologists (M.A.H., M.A.R., T.E.W., D.D.A., C.P., J.S.N.) who are approved by the Mammography Quality Standards Act and have 7–20 years of experience in interpreting mammograms participated in the observer performance experiments.

There were two reading sessions in each experiment—one with CAD and the other without CAD. The observers were asked to rate the likelihood of malignancy of the masses on a 10-point confidence rating scale under all reading conditions. In the first session, half the observers interpreted the images without CAD, and the other half interpreted them with CAD. The two reading sessions in the same experiment were separated by at least 3 weeks, and the two experiments were separated by 6 months. For all four reading sessions, the observer had unlimited time to read each case. To estimate the average reading time per case for each observer, the reading time for each case was recorded by using a stopwatch.

In the first experiment, the data set of 253 single-view mammograms was divided into a training set of 15 mammograms and a study set of 238 mammo-

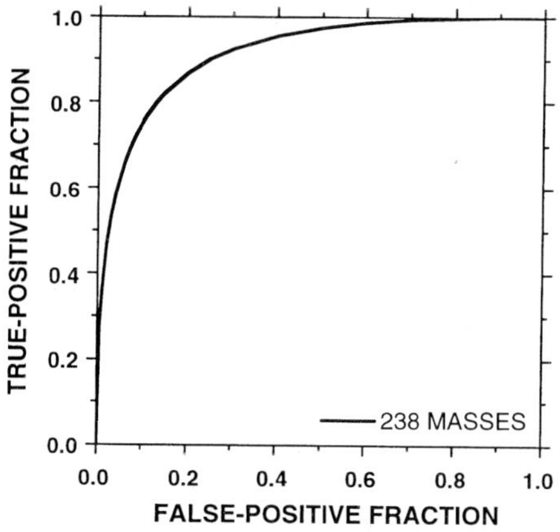

Figure 5. ROC curve for computerized classification of the 238 masses used in the observer performance study with single-view reading. The computer's ROC curve can be compared with the radiologists' ROC curves obtained from the single-view reading experiment illustrated in Figures 6 and 8.

grams (117 benign, 121 malignant). In each reading session, training was conducted before the reading of the study images. For the reading session with CAD, the fitted binormal distributions of the computer rating scores (Fig 4) for the entire data set were explained to the observer during training to familiarize the observer with the computer's rating scale. The computer rating of the mass was displayed on each image. After reading each training image, the observer was told the results of biopsy of the mass.

Each observer read the entire data set in one reading session. The order of the study images was randomized by a random number generator. The random sequence was different for each observer and for each reading session by the same observer. For the reading session with CAD, the observer was free to look at the computer rating, which was displayed on the image, either before or after estimating the likelihood of malignancy of the mass. However, each observer was asked to always read the computer rating before making a final decision. The observer was not informed of the pathologic results of any mass on the study images.

The second experiment was very similar to the first experiment. From the 238 single-view mammograms, 76 matched pairs (37 benign, 39 malignant) of craniocaudal and mediolateral oblique or lateral views were found. Another six pairs of two-view mammograms were identified from the rest of the images and used as training cases. The remaining mammograms were either single-view images or additional views of the pairs already chosen, so they were not used in this experiment. In this experiment, the observers were not informed of the pathologic results of any study case in any reading session. The 76 pairs of mammograms were read in one reading session by each observer.

For the reading session with CAD, the rating of the mass in each view was displayed on the respective image. The computer ratings of the mass on the two views were generally different. It was up to the observer to decide how to merge the two-view information. Observers were asked to give a single rating of the mass after reading both views.

ROC Analysis

The confidence ratings of each observer obtained from each reading condition were analyzed by using ROC methodology, and the classification accuracy was quantified by using the area under the ROC curve, A_z. A maximum likelihood estimation of the binormal distribution was fitted to the confidence ratings by using the LABROC program. This program provides an estimate of the A_z and of the a and b parameters of the ROC curve. The statistical significance of the difference in A_z between the reading with CAD and that without CAD was estimated with two methods: One was the Student paired t test for observer-specific paired data; the other was the Dorfman-Berbaum-Metz method for analysis of multireader, multicase ROC data (28). The statistical significance of the difference in A_z for reading single-view and two-view mammograms was estimated by using the Student paired t test for the six observers. The Student paired t test takes into account the statistical variation of readers, whereas the Dorfman-Berbaum-Metz method considers both reader variation and case sample variation by means of an analysis of variance approach. Therefore, the results of Dorfman-Berbaum-Metz analysis can be generalized to the population of readers as well as to the population of case samples.

Positive Predictive Value

An ROC curve represents the entire range of operating conditions of a diagnostic process and is independent of disease prevalence. When the disease prevalence is known, any operating point on an ROC curve can be used to derive the PPV and the corresponding false-negative fraction (false-negative fraction = 1 − true-positive fraction) on the basis of the following relationship: PPV = TPF × P(M)/[TPF × P(M) + FPF × P(B)], where TPF is the true-positive fraction, FPF is the false-positive fraction at the chosen decision threshold, and P(M) and P(B) are the prevalences of malignant and benign cases, respectively. By varying the decision threshold, the dependence of the PPV on the false-negative fraction can be derived.

Because our data set did not include masses on which biopsy had not been performed, the ROC curves obtained in this study cannot be generalized to predict the performance of the computer classifier and radiologists in clinical practice. However, to demonstrate the possible effect of CAD on the PPV in the population of masses in which biopsy is likely to be performed under the current clinical criteria, we can estimate the PPV by using the prevalence of the malignant and benign masses in this patient group. Because the PPV of masses sent for biopsy ranges from about 25% to 44% in general and from about 25% to 30% at our institution, for the purposes of our estimation, we assumed that the P(M) was 25% and the P(B) was 75% in this population. A higher prevalence of malignant cases would cause an increase in the PPV, but the trend between the PPV curves with and without CAD would be similar.

RESULTS

The ROC curve illustrating the performance of the computer classifier for the 238 study mammograms is shown in Figure 5. The ROC curve for the entire set of 253 mammograms (not shown) was almost identical to that of the 238 study cases; this indicates that the 15 training cases were typical of the 238 cases used in the study. The A_z values (± SD) for both ROC curves were 0.92 ± 0.02.

For the first experiment of reading the 238 single-view mammograms, the ROC curves for the readings by the six radiologists both without and with CAD are shown in Figures 6a and 6b, respectively. The A_z values of the six radiologists for the readings with and without CAD are listed in Table 1.

For the second experiment of reading the 76 pairs of two-view mammograms, the ROC curves for the readings by the six radiologists both without and with CAD are shown in Figures 7a and Figure 7b, respectively. The A_z values of the six radiologists in this experiment are also listed in Table 1.

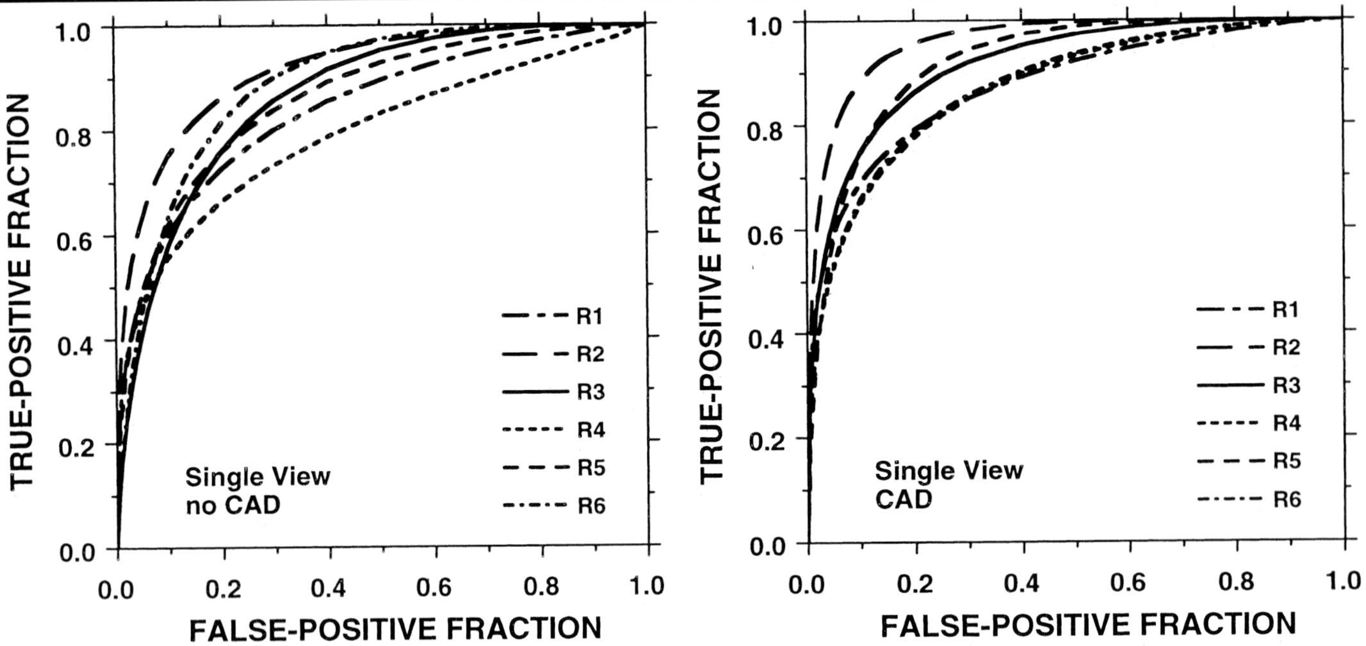

a.

b.

Figure 6. ROC curves for the six observers for single-view reading of the masses **(a)** without CAD and **(b)** with CAD. **(a, b)** *R1* = reader 1, *R2* = reader 2, *R3* = reader 3, *R4* = reader 4, *R5* = reader 5, *R6* = reader 6. Five of the six observers achieved an increase in the area under the ROC curve, A_z, with CAD.

The average ROC curve was derived from the average *a* and *b* parameters of the six individual ROC curves for a given reading condition (27). The average ROC curves for the four reading conditions are shown in Figure 8. The A_z values of the average ROC curves are listed in Table 1.

For the reading of the single-view mammograms, the performance of the computer classifier was comparable to that of the radiologist (reader 2) who had the highest classification accuracy (compare Figs 5 and 6) and higher than the average performance of the six radiologists (compare Figs 5 and 8). When the radiologists read the images with the computer aid, the classification accuracy of five radiologists improved (Table 1); the improvement in their A_z values ranged from 0.04 to 0.08. The average performance of the six radiologists became comparable to that of the computer classifier. The improvement in the radiologists' classification accuracy by using CAD was statistically significant (P = .022, Student paired *t* test; P = .020, Dorfman-Berbaum-Metz method). Reader 2 with CAD obtained an A_z value of 0.96, which was higher than that obtained by the radiologist alone or by the computer alone.

TABLE 1
Areas under the ROC Curves for the Classification of Masses with and without CAD by the Six Radiologists

Radiologist No.	A_z (Single View)* Without CAD	A_z (Single View)* With CAD	A_z (Two View)† Without CAD	A_z (Two View)† With CAD
1	0.84 ± 0.03	0.87 ± 0.02	0.90 ± 0.03	0.93 ± 0.03
2	0.92 ± 0.02	0.96 ± 0.01	0.95 ± 0.02	0.97 ± 0.02
3	0.86 ± 0.02	0.91 ± 0.02	0.92 ± 0.03	0.93 ± 0.03
4	0.79 ± 0.03	0.87 ± 0.02	0.88 ± 0.04	0.95 ± 0.03
5	0.86 ± 0.02	0.92 ± 0.02	0.93 ± 0.03	0.97 ± 0.02
6	0.89 ± 0.02	0.87 ± 0.02	0.89 ± 0.04	0.93 ± 0.03
A_z from average a, b parameters	0.87	0.91	0.92	0.96

Note.—Data are the mean ± SD.
* P = .022 for the difference between the A_z values measured with CAD and those measured without CAD, as determined by using the Student two-tailed *t* test. P = .020 for this difference, as determined by using the Dorfman-Berbaum-Metz method.
† P = .007 for the difference between A_z values measured with CAD and those measured without CAD, as determined by using the Student two-tailed *t* test. P = .026 for this difference, as determined by using the Dorfman-Berbaum-Metz method.

A trend similar to that with the single-view readings was observed with the two-view readings. The A_z value of the computer classifier for the corresponding 152 single-view masses was 0.91 ± 0.02. The classification accuracy of all six radiologists improved when they read the mammograms with the computer aid. The increase in the A_z values ranged from 0.01 to 0.07. The improvement was statistically significant (P = .007, Student paired *t* test; P = .026, Dorfman-Berbaum-Metz method). With CAD, two radiologists achieved an A_z value of 0.97, which was higher than that obtained by the radiologists alone or by the computer alone. These results indicate that the second opinion provided by the computer classifier might have strengthened the radiologists' confidence in the interpretation of some difficult cases but had less influence on the radiologists' decision when the computer made mistakes or when the radiologists were confident about their decision.

As can be seen from the data in Table 1,

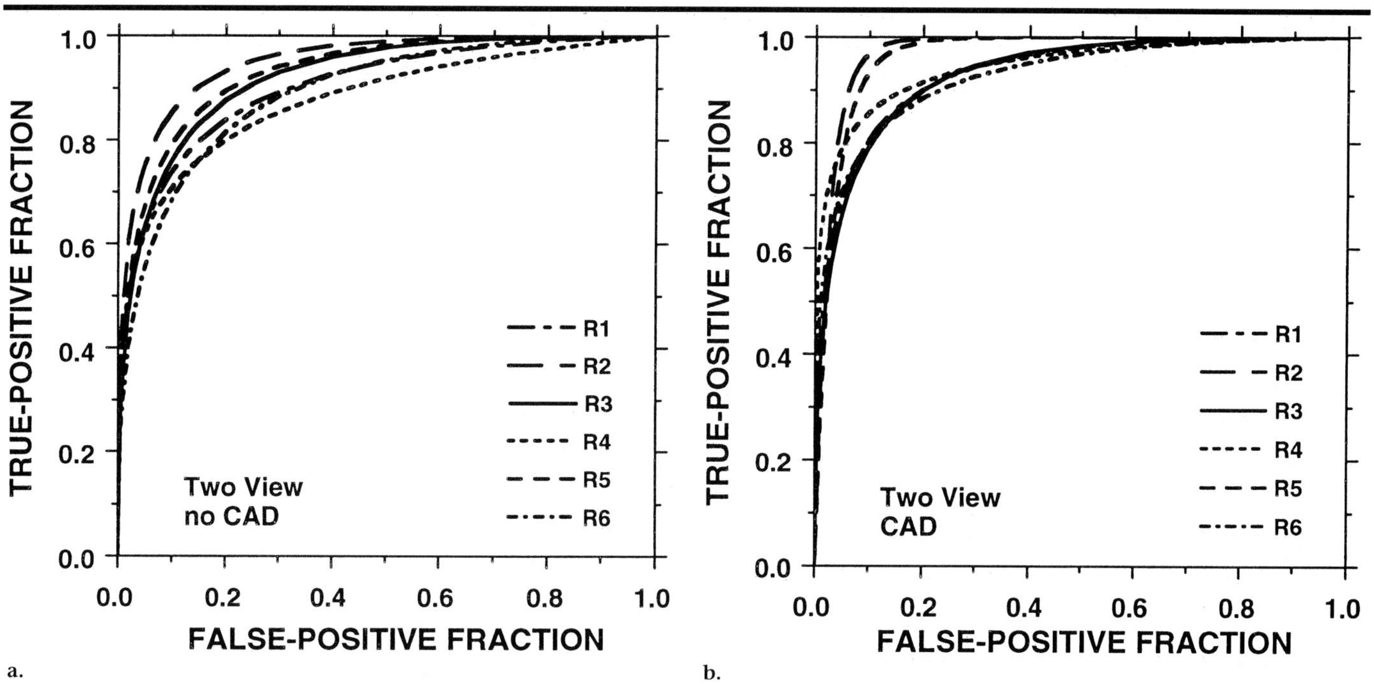

Figure 7. ROC curves for the six observers for two-view reading of the masses **(a)** without CAD and **(b)** with CAD. **(a, b)** *R1* = reader 1, *R2* = reader 2, *R3* = reader 3, *R4* = reader 4, *R5* = reader 5, *R6* = reader 6. All six observers achieved an increase in the area under the ROC curve, A_z, with CAD.

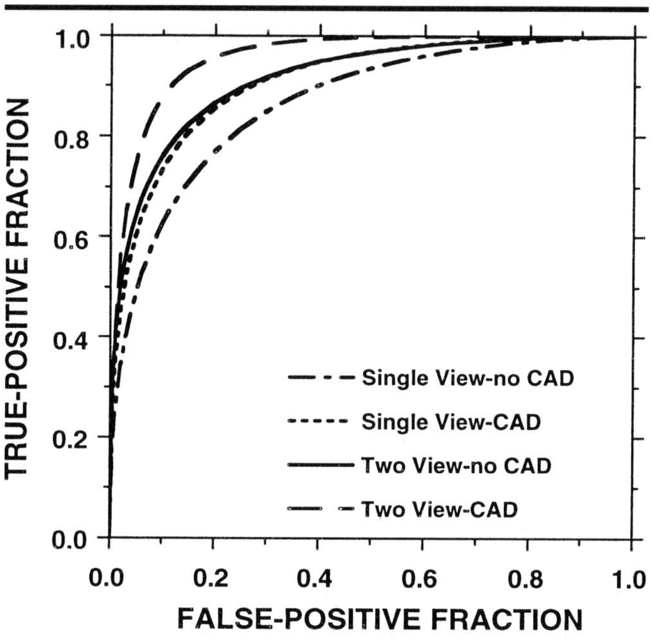

Figure 8. Average ROC curve obtained from the average *a* and *b* parameters of the six individual ROC curves for each of the four reading conditions. An improved ROC curve was achieved with CAD in both the single-view and two-view reading experiments.

the radiologists' accuracy in classifying masses by reading two-view mammograms was consistently higher than that by reading single-view mammograms ($P = .008$). This trend remained when they read the mammograms with CAD ($P = .007$). These findings are consistent with the clinical experience of the radiologists that at least two views of mammograms are needed to effectively evaluate a suspicious lesion.

The PPV as a function of the false-negative fraction was derived from the fitted ROC curves under the assumption that the prevalence of malignant masses was 25% in the population of masses sent for biopsy. The PPVs estimated for the six observers who read the two-view mammograms with and without CAD are plotted in Figure 9. CAD would provide an improvement in the PPV in the high false-negative fraction range for all observers except readers 2 and 5. The increase in the PPV at a decision threshold of "no missed malignant mass" (ie, false-negative fraction = 0) varied over a wide range; the largest gain, 39%, would be achieved by reader 2, and the smallest gain, 0%, would be achieved by reader 4.

DISCUSSION

In the observer experiment of reading two-view mammograms with CAD, we presented the computer's rating of each view separately. The decision of how to merge the computer ratings of the two views was left to the radiologist. It is likely that the radiologists took the conservative approach of using the highest malignancy rating of the two as the computer's overall rating. However, it also might have depended on whether the relative ranking between the two computer ratings agreed with the observer's opinion. In some cases, we observed that the radiologist's rating was very different from the computer's rating of either view.

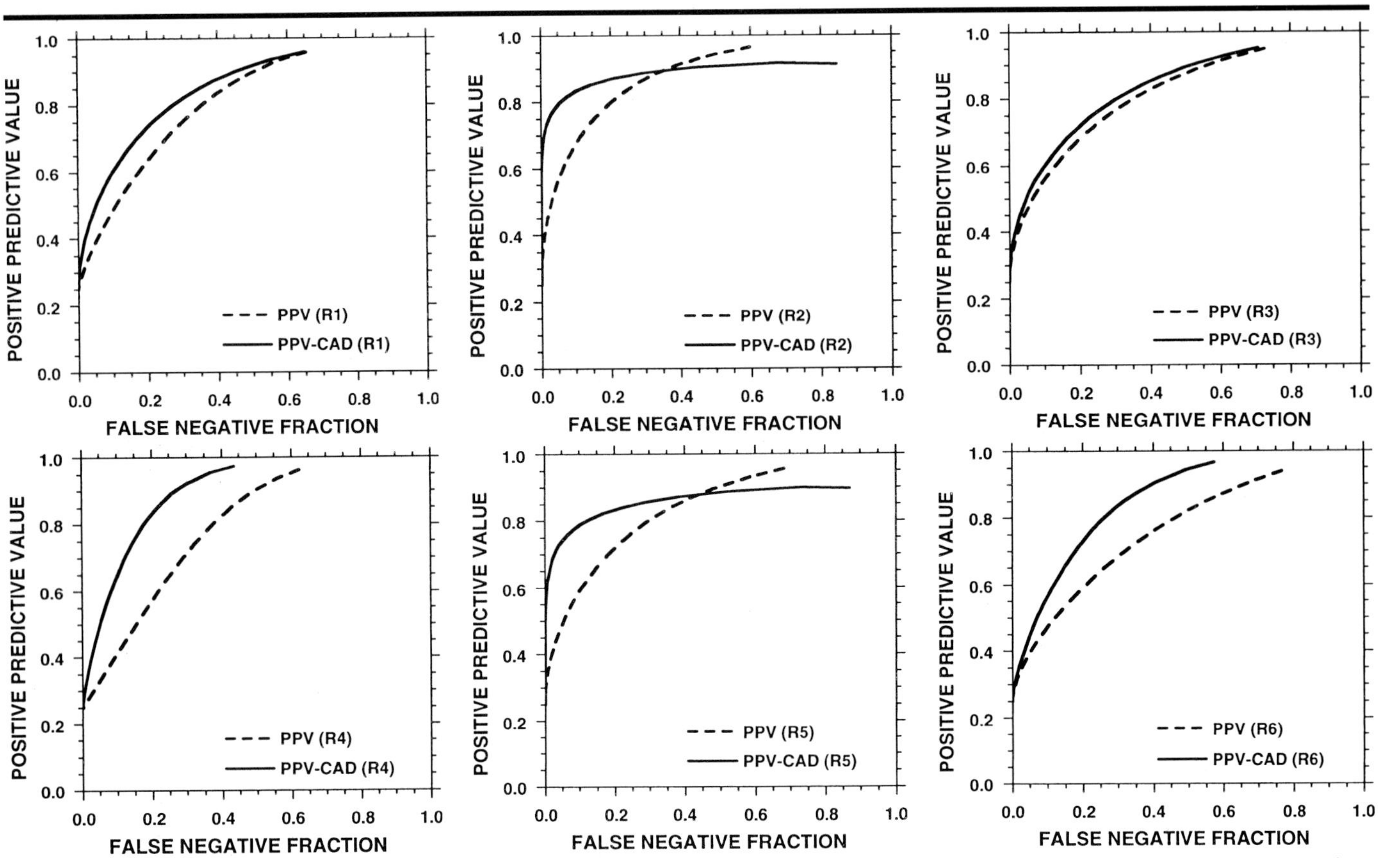

Figure 9. PPV as a function of the false-negative fraction derived from the ROC curves for the six observers (Fig 7). The PPV was predicted for a population of masses in which biopsy was likely to be performed under current clinical criteria and by assuming the prevalence of malignant masses to be 25%. *R1* = reader 1, *R2* = reader 2, *R3* = reader 3, *R4* = reader 4, *R5* = reader 5, *R6* = reader 6.

Because decision making is a complex process, the simple approach of using the highest malignant rating or the average rating from multiple views may not be the method preferred by radiologists. The separate ratings that we used in this study would provide less biased information. Further investigation is needed to determine the best approach of presenting the computer's ratings to radiologists in clinical practice.

To obtain insight into how the radiologists might use the two-view information, we compared the classification results from their true two-view reading with those from a simulated two-view reading without the computer aid. The latter results were derived from ratings of single-view readings of the same 76 pairs of mammograms interpreted in experiment 2 by assuming two strategies—one in which the highest malignancy rating between the two ratings was used, and the other in which the average of the two ratings was used (Table 2). The A_z values for these classification ratings derived from the single-view reading are listed in Table 2. The corresponding A_z values for the computer classifier are also given in Table 2 for comparison.

The A_z values for the maximal rating and the average rating were similar. Four of the radiologists obtained higher A_z values at the true two-view reading; the A_z values obtained by the remaining two radiologists were lower than those obtained at the simulated two-view reading. Although the difference did not achieve statistical significance ($P = .37$) and both readings included intraobserver variations, there seemed to be a slight trend toward the true two-view reading being more accurate than the simulated two-view reading. This may indicate that the radiologists used a more complex decision-making process to interpret the two views of the masses than that of simply maximizing or averaging the ratings from each view.

In this study, the discriminant scores of the masses given by the computer classifier were transformed into a relative malignancy rating. The relative malignancy rating scale and the distribution of the malignant and benign masses along the relative rating scale were explained to the observers in the training sessions. A relative malignancy rating scale was used because the true likelihood of malignancy of the masses could not be estimated from a small data set, as will be explained. However, the relative rating scale provided by the computer was ad-

TABLE 2
Estimation of the Malignancy Classification of 76 Masses by Two-View Reading, as Simulated from Single-View Reading of Mammograms by Radiologists without CAD

	A_z	
Radiologist No.	Maximal Rating	Average Rating
1	0.94 ± 0.03	0.93 ± 0.03
2	0.94 ± 0.03	0.94 ± 0.03
3	0.84 ± 0.05	0.86 ± 0.04
4	0.85 ± 0.04	0.83 ± 0.05
5	0.88 ± 0.04	0.89 ± 0.04
6	0.91 ± 0.03	0.92 ± 0.03
Computer	0.96 ± 0.02	0.96 ± 0.02

Note.—Data are the mean ± SD. Two strategies were used: In one, the highest of the malignancy ratings on each view was used; in the other, the average between the two ratings was used.

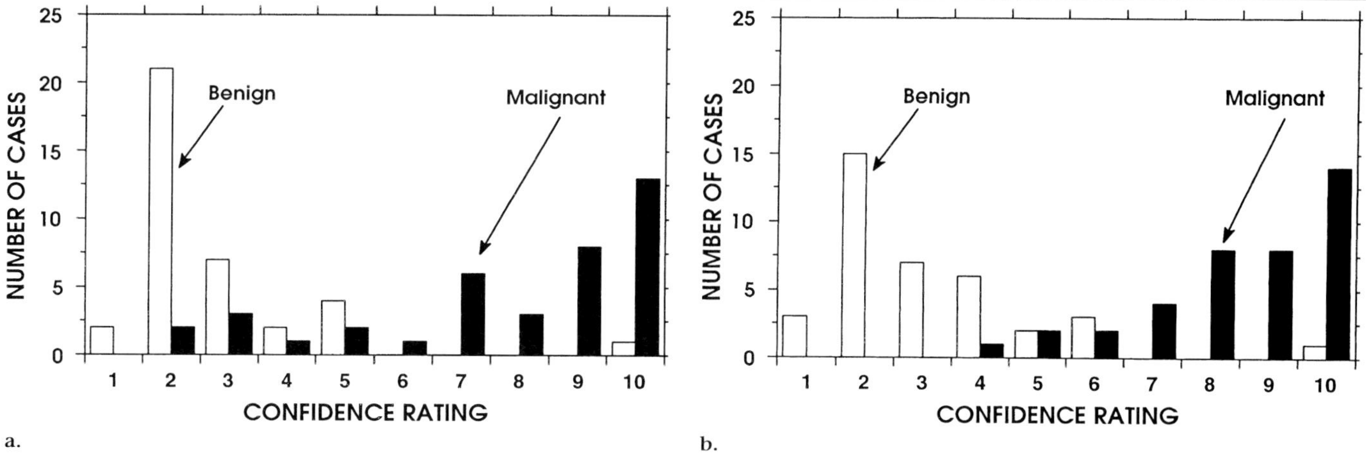

Figure 10. Histograms illustrate the confidence ratings of reader 5 obtained by reading 76 two-view mammograms **(a)** without CAD and **(b)** with CAD. The specificity of reader 5 at 100% sensitivity would increase from 5% (two of 37 masses) without CAD to 68% (25 of 37 masses) with CAD if an appropriate decision threshold were chosen.

equate for measuring the relative performance of classification with and without CAD in an ROC study.

If a computer classifier is trained and tested with very large data sets, and if both the malignant and benign cases represent random samples of the population, then the likelihood of malignancy of a classified mass can be estimated on the basis of the probability distributions of the classifier's test output scores and the prevalence of the two classes of masses in the patient population. However, with a relatively small data set, such as that used in this and other observer studies (14), there are limitations. First, the performance of a classifier trained with a small sample set may have large bias and variance (29–31). Second, the data set in this study did not include masses on which biopsy was not performed, so it did not represent a random sample of the masses in the patient population. If our classifier were applied to all cases of solid masses in clinical practice, the probability distribution of the test scores for the two classes of masses would be different from that of the current data set.

If we ignore the patient population at large, it is possible to estimate the likelihood of malignancy of a mass on the basis of the probability distribution of the classifier output scores by using the prevalence of the two classes of masses in this specific data set. However, the likelihood of malignancy derived in this way will be completely different from the true likelihood of malignancy of a mass in the patient population. This can be easily seen if one considers that the same mass with the same discriminant score will have a smaller likelihood of malignancy if it is analyzed within a data set that has a lower prevalence of malignant cases than that in the current data set.

Training the participating radiologists with a "likelihood of malignancy" derived from a small data set for the observer experiment may mislead them if they encounter a similar mass in their clinical practice. We, therefore, preferred to use a "relative malignancy rating," which is independent of the prevalences of malignant and benign masses in the data set. As long as the same classifier and the same linear transformation are used for classifying masses, the relative malignancy rating for a given mass will remain the same, regardless of the types of other masses in the data set. When a computer classifier is implemented in a clinical setting and its performance can be established in the patient population, the true likelihood of malignancy of a given mass can be estimated and provided to the radiologist. The true likelihood of malignancy may be a more informative measure for radiologists in the clinical application of CAD.

For the reading of the 76 two-view mammograms, the results of the ROC study indicated an improvement in the A_z value for all six radiologists when the computer aid was used. This indicates an overall increase in the separation of confidence rating distributions between the malignant and benign cases. The histograms in Figure 10 illustrate the distributions of confidence ratings with and without CAD for reader 5, who achieved the second greatest improvement in both the A_z value (Table 1) and the separation of malignant from benign distributions. Without CAD, this reader's ratings of the malignant cases ranged from 2 to 10. This is consistent with the fact that biopsy was performed in all masses in the data set to avoid missing the malignant cases. With CAD, there was marked improvement in the separation of the two distributions. It is possible to set a decision threshold at a confidence rating of 4, below which biopsy would not need to be performed and no malignant masses would be missed. The number of benign masses that could be identified without missing a malignant mass by setting an appropriate threshold would increase by 23 (out of 76 cases) for reader 5. Five of the six radiologists in our ROC study achieved an improvement in distinguishing benign from malignant masses, and one radiologist had no difference. Although the improvement of the five radiologists varied over a wide range, from one to 25 cases, this result indicates a strong possibility that CAD can be used to reduce the number of unnecessary biopsies.

The large variation in improvement among the radiologists may have been due to the different degrees of confidence that they had in the computer aid. As with any new diagnostic tool, this confidence is influenced by the experience the radiologist has with the tool. Although the radiologists received training before the reading sessions, the high variability in confidence was not unexpected, because this ROC study was the first instance in which they had worked with the computer aid. Their confidence levels may have also been reflected in the relatively low accuracy of classification by some radiologists with CAD compared with that of the computer classifier alone.

If a radiologist can increase his or her

confidence in the performance of a computer aid by gaining more extensive clinical experience, then he or she will likely be able to find the most effective way of merging his or her judgment with the computer's rating and thus reduce both interobserver and intraobserver variability. Because a radiologist who uses CAD can establish a meaningful decision threshold for biopsy only after becoming familiar with the sensitivity and specificity of working with CAD, the radiologists in this study were not asked to decide whether biopsy should have been performed on a mass. Rather, we focused on the evaluation of changes in the sensitivity and specificity of the radiologists' classification of masses when CAD was used.

In this ROC study, all six observers were attending radiologists with extensive experience in the interpretation of mammograms. It is possible that the computer aid may be even more useful to radiology residents or radiologists with less experience in mammography. The effect of CAD on mammographic interpretation by less-experienced readers will be a subject of investigation in future studies.

The observers were allowed unlimited time to read each case in this ROC study. To obtain an estimate of the change in reading time with CAD, we recorded the reading time of each observer in each reading session by using a stopwatch. For the single-view reading experiment, the average reading time per image without CAD varied from 4.3 seconds to 17.1 seconds (mean time for the six observers, 7.8 seconds). The average reading time per image with CAD varied from 4.2 seconds to 17.3 seconds (mean time, 7.3 seconds). For the two-view reading experiment, the average reading time per pair of images without CAD varied from 6.6 seconds to 16.0 seconds (mean time, 10.4 seconds). The average reading time per pair of images with CAD varied from 7.6 seconds to 27.1 seconds (mean time, 13.5 seconds).

The reading time essentially did not change with use of the computer aid for the single-view readings. For the two-view readings, the radiologists took longer with CAD, probably because they had to merge the two computer ratings and merge the computer ratings with their own evaluations. Further investigation is needed to determine whether there is a trade-off between the radiologist's efficiency and the method of presenting the computer rating and whether the reading time with CAD will depend on the experience that the radiologist has with the computer information.

In the observer study, we used laser-printed mammograms instead of the original mammograms for the reading experiments. A major reason is that it is difficult to keep all the original mammograms together for the entire period of the study because they are part of active patient files and thus often recalled for comparison with new studies or for other clinical reasons. Because the maximum optical density of laser-printed images was 3.1 for the laser imager used, the contrast on the printed mammograms was about 20% lower than that on the original mammograms. Although the image quality was slightly lower than that of the original, the laser-printed digitized images were judged to be adequate for reading the details of the masses by the participating radiologists. The laser-printed image set might also be considered as one that had slightly more subtle masses than the original set of images. Because the relative performance of two modalities is measured in ROC experiments, and because the readings both with and without CAD in this study were conducted with the same set of printed images, the relative performance of the two readings should be valid. It should also be noted that in order for a computer aid that uses automated image analysis to be widely accepted, direct digital mammography would have to be the imaging modality in clinical use. Laser-printed images or soft-copy monitors will be the display medium for the digital mammograms. The use of laser-printed images for this ROC study was therefore practical.

In our observer performance experiment, we found that CAD improved the radiologists' ability to distinguish malignant and benign masses. This is consistent with the results of other studies (11,14) in which a statistically significant improvement ($P < .001$ in both studies) in the radiologists' classification accuracy by using CAD was found. The results of the former study (11) further showed that the PPV of a recommendation for biopsy by the radiologists was significantly increased ($P < .001$). In our approach, the computer classifier automatically extracted image features, whereas in the other studies, the computer classifier used the radiologist's evaluation and other patient information as input. Therefore, it appears that CAD can provide a useful second opinion to radiologists, either by consistently extracting and analyzing the image features or by optimally weighting various diagnostic factors and thereby improving the consistency in the decision-making process. This suggests that a computer classifier that combines both approaches—that is, automatically extracts image features and optimally merges them with the radiologist's evaluation and patient information—may be even more effective for breast cancer diagnosis. The latter step will also improve the radiologist's utilization of the computer rating on the basis of the computer-extracted features; this utilization was found to have large interobserver variation in our ROC experiment.

In conclusion, an ROC study of the effects of CAD on radiologists' classification of malignant and benign masses on mammograms was conducted. The results showed that CAD can provide a statistically significant improvement in the classification accuracy—that is, in the A_z value—for both single-view reading ($P = .022$) and two-view reading ($P = .007$). The improved separation between the confidence ratings of the malignant masses and those of the benign masses indicates the potential that CAD may reduce the rate of biopsy of benign masses when decision thresholds are properly chosen by the radiologists. The decision threshold may vary among radiologists, as in the case of mammographic interpretation without CAD, and can be set after the radiologist working with CAD has established his or her sensitivity and specificity with this approach through clinical experience.

Further studies are needed to evaluate the effects of CAD on the accuracy of radiologist classification of masses in clinical settings in which the prevalence of malignant masses is different from that in a laboratory data set and the likelihood of malignancy of a mass can be estimated by the computer classifier. In the two-view reading ROC experiment, the reading time per case increased by about 30% with the use of CAD. The dependence of the radiologist's efficiency in reading with CAD on the presentation method and on the reader's experience in using the computer information also warrants further investigation.

Acknowledgments: The authors are grateful to Charles E. Metz, PhD for useful discussions and for the use of the LABROC and LABMRMC programs.

References

1. Landis SH, Murray T, Bolden S, Wingo PA. Cancer statistics 1998. CA Cancer J Clin 1998; 48:6–29.
2. Adler DD, Helvie MA. Mammographic biopsy recommendations. Curr Opin Radiol 1992; 4:123–129.

3. Kopans DB. The positive predictive value of mammography. AJR 1991; 158:521–526.
4. Shtern F. Digital mammography and related technologies: a perspective from the National Cancer Institute. Radiology 1992; 183: 629–630.
5. Thurfjell EL, Lernevall KA, Taube AAS. Benefit of independent double reading in a population-based mammography screening program. Radiology 1994; 191:241–244.
6. Vyborny CJ. Can computers help radiologists read mammograms? Radiology 1994; 191:315–317.
7. Chan HP, Doi K, Vyborny CJ, et al. Improvement in radiologists' detection of clustered microcalcifications on mammograms: the potential of computer-aided diagnosis. Invest Radiol 1990; 25:1102–1110.
8. Kegelmeyer WP, Pruneda JM, Bourland PD, Hillis A, Riggs MW, Nipper ML. Computer-aided mammographic screening for spiculated lesions. Radiology 1994; 191: 331–337.
9. Getty DJ, Pickett RM, D'Orsi CJ, Swets JA. Enhanced interpretation of diagnostic images. Invest Radiol 1988; 23:240–252.
10. D'Orsi CJ, Getty DJ, Swets JA, Pickett RM, Seltzer SE, McNeil BJ. Reading and decision aids for improved accuracy and standardization of mammographic diagnosis. Radiology 1992; 184:619–622.
11. Baker JA, Kornguth PJ, Lo JY, Floyd CE. Artificial neural network: improving the quality of breast biopsy recommendations. Radiology 1996; 198:131–135.
12. Chan HP, Sahiner B, Petrick N, et al. Observer performance study of radiologists' reading of mammographic masses and comparison with computerized classification (abstr). Radiology 1996; 201(P):370.
13. Chan HP, Sahiner B, Helvie MA, et al. Effects of computer-aided diagnosis (CAD) on radiologists' classification of malignant and benign masses on mammograms: an ROC study (abstr). Radiology 1997; 205(P):275.
14. Jiang Y, Nishikawa R, Schmidt RA, Metz CE, Doi K. Improving breast cancer diagnosis with computer-aided diagnosis (CAD): an observer study (abstr). Radiology 1997; 205(P):274.
15. Sahiner B, Chan HP, Petrick N, Helvie MA, Adler DD, Goodsitt MM. Classification of masses on mammograms using rubber-band straightening transform and feature analysis. Proc SPIE 1996; 2710:44–50.
16. Sahiner B, Chan HP, Petrick N, Helvie MA, Goodsitt MM. Computerized characterization of masses on mammograms: the rubber-band straightening transform and texture analysis. Med Phys 1998; 25:516–526.
17. Sahiner B, Chan HP, Petrick N, Helvie MA, Goodsitt MM. Design of a high-sensitivity classifier based on a genetic algorithm: application to computer-aided diagnosis. Phys Med Biol 1998; 43:2853–2871.
18. Ackerman LV, Gose EE. Breast lesion classification by computer and xeroradiograph. Cancer 1972; 30:1025–1035.
19. Kilday J, Palmieri F, Fox MD. Classifying mammographic lesions using computerized image analysis. IEEE Trans Med Imaging 1993; 12:664–669.
20. Pohlman S, Powell KA, Obuchowshi NA, Chilote WA, Grundfest-Broniatowski S. Quantitative classification of breast tumors in digitized mammograms. Med Phys 1996; 23:1337–1345.
21. Huo Z, Giger ML, Vyborny CJ, Wolverton DE, Schmidt RA, Doi K. Automated computerized classification of malignant and benign masses on digitized mammograms. Acad Radiol 1998; 5:155–168.
22. Haralick RM, Shanmugam K, Dinstein I. Texture features for image classification. IEEE Trans Syst Man Cybernetics 1973; 3:610–621.
23. Norusis MJ. SPSS for Windows release 6: professional statistics. Chicago, Ill: Statistical Product for Service Solutions, 1993.
24. Lachenbruch PA. Discriminant analysis. New York, NY: Hafner, 1975; 8–19.
25. Metz CE. ROC methodology in radiologic imaging. Invest Radiol 1986; 21:720–733.
26. Metz CE, Herman BA, Shen JH. Maximum-likelihood estimation of receiver operating characteristic (ROC) curves from continuously distributed data. Stat Med 1998; 17:1033–1053.
27. Metz CE. Some practical issues of experimental design and data analysis in radiological ROC studies. Invest Radiol 1989; 24:234–245.
28. Dorfman DD, Berbaum KS, Metz CE. ROC rating analysis: generalization to the population of readers and cases with the jackknife method. Invest Radiol 1992; 27:723–731.
29. Fukunaga K, Hayes RR. Effects of sample size on classifier design. IEEE Trans Pattern Analysis and Machine Intelligence 1989; 11:873–885.
30. Chan HP, Sahiner B, Wagner RF, Petrick N, Mossoba J. Effects of sample size on classifier design: quadratic and neural network classifiers. Proc SPIE 1997; 3034:1102–1113.
31. Chan HP, Sahiner B, Wagner RF, Petrick N. Classifier design for computer-aided diagnosis in mammography: effects of finite sample size. Med Phys 1997; 24:1034–1035.

Catherine S. Giess, MD
Delia M. Keating, MD
Michael P. Osborne, MD
Ruth Rosenblatt, MD

Index terms:
Breast neoplasms, calcification, 00.4535
Breast neoplasms, diagnosis, 00.32, 00.33
Breast neoplasms, surgery, 00.455, 00.458
Breast neoplasms, therapeutic radiology, 00.459

Radiology 1999; 212:829–835

Abbreviation:
DCIS = ductal carcinoma in situ

[1] From the Departments of Radiology (C.S.G., D.M.K., R.R.) and Surgery (M.P.O.), New York Presbyterian Hospital–Weill Medical College of Cornell University, Strang Cornell Breast Center, New York. Received June 17, 1998; revision requested August 6; final revision received November 17; accepted March 26, 1999. **Address reprint requests to** C.S.G., Department of Radiology, Memorial Sloan-Kettering Cancer Center, 1275 York Ave, New York, NY 10021.

Author contributions:
Guarantor of integrity of entire study, C.S.G.; study concepts and design, C.S.G., D.M.K.; definition of intellectual content, C.S.G.; literature research, C.S.G.; data acquisition, C.S.G., D.M.K.; data analysis, C.S.G.; manuscript preparation, C.S.G.; manuscript editing and review, all authors

Local Tumor Recurrence following Breast-Conservation Therapy: Correlation of Histopathologic Findings with Detection Method and Mammographic Findings[1]

PURPOSE: To correlate histopathologic findings with detection method and mammographic appearance in primary and locally recurrent breast carcinoma after breast-conservation therapy.

MATERIALS AND METHODS: Medical records and mammographic findings were retrospectively reviewed; 26 patients with 27 local recurrences after breast-conservation therapy were identified.

RESULTS: Primary histopathologic findings included six in situ and 20 invasive carcinomas. Of the 27 recurrences, 19 (70%) were at or adjacent to the lumpectomy site and eight (30%) were elsewhere in the breast. All primary ductal carcinoma in situ (DCIS) cases manifested mammographically as microcalcifications and recurred as DCIS with microcalcifications. Eleven primary invasive carcinomas (10 masses, one case of microcalcifications) were detected only mammographically, three were detected only with physical examination, and six (six masses) were detected with both. Among these 20 recurrences, 14 (five masses, nine cases of microcalcifications) were detected only mammographically, one was detected only with physical examination, and five (five masses) were detected with both. Seventeen (85%) of 20 primary invasive carcinomas recurred invasively: 16 (94%) with similar histopathologic findings and eight (47%) with similar mammographic findings.

CONCLUSION: In local recurrence after breast-conservation therapy for DCIS, histopathologic findings, detection method, and mammographic findings are usually similar. Histopathologic findings of primary invasive breast carcinoma and local recurrence are usually similar, but the detection method and mammographic findings vary. This is relevant to the interpretation of new clinical or mammographic findings following lumpectomy.

Breast-conservation therapy is widely used in the treatment of early-stage breast carcinoma, having been demonstrated to provide similar overall and disease-free survival as mastectomy (1), with the additional advantage of improved cosmesis. However, women undergoing breast-conservation therapy have a long-term risk of local recurrence, which is estimated to be approximately 1%–2.5% per year (2,3). Therefore, they must undergo continued clinical and mammographic surveillance. These two methods have been demonstrated to be complementary in the detection of local recurrence following breast-conservation therapy (4–7).

Mammography is less sensitive in the treated breast than in the untreated breast due to surgery- and radiation-induced changes in the parenchymal pattern (8). The sensitivity of mammography in this population ranges from 55% to 68% in various studies (4–7). When detected mammographically, local breast cancer recurrence has a similar appearance as cancer in the untreated breast, which is most commonly a mass, microcalcifications, or both (4–8).

The appearance and histopathologic findings of locally recurrent breast cancer compared with those of the primary lesion have been evaluated in several studies. Liberman et al (9) compared imaging and histopathologic findings of primary ductal carcinoma in situ (DCIS) with those of local recurrences in 20 patients and found that 65% of local recurrences consist of pure DCIS, with the remaining 35% containing invasive and in situ carcinoma. In 14 patients, they compared mammograms at the time of primary diagnosis with those at the time of local recurrence and found the mammographic pattern and calcification morphology to be similar in 79% and 82% of patients, respectively. Philpotts et al (10) compared the mammographic appearance of primary breast cancer with that of local recurrence and found that the lesions had a similar appearance 81% of the time. Those authors suggested that knowledge of the mammographic appearance of a patient's primary breast tumor may influence the decision to perform biopsy of a mammographic finding in the treated breast and may improve the positive predictive value of biopsy in this mammographically challenging patient population.

We reviewed the clinical, imaging, and histopathologic findings in patients who developed local recurrence following breast-conservation therapy at our institution to correlate the histopathologic findings of primary tumors and local recurrences with the detection method and imaging features.

MATERIALS AND METHODS

Retrospective review of the tumor registry and the surgical database at our institution yielded 33 local breast cancer recurrences in 32 patients who had available imaging and medical records and who had undergone breast-conservation therapy. Three patients were excluded in whom incidental, microscopic local recurrence was detected at biopsy of histologically benign microcalcifications. Three additional patients were excluded in whom no preoperative mammographic information was available. This yielded a population of 26 patients with 27 local recurrences following breast-conservation therapy, which constitute the basis of this study. All patients had mammograms at the time of local recurrence available for retrospective review. In 24 of 26 patients, mammograms at the time of primary diagnosis were also available; in the remaining two patients, reported descriptions were available. Radiographs of specimens were available and were reviewed in eight patients.

The patients were aged 28–85 years (mean, 57 years). Primary cancer in this population was diagnosed from June 1985 to December 1995; local recurrence was diagnosed from May 1990 to January 1998. The time from primary breast cancer diagnosis to local recurrence was 18–120 months (mean, 46 months). All patients were initially treated with wide local excision with or without axillary dissection. Initial tumor stage was known in 24 patients: Six had stage 0, 12 had stage I, and six had stage II disease. Two patients with invasive carcinomas smaller than 2 cm did not undergo axillary dissection due to concurrent medical problems. Margins were negative at histopathologic analysis in 18 patients, positive in one patient, and unknown in seven patients. Twenty-two patients underwent radiation therapy (one patient had treatment interrupted prior to the boost dose to the tumor bed), three refused radiation therapy, and radiation treatment information was unknown in one patient. Patients were evaluated clinically and mammographically at 6- or 12-month intervals on the basis of physician preference; during the study interval, no uniform protocol for follow-up surveillance existed at our institution. Magnification views of the lumpectomy bed were obtained at the discretion of the initial interpreting radiologist.

All available mammograms were retrospectively reviewed by two radiologists in conference (C.S.G., D.M.K.). All mammograms were considered technically adequate. Mammograms obtained at the time of primary diagnosis were reviewed simultaneously with mammograms obtained at the time of local recurrence, and findings were described by using the American College of Radiology's Breast Imaging Reporting and Data System (11).

Lesions were classified as masses, microcalcifications, or calcified masses. Primary lesions and local recurrences were classified as similar or dissimilar in appearance on the basis of these classifications; calcified masses were considered similar between primary and locally recurrent malignancies if either calcification or a mass was present mammographically. Calcified masses were classified in this manner because both masses and calcifications are primary signs of breast cancer and both may be prominent imaging features of tumors.

The location of local recurrences in the treated breast was classified as at or adjacent to the tumor bed, within the same quadrant, or in a different quadrant. According to the definition by Recht et al (3), recurrences at or adjacent to the tumor bed were considered "true recurrences or marginal misses" and those recurring in the same quadrant but at a distance from the lumpectomy site or in a different quadrant were considered "elsewhere." In this study, recurrences within 2 cm of the lumpectomy bed (marked by surgical clips or scarring) were considered to be true recurrences or marginal misses.

Medical records were reviewed (C.S.G.) to determine the clinical findings at the time of primary diagnosis and local recurrence, and histopathologic records were reviewed to determine the features of primary and locally recurrent cancers. Cancers were classified histopathologically according to the most aggressive component present; lesions containing invasive and in situ carcinoma were considered invasive. Microinvasive DCIS was classified as DCIS, but the presence of microinvasion was noted. Microinvasive DCIS was not classified as invasive carcinoma for the purpose of this retrospective study, since histopathologic definitions of microinvasion vary and since treatment in patients with microinvasive DCIS is similar to that in patients with DCIS but without microinvasion at our institution.

For the majority of tumors, size was determined histopathologically; when unavailable, size was determined mammographically. For lesions containing both invasive and intraductal carcinoma, the size of the invasive component was recorded; however, if an extensive, mammographically evident intraductal component was present, this was noted.

RESULTS

Overall, 19 local recurrences were at or adjacent to the lumpectomy bed (true recurrences or marginal misses); eight recurred elsewhere (three in the same quadrant and five in a different quadrant from the index tumor). Sixteen of the 19 local recurrences at or adjacent to the primary tumor bed had the same histopathologic diagnosis as the primary tumor, 10 of which had similar histopathologic features such as the degree of differentiation or the subtype of DCIS. In the eight tumors that recurred elsewhere in the treated breast, seven recurred with the same histopathologic diagnosis as the

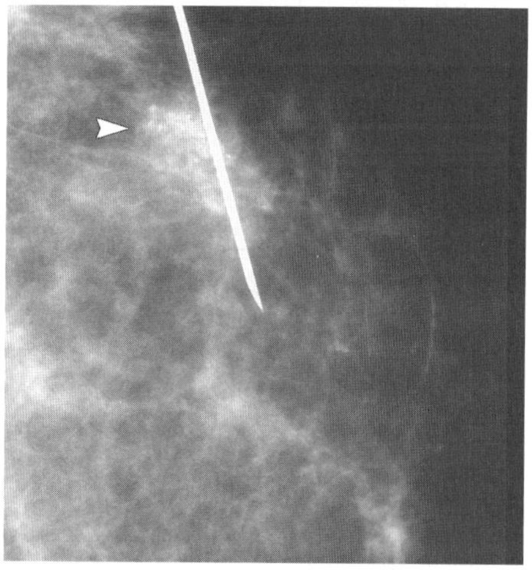

a.

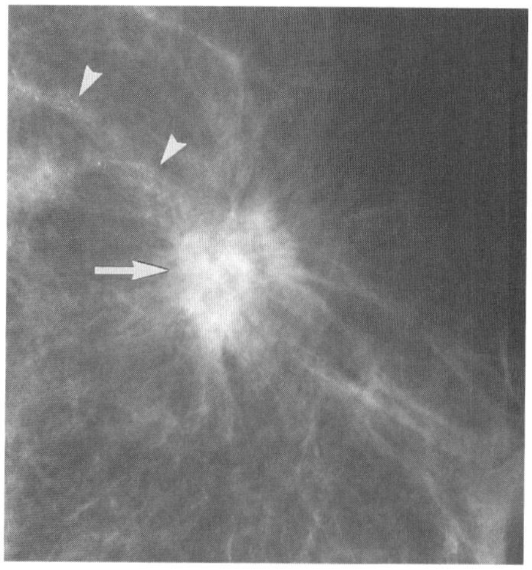

b.

Figure 1. (a) Collimated right craniocaudal mammogram obtained during a needle localization in a 52-year-old woman shows the localization needle as it extends through a cluster of pleomorphic microcalcifications (arrowhead). Histopathologic analysis yielded mixed comedo and noncomedo DCIS. (b) Collimated right craniocaudal mammogram obtained 25 months after breast-conservation therapy demonstrates new pleomorphic microcalcifications (arrowheads) in a linear distribution adjacent to the lumpectomy bed (arrow). Histopathologic analysis yielded cribriform-type DCIS with necrosis.

TABLE 1
Comparison of Imaging Findings between Primary and Locally Recurrent Breast Cancers

Imaging Finding for Primary Cancer ($N = 26$)	Imaging Findings for Locally Recurrent Cancer ($N = 27$): Similar to Primary Cancer ($n = 16$)	Imaging Findings for Locally Recurrent Cancer ($N = 27$): Dissimilar to Primary Cancer ($n = 11$)
Mass ($n = 12$)	Mass ($n = 4$)	Calcifications ($n = 7$)* Occult ($n = 1$)
Calcifications ($n = 7$)†	Calcifications ($n = 7$)‡ Calcified mass ($n = 1$)	... ...
Calcified mass ($n = 4$)	Mass ($n = 2$) Calcified mass ($n = 1$) Calcifications ($n = 1$)§	... ...
Occult ($n = 3$)	... ...	Mass ($n = 2$) Calcifications ($n = 1$)‖

Note.—Data are the number of cancers.
* Five invasive, two in situ.
† Six in situ, one invasive.
‡ Seven in situ (one patient with two recurrences).
§ In situ.
‖ Invasive.

primary tumor, two of which had similar histopathologic features. The eighth recurrence contained only DCIS, whereas the primary tumor had been invasive ductal carcinoma.

The mean size of primary tumors was 12.6 mm (range, 3–26 mm), and the mean size of local recurrences was 17.3 mm (range, 3–35 mm). One patient had a 4-mm invasive recurrence with an extensive intraductal component; her recurrence mammographically manifested as a 30-mm area of fine microcalcifications. All 26 patients with mammographically evident local recurrences had lesions considered to be Breast Imaging Reporting and Data System category 4 or 5.

Ductal Carcinoma in Situ

In six patients, the primary tumor histopathologic diagnosis was DCIS. In one of these patients, the tumor was multifocal with foci of microinvasion. One patient had widely dispersed DCIS. The remaining four patients had focal DCIS histopathologically. In all six of these patients, lesions were detected only mammographically due to microcalcifications. The morphology and distribution of the primary tumor calcifications were pleomorphic and clustered in all six patients.

These six patients had seven local recurrences. One patient had two separate recurrences; the first recurred 53 months after the primary diagnosis and the second recurred 57 months after repeat lumpectomy. All local recurrences were DCIS histopathologically and again were detected mammographically due to microcalcifications (Table 1). In four patients (five local recurrences), microcalcification morphology and distribution in local recurrences were similar to those of the primary tumor. In one patient, the primary tumor appearance was pleomorphic and clustered and the local recurrence appearance was linear and branching with a linear distribution. In one patient, the primary tumor appearance was pleomorphic and clustered and the local recurrence appearance was pleomorphic with a linear distribution (Fig 1).

Histopathologically, four of the six primary DCIS lesions contained comedo-type DCIS, one contained only noncomedo DCIS, and one contained microinvasion (subtype unspecified). All five recurrences in the four patients with primary comedo carcinoma developed at or adjacent to the lumpectomy bed; two recurrences were comedo and three were noncomedo at histopathologic analysis. In the patient with primary noncomedo carcinoma, the tumor recurred as comedo carcinoma in a different quadrant. In one patient with primary multifocal microinvasive DCIS, the tumor recurred as multifocal microinvasive DCIS in a different quadrant. The primary and local recurrence histopathologic findings are correlated with location in Table 2.

Invasive Carcinoma

Twenty patients had primary invasive breast carcinoma: 17 with ductal and three with lobular cancer at histopathologic analysis. One patient had widely dispersed DCIS in association with invasive ductal carcinoma. Eleven of 20 primary invasive carcinomas were detectable only mammographically, three were detectable only at physical examination, and six were evident with both methods.

Among the 17 mammographically evident cancers, imaging findings indicated six spiculated masses; five ill-defined masses; three spiculated masses with microcalcifications; one lobulated, ill-defined mass with microcalcifications; one case of clustered, pleomorphic microcalcifications; and one mass with unknown characteristics.

Local recurrence in these 20 patients with primary invasive malignancies was detected only mammographically in 14, only at physical examination in one, and with both methods in five. Of the 19 recurrences detected mammographically, eight manifested as noncalcified masses: Three had spiculated margins, three had ill-defined margins, and two had obscured margins. Two recurrences manifested as calcified masses, one with ill-defined, lobulated margins and one with spiculated margins. Nine recurrences manifested as microcalcifications alone, which were linear in five and pleomorphic in four cases. The distribution in these nine microcalcifications was clustered in five and segmental in four.

Seventeen (85%) of 20 patients with primary invasive carcinomas had invasive local recurrences, 16 (94%) of these 17 patients had primary cancers and local recurrences with similar histopathologic findings. The remaining three (15%) of the 20 patients had cancer that locally recurred as DCIS. Of the 16 patients sharing similar invasive histopathologic findings between primary and locally recurrent carcinoma, 11 had recurrence at or adjacent to the lumpectomy site, and five had recurrence elsewhere in the breast. The degree of histopathologic differentiation in these 16 patients was the same in nine, less well-differentiated in two, better in one, and unknown in four. The 17th patient with an invasive recurrence had primary invasive lobular carcinoma, which recurred as invasive ductal carcinoma at the lumpectomy site. In the remaining three patients with primary invasive carcinoma, cancer locally recurred as DCIS at or adjacent to the lumpectomy site in two and elsewhere in one. All three of these recurrences were detected on the basis of pleomorphic microcalcifications. Correlation of histopathologic findings with location of recurrence is detailed in Table 2.

TABLE 2
Comparison of Histopathologic Findings with the Site of Local Recurrence of Primary Breast Cancer

	Site of Local Recurrence			
	Invasive Cancer		Noninvasive Cancer	
Primary Cancer	True Recurrence or Marginal Miss	Elsewhere in Treated Breast	True Recurrence or Marginal Miss	Elsewhere in Treated Breast
Invasive (n = 20)	12	5	2	1
Noninvasive (n = 6)	0	0	5*	2

Note.—Data are the number of cancers.
* One patient with two noninvasive recurrences.

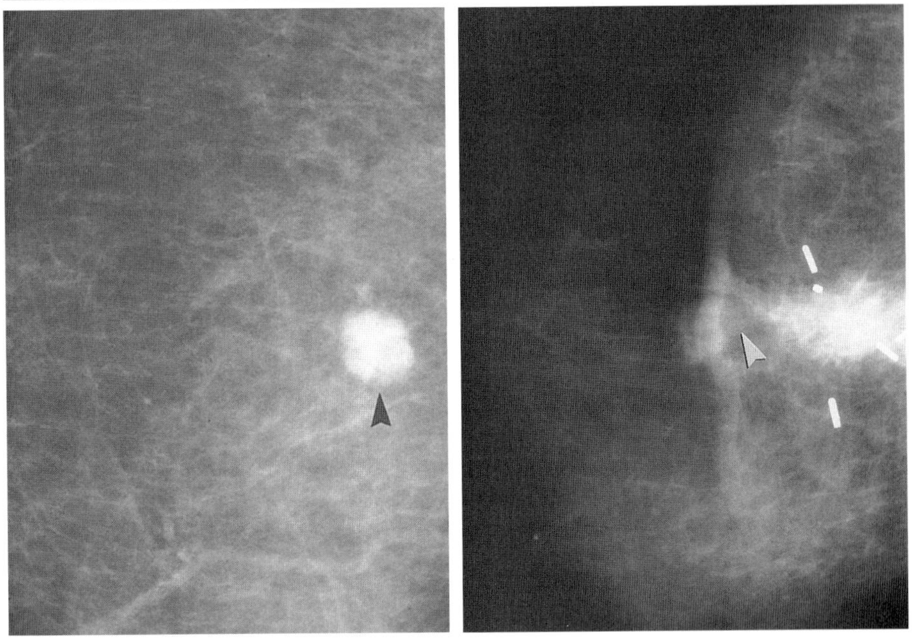

a. b.

Figure 2. **(a)** Collimated left craniocaudal mammogram obtained in a 59-year-old woman shows an ill-defined mass (arrowhead). Histopathologic analysis yielded poorly differentiated invasive ductal carcinoma. **(b)** Collimated left craniocaudal mammogram obtained 34 months after breast-conservation therapy shows an ill-defined mass (arrowhead) anterior to the lumpectomy bed, which is marked by surgical clips. Histopathologic analysis yielded recurrent poorly differentiated invasive ductal carcinoma.

Imaging features in 17 of the 20 patients with invasive carcinoma in both primary and locally recurrent tumors were similar in eight (47%) and dissimilar in nine (53%) patients. In the group with similar imaging findings between primary and locally recurrent cancers, four primary masses recurred as masses (Fig 2), one calcified mass recurred as a calcified mass, two calcified masses recurred as masses, and one case of microcalcifications recurred as a calcified mass. In the patients with dissimilar imaging findings, five primary tumors manifesting as masses recurred as microcalcifications (Fig 3), three mammographically occult primary tumors had mammographically evident recurrences (two masses, one case of microcalcifications), and one primary tumor manifesting as a mass had a mammographically occult local recurrence. These data are outlined in Table 1.

Twenty-one recurrences were treated with salvage mastectomy, and six were treated with repeat breast-conservation therapy. Follow-up data after salvage mastectomy or repeat conservation therapy was known in 24 patients: Sixteen were without evidence of disease, with a mean follow-up of 37 months (range, 8–83 months), and eight underwent salvage mastectomy within the last 8 months of the study and had no evidence of disease. Two patients were lost to follow-up after treatment of their local recurrence.

DISCUSSION

Diagnostic mammography and careful physical examination play complementary roles in the follow-up surveillance of patients who have undergone breast-conservation therapy (4–7). Since breast conservation is being widely performed for early-stage breast cancer, mammo-

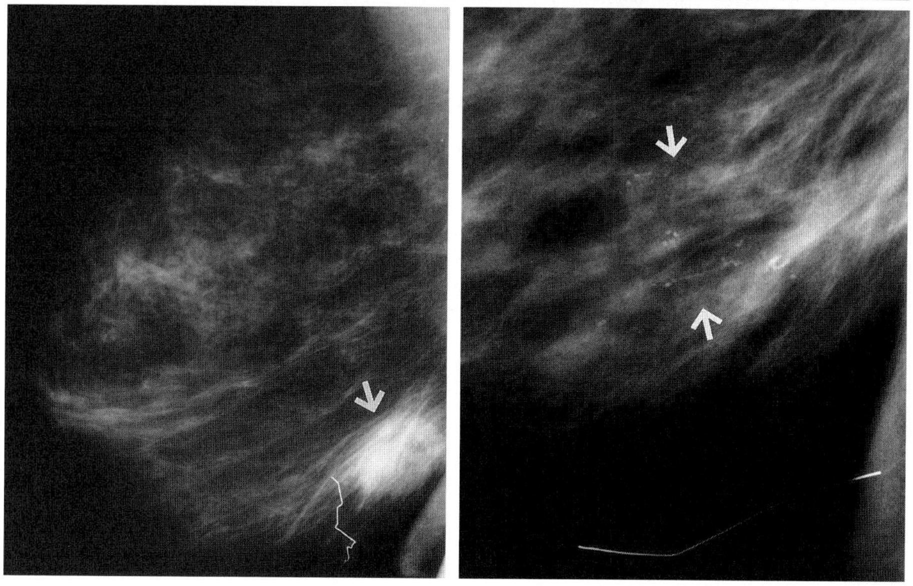

a. b.

Figure 3. **(a)** Left mediolateral oblique mammogram obtained in a 54-year-old woman demonstrates an ill-defined mass (arrow). Histopathologic analysis yielded invasive ductal carcinoma, with prominent mucin production. A metallic wire identifies the site of a previous biopsy of a benign lesion. **(b)** Collimated mediolateral oblique magnification mammogram obtained 20 months after breast-conservation therapy demonstrates numerous linear and pleomorphic microcalcifications (arrows) immediately anterior to the lumpectomy bed. Histopathologic analysis yielded recurrent invasive ductal carcinoma with comedo-type DCIS. A metallic wire identifies the cutaneous lumpectomy scar.

graphic surveillance in these patients and the early detection of local recurrence are important issues for radiologists.

When tumor recurs in a conservatively treated breast, it may recur at the lumpectomy bed (true recurrence), adjacent to it (marginal miss), or elsewhere in the treated breast (3). It is theorized that tumor recurring at or near the primary tumor site represents a true treatment failure, while tumor recurring at some distance from the primary tumor site may represent either an initially unrecognized separate tumor focus or a new primary tumor (3). This theory is supported by the similar histopathologic findings found between primary and locally recurrent tumor at or adjacent to the primary tumor bed in a study by the same group of investigators (12).

Most of our local recurrences developing at or adjacent to the primary tumor site also shared similar histopathologic findings with the primary tumor, although similar histopathologic findings were also found between most primary tumors and local recurrences developing elsewhere in the breast in our series. It is possible that these latter cases may have represented multicentric or multifocal tumor. The time to recurrence at or adjacent to the primary tumor bed has been reported to be earlier than that of tumor recurring elsewhere in the breast. In the series by Recht et al (3), the median time to recurrence for true recurrences or marginal misses was 38.5 months compared to 64.5 months for local recurrences elsewhere in the treated breast. In the series by Fowble et al (13), the median interval to recurrence for true recurrences or marginal misses was 38 months, and that for recurrences elsewhere in the treated breast was 46 months. In a different series (2), while overall 79% of local recurrences were at or within the vicinity of the primary tumor bed, over time an increasing percentage of tumors were located at a distance from the lumpectomy site. The majority of local recurrences developing after 10 years in that study were located elsewhere in the breast.

The results of these different studies are in agreement with our data, in which the median time to recurrence at or adjacent to the lumpectomy bed was 28 months (range, 18–91 months) compared with 44.5 months (range, 36–120 months) for tumors recurring elsewhere. In all of these studies, as well as our own, the majority of local tumor recurrences were at or adjacent to the lumpectomy bed (true recurrences or marginal misses). Therefore, the tumor bed must receive particularly close attention following breast-conservation therapy, with careful assessment of any new mammographic findings. Careful physical examination of the lumpectomy bed is also important, since mammographic sensitivity has been reported to be most impaired in the lumpectomy quadrant (4).

Prior to the widespread use of mammography, DCIS manifested most often as a palpable mass; currently, it most commonly manifests as microcalcifications at mammography (14,15). A number of series (16–20) have demonstrated high rates of local control and overall survival for patients with DCIS treated with breast-conservation therapy and irradiation. However, several of these studies also reported protracted cases of local recurrence in DCIS (16,17,19,20), indicating the need for long-term mammographic surveillance. When DCIS locally recurs, it usually recurs in the lumpectomy quadrant (9,15). Primary DCIS may recur as pure DCIS or invasive ductal carcinoma. In the largest of these series (20), approximately half of local recurrences were invasive and half were in situ carcinoma. Authors of several studies (6,12,21) have reported a trend toward noninvasive histopathologic findings when local recurrence is detected with mammography alone. The majority of mammographically detected recurrences in these series contained microcalcifications.

The imaging appearance of local recurrence following breast-conservation therapy for DCIS has been assessed by Liberman et al (9). In that series, primary DCIS most often recurred as DCIS and usually manifested as microcalcifications within the lumpectomy quadrant. Although the number of primary DCIS cases in our series was small ($n = 6$), all recurrences were also DCIS that manifested mammographically as microcalcifications.

Invasive carcinoma is the most frequent breast carcinoma (22). Mammographically, invasive carcinoma most often manifests as a mass with or without microcalcifications; less commonly, invasive carcinoma may manifest as microcalcifications alone (23). Treatment of early stage invasive breast cancer with lumpectomy and radiation therapy has been shown in several studies to result in good local control and overall survival rates (12,13,24). When invasive carcinoma locally recurs, the histopathologic findings of the recurrence are usually invasive as well (10,12,13,24), although at times the tumor may recur as pure DCIS.

In our series, the majority (85%) of

invasive carcinomas recurred invasively, but when they recurred as DCIS, they manifested as microcalcifications. Philpotts et al (10) compared the imaging findings of primary and locally recurrent breast cancers; they found most recurrences to be similar in imaging appearance to the primary tumor, particularly if the recurrence was within the lumpectomy quadrant. Most of the tumors in that study were invasive and recurred invasively most of the time. The imaging findings in that study contrast with our own, in which only 16 (59%) of 27 local recurrences had similarity between the mammographic appearance of the local recurrence and that of the primary tumor. Dissimilarity of appearance occurred when primary histopathologic findings were invasive, not in situ. Although most invasive tumors in our series recurred invasively, only 47% of these had a similar mammographic appearance as the primary tumor. Of note, six of the nine invasive local recurrences having a different appearance from the primary lesion manifested as only microcalcifications. In addition, the three cases of primary invasive carcinoma that recurred noninvasively contained only microcalcifications; two of these cases had an appearance dissimilar to that of the primary tumor. As microcalcifications were the only mammographic sign of local recurrence (three in situ, six invasive) in nine of 17 primary invasive carcinomas in our series, we believe that developing indeterminate microcalcifications at the lumpectomy site should be viewed with a high index of suspicion, regardless of whether the primary tumor was invasive or in situ and regardless of the appearance of the primary lesion. In this series, six (38%) of the 16 local recurrences that manifested as suspicious microcalcifications alone represented recurrent invasive carcinoma.

Two of the invasive primary carcinomas in our series were occult at initial imaging but locally recurred as a mass or as microcalcifications at mammography. Thus, mammographic surveillance was important even in patients in whom the primary tumor was occult. This has also been demonstrated by Samuels et al (25); in their study, four of six local recurrences following breast-conservation therapy in patients with occult primary tumors were mammographically visible. In the series by Schnitt et al (12), 89% of local recurrences manifesting as a new abnormality at physical examination were invasive carcinoma, while all of the local recurrences detected only as a new mammographic abnormality (all microcalcifications) contained predominantly or exclusively intraductal carcinoma. In the study by Liberman et al (9), only three patients with primary DCIS had a palpable local recurrence; however, in two of the three, the lesion contained invasive as well as in situ histopathologic findings. From these data as well as from our own, it is evident that when local recurrence is palpable, it is usually invasive.

It is surprising that the majority of our local recurrences were detected mammographically, given the decreased sensitivity of mammography shown by others in this population (4–7). The decreased sensitivity in detecting local recurrences compared with the sensitivity in detecting primary tumor has been ascribed to postoperative scarring and radiation changes (8), findings particularly pronounced in the lumpectomy quadrant.

It has been suggested that the mammographic detection of local recurrence manifesting as a mass may be more difficult than that of local recurrence manifesting as microcalcifications (10). This is supported by the series by Dershaw et al (6), in which 19 of 29 mammographically detected recurrences contained microcalcifications, and that by Orel et al (4), in which 10 of 21 mammographically detected recurrences contained microcalcifications. In the study by Orel et al (4), the majority of mammographically detected recurrences at the lumpectomy bed were detected because of the presence of microcalcifications. Similarly, 16 of 27 local recurrences in our series were mammographically detected as microcalcifications, although masses were also mammographically detectable.

There are several possible explanations for the high sensitivity of mammography in detecting local recurrence in our series. Local recurrences in our series were diagnosed more recently than those in other published series, and it is possible that the higher rate of mammographic detection is due to intervening improvements in mammographic technique since the 1970s and 1980s. Improvements in surgical and radiation therapy techniques could account for less severe surgical and radiation changes in the treated breast. Finally, heightened awareness in recent years of the need for close mammographic surveillance has allowed for the increased detection of subtle mammographic changes, which can herald local recurrence. At our institution, the current protocol for mammographic surveillance following adequate breast-conservation therapy includes biannual mammography for 2 years and annual mammography thereafter. Magnification views are obtained at the discretion of the interpreting mammographer.

A limitation of this retrospective study is the lack of information on surgical margins in seven primary tumors and information regarding the degree of histopathologic differentiation in four invasive recurrences. Surgical inking of margins was not routinely performed on specimens in prior years (3,12,16,17,19,20). In addition, as our medical center is a major referral center for the greater metropolitan area, some patients return to local centers for treatment after consultation at our institution. Therefore, some of the histopathologic material is no longer available for additional review.

In conclusion, in our series of local breast cancer recurrences following breast-conservation therapy, primary DCIS uniformly recurred as in situ carcinoma. Both primary and locally recurrent DCIS were detected solely mammographically as microcalcifications. Invasive carcinoma usually recurred invasively; less often, it recurred as in situ lesion. However, imaging features varied between primary invasive cancers and local recurrences. Although primary invasive carcinoma usually manifested clinically and/or mammographically as a mass, local recurrences in these patients were detected 45% of the time as microcalcifications alone; the majority of which represented invasive disease. This has important implications for the evaluation of new mammographic findings in the treated breast.

References

1. Jacobson JA, Danforth DN, Cowan KH, et al. Ten-year results of a comparison of conservation with mastectomy in the treatment of stage I and stage II breast cancer. N Engl J Med 1995; 332:907–911.
2. Kurtz JM, Amalric R, Brandone H, et al. Local recurrence after breast-conserving surgery and radiotherapy: frequency, time course, and prognosis. Cancer 1989; 63: 1912–1917.
3. Recht A, Silen W, Schnitt SJ, et al. Time-course of local recurrence following conservative surgery and radiotherapy for early stage breast cancer. Int J Radiat Oncol Biol Phys 1988; 15:255–261.
4. Orel SG, Troupin RH, Patterson EA, Fowble BL. Breast cancer recurrence after lumpectomy and irradiation: role of mammography in detection. Radiology 1992; 183: 201–206.
5. Hassell PR, Olivotto IA, Mueller HA, Kingston GW, Basco VE. Early breast cancer: detection of recurrence after conservative surgery and radiation therapy. Radiology 1990; 176:731–735.
6. Dershaw DD, McCormick B, Osborne MP. Detection of local recurrence after conservative therapy for breast carcinoma. Cancer 1992; 70:493–496.

7. Stomper PC, Recht A, Berenberg AL, Jochelson MS, Harris JR. Mammographic detection of recurrent cancer in the irradiated breast. AJR 1987; 148:39–43.
8. Dershaw DD. Mammography in patients with breast cancer treated by breast conservation (lumpectomy with or without radiation). AJR 1995; 164:309–316.
9. Liberman L, Van Zee KJ, Dershaw DD, Morris EA, Abramson AF, Samli B. Mammographic features of local recurrence in women who have undergone breast-conserving therapy for ductal carcinoma in situ. AJR 1997; 168:489–493.
10. Philpotts LE, Lee CH, Haffty BG, Lange RC, Tocino I. Mammographic findings of recurrent breast cancer after lumpectomy and radiation therapy: comparison with the primary tumor. Radiology 1996; 201: 767–771.
11. American College of Radiology. Illustrated breast imaging reporting and data system (BI-RADS). 3rd ed. Reston, Va: American College of Radiology, 1998.
12. Schnitt SJ, Connolly JL, Recht A, Silver B, Harris JR. Breast relapse following primary radiation therapy for early breast cancer. II. Detection, pathologic features and prognostic significance. Int J Radiat Oncol Biol Phys 1985; 11:1277–1284.
13. Fowble B, Solin LJ, Schultz DJ, Rubenstein J, Goodman RL. Breast recurrence following conservative surgery and radiation: patterns of failure, prognosis, and pathologic findings from mastectomy specimens with implications for treatment. Int J Radiat Oncol Biol Phys 1990; 19:833–842.
14. Morrow M, Schnitt SJ, Harris JR. Ductal carcinoma in situ. In: Harris JR, Lippman ME, Morrow M, Hellman S, eds. Diseases of the breast. Philadelphia, Pa: Lippincott-Raven, 1996; 355–368.
15. Stomper PC, Margolin FR. Ductal carcinoma in situ: the mammographer's perspective. AJR 1994; 162:585–591.
16. Bornstein BA, Recht A, Connolly JL, et al. Results of treating ductal carcinoma in situ of the breast with conservative surgery and radiation therapy. Cancer 1991; 67:7–13.
17. Stotter AT, McNeese M, Oswald MJ, Ames FC, Romsdahl MM. The role of limited surgery with irradiation in primary treatment of ductal in situ breast cancer. Int J Radiat Oncol Biol Phys 1990; 18:283–287.
18. Vicini FA, Lacerna MD, Goldstein NS, et al. Ductal carcinoma in situ detected in the mammographic era: an analysis of clinical, pathologic, and treatment-related factors affecting outcome with breast-conserving therapy. Int J Radiat Oncol Biol Phys 1997; 39:627–635.
19. Ray GR, Adelson J, Hayhurst E, et al. Ductal carcinoma in situ of the breast: results of treatment by conservative surgery and definitive irradiation. Int J Radiat Oncol Biol Phys 1993; 28:105–111.
20. Solin LJ, Kurtz J, Fourquet A, et al. Fifteen-year results of breast-conserving surgery and definitive breast irradiation for the treatment of ductal carcinoma in situ of the breast. J Clin Oncol 1996; 14:754–763.
21. Orel SG, Fowble BL, Solin LJ, Schultz DJ, Conant EF, Troupin RH. Breast cancer recurrence after lumpectomy and radiation therapy for early-stage disease: prognostic significance of detection method. Radiology 1993; 188:189–194.
22. Rosen PP. Invasive mammary carcinoma. In: Harris JR, Lippman ME, Morrow M, Hellman S, eds. Diseases of the breast. Philadelphia, Pa: Lippincott-Raven, 1996; 393–444.
23. Wilhelm MC, Edge SB, Cole DD, DeParedes E, Frierson HF. Nonpalpable invasive breast cancer. Ann Surg 1991; 213:600–605.
24. Grosse A, Schreer I, Frischbier HJ, Maass H, Leoning T, Bahnsen J. Results of breast conserving therapy for early breast cancer and the role of mammographic follow-up. Int J Radiat Oncol Biol Phys 1997; 38:761–767.
25. Samuels JR, Haffty BG, Lee CH, Fischer DB. Breast conservation therapy in patients with mammographically undetected breast cancer. Radiology 1992; 185: 425–427.

Mousy Type of Calcification in a Breast Fibroadenoma

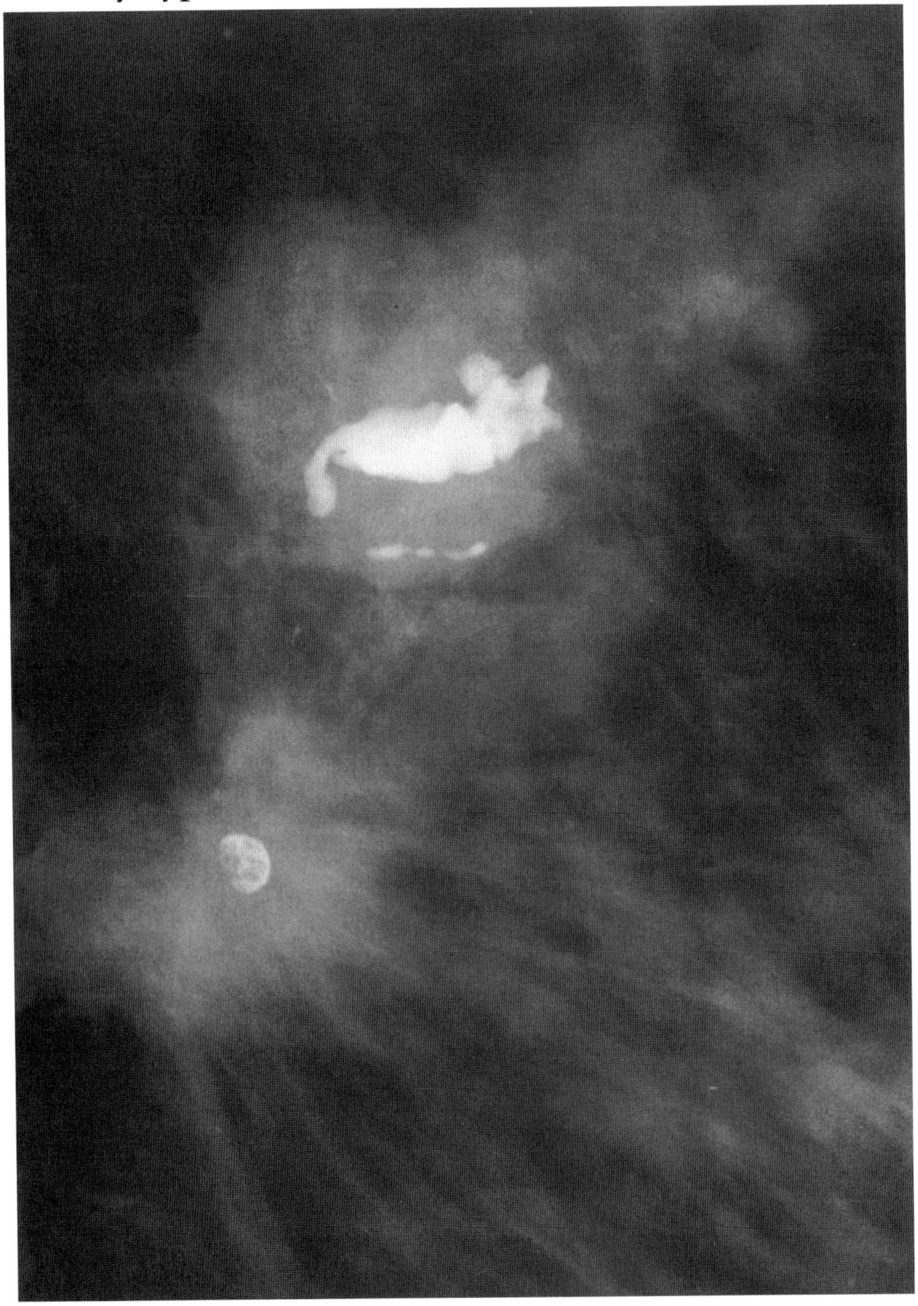

Mammogram shows a cancer, adjacent to which is a fibroadenoma containing "mouselike" calcification.

Courtesy of Richard G. Henderson, MD, Darlington, United Kingdom

Anterior Chest Wall: Frequency of Anatomic Variations in Children[1]

Lane F. Donnelly, MD
Donald P. Frush, MD
Joseph N. Foss, MD[2]
Sara M. O'Hara, MD
George S. Bisset III, MD

Index terms:
Thorax, abnormalities, 47.1496, 47.1497, 47.92
Thorax, CT, 47.1211

Radiology 1999; 212:837–840

[1] From the Department of Radiology, Division of Pediatric Radiology, Duke University Medical Center, Durham, NC. From the 1998 RSNA scientific assembly. Received July 28, 1998; revision requested October 15; revision received November 3; accepted March 16, 1999. **Address reprint requests to** L.F.D., Department of Radiology, Children's Hospital and Medical Center and the University of Cincinnati, 3333 Burnet Ave, Cincinnati, OH 45229-3039.

[2] Current address: Department of Radiology, Arnold Palmer Hospital for Children and Women, Orlando, Fla.

PURPOSE: To evaluate the frequency of anterior chest wall variations in children.

MATERIALS AND METHODS: The computed tomographic (CT) images of 200 consecutive infants and children (114 boys and 86 girls; mean age, 10.5 years; age range, 3 months to 19 years) who underwent chest CT during a 20-month period were evaluated for chest wall variations. Children who had undergone chest wall surgery or were suspected of having a chest wall abnormality were excluded. The frequency of chest wall anomalies was compared with age and sex (Fisher exact test).

RESULTS: The CT scans of 65 children (33%) depicted one or more variations in the anterior chest wall: tilted sternum ($n = 29$), prominent convexity of anterior rib or costal cartilage ($n = 19$), prominent asymmetric costal cartilage ($n = 20$), well-defined paracostal subcutaneous nodule ($n = 4$), mild pectus excavatum ($n = 4$), or mild pectus carinatum ($n = 4$). The frequency of these findings did not vary significantly with age ($P = .96$) or sex ($P = .36$).

CONCLUSION: Variations in the anterior chest wall are common, occurring in one-third of children, and should be considered normal. These asymptomatic variations should not be considered alarming when palpated at physical examination.

Because the chest wall can be involved with either malignancies or severe infections, cross-sectional imaging is often performed to evaluate palpable lesions of the chest wall discovered in children. Although such malignant processes of the chest wall are not common, the presentation for imaging of a child with a "lump" palpated at physical examination is not infrequent. In a previous study (1), in which the results were reviewed for computed tomographic (CT) and magnetic resonance (MR) imaging examinations performed in children referred for evaluation of anterior chest wall lesions, all of the palpated lumps that were asymptomatic were related to anatomic variations of no clinical importance. In our subjective experience, such variations are also seen frequently in children referred for cross-sectional imaging for other indications, when there is no question concerning a chest wall anomaly. If the frequency of chest wall variants is high, these findings should be considered normal when discovered at physical examination and should not be considered alarming to either parents or physicians. The purpose of this study was to evaluate the frequency of chest wall variations in children.

MATERIALS AND METHODS

We reviewed the CT scans of 200 consecutive children (114 boys and 86 girls; mean age, 10.5 years; age range, 3 months to 19 years) who underwent CT examination of the chest at our institution over a 20-month period to evaluate chest wall anomalies. Children who had undergone chest wall surgery or were suspected of having a chest wall abnormality were excluded from the study. No other indications prohibited inclusion in the study. The most common indications for CT examination included evaluation for pulmonary metastasis, suspicion of mediastinal mass, follow-up of lymphoma, or evaluations for pulmonary infection in an immunocompromised host, complications of pneumonia, or mediastinal

Author contributions:
Guarantor of integrity of entire study, L.F.D.; study concepts and design, L.F.D.; definition of intellectual content, L.F.D.; literature research, L.F.D.; data acquisition and analysis, all authors; manuscript preparation, L.F.D.; manuscript editing and review, all authors.

hematoma. Each child was included in the study only once, even if the child underwent multiple chest CT examinations.

All CT examinations were performed with the same type of scanner (CT HiSpeed Advantage; GE Medical Systems, Milwaukee, Wis). Because the examinations were tailored to the specific indication and patient size, the technical parameters varied. Examinations were performed without or with intravenous nonionic contrast material (2.0 mL per kilogram of body weight). Collimation ranged from 5 to 10 mm, and pitch varied from 1.0 to 1.5. All examinations were performed with the patient supine with the arms extended over the head. Breath holding was instigated when possible. All patients underwent imaging from the thoracic inlet superiorly to the level of the adrenal glands inferiorly. In all cases, images were reviewed with various window width and level settings, which always included standard mediastinal and lung settings. In each case, a data sheet pertaining to the presence or absence of chest wall variations was completed by one of four attending pediatric radiologists (L.F.D., D.P.F., S.M.O., G.S.B.) at the time the CT scans were clinically interpreted.

The CT studies in each patient were reviewed for the presence of six variations in the anterior chest wall: (*a*) tilted sternum, (*b*) prominent convexity of the anterior rib or costal cartilage, (*c*) prominent asymmetric costal cartilage, (*d*) well-defined small (<1 cm) parachondral nodule, (*e*) pectus excavatum, or (*f*) pectus carinatum (1). A tilted sternum was considered present when the sternum was not oriented in the horizontal left-to-right axis of the body (Fig 1) (1). The anterior convexity of a rib or costal cartilage was considered prominent when a solitary rib or costal cartilage demonstrated an apex anterior convexity with angulation greater than that of the adjacent superior, inferior, or contralateral ribs and costal cartilage (Fig 2) (1). A costal cartilage was considered asymmetrically prominent when the anteroposterior diameter of one cartilage was more than 3 mm larger than that of the contralateral isolevel cartilage (Fig 2). The presence of a well-defined nodule less than 1 cm in diameter was noted in the subcutaneous fat, immediately adjacent to the sternum or costal cartilage (Fig 3) (1). Pectus excavatum was considered present when the anterior chest wall was prominently concave, with the midline located more posteriorly than the adjacent, more lateral chest wall (Fig 4). Pectus carinatum was considered present when the anterior chest wall was prominently convex with the midline located more anteriorly than the adjacent, more lateral chest wall (Fig 5). A variation was considered not to be present in any case in which the presence of one of the variations was thought possibly to be related to asymmetric positioning of the patient within the scanner or asymmetric positioning of the patient's arms in relationship to the chest.

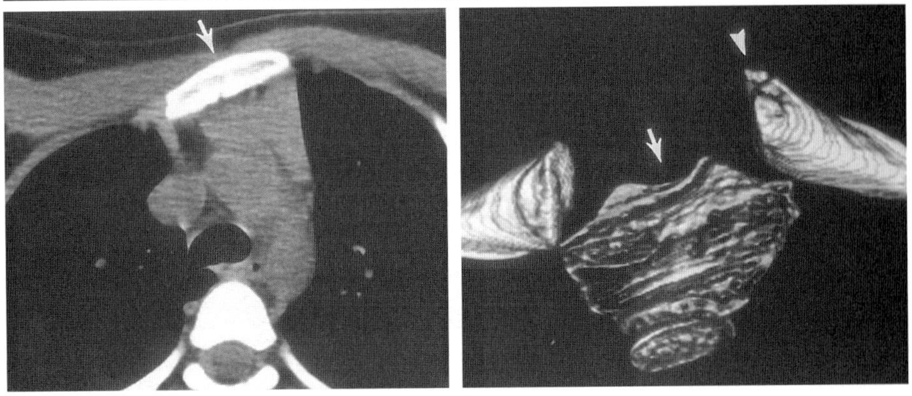

a. b.

Figure 1. Tilted sternum with associated subluxation of the left clavicular head in a 12-year-old girl. **(a)** Axial CT image shows the sternum (arrow) to be tilted with respect to the horizontal right-to-left axis of the body. The left margin of the sternum is located more anteriorly than the right margin. **(b)** Shaded-surface three-dimensional CT reconstructed image, obtained for illustrative purposes, shows tilted sternum (arrow) and anteriorly subluxated left clavicular head (arrowhead). The image is displayed as viewed in the axial plane, from the superior perspective, with the anterior region located at the top and the posterior region at the bottom of the image.

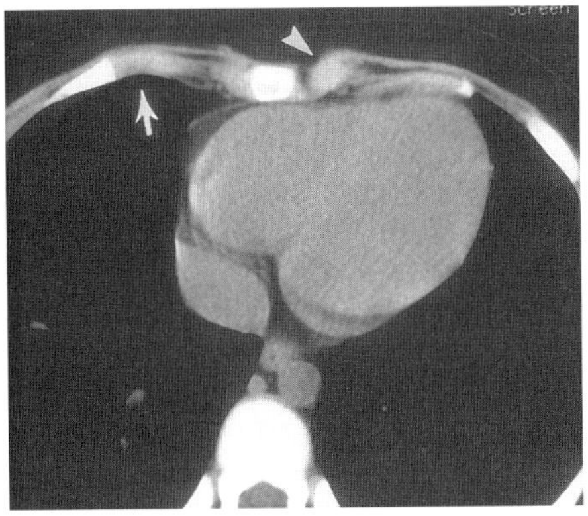

Figure 2. Right prominent anterior convex costal cartilage and left prominent costal cartilage size in a 9-year-old girl. Axial CT scan shows prominence of the anterior convexity of the right costal cartilage (arrow) and asymmetrically larger left costal cartilage (arrowhead).

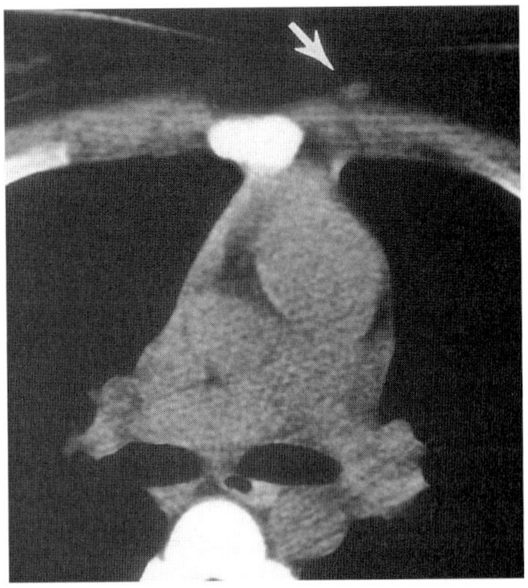

Figure 3. Small parachondral nodule in a 16-year-old boy. Axial CT scan shows a small (3-mm-diameter) nodule (arrow) in subcutaneous tissues immediately adjacent to the costal cartilage. Such nodules are believed to represent cartilaginous islands (1).

The frequency and type of anterior chest wall variations were compared between subgroups of patients on the basis of age and sex. Statistically significant differences in the frequency of variations between these subgroups was evaluated with a Fisher exact test. A *P* value of less than .05 was considered statistically significant. The findings at CT were not correlated with physical examination findings after the CT studies were reviewed.

RESULTS

The CT scans of 65 (33%) of the 200 patients depicted variations of the anterior chest wall. Variations included tilted

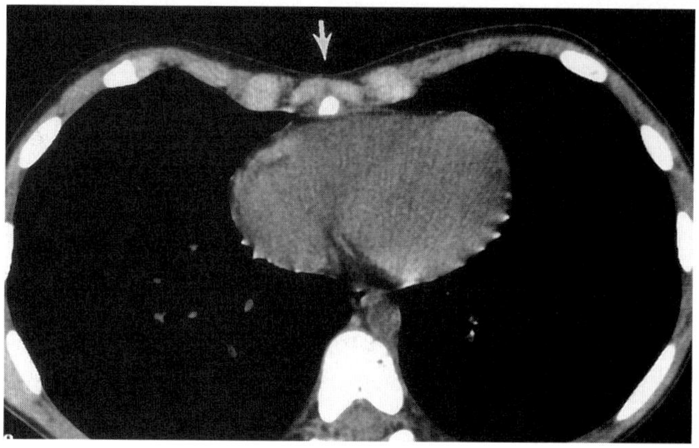

Figure 4. Pectus excavatum in a 7-year-old girl. Axial CT scan shows anterior chest wall to be concave. The midline chest wall (arrow) is located more posteriorly than the more lateral chest wall.

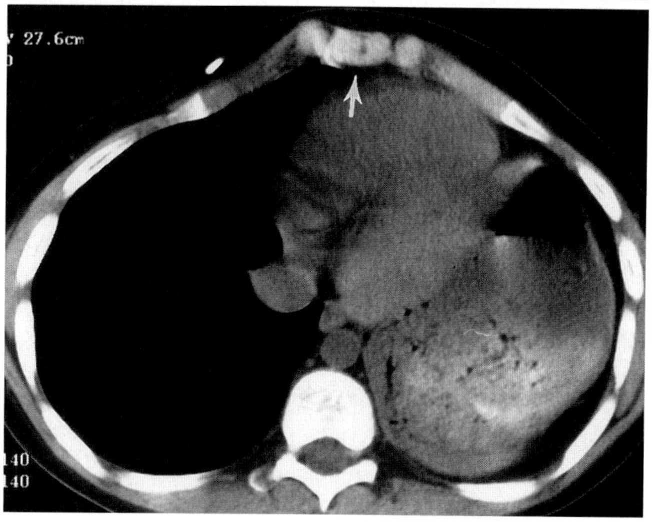

Figure 5. Pectus carinatum in a 13-year-old boy. Axial CT scan shows apex anterior convexity of anterior chest. The midline chest wall (arrow) is located more anteriorly than the more lateral chest wall. The left hemidiaphragm is elevated secondary to acute phrenic nerve involvement by mediastinal lymphoma. The high-attenuation linear structure in the subcutaneous tissues of the right anterior chest wall represents a central venous catheter.

sternum (n = 29), prominent convexity of anterior rib or costal cartilage (n = 19), prominent asymmetric costal cartilage (n = 20), well-defined paracostal subcutaneous nodule (n = 4), mild pectus excavatum (n = 4), and mild pectus carinatum (n = 4). More than one variation was noted in 15 of the 65 patients.

The frequency of asymmetric variations among subgroups of patients was evaluated. Variations were depicted in 34 (30%) of the 114 boys and 31 (36%) of the 86 girls. The mean age for patients with variations was 10.8 years as compared to 10.0 years for patients without variations. Among the 200 children, CT scans depicted variations in 13 (33%) of the 39 patients aged 3 months to 3 years, 16 (30%) of the 54 patients aged 4–8 years, 15 (33%) of the 46 patients aged 9–13 years, and 21 (34%) of the 61 patients aged 13–19 years. There was no statistically significant trend between frequency of variations and age (P = .96) or sex (P = .36).

DISCUSSION

Because evaluation of abnormalities of the chest wall can be difficult by means of physical examination (2) or radiography (1–7), cross-sectional imaging with either CT or MR imaging is often performed when a chest wall abnormality is suspected. Demonstration of abnormalities of the anterior chest wall at radiography can be more difficult in children than in adults because the bulk of the anterior chest wall is made of nonossified cartilage in children. MR imaging and CT are sensitive in the demonstration of aggressive chest wall lesions, including bone destruction, irregular soft-tissue mass, and pleural effusion (1,3,6,7).

In children, multiple aggressive lesions may involve the ribs and chest wall (3). These include malignancies such as Ewing sarcoma, osteosarcoma, neuroectodermal tumors, leukemia, and metastatic neuroblastoma, and aggressive inflammatory conditions such as osteomyelitis and Langerhans cell histiocytosis (3). In the imaging literature concerning the chest wall in children, most studies have dealt with imaging findings in these aggressive conditions or with pectus excavatum (8–10). Although the normal calcification patterns of costal cartilage in adults older than 30 years have been described (11), other characteristics concerning variations in shape and configuration of the anterior chest wall have not been described, to our knowledge.

In a previous study, a population of children suspected of having anterior chest wall lesions was evaluated with cross-sectional imaging (1). In that study, all patients who had clinically important abnormalities, such as malignancy or infection, indicated pain or tenderness at physical examination. In asymptomatic children, however, the cause of the palpable abnormality was always a benign variation in the anterior chest wall. Therefore, benign history and physical examination results have a high negative predictive value for excluding important abnormalities. In this study, we evaluated a population of children who were not suspected of having chest wall abnormalities and underwent CT of the chest for other indications. One-third of the children had these variations in the anterior chest wall. These findings (in the population of children in our study, who were considered to have normal chest walls) are probably not different from those in the patients who were referred with palpable "bumps" in the previous study (1). The only difference may be that in the latter group, these variations were brought to attention by the child, parent, or physician after noticing the area at physical inspection.

Slight variations in the configuration of the costal cartilage, ribs, and sternum are commonly encountered in children and should be considered normal. When these variations in anatomy are encountered at physical examination, they should not be considered alarming. Unless the patient has pain or an underlying illness that predisposes them to a chest wall process (such as immunodeficiency, previous chest wall surgery, or a source of metastatic disease), cross-sectional imaging or ultrasonography is most likely not necessary.

Because of the potential for asymmetric somatic growth to play a role in the frequency of such normal variations in children, we suspected that there might be a higher frequency in children during ages of rapid growth. However, there were no age groups in which there was a higher frequency of variations. In addition, there was no statistically significant difference in the frequency between boys and girls. In all age and sex groups, the frequency was always approximately 33%.

The majority of variations encountered in this study were mild in degree and would not have raised the possibility of a pertinent abnormality with most radiologists. Our goal was not to suggest that there is an epidemic of chest wall variations suddenly elucidated by our interpretations of CT scans. We emphasize that we are not advocating the use of CT to evaluate for these normal variations. Our goal was to use information available on CT studies performed for other reasons to evaluate the frequency of such variations. It is only when such a variation is detected at physical examination and raises the issue of a pathologic process that knowledge of these aberrations has clinical relevance.

In conclusion, variations in the anterior chest wall are common, occurring in one-third of children, and should be considered normal. Findings in a previous study (1) have shown that normal variants of the chest wall, which are of no clinical importance, are usually the cause of asymptomatic "bumps" that are recommended for imaging evaluation. The high frequency of these normal aberrations should be considered when contemplating imaging in a child with an asymptomatic chest wall "lump."

Acknowledgment: We thank David M. Delong, PhD, for his help with the statistical analysis.

References

1. Donnelly LF, Taylor CNR, Emery KH, Brody AS. Asymptomatic, palpable, anterior chest wall lesions in children: is cross-sectional imaging necessary? Radiology 1997; 202:829–831.
2. Hatfield MK, Gross BH, Glazer GM, Martel W. Computed tomography of the sternum and its articulations. Skeletal Radiol 1984; 11:197–203.
3. Faro SH, Mahroubi S, Ortega W. CT diagnosis of rib anomalies, tumors, and infection in children. Clin Imaging 1993; 17:1–7.
4. Brossmann J, Stabler A, Preidler KW, Trudell D, Resnick D. Sternoclavicular joint: MR imaging–anatomic correlation. Radiology 1996; 198:193–198.
5. Goodman LR, Teplick SK, Kay H. Computed tomography of the normal sternum. AJR 1983; 141:219–223.
6. Destouet JM, Gilula LA, Murphy WA, Sagel SS. Computed tomography of the sternoclavicular joint and sternum. Radiology 1981; 138:123–128.
7. Gouliamos AD, Carter BL, Emami B. Computed tomography of the chest wall. Radiology 1980; 134:433–436.
8. Maddern IR, Goodman LR, Almassi GH, Haasler GB, McManus RP, Olinger GN. CT after reconstructive repair of the sternum and chest wall. Radiology 1993; 186:665–670.
9. Lancaster L, McIlhenny J, Rodgers B, Alford B. Radiographic findings after pectus excavatum repair. Pediatr Radiol 1995; 25:452–454.
10. Ellis DG. Chest wall deformities in children. Pediatr Ann 1989; 18:161–165.
11. Ontell FK, Moore EH, Shepard JA, Shelton DK. The costal cartilage in health and disease. RadioGraphics 1997; 17:571–577.

Isabelle Trop, MD
Josée Dubois, MD
Laurent Guibaud, MD
Andrée Grignon, MD
Heidi Patriquin, MD
Catherine McCuaig, MD
Laurent A. Garel, MD

Soft-Tissue Venous Malformations in Pediatric and Young Adult Patients: Diagnosis with Doppler US[1]

Index terms:
Arteriovenous malformations, 9*.14[2]
Neoplasms, in infants and children, 9*.14, 9*.83
Soft tissues, neoplasms, 9*.14, 9*.83
Soft tissues, US, 9*.12983
Veins, US, 9*.12983
Venography, 9*.124

Radiology 1999; 212:841–845

Abbreviation:
VM = venous malformation

[1] From the Departments of Medical Imaging (I.T., J.D., L.G., A.G., H.P., L.A.G.) and Dermatology (C.M.), Hôpital Sainte-Justine, 3175 Côte-Sainte-Catherine, Montréal, Québec, Canada H3T 1C5. Received July 17, 1998; revision requested August 27; final revision received November 13; accepted February 22, 1999. **Address reprint requests to** J.D. (e-mail: *joseedubois@compuserve.com*).

[2] 9*. Vascular system, location unspecified

PURPOSE: To describe the diagnostic features, appearance, and vascularization pattern of venous malformations (VMs) at Doppler ultrasonography (US).

MATERIALS AND METHODS: Between February 1991 and May 1997, 51 soft-tissue VMs were studied with Doppler US in patients between 1 day and 21 years of age (mean age, 9 years). These VMs were located in the maxillofacial region (n = 19), trunk (n = 5), and upper (n = 10) and lower (n = 17) extremities. Twenty–three VMs had venographic confirmation, seven had only histologic confirmation, and 21 had both venographic and histologic confirmation. US was performed with 7.5- or 7–10-MHz linear transducers, a low pulse repetition frequency (mean, 1,680 Hz), and the lowest wall filter (25–50 Hz).

RESULTS: At gray-scale US, VMs appeared as hypoechoic, heterogeneous lesions in 82% of cases. All lesions displayed compressibility. In eight lesions (16%), phleboliths were identified, thus confirming the diagnosis of VM. Analysis of vascular flow revealed monophasic, low-velocity flow in 40 VMs (78%), with an average flow velocity of 0.22 kHz. Biphasic flow was noted at the periphery of three lesions, which is indicative of a mixed capillary-venous malformation. The remaining eight lesions did not display any flow.

CONCLUSION: In pediatric patients, Doppler US is a noninvasive, easily available, and rapid mode of investigation of vascular lesions and can help confirm the diagnosis of VM when it shows a characteristic flow pattern.

Venous malformations (VMs) are part of a spectrum of benign vascular lesions commonly found in the pediatric population. These lesions occasionally may be difficult to distinguish solely on the basis of their clinical appearance. In 1982, Mulliken and Glowacki (1) classified congenital vascular anomalies into true hemangiomas and various vascular malformations on the basis of their histologic features.

Vascular malformations are true congenital lesions, which by definition are always present at birth, although they are not always detected (2). They are classified according to the main channel type present: capillary, lymphatic, arterial, venous, or mixed (1). These lesions do not occur in one sex more than the other. They often grow in proportion to the child and can display periods of active growth. Vascular lesions have been categorized further into low- and high-flow types (3) on the basis of the hemodynamic characteristics of the lesions, a distinction that is important in the choice of management strategies. By definition, vascular malformations do not regress spontaneously.

VMs often can be diagnosed on the basis of clinical characteristics: They are bluish, easily compressible, cold, and increase in size with maneuvers aimed at increasing venous pressure (2). However, malformations occasionally may manifest atypical features, and ancillary studies are needed to confirm the diagnosis. A precise diagnosis will lead to the most appropriate treatment; the standard for the diagnosis of VM is venography or biopsy. To our knowledge, the role of Doppler ultrasonography (US) has not been reported. The aim of this study, therefore, is to emphasize the value of Doppler US in the diagnosis of soft-tissue VMs in pediatric and young adult patients.

Author contributions:
Guarantors of integrity of entire study, J.D., I.T.; study concepts, J.D.; study design, I.T., J.D., L.A.G., H.P.; definition of intellectual content, I.T., J.D.; literature research, I.T., J.D.; clinical studies, all authors; data acquisition, I.T., J.D., L.G., A.G.; data analysis, I.T., J.D., L.G.; manuscript preparation, I.T., J.D., L.A.G., H.P.; manuscript editing, I.T., J.D., L.A.G., H.P., C.M.; manuscript review, all authors

MATERIALS AND METHODS

Between February 1991 and May 1997, 51 VMs in 51 patients (31 female patients, 20 male patients; age range, 1 day to 21 years; mean age, 9 years) were examined by means of gray-scale US and Doppler US in our institution. The lesions were distributed as follows: 19 in the maxillofacial region, five in the trunk, 10 in the upper extremities, and 17 in the lower extremities. Twenty-seven (53%) of the VMs reviewed had been noticed from birth. Eight additional lesions appeared during the first 2 years of life. The remaining 16 VMs appeared at an older age, often in relation to puberty (n = 10) or an episode of trauma (n = 6). At the conclusion of the study period, all examinations were reviewed retrospectively and independently by two investigators (J.D., I.T.). Cases of discrepancy (few) were resolved by a third investigator (L.G.).

Children were referred from our dermatology and vascular malformations clinics by the attending clinician dermatologist, with a presumptive clinical diagnosis of VM. We excluded the patients with Klippel-Trénaunay-Weber syndrome. Our series included patients with VMs only. Patients were referred routinely for US evaluation of a soft-tissue mass clinically suspicious for VM. This diagnosis was proved in all patients: Twenty-three VMs had confirmation only by direct puncture for venography, seven had only histologic confirmation, and 21 had both venographic and histologic confirmation.

Venography was performed percutaneously with direct intralesional puncture and administration of iohexol ([180 mg of iodine per milliliter] Omnipaque; Nycomed, Brampton, Ontario). The venographic criteria used for the diagnosis of VM were those described by Burrows et al (3): ectatic, dilated vascular spaces that demonstrate prolonged pooling of contrast material, with dilated draining veins without arteriovenous shunting or enlarged arterial feeders. Tissue staining was absent or faint and brief.

Biopsy was performed in 28 lesions. For 13 patients, this was performed in an attempt to excise the lesion before referral to our service. Seven patients underwent excision of their lesion after sclerotherapy for treatment of cosmetic and functional impairments. Eight patients had biopsy performed secondary to the treating surgeon's decision (most of these were at the beginning of the study). Histologic analysis confirmed the presence of the ectatic, dilated venous channels characteristic of VM.

US examinations were performed with color Doppler equipment: a Quantum II machine (Siemens, Issaquah, Wash) with a 7.5-MHz linear gray-scale and Doppler transducer or an Ultramark 9 HDI unit (Advanced Technology Laboratories, Bothell, Wash) with a 7–10-MHz linear transducer. A 1-cm-thick standoff pad was used when judged necessary. Examinations were performed by pediatric radiologists (J.D., A.G., L.A.G., H.P.).

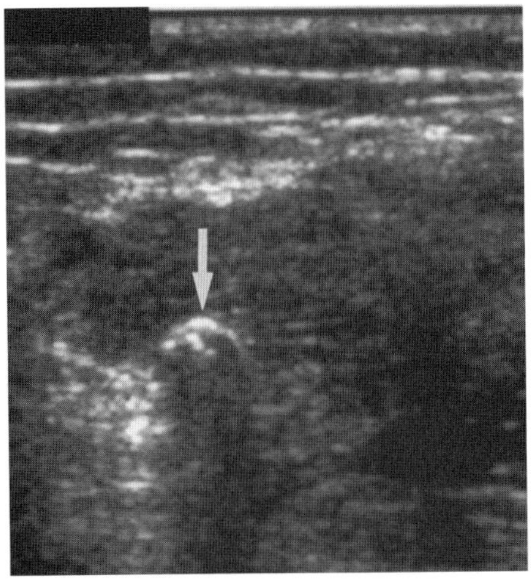

Figure 1. Transverse gray-scale US image of a VM in the thigh in a 12-year-old girl shows isoechoic, heterogeneous architecture with a phlebolith (arrow).

All lesions were analyzed according to the following feature characteristics. Echogenicity was assessed as hypo-, iso-, or hyperechoic in comparison with the surrounding subcutaneous tissue. The presence of echogenic shadowing elements, characteristic of calcifications, was noted (Fig 1). Internal architecture was classified as homogeneous or heterogeneous, and the presence of anechoic cavities was noted. In addition, the length, width, and depth were measured by using electronic calipers for all lesions with well-defined borders. Finally, the presence of compressibility was assessed for all lesions, first by means of gentle and then more firm manual probe pressure.

Color Doppler US was performed by using a restricted field of interest and by scanning the entire lesion. Parameters were set at the lowest Doppler gain settings necessary to prevent aliasing; pulse repetition frequencies varied between 615 and 3,704 Hz (average setting, 1,680 Hz), and wall filters were 25–50 Hz. Doppler recordings were obtained from the area displaying the highest vascularity for all lesions. The area of highest vascularization identified with color flow signal was selected, and Doppler shifts were ascertained with pulsed Doppler. The presence or absence of flow was noted, and when present, the quality of the flow was categorized as monophasic or biphasic.

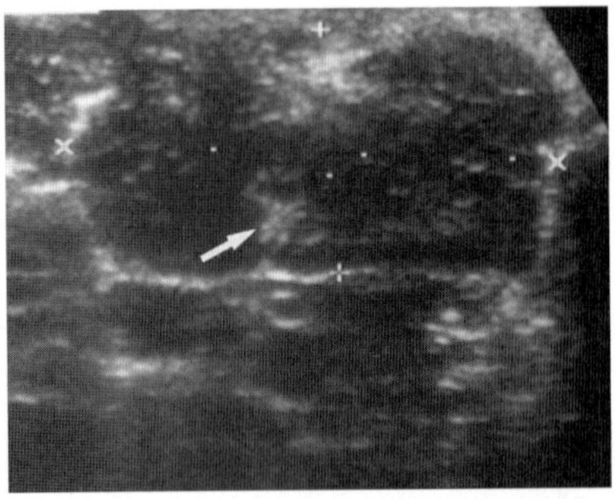

a.

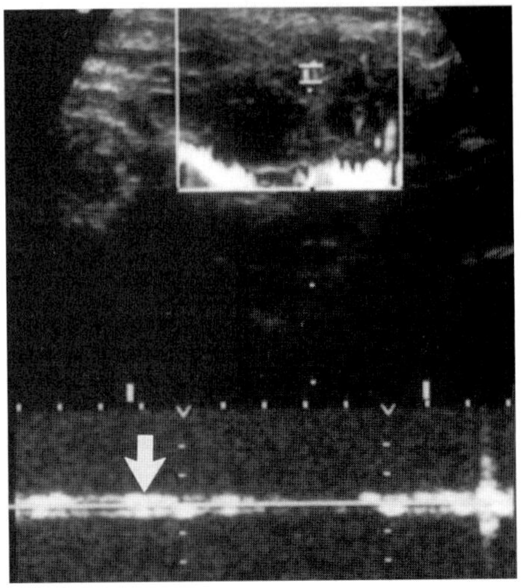

b.

Figure 2. Transverse US images of an anterior VM in the neck in an 8-year-old girl. **(a)** Gray-scale US image displays characteristic hypoechoic, heterogeneous architecture (arrow). The margins of the lesion are delineated by the electronic calipers. **(b)** Pulsed Doppler US image reveals monophasic (arrow) venous flow diagnostic of VM.

RESULTS

At gray-scale US, VMs appeared as hypoechoic, heterogeneous lesions in all (Fig 2) but nine patients (42 of 51 [82%]). The nine atypical VMs appeared isoechoic (n = 4 [8%]) or hyperechoic (n = 5 [10%]) with respect to the surrounding subcutaneous tissue but displayed a heterogeneous echo texture in all but one patient (98%). When possible (n = 28), lesions were measured; factors that precluded measurement include the presence of very irregular, infiltrative borders and the presence of very large lesions that could not be imaged entirely at once on the screen (eg, a 25 × 9-cm trunk

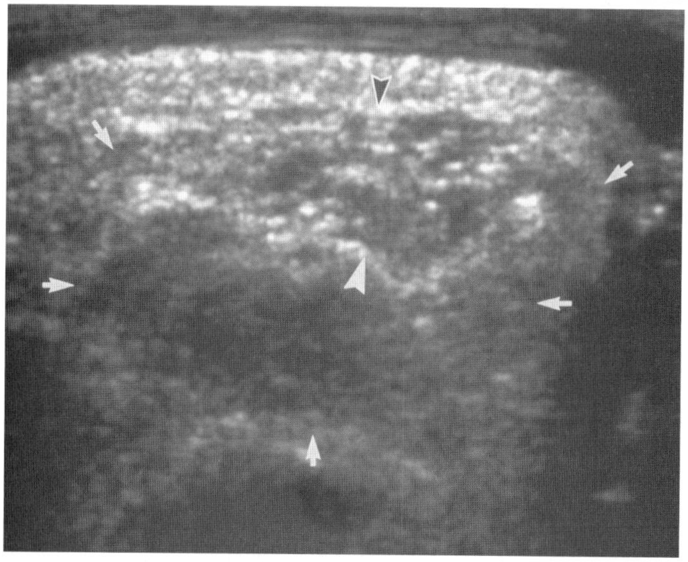

a.

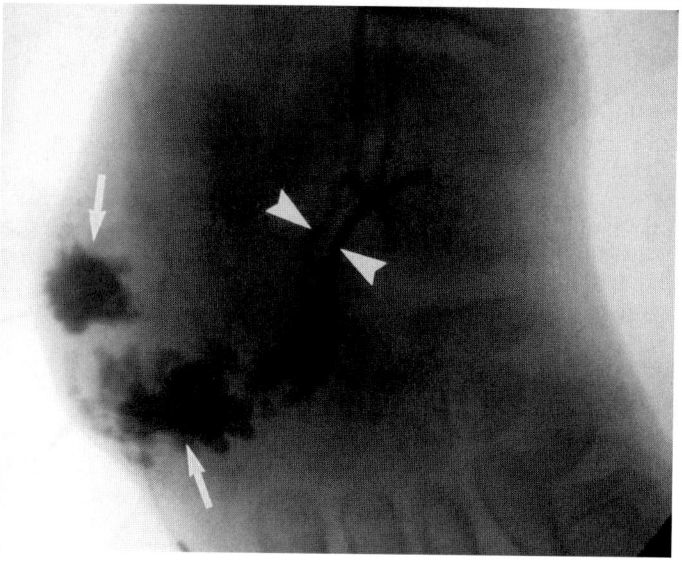

c.

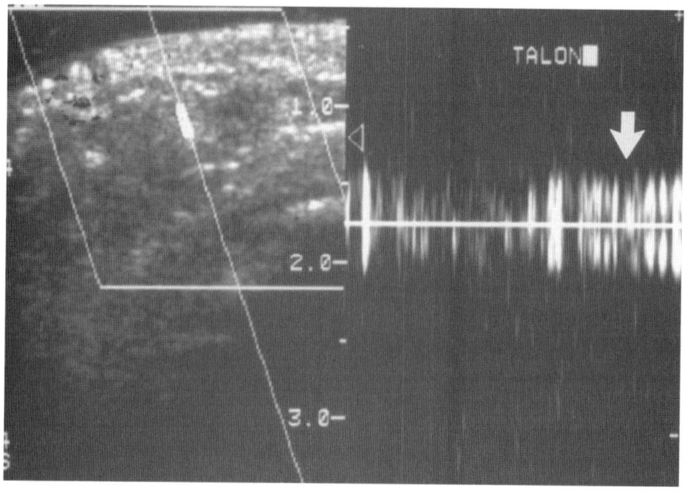

b.

Figure 3. Images of a VM in the heel in a 4-year-old girl. **(a)** Transverse gray-scale US image displays atypical architecture with zones of hyperechogenicity (arrowheads) relative to the surrounding subcutaneous tissue. The margins of the VM are delineated by arrows. **(b)** Transverse pulsed Doppler US image reveals monophasic (arrow) venous flow of 0.1 kHz, which is diagnostic of VM. **(c)** Oblique direct intralesional venogram outlines numerous venous lakes (arrows), with well-demonstrated draining veins (arrowheads). No arterial structures are visible.

lesion in a 9-year-old girl). At US, the average volume of measured lesions was 7.4 cm^3 (volume range, 0.06–71.3 cm^3). Hyperechoic foci with posterior acoustic shadowing, which represented calcifications as confirmed by means of a conventional radiograph or computed tomographic (CT) scan, could be detected in eight lesions (16%). Tubular, anechoic structures, suggestive of vascular channels, were identified within two lesions (4%). All lesions were compressible at testing. The echogenicity was independent of the presence or absence of flow.

At Doppler analysis, the deepest recording was obtained at 27 mm from the skin surface. Pulsed Doppler studies revealed monophasic low-velocity flow in 40 VMs (78%) (Fig 3) and biphasic low-velocity flow in three lesions (6%) (Fig 4), and no flow was detectable in the remaining eight lesions (16%) (Fig 5). This can represent either true absence of flow, due to spontaneous thrombosis of all or part of the VM (often associated with pain), or very slow venous flow, not detectable despite the most sensitive parameters available on our machines. The average flow velocity measured in the 43 VMs was 0.22 kHz (range, 0.01–0.6 kHz). Biphasic signal representing arterial flow was recorded from the periphery of three lesions, which characterized a mixed vascular malformation with a capillary component—namely, a capillary-venous malformation. There was no difference in the appearance of VMs in relation to their location.

DISCUSSION

The diagnosis of VM often can be strongly suspected on the basis of clinical characteristics: They are bluish, cold, easily compressible, and increase in size with maneuvers to increase venous pressure (2,4). When there is no frank bluish hue and the overlying skin appears normal, a VM first must be differentiated from the high-flow vascular malformations and hemangiomas; other possible differential diagnoses include lymphangiomas, resolving hematomas, or neoplastic conditions. Some of these malignant lesions could be compressible, such as liposarcomas, alveolar soft-tissue sarcomas, or angiosarcomas, but these are rare tumors in children and can be differentiated from VMs because most of them manifest an arterial component at Doppler US.

Because deep vascular lesions produce no repercussion on the overlying skin, it often is impossible to assess adequately, on the basis of clinical grounds alone, the presence or the absence of pulsatile flow. The identification of pulsatile flow indicates the presence of a strong arterial component and thereby supports diagnoses such as hemangioma or arteriovenous malformation and rules out the diagnosis of VM. Neoplastic lesions, especially rhabdomyosarcoma and neuroblastoma metastases in this young population, also display an arterial component in most instances.

When not clearly diagnosed at physical

examination alone, vascular malformations can be investigated with various imaging modalities. Conventional radiographs, though generally of little use, are invaluable if they demonstrate the presence of phleboliths, as these are pathognomonic of VM (3). CT and magnetic resonance (MR) imaging provide good anatomic detail, with precise delineation of the extent of lesions and the relation to surrounding structures (5). CT is more sensitive than conventional radiography in the depiction of calcifications. MR imaging is helpful in that it can further characterize the type of flow present when flow void is identified (5,6). Despite their great sensitivity, however, neither of these modalities provide information specific enough to allow a precise diagnosis.

Angiography can be invaluable in delineating the feeding and draining vessels and in defining the hemodynamics of vascular lesions. However, angiography is noncontributory in the diagnosis of VM, as findings are generally normal (3). The characteristic features of VM are noted after direct intralesional puncture and lesion opacification, with the demonstration of tortuous, dilated venous channels, without arteriovenous communication (3). Thus, angiography can help rule out high-flow vascular malformations, with their arterial components.

Gray-scale US can help in the diagnosis of VMs and other soft-tissue masses in various ways (7,8). As mentioned previously, the detection of phleboliths will provide a precise diagnosis of VM. However, few VMs display intralesional calcifications (eight lesions [16%] in this study), which diminishes the usefulness of this criterion.

Echo texture also can help in narrowing the differential diagnosis. The majority of venous lesions (82%) that we studied were hypoechoic relative to the surrounding subcutaneous tissue and manifested heterogeneous architecture. Echogenicity alone will not be helpful in eliminating vascular malformations or hemangiomas, as these lesions also are hypoechoic and heterogeneous relative to surrounding tissue (7,8). Such a pattern, however, is different from that of lymphangiomas and allows differentiation.

Lymphangiomas come in two forms: macrocystic and microcystic. Macrocystic lymphangiomas appear as large, anechoic cavities separated by septa at US (8). None of the VMs that we reviewed demonstrated such cystic cavities; only two of the 51 lesions showed evidence of elongated, anechoic structures that easily could be demonstrated to represent vascular structures.

Conversely, microcystic lymphangiomas consist of a myriad of microscopic cavities, which give rise to a hyperechoic texture in relation to the surrounding subcutaneous tissue, owing to the large number of interfaces encountered by the ultrasound beam (8). Only five (10%) of the lesions that we reviewed manifested a hyperechoic texture when compared with surrounding tissue. All of the nine atypical VMs displayed monophasic flow at Doppler US; lymphangiomas, on the other hand, are globally avascular, apart from the septa, from which a mixed type of vascular flow, both venous and arterial, occasionally can be recorded (8).

Doppler US offers great promise in the differentiation of soft-tissue vascular lesions (9–11). We recently have reported the Doppler features characteristic of hemangiomas (12): high vessel density (defined as more than five structures per square centimeter) and a peak arterial Doppler shift of 2 kHz or more. The application of these criteria resulted in a sensitivity of 84% (59 of 70 hemangiomas) and a specificity of 98% (45 of 46 hemangiomas) in the Doppler diagnosis of hemangiomas. Hübsch et al (10) described the appearance of arteriovenous malformations at pulsed and color-coded

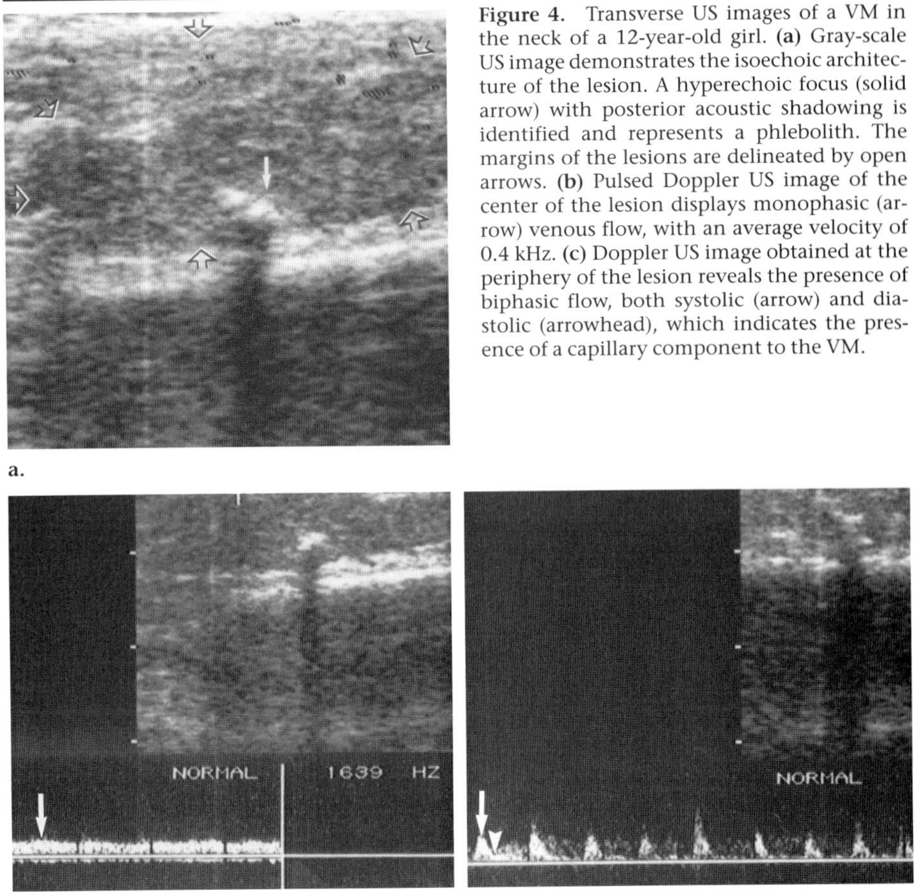

a. b. c.

Figure 4. Transverse US images of a VM in the neck of a 12-year-old girl. **(a)** Gray-scale US image demonstrates the isoechoic architecture of the lesion. A hyperechoic focus (solid arrow) with posterior acoustic shadowing is identified and represents a phlebolith. The margins of the lesions are delineated by open arrows. **(b)** Pulsed Doppler US image of the center of the lesion displays monophasic (arrow) venous flow, with an average velocity of 0.4 kHz. **(c)** Doppler US image obtained at the periphery of the lesion reveals the presence of biphasic flow, both systolic (arrow) and diastolic (arrowhead), which indicates the presence of a capillary component to the VM.

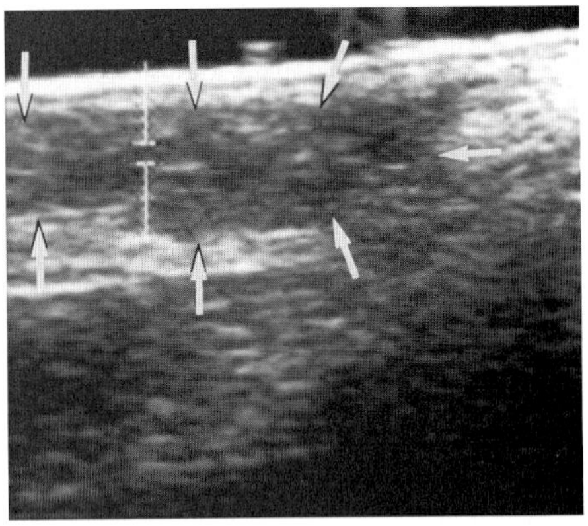

Figure 5. Transverse gray-scale US image of a VM of the lip in a 10-year-old boy demonstrates typical hypoechoic, heterogeneous architecture. No Doppler flow was recorded from the lesion. Arrows demonstrate the margins of the lesion.

Doppler US and demonstrated that US can be of great help in the diagnosis of soft-tissue vascular lesions.

Three (6%) of the 51 lesions in our series showed a biphasic component to their vascular flow. In lesions with biphasic vascular flow, a mixed vascular malformation is likely, such as capillary-venous or lymphatic-capillary-venous malformations (1). Pure monophasic flow often can be recorded from other sites within the lesion. The arterial signal remains of low velocity, and there is no confusion possible with the high-flow vascular malformations.

In 16% (eight of 51) of the VMs reviewed, no detectable flow was recorded. The absence of flow may reflect thrombosis of the malformation at the time of thrombophlebitis, usually accompanied clinically by pain. The absence of recordable flow also could be an indication of the limitations of the equipment.

Other entities that can mimic VMs clinically include hematomas. A history of trauma and the absence of venous flow will help separate the two entities in the majority of cases. It also is easy to exclude the diagnoses of rhabdomyosarcoma and neuroblastoma metastases, because soft-tissue neoplastic lesions are not compressible (7). Furthermore, Doppler analysis often can demonstrate the presence of arterial and venous flow, with arteriovenous fistulas, in these malignancies.

In conclusion, US can help in the diagnosis of clinically atypical VMs. We suggest the following criteria for the US diagnosis of VM. At gray-scale US, VMs are hypoechoic, heterogeneous lesions in which phleboliths may be detected (pathognomonic if present), and they display compressibility. At Doppler analysis, monophasic, low-velocity venous signal is encountered. The presence of slow arterial flow can suggest a mixed form of vascular malformation. In the future, it will be interesting to perform a prospective study to determine the sensitivity and specificity of the various imaging modalities in the diagnosis of hemangiomas and vascular malformations.

References

1. Mulliken JB, Glowacki J. Hemangiomas and vascular malformations in infants and children: a classification based on endothelial characteristics. Plast Reconstr Surg 1982; 69:412–420.
2. Fishman SJ, Mulliken JB. Hemangiomas and vascular malformations of infancy and childhood. Pediatr Clin North Am 1993; 40:1177-1200.
3. Burrows PE, Mulliken JB, Fellows KE, Strand RD. Childhood hemangiomas and vascular malformations: angiographic differentiation. AJR 1983; 141:483–488.
4. Letson GD, Greenfield GB, Heinrich SD. Evaluation of the child with a bone or soft-tissue neoplasm. Orthop Clin North Am 1996; 27:431–451.
5. Totty WG, Murphy WA, Lee JKT. Soft-tissue tumors: MR imaging. Radiology 1986; 160:135–141.
6. Meyer JS, Hoffer FA, Barnes PD, Mulliken JB. Biological classification of soft-tissue vascular anomalies: MR correlation. AJR 1991; 157:559–564.
7. AbiEzzi SS, Miller LS. The use of ultrasound for the diagnosis of soft-tissue masses in children. J Pediatr Orthop 1995; 15:566–573.
8. Sintzoff SA Jr, Gillard I, Van Gansbeke D, Gevenois PA, Salmon I, Struyven J. Ultrasound evaluation of soft-tissue tumors. J Belge Radiol 1992; 75:276–280.
9. Foley WD, Erickson SJ. Color Doppler flow imaging. AJR 1991; 156:3–13.
10. Hübsch P, Trattnig S, Kainberger FM, Barton P, Karnel F. Imaging of peripheral arteriovenous malformations using color-coded Doppler sonography. Ultraschall Med 1991; 12:87–90. [German]
11. Bruns J, Lussenhop S, Behrens P. Ultrasound imaging of soft tissue tumors of the extremities and para-articular soft tissue changes. Ultraschall Med 1994; 15:74–80. [German]
12. Dubois J, Patriquin HB, Garel L, et al. Soft-tissue hemangiomas in infants and children: diagnosis with Doppler sonography. AJR 1998; 171:247–252.

Gastrointestinal Tract Bug

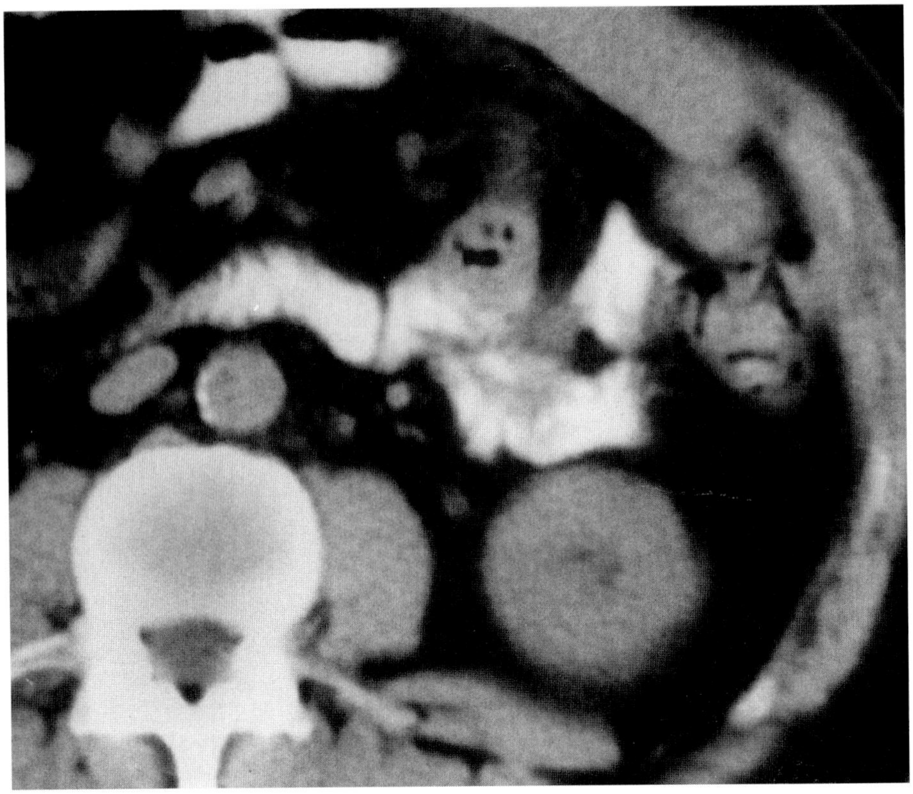

Courtesy of Samuel Hamilton, MD, Dublin, Ireland

Rosanna Pallotta, MD
Tamara Ehresmann, MD
Mario Roggini, MD
Paola Fusilli, MD

Index terms:
Bones, growth and development
Bones, osteochondrodysplasias, 40.151
Children, skeletal system, 40.151
Infants, skeletal system, 40.151

Radiology 1999; 212:847–852

[1] From the Department of Medicine and Aging Sciences, Regional Service for Diagnosis, Prevention and Care of Birth Defects, G. D'Annunzio University School of Medicine, Chieti, Italy (R.P., T.E., P.F.), and the Department of Radiology, University La Sapienza, Rome, Italy (M.R.). Received January 19, 1998; revision requested February 18; final revision received November 16; accepted February 22, 1999. **Address reprint requests to** R.P., P.zza della Rinascita 75, 65122 Pescara, Italy (e-mail: *pallotta@unich.it*).

Author contributions:
Guarantor of integrity of entire study, R.P.; study concepts and design, R.P.; definition of intellectual content, R.P.; literature research, T.E.; clinical studies, all authors; data acquisition, M.R.; data analysis, all authors; manuscript preparation, R.P., T.E., P.F.; manuscript editing, T.E., P.F.; manuscript review, R.P.

Kyphomelic Dysplasia: Clinical and Radiologic Long-term Follow-up of One Case and Review of the Literature[1]

The authors describe the 17-year follow-up of the (to their knowledge) only adult and only female patient affected with kyphomelic dysplasia so far described in the literature, with assessment of the phenotypic, orthopedic, and radiologic progression of this syndrome.

The term "kyphomelic dysplasia" was used in 1983 (1) to describe a generalized prenatal skeletal disease that causes a peculiar dwarfism that is clinically and radiologically characterized by the following: a disproportionately short stature, rhizomesomelic shortening with lateral bowing of the long bones, flared irregular metaphyses, a short narrow chest, mild dysmorphic facial features, improvement of bone changes with advancing age, and normal psychomotor development.

Inheritance of this syndrome is autosomal recessive. To our knowledge, 13 cases of kyphomelic dysplasia have been reported up to now (1–9); three pairs of these patients were siblings (3,4,8). Striking anamnestic, clinical, and radiologic analogies between the patient reported on by Temple et al (5) and the patient reported on by Maffulli et al (6) led us to suspect that this patient was the same child. For this reason, the actual number of cases reported in the literature (to our knowledge) is 12. Four of these patients died within the first 13 months of life (3,4,7), and only four of the remaining patients were followed up, for a maximum of 7 years and 5 months (5,8–10).

For 17 years, we observed who we believe to be the only female patient affected with kyphomelic dysplasia. This patient was previously reported on by Rezza et al (3), and at present, she is, to our knowledge, the only adult affected with this skeletal disease referred to in the literature.

Case Report

The patient (Fig 1) and her eldest brother, who died at age 7 months, were originally described by Rezza et al (3) as two cases of kyphomelic dysplasia. The condition of both of them was erroneously diagnosed as achondroplasia. The patient was referred to us for observation when she was aged 3 years, and we are continuing her follow-up. To show better evidence of the sequential changes that occur in kyphomelic dysplasia over time, from childhood to adulthood, we completed the radiologic investigation of this patient's condition that was previously reported (3), starting from the patient's first months of life.

The results of radiologic examination of the patient at age 9 months 15 days revealed slight frontal bossing and a low nasal bridge, moderate occipital flattening, a reduced posterior fossa, a normal Turkish saddle, a slightly hypoplastic superior maxilla, a narrow thoracic cage, cervical accessory ribs, short cupped ribs (Fig 2a), short femora bowed at the proximal third with anterior bowing, short tibiae with slight anterior bowing, short fibulae, coxa vara and genu varum, and metaphyseal flaring (Fig 2b).

At age 2.1 years, the patient's humeri were short and stubby, the radii and ulnae were short and bowed at the medial third, and the ulnae were shorter than the radii, with metaphyseal flaring (Fig 3a). In the lower extremities, the most striking findings were small iliac wings, coxa vara and genu varum, metaphyseal flaring, and cortical thickening (Fig 3b).

At age 3.1 years, the radiographs obtained in the patient showed short, anterior cupped ribs, normal interpediculate and intervertebral distances, and a horizontally shaped sacrum. Furthermore, the radial bowing was slightly reduced, but the ulnae were still shorter than the radii. The iliac wings remained small, but the acetabula were flattened; coxa vara and genu varum still existed. The femoral bowing was dramatically improved (Fig 4). The tibiae were shorter than the fibulae and showed bilateral medial cortical thickening with increased metaphyseal flaring.

At clinical examination at age 6.10 years (Fig 1a), the patient had a normal head with a slight pterygium colli, a long philtrum, a narrow chest, short upper and lower limbs with proximal bowing and limited extension of the elbow and knee joints, slightly prominent knees, a straight spine with a prominent sacral region, and a waddling gait. Her hands and feet were normal in shape and length. She had a short stature although her parents' heights were in the 50th percentile range for heights in the south Italian population. Her auxometric parameters were as follows: total height, 100 cm (<3rd percentile); upper proximal segment of the arm (acromion to distal medial border of olecranon), 12 cm (<<3rd percentile); forearm length (olecranon to distal lateral process of the radius), 13 cm (<<3rd percentile); upper leg length (greater trochanter to proximal lateral tibial condyle), 23.5 cm (<<3rd percentile); lower leg length (proximal lateral condyle of the tibia to sole of the foot), 19 cm (<<3rd percentile); chest circumference, 51 cm (3rd to 25th percentile); biacromial distance, 27.5 cm (75th percentile); and biiliac distance, 21 cm (75th percentile).

Radiographs obtained in the patient at age 6.10 years showed a normal skull; an unchanged thorax, dorsolumbar straightness with slight scoliosis and a pronounced backward angulation of the sacrum; normal width of the spinal canal; a normal pelvis; coxa vara stressed by lateral bowing of the femoral diaphysis; short, sharply angled broad femora with wide, slightly irregular metaphyses (Fig 5a); and unchanged tibiae and fibulae (Fig 5b). The remaining long bones were short and slightly bowed.

At age 10.6 years (Fig 1b) the patient's clinical features were unchanged. The radiologic findings in the patient at age 11 years indicated radii and particularly ulnae that were shortened and slightly bent at the medial third (Fig 6a), unchanged iliac wings, and moderately bowed femora at the proximal third. The coxa vara, metaphyseal flaring, and femoral bowing had improved (Fig 6b). The results of rheumatologic and metabolic analyses performed in the patient were negative. She was lost to further follow-up for nearly 7 years.

The radiologic findings of the thorax, pelvis, and limbs in the patient at age 18 years were nearly unchanged. At age 19 years, the patient's femoral bowing had almost completely regressed (Fig 7), and she decided to undergo lengthening of the femora, tibiae, and fibulae.

Since the radiologic examination at age 19 years, the patient's medical history has been uneventful, except for sporadic lumbosacral pains. According to medical history data, her sexual development has been normal. At age 20 years, the patient reached a final adult height of 134 cm, which was further increased by 13 cm as a result of Ilizarov lengthening. The rhizomesomelic shortening is mostly evident in the upper limbs, which appear quite straight. The limited extension at the knee, which worsened because of a chondropathy, as confirmed by using magnetic resonance imaging, and the dorsolumbar straightness (Fig 8) are still present. The vertebral bodies appear to be slightly increased in height; the pedicles and interpediculate distances are normal. Several sclerotic areas and osteophytes are present. The only persistent facial

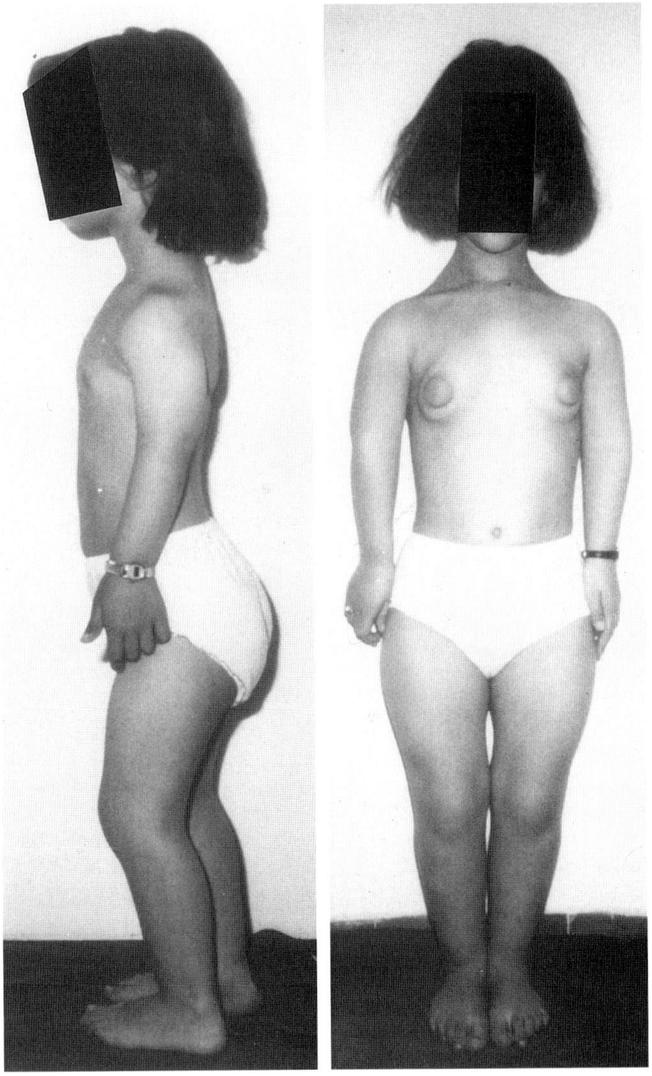

a. b.

Figure 1. **(a, b)** Photographs of the proband at **(a)** age 6.10 years and **(b)** age 10.6 years. In **a**, note the shortening of the limbs and the limited extensions of the elbow and knee.

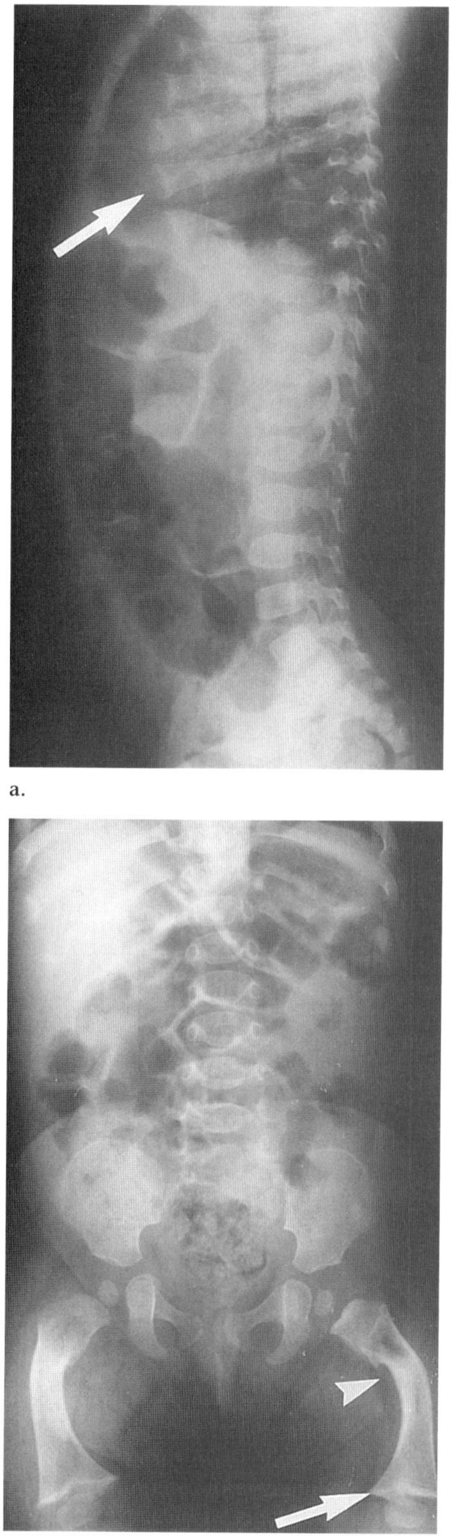

a.

b.

Figure 2. (a) Lateral and (b) frontal radiographs obtained in the study patient at age 9 months 15 days show (a) short ribs with cupped anterior ends (arrow), as well as (b) stubby femora (arrowhead) bowed at the proximal third and a flared metaphysis (arrow).

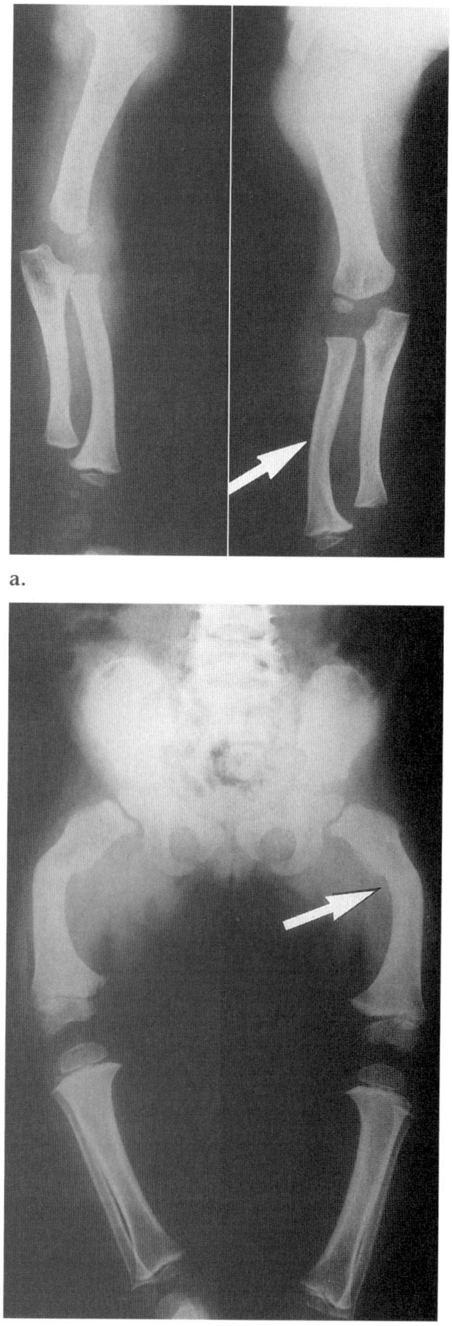

a.

b.

Figure 3. (a, b) Frontal radiographs obtained in the study patient at age 2.1 years. (a) Radiographs show shortened long bones, particularly the radii and ulnae, bowed radii (arrow), and slight metaphyseal flaring. (b) Radiograph shows femora (arrow) bowed at the proximal third, short tibiae and fibulae, and metaphyseal flaring.

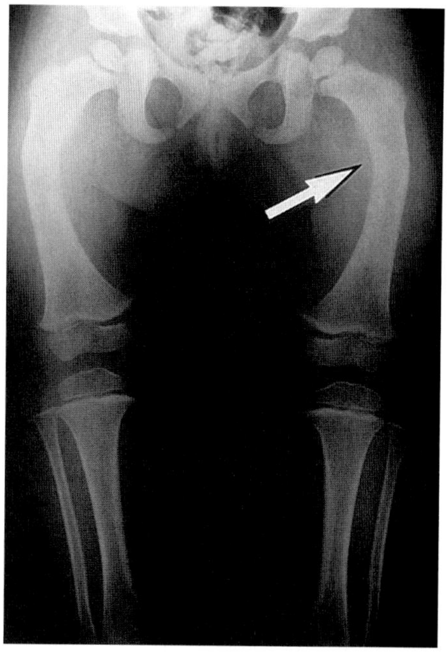

Figure 4. Frontal radiograph obtained in the study patient at age 3.1 years shows dramatic improvement of the femoral bowing (arrow).

abnormality is the elongated philtrum. The results of a metacarpophalangeal profile showed no marked abnormality. On the basis of our recent experiences with this patient, she appears to have sound intelligence. For more than 2 years, she has developed obesity localized in the buttocks and thighs.

Discussion

The follow-up of this patient for 17 years has enabled us to establish a better clinical and developmental picture of kyphomelic dysplasia to adulthood. To our knowledge, the case of kyphomelic dysplasia described herein is the only adult patient reported on up to now, because all of the 11 cases of this skeletal dysplasia described to date have been in children. Furthermore, she is, to our knowledge, the only woman with this abnormality referenced in the literature, which reflects the predominance of male versus female patients with this condition.

In 1976, Khajavi et al (2) identified, among subjects with dwarfism characterized by congenital bowing of long bones, two sporadic cases that were distinguished by a greater diaphyseal angulation of long bones, which appeared short and flared in the metaphyseal region. These patients lacked craniosynostosis, diffuse osteoporosis, and skeletal anomalies in the limb-girdle region and spine. They were classified as having "short-limbed camptomelic syndrome, normocephalic type," with a possible autosomal recessive inheritance.

Two years later, Hall and Spranger (8) reported on a "probable familial disorder

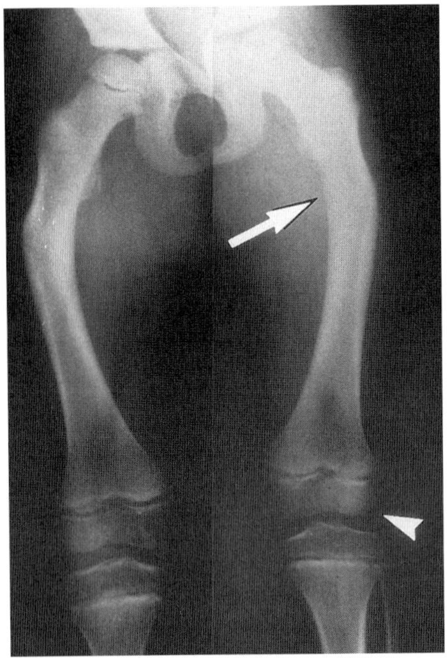

a.

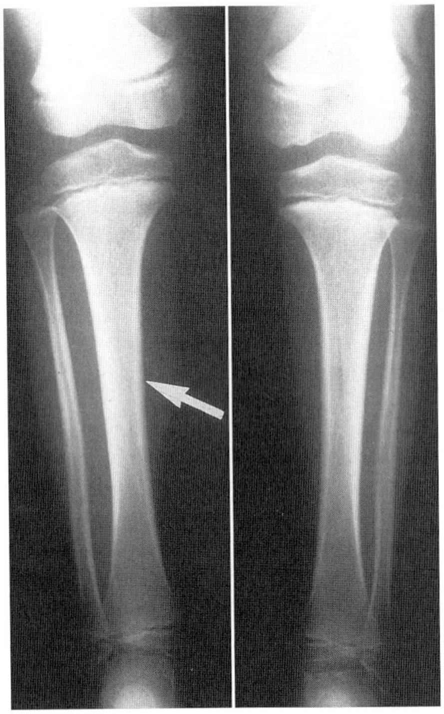

b.

Figure 5. **(a, b)** Frontal radiographs obtained in the study patient at age 6.10 years show **(a)** improvement of the femoral bowing (arrow) and slightly flattened condyles (arrowhead), as well as **(b)** straight tibiae (arrow) with cortical thickening.

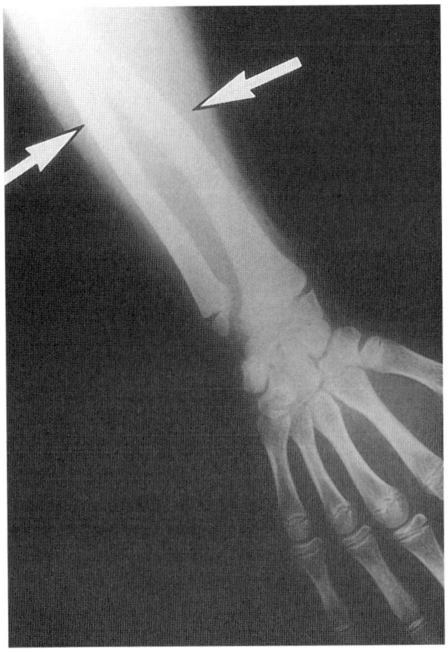

a.

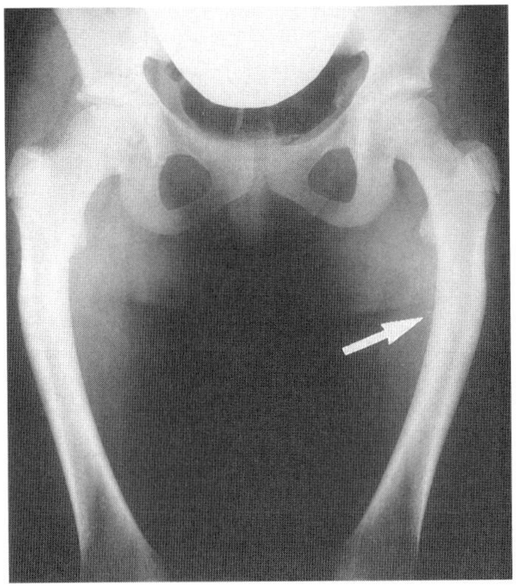

b.

Figure 6. **(a, b)** Frontal radiographs obtained in the study patient at age 11 years show **(a)** short radius and ulna bowed at the medial third (arrows), and **(b)** femora (arrow) moderately bowed at the proximal third.

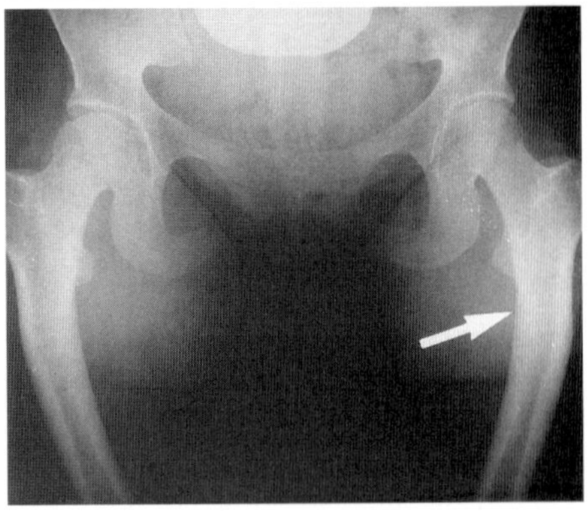

Figure 7. Frontal radiograph obtained in the study patient at age 19 years shows nearly complete regression of the femoral bowing (arrow).

characterized by severe congenital bowing and rhizomelic/mesomelic shortening with good prognosis" in two brothers. The radiologic findings, which improved dramatically during these patients' first 6 years of life, joint limitation, normal psychomotor development, and the affected siblings supported a distinct, possibly autosomal recessive pseudocamptomelic condition with an unknown natural course.

In 1983, Maclean et al (1) identified a fifth case of this entity, and because of the severity of femoral involvement, called the condition "kyphomelic dysplasia." This term was criticized as being inappropriate (3,4), and the inheritance, which was interpreted as x linked because all of the identified cases were in male patients (1), was assessed to be autosomal recessive (3).

The anamnestic and clinical characteristics of all the cases reported in the literature are shown in the Table. The radiologic anomalies appear to be the same in all the patients, and in our opinion, they enable an easy differentiation of the diagnosis, particularly from the frequently occurring rhizomesomelic dwarfism, achondroplasia. The peculiar changes that distinguish kyphomelic dysplasia from achondroplasia are largely a normocephalic skull, bowing of long bones, particularly those of the femora, an absence of the posterior concavity and of the anterior wedging of the vertebral bodies, a lack of progressive narrowing of the interpediculate distances and spinal canal diameters, and proportionate hands.

At birth, the lateral bowing and shortness of limbs (in 12 of 12 cases) are already coexistent with a skull with normal dimensions (in 10 of 10 cases) and normal facies. The pterygium, which was seen only in the female patient who we followed up, is due to cervical accessory ribs. The spine of the longer surviving patients who reach walking age (3,5,6,8,9) is straight, and patients reportedly have a waddling gait. True (2,9) or mild (1,3,5) platyspondylisis at radiologic examination also has been observed.

In the patient we observed, the vertebral bodies in adulthood are normal. There is sacralization of the fifth lumbar vertebra; the pedicles and interpediculate distances appear to be in the normal range. It has been determined that the typical improvement of the long bones

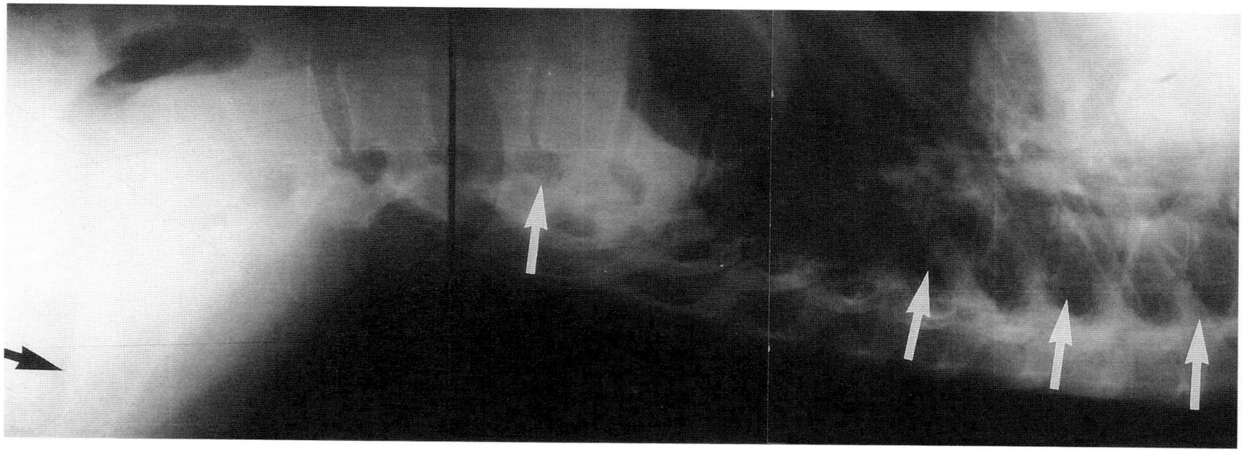

Figure 8. Lateral radiograph of the spine in the study patient at age 20 years. Note the straightness (white arrows) of the thoracic and lumbar spine (ie, loss of lumbar lordosis). The lumbar vertebral bodies are slightly increased in height. The horizontal orientation of the sacrum (black arrow) also is seen.

Anamnestic, Clinical, and Radiologic Features in 12 Patients Described in the Literature

	Reference Case										
	Khajavi et al (2)	Hall and Spranger (8)	Maclean et al (1)	Rezza et al (3)	Viljoen et al (9)	Temple et al (5)	Maffulli et al (6)	Turnpenny et al (4)	Corder et al (7)	Total No. of Cases	Current Case
No. and sex of patients	2 M	2 brothers	1 M	2 (brother and sister)	1 M	1 M	1 M*	2 brothers	1 M	11 M/1 F	. . .
Consanguinity	?	?	–	Probably	–	–	–	+	–	2/6	. . .
Age at first observation	. . .	4.0 mo/6.0 y	Birth	–/10.0 mo	Birth	3.0 mo	3.4 y	2.0 mo/Birth	2.0 mo	. . .	3.0 y
Age at last observation	. . .	7.5 y/–	6.0 mo	–/3.0 y	4.6 y	6.0 y	6.1 y	. . ./13.0 mo	. . .	. . .	20.0 y
Death	. . .	. . .	. . .	7 mo/. . .	. . .	. . .	. . .	2.0 mo/13.0 mo	2.0 mo	4/12	. . .
Normal mental development	. . .	+/+	+	+/+	+	+		. . ./+	+	9/9	+
Normal karyotype	. . .	. . .	+	. . ./+	. . .	+		. . .	. . .	3/3	. . .
Normal serum level of calcium and phosphor	. . .	+/+	+	. . ./+	+	+		. . ./+	. . .	7/7	+
Improvement with age	. . .	+/+	+	. . ./+	+	+		. . ./+	. . .	7/7	+
Bones and joints											
Rhizomesomelic dwarfism	+/+	+/+	+	+/+	+	+		+/+	+	12/12	+
Bowing of femora	+/+	+/+	+	+/+	+	+		+/+	+	12/12	+–
Humeri	+/+	+/–	. . .	+/+–	+	–		–/–	+	7/11	–
Tibiae	+/+	+/–	+	–/+–	+	–		+/+	+	9/12	–
Radii	–/+	+/–	. . .	+/+	+	–		+/+	+	8/11	+–
Large and irregular metaphysis	+/+	+/–	+	+/+	+	+		+/+	+	11/12	+
Irregular epiphyseal ossification	+/+	. . .	. . .	. . ./+	. . .	+		. . .	. . .	4/4	. . .
Limited joint movements:											
Hips	. . .	. . .	+	. . .	+	+		+/+	+	6/6	+
Elbows	. . .	+/+	. . .	. . ./+	. . .	. . .		+/+	+	6/6	+
Knees	. . .	+/+	+	. . ./+	. . .	+		+/+	+	8/8	+
Normocephaly	+/+	+/+	+	+/+	+	+		. . ./+	. . .	10/10	+
Narrow shoulders	. . .	+/+	. . .	. . .	. . .	–		+/+	–	4/6	+
Narrow chest	. . .	+/+	+	+/+	. . .	+		+/+	+	9/9	+
Short ribs with cupped anterior ends	. . .	+/. . .	+	+/+	. . .	+		+/+	+	8/8	+–
Platyspondylisis	+/+	. . .	+	+/+–	+	+		–/–	–	7/10	–
Lumbodorsal kyphosis	. . .	+/+	?	?/+	–	+		?/?	. . .	4/5	+
Increased acetabular angles	+/+	. . .	+	. . ./–	+	+		–/–	. . .	5/8	–
Other											
Skin dimpling over bony prominences	. . .	. . .	+	. . .	+	+		. . ./+	+	5/5	–

Note.—+ = present, – = absent, +– = mild, ? = uncertain.
* This is the same patient described by Temple et al in reference 5.

and ribs after birth is probably due to a faulty metabolic interaction between the mother and fetus (8); however, no abnormalities of the calcium-to-phosphorus ratio metabolism were detected (1,3,4,5,8) in our experience. The multiple joint limitation at the hip (1,3,5,6), elbows (3,8), and knees (1,3,5,6,8) is still unexplained. Excluding the younger patients (1,4,7), the one patient (5,6) in whom contracture bands of the posterior part of the knee made evaluation difficult, and the case of Viljoen et al (9), both the patients referred by Hall and Spranger (8) and the patient we observed had a prominent knee. The patient we observed still has limited flexor extension at both knees and has developed articular anomalies as she has grown older.

On the basis of the clinical data, there may be an underlying immunodeficiency, which, combined with the presence of a narrow thoracic cage, may cause precocious death. Two patients died of pneumonia in their first months of life (3,4), and repeated respiratory infections with distress were reported during the first years of life in other patients (1,4,5). The immune status of these patients had not been evaluated. One patient has a severe combined immunodeficiency and red cell aplasia (7).

Because of the three pairs of affected siblings (3,4,8) described in the literature, one pair of whom had consanguineous parents (4), the inheritance of kyphomelic dysplasia is assumed to be autosomal recessive. Without gene locus identification, prenatal diagnosis of this syndrome is based on ultrasonographic findings. With long-term follow-up, we assessed the phenotypic, orthopedic, and radiologic progression of this syndrome.

Acknowledgments: We thank orthopedists Silvio Boero, MD, G. Gaslini Institute, Genova, who performed the limb lengthening, and Sergio Margiotta, MD, Hospital of Popoli, Pescara, Italy, for careful collaboration in the treatment of our patient.

References

1. Maclean RN, Prater WK, Lozzio CB. Brief clinical report: skeletal dysplasia with short angulated femora (kyphomelic dysplasia). Am J Med Genet 1983; 14:373–380.
2. Khajavi A, Lachmann R, Rimoin D, et al. Heterogeneity in the camptomelic syndromes: long and short bone varieties. Pediatr Radiol 1976; 120:641–647.
3. Rezza E, Iannaccone G, Lendvai D. Familial congenital bowing with short thick bones and metaphyseal changes, a distinct entity: report of the clinical and radiological findings in two siblings. Pediatr Radiol 1984; 14:323–327.
4. Turnpenny PD, Dakwar RA, Boulos FN. Kyphomelic dysplasia: the first 10 cases. J Med Genet 1990; 27:269–272.
5. Temple IK, Thompson EM, Hall CM, Bridgeman G, Pembrey ME. Kyphomelic dysplasia. J Med Genet 1989; 26:457–468.
6. Maffulli N, Blakeway C, Fixsen JA. Long-term follow-up of a case of kyphomelic dysplasia. Orthopedics 1993; 16:86–89.
7. Corder WT, Hummel M, Miller C, Wilson NW. Association of kyphomelic dysplasia with severe combined immunodeficiency. Am J Med Genet 1995; 57:626–629.
8. Hall BD, Spranger JW. Familial congenital bowing with short bones. Radiology 1979; 132:611–614.
9. Viljoen D, Beighton P. Kyphomelic dysplasia: further delineation of the phenotype. Dysmorphol Clin Genet 1988; 1:136–141.
10. O'Reilly MAR, Hall CM. Kyphomelic dysplasia (letter). J Med Genet 1994; 31:423.

David M. Warshauer, MD
Joseph K. T. Lee, MD

Index terms:
Celiac disease, 74.7611
Enteritis, 74.291
Fibrosis, cystic, 74.1496
Intestines, CT, 70.12112, 70.12115
Intestines, diseases, 70.31, 70.32, 70.33, 70.73, 70.7611
Intestines, MR, 70.12143
Intussusception, 70.73
Lymphatic system, hyperplasia, 99.329
Surgery, complications, 74.458

Radiology 1999; 212:853–860

[1] From the Department of Radiology, University of North Carolina School of Medicine, Campus Box 7510, Rm 2016 Old Clinic Bldg, Manning Dr, Chapel Hill, NC 27599-7510. Received September 9, 1998; revision requested November 3; revision received December 9; accepted February 2, 1999. **Address reprint requests to** D.M.W. (e-mail: *dmw@pop.unc.edu*).

Author contributions:
Guarantor of integrity of entire study, D.M.W.; study concepts and design, D.M.W.; definition of intellectual content, D.M.W.; literature research, D.M.W.; clinical studies, D.M.W.; data acquisition and analysis, D.M.W., J.K.T.L.; statistical analysis, D.M.W.; manuscript preparation, editing, and review, D.M.W., J.K.T.L.

Adult Intussusception Detected at CT or MR Imaging: Clinical-Imaging Correlation[1]

PURPOSE: To determine the clinical presentation in cases of adult intussusception demonstrated at computed tomography (CT) or magnetic resonance (MR) imaging and to correlate the imaging appearance with clinical diagnosis.

MATERIALS AND METHODS: Retrospective review of CT and MR images and clinical records of all patients with an intussusception demonstrated on CT or MR images from January 1, 1991, through April 30, 1998.

RESULTS: Thirty-three patients had one or more intussusceptions demonstrated on CT (n = 30) or MR (n = 3) images. Twenty-nine patients had enteroenteric intussusceptions, and four had intussusceptions involving the colon. Ten patients (30%) had a neoplastic lead point, including all four of the intussusceptions involving the colon (benign mass, n = 3; malignant mass, n = 7). In 23 cases (70%), no neoplastic lead point was identified. A variety of causes were implicated in these cases, with 16 cases (48%) classified as idiopathic. Enteric intussusceptions in the nonneoplastic group were shorter in length (median, 4 vs 10.8 cm; P = .002), smaller in diameter (median, 3 vs 4 cm; P = .002), and less likely to be associated with obstruction (4.3% vs 50%; P = .02).

CONCLUSION: Less than one-third of adult intussusceptions demonstrated at CT or MR imaging were caused by a neoplastic lead point. Almost half of adult cases in this series were idiopathic.

Intussusception in the adult is rare. It is estimated to compose 5% of all intussusceptions and cause 1% of all bowel obstructions and 0.003%–0.02% of all hospital admissions (1). Results of prior studies (1–8) based on discharge diagnosis or surgical result have found that 80%–90% of adult cases have an underlying cause. Neoplasm was the most common cause in these series and was found in approximately 65% of adult cases (Table 1).

Intussusception is well diagnosed by means of computed tomography (CT) or magnetic resonance (MR) imaging (9–12). The appearance of a bowel-within-bowel configuration with or without contained fat and mesenteric vessels is pathognomonic. Our recent experience with cross-sectional imaging methods suggests that intussusceptions discovered on CT or MR images are more likely to have a nonneoplastic cause than previously thought. We undertook this study to determine the cause in cases of intussusception diagnosed at CT or MR imaging. We also examined potential imaging and clinical differences between intussusceptions with and those without a neoplastic lead point.

MATERIALS AND METHODS

Patients

A free-text search for the letter string "intuss" was performed on all CT and body MR imaging reports from January 1, 1991, through April 30, 1998. Fifty-three patients were identified and their studies reviewed (D.M.W., J.K.T.L.). The presence of an intussusception was determined if a bowel-within-bowel appearance was noted on at least two axial or longitudinal sections. Thirty-five patients were identified as having one or more intussusceptions meeting these criteria.

To identify additional patients who may have undergone CT or MR imaging that showed intussusception but in whom the intussusception was missed, a search of patient records with a discharge diagnosis of intussusception was also performed. This revealed one patient in whom an intussusception was visible on MR images but had not been noted in the initial report. This patient met the previously listed criteria and was then added to our sample.

One additional patient who met the same criteria was included in our study group after a review of teaching files for the dates noted. In this case, a transient intussusception was noted at CT but inadvertently had not been mentioned in the initial report.

The 37 patients thus identified composed 0.2% (37 of 16,399) of all patients undergoing abdominal CT or abdominal MR imaging during the time interval studied. Four of the 37 identified patients were in the pediatric or adolescent age group (ages 1, 4, 10, and 14 years) and were not considered further in this analysis. The remaining 33 patients (24 male patients, nine female patients; age range, 18–84 years; median age, 41 years) constituted our study population.

Clinical Data and Pathogenesis

Demographic data and clinical information were obtained by reviewing the patients' charts (D.M.W.). The presence of abdominal symptoms was recorded along with findings at physical examination. The presence of guaiac-positive stools and the patient's preimaging hematocrit values were also recorded if obtained within 2 weeks of imaging. The pathogenesis of the intussusception was established by means of clinical follow-up, chart review, and review of surgical and histologic findings. If no local or systemic explanation for the intussusception was noted, the diagnosis was classified as idiopathic.

CT and MR Imaging

CT studies were performed with use of a Somatom Plus 24, Somatom Plus S, or Somatom Plus 4 CT Scanner (Siemens Medical Systems, Iselin, NJ). In 22 patients, the scan was obtained by using helical mode. Twenty-nine of the 30 CT examinations were performed with 100–150 mL of intravenously injected iohexol or diatrizoate meglumine (Omnipaque 300 or Hypaque; Nycomed Amersham, Princeton, NJ). Orally administered contrast material (280–1,080 mL) was used for all of the CT examinations and was either dilute barium (Cheetah Barium Sulfate Suspension, Lafayette Pharmaceuticals, Lafayette, Ind or E-Z-Cat, E-Z-Em, Westbury, NY) or dilute Gastrografin (Bracco Diagnostics, Princeton, NJ).

MR imaging studies were performed with use of a 1.5-T Magnetom SP or 1.5-T Vision system (Siemens Medical Systems). In all three of the MR imaging studies, contrast material (Magnevist; Berlex Laboratories, Wayne, NJ) was injected intravenously. No contrast material was administered orally for any of the MR imaging studies.

CT and MR images were evaluated by consensus reading of two experienced abdominal radiologists (D.M.W., J.K.T.L.). The appearance and number of intussusceptions and the type of bowel involved (enteroenteric, enterocolic, colocolic) were recorded as were the length and diameter of the intussuscipiens. Small-bowel obstruction was deemed present if multiple bowel loops proximal to the intussusception were dilated to a diameter of 3 cm or greater and bowel loops distal to the intussusception were decompressed to 1.5 cm or less in diameter.

Data Analysis

Basic descriptive statistics—median, range, and 25th and 75th percentiles—were calculated for patient demographic and clinical data, as well as for radiologic findings. Comparison of continuous data—age, hematocrit value, and length and diameter of the intussusception—between groups with a neoplastic lead point and those without a neoplastic lead point was performed by using the Mann-Whitney *U* test. This nonparametric statistic was chosen rather than a standard *t* test owing to the non-Gaussian distribution of the data discovered during analysis. Comparison of categorical data (sex, race, presence of small-bowel obstruction, presence of adenopathy, etc) between groups was performed by using the χ^2 test. The Fisher exact test was applied in 2 × 2 analysis tables when any expected values in a cell were less than 5. A *P* value less than .05 was required for rejection of the null hypothesis. STATVIEW 5 software (SAS Institute, Cary, NC) was used for the statistical analysis.

RESULTS

Patient Data

Thirty-three adult patients were identified as having one (n = 27), two (n = 4), or three (n = 2) visible intussusceptions meeting the inclusion criteria. In 30 patients, the intussusceptions were identified at CT; in three patients, the intussusceptions were noted at MR imaging. Three patients were identified in 1993, four in 1994, five in 1995, four in 1996, nine in 1997, and eight in 1998.

TABLE 1
Type and Cause of Adult Intussusception

Parameter	Totals from Eight Clinical Series*	Total from This Study
No. of years surveyed	149	7.3
No. of cases	236	33
Type		
Enteric	125 (53)	29 (88)
Colic†	111 (47)	4 (12)
Neoplastic		
Malignant	93 (39)	7 (21)
Benign	63 (27)	3 (9)
Nonneoplastic		
Idiopathic	29 (12)	16 (48)‡
Meckel diverticulum	14 (6)	0
Celiac disease	0	1 (3)
Postoperative complications or adhesions	27 (11)	1 (3)
Local inflammation	2 (1)	3 (9)
Lymphoid hyperplasia	2 (1)	1 (3)
Cystic fibrosis	0	1 (3)
Scleroderma	1 (<1)	0
Miscellaneous	5 (2)	0

Note.—Data are the number of cases, except for the number of years surveyed. Data in parentheses are the percentage of the total number of cases in the column.

* The clinical series were published in 1981–1997 (1–8). Two studies (2,6) excluded patients with postoperative intussusceptions and included only patients with intussusception documented at laparotomy or autopsy. One study (1) included only patients with surgically proved intussusception. Two studies (2, 6) included patients 15 years or older. One study (3) included patients 16 years or older. One study (8) included patients more than 16 years old.

† Category includes both enterocolic and colocolic intussusception.

‡ Data include patients with associated distant inflammation (n = 5) and a patient with recent abdominal trauma.

Clinical Data

Twenty-nine of the patients had abdominal symptoms at the time of imaging. Abdominal pain was the most common complaint and was noted in 24 (73%) patients. Abdominal physical examination results were unremarkable in 11 patients. Tenderness or guarding were noted in the right or left upper quadrant (n = 4), in the right or left lower quadrant

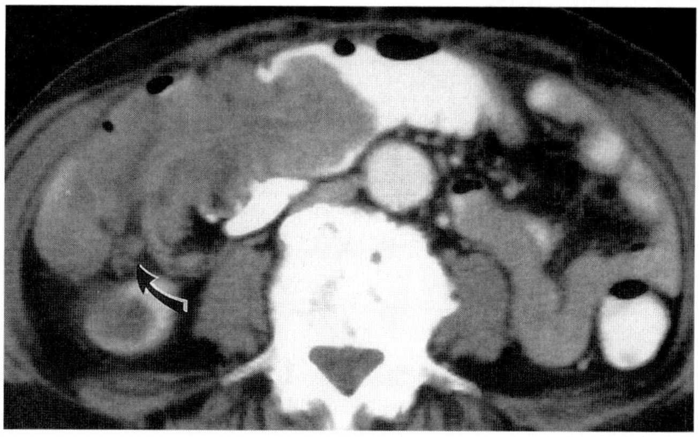

Figure 1. Colocolic intussusception with a neoplastic lead point. Axial CT scan obtained in an 84-year-old man with colon cancer developing in a villous adenoma shows the longitudinal bowel-in-bowel appearance with mesenteric fat and vessels being drawn into the intussusception (arrow).

(n = 3), in the left costovertebral angle region (n = 1), and in a diffuse or unlocalized pattern (n = 7). An abdominal mass was palpated in seven patients. Two patients demonstrated abdominal distention. Stool was checked for occult blood within 2 weeks after CT or MR imaging in 19 of the 33 patients and results were positive in eight patients. Hematocrit values were evaluated within 2 weeks after imaging in 30 patients and showed a median value of 35.5 (25th percentile = 28.9, 75th percentile = 40.5).

Appearance at CT or MR Imaging

Forty-one intussusceptions were observed in the 33 patients. The diagnosis of intussusception was made by observing an axial bowel-within-bowel appearance in 22 intussusceptions, by noting a longitudinal bowel-within-bowel appearance in four intussusceptions, and by seeing the intussusception on both axial and longitudinal sections in 15 intussusceptions. In addition to the bowel-within-bowel appearance, 28 intussusceptions demonstrated fat within the bowel lumen adjacent to the intussusceptum. The appearance of mesenteric vessels being drawn into the intussusception was noted in 22 intussusceptions.

There were 37 cases of enteroenteric intussusception and four cases of either colocolic or ileocolic intussusception. The median length of the intussusceptions was 4.8 cm (25th percentile = 3.2, 75th percentile = 9.1). The median diameter of the intussusceptions was 3.4 cm (25th percentile = 2.8, 75th percentile = 4.0). Obstruction was present in only four patients.

Mesenteric adenopathy was noted in two cases in which there was a malignant neoplasm acting as a lead point for intussusception: in one case of reactive lymphoid hyperplasia and in one case of Crohn disease that was distant from the site of intussusception.

Pathogenesis

A neoplastic lead point was responsible for 12 intussusceptions in 10 patients. In seven patients, the lead point was a malignant neoplasm (Fig 1). Three patients had metastatic disease (large cell lung cancer and colon cancer metastatic to small bowel and squamous cell lung cancer metastatic to large bowel) and three patients had a primary bowel malignancy (two cases of adenocarcinoma of the colon and one of adenosquamous colon cancer). Immunoblastic lymphoma was diagnosed at resection in one patient (Fig 2). Four of the seven patients with a malignant lead point had either a colocolic or ileocolic intussusception.

In three intussusceptions in three patients, the lead point was a benign neoplasm, and in all three patients the intussusception was enteroenteric. There was one case each of an adenomatous polyp, a hamartomatous polyp, and a Peutz-Jeghers polyp.

Twenty-three patients had 29 intussusceptions with no identifiable neoplastic lead point. All nonneoplastic intussusceptions were enteroenteric. In seven of these patients, a possible cause for the intussusception could be found. One patient had cystic fibrosis. One patient with three intussusceptions seen at CT had celiac disease diagnosed at small-bowel biopsy; this patient has previously been reported on (13). One patient with two intussusceptions had reactive lymphoid hyperplasia producing mesenteric adenopathy. In three patients, there was local inflammation from pancreatitis (n = 2) or mesenteric panniculitis (n = 1) (Fig 3). One of the patients with pancreatitis had submucosal hemorrhage at endoscopic biopsy. In one patient, the intussusception occurred 3 months following ileocecectomy with ileoascending colon anastomosis (Fig 4).

In 16 of the 23 patients with nonneoplastic intussusception, no clear cause for the intussusception was noted, and the intussusceptions were classified as idiopathic. In five of the patients in this group, an inflammatory process—pancreatitis, appendicitis, cholecystitis, Crohn disease, or nonspecific ileal inflammation—was noted in the abdomen but was not contiguous with the intussusception. All five of these patients underwent abdominal-pelvic surgery a mean of 13 days following the initial CT: cholecystectomy (n = 2), cholecystectomy with pancreatic cystoduodenostomy and pyloroplasty (n = 1), appendectomy (n = 1), and exploratory laparotomy with lysis of adhesions (n = 1). No intussusception or small-bowel mass was noted at surgery in any of the patients. Follow-up CT was performed in one of the five patients approximately 14 months after initial imaging, but no intussusception was noted. Two of the five patients underwent repeat CT through the area of intussusception at the time of initial CT, but the intussusception was not demonstrated the second time. Three of the five patients underwent small-bowel follow-through 1, 2, and 5 days after initial CT, and again no intussusception was noted nor was a small-bowel mass identified.

In one patient, intussusception was observed after blunt abdominal trauma. At surgery, a small liver laceration was seen with bile staining of intraperitoneal structures; however, no bowel injury was noted.

In the 10 remaining patients with idiopathic intussusception, no intraabdominal process was noted nor was other cause suggested (Figs 5, 6). One patient in this group underwent exploratory pelvic laparoscopy with lysis of adhesions. No mention, however, was made of any small-bowel disease. One patient underwent repeat CT immediately following the initial CT examination, but this showed no intussusception or mass lesion. This patient had also undergone two prior CT examinations 5 and 7 months earlier that

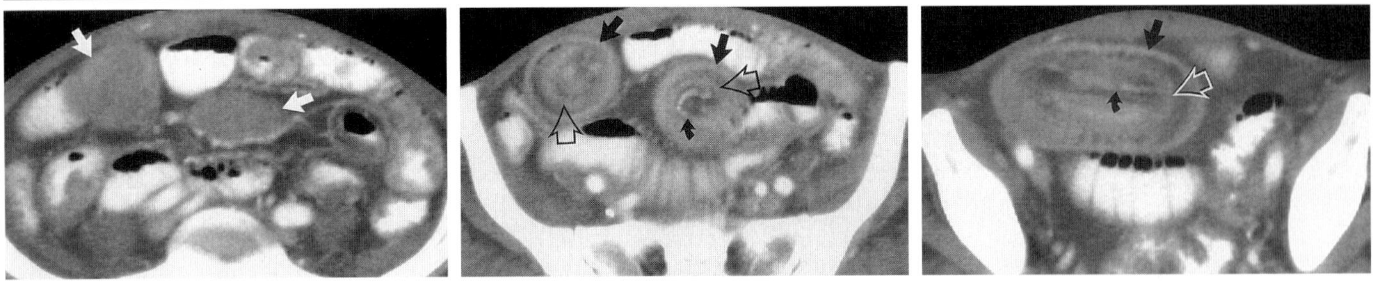

a. b. c.

Figure 2. Axial CT scans obtained in a 44-year-old man show enteroenteric intussusception caused by immunoblastic lymphoma. **(a)** Image shows mesenteric and bowel-associated masses (arrows). **(b, c)** Images show enteroenteric intussusception forming a loop within the pelvis. The intussuscipiens (solid straight arrows), intussusceptum (open arrows), and mesenteric vessels within the intussusceptum (curved arrows) are shown. Images are 8-mm-thick axial sections; **a** and **b** were obtained 2.4 cm apart, and **b** and **c** were obtained 3.2 cm apart.

did not show intussusception, although a CT scan obtained at another institution 1 year earlier had shown a transient small intussusception. Three additional patients underwent follow-up CT a mean of 144 days following initial CT, but no intussusception was demonstrated at repeat imaging. Three patients underwent small-bowel follow-through within 7 days of initial CT, but in none of these patients was either an intussusception or a small-bowel mass identified.

Clinical follow-up was performed by means of telephone interview in seven of the 10 cases, either directly with the patient (five patients) or with the patient's physician (two patients). This was performed a mean of 7 months (range, 2–20 months) following initial CT. Only one of the seven patients noted recurrent abdominal pain, and this patient was thought to have irritable bowel syndrome. Two patients noted gastrointestinal bleeding, but in one this was thought to be due to internal hemorrhoids. No explanation for the episode of intussusception was noted in any of the seven patients. Clinical follow-up was performed by means of chart review in the remaining three patients, who could not be contacted by phone. In two patients, examined 2 months and 20 months following initial CT, there was no mention of abdominal symptoms. In one patient, examined 1 week following CT, abdominal symptoms were thought to be secondary to gastritis.

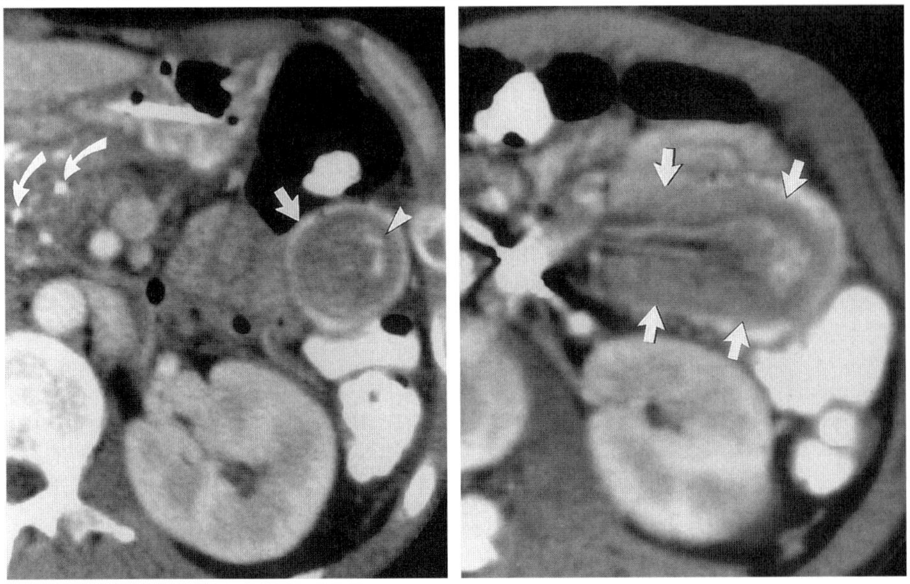

a. b.

Figure 3. Axial CT scans obtained in a 42-year-old man show transient intussusception associated with local inflammation from pancreatitis. **(a)** At the level of the pancreatic head, the intussusceptum (arrowhead) is seen within the intussuscipiens (straight arrow). Note the calcifications (curved arrows) in the region of the pancreatic head and infiltration of anterior pararenal space fat. **(b)** Image obtained 5.2 cm caudad to **a** shows mesenteric vessels, fat, and bowel (arrows) entering the intussuscipiens. Small-bowel follow-through performed 1 day following CT showed fold thickening in the duodenum and proximal jejunum but no intussusception. CT performed 1 month later also showed no intussusception.

Clinical-Pathologic Correlation

There was no significant difference in sex in patients with a neoplastic lead point and those without a neoplastic lead point. Patients with a neoplastic lead point were, however, significantly older (median, 47.5 years [25th percentile = 40.0, 75th percentile = 67] for neoplastic vs 39.0 years [25th percentile = 23.0, 75th percentile = 47.0] for nonneoplastic; P = .036). There was no significant difference in the frequency of abdominal symptoms between groups with a neoplastic lead point and those without a neoplastic lead point. Although the hematocrit value was significantly lower in patients in the neoplastic group (median hematocrit value = 27.6 [25th percentile = 24.3, 75th percentile = 33.8] for neoplastic vs 39.0 [25th percentile = 33.1, 75th percentile = 42.3] for nonneoplastic; P = .004), there was no significant difference in frequency of guaiac-positive stools (Table 2).

Radiologic-Pathologic Correlation

All colocolic or ileocolic intussusceptions in this series (n = 4) were secondary to a neoplastic lead point. However, only eight of 37 enteroenteric intussusceptions were due to neoplasm. Enteroenteric intussusceptions with a neoplastic lead point were significantly longer than nonneoplastic intussusceptions (median, 10.8 cm [25th percentile = 7.5, 75th

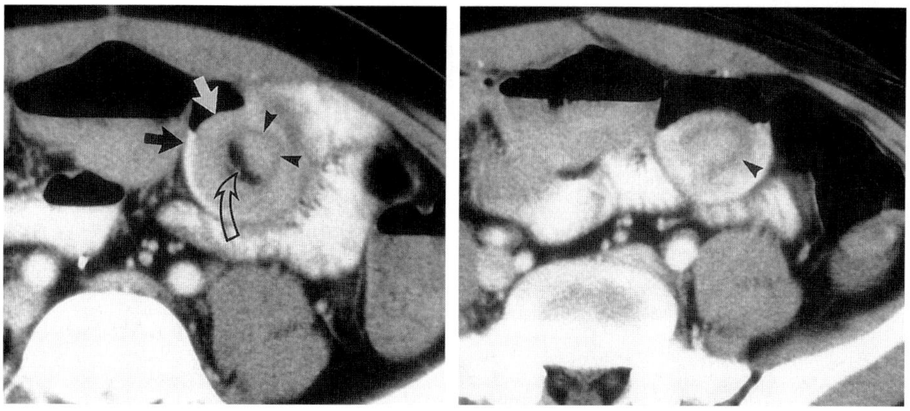

a. b.

Figure 4. (a, b) Axial CT scans obtained in a 26-year-old man show enteroenteric intussusception associated with recent surgery. The patient had undergone ileocecectomy with ileoascending colon anastomosis 3 months previously for Crohn disease. The intussuscipiens (black arrow), intussusceptum (white arrow), fat (open arrow) within the intussusceptum, and a lower attenuation rim thought to represent the muscularis externa (arrowheads) of the intussusceptum are shown. The patient underwent repeat surgery on the day the scan was obtained. Although an intussusception was not demonstrated at surgery, ischemic changes were seen in the neoterminal ileum. Images are 8 mm thick and were obtained 1.6 cm apart.

TABLE 2
Comparison of All Intussusceptions with or without a Neoplastic Lead Point

Cause	No. of Patients	Median Age (y)	No. of Patients with Multiple Intussusceptions	Type and No. of Intussusceptions*	No. of Patients with Abdominal Pain	Median Hematocrit Value
Neoplastic	10	47.5	1	Enteric 8, colic 4	6	27.6
Nonneoplastic	23	39	5	Enteric 29, colic 0	18	39
P value	...†	.036	NS	.005	NS	.004

Note.—*P* values are listed only where the value was less than .05. NS = not significant.
* Colic category includes enterocolic and colocolic intussusception.
† No comparison was made.

percentile = 17.4] for neoplastic vs 4.0 cm [25th percentile = 3.0, 75th percentile = 6.1] for nonneoplastic; $P = .002$). Furthermore, no neoplastic intussusceptions were shorter than 3.6 cm, while 41% of nonneoplastic intussusceptions were shorter than 3.6 cm.

Similarly, enteroenteric intussusceptions with a neoplastic lead point had a significantly larger diameter than that of nonneoplastic intussusceptions (median, 4.0 cm [25th percentile = 3.7, 75th percentile = 4.5] for neoplastic vs 3.0 cm [25th percentile = 2.7, 75th percentile = 3.7] for nonneoplastic; $P = .002$). No neoplastic intussusceptions were smaller than 3.4 cm in diameter, whereas 66% of nonneoplastic intussusceptions were. Bowel obstruction was significantly more common in the enteroenteric intussusceptions secondary to a neoplastic lead point and occurred in three of six patients with neoplastic lead points versus one of 23 patients with nonneoplastic intussusception (Fisher exact test; $P = .02$) (Table 3; Figs 7, 8).

DISCUSSION

Adult intussusception is unusual, and its cause is varied (1,14). The majority of published studies are in the surgery literature and are based on discharge diagnosis and result at surgery. Table 1 summarizes the results of eight such studies published in 1981–1997 (1–8). Although there is variation, the majority of these and earlier studies (15,16) show nearly equal numbers of enteric versus colic intussusceptions with 80%–90% of adult cases having a demonstrable cause. Approximately 65% are due to neoplasm with a somewhat higher rate in intussusceptions involving the colon than those that involve only the small bowel. Malignant tumors are more common than benign tumors in the colon, with the reverse being true in the small bowel (14). Nonneoplastic causes compose the remaining 15%–25% of cases with a known cause and include adhesions and postoperative complications, Meckel diverticula, lymphoid hyperplasia and adenitis, trauma, celiac disease, duplications, and Henoch-Schönlein purpura.

In contradistinction to these studies, our data suggest that intussusceptions discovered in the adult patient at CT or MR imaging are predominantly enteroenteric in type and more often nonneoplastic in cause. Only 30% of the patients in this study had a neoplastic lead point, although it is important to note that this included all four patients with intussusceptions involving the colon. Over two-thirds of the patients in our study had intussusceptions without a neoplastic lead point. Although a cause can be suggested in many of these cases, almost half (48%) of all cases were idiopathic.

The increased prevalence of transient nonobstructing enteric intussusception noted in this study probably more closely reflects the true physiologic situation. Previous studies (1–8) that required either surgical confirmation or substantial enough clinical effect for coding as a discharge diagnosis are clearly biased toward more marked and fixed lesions. Previous studies in the radiology literature (9,17) may have suffered from a similar bias, although the case ascertainment methodology is not spelled out. In studies by Merine et al (9) and Gayer et al (17), 20 of 25 patients underwent surgery, and 19 of 25 had neoplastic causes of the intussusception.

Although intussusception is most commonly thought of as secondary to mechanical factors (ie, a mass attached or in the bowel wall or a kink in the bowel wall is pulled forward by normal peristalsis with resultant invagination of the involved wall), functional disturbances also can cause intussusception without gross mural abnormality. Celiac disease is a prime example of this effect, in which gluten sensitivity causes muscular flaccidity followed by transient intussusception (13,18). Diarrheal diseases with resultant abnormal bowel motility also have been cited as the cause for the increased prevalence of nonneoplastic adult intussusception in tropical regions (19–21). In one study from Papua, New Guinea, 66% (21 of 32) of cases had no detectable associated disease (20).

We suspect that the increased number of nonneoplastic cases in our study re-

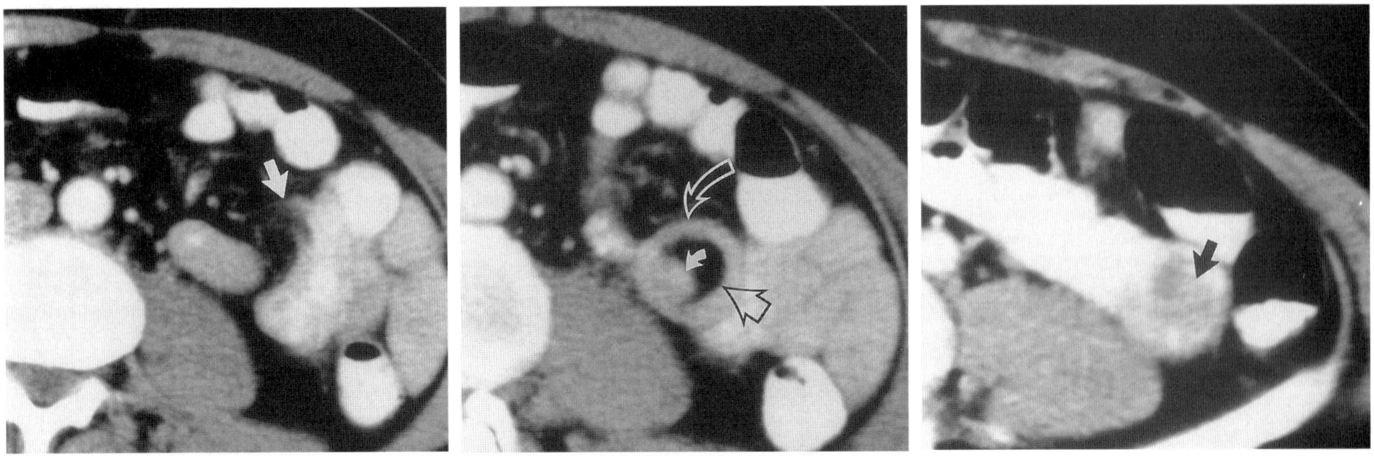

a. b. c.

Figure 5. Axial CT scans obtained in a 47-year-old man without symptoms show idiopathic enteroenteric intussusception. **(a)** Image demonstrates vessels (arrow) entering the intussusception. **(b)** Image demonstrates fat (open black arrow) pulled into the intussusception (open white arrow) adjacent to a redundant portion of the intussusceptum (solid white arrow). **(c)** Image is the last section on which the intussusceptum (arrow) is visible and was obtained 4 cm below **b**. Results of small-bowel follow-through performed 4 days later were unremarkable. Repeat CT 8 months later showed no evidence of bowel lesion or intussusception. **a** and **b** are contiguous 1-cm-thick axial sections.

flects the presence of minor transient disturbances in bowel motility without clinical importance. Most of these cases would not have come to attention were it not for CT being performed to evaluate unrelated disease or symptoms. An analogy can be drawn to swallowing. Although substantial disturbances in pharyngeal function can result in clinically important aspiration, it is not uncommon for each of us to aspirate slightly. Such minor and infrequent aspiration is of no clinical importance.

Our finding of an increased prevalence of nonneoplastic intussusception is important in that it suggests that not all adult enteric intussusceptions diagnosed at CT or MR imaging require aggressive work-up. Although in previous studies (9,17) CT has been unreliable in directly distinguishing a neoplastic lead point from thickened or edematous bowel wall, several differences between patient groups with and without a neoplastic lead point were noted in this study. Patients with a nonneoplastic cause were significantly younger than those with small-bowel neoplasia and had significantly higher hematocrit values. Nonneoplastic enteroenteric intussusceptions were also significantly shorter, smaller in diameter, and less likely to be associated with obstruction than those with a neoplastic lead point. Furthermore, no neoplastic enteric intussusceptions were shorter than 3.6 cm or smaller than 3.4 cm in diameter, whereas 41% and 66% of nonneoplastic intussusceptions were shorter and smaller than these cutoff values. Obstruction was uncommon in the nonneoplastic group and occurred in only one patient. Nonneoplastic intussusceptions were also transient. Repeat CT sections through the involved bowel that were obtained either immediately or after a longer interval usually failed to demonstrate an intussusception.

Taken together, these findings suggest that aggressive work-up need not be undertaken in younger patients with transient, short, small, nonobstructing enteroenteric intussusception. This recommendation is supported by a recent description of five cases of transient nonobstructing intussusception seen at CT (22). In that study, the lesions were all enteroenteric intussusceptions unassociated with obstruction or substantial dilatation in the

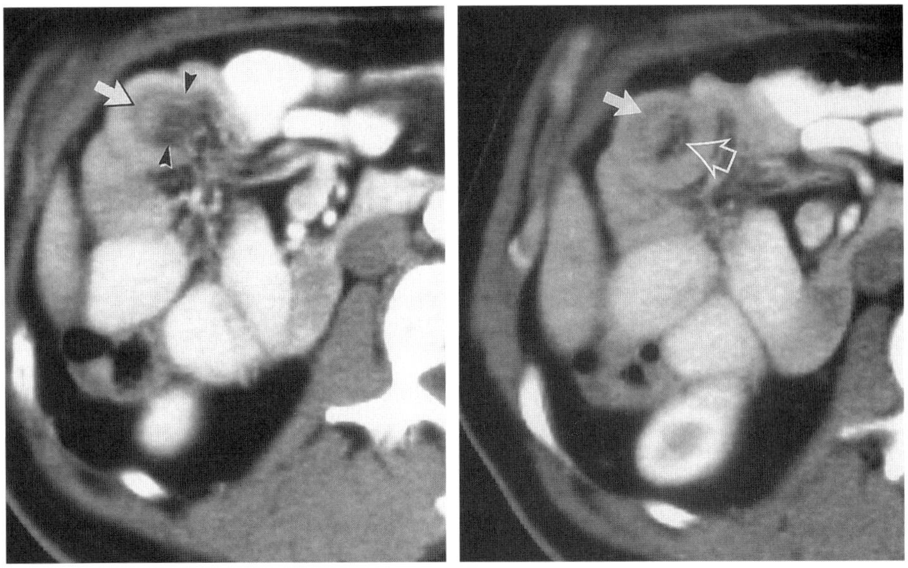

a. b.

Figure 6. **(a, b)** Axial CT scans obtained in a 61-year-old man with back pain show idiopathic enteroenteric intussusception. Images demonstrate mesenteric vessels and fat (arrowheads) entering the intussusception, fat (open arrow) within the intussusceptum, and a lower attenuation line thought to correspond to the muscularis externa (solid arrows) of the intussusceptum. Results of small-bowel follow-through 2 days later showed no definite mass or intussusception. Repeat CT 1 month later also showed no small-bowel mass or intussusception. The patient was asymptomatic at subsequent clinical follow-up. Images **a** and **b** are contiguous 8-mm-thick sections.

TABLE 3
Comparison of Enteroenteric Intussusceptions with or without a Neoplastic Lead Point

Cause	No. of Patients	No. of Intussusceptions	No. of Obstructions Noted	Median Length of Intussusception (cm)	Median Diameter of Intussusception (cm)
Neoplastic	6	8	3	10.8	4
Nonneoplastic	23	29	1	4	3
P value	. . .*	. . .*	.02	.002	.002

Note.—*P* values are listed only where the value was less than .05.
* No comparison was made.

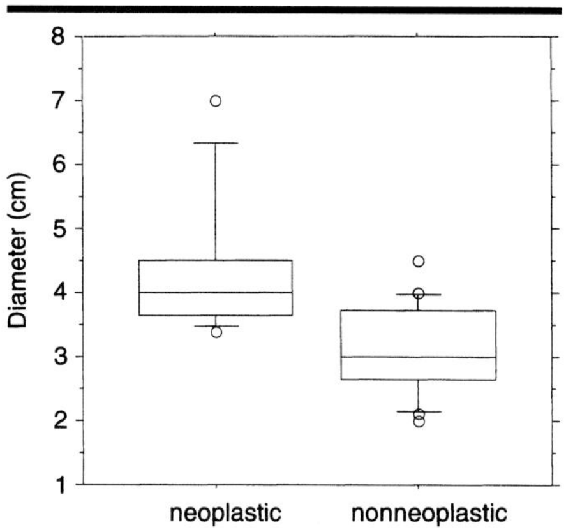

Figure 7. Box plot of intussusception diameter for enteroenteric intussusceptions with a neoplastic lead point and those without. Nonneoplastic intussusceptions were significantly smaller in diameter ($P = .002$) than intussusceptions with a neoplastic lead point. Horizontal lines indicate 10th, 25th, 50th (median), 75th, and 90th percentiles. Values above the 90th and below the 10th percentiles are plotted as points.

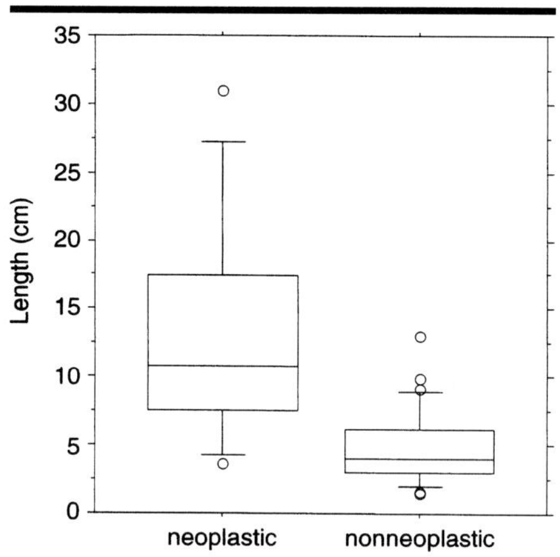

Figure 8. Box plot of intussusception length for enteroenteric intussusceptions with and those without a neoplastic lead point. Nonneoplastic intussusceptions were significantly shorter ($P = .002$) than intussusceptions with a neoplastic lead point. Horizontal lines indicate 10th, 25th, 50th (median), 75th, and 90th percentiles. Values above the 90th and below the 10th percentiles are plotted as points.

involved loop. The length of the intussusceptions was not discussed.

It is interesting that there was not a difference in abdominal symptoms between neoplastic and nonneoplastic groups in our study. We suspect that this is probably because of the ubiquitous and nonspecific nature of abdominal complaints.

Our study results suggest that the overall diagnosis of intussusception at CT and MR imaging may be becoming more common. From 1991 through 1996, 16 patients were examined in our study. From 1997 through April of 1998, an additional 17 patients were examined. This increase may in part be artifactual, reflecting our increased scrutiny of bowel. Part, however, may be due to improvements in technology, with spiral scans now able to cover the entire abdominal cavity in a single breath hold. This faster scanning allows transient events to be imaged in their entirety before they change position or resolve.

Several concerns should be noted regarding this study. There is the question of whether the diagnosis of intussusception at CT or MR imaging is valid without surgical proof. Because the diagnosis depends on the physical relationship of bowel loops and not a histologic diagnosis, we believe that the CT diagnosis is accurate. This view is supported in the literature (9–11). For increased assurance, we took only cases in which the intussusception could be identified clearly on at least two separate sections. The frequent finding of fat within the intussusception (seen in 76% of patients [68% of intussusceptions] in this study) and of mesenteric vessels entering the involved loop (seen in 61% of patients [54% of intussusceptions]) also supports the validity of our diagnosis.

We were also concerned in this study that we could be missing cases, that is, that our results may underestimate the frequency of incidental nonneoplastic intussusception, as these may not have been observed and noted on the report or some may not have shown a classic bowel-in-bowel configuration. This is a potential difficulty and cannot entirely be discounted. Our data, therefore, should be viewed as showing minimum frequency that, if anything, underestimates the actual occurrence rate.

Another potential problem was the possibility of misallocating diagnoses. For example, might some of our idiopathic group actually have mild adhesions, enteritis, or dysmotility? More important, was our follow-up adequate to exclude the presence of small tumors? Although misallocation is possible as the small bowel is difficult to evaluate, it should be noted that for the 16 nonneoplastic cases without clear local explanation (idiopathic plus distant inflammation and trauma groups), seven patients underwent surgery, seven had negative findings on immediate or delayed repeat CT scans, and six had negative small-bowel follow-through results. Clinical follow-up in those patients who had not undergone surgery disclosed no alternative diagnoses, and in only one case was recurrent abdominal pain noted, which was thought to be secondary to irritable bowel syndrome. Although perhaps less than ideal, clinical and radiologic follow-up is probably the best that can be achieved, as it is difficult to justify surgery or invasive testing in these patients with relatively few symptoms.

A final potential difficulty lies in the relatively small number of patients in this study. Although we found significant differences between neoplastic and nonneoplastic groups, it will be important to confirm these findings in larger or multiple series.

In summary, less than one-third of adult intussusceptions demonstrated at CT or MR imaging were caused by a neoplastic lead point. A variety of other causes were implicated in the remaining patients, with almost half of adult cases in this series being idiopathic. Enteroenteric intussusceptions with a nonneoplastic cause were shorter, smaller in diameter, and less likely to be associated with obstruction or anemia than intussusceptions secondary to neoplasm. Our study results suggest that extensive work-up in cases of transient, short, small enteric intussusceptions may be unnecessary in the patient without symptoms.

Acknowledgment: We thank Keith E. Muller, PhD, Associate Professor, Department of Biostatistics, University of North Carolina, for his review of the statistical analysis.

References

1. Azar T, Berger DL. Adult intussusception. Ann Surg 1997; 226:134–138.
2. Nagorney DM, Sarr MG, McIlrath DC. Surgical management of intussusception in the adult. Ann Surg 1981; 193:230–236.
3. Coleman MJ, Hugh TB, May RE, Jensen MJ. Intussusception in the adult. Aust N Z J Surg 1981; 51:179–180.
4. Agha FP. Intussusception in adults. AJR 1986; 146:527–531.
5. Carter CR, Morton AL. Adult intussusception in Glasgow, UK. Br J Surg 1989; 76:727.
6. Reijnen HA, Joosten HJ, de Boer HH. Diagnosis and treatment of adult intussusception. Am J Surg 1989; 158:25–28.
7. Hamaloglu E, Yavuz B. Intussusception in adults. Panminerva Med 1990; 32:118–121.
8. Begos DG, Sandor A, Modlin IM. The diagnosis and management of adult intussusception. Am J Surg 1997; 173:88–94.
9. Merine D, Fishman EK, Jones B, Siegelman SS. Enteroenteric intussusception: CT findings in nine patients. AJR 1987; 148:1129–1132.
10. Lorigan JG, DuBrow RA. The computed tomographic appearances and clinical significance of intussusception in adults with malignant neoplasms. Br J Radiol 1990; 63:257–262.
11. Iko BO, Teal JS, Siram SM, Chinwuba CE, Roux VJ, Scott VF. Computed tomography of adult colonic intussusception: clinical and experimental studies. AJR 1984; 143:769–772.
12. Marcos HB, Semelka RC, Worawattanakul S. Adult intussusception: demonstration by current MR techniques. Magn Reson Imaging 1997; 15:1095–1098.
13. Strobl PW, Warshauer DM. CT diagnosis of celiac disease. J Comput Assist Tomogr 1995; 19:319–320.
14. Felix EL, Cohen MH, Bernstein AD, Schwartz JH. Adult intussusception: case report of recurrent intussusception and review of the literature. Am J Surg 1976; 131:758–761.
15. Stubenbord W, Thorbjarnarson B. Intussusception in adults. Ann Surg 1970; 172:306–310.
16. Brayton D, Norris W. Intussusception in adults. Am J Surg 1954; 88:32–43.
17. Gayer G, Apter S, Hofmann C, et al. Intussusception in adults: CT diagnosis. Clin Radiol 1998; 53:53–57.
18. Cohen MD, Lintott DJ. Transient small bowel intussusception in adult coeliac disease. Clin Radiol 1978; 29:529–534.
19. Atri SC, Singh AK, Naithani YP. Adult intussusception in Allahabad. J Indian Med Assoc 1983; 81:155–158.
20. Hadley GP, Simpson RL. Adult intussusception in the tropics. Br J Surg 1983; 70:281.
21. Ademiluyi SA. Intussusception in Nigerian adults. J Natl Med Assoc 1987; 79:873–876.
22. Catalano O. Transient small bowel intussusception: CT findings in adults. Br J Radiol 1997; 70:805–808.

Laura R. Carucci, MD
Marc S. Levine, MD
Stephen E. Rubesin, MD
Igor Laufer, MD

Index terms:
Stomach, neoplasms, 72.30
Stomach, varices, 72.75

Radiology 1999; 212:861–865

[1] From the Department of Radiology, Hospital of the University of Pennsylvania, 3400 Spruce St, Philadelphia, PA 19104. Received November 24, 1998; revision requested December 30; revision received January 25, 1999; accepted March 3. **Address reprint requests to** M.S.L.

Author contributions:
Guarantor of integrity of entire study, M.S.L.; study concepts, M.S.L.; study design, M.S.L., L.R.C.; definition of intellectual content, M.S.L., L.R.C., S.E.R., I.L.; literature research, L.R.C.; clinical studies, M.S.L., S.E.R., I.L.; data acquisition, L.R.C.; data analysis, L.R.C., M.S.L.; manuscript preparation, L.R.C., M.S.L.; manuscript editing, M.S.L., S.E.R., I.L. manuscript review, S.E.R., I.L.

Tumorous Gastric Varices: Radiographic Findings in 10 Patients[1]

PURPOSE: To determine the appearance of tumorous gastric varices on double-contrast barium studies and whether these varices have characteristic radiographic features.

MATERIALS AND METHODS: Review of radiology files revealed 86 patients with gastric varices diagnosed during double-contrast upper gastrointestinal tract examinations. Of these 86 patients, 12 (14%) had a conglomerate mass of varices, or tumorous varices. Five of the 12 patients had proved gastric varices and five were presumed to have varices on the basis of additional diagnostic test results, clinical follow-up findings, or both. Radiographs from these 10 patients were reviewed retrospectively to determine the size, location, and morphologic features of these lesions.

RESULTS: Tumorous varices had a mean size of 6.8 cm (range, 3–11 cm). They involved the posteromedial border of the gastric fundus in eight patients, the central cardiac region in one, and the anterolateral-inferior fundal border in one. Viewed in profile, the varices appeared as smooth submucosal masses with undulating contours and discrete borders. Viewed en face, the varices manifested as a conglomerate of thickened, tortuous folds that faded peripherally into the adjacent mucosa.

CONCLUSION: Tumorous gastric varices manifest as remarkably similar findings on double-contrast barium studies, usually appearing en face as a conglomerate of thickened, lobulated folds and in profile as smooth, undulating, submucosal masses on the posteromedial border of the gastric fundus. It is important to be aware of the characteristic features of tumorous gastric varices on double-contrast studies so that they are not mistaken for neoplastic lesions in the stomach.

When varices occur in the stomach, they classically appear on barium studies as multiple rounded, submucosal nodules that have been likened to the appearance of a bunch of grapes in the gastric fundus (1). Occasionally, however, a conglomerate mass of varices, or tumorous varices, may manifest as a large, polypoid, fundal mass that can be mistaken radiographically for a neoplastic lesion (1–11). Although most of these have been anecdotal case reports, many authors believe that it is difficult or impossible to differentiate tumorous varices from a polypoid carcinoma, lymphoma, or gastrointestinal stromal tumor (leiomyosarcoma) on barium studies (3,4,6,8). We have encountered a number of patients with a conglomerate mass of fundal varices during double-contrast upper gastrointestinal tract examinations. This investigation was therefore undertaken to determine the appearance of tumorous gastric varices on double-contrast barium studies in a series of patients with this finding and to determine whether these varices have characteristic radiographic features.

MATERIALS AND METHODS

A review of computerized radiology files at our university hospital revealed 54 patients with gastric varices that were diagnosed at double-contrast upper gastrointestinal tract examinations (patients swallowed a barium sulfate solution [E-Z–HD; E-Z–Em, Westbury, NY; 120 mL]) during a 10-year period between 1988 and 1998. A review of radiology files at our affiliate, the Veterans Affairs Medical Center of Philadelphia, revealed another 32 patients

Summary of Predisposing Clinical Conditions, Status of Esophageal Varices, and Other Diagnostic Tests in 10 Patients with Tumorous Varices

Patient No.	Condition	Esophageal Varices Present	Presence of Gastric Varices			
			Endoscopy	CT	US	Angiography
1	Alcoholic cirrhosis	No	Imaging not done	Yes	Splenomegaly	Imaging not done
2	Hepatitis B, abnormal liver function test results	No	No	Imaging not done	Cirrhosis	Imaging not done
3	Hepatitis C	No	No	Imaging not done	Cirrhosis	Imaging not done
4	Recurrent pancreatitis	Yes	Imaging not done	Imaging not done	Imaging not done	Imaging not done
5	Cirrhosis, hepatitis C	No	Yes	Imaging not done	Imaging not done	Yes
6	Cirrhosis, portal hypertension	No	Imaging not done	Imaging not done	Imaging not done	Imaging not done
7	Alcoholic hepatitis	Yes	Imaging not done	Yes	Imaging not done	Imaging not done
8	Liver failure	Yes	Imaging not done	Cirrhosis	Cirrhosis, ascites	Imaging not done
9	Liver failure	Yes	Yes	Cirrhosis	Imaging not done	Yes
10	Hepatitis, portal hypertension	Yes	Yes	Imaging not done	Imaging not done	Yes

with gastric varices that were diagnosed during a 5-year period between 1993 and 1998. Of these 86 patients with radiographically diagnosed gastric varices, 74 (86%) had typical findings of varices on double-contrast studies with multiple rounded, submucosal nodules or serpentine folds in the gastric fundus. The remaining 12 patients (14%) had a conglomerate mass of varices, or tumorous varices, that manifested as a polypoid fundal mass rather than as multiple submucosal nodules or serpentine folds. In a subsequent review of medical, radiology, and endoscopy records, five of these 12 patients were proved to have gastric varices and five were presumed to have varices on the basis of clinical, radiologic, and/or endoscopic follow-up data (Table). The remaining two patients did not have adequate follow-up. Our study group comprised the 10 patients proved or presumed to have gastric varices.

All 10 patients had preexistent conditions known to predispose them to the development of gastric varices (see Results). Eight patients had findings of additional diagnostic testing that supported or confirmed the diagnosis of gastric varices, including endoscopy in five patients, abdominal computed tomography (CT) in four, abdominal ultrasonography (US) in four, and angiography in three (see Results). Although two patients did not undergo additional diagnostic testing, one had known portal hypertension and the other had chronic pancreatitis and pseudocyst formation with presumed splenic vein obstruction.

The images from double-contrast upper gastrointestinal tract examinations of these 10 patients with tumorous gastric varices were reviewed retrospectively by two gastrointestinal radiologists (M.S.L., I.L.) together to determine the size, location, and morphologic features of the varices.

RESULTS

Clinical Findings

The mean age of these 10 patients was 54.9 years (age range, 22–73 years). Nine were men, and one was a woman. All 10 patients had clinically documented conditions known to predispose them to the development of gastric varices, including hepatitis in five patients, portal hypertension in two, cirrhosis in three, liver failure in two, and pancreatitis in one (Table). Five patients presented with symptoms of acute upper gastrointestinal bleeding (hematemesis or melena).

Radiographic Findings

The conglomerate masses of gastric varices in these 10 patients had a mean size of 6.8 cm (range, 3–11 cm). The varices involved the posteromedial border of the gastric fundus in eight patients (six varices extended superiorly to the fundal apex and two extended inferiorly to the lower fundus), the central cardiac region in one, and the anterolateral-inferior border of the fundus in one. Thus, 80% of patients had varices that involved the posteromedial border of the gastric fundus and usually extended to the fundal apex. When viewed in profile, these tumorous varices appeared as smooth submucosal masses with an undulating contour and discrete borders (Figs 1a, 2a, 3a). When viewed en face, the varices were manifest as a conglomerate of thickened, tortuous folds that faded peripherally into the adjacent mucosa (Figs 1b, 2b, 3b). These tumorous varices therefore had a characteristic appearance both en face and in profile on double-contrast studies.

In five (50%) of the 10 patients with tumorous varices, barium studies also revealed serpentine longitudinal folds in the lower third or half of the thoracic esophagus that were compatible with esophageal varices.

Other Diagnostic Tests

Endoscopic results confirmed the presence of tumorous varices in three of the five patients who underwent endoscopy (Table). In the remaining two patients, gastric varices were not seen at endoscopy. In two patients, CT scans revealed typical findings of gastric varices, with lobulated fundal masses that enhanced to the same degree as the great vessels after intravenous contrast material administration (Fig 1c). In two other patients, nonenhanced CT scans revealed cirrhosis and portal hypertension. Abdominal US revealed cirrhosis in two patients, cirrhosis and ascites in one, and splenomegaly in one. Finally, angiographic results confirmed the presence of gastric varices in all three patients who underwent this procedure.

In summary, the presence of gastric varices was proved with endoscopy, CT, angiography, or all three methods in five patients. The remaining five patients were presumed to have gastric varices because of a history of end-stage liver disease or cirrhosis, or both in four (with findings of cirrhosis at US in three) and a history of recurrent pancreatitis in one.

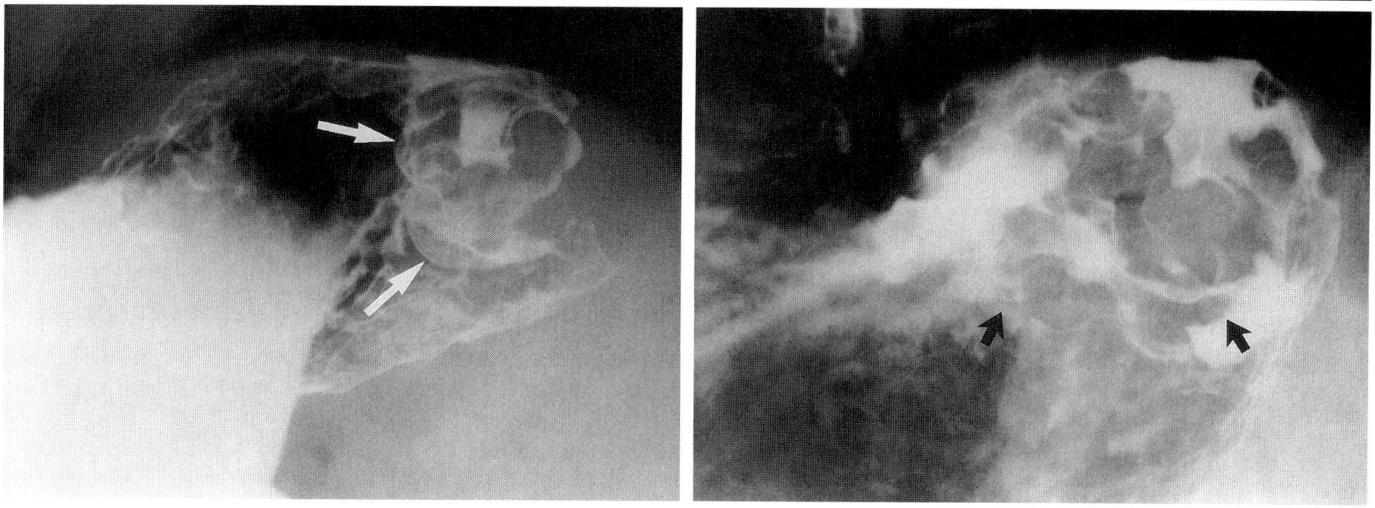

a. b.

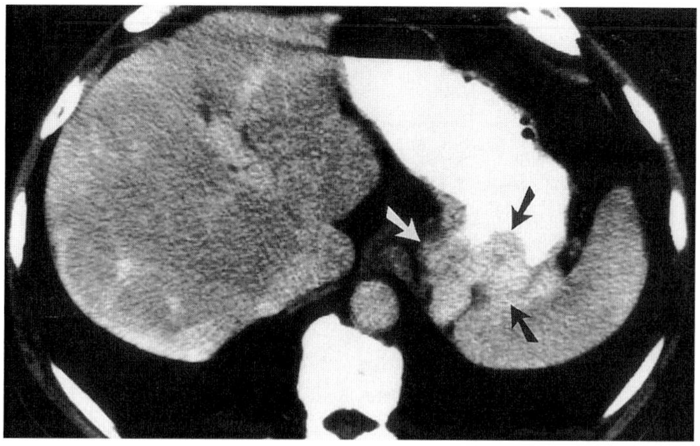

c.

Figure 1. Tumorous gastric varices in a 67-year-old man with alcoholic cirrhosis. **(a)** Lateral double-contrast barium radiograph shows a smooth, undulating, submucosal mass (arrows) in profile on the posteromedial border of the gastric fundus. **(b)** Oblique radiograph shows a conglomerate of thickened, lobulated folds (arrows) that fade peripherally into adjacent mucosa. These findings are characteristic of tumorous varices. **(c)** Contrast-enhanced axial CT scan shows a lobulated mass (arrows) on posteromedial border of the fundus that enhances to the same degree as the great vessels. These findings are typical of gastric varices on CT scans.

DISUSSION

Conglomerate masses of gastric varices, or tumorous varices, have traditionally been considered a rare finding of radiologic or endoscopic examinations. In our series, however, tumorous varices were found to represent 14% of all gastric varices diagnosed on double-contrast barium studies. In a previous series, tumorous varices represented nearly 10% of all gastric varices diagnosed at endoscopy (12). These conglomerate masses of gastric varices therefore appear to be more common findings on barium studies or at endoscopy than has generally been recognized.

It is important to be aware of the clinical implications of tumorous varices, as they are more likely to bleed than other forms of gastric varices (13,14). In our study, 50% of patients with tumorous varices presented with symptoms of acute upper gastrointestinal tract bleeding. In previous studies, signs of bleeding have been found at endoscopy in approximately 35% of patients with tumorous varices versus in only 6%–7% of all patients with gastric varices (13,14). These individuals must therefore be followed up closely because of their greater risk of gastrointestinal tract bleeding than patients with smaller, more typical gastric varices.

The overall reported sensitivity of endoscopy in the detection of gastric varices has ranged from 40% to 80% (10,12,15). Conglomerate masses of varices may be even more difficult to detect at endoscopy than most gastric varices. In one series (10), the lesions were misdiagnosed at endoscopy in two of three patients with tumorous varices diagnosed on double-contrast studies.

Unlike esophageal varices, which typically have a bluish hue at endoscopy because of their superficial location beneath the esophageal mucosa, gastric varices tend to have a subserosal location, so a bluish hue may not be present (8,16). Also, gastric varices are often obscured by overlying gastric rugae (14). As a result, tumorous varices may be mistaken at endoscopy for other submucosal masses or a conglomerate of thickened folds. In fact, several deaths have been reported as a result of catastrophic bleeding due to endoscopic biopsy or attempted surgical resection of unrecognized varices (3,17). It is therefore important to be aware of the limitations of endoscopy in diagnosing tumorous varices and of the potential danger of obtaining endoscopic biopsy specimens in these patients.

Although most gastric varices are associated with typical findings on barium studies, tumorous varices have been mistaken on radiographs for polypoid carcinomas, gastrointestinal stromal tumors, or other neoplastic lesions (1–11). Some authors (3,4,6,8) have used terms such as "mimicry" and "deception" to emphasize this difficulty in differentiating conglomerate masses of fundal varices from true neoplasms. In these previously reported cases, it is important to recognize that most of the patients had single-contrast barium studies on which the varices appeared as nondescript masses in the gastric fundus.

In our study, however, tumorous varices had a characteristic location and appearance on double-contrast studies. The varices were typically located on the posteromedial border of the gastric fundus at

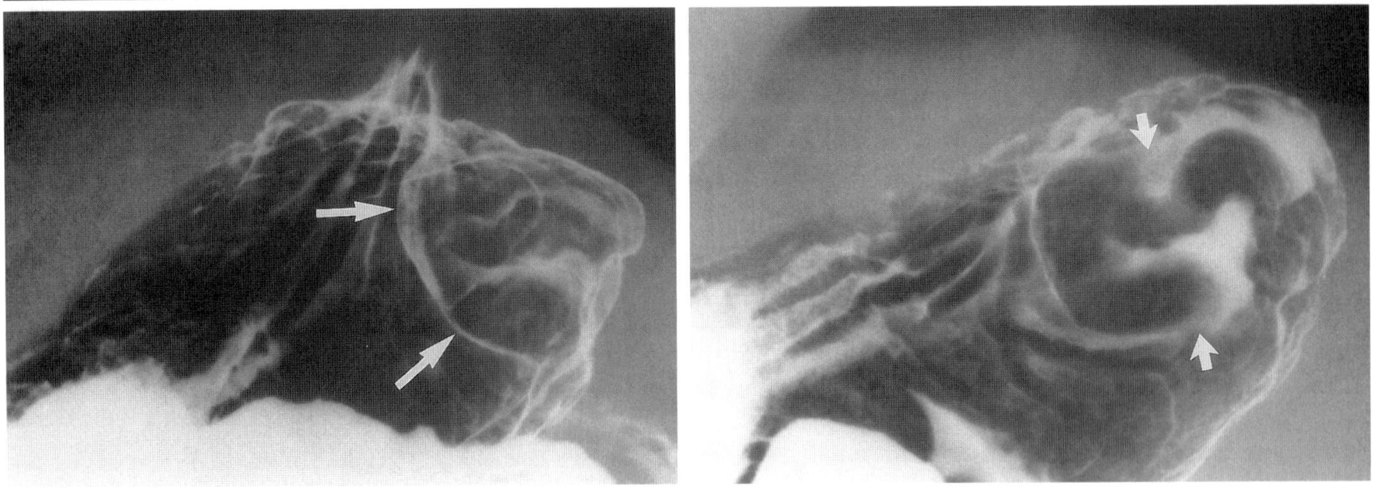

a. b.

Figure 2. Tumorous gastric varices in a 39-year-old man with cirrhosis. **(a)** Lateral double-contrast barium radiograph shows a smooth submucosal mass (arrows) in profile on the posteromedial border of the fundus. **(b)** Oblique radiograph shows markedly thickened, lobulated folds (arrows) in fundus that fade peripherally into adjacent mucosa.

or near the fundal apex. Moreover, the varices had remarkably similar radiographic findings, appearing in profile as smooth submucosal masses with an undulating contour and discrete borders and en face as a conglomerate of thickened, tortuous folds that faded peripherally into the adjacent mucosa (Figs 1–3). In 50% of patients, the diagnosis was supported on barium studies by the presence of associated varices in the esophagus. Our experience therefore suggests that, on double-contrast studies, tumorous gastric varices have characteristic features that enable their differentiation from true neoplasms in most patients.

When tumorous gastric varices are suspected on barium studies, other diagnostic imaging, including contrast material-enhanced CT and angiography, may be required to confirm the presence of varices (18). Recently, endoscopic US has also been advocated as a useful technique for the diagnosis of gastric varices (19–21). In fact, some authors believe that endoscopic US is superior to endoscopy for detecting these lesions (20,21).

The lack of definitive confirmation of the diagnosis of varices represents a limitation of our study, as the presence of tumorous gastric varices was proved with endoscopy, CT, and/or angiography in five of 10 patients. Although the remaining five patients did not have documented varices, four had end-stage liver disease and/or cirrhosis and one had recurrent pancreatitis. These five patients were therefore presumed to have gastric varices on the basis of the clinical data.

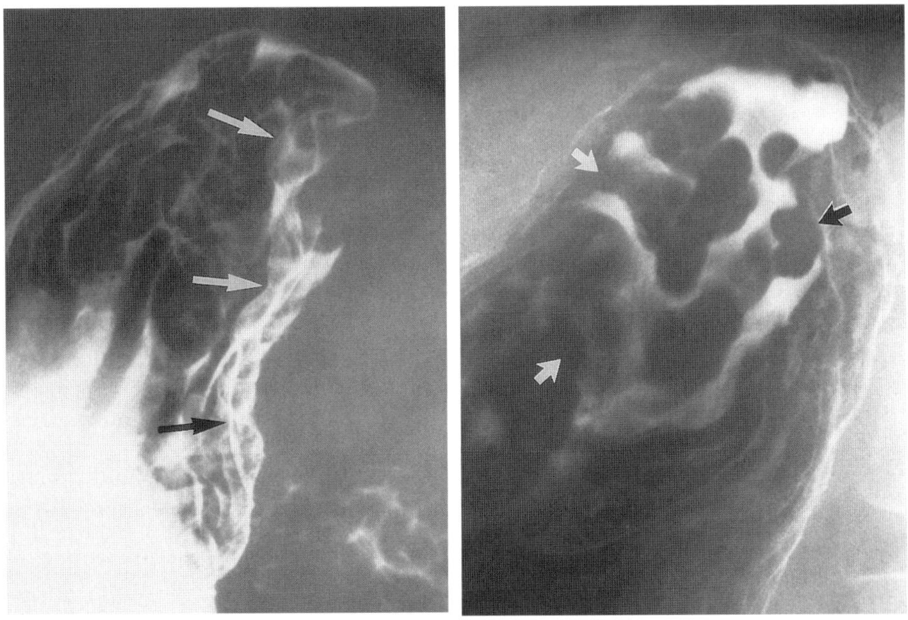

a. b.

Figure 3. Tumorous gastric varices in a 57-year-old man with portal hypertension. **(a)** Lateral double-contrast barium radiograph shows a smooth, flat, undulating submucosal mass (arrows) in profile on the posteromedial border of the gastric fundus. This patient had the largest mass of fundal varices encountered in our series. **(b)** Oblique radiograph shows a conglomerate of thickened, lobulated folds (arrows) that fade peripherally into adjacent mucosa.

Despite the classic teaching that patients with isolated gastric varices have splenic vein obstruction rather than portal hypertension, it has previously been shown that these individuals are more likely to have portal hypertension as the pathophysiologic basis for the varices, even in the absence of esophageal varices (11). In our series, all five patients with isolated gastric varices on barium studies had liver disease and/or portal hypertension as the cause of the varices. Although this is a small number of patients, our findings suggest that tumorous varices in the stomach (without esophageal varices) are more likely to be caused by portal hypertension than by splenic vein obstruction.

In conclusion, a conglomerate mass of gastric varices was found in 14% of all patients with radiographically diagnosed gastric varices, so tumorous varices are more common lesions than has generally been recognized. Tumorous varices manifest as remarkably similar findings on double-contrast barium studies, usually appearing en face as a conglomerate of thickened, lobulated folds and in profile as smooth, undulating, submucosal masses on the posteromedial border of the gastric fundus. It is important to be aware of the characteristic features of tumorous gastric varices on double-contrast studies so that they are not mistaken for neoplastic lesions in the stomach.

References

1. Levine MS. Varices. In: Gore RM, Levine MS, Laufer I, eds. Textbook of gastrointestinal radiology. Philadelphia, Pa: Saunders, 1994; 499–511.
2. Evans JA, Delany F. Gastric varices. Radiology 1953; 60:46–51.
3. Wohl GT, Shore L. Lesions of the cardiac end of stomach simulating carcinoma. AJR 1959; 82:1048–1057.
4. Belgrad R, Carlson HC, Payne WS, Cain JC. Pseudotumoral gastric varices. AJR 1964; 91:751–756.
5. Swischuk LE. Gastric varices presenting as "pseudotumors" of the cardia. Am J Dig Dis 1967; 12:839–844.
6. Kaye JJ, Stassa G. Mimicry and deception in the diagnosis of tumors of the gastric cardia. AJR 1970; 110:295–303.
7. Rice RP, Thompson WM, Kelvin FM, et al. Gastric varices without esophageal varices: an important preendoscopic diagnosis. JAMA 1977; 237:1976–1979.
8. Marshall JP, Smith PD, Hoyumpa AM. Gastric varices: problems in diagnosis. Am J Dig Dis 1977; 22:947–955.
9. Anderson MF, Dunnick NR. Pseudotumor caused by gastric varices. Dig Dis 1977; 22:929–932.
10. Muhletaler C, Gerlock J, Goncharenko V, et al. Gastric varices secondary to splenic vein occlusion: radiographic diagnosis and clinical significance. Radiology 1979; 132: 593–598.
11. Levine MS, Kieu K, Rubesin SE, et al. Isolated gastric varices: splenic vein obstruction or portal hypertension? Abdom Imaging 1991; 15:188–192.
12. Okuda K, Yasumoto M, Goto A, Kunisaki T. Endoscopic observations of gastric varices. Am J Gastroenterol 1973; 60:357–365.
13. Hashizume M, Kitano S, Yamaga H, et al. Endoscopic classification of gastric varices. Gastrointest Endosc 1990; 36:276–280.
14. Thakeb F, Salem SA, Abdallah M, El Batanouny M. Endoscopic diagnosis of gastric varices. Endoscopy 1994; 26:287–291.
15. Malde HM, Kedar RP, Chadha D. Isolated gastric varices: ultrasound detection. Abdom Imaging 1993; 18:229–231.
16. Sauerbruch T, Kleber G. Upper gastrointestinal endoscopy in patients with portal hypertension. Endoscopy 1992; 24:45–51.
17. Smookler BH. Gastric varices: characteristics and clinical significance. Gastroenterology 1956; 31:581–587.
18. Balthazar EJ, Megibow AJ, Naidich D, LeFleur RS. Computed tomographic recognition of gastric varices. AJR 184: 142: 1121–1125.
19. Boyce GA, Sivak MV, Rosch T, et al. Evaluation of submucosal upper gastrointestinal tract lesions by endoscopic ultrasound. Gastrointest Endosc 1991; 37:449–454.
20. Boustiere C, Dumas O, Jouffre C, et al. Endoscopic ultrasonography classification of gastric varices in patients with cirrhosis: comparison with endoscopic findings. J Hepatol 1993; 19:268–272.
21. Burtin P, Cales P, Oberti F, et al. Endoscopic ultrasonographic signs of portal hypertension in cirrhosis. Gastrointest Endosc 1996; 44:257–261.

Evelyne M. Loyer, MD
Hsiao Chin, MD[2]
Ronelle A. DuBrow, MD
Cynthia L. David, MD
Farzin Eftekhari, MD
Chusilp Charnsangavej, MD

Index terms:
Bile ducts, neoplasms, 76.321
Computed tomography (CT), contrast enhancement, 76.12113, 76.12114
Computed tomography (CT), helical, 76.12115
Liver, CT, 76.12111, 76.12113, 76.12114, 76.12115
Liver neoplasms, 76.321, 76.323

Radiology 1999; 212:866–875

Abbreviations:
HAP = hepatic arterial phase
HCC = hepatocellular carcinoma
PVP = portal venous phase

[1] From the Department of Diagnostic Radiology, the University of Texas M. D. Anderson Cancer Center, Box 57, 1515 Holcombe Blvd, Houston, TX 77030. Received January 7, 1998; revision requested March 6; final revision received November 23; accepted March 8, 1999. **Address reprint requests to** E.M.L. (e-mail: *eloyer@di.mdacc.tmc.edu*).

[2] Current address: Department of Radiology, Memorial City Hospital, Houston, Tex.

Hepatocellular Carcinoma and Intrahepatic Peripheral Cholangiocarcinoma: Enhancement Patterns with Quadruple Phase Helical CT—A Comparative Study[1]

PURPOSE: To define the hemodynamic features of hepatocellular carcinoma (HCC) and intrahepatic cholangiocarcinoma by using quadruple phase helical computed tomography (CT) and determine the value of this information in characterizing tumors.

MATERIALS AND METHODS: Helical CT of the liver was performed in 45 patients with newly diagnosed HCC or peripheral cholangiocarcinoma. Scans were obtained before and 25 seconds, 70 seconds, and 2–6 minutes after the start of the contrast material injection. The intensity and spatial distribution of contrast material uptake were evaluated during all phases. Time-attenuation curves were established for each lesion. Relative attenuation and lesion conspicuity were assessed. A diagnostic confidence level was assigned to each lesion.

RESULTS: In the majority of HCC lesions, a single, early peak of enhancement followed by a continuous decrease in tumor attenuation over time was seen. The greatest tumor conspicuity occurred during the delayed phase. In cholangiocarcinoma, tumor attenuation increased during the delayed phase. In the majority of lesions, the greatest tumor conspicuity was seen during the portal venous phase. In both tumor types, the diagnostic confidence level improved when the delayed phase was used.

CONCLUSION: The variation over time in the intensity of contrast enhancement in HCC and cholangiocarcinoma differs sufficiently to make this a useful diagnostic criterion. The delayed phase is particularly important because it amplifies this difference.

The enhancement characteristics of hepatic tumors at dynamic computed tomography (CT) are influenced by their histologic type. The capability of helical CT to enable scanning of the entire liver sequentially during the hepatic arterial and portal venous phases (HAP and PVP, respectively) of enhancement affords the opportunity to study the temporal evolution of the contrast enhancement of hepatic tumors and to use this information to predict, to some extent, the pathologic diagnosis. Nodular hepatocellular carcinoma (HCC) and peripheral cholangiocarcinoma exhibit very different pathologic features and have been shown to have different patterns of enhancement (1–6). In this study, we compared the enhancement patterns of HCC and peripheral cholangiocarcinoma by using quadruple phase helical CT. Our purpose was to define the evolution of enhancement of each tumor type over time by using helical CT and determine the usefulness of this information for tumor characterization.

Author contributions:
Guarantor of integrity of entire study, E.M.L.; study concepts, C.C.; study design, E.M.L., C.C.; definition of intellectual content, C.C.; literature research, H.C.; clinical studies, all authors; data acquisition, H.C., R.A.D., E.M.L., C.L.D., F.E.; data analysis, all authors; manuscript preparation and editing, H.C., E.M.L.; manuscript review, C.C., E.M.L., R.A.D.

MATERIALS AND METHODS

Forty-five consecutive patients (26 men, 19 women; age range, 22–75 years; mean age, 66 years) with newly diagnosed nodular HCC or peripheral cholangiocarcinoma underwent imaging between April 1995 and February 1996 by means of a uniform quadruple phase helical CT technique. All of these patients had biopsy-proved HCC or cholangiocarcinoma. Twenty-five patients had HCC, 19 patients had cholangiocarcinoma, and one patient had mixed HCC and cholangiocarcinoma. The dominant lesion, and at least one smaller lesion when the disease was multifocal, was characterized. Lesions were classified by size into one of the following three groups: 5 cm or larger, at least 2 cm but smaller than 5 cm, or smaller than 2 cm (mean, 5.7 cm).

All scans were obtained by using a CT HiSpeed Advantage scanner (GE Medical Systems, Milwaukee, Wis). First, nonenhanced axial scans with 10-mm collimation were acquired. Then, contrast material–enhanced helical CT of the entire liver was performed during a single breath hold by using 7–10-mm collimation with a 1.0:1.0 or 1.5:1.0 pitch in a craniocaudal direction. The scanning sequences were initiated 25 seconds, 70 seconds, and 2-6 minutes (mean, 3 minutes 10 seconds) after the start of the intravenous injection of 150 mL of 60% nonionic contrast material (iohexol [Omnipaque 300]; Nycomed, Princeton, NJ) at a rate of 2.5 mL/sec. This rate was chosen because it can be achieved consistently. This scanning protocol provided three sets of scans that corresponded to the HAP (25 seconds), PVP (70 seconds), and delayed phase (2-6 minutes) of contrast enhancement. The time required to acquire each set of scans was 20–30 seconds. Because this technique did not add any risk compared with conventional abdominal CT, and because at our institution patients sign a general consent form that covers all diagnostic studies, neither institutional review board approval nor informed consent was considered to be necessary.

The lesions were assessed objectively and subjectively. In the objective analyses, the CT attenuation coefficients of tumors were measured during four different phases. The regions of interest were chosen by one radiologist (H.C.). The enhancement of the heterogeneously enhancing lesions was evaluated in the areas where there was more homogeneous enhancement. Film hard-copy images were reviewed by at least three of the radiologists (E.M.L., R.A.D., C.L.D., F.E., C.C.) who participated in the study. If more than one region of interest was selected in large heterogeneously enhancing tumors, then the region of interest used for analysis was chosen by consensus. Measurements of the solid component of the tumor and of the normal liver parenchyma were obtained from the same areas on the four scans (obtained during the four different phases). By using these data, time-attenuation curves and curves of differences in attenuation between the tumor and liver parenchyma were established.

The attenuation values of uninvolved liver parenchyma measured in both tumor types were compared by using the Mann-Whitney test. *P* values were computed by using Stat Exact software (Cytel, Cambridge, Mass). A *P* value of less than .05 denoted statistical significance.

In the subjective analyses, tumor attenuation was graded with respect to the surrounding liver parenchyma. Five radiologists (E.M.L., H.C., R.A.D., C.L.D., F.E., C.C.) interpreted the scans and established a consensus grade without knowledge of the tissue diagnosis. The scans were evaluated with both narrow (window width, 100 HU; window level, 60–90 HU) and soft-tissue (width, 400 HU; level, 70–80 HU) window settings. On all four sets of scans, the lesions were classified as hyperattenuating, isoattenuating, or hypoattenuating relative to the adjacent parenchyma. Heterogeneously enhancing lesions were classified as hyperattenuating when most of the solid tumor was enhancing.

The lesions that were hyperattenuating or hypoattenuating were further subdivided into the following three categories according to their conspicuity: 1, barely visible against the surrounding liver parenchyma; 2, intermediately obvious; or 3, extremely obvious. Consequently, the following seven categories were defined: hyperattenuating 3, hyperattenuating 2, hyperattenuating 1, isoattenuating, hypoattenuating 1, hypoattenuating 2, hypoattenuating 3. Lesions with the highest relative attenuation were described as hyperattenuating 3, and those with the lowest relative attenuation were described as hypoattenuating 3. Each lesion was assigned to four categories, one for each set of scans, which together expressed a qualitative assessment of the tumor attenuation and conspicuity over time. By using these data, a curve of the relative attenuation of the tumor over time was established for each lesion.

Ancillary findings also were documented and included the presence of a capsule, tumor thrombus, arterioportal shunting, cirrhosis, ascites, adenopathy, biliary obstruction, calcification, and/or necrosis. A diagnosis of each case was established by consensus on the basis of the subjective appreciation of the enhancement pattern, morphologic characteristics, and ancillary findings. A confidence level for each diagnosis was then assigned.

To determine the importance of the delayed phase, the studies were reviewed a second time, after a delay of 2 months, by using the scans obtained before contrast material administration and those obtained during the HAP and PVP. Diagnoses were established a second time, and the diagnostic confidence levels were assigned and compared with the confidence levels reached when all four phases were used initially.

RESULTS

Hepatocellular Carcinoma

Morphologic features.—We analyzed 40 HCC lesions in 25 patients. Twenty-two lesions were 5 cm or larger, 10 were 2 cm or larger but smaller than 5 cm, and eight were smaller than 2 cm. The tumor was unifocal in 13 (52%), multifocal with a dominant mass in 10 (40%), and multifocal without a dominant mass in two (8%) patients. A mosaic pattern was present in seven (28%), a capsule was seen in 16 (64%), and necrosis characterized by an area of attenuation close to that of water was seen in 10 (40%) patients. Portal or hepatic vein thrombosis was seen in 10 patients (40%), and arterioportal shunting was seen in two (8%). Radiologic evidence of cirrhosis was present in five (20%) patients. Other features included the following: ascites in 10 (40%) patients, lymphadenopathy in eight (32%) patients, focal biliary dilatation in two (8%) patients, and calcification in two (8%) patients.

Enhancement characteristics.—The CT attenuation measurements revealed a pattern of enhancement characterized by a single peak of enhancement during the HAP and/or PVP followed by a decrease in attenuation over time in 38 (95%) of the 40 lesions (Fig 1). The mean attenuation values during the precontrast phase, HAP, PVP, and delayed phase were 33, 61, 90, and 69 HU, respectively. The highest attenuation coefficients were measured on the PVP scans in 30 lesions, on the PVP and HAP scans in eight lesions, and on the HAP scans alone in none. Attenuation measurements demonstrated no enhancement in two lesions. There was no difference in the delay time of enhancement when the size of the lesions was considered. On average, the CT attenuation of tumors during the PVP increased 180% compared with those during the precontrast phase. A decrease in contrast enhancement over time was seen in all but one lesion.

Although attenuation measurements on the delayed phase scans were, in general, higher than those on the HAP scans, they were lower than those on the PVP scans by 20 HU or more in 21 lesions and by less than 20 HU in 15 lesions. The attenuation during the delayed phase was equal to that during the PVP in three lesions. In one lesion, the attenuation was higher during the delayed phase, but only by 13 HU. The difference in attenuation coefficients between the tumor and the surrounding liver parenchyma was highest during the PVP and/or delayed phase in 29 lesions, during the HAP and PVP in four lesions, and during the HAP only in one lesion. In six lesions, the differences in attenuation between the tumor and the normal liver parenchyma were similar during all phases.

In the subjective analysis, the lesions were classified into two groups based on the presence (group 1) (Fig 2) or absence (group 2) of hyperattenuation relative to the liver parenchyma. The lesions in both groups, however, were similarly characterized by a decrease over time in tumor attenuation relative to the liver parenchyma (Fig 2). There were 30 (75%) lesions in group 1. Sixteen lesions were 5 cm or larger, 10 lesions were at least 2 cm but smaller than 5 cm, and four lesions were smaller than 2 cm.

On the precontrast scans, all lesions were either isoattenuating (n = 13) or hypoattenuating (n = 17) relative to the surrounding liver parenchyma. After intravenous contrast material enhancement, all lesions became hyperattenuating. Enhancement relative to the surrounding liver appeared to be at its maximum during the HAP in 18 lesions (60%), during the PVP in eight (27%) lesions, and during both phases in four (13%) lesions (Fig 3a). In the four latter cases, the degree of enhancement achieved during the HAP persisted to be unchanged during the PVP. This peak in relative attenuation was followed in all cases by a continuous decrease in relative attenuation (Fig 3a). There was no difference in the evolution of contrast material uptake when the size of the lesions was considered.

There were 10 (25%) lesions in group 2. Six lesions were 5 cm or larger, and four were smaller than 2 cm. On the precontrast scans, all lesions were either isoattenuating (n = 4) or hypoattenuating (n = 6). Following intravenous contrast material enhancement, none of these lesions became hyperattenuating; they remained isoattenuating or hypoattenuating relative to the liver parenchyma. The attenuation scores (Fig 3b), however, indicated a change in the relative tumor attenuation over time. Three lesions had a relative increase in attenuation during the HAP, and one lesion had an increase in attenuation during the PVP; the peaks of enhancement in both these groups of lesions were followed by a decrease in attenuation thereafter. In six lesions, only a decrease in the relative tumor attenuation was observed over time; this occurred during the PVP and delayed phase (Fig 3b). A comparison with the objective attenuation measurements in these six lesions, however, showed that a peak of enhancement did occur during the PVP in three lesions and during the HAP and PVP in one lesion. Attenuation measurements confirmed the absence of enhancement in two of these six tumors.

Overall, in the subjective analysis, a single peak of enhancement was seen in 34 (85%) of the 40 lesions. The lowest relative tumor attenuation was observed on the scans obtained during the delayed phase in 31 (78%) lesions. The attenuation was lowest during the delayed phase alone in 23 (58%) lesions. In 17 lesions (42%), the lowest relative tumor attenuation was observed during more than one phase; the delayed phase was one of these phases in eight of these cases. Tumor conspicuity varied with the phase of enhancement and was judged to be maximal during one phase or frequently during two phases, but rarely during three of the four phases. The delayed phase was among the phases chosen for its highest conspicuity in 30 lesions (75%), whereas the HAP, PVP, or precontrast phase was among the phases chosen respectively, in six, 16, and three lesions.

In 16 (40%) lesions, a capsule was identified and the time of enhancement of the capsule differed from that of the tumor. The capsule was seen on the precontrast study as a hypoattenuating, often incomplete ring in six lesions. It was

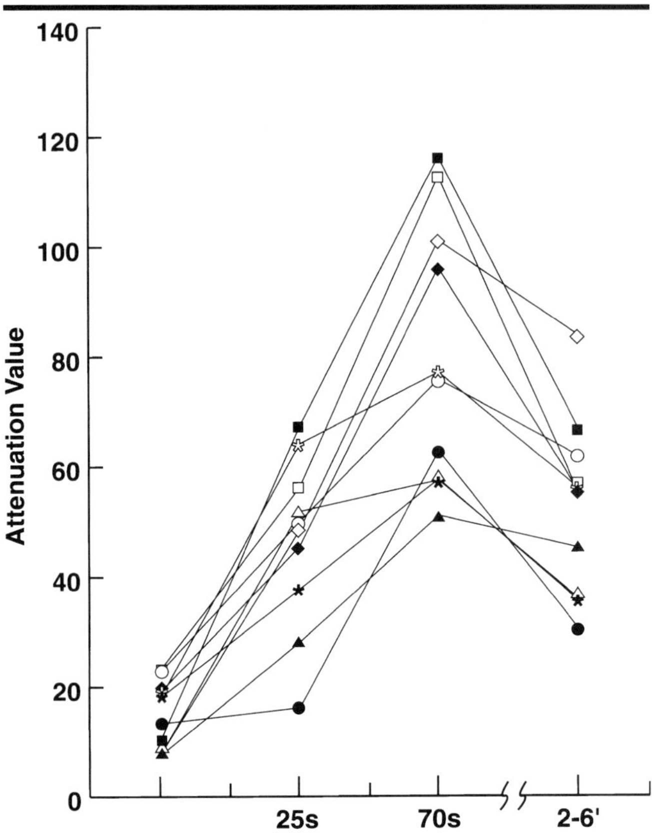

Figure 1. Graph illustrating objective analysis of HCC lesions. □, ○, ◆, ◇, open asterisk, *, ●, ■, △, and ▲ represent the attenuation values of the 10 tumors. Time-attenuation curves for 10 tumors measuring at least 2 cm but less than 5 cm show a single peak of enhancement during the PVP followed by a decrease in attenuation over time. The time-attenuation curves for the tumors 5 cm or larger and for tumors smaller than 2 cm were similar to these.

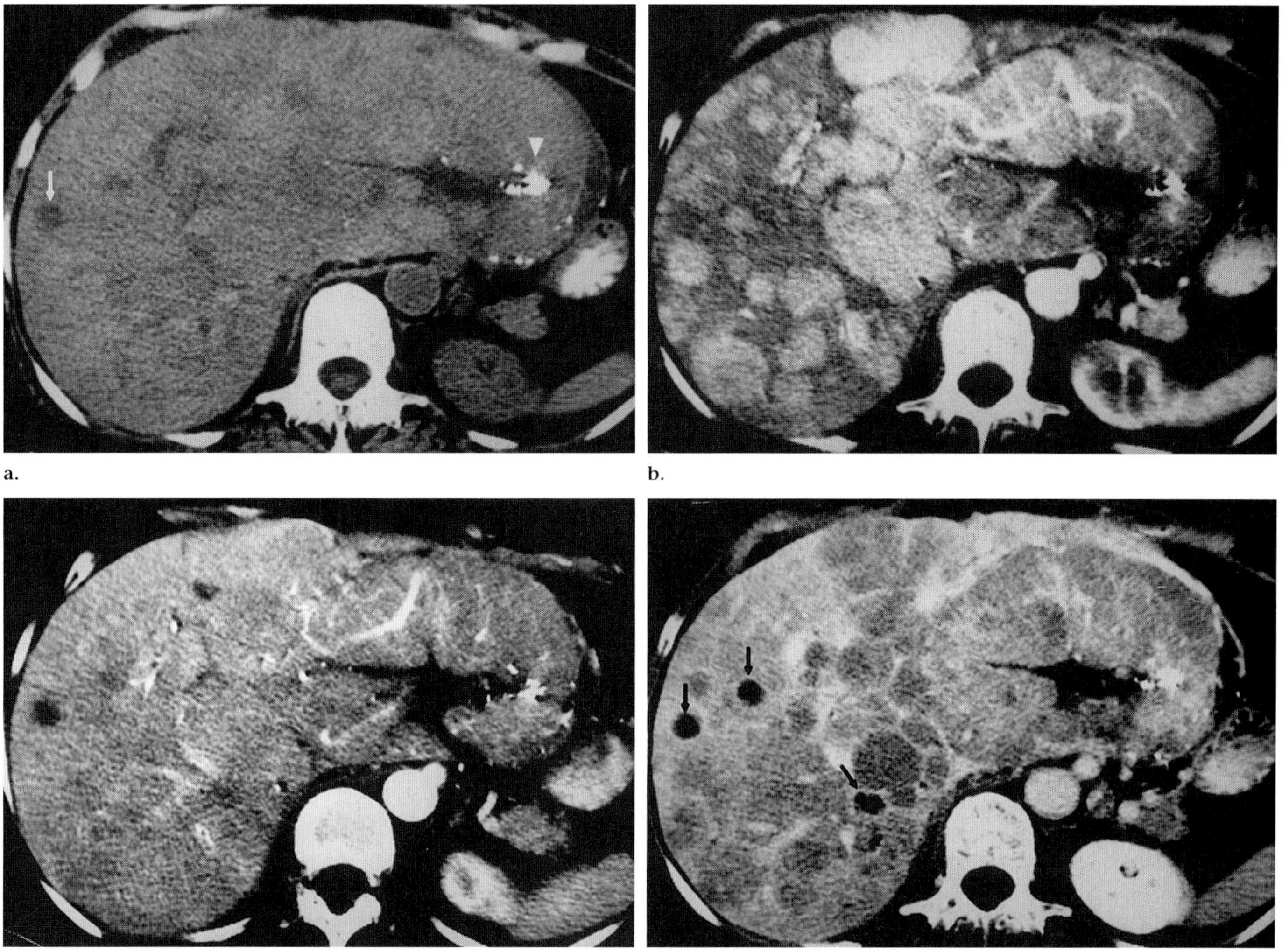

a. b. c. d.

Figure 2. (**a–d**) Axial abdominal CT scans obtained during the (**a**) precontrast phase, (**b**) HAP, (**c**) PVP, and (**d**) delayed phase demonstrate the HCC enhancement pattern. (**a**) Precontrast scan shows enlargement of the liver. There is loss of the normal vascular anatomy but no definite focal change in attenuation. During the subjective evaluation, this tumor was judged to be isoattenuating. One small tumor nodule (arrow) is of lower attenuation than the surrounding liver parenchyma. The high-attenuating material (arrowhead) in the left lobe is a result of prior chemoembolization. (**b**) HAP scan shows marked increase in relative tumor attenuation and conspicuity. The dominant mass in the left lobe and the tumor nodules were judged to be hyperattenuating 3. (**c**) PVP scan shows decrease in relative tumor attenuation and conspicuity. The tumor was judged to be isoattenuating. (**d**) Delayed phase scan shows further decrease in relative tumor attenuation and increase in conspicuity. The tumor was judged to be hypoattenuating 3. The areas of very low attenuation (arrows) correspond to tumor nodules demonstrating a more pronounced loss of contrast.

also seen as a hypoattenuating ring during the HAP in five of these six lesions. The capsule was seen as an enhancing rim during the PVP in seven lesions and during the delayed phase in all 16 lesions.

The diagnosis of HCC was established in 24 (96%) of the 25 patients on the basis of morphologic and subjective analysis of the enhancement characteristics. When the cases were reviewed a second time by using the same scoring system but without the aid of the delayed phase scans, the correct diagnosis was made again in the same 24 patients. Although there was no difference in the diagnostic accuracy, the diagnostic confidence level was greater in 14 (56%) cases when the delayed phase scans were available.

Intrahepatic Peripheral Cholangiocarcinoma

Morphologic features.—A total of 42 cholangiocarcinoma lesions in 19 patients were assessed. Sixteen lesions were 5 cm or larger, 13 lesions were at least 2 cm but smaller than 5 cm, and 13 lesions were smaller than 2 cm. The disease was unifocal in six patients (32%) and multifocal in 13 (68%) patients. In 12 of the 13 patients with multifocal lesions, the dominant mass was larger than 5 cm. Tumor necrosis characterized by an area of attenuation similar to the attenuation of water was present in four patients. Biliary dilatation was seen in seven (37%), underlying cirrhosis was seen in four (21%), and ascites was seen in four (21%) patients. Lymphadenopathy was seen in 12 (63%) patients. Neither calcification, tumorous capsule, tumor thrombus, nor arterioportal shunting was seen in any patient.

Enhancement characteristics.—CT attenuation measurements indicated tumoral enhancement in all lesions, with maximum enhancement during the PVP and/or delayed phase (Fig 4). On average, CT attenuation increased by 132% during the PVP

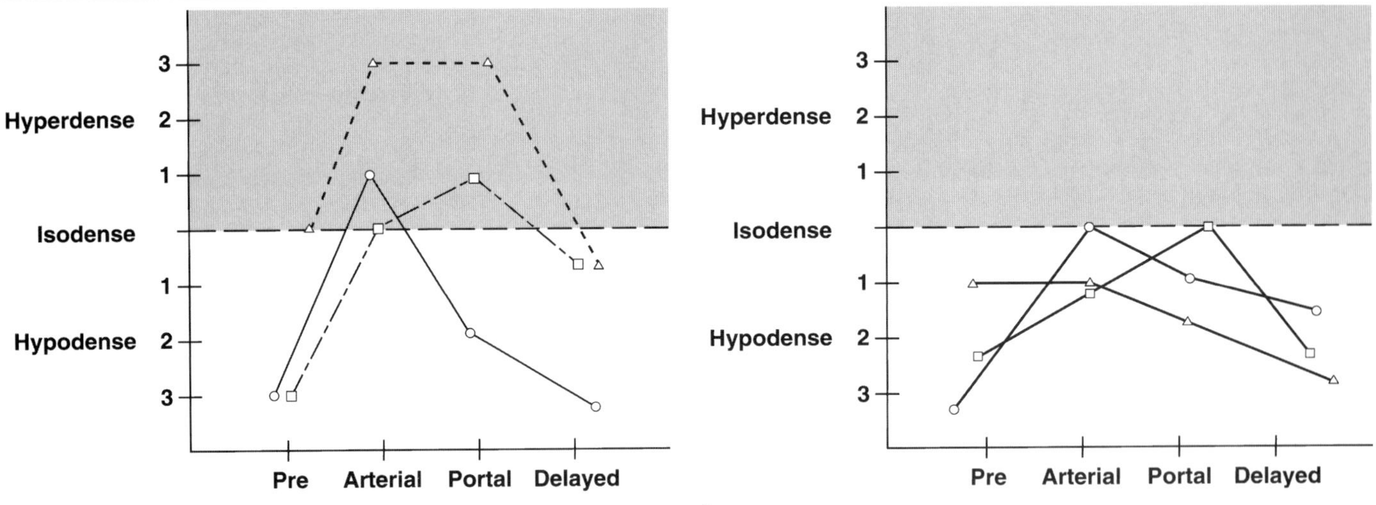

a. b.

Figure 3. Graph illustrating subjective analysis of HCC lesions. The relative tumor attenuation over time is represented. The y axis reflects the conspicuity of the lesions. *Hypodense 3* and *Hyperdense 3* indicate maximal conspicuity of hypoattenuating and hyperattenuating lesions, respectively; *Hypodense 1* and *Hyperdense 1* indicate the lowest conspicuity. Schematic curves for representative lesions in each group are shown. **(a)** In group 1, all of the tumors became hyperattenuating relative to the surrounding parenchyma. Peak enhancement is followed by a continuous decrease in tumor attenuation. The intensity of enhancement varies, as does the time to peak enhancement; maximal enhancement occurred during the HAP in 18 lesions (○), during the PVP in eight lesions (□), and during both phases in four lesions (△). **(b)** In group 2, all of the tumors remained hypoattenuating relative to the surrounding parenchyma. However, a relative increase in attenuation was appreciated during the HAP (○) in three lesions and during the PVP (□) in one lesion. Although less intense, the relative tumor attenuation curves for these lesions were similar in shape to the curves for group 1. In six lesions, only a decrease in the relative tumor attenuation during the PVP and delayed phase (△) was seen.

compared with the attenuation during the precontrast phase. The mean CT attenuations during the precontrast phase, HAP, PVP, and delayed phase were 23, 31, 56, and 61 HU, respectively. Measurement of CT attenuation on the delayed phase scans indicated a persistence of or further increase in tumoral enhancement. Attenuation measurements during the delayed phase were higher than those during the PVP in 31 (74%) lesions (by more than 20 HU in five lesions, by 10–20 HU in 11 lesions, and by less than 10 HU in 15 lesions). A decrease in the objective measurement was seen in 11 lesions (26%), but it was a difference of only 2–4 HU. The difference in attenuation between the tumor and surrounding liver parenchyma was maximal during the PVP.

Mean Attenuation Coefficients of the Normal Liver Parenchyma in Patients with HCC and in Patients with Cholangiocarcinoma

Carcinoma Group	Precontrast Phase	HAP	PVP	Delayed Phase
HCC	47	62	105	96
Cholangiocarcinoma	38	48	98	79

All values are in Hounsfield units.

The results of subjective analysis showed that all lesions were either hypoattenuating (35 lesions) or isoattenuating (seven lesions) on the precontrast scans. After intravenous contrast material enhancement, three lesions became hyperattenuating and three lesions became isoattenuating. The other 36 lesions remained predominantly hypoattenuating during the HAP and PVP (Fig 5). In 18 lesions, however, the attenuation scores indicated that despite persistent hypoattenuation, the relative tumor attenuation actually increased during the HAP (Fig 6). The attenuation scores remained similar to those during the precontrast study in 21 lesions and decreased in three lesions (Fig 6). The lowest relative tumor attenuation was seen during the PVP in 36 (86%) of the 42 lesions. In contrast, the delayed phase compared with the PVP was characterized by an increase in relative tumor attenuation in 27 lesions (64%) (Fig 6a), no change in 12 lesions (Fig 6b), and a decrease in relative attenuation in three lesions. In addition, in 14 lesions, the distribution of contrast material in the lesion migrated centrally during the delayed phase; this bull's eye pattern is also seen with adenocarcinoma but not with HCC. Lesion conspicuity varied according to the enhancement phase and was judged to be maximal during the PVP in 36 (86%) lesions.

In all 19 patients, the diagnosis of cholangiocarcinoma was predicted accurately on the basis of morphologic characteristics and subjective analysis of enhancement. When the scans were reviewed a second time by using the same scoring system but without the benefit of the delayed phase scans, the diagnosis was made correctly in 18 patients. Confidence in the diagnosis was greater in nine patients (47%) when the delayed phase scans were available.

Mixed HCC and Cholangiocarcinoma

One lesion had mixed characteristics at CT. According to subjective analysis, the relative attenuation increased continuously over time. By using only the precontrast phase, HAP, and PVP scans, this lesion was judged to be HCC. The delayed phase scans showed a further increase in attenuation, which suggested the diagnosis of cholangiocarcinoma. The pathologic diagnosis was mixed HCC and cholangiocarcinoma.

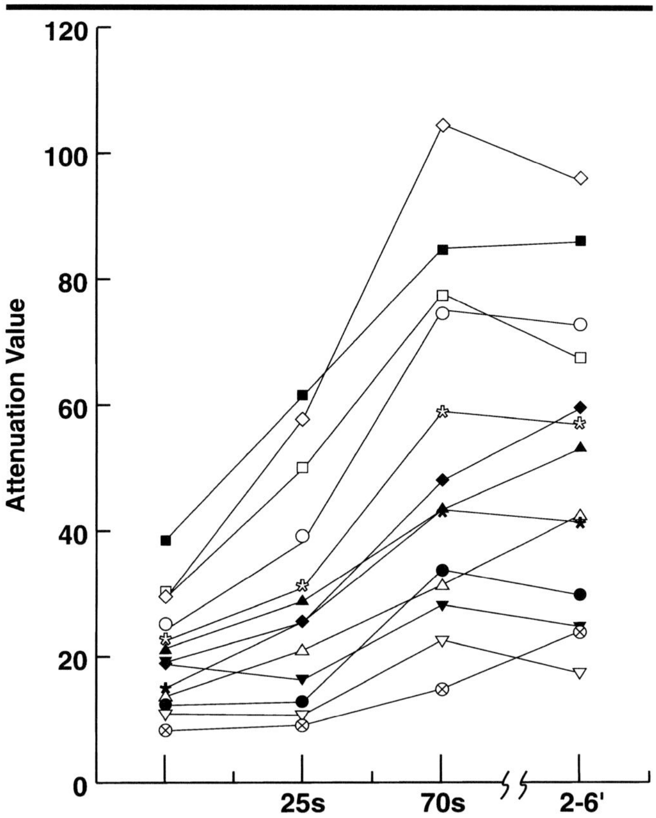

Figure 4. Graph illustrating objective evaluation of cholangiocarcinoma. ■, □, ◇, ○, open asterisk, ▲, ▼, ◆, *, △, ●, ▽, and ⊗ represent the attenuation values of the 13 tumors. Time-attenuation curves for 13 tumors measuring at least 2 cm but less than 5 cm show a tendency toward increased attenuation over time. Note that the y axis differs from that in Figure 1. The time-attenuation curves for tumors equal to or larger than 5 cm and for tumors smaller than 2 cm were identical to these.

Attenuation of Nontumorous Liver Parenchyma

The attenuation values of uninvolved liver were higher in the HCC group than in the cholangiocarcinoma group (Table). These differences were found to be significant during the precontrast (Mann-Whitney test, $P = .015$) and delayed (Mann-Whitney test, $P = .028$) phases and showed a trend during the HAP (Mann-Whitney test, $P = .088$).

DISCUSSION

Tumor enhancement may be characterized by intensity, spatial distribution of contrast material, and most important, the evolution over time of both of these parameters. In this study, we focused on the temporal evolution of contrast material uptake by HCCs and peripheral cholangiocarcinomas. We assessed the changes over time in relative tumor attenuation (subjective evaluation), in the attenuation coefficient values of the tumors (objective evaluation), and in the spatial distribution of contrast material.

The results obtained with subjective grading and objective measurement of attenuation coefficients differed in some aspects. With HCCs, on the basis of subjective measurements, peak enhancement occurred during the HAP in 21 (52%) lesions, whereas with objective measurements, it occurred during the PVP in 38 (95%) lesions. Both sets of data, however, showed a single, early peak of enhancement followed by a continuous decrease in attenuation. This was observed by using subjective measurements in 34 (85%) tumors and by using attenuation measurements in 38 (95%) tumors.

With cholangiocarcinomas, enhancement could be defined by using attenuation measurements, but was more difficult to appreciate by using subjective analysis because the majority of the lesions remained hypoattenuating during the HAP and PVP. Both the objective and subjective data, however, demonstrated a similar tendency for delayed accumulation of contrast material as opposed to the washout seen with HCC. This accumulation was seen by using subjective measurements in 27 (64%) lesions and by using attenuation measurements in 31 (74%) lesions.

The apparent discordance between the subjective and objective evaluations can be explained. Subjective evaluation involves the visual appreciation of the difference in attenuation between the liver parenchyma and tumor and is dependent on the enhancement of the normal liver parenchyma as well as that of the tumor. With HCC, the attenuation of the tumor during the PVP is maximal, but it is lower than that of the surrounding liver parenchyma; therefore, the tumor appears to be hypoattenuating. In contrast, during the HAP, the attenuation measurement of the tumor is equal to or higher than that of the surrounding liver parenchyma; therefore, the tumor appears to be isoattenuating or hyperattenuating even though the absolute tumor attenuation measurement is lower than that during the PVP.

With cholangiocarcinoma, the tumor attenuation is lower than that of the surrounding liver parenchyma during all phases; therefore, the tumor remains hypoattenuating according to subjective analysis. Although enhancement during the PVP is not appreciated because of the high attenuation of the surrounding liver parenchyma, it may be appreciated during the delayed phase as the attenuation of the surrounding liver parenchyma decreases.

Our findings with respect to the enhancement of HCC concur with those of studies by Araki et al (3) and Hosoki et al (7,8), who also used measurements of tumor attenuation coefficients after contrast material injection to show that tumoral enhancement follows a time-attenuation curve that ascends and descends rapidly. In these studies, maximal enhancement occurred during the HAP. In our study, the highest attenuation coefficients were measured during the PVP. This difference is possibly related to a more rapid administration of contrast material in these studies than that in our protocol.

A similar temporal evolution of enhancement in HCCs has also been described by using subjective evaluations. Honda et al (9) assessed tumoral enhancement at 45 seconds and 6 minutes after contrast material injection. Thirty-eight (56%) of 68 lesions showed diffuse, pe-

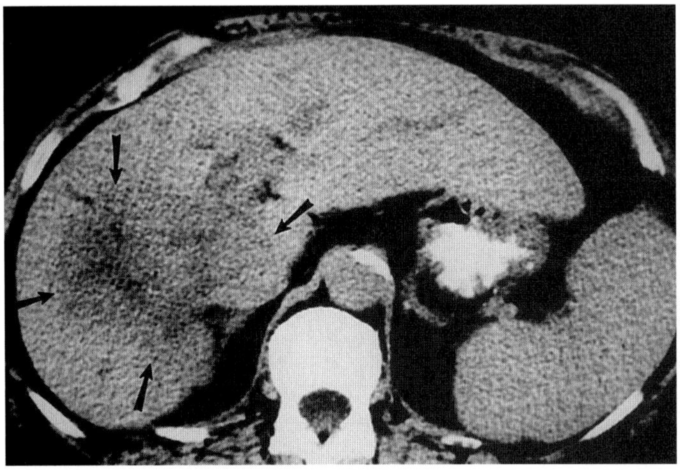

a.

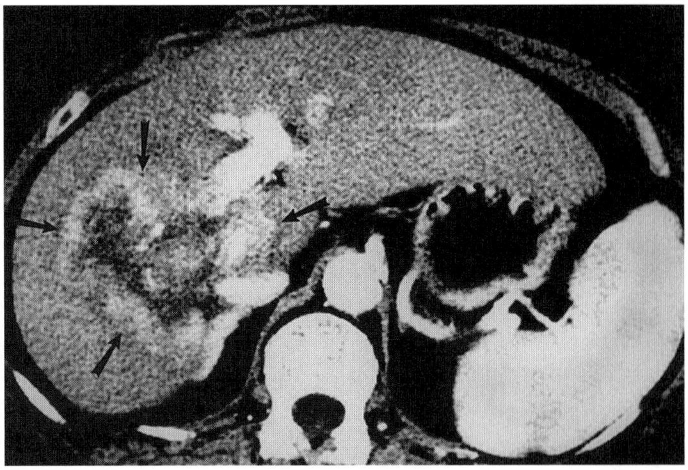

b.

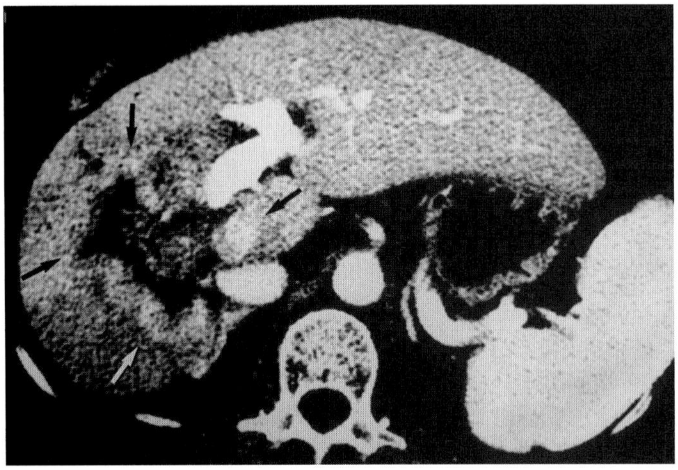

c.

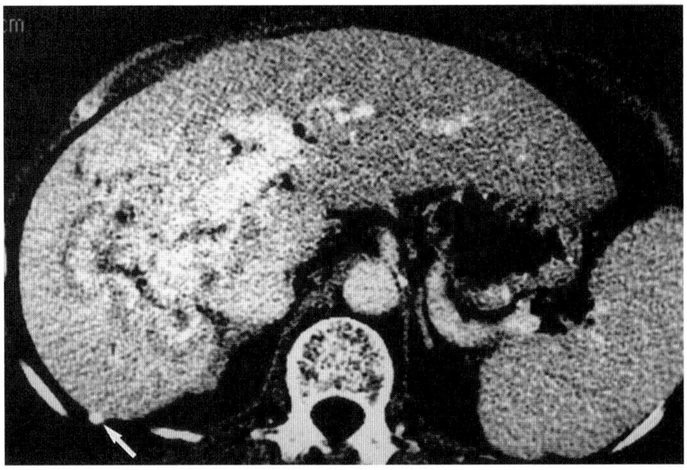

d.

Figure 5. **(a–d)** Axial abdominal CT scans obtained during the **(a)** precontrast, **(b)** HAP, **(c)** PVP, and delayed phase demonstrate the enhancement pattern of cholangiocarcinoma. **(a)** Precontrast scan shows an area of ill-defined hypoattenuation (arrows) in the right lobe. The mass was judged to the hypoattenuating 2 in the subjective assessment. **(b)** HAP scan shows peripheral enhancement (arrows). The attenuation of most of the tumor, however, similar to that on the precontrast study (**a**), is hypoattenuating 2. **(c)** PVP scan shows the mass (arrows) to have decreased relative attenuation and increased conspicuity. This tumor was judged to be hypoattenuating 3 in the subjective evaluation. **(d)** Delayed phase scan shows increased relative tumor attenuation with central migration of contrast material. This tumor was judged to be hyperattenuating 3 in the subjective evaluation. An enhancing capsular vein (arrow) also is seen.

ripheral, or mixed enhancement during the early phase and apparent decreased attenuation during the delayed phase. Twenty-eight (41%) of the 68 lesions did not show enhancement, and two (3%) lesions increased in attenuation on the delayed phase scans. The long interval between the two scanning phases, however, raises the possibility that enhancement, which is transient, might have been missed in some of these tumors. Cho et al (10) evaluated the scans obtained in 84 HCC lesions during the HAP (20–45 seconds), PVP (55–90 seconds), and delayed (2–4 minutes) phases of contrast enhancement. Seventy-three (87%) of these lesions showed moderate to marked hyperattenuation during the HAP, and 67 (80%) were hypoattenuating during the delayed phase. Similarly, Takayasu et al (11) evaluated 18 HCCs smaller than 3 cm and found a single peak of enhancement. They described this pattern as low attenuating on nonenhanced scans, high attenuating on early enhanced scans, and low attenuating on late enhanced scans. This pattern was seen in 16 (89%) of the lesions.

Most frequently in HCC, relative hyperattenuation is maximal during the HAP, but peak enhancement during the PVP or during the overlapping HAP and PVP can occur, as it did in some of our cases (22% and 10% of lesions, respectively, when they were evaluated subjectively). Variations in the time to peak enhancement among lesions have been reported by other investigators (10,12) as well. Improved rates of detecting HCCs by using biphasic contrast-enhanced helical CT were reported by Baron et al (12); this suggests that the use of both the HAP and PVP optimizes the examination of patients suspected of having HCC. Although we did not study the sensitivity of our technique, the results of our study also suggest that the use of both phases is important in this patient population because the time to maximal enhancement is not constant.

The results of our study confirm the value of the delayed phase in the detection and characterization of HCCs. Capsular or septal enhancement, when present,

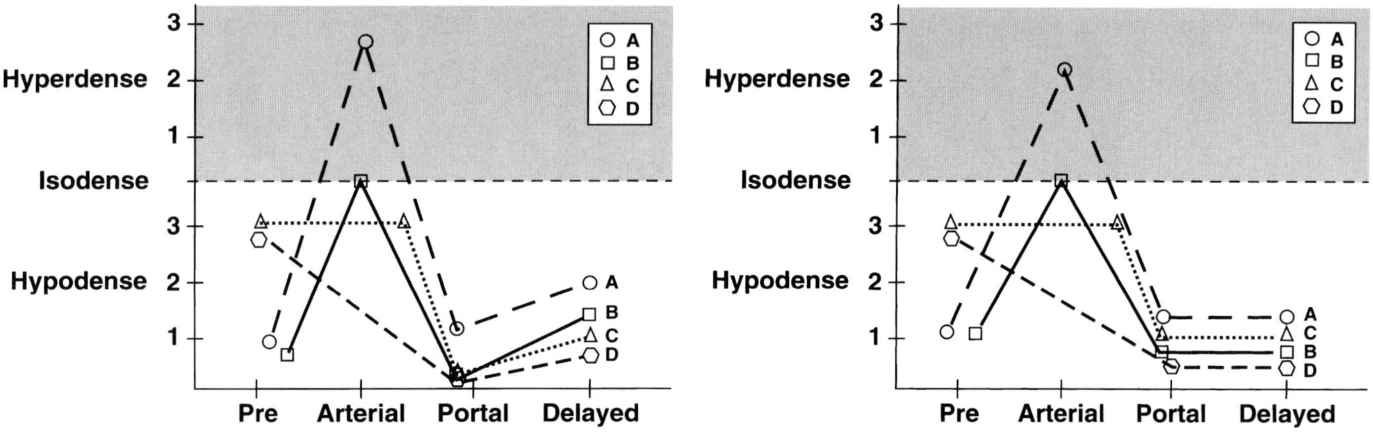

a.

b.

Figure 6. Graph illustrating subjective analysis of cholangiocarcinoma. **(a, b)** The y axis reflects the conspicuity of the lesions. *Hypodense 3* and *Hyperdense 3* indicate maximal conspicuity for hypoattenuating and hyperattenuating lesions, respectively; *Hypodense 1* and *Hyperdense 1* indicate the lowest conspicuity. Schematic curves for the representative lesions are shown. Peak enhancement occurred during the HAP in 18 tumors (○ and □). The remaining 24 tumors did not appear to enhance during the HAP (△ and ⬡). **(b)** All cholangiocarcinoma lesions were characterized by a decrease in relative attenuation during the PVP. Unlike in HCC lesions, a further decrease in relative attenuation was not seen during the delayed phase, but rather an increase in relative attenuation occurred in 27 lesions (○, □, △, and ⬡ in **a**). The relative tumor attenuation remained stable in 12 lesions (○, □, △, and ⬡ in **b**). A decrease in relative tumor attenuation during the delayed phase (not shown) was seen in three of 42 tumors.

occurs during this phase (4,10,13). In our study, capsular enhancement was seen during the delayed phase in 16 lesions; it was seen during the PVP in seven lesions. Hypoattenuation of tumors during the delayed phase has been reported in 88% and 80% of lesions in two different studies (10,14). This phase assisted in the detection of 13% of lesions in the study by Honda et al (14). Hwang et al (15) showed that a small number of lesions may be seen during the delayed phase only. In our study, loss of contrast during the delayed phase was seen subjectively in 85% and objectively in 95% of lesions. When delayed phase scans were available, the diagnostic confidence increased in 56% of the patients.

Although lesion conspicuity was not the focus of this study, we assessed this parameter with both subjective grading and attenuation measurements. With both methods, we found that the conspicuity of HCCs was highest during the delayed phase and poor during the HAP. The reason for the poor enhancement during the HAP compared with that in prior reports may be twofold. We used an injection rate of 2.5 mL/sec, which is slower than the rates used by some of the other investigators. More important, the average tumor size in our population was 5.7 cm; only eight of 40 lesions were smaller than 2 cm, and four were 2 cm. The value of the HAP in the detection of small as well as large HCC lesions has been shown (12), but in general, this phase is more useful in the detection of small tumors (10,16,17). In our study, of the six lesions that were best seen on HAP scans, four were smaller than 2 cm.

Our findings on the enhancement of peripheral cholangiocarcinomas also concur with those of other researchers (5,18–20). Cholangiocarcinomas are most frequently hypoattenuating during the early phases of contrast material administration but show relatively increased attenuation on delayed phase scans (19). Cholangiocarcinomas may be hyperattenuating during the early phase of contrast enhancement, as they were in three of our cases, but this is uncommon (18,19). In our study, a delayed increase in attenuation was found subjectively in 27 (64%) lesions and objectively in 31 (74%) lesions. Three lesions showed a decrease in relative tumor attenuation during the delayed phase. Lacomis et al (5) showed that delayed tumor enhancement on scans obtained 6–36 minutes after contrast material injection may aid in the detection and characterization of cholangiocarcinomas. The tumor was seen on the delayed phase scans only in three of the 47 patients in their study (5). This pattern of delayed enhancement is indistinguishable from that observed in metastatic adenocarcinoma and may be due in part to the fibrous stroma of these tumors.

The spatial distribution of contrast material within tumors during the delayed phase may prove to be useful in evaluating cholangiocarcinomas. Peripheral enhancement on early phase scans and central enhancement surrounded by a peripheral low-attenuating area (ie, bull's eye) on delayed phase scans are known patterns of enhancement with adenocarcinomas (6,21) and have been reported with cholangiocarcinoma (21,22). In 14 of the cholangiocarcinomas that we evaluated, enhancement was initially seen at the periphery of the lesion and later in the center of the lesion with a hypoattenuating rim. Overall, we found that the use of the delayed phase increased diagnostic confidence in 47% of the patients with cholangiocarcinoma.

In conclusion, the evolutions over time of the relative CT attenuation of HCCs and of peripheral cholangiocarcinomas differ sufficiently to be a differential diagnostic criterion. Adenocarcinoma and cholangiocarcinoma cannot, however, be differentiated on the basis of their enhancement patterns. A quadruple phase spiral CT technique appears to be optimal for the characterization of primary hepatic tumors. This technique ensures the demonstration of peak HCC lesion enhancement despite individual variation in the time to maximal enhancement. With cholangiocarcinoma, the technique allows demonstration of the delayed increase in tumor attenuation. The delayed phase is particularly helpful because it exposes the opposite enhancement trends of the two tumor types (Fig 7). Enhancement of the capsule or septa, when present, in HCC and of the central migration of contrast material in cholangiocarcinoma are also demonstrated during this phase. The de-

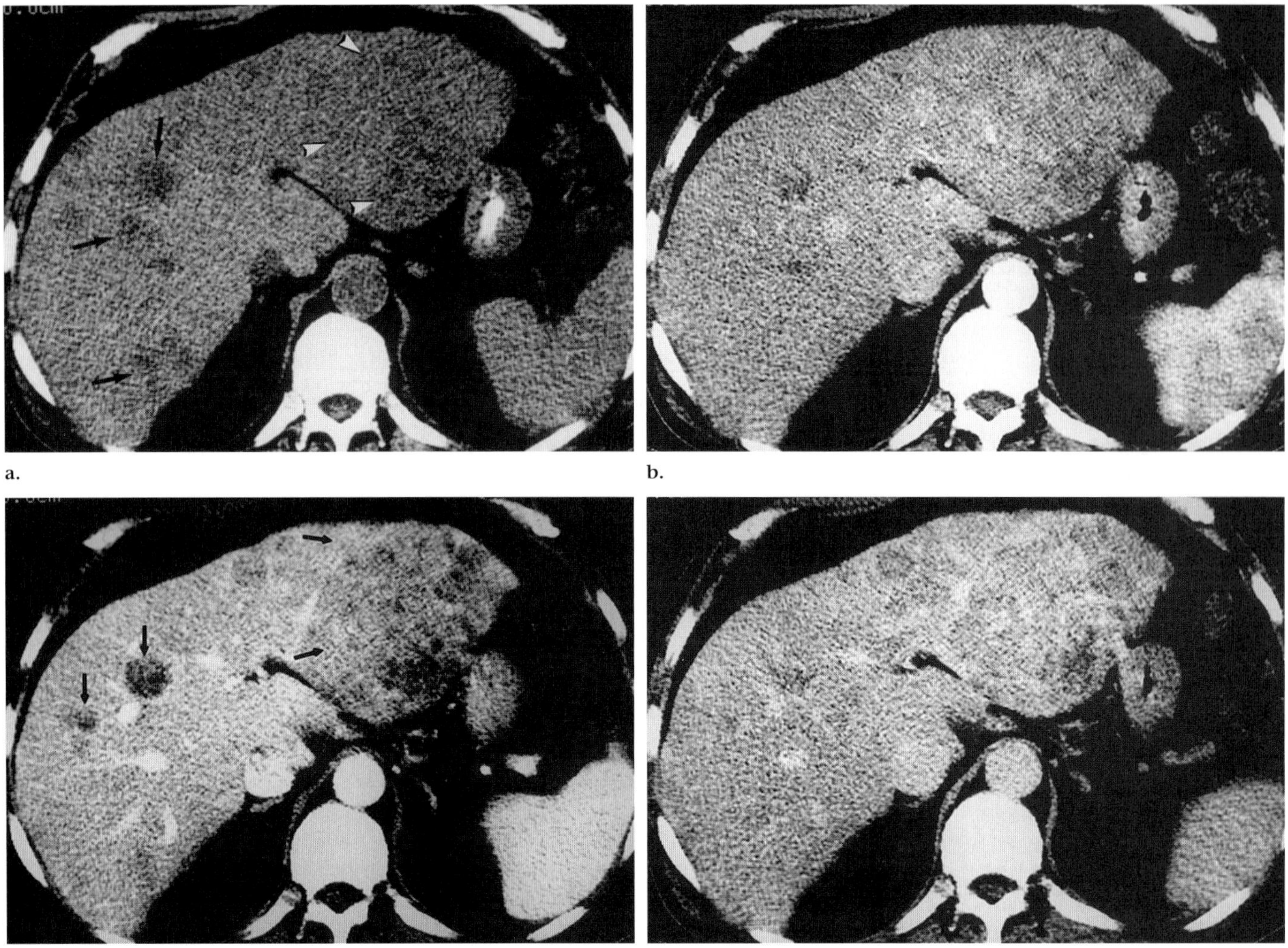

a. b. c. d.

Figure 7. (a–d) Axial abdominal CT scans obtained during the (a) precontrast phase, (b) HAP phase, (c) PVP phase, and (d) delayed phase demonstrate the value of the delayed phase. (a) Precontrast scan shows ill-defined area of low attenuation (arrowheads) occupying the lateral segment of the left liver lobe, with changes in the contour. Several hypoattenuating nodules (arrows) are seen in the right lobe. The tumor was judged to be hypoattenuating 2 in the subjective assessment. (b) HAP scan shows increased relative tumor attenuation and decreased conspicuity. The tumor was judged to be hypoattenuating 1 in the subjective evaluation. (c) PVP scan shows decreased relative attenuation of tumor nodules (arrows) and increased conspicuity. The tumor was judged to be hypoattenuating 2 in the subjective evaluation. (d) Delayed phase scan shows an increase in relative tumor attenuation. The tumor was judged to be hypoattenuating 1 in the subjective evaluation. Because this usually was not seen with HCC, the diagnosis of cholangiocarcinoma or adenocarcinoma is more likely.

lays do not need to be longer than 6 minutes (delayed time was <2 minutes 30 seconds in 20 patients), because the focus is not on an individual phase but rather on the overall pattern of enhancement over time. This short delay time allows the patient to remain on the table until completion of the examination.

Knowledge of the described characteristic patterns of enhancement will help in the evaluation of lesions that are atypical during one or more individual phases, because the overall pattern is often preserved. The results of our study also indicate that the technique of contrast material administration and the scanning delay are very important parameters to consider in the interpretation of single phase CT scans, because the expected enhancement of a particular type of lesion will vary substantially with the phase of enhancement. Finally, the observation that the uninvolved liver parenchyma has higher attenuation in the HCC group may be related to underlying cirrhosis and iron deposits in the liver of these patients.

Acknowledgment: The authors thank Elihu Estey, MD, for performing statistical analysis and Debbie Smith for secretarial assistance.

References

1. Shugihara S, Kojiro M. Pathology of cholangiocarcinoma. In: Okuda K, Ishak KG, eds. Neoplasms of the liver. Tokyo, Japan: Springer-Verlag, 1987; 143–158.
2. Kojiro M, Nakashima T. Pathology of hepatocellular carcinoma. In: Okuda K, Ishak KG, eds. Neoplasms of the liver. Tokyo, Japan: Springer-Verlag, 1987; 81–103.
3. Araki T, Itai Y, Furi S, Tasaka A. Dynamic CT densitometry of hepatic tumors. AJR 1980; 135:1037–1043.
4. Itai, Y, Ohtomo K, Kokubo T, et al. CT of hepatic masses: significance of prolonged and delayed enhancement. AJR 1986; 146: 729–733.
5. Lacomis JM, Baron RL, Oliver JH III, et al. Cholangiocarcinoma: delayed CT contrast enhancement patterns. Radiology 1997; 203:98–104.
6. Muramatsu Y, Takayasu K, Moriyama N, et al. Peripheral low-density area of hepatic tumors: CT-pathologic correlation. Radiology 1986; 160:49–52.
7. Hosoki T, Chatani M, Mori S. Dynamic

computed tomography of hepatocellular carcinoma. AJR 1982; 139:1099–1106.
8. Hosoki T, Toyonaga Y, Araki Y, Mori S. Dynamic computed tomography of isodense hepatocellular carcinoma. J Comput Assist Tomogr 1984; 8:263–268.
9. Honda H, Ochiai K, Adachi E, et al. Hepatocellular carcinoma: correlation of CT, angiographic, and histopathologic findings. Radiology 1993; 189:857–862.
10. Cho JS, Kwag JG, Oh YR, et al. Detection and characterization of hepatocellular carcinoma: value of dynamic CT during the arterial dominant phase with uniphasic contrast medium injection. J Comput Assist Tomogr 1996; 20:128–134.
11. Takayasu K, Furukawa H, Wakao F, et al. CT diagnosis of early hepatocellular carcinoma: sensitivity, findings and CT-pathologic correlation. AJR 1995; 164:885–890.
12. Baron RL, Oliver JH III, Dodd GD III, et al. Hepatocellular carcinoma: evaluation with biphasic, contrast-enhanced, helical CT. Radiology 1996; 199:505–511.
13. Lalonde L, van Beers B, Jamart J, et al. Capsule and mosaic pattern of hepatocellular carcinoma: correlation between CT and MR imaging. Gastrointest Radiol 1992; 17:241–244.
14. Honda H, Matsuura Y, Onitsuka H, et al. Differential diagnosis of hepatic tumors (hepatoma, hemangioma, and metastasis) with CT: value of two-phase incremental imaging. AJR 1992; 159:735–740.
15. Hwang GJ, Kim MJ, Yoo SK, et al. Nodular hepatocellular carcinomas: detection with arterial-, portal-, and delayed-phase images at spiral CT. Radiology 1997; 202:383–388.
16. Hollet MD, Jeffrey RB Jr, Nino-Murcia M, et al. Dual-phase helical CT of the liver: value of arterial phase scans in the detection of small (<1.5 cm) malignant hepatic neoplasms. AJR 1995; 164:879–884.
17. Choi BI, Cho JM, Han JK, et al. Spiral CT for the detection of hepatocellular carcinomas: relative value of arterial- and late-phase scanning. Abdom Imaging 1996; 21:440–444.
18. Choi BI, Park JH, Kim YI, et al. Peripheral cholangiocarcinoma and clonorchiasis: CT findings. Radiology 1988; 169:149–153.
19. Honda H, Onitsuka H, Tasumori K, et al. Intrahepatic peripheral cholangiocarcinoma: two-phased dynamic incremental CT and pathologic correlation. J Comput Assist Tomogr 1993; 17:397–402.
20. Thorsen MK, Quiroz F, Lawson TL, et al. Primary biliary carcinoma: CT evaluation. Radiology 1984; 152:479–483.
21. Itai Y, Araki T, Furui S, et al. Differential diagnosis of hepatic masses on computed tomography, with particular reference to hepatocellular carcinoma. J Comput Assist Tomogr 1981; 5:834–842.
22. Ros PR, Buck JL, Goodman ZD, et al. Intrahepatic cholangiocarcinoma: radiologic-pathologic correlation. Radiology 1988; 167:689–693.

Neil M. Rofsky, MD
Vivian S. Lee, MD, PhD
Gerhard Laub, PhD
Michael A. Pollack, MD
Glenn A. Krinsky, MD
David Thomasson, PhD
Michael M. Ambrosino, MD
Jeffrey C. Weinreb, MD

Index terms:
Abdomen, MR, 70.121412, 70.121415, 70.121419, 70.12143
Magnetic resonance (MR), technology, 70.121412, 70.121415, 70.121419

Radiology 1999; 212:876–884

Abbreviations:
CNR = contrast-to-noise ratio
GRE = gradient echo
MIP = maximum intensity projection
SNR = signal-to-noise ratio
2D = two-dimensional
3D = three-dimensional

[1] From the Department of Radiology, New York University Medical Center, MRI-Basement, Schwartz Bldg, 530 First Ave, New York, NY 10016 (N.M.R., V.S.L., M.A.P., G.A.K., M.M.A., J.C.W.), and Siemens Medical Systems (G.L., D.T.). Received October 1, 1998; revision requested November 11; revision received December 28; accepted April 1, 1999. **Address reprint requests to** N.M.R.

Author contributions:
Guarantors of integrity of entire study, N.M.R., V.S.L.; study concepts, N.M.R., D.T., J.C.W.; study design, N.M.R.; definition of intellectual content, N.M.R., G.L., J.C.W.; literature research, N.M.R., D.T.; clinical studies, N.M.R., V.S.L., G.A.K.; experimental studies, N.M.R., M.A.P., G.L., D.T.; data acquisition, M.A.P.; data analysis, V.S.L., N.M.R.; statistical analysis, V.S.L., M.M.A.; manuscript preparation, N.M.R., V.S.L.; manuscript editing, V.S.L., G.A.K., J.C.W.; manuscript review, V.S.L., G.L., G.A.K., J.C.W.

Abdominal MR Imaging with a Volumetric Interpolated Breath-hold Examination[1]

PURPOSE: To compare a T1-weighted, three-dimensional (3D), gradient-echo (GRE) sequence for magnetic resonance (MR) imaging of the body (volumetric interpolated breath-hold examination, or VIBE) with a two-dimensional (2D) GRE breath-hold equivalent.

MATERIALS AND METHODS: Twenty consecutive patients underwent 1.5-T MR imaging. The examinations included pre- and postcontrast (20 mL gadopentetate dimeglumine) fat-saturated 2D GRE breath-hold imaging and fat-saturated volumetric interpolated breath-hold imaging before, during (arterial phase), and after injection, with thin (2-mm source images) and thick (8-mm reconstruction images) sections. The three images were compared qualitatively and quantitatively (signal-to-noise ratio [SNR] and contrast-to-noise ratio [CNR]).

RESULTS: Qualitatively, the 2-mm source images had poorer pancreatic edge definition on precontrast images compared with the other two data sets ($P < .05$). On gadolinium-enhanced images, scores for clarity of pancreatic edge, number of vessels visualized, and arterial ghosting were significantly lower for the postcontrast 2D GRE images. Quantitatively, SNR measurements in the liver, aorta, and renal cortex on pre- and postcontrast images were significantly higher for the 8-mm reconstruction images than for the 2D GRE or 2-mm source images ($P < .05$). Aorta-to-fat CNR was significantly higher on the 8-mm reconstruction images.

CONCLUSION: Fat-saturated volumetric interpolated breath-hold images have quality comparable to that of conventional fat-saturated 2D GRE images.

Fast T1-weighted imaging with gradient-echo (GRE) sequences has rapidly become a cornerstone of body magnetic resonance (MR) imaging because it can produce high-spatial-resolution images that provide excellent anatomic detail (1–3). The ability to acquire data sets within very short times (<25 seconds) allows imaging to be performed within a breath hold, thereby reducing artifacts related to respiratory and other bulk motion. For dynamic contrast material–enhanced MR imaging, faster sequences enable precise timing of data acquisition during selected periods of enhancement (eg, hepatic arterial phase vs portal venous phase). This precision can be vital both to the detection of lesions that are visible only during certain short periods of enhancement and to lesion characterization (2–7). Present strategies for fast T1-weighted body MR imaging have been dominated by two-dimensional (2D) imaging.

For 2D breath-hold techniques in the abdomen, the quality and efficacy of imaging is limited by the need to acquire enough sections to cover a relatively large region, typically at least 160–200 mm. This must be accomplished with the finite number of sections that can be obtained in less than 25 seconds and thus requires use of relatively thick sections (8–10 mm). With 2D GRE pulse sequences in the abdomen, subcentimeter lesions could be missed or insufficiently characterized owing to partial volume averaging and low contrast-to-noise ratio (CNR) (8).

Short acquisition times place serious constraints on imaging; increased anatomic coverage comes at the expense of decreased spatial resolution and may require use of higher bandwidths that reduce the signal-to-noise ratio (SNR). In addition, fat-saturation methods, which can improve CNR on contrast-enhanced images, require additional imaging time. The application of fat saturation to GRE imaging on a routine basis has not been popular since most strategies do not provide adequate anatomic coverage in the time frame of breath-hold imaging.

Three-dimensional (3D) Fourier transform GRE imaging has potential advantages over 2D imaging. In comparison with traditional 2D GRE sequences, properly structured 3D GRE sequences have the capacity to provide thinner sections, no gaps, fat saturation, higher SNR, and comparable image contrast in the same breath-hold time frame. Furthermore, with appropriately thin sections and accurate timing, the same data set could be used to generate high-quality MR angiograms and thus provide added value. Therefore, 3D GRE imaging has the potential to yield a comprehensive evaluation of the upper abdomen. However, previous efforts with 3D GRE imaging have been hindered by relatively limited resolution and anatomic coverage (6,7,9).

In this study, we evaluated an alternative approach to 3D GRE imaging that addresses those limitations. We call the technique "volumetric interpolated breath-hold examination," or VIBE. With volumetric interpolated breath-hold imaging, data sets that have nearly isotropic resolution in three dimensions (on the order of 2-mm voxel size) can be obtained while preserving adequate anatomic coverage and uniform fat saturation within a breath hold.

We propose the volumetric interpolated breath-hold examination is a versatile and efficient approach to body MR imaging. The goals of this study were to assess the feasibility of implementing the approach; to compare the SNR, CNR, and fat saturation of the sequence to those with a more conventional 2D GRE sequence; and to illustrate reconstruction and angiographic possibilities with this 3D volumetric imaging method.

MATERIALS AND METHODS

Patients and Protocol

Twenty consecutive patients (10 women and 10 men; average age, 61 years; age range, 36–73 years) referred for abdominal MR imaging were examined with a 1.5-T system (Vision; Siemens Medical Systems, Iselin, NJ) with maximum gradient strength of 25 mT/m and rise time of 600 µsec with a torso phased-array coil. Informed consent was obtained from all patients before imaging, and the study was sanctioned by the institutional review board. A 22-gauge intravenous catheter was placed in an antecubital or forearm vein before the start of the study and attached to an MR-compatible power injector (Spectris; MedRad, Pittsburgh, Pa).

Breath-hold 2D axial T1-weighted fat-saturated images and breath-hold 3D T1-weighted fat-saturated volumetric interpolated breath-hold images were obtained before contrast material administration. For all sequences, patients were instructed to suspend respiration at end expiration. According to the method detailed by Earls et al (10), a timing image was then obtained with a test dose of 1 mL gadopentetate dimeglumine (Magnevist; Berlex Laboratories, Wayne, NJ) followed by 20 mL saline solution, both injected at a rate of 2 mL/sec. This allowed estimation of patient circulation time (bolus transit time from arm vein to abdominal aorta) and was used to ensure acquisition of optimal arterial phase images.

Dynamic imaging was performed with 19 mL gadopentetate dimeglumine. During dynamic imaging, three identical acquisitions with the fat-saturated volumetric interpolated breath-hold sequence were performed in quick succession (20–30 seconds between each to allow patients to catch their breath). The first acquisition was timed for arterial enhancement. After the third acquisition, postcontrast 2D fat-saturated imaging (with parameters identical to those in the precontrast 2D fat-saturated sequence) was performed.

MR Sequences and Parameters

The field of view, craniocaudal coverage, and the number of in-plane phase-encoding steps were tailored for each patient, and they were kept constant in the 2D fat-saturated GRE and fat-saturated volumetric interpolated breath-hold sequences for each individual. A bandwidth of 488 Hz per pixel was used in both sequences.

Two-dimensional GRE.—This is a fast low-angle shot, or FLASH, GRE sequence in which periodic chemically selective fat-saturation pulses have been incorporated. The field of view was 300–370 mm with a rectangular configuration in the phase-encoding (anteroposterior) dimension. The rectangular field of view was modified to accommodate the individual's body habitus. An initial matrix of 160 × 256 was used to yield in-plane spatial resolution of 2.3 × 1.4 mm or less and was modified to 125 phase-encoding steps with the rectangular field of view.

A 2D fat-saturation strategy was used in which two fat-saturation pulses were applied every 20 sections. The first pulse was applied at the beginning of the line acquisition (phase encoding) for the first section, and the second was applied after the line data from 10 sections were obtained. This strategy was repeated until the matrix was complete. This yielded an effective combination of fat saturation and anatomic coverage (20 sections) in the time frame of a breath hold. Although this fat-saturation strategy was experimental, it has since become commercially available. The section thickness was 5 mm with no gap between sections ($n = 3$) or 8 mm ($n = 17$) with no gap between sections ($n = 15$) or a 20% gap ($n = 2$). This allowed craniocaudal coverage of 100, 160, and 200 mm, respectively.

The 2D sequence was performed with repetition time msec/echo time msec of 180/2.8 with 80° flip angle, and 20 sections were generated during a breath hold of less than 23 seconds. The precise acquisition time depended on the rectangular field of view used.

Fat-saturated volumetric interpolated breath-hold examination.—In this application, a 3D radio-frequency–spoiled GRE sequence with isotropic or nearly isotropic spatial resolution was implemented. For this purpose, a symmetric echo was used in the read direction with a bandwidth of 488 Hz per pixel and 160 readout points. The k space was filled with 160 points along k_y and 40 points along k_z. Interpolation was performed in the section-select direction, as shown in Figure 1, which resulted in 80 partitions. Each partition was interpolated to a 256 square matrix. This strategy was selected to reduce the voxel size and maintain a short imaging time. As is typical of 3D sequences, there was no intersection gap. The field of view was 300–370 mm with a rectangular configuration in the phase-encoding (anteroposterior) dimension matched to that in the 2D fat-saturated sequence of a particular patient. An initial matrix of 160 × 160 data points was used to yield in-plane spatial resolution of less than 2.3 × 2.3 mm depending on the choice of field of view. The imaging matrix was 256 × 256 with a pixel size of less than 1.5 mm. The slab thickness was 160–200 mm divided into 80 partitions with a partition thickness of 2.0–2.5 mm.

In standard 3D Fourier transform imaging, the spatial resolution in the section-select direction is determined on the basis of the maximum spatial frequency, k_z, along the section-select direction. Typically, symmetric imaging in k space is performed. However, in a fashion similar to asymmetric echo sampling in the readout direction, the number of phase-encoding steps in the section-select direction can be reduced by means of asymmetric sampling in k_z. Consequently, asymmetric sampling along with sinc interpolation (zero filling) allows a reduction in the number of phase-encoding steps and therefore a reduction in overall imaging time. The loss in SNR, which goes along with a reduction in imaging time, is partially compensated by noise reduction filters that may be applied to the raw data.

This sequence incorporated a sequential phase-encode order in the k_y direction and a centric phase-encode reordering in the k_z direction (partitions loop). A chemically selective fat-saturation pulse was applied just before each partitions loop. The partitions loop was centric reordered to optimize fat-saturation uniformity. This fat-saturation strategy has been available in a previous commercially available 3D sequence (Siemens Medical Systems).

The 3D sequence was performed with the following parameters: 4.2/1.8 with 12° flip angle, 40 partitions were generated in a breath hold of less than 24 seconds, depending on the rectangular field of view. The 12° flip angle was selected after comparing liver-to-spleen CNR with multiple flip angles in eight patients before this study (unpublished data). The 3D volumetric interpolated breath-hold examination was performed before, during, and after administration of gadopentetate dimeglumine, with 20 seconds between each breath-hold acquisition.

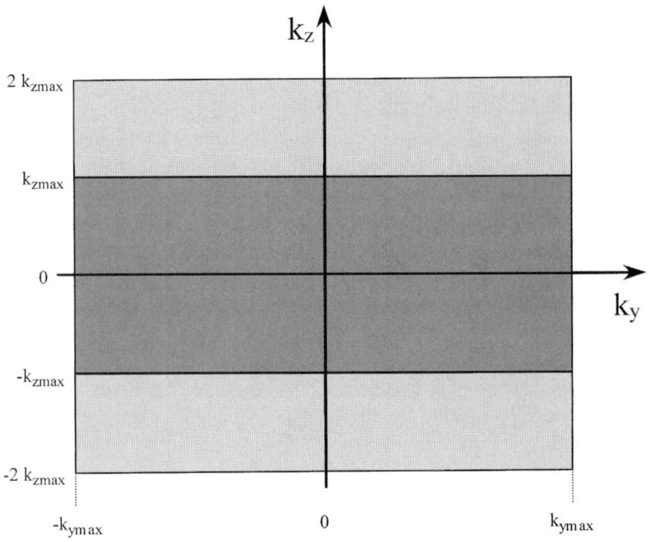

Figure 1. Schematic shows a k-space acquisition in the volumetric interpolated breath-hold examination. The dark gray area is filled with $N_y \times N_z$ data points. The remaining light gray area is filled with zeros to provide smaller voxel size. The actual spatial resolution is defined by k_{ymax} along the y direction and k_{zmax} along the z direction. k_{ymax} corresponds to 80 frequency-encoding samples, and k_{zmax} corresponds to 20 partition-encoding gradients.

Image Processing

Postprocessing of the fat-saturated volumetric interpolated breath-hold images was performed on a commercially available MR workstation, a satellite console of the MR unit. Reformations of the data sets before and after contrast material administration were performed by one investigator (M.A.P) who was not involved with the qualitative comparison. These reformations included axial 2-mm-thick sections obtained at intervals of 5–8 mm to match the locations of the 20 sections obtained with the 2D fat-saturated sequence. The fat-saturated volumetric interpolated breath-hold data sets were also reformatted as 5–8-mm-thick sections (no gap) and matched in position to the 2D fat-saturated images.

In addition, sagittal and coronal multiplanar reconstruction images were generated and reviewed interactively on the console, and selected images were acquired as deemed necessary by the interpreting radiologist. Similarly, maximum intensity projection (MIP) images were generated interactively from postcontrast fat-saturated volumetric interpolated breath-hold images with use of restricted volumes of interest, and hard copies of selected MIP images were obtained.

Data Analysis: Quantitative Assessment of Image Quality

Blinded to imaging results, a single investigator (M.A.P.) performed region-of-interest analysis for each of the six sets of images for each of the 20 patients: pre- and postcontrast 2D fat-saturated images, pre- and postcontrast 2-mm fat-saturated volumetric interpolated breath-hold source images, and pre- and postcontrast 8-mm fat-saturated volumetric interpolated breath-hold reconstruction images. The postcontrast 2-mm data that were quantitatively analyzed were obtained in the third of three postcontrast acquisitions performed just before the postcontrast 2D fat-saturated sequence. This was done to minimize differences in contrast media dynamics.

For each patient, matching regions of interest were placed over the liver, pancreas, spleen, retroperitoneal fat, subcutaneous fat, renal cortex, aorta, and air outside the patient's body. Care was taken to place regions within normal-appearing portions of each organ and away from intraparenchymal blood vessels. Means and SDs of signal intensity were recorded. On the basis of these measurements, the following parameters were computed: liver, renal cortex, and aorta SNRs, and liver-to-spleen, liver-to–retroperitoneal fat, pancreas-to-fat, renal cortex-to-fat, and aorta-to-fat CNRs. Signal noise was estimated on the basis of the SD of signal intensity measured in the region of interest outside the patient's body. For each sequence of reformatted data sets, regions of interest were placed at comparable section positions.

CNRs were calculated as $|SI_{tissueA} - SI_{tissueB}|/SD_{noise}$, where SI is signal intensity; tissue A is liver, pancreas, renal cortex, or aorta; and tissue B is spleen or retroperitoneal fat.

Data Analysis: Qualitative Analysis of Image Quality

Three independent reviewers (N.M.R., V.S.L., G.A.K.), who were blinded to patient and sequence information, viewed sets of 20 images in a random fashion. Each set consisted of the 20 images obtained with a given sequence displayed on a single sheet of film. There were three precontrast and three postcontrast sets (2D fat-saturated images, 2-mm fat-saturated volumetric interpolated breath-hold source images, or 8-mm reconstruction images) for a total of six sets per patient. Thus, 120 images per patient were evaluated, 20 images at a time.

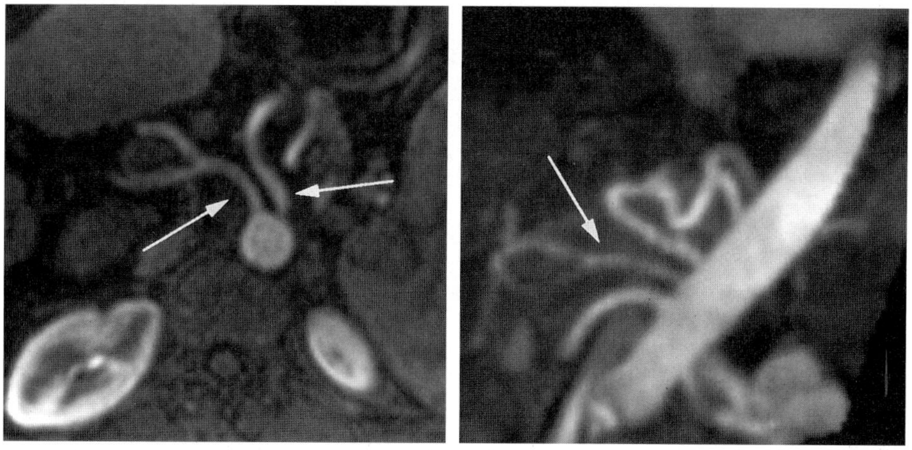

a. b.

Figure 2. Fat-saturated volumetric interpolated breath-hold images from the same data set obtained during the arterial phase of contrast material administration in a patient with cirrhosis. **(a)** Axial 2-mm fat-saturated volumetric interpolated breath-hold source image (4.2/1.8 with 12° flip angle) was obtained near the level of the celiac axis origin. Note that two vessels (arrows) originate from the anterior aspect of the abdominal aorta. **(b)** MR angiogram was created by means of the MIP technique with a restricted volume of interest and presented in an oblique orientation. This image effectively demonstrates the variant anatomy of an independent origin of the hepatic artery (arrow); the celiac axis and superior mesenteric artery origins are depicted above and below, respectively.

Image quality was assessed by scoring the following parameters on a scale of 1–5, with 5 representing the highest quality image or the least degradation by artifact. The parameters included clarity of liver edge, clarity of pancreas edge, ghosting, clarity of vessels, uniformity of fat saturation centrally (within the peritoneum and retroperitoneum) and peripherally (subcutaneous fat), number of vessels identified, and arterial ghosting.

The following scale was used to evaluate clarity of the liver and pancreas edge: 1, unreadable; 2, extreme blur; 3, moderate blur; 4, mild blur; and 5, sharp. For ghosting, the following scale was used: 1, unreadable study; 2, more than three ghosts; 3, two ghosts; 4, one ghost; 5, no ghosting. For fat saturation, the approximate percentage of area that demonstrated uniform fat saturation was graded as follows: 1, no fat saturation; 2, 0%–24% fat saturation; 3, 25%–49%; 4, 50%–74%; and 5, 75%–100%. For the number of vessels seen, readers were instructed to attempt to identify as many of the following vessels as possible: right, left, and middle hepatic veins; main portal vein; right and left portal veins; and right and left segmental veins (total of 10 vessels). The number identified was then converted to a scale of 1–5 as follows: 1, no vessels; 2, one to three vessels; 3, four to seven vessels; 4, seven to nine vessels; 5, 10 vessels.

Statitical Analysis

Comparisons of SNR and CNR with the three imaging sequences both before and after contrast material administration were made by means of one-way analysis of variance (EXCEL; Microsoft, Redmond, Wash). For those parameters with which a statistically significant difference ($P < .05$) was observed, comparisons between pairs of methods were then made by means of a two-tailed Student *t* test.

With subjective ratings of image quality, the Kendall coefficient of concordance was used to evaluate the degree of agreement among the three readers, and then the Friedman nonparametric test for related samples (SPSS 6.1; SPSS, Chicago, Ill) was used to assess for statistically significant differences among the three methods. With parameters for which a statistically significant difference in ratings was observed, a comparison between pairs of techniques was made by means of the Wilcoxon rank sum test.

RESULTS

All patients tolerated the MR examination and performed adequate breath holds for diagnostic evaluations. Representative fat-saturated volumetric interpolated breath-hold images, including the 2-mm source images, 8-mm multiplanar reconstruction images, and selected MIP images, are shown in Figures 2–4.

Quantitative Results

Average values for quantitative measurements of SNR and CNR on the images are given in the Table.

For pre- and postcontrast studies, SNR measurements in the liver, aorta, and renal cortex were significantly higher on the 8-mm fat-saturated volumetric interpolated breath-hold reconstruction images than on the 2D fat-saturated or 2-mm fat-saturated volumetric interpolated breath-hold source images ($P < .05$). There was no statistically significant difference between the 2D fat-saturated and 2-mm source images.

Although the difference did not achieve a threshold of a P value less than .05 for statistical significance, a consistent trend in CNR was observed in which the 8-mm reconstruction images had higher liver-to-fat, pancreas-to-fat, and renal cortex–to-fat CNR on both on pre- and postcontrast studies. Aorta-to-fat CNR was significantly higher on the 8-mm reconstruction images compared with images obtained with the other two methods on only postcontrast images.

Qualitative Results

The Kendall coefficient of concordance, used to evaluate the degree of agreement among the three readers, showed that there was no significant difference at a level of significance of a P value less than .05. Average values for subjective measures of image quality are shown in the Table. Overall, the qualitative values support the quantitative results. Average ratings exceeded a value of 4 (on a scale of 1–5 with 5 representing highest quality) for all techniques both before and after contrast material administration. For precontrast images, differences in clarity of the pancreas edge achieved statistical significance ($P < .05$) with values for the 2-mm fat-saturated volumetric interpolated breath-hold source images, which were significantly lower than those for images obtained with the other techniques (Fig 5). The remaining image quality parameters were not significantly different among the three methods before contrast material administration (Fig 5).

For contrast-enhanced studies, measurements of clarity of the pancreas edge, number of vessels visualized, and arterial ghosting were significantly lower for the

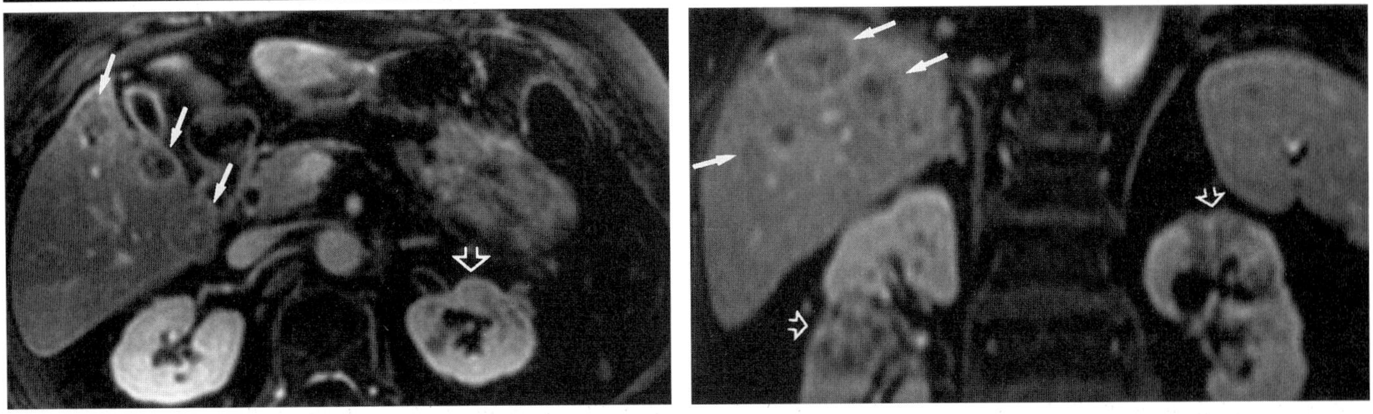

a.

b.

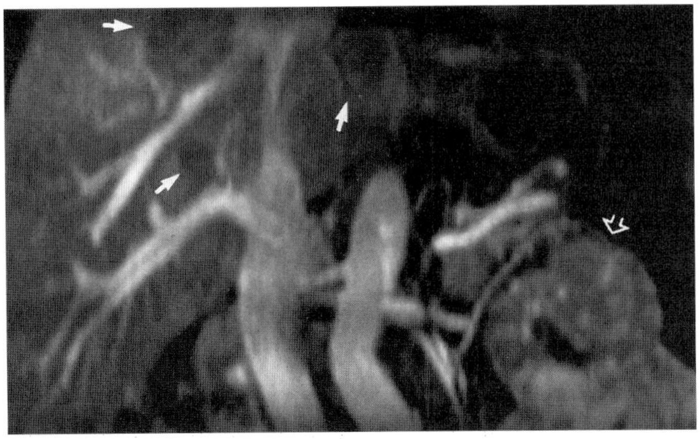

c.

Figure 3. Portal phase fat-saturated volumetric interpolated breath-hold images from the same data set in a patient with widespread metastatic disease. **(a)** Axial 2-mm fat-saturated volumetric interpolated breath-hold source image (4.2/1.8 with 12° flip angle) was obtained during the portal venous phase of contrast material administration. Liver (solid arrows) and left renal (open arrow) metastases are evident. **(b)** Coronal 8-mm reconstruction image provides an alternative perspective for evaluation and shows other liver (solid arrows) and renal (open arrows) metastases. **(c)** MIP image with restricted volume demonstrates the relationship of the metastases (solid arrows) to the intrahepatic vessels, which is useful for presurgical and preinterventional planning. A large left renal metastasis (open arrow) is seen projecting off the upper pole.

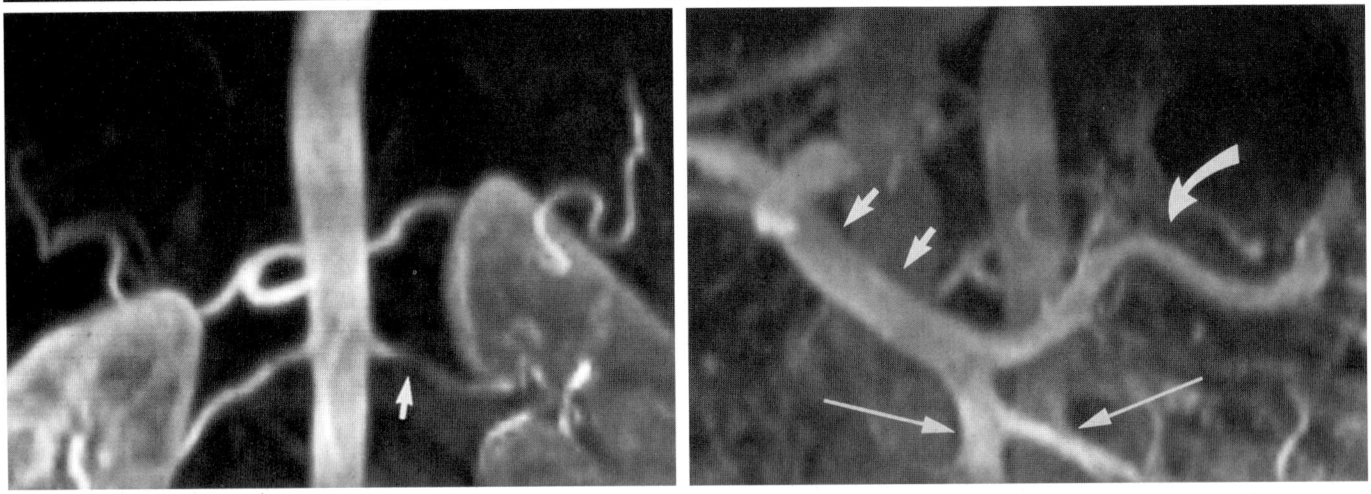

a.

b.

Figure 4. Fat-saturated volumetric interpolated breath-hold MIP images (4.2/1.8 with 12° flip angle) generated from axial 2-mm source images obtained during the arterial and portal venous phases after contrast material administration. **(a)** Arterial phase coronal MIP image demonstrates an incidental left renal arterial stenosis (arrow). Residual contrast material from the test dose is depicted in the renal collecting systems. **(b)** Portal venous phase coronal MIP image demonstrates both venous and arterial anatomy. The mesenteric veins (long straight arrows), the splenic vein (curved arrow), and the portal vein (short straight arrows) are the most conspicuous vessels.

2D fat-saturated images than for the 2-mm fat-saturated volumetric interpolated breath-hold source images or the 8-mm reconstruction images. Despite the lower quality result for arterial ghosting on the 2-mm fat-saturated volumetric interpolated breath-hold source images and the 8-mm reconstruction images, MR angiograms with excellent quality were gener-

Average Values for Pre- and Postcontrast Signal Intensity and Subjective Image Parameters

Image Parameter	2D Fat-saturated Images	Fat-saturated Volumetric Interpolated Breath-hold Examination: 2-mm Source Images	Fat-saturated Volumetric Interpolated Breath-hold Examination: 8-mm Reconstruction Images	*P* Value*
Precontrast				
SNR				
Liver	23.6 ± 12.0	24.4 ± 10.4	37.1 ± 17.8	<.001†
Aorta	10.3 ± 3.5	12.3 ± 4.7	18.9 ± 10.7	<.001†
Renal cortex	28.7 ± 10.8	30.8 ± 12.4	43.0 ± 16.0	<.001†
CNR (to fat)				
Liver	17.3 ± 9.9	15.4 ± 7.5	21.7 ± 12.1	.13
Pancreas	19.3 ± 8.6	14.7 ± 7.1	19.3 ± 9.0	.14
Renal cortex	22.4 ± 9.3	21.8 ± 9.4	27.3 ± 10.2	.15
Aorta	4.0 ± 4.1	3.3 ± 5.2	3.4 ± 8.9	.93
Postcontrast				
SNR				
Liver	40.3 ± 28.4	44.5 ± 18.4	62.4 ± 29.3	.022†
Aorta	45.2 ± 32.4	55.2 ± 20.1	75.7 ± 19.8	.001†
Renal cortex	81.2 ± 79.6	91.0 ± 35.5	126.6 ± 54.1	.046†
CNR (to fat)				
Liver	28.8 ± 23.0	29.7 ± 16.6	40.9 ± 23.3	.142
Pancreas	29.8 ± 21.8	31.8 ± 12.3	41.4 ± 12.1	.057
Renal cortex	69.7 ± 74.5	76.2 ± 31.5	105.1 ± 46.0	.094
Aorta	33.7 ± 27.5	40.4 ± 17.6	54.3 ± 16.0	.010†
Subjective				
Precontrast				
Clarity of liver edge	4.45 ± 0.7	4.28 ± 0.6	4.51 ± 0.6	.17
Clarity of pancreas edge	4.47 ± 0.8	4.11 ± 0.8	4.39 ± 0.7	.02‡
Fat suppression	4.07 ± 0.8	4.26 ± 0.7	4.49 ± 0.7	.08
Number of vessels	4.32 ± 0.7	4.39 ± 0.7	4.43 ± 0.6	.71
Arterial ghosting	4.90 ± 0.3	4.96 ± 0.2	4.91 ± 0.3	.88
Postcontrast				
Clarity of liver edge	4.41 ± 0.7	4.36 ± 0.6	4.60 ± 0.5	.15
Clarity of pancreas edge	4.12 ± 0.6	4.30 ± 0.7	4.51 ± 0.7	.02§
Fat suppression	4.63 ± 0.6	4.58 ± 0.5	4.61 ± 0.5	.58
Number of vessels	4.25 ± 0.9	4.34 ± 0.6	4.63 ± 0.6	.04
Arterial ghosting	4.40 ± 0.7	4.86 ± 0.4	4.54 ± 0.6	.01‖

Note.—Data are the mean ± SD.

* *P* values for pre- and postcontrast data are based on analysis of variance.

† For all cases with $P < .05$, Student *t* test was performed for each pair of imaging methods, and no significant difference was found between the 2D images and 2-mm source images.

‡ For all cases with $P < .05$, Wilcoxon rank sum test was performed for each pair of imaging methods, and no significant difference was found between the 2D images and 8-mm reconstruction images.

§ Wilcoxon rank sum test demonstrated no significant difference between the 2D images and 2-mm source images.

‖ Wilcoxon rank sum test demonstrated a statistically significant difference between each pairing of images obtained with the three imaging methods.

ated (Fig 4). Differences in all other parameters were not significant among the three approaches (Fig 6).

DISCUSSION

Volumetric interpolated breath-hold imaging represents an MR technique directed toward minimizing partial volume effects and maximizing image contrast, a universal goal of all imaging technologies. With the volumetric interpolated breath-hold imaging approach, sections thinner than those currently in use for body MR are possible; thus, partial volume effects can be minimized, and the evaluation of very small masses is more feasible. In addition, as voxels approach nearly isotropic resolution, options for postprocessing broaden. Nearly isotropic voxels (on the order of 2 mm) allow multiplanar reconstruction images to be generated in any desired plane. Such reconstructions have in-plane resolution closely approximating that possible with separately acquired 2D images. The usefulness of thin-section volumetric interpolated breath-hold imaging ultimately relies on generation of images of sufficient quality.

Our quantitative and qualitative results show that images obtained with the fat-saturated volumetric interpolated breath-hold sequence are comparable to or better than those obtained with the 2D fat-saturated GRE sequence. The prohibitive reduction in SNR that accompanies use of very thin sections with 2D techniques seems mitigated with fat-saturated volumetric interpolated breath-hold imaging, perhaps owing to the inherent improvement in SNR with 3D techniques and possibly by means of the judicious selection of flip angle (11). In our study, the flip angle was selected to optimize liver-to-spleen CNR. This may account for the slightly greater precontrast pancreas-to-fat CNR observed on 2D fat-saturated images compared with that on the 2-mm fat-saturated volumetric interpolated breath-hold source images or the 8-mm reconstruction images (Table). Given the shorter T1 of the pancreas, it is likely that a larger flip angle could have been selected for the 3D sequence to optimize pancreas-to-background CNR.

We recognize that on a strictly scientific basis, it would have been useful to obtain arterial phase postcontrast studies for both the 2D and 3D approaches and compare these. Such a comparison would have required a separate imaging session to acquire distinct arterial phase images for both approaches, and we believed that the additional time and contrast material exposure was not warranted. The data we acquired for both the precontrast and delayed postcontrast images show the efficacy of the 3D approach. We do not believe that the arterial phase evaluations would have any other differences. Moreover, meaningful multiplanar reformation and MIP images possible with the 3D approach cannot be obtained with the 8-mm-thick sections needed for adequate anatomic coverage with the 2D approach.

Our strategy of using an intermittent fat-saturation pulse for both 2D and 3D techniques enabled fat saturation with minimum added imaging time. Fat saturation improves CNR (12–15) and reduces the potential degradation of image quality resulting from motion-related artifacts. Saturation of fat also improves the depiction of enhanced vascular structures on gadolinium-enhanced MR angiograms. We note that volumetric interpolated breath-hold imaging can also be performed without fat saturation, such as when insufficient magnetic field homogeneity precludes effective frequency-selected fat saturation.

At the time this article was written, there were only a handful of reports about 3D fast GRE acquisitions for abdominal imaging (6,7,16,17). Results in these studies were limited by relatively poor spatial resolution, insufficient anatomic coverage, or both. For example, Soyer et al (6) reported results with a 3D GRE technique that allowed 12 partitions in a 21-second breath hold or 20 partitions in a 30-second breath hold with a 128 × 256 matrix. In that study, partition thickness was 10 mm and therefore the 21-second breath hold could provide only 120 mm of craniocaudal coverage. Such applications of 3D imaging do not provide clear advantages over conventional 2D GRE imaging. Recently, the use of thin-section 3D imaging was described for evaluation of the kidneys in which a limited slab thickness preserved breath-hold capacity (18).

In our study, improved imaging efficiency has been pursued by taking advantage of pulse sequence and reconstruction tools that are unique to 3D sequence structures. By means of zero filling in the section-select direction, we achieved interpolated data that reduced the voxel dimension by a factor of two. By combining these strategies with use of extremely short repetition times (the latter made possible with commercially available high-performance gradients), the fat-saturated volumetric interpolated breath-hold sequence provided volumetric images with 2-mm effective partition thickness within the time frame of a breath hold. With the smaller voxel size, our preliminary observations predict a corresponding improvement in the detection and characterization of small lesions. A scientific study that evaluates the impact of voxel size on lesion detection and characterization is needed.

Results in prior work have shown that zero-filling interpolation (19) and section doubling (20) can reduce partial volume artifacts on 3D MR angiograms. Previously, these techniques have not, to our knowledge, been pursued for body imaging. The precise effects of zero filling on section-select resolution can be complex (21). We expect that the section-select resolution we achieved with interpolation is slightly less than that achieved by doubling the number of partitions without interpolation; however, the latter requires a time penalty and in many cases will eliminate the possibility of breath-hold imaging.

The temporal dynamics of sequential,

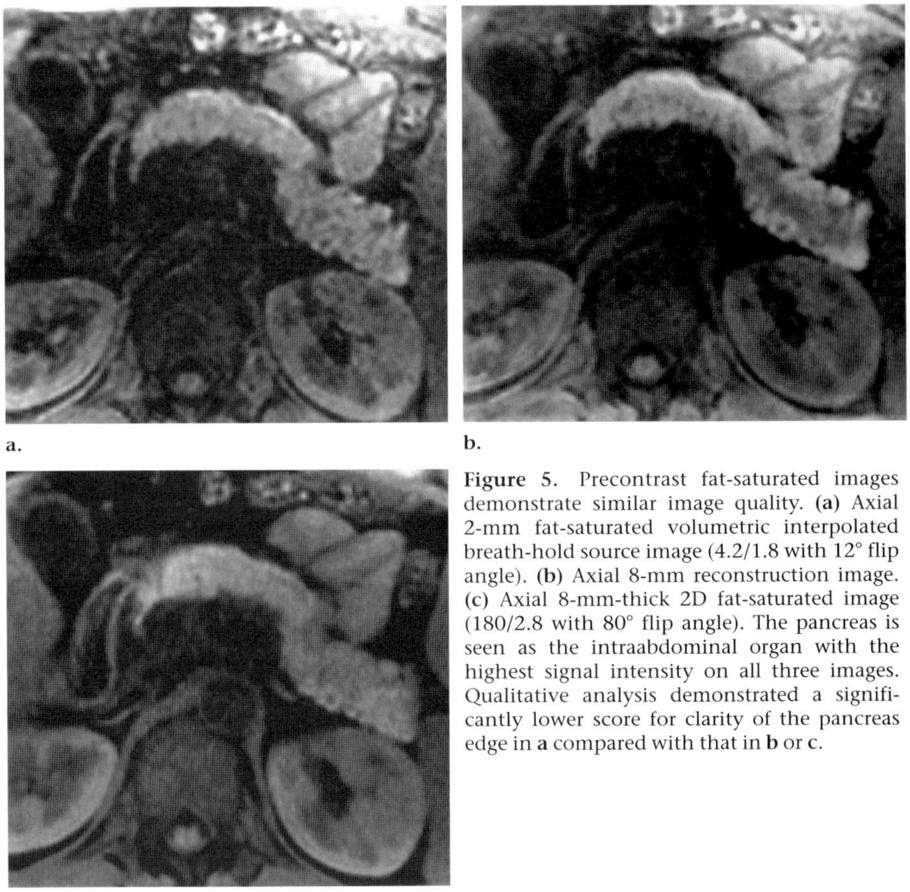

a. b. c.

Figure 5. Precontrast fat-saturated images demonstrate similar image quality. **(a)** Axial 2-mm fat-saturated volumetric interpolated breath-hold source image (4.2/1.8 with 12° flip angle). **(b)** Axial 8-mm reconstruction image. **(c)** Axial 8-mm-thick 2D fat-saturated image (180/2.8 with 80° flip angle). The pancreas is seen as the intraabdominal organ with the highest signal intensity on all three images. Qualitative analysis demonstrated a significantly lower score for clarity of the pancreas edge in **a** compared with that in **b** or **c**.

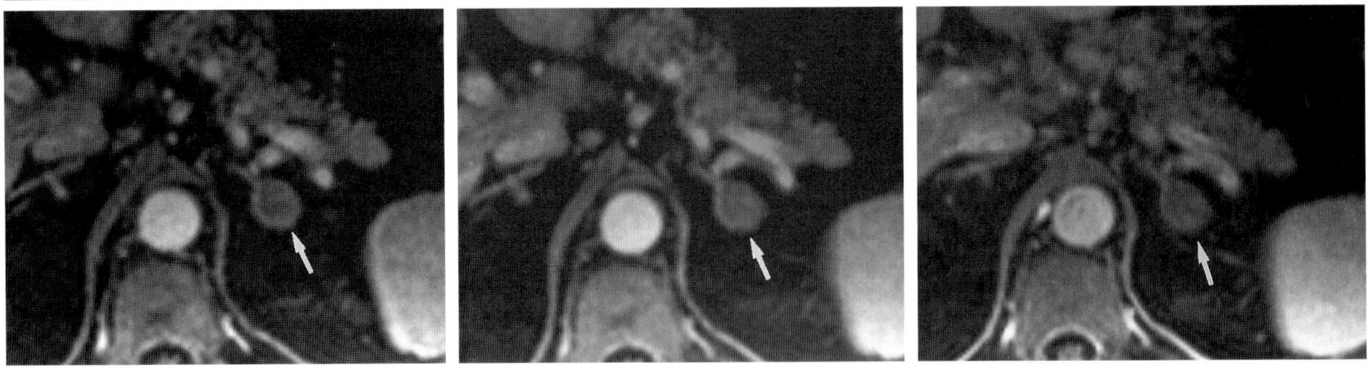

a. b. c.

Figure 6. Delayed postcontrast fat-saturated images in a patient with an incidental left adrenal adenoma (arrow in **a–c**). **(a)** Axial 2-mm fat-saturated volumetric interpolated breath-hold source image (4.2/1.8 with 12° flip angle). **(b)** Axial 8-mm reconstruction image. **(c)** Axial 8-mm-thick 2D fat-saturated image (180/2.8 with 80° flip angle). Quantitative results showed significantly higher SNR measurements for the liver, aorta, and renal cortex in **b** compared with those in **a** or **c**. However, image quality appears similar.

contrast-enhanced studies bring out important differences between 2D and volumetric interpolated breath-hold imaging techniques. With use of a 2D imaging approach, separate acquisitions are required to obtain alternative imaging planes; thus, image contrast varies with the temporal dynamics of contrast media distribution and therefore with the plane of each separate acquisition. In contradistinction, multiplanar reconstruction images from volumetric interpolated breath-hold data contain image contrast identical to that obtained in the initial acquisition plane. Thus, volumetric interpolated breath-hold examinations can offer images in any obliquity from the data sets obtained during critical phases of enhancement (arterial and portal venous phases of liver enhancement, for example). We predict that the use of multiplanar reconstruction techniques to reformat dynamically acquired volumetric data sets will translate into improved lesion detection and characterization. Verification of this prediction requires further study.

There are additional practical implications for breath-hold volumetric imaging in the body. Multiplanar reconstruction images of volumetric data sets can be used to improve localization of lesions and pretherapeutic planning. For example, for patients who may undergo radio-frequency or cryoablation of liver masses, assessment of proximity of lesions to nearby biliary and vascular structures can be vital. In addition, volumetric imaging can improve definition of segmental anatomy and help the planning of segmental resection of liver masses (22–24). Similarly, the feasibility of partial nephrectomy can be aided by means of precise localization of the masses (25–27).

With use of timing imaging to ensure acquisition of a volumetric data set during peak arterial enhancement, the arterial phase volumetric interpolated breath-hold images that are used to evaluate parenchymal disease can also be manipulated to obtain angiographic images. Postcontrast volumetric interpolated breath-hold images can be reconstructed by using MIP algorithms (Figs 2–4), thereby incorporating the advantages of gadolinium-enhanced 3D MR angiography (10,28–30). The effective demonstration of arterial and venous anatomy is important in the staging of tumors such as renal and pancreatic neoplasms. With volumetric interpolated breath-hold imaging, this can be accomplished by using the same data sets from which cross-sectional axial images are prospectively obtained. Finally, there may be fortuitous angiographic findings demonstrated on angiograms obtained with the volumetric interpolated breath-hold sequence (eg, renal artery stenoses or splenic artery aneurysms) that can lead to early diagnoses and possible elimination of the need for additional tests.

We recognize that the large number of images generated with such a volumetric approach can present challenges for interpretation and also affect data storage considerations. An option for presentation of data is to make hard copies of selected acquisitions as limited reformatted images (eg, 20 images per acquisition consisting of 8-mm reformatted sections). Aside from minimizing film, shipping, and storage costs, images reformatted at larger section thicknesses also provide improved SNR compared with that on the original thin-section images, as we have shown. Similar results have been reported previously (31). While improved SNR could translate into improved image aesthetics, the reformation images reintroduce greater partial volume averaging effects. Therefore, to capture the true benefits of thin-section imaging, a review of source images is important for interpretation. The volumetric approach to imaging may thus lend itself to direct interpretation at the workstation and allow the user to "sweep" through the data sets in standard and oblique planes.

The volumetric interpolated breath-hold imaging sequence was modified from 3D sequences originally structured for gadolinium-enhanced MR angiography. It differs from the MR angiographic sequences by replacing an asymmetric echo in the read direction with an echo that is symmetric; this change improves the in-plane spatial resolution. The sequence also differs by including a decreased flip angle to better address abdominal imaging contrast. It is possible for the reader to attempt 3D body imaging with section-interpolated MR angiographic sequences; however, our initial observations with them prompted the aforementioned changes. The pursuit of alternate zero-fill strategies offers opportunities for further research and potential improvements in volumetric interpolated breath-hold techniques.

In summary, the volumetric interpolated breath-hold examination offers a more comprehensive and efficient approach to body MR imaging. We demonstrated the feasibility of the fat-saturated examination in the clinical setting, showed its comparability in image quality to that with a more conventional fat-saturated 2D GRE imaging strategy, and illustrated examples of its reconstruction and angiographic capabilities. If further studies document that volumetric interpolated breath-hold examination improves the accuracy and utility of body MR imaging, the technique might replace other breath-hold, T1-weighted imaging strategies.

References

1. Semelka RC, Simm FC, Recht M, Deimling M, Lenz G, Laub GA. T1-weighted sequences for MR imaging of the liver: comparison of three techniques for single-breath, whole-volume acquisition at 1.0 and 1.5 T. Radiology 1991; 180:629–635.
2. Hamm B, Thoeni RF, Gould RG, et al. Focal liver lesions: characterization with nonenhanced and dynamic contrast material-enhanced MR imaging. Radiology 1994; 190:417–423.
3. Low RN, Francis IR, Herfkens RJ, et al. Fast multiplanar spoiled gradient-recalled imaging of the liver: pulse sequence optimization and comparison with spin-echo MR imaging. AJR 1993; 160:501–509.
4. Peterson MS, Baron RL, Murakami T. Hepatic malignancies: usefulness of acquisition of multiple arterial and portal venous phase images at dynamic gadolinium-enhanced MR imaging. Radiology 1996; 201:337–345.
5. Yamashita Y, Miyazaki T, Hatanaka Y, Takahashi M. Dynamic MRI of small renal cell carcinoma. J Comput Assist Tomogr 1995; 19:759–765.
6. Soyer P, de Givry SC, Gueye C, Lenormand S, Somveille E, Scherrer A. Detection of focal hepatic lesions with MR imaging: prospective comparison of T2-weighted fast spin-echo with and without fat suppression, T2-weighted breath-hold fast spin-echo, and gadolinium chelate-enhanced 3D gradient-recalled imaging. AJR 1996; 166:1115–1121.
7. Murakami T, Tsuda K, Nakamura H, et al. 3DFT-FLASH MR imaging of pancreatic cancer with gadopentetate dimeglumine. Acta Radiol 1996; 37:190–194.
8. Carlson J, Crooks L, Ortendahl D, Kramer DM, Kaufman L. Signal-to-noise ratio and section thickness in two-dimensional versus three-dimensional Fourier transform MR imaging. Radiology 1988; 166:266–270.
9. Frahm J, Haase A, Matthaei D. Rapid three-dimensional MR imaging using the FLASH technique. J Comput Assist Tomogr 1986; 10:363–368.
10. Earls JP, Rofsky NM, DeCorato DR, Krinsky GA, Weinreb JC. Breath-hold single-dose gadolinium-enhanced three-dimensional MR aortography: usefulness of a timing examination and MR power injector. Radiology 1996; 201:705–710.
11. Mills TC, Ortendahl DA, Hylton NM, Crooks LE, Carlson JW, Kaufman L. Partial flip angle MR imaging. Radiology 1987; 162:531–539.
12. Semelka RC, Shoenut JP, Kroeker MA, MacMahon RG, Greenberg HM. Renal lesions: controlled comparison between CT and 1.5-T MR imaging with nonenhanced and gadolinium-enhanced fat-suppressed spin-echo and breath-hold

FLASH techniques. Radiology 1992; 182: 425–430.
13. Semelka RC, Hricak H, Bis KG, Werthmuller WC, Higgins CB. Liver lesion detection: comparison between excitation-spoiling fat suppression and regular spin-echo at 1.5T. Abdom Imaging 1993; 18: 56–60.
14. Mitchell DG, Vinitski S, Saponaro S, Tasciyan T, Burk DL Jr, Rifkin MD. Liver and pancreas: improved spin-echo T1 contrast by shorter echo time and fat suppression at 1.5 T. Radiology 1991; 178:67–71.
15. Helmberger T, Mergo PJ, Stoupis C, Torres GM, Burton SS, Ros PR. Improved technique for pancreatic MRI: value of oblique fat suppression imaging with oral barium administration. J Comput Assist Tomogr 1998; 22:391–397.
16. Soyer P, Dufresne AC, Somveille E, Scherrer A. Focal nodular hyperplasia of the liver: assessment of hemodynamic and angioarchitectural patterns with gadolinium chelate-enhanced 3D spoiled gradient-recalled MRI and maximum intensity projection reformatted images. J Comput Assist Tomogr 1996; 20:898–904.
17. Murakami T, Nakamura H, Tsuda K, et al. Treatment of hepatocellular carcinoma by chemoembolization: evaluation with 3DFT MR imaging. AJR 1993; 160:295–299.
18. Rofsky NM, Bosniak MA. MR imaging in the evaluation of small (≤3.0 cm) renal masses. Magn Reson Imaging Clin N Am 1997; 5:67–81.
19. Du YP, Parker DL, Davis WL, Cao G. Reduction of partial-volume artifacts with zero-filled interpolation in three-dimensional MR angiography. JMRI 1994; 4:733–741.
20. Hylton NM, Simovsky I, Li AJ, Hale JD. Impact of section doubling on MR angiography. Radiology 1992; 185:899–902.
21. Hurst GC, Hua J, Simonetti OP, Duerk JL. Signal-to-noise, resolution, and bias function analysis of asymmetric sampling with zero-padded magnitude FT reconstruction. Magn Reson Med 1992; 27:247–269.
22. Soyer P, Bluemke DA, Bliss DF, Woodhouse CE, Fishman EK. Surgical segmental anatomy of the liver: demonstration with spiral CT during arterial portography and multiplanar reconstruction. AJR 1994; 163:99–103.
23. Gazelle GS, Haaga JR. Hepatic neoplasms: surgically relevant segmental anatomy and imaging techniques. AJR 1992; 158: 1015–1018.
24. Fasel JH, Selle D, Evertsz CJ, Terrier F, Peitgen HO, Gailloud P. Segmental anatomy of the liver: poor correlation with CT. Radiology 1998; 206:151–156.
25. Gschwend JE, Vogel U, Bader C, Mattfeldt T, Hautmann RE. Predictive value of magnetic resonance imaging and computerized tomography for conservative renal surgery in an ex vivo tumor enucleation study followed by step-sectioning. J Urol 1996; 155:451–454.
26. Scattoni V, Colombo R, Nava L, et al. Imaging of renal cell carcinoma with gadolinium-enhanced magnetic resonance: radiological and pathological study. Urol Int 1995; 54:121–127.
27. Chernoff DM, Silverman SG, Kikinis R, et al. Three-dimensional imaging and display of renal tumors using spiral CT: a potential aid to partial nephrectomy. Urology 1994; 43:125–129.
28. Prince MA. Body MR angiography with gadolinium contrast agents. Magn Reson Imaging Clin N Am 1996; 4:11–24.
29. Hany TF, Debatin JF, Leung DA, Pfammatter T. Evaluation of the aortoiliac and renal arteries: comparison of breath-hold, contrast-enhanced, three-dimensional MR angiography with conventional catheter angiography. Radiology 1997; 204:357–362.
30. Shirkhoda A, Konez O, Shetty AN, Bis KG, Ellwood RA, Kirsch MJ. Mesenteric circulation: three-dimensional MR angiography with a gadolinium-enhanced multiecho gradient-echo technique. Radiology 1997; 202:257–261.
31. Li D, Haacke EM, Tarr RW, Venkatesan R, Lin W, Wielopolski P. Magnetic resonance imaging of the brain with gadopentetate dimeglumine-DTPA: comparison of T1-weighted spin-echo and 3D gradient-echo sequences. JMRI 1996; 6:415–424.

Lane F. Donnelly, MD
James R. MacFall, PhD
H. Page McAdams, MD
J. Marc Majure, MD
Jean Smith, MS
Donald P. Frush, MD
Paul Bogonad, PhD
H. Cecil Charles, PhD
Carl E. Ravin, MD

Cystic Fibrosis: Combined Hyperpolarized ^{3}He-enhanced and Conventional Proton MR Imaging in the Lung—Preliminary Observations[1]

Index terms:
Fibrosis, cystic, 60.252
Helium, 60.12147
Lung, MR, 60.12143
Magnetic resonance (MR), contrast enhancement, 60.12143
Magnetic resonance (MR), nuclei other than H, 60.12147

Radiology 1999; 212:885–889

Abbreviations:
CF = cystic fibrosis
FEV_1 = forced expiratory volume in 1 second
FVC = forced vital capacity
SE = spin echo
SI = signal intensity

[1] From the Departments of Radiology, Division of Pediatric Radiology (L.F.D., J.R.M., H.P.M., J.S., D.P.F., P.B., H.C.C., C.E.R.) and Pediatrics, Division of Pulmonary Medicine (J.M.M.), Duke University Medical Center, Durham, NC. From the 1998 RSNA scientific assembly. Received September 17, 1998; revision requested November 10; revision received November 19; accepted March 29, 1999. **Address reprint requests to** L.F.D., Department of Radiology, Children's Hospital Medical Center and the University of Cincinnati, 3333 Burnet Ave, Cincinnati, OH 45229-3039.

Author contributions:
Guarantors of integrity of entire study, L.F.D., J.R.M.; study concepts, L.F.D., J.R.M., H.P.M., D.P.F., J.M.M.; study design, L.F.D., J.R.M., H.P.M.; literature research, all authors; clinical studies, all authors; data acquisition, all authors; data analysis, L.F.D., H.P.M., D.P.F.; manuscript preparation, L.F.D.; manuscript editing and review, all authors.

Four patients with cystic fibrosis (CF) were examined with combined hyperpolarized helium 3–enhanced and conventional proton magnetic resonance (MR) imaging. After inhalation of the polarized ^{3}He gas, single breath-hold, gradient-echo images (resonant frequency of ^{3}He) were obtained to depict lung ventilation. Conventional T2-weighted fast spin-echo (hydrogen) images were also obtained to depict morphologic abnormalities. ^{3}He images were successfully and reproducibly generated that showed both morphologic abnormalities and, often more extensive, ventilation abnormalities. ^{3}He MR imaging may provide a method for evaluating progression of pulmonary disease in patients with CF.

Image scoring systems have been used clinically and as a research tool to objectively evaluate the progression of lung disease in patients with cystic fibrosis (CF) (1–7). The goal is to facilitate objective evaluation of existing and newly developed therapeutic regimens, such as gene therapy and mucolytic agents (1–7). Current options for pulmonary evaluation in patients with CF include chest radiography, thin-section computed tomography (CT), pulmonary function testing, and single photon emission CT (SPECT) for pulmonary perfusion or ventilation imaging (1–7). Pulmonary function tests help analysis of global lung function. Unfortunately, CF may cause focal nonuniform lung injury, which is not accurately depicted by means of an assessment of global function. For this reason, imaging studies have been used primarily to develop scoring systems with which to monitor progression of disease (1–7).

Thin-section CT and chest radiography are performed to evaluate morphologic changes of CF to determine the severity of disease. Findings in multiple studies in patients with CF suggest thin-section CT is superior to chest radiography for the evaluation of lung disease, such as bronchiectasis, peribronchial thickening, mucus plugging, and emphysema (1–4). Thin-section CT is also more sensitive for early lung changes. However, there has been concern that the morphologic changes seen at thin-section CT and chest radiography may not reflect early functional pulmonary disease, which has been depicted at SPECT perfusion or ventilation imaging. Functional imaging may offer a more sensitive way with which to detect early changes of CF in patients with minimal disease (1,6,8). Morphologically normal lung can at times demonstrate marked functional abnormalities at ventilation and perfusion imaging (1,8). This is of particular importance in the evaluation of progression in young patients with minimal disease and no or minimal findings at thin-section CT. Since many protocols that evaluate new therapies involve young children with minimal or no lung disease, the detection of early lung changes in CF is critical. Functional and morphologic evaluation can be performed with a combination of both thin-section CT and SPECT, but the cost and radiation dose associated with both examinations is prohibitive, especially when these examinations are performed serially.

The optimal single imaging modality with which to grade progression of the pulmonary changes seen in patients with CF would provide both morphologic and functional information and, because of the sequential nature of following up of progression of disease, would not use radiation. Use of combined hyperpolarized helium 3–enhanced and conventional proton magnetic resonance (MR) imaging may meet these criteria. By imaging with a hyperpolarized ventilation contrast agent, such as ^{3}He, high signal intensity (SI) can be generated within the pulmonary air spaces. In patients with CF, ^{3}He MR imaging may provide both functional information related to airway occlusion and absent ventilation, as has been previously demonstrated with SPECT (1), and anatomic information by means of conventional proton-based, fast spin-echo (SE) imaging. The purpose of this study was to evaluate the preliminary findings with combined ^{3}He and proton MR imaging in four patients with CF.

Materials and Methods

Four young adult patients with CF (two men and two women; age range, 18–24 years; mean age, 20 years) and moderate to severe lung disease underwent hyperpolarized ^{3}He MR imaging. The study was approved by our institutional review board, and all studies were performed with written informed consent. Hyperpolarized ^{3}He MR images were obtained on a 1.5-T imager (Signa, revision 5.6; GE Medical Systems, Milwaukee, Wis) equipped with a broadband receiver that can adjust the radio frequency for the gyromagnetic ratio of both ^{3}He (3,456.31 Hz/G) and hydrogen (4,257.26 Hz/G). A specially designed quadrature transmit-receive torso surface coil (26 cm long), which does not interfere with hydrogen imaging with the body coil, was constructed for ^{3}He imaging (Medical Advances, Milwaukee, Wis).

Initially, with the ^{3}He torso coil in place, conventional proton-based MR images were obtained throughout the chest with use of the body coil. Fast SE intermediate- and T2-weighted images were obtained in the coronal plane (repetition time msec/echo time msec = 3,000/80, 6-mm section thickness, 2-mm gap, 128 × 256 matrix, 32-cm field of view, one signal acquired, respiratory gating). After acquisition of the proton images and without moving the patient or the ^{3}He torso coil, hyperpolarized ^{3}He images were obtained with use of the ^{3}He torso coil.

^{3}He gas was hyperpolarized by means of a process that involves a collision exchange between rubidium and helium gases mixed together, heated to 180°C, and subjected to high-intensity laser illumination for several hours (9). When the container is cooled to room temperature, the rubidium is absorbed on the surface of the production container with residual concentrations of less than one in 100,000,000,000 atoms per cubic centimeter. The helium gas was polarized by using a prototypic unit (Magnetic Imaging Technologies, Durham, NC). Unit calibration tests demonstrated 9%–11% polarization of the helium after the process. After the ^{3}He was polarized and cooled, it was placed in a delivery apparatus—a plastic bag with an attached tube containing a simple plastic stopcock on-off valve. The bag had a maximum capacity of 1 L. The bag was filled to between 0.7 and 0.9 L. Subjects were instructed to inhale the gas and hold their breath.

Immediately after the patients inhaled the ^{3}He gas, gradient-echo images were obtained in the coronal plane (9.5/3.0 with 8° flip angle, single breath hold, 6-mm section thickness, 2-mm gap, 128 × 256 matrix, 32-cm field of view, one signal acquired). ^{3}He gas inhalation and MR imaging were repeated in each subject to evaluate reproducibility.

During the examination, the patient's respiratory rate, pulse rate, and blood oxygenation levels were monitored. The patient's ability to cooperate with the examination was noted as were any changes in these vital signs during the study.

For comparison, the conventional proton fast SE and ^{3}He images were printed with identical anatomic levels side by side. This aided interpretation of absent ventilation on the ^{3}He images by defining the expected extent of the lung. Grading systems were constructed to help interpret both the ^{3}He images and the conventional proton images. Each lung was divided into six zones that were independently graded. Three lung regions were based on superior to inferior thirds: upper, middle, and lower. Each region was then divided into an anterior and posterior zone, which yielded a total of six zones per lung.

Each lung zone was given a functional score based on the degree of ventilation as seen on the ^{3}He MR images. Scores were based on the percentage of lung ventilated (percentage ventilation = area enhanced/total area of zone). Scores ranged from 0 (normal) to 4 (less than 25% of lung zone ventilated) (Table 1). The potential scores per patient (12 lung zones) ranged from 0 to 48. The ^{3}He MR studies of two healthy male volunteers, who had no history or symptoms of pulmonary disease, showed diffuse homogeneous SI throughout the lungs (Fig 1). These studies were used as a normal reference. Imaging in the healthy volunteers was also approved by our institutional review board.

Each lung zone was also graded for the presence of morphologic abnormalities as depicted on the conventional fast SE images. A score from 0 to 4 was given for both the presence of bronchial abnormalities and acinar replacement, with both scores based on the portion of the lung zone involved (Table 2). Bronchial abnormalities included peribronchial thickening, mucus plugging, and bronchiectasis. Peribronchial thickening was defined as the presence of increased linear SI in pairs in the anatomic distribution of the bron-

TABLE 1
Scoring System for Lung Function Based on Percentage of Lung Ventilated as Seen on ^{3}He MR Images

Grade	Percentage Ventilation
0*	100
1	76–99
2	51–75
3	26–50
4†	1–25

* Normal.
† Severe disease.

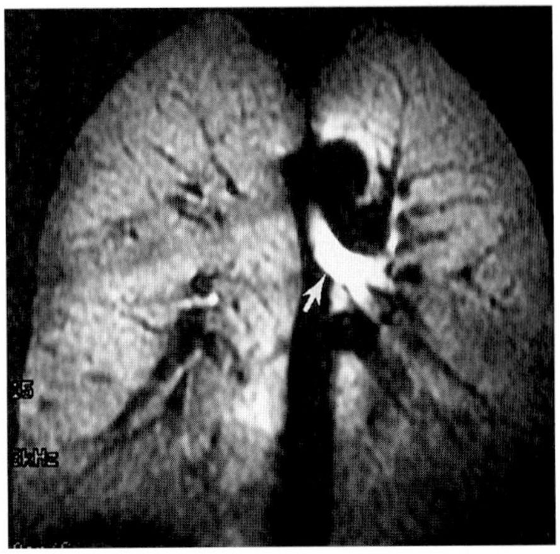

Figure 1. Normal ^{3}He MR image in a 53-year-old male volunteer. Coronal gradient-echo image (9.5/8 with 8° flip angle) through the posterior lung shows homogeneous high SI diffusely throughout the lungs. High SI from the hyperpolarized ^{3}He is seen within the left main bronchus (arrow).

TABLE 2
Scoring System for Morphologic Abnormalities as Seen on Conventional Fast SE MR Images

Grade	Percentage Involvement: Bronchial*	Percentage Involvement: Acinar Replacement*	Lymphadenopathy
0	No SI	No SI	None
1	1–25	1–25	Hilar (<1 cm diameter)
2	26–50	26–50	Hilar (>1 cm diameter)
3	51–75	51–75	Subcarinal
4	76–100	76–100	Other mediastinal

* Portion of zone involved.

TABLE 3
Comparison between MR Image Scores, Chest Radiograph Scores, and Pulmonary Function Test Results in Four Patients with CF

Modality and Score	Subject No. 1	2	3	4
Total MR imaging (maximum, 144)	39 (27)	50 (35)	52 (36)	66 (46)
Functional ^{3}He MR imaging (maximum, 48)	29 (60)	25 (52)	31 (65)	25 (52)
Morphologic MR imaging (maximum, 96)	10 (10)	25 (26)	21 (22)	41 (43)
FEV_1 (percentage of predicted value)	62	29	39	30
Brasfield chest radiograph (maximum, 25)	8	16	12	17

Note.—Numbers in parentheses are percentage of maximum score.

chi. Mucus plugging was defined as the presence of punctate areas of increased T2-weighted SI within the anatomic distribution of the bronchi. Bronchiectasis was defined as an abnormal increase in the caliber of the bronchi. Acinar replacement was defined as the presence of lung consolidation, collapse, or bullous change that replaced areas of aerated lung. Lung consolidation was defined as the presence of geographic areas of increased T2-weighted SI in the anatomic location of expected absence of SI in aerated lung. Likewise, lung collapse was determined on the basis of areas of increased SI associated with volume loss. Bullous change was defined as the presence of large cavities with walls having increased T2-weighted SI. In each zone, the potential score was 0 to 8. Lymphadenopathy was also determined as the presence of focal increased T2-weighted SI in the hila or subcarinal region or elsewhere in the mediastinum. The degree of lymphadenopathy was graded from 1 to 4 (Table 2). Therefore, the possible scores per patient (12 zones plus lymphadenopathy) ranged from 0 to 100, with higher scores indicating more abnormality. A total combined functional and morphologic score also given for each patient had a range of 0 to 148.

The MR imaging studies were reviewed simultaneously by two radiologists (L.F.D., H.P.M.), who reached conclusions by consensus. The reviewers were blinded to results of the pulmonary function tests and chest radiography. The two ^{3}He MR imaging data sets obtained in each patient were each scored separately and compared to evaluate reproducibility. The functional ^{3}He and morphologic conventional proton scores (percentage of total possible score) were compared for each lung zone. The mean ^{3}He MR imaging score for the four examinations was also calculated for each lung zone.

In each patient, scores were compared with findings at chest radiography and pulmonary function testing (Table 3). Chest radiographs were scored for the severity of disease on the basis of the scoring system described by Brasfield et al (4,5). The potential Brasfield scores ranged from 0 (normal) to 25 (severe disease) (4,5). Findings at MR imaging were also compared with those at pulmonary function testing in each subject. Parameters evaluated included the forced vital capacity (FVC) and forced expiratory volume in 1 second (FEV_1). The percentage of predicted values was calculated for each pulmonary function parameter by means of the Knudson equations (10).

Results

The four patients tolerated the five MR imaging examinations without adverse effects, and all were able to cooperate to yield high-quality images. There were no changes in vital signs, and blood oxygen saturation did not decrease by more than 10% while the hyperpolarized ^{3}He images were obtained. The overall scores are summarized in Table 3.

In all subjects, areas of absent lung ventilation were depicted on the hyperpolarized ^{3}He MR images. These areas of absent ventilation ranged from wedge-shaped peripheral defects to entire lung zones (Figs 2, 3). The ^{3}He lung zone scores ranged from normal ventilation (score, 0) to completely absent ventilation (score, 4). Total ^{3}He ventilation scores ranged from 18 (38% of maximum score) to 31 (65% of maximum score) (Table 3). In all subjects, the lack of ventilation was most severe in the upper posterior lung zones, and ventilation was most normal in the lower lung zones. The mean ^{3}He score for the upper posterior lung zone in the four subjects was 3.9. The mean score for the lower lung zones was 1.2. Concerning reproducibility, the individual lung zone scores were identical in all subjects for the two ^{3}He data sets obtained at each examination.

On the conventional fast SE images, the morphologic scores for individual lung zones ranged from 0 (normal) to 8 (most severe disease). Lymphadenopathy was present in all subjects (Fig 2), with scores ranging from 1 to 4. The total morphologic score per subject ranged from 10 (10% of maximum score) to 41 (43% of maximum score) (Table 3).

In a comparison of the percentage of maximum score for the functional ^{3}He image and morphologic conventional image scores for individual lung zones, ^{3}He ventilation scores indicated more severe disease than did the morphologic scores in 29 (60%) of the 48 lung zones evaluated (Fig 2). The severity of disease indicated by the ^{3}He image scores was equal to that indicated by the morphologic conventional image scores in 19 (40%) lung zones (Fig 3). In no zones was the morphologic score higher than the ^{3}He ventilation score. In many of the lung zones, the degree of absent ventilation was severe despite minimal morphologic changes (Fig 2). In addition, the percentage of maximum total ^{3}He scores was greater than that of the morphologic scores in all cases (Table 3).

In the four patients, there was general correlation between the total MR imaging scores, the Brasfield chest radiograph scores, and the pulmonary function test results (Table 3). The small number of subjects precluded statistical analysis. The FVC was 3.03 L (88% of predicted value) for subject 1, 1.74 L (51% of predicted value) for subject 2, 3.18 L (75% of predicted value) for subject 3, and 2.60 L (58% of predicted value) for subject 4. The FEV_1 was 1.96 L (62% of predicted value) for subject 1, 0.89 L (29% of predicted value) for subject 2, 1.55 L (39% of predicted value) for subject 3, and 1.28 L (30% of predicted value) for subject 4.

Discussion

MR imaging based on the evaluation of hydrogen protons has become the imaging modality of choice for evaluation of many organ systems and disease states. However, the role of MR imaging in the evaluation of pathologic lung conditions has been extremely limited as a result of the low concentration of hydrogen protons in normal lung tissue, which results in very low SI. One of the factors contributing to this lack of SI is that only a minority (one proton in 10,000,000 atoms) becomes polarized when an external magnetic field is applied (9). As a result of imaging with a hyperpolarized ventilation contrast agent, high SI can be generated within the pulmonary airspaces. Imaging with hyperpolarized ^3He, available on a research basis in forms with as much as 30% polarized molecules (9,11), offers a potential increase in signal-to-noise ratios of 100,000 times the values for proton imaging. The ^3He can be imaged by adapting a conventional MR imaging system by tuning the radio frequency from the resonant frequency of hydrogen to that of helium (9,11). Because SI is generated by the hyperpolarized substance and is not related to T1 recovery time, very short repetition times can be used, which result in very quick image generation. Images of a subject's entire lungs have been generated in as few as 10 seconds (9). High-spatial-resolution images have been safely obtained in healthy volunteers by having the subjects inhale hyperpolarized ^3He while lying inside a conventional MR imaging unit (9,11). The value of ^3He MR imaging in patients with pathologic lung conditions has not yet been defined (11).

In this study, high-quality images of the lung were generated in all subjects, even in the presence of moderate to severe pulmonary disease from CF. Because of the short time of acquisition for the ^3He images, all of the subjects were able to cooperate with the length of breath holding required. We did not test the ability of young children to cooperate with this examination. The time of breath holding for ^3He MR imaging is approximately 10 seconds. For CT examinations, we have had success with breath holding for longer times in children as young as 4 years and routinely in children older than 6 years. Therefore, we would not anticipate difficulty with cooperation for ^3He MR imaging except with very young children. For very young children, it may be possible to achieve ^3He MR imaging by using a "stop ventilation" technique (12). None of our patients demonstrated any signs of respiratory compromise related to the administration of the ^3He gas. Therefore, no technical or safety issues seem to prohibit the evaluation of patients with CF by means of ^3He MR imaging. In addition, in this small series, results of ^3He MR imaging were reproducible, with identical imaging findings in two separate data acquisitions.

In all subjects, abnormalities of both ventilation and morphology were readily detected. In the majority of individual lung zones and for all total ^3He scores, the ^3He functional MR image scores demon-

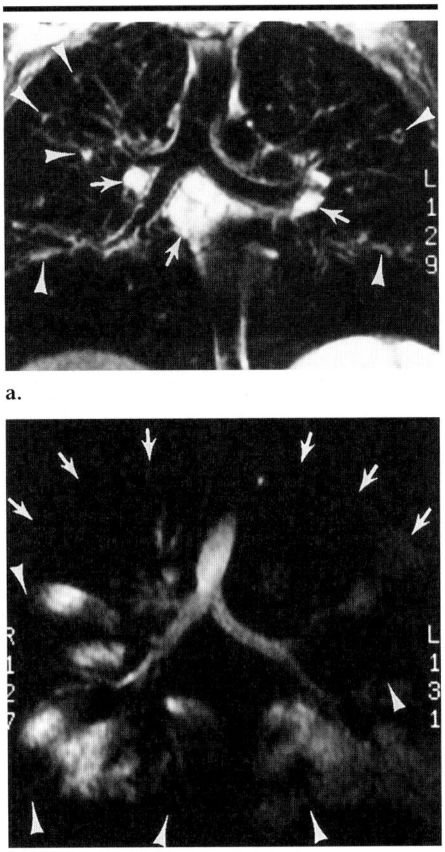

Figure 2. Subject 2. Severe ventilation defects are disproportionately greater in distribution than are morphologic abnormalities in a 24-year-old woman with CF. **(a)** Coronal conventional fast SE MR image (3,000/80) at the level of the trachea shows areas of mildly increased linear and punctate nodular SI (arrowheads) within the upper and middle lung zones bilaterally, as well as bilateral hilar and subcarinal lymphadenopathy (arrows). **(b)** Coronal ^3He gradient-echo MR image (9.5/8 with 8° flip angle) shows complete (right) and nearly complete (left) absence of SI within the upper lungs (arrows). There are also large areas of absent SI within the middle and lower lungs (arrowheads).

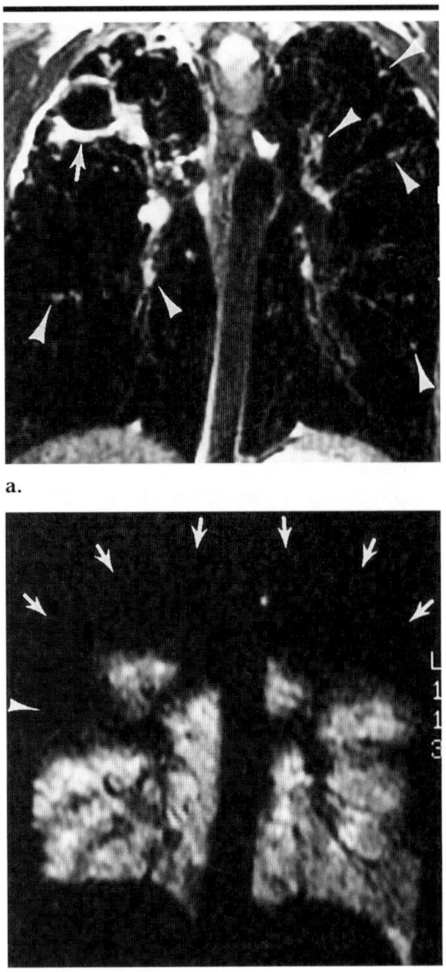

Figure 3. Subject 1. Severe functional and morphologic abnormalities in a 20-year-old woman with CF. **(a)** Coronal conventional fast SE MR image (3,000/80) through the posterior lung shows bullous change (arrow) and increased linear and nodular SI (arrowheads) involving the upper and lower lobes bilaterally. **(b)** Coronal ^3He gradient-echo MR image (9.5/8 with 8° flip angle) shows complete absence of SI in the upper lung bilaterally (arrows). There is also a large, wedge-shaped area of absent SI (arrowhead) within the lateral portion of the right middle lung.

strated more severe findings than did the scores for changes on conventional morphologic MR images. In many lung zones, severe ventilation abnormalities were seen despite minimal morphologic abnormalities. Morphologic changes at chest radiography and thin-section CT have been used as the basis for following up patients with CF for progression of disease (1–5). However, a study (1) comparing functional information obtained at pulmonary perfusion SPECT with morphologic changes seen at thin-section CT suggested that functional changes may be present prior to the occurrence of morphologic changes. Our preliminary results and the results of the previous study (1) suggest that functional abnormalities may be more sensitive to pulmonary changes of CF than are morphologic changes. Because many treatment protocols involve young children with minimal or no apparent lung disease, the ability to detect early changes in CF is critical for a modality to be used in following up progression of disease.

The standard of reference for evaluation of morphologic changes in CF is thin-section CT (1–3). To our knowledge, conventional hydrogen proton MR imaging has not been previously described as a method with which to evaluate morphologic changes in patients with CF. This is most likely related to the previously limited use of MR imaging in pulmonary imaging. However, with both the increasing speed at which fast SE images can be generated and improved techniques of respiratory gating, our preliminary results show promising potential for MR imaging to be accurate in this capacity. However, the unknown accuracy of MR imaging for depicting morphologic pulmonary changes is a limitation of our study. Further studies are needed that compare findings with combined ^{3}He and proton MR imaging to those with thin-section CT.

Because both functional and morphologic information concerning the pulmonary status of patients with CF can be generated on hyperpolarized ^{3}He MR imaging studies in a safe, reproducible, and technically feasible manner and because radiation is not used, ^{3}He MR imaging may be an ideal way of serially evaluating patients with CF for progression of disease. We believe our preliminary results warrant further investigation, including application of this technology in the cases of younger patients with CF and minimal lung disease.

Acknowledgments: We thank J. Antonio Jackson, Craig Kornegay, BS, Brad Wheeler, BS, David Zollinger, BS, and Geri Zollinger, MS, from Magnetic Imaging Technologies for their assistance with the ^{3}He gas polarizing system, and Ralph Hashoian from Medical Advances for his design of the ^{3}He radio-frequency coil.

References

1. Donnelly LF, Gelfand MJ, Brody AS, Wilmont RW. Comparison between morphologic changes seen on high-resolution CT and regional pulmonary perfusion seen on SPECT in patients with cystic fibrosis. Pediatr Radiol 1997; 27:920–925
2. Bhalla M, Turcios N, Aponte V, et al. Cystic fibrosis: scoring system with thin section CT. Radiology 1991; 179:783–788.
3. Nathanson I, Conboy K, Murphy S, Afshani E, Kuhn JP. Ultrafast computerized tomography of the chest in cystic fibrosis: a new scoring system. Pediatr Pulmonol 1991; 11:81–86.
4. Brasfield D, Hicks G, Soong SJ, Peters J, Tiller RE. Evaluation of scoring system of the chest radiograph in cystic fibrosis: a collaborative study. AJR 1980; 134:1195–1198.
5. Brasfield D, Hicks G, Soong S, Tiller R. The chest roentgenogram in cystic fibrosis: a new scoring system. Pediatrics 1979; 63: 24–29.
6. Piepsz A, Wetzburger C, Spehl M. Critical evaluation of lung scintigraphy in cystic fibrosis. J Nucl Med 1980; 21:909–913.
7. Weatherly MR, Palmer CG, Peters ME, et al. Wisconsin cystic fibrosis chest radiograph scoring system. Pediatrics 1993; 91: 488–495.
8. Noma S, Moskowitz GW, Herman PG, Khan A, Rojas KA. Pulmonary scintigraphy in elastase-induced emphysema in pigs: correlation with high-resolution computed tomography and histology. Invest Radiol 1992; 27:429–435.
9. MacFall JR, Charles HC, Black RD, et al. Human lung air spaces: potential for MR imaging with hyperpolarized He-3. Radiology 1996; 200:553–558.
10. Knudson RJ, Lebowitz MD, Holberg CJ, Borrows B. Changes in the normal expiratory flow-volume curve with growth and aging. Am Rev Respir Dis 1983; 127:725–734.
11. Kauczor HU, Hofmann D, Kreitner KF, et al. Normal and abnormal pulmonary ventilation: visualization at hyperpolarized He-3 MR imaging. Radiology 1996; 201: 564–568.
12. Long FR, Castile RG, Hogan MJ, Brody AS, Shiels WE II. Improved high-resolution CT of the lung in infants and very young children by using a "stop ventilation" technique (abstr). Pediatr Radiol 1998; 28:656.

Pulmonary Perfusion: Respiratory-triggered Three-dimensional MR Imaging with Arterial Spin Tagging—Preliminary Results in Healthy Volunteers[1]

David A. Roberts, MD, PhD
Warren B. Gefter, MD
Joshua A. Hirsch, MD
Rahim R. Rizi, PhD
Lawrence Dougherty, PhD
Robert E. Lenkinski, PhD
John S. Leigh, Jr, PhD
Mitchell D. Schnall, MD, PhD

Index terms:
Lung, MR, 60.121412, 60.121417
Lung, perfusion, 60.91
Lung, ventilation, 60.91

Radiology 1999; 212:890–895

Abbreviations:
RF = radio frequency
SI = signal intensity
SNR = signal-to-noise ratio

[1] From the Department of Radiology, University of Pennsylvania Medical Center, 1 Silverstein, 3400 Spruce St, Philadelphia, PA 19104-4283. Received March 5, 1998; revision requested June 5; final revision received October 27; accepted March 16, 1999. Supported in part by a seed grant from the Society for Thoracic Radiology. **Address reprint requests to** D.A.R. (e-mail: *roberts@oasis.rad.upenn.edu*).

Author contributions:
Guarantor of integrity of entire study, D.A.R.; study concepts, D.A.R., J.S.L.; study design, D.A.R., M.D.S., R.E.L.; definition of intellectual content, M.D.S., D.A.R., J.S.L.; literature research, D.A.R.; clinical studies, D.A.R., R.E.L., L.D., M.D.S.; data acquisition, J.A.H., D.A.R., R.R.R.; data analysis, D.A.R., R.R.R.; statistical analysis, D.A.R.; manuscript preparation and editing, D.A.R.; manuscript review, R.R.R., W.B.G., R.E.L., M.D.S.

The authors used a spin-tagging method of magnetic resonance perfusion imaging to measure pulmonary perfusion in eight healthy volunteers with use of a respiratory-triggered three-dimensional pulse sequence. The average signal intensity (SI) decrease upon arterial labeling was 24%. The perfusion SI increased by 21% after exercise (P = .02). Focal blood flow abnormalities were observed in a patient with chronic obstructive pulmonary disease.

The imaging of pulmonary perfusion has many important applications in medicine and has proved useful in the diagnosis of pulmonary vascular disease and in the evaluation of disease in patients with emphysema. Pulmonary embolism is a major cause of morbidity and mortality in the United States (1). Data indicate that there is an increase in the mortality of patients who are not appropriately treated for pulmonary embolism, indicating the critical need for accurate diagnosis of this disease (2). The diagnosis of pulmonary embolism is based on the demonstration of decreased or absent blood flow in a focal region of the lung without a corresponding ventilation abnormality. Currently, the most commonly used noninvasive imaging method is radionuclide ventilation-perfusion scanning. Although normal or grossly abnormal ventilation-perfusion scans provide extremely useful clinical information, there is an unacceptably high frequency of equivocal results that necessitates further evaluation (3). Although pulmonary angiography is a highly accurate and safe method, there is evidence that it is underused, perhaps due to its relative expense and invasiveness (4,5). The development of an accurate, noninvasive method of pulmonary perfusion imaging would constitute an advance in patient care.

Magnetic resonance (MR) imaging of the lung parenchyma is intrinsically difficult due to the large degree of microscopic magnetic field inhomogeneity, which causes the observed transverse relaxation time (T2*) to be extremely short (6,7). However, the recent development of gradient-echo pulse sequences with extremely short echo time and projection reconstruction techniques has allowed investigators to image the pulmonary parenchyma (8–10). Recently, several MR methods of pulmonary perfusion imaging have been described (11–16). To date, the MR methods described have been breath-hold techniques that are based on dynamic observation of the pulmonary magnetization after either injection of a bolus of paramagnetic contrast agent (13,15,16) or spatially selective inversion of the mediastinum (12,14). An alternative noninvasive technique exploits differences in signal intensity (SI) between different cardiac phases (11). Although promising, these methods necessitate breath-holding maneuvers, which are often impossible for patients with pulmonary disease. In addition, injection of a contrast agent for the perfusion study introduces additional risk and expense.

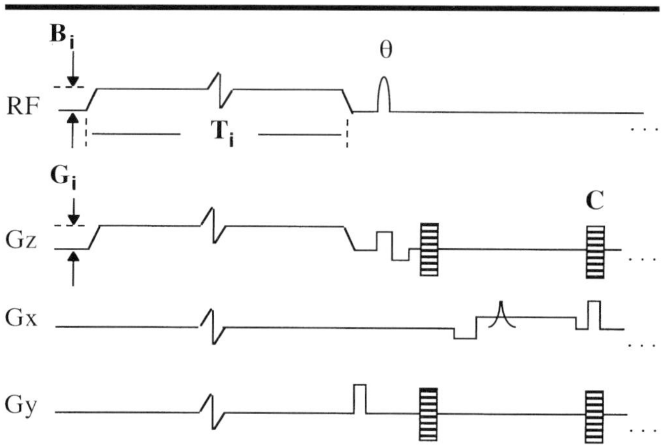

Figure 1. Schematic depicts the three-dimensional, compact, gradient-echo pulse sequence used to acquire MR perfusion image data. It shows the RF and gradient (*Gx*, *Gy*, and *Gz*) waveforms. An arterial labeling RF pulse is applied in the presence of a gradient during the interpulse interval to provide continuous magnetic labeling of pulmonary arterial blood flow. The amplitude, B_i, of the RF pulse is 24 mG, and the duration of the pulse, T_i, is 40 msec. The flip angle, θ, is 30°. The time axis is not to scale. *C* = crusher gradient, G_i = inversion gradient.

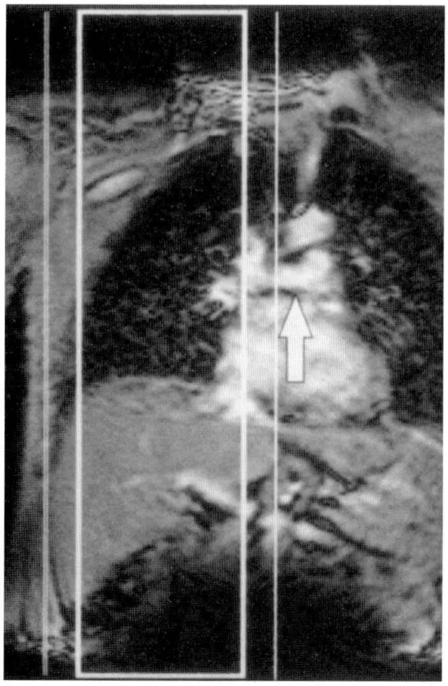

Figure 2. T1-weighted localizer MR image illustrates the experimental design of the perfusion measurement and the locations of the planes of arterial labeling for the inversion image (line on the right) and for the magnetization transfer control image (line on the left) relative to the image volume (rectangle). Under the conditions used in this experiment, the labeling RF pulse created a band of saturation approximately 0.6 mm thick, as indicated by the lines. Arterial blood in the right pulmonary artery (arrow) was labeled during acquisition of the inversion image.

The quality of subsequent MR angiograms is also reduced by contrast material injection owing to reduced background suppression, which causes a reduction in the contrast-to-noise ratio.

The arterial spin-tagging method of perfusion imaging is based on the steady-state magnetic labeling of the arterial water supplying an organ (17,18). This results in a measurable change in the steady-state magnetization from which values for tissue-specific perfusion can be calculated. This method has been applied successfully in both animal and human studies (17–23). To our knowledge, the application of this method to the study of pulmonary perfusion has not been reported. In this study, we evaluated use of a three-dimensional, respiratory-triggered implementation of this technique to depict regional pulmonary perfusion in healthy subjects without the need for breath holding.

Materials and Methods

Human Subjects

This study was conducted according to a protocol approved by our institutional review board. Informed consent was obtained from all volunteers after the nature of the study was fully explained. Eight healthy adult subjects (three men, five women; age range, 21–33 years; average age, 27 years ± 5 [SD]) participated in this study. None of the subjects had a history of pulmonary disease, and all were nonsmokers.

Image Acquisition

MR imaging data were acquired with a 1.5-T imaging system equipped with high-power gradients (Echospeed Signa, revision 5.6 software; GE Medical Systems, Milwaukee, Wis). The gradients had a peak amplitude of 2.2 G/cm. For monitoring purposes, cardiac electrodes were placed on the chest wall, and a respiratory excursion transducer was looped around the chest. A quadrature birdcage coil encompassing the entire body was used for signal transmission. To maximize the signal-to-noise ratio (SNR), a phased-array coil was placed around the thorax for signal reception that consisted of anterior and posterior two-element arrays. An automated gradient shim was performed, and the radio-frequency (RF) synthesizer frequency was centered on the proton water resonance frequency.

The pulse sequence used to acquire data appears in Figure 1. It is a three-dimensional, compact, gradient-echo pulse sequence that incorporates an asymmetric, truncated sinc RF slab excitation pulse of 1.28-msec duration. The following imaging parameters were used: repetition time msec/echo time msec of 50/716–760 with 30° flip angle, 7–10-mm section thickness, 40–48-cm field of view, and 256 × 64 × 16 matrix. The nominal in-plane resolution was approximately 2 × 8 mm. To minimize the echo time, a fractional echo was acquired with a 64-kHz receiver bandwidth. A sagittal volume was excited that included the right lung, as indicated in Figure 2. Trapezoidal gradient and RF pulses were placed in the interpulse interval to label blood flow according to the principle of flow-induced adiabatic fast passage (24,25). The offset frequency of the labeling pulse was adjusted in each case so that the location of the plane of arterial labeling intersected the right pulmonary artery (Fig 2). In all subjects, the right pulmonary artery was readily identified on the scout localizer image by both the radiologist (D.A.R.) and technologist. The amplitude of the labeling RF pulse, B_i, was 24 mG, and its duration was 40 msec, corresponding to a duty cycle of 80%. The amplitude of the inversion gradient, G_i, was 0.1 G/cm. Under these conditions, the labeling RF pulse created a band of saturation approximately 0.6 mm thick, as indicated by the lines in Figure 2. On the basis of measurements obtained on our localizer images, the average diameter of the right pulmonary artery was 1.6 cm. Assuming that the right pulmonary artery receives half the normal cardiac output of 5 L/min, then the estimated average velocity of flow is 8.3 cm/sec. This yields an adiabaticity factor (21) for the inversion of 2.8, yielding an estimated degree of inversion of 95%. As the duty cycle is 80%, this yields an estimated net inversion efficiency of 76%. This likely represents an overestimation of the degree of inversion as higher velocities occur during the cardiac cycle that yield lower inversion efficiencies. Although one would ideally like to achieve 100% inversion efficiency to maximize the observed SI change, this was the highest achievable value to remain within limitations of the specific absorption rate.

The pulse sequence was triggered to the respiratory cycle, as shown in Figure 3. The excitation and arterial labeling RF pulses and gradients were applied continuously to maintain a steady-state condition. However, data acquisition was performed during only the end-expiratory phase of the respiratory cycle, as indicated by the black bars in the diagram. Sixteen slab encodings were acquired at end expiration, requiring a temporal window of 800 msec. This approach maximized the signal from the lung, which was observed to be higher at end expiration.

Magnitude image data were acquired in the presence of arterial labeling (inversion) and under control conditions in which the amplitude of the label RF was set to zero (control). To correct for magnetization transfer effects of the labeling RF pulse (26), an additional acquisition (magnetization transfer control) was performed in which the plane of arterial labeling was located in a symmetric location on the opposite side of the image volume, as shown in Figure 2. This geometry reproduced the off-resonance effects of the pulse in the absence of arterial labeling and allowed estimated correction for these effects. The entire data acquisition typically required less than 15 minutes.

This method, as described, does not provide an absolute quantitation of perfusion. Instead, images are produced of the relative regional SI change induced by means of arterial labeling. For this reason, accurate knowledge of the degree of arterial inversion at the level of the pulmonary artery is not important for the detection of spatial defects in a given individual. However, this does become important when attempting to compare results obtained in the same individual at different points in time.

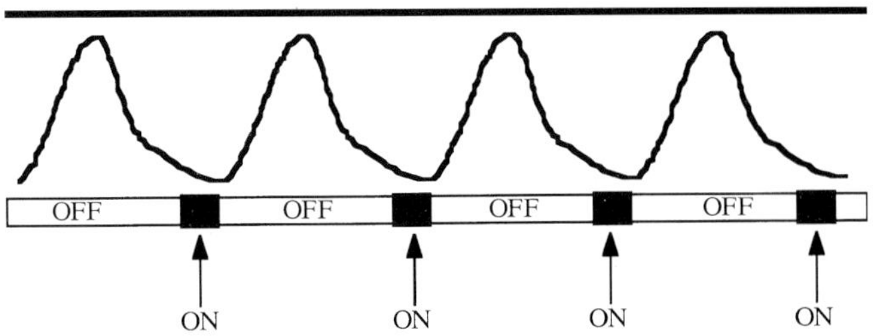

Figure 3. Schematic depicts respiratory triggering performed by monitoring the patient's chest excursion. The trigger was set so data acquisition was enabled during only the end-expiratory phase of the respiratory cycle (■).

Exercise Studies

Subjects (n = 8) were instructed to exercise by performing a leg-raising maneuver until the point of exhaustion. The basal heart rate and the heart rate immediately after exercise were recorded. Perfusion data were acquired before and after exercise. Comparison of the heart rate and the pre- and postexercise data was performed by means of the paired Student t test. In one patient, images obtained after exercise were corrupted by motion artifact and were excluded. Therefore, postexercise data were available in only seven patients.

Data Analysis

All data analysis was performed off-line on a workstation (Silicon Graphics, Mountain View, Calif) by using the Interactive Data Language (Research Systems, Boulder, Colo). Calculation of the perfusion images typically required 10 minutes per patient, including both data transfer to the workstation and subsequent analysis. The total time necessary to produce perfusion images of the right lung was 30 minutes.

Prior to formation of magnitude image subtraction data, the inversion image data were corrected for off-resonance effects of the labeling RF. A region of interest was drawn interactively around the lung in each image in the control and magnetization transfer control data sets. Pixels composing pulmonary parenchyma were then identified by means of segmentation of the magnitude image data within these regions of interest by using an upper threshold of 150. This value was chosen empirically, as segmentation at this level eliminated contributions from the pulmonary arteries in all patients. Note that this form of segmentation does not eliminate contributions from the bronchi, which are expected to have zero SI as they contain air. This represents a small error in the analysis. The degree of magnetization transfer saturation, S, caused by the labeling pulse in pulmonary parenchyma was computed as the ratio of the average SI with the pulse divided by the average SI without the pulse. This was computed for each section in the magnetization transfer control acquisition as a function of distance, z', from the plane of the lateral labeling pulse. It is important to note that the physical location of the plane used to determine the degree of saturation was different from the corresponding plane in the inversion data set. Therefore, a point-by-point correction could not be performed. The computation yielded a correction factor, $S'(z')$, for magnetization transfer effect as a function of z'. Assuming that the lung is spatially homogeneous in its off-resonance properties, the appropriate correction factor for arterial spin-tagging images is $S(z) = S'(z')$, where z is the distance of an arterial spin-tagging image from the plane of arterial labeling. In some cases, the extreme medial or lateral images in the volume contained so little lung parenchyma that an accurate calculation could not be performed. In these cases, no correction was performed ($S[z] = 1.0$).

Images of the regional percentage SI change after correction for off-resonance effects (Δ_{CORR}) induced upon arterial labeling in a section located a distance, z, from the plane of arterial labeling were calculated as

$$\Delta_{CORR}(x, y, z) = 100 \times \{M_c(x, y, z) - [M_i(x, y, z)/S(z)]/M_c(x, y, z)\},$$

where M_c and M_i are the magnitude SI in images acquired under control conditions (no labeling RF) and under conditions of arterial labeling, respectively. This calculation was not performed in pixels on the control image in which the SI was zero. In these pixels, the value of Δ_{CORR} was set to zero.

The SI in the control image was determined by computing the average value in

Perfusion Data in Eight Healthy Subjects

Subject No.	SNR in Control Image	Percentage SI Change before Exercise: Between Inversion and Control Images	Percentage SI Change before Exercise: After Correction for Off-Resonance Effects	Percentage SI Change after Exercise: Between Inversion and Control Images	Percentage SI Change after Exercise: After Correction for Off-Resonance Effects
1	25	36	26	37	26
2	60	36	26	47	38
3	57	29	22	38	24
4	49	30	24	33	27
5	67	30	22	37	28
6	58	29	23	38	31
7	40	34	26	37	28
8	29	34	25	(NA)	(NA)
Total (mean ± SD)	48 ± 15	32 ± 3	24 ± 2	38 ± 4	29 ± 5

Note.—NA = not applicable. Pixels composing the lung parenchyma were identified by means of simple thresholding after a region of interest was placed around the lung. This eliminated contributions from large central vessels.

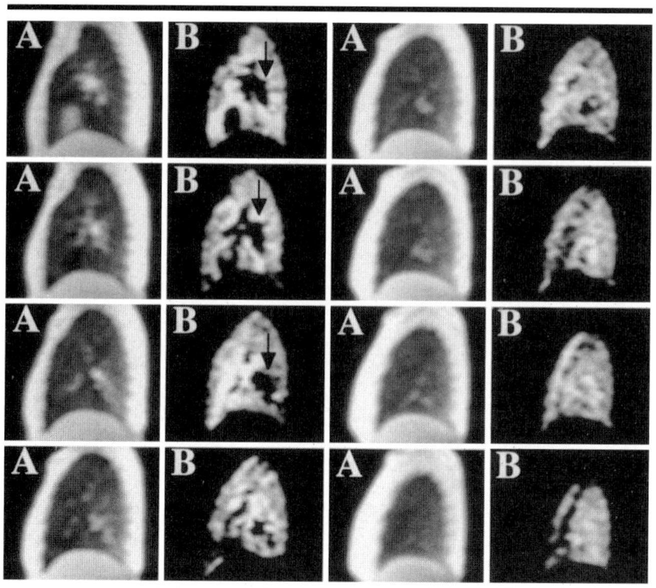

Figure 4. Images depict results of the arterial spin-tagging perfusion measurement technique in a resting healthy volunteer. *A*, Sagittal MR images of the corrected percentage SI change after correction for off-resonance effects induced by arterial labeling appear next to *B*, the corresponding control images. The SI changes are scaled from 0 (black) to 80% (white). Small SI changes in the chest wall have been excluded from display by means of segmentation. The section location progresses from most medial (top left) to most lateral (bottom right). Black defects (arrows in the second column) shown in some of the blood flow images (*B*) represent central pulmonary arteries that have been excluded from the analysis as have pulmonary veins and bronchi.

a small region of interest placed around the peripheral aspect of the lung in the central section. The noise was computed as the SD in a small region of interest outside the body, in the upper left corner of the same section. This location was chosen to minimize the effect of potential respiratory motion artifacts on the noise calculation. The SNR was then computed as their ratio.

Values for the mean SI change in pulmonary parenchyma were computed as follows: (*a*) a region of interest was interactively placed around the lung in each of the control images, and (*b*) segmentation within this region was then performed with use of an upper threshold of 150 to identify pixels composing lung parenchyma. Inspection of the segmented images showed that this eliminated contributions from the central pulmonary arteries.

Results

Statistical analysis of the perfusion data acquired in eight subjects appears in the Table. The average SNR obtained in the lung parenchyma in eight subjects was 48 ± 15 (mean ± SD). The average percentage SI change at rest before and after correction for off-resonance effects was 32% ± 3 and 24% ± 2, respectively (n = 8). These data demonstrate that approximately one-third of the observed SI change is due to off-resonance effects, most of which arise from sections closest to the plane of arterial labeling. Typical results obtained from a healthy volunteer at rest appear in Figure 4. In all subjects, readily observable changes in the pulmonary magnetization were observed to the level of the pleura. Only minimal respiratory motion artifacts were observed.

Results of exercise testing also appear in the Table. The average heart rate was 60 beats per minute ± 6 and 93 beats per minute ± 12 before and after exercise, respectively ($n = 7$, $P = .001$). The average percentage SI change after correction for off-resonance effects before and after exercise was 24% ± 2 and 29% ± 5, respectively (P = .02). Thus, there was a 21% increase in the observed SI change after exercise.

We also obtained preliminary data in a patient with chronic obstructive pulmonary disease (Fig 5). The reformatted sagittal computed tomographic (CT) images reveal bullous disease, which asymmetrically affects the right upper and middle lobes, with relative sparing of the right lower lobe (Fig 5, top row). Despite the presence of bullous disease, an SNR of approximately 11:1 was obtained in the affected parts of the lung on the control images (Fig 5, middle row). The arterial spin-tagging perfusion images demonstrated marked hypoperfusion in a distribution that closely paralleled the distribution of chronic obstructive pulmonary disease (Fig 5, bottom row). Hypoperfusion was observed to the extreme lateral aspect of the lung, where off-resonance effects were quite small.

Discussion

Despite its relatively low SNR, the human lung otherwise represents an ideal organ for application of the arterial spin-tagging method of perfusion imaging. In addition to having a well-defined arterial blood supply, the lung also possesses an extremely large tissue-specific perfusion and blood volume. Each lung receives approximately one-half the cardiac output, yielding a typical volumetric flow rate of 2,500 mL/min in a 70-kg person. The right lung weighs approximately 625 g (27), yielding a tissue-specific perfusion of 4.0 $mL \cdot g^{-1} \cdot min^{-1}$. This value is more than four times larger than the values reported for human gray matter (28). In addition, the lung also has a relatively large blood volume compartment (29–31). In contrast to prior implementations of this technique, we made no attempt to suppress the intravascular compartment as this is extremely difficult due to the short transverse relaxation time. As a consequence, the observed SI changes at arterial labeling are a function of not only perfusion but also the blood volume and the artery-to-capillary transit time (26). Specifically, assuming an apparent T1 of 1.0 seconds, a partition coefficient of 1.0, and an effective degree of labeling of 65%, the predicted SI change based on perfusion alone should be approximately 8%, accounting for approximately one-third of the SI changes observed in this study. The majority of the observed SI changes are probably due to blood volume effects. These factors make the absolute quantitation of pulmonary perfusion difficult with this approach.

However, the presence of thromboembolic disease leads to decreases in pulmonary perfusion and blood volume while at the same time prolonging the transit time. All of these changes are expected to lead to a marked reduction in the observed SI change upon arterial labeling. Therefore, the arterial spin-tagging method should be especially sensitive to the presence of pulmonary thromboembolic disease. This may have important clinical implications as recent data suggest that as many as 30% of patients with pulmonary emboli have involvement at the subsegmental level or below (32). This area has been difficult to evaluate with cross-sectional imaging techniques (33,34).

The assumption of a spatially uniform off-resonance characteristic in the lung represents a potential source of error. It is indeed probable that in the presence of disease there are marked regional variations in the magnetization transfer properties of the lung that would invalidate this assumption. The use of amplitude-modulated control irradiation would eliminate this as a potential source of error; however, such pulses could not be implemented at present owing to limitations of the RF amplifier.

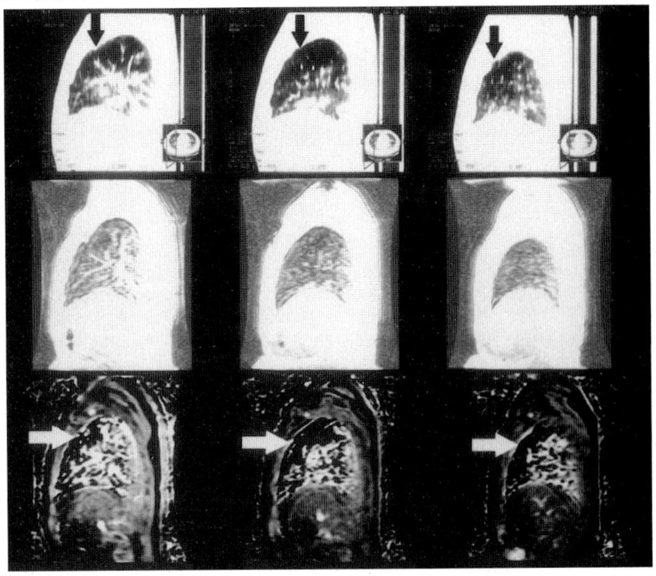

Figure 5. Top row: Reformatted, sagittal, nonenhanced CT images obtained in a patient with underlying chronic obstructive pulmonary disease reveal asymmetric bullous disease (arrows) preferentially affecting the right upper and middle lobes. Middle row: Despite the presence of bullous disease, the SNR in the affected areas was 11:1 on the control images. Bottom row: The corresponding arterial spin-tagging perfusion images demonstrate focal defects (arrows) in perfusion that correlate well with the distribution of involvement depicted at CT.

The spin-tagging pulse labels all blood flow occurring at the level of the pulmonary hilum. Therefore, the perfusion images reflect contributions from both the pulmonary and bronchial arteries. This is an important difference from radionuclide ventilation-perfusion scanning in which, in the absence of shunt formation, uptake reflects only pulmonary arterial flow. Results obtained with the arterial spin-tagging technique may differ from those obtained on ventilation-perfusion scans, especially in patients with chronic lung disease in whom prominent bronchial collateral vessels may exist. In addition, this may decrease the sensitivity of this method for the detection of pulmonary embolism as bronchial supply to the affected segment may persist.

The arterial spin-tagging method may be used to obtain noninvasive images of pulmonary blood flow without the need for patient breath holding. The arterial spin-tagging technique is entirely noninvasive and eliminates the risks and expense associated with contrast material administration. In comparison with previously described MR techniques for pulmonary perfusion imaging (11,12,14), this technique does not require breath holding, a task that is often impossible for patients with pulmonary disease. In fact, this method is ideally suited to the evaluation of disease in patients receiving artificial ventilation as nearly perfect respiratory triggering may be achieved in this setting. As a steady-state technique, it theoretically allows a greater effect of arterial labeling to build up during the acquisition. Alternative MR pulmonary perfusion imaging techniques that require the intravenous injection of paramagnetic contrast agents have also been described (13,16). These methods suffer from the need for breath holding, a task that is often impossible for patients with clinically important pulmonary disease. Although pulmonary MR angiography has been shown to be a highly accurate and safe method for the diagnosis of pulmonary embolism, the need to inject gadolinium for the perfusion study inevitably reduces the quality of subsequent MR angiograms owing to decreased background suppression. In addition, the accuracy of pulmonary MR angiography at the subsegmental level and below is not known (34). There is evidence that a major fraction of pulmonary emboli occur at the subsegmental level or below (32). As the spin-tagging method does not involve contrast material injection, this technique may become useful as a means of focusing the MR angiographic examination in a specific region of the lung, thereby potentially increasing the spatial resolution and diagnostic yield of pulmonary MR angiograms and allowing the diagnosis of subsegmental pulmonary embolism. In addition, in conjunction with recently developed noninvasive methods of MR ventilation imaging (35,36), it has the potential to constitute a component of an entirely noninvasive, high-spatial-resolution form of MR ventilation-perfusion imaging.

The clinical utility of the arterial spin-tagging method, although promising, may be limited by several technical factors. Specifically, its success rate and accuracy in a patient population are unknown. Techniques must be developed to allow perfusion imaging of the left lung, where effects due to cardiac motion and intracardiac labeling of blood flow must be addressed. Such techniques may lead to increases in acquisition time. The arterial spin-tagging method in isolation is likely to suffer from indeterminate results in the clinical setting of pulmonary embolism for the same reasons that radionuclide scanning does. Despite these limitations, it is reasonable to conjecture that this method, coupled with high-spatial-resolution MR angiography and ventilation imaging, may form an important part of an integrated functional and anatomic MR examination of the lung.

Acknowledgments: The authors are grateful to David Alsop, PhD, and Leon Axel, PhD, MD, from the Department of Radiology, University of Pennsylvania Medical Center for helpful discussion and advice. We are also grateful to Zahi Fayad, PhD, from the Department of Radiology, Mount Sinai Medical Center, New York, NY, for stimulating discussion. Valuable technical assistance was provided by Norman Butler, MRT.

References

1. Roberts HR, Adel S, Bernstein EF, et al. Prevention of venous thrombosis and pulmonary embolism. JAMA 1986; 256:744–749.
2. Benotti R, Ockene IS, Alpert JS. The clinical profile of unresolved pulmonary embolism. Chest 1983; 84:669–678.
3. The PIOPED Investigators. Value of the ventilation/perfusion scan in acute pulmonary embolism: results of the Prospective Investigation of Pulmonary Embolism Diagnosis (PIOPED). JAMA 1990; 263:2753–2759.
4. Sostman HD, Ravin CE, Sullivan DC, Mills SR, Glickman MG, Dorfman GS. Use of pulmonary angiography for suspected pulmonary embolism: influence of scintigraphic diagnosis. AJR 1982; 139:673–677.
5. Hudson ER, Smith TP, McDermott VG, et al. Pulmonary angiography performed with iopamidol: complications in 1,434 patients. Radiology 1996; 198:61–65.
6. Bergin CJ, Glover GH, Pauly JM. Lung parenchyma: magnetic susceptibility in MR imaging. Radiology 1991; 180:845–848.
7. Bergin CJ, Glover GM, Pauly J. Magnetic resonance imaging of lung parenchyma. J Thorac Imaging 1993; 8:12–17.
8. Bergin CJ, Pauly JM, Macovski A. Lung parenchyma: projection reconstruction MR imaging. Radiology 1991; 179:777–781.
9. Mayo JR, MacKay A, Muller NL. MR imaging of the lungs: value of short TE spin-echo pulse sequences. AJR 1992; 159:951–956.
10. Alsop DC, Hatabu H, Bonnet M, Listerud J, Gefter W. Multi-slice, breathhold imaging of the lung with submillisecond echo times. Magn Reson Med 1995; 33:678–682.
11. Mayo JR, Whittall K, Xiang Q, MacKay A. Peripheral pulmonary blood flow detected with MR imaging (abstr). Radiology 1994; 194(P):311.
12. Hatabu H, Wielopolski PA, Edelman RR. Pulmonary perfusion MR imaging with ultrashort TR/TE GRE sequence and signal targeting with alternating RF (abstr). Radiology 1995; 197(P):231–232.
13. Hatabu H, Gaa J, Kim D, Li W, Prasad PV, Edelman RR. Pulmonary perfusion: qualitative assessment with dynamic contrast-enhanced MRI using ultra-short TE and inversion recovery turbo FLASH. Magn Reson Med 1996; 36:503–508.
14. Edelman RR, Hatabu H, Tadamura E, Kim D, Prasad PV, Buxton RB. Pulmonary perfusion: noninvasive imaging and quantification by magnetic resonance (abstr). In: Proceedings of the Fourth Meeting of the International Society for Magnetic Resonance in Medicine. Berkeley, Calif: International Society for Magnetic Resonance in Medicine, 1996; 1314.
15. Haraldseth O, Kvaerness J, Amundsen T, Waage A, Bjermer L. MR perfusion imaging of the human lung (abstr). In: Proceedings of the Fourth Meeting of the International Society for Magnetic Resonance in Medicine. Berkeley, Calif: International Society for Magnetic Resonance in Medicine, 1996; 15.
16. Hatabu H, Gaa J, Kim D, Li W, Prasad PV, Edelman RR. Pulmonary perfusion and angiography: evaluation with breathhold enhanced three-dimensional fast imaging steady-state precession MR imaging with short TR and TE. AJR 1996; 167:653–655.
17. Detre JA, Leigh JS, Williams DS, Koretsky AP. Perfusion imaging. Magn Reson Med 1991; 22:1–9.
18. Williams DS, Detre JA, Leigh JS, Koretsky AP. Magnetic resonance imaging of perfusion using spin inversion of arterial water. Proc Natl Acad Sci USA 1992; 89:212–216.
19. Williams DS, Zhang W, Koretsky AP, Adler S. MRI of perfusion in the kidney in vivo using spin inversion of arterial water (abstr). In: Proceedings of the 12th Annual Scientific Meeting of the Society of Magnetic Resonance in Medicine. Berkeley, Calif: Society of Magnetic Resonance in Medicine, 1993; 641.
20. Walsh EG, Minematsu K, Leppo J, Moore SC. Radioactive microsphere validation of a volume localized continuous saturation perfusion measurement. Magn Reson Med 1994; 31:147–153.
21. Roberts DA. Magnetic resonance imaging of perfusion in humans using spin-tagging of arterial water. Thesis. University of Pennsylvania, Philadelphia, Pa, 1994.
22. Detre JA, Zhang W, Roberts DA, et al. Perfusion imaging using arterial spin-tagging. NMR Biomed 1994; 7:75–82.
23. Roberts DA, Detre JA, Bolinger L, et al. Renal perfusion in humans: MR imaging with spin-tagging of arterial water. Radiology 1995; 196:281–286.
24. Dixon WT, Du LN, Faul DD, Gado M, Rossnick S. Projection angiograms of blood labeled by adiabatic fast passage. Magn Reson Med 1986; 3:454–462.
25. Lee HK, Nalcioglu O, Moran PR. Spatially-resolved flow velocity measurements and projection angiography by adiabatic passage. Magn Reson Imaging 1991; 9:115–127.
26. Zhang W, Williams DS, Detre JA, Koretsky AP. Measurement of brain perfusion by volume-localized NMR spectroscopy using inversion of arterial water spins: accounting for transit time and cross-relaxation. Magn Reson Med 1992; 25:362–371.
27. Warwick R, Williams PL, eds. Gray's anatomy. 35th British ed. Philadelphia, Pa: Saunders, 1973; 1196.
28. Roberts DA, Detre JA, Insko EK, Bolinger L, Leigh JS Jr. Quantitative magnetic resonance imaging of human brain perfusion at 1.5 T using steady-state inversion of arterial water. Proc Natl Acad Sci USA 1994; 91:33–37.
29. Maloney J. Radioisotope technique for measuring regional blood volume in the lung. Int J Appl Radiat Isot 1972; 23:87–91.
30. Harris P, Heath D, eds. The human pulmonary circulation. Edinburgh, Scotland: Churchill-Livingstone, 1986; 103–106.
31. Guyton AC. Textbook of medical physiology. 7th ed. Philadelphia, Pa: Saunders, 1986; 288–289.
32. Oser RF, Zuckerman DA, Gutierrez FR, Brink JA. Anatomic distribution of pulmonary emboli at pulmonary angiography: implications for cross-sectional imaging. Radiology 1996; 199:31–35.
33. Remy-Jardin M, Remy J, Deschildre F, et al. Diagnosis of pulmonary embolism with spiral CT: comparison with pulmonary angiography and scintigraphy. Radiology 1996; 200:699–706.
34. Meaney JF, Weg JG, Chenevert TL, Stafford-Johnson D, Hamilton BH, Prince MR. Diagnosis of pulmonary embolism with magnetic resonance angiography. N Engl J Med 1997; 336:1422–1427.
35. Middleton H, Black RD, Saam B, et al. MR imaging with hyperpolarized 3-He gas. Magn Reson Med 1995; 33:271–275.
36. Edelman RR, Hatabu H, Tadamura E, Li W, Prasad PV. Noninvasive assessment of regional ventilation in the human lung using oxygen-enhanced magnetic resonance imaging. Nat Med 1996; 2:1236–1239.

Pulmonary Arterial Resistance: Noninvasive Measurement with Indexes of Pulmonary Flow Estimated at Velocity-encoded MR Imaging—Preliminary Experience[1]

Elie Mousseaux, MD, PhD
Jean Pierre Tasu, MD, PhD
Odile Jolivet, PhD
Gérard Simonneau, MD
Jacques Bittoun, MD, PhD
Jean-Claude Gaux, MD

Index terms:
Hypertension, pulmonary, 564.78
Magnetic resonance (MR), phase imaging, 564.12144
Pulmonary arteries, abnormalities, 564.78
Pulmonary arteries, flow dynamics, 564.78

Radiology 1999; 212:896–902

Abbreviations:
PVR = pulmonary vascular resistance
SEE = standard error of the estimate

[1] From the Department of Cardiovascular Radiology, Hôpital Broussais, 96 rue Didot, 75014 Paris, France (E.M., O.J., J.C.G.); Institut National de la Santé et de la Recherche Médicale (INSERM) U494, Centre Hospitalier Universitaire (CHU) Pitié-Salpêtrière, Paris, France (E.M., O.J.); Unité de Recherche Associée (URA), Centre National de la Recherche Scientifique (CNRS) 2212, Centre luter Etablissement de Résonance Magnétique (CIERM), Hôpital de Bicêtre, Le Kremlin Bicêtre, France (J.P.T., J.B.); and the Department of Respiratory Disease, Hôpital Antoine Béclère, Clamart, France (G.S.). From the 1998 RSNA scientific assembly. Received May 29, 1998; revision requested July 16; final revision received November 20; accepted February 22, 1999. **Address reprint requests to** E.M. (e-mail: *mousseaux@hbroussais.fr*).

Author contributions:
Guarantors of integrity of entire study, J.B., J.C.G.; study concepts, E.M., O.J., G.S.; study design, E.M., J.P.T.; definition of intellectual content, E.M., J.P.T., O.J.; literature research, J.P.T., E.M.; clinical studies, G.S., E.M.; experimental studies, J.P.T., E.M.; data acquisition, J.P.T., E.M.; data analysis, E.M., J.P.T., G.S.; statistical analysis, E.M., J.P.T.; manuscript preparation, E.M., J.P.T., O.J.; manuscript editing, E.M., O.J.; manuscript review, all authors.

Cardiac output and pulmonary vascular resistance (PVR) were measured in 19 patients by means of catheterization of the right side of the heart. Results were compared with the cardiac output and indexes of pulmonary arterial blood flow estimated with velocity-encoded magnetic resonance (MR) imaging. Correlations were good between estimates with right-sided heart catheterization and those with velocity-encoded MR imaging. By providing accurate pulmonary arterial blood flow measurements, velocity-encoded MR imaging allowed distinction of patients with high PVR from subjects with normal PVR.

A noninvasive method that provides reliable estimates of pulmonary arterial pressure, cardiac output, and pulmonary vascular resistance (PVR) would be helpful for measuring hemodynamic parameters in patients with chronic pulmonary hypertension and for detecting and monitoring the disease. Focused echocardiographic Doppler examination can provide data about tricuspid and pulmonary valve regurgitations suitable for producing reliable estimates of pressures in 53%–97% of patients (1,2). However, there remains a need for a reliable method of assessing cardiac output and PVR with Doppler echocardiography, especially in patients with right-sided heart disease.

It is possible to directly and accurately measure stroke volume of the right and left ventricles and the corresponding cardiac output with velocity-encoded magnetic resonance (MR) imaging in the main pulmonary artery or in the ascending aorta (3–9). At velocity-encoded MR imaging in patients with pulmonary hypertension, pulmonary arterial flow measurements have indicated very inhomogeneous velocity profiles, large volumes of retrograde flow, and low distensibility of the main pulmonary artery (5,7,10). Results of velocity-profile analyses within the pulmonary artery and throughout the cardiac cycle at velocity-encoded MR imaging also suggest that quantification of selected parameters of blood flow may be used as a noninvasive method for estimating PVR.

The natural logarithm of the percentage of pulmonary retrograde flow obtained at velocity-encoded MR imaging was found to be proportional to PVR (5). As previously found in Doppler studies (11,12), the acceleration time, defined in velocity-encoded MR imaging as the time from the onset of flow to the peak velocity, was much shorter in patients with primary pulmonary hypertension than it was in healthy volunteers (7), and it was inversely correlated with mean pulmonary arterial pressure (7,13). In other Doppler studies (14,15), however, the acceleration time was found to be a poor predictor of pulmonary arterial pressure or PVR. During ejection, the right ventricle generates pulsatile pressure and flow waves that interact with and are modified by characteristics of the distensible pulmonary arterial circulation.

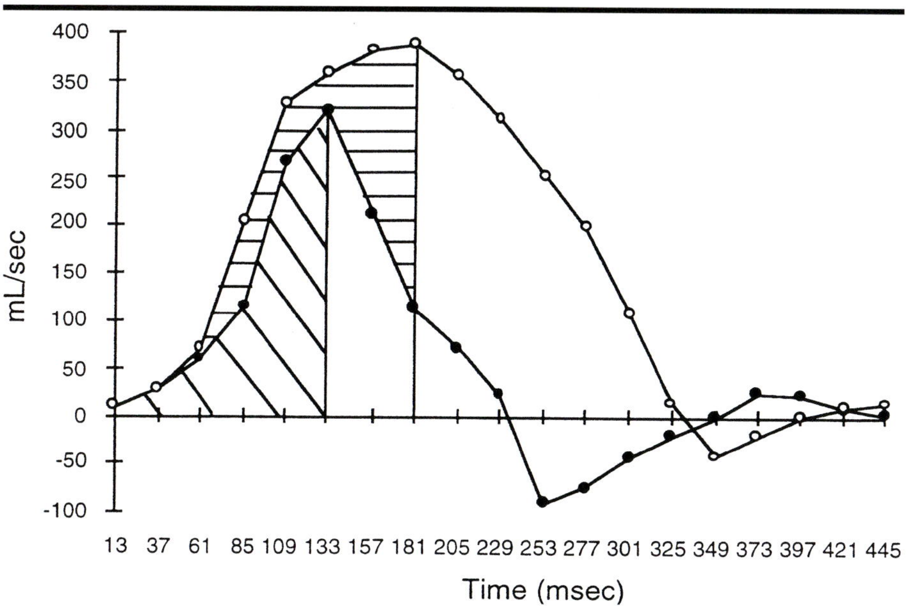

a.

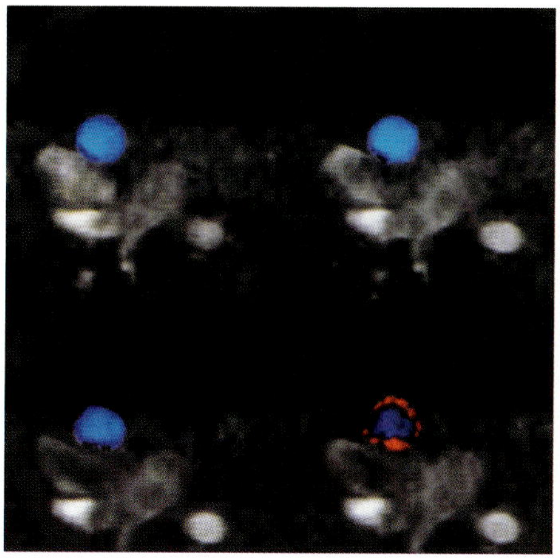

b.

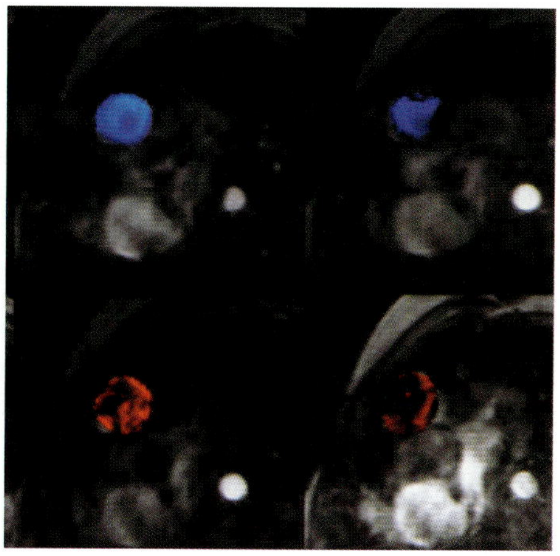

c.

Figure 1. **(a)** Graph depicts pulmonary flow rates throughout the cardiac cycle and the corresponding acceleration volumes (lined areas) in a patient with normal PVR (○) and one with high PVR (●). In **(b)** a patient with normal PVR and **(c)** a patient with high PVR, double-oblique images obtained with electrocardiography-gated velocity-encoded MR imaging perpendicular to the main pulmonary artery, 10–15 mm above the pulmonary valves, depict the corresponding pulmonary flow patterns at 133 msec (top left), 181 msec (top right), 253 msec (bottom left), and 325 msec (bottom right). The patients have the same heart rate. These images are a result of superimposition of a velocity-encoded region of interest (color coded in blue or red) in the cross-sectioned main pulmonary artery on magnitude images (color coded in black or white). Note the lower acceleration volume in **c**—associated with the short acceleration time, increased cross-sectional area, low peak antegrade flow (blue), and large retrograde flow (red) beginning soon after the peak—compared to that in **b**.

The present study was performed to describe and assess the accuracy of indexes of PVR measurements obtained at velocity-encoded MR imaging on the basis of estimations of the instantaneous main pulmonary arterial blood flow and wave form morphology. The accuracy of estimates of cardiac output at velocity-encoded MR imaging was also evaluated and used to assess the measurements of instantaneous pulmonary arterial blood flow. Thus, the present study was designed to determine whether velocity-encoded MR imaging within a single cross-sectional area of the pulmonary artery can provide reliable measurements of cardiac output and PVR, which are recognized as prognostic hemodynamic factors in patients with pulmonary hypertension.

Cardiac output and various indexes derived from pulmonary arterial blood flow were estimated in patients by means of velocity-encoded MR imaging, and results were compared with cardiac output and PVR values obtained by means of catheterization of the right side of the heart. The indexes derived at velocity-encoded MR imaging were also estimated within the main pulmonary artery and the ascending aorta in healthy volunteers, and those data were compared with the findings obtained in patients with and patients without pulmonary hypertension.

Materials and Methods

Subjects

The study was approved by the ethical review board of our institution, and all subjects gave their informed consent.

Volunteers.—Ten healthy volunteers without history of cardiovascular events (four women, six men; age range, 20–33 years; mean age, 25 years) were examined with velocity-encoded MR imaging.

Patients.—Nineteen patients (eight women, 11 men; age range, 20–65 years; mean age, 38 years) gave their informed consent for right-sided heart catheterization and MR imaging; the procedures were performed within 48 hours of each other (mean, 28 hours). No change in drug treatment and no clinically important evolution of the disease occurred in the interval between the two examinations. Indications for cardiac catheterization were the assessment of primary (n = 10) and secondary (n = 5) pulmonary hypertension and the follow-up of cardiac transplants (n = 4). The patients were assigned to one of two groups based on the PVR findings after right-sided heart catheterization. Group 1 patients (n = 12) had a PVR of more than 6 mm Hg · min · L^{-1}; all 10 patients with primary pulmonary hypertension were in this group. Group 2 patients (n = 7) had a PVR of less than 6 mm Hg · min · L^{-1}.

MR Flow Techniques

MR imaging was performed on a 1.5-T system (Signa; GE Medical Systems, Milwaukee, Wis). In the healthy volunteers, two series of localizer images were obtained in the axial and coronal planes. Then two images were acquired for velocity measurements. The first was in a double-oblique section perpendicular to the direction of the ascending aorta at the level of the pulmonary bifurcation, and the second was in a double-oblique section perpendicular to the main pulmonary artery, 10–15 mm above the pulmonary valves. Only one set of velocity measurements was acquired for each patient, perpendicular to the main pulmonary artery.

In the present study, the three-dimensional Fourier method for velocity-encoded MR imaging was achieved by means of four velocity-encoded gradient steps in the direction of the section-selection gradient followed by zero-filling interpolation along the 256 points of the velocity dimension around the four central planes of the acquisition (16). The parameters of the sequence included repetition time of 21 msec and echo time of 12 msec, a field of view of 32 cm, an acquisition matrix of 128 × 256 visualized in 256 × 256, and a constant 60° flip angle. The velocity-encoding gradient was adjusted so that velocities from 1.5 to −1.5 m/sec were measured without aliasing. Depending on the heart rate, 25–35 time frames were acquired with electrocardiographic gating during the first 80% of the cardiac cycle. Each velocity-encoded MR study was acquired in 4–8 minutes, according to the heart rate.

Quantitative Analysis of Flow at Velocity-encoded MR Imaging

The reconstructed velocity images were color coded. The color scale range was from 1.5 to −1.5 m/sec during systole and from 0.35 to −0.35 m/sec during diastole, to optimize the lowest velocities and provide optimal differentiation between structures on the velocity image. The observer was provided with simultaneous displays of the magnitude and corresponding velocity images for each phase of the cardiac cycle. Use of a semiautomated process helped the operator to precisely superimpose a region of interest on the vessel section at each phase of the cardiac cycle.

Stroke volume and output calculations.—In the ascending aorta and main pulmonary artery, left and right ventricular stroke volumes were estimated by means of integration of the flow velocity over the vessel section and then over the cardiac cycle. The output of both ventricles was then estimated by multiplying the corresponding stroke volume by the heart rate. The heart rate was averaged for each series over the 512 cardiac cycles of the acquisition period.

Calculation of hemodynamic indexes.—The curve of pulmonary arterial flow rate as a function of time over the cardiac cycle was used to estimate the antegrade and retrograde flow volumes and the percentage of retrograde flow. Thus, the pulmonary regurgitation fraction was defined as the ratio of the retrograde to the antegrade flow volumes. The acceleration time was defined as the time from the onset of flow to the peak velocity (Fig 1). Three other criteria were also analyzed: the maximal change in flow rate during ejection, defined as the maximal value of the ascending slope of the flow rate; the acceleration volume, estimated by integrating the flow rate of the vessel from the onset of ejection flow to the peak velocity; and the ratio of these two criteria.

Right-sided Heart Catheterization

In the patients, a thermodilution Swan-Ganz balloon catheter (Controlcath; Baxter Healthcare, Irvine, Calif) was advanced into a main pulmonary artery after puncture of a brachial or jugular vein. Cardiac output and stroke volume were measured with use of standard methods for 4 minutes on three to five occasions, and the results were averaged. Also recorded were pulmonary pressures, stroke volume (cardiac output divided by heart rate), and PVR (in millimeters of mercury × minute per liter) (derived from the difference in mean pulmonary pressure and capillary wedge pressure divided by the cardiac output).

Statistical Analysis

All velocity-encoded MR imaging measurements were performed independently by two operators (E.M., J.P.T.) and repeated by one operator (E.M.) 2 months later to assess the inter- and intraobserver agreement, respectively. Each operator estimated velocity-encoded MR imaging measurements blindly, and neither operator was aware of the right-sided heart catheterization results. The estimates of left and right ventricular stroke volume and cardiac output obtained at velocity-encoded MR imaging and thermodilution were compared by means of linear regression analysis and calculation of the standard error of the estimate (SEE). The relationship between the mean and the difference of measurements was used to complement the linear regression analyses. Paired Student t tests were also performed for such comparisons. Linear regression analysis was used to compare PVR measurements obtained at right-sided heart catheterization and the indexes of pulmonary blood flow derived at velocity-encoded MR imaging. The flow-derived indexes obtained at velocity-encoded MR imaging in the pulmonary arteries in groups 1 and 2 and healthy volunteers and within the ascending aorta in the healthy volunteers were compared by means of analysis of variance. Index values were given as the mean plus or minus one SEE. A P value less than .05 was considered significant.

TABLE 1
Intra- and Interobserver Reproducibility of Velocity-encoded MR Imaging Estimates of Stroke Volume in Healthy Volunteers

Linear Regression Analysis	Stroke Volume: Left Ventricular	Stroke Volume: Right Ventricular
	Intraobserver Reproducibility	
Correlation (r)	0.99	0.98
Slope of the equation*	1.04	0.98
Mean difference ± SD		
Milliliters	2 ± 3	1 ± 5
Percentage	0.2 ± 3.0	0.5 ± 3.0
	Interobserver Reproducibility	
Correlation (r)	0.98	0.98
Slope of the equation†	0.99	0.96
Mean difference ± SD		
Milliliters	2 ± 4	1 ± 5
Percentage	0.2 ± 4.0	5 ± 4

* Measurement 1 in x, 2 in y.
† Observer 1 measurement 1 in x, observer 2 in y.

Results

Cardiac Output and Stroke Volume

Healthy volunteers.—The mean right and left ventricular stroke volumes were 95 mL ± 24 and 91 mL ± 22, respectively. The corresponding values normalized for the body surface area were 52 mL/m^2 ± 13 and 50 mL/m^2 ± 11, respectively. The cardiac output, which takes into account possible variations in heart rate, was 6.65 L/min ± 1.7 for the pulmonary circulation and 6.37 L/min ± 1.54 for the systemic circulation. The corresponding values normalized for the body surface area were 3.63 L/min/m^2 ± 0.91 and 3.48 L/min/m^2 ± 0.84, respectively. The mean ratio of right to left stroke volumes for healthy subjects was 1.04 mL ± 0.11. The amounts of pulmonary or aortic blood flow during an average cardiac cycle were well correlated (pulmonary stroke volume, 0.96 × aortic stroke volume + 7 [r = 0.93; SEE = 6 mL]). Intra- and interobserver reproducibilities for stroke volume measurement are shown

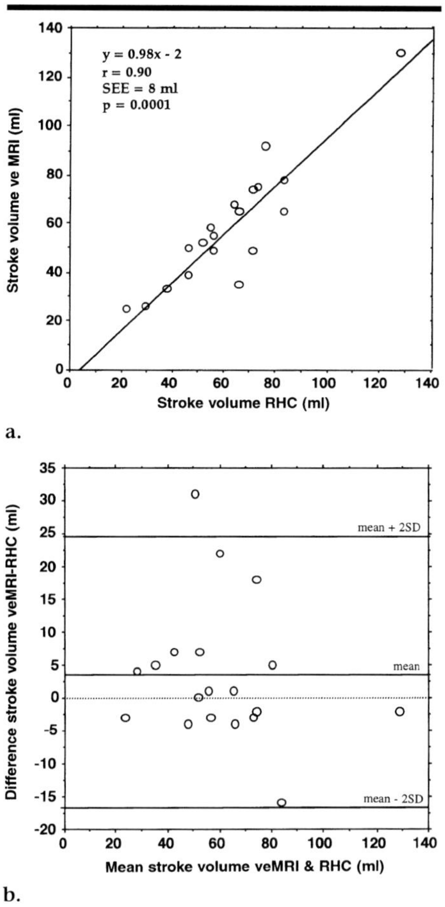

Figure 2. **(a)** Plot of linear regression between estimates of stroke volume obtained at thermodilution during right-sided heart catheterization (*RHC*) and at velocity-encoded MR imaging (*veMRI*). **(b)** Plot of the difference between the two measurements (y axis) versus the mean of these measurements (x axis). Correlation was high between estimates of stroke volume.

in Table 1. The differences between stroke volume measurements of the same observer or between measurements of two observers were not statistically different from zero.

Patients.—The heart rate recorded during velocity-encoded MR imaging (84 beats per minute ± 16) was very close to that recorded during right-sided heart catheterization (83 beats per minute ± 15). Right ventricular stroke volumes obtained with velocity-encoded MR imaging (59 mL ± 25) were not statistically different from those obtained by means of thermodilution (62 mL ± 23). Mean cardiac output was 4.62 L/min ± 1.53 at velocity-encoded MR imaging and 4.93 L/min ± 1.35 at right-sided heart catheterization. Figure 2a shows the regression analysis for stroke volumes obtained at right-sided heart catheterization and velocity-encoded MR imaging (observer 1 measurement). Figure 2b shows the differences between measurements versus the mean of measurements. These differences between measurements were not statistically different from zero and were not correlated with the mean of measurements. The results obtained by observer 1 were close to those by observer 2 (r = 0.98, the mean stroke volume at velocity-encoded MR imaging was 0.96 that at right-sided heart catheterization minus one, SEE = 4 mL). Correlation was good between estimates of cardiac output at velocity-encoded MR imaging (y) and at right-sided heart catheterization (x) ($y = 0.89x$ + 0.2 L/min, r = 0.87, SEE = 0.59 L/min). The average difference between the two methods was 0.40 L/min ± 0.74. The difference between measurements with both methods was not statistically different from zero.

Indexes of PVR

Results in the two patient groups for measurements at right-sided heart catheterization and velocity-encoded MR imaging are given in Table 2. The correlation coefficients and regression linear curve between PVR and each hemodynamic index (acceleration time, acceleration volume, and the ratio of maximal change in flow rate during ejection to acceleration volume) are shown in Figure 3. Inverse correlations were found between PVR and acceleration time or acceleration volume. PVR was directly correlated with the ratio of maximal change in flow rate during ejection to acceleration volume. Finally, the correlations were poor between PVR and the pulmonary regurgitation fraction (r = 0.23) or the maximal change in flow rate during ejection (r = 0.13).

Hemodynamic Indexes

Hemodynamic parameters for the patients and healthy volunteers are presented in Table 2. Acceleration time in the pulmonary artery was significantly shorter in group 1 than in group 2 or the healthy volunteers. Acceleration times estimated in the ascending aorta in healthy volunteers were close to those measured in the pulmonary artery in group 1. There was no significant difference in the estimates of stroke volume in the pulmonary artery and ascending aorta, but the acceleration volume in the ascending aorta was significantly lower than that in the pulmonary artery. Regarding maximal change in flow rate during ejection, there was no significant difference between pulmonary arterial measurements in the two groups and healthy volunteers, but measurements in the aorta in healthy volunteers were significantly higher than those in the pulmonary artery of patients in groups 1 and 2 and the healthy volunteers.

The best hemodynamic parameter for differentiating between groups 1 and 2 was the ratio of maximal change in flow rate during ejection to acceleration volume in the pulmonary artery. Figure 3c shows that data for only one group 1 patient overlapped those for the group 2 patients with high PVR. Estimates of the ratio in the ascending aorta of healthy volunteers were also between those in the pulmonary artery for groups 1 and 2. Figure 4 illustrates the correlation between the ratios measured by the two observers. The mean difference between observers was 12 sec^{-2} ± 39, which was not statistically different from zero. Furthermore, no significant relationship was found between mean measurements of the two observers and the difference between these measurements. The correlation coefficient and slope of the curve for intraobserver reproducibility were 0.99 and 1.03, respectively, and the SEE was 20 sec^{-2}.

Discussion

The main findings in this study are as follows. (*a*) In patients with and patients without pulmonary hypertension, velocity-encoded MR imaging provided measurements of pulmonary flow volume and right-sided cardiac output similar to those obtained by means of thermodilution at right-sided heart catheterization. In healthy volunteers, velocity-encoded MR imaging also provided measurements of pulmonary flow volume and right-sided cardiac output similar to those obtained in the ascending aorta in the patients at right-sided heart catheterization. (*b*) The ascending phase of the pulmonary arterial inflow volume estimated at velocity-encoded MR imaging can give new hemodynamic indexes that are proportional to PVR. The ratio of the maximum slope for the ascending inflow rate (maximal change in flow rate during ejection) to the acceleration volume was inversely correlated with PVR (r = 0.89). (*c*) This ratio can be used to distinguish patients with high PVR (≥6 mm Hg · min · L^{-1}) from patients with nearly normal PVR or healthy volunteers.

Few studies of measurement of cardiac output with velocity-encoded MR imaging have provided results close to those obtained with well-accepted invasive techniques such as thermodilution (6–9,17) or use of the Fick principle (8,9).

TABLE 2
Findings in Patients with and Patients without Pulmonary Hypertension and Normal Values in Healthy Volunteers

	Right-sided Heart Catherization			Velocity-encoded MR Imaging				
Patient No./Sex/ Age (y) and Other Findings	Cardiac Output (L/min)	Mean Pulmonary Arterial Pressure (mm Hg)	Pulmonary Vascular Resistance (mm Hg · min · L^{-1})	Cardiac Output (L/min)	Acceleration Time (msec)	Acceleration Volume (mL)	Maximal Change in Flow Rate during Ejection (mL/sec^2)	Ratio (sec^{-2})*
Patients with pulmonary hypertension								
1/F/65	5.00	65	11	5.47	73	17	7,475	427
2/F/27	4.96	65	12	3.25	74	10	4,728	484
3/M/42	5.39	60	10	4.65	74	11	4,875	456
4/F/24	4.29	54	11	3.64	75	15	6,878	469
5/M/34	5.77	60	9	3.26	88	23	8,554	369
6/F/20	4.80	53	9	4.83	108	16	6,661	415
7/M/36	5.22	61	9	6.05	70	17	8,994	533
8/F/29	2.34	62	22	2.82	67	7	4,764	654
9/F/56	4.75	63	11	4.83	144	18	8,889	487
10/F/33	3.17	74	20	2.77	93	13	8,800	800
11/F/47	3.12	82	23	2.19	65	8	4,230	559
12/M/49	5.22	54	8	4.46	115	21	6,443	306
Mean ± SD	4.5 ± 1.1	63 ± 8	13 ± 5	4.02 ± 1.2	8.7 ± 24	15 ± 5	6,774 ± 1,799	497 ± 131
Patients without pulmonary hypertension								
13/F/47	5.11	37	5	4.62	107	22	8,475	387
14/F/56	6.58	21	3	6.49	134	36	7,242	202
15/M/46†	5.30	13	1	5.28	93	19	5,436	283
16/M/47†	3.60	24	1	3.81	145	27	6,187	231
17/M/44†	8.30	25	2	8.41	140	40	6,955	175
18/M/42†	4.71	17	1	4.59	122	25	6,064	238
19/M/37	6.57	27	3	6.42	160	37	5,769	154
Mean ± SD	5.7 ± 1.5	23 ± 8	2.0 ± 1.5	5.66 ± 1.50	128 ± 23	29 ± 8	6,589 ± 1,045	238 ± 78
Healthy volunteers (mean ± SD)								
Pulmonary artery	NA	NA	NA	6.65 ± 1.70	134 ± 19	42 ± 12	7,176 ± 2,720	178 ± 62
Ascending aorta	NA	NA	NA	6.37 ± 1.54	89 ± 13	26 ± 6	9,483 ± 2,248	373 ± 103
Analysis of variance for intergroup comparison‡	NA	NA	NA	NS	$P < .001$	$P < .001$	$P < .02$	$P < .001$

Note.—NA = not applicable, NS = not significant. Data for healthy volunteers are the mean ± SD.
* Ratio of maximal change in flow rate during ejection to acceleration volume.
† Patients with cardiac transplant.
‡ Comparison between patients with and patients without pulmonary hypertension.

Small differences between measurements of right-sided cardiac output or stroke volume with velocity-encoded MR imaging or thermodilution were found in the present study; these differences were similar to those in the previous studies. The differences may be due to the absence of simultaneous measurements, which emphasizes the spontaneous variability of cardiac output in patients (18,19) and the known limitations of the thermodilution technique for assessment of low cardiac output (19). An advantage of velocity-encoded MR imaging over thermodilution for estimation of cardiac output is that it is noninvasive and depends less on changes in stroke volume from one cardiac cycle to another (in the present study, measurements were averaged over 512 consecutive cardiac cycles).

The estimates of pulmonary flow volume and flow-time curves with velocity-encoded MR imaging gave hemodynamic parameters that are inversely or directly proportional to PVR. The decrease in acceleration time was first proposed as a criterion for pulmonary arterial hypertension or increased PVR in Doppler studies (11,20,21). The increased magnitude and earliness of the reflection wave may cause premature closure of the pulmonary valve in patients with high chronic pulmonary arterial pressure. Results at velocity-encoded MR imaging have shown a good inverse correlation ($r = 0.90$) between mean pulmonary arterial pressure and acceleration time (7) in patients with severe primary pulmonary hypertension and mean pulmonary arterial pressures of 40–83 mm Hg. Patients without primary pulmonary hypertension were also included in the present study, and we found a significant correlation between acceleration time and PVR ($r = 0.65$). The pulmonary acceleration time was also significantly lower in patients with high PVR than in those with nearly normal PVR or in healthy volunteers.

The acceleration volume was inversely correlated with PVR ($r = 0.78$), and the correlation with this parameter was better than that for the relation between acceleration time and PVR. Patients with high PVR were also clearly distinguished from those with low PVR on the basis of estimates of acceleration volume. This parameter emphasizes the shorter acceleration time and the lower pulmonary blood flow throughout this period in patients with pulmonary hypertension. The acceleration volume, which is influenced by the right ventricular contractile forces, may represent the initial mass of pulsatile blood encountering the elastic properties of the pulmonary arterial tree and opposing inertial forces and reflection waves. This resistance to ejected blood flow in cases of pulmonary hypertension leads to premature peak systolic blood flow and early retrograde flow, which begins just after peak blood flow and increases until end systole (5,7,10,22).

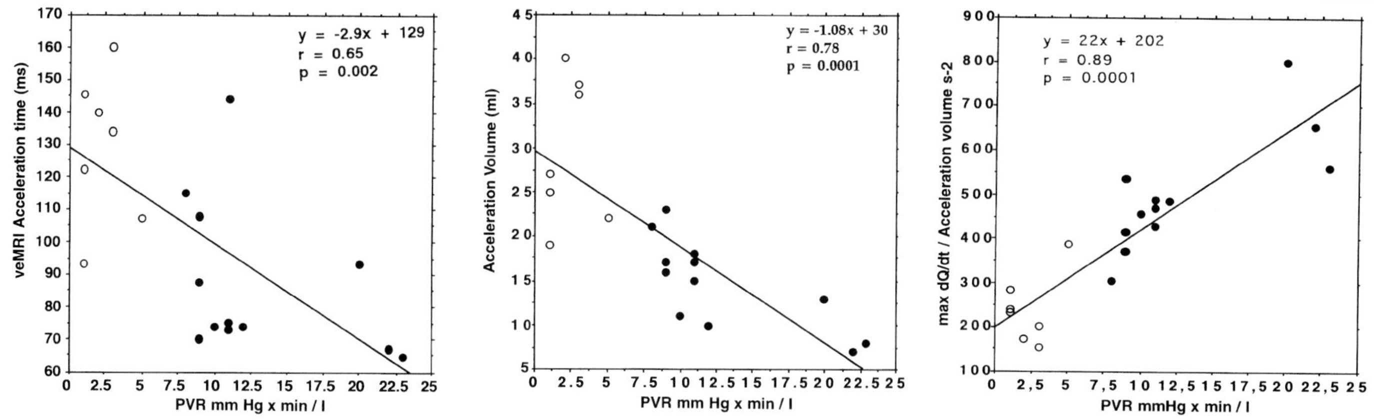

a. b. c.

Figure 3. (a–c) Graphs depict linear correlation between PVR and three successive velocity-encoded MR imaging (*veMRI*) indexes: **(a)** acceleration time, **(b)** acceleration volume, and **(c)** ratio of maximal change in flow rate during ejection (*max dQ/dt*) to acceleration volume in patients with high PVR (●) and patients with normal PVR (○). Correlation between PVR estimated by means of right-sided heart catheterization (*x*) and indexes of pulmonary arterial blood flow at velocity-encoded MR imaging (*y*) could be high, especially with use of the ratio of maximal change in flow rate during ejection to acceleration volume.

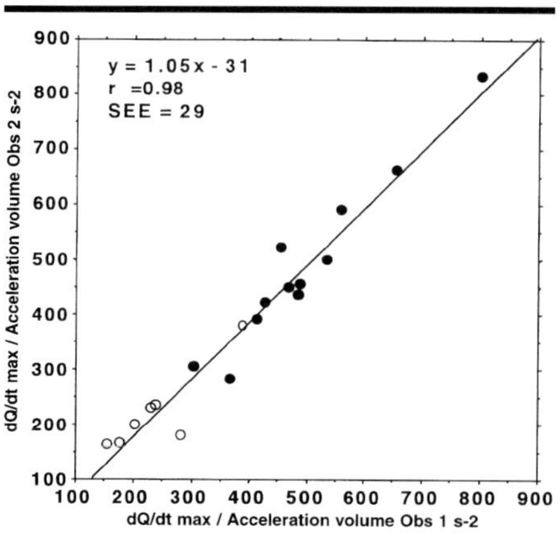

Figure 4. Plot depicts linear regression between estimates by observers 1 and 2 (*Obs 1, Obs 2*) of the ratio of maximal change in flow rate during ejection (*dQ/dt max*) to acceleration volume in patients with high PVR (●) and in patients with normal PVR (○). In this study, interobserver reproducibility was good for estimates of the ratio, which was found to be the best index of PVR at velocity-encoded MR imaging.

These flow profile characteristics during the cardiac cycle were also found in the present study. However, unlike in previous velocity-encoded MR imaging studies, there was a poor correlation between retrograde flow and PVR.

Maximum acceleration, estimated as the first temporal derivative of Doppler velocity, has been described as a good inotropic index of the left ventricle with low load and heart-rate dependence when blood velocity is analyzed within the ascending aorta (23–27) or of the right ventricle when blood velocity is analyzed within the pulmonary artery (28). However, acceleration also depends on the distensibility of the vessel at its origin from the heart and on changes in the velocity profile during the early phase of ejection. Both the distensibility of the vessel and the velocity profile changes can be taken into account on the basis of maximal change in flow rate during ejection rather than on acceleration. Because PVR has a high dependence on volume load, the lack of correlation between the maximal change in flow rate during ejection for pulmonary flow and PVR confirms the low dependence of this parameter on volume load. Maximal change in flow rate during ejection has also been used to normalize the acceleration volume by means of an inotropic index.

In this study, the ratio of maximal change in flow rate during ejection to acceleration volume was well correlated with PVR ($r = 0.89$). It is thus a suitable parameter that is directly related to PVR. The ratio was much higher in group 1 than in group 2 ($P < .001$). Only one group 2 patient, with a PVR of 5 mm Hg · min · L^{-1} (patient 13 in Table 2), had a ratio of maximal change in flow rate during ejection to acceleration volume (387 sec^{-2}) that overlapped the values for group 1. Acceleration volume and the ratio of maximal change in flow rate during ejection to acceleration volume were significantly lower in the ascending aorta flow than in the pulmonary arterial flow in healthy volunteers, even though the right and the left ventricular stroke volumes were similar, whereas the aortic maximal change in flow rate during ejection was higher. The ratios of maximal change in flow rate during ejection to acceleration volume in the ascending aorta in healthy volunteers were also close to the values for group 1 patients with high PVR.

Although systemic resistance was not assessed in our healthy volunteers younger than 30 years, it is likely to be close to the PVR of group 1 patients (13 mm Hg · min · $L^{-1} \pm 5$). Thus, an increase in PVR gives rise to forces opposing the pulsatile ejected volume in the pulmonary artery that produce the acceleration time, acceleration volume, and ratio of maximal change in flow rate during ejection to acceleration volume in the ascending phase of the aortic inflow in healthy volunteers. Further experimental studies with simultaneous measurements of input impedance, PVR, and flow measurement within the pulmonary artery with velocity-encoded MR imaging will provide a better understanding of the meanings of acceleration volume and the ratio of maximal change in flow rate during ejection to acceleration volume. These hemodynamic parameters at velocity-encoded MR imaging are mainly reflections of the right ventricular afterload, however, which is accepted as a good indicator of poor outcome in patients with primary pulmonary hypertension (29).

Intra- and interobserver reproducibilities were good in the present study for measurements of cardiac output and stroke volume and index estimates derived from the flow-rate curve throughout the cardiac cycle at velocity-encoded

MR imaging. This can be attributed to the semiautomatic analysis that was used. High flow signal intensities were depicted on magnitude images of great vessels obtained in patients with high velocities during systole, owing to the time-of-flight effect and very homogeneous velocity distribution. On either magnitude or velocity images, use of a thresholding method can help observers define the vessels more independently than they can by simply placing a circular region of interest as close as possible to the vascular wall. The Fourier method used for velocity-encoded MR imaging gave velocity values close to the aliasing velocity that were as accurate as those for velocities close to zero.

In conclusion, the mechanical relationship between the right ventricle and the pulmonary circulation has not been extensively studied, to our knowledge. The paucity of studies is essentially due to the need to use invasive techniques, but these cannot be justified ethically for the majority of patients. Estimates of pulmonary blood flow at velocity-encoded MR imaging should allow assessment of cardiac output and blood-flow–derived indexes of PVR in patients with right-side heart disease or primary or secondary pulmonary hypertension. This completely noninvasive approach should increase our understanding of the pathophysiologic changes affecting the pulmonary circulation of patients with various pulmonary diseases and should help in the follow-up of hemodynamic changes associated with medical therapies such as long-term vasodilator treatment in patients with primary pulmonary hypertension. Additional studies with different MR imaging systems, different velocity-encoded MR techniques, and inclusion of the appropriate spectrum of patients with pulmonary hypertension should be undertaken to validate the present results.

References

1. Abramson SV, Burke JB, Pauletto FJ, Kelly JJ Jr. Use of multiple views in the echocardiographic assessment of pulmonary artery systolic pressure. J Am Soc Echocardiogr 1995; 8:55–60.
2. Borgeson DD, Seward JB, Miller FA Jr, Oh JK, Tajik AJ. Frequency of Doppler measurable pulmonary artery pressures. J Am Soc Echocardiogr 1996; 9:832–837.
3. Kondo C, Caputo GR, Semelka R, Foster E, Shimakawa A, Higgins CB. Right and left ventricular stroke volume measurements with velocity-encoded cine MR imaging: in vitro and in vivo validation. AJR 1991; 157:9–16.
4. Mogelvang J, Stahlberg F, Sondergaard L, Thomsen C, Lindvig K, Henriksen O. Determination of cardiac output by magnetic resonance imaging. Am J Noninvasive Cardiol 1992; 6:201–204.
5. Kondo C, Caputo GR, Masui T, et al. Pulmonary hypertension: pulmonary flow quantification and flow-profile analysis with velocity-encoded cine MR imaging. Radiology 1992; 183:751–758.
6. Sondergaard L, Hildebrandt P, Lindvig K, et al. Valve area and cardiac output in aortic stenosis: quantification by magnetic resonance velocity mapping. Am Heart J 1993; 126:1156–1164.
7. Tardivon AA, Mousseaux E, Brenot F, et al. Quantification of hemodynamics in primary pulmonary hypertension with magnetic resonance imaging. Am J Respir Crit Care Med 1994; 150:1075–1080.
8. Hundley WG, Li HF, Hillis LD, et al. Quantitation of cardiac output with velocity-encoded, phase-difference magnetic resonance imaging. Am J Cardiol 1995; 75:1250–1255.
9. Hundley WG, Meshack BM, Willett DL, et al. Comparison of quantitation of left ventricular volume, ejection fraction, and cardiac output in patients with atrial fibrillation by cine magnetic resonance imaging versus invasive measurements. Am J Cardiol 1996; 78:1119–1123.
10. Bogren H, Klipstein R, Mohiaddin R, et al. Pulmonary artery distensibility and blood flow patterns: a magnetic resonance study of normal subjects and of patients with pulmonary arterial hypertension. Am Heart J 1989; 118:990–999.
11. Kitabatake A, Inoue M, Asao M, et al. Noninvasive evaluation of pulmonary hypertension by a pulsed Doppler technique. Circulation 1983; 68:302–309.
12. Kosturakis D, Goldberg SJ, Allen HD, Loeber C. Doppler echocardiographic prediction of pulmonary arterial hypertension in congenital heart disease. Am J Cardiol 1984; 53:1110–1115.
13. Wacker CM, Schad LR, Gehling U, et al. The pulmonary artery acceleration time determined with the MR-RACE-technique: comparison to pulmonary artery mean pressure in 12 patients. Magn Reson Imaging 1994; 12:25–31.
14. Nanna M, Lin SL, Tak T, et al. Inaccuracy of Doppler estimates of pulmonary artery pressure using pulmonary flow acceleration time. Can J Cardiol 1990; 6:19–23.
15. Ebeid MR, Ferrer PL, Robinson B, Weatherby N, Gebland H. Doppler echocardiographic evaluation of pulmonary vascular resistance in children with congenital heart disease. J Am Soc Echocardiogr 1996; 9:822–831.
16. Bittoun J, Bourroul E, Jolivet O, et al. High-precision MR velocity mapping by 3D-Fourier phase encoding with a small number of encoding steps. Magn Reson Med 1993; 29:674–680.
17. Sondergaard L, Lindvig K, Hildebrandt P, et al. Quantification of aortic regurgitation by magnetic resonance velocity mapping. Am Heart J 1993; 125:1081–1090.
18. Rich S, D'Alonzo GE, Dantzker DR, Levy PS. Magnitude and implications of spontaneous hemodynamic variability in primary pulmonary hypertension. Am J Cardiol 1985; 55:159–163.
19. Hillis LD, Firth BG, Winniford MD. Analysis of factors affecting the variability of Fick versus indicator dilution measurements of cardiac output. Am J Cardiol 1985; 56:764–768.
20. Turkevich D, Groves BM, Micco A, Trapp JA, Reeves JT. Early partial systolic closure of the pulmonic valve relates to severity of pulmonary hypertension. Am Heart J 1988; 115:409–418.
21. Mallery JA, Gardin JM, King SW, Ey S, Henry WL. Effects of heart rate and pulmonary artery pressure on Doppler pulmonary artery acceleration time in experimental acute pulmonary hypertension. Chest 1991; 100:470–473.
22. Laskey WK, Ferrari VA, Palevsky HI, Kussmaul WG. Pulmonary artery hemodynamics in primary pulmonary hypertension. J Am Coll Cardiol 1993; 21:406–412.
23. Noble MI, Gabe IT, Trenchard D, Guz A. Blood pressure and flow in the ascending aorta of conscious dogs. Cardiovasc Res 1967; 1:9–20.
24. Bennett ED, Else W, Miller GA, Sutton GC, Miller HC, Noble MI. Maximum acceleration of blood from the left ventricle in patients with ischaemic heart disease. Clin Sci Mol Med 1974; 46:49–59.
25. Bennett ED, Barclay SA, Davis AL, Mannering D, Mehta N. Ascending aortic blood velocity and acceleration using Doppler ultrasound in the assessment of left ventricular function. Cardiovasc Res 1984; 18:632–638.
26. Wallmeyer K, Wann LS, Sagar KB, Kalbfleisch J, Klopfenstein HS. The influence of preload and heart rate on Doppler echocardiographic indexes of left ventricular performance: comparison with invasive indexes in an experimental preparation. Circulation 1986; 74:181–186.
27. Spencer KT, Lang RM, Neumann A, Borow KM, Shroff SG. Doppler and electromagnetic comparisons of instantaneous aortic flow characteristics in primates. Circ Res 1991; 68:1369–1377.
28. Heerdt PM, Pond CG, Kussman MK, Triantafillou AN. Use of a Doppler pulmonary artery catheter for continuous measurement of right ventricular pump function and contractility during single lung transplantation. J Heart Lung Transplant 1993; 12:682–688.
29. Eysmann SB, Palevsky HI, Reichek N, Hackney K, Douglas PS. Two-dimensional and Doppler-echocardiographic and cardiac catheterization correlates of survival in primary pulmonary hypertension. Circulation 1989; 80:353–360.

Simon J. Graham, PhD
R. Mark Henkelman, PhD

Index terms:
Brain, abnormalities, 10.871
Brain, MR, 10.121417
Brain, white matter, 10.121417
Magnetic resonance (MR), magnetization transfer contrast, 10.121417
Sclerosis, multiple, 10.871

Radiology 1999; 212:903–910

Abbreviations:
GRE = gradient echo
MT = magnetization transfer
RF = radio frequency
TR = repetition time

[1] From the Departments of Medical Biophysics (S.J.G., R.M.H.) and Medical Imaging (R.M.H.), University of Toronto, Ontario, Canada, and Imaging and Bioengineering Research, Sunnybrook and Women's College Health Sciences Centre, 2075 Bayview Ave, Toronto, Ontario, Canada M4N 3M5. Received September 10, 1998; revision requested November 3; revision received December 2; accepted March 1, 1999. Supported in part by the Terry Fox Foundation and GE Medical Systems of Canada. **Address reprint requests to** S.J.G. (e-mail: *sgraham@sten.sunnybrook.utoronto*).

Author contributions:
Guarantor of integrity of entire study, R.M.H.; study concepts and design, R.M.H., S.J.G.; definition of intellectual content, R.M.H., S.J.G.; literature research, S.J.G., R.M.H.; experimental studies, S.J.G.; data acquisition and analysis, S.J.G.; statistical analysis, S.J.G.; manuscript preparation and editing, S.J.G.; manuscript review, R.M.H.

Pulsed Magnetization Transfer Imaging: Evaluation of Technique[1]

With use of an established physical model, numeric simulations were performed to evaluate current imaging protocols for the two primary applications of magnetization transfer: cerebral magnetic resonance angiography and neuroimaging of white matter disease. The authors found that the current technique is appropriate in the former but suboptimal in the latter. Further clinical investigations could potentially improve magnetization protocols for neuroimaging.

Magnetization transfer (MT) is well known to improve contrast for selective tissues on clinical magnetic resonance (MR) images. Its principal uses are in cases of (*a*) cerebral MR angiography, in which MT enhances the detectability of small vessels by improving the signal suppression of static brain tissues without affecting blood (1,2), and (*b*) white matter disease (eg, multiple sclerosis), in which MT enhances lesion conspicuity (3), allows characterization of normal-appearing white matter (4,5), and provides a correlate measure of cognitive decline (6). Other MT applications (eg, musculoskeletal [7] and head and neck [8] imaging of tumors) are also being developed.

Qualitatively, the MT effect is easily described. When radio-frequency (RF) energy is applied several kilohertz off resonance from the Larmor frequency of the water molecules in tissues, longitudinal magnetization associated with tissue proton macromolecules (the semisolid pool) is preferentially saturated in comparison with water protons (the liquid pool), which normally provide the dominant signal intensity in clinical MR imaging. Exchange of longitudinal magnetization between the pools, via macromolecular sites such as hydroxyl or amide groups (9,10), causes signal reduction in the liquid pool. For a variety of tissues, this MT effect is typically 10%–50% of the signal intensity obtained at clinical imaging when MT pulses are not applied (11). Quantitatively, however, the MT effect is a complicated function of the relaxation times and absorption line shapes of the semisolid and liquid pools, their respective volume fractions, and the efficiency of MT exchange. Notwithstanding this complexity, quantitative understanding of MT provides important physical insight regarding how MT image contrast is generated for specific pulse sequences. From the fundamental MT and relaxation properties of tissues, the optimal contrast can be determined for specific clinical applications. Early in the development of MR imaging, similar analyses were performed to optimize T1- and T2-weighted contrast (12,13).

In the past decade, progress has been made in describing the MT properties of tissues mathematically. Initially, a two-pool model was developed to characterize the MT effect in an aqueous agar gel system under continuous RF irradiation off resonance (14). This model also applies for many clinically relevant tissues (gray matter, white matter, muscle, liver, and blood) when irradiation of the semisolid pool is correctly specified (11,15). More recently, the model was extended to include saturation pulses of short duration, which are used in clinical MT imaging to minimize patient power absorption and imaging time (16). In this study, we used this method to evaluate MT imaging protocols for two applications: static signal suppression in cerebral MR angiography and optimization of contrast in white matter disease. In particular, there is need for such an evaluation in white matter neuroimaging; the reported MT effect for normal white matter ranges from 16% (17) to 60% (18), which suggests that there are wide variations in the effectiveness of clinical MT protocols.

Simulations were performed for spoiled gradient-echo (GRE) imaging, a pulse sequence often used in conjunction with MT. The predicted signals, based on measurements of the MT and relaxation properties of excised tissues at body temperature, were compared with those in the literature.

Materials and Methods

MR Parameters of Tissues

To simulate the MR signals produced at pulsed MT imaging, several fundamental MR parameters must be estimated for the tissues of interest. Proton-density estimates for blood and gray and white matters were obtained from previously reported water content measurements (19), and for the latter two tissues, these estimates were modified to exclude the vascular component (20). Whereas numerous reports of the relaxation properties of tissues exist, MT parameters have previously been measured at room temperature only (11,15) and may not reflect physiologic conditions. Therefore, initial experiments at body temperature were performed with ex vivo tissues to measure MR parameters for simulation purposes. Blood was obtained from a single human subject, with the approval of our local ethics committee and with informed consent, and was oxygenated by means of vigorous shaking in air. Homogeneous samples of gray matter from the parietal cortex and white matter from the corpus callosum were excised from freshly slaughtered cattle. Samples were approximately 0.5 cm^3 in volume and were placed in sealed borosilicate glass tubes (10-mm outside diameter). No other sample preparation was performed. All measurements were initiated within 90 minutes after tissues were extracted. Because such measurements are typically quite precise, experiments were repeated with only two samples of each tissue to assess reproducibility.

Experiments were conducted at 1.5 T by using a superconducting magnet with a bore diameter of 20 cm (Nalorac Cryogenics, Martinez, Calif), controlled with a programmable console (SMIS, Surrey, England). Samples were maintained at body temperature with heated forced air. Experiments were performed without imaging to measure bulk sample properties. The rectangular pulse duration was approximately 10 μsec for a 90° pulse. Three MR experiments were performed: (*a*) a Carr-Purcell-Meiboom-Gill, or CPMG, sequence (21,22) to measure T2 (repetition time [TR] of 10,000 msec, 1-msec echo spacing, 5,000 even echoes sampled, four signals averaged); (*b*) an inversion-recovery sequence (21) to measure T1 relaxation (31 inversion time intervals spaced logarithmically from 1 to 32,000 msec, free induction decay amplitude acquired at each inversion time interval, two signals averaged, 10,000 msec between 90° and inversion pulses); and (*c*) continuous-wave RF irradiation off resonance (14) to measure the MT effect (5-second duration, 27 frequencies off resonance spaced logarithmically from 0.01 to 225 kHz, seven continuous-wave irradiation amplitudes increasing from pulse amplitude, or f_1, of 83 Hz by factors of two). Because the duration of the MT experiments was approximately 84 minutes, the total set of MT data for blood was obtained by measuring seven well-mixed blood samples for 12 minutes each to eliminate potential error due to sedimentation of red blood cells. Measurements of the sample temperature indicated that negligible RF power absorption occurred during the course of these experiments (data not shown).

Analysis of these data first involved estimation of average relaxation times, or <T1> and <T2>, for each tissue by means of monoexponential fits to the relaxation data. For white matter, average T2 was estimated by means of a weighted sum of relaxation times obtained from a biexponential fit. MT parameters and relaxation times for the liquid pool *A*, $T1_A$ and $T2_A$, were estimated from a least squares fit of the MT data to an established two-pool model describing the MT effect for continuous-wave RF irradiation (14) and knowledge of the average T1 and T2 values. An iterative procedure was included to estimate the absorption line shape of the semisolid pool (15), and it was performed at each irradiation frequency off resonance. (T1 for the semisolid pool *B*, $T1_B$, was not estimated precisely from the data and was assumed to be 1,000 msec for all tissues. This assumption is justified because the $T1_B$ value has little influence on pulsed MT simulations [16]. Sensitivity analysis [data not shown] indicated that a 10% change in $T1_B$ produced a change of approximately 0.1% in MT effect.) All errors were reported either as the average SD obtained from the fitting procedure or as half the difference between the mean parameter estimates for the two samples of each tissue, whichever was largest.

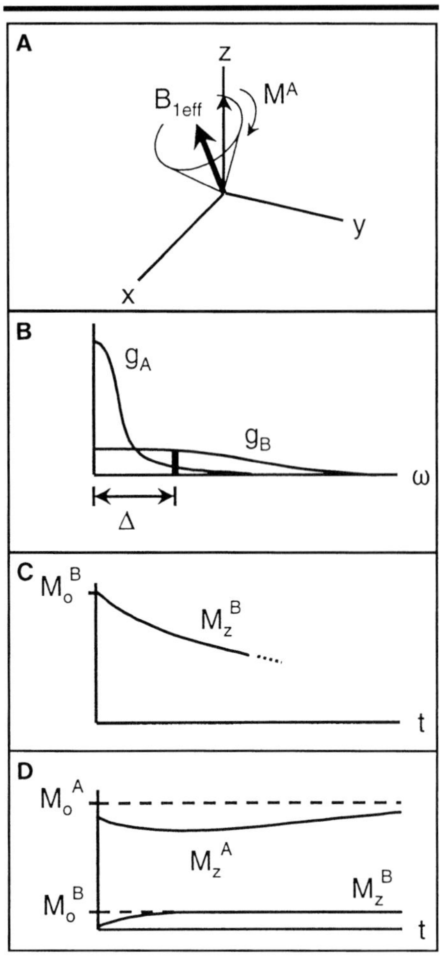

Figure 1. Schematics depict pulsed MT with excitation, absorption, saturation, and evolution, or EASE. *A*, Excitation of the liquid pool magnetization. B_{1eff} = effective B_1 field, M^A = magnetization in the liquid pool. *B*, Absorption line shapes for the liquid pool (g_A) and the semisolid pool (g_B). Δ = frequency off resonance, ω = frequency. In *C* and *D*, M_o^A = relative size of the liquid pool, M_o^B = relative size of the semisolid pool, M_z^A = saturation (attenuation) of longitudinal magnetization in the liquid pool, M_z^B = saturation (attenuation) of longitudinal magnetization in the semisolid pool, t = time. *C*, Saturation of the semisolid pool. *D*, Evolution of both pools after completion of an MT pulse. (See Materials and Methods for details.)

Pulsed MT with Excitation, Absorption, Saturation, and Evolution, or "EASE"

Simulation of pulsed MT contrast requires an understanding of four key concepts: excitation, absorption, saturation, and evolution. These concepts are illustrated in Figure 1, and mathematic treatment is provided elsewhere (16). In response to an MT pulse, magnetization in the liquid pool, M^A, nutates about the associated effective B_1 field in a manner

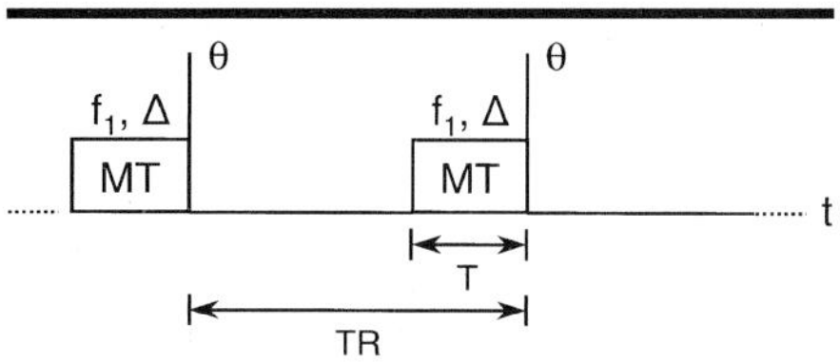

Figure 2. Schematic depicts simplified spoiled GRE sequence including MT pulses. Key parameters influencing contrast are MT pulse amplitude, f_1; frequency off resonance, Δ; imaging flip angle, θ; and repetition time, *TR*. The minimum TR interval is compromised by the time duration, *T*, required for MT saturation. t = time.

very similar to the well-known RF excitation described with the Bloch equations (Fig 1, *A*). The associated decrease in longitudinal magnetization can be mistaken with MT and is known as the direct effect. Absorption of RF energy by both pools, however, is characterized by the absorption line shapes, g_A and g_B, and the MT pulse amplitude, f_1, applied at a given frequency offset from resonance, Δ (Fig 1, *B*). Because the semisolid pool has a very small T2 value (approximately 10 μsec), the line shape g_B is much broader than that of g_A, and absorption occurs preferentially in the semisolid pool and becomes less efficient (requires more power) as the offset frequency increases. Fast T2 relaxation in the semisolid pool also ensures that RF absorption manifests as saturation (attenuation) of longitudinal magnetization, M_z^B, with negligible generation of transverse magnetization (Fig 1, *C*). When the MT pulse is turned off, magnetization in both pools evolves owing to T1 recovery and MT exchange, characterized by a rate constant, *R* (Fig 1, *D*). The equilibrium magnetization in the liquid pool is taken as unity, whereas the relative size of the semisolid pool is indicated as M_o^B. The evolution occurs in two phases: a fast phase, dominated by the rate *R*, in which the liquid pool replenishes the longitudinal magnetization in the semisolid pool quite rapidly, and a slow phase, dominated by $T1_A$, in which the coupled system returns to equilibrium.

The signal decrease in the liquid pool due to one MT pulse is typically only several percent, but repetitive application of MT pulses produces a pronounced net decrease over time. In general, the net signal decrease in the liquid pool due to MT exchange depends on (*a*) the product of *R* and the fractional size of the semisolid pool with respect to the liquid pool, M_o^B, divided by the rate of T1 recovery in the liquid pool (23) and (*b*) the MT pulse parameters: pulse amplitude, duration, offset frequency, and repetition time.

Pulsed MT Imaging

Although the excitation, absorption, saturation, and evolution principles are applicable to arbitrary pulse sequences, MT pulses used with spoiled GRE imaging are of primary interest because this combination currently receives the most clinical application. The pulse sequence used in simulations in this study contained three distinct elements (Fig 2): MT pulse plus spoiler gradient (with total time duration, *T*); small flip angle excitation characterized by the angle, θ, which produces transverse magnetization for the liquid pool but has negligible effect on the semisolid pool; and TR, which incorporates time for spatial encoding and evolution of image contrast. (The inclusion of MT pulses inevitably compromises the minimum TR achievable with spoiled GRE imaging). Transverse magnetization is assumed to be completely spoiled prior to application of the subsequent MT saturation pulse.

Simulations were conducted (MATLAB; MathWorks, Natick, Mass) with use of the standard MT pulse implemented at 1.5 T (Signa; GE Medical Systems, Milwaukee, Wis) (pulse envelope described by an apodized, single-lobe sinc function of 14-msec duration and 150-Hz bandwidth). Therefore, image contrast depended on four parameters: MT pulse amplitude, f_1, and offset frequency, Δ, and the conventional spoiled GRE parameters, θ and TR. To investigate the relative importance of each of these parameters and the associations between them, simulations were performed for each clinical application by using a broad range of possible imaging protocols (f_1, 0.2–1.0 kHz; Δ, 0.5–4.0 kHz; θ, 5°–40°; TR, 20–125 msec). The spoiled GRE signal intensity without MT pulses, SI, was also calculated according to the appropriate equation (24):

$$\mathrm{SI} = [\sin\theta(1 - e^{-\mathrm{TR}/\mathrm{T1}_A})]/[1 - \cos\theta e^{-\mathrm{TR}/\mathrm{T1}_A}],$$

with the equilibrium magnetization for the liquid pool again taken as unity.

Simulations of Cerebral MR Angiography

The pulse sequence shown in Figure 2 is easily used to simulate imaging contrast for cerebral MR angiography. Current state-of-the-art clinical imaging protocols combine pulsed MT, multiple offset thin-slab acquisition, or MOTSA (25); application of the three-dimensional fast spoiled GRE sequence; and tilted, optimized, nonsaturating, excitation, or TONE, pulses for ramped small flip angle excitation across each slab (26). A typical slab thickness of 20 mm was assumed, and the ratio of θ values at the entrance and exit of the slab was 1:2.2 according to clinical prescriptions (27). Time-of-flight contrast between flowing blood and static tissues was assessed for vessels in the center of the slab. While magnetization associated with static tissues was allowed to reach steady state, blood was assumed to flow uniformly perpendicular through the slab and thus was subject to markedly fewer MT pulses and ramped RF excitation, which is dependent on blood velocity and TR (25). To assess image contrast for small 0.5-mm-diameter vessels, an empirical model relating vessel diameter and blood velocity was used (28) that predicted an average flow velocity of 37 mm/sec.

Because MR angiographic applications are subject to imaging time constraints, simulations were performed with TRs of 45 msec and 26 msec without MT pulses for comparison. These conditions represent the minimum TR values obtainable in a previous clinical study (27). Blood at the center of the image slab therefore received either six or 10 excitations with or without MT, respectively. In the absence of MT, over the middle half of the slab, the blood signal varied plus or minus 20% from the value at the center, assuming a flip angle of 25°.

To compare the efficiency of cerebral MR angiography with different MT pulse parameters and without MT, the signal difference between blood and static tissue was calculated and divided by the square root of TR. This figure of merit is proportional to the signal-difference–to-noise ratio independent of acquisition time. The calculation accounts for the increase in minimum imaging time that occurs when MT pulses are used, which could in principle be used to perform signal averaging when MT pulses are absent.

Simulations of White Matter Neuroimaging

In this example, simulations were performed with a TR value of 20 msec, which approximates the minimum TR that is currently achievable when MT pulses are included, and also for a TR value of 125 msec, a typical value used for MT imaging of multiple sclerosis (5). Results of imaging protocols were compared on the basis of the MT ratio difference between white and gray matters per square root of TR, in which the MT ratio was expressed as the percentage signal decrease due to MT relative to the signal achieved without MT at the same TR value.

Results

MR Parameters of Tissues

Estimated relative proton density and estimated relaxation time and MT parameters obtained by means of measurements at body temperature are summarized in the Table for ex vivo blood, gray matter, and white matter tissues. The estimates show the expected general relationships. The $T1_A$ and $T2_A$ values for white matter were reduced with respect to those of gray matter and correlate with the reduced proton density and water content in white matter (29). The relaxation times for blood are characteristically large, and in particular the $T2_A$ value of 310 msec was representative of oxygenated rather than deoxygenated blood, similar to previous measurements (30,31). Considering the MT parameters, the semisolid pool is largest for white matter and smallest for blood, and the MT rate constants have the same ranking as those in a previous study (11). Interestingly, the rate constants were found to be larger by a factor of two than those measured at room temperature (11). This observation is important because it emphasizes that previous estimates of MT parameters from data acquired at room temperature are inappropriate when used to predict contrast in vivo. The specific mechanism responsible for the temperature dependence of MT exchange remains to be determined, although diffusion probably plays a role.

In Figure 3, the extracted (15) absorption line shape, g_B, is plotted for each tissue versus offset frequency, Δ. The area under each line shape equals one and for clarity, error bars (obtained by varying χ^2 for the fit by ±1 SD) are indicated for white matter only. The absorption line shape for blood is much narrower than those for gray and white matters, displaying a fivefold larger amplitude on resonance (Δ = 0) and a half width at half maximum of approximately 500 Hz. The line shapes for white and gray matters are equivalent within experimental error and still have appreciable amplitude at 10 kHz off resonance (data not shown).

Estimated Relaxation Times and MT Parameters for ex Vivo Tissues at Body Temperature (B_o = 1.5 T)

Tissue	Estimated Relative Proton Density	Liquid Pool $T1_A$ (msec)	Liquid Pool $T2_A$ (msec)	Relative Size of Semisolid Pool, M_o^B (%)	Rate, R (sec^{-1})
Blood	1.00	1,440 ± 100	312 ± 30	2.0 ± 0.1	38 ± 7
Gray matter	1.00	1,390 ± 60	111 ± 5	3.7 ± 0.1	61 ± 4
White matter	0.83	710 ± 60	76 ± 2	10.6 ± 0.1	44 ± 3

Note.—Data are the mean ± SD.

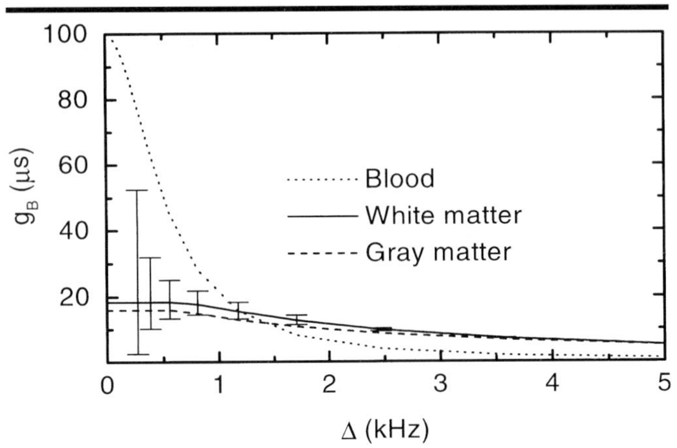

Figure 3. Schematic depicts estimated absorption line shapes of the semisolid pool, g_B, for ex vivo blood, white matter, and gray matter at body temperature. The area of each line shape is normalized to one, and for clarity, error bars (obtained by varying χ2 for the fit by ±1 SD) are shown for only white matter. The absorption line shape for blood is much narrower than that for white or gray matter. Δ = frequency off resonance.

Cerebral MR Angiography

Imaging efficiency characterized by the signal difference ΔM_{xy} (blood signal minus static tissue signal) per square root of time is shown in Figure 4 for a range of MT imaging protocols at TRs of 45 msec (thick lines) and for protocols of 26 msec (thin lines) without MT pulses. For clarity, only MT protocols that were quite close to maximizing the signal difference per square root of time are shown. White matter was taken as the static tissue because it has a much shorter T1 than does gray matter and is more difficult to suppress. Figure 4, top, which illustrates the relationship with flip angle, indicates that use of an MT pulse of modest amplitude (f_1 = 450 Hz, Δ = 1.2 kHz) resulted in an improvement of 11% in signal difference per square root of time compared with that for imaging without an MT pulse. Because the MT pulse increases the available minimum TR (in this case, 45 vs 26 msec), the imaging flip angle must be increased for maximum efficiency, from 25° without MT pulses to 30° with MT pulses. The gain in efficiency is only weakly dependent on MT pulse amplitude and off-resonance frequency (Fig 4, middle and bottom, thick lines), requiring f_1 and Δ values above thresholds of only approximately 300 Hz and 1.5 kHz, respectively.

The dotted line in Figure 4, bottom, indicates the predicted signal difference per square root of time if neither blood nor static tissue exhibited MT exchange (ie, the signal difference due to only the direct effect in the two tissues). A substantial portion of the signal difference was due to the direct effect for frequencies off resonance below approximately 1.5 kHz. At larger frequencies off resonance, however, the direct effect diminished and tended toward the signal difference obtained without MT pulses, which indicated that the maximum gain in sensitivity occurred when MT exchange was maximized and the direct effect was minimized.

Gray Matter–to–White Matter Contrast

A similar family of curves is shown in Figure 5, which illustrates the MT ratio difference between white and gray matters per square root of time for different

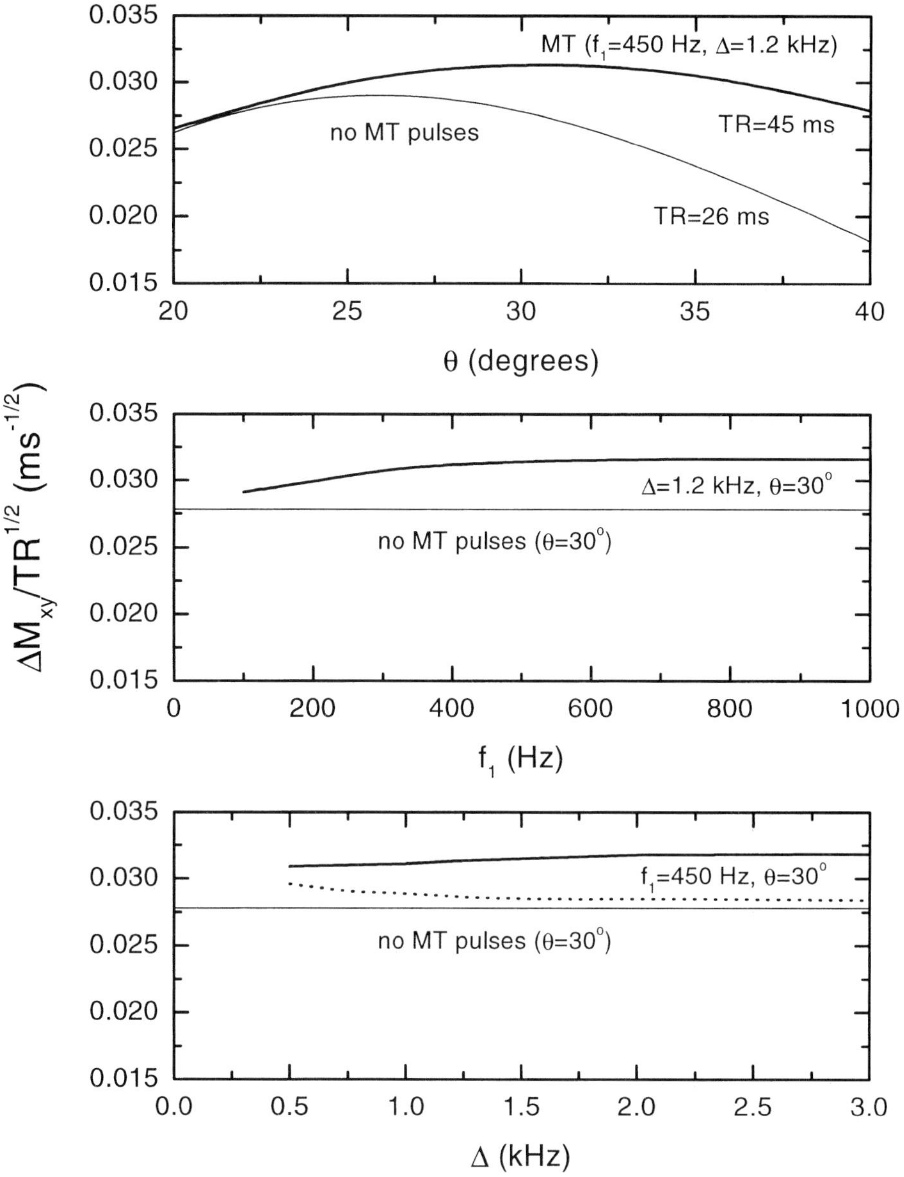

Figure 4. Schematics depict signal difference, ΔM_{xy}, (blood signal minus static tissue signal) per square root of TR for a range of MT protocols that are near optimum (TR = 45 msec [thick line]). Relationships are shown with top, flip angle, θ; middle, MT pulse amplitude, f_1; and bottom, frequency off resonance, Δ. Imaging without MT pulses is indicated by thin lines (TR = 26 msec). Bottom: The dotted line is obtained when none of the tissues of interest exhibits MT exchange.

MT protocols with TRs of 20 and 125 msec. Again, only protocols producing MT ratio differences that were close to the most efficient at each TR value are shown. The maximum MT ratio difference was slightly less at longer TR (16% for TR of 20 msec, with respect to gray matter, 11% for TR of 125 msec [data not shown]). Expressed per square root of time, therefore, the MT ratio difference generated at TR of 20 msec was more efficient by a factor of approximately 3.6. The flip angle value for maximum MT was smaller at TR of 20 msec (θ = 15°) and required adjustment within 5° for best efficiency, whereas θ values for TR of 125 msec provided good sensitivity from 20° to 40° (Fig 5, top). A similar effect was exhibited with respect to MT pulse amplitude and frequency off resonance (Fig 5, middle and bottom). The maximum MT ratio difference at TR of 20 msec required f_1 amplitudes of approximately 300–500 Hz at 1.5–2.5 kHz off resonance, whereas TR of 125 msec required f_1 greater than approximately 500 Hz at 1.5–4.0 kHz off resonance.

In Figure 5, bottom, dotted lines illustrate the MT ratio difference that would be observed if the direct effect of RF absorption on the liquid pool was neglected. For the optimized imaging protocols at each TR value, MT exchange accounted for approximately 95% of the signal difference between white and gray matters.

Discussion

With a detailed understanding of MT exchange, simulations can be used to evaluate the MT contrast produced with imaging protocols for various clinical applications. This approach fulfills a practical need. Simulations can be more comprehensive than actual imaging experiments, have no initial effect on local MR imaging resources, and usually do not require patient databases. They can also be used to investigate protocols that are currently unachievable with clinical imagers and parameters that are difficult or impossible to measure physically (eg, dotted lines in Figs 4, bottom and 5, bottom). Thus, simulations can provide impetus for improved MR imaging technology. They are, however, simplifications of reality. How should the simulation results in this study influence clinical practice? For the two applications investigated, investigators in previous clinical studies have attempted to optimize MT technique for cerebral MR angiography (27) and assessment of white matter disease (18,32).

Cerebral MR Angiography

Previously, Goodrich et al (27) compared results with multiple offset thin-slab acquisition, or MOTSA, plus tilted, optimized, nonsaturating, excitation, or TONE, methods with MT pulses to those without MT pulses, with use of the same TR values investigated in our study and the same MT pulse envelope. For fixed MT pulse amplitude and frequency off resonance (f_1 = 470 Hz, Δ = 1.2 kHz), various tilted, optimized, nonsaturating, excitation pulse flip angles and slab thicknesses were investigated. For 10 patients, the largest peak signal-difference–to-noise ratio with MT for 0.5- to 0.75-mm-diameter vessels occurred with a slab thickness of 16 mm and represented a gain of 29% compared to results with analogous imaging without MT pulses. When expressed as signal-difference–to-noise ratio per unit time, these two imaging protocols were in fact roughly equivalent in efficiency. In comparison, the simulations predicted 45% increased signal difference when MT pulses were used compared with when MT pulses were absent and predicted a modest gain in signal difference per unit time of 11%. Considering the inherent assumptions in the simulations, the simulation and clinical results were in quite good agreement. Furthermore, the simulation results indicate that vessel contrast is quite insensitive to the choice of MT protocol and suggest that appropriate technique is currently used in this clinical application (27). MT pulse amplitudes above a threshold of 400 Hz and offset frequencies above 1.5 kHz all prove satisfactory.

Imaging of White Matter Disease

McGowan et al (32) developed an MT imaging protocol that has been adopted in numerous neuroimaging studies (3,5,33). In initial experiments, sinc pulses were used, with nominal bandwidth of 100 Hz and duration of 19 msec; from investigations of several different f_1 amplitudes, f_1 of 160 Hz was found to produce the largest MT effect for frequency offsets ranging from 3 to 15 kHz. This MT pulse was coupled with GRE imaging (TR of 100 msec, minimum echo time, θ of approximately 10°) to achieve primarily proton-density contrast in the absence of MT pulses. The average specific absorption rate of this pulse sequence was approximately 2.0 W/kg and generated an average MT ratio for normal white matter of 43% ± 1 (mean ± SD) (33). Alternatively, Finelli et al (18) proposed a technique with a 10-msec single-period sinusoid envelope and f_1 of 700 Hz and Δ of 4 kHz coupled with a more rapid spoiled GRE sequence (TR of 25 msec, echo time of 4.4 msec, and flip angle of 6°). In this case, the average specific absorption rate was 4.0 W/kg, which produced an MT ratio of 59% ± 2 in normal white matter.

The large difference in MT ratios obtained with these two different imaging protocols can be easily explained theoretically. For a single ideal MT pulse that completely saturates the semisolid pool and leaves the liquid pool unaffected, the critical time, or t_{crit}, can be calculated when maximum signal decrease occurs in the liquid pool owing to MT exchange (16). From the Table, the critical time is approximately 100 msec for blood and approximately 70 msec for gray and white matters. The MT pulse repetition period should, therefore, be much less than the critical time to accumulate the MT effect efficiently over many pulses. Thus, imaging with shorter TR interval produces larger MT ratio values. If TR is much greater than the critical time, then MT effect is accumulated inefficiently; pulse power must be markedly increased to produce more direct effect. It is only because T1 recovery in the liquid pool

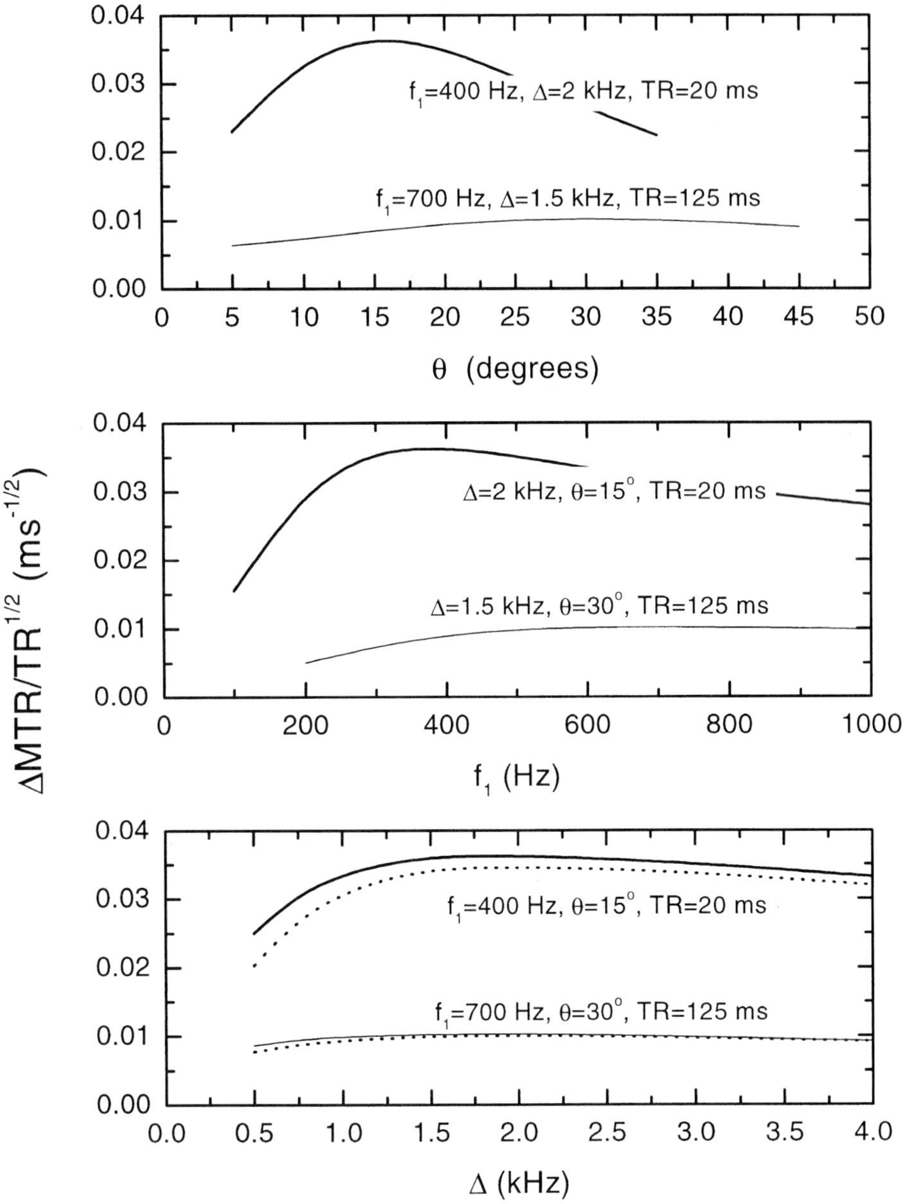

Figure 5. Schematics depict MT ratio difference, *ΔMTR* (white matter minus gray matter) per square root of TR for MT protocols near optimum efficiency at TRs of 20 msec (thick line) and 125 msec (thin line). Relationships are shown with top, flip angle, *θ*; middle, MT pulse amplitude, f_1; and bottom, frequency off resonance, *Δ*. Bottom: The dotted lines predict the MT ratio difference obtained if the direct effect is neglected.

occurs more rapidly than MT exchange under these conditions that appreciable MT ratio values are obtained at longer TR (16).

The simulation results suggest an alternative MT imaging protocol for neuroimaging to that previously advocated. Both McGowan et al (32) and Finelli et al (18) focused on maximizing the MT effect for white matter. However, if white matter MT is maximized, then it may also be maximized for white matter that is partially demyelinated or exhibits partial axonal loss. What is ultimately important is the MT ratio contrast between normal white matter and white matter lesions. With use of gray matter to represent axonal loss, we found that MT ratio contrast is maximized between white and gray matters with technique that does not provide the maximum MT effect in both tissues. Furthermore, this protocol, found by means of simulation (f_1 = 400 Hz, Δ = 2 kHz, θ = 15°, TR = 20 msec), exhibits an average specific absorption rate less than 4.0 W/kg when compared with that of Finelli et al (18).

General Recommendations

The results from these simulations were obtained on the basis of a number of simplifying assumptions. In particular, (*a*) MR properties of ex vivo tissues at body temperature were used to approximate those of living tissues in physiologic conditions, with bovine gray and white matters substituted for the human analogues; (*b*) T2* effects were neglected; (*c*) owing to the lack of detailed MR measurements of the MR properties of white matter lesions (which are variable in character), gray matter was used as a substitute; and (*d*) time-of-flight signal enhancement for blood accounted neither for vessel narrowing, branching, and tortuosity nor for the nonlocalized MT saturation in clinical application (27) (ie, where each MT pulse actually saturates the entire head, not just a single slab). The error introduced by these assumptions is difficult to assess. Assumption *d*, however, means that flowing blood is likely subject to more MT and imaging pulses than were simulated. This could account for the theoretically greater MT over that actually observed clinically (27).

Nevertheless, the simulation results were sufficiently compelling that they highlight the need to optimize MT imaging protocols by means of clinical studies and to investigate image contrast further in patient populations. For cerebral MR angiography, results in such studies have produced good MT imaging technique (27). There are several basic guidelines for conducting such investigations that are easily implemented in any MR imaging laboratory.

1. Choose the minimum TR that allows an acceptable specific absorption rate. Use of MT pulses alters the flip angle θ that produces best image contrast per unit time, so image quality must be investigated as a function of θ. This can be performed adequately with use of the standard MT pulse provided with the MR imager. Noise levels should be reduced to acceptable levels by means of signal averaging.

2. Choose an MT pulse: Both binomial on-resonance and shaped off-resonance pulses are acceptable. Findings in previous simulations and clinical studies indicate that appreciable MT effect can be obtained by means of both binomial on-resonance and shaped off-resonance pulses (16,18,34). The direct effect must be minimized in both cases, which is simpler with shaped pulses because they are less sensitive to static field inhomogeneity (34). For different shaped pulses, MT effect scales linearly with average pulse power (16,35); standard choices, such as sinc or Gaussian pulse envelopes should provide desired MT contrast within current specific absorption rate limits. To minimize the required power, the off-resonance frequency should be chosen just large enough to produce negligible direct effect, and results of simulations indicate that offset frequencies of 1.5–2.0 kHz are appropriate.

3. Investigate image contrast as a function of MT pulse amplitude. Weak MT pulses produce poor MT image contrast, whereas excess power produces undesirable direct effect. For neuroimaging, findings in this study suggest that the desirable MT pulse amplitude is insensitive to the imaging flip angle, so that θ determined in guideline 1 should be sufficient. If MT pulse amplitude must be increased, then the TR value may also have to be increased slightly for specific absorption rate to remain acceptable, and guideline 1 should be revisited.

The simulation results also suggest that the MT protocol for cerebral MR angiography is flexible (a range of MT pulse parameters produce equivalent contrast). It may be possible to determine the best MT protocol for imaging white matter disease and then to use this protocol for cerebral MR angiography without much loss of efficiency. Such an approach would facilitate pulse sequence implementation but requires verification with further study.

Other Pulse Sequences

This study focused on use of MT pulses with spoiled GRE imaging, the predominant pulse sequence used in MT protocols. However, appreciable deliberate MT effect can also be generated with spin-echo imaging (34) as long as enough interleaved sections are acquired per TR interval to ensure that MT pulses are applied with a period much less than the critical time. This pulse sequence is more complicated to simulate because some saturation of the semisolid pool is caused by refocusing pulses at varying frequencies off resonance during multisection interleaving (36). An accurate comparison of pulsed MT with spoiled GRE versus spin-echo pulse sequences is beyond the scope of this article. Interestingly, use of MT pulses with fast spin-echo imaging produces little deliberate (17) MT effect, because the echo train length typically exceeds the critical time. However, unintended MT contrast is also produced when fast spin-echo imaging is performed without an MT saturation pulse, owing to the many refocusing pulses (36,37). This suggests that calculation of MT ratios is inadvisable with use of fast spin-echo imaging.

In conclusion, simulation results indicate that current use of MT in imaging protocols is close to optimal for cerebral MR angiography, whereas neuroimaging protocols can likely be made more effective. It is hoped that this report will encourage clinical neuroradiologists to investigate improvement of MT protocols for white matter lesions.

References

1. Pike GB, Hu BS, Glover GH, Enzmann DR. Magnetization transfer time-of-flight magnetic resonance angiography. Magn Reson Med 1992; 25:372–379.
2. Furst G, Hofer M, Steinmetz H, et al. Intracranial stenoocclusive disease: MR angiography with magnetization transfer and variable flip angle. AJNR 1996; 17: 1749–1757.
3. Grossman RI, Gomori JM, Ramer KN, Lexa FJ, Schnall MD. Magnetization transfer: theory and clinical applications in neuroradiology. RadioGraphics 1994; 14:279–290.
4. Filippi M, Campi A, Dousset V, et al. A magnetization transfer imaging study of normal-appearing white matter in multiple sclerosis. Neurology 1995; 45:478–482.
5. Van Buchem M, McGowan JC, Kolson DL, Polansky M, Grossman RI. Quantitative volumetric magnetization transfer analysis in multiple sclerosis: estimation of macroscopic and microscopic disease burden. Magn Reson Med 1996; 36:632–636.
6. Rovaris M, Filippi M, Falautano M, et al. Relations between MR abnormalities and patterns of cognitive impairment in multiple sclerosis. Neurology 1998; 50:1601–1608.
7. Li KCP, Hopkins KL, Moore SG, et al. Magnetization transfer contrast MRI of musculoskeletal neoplasms. Skeletal Radiol 1995; 24:21–25.
8. Markkola AT, Aronen HJ, Paavonen T, et al. Spin lock and magnetization transfer imaging of head and neck tumours. Radiology 1996; 200:369–375.
9. Kucharczyck W, MacDonald PM, Stanisz GJ, Henkelman RM. Relaxivity and magnetization transfer of white matter lipids at MR imaging: importance of cerebrosides and pH. Radiology 1994; 192:521–529.
10. Liepinsh E, Otting G. Proton exchange rates from amino acid side chains: implications for image contrast. Magn Reson Med 1996; 35:30–42.
11. Morrison C, Henkelman RM. A model for magnetization transfer in tissues. Magn Reson Med 1995; 33:476–482.
12. Henkelman RM, Hardy P, Poon PY, Bronskill MJ. Optimal pulse sequence for imaging hepatic metastases. Radiology 1986; 161:727–734.
13. McVeigh ER, Henkelman RM, Bronskill MJ. Optimization of survey protocols for MRI. Magn Reson Med 1990; 13:177–191.
14. Henkelman RM, Huang X, Xiang Q, Stanisz GJ, Swanson SD, Bronskill MJ.

Quantitative interpretation of magnetization transfer. Magn Reson Med 1993; 29: 759–766.
15. Li JG, Graham SJ, Henkelman RM. A flexible magnetization transfer line shape derived from tissue experimental data. Magn Reson Med 1997; 37:866–871.
16. Graham SJ, Henkelman RM. Understanding pulsed magnetized transfer. JMRI 1997; 7:903–912.
17. Van Waesberghe JHTM, Castelijns JA, Lazeron RHC, Lycklama à Nijeholt GJ, Barkhof F. Magnetization transfer contrast (MTC) and long repetition time spin-echo MR imaging in multiple sclerosis. Magn Reson Imaging 1998; 16:351–358.
18. Finelli DA, Hurst GC, Amantia P Jr, Gullapali RP, Apicella A. Cerebral white matter: technical development and clinical applications of effective magnetization transfer (MT) power concepts for high-power, thin-section, quantitative MT examinations. Radiology 1996; 199:219–226.
19. Ernst T, Kreis R, Ross BD. Absolute quantitation of water and metabolites in the human brain. I. Compartments and water. J Magn Reson 1993; 102(series B):1–8.
20. Woodbury DM. Physiology of body fluids. In: Ruch TC, Patton HD, Scher AM, eds. Physiology and biophysics: circulation, respiration, and fluid balance. 20th ed. Philadelphia, Pa: Saunders, 1974.
21. Carr HY, Purcell EM. Effects of diffusion on free precession in nuclear magnetic resonance experiments. Phys Rev 1954; 94:630–638.
22. Meiboom S, Gill D. Modified spin-echo method for measuring nuclear relaxation times. Rev Sci Instr 1958; 29:688–691.
23. Henkelman RM, Morrison CS. A model of magnetization transfer for various tissues in vitro (abstr). In: Proceedings of the Third Meeting of the International Society for Magnetic Resonance in Medicine. Berkeley, Calif: International Society for Magnetic Resonance in Medicine, 1995; 108.
24. Van der Meulen P, Groen JP, Tinus AMC, Bruntink G. Fast field echo imaging: an overview and contrast calculations. Magn Reson Imaging 1988; 6:355–368.
25. Parker DL, Yuan C, Blatter DD. MR angiography by multiple thin slab acquisition. Magn Reson Med 1991; 17:434–451.
26. Atkinson D, Brant-Zawadski M, Gillan G, Purdy D, Laub G. Improved MR angiography: magnetization transfer suppression with variable flip angle excitation and increased resolution. Radiology 1994; 190: 890–894.
27. Goodrich KC, Blatter DD, Parker DL, Du YP, Meyer KJ, Bernstein MA. A quantitative study of ramped radio frequency, magnetization transfer, and slab thickness in three-dimensional time-of-flight magnetic resonance angiography in a patient population. Invest Radiol 1996; 31: 323–332.
28. Du YP, Parker DL, Davis WL, Cao G, Buswell HR, Goodrich KC. Experimental and theoretical studies of vessel contrast-to-noise ratio in intracranial time-of-flight MR angiography. JMRI 1996; 1:99–108.
29. Fullerton GD. Physiologic basis of magnetic relaxation. In: Stark DD, Bradley WG Jr, eds. Magnetic resonance imaging. 2nd ed. St Louis, Mo: Mosby–Year Book, 1992.
30. Thulborn KR, Waterton JC, Matthews PM, Radda GK. Oxygenation dependence of the transverse relaxation time of water protons in whole blood at high field. Biochem Biophys Acta 1982; 288:354–361.
31. Wright GA, Hu BS, Macovski A. Estimating oxygen saturation of blood in vivo with MR imaging at 1.5T. JMRI 1991; 1:275–283.
32. McGowan JC, Schnall MD, Leigh JS. Magnetization transfer imaging with pulsed off-resonance saturation: variation in contrast with saturation duty cycle. JMRI 1994; 4:79–82.
33. Loevner LA, Grossman RI, Cohen JA, Lexa FJ, Kessler D, Kolson DL. Microscopic disease in normal-appearing white matter on conventional MR images in patients with multiple sclerosis: assessment with magnetization-transfer measurements. Radiology 1995; 195:511–515.
34. Pike GB, Glover GH, Hu BS, Enzmann DR. Pulsed magnetization transfer spin-echo MR imaging. JMRI 1993; 3:531–539.
35. Hua J, Hurst GC. Analysis of on- and off-resonance magnetization transfer techniques. JMRI 1995; 5:113–120.
36. Santyr GE. Magnetization transfer effects in multislice MR imaging. Magn Reson Imaging 1993; 11:521–532.
37. Constable RT, Anderson AW, Zhong J, Gore JC. Factors influencing contrast in fast spin-echo MR imaging. Magn Reson Imaging 1992; 10:497–511.

Letters to the Editor

ROC Curve Analysis in the Evaluation of Contrast-enhanced Color Doppler US

From:
Jonathan Winehouse, FRCS,* Michael Douek, FRCS,* and William Lees, FRCR†
Departments of Surgery* and Radiology,† Royal Free and University College Medical School
67-73 Riding House Street, London W1P 7LD, United Kingdom

Editor:
We read with interest the article by Dr Huber and colleagues (1) in the August 1998 issue of *Radiology* that elegantly describes a computer-assisted method for quantifying contrast material–enhanced color Doppler ultrasound signals from both malignant and benign breast lesions.

To assess the sensitivity and specificity (diagnostic accuracy) of contrast-enhanced color Doppler ultrasonography (US), Dr Huber and colleagues' patient grouping was divided by using the median value of the color pixel density as a cutoff point. A χ^2 test was then applied to determine a statistical difference in color pixel density between benign and malignant lesions.

Our concerns with this aspect of the method are twofold. First, one is unable to anticipate a clinically useful cutoff point prior to analysis; to do so is assumptive and therefore completely arbitrary. Second, this method ignores an important outcome gained in part from the use of paired control subjects (2,3), that is, whether contrast-enhanced examination can be shown to have a true advantage over conventional color Doppler US.

We have also been working with the US contrast agent SH U 508A (Levovist; Schering, Berlin, Germany) (4) along similar lines, and our results with 58 patients (16 recurrences) demonstrated a diagnostic accuracy of 90% for this agent in differentiating breast cancer recurrence from scar tissue—a significant and highly useful improvement over conventional color Doppler US (diagnostic accuracy, 80%; $P = .038$). We in effect compared peak (enhanced) color pixel densities with baseline (nonenhanced) color pixel densities with the use of receiver operating characteristic (ROC) curves (Figure). This method also uses the paired nature of the study group (enhanced vs nonenhanced) and therefore more accurately demonstrates any difference that may be produced by the addition of a contrast agent. In addition, useful cutoff points along the ROC curves can be easily defined for both contrast-enhanced and nonenhanced baseline scans. The method we used has been fully described in previous issues of *Radiology* (2,3).

We believe that the results from these studies may be more accurately reflected with ROC curve analysis, and we would therefore like to draw our colleagues' attention to these articles.

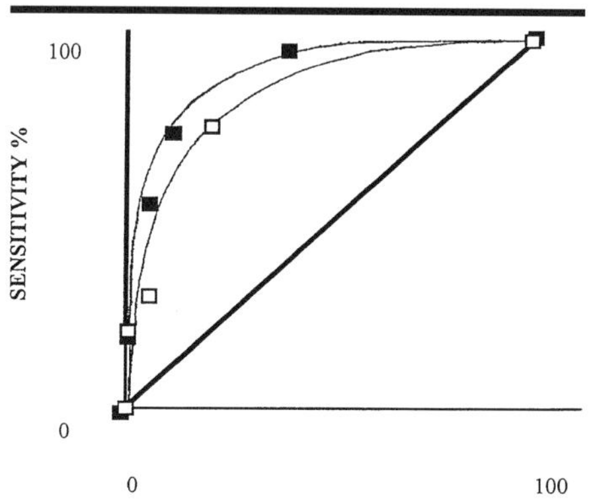

ROC curves comparing nonenhanced and contrast-enhanced color Doppler US scans in patients with suspected breast cancer recurrence. Solid line = no test discrimination, ■ = peak color pixel density (enhanced), □ = baseline color pixel density (nonenhanced).

References

1. Huber S, Helbich T, Kettenbach J, Dock W, Zuna I, Delorme S. Effects of a microbubble contrast agent on breast tumors: computer-assisted quantitative assessment with color Doppler US—early experience. Radiology 1998; 208:485–489.
2. Hanley JA, McNeil BJ. The meaning and use of the area under a receiver operating characteristic (ROC) curve. Radiology 1982; 143:29–36.
3. Hanley JA, McNeil BJ. A method of comparing the areas under receiver operating characteristic curves derived from the same cases. Radiology 1983; 148:839–843.
4. Douek M, Winehouse J, Deng J, et al. Differentiation of breast cancer recurrence from scar tissue by contrast-enhanced colour Doppler ultrasound. Presented at the Annual Meeting of the Royal Society of Medicine, London, November 4, 1998.

Dr Huber and colleagues respond:

We are pleased by the interest in our article (1). Dr Winehouse and colleagues remark that using the median as a cutoff point is arbitrary and that an ROC analysis would help to determine an appropriate cutoff level. This is a frequent comment, and we have already discussed this point with one of the reviewers of the article. We perform ROC analyses frequently in our studies, but we intentionally refrained from doing so in this particular instance. We call to mind that, as the title indicates, this is very preliminary work. Here, we intended to point out where current methodologic limitations lie rather than to determine the ultimate diagnostic value of this method. Our sample consisted of 31 patients with malignant and 16 with benign lesions.

We agree that there is a paired nature in the study group. This means that the result of the examination in a given patient may, for example, be false-negative with the nonenhanced and true-positive with the enhanced technique, or it may shift from true-negative to false-positive. It indeed would be interesting to examine how the classification changes in an individual patient. Unfortunately, the χ^2 test does not answer this question, nor does the ROC analysis. ROC analysis does nothing more than plot specificity against sensitivity with different cutoff values. When two methods or criteria are compared, specificity and sensitivity are calculated separately for each method, but the diagnoses achieved in individual patients are not compared. Indeed, ROC analysis enables a more systematic and differentiated comparison of two methods, but by no means does it use the paired nature of the study group. While Dr Winehouse and colleagues may disagree, having cited the articles by Hanley and McNeil (2,3), we still believe this is true for the commonly used ROC analysis.

The method described by Hanley and McNeil (3) clearly differs from the usually applied ROC analysis. Here, the authors indeed attempt to adapt the ROC approach to data sets with different data derived from the same cases. The clear drawback is, however, that it is highly complex and in our opinion not sufficiently robust to avoid statistical artifacts. Furthermore, it will be extremely difficult to trace any artifacts back to the original data. When different methods and criteria are compared, they are commonly applied to the same samples. Although published in 1983, the method described in this article has not yet achieved the range of a standard approach for this very common problem. Thus, we believe that standard statistical approaches familiar to the reader should be used to ensure that the results are understood and also amenable to criticism.

Our main reason for not using ROC analysis was the small sample. In our case, the distribution of values could not be expected to be stable enough to be proved the same when more patients were added. Therefore, "fitting" the cutoff value to the study sample by ROC analysis would clearly run the risk that falsely high significance levels would be calculated and that the results would appear better than they actually were. Splitting the group by using simply the median as a cutoff point is the procedure of choice because of the preliminary nature of the study imposed by the small study sample and the retrospective nature of the analysis. The procedure does run the risk that the significance levels are underestimated, but it is probably more honest. If a true prospective study is planned—that is, with predefined cutoff values derived from preliminary studies—we believe it is justified then to tailor the thresholds to clinical needs.

References

1. Huber S, Helbich T, Kettenbach J, Dock W, Zuna I, Delorme S. Effects of a microbubble contrast agent on breast tumors: computer-assisted quantitative assessment with color Doppler US—early experience. Radiology 1998; 208:485–489.
2. Hanley JA, McNeil BJ. The meaning and use of the area under a receiver operating characteristic (ROC) curve. Radiology 1982; 143:29–36.
3. Hanley JA, McNeil BJ. A method of comparing the areas under receiver operating characteristic curves derived from the same cases. Radiology 1983; 148:839–843.

Sabine Huber, MD, Ivan Zuna, PhD, and Stefan Delorme, MD
Department of Radiology, Lainz Hospital
Wolkersbergenstrasse 1, 1130 Vienna, Austria

Erratum

"Pulmonary Emphysema: Imaging Assessment of Lung Volume Reduction Surgery." Radiology 1999; 212:1–3.

Page 1, second column, line 22, sentence should have read as follows:

Virtually every day, radiologists see chest radiographs that show **attenuation** of upper lung zone vessels, which is the most common chest radiographic sign of the characteristic upper zone distribution of centrilobular pulmonary emphysema in tobacco abusers.

In Memoriam

Dr Harry W. Fischer, Professor Emeritus of Radiology and former chairman of the Department of Radiology at the University of Rochester (NY), died at his home in Frankfort, Michigan, on November 1, 1998, of long-term complications of a stroke in 1992 that left him hemiplegic and aphasic. He was born in 1921 in St Louis, Missouri.

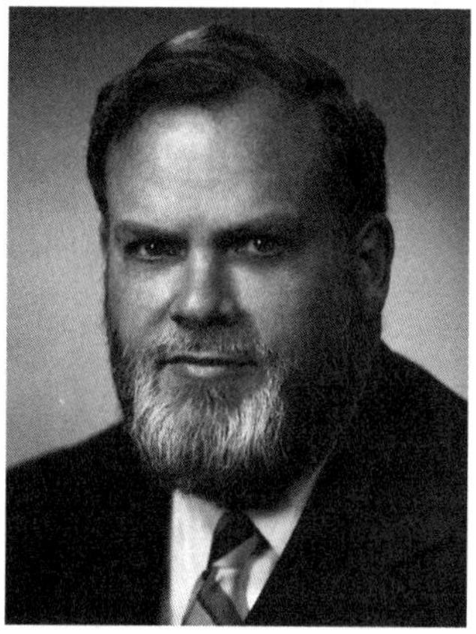

Harry W. Fischer, MD
1921–1998

He received his BS degree from the University of Chicago (Ill) in 1943, the same year he married his high school sweetheart, Kay Jarvis. Two years later, he received his MD degree from the University of Chicago. After discharge from the U.S. Navy in 1948, he entered a surgery residency under the direction of Evarts Graham, MD, at Washington University (St Louis, Mo). During his final year of residency, he had poliomyelitis, which left him with neuromuscular deficits that made a career in surgery impossible.

Changing careers, Harry became a radiology resident at St Louis (Mo) University from 1952 to 1954. After 2 years in private practice, including a 1956 appointment at the Institute of Medical Education and Research at St Louis (Mo) City Hospital, he began his academic radiology career at the University of Iowa Hospitals (Iowa City) in 1956. That was where I (J.R.T.) first met Harry Fischer, at the start of my residency. We became close friends and colleagues, a partnership that lasted until his death. Our long friendship provides the basis for many of the personal insights in this writing.

At Iowa, Harry firmly established himself as one of the few medically trained basic researchers in radiology at that time. Using his surgical experience and skills, he established the experimental dog laboratory at the Department of Radiology. There, he pioneered the procedural technique and use of contrast agents for imaging of the lymphatic system. In 1961, Harry published one of the first images in a human in whom the new intralymphatic contrast agent was used to demonstrate a metastasis from a malignant melanoma to an inguinal lymph node. At the same time, he began his long-term research program in other contrast agents.

The years that I spent at University of Iowa (1958–1966) provided first-hand experience in researching imaging contrast agents with Harry. This was also one of the most pleasant and hilarious periods of our friendship. It was always a challenge to the residents when the laboratory animal film images were shown at the weekly image conferences, which resulted in great fun and good humor.

By 1963, Harry was chief of diagnosis in the department headed by Eugene F. Van Epp, MD, and he established many practice organizational changes. He started the "officer of the day" method for consulting with clinicians and divided the reading exercises into general and subspecialty areas. He also involved residents in animal and contrast agent research. This launched his interest in departmental organization and design, which ultimately resulted in a book (*Radiology Departments: Planning, Operation, and Management*. Ann Arbor, Mich: Edwards Brothers, 1982) and four international seminars on the subject.

In 1966, Walter W. Whitehouse, MD, recruited Harry to the University of Michigan (Ann Arbor). He became chief of the new radiology outpost at Wayne County Hospital (Eloise, Mich), where he set up an extensive animal and contrast agent research laboratory and recruited a stellar staff who ultimately became leaders in American angiography: Kyung Cho, MD, Vincent Chuang, MD, Helen C. Redman, MD, and Stewart Reuter, MD.

My (H.C.R.) association with Harry also provides material for a portion of this memorial. At Wayne County, I was responsible for the large research laboratory he established and spent many hours there working on his contrast agent projects and on my own research on blood flow modification and measurement. I received encouragement and support from him every step of the way.

Harry was active in the hospital, as well, and served as chief of staff for several years. He made quite a splash at Wayne County when he purchased an elderly right-hand-drive Rolls Royce sedan that he drove to and from work. The eye-catching car cruised serenely on the freeway with no driver apparently in control in the left front seat!

He was interested in all aspects of the residents' lives and entertained them and the faculty at his home. One memorable party was based on the making of fresh apple cider. It was a lovely fall day in Ann Arbor, and the leaves were colorful. Harry had an old cider press and lots of apples, and he put the residents to work making fresh, delicious cider. The end result surprised many!

In 1971, Harry was recruited to become chairman of radiology at the University of Rochester. This was a "natural" for Harry, because (*a*) by now he was a national expert in contrast agent research, and Rochester was a serious research institution; (*b*) a new Strong Memorial Hospital was under construction, and he could help form a state-of-the-art department; and (*c*) he and Robert N. Joynt, MD, PhD, neurology department chairman and, later, dean, had been close colleagues and friends at Iowa.

Harry set out to develop further one of the top investigational research departments in the country. Raymond Gramiak, MD, a research pioneer in ultrasonography, was already there. Among others of the new staff were radiologists and others with PhD degrees who subsequently made major contributions to radiology in the fields of physics, contrast agent development, and clinical imaging research. Perhaps the most notable were Beverly Wood, MD, in pediatric imaging; Jovitas Skucas, MD, in gastrointestinal imaging; Robert Spataro, MD, and Richard Katzberg, MD, in genitourinary imaging; Robert O'Mara, MD, in nuclear radiology; Thomas Morris, PhD, in physiology; and Donald Plewes, PhD, in physics.

He ran the department with an old fashioned "iron hand," but he did so with fairness and wonderful, wry humor. At least the residents, staff, and all others he worked with knew at all times where he was coming from. He developed a monograph on the philosophy of radiology research and practice to help get residents into the right frame of mind at the outset. In every resident class, at least half already had a PhD degree, so future research had a strong personnel base. He also was proud of his primers for residents, *The Radiologist's First Reader* (1988) and *The Radiologist's Second Reader* (1992), both published by Book Crafters (Chelsea, Mich).

The other aspect, besides research, that characterized this department was its international flavor. This went back to Harry's 3-month trip to Europe in 1965 under the auspices of the Commonwealth Fund, which led to many long-standing friendships and professional associations. These were his source to recruit excellent European radiologists, who brought new viewpoints and skills to Rochester. He also recruited radiologists from Australia and New Zealand. Many of these were, or later became, leaders of radiology in their countries.

He had a big vision: that radiology would come to have a solid scientific basis. He was an insistent needler of people at meetings who presented flamboyant claims and conclusions based on weak scientific evidence. His devotion to sound research was well known.

He was a prolific author and contributor to over 150 articles and 15 textbooks. Most were about basic contrast agent research: physiology, mechanisms of action, toxicity, and utility. He became one of the foremost international experts on contrast agents and served on the editorial boards of *Radiology* and *Investigative Radiology* and edited articles for *Cancer* and the *Journal of the American Medical Association.* He was active in many organizations, including the Radiological Society of North America.

He also contributed time and expertise to governmental and other national organizations. These included the U.S. Food and Drug Administration (FDA) Radiopharmaceuticals Advisory Committee, U.S. Pharmacopeia (USP) Committee of Revision, USP Advisory Panel on Diagnostic Agents (Nonradioactive) and Radiological Contrast Agents (chairman), National Institutes of Health Study Section on Diagnostic Radiology, American College of Radiology Commission on Drugs, Commission on Public Health and Radiation Protection (chairman), National Council on Radiation Protection Scientific Committee on Quality Assurance and Measurements in Diagnostic Radiology, and FDA Committee on Radiologic Equipment.

His many accomplishments were acknowledged both here and abroad. He was an honorary member of the Swedish Society of Medical Radiology and the Radiological Society of Finland, as well as an honorary fellow of the Royal Australasian College of Radiologists. The Association of University Radiologists awarded him its Gold Medal in 1981. In 1995, he was awarded the Gold Medal of the Society of Uroradiology and also received an honorary degree from the University of Gothenburg, Sweden. The Radiological Society of North America dedicated its *1995 Scientific Program* to him. The University of Chicago named him a Distinguished Alumnus in 1982. In 1989, the Harry Fischer Award for Excellence in Contrast Media Research was established by the Contrast Media Research Society. There also is a research fund in his name at the University of Rochester.

His major influence will continue through the young researchers he mentored and started on their careers. He was responsible for injecting a substantial bolus of strong science into radiology over the years.

He will be dearly missed by his family and a great number of colleagues. During the last 6 years of his life, he had a difficult time accepting the loss of control caused by his stroke. His wife, Kay, never faltered, however, and kept him going with her optimistic view of life and strong devotion to Harry.

Here's to Harry Fischer—long may the influence of his scientific research on radiology persist.

He is survived by his wife, Kay, and his four children and their families.

John R. Thornbury, MD, and Helen C. Redman, MD

Abstracts of Current Literature

Cardiovascular System

Prevalence of Congenital Cardiovascular Malformations in Children of Human Immunodeficiency Virus–infected Women: The Prospective P²C² HIV Multicenter Study. Wyman W. Lai, Steven E. Lipshultz, Kirk A. Easley, et al. *J Am Coll Cardiol* 1998; 32:1749–1755. (W.W.L., Division of Pediatric Cardiology, Mount Sinai Medical Center, 1 Gustave L. Levy Pl, Box 1201, New York, NY 10029-6574)

Objectives: The purpose of the study was to assess the effects of maternal HIV-1 (human immunodeficiency virus) infection and vertically transmitted HIV-1 infection on the prevalence of congenital cardiovascular malformations in children. *Background:* In the United States, an estimated 7000 children are born to HIV-infected women annually. Previous limited reports have suggested an increase in the prevalence of congenital cardiovascular malformations in vertically transmitted HIV-infected children. *Methods:* In a prospective longitudinal multicenter study, diagnostic echocardiograms were performed at 4–6-month intervals on two cohorts of children exposed to maternal HIV-1 infection: 1) a Neonatal Cohort of 90 HIV-infected, 449 HIV-uninfected and 19 HIV-indeterminate children; and 2) an Older HIV-Infected Cohort of 201 children with vertically transmitted HIV-1 infection recruited after 28 days of age. *Results:* In the Neonatal Cohort, 36 lesions were seen in 36 patients, yielding an overall congenital cardiovascular malformation prevalence of 6.5% (36/558), with a 8.9% (8/90) prevalence in HIV-infected children and a 5.6% (25/449) prevalence in HIV-uninfected children. Two children (2/558, 0.4%) had cyanotic lesions. In the Older HIV-Infected Cohort, there was a congenital cardiovascular malformation prevalence of 7.5% (15/201). The distribution of lesions did not differ significantly between the groups. *Conclusions:* There was no statistically significant difference in congenital cardiovascular malformation prevalence in HIV-infected versus HIV-uninfected children born to HIV-infected women. With the use of early screening echocardiography, rates of congenital cardiovascular malformations in both the HIV-infected and HIV-uninfected children were five- to ten-fold higher than rates reported in population-based epidemiologic studies but not higher than in normal populations similarly screened. Potentially important subclinical congenital cardiovascular malformations were detected.

Authors' Abstract

Reasons for selecting abstract:

- Important clinical problem
- Effect of HIV and status on offspring

Selected by *Robert M. Steiner, MD*
New York Methodist Hospital–Weill Medical College of Cornell University, New York, NY

A Prospective Randomized Trial of Prevention Measures in Patients at High Risk for Contrast Nephropathy: Results of the P.R.I.N.C.E. Study. Melissa A. Stevens, Peter A. McCullough, Kenneth J. Tobin, et al. *J Am Coll Cardiol* 1999; 33:403–411. (From the Division of Cardiology, William Beaumont Hospital, Royal Oak, Mich)

Objectives: This study was done to test the hypothesis that a forced diuresis with maintenance of intravascular volume after contrast exposure would reduce the rate of contrast-induced renal injury. *Background:* We have previously shown a graded relationship with the degree of postprocedure renal failure and the probability of in-hospital death in patients undergoing percutaneous coronary intervention. Earlier studies of singular prevention strategies (atrial natriuretic factor, loop diuretics, dopamine, mannitol) have shown no clear benefit across a spectrum of patients at risk. *Methods:* A prospective, randomized, controlled, single-blind trial was conducted where 98 participants were randomized to forced diuresis with intravenous crystalloid, furosemide, mannitol (if pulmonary capillary wedge pressure <20 mm Hg), and low-dose dopamine ($n = 43$) versus intravenous crystalloid and matching placebos ($n = 55$). *Results:* The groups were similar with respect to baseline serum creatinine (2.44 ± 0.80 and 2.55 ± 0.91 mg/dl), age, weight, diabetic status, left ventricular function, degree of prehydration, contrast volume and ionicity, and extent of peripheral vascular disease. The forced diuresis resulted in higher urine flow rate (163.26 ± 54.47 vs. 122.57 ± 54.27 ml/h) over the 24 h after contrast exposure ($p = 0.001$). Two participants in the experimental arm versus five in the control arm required dialysis, with all seven cases having measured flow rates <145 ml/h in the 24 h after the procedure. The mean individual change in serum creatinine at 48 h, the primary end point, was 0.48 ± 0.86 versus 0.51 ± 0.87, in the experimental and control arms, respectively, $p = 0.87$. There were no differences in the rates of renal failure across six definitions of renal failure by intent-to-treat analysis. However, in all participants combined, the rise in serum creatinine was related to the degree of induced diuresis after controlling for baseline renal function, $r = -0.36$, $p = 0.005$. The rates of renal failure in those with urine flow rates greater than 150 ml/h in the postprocedure period were significantly lower, 8/37 (21.6%) versus 28/61 (45.9%), $p = 0.03$. *Conclusions:* Forced diuresis with intravenous crystalloid, furosemide, and mannitol if hemodynamics permit, beginning at the start of angiography provides a modest benefit against contrast-induced nephropathy provided a high urine flow rate can be achieved.

Authors' Abstract

Reasons for selecting abstract:

- Adverse reactions with contrast media
- Preventive measures for adverse effects of contrast media

Selected by *Robert M. Steiner, MD*
New York Methodist Hospital–Weill Medical College of Cornell University, New York, NY

Real-Time Measurement of Radiation Exposure to Patients during Diagnostic Coronary Angiography and Percutaneous Interventional Procedures. Jack T. Cusma, Malcolm R. Bell, Merrill A. Wondrow, et al. *J Am Coll Cardiol* 1999; 33:427–435. (From the Mayo Foundation and Clinic, Rochester, Minn)

Objectives: The aim of this study was to accurately assess the radiation exposure received by patients during cardiac catheterization in a large sample representative of the current state of practice in cardiac angiography. *Background:* Radiation exposure to patients and laboratory staff has been recognized as a necessary hazard in coronary angiography. The effects on x-ray exposure of the increased complexity of coronary angiographic procedures and, in particular, the increasing use of coronary artery stenting, have not been adequately addressed in previous studies. *Methods:* X-ray exposure measurements were performed on a consecutive series of 972 patients undergoing 992 diagnostic and interventional studies in the Mayo Clinic catheterization laboratory within an eight week period in late 1997. Data were acquired from 706 diagnostic procedures and 286 interventional procedures using a real-time exposure measurement system to continuously calculate and record the exposure rate and total exposure, reflecting all parameters relevant to the specific patient and procedure situation. *Results:* The median exposure for all 992 procedures was 41.8 mC/kg (162.1 R); the corresponding values for diagnostic and interventional procedures were 34.9 and 95.6 mC/kg, respectively (135.3 vs. 370.5 R). There were significant differences in the fluoroscopy exposure time between diagnostic and interventional procedures: 4.7 min vs. 21.0 min. Heavier patients (>83 kg) received x-ray exposures at a significantly higher rate than did lighter patients (<83 kg) during both fluoroscopy and cine; 44.9 mC/kg/min (173.9 R/min) vs. 27.9 mC/kg/min (108.3 R/min) for cine exposure rate and 2.3 mC/kg/min (8.8 R/min) vs. 1.5 mC/kg/min (5.8 R/min) for fluoroscopy exposure rate. *Conclusions:* Changes in practice have led to higher values for patient x-ray radiation exposures during cardiac catheterization procedures. The real-time display and recording of x-ray exposure facilitates the reduction of exposure in the catheterization laboratory.

Authors' Abstract

Reason for selecting abstract:

- Radiation exposure during frequently performed studies

Selected by *Robert M. Steiner, MD*
New York Methodist Hospital–Weill Medical College of Cornell University, New York, NY

Pediatrics

Atypical Chronic Lung Disease Patterns in Neonates. Lama Charafeddine, Carl T. D'Angio, Dale L. Phelps. *Pediatrics* 1999; 103:759–765. (From the Department of Pediatrics, Division of Neonatology, University of Rochester School of Medicine, Children's Hospital at Strong, Rochester, NY)

Objective: To determine, in the postsurfactant era, the incidence and clinical characteristics of infants with atypical versus traditionally defined bronchopulmonary dysplasia (BPD) among premature infants with birth weights <1251 g. *Design:* Retrospective cohort study. *Setting:* A single regional neonatal intensive care unit (level III/IV). *Patients:* Two hundred thirty-two premature infants <1251 g at birth consecutively admitted during a 2-year period. *Main Outcome Measure:* Incidence of classic BPD and atypical chronic lung disease (CLD) (occurring without preceding respiratory distress or after recovery from respiratory distress). *Results:* Among 177 infants <1251 g who survived to 28 days, 27 (15%) had atypical CLD and 61 (34.5%) had classic BPD. Atypical CLD infants were significantly heavier and more mature than classic BPD infants (mean birth weights, 922 ± 152 g vs 854 ± 173 g; and mean gestational age, 26.8 ± 1.3 weeks vs 26.1 ± 1.6 weeks). Median duration of ventilator support (31 days; range, 2 to 127 vs 42 days; range, 4–145 days) and oxygen therapy (30 days; range, 11 to 163 vs 48 days; range, 19–180 days) were shorter in atypical CLD infants than in classic BPD infants. *Conclusion:* Atypical CLD comprised 31% of total cases of CLD. Atypical CLD appears to be less severe than classic BPD. These data suggest that initial, acute lung injuries are not the sole antecedents of neonatal CLD.

Authors' Abstract

Reason for selecting abstract:
- Variable patterns of lung disease and respiratory distress

Selected by *Beverly P. Wood, MD*
University of Southern California School of Medicine, Los Angeles

Comprehensive Management of Dysfunctional Voiding. Seth L. Schulman, Carol K. Quinn, Natalie Plachter, et al. *Pediatrics* 1999; 103(3); *http://www.pediatrics.org/cgi/content/full/103/3/e31.* (From the Department of Pediatrics, Children's Hospital of Philadelphia, University of Pennsylvania School of Medicine, Philadelphia)

Objective: Dysfunctional voiding is a major problem leading to daytime-wetting and recurrent urinary tract infection (UTI). Our center is devoted to treating children with dysfunctional voiding. We offer a multidisciplinary approach with a pediatric nephrologist, nurse practitioners, and a psychologist. This article is the first to describe the efficacy of this approach on a large population of American children. *Patients:* Between 1992 and 1995, 366 children with symptoms of voiding dysfunction were referred for urodynamic studies. Criteria were based on the child's age, symptoms, and failure to respond to empirical therapy. Females made up 77% of the population, and the mean age at referral was 8.5 years (range, 4 to 18 years). Day-wetting occurred in 312 (89%), night-wetting in 278 (79%), recurrent UTI in 218 (60%), and vesicoureteral reflux (VUR) in 48 (20%) of those undergoing voiding cystourethrography. *Results:* A minimum of 6 months' follow-up data (mean, 22 months) is available on 280 children (77% studied). Urge syndrome was the predominant urodynamic finding in 52%, followed by bladder sphincter dysfunction in 25%. Treatment consisted of antibiotic prophylaxis (59%), anticholinergic medication (49%), biofeedback (25%), and psychological counseling (15%). Of the 222 children with daytime-wetting (45%), 100 are cured (off all medication, no wetting) and 82 (37%) are improved (on medication or >50% reduction in symptoms). Improvement or cure was seen in 69% of children with night-wetting. Of the 199 children with UTI, 127 (64%) never developed another infection. Vesicoureteral reflux resolved in 16 of 30 (53%) children undergoing repeat voiding cystourethrography. *Conclusion:* Our comprehensive approach demonstrates a favorable outcome that promises to reduce the medical and psychological morbidity seen in patients with voiding dysfunction.

Authors' Abstract

Reasons for selecting abstract:
- Relation to recurrent urinary tract infection and daytime-wetting
- Voiding cystourethrogram findings

Selected by *Beverly P. Wood, MD*
University of Southern California School of Medicine, Los Angeles

Cranial Ultrasound Abnormalities Identified at Birth: Their Relationship to Perinatal Risk and Neurobehavioral Outcome. Marylou Behnke, Fonda Davis Eyler, Cynthia Wilson Garvan, et al. *Pediatrics* 1999; 103(4); *http://www.pediatrics.org/cgi/content/full/103/4/e41.* (From the Department of Pediatrics, University of Florida, Gainesville)

Objectives: Minor cranial ultrasound abnormalities, such as mild ventricular enlargement, choroid plexus cysts, and subependymal cysts, have been identified in 3% to 5% of the newborn population. Although clinicians generally consider these abnormalities to be insignificant for the outcome of the newborn, few convincing data have been published to support this optimism. The objectives of this study were to identify potential risk factors associated with the identification of cranial ultrasound abnormalities at birth and to determine if the abnormalities were related to neurobehavioral sequelae in the newborn. *Methods:* Three hundred eight women were enrolled in this prospective, longitudinal maternal-infant health and development study either at the time they entered the public health care system for prenatal care or at delivery if they had no prenatal care. Each woman participated in an in-depth psychosocial interview at the end of each trimester of pregnancy. Retrospective chart review by experienced medical personnel was used to compile data for the Hobel perinatal risk score for each study participant after delivery. Offspring underwent cranial ultrasound evaluation, the Amiel-Tison Neurologic Assessment, and the Brazelton Neonatal Behavioral Assessment Scale within 96 hours of birth by experienced examiners blinded to any maternal-infant history. *Results:* Of the 308 women originally enrolled in the study, 301 delivered living infants. Of these, 266 infants (88%) underwent a cranial ultrasound evaluation and are the subject of this article. For the purposes of the current study, infants were divided into those with normal (n = 239) and those with abnormal (n = 27) ultrasound results. Abnormal ultrasound results included the following lesions: subependymal cyst (n = 13); mild ventricular enlargement (n = 6); choroid plexus cysts (n = 3); a combination of cysts and increased ventricular size (n = 2); a 7-mm midline cyst in the superior posterior portion of the third ventricle (n = 1); subependymal hemorrhage and ventricular enlargement (n = 1); and increased ventricular size, subependymal hemorrhage and cysts, and two small, right thalamic calcifications (n = 1). There were no significant differences between those with an abnormal ultrasound and those with a normal ultrasound for birth weight, length, gestational age, rate of prematurity, frequency of nulliparity, or frequency of small for gestational age infants. However, infants with an abnormal ultrasound had a significantly smaller mean head circumference than those with a normal ultrasound (34.5 ± 1.9 cm vs 33.7 ± 1.9 cm). The infants with an abnormal ultrasound had a higher median prenatal (50 vs 45), neonatal (14 vs 8), and total (94 vs 77) Hobel risk score but not a higher labor-delivery score. There were no significant differences when these groups were compared on additional risk factors not included in the Hobel scoring system such as race and socioeconomic status. In addition, mothers who used a greater number of drugs during the first trimester of pregnancy were more likely to have an infant with an abnormal ultrasound at birth such that the probability of having an abnormal ultrasound rose to 22% by the time the pregnant women were using four drugs. Neurologic examinations revealed no differences between the infants with normal and abnormal ultrasounds. There were also no group differences for five of the seven Brazelton cluster scores, the excitable or depressed clusters, or eight of the nine qualifier scores. However, infants with abnormal ultrasounds performed significantly better on the habituation (7.3 ± 0.8 vs 6.6 ± 1.5) and autonomic regulation (6.5 ± 0.8 vs 6.0 ± 1.0) clusters but more poorly on the cost of attention qualifier score (4.9 ± 1.2 vs 5.5 ± 1.2) on the Brazelton Neonatal Behavioral Assessment Scale. *Conclusion:* Infants with an abnormal cranial ultrasound at birth had higher perinatal risk scores. Additionally, we conclude that the abnormalities identified on cranial ultrasound within the first 96 hours of life were most likely benign with no clinical significance in the immediate neonatal period. However, because of the finding of several subtle differences in behavior, follow-up beyond the neonatal period would be advisable to determine if any late-onset abnormalities occur.

Authors' Abstract

Reasons for selecting abstract:
- Neurologic outcome
- Large infant cohort

Selected by *Beverly P. Wood, MD*
University of Southern California School of Medicine, Los Angeles

Classified Services

POLICY

As a service to its readers, *Radiology* accepts classified advertising, and every effort is made to ensure that the ads are relevant to the practice of radiology. Acceptable categories include positions available, positions sought, fellowships, announcements of postgraduate courses or symposia, practices for sale, medical facilities for rent or sale, used radiologic equipment and apparatus for sale, medical employment bureau advertising, academic posts to be filled, available posts for interns and residents, and malpractice insurance. We retain the right to refuse any advertisement considered not relevant, and respondents are advised to investigate each offer since we cannot assume responsibility for the offers or claims of advertisers.

RATES (per month, per insertion)

Line ads in *Radiology* (no agency commission)

50 words or less $100.00

51–100 words $145.00

Each word over 100—$1.00 per word.

Box Number—$30.00 additional per each insertion (this service is optional).

TERMS

Payment must accompany order.* Make checks payable to **Radiological Society of North America.** We accept American Express, VISA, Mastercard, and Diners Club for classified ads. Call for details. Send payment to:

RSNA, Radiology Classified Ad Department
Accounts Payable, 820 Jorie Boulevard
Oak Brook, IL 60523-2251 USA.

*Purchase Order Numbers are accepted with prior approval.

Please mark each issue:

❒ Jan ❒ Feb ❒ Mar ❒ Apr ❒ May ❒ June
❒ July ❒ Aug ❒ Sept ❒ Oct ❒ Nov ❒ Dec

Send invoice and tearsheet to:

____
____
____
____

Advertisers who cancel ads will not receive refunds.

DEADLINE

Copy must be received by the **20th of the second month preceding issue**. Please submit copy typed and double-spaced. An initial or an abbreviation equals one word. A telephone number with area code equals one word.

CLASSIFIED DISPLAY ADVERTISING

Black and white frequency rates are based on the total number of insertions used within a 12-month period from date of first insertion. (Unit prices are shown below.)

Ad Space	Size	1X	6X	12X
1 page	7" x 9-1/2"	$2350	2270	2190
2/3 pg vert	4-1/2" x 9-1/2"	$2000	1930	1860
1/2 pg horzt	7" x 4-1/2"	$1550	1490	1430
1/2 pg vert	3-3/8" x 9-1/2"	$1550	1490	1430
1/2 pg island	4-1/4" x 7-1/2"	$1550	1490	1430
1/3 pg vert	2-1/4" x 9-1/2"	$1100	1050	1000
1/3 pg square	4-1/2" x 4-1/2"	$1100	1050	1000
1/4 page	3-3/8" x 4-1/2"	$ 900	860	820
1/6 page	2-1/4" x 4-1/2"	$ 650	630	610
1/9 page	2-1/4" x 3"	$ 450	430	410

Preferred materials are composite negatives, right-reading, emulsion side down. (Conversion materials such as positive film, repro proofs, and camera-ready artworks are acceptable; there may be an additional charge.)

Customer supplied negative: cost as noted
Customer supplied copy to be set and ad prepared: add 20%

Call Production Department for additional information. Address for correspondence, insertion orders, copy, proofs, box number, and payment:

***Radiology* Advertising Production Office**
820 Jorie Boulevard
Oak Brook, IL 60523-2251

To respond to a box number ad, send your CV and/or any other information to the above address; on the front of the envelope, please indicate the appropriate box number.

For further information:
Patrick Williamson, *Advertising Coordinator*
630.571.7817
630.571.7837 (fax)

Positions Available

THE DEPARTMENT OF RADIOLOGY AT THE UNIVERSITY OF ALABAMA AT BIRMINGHAM—Is actively recruiting an interventional radiologist. The section of Vascular and Interventional Radiology provides services for 1,100-beds at the University and Veteran's Administration Hospitals and performs over 5,500 procedures per year. Currently there are three full-time faculty members. Facilities include a Siemens Multistar TOP and two Philips angio suites currently under construction. Applicants must be Board-certified in diagnostic radiology, have a CAQ in vascular and interventional radiology (or eligible for a CAQ), and eligible for licensure in the state of Alabama. Duties include medical student and resident teaching, radiology service and clinical research. Academic rank and tenure status will depend upon qualifications and experience. Interested candidates should submit their CV to Robert J. Stanley, MD, Department of Radiology, University of Alabama at Birmingham, AL 35233. The University of Alabama at Birmingham is an affirmative action/equal opportunity employer.

THE UNIVERSITY OF KENTUCKY—Is seeking a full-time, tenured line, open rank academic thoracic radiologist. Must be Board-eligible; certification preferred. Duties would also include interpretation of film for evaluation of occupational lung disease. Responsibilities include patient care, medical student and resident teaching, and regularly scheduled interdepartment conferences. Opportunity to pursue clinical research. Please mail or fax letter of interest and curriculum vitae to James C. Reed, MD, Chairman, Department of Radiology, HX304, UK Medical Center, Lexington, KY 40536-0084; fax 606-257-6014. UK is an equal opportunity employer.

ASHEVILLE, NC— A Board-certified radiologist is needed to help with night, weekend day, and holiday call coverage of 21-person group practice in major referral center. Partnership track available with excellent time off and benefits package in beautiful mountain vacation area. Send CV to Ms Sue Spivey, P.O. Box 2959, Asheville, NC 28802

RADIOLOGISTS (ALL TYPES)—Kendall and Davis has numerous radiology openings nationwide. For a detailed description of these positions, check out our website at *www.KENDALL andDAVIS.com*, or if you prefer, call Judi Phillips at 800-950-1551 or fax your CV to 314-843-2262. Sorry, no J-1 positions available.

NIGHT RADIOLOGISTS—Bay Imaging Consultants Medical Group, Inc, a large San Francisco Bay area private practice radiology group with multiple outpatient and hospital sites, is seeking night radiologists for the night rotation. The night rotation is comprised of 12-hour rotations from 7:00pm to 7:00am. Must be Board-certified. Competitive salary. Start date as soon as possible. Please submit your CV, a cover letter and the names of three references to Human Resources, 175 Lennon Ln, Suite 100, Walnut Creek, CA 94598. EOE.

EXPERIENCED BOARD-CERTIFIED DIAGNOSTIC RADIOLOGIST—Join 15 radiologists in a highly successful group covering multiple hospitals and OP facilities. High volume practice includes all aspects of general radiology. Specific interest in body MR, US, and nuclear medicine preferred. Partnership tract includes excellent compensation/benefit package including paid vacation, malpractice & health insurance pension with CME and moving allowance. Very progressive medical community located 90 miles from Dallas in East Texas. Send CV to Larry Smith, Practice Administrator, Tyler Radiology Assoc, 1407 S Fleishel, Suite 301, Tyler, TX 75701 or fax to 903-593-0559.

DIAGNOSTIC RADIOLOGIST—With stable five-person group in Duluth, MN. Candidate must be proficient in all aspects of diagnostic imaging, routine angiography and interventional procedures. Fellowship training strongly preferred. Position leads to partnership. Apply to Calvin C. Loken, MD, 924 E Superior St, Suite 109, Duluth, MN 55802.

THE UNIVERSITY OF TENNESSEE, MEMPHIS—Is actively recruiting for a radiologist specializing in cross-sectional imaging. The Radiology Department provides services for 1,600 adult and pediatric beds in an urban medical center which includes the Regional Medical Center at Memphis and its Level I trauma center, the tertiary UT/Bowld Hospital and its active renal, liver and pancreas transplant service, the Memphis VA Medical Center, the LeBonheur Children's Hospital and the Jude Cancer Research Institute. Applicants must be Board-certified or eligible in diagnostic radiology, fellowship-trained in body imaging and eligible for licensure in the state of Tennessee. Sub-specialty training is preferable but not required. Appointment will be at the Assistant to Associate level depending upon experience and qualifications. Interested applicants should respond with a letter of interest, current curriculum vitae and the names and addresses of three references to Robert E. Gold, MD, Chair, Department of Radiology, The University of Tennessee, Memphis, 800 Madison Ave, Memphis, TN 38163. The University of Tennessee is an equal opportunity/affirmative action/Title IX/Section 504/ADA employer.

RADIOLOGY, SALEM, OR—Northwest Permanente, PC, a physician managed, multispecialty group serving the members of Kaiser Permanente in the northwest division, has an excellent opportunity beginning in 1999 for a BC/BE radiologist to join two radiologists at our medical facilities in Salem, OR capital city. Located 45 miles South of Portland, our Salem 40-physician multispecialty group currently offers professional services to 43,000 plan members in the area. Our need is for a general radiologist whose skills include CT, US, fluoroscopy and mammography. Northwest Permanente has a total of 32 radiologists at our clinics and affiliated hospitals in the Portland metropolitan area and Salem providing quality care to over 430,000 plan members in Oregon and Washington. Ours is a collegial and stimulating practice in one of the most successful managed care programs in the country. In addition to a lifestyle inherent to the beautiful Pacific Northwest, we offer a predictable work schedule, and a competitive salary and benefit package which includes professional liability coverage, a comprehensive pension program, sabbatical leave and more. For additional information please forward CV to R.A. Clark, Director, Physician Resources, Northwest Permanente, PC, 500 NE Multnomah, Suite 100, Portland, OR 97232-2099. EOE.

GEORGIA—Immediate opening for Board-certified radiologist to join a six-member group expanding to seven due to practice growth. Group covers three hospitals and a brand new 5200 sq ft outpatient imaging center with state-of-the-art equipment, including Acuson Sequoia Ultrasound, three Helical CT scanners, ADAC variable head nuclear medicine camera and GE Horizon 1.5 Tesla MRI. Position is a partnership track with excellent benefits and salary, located 90 minutes south of Atlanta. Please send CV to Scott M. Stephen, MD, 748 F North Houston Rd, Warner Robins, GA 31093 or fax to 912-922-6116. For further information, call Kim at 912-922-5214.

TIFTON, GA—A three-man radiology group in South Georgia seeks general radiologist with special interest/training in MR or interventional radiology. Partnership track position to begin July 2000. Generous time off. Two hours to Atlantic or Gulf. Send CV to Dr Kelley P. Douglas, Tifton Radiology, PC, 1495 Kennedy Rd, Tifton, GA 31794 or fax to 912-386-4495.

THE DEPARTMENT OF REGIONAL RADIOLOGY AT THE CLEVELAND CLINIC FOUNDATION—Cleveland, Ohio, is in the process of recruiting ABR-certified general diagnostic radiologists to practice in community hospitals and ambulatory care facilities, which are part of the Cleveland Clinic Health System. The department consists of 20 staff radiologists servicing four community hospitals and seven ambulatory care facilities/surgi centers. Approximately 278,000 examinations were performed at the sites in 1998. The hospital departments and outpatient facilities are fully networked (imaging and RIS) with the Cleveland Clinic Foundation main campus radiology department, which is staffed by 48 subspecialty radiologists. If this opportunity is appealing to you, please contact Gregory P. Borkowski, MD, FACR, Chairman, Regional Radiology Practice, The Cleveland Clinic Foundation, Department of Radiology, Hb-6, 9500 Euclid Ave, Cleveland, OH 44195; phone 216-444-6625, fax 216-445-4432, e-mail *borkowg @cesmtp.ccf.org.*

DIRECTOR OF BREAST IMAGING—Suburban LA hospital seeks breast imager to direct large breast imaging center affiliated with a 400-bed in-patient facility. Has screening, diagnostic mammography services, ultrasound, ABBI, mammotome, and access to MRI. Must be Board-certified in radiology and capable of performing other routine radiographic studies. Please reply to Box R-107.

EVENING/WEEKEND DIAGNOSTIC RADIOLOGISTS—Midwest group seeking Board-certified (eligible) individuals to rotate coverage. General, CT, US, nuclear medicine skills needed. Basic angio helpful. Salaried positions; 810-412-9944, ask for Judi.

MINNESOTA: BUSY MINNESOTA RADIOLOGY PRACTICE—Dakota Clinic, a 175-physician-owned multispecialty clinic based in Fargo, ND, is seeking a BE/BC radiologist for our Thief River Falls, MN division for the summer of 2000. Located in northwest Minnesota, this 16-physician group is looking to replace its retiring radiologist with an eager individual proficient in general, CT, MRI and nuclear radiology. Enjoy a new 50,000 square foot state-of-the-art clinic and modern hospital. We offer a competitive salary and benefits package with stockholdership available after two years. Thief River Falls, the home of Arctic Cat snowmobiles, is a growing community of 9,000 with a service area of 45,000. This family-oriented community offers excellent schools, low crime, hunting, fishing and easy access to Minnesota lakes. To learn more about this opportunity, mail, fax or e-mail your CV to Dick Reis, Physician Recruitment Manager, Dakota Clinic Ltd, 1702 S University Dr, Fargo, ND 58103. Fax 701-280-3229, e-mail *dreis @dakcl.com*, toll-free number 1-800-882-7310. Dakota Clinic: *www.dakotaclinic.com.*

NEURORADIOLOGIST—The University of Michigan at Ann Arbor is seeking an academic neuroradiologist. Call or e-mail Dr. Gebarski for details at 734-936-4484; *gebarski@umich.edu.*

WANTED: BOARD-CERTIFIED RADIOLOGISTS IN NE PENNSYLVANIA—Radiological Consultants, Inc, has a demand for several radiologists secondary to both retiring members as well as an expanding service area. We are group of 17 radiologists in northeast Pennsylvania covering two hospitals in Scranton, one hospital in Wilkes Barre, one hospital in Nanticoke, as well as an MRI center which houses two 1.5 Tesla magnets as well as an open 0.3 Tesla magnet. We are currently targeting fellowship-trained or an equivalent experienced radiologist. Competitive salary and benefits are being offered for this excellent opportunity. Reply to Radiological Consultants, Inc, c/o John J. Culliney, MD, 751 Keystone Industrial Park, Dunmore, PA 18512. Phone 717-346-8272 or fax CV to 717-346-4872.

MAMMOGRAPHER IN CENTRAL JERSEY—Group of five hospital-based private practice radiologists seeking fellowship-trained mammographer for new state-of-the-art women's center including stereotactic biopsy. Partnership opportunity. Please contact Dr. McManus, 732-886-4445.

PEORIA RADIOLOGY ASSOCIATES, PC—Is currently recruiting two general radiologists for one of our satellite institutions. This represents a unique career opportunity to join a large private subspecialty radiology group with close university affiliation. This is a partnership track offer. Peoria Radiology Associates, PC, is a 25-person, highly subspecialized group that has an active teaching program including radiology residents and fellowships in neuroradiology, breast imaging and interventional radiology. There is an excellent compensation and benefit package. Clinical responsibilities include all areas of medical imaging, including MRI and possibly some interventional radiology. All inquiries will be held confidential. Please indicate whether you wish to be contacted at home or at work. Please reply with CV to Kay Springer, Peoria Radiology Associates, PC, 530 NE Glen Oak Ave, Peoria, IL 61637, or fax 309-655-2951.

THE UNIVERSITY OF CINCINNATI, DEPARTMENT OF RADIOLOGY—Seeks qualified candidates for non-tenure track positions at the assistant or associate professor level, rank commensurate with experience. Opportunities are available for physicians with subspecialty interest in one or more of the following areas: general body imaging, abdominal, thoracic, breast imaging, body MRI, and angio/interventional. Fellowship training is preferred but not required. Must be ABR/AOBR-certified and have, or be eligible for, an Ohio medical license. Applicants should be interested in pursuing a combined academic/clinical career. Responsibilities include clinical patient care and teaching/supervision of residents, fellows and students. Participation in basic and clinical research is supported. Letters of inquiry and CV should be forwarded to Ms Shira Karns, Radiology Business Office, 2600 Euclid Ave, Cincinnati, OH 45219. The University of Cincinnati is an AA/EOE/ADA employer. Women, minorities, persons with disabilities, Vietnam era and disabled veterans are encouraged to apply. UC is a smoke-free work environment.

DYNAMIC RADIOLOGY GROUP—In beautiful Pacific NW seeking a generalist with specialty expertise. 380+-bed, level II trauma center. Partnership track. Great community; affordable living; close to skiing, fishing, boating, wilderness. Qualified applicants please send CV to Ronald J. Cocchiarella, MD, 801 W 5th Ave, #205, Spokane, WA 99204 or fax 509-747-1180.

PEDIATRIC RADIOLOGIST—Rainbow Babies and Children's Hospital of the University Hospitals of Cleveland, Case Western Reserve School of Medicine, is seeking a fellowship-trained academic pediatric radiologist at the assistant or associate professor level. Rainbow Babies is a 244-bed facility. The department performs approximately 43,000 exams/yr. The applicant will join five other pediatric radiologists. Candidates must be certified by the American Board of Radiology and must have or be eligible to sit for the certificate of added qualifications in pediatric radiology. Compensation and fringe benefits are competitive. Address inquiries to Carlos J. Sivit, MD, Director, Pediatric Radiology, Rainbow Babies and Children's Hospital, 11100 Euclid Ave, Cleveland, OH 44106-5056; 216-844-1172; fax 216-844-5474; e-mail *sivit@uhrad.com*.

VASCULAR/INTERVENTIONAL RADIOLOGIST—Portland, OR. Northwest Permanente, PC, a physician-managed multi-specialty group serving over 440,000 members of Kaiser Permanente in the Northwest has an excellent opportunity in the Portland area for a Board-certified radiologist with fellowship training or extensive clinical experience in angiography or interventional radiology. Our practice includes opportunities to be involved in interpretation of neurological and peripheral vascular MRA and performances of TIPS, uterine artery embolizations, hepato-biliary and general body intervention and vascular stenting with an opportunity to develop a stent-graft program. Our program in Oregon and Washington offers a collegial and professionally stimulating environment in one of the most successful managed care systems in the

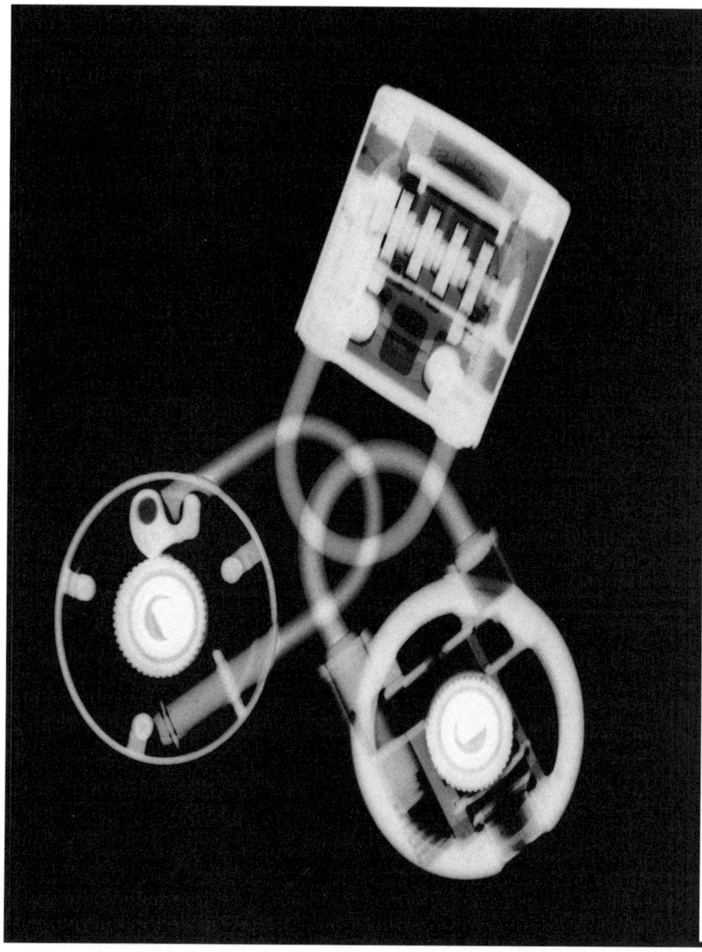

gy. The candidate must have experience in a broad range of diagnostic and therapeutic interventional procedures. Board certification is required as well as being interventional CAQ-certified or eligible. An interest in non-invasive vascular imaging is also desirable. Reply to Kenneth Matasar, MD, FACR, Chairman, Diagnostic Radiology, William Beaumont Hospital, 3601 West 13 Mile Road, Royal Oak, MI 48073. Fax 248-551-5490.

ANGIO-INTERVENTIONAL/GENERAL RADIOLOGIST—Private practice of five, with four outpatient clinics and a new 230-bed active community hospital seeking general radiologist with angio/interventional capability. Excellent pay, liberal benefits, minimal call. Position to be filled immediately. Fax resume to 313-581-6464.

GENERAL RADIOLOGIST, LAS VEGAS, NV—Expanding, stable and progressive 13-member outpatient practice is seeking two BC fellowship-trained radiologists for two excellent partnership track positions in one of the fastest growing cities in the United States. The practice runs three of the largest state-of-the-art imaging centers in the nation and includes six MRIs, four CT scanners, two angio suites, nuclear medicine, mammography and US. Strong general radiology skills needed (no interventional skills required). Interest in mammography would be beneficial for one position, but not required. These positions currently involve no call and no angio coverage. Positions are available immediately, but start date is flexible to summer of 2000. Please send CV to Dr Chang, 2950 S Maryland Pkwy, Las Vegas, NV 89109.

METRO ST. LOUIS—Well-established, large private practice group continuing to expand is recruiting two new radiologists for partnership track. Candidate should be ABR-certified; fellowship training is highly desirable. Our new radiologists would be expected to make an impact by continuing to develop new imaging approaches and state-of-the-art techniques for our hospital and outpatient practice. We currently staff three busy suburban hospitals and own and operate three additional free-standing imaging centers. Salary and benefits are very competitive. For more information, contact Darryl Zuckerman, MD, Department of Radiology, St. Joseph Health Center, 300 First Capitol Dr, St. Charles, MO 63301; phone 314-947-5444, fax 314-947-9860.

SEATTLE POSITION AVAILABLE—Move to Seattle and the beautiful Pacific Northwest. Growing private practice in a desirable Seattle suburb seeks thirteenth full-time radiologist. Inpatient/outpatient setting with a 250-bed multispecialty hospital and several imaging centers. Individual sought with experience and skills in neuro and musculoskeletal MRI. Presently two magnets (including Siemens Vision 1.5T with Echo Planer Imaging), third installation planned. Would also participate in other general radiology rotations and equal call. Partnership track, competitive benefits and salary. Please direct inquiries to Steve Sperling, MD, Overlake Hospital Medical Center, 1035 116th Ave NE, Bellevue, WA 98004; 425-688-5537.

RADIOLOGY OPPORTUNITIES—Watson Clinic LLP is a 175-physician multispecialty group seeking two radiologists. Join 14 radiologists in this fully diversified practice which includes MRI, CT, mammogram, DEXA, GI/IVP, U/S and interventional work at a 660-bed tertiary care hospital two blocks south of the clinic. One position available to join one other in mammography. Ability to perform stereotactic needle biopsies required. Additional practice opportunity available in CT/body imaging. We offer early partnership, salary guarantee with production incentive, excellent benefits package and paid malpractice insurance. Please send a CV to Professional Services, Watson Clinic, LLP, 1600 Lakeland Hills Blvd, Lakeland, FL 33804; phone 800-854-7786, fax 941-680-7951.

THE NEURORADIOLOGY SECTION AT THE UNIVERSITY OF ALABAMA AT BIRMINGHAM—Is recruiting two Board-certified neuroradiologists (CAQ-certified) to join four neuroradiologists. Coverage for UAB Hospital, VAH and Kirklin Clinic includes 24,000 procedures annually, teaching house staff and research. The radiology department in the medical center has 4 GE CT/I helical scanners, and 4 MRI scanners: two GE Signa 1.5T, one Siemens Expert 1T and one GE Signa 1T; and one biplane Siemens Neurostar angiography room. Contact Dr Robert Stanley, Department of Radiology, University of Alabama at Birmingham, Birmingham, AL 35233; phone 205-934-9577, fax 205-934-8110. UAB is an equal opportunity employer.

RADIOLOGIST, PORTLAND, OR—Our well-established eight-member group has an immediate opening for a Board-certified radiologist with additional training in body imaging or interventional radiology. Other fellowship training considered. We anticipate the position to lead to partnership in 2 to 3 years. We practice at a major central city hospital with a large pediatric program and a Level I trauma center. Salary and benefits are competitive. Send CV to Blaine Kozak, MD, or fax to 503-413-2554. Call 503-413-4032 or e-mail *bkozak@lhs.org*.

SEEKING A BOARD-CERTIFIED RADIOLOGIST—To join a progressive multi-hospital group practice in beautiful western Maryland. All modalities including '98 GE Horizon 1.5T MRI and Digital Siemens Angio Suite. Interventional training or experience preferred. Excellent compensation toward partnership. Contact Jong Kim, MD, Sacred Heart Hospital, Radiology Department, 900 Seton Dr, Cumberland, MD 21502, phone 301-723-5133.

NUCLEAR MEDICINE—Portland, OR. Northwest Permanente, PC, a physician-managed multispecialty group serving over 440,000 members of Kaiser Permanente in the Northwest has an excellent opportunity in the Portland area for a radiologist, Board-certified or eligible in nuclear medicine. Our program in Oregon and Washington offers a collegial and professionally stimulating environment in one of the most successful managed care systems in the country, plus a quality lifestyle in the Northwest. In addition, we provide a competitive salary and benefit package which includes a generous retirement program, sabbatical leave, professional liability coverage and more. Please forward CV to N.M. Clark, Director, Professional Resources, Northwest Permanente, PC, 500 NE Multnomah, Ste 100, Portland, OR 97232-2099. EOE.

THE SECTION OF NEURORADIOLOGY IN THE DEPARTMENT OF RADIOLOGY AT THE CLEVELAND CLINIC FOUNDATION—Is offering two full-time staff positions due to rapid growth of their practice. Candidates should be Board-certified radiologists who have completed a fellowship, preferably two years, in an accredited neuroradiology program, and who are CAQ-certified or eligible. A strong background in academic radiology, cerebral angiography, myelography, CT, MR and MR angiography is required. (Clinical interest in functional MR is particularly valuable.) The neuroradiology section provides a well-balanced team atmosphere with existing expertise in pediatric neuroradiology, interventional neuroradiology and cerebrovascular disease, spine imaging and an MR research center supported by three PhD level staff physicists and two (PhD and masters level) biostatisticians. A research center with a large commitment to vascular disease is available for basic investigations in interventional neuroradiology; clinical research protocols for all facets of neurointervention are already in place. Applications will be accepted until positions are filled. For more information, please contact Thomas J. Masaryk, MD, Section Head, Neuroradiology, Department of Radiology, Hb-6, 9500 Euclid Ave, Cleveland, OH 44195; e-mail *masaryk@ccisd2.ccf.org*. Phone 216-444-6653. Equal opportunity/affirmative action employer.

ABDOMINAL RADIOLOGIST AT THE CLEVELAND CLINIC FOUNDATION—The section of abdominal imaging at the Cleveland Clinic Foundation has two openings starting immediately, one to fill an open position and another to meet expanding clinical demands. We are currently a seven-member section interpreting abdominal CT, ultrasound, vascular ultrasound, luminal GI studies, GU studies, abdominal MRI as well as performing common abdominal interventions, including biopsies and abscess drainages. The practice is busy, performing over 20,000 CTs, 18,000 ultrasounds, 500 abdominal MRs and 1,000 interventions last year. We serve a highly trained and sophisticated group of gastroenterologists, oncologists, and surgeons sub-specializing in colon and rectum, hepato-pancreatico-biliary surgery, urology and gynecology. Equipment is state-of-the-art CT, including a new multi-row scanner, ultrasound and MRI. Cross-sectional imaging is fully networked and image interpretation is all work station based. The medical center is a multi-specialty group practice that is rapidly expanding on the main campus as well as in the community. Fellowship training in abdominal imaging and ABR certification is required. Salary and benefits are very competitive. Contact Mark E. Baker, MD, Head, Section of Abdominal Imaging, Division of Radiology, Hb-6, The Cleveland Clinic Foundation, 9500 Euclid Ave, Cleveland, OH 44195; 216-444-6638.

INTERVENTIONAL RADIOLOGIST—Memorial Sloan-Kettering Cancer Center (MSKCC) has a faculty position open in the Vascular/Interventional section, which performs all types of vascular/interventional procedures related to the care of patients with cancer. This includes a very active role in hepatobiliary, genitourinary, and venous access procedures. The service is experiencing significant growth in ablative and minimally invasive methods of treating cancer, and excellent research opportunities exist at this Cornell University Medical College affiliate. Applicants should be Board-certified with a CAQ in VIR. Appointment at Assistant or Associate level, commensurate with experience and accomplishments. Please send a curriculum vitae and letter of interest to Karen T. Brown, MD, Department of Radiology, Memorial Sloan-Kettering Cancer Center, 1275 York Ave, New York, NY 10021; fax 212-717-3325. MSKCC is an equal opportunity employer/affirmative action employer. Women and minorities are encouraged to apply; *www.mskcc.org*.

PEDIATRIC RADIOLOGIST—The Department of Radiology at the University of Rochester Medical Center/Strong Memorial Hospital has a full-time faculty position available for a fellowship-trained pediatric radiologist. Approximately 35,000 pediatric examinations are performed each year by three and one-half pediatric radiologists at The Children's Hospital at Strong. General imaging is performed as well as CT, ultrasound, and body MRI. Send cover letter and CV to Nina Klionsky, MD, 601 Elmwood Ave, Rochester, NY 14642, fax 716-758-8290, e-mail *nina_klionsky@urmc.rochester.edu*. The University of Rochester is an equal opportunity employer.

SOUTHERN OREGON—Opportunity for Board-certified radiologists to join a group of five well-established radiologists. The practice includes two hospitals and outpatient facilities. Experience in all modalities and mammography certification necessary. Fellowship training is desired. Partnership track optional. Excellent lifestyle with many outdoor activities from the Pacific coast to the Oregon Cascades. Great family environment. Send CV to Larry Strickland, Administrator, Roseburg Radiologists, PC, PO Box 1547, Roseburg, OR 97470.

MASSACHUSETTS—Immediate opening for Board-certified diagnostic radiologist to join progressive 14-person group just south of Boston. Partnership or per diem arrangement is possible. Strong interest in breast imaging preferred, but not essential. Please contact Peter H. Gordon, MD, Good Samaritan Medical Center, 235 N Pearl St, Brockton, MA 02301. *phgordon@massmed.org*

NUCLEAR MEDICINE/RADIOLOGIST—The Mount Auburn Hospital Department of Radiology has an opening for a staff radiologist to direct the Division of Nuclear Medicine. The hospital is a community teaching hospital affiliated with Harvard Medical School. The radiology department sponsors a fully accredited residency in diagnostic radiology. Requirements for position include Board certification, a fellowship in nuclear medicine, eligibility/certification for CAQ in nuclear medicine, and an interest in investigative nuclear medicine. Interested candidates should fax their curriculum vitae to Michael J. Shortsleeve, MD, Chairman, Department of Radiology, Mount Auburn Hospital, 330 Mount Auburn St, Cambridge, MA 02238; phone 617-499-5070, fax 617-499-5138.

SECTION HEAD-WOMEN'S IMAGING—The Department of Radiology at the SUNY Health Science Center at Syracuse seeks an individual to serve as Section Head of Women's Imaging. The SUNY Health Science Center is a 380-bed tertiary care academic health center in Syracuse, NY, a short drive from the Adirondack Mountains and Lake Ontario. Our 25-member subspecialized radiology group provides service to the main campus, one satellite office and three private imaging centers. Candidates must be Board-certified with fellowship training in mammography, breast ultrasound, stereotactic biopsies, needle localizations and OB/GYN ultrasound. Responsibilities include teaching, research, publication and patient care. The level of faculty appointment and salary will depend upon the applicant's experience and academic productivity. Applicants should respond with a letter of interest and copy of their current CV to John F. Cardella, MD, Chairman, Department of Radiology, SUNY Health Science Center, 750 E Adams St,

Syracuse, NY 13210 or *cardellj@mailbox.hscsyr.edu.* SUNY Health Science Center is a smoke-free campus, an equal opportunity/affirmative action employer and encourages minority and female applicants to apply.

THE UNIVERSITY OF KENTUCKY DEPARTMENT OF DIAGNOSTIC RADIOLOGY—Is recruiting a Board-certified radiologist, fellowship-trained or comparable experience in breast imaging. Duties will include directing activities in comprehensive breast care center, developing a network of screening centers and a strong interest in education and research. Rank based on experience. This position also includes some general radiology to provide coverage of radiology network. Please send or fax letter of interest, along with curriculum vitae to James C. Reed, Chairman, Department of Diagnostic Radiology, A110 Kentucky Clinic, University of Kentucky Medical Center, Lexington, KY 40536-0284. Fax 606-257-6014. UK is an equal opportunity employer.

THE RADIOLOGY DEPARTMENT AT THE UNIVERSITY OF PENNSYLVANIA MEDICAL CENTER—Has the following position available: a faculty appointment in the University of Pennsylvania at the assistant professor, associate professor or professor of radiology level. The position is in the ultrasound and computed body tomography sections. The level of the position will be determined by the applicant's experience and expertise. Applicants must be Board-certified in radiology and have experience in ultrasound and computed tomography. The minimum experience needed is a US/CT fellowship. The University of Pennsylvania is an equal opportunity/affirmative action employer. Minority and women candidates are encouraged to apply. Please contact Beverly G. Coleman, MD, Director, Ultrasound Imaging, Radiology Department, University of Pennsylvania Medical Center, 3400 Spruce St, Philadelphia, PA 19104; phone 215-662-3466, fax 215-349-5627, e-mail *coleman@oasis.rad.upenn.edu.*

CHIEF OF RADIOLOGY/ARIZONA—Prosperous regional medical center seeks a director for radiology services that are expanding in volume and modalities. Department is equipped with the latest in technology. Imaging services include MRI, CT, nuclear, mammography, plain film and interventional studies. Location is a lake resort community of 45,000 in Arizona. Call David King (King Search, Inc) at 800-990-0780, 770-886-0780 or fax 770-886-9522. Send CV to King Search & Consulting, Inc, 1380 Zephyr Ct, Cumming, GA 30041. *Kingsearch@msn.com.*

GENERAL RADIOLOGIST—The Department of Radiology at Indiana University School of Medicine seeks academically oriented general radiologist for faculty position in a small university-affiliated hospital. In addition to plain film, the hospital provides MRI, CT, nuclear medicine and US. Approximately 37,000 exams are performed annually. Tenure or clinical track dependent upon qualifications. Minimum requirements include MD with Board certification in radiology and eligibility for licensure in Indiana. Please reply with curriculum vitae to Mervyn D. Cohen, MD, Indiana University Hospital, Room UH 0663, 550 N University Blvd, Indianapolis, IN 46202-5253, or e-mail *jamriley@iupui.edu.* Indiana University is an equal opportunity/affirmative action employer.

NEURO AND MUSCULOSKELETAL RADIOLOGISTS—Excellent opportunity for well-trained BC/BE radiologists to join successful 10-member hospital-based group practice located in northeast Ohio. One full-time neuroradiologist and one full-time musculoskeletal radiologist are needed. There are partnership track positions with excellent salary and benefits. Please send CV to Trumbull Radiologists, Inc, c/o Marge Deley, Business Manager, 2588 Elm Rd, Cortland, OH 44410; 330-372-5859; fax 330-372-5901.

BREAST IMAGING RADIOLOGIST—The Department of Radiology at the Medical College of Georgia is seeking an ABR-eligible or -certified breast imaging radiologist for a full-time or part-time faculty position opening in July 1999. Fellowship training or extensive experience preferred but not mandatory. The successful candidate will direct and practice in a

NORTHEAST
PROVIDENCE, RHODE ISLAND
SUPER OPPORTUNITY WITH
BEST OF ACADEMIC AND PRIVATE PRACTICE

- 3 Hospitals (3 MRI's)
- 10 Private Offices (3 MRI's)
- Residents, Fellows, Medical Students
- Brown University School of Medicine Appointment

Women's Imager – to perform mammography, OB Ultrasound and General Radiology.
Pediatric Radiologist – must have CAQ in Pediatric Radiology and willing to also do General Radiology.
General Radiologist – able to work outpatient imaging centers and either do General Radiology or ER Radiology in hospital settings.

Over 600,000 exams per year; 50 plus radiologists; academics; ownership; security, early partnership, great salaries.

Send letter of intent/curriculum vitae to:
John J. Cronan, M.D., Chairman
Department of Diagnostic Imaging
Brown University School of Medicine
Phone: (401) 444-5184 Fax: (401) 444-5017
E-Mail: JCronan@Lifespan.org

this population, as well as contracting with several other smaller hospitals. This is a general practice utilizing conventional imaging in addition to spiral CT, mobile MRI, ultrasound, mammography, nuclear medicine and some intervention procedures. Sterling is located two hours northeast of Denver on Interstate 76. It has a strong economy and is a great place to raise a family. There are parks, fairs, hunting, boating, fishing opportunities, an 18-hole golf course and a country club. Please mail CV to Sherry Kozero-Roth, Physician Recruiting, 1801 16th St, Greeley, CO 80631 or fax 970-350-6431.

CAQ-ELIGIBLE NEURORADIOLOGIST—Needed to join large, subspecialized private practice. Partnership track. Majority of time to be spent in neuroradiology. Experience/interest in functional MRI and MR spectroscopy is desirable. Practice currently covers five hospitals and multiple imaging centers with state-of-the-art equipment. Send CV to John Walter, MD, 1500 Expo Pkwy, Sacramento, CA 95815, fax 916-920-4434, e-mail *jwalter@ns.net.*

IMMEDIATE OPENING—For a fellowship-trained radiologist to join large, subspecialized private practice. Partnership track. Majority of time to be spent in body cross-sectional imaging. Practice currently covers five hospitals and multiple imaging centers with state-of-the-art equipment. Send CV to John Walter, MD, 1500 Expo Pkwy, Sacramento, CA 95815, fax 916-920-4434, e-mail *jwalter@ns.net.*

MUSCULOSKELETAL RADIOLOGIST—A six-member group in western Colorado seeking fellowship-trained MS radiologist. A 300-bed hospital serving 14 busy orthopedic surgeons. Partnership track with generous income and vacation. Growing community with lifestyle inherent to Rocky Mountain West. Respond to Reed Bumgarner, MD, 2530 N Eighth St, Ste#101, Grand Junction, CO 81501, 970-244-7067.

FACULTY POSITIONS IN BREAST RADIOLOGY—The Department of Radiology at the University of South Florida (USF) College of Medicine is seeking two breast imaging radiologists at the assistant/associate professor level and both positions may be tenure earning. These positions are based at the H. Lee Moffitt Cancer Center and Research Institute at USF, an NCI-designated cancer center. Clinical practice is divided between a multidisciplinary diagnostic breast center and a separate screening center. Breast imaging modalities include seven conventional mammography units, dedicated breast sonography, two stereotactic biopsy units, breast MRI, and investigational direct digital mammography. Both positions include clinical service, teaching of radiology residents and fellows, participation in clinical investigations, and other scholarly activities. Applicants should have an MD degree, be Board-certified in diagnostic-radiology, and have a minimum of 1 year fellowship training or practice experience in their subspeciality discipline, with expertise in all modalities of practice. Salary and rank are commensurate with qualifications and experience. A valid Florida medical license is required prior to beginning employment. One position will begin January 1, 2000 and the other starts on or after July 1, 2000. Applications or nominations for these positions should be addressed to Robert Clark, MD, Chairman, Department of Radiology, H. Lee Moffitt Cancer Center and Research Institute at USF, 12902 Magnolia Drive, Tampa, FL 33612. Phone 813-972-8425, fax 813-979-7231, e-mail *clark@moffitt.usf.edu.* Application deadline is October 29, 1999. USF is an Equal Opportunity/Affirmative Action/Equal Access Institution. For disability accommodations, contact Claudette Cigarran at 813-974-2538, TDD 974-2218, a minimum of five working days in advance.

spectroscopy and diffusion/perfusion imaging helpful. Contact Jonathan Breslau, MD, Box T, 1500 Expo Parkway, Sacramento, CA 95815. E-mail to *recruit@radiological.com*. Fax 916-920-4434. Phone 916-646-8427.

NIGHT RADIOLOGIST—Needed for teleradiology only in the suburban Maryland area. May work from home if desired. Hours are 11 pm to 8 am. Ultrasound, CT, nuclear medicine, and MRI. Excellent salary and benefit package. If interested, please fax CV to Paul L. Sandler at 301-590-8961 or please call 301-590-2650 for further information.

NORTHERN CALIFORNIA—Diagnostic radiologist with body imaging fellowship/additional training a plus. Offering partnership track. Position requires familiarity with all modalities including mammography, MRI, nuclear medicine and angio. Practice includes coverage of two major medical centers and a group-owned outpatient imaging center. Send CV to Marcia Hinkle Diaz, MD, or Linda Adams, 2020 Court St, Redding, CA 96001. Phone 530-243-9295; fax 530-243-8502.

NORTHERN CALIFORNIA—Neuroradiologist position, fellowship-trained. Offering partnership track. Position requires familiarity with all modalities including angio, MRI, nuclear medicine. Practice includes coverage of two major medical centers and a group-owned outpatient imaging center. Send CV to Marcia Hinkle Diaz, MD or Linda Adams, 2020 Court St, Redding, CA 96001. Phone 530-243-9295; fax 530-243-8502.

DULUTH, MN—ABR-certified general diagnostic radiologist needed to join a group of 14. Expertise required in fluoroscopy, CT, ultrasound, MRI, mammography and plain films, as well as in CT and US guided biopsy. Special interest in musculoskeletal imaging welcomed. SMDC is a 300-physician multispecialty group with three hospitals and 25 clinic locations serving a referral population of 460,000 in northeastern Minnesota, northern Wisconsin and upper Michigan. Duties involve provisional reading of CT images via teleradiology systems from other hospitals. Research and teaching opportunities are also available. Our location on Lake Superior offers more than beautiful lake vistas, access to the Apostle Islands, pristine inland lakes and the Boundary Waters Wilderness, or ski resorts and championship golf courses; it also is home to three universities and a vibrant arts community—everything you need to enjoy your vocation and avocations. Contact or send your CV in confidence to Marci Jackson, 800-342-1388, 218-725-3177, or fax 218-722-9952. SMDC Physician & Provider Recruitment, St Mary's/Duluth Clinic Health System, 400 E Third St, Duluth, MN 55805. E-mail *provider@smdc.org*. Visit our website at *www.smdc.org* and *www.duluth.com*. EOE, A/A. Sorry, no J-1 waivers available.

NEURORADIOLOGIST—The Department of Radiology at the Albany Medical Center is seeking a Board-certified, CAQ-eligible or certified neuroradiologist (NY state license required to practice). At present there are three full-time neuroradiologists and a PhD of spectroscopy. State-of-the-art equipment includes two 1.5T Signa MR systems, 3 GE helical CT scanners including Light Speed and bi-plane DSA. Successful candidates will receive an academic appointment commensurate with experience at the Albany Medical College, which offers a generous compensation and benefits package. The Albany Medical Center is a major tertiary care facility located in upstate New York, within driving distance of Boston and New York City. Albany Medical Center actively seeks applications from women and minorities and is an EEO/AA employer. Please send CV to William A. Wagle, MD, Head of Neuroradiology, Department of Radiology (MC-113), Albany Medical College, 47 New Scotland Ave, Albany, NY 12208. Phone 518-262-3277, fax 518-262-4210.

TEXAS TECH UNIVERSITY, EL PASO—Department of Radiology seeks a Board-eligible or certified radiologist. This is an interesting and challenging position in a county hospital that is the trauma center for a community of 650,000 and the primary inpatient and outpatient caregiver for a large indigent and underserved population of 250,000. Our equipment is current with a new MRI, second CT scanner, and combined cardiovascular machine soon to be installed. Our mammography program is a center of excellence. Our ultrasound and mammography sections are ACR-accredited. This is an ideal position for a recent trainee who desires to affiliate with a medical school and become part of an active clinical service. Salary is commensurate with training and experience. Benefits including retirement are generous. El Paso is a delightful city of 650,000 people with a year-round warm, dry climate and the ease of southern living. Send correspondence to Dr Lloyd K. Mark, Professor and Regional Chairman, Department of Radiology, Texas Tech University HSC at El Paso, 4800 Alberta St, El Paso, TX 79905. Fax to 915-545-6607, e-mail to *radelkm@ttuhsc.edu* or call 915-545-6845.

TEXAS TECH UNIVERSITY HEALTH SCIENCES CENTER—At El Paso, TX, Department of Radiology, seeks a Board-certified Regional Chairman with academic background. Thomason Hospital is a 225-bed county facility staffed by Texas Tech Medical School Faculty. The recently renovated, enlarged and fully equipped radiology department, featuring the entire complement of modern technology, performs approximately 125,000 exams annually. Individuals with excellent administrative, leadership skills along with clinical expertise in general or subspecialty diagnostic areas are encouraged to apply. The successful candidate will be eligible for appropriate faculty rank at Texas Tech School of Medicine. El Paso is a growing border community of 650,000 with excellent climate and opportunities for recreational activities. Please respond to Darius A. Boman, MD, Chairman, Search Committee, Department of Pathology, Texas Tech University HSC, 4800 Alberta Ave, El Paso, TX 79905. E-mail *adoelkf@ttuhsc.edu*. Equal opportunity/affirmative action employer. ADA compliance.

UCSD SCHOOL OF MEDICINE—The Department of Radiology is seeking a vascular/interventional radiologist to participate in clinical, teaching and research programs. Qualifications required include Board eligibility/certification, California medical license, 1-year fellowship in vascular/interventional radiology. Faculty-level experience desirable. Rank, series and salary to be determined based on qualifications and experience in accordance with UC policy. The University of California, San Diego, is an equal opportunity/affirmative action employer. All curricula vitae received prior to November 15, 1999 or thereafter until position is filled will be given full consideration. Send to Anne C. Roberts, Professor of Clinical Radiology, Department of Radiology-8756, UCSD Medical Center, 200 W Arbor Dr, San Diego, CA 92103-8756.

NEURORADIOLOGIST—The Department of Radiology at the University of Minnesota has a full-time position available in the neuroradiology section at the rank of associate or assistant professor, clinical track or tenure track. Minimum requirements are Board certification in radiology, a minimum of 2 years post-residency in all facets of neuroradiology, as well as graduate and undergraduate medical instruction. Experience in interventional and/or head and neck neuroradiology is desirable. The successful candidate must have demonstrated involvement in quality research, publications in peer-reviewed journals and effectiveness in teaching and mentoring. Research experience in functional MRI, MR spectroscopy, and/or interventional MR is desirable. Salary is negotiable and competitive, and is dependent upon scholarly productivity and post-MD experience. Applicants must be licensed or able to obtain a license to practice medicine in the state of Minnesota before appointment date. Applications will be accepted until position is filled. Send letters to Dr Chip Truwit, Director of Neuroradiology, Department of Radiology, Box 292 Mayo Bldg, University of Minnesota, 420 Delaware St SE, Minneapolis, MN 55455. The University of Minnesota is an equal opportunity educator and employer.

THE PENN STATE UNIVERSITY COLLEGE OF MEDICINE—Penn State Geisinger Health System, Department of Radiology, Milton S. Hershey Medical Center, is currently recruiting full-time faculty for the following areas: neuroradiology/neurointerventional radiology (two faculty), and body imaging (two faculty). The acquisition of new contracts and growing clinical demand has created a need for four radiologists. The Milton S. Hershey Medical Center is located in scenic Hershey, PA. It is a 500-bed tertiary care academic health center 14 miles from the state capital of Harrisburg. The campus is also home to the Pennsylvania State University College of Medicine. Our AHC and department of radiology afford: a 130-bed children's hospital; access to the Penn State Geisinger Health System, the third-largest group practice in the United States; access to a system-owned HMO offering two tertiary and one community care centers; 80 clinical practice sites system-wide; a 40-county service area; a solid payor mix (only 17.6% is managed care business); access to an expanding physician-led health system comprised of 1,000 multispecialty providers; state-of-the-art technology; excellent clinical and research capabilities; 180,000 annual imaging studies; 25 attending, 23 residents and five fellow radiologists. Eligible candidates must have a keen interest in teaching, have completed an accredited radiology residency, be Board-certified or Board-eligible, and possess or be able to obtain a Pennsylvania state medical license. The level of faculty appointment and salary will be commensurate with the individual's experience and training. Interested applicants should forward their curriculum vitae to John E. Madewell, MD, Professor and Chair, Department of Radiology, H066, The Milton S. Hershey Medical Center, 500 University Dr, Hershey, PA 17033. Phone 717-531-8044, fax 717-531-5596. Penn State College of Medicine/Penn State Geisinger Health System is committed to affirmative action, equal opportunity and the diversity of its workforce.

VASCULAR AND INTERVENTIONAL RADIOLOGY POSITION—The Vascular/Interventional Radiology Section at the Cleveland Clinic Foundation. We are currently recruiting a sixth full-time vascular/interventional radiologist to join our expanding practice. Training in peripheral vascular and dialysis access interventions, TIPS, hepatobiliary, genitourinary and embolotherapy procedures is required. The candidate should have an interest in clinical and/or basic science investigations. Candidates must also be Board-certified in diagnostic radiology, eligible for membership in the SCVIR, and able to obtain an Ohio medical license. The Cleveland Clinic Foundation is a 1,000-bed teaching hospital with a long history of exceptional care for patients with cardiovascular, hepatobiliary, renal and oncologic diseases. Diagnostic imaging and interventional equipment are state-of-the-art, including six angiography labs and an active peripheral MRA program. For further information, please contact Reba Gaddis, Division of Radiology, The Cleveland Clinic Foundation, Hb-6, 9500 Euclid Ave, Cleveland, OH 44195; e-mail *gaddisr@ccf.org*.

VASCULAR/INTERVENTIONAL RADIOLOGIST—Medical University of South Carolina Department of Vascular and Interventional Radiology is seeking a fellowship-trained vascular and interventional radiologist. The practice is rapidly expanding and performs all aspects of diagnostic and interventional radiology procedures, including CT angiography. The division currently provides services for over 3,000 patients/year and expansion into a new vascular center is planned. An animal angio lab is available for research. Faculty appointment will be at the assistant professor level. For information, contact (by October 15, 1999) Renan Uflacker, MD, c/o Melanie Jackson, MUSC Department of Radiology, 169 Ashley Ave, PO Box 250322, Charleston, SC 29425. Phone 843-792-5387, e-mail *uflackrp@musc.edu*. MUSC is an equal opportunity employer.

EASTERN PA—Independent group seeking two radiologists with added interest in angiointerventional, neuroradiology, and/or MRI for partnership track positions. Practice includes stable inpatient and outpatient imaging environments in a growing family-oriented community one hour from Philadelphia and two hours from NYC. Apply to Jeffrey Blinder, MD, Sacred Heart Hospital, Department of Radiology, 421 Chew St, Allentown, PA 18102. Phone 610-776-5308; fax 610-776-4671.

CALIFORNIA CENTRAL COAST—Full service, well-established and growing outpatient imaging center. State-of-the-art equipment. No call or weekends. Part-time or full-time needed. Excellent pay and benefits. Recent neuroradiology or MRI fellowship helpful. 1100 Monterey St, Suite #210, San Luis Obispo, CA 93401. E-mail *fvern@aol.com*.

THORACIC RADIOLOGY FACULTY POSITION—The Department of Radiology at the University of Vermont/Fletcher Allen Health Care is recruiting a new full-time faculty member for the division of thoracic radiology at the assistant or associate professor level. The candidate must be Board-certified in diagnostic radiology and have completed a 1-year fellowship in thoracic imaging. The candidate must be familiar with all aspects of thoracic imaging including conventional and computed chest radiography, CT, MRI, image-guided transthoracic needle biopsy and percutaneous catheter drainage procedures. Candidates with experience and strong interest in chest and cardiac MRI will be preferred. The department has state-of-the-art equipment including three GE helical CT scanners and two GE 1.5T MRI scanners. Computed radiography will be installed in the fall of 1999. The candidate will be expected to participate in the training of 12 radiology residents and three cross-sectional imaging fellows, and along with other divisional faculty, will be responsible for several weekly and monthly interdisciplinary conferences. Active participation in clinical research both within the division and in collaboration with affiliated departments is expected. Eligibility for Vermont medical licensure is required. Women and minority candidates are encouraged to apply. The deadline for the receipt of applications is October 31, 1999. Interested applicants should forward their CV to and contact Jeffrey Klein, MD, Director, Thoracic Radiology, University of Vermont College of Medicine, Fletcher Allen Health Care, Department of Radiology, 111 Colchester Ave, Burlington, VT 05401. Phone 802-656-2327; fax 802-656-4822; e-mail *jeffrey.klein@vtmednet.org*. Fletcher Allen Health Care and the University of Vermont are equal opportunity/affirmative action employers.

EXCELLENT PARTNERSHIP OPPORTUNITIES IN UPSTATE NEW YORK—Growing, amiable 20-physician practice seeks three Board-certified radiologists (general, nuclear medicine or interventional). Full-time, part-time and night shift options available. Specialized practice serving three hospitals and seven offices. Family-oriented community with top-rated public/private schools and the State University of New York at Binghamton. Binghamton is a safe, affordable small city with access to a wide range of year-round activities and close proximity to large metropolitan areas. To apply, please fax cover letter and curriculum vitae to 607-729-0031, attention Dr Michael Grenis; phone 607-729-1999.

KENTUCKY—Nine-member private practice group seeks full-time Board-certified radiologist to join busy hospital and office practice. Fellowship training preferred but not required. All imaging modalities including MRI and angio/intervention. Excellent equipment including 1.5T GE Horizon w/EPI. Pleasant, family-oriented community of approximately 90,000 on Ohio River in western Kentucky with low crime, excellent schools and cultural amenities. Send CV to D.K. Roberts, Radiology PSC, Mayfair Square, Owensboro, KY 42301. Phone 270-684-3224.

PEDIATRIC RADIOLOGIST, DENVER, CO—Private practice position, to join two pediatric CAQ-Boarded radiologists in subspecialized radiology group. Expanding pediatric practice (8% increase in 1998). Pediatric neuroradiology experience a plus. No angiography required. Tertiary care pediatrics with large NICU, PICU, inpatient and outpatient service. Full range of pediatric subspecialists on staff. Expanding pediatric services at additional hospitals. Position offers 50%–75% pediatric radiology with strong growth potential, conducive environment, and great colleagues. Competitive compensation and benefits offered. Contact Drs Gerry Horgan or Garret Gannuch at 303-839-6880 or fax your CV to 303-226-7228.

DIAGNOSTIC RADIOLOGIST—Group of five radiologists in northern Philadelphia suburbs is seeking a recently trained, Board-certified radiologist with MR fellowship. Also must be proficient in all aspects of diagnostic imaging. Interventional skill is desirable. Competitive salary leading to early partnership. Send CV to Sayed M. Hashemi, MD, Department of Radiology, North Penn Hospital, Lansdale, PA 19446, or fax to 215-361-4872.

ORLANDO—Large, rapidly expanding Orlando radiology group of 30 radiologists currently seeking several Board-certified general radiologists for immediate or July 2000 employment. Positions include general radiologist with special skills in mammography; general radiologist with special interest in interventional procedures; general radiologist with special interest in MRI, particularly cardiac imaging; general radiologist with broad general experience. Board-certified or Board-eligible. Fellowship-trained a plus, but not required. Partnership track, excellent benefits and generous vacation policy. Information about part-time positions available upon request. Send CV and references to Susan L. Rebsamen, MD, PO Box 150505, Altamonte Springs, FL 32715, or fax 407-767-0608, or e-mail *susank@iag.net*.

BREAST IMAGING—A progressive 21-radiologist private practice group in coastal Orange County, California is seeking an additional breast imaging specialist with fellowship training. This full partnership track position with exceptional compensation and benefits would involve approximately 75% mammography and 25% general radiology (excluding angiography) with some evening and weekend call. Our high volume, state-of-the-art breast facility includes five mammography and two ultrasound units, a prone biopsy table and a dexa unit. Please send CV with inquiry to Winston Whitney, MD, Department of Radiology, Hoag Memorial Hospital, PO Box 6100, Newport Beach, CA 92658-6100.

FACULTY POSITION IN BREAST IMAGING, JOHNS HOPKINS MEDICAL INSTITUTIONS—The Department of Radiology at Johns Hopkins Medical Institutions has a faculty position opening in the division of breast imaging at the clinical instructor, assistant professor or associate professor level. The department currently performs approximately 35,000 breast imaging and 1,700 interventional studies per year at facilities that include the Johns Hopkins Breast Imaging Center (a university hospital-based outpatient facility) and a suburban multi-specialty outpatient center (The Johns Hopkins Greenspring Clinic). The Johns Hopkins Breast Imaging Center has five mammography units, a full breast digital mammography unit, two ultrasound units, a stereotactic core biopsy unit, and an ABBI system. In addition, breast MRI and nuclear breast imaging are also performed. The Greenspring Clinic has three mammography units, two ultrasound units and a stereotactic core biopsy system. Research programs include multi-institutional clinical trials, JHU-based clinical trials, basic molecular and gene therapy, breast cancer/imaging research program and biomedical engineering/technology development in breast imaging. Comprehensive training is given in all areas of breast imaging to radiology residents and breast imaging fellows. Applicants must be Board-certified with good recommendations. Breast imaging fellowship or appropriate experience is required. Interested individuals should contact Laurie L. Fajardo, MD, Visiting Professor of Radiology, Vice Chair, Clinical Research, Director of Breast Imaging, Johns Hopkins University, 601 N Caroline St, PO Box 0814, Baltimore, MD 21287. Phone 410-955-7095; fax 410-614-1079; e-mail *lfajardo@helix.rad.jhu.edu*. The Johns Hopkins University is an affirmative action/equal opportunity employer.

WILMINGTON, NC—60-physician multi-specialty group seeks BC/BE radiologist to start new department. Full or part-time position. Our group provides full scope services for 350,000 population referral area. Wilmington is one of North Carolina's most desirable areas, boasting a strong industrial base, 10,000-student university campus, miles of beautiful beaches, and family-oriented activities including year-round sailing, golfing, fishing, biking and tennis. Physician equity, outstanding compensation and benefits. EOE. Call Kathy Gresham at 919-755-1789 or send CV to Wilmington Health Associates, 1202 Medical Center Drive, Wilmington, NC 28401. Fax 919-755-1789; e-mail *kwgresham@aol.com*.

EVENING RADIOLOGIST—Progressive 35-member group serving four hospitals in Memphis, TN is seeking a full-time radiologist to provide general diagnostic radiology, CT, ultrasound and emergency nuclear medicine procedures. No special or interventional procedures required. Attractive position with excellent salary and fringe benefits. Please fax CV and cover letter to 901-747-1001 or e-mail *imaging@magibox.net* or mail to Mid-South Imaging & Therapeutics, PA, 6305 Humphreys Blvd, Suite 205, Memphis, TN 38120.

DIAGNOSTIC RADIOLOGIST, BODY IMAGER—Tulane University Medical Center is seeking a fellowship-trained body imager. Successful completion of fellowship training is required. MRI, CT, angiography, interpretation and consultation are intregral parts of the position. Salary and academic rank will be commensurate with experience and qualifications. Applicants must be ABR-certified and eligible for LA licensure. Tulane University is an EEO/AA employer and encourages applications from qualified women and minority candidates. Please contact Edward H. De Mouy, MD, Chairman, Department of Radiology SL-54, Tulane University Medical Center, 1430 Tulane Ave, New Orleans, LA 70112.

PEDIATRIC RADIOLOGIST—Tulane University Medical Center is seeking a qualified individual for a faculty position in the section of pediatric radiology. Successful completion of accredited fellowship training is required. MRI, CT, film interpretation and consultation are integral parts of the position. Salary and academic rank will be commensurate with experience and qualifications. Applicants must be ABR-certified and eligible for LA licensure. Tulane University is an EEO/AA employer and encourages applications from qualified women and minority candidates. Please contact Edward H. De Mouy, MD, Chairman, Department of Radiology SL-54, Tulane University Medical Center, 1430 Tulane Ave, New Orleans, LA 70112.

MUSCULOSKELETAL RADIOLOGIST—18-member private practice radiology group in Denver, CO is seeking a Board-certified, fellowship-trained musculoskeletal radiologist with strong general radiology skills for partnership track position. Please send CV including references to Clint Anderson, MD, 8380 N Zuni, Suite 100, Denver, CO 80221, or fax to 303-430-1162.

MULTIPLE POSITIONS AVAILABLE—Large, well-established private practice group is expanding to an additional hospital site and seeking multiple radiologists with fellowship training in angio/interventional, neuroradiology, imaging (MRI, CT, US), nuclear medicine, pediatric radiology and mammo/women's imaging. Lehigh Valley Health Network includes a 600-bed tertiary care university-affiliated hospital as well as a nearby 200-bed community hospital. LVHN is located in the Allentown/Bethlehem, PA area, one hour from Philadelphia and one-and-a-half hours from NYC. Offering competitive salary and benefits package leading to full partnership. Send CV to Robert Kricun, MD, Chairman, Department of Radiology, Lehigh Valley Hospital, c/o Physician Recruiting, 2166 S 12th St, Allentown, PA 18103. Fax 610-402-7014. Call 610-402-7008 for more information.

20-PHYSICIAN SUBSPECIALIZED PRIVATE PRACTICE GROUP—is seeking Board-certified radiologists for a rapidly expanding practice. Established in 1954, the group provides services at locations that include a large university hospital, small community hospitals and a large private imaging center. Fellowship training preferred in body imaging, pediatric, nuclear, mammography, musculoskeletal or interventional radiology. Partnership track positions allow for possible coastal, river or bay living with excellent pay and vacation. State-of-the-art equipment in a congenial democratic group. For information, contact Lysle K. Ailstock, MD, (*ailstock @easternrad.com*), Eric J. Finical, MD (*eric61@ecu .campuscwix.net*), or Timothy J. Clark, MD (*clark@easternrad.com*), or fax 252-758-9995.

CENTRAL NEW YORK—Small private practice group seeks ABR-certified/eligible radiologist for partnership track position. Generous salary with substantial time off. All modalities. Limited interventional. New CT, MR and teleradiology. Inquiries to Andrew McDonnell, MD, Corning Hospital, 176 Denison Pkwy East, Corning, NY 14830, or fax 607-937-7647.

BODY IMAGING AND WOMEN'S IMAGING RADIOLOGISTS—Fairfax Radiological Consultants is a large, expanding subspecialized radiology group in the northern Virginia suburbs of Washington DC. We are seeking several fellowship-trained individuals with strong skills in either women's imaging or body imaging (CT/US and MRI). We offer unique opportunities for partnership track positions in a subspecialized private practice that includes a very busy full-service 650-bed suburban tertiary care hospital and multiple outpatient imaging centers. These include a full-service breast imaging center, a dedicated ultrasound center, MRI center and multi-modality centers that include spiral CT. Direct inquiries and CVs to Roberta Illy, Human Resources Director, PO Box 3650, Merrifield, VA 22116. Phone 703-698-4444; fax 703-698-4451. EOE.

ASSOCIATE CHAIR IN RADIOLOGY—The University of Florida Health Science Center, Jacksonville invites applications and nominations for the position of associate chair for the Jacksonville campus, Department of Radiology. The associate chair is the senior academic position at the University of Florida Health Science Center at Jacksonville, FL, with full responsibility for the academic and administrative functions of the department. The associate chair also serves as chief of the department of radiology at University Medical Center, a 517-bed teaching hospital and urban campus of the University of Florida. There is an accredited radiology residence program. The appointment in this tenure-track position will be at the level of professor and associate chairman, or associate professor and associate chairman. Salary and benefits are excellent. Candidates must be Board-certified; a record

Chair, Department of Radiology

The College of Medicine of the State University of New York Health Science Center at Brooklyn (Downstate) invites nominations and applications for the position of Professor and Chair of the Department of Radiology.

The Department of Radiology has 25 full-time faculty members and a fully accredited residency program including 24 residents. Major subspecialties of the Department are: Genitourinary, Pediatric Radiology, Ultrasound, Chest, Neuroradiology, Nuclear Medicine, CT/MRI, GI Radiology, Mammography and Interventional Radiology.

The Department has a large clinical program involving Kings County Hospital Center, the second largest municipal hospital in the country with a level 1 trauma center, University Hospital of Brooklyn, and the Brooklyn VA Hospital.

The College seeks a dynamic and visionary academic leader with a commitment to excellence in education, research, and patient care. The successful candidate must be Board certified and qualified for appointment at the rank of Professor of Radiology. The candidate should have a record of accomplishment in education and scholarly activities and proven abilities in administration and management in an academic setting.

Applications and nominations may be submitted for confidential review to:
James E. Cottrell, MD
Chair, Radiology Search Committee
SUNY-Health Science Center at Brooklyn
450 Clarkson Ave, Box 97
Brooklyn, NY 11203

HEALTH SCIENCE CENTER AT BROOKLYN · STATE UNIVERSITY OF NEW YORK
COLLEGE OF MEDICINE

of academic and administrative leadership is essential. Interested candidates are requested to submit a CV and the names/addresses of three references by the recruiting deadline of October 30, 1999 to George R. Wilson III, MD, Chair, Search Committee, UFHSC/J, 655 W 8th St, Jacksonville, FL 32209. The anticipated starting date for this position is January 1, 2000. The University of Florida is an affirmative action/equal opportunity employer.

BOSTON—Rapidly growing private teleradiology practice seeks Board-certified musculoskeletal radiologist. Pleasant work environment, no night or weekend call and flexible work schedule. Excellent compensation package and partnership opportunity. Expected start date July 2000 or sooner. Fax cover letter/CV to 617-969-1372.

THE DEPARTMENT OF RADIOLOGY, VIRGINIA COMMONWEALTH UNIVERSITY—Medical College of Virginia campus, Richmond, VA seeks candidates for several faculty positions in diagnostic radiology. These include positions in angiography/interventional radiology, neuroradiology, interventional neuroradiology, breast imaging and trauma/emergency department radiology. ABR certification or eligilbility required as well as CAQ, where applicable. Fellowship training and interest in teaching and research are preferred. MCV Hospital is a 1,058-bed facility and a Level I trauma center. Individuals should have experience working in a culturally diverse environment. Academic rank and salary commensurate with experience. For position description, or to submit CV, write James L. Tatum, MD, Department of Radiology, PO Box 980470, Richmond, VA 23298-0470. Phone 804-828-6600; fax 804-828-6129. VCU/MCV is an equal opportunity/affirmative action employer. Women, minorities and persons with disabilities are encouraged to apply.

FLORIDA GULF COAST—Group of eight radiologists seeks a fellowship (musculoskeletal, MRI or neuro) trained radiologist to start approximately July 2000. Partnership track. Send CV with cover letter to Radiology Associates, Attn: Recruitment, PO Box 17549, Pensacola, FL 32522. Fax 850-469-8102; e-mail *fradassoc@aol.com.*

INTERVENTIONAL RADIOLOGIST—The VA Medical Center at Memphis, TN is seeking an interventional radiologist, fellowship desirable. BE/BC in diagnostic radiology. Affiliated with the University of Tennessee, interventionalist would be involved in fellowship and residency training with ample research opportunities. Regional Medical Center has all imaging modalities and two new angiography suites purchased to be installed. Comprehensive PACS installation underway. New MRI with cardiovascular capabilities installed June 1999. Contact John Ware, MD, Chief, Radiology Service, Department of Veterans Affairs, 1030 Jefferson Ave, Memphis, TN 38104. Fax 901-577-7466.

PHYSICIAN: THE NUCLEAR MEDICINE SERVICE—At Hunter Holmes McGuire VA Medical Center/Medical College of Virginia, Virginia Commonwealth University, Richmond, VA is seeking a nuclear medicine physician, preferably a nuclear radiologist, to share duties at the VA and Virginia Commonwealth University-Medical College of Virginia Hospitals. ABNM and/or nuclear radiology Board certification is required. Interested applicants may request an application by contacting Larry D. James, Human Resources Management Service at 804-675-5311. CVs should be forwarded to Timothy Burke, MD, Chief, Nuclear Medicine Service, VA Medical Center, 1201 Broad Rock Blvd, Richmond, VA 23249. Applicant may be subject to drug testing. An equal opportunity/affirmative action employer. Women, minorities and persons with disabilities are encouraged to apply.

THE UNIVERSITY OF MISSISSIPPI MEDICAL CENTER—Department of Radiology is seeking a full-time Board-certified general radiologist, imaging fellowship preferred. Interested parties should submit a CV to Brent Harrison, MD, Department of Radiology, University of Mississippi Medical Center, 2500 State St, Jackson, MS 39216. EOE, M/F/D/V.

THE UNIVERSITY OF MISSISSIPPI MEDICAL CENTER—Department of Radiology seeks a fellowship-trained interventional neuroradiologist. Established interventional practice. Compensation commensurate with qualifications. Interested parties should contact Brent Harrison, MD, University of Mississippi Medical Center, Department of Radiology, 2500 State St, Jackson, MS 39216. Phone 601-984-2515. EOE, M/F/D/V.

DENVER HEALTH MEDICAL CENTER—Department of Radiology, and the School of Medicine, University of Colorado Health Sciences Center are recruiting for a Board-certified radiologist with at least 1 year accredited fellowship in body imaging. The position would encompass resident teaching and clinical work in the fields of ultrasound and body CT and MRI with academic time provided for clinical research and presentations. The department of radiology has recently been renovated and equipment is state-of-the-art. Salary and academic rank commensurate with experience. This is a joint position with primary clinical responsibilities at Denver Health Medical Center, the regional level I trauma center, located in the heart of the Rocky Mountains. The workplace provides a busy and stimulating clinical and academic environment, whereas the surrounding Colorado outdoors provides ample recreational opportunities when work is over. Interested candidates should send their CV to Randall M. Patten, MD, Director, Radiology, Department of Radiology, Mail Code 0024, Denver Health Medical Center, 777 Bannock St, Denver, CO 80204-4507. Phone 303-436-7614; fax 303-436-6022; e-mail *rpatten@dhha.org.* The University of Colorado Health Sciences Center and DHMC are affirmative action/equal opportunity employers and invite applications from all qualified candidates. Applications accepted until the position is filled.

DENVER HEALTH MEDICAL CENTER—Department of Radiology, and the School of Medicine, University of Colorado Health Sciences Center are recruiting for a Board-certified radiologist with at least 1 year accredited fellowship in interventional radiology. The position would encompass resident teaching and clinical work in the fields of angiography and interventional radiology with academic time provided for clinical research and presentations. The department of radiology has recently been renovated and equipment is state-of-the-art. Salary and academic rank commensurate with experience. This is a joint position with primary clinical responsibilities at Denver Health Medical Center, the regional level I trauma center, located in the heart of the Rocky Mountains. The workplace provides a busy and stimulating clinical and academic environment, whereas the surrounding Colorado outdoors provides ample recreational opportunities when work is over. Interested candidates should send their CV to Charles Ray, Jr, MD, Chief, Interventional Radiology, Department of Radiology, Mail Code 0024, Denver Health Medical Center, 777 Bannock St, Denver, CO 80204-4507. Phone 303-436-7614; fax 303-436-6022; e-mail *cray@dhha.org.* The University of Colorado Health Sciences Center and DHMC are affirmative action/equal opportunity employers and invite applications from all qualified candidates. Applications accepted until the position is filled.

RADIOLOGY—Busy 10-member group in Orange County, California seeks general radiologist, for inpatient and outpatient work. Skills in body imaging (CT, MRI, ultrasound) or nuclear medicine would be helpful. Fellowship would be desirable but not required. Full-time preferred but would consider part-time. Some night/weekend work. Must function well in busy environment. No interventional. Please send CV to Box R-114.

PROGRESSIVE 14-PERSON GROUP—Seeks a recently fellowship-trained individual preferably with expertise in body MR. The group covers four hospitals, each with state-of-the-art equipment, and reads from six MRI centers. Generous salary and benefits leading to full and equal partnership. Please send CV to Thomas Magee, MD, Department of Radiology, Menorah Medical Center, 5721 W 119th St, Overland Park, KS 66209. Fax 913-498-6699.

NUCLEAR MEDICINE RADIOLOGIST—Group of 10 radiologists in Orange County, California seeks general radiologist. Certified ABNM or Nuclear Medicine Special Competence ABR with current competence in nuclear diagnosis and therapy. Will do nuclear medicine for general radiology. Cross-sectional imaging skills desirable. Immediate opening. Please send CV to Box R-115.

DENVER HEALTH MEDICAL CENTER—Department of Radiology, and the School of Medicine, University of Colorado Health Sciences Center are recruiting for a Board-certified radiologist with experience or accredited fellowship in trauma and musculoskeletal radiology. The position would encompass resident teaching and clinical work in the fields of emergency and orthopedic radiology. We have very active, innovative and cooperative colleagues in both the emergency medicine and orthopedic surgery departments. The department of radiology has recently been renovated and equipment is state-of-the-art. Salary and academic rank commensurate with experience. This is a joint position with primary clinical responsibilities at Denver Health Medical Center, the regional level I trauma center, located in the heart of the Rocky Mountains. The workplace provides a busy and stimulating clinical and academic environment, whereas the surrounding Colorado outdoors provides ample recreational opportunities when work is over. Interested candidates should send their CV to Randall M. Patten, MD, Director, Radiology, Department of Radiology, Mail Code 0024, Denver Health Medical Center, 777 Bannock St, Denver, CO 80204-4507. Phone 303-436-7614; fax 303-436-6022; e-mail *rpatten@dhha.org*. The University of Colorado Health Sciences Center and DHMC are affirmative action/equal opportunity employers and invite applications from all qualified candidates. Applications accepted until the position is filled.

POSTDOCTORAL POSITION—To investigate function and dysfunction of the human oncoprotein MDM2. Applications are invited from recent graduates for a postdoctoral position in a laboratory involved in understanding molecular biology of tumorigenesis and role of the human oncoprotein MDM2 in the etiology of cancer (see EMBO J, 1998, 17:p2513). This position is to investigate the biochemical mechanism of human MDM2-mediated growth regulation in normal cells. Individuals with expertise in cDNA technology, DNA sequencing, mammalian cell culture systems or expression analysis in transgenic mice are especially encouraged to apply. Salary is negotiable. Send complete curriculum vitae and arrange for three letters of reference to be sent directly to Swati Palit Deb, PhD, Associate Professor, Department of Cancer Biology, Comprehensive Cancer Center of Wake Forest University, Medical Center Blvd, Winston-Salem, NC 27157-1082. Fax 336-716-0255; e-mail *swdeb@wfubmc.edu*. AA/EOE.

RADIOLOGIST, WESTERN MASSACHUSETTS—Large multi-specialty group practice seeks a full-time BC general radiologist to join four others in covering this multi-site practice. Must be flexible and proficient in mammography, CT and fluoroscopy as well as plain films. MRI, doppler and vascular imaging a plus. No angio. Primarily days with one evening per week and every fifth weekend. No overnight on-call. No hospital responsibilities. Potential for shareholder status in third year. Located in the beautiful Pioneer Valley and five college area, there is an abundance of cultural, educational and recreational opportunities. For more information, send CV to David Marinelli, MD, Chief of Radiology, Medical West Associates, 444 Montgomery St, Chicopee, MA 01020, fax 413-598-7115. Or call Joanne Alderman, Manager of Provider Support, 800-457-6145.

MUSCULOSKELETAL RADIOLOGIST—The University of Texas Health Science Center at San Antonio seeks a Board-certified radiologist with fellowship training in musculoskeletal radiology for a faculty position at the rank of assistant professor. American Board of Radiology certification is required. Faculty attend at University Health System Hospital (600 beds) and the South Texas Veteran Health Care System at the Audie Murphy Memorial Veterans Hospital (450 beds). The hospitals are regional referral centers for trauma, oncology, surgery, general medicine, organ transplantation and state-of-the-art spinal cord injury center. Salary is commensurate with qualification. The University of Texas HSC at SA is an equal employment opportunity/affirmative action employer. Send curriculum vitae and names and addresses of three references to Stewart R. Reuter, MD, JD, Professor and Chairman, Department of Radiology, 7703 Floyd Curl Drive, San Antonio, TX 78284.

NORTH TEXAS—General radiologist with interventional experience. Join a five-person radiology group which is part of a large multispecialty group. Large primary care, specialty and surgical referral based continue to grow. Practice general radiology (all modalities) with an opportunity to do interventional work. Each radiologist performs 17,000 exams/year. This community of 100,000 (service area of 275,000) continues to enjoy a strong and diverse economic base. It also offers excellent schools, affordable housing, and many social and recreational amenities. Located two hours from Dallas/Ft. Worth. A very competitive salary, production, partnership track, and a full benefits schedule are offered. Call Ken Sammut at 888-372-9415 or fax your CV to 610-361-7585. E-mail *ksammut@cejka.com*. ID#6660RA. Visit our website at *www.cejka.com*.

RADIOLOGIST, ONTARIO—Hamilton Health Sciences Corporation (HHSC) has plans to recruit several radiologists within the next year. HRA is a group of 30 radiologists supplying radiological services to the three sites of the Hamilton Health Sciences Corporation (i.e. Chedoke/McMaster Hospital, Hamilton General site and Henderson General site) as well as several private offices in the Hamilton-Wentworth area. There is an ongoing commitment to the academic programs of McMaster University both at undergraduate and residency levels. Recent approval has been given for two additional MRI scanners. Openings exist for individuals with training and expertise in neuroradiology, interventional, MRI and ultrasound as well as for general radiologists. Must have fellowship in diagnostic radiology, Royal College of Physicians and Surgeons of Canada or equivalent, and have or be eligible for Ontario license. Starting remuneration is competitive leading to early partnership. Interested candidates should send their CV to Dr G. Thomson, Chief Radiologist, Henderson Site, 711 Concession St, Hamilton, ONT L8L 2X2 Canada. Phone 905-527-4322 ext 2298; fax 905-575-2660.

BREAST IMAGING OPPORTUNITY—A busy breast imaging center in Seattle is recruiting for a BC/BE radiologist with fellowship training or equivalent experience in breast imaging. The practice includes screening and diagnostic mammography, breast ultrasound and all breast related interventional procedures. Send CVs to 1221 Madison Ave, Seattle, WA 98104, attention Strode Weaver. For questions, call Strode Weaver at 206-215-3535.

CROSS-SECTIONAL IMAGER—24-radiologist group in the Pacific Northwest seeking cross-sectional imager with fellowship training in US/CT/MRI for partnership track position. Duties include general radiology. Excellent salary and benefits. Contact Cindy Price, Tacoma Radiology, PO Box 1535, Tacoma, WA 98401. Fax 253-383-3919 or e-mail *cprice@tacomarad.com*.

NUCLEAR MEDICINE—Large group in the Pacific Northwest seeking fourth fellowship-trained nuclear medicine specialist for partnership track position. Duties include general radiology. Excellent salary and benefits. Contact Cindy Price, Tacoma Radiology, PO Box 1535, Tacoma, WA 98401. Fax 253-383-3919, or e-mail *cprice@tacomarad.com.*

CHAIR, DEPARTMENT OF RADIOLOGICAL SCIENCES, UCLA SCHOOL OF MEDICINE—The UCLA School of Medicine has initiated a search for a chairperson for the department of radiological sciences. Candidates should have a strong commitment to, and capacity for leadership of the clinical and research activities of a strong academic faculty. The department has more than 60 faculty, approximately 40 residents in training and three ACGME-accredited fellowship programs. Clinical, diagnostic and interventional imaging services are provided in several inpatient and outpatient facilities at UCLA Medical Center in Westwood and the Santa Monica-UCLA Medical Center. Approximately 350,000 procedures are performed annually. Inquiries or applications should be addressed to the Chair of the Search Committee, H. Rodney Withers, MD, DSc, Department of Radiation Oncology, UCLA Medical Center, Los Angeles, CA 90095-1714. UCLA is an equal opportunity/affirmative action employer.

TWO OPENINGS—Seeking a recently fellowship-trained neuroradiologist, body imager and/or pediatric radiologist for two openings. Great first-year salary. 1 year to partnership. Full benefits, equal call, equal vacation. Diagnostic Imaging Associates is a hospital and outpatient based group of six going to eight. Respond to Robin E. Osborn, DO, PO Box 1365, Springfield, OH 45501 or phone 937-399-6597.

ASSISTANT/ASSOCIATE PROFESSOR—Full-time faculty position available September 1, 1999. The Department of Radiology at the University of Wisconsin Medical School, Madison is seeking a fellowship-trained radiologist with experience in women's imaging and/or abdominal imaging who is interested in pursuing an academic career. The ideal candidate would have a primary focus in women's imaging with additional skills in abdominal radiology. Duties include medical student and resident teaching, radiology service and clinical research. Candidates must be Board-certified in diagnostic radiology. Cover letter and resume should be made in application to Patrick Turski, MD, Professor and Chairman, Department of Radiology, E3/311, Clinical Science Center, 600 Highland Ave, Madison, WI 53792-3252. Unless confidentiality is requested in writing, information regarding the applicants must be released upon request. Finalists cannot be guaranteed confidentiality. An equal opportunity/affirmative action employer.

DIRECTOR OF INTERVENTIONAL NEURORADIOLOGY—Outstanding opportunity to develop and direct an interventional neuroradiology service in an academically oriented 30-person private practice radiology group in a tertiary center of 1,000 beds serving immediate population of 500,000 and associated population of 1,500,000. Prospective individual will have the strong support and cooperation of radiology, neurosurgery, neurology, otolaryngology and hospital administration to establish a first-class clinical service. A dedicated state-of-the-art neurointerven-tional suite is budgeted and the prospective individual will be involved in its design. Practice is located in South Florida, in one of the most rapidly growing regions of United States, enjoying year-round sun, ocean and recreation, as well as full cultural amenities. Applicants should send their curriculum vitae to Bruce Braffman, MD, Director of Neuroradiology, 9050 Pines Blvd, Suite 200, Pembroke Pines, FL 33024.

VASCULAR/INTERVENTIONAL RADIOLOGIST—The Department of Radiology at the College of Physicians and Surgeons of Columbia University is seeking an ABR-certified, fellowship-trained vascular/interventional radiologist for a full-time faculty position. Position includes all areas of vascular and interventional radiology. Responsibilities include patient care, active participation in resident and fellowship education and participation in clinical and/or basic research. Salary and academic rank will be commensurate with experience and qualifications. Candidate must be able to obtain a NYS medical license; narcotics license desirable. Please direct inquiries to Philip O. Alderson, MD, Chairman, Columbia University, Department of Radiology, 177 Fort Washington Ave, MHB 2-131, New York, NY 10032. Columbia University is an affirmative action/equal opportunity employer. Women and minorities are encouraged to apply.

NEURORADIOLOGIST—The Department of Radiology at the College of Physicians and Surgeons of Columbia University is seeking a fellowship-trained, CAQ-certified or eligible neuroradiologist for a full-time faculty position. Position requires hands-on experience in CT and MRI scanning and angiographic procedures. Responsibilities include patient care, active participation in clinical and/or basic research. Salary and academic rank will be commensurate with experience and qualifications. Candidate must be able to obtain a NYS medical license; narcotics license desirable. Please direct inquiries to Philip O. Alderson, MD, Chairman, Department of Radiology, Columbia University, 177 Fort Washington Ave, MHB 2-131, New York, NY 10032. Columbia University is an affirmative action/equal opportunity employer. Women and minorities are encouraged to apply.

BREAST IMAGING—The largest radiology group located on the desirable west coast of Florida is seeking a fellowship-trained radiologist with experience in breast imaging. This qualified radiologist will be asked to lead the breast imaging and mammography functions in our large multi-location practice in Tampa, FL. We offer an excellent salary and benefits package for this position, which leads to partnership. If interested in this unique opportunity, please fax your CV to Michael J. Foley, MD at 813-622-7589.

INTERVENTIONAL RADIOLOGY—A fellowship-trained radiologist is needed to join Florida's largest west coast radiology group. This opportunity is for placement in the Bradenton/Sarasota area at one of the premiere hospitals in the region. The position leads to partnership and offers an excellent salary and benefits package. If interested, please fax your CV to Michael J. Foley, MD at 813-622-7589.

NEURORADIOLOGIST—The largest radiology group on the desirable west coast of Florida is seeking a neuroradiologist to join our group. This candidate should be fellowship-trained and Board-certified and CAQ-certified/eligible. Our growing practice covers multiple hospital and outpatient imaging facilities. We offer an excellent salary and benefits package, which leads to partnership. If interested in this unique opportunity, please fax your CV to Michael J. Foley, MD at 813-622-7589.

MUSCULOSKELETAL RADIOLOGIST—The largest radiology group on the beautiful west coast of Florida is seeking a radiologist who is fellowship-trained in musculoskeletal/body imaging. We offer an excellent salary and benefits package that leads to partnership. If interested in this unique opportunity, please fax your CV to Michael J. Foley, MD at 813-622-7589.

TELERADIOLOGY/NIGHTHAWK—Outstanding position for the right individual. Nighttime/third-shift coverage. Excellent benefits and salary. Make your own schedule. Successful practice with fellowship-trained radiologists in all subspecialties. Dynamic, growing metro area on the gulf coast of Florida. Please contact Dr Serge Djukie or Phyllis Marie at 813-626-1722, ext 232 or fax CV to 813-622-7589.

GENERAL RADIOLOGIST—The largest radiology group on the beautiful west coast of Florida is seeking a general radiologist who is fellowship-trained in MRI/body imaging or nuclear medicine. We offer an excellent salary and benefits package that leads to partnership. If interested in this unique opportunity, please fax your CV to Michael J. Foley, MD at 813-622-7589.

GROUP HEALTH PERMANENTE, SEATTLE, WA—currently has three openings. We are seeking a diagnostic radiologist with a fellowship in nuclear medicine, a Board-certified interventional radiologist and a neuroradiologist. Candidates should have ultrasound, mammography, CT and body MRI experience. We are a well-established physician-managed multispecialty group recently affiliated with the Kaiser Permanente system. Interesting referral practice with a predictable call schedule offers time to enjoy the Pacific Northwest. For further information, visit our website at *www.ghc.org* or call 800-543-9323. Fax CV and cover letter to 206-448-6191. Equal opportunity employer.

RADIOLOGIST, PORTLAND, OR—Northwest Permanente, PC, a stable, physician-managed multispecialty serving over 440,000 members of Kaiser Permanente in the Northwest, has an excellent opportunity for a Board-certified general radiologist to join our 30-member radiology department in the Portland metropolitan area. We are seeking a general radiologist with fellowship training or extensive clinical expertise in body imaging. Our program in Oregon and Washington provides a collegial and professionally stimulating environment in one of the most successful managed-care systems in the country. In addition to a quality lifestyle inherent to the beautiful Pacific Northwest, we offer a competitive salary and benefit package which includes a generous retirement program, sabbatical leave, professional liability coverage and more. Please forward CV to R.A. Clark, Director, Professional Resources, Northwest Permanente, PC, 500 NE Multnomah, Suite 100, Portland, OR 97232-2099. EOE.

ACADEMIC OPPORTUNITY—The University of Kentucky is seeking a full-time, tenured line academic neuroradiologist with interventional neuroradiology expertise. Must be willing to cross cover in other areas. Responsibilities include patient care, medical student and resident teaching and regularly scheduled interdepartment conferences. Must be CAQ-certified or eligible for certification. Senior membership in the ASNR desired. Opportunity for research with nationally known Alzheimer's Research Center with busy neurosurgery department. Please mail or fax letter of interest and curriculum vitae to James C. Reed, MD, Chairman, Department of Radiology, HX304, UK Medical Center, Lexington, KY 40536-0084; fax 606-257-6014. UK is an equal opportunity employer.

SEATTLE AREA—Radia Medical Imaging is a 40-member radiology practice concentrated in the greater Seattle area. We serve five hospitals, one large multi-specialty clinic and own and operate a series of well-established outpatient clinics. The Seattle area is consistently rated as one of the top areas of the country to live and work, with an abundance of outdoor recreation, a progressive metropolitan area and a robust economy. We are a rapidly growing practice and seeking a few top radiologists to join our team. For a list of our most current openings as well as more information on our practice, visit our website at *www.radiax.com*. Send CV attention Mark Churchill, 728 134th St, SW, #120, Everett, WA 98204. E-mail to *markchurchill@radiax.com*. Fax 425-297-6250.

NEURORADIOLOGIST—Arizona progressive, respected group of 35 seeks seventh neuroradiologist for partnership position. 70+% of work and call only in neuroradiology. Coverage for four hospitals and four group-owned imaging centers. Send CV to Search Committee, PO Box 12249, Tucson, AZ 85732-2249 or fax to 520-318-6139.

THE SECTION OF NUCLEAR MEDICINE—in Diagnostic Radiology at the University of Kentucky Medical Center is offering a full-time faculty position that includes responsibilities as Chief of Nuclear Medicine. Candidates should be Board-certified in diagnostic radiology with special competence in nuclear radiology. Can be Board-certified in both diagnostic radiology and nuclear medicine. A strong interest and evidence in academic nuclear medicine is required, with grant experience desired. Applicant must have significant clinical experience and willingness to participate in other sections of diagnostic radiology. Academic rank based on experience and qualifications. Send CV and letter of interest to James C. Reed, MD, Chairman, Diagnostic Radiology, University of Kentucky, 800 Rose St, Lexington, KY 40536-0084, or fax 606-257-6014. UK is an EOE employer.

Fellowships

FELLOWSHIP IN IMAGING/ANGIO-INTERVENTIONAL—A 1-year fellowship program at Lehigh Valley Hospital in Allentown, PA is available beginning July 1, 2000. LVH is a 650-bed acute care, university affiliated hospital. The fellowship program offers training in CT (head and body), ultrasound, MR, angiography, and interventional radiology. For further information contact Elliot Shoemaker, MD, Department of Radiology, Lehigh Valley Hospital, PO Box 689, Allentown, PA 18105-1556 or telephone 610-402-8088 for fax 610-402-1023.

THE DEPARTMENT OF RADIOLOGY OF THE BRIGHAM AND WOMEN'S HOSPITAL-HARVARD MEDICAL SCHOOL—Offers 1 or 2-year fellowship positions in the following areas: 1) cardiovascular and interventional, 2) neuroradiology, 3) abdominal, 4) abdominal interventional, 5) magnetic resonance, 6) women's imaging, 7) oncoradiology, 8) chest, 9) bone, 10) nuclear medicine, 11) computer science, 12) mammography, 13) EW. For more information please send curriculum vitae specifying your area of interest to Steven E. Seltzer, MD, Chairman, Department of Radiology, Brigham and Women's Hospital, 75 Francis St, Boston, MA 02115. Harvard Medical School and Brigham and Women's Hospital are equal opportunity, affirmative action employers.

INDIANA UNIVERSITY SCHOOL OF MEDICINE FELLOWSHIPS—The Department of Radiology at Indiana University in Indianapolis offers fellowships in abdominal imaging, breast imaging, chest imaging, musculoskeletal imaging, neuroradiology, nuclear medicine, pediatric radiology, and vascular and interventional radiology. Indiana has a 40-member teaching faculty, state-of-the-art equipment, a large clinical practice (over 400,000 patient examinations per year), and active research. For more information please visit our web site at *www.indyrad.iupui.edu*. Must obtain license to practice medicine in the state of Indiana. Grant (award) type/term/amount: competitive; 1-2-years. Department funding, contact Kathie Pedersen, Indiana University Hospital 0279, 550 N University Blvd, Indianapolis, IN 46202-5253; telephone 317-274-1840, fax 317-274-1848, e-mail *kmpeders @iupui.edu*. Deadlines: n.a. Key words: abdominal imaging, breast imaging, chest imaging, musculoskeletal imaging, neuroradiology, nuclear medicine, pediatric radiology, vascular and interventional radiology. Award amount key: n.a. Links: go to RFP/A.

NEURORADIOLOGY FELLOWSHIP, UNIVERSITY OF MICHIGAN—Due to expansion of our program, the University of Michigan at Ann Arbor is opening two new neuroradiology fellowship positions. One position each is available starting July 1999 and July 2000. For more information, please contact Dr. Gebarski at 734-936-4484. (*gebarski@umich.edu)*

NEURORADIOLOGY FELLOWSHIP POSITION FOR JULY 2000—A 1 or 2-year neuroradiology fellowship accredited by the ACGME. Training includes all aspects of neuroradiology, head and neck radiology and participation in interventional neuroradiology procedures. A one-month elective away is offered in pediatric neuroradiology or interventional for those in the 2nd-year. The hospital has state-of-the-art equipment: 1) three helical GE CT scanners, 2) two GE 1.5T Signa MR scanners, echospeed on one scanner and plans to upgrade to echospeed on the other, and 3) new biplane Toshiba neuroangiography unit. The outpatient center has an echospeed 1.5T Signa MR scanner with plans for addition of another MR scanner and helical CT scanner. There are five full-time neuroradiology, three PhD physicists and three visiting research faculty. The neuroradiology section conducts many research projects, including those in functional MRI. Research facilities include small and large animal surgical suites, chemistry, physiology, and physics laboratories. In addition, a 2.0T, 30cm bore MRI animal scanner is available in the NMR Medical Center Laboratory. Direct inquiries to Henry Wang, MD, PhD, Department of Radiology, University of Rochester Medical Center, 601 Elmwood Ave, Box 648, Rochester, NY 14642; phone 716-273-4133, fax 716-473-4861, e-mail *henry_wang @urmc.rochester.edu*. The University of Rochester is an equal opportunity employer.

FELLOWSHIPS AT THE UNIVERSITY OF ROCHESTER SCHOOL OF MEDICINE—The Department of Radiology at the University of Rochester Medical Center has openings for fellowships in pediatric radiology, body imaging, neuroradiology, angiography and interventional radiology, and musculoskeletal radiology for July 2000. Strong Memorial Hospital is a tertiary care teaching facility performing 195,000 radiologic procedures/year in a single location. Please direct your inquiry and send your curriculum vitae to Arvin E. Robinson, MD, Chair, Department of Radiology, Box 648, University of Rochester Medical Center, Rochester, NY 14642-8648; phone 716-275-2733. The University of Rochester is an equal opportunity employer.

A 6-MONTH OPEN MRI FELLOWSHIP - SAN FRANCISCO BAY AREA—Potential to join radiology group after fellowship. Currently three radiologists reading for three open magnets; soon to expand to five open magnets. Competitive pay and benefits. Please fax CV to 510-784-1142 attn Peter Rothschild, MD.

BODY IMAGING FELLOWSHIP —University of Vermont/Fletcher Allen Health Care, Burlington, VT. One-year fellowship position in body imaging available at University of Vermont commencing July 2000. The fellowship program is based at Fletcher Allen Health Care, a 500-bed tertiary-care teaching hospital offering the full range of medical and surgical specialty care and a Comprehensive Cancer Center (as designated by NCI). The fellowship has excellent exposure to all facets of imaging including body CT, ultrasound (including obstetric, pediatric, and vascular ultrasound), and body and musculoskeletal MRI. Extensive experience in CT and ultrasound-guided interventional procedures is also part of the training. Equipment includes three GE HiSpeed helical CT scanners, two state-of-the-art GE MR units, eight US rooms with GE or Acuson equipment, and PACS/3D workstations. The Medical Center offers a collegial environment, and Burlington is truly one of the best small cities in the United States. FACH is an equal opportunity/affirmative action employer. Please address all inquiries to Robert K. Zeman, MD, Professor and Chairman, Dept of Radiology, Fletcher Allen Health Care, MCHV Campus-Patrick 113, 111 Colchester Ave, Burlington, VT 05401; 802-656-3592.

THE UNIVERSITY OF MASSACHUSETTS MEDICAL CENTER—Offers fellowship positions in neuroradiology, vascular/interventional and body imaging/MRI. The University of Massachusetts includes a medical school and a 388-bed hospital and trauma center located 40 miles west of Boston. The radiology department performs approximately 200,000 exams per year. State-of-the-art equipment includes two vascular/interventional, two CT and two 1.5Tesla MRI units. The positions include teaching of medical students and residents with opportunities for research and conference attendance. The neuroradiology and vascular/interventional fellowships are approved by ACGME. For information, contact John Knorr, DO, for neuroradiology, Ducksoo Kim, MD, for vascular/interventional, and Ashley Davidoff, MD, for body imaging at University of Massachusetts Medical Center, Department of Radiology, 55 Lake Ave N, Worcester, MA 01655; 508-856-2215.

MEMORIAL SLOAN-KETTERING CANCER CENTER, DEPARTMENT OF RADIOLOGY—Offers fellowship positions. Body imaging (1-year, five positions) fellowship provides extensive experience in body CT, body MRI and ultrasound, including imaging of chest/abdomen/pelvis/extremities in adult and pediatric patients. State-of-the-art equipment includes six CT scanners, three 1.5T MRI scanners, and six ultrasound units. Director: David Panicek, MD. Breast imaging (six months, plus six months of body imaging; five positions) provides comprehensive training in all aspects of breast diagnosis (mammography, sonography, MRI, screening and diagnosis) and intervention (including ultrasound and stereotactic biopsy). Director: David Dershaw, MD. Other fellowships include nuclear medicine (2-years; contact Steven Larson, MD, at MSKCC), and combined New York Presbyterian/MSKCC fellowships in neuroradiology (2-years; contact Michael Deck, MD, at NYP) and vascular/interventional radiology (1-year; contact Thomas Sos, MD, at NYP). Excellent opportunities for research exist at this Cornell University Medical College affiliate, with competitive salary and benefits. Request brochure and application from David Panicek, MD, Department of Radiology, Memorial Sloan-Kettering Cancer Center, 1275 York Avenue, New York, NY 10021; e-mail *panicekd@mskcc.org*. Website *http://www.mskcc.org*. An equal opportunity employer.

MRI FELLOWSHIP—A 1-year fellowship program at the outpatient imaging center of the University of Rochester is available beginning July 2000. The outpatient center performs over 6500 MR exams per year using a 1.5T echo-planar magnet. The fellowship program offers training in neuro, musculoskeletal and body MRI. Fellows will receive an excellent clinical experience and are required to perform research that culminates in publication. Candidates must be ABR-eligible or certified and have a NY license. For further information, contact Steven P. Meyers, MD, PhD, Department of

FELLOWSHIP, VASCULAR/INTERVENTIONAL—The Department of Radiology, University Hospital at SUNY College of Medicine, Syracuse, announces the unexpected opening of an ACGME-accredited fellowship position in interventional radiology for July 1, 2000. The fellowship program covers two teaching hospitals, where in excess of 4,000 vascular and non-vascular examinations are performed. Contact Dr Kenneth D. Murphy, Director, Vascular/Interventional Radiology, University Hospital, SUNY-Syracuse, 750 E Adams St, Syracuse, NY 13210. Phone 315-464-7439; fax 315-464-7458; e-mail *murphyk@mailbox.hscsyr.edu*. State University of New York, Syracuse is an equal opportunity employer.

FELLOWSHIP IN ABDOMINAL IMAGING AND INTERVENTIONS—The Department of Radiology, Massachusetts General Hospital and Harvard Medical School offers a 2-year fellowship in abdominal imaging and interventional radiology beginning July 1, 2001. Training covers all aspects of abdominal imaging (fluoroscopy, ultrasound, CT and MR) and nonvascular interventions in the GI/GU tract. This is an accredited interventional fellowship that includes elective time to allow a fellow to take the vascular/interventional CAQ exam. Ample time is made available for both clinical and laboratory research in the above areas during the second year. Candidates should be ABR-eligible or ABR-certified. Address inquiries to Peter R. Mueller, MD, Department of Radiology, Massachusetts General Hospital, 55 Fruit St, Boston, MA 02114. An equal opportunity employer.

HENRY FORD HOSPITAL—Has an unexpected opening for cross-sectional fellowship starting July 1, 2000. The fellowship consists of MRI-body and neuro, including MRA, spiral CT, including abscess drainage and biopsy, and abdominal, vascular, obstetrical and pelvic ultrasound. Equipment includes three MRI scanners, five CT machines and numerous ultrasound units. Please direct inquiries to Michael A. Sandler, MD, Department of Diagnostic Radiology, Henry Ford Hospital, Detroit, MI 48202. Phone 313-916-1355; fax 313-916-1106; e-mail *michaels@rad.hfh.edu*.

MUSCULOSKELETAL FELLOWSHIP—A 1-year fellowship position at the University of Texas Southwestern Medical Center is available beginning July 1, 2000. This position includes all imaging modalities related to musculoskeletal imaging, including MRI. There are currently three faculty members within the section, and the section covers both hospital-based and ambulatory care services. Opportunities for research are available. Inquiries should be directed to Dianna Otterstad, Fellowship Coordinator at Department of Radiology, UT Southwestern Medical Center, 5323 Harry Hines Blvd, Dallas, TX 75235-8896, or e-mail *dianna.otterstad@email.swmed.edu*.

NEURORADIOLOGY FELLOWSHIP—The Mallinckrodt Institute of Radiology has an unexpected opening for a fellowship position starting July 1, 2000, with clinical, research and teaching duties. This ACGME-accredited program is staffed by 13 subspecialized neuroradiologists who cover both adult and pediatric hospitals. Applicant must be Board-certified and must have completed their residency in radiology by starting date. Interested candidates may contact Daniel K. Kido, MD, Neuroradiology Section, Mallinckrodt Institute of Radiology, Washington University School of Medicine, 510 S Kingshighway Blvd, St Louis, MO 63110. Phone 314-362-5950; fax 314-362-4886.

FELLOWSHIPS IN PEDIATRIC RADIOLOGY—The Department of Diagnostic Imaging and Radiology, Children's National Medical Center, Washington, DC is soliciting applications for postgraduate fellowship training in pediatric radiology commencing July 2000 and July 2001. The department performs over 65,000 examinations annually in one of the four largest children's hospitals and ambulatory practices in North America. The department has 10 faculty and many fellows and resident trainees. Imaging services and training include state-of-the-art radiography, fluoroscopy, ultrasound, nuclear medicine, cardiovascular imaging, interventional radiology, computed tomography and magnetic resonance imaging. There are many opportunities for rewarding careers in pediatric radiology in either academic or practice environments. If you wish to receive more information about the fellowship or careers in pediatric radiology, please contact David C. Kushner, MD, FACR, Chairman, Diagnostic Imaging and Radiology, Children's National Medical Center, 111 Michigan Ave, NW, Washington, DC 20010. Telephone 202-884-5430; fax 202-884-3644.

For Sale

FOR SALE—Radiologic teaching file of the late William Meszaros, MD, consisting of 2,145 cases and 48 boxes of slides. Extensive cardiac and bone sections. For more information, call 847-381-6430, or write to Mrs William Meszaros, 418 Park Barrington Dr, Barrington, IL 60010.

RSNA®
RSNA Executive Offices • 820 Jorie Boulevard
Oak Brook, IL 60523 • (630) 571-2670

Bulletin Board — September 1999

✓ More "Hot Topics" for RSNA '99
✓ IHE To Become Major *info*Rad Focus
✓ Review Your Membership Directory Listing

■ The ongoing "Hot Topics" presentation will once again be part of this year's RSNA Scientific Assembly and Annual Meeting. The "Hot Topics" format was created in order to gather the most up-to-date scientific information for the RSNA Scientific Assembly and Annual Meeting. If you have performed research that was too recent to have been submitted by the April 15 deadline, please call (630) 571-7877 to request an application for your "hot topic." The deadline for submissions is October 28, 1999.

■ Integration will be the byword in *info*RAD at RSNA '99. The Integrating the Healthcare Enterprise (IHE) initiative has generated a series of program events clustering around the theme of integration that provides a major new focus for *info*RAD. At the heart of these activities will be the initial IHE Year 1 Demonstration, a joint effort with the Healthcare Information and Management Systems Society (HIMSS). This multi-vendor interoperability demonstration will feature major players in imaging and information systems exchanging information in an open, standards-based environment that simulates real-life clinical scenarios. The demonstration will run continuously at 15-minute intervals during the business hours of *info*RAD.

■ RSNA members should review their listings in the 1999 RSNA Membership Directory and submit changes and/or corrections through a new change-of-address form in the Membership area of RSNA Link. Follow the link to "Membership" on the home page or go directly to www.rsna.org/about/membership/changeofaddress.html. When you fill out this form, your information goes directly by e-mail to the membership department at RSNA headquarters. You may also submit changes and corrections via regular mail to, Manager of Membership Records, RSNA, 820 Jorie Blvd, Oak Brook, IL 60523. Changes received by December 31, 1999 will be included in the 2000 directory.

■ The following is a list of applicants for RSNA membership, published as provided by the bylaws of the Society. Society members are asked to review these names. Should a member have a question concerning the eligibility of an applicant, within 30 days of the publication of this list, the member should request that the applicant's membership be withheld pending investigation and reconsideration by the Membership and Credentials Board. Please mark your signed letter of protest "Confidential" and address it to Secretary-Treasurer, RSNA, 820 Jorie Blvd, Oak Brook, IL 60523. Please note that listed here are only the locations in which the prospective members reside and the counselors for those areas.

ALABAMA
Counselor: Robert E. Koehler, MD
Brenda C. Grabb, MD, Birmingham

CALIFORNIA
Counselors: Deborah S. Ablin, MD
Kenneth W. Chin, MD
Nancy A. Ellerbroek, MD
Gary R. Hansen, MD
Eric W. Olcott, MD
Dolores H. Pretorius, MD
Carl J. Rossi, MD, Loma Linda
Stuart L. Stein, MD, Palo Alto

FLORIDA
Counselor: John A. Arrington, MD
Edward J. James, MD, Parkland

ILLINOIS
Counselors: Boyd E. Nelson, MD
Milton L. Paige, MD
Paula C. Kezdi-Rogus, MD, Westmont

MARYLAND
Counselor: Henry A. Munitz, MD
Deborah M. Prescott, DVM, PhD, Gaithersburg

MASSACHUSETTS
Counselor: Robert H. Cleveland, MD
Edward J. Hogan, MSEE, North Billerica

NEW JERSEY
Counselor: Karen L. Karlson, MD
Noam S. Eshkar, MD, Upper Montclair
Ira R. Stark, DO, Stratford

NORTH CAROLINA
Counselor: James A. Fagan, MD
Eithne T. Burke, MB, Chapel Hill
Kevin J. Kerlin, MD, Goldsboro

PENNSYLVANIA
Counselors: Nilima Dash, MD
Kathryn A. Evers, MD
John E. Madewell, MD
Thomas J. Quinn, MD, Devon
Dominik Weishaupt, MD, Philadelphia

TENNESSEE
Counselor: Joseph J. Busch, MD
Glenn F. Nabors, MD, Hendersonville

WISCONSIN
Counselor: Thomas F. Berns, MD
Lonie R. Salkowski, MD, Menomonee Falls

CANADA

NOVA SCOTIA
Counselor: Robert A. Vandorpe, MD
Timothy W. Clark, MD, Halifax
Anne Doiron, MD, Moncton

CORRESPONDING
Kazuo Awai, MD, Japan
Arindam Bharadwaz, MBBS, India
Philippe J. Cluzel, MD, France
Mahmoud L. El Sheikh, MD, Egypt
Hisashi Fujimoto, MD, Japan
Lorenzo A. Guendel, MD, Ravensburg
Tariq A. Hameed, MBBS, Pakistan
Jean Y. Meuwly, MD, Switzerland
Gustavo R. Mysler, MD, Argentina
Shunsuke Nosaka, MD, Japan
John K. Pereira, MD, Australia
Hazar A. Tabban, Jr, MBBCh, Saudi Arabia
Mari Tokunaga, MD, Japan
Syed F. Ul-Haq, MBBS, Pakistan
Guido Verhoek, MD, Switzerland
Takashi Yamamoto, MD, Japan

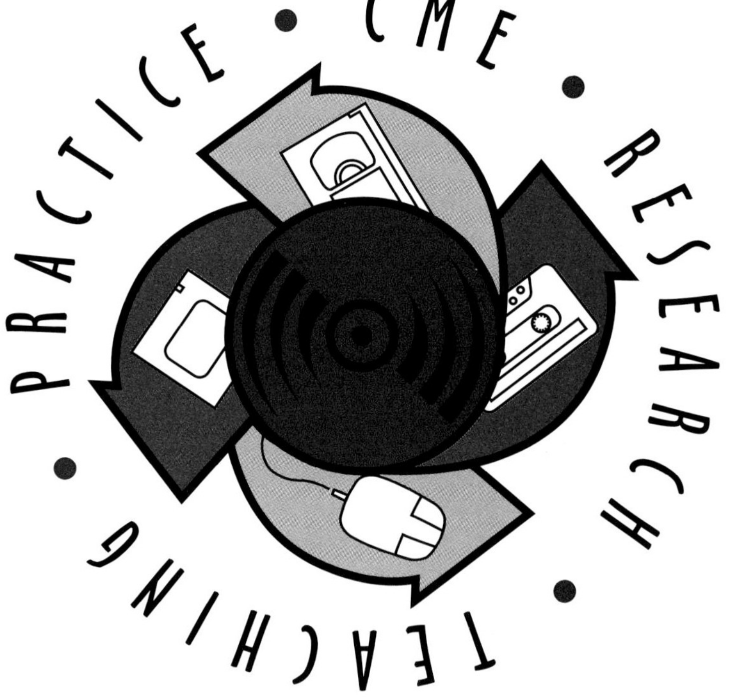

Physics

Education Center Resources

September 1999

RSNA® | Radiological Society of North America, Founded in 1915

Featured Topics

- Laser Biophysics
- Photodynamic Therapy
- Film Processing
- Basic Physics of Digital Imaging and Computed Radiography

New Service

The entire 1998–1999 Education Center Resources Catalog is now available on the RSNA *Link*, the Web site of the Radiological Society of North America, on the Internet.

You can reach us through the World Wide Web (WWW) by entering the uniform resource locator: http://www.rsna.org

We invite you to browse through the catalog, search for specific courses of interest, then simply order via our fax or 800 phone number.

Detach and store for your future use.

The following 12 Physics titles are now available in the Education Center Resources Library. All videotapes are available for purchase or rental. (U.S., Canada, and Mexico). All video programs may be purchased in NTSC, PAL, and SECAM television standards. Slides and audiotapes are available for purchase only.

For more information, call or fax the RSNA Education Center Resources at the numbers listed on the order form. To order by mail, use the form on the back.

NEW!

Laser Biophysics *RSP 728*

Patrick J. Clark

This course presents a comprehensive overview of laser generation, propagation, application, control and safety, and develops the theory of coherent light and the mechanism for selective chromophore activation in tissue. *Learning objectives:* (1) Discuss the physical properties of laser light. (2) Summarize its application in chromophore activation. (Patrick J. Clark is on the speakers' forum for Laserscope and Coherent.)

VHS *M$140, N$160*

Not available in slide/audiotape

NEW!

Photodynamic Therapy *RSP 729*

Fred W. Hetzel, PhD

Wavelengths which have specific responses in organic targets are chosen for this selectivity just as the photodynamic drug itself is chosen for selectivity. *Learning objective:* Explain the limitations associated with laser chromophore activation relative to a differential response between activation of exogenous drug chromophore vs indigenous chromophores in organic constituents. (Fred W. Hetzel is a lecturer for Laserscope.)

VHS *M$140, N$160*

Not available in slide/audiotape

Film Processing, Processor Quality Control, and Artifacts *RSP 476*

Arthur G. Haus

Susan M. Jaskulski, RT (R) (M)

171 slides/2 audiotapes *M$205, N$225*

Not available on videotape

Physics and Technology of Interventional Fluoroscopic Equipment *RSP 661*

Stephen Balter, PhD

72 slides/2 audiotapes *M$205, N$225*

Not available on videotape

Update on Fluoroscopic Equipment and Test Procedures *RSP 664*

Phillip L. Rauch, MS

Keith J. Strauss, MS

146 slides/2 audiotapes *M$205, N$225*

Not available on videotape

Basic Physics of Digital Imaging and Computed Radiography *RSP 615*

Douglas M. Tucker, PhD

John C. Weiser, PhD

108 slides/2 audiotapes *M$205, N$225*

VHS *M$205, N$225*

To order call (800) 272-2920 or FAX (630) 990-9958
(Outside U.S., phone (630) 990-9941)

M/N = Member/Nonmember prices

High-Dose Fluoroscopy *RSP 549*
M. Victoria Marx, MD
J. Thomas Payne, PhD

VHS *M$205, N$225*
Not available in slide/audiotape

AAPM/RSNA Tutorial on Equipment Selection: Fluoroscopic Systems, Including Interventional Fluoroscopy *RSP 582*
Richard L. Morin, PhD
Joel E. Gray, PhD
Stuart E. Braverman, MD
Andrew K. Poznanski, MD
John G. Stears, RTR
Ernst Ammann, Dr Ing
John A. Rowlands, PhD
Keith J. Strauss, MS

VHS, 2 videotapes *M$205, N$225*
Not available in slide/audiotape

Film Processing, Processor Quality Control, and Artifacts *RSP 476*
Arthur G. Haus
Susan M. Jaskulski, RT (R) (M)

171 slides/2 audiotapes *M$205, N$225*

AAPM/RSNA Physics Tutorial for Residents: Basic Nuclear Medicine Physics *PM 9700*
Mark T. Madsen, PhD, moderator
James A. Patton, PhD
Mark W. Groch, PhD
James A. Pronto, MS
Douglas J. Simpkin, PhD
Nicole T. Ranger, Msc
Mark S. Rzeszotarski, PhD

Slides *US: M$255, N$275*
Outside US: M$280, N$300

AAPM/RSNA Physics Tutorial for Residents: Basic X-ray Physics *PM 9600*
Cynthia H. McCollough, PhD

Frank Zink, PhD
J. Anthony Seibert, PhD
Jerrold Bushberg, PhD
Marlene H. McKetty, PhD

Slides *US: M$255, N$275*
Outside US: M$280, N$300

AAPM/RSNA Physics Tutorial: The Physics of Screen-Film Radiography *PM 9500*
E. Russell Ritenour, PhD
Arthur G. Haus
E. Lee Kitts, Jr, PhD
Gary T. Barnes, PhD
Joel E. Gray, PhD
Carl J. Vyborny, MD, PhD

Slides *US: M$255, N$275*
Outside US: M$280, N$300

Place
Stamp
Here

TO: RSNA EDUCATION CENTER RESOURCES
PO BOX 5316
OAK BROOK, IL 60522-5316
USA

FOLD HERE

Order Form

You may mail or fax this form. To fax your order, dial 630-990-9958. Please print.

☐ *RSNA Member* ☐ *Nonmember*

NAME

RSNA MEMBER # (REQUIRED FOR MEMBER PRICING)

ADDRESS

CITY

STATE/COUNTRY

ZIP

PHONE

FAX

Order Information (for purchase and rentals)

Course Number	*Showing Date (Rental Only)*	*Format (Purchase Only)*	*Price*

FOLD HERE

Check one:

☐ *Rental*

☐ *Purchase*

Subtotal ______

Shipping & Handling ______

Total ______

Shipping Information

United States

1 program = $7
2 – 3 programs = $10
4 – 6 programs = $20
7 programs and up = $30

Rental

No charge for shipping to renter. Renter is responsible for return shipping charges.

Outside United States

1 program = $10
Each additional program = $5
All orders from outside the U.S. must be prepaid, either by MasterCard, VISA, AMEX or Diners Club or a check in U.S. dollars, drawn on a U.S. bank.

Payment Information

☐ Payment by check

☐ Payment by credit card: ☐ VISA ☐ MasterCard ☐ AMEX ☐ Diners Club

CARD NUMBER

SIGNATURE

EXP. DATE

For faster service, phone (800) 272-2920 or fax (630) 990-9958 (Outside U.S., phone (630) 990-9941).

Foto-Comm Corporation is the distributor of RSNA Education Center Resources.

RAD

~~out~~sourcing?

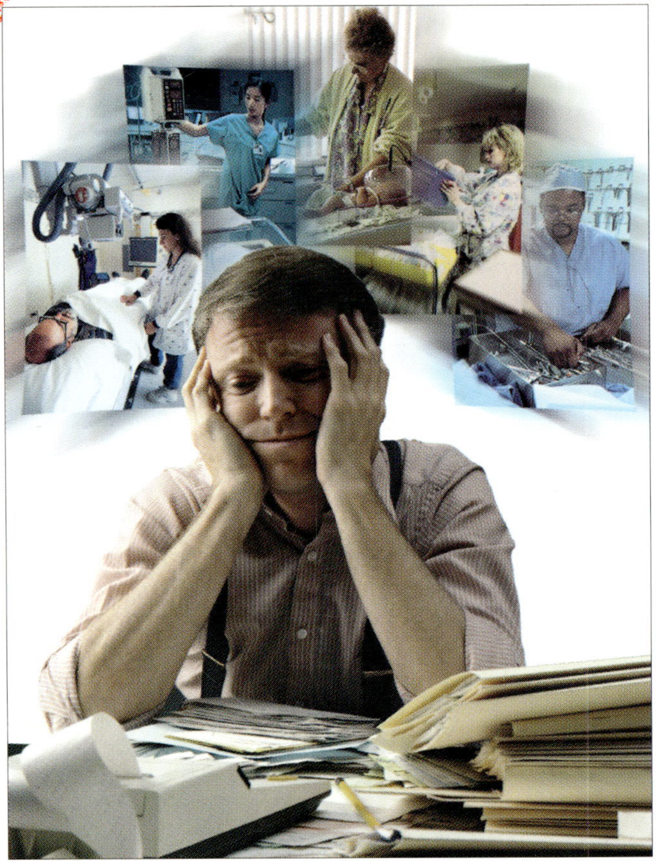

no, *re*sourcing

- Why do you suppose so many leading hospitals have chosen to off-load management of service for all their clinical equipment (biomedical as well as imaging, regardless of vendor) to a single source – GE's CompreCare?

  Because increasingly, customers are redefining "outsourcing" as "**re - sourcing**".

- **As demands grow, with revenue unpredictable,** clinical staff is stretched even thinner. With limited human resources, wise administrators have determined they'd rather have their people focus upon their core competencies where it counts most – in providing quality patient care.

- Wherever skilled and reliable help is available, customers tell us that it pays to eliminate distractions. Let GE handle infrastructure and support tasks.

- **In short, the key issue today is "Resourcing"... selective deployment of strategic resources – human and technological – to build the strongest team possible.** Isn't that what CompreCare provides?

And when you think ~~out~~(re)sourcing – think GE.

Because CompreCare is only one of many resourceful solutions we can offer you to make your team unbeatable.

rethink. rework. *re*source.

GE Medical Systems
We bring good things to life.